MW00388916

Nuclear Medicine
Diagnosis and Therapy

Nuclear Medicine
Diagnosis and Therapy

Edited by

John C. Harbert, M.D.
Emeritus Professor of Medicine
and Radiology
Georgetown University School of Medicine
Washington, DC

William C. Eckelman, Ph.D.
Chief, PET Department
The Clinical Center
National Institutes of Health
Bethesda, MD

Ronald D. Neumann, M.D.
Chief, Department of Nuclear Medicine
The Clinical Center
National Institutes of Health
Bethesda, MD

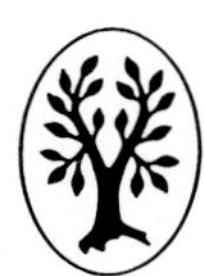

1996
Thieme Medical Publishers, Inc., New York
Georg Thieme Verlag, Stuttgart • New York

Thieme Medical Publishers, Inc.
381 Park Avenue South
New York, New York 10016

Nuclear Medicine: Diagnosis and Therapy
John C. Harbert, M.D.
William C. Eckelman, Ph.D.
Ronald D. Neumann, M.D.

Library of Congress Cataloging-in-Publication Data

Nuclear medicine: diagnosis and therapy/edited by John C. Harbert,
William C. Eckelman, Ronald D. Neumann.
p. cm.
Includes bibliographical references and index
ISBN 0-86577-570-2 (TMP: hardcover). —ISBN 3-13-101121-1 (GTV: hardcover)
1. Nuclear Medicine. I. Harbert, John Charles, 1937-
II. Eckelman, William C. III. Neumann, Ronald Daniel.
[DNLM: 1. Nuclear Medicine. 2. Radionuclide Imaging.
3. Radioisotopes—therapeutic use. WN 440 N9657 1996]
R895.N813 1996
616.07′575–dc20
DNLM/DLC
for Library of Congress 95-20599
CIP

Important note: Medicine is an ever-changing science. Research and clinical experience are continually broadening our knowledge, in particular our knowledge of proper treatment and drug therapy. Insofar as this book mentions any dosage or application, readers may rest assured that the authors, editors, and publishers have made every effort to ensure that such references are strictly in accordance with the state of knowledge at the time of production of the book. Nevertheless, users are requested to carefully examine the manufacturers' leaflets accompanying each drug to check on their own responsibility whether the dosage schedules recommended therein or the contraindications stated by the manufacturers differ from the statements made in the present book. Such examination is particularly important with drugs that are either rarely used or have been newly released on the market.

Printed in the United States of America.

5 4 3 2 1

TMP ISBN 0-86577-570-2
GTV ISBN 3-13-101121-1

Contents

Section Two: Clinical Sciences

Contributors

Mary P. Andrich, M.D.
Center for Biologics Evaluation and Research
FDA
Rockville, MD

James A. Arrighi, M.D.
Assistant Professor of Medicine and Radiology
Yale University School of Medicine
New Haven, CT

Harold L. Atkins, M.D.
Professor of Medicine
Department of Medicine
Brookhaven National Laboratory
Upton, NY

Stephen L. Bacharach, Ph.D.
Department of Nuclear Medicine
The Clinical Center
National Institutes of Health
Bethesda, MD

Bruce J. Baum, D.M.D., Ph.D.
Clinical Director
Chief, Clinical Investigation and Patient Care Branch
National Institute of Dental Research
National Institutes of Health
Bethesda, MD

John D. Boice, Jr., Sc.D.
Chief, Radiation Epidemiology Branch
National Cancer Institute
National Institutes of Health
Bethesda, MD

A.P. Callahan
Nuclear Medicine Group
Health and Safety Research Division
Oak Ridge National Laboratory
Oak Ridge, TN

Jorge A. Carrasquillo, M.D.
Deputy Chief, Department of Nuclear Medicine
The Clinical Center
National Institutes of Health
Bethesda, MD

Richard E. Carson, Ph.D.
PET Department
The Clinical Center
National Institutes of Health
Bethesda, MD

Clara C. Chen, M.D.
Department of Nuclear Medicine
The Clinical Center
National Institutes of Health
Bethesda, MD

Lisa Langlois Coronado, B.S.
Deputy Radiation Safety Officer
Genetics Institute, Inc.
Cambridge, MA

Bert M. Coursey, Ph.D.
Group Leader, Radiation Interactions and Dosimetry
National Institute of Standards and Technology
Gaithersburg, MD

Gyorgy Csako, M.D.
Department of Clinical Chemistry
The Clinical Center
National Institutes of Health
Bethesda, MD

Margaret E. Daube-Witherspoon, Ph.D.
PET Department
The Clinical Center
National Institutes of Health
Bethesda, MD

Giovanni Di Chiro, M.D.
Chief, Neuroimaging Branch
NINDS
National Institutes of Health
Bethesda, MD

Vasken Dilsizian, M.D.
Department of Nuclear Medicine
The Clinical Center
National Institutes of Health
Bethesda, MD

William C. Eckelman, Ph.D.
Chief, PET Department
The Clinical Center
National Institutes of Health
Bethesda, MD

Martin Erlichman, M.S.
Office of Health Technology Assessment
Agency of Health Care Policy and Research
Rockville, MD

Ted W. Fowler, M.S.P.H., C.H.P.
U.S.E.P.A.
National Air and Radiation
Environmental Laboratory
Montgomery, AL

Philip C. Fox, D.D.S.
National Institute of Dental Research
National Institutes of Health
Bethesda, MD

Michael J. Fulham, M.B., B.S., F.R.A.C.P.
Director of the PET Department and Staff
Neurologist
The Royal Prince Alfred Hospital
Camperdown NSW 2050
Sydney, Australia

Michael V. Green, M.S.
Department of Nuclear Medicine
The Clinical Center
National Institutes of Health
Bethesda, MD

John C. Harbert, M.D.
Emeritus Professor of Medicine and Radiology
Georgetown University School of Medicine
Washington, DC

Peter Herscovitch, M.D.
PET Department
The Clinical Center
National Institutes of Health
Bethesda, MD

Robert P. Hirsch, Ph.D.
Chairman, Department of Health Care Sciences
The George Washington University
School of Medicine and Health Sciences
Washington, DC

Thomas Holohan, M.D., F.A.C.P.
Director, Office of Health Technology Assessment
Agency for Health Care Policy and Research
Rockville, MD

Lynn Evans Jenkins, M.S.
Health Physicist
Radiation Safety Branch
National Institutes of Health
Bethesda, MD

F.F. (Russ) Knapp, Jr., Ph.D.
Group Leader, Nuclear Medicine Group
Health and Safety Research Division
Oak Ridge National Laboratory
Oak Ridge, TN

John McAfee, M.D.
Department of Nuclear Medicine
The Clinical Center
National Institutes of Health
Bethesda, MD

Barbara J. McNeil, M.D.
Director, Department of Health Care Policy
Harvard Medical School
Boston, MA

S. Mirzadeh, Ph.D.
Nuclear Medicine Group
Health and Safety Research Division
Oak Ridge National Laboratory
Oak Ridge, TN

Ronald D. Neumann, M.D.
Chief, Department of Nuclear Medicine
The Clinical Center
National Institutes of Health
Bethesda, MD

Chang H. Paik, Ph.D.
Department of Nuclear Medicine
The Clinical Center
National Institutes of Health
Bethesda, MD

Patrick J. Peller, M.D.
Division of Nuclear Medicine
Lutheran General Hospital
Park Ridge, Ill

David C. Price, M.D.
Professor of Radiology and Medicine
Chief, Clinical Nuclear Medicine
Department of Radiology
The Medical Center at the University of California
San Francisco, CA

James C. Reynolds, M.D.
Department of Nuclear Medicine
The Clinical Center
National Institutes of Health
Bethesda, MD

Mark Rotman, Pharm. D., M.S., B.C.N.P.
Department of Nuclear Medicine
The Clinical Center
National Institutes of Health
Bethesda, MD

Carolyn M. Rutter, Ph.D.
Department of Health Care Policy
Harvard Medical School
Boston, MA

Jürgen Seidel, Ph.D.
Department of Nuclear Medicine
The Clinical Center
National Institutes of Health
Bethesda, MD

J. Seidman
Department of Nuclear Medicine
The Clinical Center
National Institutes of Health
Bethesda, MD

Salman Siddiqi
Research Fellow
Becton Dickinson Diagnostic Instruments
and Systems
Sparks, MD

H. Dirk Sostman, M.D.
Chair, Radiology Department
Cornell Medical School
New York, NY

Joseph Steigman, Ph.D.
Professor Emeritus of Radiology
and Biochemistry
Division of Nuclear Medicine
Downstate Medical Center
Brooklyn, NY

Frans J. Th. Wackers, M.D.
Professor of Radiology and Medicine
Yale University School of Medicine
New Haven, CT

William J. Walker, Ph.D., C.H.P.
Chief, Radiation Safety Branch and Radiation
Safety Officer (Retired)
National Institutes of Health
Bethesda, MD

Ronald E. Weiner, Ph.D.
Associate Professor of Nuclear Medicine
University of Connecticut Health Center
Farmington, CT

John N. Weinstein, M.D.
Chief, Division of Cancer Biology
and Diagnosis
National Cancer Institute
National Institutes of Health
Bethesda, MD

Harvey Zeissman, M.D.
Chief, Division of Nuclear Medicine
Georgetown University Hospital
Washington, DC

Preface

Technologic advances are faster paced in nuclear medicine than in most specialties of medicine. This is partly because nuclear medicine is a young medical science and partly because so many participants from such other fields as physics, chemistry, engineering, and computer science continually provide us with sophisticated technology needing to be adapted to medical use. We have tried in this book to reflect these advances while retaining all of the important elements that form the field of nuclear medicine.

The numerous advances in the technologic aspects of nuclear medicine that have occurred since the publication of *Textbook of Nuclear Medicine,* in 1984, and its companion, *Nuclear Medicine Therapy,* in 1987, have been carefully reviewed and constitute most of the changes in this text. Noteworthy basic science advances are contained in the chapters on imaging systems, modeling, computer systems, and radiopharmaceutical chemistry. The profound pace of change in clinical nuclear practices is reflected in the chapters devoted to cardiovascular nuclear medicine, neurologic nuclear medicine tests and those pages devoted to nuclear medicine applications for oncology in particular. The result, we believe, is a more useful general textbook for residents and students of nuclear medicine and as a reference for active practitioners of nuclear medicine as well as clinicians who utilize nuclear medicine services.

John C. Harbert, M.D.
William C. Eckelman, Ph.D.
Ronald D. Neumann, M.D.

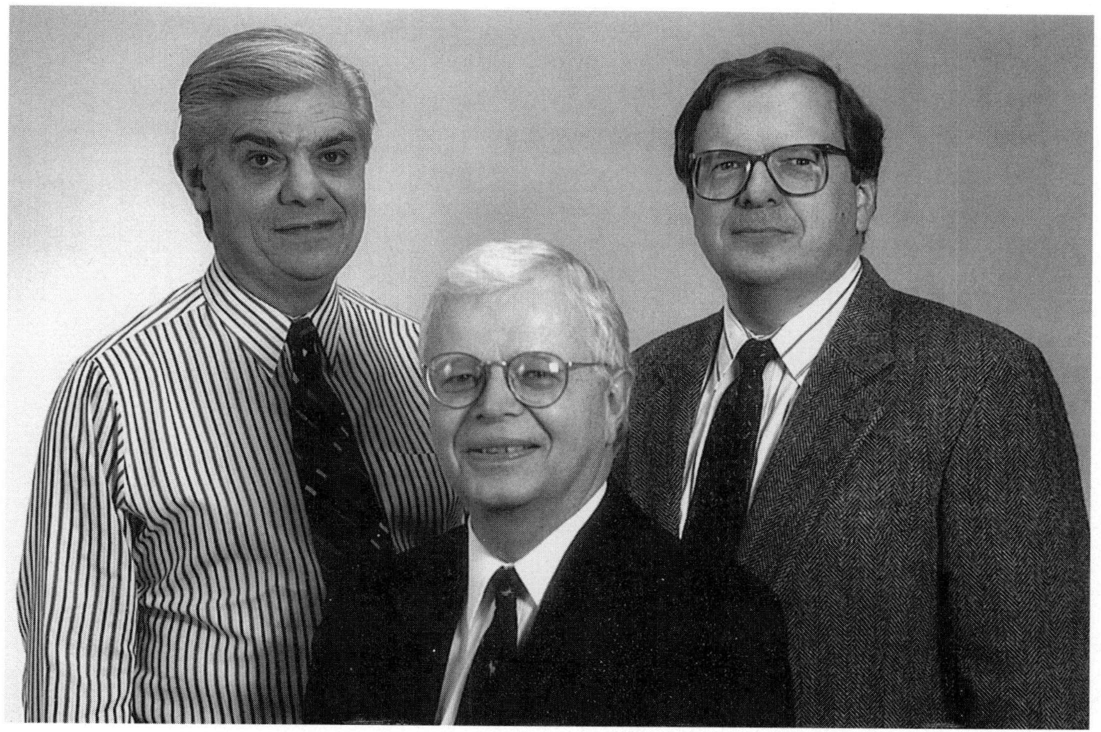

W.C.E. J.C.H. R.D.N.

Acknowledgements

The task of writing and compiling as much information as is contained in this volume required collaboration of many colleagues, all of whom have the editors' deep gratitude. For their valuable assistance, we particularly want to thank our esteemed contributors and several additional colleagues: Drs. Eva B. Dubovsky, Masoud Madj, David Brown, David Dalzell, James Seabold, Letty G. Lutzker, Lawrence E. Holder, Scott F. Rosebrough, Alan N. Schwartz, Walton W. Schreeve, Robert A. Ralph, David C. McCullough, Erica George, Homer B. Hupf, Mike Stabin, Michael Winston, Jeffrey A. Norton, L. Dade Lunsford and Roger Secker-Walker.

Special thanks are given to Jan Paluch, Margaret Green and L.C. Chen for assistance in the preparation of the manuscript, and to Steve Galen for his support during the planning and approval phase of this project.

The editors gratefully acknowledge the contribution of the Society of Nuclear Medicine in allowing the reproduction of numerous figures and tables from *The Journal of Nuclear Medicine.*

Particular gratitude goes to our wives and family members who suffered with us during the many hours devoted to this project.

J.C.H.
W.C.E.
R.D.N.

Section One

Basic Sciences

1 Atomic and Nuclear Structure

John C. Harbert

MATTER AND ENERGY

Structure of Matter

Although the corpuscular nature of matter had been speculated in antiquity, an understanding of matter was only philosophical and provided no basis for experimental proof. At the end of the 18th century, Lavoisier postulated the existence of molecules of definite chemical composition, which could be reduced to simpler substances that then could not be further reducible by classic chemical methods.

In the following century, Dalton verified that the ratio of elements within molecules varied discretely and that the numeric relationship between elements in molecules represented whole numbers. For example, in the group of hydrocarbons 12 g of carbon and 4 g of hydrogen form 1 mol of methane, 24 g of carbon and 6 g of hydrogen form 1 mol of ethane, and 24 g of carbon and 4 g of hydrogen form 1 mol of ethylene.

Subsequent developments that reinforced the concept of the atom were contributed by Gay-Lussac (law of gas volumes, 1809), Avogadro (Avogadro's number, 1811), Faraday (electrolysis, 1833), Cannizzaro (atomic weights, 1858), Meyer and Mandeleev (periodic table, 1870), and Perrin (Brownian motion, 1908).

Based initially on atomic weights, Mendeleev's classification of the elements indicated a periodic recurrence of similar chemical properties. This categorization reveals an admirable degree of precision when one considers that Mendeleev was without knowledge of several important facts about matter, particularly data derived from mass spectrometry. Inconsistencies in the periodic chart were later clarified by arraying the elements in order of increasing atomic number rather than weight (Fig. 1).

Rutherford's Atom

The understanding of matter further evolved following experiments by Lord Rutherford in 1911. He directed a narrow beam of alpha particles at a thin, gold foil and observed that some of the alpha particles passed through in a straight line while others were deflected through large scattering angles. In fact, some alpha particles were deflected 180° backward. These particles were apparently the result of head-on collisions with the foil nuclei. These observations suggested to Rutherford that matter is discontinuous, the atom is positively charged, and the charge is localized to a small volume whose size he was able to estimate from the alpha particle charge and the scattering angle.

The atom imagined by Rutherford was analogous to a planetary system, still a useful comparison. The atom may be thought of as having a small, dense, central nucleus consisting of Z protons—each with unit positive charge—and N neutrons, the sum of which equals the *atomic mass number A*. The radius of the nucleus is related to its atomic mass:

$$r = r_0 A^{1/3}$$

where r_0 is a constant equal to 1.2×10^{-15} m. Thus, the radius of a carbon nucleus equals 2.2×10^{-15} m.

The electrons, which contribute negligibly to the atom's mass, are organized about the nucleus in spherical orbital *shells*, each with unit negative charge and equal in number to the number of protons. The radius of the outer orbital shell of the atom is approximated by

$$r_a = 0.6 \times 10^{-10} (A/\rho)^{1/3}\text{m}$$

where ρ is the density of the material in its solid form. Thus atoms vary in diameter from about 0.6×10^{-10} m for hydrogen to about 1.7×10^{-10} m for the largest atoms, not a great variation in size. With the mass of an electron 1/1836 that of a proton, an apt spatial analogy of the nucleus to its electrons would be a golf ball surrounded by a few pinheads circling 1 km out in space. By far, the greatest volume of matter, even in heavy metals, is empty space, which helps explain why radiation traveling through matter may penetrate a long way before interacting with an atomic nucleus or electron.

Rutherford's atom presented certain inconsistencies. For example, according to classical mechanics, negatively charged electrons orbiting positively charged nuclei as Rutherford postulated would spiral inward with ever-decreasing radius, decelerate, and emit energy. Clearly this does not happen.

Bohr's Atom

In 1913, Niels Bohr provided a more satisfactory model of the atom, based on quantum mechanics, wherein the electrons occupy positions at well-defined distances from the nucleus (stable orbits). This is essentially the structure of the atom as we understand it today. Changes in energy state

PERIODIC TABLE OF THE ELEMENTS

1 H 1.00797																	2 He 4.0026
3 Li 6.939	4 Be 9.0122											5 B 10.811	6 C 12.01115	7 N 14.0067	8 O 15.9994	9 F 18.9984	10 Ne 20.183
11 Na 22.9877	12 Mg 24.305											13 Al 26.98154	14 Si 28.0855	15 P 30.97376	16 S 32.064	17 Cl 35.453	18 Ar 39.948
19 K 39.0983	20 Ca 40.08	21 Sc 44.9559	22 Ti 47.90	23 V 50.942	24 Cr 51.996	25 Mn 54.9380	26 Fe 55.847	27 Co 58.9332	28 Ni 58.71	29 Cu 63.546	30 Zn 65.38	31 Ga 69.72	32 Ge 72.59	33 As 74.9216	34 Se 78.96	35 Br 79.904	36 Kr 83.80
37 Rb 85.467	38 Sr 87.62	39 Y 88.9059	40 Zr 91.22	41 Nb 92.9064	42 Mo 95.94	43 Tc 98.9062	44 Ru 101.07	45 Rh 102.9055	46 Pd 106.4	47 Ag 107.868	48 Cd 112.41	49 In 114.82	50 Sn 118.69	51 Sb 121.75	52 Te 127.60	53 I 126.9045	54 Xe 131.30
55 Cs 132.9054	56 Ba 137.33	57 La 139.9055	72 Hf 178.49	73 Ta 180.948	74 W 183.85	75 Re 186.2	76 Os 190.2	77 Ir 192.22	78 Pt 195.09	79 Au 196.9665	80 Hg 200.59	81 Tl 204.37	82 Pb 207.19	83 Bi 208.9808	84 Po (209)	85 At (210)	86 Rn (222)
87 Fr (223)	88 Ra 226.0254	89 Ac (227)	104 (Rf) (261)	105 (Ha) (262)	106 (263)												
				58 Ce 140.12	59 Pr 140.9077	60 Nd 144.24	61 Pm (145)	62 Sm 150.4	63 Eu 151.96	64 Gd 157.25	65 Tb 158.9254	66 Dy 162.50	67 Ho 164.9304	68 Er 167.26	69 Tm 164.0342	70 Yb 173.04	71 Lu 174.97
				90 Th 232.0381	91 Pa 231.0359	92 U 238.029	93 Np 237.0482	94 Pu (244)	95 Am (243)	96 Cm (247)	97 Bk (247)	98 Cf (251)	99 Es (254)	100 Fm (257)	101 Md (258)	102 No (259)	103 (Lr) (257)

Figure 1. Periodic table of the elements.

are required for an electron to move from one level to another. Energy is required to raise an electron from an inner, more-stable orbit to an outer, less-stable orbit. These levels are fixed, so that discrete increments of energy are required for each orbital transition. The energy required is equal to the difference in the *binding energies* of the two orbits between which the electron moves. Bohr determined that this energy difference would be equal to $\hbar\nu$, where $\hbar$ is Planck's constant, or 6.62×10^{-34} J · s and ν is the frequency of the emitted radiation in s^{-1}.

The orbital shells are denominated by the principal quantum number n, which relates to the energy state of the electron, and by letters for the orbital shells (Table 1). Each orbital shell has a number of subshells, denominated by Roman numerals, with the electron capacities shown in Table 1 and Figure 2. When the atom is at *ground state*, ie, the state with the least energy, all or most of the inner orbital shells are filled before the outer shells are filled. The maximum number of electrons found in any shell is a function of the quantum number n and is given by $2n^2$. The outer shell never contains more than eight electrons. These are termed the valence electrons and determine to a large extent the chemical properties of the atom. Other quantum numbers are assigned for the angular momentum, magnetic moment, and spin direction of the electron. According to the Pauli exclusion principle, no two electrons in any atomic system have identical values for all four quantum numbers.

Table 1. Denomination and Capacity of Electron Shells

PRINCIPLE QUANTUM NUMBER (n)	PRIMARY SHELL	ELECTRONS PER SUBSHELL							TOTAL CAPACITY
		I	*II*	*III*	*IV*	*V*	*VI*	*VII*	
1	K	2	—	—	—	—	—	—	2
2	L	2	2	4	—	—	—	—	8
3	M	2	2	4	4	6	—	—	18
4	N	2	2	4	4	6	6	8	32
5	O	2	2	4	4	6	6	8	32
6	P	2	2	4	4	*	*	*	32
7	Q	2	*	*	*	*	*	*	32

*These subshells are available to electrons in excited states, but are not needed by atoms in the ground state.

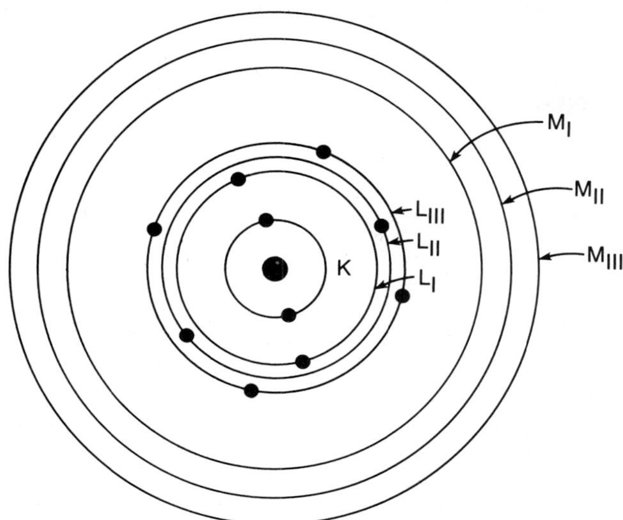

Figure 2. Schematic representation of a neon atom. The *M* subshells contain only electrons that have been excited by the addition of energy and raised from a *K*- or *L*-shell.

Mass and Energy

Kinetic energy is the energy that a body or particle possesses by virtue of its movement. Classically, this energy is expressed as

$$T = 1/2\ mv^2$$

This expression applies when the velocity v is small compared with that of light. As a particle approaches the speed of light, the variation of mass with velocity becomes appreciable, the mass increasing with increasing velocity:

$$m = \frac{m_0}{\sqrt{1 - v^2/c^2}}$$

where m_0 is the rest mass. Mass and energy are equivalent, related by Einstein's equation:

$$E = mc^2$$

The total energy of a particle, then, is the sum of the energy that it has by virtue of its mass and its kinetic energy:

$$E = \frac{m_0c^2}{\sqrt{1 - v^2/c^2}}$$

As the velocity of a particle approaches the speed of light, the mass increases by an amount equal to the increase in T. The variation of mass with velocity is important when dealing with such accelerated particles as protons or deuterons in cyclotrons.

Units of Mass and Energy

In the *Système International d'Unités* (SI), the basic unit of mass is the kilogram (kg) and the derived unit of energy is the joule (J), or that amount of energy required to accelerate 1 kg to a velocity of 1 $m \cdot s^{-1}$ (Appendix A). For events occurring on the atomic scale, however, more appropriate units are used. Energy of particles and of electromagnetic radiation is most often expressed in units of electron volts (eV), which correspond to the energy acquired by an electron accelerated across a potential difference of 1 V (1.6×10^{19} J). The basic unit of mass is the *unified atomic mass unit* (u), sometimes called the universal mass unit. By convention u is defined as 1/12 the mass of ^{12}C including its electrons.*

The equivalence between mass and energy cannot be determined by classic chemistry because the variation in mass that occurs in chemical reactions is extremely small. One must observe the larger mass changes encountered in nuclear reactions to appreciate these differences. Thus the classic concept of conservation of matter has been replaced by the law of conservation of energy and the law of the equivalence between mass and energy, expressed in Einstein's equation $E = mc^2$, where c is the velocity of light in a vacuum 3×10^8 $m \cdot s^{-1}$. The transformation of 1 u into energy yields 931.5 MeV; an electron at rest is equivalent to 0.511 MeV. Other mass equivalents are given in Table 2. Appendix A lists several additional units, constants, and useful conversion formulae.

The energy released by mass conversion occurs most often in the form of electromagnetic radiation, especially photons. These are oscillating electrical and magnetic fields without mass, traveling in a vacuum at the speed of light. Electromagnetic radiation is characterized by wavelength λ and frequency ν related by

$$\lambda\ \nu = c$$

where λ is expressed in Angstrom units (10^{-10} m). Photon energy is represented by the following equation:

$$E = \hbar\ \nu$$

where $\hbar$ = Planck's constant (6.626×10^{-34} J $\cdot$ s, or 4.135×10^{-15} eV $\cdot$ s). The wavelength λ is related to photon energy by

$$\lambda = \frac{1.24 \times 10^{-6}}{E}$$

where λ is in meters and E is in electron volts.

By convention, photons that arise from nuclear transformations are called *gamma* (λ)-rays, and photons that arise from extranuclear sources are called *x-rays*.

Electrons

J.J. Thomson demonstrated in 1895 that cathode-ray tubes function by means of a flux of very small particles of negative electrical charge—now known to be electrons—striking

*A slightly different unit, the atomic mass unit (amu), is used frequently in chemistry and is based upon the average weight of the isotopes of oxygen. One unified atomic mass unit equals 1.00083 amu.

Table 2. Rest Mass and Energy of Nucleons and Electrons

PARTICLE	SYMBOL	CHARGE	MASS (u)*	ENERGY (MeV)
Proton	p	+1	1.007276	938.27
Neutron	n	0	1.008665	939.57
Electron	e	−1	0.000548	0.511
α-particle	α	+2	4.0015	3727.4

*u = 1.66054×10^{-27} kg.

a metal anode. The mass of the electron is 9.1×10^{-30} kg, with a charge of 1.602×10^{-19} C. A similar particle, with equal mass but positive charge, was discovered by Anderson in 1932 and called a positive electron, or *positron*. The positron does not exist free in nature because, soon after being formed, it combines with an electron and both are *annihilated*. Their combined rest masses, corresponding to 1.022 MeV, are converted to two 0.511-MeV photons, which are emitted in opposite directions.

Electron Energy Levels

Electrons are bound to the atom within their various orbital shells. Each shell and subshell has a characteristic binding energy, which can be determined by nuclear spectrometry. In an atom at the ground state, the electron energy level is at a minimum and said to be stable. In a hydrogen atom, the binding energy E_b of its single electron is given by

$$E_b = \frac{-13.6}{n^2} \text{ eV}$$

where the value −13.6 is the *mean ionization potential* and n is the principal quantum number (Table 1). In the case of hydrogen, which has a single orbital shell, n equals 1 and E_b equals −13.6 eV. The mean ionization potential I represents the average energy required to remove an orbital electron (ionization), which forms an *ion pair* consisting of the negatively charged electron and the positively charged atom. The binding energies of inner electrons are always greater than those of outer electrons. Because ionization occurs most frequently in the outer orbital shells of multielectron atoms, where the binding energies are less, any specific ionizing event may require much less energy than the mean potential.

These concepts are illustrated in Figure 3, which depicts the orbital shells of ^{99m}Tc as though they were various levels in a well. The binding energies, given at the right, represent the amount of energy needed to lift an electron at that particular level out of the well. If an electron in the K shell interacts with and acquires the energy of an incident 20.98-keV photon, it would not gain enough energy to escape the atom, but would be elevated to the N subshell (dotted line). The atom would then be in an *excited* state, ie, the atom contains excess energy above its ground state. Numerous transition pathways exist whereby the atom could "deexcite" and return to its ground state. One possible pathway is depicted in the series of solid arrows showing transitions $N_I \rightarrow M_V \rightarrow L_{II} \rightarrow K_I$. During this process, three photons of 0.18, 2.55, and 18.25 keV, respectively, are given off, representing the energy differences between transitions. This process of deexcitation, in which several photons are emitted in random directions, is called a *cascade* and usually occurs in nanoseconds. Only certain transitions are allowed. Thus, if the K electron received only 15 keV, it would not be sufficient to excite the atom. If an L_I electron received this 15 keV, however, it would be ejected from the atom with 15.00 − 3.04 = 11.96 keV of kinetic energy, which would ionize the atom in the process. Subsequently, this L_I vacancy would be filled by electrons from higher levels, each transition resulting in the emission of a photon equal in energy to the difference

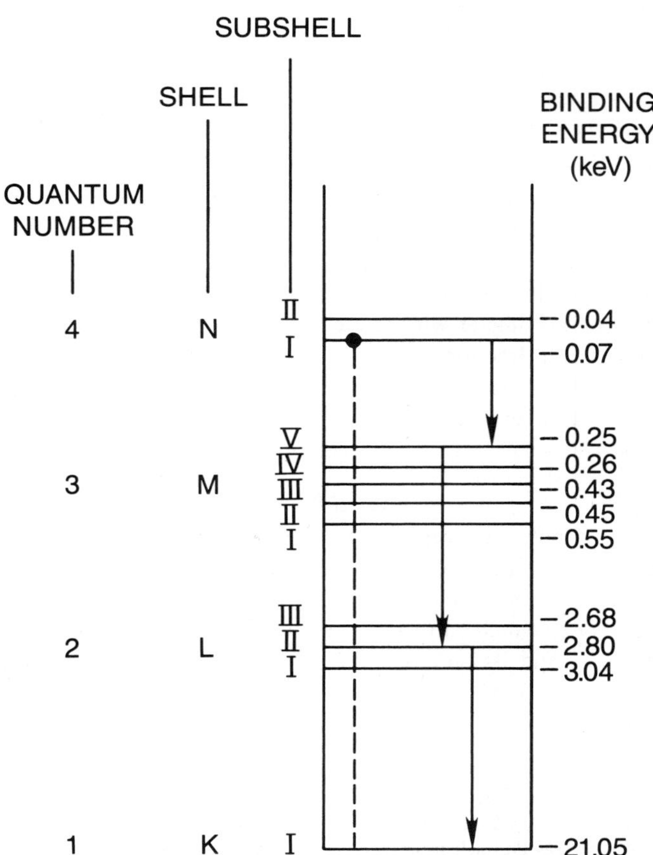

Figure 3. Diagram illustrating the electron binding energies for ^{99m}Tc. See text for explanation.

between its previous and new levels until the atom deexcites and emits 3.04 keV of energy in the form of photons.

Ionization by removal of an outer electron may require only a few electron volts, whereas to remove an inner electron from a large atom may require up to 100 keV (E_b increases with increasing Z). The deexcitation process, however, is the same. Higher-energy photons are called "characteristic" x-rays because their energies identify the orbital transition that produced them. Characteristic x-rays are also named by the transition process that creates them. If a free electron falls into a K vacancy, a K-characteristic x-ray is emitted, and the atom deexcites with a single photon emission equal in energy to the binding energy of the K-orbital electron. If the K-shell vacancy is filled by an L_l electron, a K_α x-ray (equal to the difference in binding energies of the K- and L-orbital electron) is emitted; if the vacancy is filled by an M electron, a K_β x-ray, and so forth. L-shell vacancies filled by M and N electrons emit L_α and L_β x-rays, respectively. The outermost shell vacancies are filled by free electrons in the environment. Because they are unique for each element, analysis of unknown sample elements is often performed by nuclear excitation and analyzing the characteristic x-rays emitted.

The excited atom has an alternative means of deexcitation by giving off *Auger electrons*. Part of the energy of excitation may be imparted to an orbital electron (usually in the outer orbits), which, when ejected from the atom, carried with it the energy absorbed minus the binding energy of the vacant subshells. The kinetic energy T of these Auger electrons is

$$T = E - E_b$$

The Auger process leaves an electron shell vacancy, which is filled by an electron from a higher shell or by a free electron, and further emission of characteristic x-rays occurs. The *Auger yield* is the fraction of vacancies that, when filled, results in the emission of Auger electrons vs characteristic x-rays. It is higher with lighter elements. The *fluorescence yield* is the fraction of vacancies that, when filled, results in photon emission (see Fig. 10). The fluorescence yield increases with increasing Z.*

The Nucleus

In its simplest conceptualization, the nucleus is composed of neutrons and protons, collectively known as *nucleons* (Table 2). The nucleus is described in terms of its mass number A, which corresponds to the sum of its neutrons and protons, and its atomic number Z, which is equal to the number of protons and to the number of orbital electrons in the nonionized state. The atom is called a *nuclide* and is symbolized

$$^A_ZX$$

where X is the element symbol. For example, hydrogen is expressed as $^1_1$H, and deuterium, which has a proton and a neutron, as $^2_1$H. In the medical literature and by convention in this book, the mass number is superscripted before the elemental symbol, eg, ^{2}H. The subscript is often deleted since the atomic number can be determined from the chemical symbol (see Fig. 1 and Appendix C). Nuclides with the same Z but different A are called *isotopes*. Since chemical properties depend upon the atomic number, which determines the number of orbital electrons, isotopes have essentially identical chemical properties. Most elements found in nature have more than one isotope. Some examples of natural isotopes are listed in Table 3.

Table 3. Examples of Natural Isotopes

ELEMENT	ISOTOPES	u	% ABUNDANCE
H	$^1_1$H	1.008145	99.98
	$^2_1$H	2.014741	0.02
O	$^{16}_8$O	16.00000	99.759
	$^{17}_8$O	17.00453	0.037
	$^{18}_8$O	18.00488	0.204
Cl	$^{35}_{17}$Cl	34.98006	75.4
	$^{37}_{17}$Cl	36.97767	24.6
U	$^{234}_{92}$U	234.1129	0.006
	$^{235}_{92}$U	235.1156	0.712
	$^{238}_{92}$U	238.1241	99.282

The arrangement of nucleons within the nucleus is not fully understood. Of the several models proposed to conceptualize the structure of the nucleus, the *shell model* depicts the nucleons moving in orbits about one another in a manner similar to the movement of electrons about the nucleus in Bohr's model of the atom. The most stable arrangement for the nucleons is the *ground state*. When the energy level is raised above the ground state, eg, following radioactive decay, the nucleus is said to be either excited or *metastable*. Excitation is a transient state lasting less than 10^{-12} seconds; metastability is an excited state lasting longer, ie, minutes or hours. In either case, energy in the form of photons or conversion electrons is given off to return the nucleus to the ground state.

Another way of conceptualizing nuclear energy levels is provided by the energy "well" shown in Figure 4. The nucleus has an internal organization of energy levels that are in some respects analogous to, though much higher than, the energy levels of orbital electrons. The nucleus can be excited when a nuclear constituent is raised above its ground energy level. When it falls back to the ground state, energy is liberated in the form of photons with energy equal to the difference between the two nuclear energy levels. Radioac-

*Auger electrons are denoted by e_{abc} where a denotes the shell with the original vacancy, b denotes the shell from which the vacancy was filled, and c denotes the shell from which the Auger electron was emitted. For example, an Auger electron denoted e_{KLM} arose from the M shell in response to a K-shell vacancy filled by an L-shell electron.

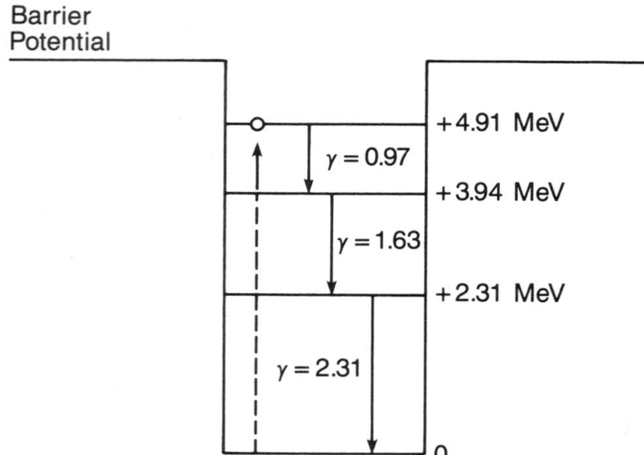

Figure 4. Energy level diagram representing excess nuclear energy. See text for description.

tive nuclei may be naturally unstable or they may be made radioactive by bombardment with high-energy photons, neutrons, or accelerated particles. Figure 4 shows ^{14}N after photon bombardment, which creates an unstable nucleus 4.91 MeV above the ground state. One possible means of deexcitation is *isomeric transition*, in which the cascade of gamma photons is emitted as indicated. *Isomers* possess the same Z and A, but different energy states. Nuclides of the same A but different Z are called *isobars*. *Isotones* have the same number of neutrons, but different A and Z (Fig. 5).

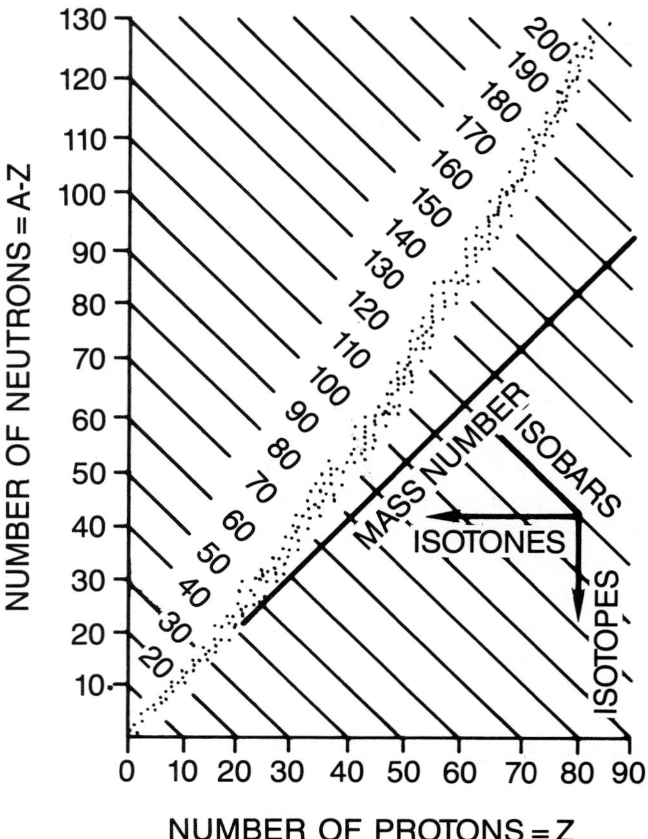

Figure 5. Nuclear composition of the natural elements. The ratio of neutrons to protons increases with increasing atomic number.

Nuclear Stability

Another obstacle of Rutherford's theory of the atom was an explanation of nuclear stability in view of the coulombic forces exerted by the protons' tending to repel one another. It is now known that nuclear stability is achieved by the *strong nuclear force*, which is immensely stronger than electrostatic or gravitational forces and which operates only over very short distances ($\sim 10^{-15}$ m) as found in the nucleus. This force is thought to be exerted by the newly discovered W particles, which are in perpetual agitation between neutrons and protons.

The strong nuclear force operates between both protons and neutrons. Thus, protons attract one another through the strong nuclear force and, at the same time, repel one another through coulombic forces. The net effect is an attractive force that binds the nucleons to form the nucleus. As the number of protons increases, the strength of the coulombic force increases, which tends to break the nucleus apart. To counteract the increasing coulombic force, more neutrons are needed to maintain stability, since they are affected only by the attractive strong nuclear force. As shown in Figure 5, only the lighter nuclei have approximately equal numbers of neutrons and protons. All of the heavier nuclei have excess neutrons needed to achieve nuclear stability. Eventually the repulsive forces between protons cannot be offset by additional neutrons. Thus above $Z = 83$, all nuclei are unstable.

Since energy is equivalent to mass, the mass equivalent of the nuclear binding energy E_b can be determined and this is known as atomic *mass defect*. The mass defect is the difference between the weight of the nucleus and the sum of the weights of its component nucleons:

$$E_b = 931.5\ [(Zm_p + Nm_n + Zm_e) - M]$$

where 931.5 represents MeV/u, Z is the number of protons and electrons, N is the number of neutrons, and M is the atomic mass (not the nuclear mass). As an example, consider the binding energy of $^{16}_{8}O$.

$$E_b = 931.5\ [(8 \times 1.007276) + (8 \times 1.008665) + (8 \times 0.000548) - 16.0000] = 122.876 \text{ MeV}$$

The energy binding of the nucleus (and the electrons) is the energy required to separate it into its constituent nucleons. Figure 6 presents the mean nuclear binding energy in relation to the mass number. Note that the average E_b per nucleon is about 8 MeV and the highest binding energies (most stable nuclei) occur with atoms with mass numbers between 40 and 80.

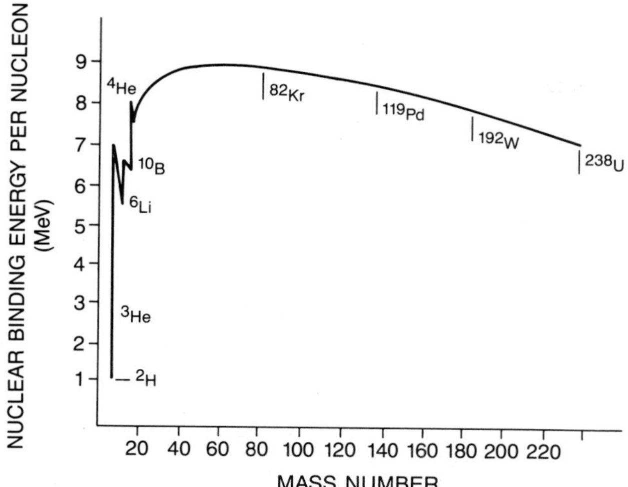

Figure 6. Average nuclear binding energy (MeV) per nucleon as a function of mass number. The fractional activity remaining at any time, t, is a function of the decay constant, λ.

RADIOACTIVITY

In 1896, Henri Becquerel observed that uranium ore was capable of blackening photographic plates and ionizing gases. In 1898, Marie and Pierre Curie named this phenomenon radioactivity and demonstrated its occurrence in radium, polonium, and thorium (besides uranium). Not until some years later did Rutherford and Soddy explain radioactivity as a process of transmutation of an unstable element to another element through the emission of radiation. Alpha particles were detected by Rutherford, who later identified them as helium nuclei, ${}^{4}_{2}He$.

Natural radionuclides, ie, those associated with radioactive elements found in nature, all decay with emissions of alpha, beta, or gamma radiation or, in some cases, by nuclear fission. Most of these natural radionuclides belong to "radioactive families," which include the actinium, thorium, and uranium families. A family exists when one radionuclide decays to a second radionuclide, and so forth, until a stable nuclide is formed. Parent radionuclides of these families all have atomic numbers greater than 82. These so-called *primordial* radionuclides decay very slowly ($\approx 10^8$ to 10^{10} years). It could not be otherwise because they have existed since the formation of our galaxy and all primordial short-lived radionuclides have disappeared. Some radionuclides, such as ${}^{40}K$ (1.3×10^9 years) and ${}^{87}Rb$ (5.2×10^{10} years) do not belong to families, but do have very long half-lives. Several *cosmogenic* radionuclides have shorter half-lives. An example is ${}^{14}C$ (5730 years) which is being created continuously in the atmosphere through bombardment of stable nitrogen nuclei by cosmic rays. This radionuclide forms the basis of carbon-dating techniques. When carbon becomes fixed in terrestrial organic material, the addition of new ${}^{14}C$ ceases. The concentration of ${}^{14}C$ in nonliving matter compared with contemporary concentrations is related by the half-life of ${}^{14}C$ to its age. All other radionuclides found in the environment originate from man-made sources. An excellent discussion of this subject may be found in NCRP Report No. 50.[2]

Radioactive Decay

Radioactive decay is the process whereby a nucleus that contains an excess of energy undergoes a transformation to a more stable state by emitting energy in the form of elementary particles or electromagnetic radiation. For every radioactive nuclide, a probability of decay exists. The relationship between this probability and the number of atoms in a large sample that will decay in some given time is called the "radioactive decay law." It states that the rate of change in the number of atoms ($-dN/dt$) is given by the product of the number of atoms N and the *radionuclide decay constant* λ:

$$-dN/dt = \lambda N$$

The negative sign indicates that N is decreasing with time. The integral form of this equation gives the radioactive decay law:

$$N_t = N_0 e^{-\lambda t}$$

where N_t is the number of atoms at time t, and N_0 is the number of atoms at $t = 0$.

The *half-life* ($T_{1/2}$) is the parameter that is usually measured and may be used to identify a radionuclide. The half-life is the time required to reach 1/2 N_0:

$$1/2\ N_0 = N_0 e^{-\lambda T_{1/2}}$$

which leads to

$$T_{1/2} = \frac{\ln 2}{\lambda} = \frac{0.693}{\lambda}$$

and

$$\lambda = 0.693/T_{1/2}$$

The average time a radionuclide survives is the *mean life* τ and is given by

$$\tau = 1/\lambda = 1.44\ T_{1/2}$$

This quantity is more often used in radiation dosimetry (Chapter 12).

Radioactive decay rates can be slightly altered under certain very rare circumstances. For example, changing the chemical composition of some molecules or altering the atom's ionization state can measurably alter the decay rate (by changing the physical positions of atomic electrons that may be involved in the radioactive decay process). For the most part, however, these changes are minuscule.

Activity

The activity A of a radioactive sample is the number of atoms undergoing transformation per unit time dN/dt. Since the activity decreases at the same rate as N_t, a similar relationship exists:

$$A_t = A_0 e^{-\lambda t}$$

The unit of radioactivity is the bequerel (Bq), which corresponds to a decay rate of one disintegration per second (dps). In older literature radioactivity is expressed in curies. The curie (Ci) equals 3.7×10^{10} dps, or 2.22×10^{12} disintegrations per minute (dpm). The curie was adopted because it was thought to represent the activity in exactly 1 g of ^{226}Ra, a readily available radioactive material. As measurements improved, this value was found to be in error by about 1%. Because the bequerel is a small amount of activity for the applications encountered in nuclear medicine, the kilobequerel (kBq) (2.7×10^{-8} Ci) and megabequerel (MBq) (2.7×10^{-5} Ci) are used more frequently. In this text, activity is expressed in both units.

The mass M of a carrier-free radionuclide represented by an activity of 1 Ci varies with the half-life. It is given by

$$M\ (\text{g/Bq}) = \frac{k \cdot T_{1/2} \cdot A}{N_A}$$

where k is a constant that depends upon the units in which the half-life is expressed and N_A is Avogadro's number, or 6.022×10^{23} nuclei per mole. The *specific activity* expresses the activity of a radionuclide relative to the total elemental mass in a mixture of radioactive and stable atoms (eg, the amount of ^{131}I in a mixture with stable ^{127}I) and is usually expressed in curies per mole or becquerels per mole of the element. For carrier-free radionuclides, ie, the sample is unmixed with any other nuclear species, the specific activity can be calculated from

$$\text{specific activity} \equiv \frac{\text{activity}}{\text{mass}} = \frac{\lambda N}{NM/A_A} = \frac{\lambda A_A}{M}$$

where N = the number of radioactive nuclei, M = molecular weight of the sample, A_A = Avogadro's number (6.022×10^{23} nuclei per mole), and $\lambda = 0.693/T_{1/2}$.

It must be remembered that the source disintegration rate does not necessarily equal the radiation emission rate. Often radiations of a particular type or energy are emitted in only a fraction of all disintegrations. For example, ^{113m}In decays with the emission of its 391-keV gamma emission in only 62% of disintegrations (Appendix B). Measures of the emission rate would thus underestimate activity by about 38%. Therefore, it is essential to know a radionuclide's *decay scheme*. Many of these are given in Appendix B and in References 3 and 4.

The growth of daughter products in radioactive families is discussed in Chapter 10.

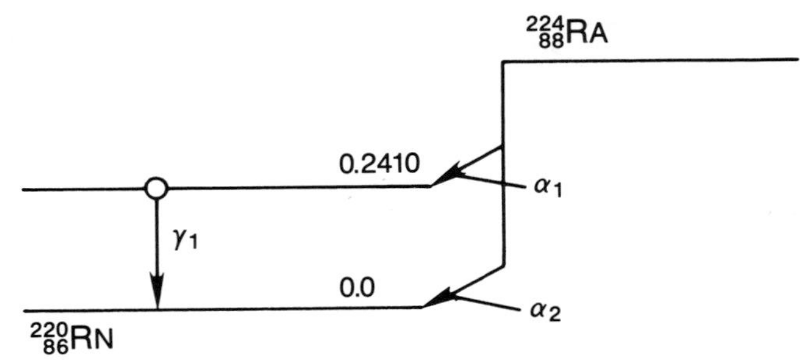

TRANSITION	MEAN NUMBER/ DISINTEGRATION	TRANSITION ENERGY (MeV)
ALPHA 1	0.0520	5.5427
ALPHA 2	0.9480	5.7837
GAMMA 1	0.0520	0.2410

Figure 7. Simplified decay scheme of ^{224}Ra. Half-life = 3.64 days. (From Reference 4.)

DECAY PROCESSES

All radionuclides used in nuclear medicine are artificially produced in either reactors or particle accelerators (see Chapter 9). The excess nuclear energy that they contain is eliminated by six different processes, which generically are termed radioactive decay. These processes are described by the decay scheme, which is unique for each radionuclide and describes not only the mode of decay but also the energy carried off with each nuclear transition and the probability of decay by that transition (Appendix B). Since most radionuclides have several possibilities of decay by which they reach ground state, these decay schemes may be quite complex.

Alpha Decay

Alpha (α) particles are helium nuclei consisting of two neutrons and two protons. They are emitted with discrete energies in the range of 4 to 8 MeV and are often accompanied by photon emissions. The decay of ^{224}Ra, shown schematically in Figure 7, is written as

$$^{224}_{88}\text{Ra} \rightarrow {}^{220}_{86}\text{Rn} + {}^{4}_{2}\alpha + \text{E}$$

In this example, alpha particles of two different energies are emitted, α_1 with 5.54 MeV in about 5% of disintegrations and α_2 with 5.78 MeV in about 95% of disintegrations. The particle α_1 is accompanied by a photon emission of 0.241 MeV. In both decay modes, the nucleus loses 5.78 MeV of energy, decreasing its atomic weight by 4 and atomic number

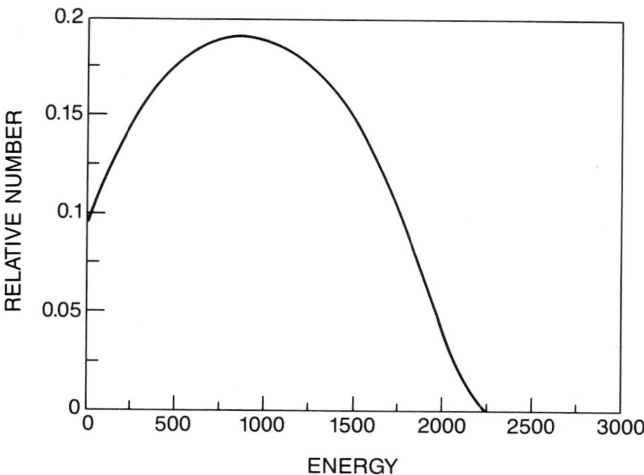

Figure 8. Beta spectrum of ^{90}Y. Beta-ray energies in KeV. $\bar{E}_{\beta^-}$ = 934 keV; $E_{\beta max}$ = 2283 keV.

by 2. The energetics of alpha disintegration may be generalized for any nuclide X disintegrating to Y:

$$ {}^{A}_{Z}X \rightarrow [{}^{A-4}_{Z-2}Y] + [{}^{4}_{2}\alpha] + E $$

Isobaric Transitions

Most radionuclides are unstable by virtue of a neutron:proton imbalance: either too many neutrons or too many protons. Most nuclei do not have enough energy to eject a nucleon. A much more common mode of decay is to eject a charged electron, either beta particle (β^-) or positron (β^+), thus converting neutrons into protons or protons into neutrons, respectively. In these transitions, the atomic number changes, but the atomic mass remains the same—thus the denomination *isobaric transitions*. In general, nuclides with excess neutrons transform by beta decay and nuclides with proton excess decay by positron emission or *electron capture*.

Beta Decay

Beta emission, which was described by Fermi in 1934, can be represented by the following notation:

$$ {}^{A}_{Z}X \rightarrow {}^{A}_{Z+1}Y + {}^{0}_{-1}e + E_{\nu} + E_{\beta} $$

In this case a neutron is transformed into a proton, a negative electron is emitted, and the atomic number increases by 1. Unlike alpha and gamma emissions, beta emissions do not have discrete energies. The kinetic energies of beta particles emitted from the same radionuclide vary from a little above zero to a maximum E_{max}, which is characteristic of the nuclide (Fig. 8). Because the total loss of energy by the nucleus in each disintegration (the *decay energy, Q*) must be discrete (ie, unvarying), an additional energy dissipation process must be postulated. Pauli hypothesied that another, undetected particle emitted with the beta particle must carry the necessary energy to preserve energy conservation. This "particle" ν, called the *neutrino*, has no mass or charge. Hence, it interacts weakly with matter and goes unobserved except through elaborate detection techniques. Its half-value thickness in lead is ten times the distance between the moon and the earth!

Table 4. Some Sources of β^- Emissions

NUCLIDE	HALF-LIFE	E_{max} (MeV)
^{3}H	12.35 y	0.0186
^{14}C	5730 y	0.156
^{32}P	14.29 d	1.710
^{35}S	87.4 y	0.167
^{36}Cl	3.01×10^5 y	0.709
^{45}Ca	163 d	0.257
^{63}Ni	96 y	0.066
^{89}Sr	50.5 d	1.492
^{90}Y	64.0 h	2.283
^{99}Tc	2.111×10^5 y	0.292
^{147}Pm	2.62 y	0.224

The mass difference between X and $(Y + \beta-)$ is $E_{max} = E_{\beta} + E_{\nu}$. This process of decay is also accompanied by the release of antineutrinos, but they can be neglected because they also go undetected.

The distribution of beta energies is important because they have a short range in tissue and thus deposit their energy close to their point of origin. For dosimetry purposes, whenever the energy deposited in tissue is calculated, the mean beta energy $\bar{E}_{\beta}$ is given. This value is usually about 40% of E_{max}. Some examples of "pure" β^- emitters are given in Table 4.

Decay schemes involving beta emission may be simple, as in the case of ^{14}C decay (Fig. 9), or complex, as in the case of ^{99}Mo, in which beta particles with several E_{max} values

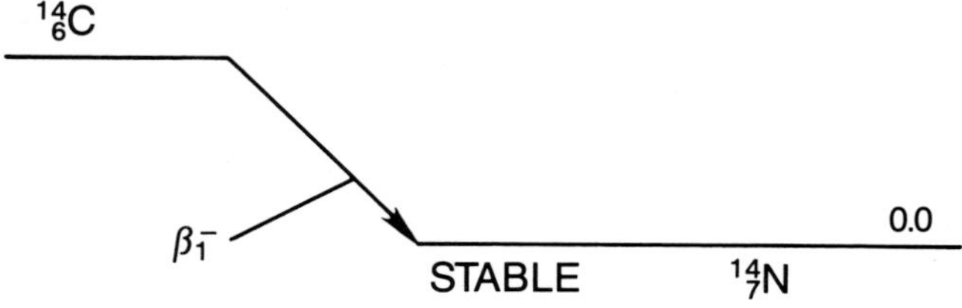

TRANSITION	MEAN NUMBER/ DISINTEGRATION	TRANSITION ENERGY (MeV)
BETA MINUS 1	1.0000	0.1561

Figure 9. Decay scheme of ^{14}C. Half-life = 5730 years. (From Reference 6.)

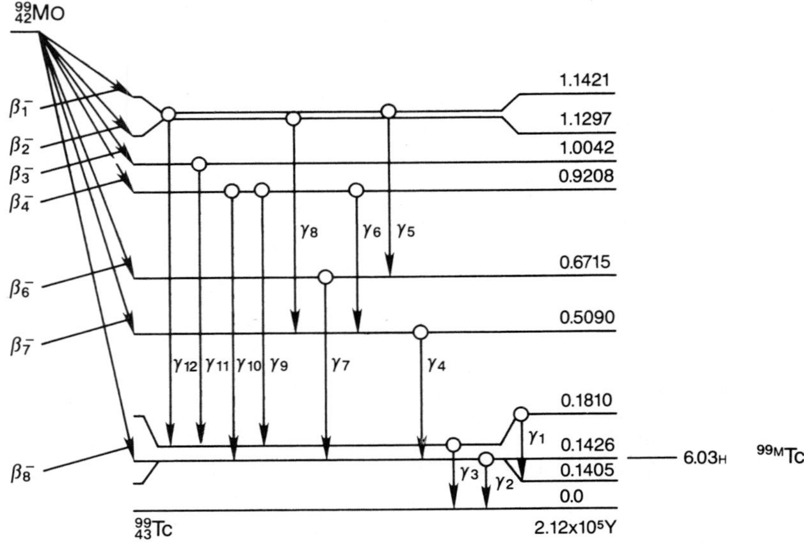

RADIATION	MEAN NUMBER/ DISINTE-GRATION N_i	MEAN ENERGY/ PARTICLE E_i (MeV)	RADIATION	MEAN NUMBER/ DISINTE-GRATION N_i	MEAN ENERGY/ PARTICLE E_i (MeV)
BETA MINUS 1	0.0012	0.0658	GAMMA 4	0.0143	0.3664
BETA MINUS 3	0.0014	0.1112	GAMMA 5	0.0001	0.3807
BETA MINUS 4	0.1850	0.1401	GAMMA 6	0.0002	0.4115
BETA MINUS 6	0.0004	0.2541	GAMMA 7	0.0005	0.5289
BETA MINUS 7	0.0143	0.2981	GAMMA 8	0.0002	0.6207
BETA MINUS 8	0.7970	0.4519	GAMMA 9	0.1367	0.7397
GAMMA 1	0.0130	0.0405	K INT CON ELECT	0.0002	0.7186
K INT CON ELECT	0.0428	0.0195	GAMMA 10	0.0479	0.7782
L INT CON ELECT	0.0053	0.0377	K INT CON ELECT	0.0000	0.7571
M INT CON ELECT	0.0017	0.0401	GAMMA 11	0.0014	0.8231
GAMMA 2	0.0564	0.1405	GAMMA 12	0.0011	0.9610
K INT CON ELECT	0.0058	0.1194	K ALPHA-1 X-RAY	0.0253	0.0183
L INT CON ELECT	0.0007	0.1377	K ALPHA-2 X-RAY	0.0127	0.0182
GAMMA 3	0.0657	0.1810	K BETA-1 X-RAY	0.0060	0.0206
K INT CON ELECT	0.0085	0.1600	KLL AUGER ELECT	0.0087	0.0154
L INT CON ELECT	0.0012	0.1782	KLX AUGER ELECT	0.0032	0.0178
M INT CON ELECT	0.0004	0.1806	LMM AUGER ELECT	0.0615	0.0019
			MXY AUGER ELECT	0.1403	0.0004

Figure 10. Principal decay scheme of ^{99}Mo. Half-life = 66 hours. (From Reference 6.)

may be emitted along with gamma rays in decaying ^{99m}Tc (Fig. 10). In standard nuclear notation:

$$^{A}_{Z}X \xrightarrow{\beta-} {}^{A}_{Z+1}Y^* \xrightarrow{\gamma} {}^{A}_{Z+1}Y$$

where * refers to a nucleus in an excited state.

In the case of ^{99}Mo, eight beta decay possibilities are shown in Figure 10. In every case the ^{99}Tc nucleus is left in an excited state, ie, the beta particles and neutrinos have not carried off sufficient energy to reach the ground state. This energy is given off in the form of gamma rays within nanoseconds of the beta emission. In contrast with beta particles, gamma rays are emitted with discrete energies. In about 87% of disintegrations, the ^{99}Tc nucleus is left in a metastable state (^{99m}Tc), decaying with a half-life of 6 hours. Metastable states will be discussed later in this chapter.

Positron Decay

A proton can be converted to a neutron in two ways. One is by the formation and ejection of a positron, in which the

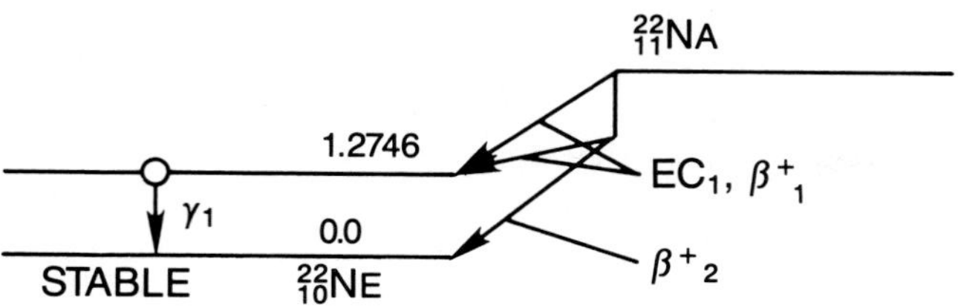

TRANSITION	MEAN NUMBER/ DISINTE-GRATION	TRANSITION ENERGY (MeV)
ELECT CAPT 1	0.0940	1.5680
GAMMA 1	1.0000	1.2746
BETA PLUS 1	0.9060	0.5460
BETA PLUS 2	0.0006	1.8210

Figure 11. Simplified decay scheme of ^{22}Na. Half-life = 2.6 years. (From Reference 6.)

atomic number decreases by 1. The nuclear transformation is denoted

$$^{A}_{Z}X \xrightarrow{\beta+} {}^{A}_{Z-1}Y + {}^{0}_{+1}e^{+} + E_{\beta+} + E_{\nu}$$

The excess nuclear energy is thus reduced by an amount equivalent to the positron mass, 0.511 MeV, plus the kinetic energy of the positron and the neutrino. Any excess energy remaining is then usually given off in the form of photon emissions (Fig. 11). Positrons have an energy spectrum similar to that of beta particles. The positron cannot exist long in nature, but soon combines with an electron to annihilate and form two 0.511-MeV photons, which are given off at 180° (see Fig. 16). It is these annihilation photons that are detected in positron emission tomography (PET).

To decay by positron emission, the parent radionuclide must have a mass greater than its daughter by at least two electron rest masses. To form the positron, its antiparticle, an electron, must also be formed. This formation requires the mass equivalence of 1.022 MeV of energy. The vertical line representing positron decay in the decay scheme of Figure 11 represents this 1.022 MeV of energy.

Electron Capture (EC)

The other mechanism whereby a proton is converted to a neutron is by nuclear capture of an orbital electron. The electrons may be thought of as oscillating in their orbits. In these oscillations, some electrons, particularly those in the inner *K* and *L* shells, may be captured by the nucleus, where the electron charge effectively neutralizes a proton. The excess nuclear energy is given off by the formation and ejection of neutrinos, which go undetected. As the electron vacancy is filled by electrons from other orbits, deexcitation occurs through emission of characteristic x-rays. Iron-55 and ^{181}W are radionuclides that decay in this manner. The kinetics of electron capture may be written

$$^{A}_{Z}X + e^{-} \rightarrow {}^{A}_{Z-1}Y + E_{\nu} + E_{b}$$

where E_b is the orbital binding energy of the captured electron.

Neutron-deficient nuclei with less than 1.022 MeV excess energy usually decay exclusively by EC. Nuclei with more than 1.022 MeV excess energy may decay by either positron emission or EC. In general, nuclei of lighter atomic weight decay by positron emission while heavier nuclei decay by EC. In heavier nuclei, the orbital electrons are closer to the nucleus, which increases the probability of capture. In many cases, the nucleus remains in an excited state (designated by an asterisk) and returns to its ground state through gamma-ray emission:

$$^{A}_{Z}X + e^{-} \rightarrow {}^{A}_{Z-1}Y^{*} \rightarrow {}^{A}_{Z-1}Y + \gamma$$

Medically important radionuclides that decay by EC and by electron capture plus gamma emission (EC, γ) include ^{67}Ga, ^{111}In, ^{123}I, and ^{125}I.

Isomeric Transitions

As already seen, many radionuclides emit gamma rays to bring the nucleus to its ground state. This is called *isomeric transition*, because the atoms have the same *A* and *Z* before and after decay. When a delay occurs between the first decay event and the second, the nuclide is said to be *metastable* and is designated with an m after the mass number. Technetium-99m is the most common example encountered in nuclear medicine (Fig. 12). In the case of ^{99m}Tc, the parent ^{99}Mo, with a half-life of 66 hours, decays by beta emission, 82% of which results in ^{99m}Tc with an energy level of 0.142 MeV. This excited nucleus decays with a 6-hour half-life by one of two processes: in 98.6% of disintegrations a two-step cascade yields 2- and 140-keV gamma rays; in the other 1.4% of disintegrations, a single 142-keV gamma ray is emitted. Because technetium and molybdenum are chemically different, they can be easily separated to yield a radionuclide that has a short half-life, emits no beta particles, and yields a high percentage of useful gamma rays. Some useful gamma-ray sources are listed in Table 5.

Internal Conversion

This process is an alternative to gamma emission and occurs frequently with metastable radionuclides. The excited nucleus imparts its excitation energy to an orbital electron called a *conversion electron*, which is ejected from the atom. Any excess nuclear excitation energy that exceeds the orbital binding energy is imparted to the conversion electron as kinetic energy. The orbital vacancy is then filled from periph-

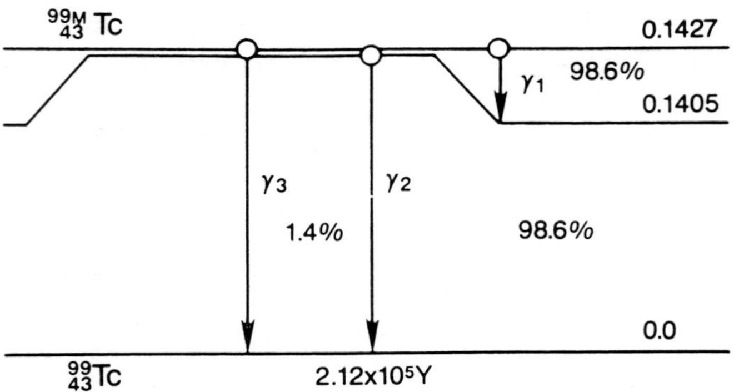

TRANSITION	MEAN NUMBER/ DISINTE- GRATION	TRANSITION ENERGY (MeV)
GAMMA 1	0.9860	0.0021
GAMMA 2	0.9860	0.1405
GAMMA 3	0.0140	0.1426

Figure 12. Simplified decay scheme of ^{99m}Tc. Half-life = 6.0 hours. See Appendix B for more complete decay scheme.

eral or free electrons with the emission of characteristic x-rays or Auger electrons.

As described in the example of ^{99m}Tc, the metastable nuclide can decay by two processes. Internal conversion occurs with both decay schemes. Approximately 10% of the 140-keV gamma rays are converted, and the ratio of orbital electrons undergoing conversion is K:L:(M + N) = 913:118:39 per 10^4 disintegrations (see Appendix B). Note that from Figure 10 ^{99}Mo emits conversion electrons of ten different energies. The complete emission spectrum of ^{99m}Tc then shows not only the 142-, 140-, and 2-keV gamma rays, but also the K, L, M, and N x-rays and a variety of Auger electrons. The latter are analogous to conversion electrons except that the incident photons arise from orbital shells rather than the nucleus. They are important only from a radiation dosimetry standpoint because, while they are not detected externally, they nevertheless contribute to absorbed radiation.

Conversion electrons behave like beta particles in matter, with energy equal to the nuclear excitation energy minus the orbital binding energy. For ^{99m}Tc, the energy imparted to a K conversion electron is

$$E_{eK} = 142 - 21 = 121 \text{ keV}$$

or

$$E_{eK} = 140 - 21 = 119 \text{ keV}$$

The observable difference between beta particles and conversion electrons is that the latter are emitted with nearly discrete energies, rather than in a continuous spectrum of energies as shown in Figure 8.

Table 5. Some Gamma Ray Sources

NUCLIDE	HALF-LIFE	ENERGY (MeV)	ABUNDANCE (%)
^{22}Na	2.602 y	1.274	99.9
^{51}Cr	27.7 d	0.320	10
^{57}Co	271 d	0.122	86
^{60}Co	5.27 y	1.332	100
		1.173	100
^{88}Y	106.6 d	0.898	93.7
		1.836	99.3
^{137}Cs	30.17 y	0.662	85
^{241}Am	432 y	0.060	36

Nuclear Fission

Heavy radionuclides such as ^{235}U, ^{237}Np, ^{239}Pu, and ^{252}Cf undergo spontaneous fission, which results in two smaller nuclei and the emission of two or three fission neutrons. The masses of the two *fission fragments* occur typically in a 60:40 ratio. For example, $^{99}_{40}$Zr:

$$^{235}_{92}\text{U} + {}^{1}_{0}\text{n} \rightarrow [^{236}_{92}\text{U}] + 2\,{}^{1}_{0}\text{n} + E \quad (\nearrow {}^{99}_{40}\text{Zr},\ \swarrow {}^{135}_{52}\text{Te})$$

The excess energy E, usually 200 to 300 MeV per fission fragment, is initially imparted to the fragments and neutrons as kinetic energy and ultimately dissipated as heat. Most of the fission fragments have excess neutrons and decay further by beta decay. Fission is of interest to nuclear medicine (1) because most fission fragments are radioactive and provide a source of inexpensive, high specific-activity tracer nuclides (eg, ^{131}I, ^{133}Xe, ^{99}Mo) and (2) because the neutrons liberated in the fission process may be used to produce radionuclides by *neutron activation* of targets inserted into the reactor core. These processes are discussed in Chapter 9.

INTERACTION OF RADIATION WITH MATTER

All types of radiation have energy, whether inherent, as in the case of electromagnetic radiation, or kinetic, as in the case of moving particles. When radiation interacts with matter, this energy is transferred to the atoms of the material through which it passes. The mechanisms whereby radiation is absorbed are of fundamental interest because they form the basis of both radiation detection and an understanding of the biologic effects that radiation induce.

The transfer of energy from a particle or photon to the absorbing material occurs primarily through two mechanisms: *ionization* and *excitation*. Ionization is the process whereby an orbital electron is removed from an atom or molecule, resulting in an ion pair: a negative electron and a positively charged atom or molecule. Excitation leaves the atom or molecule in an excited state without ejecting an electron. The end result of excitation is the ultimate dissipation of energy as light, heat, or chemical reactions.

Interactions of Alpha and Heavy Charged Particles

The forces acting between heavy charged particles, such as alpha particles, and matter are coulombic or electrostatic forces between their positive charge and the negative charge of orbital electrons in the absorber matter. The force F between two particles of charge q and q' is inversely proportional to the square of the distance between them:

$$F = \frac{q\,q'}{d^2}$$

If the charges are alike, the force is repelling; if they are opposite, it is attractive. Thus, when a charged particle moves through matter, the interactions with orbital electrons and nuclei are not mechanical collisions, but coulombic deflections (Fig. 13). Since the number of particles per unit volume is proportional to the density, more interactions per unit path length occur in denser materials than in lighter ones. The energy imparted by the charged particle to the absorber atoms through ionization and excitation is ultimately dissipated in the production of characteristic x-rays, light photons, and heat.

The four principal interactions between heavy charged particles and matter are (1) elastic collisions with atomic nuclei, which result in bremsstrahlung radiation (discussed in the next section); (2) excitation of atomic electrons, which results in characteristic x-rays and Auger electrons; (3) ionization by collision with atomic electrons and the formation of ion pairs; and (4) catastrophic collisions with absorber nuclei. Usually, ejected electrons are outer orbital electrons, which require only small amounts of energy to overcome their binding energy. Except for catastrophic collisions with nuclei, which occur rarely because of their small size, only a small fraction of the particle's energy is lost with each interaction, principally through ionization. An alpha particle, for example, loses approximately 34 eV per ion pair formed in air. Thus a 2-MeV alpha particle interacts about 6×10^4 times before slowing down sufficiently to pick up orbital electrons and finally coming to rest as a neutral helium atom. Occasionally, a *secondary electron* is ejected with sufficient force for it to behave as a beta particle, which causes secondary ionizations. Such particles are referred to as delta (δ) rays. In solid matter most of the energy loss of heavy charged particles occurs through delta rays.

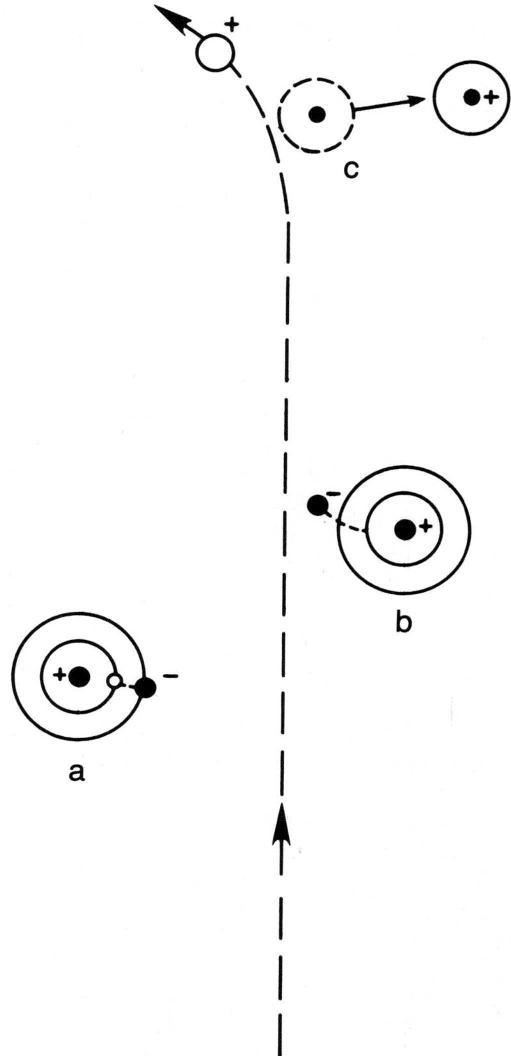

Figure 13. Path of heavy charged particle in matter. Excitation (a) and ionization (b) do not deflect the alpha-particle path. Close approach to an absorber nucleus (c) causes deflection of the alpha particle and the nucleus, which may in turn produce ionization.

The description of the loss of energy in a medium gives rise to a number of important concepts. The *total* energy lost per unit length of path traversed, including both radiation and collision losses, is the *linear stopping power* (S_l), expressed in MeV/cm:

$$S_l = \frac{-\mathrm{d}E}{\mathrm{d}x}$$

Since S_l is directly proportional to N and Z, high atomic number and high-density materials will have the greatest stopping power.

S_l is closely related to the *linear energy transfer* (LET), which relates to the energy deposited *locally* in the absorber per unit path length. In most biologic materials, little energy

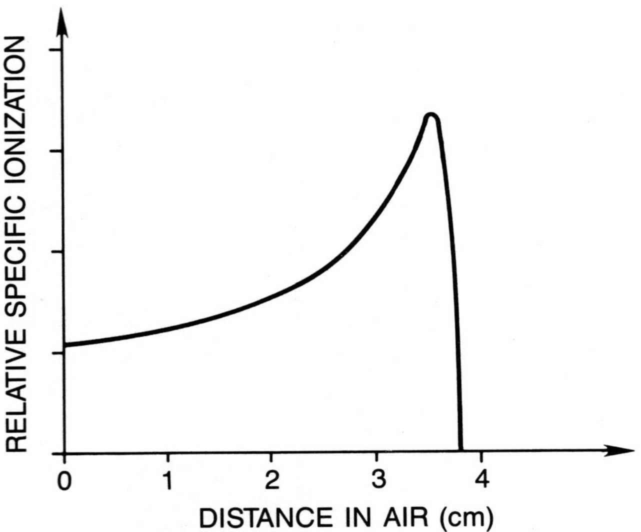

Figure 14. Specific ionization of an alpha particle as a function of path length. The peak just before the end of the particle track is the Bragg peak.

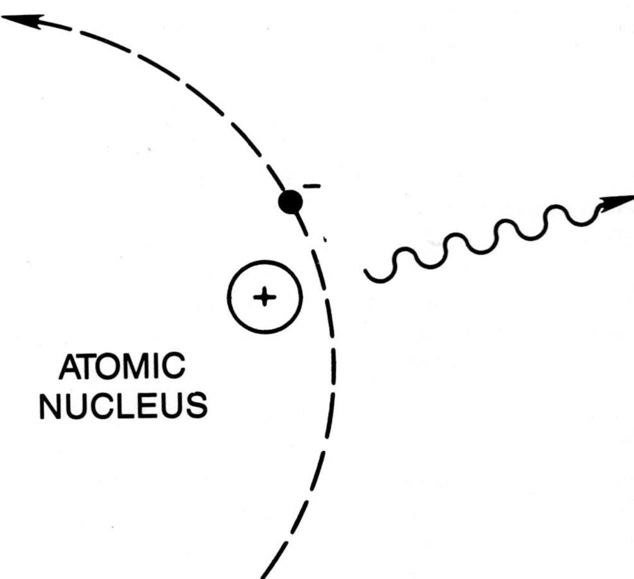

Figure 15. Production of bremsstrahlung. See text for explanation.

is lost by bremsstrahlung production; thus the values of S_l and LET are nearly equal. The LET is important in radiation biology because it reflects the tissue damage done by type of particle. Because of the relatively short path length of heavy charged particles, the LET is high relative to other forms of radiation of the same energy. Alpha particles, for example, travel a few centimeters in air and a few micrometers in tissue.

The rate of energy loss depends on the particle charge, the density of the medium, and the velocity of the particle. The *specific ionization* (SI) refers to the number of ionization events per unit distance. The increase in specific ionization as the particle slows near the end of its track is known as the *Bragg effect* (Fig. 14). The rapid fall in the SI after the Bragg peak represents the sudden decrease in specific ionization as the charge is neutralized by the addition of orbital electrons.

The ratio of LET to specific ionization gives the *average energy expended per ionizing event* (*W*)

$$W = \text{LET/SI}$$

The value of *W* for air is approximately 33.97 eV per event.

Another concept is the *ionization potential* (*I*), which represents the average energy required to produce ion pairs, an average obtained from all of the orbital electron shells. *W* is always greater than *I* because almost half of a particle's energy is dissipated in excitation events that do not result in ionization. Both *W* and *I* decrease with increasing *Z* of the absorber material because of the greater number of outer orbital electrons of lower binding energy. For example, $W = 33.97$ eV for air ($Z = 7.6$) and $W = 2.9$ eV for germanium ($Z = 32$) used in semiconductor detectors. The greater number of ion pairs per MeV of particle energy accounts for the greater detector efficiency of materials with higher *Z*.

Interactions of Beta Particles

Electrons undergo the same interactions in matter as heavy charged particles. For considerations in nuclear medicine, beta particles and positrons interact with matter identically, but certain differences occur in the process of energy loss for electrons compared with that for heavy charged particles. First, a larger energy loss per interaction generally occurs because the masses of the incident electron and the orbital electron are the same. On the other hand $-dE/dx$ is lower for electrons because of their small size. Consequently, the electron range is greater than that of heavy charged particles.

The path of an electron is likely to vary greatly because of a greater likelihood that an interaction will result in a large angular deflection. The path of heavy charged particles, on the other hand, is usually straight and nearly the same for all particles having the same charge and velocity.

Beta particles also lose energy by the production of *bremsstrahlung*, or "braking radiation." When an electron approaches an atomic nucleus, the strong attraction for the nucleus decelerates the particle (Fig. 15). When the kinetic energy of a charged particle exceeds its rest mass energy, the excess energy is eliminated through photon emission. This process, which holds for all particles, becomes particularly important for electrons because their rest mass energy is only 0.511 MeV. The intensity of bremsstrahlung production is proportional to the square of the atomic number *Z* of the material and the particle's charge *z* and inversely proportional to the square of the particle's mass *M* or Z^2z^2/M^2. Thus electrons are more likely to produce bremsstrah-

Table 6. Beta-Particle Ranges in Air and Water

	E_{max} (MeV)	AIR (cm)	WATER (cm)
^{3}H	0.018	5	0.0006
^{14}C	0.156	22	0.03
^{32}P	1.70	610	0.8

Data from Reference 6.

lung than alpha particles because of their smaller mass, despite their lesser charge. Electrons striking dense material produce more photons than those striking lighter material. This process accounts for the production of x-rays in an x-ray tube. Bremsstrahlung also is used to detect the presence of such highly energetic beta particles as ^{32}P (E_{max} = 1.71 MeV) in tissue. The bremsstrahlung spectrum is continuous, similar to the distribution shown in Figure 8. The energy depends upon the velocity of the particle and the deceleration produced by each encounter.

Because bremsstrahlung production increases by Z^2 of the absorber, high-Z materials do not provide the best shielding for beta-emitting radionuclides. Thus lead should not be used to contain energetic beta emitters because, while the beta particles will not escape, the bremsstrahlung produced in the container or shielding material may. Plastic and glass provide better shielding than lead because beta-particle absorption is adequate and bremsstrahlung production is minimal.

In any absorbing medium, the mean path length of beta particles exceeds the range of heavy charged particles. Measured by absorption thickness, the range of beta particles varies even for particles of the same energy (eg, conversion electrons) because of their irregular track characteristics. For comparison, the maximum ranges of ^{3}H, ^{14}C, and ^{32}P beta particles are shown in Table 6.

Cerenkov radiation also is produced by beta particles. These radiations are light photons, emitted by energetic electrons whose velocity is greater than the speed of light in the medium in which they are traveling. This phenomenon, which is responsible for the bluish white light emitted around the core of swimming pool reactors, is discussed in more detail in Chapter 2.

A third radiation process comes about through positron annihilation. When positrons are emitted from the nucleus, they produce excitation, ionization, bremsstrahlung, etc., just as electrons do. As they slow down, however, they do not wander freely in the absorbing material as do electrons. They combine with a free electron and annihilate to form two 0.511-MeV photons equal to the rest mass of the two particles. The photons are given off at angles 180° to each other, as shown in Figure 16. This phenomenon can be used to detect the location of the positron emitter. The positron travels only a few millimeters in tissue before annihilating; therefore, relatively precise localization can be determined by placing two opposing detectors, connected through a coincidence circuit, on either side of the source. Since the 180° directionality of the simultaneous photons is constant, only one of the detectors need be collimated to localize the plane of annihilation.

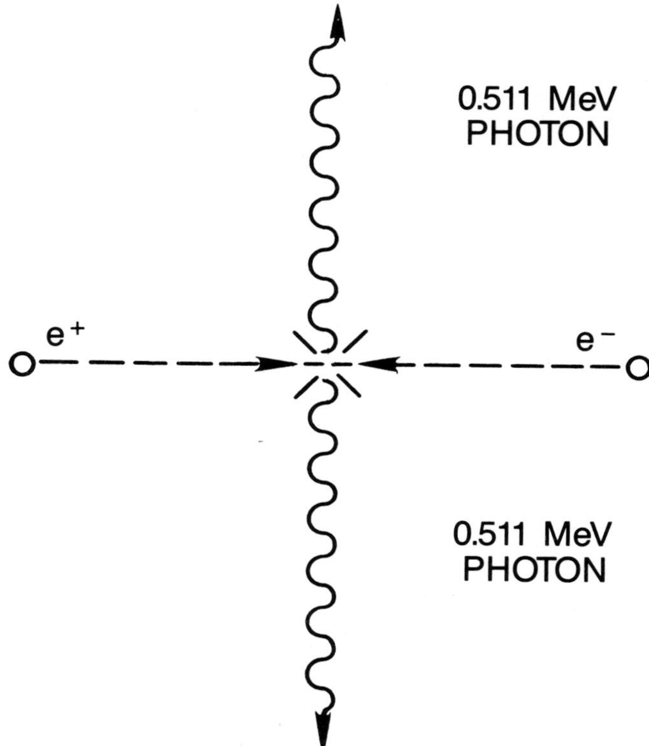

Figure 16. Positron annihilation.

Interactions of Photons

The interaction of all uncharged particles, including neutrons, neutrinos, and photons, is largely the same and quite different from interactions involving charged particles. The photons of importance include gamma rays, x-rays, and bremsstrahlung, which have different denominations only by virtue of their origin: gamma rays from nuclei, x-rays from the atom—usually from orbital electrons, and bremsstrahlung from free particles.

While photons appear to be influenced by the electromagnetic fields of electrons and nuclei, their only interaction is by direct impact upon them. Three principal mechanisms explain how photons are absorbed or *attenuated*: photoelectric absorption, Compton scatter, and pair production. All of these events lead to complete or partial transfer of energy from the gamma ray to the absorber electrons.

Photoelectric Absorption

This phenomenon occurs when all of the photon's energy is absorbed by the atom, which, in the process, ejects an

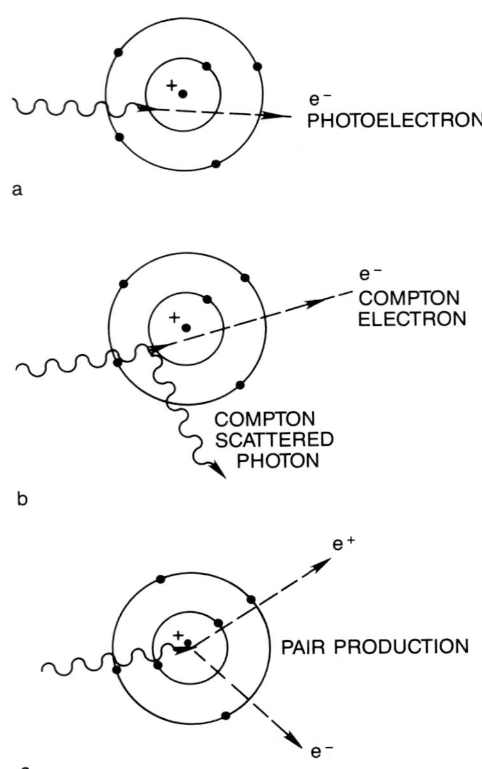

Figure 17. Principal photon interactions in matter.

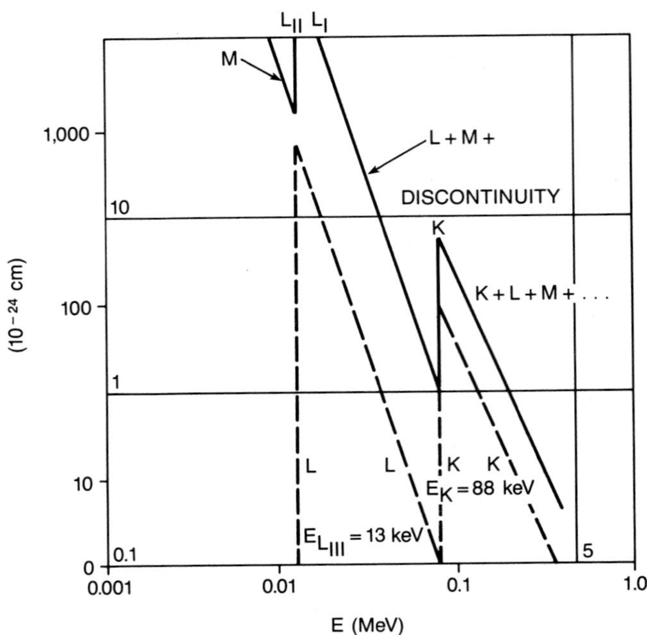

Figure 18. Probability of photon absorption (coefficient of absorption in cm^{-1} as shown in the ordinate) in lead by the photoelectric effect as a function of photon energy.

orbital electron, usually from the K or L shells (Fig. 17a). If the energy E_γ of the incident photon is greater than the electron's binding energy E_b, the electron leaves its orbit with kinetic energy:

$$T_e = E_\gamma - E_b$$

Photoelectric absorption is a process that involves whole atoms and does not occur with free electrons. The atom is ionized and the *photoelectron* than behaves in matter as would an Auger electron or a beta particle. The vacancy in the orbital shell is then filled by higher orbital electrons and by emission of characteristic x-rays and Auger electrons as described earlier.

When the incident photon energy exceeds the binding energies of orbital electrons, probability favors the inner orbital electrons undergoing the photoelectric effect. This probability is expressed graphically in Figure 18, in which the photoelectric cross section (probability of absorption) in barns is shown as a function of the photon energy in a lead absorber.

The dashed lines represent the absorption cross sections for the K and L orbital shells, and the solid lines represent cross sections for combinations of shells. For example, the binding energy for an L_3 orbital electron is 13 keV. Absorption of photons below this energy by an L_3 electron is practically nil. As the incident gamma-ray energy reaches this energy, the probability of absorption by photoelectric effect increases suddenly and then falls off sharply with increasing energies until the *K edge* or *K discontinuity* is reached. At this point another sudden increase in photoelectric absorption occurs, now by the K electrons with a binding energy of 88 keV. The photon preference is always for the inner electrons.

In Figure 19, the linear absorption coefficients are shown for a sodium iodide crystal as a function of gamma-ray energy. It can be seen that the photoelectric effect predominates in sodium iodide crystals for energies below about 250 keV. In general, the photoelectric effect increases with increasing Z of the absorber and decreases with increasing gamma-ray energies. The photoelectric effect is approximately proportional to Z^3/E_γ^3. This strong dependence on Z indicates why high-Z materials are favored in gamma-ray detectors and shielding.

Compton Scattering

A second mechanism of gamma-ray absorption is Compton scattering, in which an incident photon is deflected by an electron in the absorber medium, imparting some of its energy to the electron, which then becomes a *recoil electron* (Fig. 17b). The photon is scattered at an angle Θ to the incident direction and it can be shown that the new photon energy E'_γ is proportional to the scattering angle

$$E'_\gamma = \frac{E_\gamma}{1 + \frac{E_\gamma}{m_0c^2}(1 - \cos\theta)}$$

where m_0c^2 is the electron rest mass energy, or 0.511 MeV. The kinetic energy of the recoil electron is then

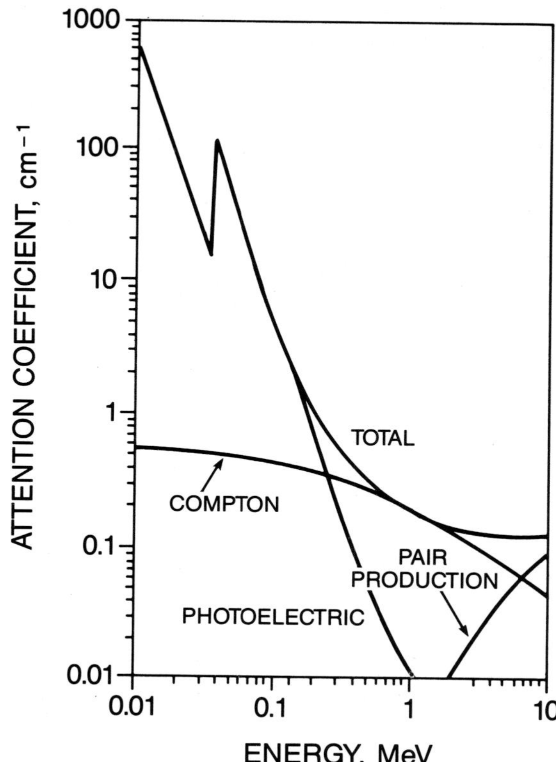

Figure 19. Attenuation coefficients as a function of photon energy in a NaI crystal.

$$T_e = E_\gamma - E'_\gamma$$

Compton scattering is responsible for many of the characteristics of gamma pulse-height spectra and is discussed in detail in Chapter 3. The Compton scatter component of gamma-ray attenuation decreases slowly with increasing photon energy and with increasing Z of the absorber.

Pair Production

When an energetic photon passes near an atomic nucleus, the photon may annihilate and form an electron-positron pair (Fig. 17c). The minimum energy required for this interaction is 2 m_0c^2, or 1.022 MeV. The remaining energy is divided between the two particles as kinetic energy:

$$E_\gamma = 2m_0c^2 + T_{e^-} + T_{e^+}$$

The positron soon combines with an electron in the absorber and annihilates to form two 0.511-MeV photons, which are given off at 180° angles. The cross section of pair production increases with increasing Z of the absorber and logarithmically with the gamma energy (Fig. 19).

Of these three processes, only the photoelectric effect results in all or nearly all of the incident photon energy being deposited in the absorber. In Compton scattering, the total energy of the incident photon is absorbed only if the scattered photons are completely absorbed as well. Since the probability of all of these interactions increases with increasing Z, it is evident that high-Z materials, such as lead (Z = 82), provide the best shielding for gamma rays.

There are two other photon interactions that are of interest even though they contribute little to gamma-ray attenuation encountered in nuclear medicine: *Rayleigh scattering* and *photonuclear reactions*.

Rayleigh Scattering

Rayleigh scattering, or *coherent scattering*, is an interaction between a photon and an atom as a whole. Because of the large atomic mass, there is practically no recoil energy absorbed by the atom. The photon is absorbed and reemitted with approximately the same energy, but in a random direction. Thus this mechanism contributes little to energy absorption but may contribute significantly to the attenuation of a photon beam. It is important to CT scanning. Rayleigh scattering occurs principally at low photon energies (<50 keV).

Photonuclear Reactions

At very high photon energies (>2 MeV), photons may be absorbed by atomic nuclei with the ejection of a nucleon: a proton, neutron, or alpha particle. Since the (γ,n) reaction predominates, neutron-deficient nuclei are formed. These are usually radioactive and decay by positron emission. Photonuclear reactions are of some theoretical interest as a means of radionuclide production but have no importance in photon attenuation in nuclear medicine.

Attenuation of Photon Beams

The measure of photon absorption is given by the *linear attenuation coefficient* μ, which has units of cm^{-1}. The fractional decrease in photon beam intensity $\Delta I/I$ by an absorber of thickness x is given by

$$\frac{\Delta I}{I} = -\mu\, x$$

Integrating for some thickness x:

$$I = I_0 e^{-\mu x}$$

where I is the photon beam intensity in counts per second after passing through the absorber and I_0 is the incident beam intensity.

This equation may be expressed in terms of the density of the absorber or the *mass attenuation coefficient* in cm^2/g as

$$I = I_0 e^{-\mu m}$$

since

$$\mu_m = \mu/\rho$$

The linear attenuation coefficient μ represents the cross section of interaction for all three gamma absorption processes illustrated in Figure 19. Here the attenuation of gamma rays in cm^{-1} is plotted as a function of gamma-ray energy in MeV. The total attenuation is plotted as a solid line, which is the product of attenuation by photoelectric effect, Compton scattering, and pair production.

REFERENCES

1. Kaye GWC, Laby TH. *Tables of Physical and Chemical Constants and Some Mathematical Functions*. London: Longman Group, 1973.
2. NCRP. Environmental Radiation Measurements. Report No. 50. Washington DC: National Council on Radiation Protection and Measurements, 1976.
3. Lederer CM, Shirley VS, Eds. *Table of Isotopes*. 7th Ed. New York: John Wiley & Sons, 1978.
4. Dillman LT, VonderLage FC. Radionuclide Decay Schemes and Nuclear Parameters for Use in Radiation-Dose Estimation. M1RD Pamphlet No. 10. New York: Society of Nuclear Medicine, 1975.
5. NCRP. Structural Shielding Design and Evaluation for Medical Use of X-Rays and Gamma Rays of Energies up to 10 MeV. Report No. 49. Washington DC: National Council on Radiation Protection and Measurements, 1976.
6. Weber DA, Eckerman KF, Dillman LT, Ryman JC. MIRD: Radionuclide Data and Decay Schemes New York. New York: The Society of Nuclear Medicine, 1989.

2 Radiation Detector Systems

John C. Harbert, Bert M. Coursey

The detection of radioactivity is based on the interaction of radiation with matter involving the absorption processes discussed in Chapter 1. Radiation can be measured calorimetrically by detecting the amount of heat absorbed in a detector medium, but most detectors depend on the ionization that occurs when photons and nuclear particles are absorbed within the detector. Detection systems are classified in three ways: (1) by the medium in which the interaction takes place, ie, liquid, solid, or gas; (2) by the nature of the physical phenomenon prouced, ie, excitation, ionization, or chemical change; or (3) by the type of electronic pulse generated, ie, by a pulse amplitude that is constant or else is proportional to the energy of the incident radiation. Examples of radiation detection systems based on chemical changes include film emulsions and thermoluminescent dosimeters. Along with the associated electronics used to register the interactions, detection systems make up an impressive array of apparatus.

GAS-FILLED DETECTORS

Gas-filled ionization chambers are among the earliest nuclear radiation detectors and have many important uses in nuclear medicine. The three most common types are (1) ionization chambers used for personnel dosimeters, radiopharmaceutical dose calibrators, and laboratory monitors; (2) proportional counters for measuring charged particles; and (3) Geiger-Müller tubes for measuring ambient radiation.

These detectors all operate on the same general principle: the ability of ionized gas within an electrically charged enclosure to alter the voltage potential between two electrodes. The general design of these chambers is schematically represented in Figure 1. A gas-filled chamber made of some conducting material, which serves as the cathode, is connected to a well-insulated central anode through a resistance-capacitance (R-C) circuit across which a voltage *V* has been applied. Ionizing radiation entering the chamber produces electrons and positively charged ion pairs from the gas atoms. These are collected by the central anode and outer chamber walls, respectively, because of the direction of the electrical field. The change in charge (pulse height) on the capacitor *C* per radiation detected is proportional to the number of ions collected. The pulse height as a function of the voltage *V* applied across the electrodes is shown in Figure 2 for two charged particles of different energy. The curves reflect the capacitance that would be generated by the two ionizing events.

These curves are divided into four recognizable regions. In region I, the voltage applied produces an electric field too weak to attract many ion pairs to the electrodes before they recombine to neutral atoms. Recombination occurs when negative and positive ions combine and neutralize one another before reaching the electrodes. Their contribution to the measured *pulse height* (signal amplitude) is thus negated. As the voltage is increased, the drift velocity of the ions increases, reducing the time available for recombination. The fraction of the charge collected therefore increases. This region has little utility for most detector systems.

In region II, further increases in voltage have little effect on the pulse height because all of the ions produced by each radiation event are collected and none recombines. This plateau, where the pulse height remains relatively constant with changes in applied voltage, is called the *ionization* region, and the charge necessary for operation in this region is known as the *saturation current.* In this region, the pulse height is proportional to the energy deposited in the chamber by the incident radiation, although the signal output requires considerable amplification to drive a scaler or pulse-height analyzer. For example, the energy expended (*W*) in producing a single ion pair in air is about 34 eV. A 1-MeV beta particle thus would produce about $10^6/34 \approx 3 \times 10^4$ ion pairs. In typical ionization chambers this will yield a pulse amplitude of about 5×10^{-5} V. Signals this weak require relatively sophisticated amplifiers and pulse-processing electronics.[1] For this reason, detectors operated in this region are seldom used for measuring individual events, but rather are used for measuring radiation flux (particles/cm^2/s).

As voltage is increased further, the charge collected is increased by a multiplication factor due to the phenomenon of *gas amplification* (region III, Fig. 2). The electrons formed in the primary ionizing event are now accelerated sufficiently to cause secondary ionization of the neutral gas molecules as they speed toward the collecting electrodes and thus add to the collected charge. The secondary ions may also acquire enough energy to ionize more neutral atoms so that a *cascade* effect is produced. The factor by which ionization is increased is called the *gas amplification factor.* It may reach as high as 10^4 to 10^6. In the portion of region III used for particle detection, the pulse height remains dependent upon

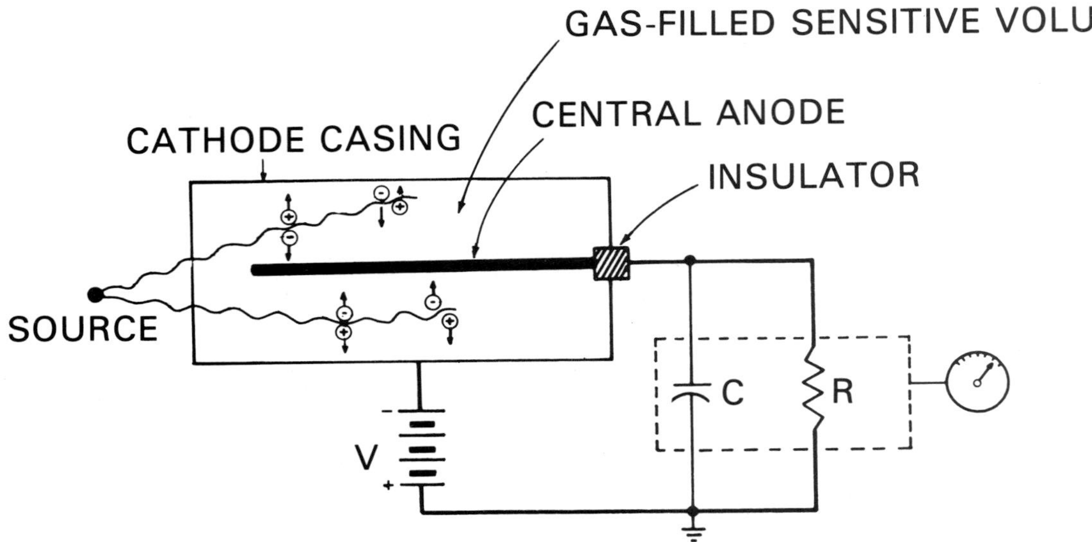

Figure 1. Diagram of a gas-filled detector.

the initial energy of the ionizing particle, provided all of the energy is absorbed within the detector. This area is called the *proportional* region. As voltage is increased at the upper end of this region, the two curves come together, ie, the pulse height now becomes more dependent upon the voltage applied than upon the energy of the ionizing radiation. This area is called the region of *limited proportionality.* It is not important in the measurement of ionizing radiations.

In region IV, pulse height is entirely independent of radiation energy. The upper limit of gas amplification is here limited by the type of gas used and the design characteristics of the chamber. A plateau is again reached. This area is known as the Geiger-Müller region. Above this region, *continuous discharge* occurs within the chamber. This phenomenon is discussed in more detail in the next section.

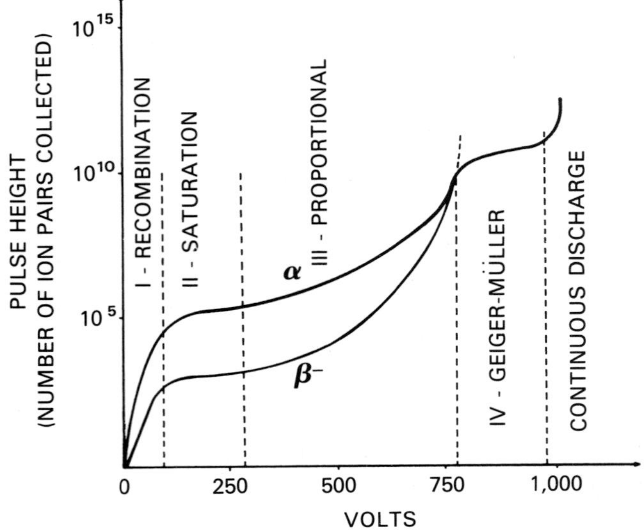

Figure 2. Characteristic pulse-height curves produced by beta and alpha particles as a function of applied voltage in a gas-filled detector.

Ionization-Chamber Detectors

The broadest applications of ionization chamber detectors are found in health physics, where they are used to measure the intensity of environmental radiation or cumulative doses of radiation. These detectors often contain dry air at atmospheric pressure, enclosed within a cylindrical chamber, as shown in Figure 1. Saturation voltage is maintained between the electrodes, usually by a battery, so that they operate in region II of Figure 2. The saturation voltage must be determined for each instrument because it varies with the size and shape of the detector, the spacing of the electrodes, and the type of gas used. Ionization chambers may be used to measure all types of ionizing radiation. Since the pulse height is proportional to the radiation energy deposited within the detector, they may be operated in a *pulse mode* in conjunction with electronic equipment designed for pulse-height analysis. They are seldom used in this manner, however, because the time for ion collection on the electrodes is long ($\sim 10^{-3}$ seconds) and the pulse amplitude is so low that a high level of "noise" (spurious counts unrelated to the radiation measured) is inherent in the system. They are most often used in *current mode or mean-level* operation to measure radiation of relatively high intensity where the current measured is proportional to the radiation flux emitted from some radiation source. The output of such a detector is the deflection of a ratemeter that integrates individual pulses over a selectable time interval. An example is the "Cutie Pie," a portable dose ratemeter in which ambient radiation (exposure rate) is read directly from a meter calibrated in roentgens* per hour (R/h) (Fig. 3).

*See Appendix A for definition of a roentgen.

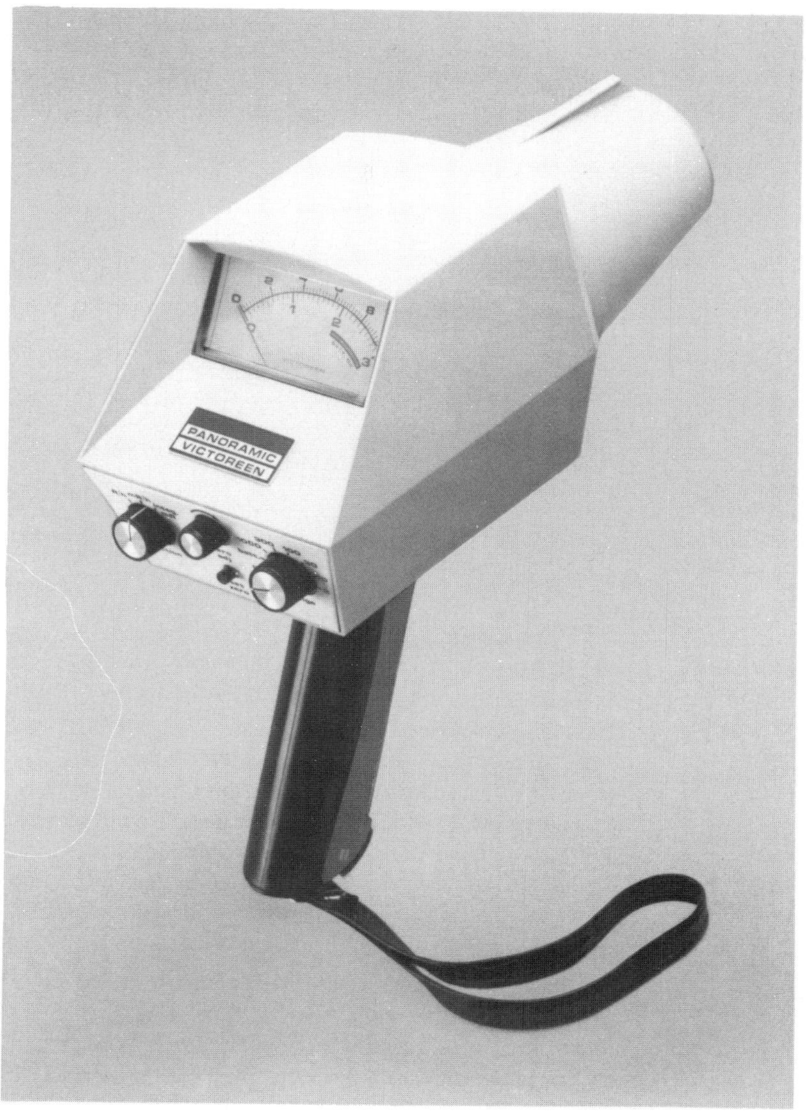

Figure 3. "Cutie Pie" portable dose ratemeter. External voltage is provided by batteries. The cylindrical ionization chamber is usually provided with a protective cap that can be removed to measure low-energy radiation.

The sensitivity of ionization chamber survey meters is strongly influenced by the energy of the radiation detected. Low-energy photons and beta particles are attenuated by the chamber walls and high-energy photons pass right through the detector gas, thereby reducing detector efficiency. A typical survey meter response curve to photons is shown in Figure 4.

Another common ionization chamber is the pocket dosimeter, which measures the quantity of radiation delivered over a certain time period, typically hours or days (Fig. 5). The dosimeter is charged to a predetermined voltage V_1 by a battery-powered charging system. As ions are produced by incident radiation, they are collected by the electrodes, gradually reducing the original voltage between the electrodes. At the end of the exposure period, the reduced voltage V_2 is measured by an electrometer, and the difference is proportional to the radiation dose calibrated in gray or rad. Direct-reading dosimeters are modifications of the Lauritzen electroscope, which consists of a gas-filled chamber with heavy-duty enclosure and a specially adapted central collecting anode. The anode consists of a gold-plated quartz fiber attached to the collector anode. When the dosimeter is charged by a battery, electrostatic forces repel the quartz fiber from the anode. As the charge between the electrodes is neutralized by ionizing radiation, the electrostatic force diminishes and the fiber returns to its resting position. The position of the fiber is viewed through a lens system, which also focuses on a scale calibrated in roentgens or milliroentgens. Thus, at any time, the wearer can determine the integrated dose of radiation exposure.

One of the most common gas-filled detectors is the "dose calibrator," which consists of a large-volume sealed ionization chamber. Most dose calibrators are pressurized to several atmospheres with argon or xenon gas to increase density and the gamma-ray response in the region 100 keV to 1 MeV. These chambers have a central well large enough to accept vials or syringes of up to about 100-mL capacity for determining activity to be administered to patients (Fig. 6).

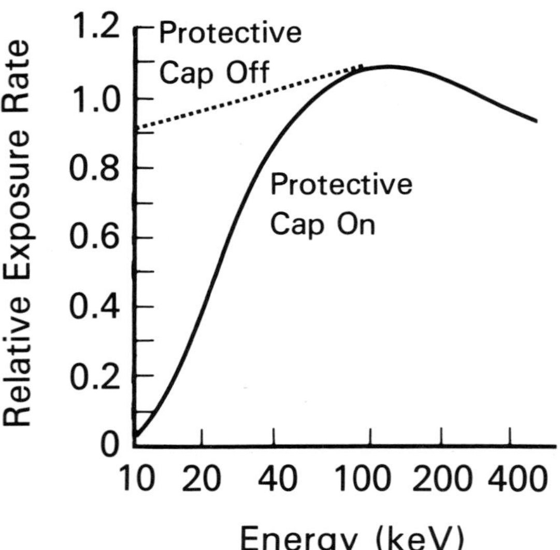

Figure 4. Energy-response curve to photons of an ionization-chamber survey meter with removable protective cap.

They are calibrated for several radionuclides, and the readout is given directly in MBq or mCi, automatically corrected for decay scheme and energy of the principal gamma emissions. Special features may be added to give a readout in terms of concentration, eg, MBq/mL. Special programs also calculate the hourly decay of a radionuclide so that the proper volume to be administered for a given activity can be determined for any hour of the working day.

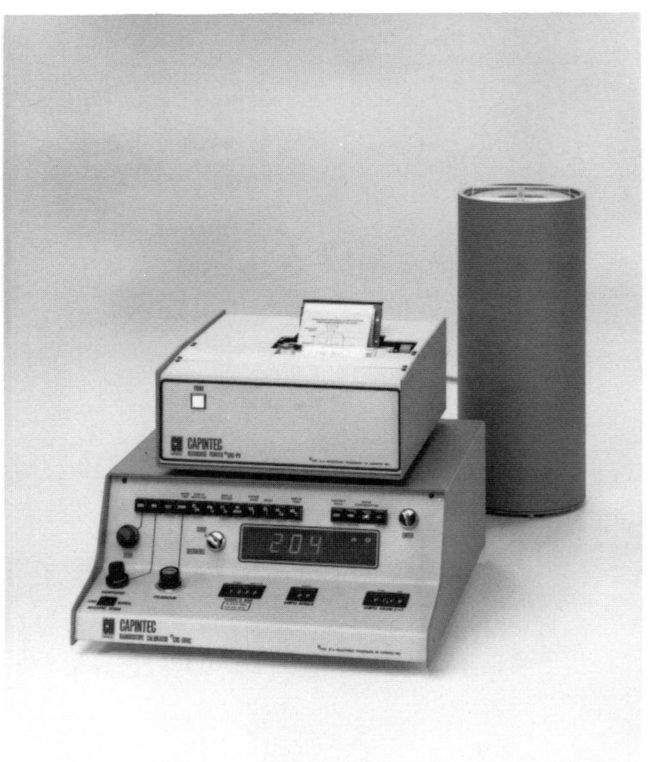

Figure 6. Modern dose calibrator.

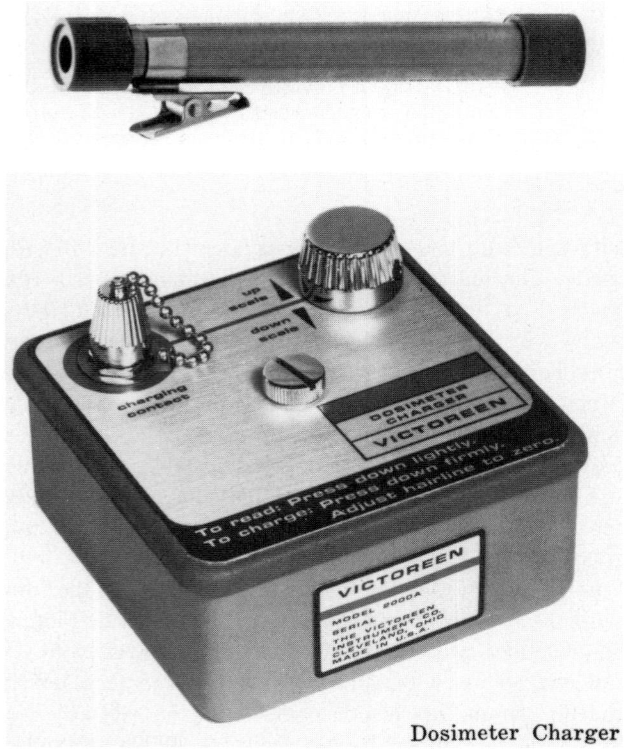

Figure 5. Pocket dosimeter and charging system.

Dose calibrators are now used almost universally in nuclear medicine laboratories as a check against the radiopharmaceutical manufacturer's assay and/or as a final quality control check on the accuracy of patient doses. While ionization chambers are not very sensitive to gamma rays, the relatively large activities encountered in nuclear medicine applications overcome this limitation.

Proportional Counters

In these detectors, the voltage applied between the collector electrodes is sufficient to produce gas amplification factors as high as 10^6. This yields pulse heights that require less elaborate amplification circuitry than is required for region II counters. Proportionality between radiation energy and pulse height is maintained, allowing accurate spectrometry.[2] A common adaptation is the *gas flow proportional counter.* It is used for detecting beta and alpha radiation in samples inserted directly into the ionization chamber (Fig. 7). The gas is supplied from cylinders of compressed gas mixtures, which continuously replenish the gas that escapes from the entry port. These systems are generally operated in the pulse mode and are calibrated against known standards of the same radionuclide as the unknown samples. Their principal application in nuclear medicine is in gas chromatography, in which compounds labeled with ^{3}H and ^{14}C are converted

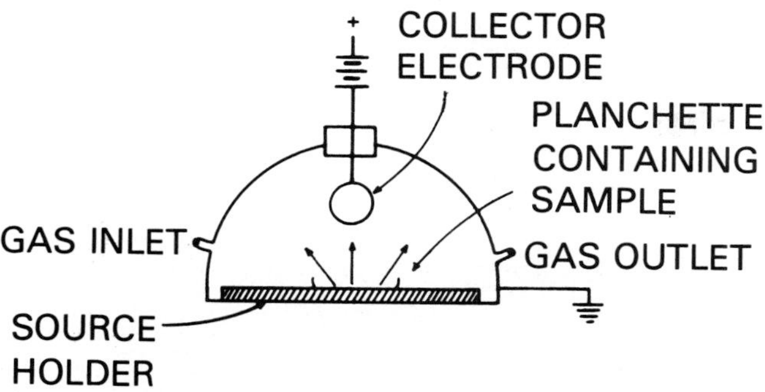

Figure 7. Gas flow proportional counter with 2π geometry, a loop wire anode, and hemispherical cathode.

to ^3H_2O or $^{14}CO_2$ and passed through proportional counters for measurement.[3]

Geiger-Müller (G-M) Tubes

When the ion chamber is operated in region IV, the dependence between radiation energy and pulse height is lost. Electrons now strike the central anode with sufficient force to produce ultraviolet photons. These photons strike other electrons within the gas and walls of the chamber, causing *Townsend avalanches* of billions of ion pairs all along the anode. Gradually, a barrier of slow-moving positive ions builds up around the central wire anode. This barrier serves to stop the avalanche by capturing additional electrons before they reach the anode. Geiger-Müller tubes are suitable for measuring all types of ionizing radiation, including weak x-rays and charged particles. They are also useful in detecting low-level radiation from radionuclide spills that occur in the laboratory. The large pulse heights (several volts) require only simple amplifier circuitry. On the other hand, the independence of radiation energy and pulse height does not allow discrimination between various kinds of radiation. All pulses from a G-M tube are essentially the same amplitude, regardless of the number of ions produced in the initial ionizing event. Because of the slow drift of positive ions to the outer cathode, the counting rate of detection is severely limited (about 20,000 counts per second, cps). Consequently, G-M tubes are not usually used for calibration purposes or for quantifying activity.

The high sensitivity of G-M tubes derives from the fact that only a single ion pair is required to trigger the discharge. When this discharge occurs, the avalanche induced proceeds all along the central collecting anode, causing a complete breakdown throughout the tube. For the counter to recover, a *quenching* mechanism must be provided to stop the discharge. The most efficient quenching agents are organic molecules such as ethyl alcohol. These molecules are broken down by secondary photons produced in the discharge and consequently absorb sufficient energy to stop it. If the high voltage is increased above the Geiger plateau, the ion pairs receive so much energy that the quenching effect cannot absorb enough energy and the tube goes into continuous discharge. When this happens, the organic molecules are broken down at a rapid rate, and the tube may be quickly ruined unless voltage is reduced.

Even so, tubes containing organic molecules have a limited working life (about 10^{10} pulses). Most modern tubes contain halogen gases as quenching agents, usually chlorine or bromine. In the case of halogen molecules, the atoms recombine upon completion of the discharge, thus reducing or eliminating the problem of depletion and greatly lengthening tube life. There is a trade-off, however. Because halogens are less effective than organic molecules as quenching agents, the G-M plateau is both shortened (from about 300 to 150 V) and steepened (from 2 to 10% slope). As a consequence, the sensitivity varies much more sharply with fluctuations in high voltage.

Most G-M tubes used as survey instruments are enclosed in a sturdy case of aluminum or stainless steel. They may have an end or side window and frequently have a very thin, low-density window ($\sim$1.5 mg/cm^2) made of mica or mylar so that beta particles can enter the chamber. For detecting gamma rays, the window thickness is generally less critical. The tube is usually attached to a cord for easy probing while the battery, ratemeter, and audible "clicker" are contained in a convenient carrying case (Fig. 8).

Calibration of Ionization Chambers

Most ionization chambers are calibrated in R/hr. Those with very thin windows operate at atmospheric pressure and require periodic calibration using a standard source of known activity. Several radionuclide sources may be used; ^{137}Cs (using the ^{137m}Ba gamma ray) and ^{60}Co are examples. The ionization chamber is placed at a measured distance d from the source, and the meter deflection is noted. The dose rate I_0 in R/hr is determined from the relation:

$$I_0 = \frac{\Gamma A}{d^2}$$

where Γ is the *exposure rate constant* in appropriate units, eg, R · cm^2/mCi · hr, A is the activity in mCi, and d is the distance in centimeters. The distance used is usually 1 m or sufficient distance between source and detector to consider the source a point source and the detector a point detector. Most ion chambers are purchased with certificates specifying this distance.

Table 1 lists values of Γ for some common radionuclide sources. The exposure rate constant includes the exposure rates from photons of the characteristic x-rays and internal bremsstrahlung, if any, along with the exposure rate from the gamma rays. It is assumed that only photons passing directly from the source to the detector contribute to the exposure and that scattered photons may be neglected.

The constant Γ is used only with point sources. Exposure rate constants for line, sheet, or disk sources are more complicated and are usually determined using computer software packages that are widely available.

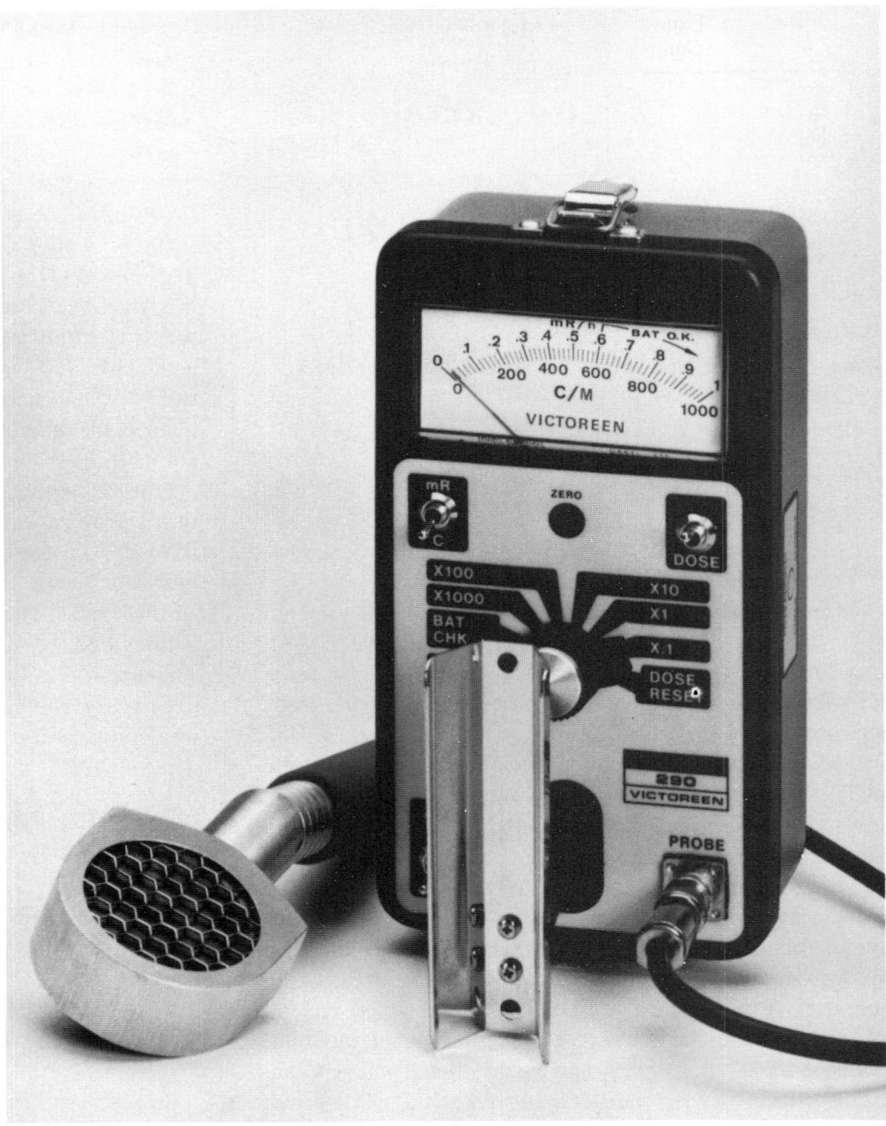

Figure 8. Survey meter with G–M tube.

Integrating dose meters such as the pocket dosimeter are calibrated in the same manner by using a timed exposure measured in cGy or rad. For x- and gamma rays, roentgen and rad are considered to be roughly equivalent.

SCINTILLATION DETECTORS

In comparison with gas-filled detectors, scintillation detectors have two principal advantages that account for their widespread use in nuclear medicine: they are capable of much higher counting rates than pulse ionization chambers because of fast resolving times and they are much more efficient for gamma-ray detection while preserving pulse-height proportionality. These detetors have a relatively short history; modern detectors were only introduced in the late 1940s. The basic elements of a scintillation detector system using a thallium-activated sodium iodide NaI(Tl) crystal are shown in Figure 9. Ionizing radiation is absorbed in the scintillator, and its energy is converted to light photons, hence the term *scintillation crystal*. Some of these photons strike the photocathode of an *electron multiplier* tube (EMT), also known as a photomultiplier (PM) tube. Electrons ejected by the photocathode are amplified by a series of dynodes in the PM tube to form a voltage output pulse proportional in height to the energy of the ionizing event. This signal is then amplified and shaped prior to processing by several possible display formats. The general system is versatile and forms the basis for most radiation detector systems used in nuclear medicine.

Sodium Iodide Crystals

While scintillation crystals may be used for detecting any type of ionizing radiation, this discussion considers primarily gamma-ray detection. Many different materials fluoresce when exposed to ionizing radiation, and each has its own particular characteristics, eg, wavelength emission, decay

Table 1. Exposure-Rate Constants for Selected Gamma-Ray Sources

RADIONUCLIDE	γ ENERGIES (MeV)	EXPOSURE-RATE CONSTANT (R · cm²/mCi · h)
^{137}Cs	0.6616	3.23
^{51}Cr	0.3200	0.184
^{60}Co	1.173–1.322	13.1
^{99m}Tc	0.140	1.2
^{198}Au	0.4118–1.088	2.3
^{125}I	0.0355	0.04
^{131}I	0.285–0.637	2.3
^{192}Ir	0.1363–1.062	3.9
^{226}Ra in equilibrium	0.0465–2.440	9.068*

*This value includes no filtration. The usual value of 8.25 is for a filter of 0.5 mm platinum and includes secondary radiations generated in the platinum filter.

Modified from NCRP Report No. 41.[4]

time, and density.[3,6] Several inorganic scintillators are listed in Table 2. Sodium iodide crystals are particularly useful in gamma-ray detection because of their high density, created by high iodine content (85% by weight) with high atomic number (Z = 53). Most scintillation crystals are hot pressed or extruded into their desired shape. This results in a strong polycrystalline material that has the same scintillation efficiency and transparency as if it were a single crystal grown from solution. While NaI(Tl) crystals are slower (longer light decay time) than most organic phosphors, they are sufficiently fast for most nuclear medical applications, the light yield is high, and the spectral wavelength emission is well matched to the bialkali photocathodes used in most EM tubes.

Gamma rays striking the crystal are absorbed by the three processes described in Chapter 1: the photoelectric effect, Compton scattering, and pair production. The photoelectric effect predominates at low energies but falls off rapidly above 90 keV.

In each absorption process, photon energy is imparted to orbital electrons within the crystal lattice. This raises the electron from the valence band to a conduction band, where the electron is free to move from atom to atom across a crystal plane (Fig. 10). In materials classified as insulators or semiconductors, electrons have discrete energy bands that they must occupy. The region between that valence band and the conduction band is a *forbidden band* which electrons cannot occupy in a pure crystal. When the electron gains sufficient energy to raise it to the conduction band, it is free to wander within the crystal lattice until it comes across an unfilled orbital shell (electron hole) in the valence band. When this occurs, the electron quickly returns to the valence band and, in doing so, emits a fluorescent photon. This process requires approximately 10^{-12} s.

In pure sodium iodide, the energy gap between the valence and conduction bands is so great that the fluorescent photon emitted is beyond the visible light range and therefore not suitable for the scintillation process. To overcome this, the crystal is doped with an impurity, known as an *activator.* Thallium is added in approximately 10^{-3} mol fraction during crystal growth. The thallium atoms create special sites in the crystal lattice that serve to facilitate excitation. The excited energy levels of thallium lie within the forbidden band so that less energy is required to raise the electron out of the valence band. This transition now gives rise to a lower-energy photon (about 3 eV) that lies within the visible light range and is efficiently detected by the photocathode.

In NaI(Tl) crystal one electron-hole pair is created for each approximately 20 eV of photon energy absorbed. Thus

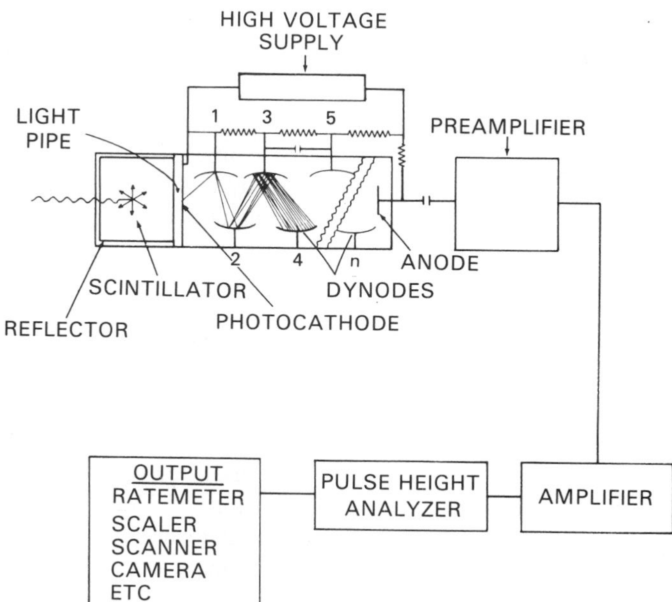

Figure 9. Scintillation detector systems with a light pipe coupling the NaI(Tl) scintillation crystal to the electron multiplier tube and associated electronics.

Table 2. Properties of Some Solid Scintillators

MATERIAL	WAVELENGTH OF MAXIMUM EMISSION (nm)	DECAY CONSTANT (μs)*	SCINTILLATION CUTOFF WAVELENGTH (nm)	INDEX OF REFRACTION	DENSITY (g/cm^3)	HYGRO-SCOPIC	γ SCINTILLATION CONVERSION EFFICIENCY (%)
NaI(Tl)	410	0.23	320	1.85	3.67	Yes	100
CaF_2(Eu)	435	0.94	405	1.44	3.18	No	50
CsI(Na)	420	0.63	300	1.84	4.51	Yes	85
CsI(Tl)	565	1.0	330	1.80	4.51	No	45
^{6}LiI(Eu)	470–485	1.4	450	1.96	4.08	Yes	35
TlCl(Be,I)	465	0.2	390	2.4	7.00	No	2.5
CsF	390	0.005	220	1.48	4.11	Yes	5
BaF_2	325	0.63	134	1.49	4.88	No	10
$Bi_4Ge_3O_{12}$	480	0.30	350	2.15	7.13	No	15
KI(Tl)	426	0.24/2.5	325	1.71	3.13	Yes	24
$CaWO_4$	430	0.9–20	300	1.92	6.12	No	14–18
$CdWO_4$	530	0.9–20	450	2.2	7.90	No	17–20

Data from Reference 19 and Harshaw Chemical Co.

a 1-MeV gamma ray would yield 5×10^4 electron-pair holes. However, not all pairs form light photons. Sodium iodide crystals are about 12% efficient.[8] Therefore, only about 6×10^3 photons are produced. The number of light photons emitted is directly proportional to the gamma-ray energy, assuming the gamma ray has been completely absorbed within the crystal. If part of the energy escapes from the crystal, as frequently occurs with Compton scattering, fewer light photons will be produced, and the resulting output pulse will be less than the energy of the incident photon. This energy loss creates the Compton region of the gamma-ray spectrum. The entire deexcitation process within a NaI(Tl) crystal requires approximately 0.2 μs. This is known as the *decay time* of the crystal. Even with such short decay times, very high counting rates may result in overlapping events that create output pulses too high for the photon energy absorbed.

In the design of crystals, it is important for a large fraction of the light produced to reach the photocathode. Because NaI is highly refractive, crystals are often roughened to reduce the reflection between the crystal and the light pipe. Both the crystal and the circumference of the light pipe are coated with a highly reflective substance, usually Al_2O_3 or MgO, to reflect maximum light to the photocathode. NaI(Tl) crystals are hygroscopic and must be hermetically sealed. Absorption of moisture and oxygen discolors the crystal, which increases

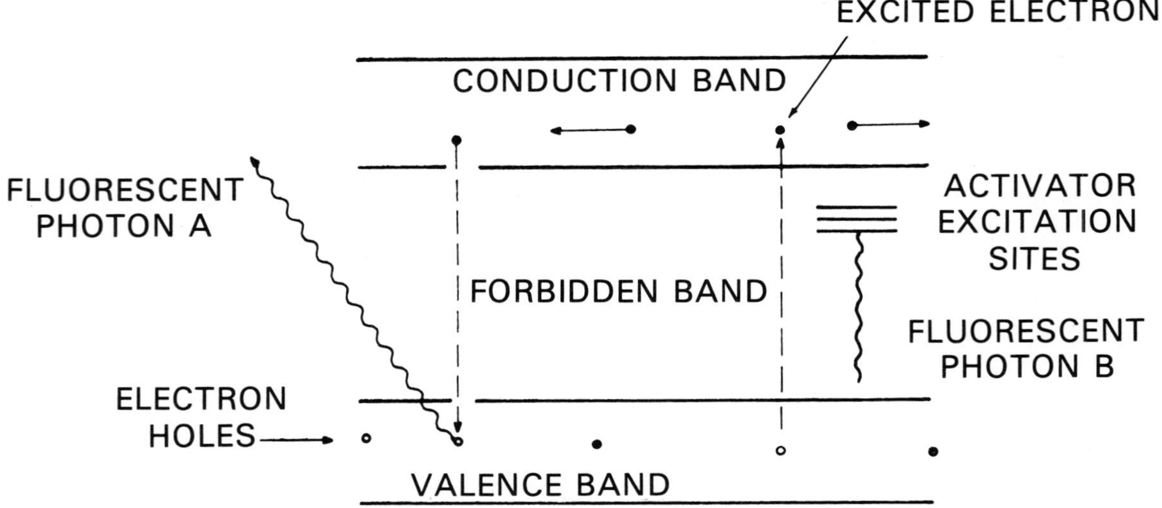

Figure 10. Ionization process in crystal lattice showing mechanism of fluorescence production. Photon A is produced when a free electron in the conduction band of pure NaI fills an electron hole. Photon B is emitted when an electron from one of the activator excitation levels fills an electron hole. The lower energy of photon B falls in the visible light range.

internal light absorption. In many cases, the EM tube is sealed directly to the crystal. In other cases, such as the gamma camera, the EM tube is separated from the crystal. In this case, a plastic light pipe is optically coupled to the crystal and the EM tube with silicone grease. In high-quality scintillator systems, the optical efficiency approaches unity.[3]

The efficiency of the scintillation process is also temperature related to some extent.[1] It is therefore important that the room operating temperature remain the same between the time of counting a standard and an unknown sample.

In PET and CT scanners, scintillation crystals of bismuth germanate, $Bi_4Ge_3O_{12}$ (often abbreviated BGO), have largely replaced NaI(Tl) crystals, because their high density (7.13) and high Z (83) permit the use of small, more-efficient crystals that improve scanner resolution.[13] Unfortunately, the light yield is relatively low, being only about 10% that of NaI at room temperatures. This is of little importance in CT scanners, where because of the high x-ray flux they are operated in the current mode rather than pulse mode.

LIQUID SCINTILLATORS

The use of a liquid scintillator offers a singular advantage: it allows complete mixing of the radioactive sample in the detector volume, thereby achieving virtual 4π geometry and eliminating absorption in the counter walls between sample and detector. Liquid-scintillation counting is therefore especially useful for weak beta-particle emitters such as ^{3}H, ^{14}C, and ^{35}S. For higher energy beta emitters, such as ^{32}P, ^{89}Sr, and ^{90}Y, the counting efficiency approaches 100%. Liquid-scintillation counters work equally well for photon-emitting nuclides (^{99m}Tc, ^{111}In, ^{201}Tl), but they are rarely used for this purpose because gamma counters [NaI(Tl)] are usually available and they are not susceptible to sample quenching of the scintillation response.

Liquid scintillators formulated for use in health sciences applications have four main components: solvent, primary fluor, secondary fluor, and surfactant.

Solvent

The solvent makes up the bulk of the scintillating matrix. It absorbs the energy of the ionizing radiation event and transfers it to adjacent solvent molecules as shown in Figure 11. The most efficient energy transfer process in the solvent is radiationless energy transfer from one solvent molecule to the next involving the first molecular singlet excited state. This pathway is favored in aromatic solvents that contain multiple conjugated double bonds. In the early days benzene and dioxane-naphthalene mixtures were used for this purpose, but they have been completely replaced with safer and more efficient solvents. In the 1970s and 1980s liquid scintillators were formulated with toluene, *p*-xylene, and then pseudocumene. The most recent class of materials uses diisopropylnaphthalene (DIN) or similar high-molecular weight, low-vapor-pressure aromatics. These new materials offer lower toxicity, higher flash points, and improved scintillator efficiency.

Primary Fluor

The primary fluor (solute) is present in concentrations of 5 g/L solvent. It absorbs radiant energy from the solvent and emits a light photon in the near UV (360 to 390 nm). A typical primary fluor is PPO (2,5-diphenyloxazole). Its absorption and emission spectra are shown in Figure 12. Some other common fluors are shown in Table 3.

Secondary Fluor

The secondary fluor, also called a wavelength shifter, absorbs the photon from the primary fluor and reemits it at a longer wavelength (410 to 420 nm). This is in the visible region and gives scintillators their characteristic blue fluorescent hue. One of the most common secondary fluors is POPOP 1,4-bis[2-(5-phenyloxazolyl)]-benzene, which shifts the fluorescence maxima of PPO from 380 to 420 nm. The secondary was originally in the formulations to shift the signal to better match the EM response. This is unnecessary with newer EMs, but the secondary is still useful because it diminishes the effect of color quenching by the sample.

Surfactant

Scintillators with only the solvent and fluor(s) are used in neutron detectors, high-energy physics experiments, large-volume whole-body counters, etc. However, for scintillators to be useful for assaying samples, one must be able to incorporate the (usually aqueous) sample into the aromatic solvent. In the 1950s this was accomplished with a secondary solvent such as ethanol or dioxane that would increase miscibility with water. These materials caused enormous difficulties with sample precipitation and phase separation and were long ago discarded in favor of surfactants, an example of which is shown in Figure 13. The usual surfactant has an alkyl chain that is soluble in the aromatic solvent and an ethoxy chain that is soluble in water. Exact formulations are proprietary, but a 2:1 solvent-to-surfactant mixture will give a scintillator that can incorporate fairly large amounts of water. Many materials form a rigid gel at 50% water.

Many excellent commercial premixed scintillators have been developed for specific applications. The data sheets with these give the limitations for different types of samples. No single scintillator is appropriate for all samples and applications. Many of the present commercial scintillators are marketed as "disposable" and, while there is little doubt that they are significantly safer than the older toluene-based materials, local regulations may still prescribe how liquid-scintillator wastes should be collected and disposed of (see Chapter 14).

Physics of the Liquid Scintillation Process

The key physical and photophysical processes in the liquid scintillator are well understood and are described in detail in references 17, 18, and 24. A schematic of the vial and

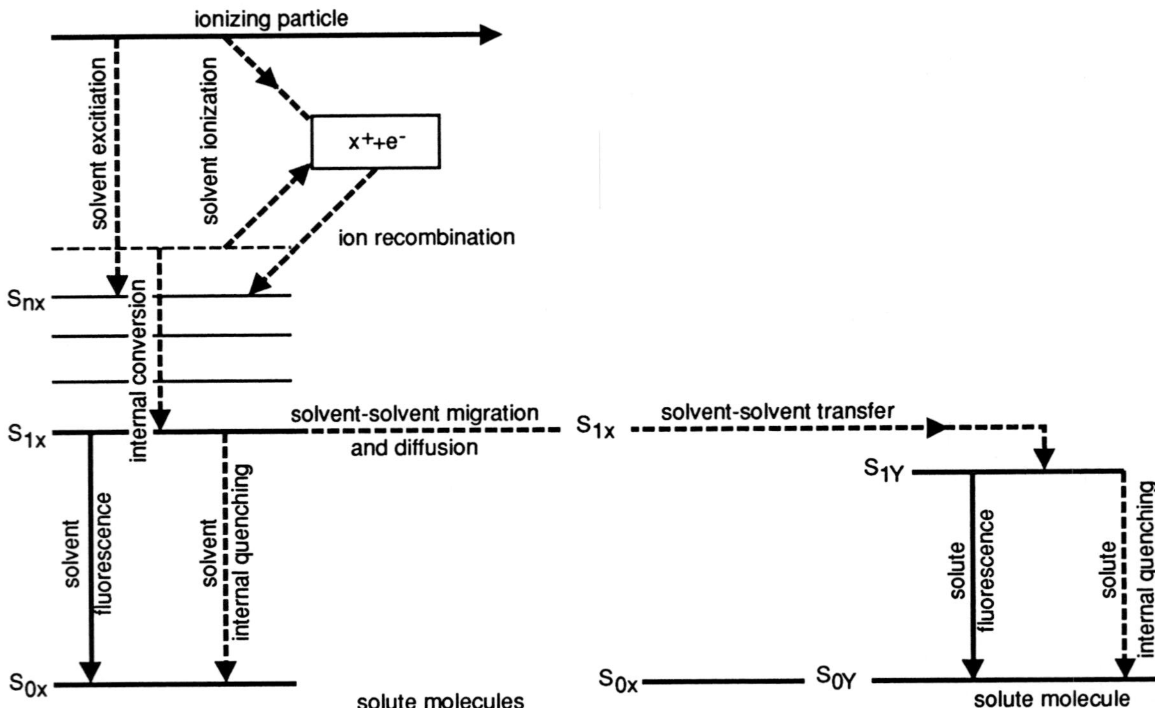

Figure 11. The scintillation process in a binary solution of aromatic molecules consisting of a solvent (such as toluene) and a solute (fluor such as PPO). The *S* values represent the molecular excited states of the solvent (with the subscript X) and the solute (subscript Y). For each type of molecule there is a singlet manifold of excited states S_n; the first single excited state is S_1 and the ground state is S_0. Under the best conditions, only 4% of the energy of the ionizing particle is converted to fluorescent energy in the solute (schematic from Reference 24).

EMs is shown in Figure 14. Light photons from the vial impinge on the photocathode where they are converted to photoelectrons, which are in turn collected at the first dynode.

Because the system is quantifying the amount of visible light incident on the EM tubes, it is clear that (1) processes that enhance the signal output from the scintillator must be maximized; (2) processes that "quench" the light output must be minimized; and (3) competing factors that cause stray light to be included in the signal must be minimized.

An overall *figure of merit* for the system has been defined as the number of photoelectrons collected at the first dynode of one tube per keV of energy deposited in the scintillator. The figure of merit (η) has been given by Coursey and Mann[22] in a form that demonstrates the three basic elements of the scintillation process:

1. the production of primary photons by excitation of the scintillator;
2. the light-collection efficiency; and
3. the phototube response.

$$\eta_E = \frac{\left[\frac{S_E \cdot E_\beta}{\hbar\bar{\nu}}\right][G][mCg]}{E_\beta},$$

where E_β = energy of beta particle; S_E = scintillation yield, the fraction of electron energy converted to light energy;[17] $\hbar\bar{\nu}$ = average energy of emitted photons; G = light-collection efficiency, that fraction of the photons generated in step (1) that arrives at the photocathode; $m\ C\ g$ = EM tube response, the fraction of photons arriving at the photocathode, that result in photoelectrons arriving at the first dynode; where m = spectral matching factor, which has a value between 0 and 1 and is a measure of the overlap of the emission spectrum of the scintillator and the absorption spectrum of photocathode, C = maximum photoelectric efficiency of the photocathode, also called the "quantum efficiency," and q = photoelectron-collection efficiency at the first dynode. Some nominal values for these parameters for an unquenched tritium standard in the standard two-EM commercial liquid-scintillation counter have been estimated by Coursey and Mann,[22] and are given in Table 4. Tritium has a maximum beta energy of 18 keV and an average of 5 keV. Thus, on average 5000 eV of energy is deposited over a range 0.8 μm in the solvent. Since the ionization potentials for most of the molecules are less than 6 eV, the tritium beta particles do considerable local damage along that short path. Most of this energy is dissipated as heat; only 71 photons are emitted by the primary fluor. These photons will be absorbed and reemitted several times before they escape the vial. Three processes are particularly important: delayed light emission, chemical quenching, and color quenching.

The prompt signal from liquid scintillators is one of their

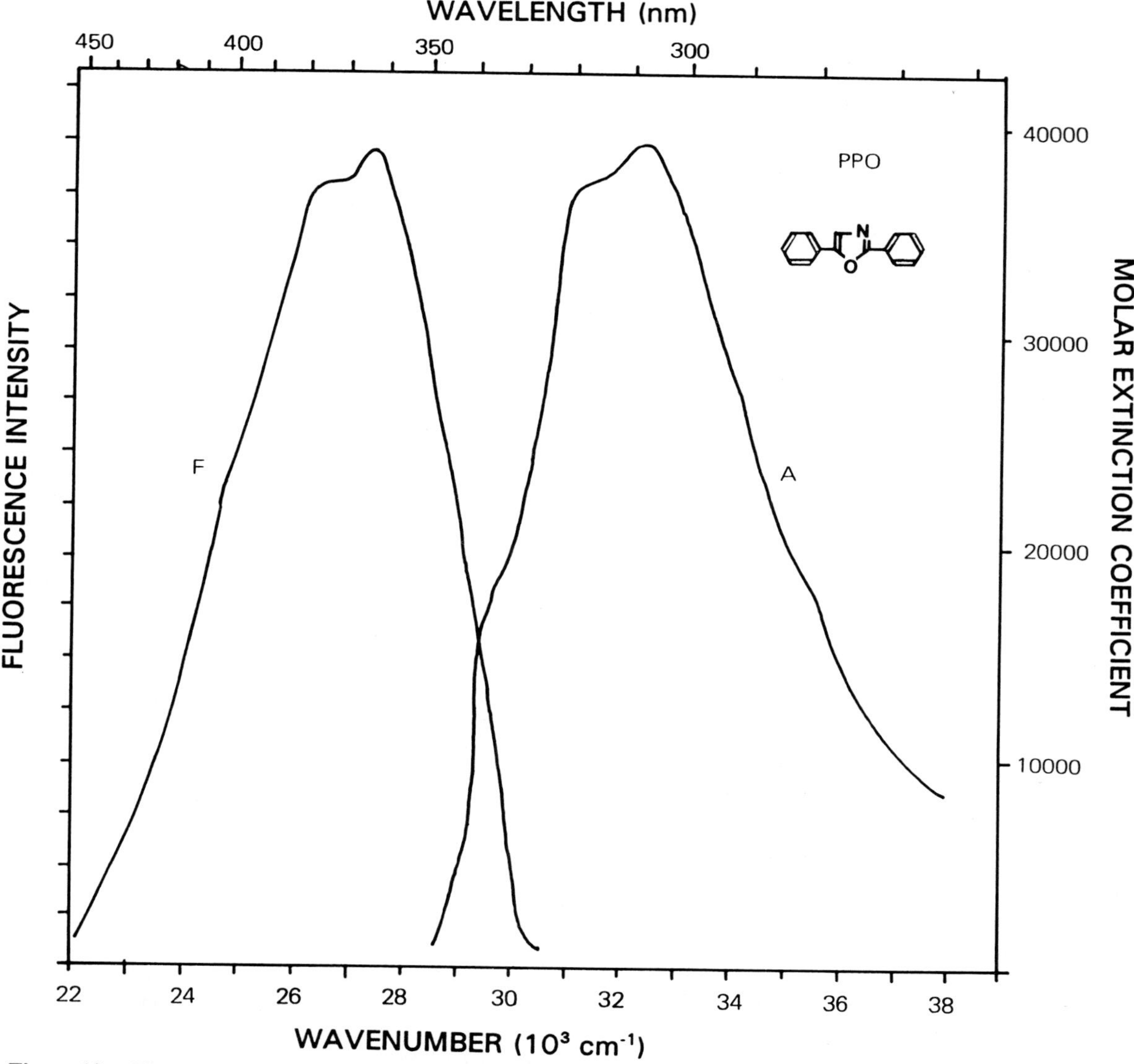

Figure 12. Fluorescence and absorption spectra for PPO (2,5-diphenyloxazole). Ideal scintillators have a large difference between the peak maxima for fluorescence and absorption (the Stokes shift). This minimizes reabsorption of fluorescent photons, a process known as self-quenching. A = Absorption spectrum. F = Fluorescence spectrum.

chief advantages over inorganic crystals (typically 3 ns for organics compared to 230 ns for NaI(Tl).[19] With the aromatic systems selected, the photon emissions come from deexcitations of molecular singlet states. Molecular triplet states have much longer life–times. If a significant amount of the energy is tied up in the excited triplets, it will lengthen the tail on the pulse and complicate the electronic pulse processing. This property is used to advantage in newer liquid scintillation counting systems that distinguish alpha and beta events. The slow moving alpha particles do even more damage along the particle track than betas, resulting in a greater number of excited triplets. Pulse-shape techniques can thus be used to distinguish alpha- from beta-particle pulses, and some liquid scintillation counters have been built for this specific application.[25]

Chemical quenching refers to a series of processes that prevent emission of photons by the primary fluor. Any other molecular components in the scintillator can compete with the main processes shown in Figure 11. Molecular oxygen, O_2, present from air dissolved in the scintillator, is one of the chief chemical quenchers, but usually no attempt is made to deaerate the samples. Impurities in the scintillator constituents or the sample can also serve as alternate deexcitation pathways that do not lead to fluorescent photons.

Color quenching is a shorthand notation for several processes that reduce the number of photons from the secondary fluor that arrive at the vial wall. Thus color quenching is caused by any chromophores that absorb photons from either the primary or secondary fluor. Hemoglobin is a good example of a color quenching agent that may be present in the sample to be assayed.

Several processes can lead to elevated background signals.

Table 3. Properties of Some Organic Fluors (Solutes) Commonly Used in Liquid Scintillation Counting

SOLUTE	CHEMICAL STRUCTURE	q	m	t (ns)	λ (nm)	SOLUBILITY (TOLUENE) (g L^{-1}, 20°C)
TP *p*-Terphenyl	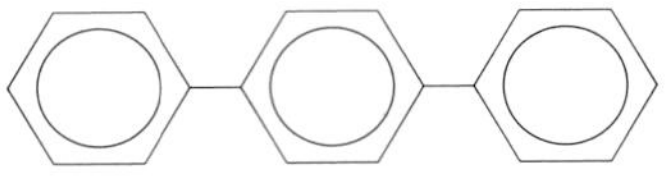	0.93	0.97	1.0	342	8.6
PPO 2,5-Diphenyloxazole	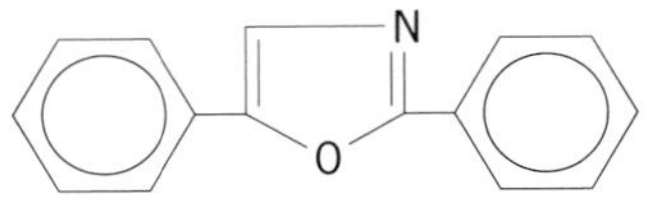 N, O	1.00	0.97	1.4	375	414
POPOP 1,4-Di-[2-(5-phenyloxazolyl)]-benzene	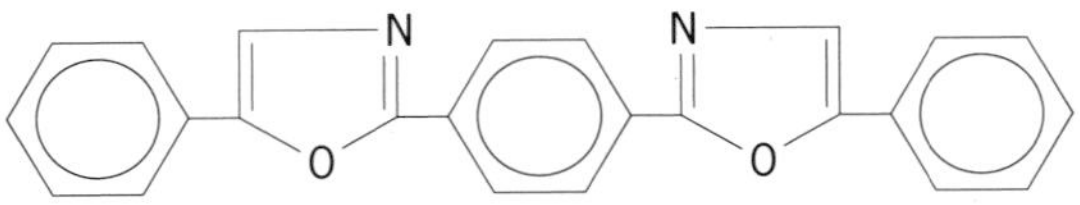 N, O, N, O	0.93	0.83	1.5	415	2.2
M_2-POPOP 1,4-Di-[2-(4-methyl-5-phenyloxazolyl)]-benzene	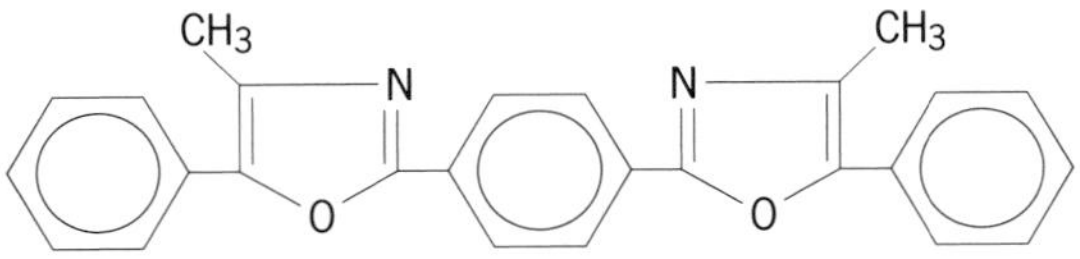 CH3, N, O, N, O, CH3	0.93	0.78	1.7	427	3.9
PBD 2-Phenyl-5-(4-biphenylyl)-1,3,4-oxadiazole	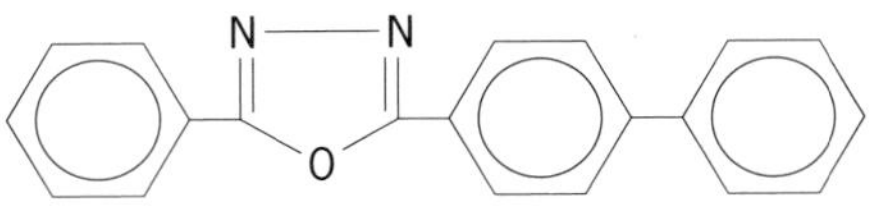 N—N, O	0.83	0.96	1.1	375	12
tert-Butyl-PBD 2-(4′-*t*-Butylphenyl)-5-(4″-biphenylyl)-1,3,4-oxadiazole	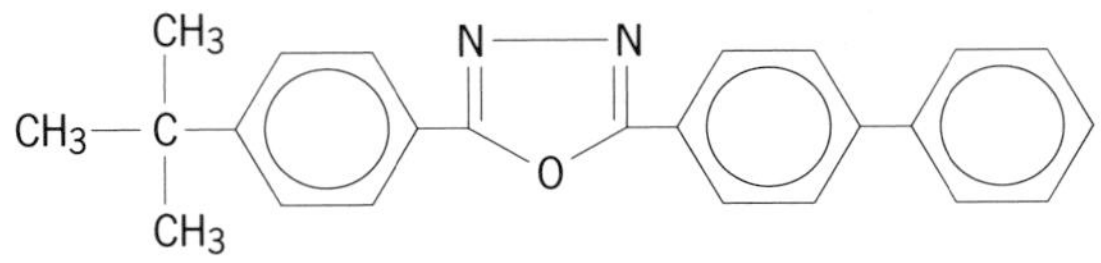 CH3, CH3—C, CH3, N—N, O	0.85	0.95	1.2	385	119

Relative fluorescent quantum efficiencies (q), spectral matching factors (m), fluorescent lifetimes (t), average fluorescent emission wavelengths (λ), and solubilities.

From NCRP Report 58.

These are discussed in detail by Horrocks[17] and Peng.[16] These include *chemiluminescence* in the sample, fluorescence from the glass sample vials, and thermal noise from the EM tubes. These can easily lead to rates in excess of 10,000 counts per minute in each phototube. This background can be drastically reduced by using two EM tubes and imposing a coincidence requirement, that is, both tubes must detect the event (within some resolving time such as 20 nanoseconds). This reduces the background to 50 counts per minute or less.

This coincidence requirement does, however, lower the efficiency slightly. If we return to the tritium example, with only 71 primary photons emitted, there is a rather high probability that one or the other of the EMs will miss the decay event altogether. That is why the detection efficiency, counts recorded/decay events, is only 63% for unquenched scintillators. Higher-energy beta emitters (^{14}C, ^{45}Ca) give correspondingly higher numbers of light photons, and the chances for coincident detection improves. Figure 15 gives detection efficiency vs maximum beta-particle energy.

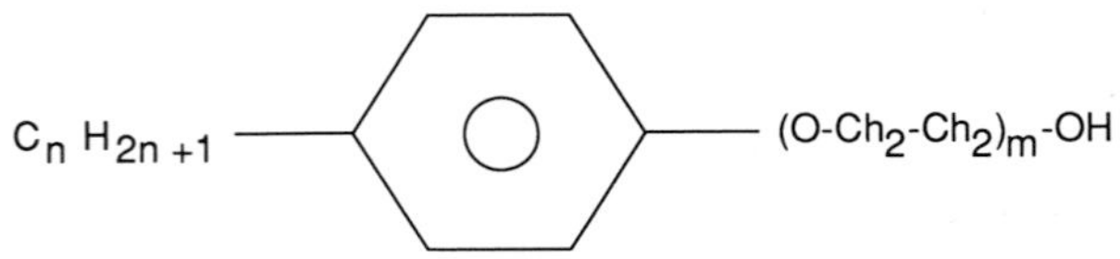

$$C_nH_{2n+1}-C_6H_4-(O\text{-}Ch_2\text{-}Ch_2)_m\text{-}OH$$

Figure 13. General structure of Triton X100, a typical surfactant used for incorporating water into an aromatic organic solvent, $m = 9$ and $n = 8$.

Except for the pulse-shaping and coincidence-discrimination techniques mentioned above, the pulse processing and electronics for commercial liquid scintillation counters are much the same as for gamma counters employing NaI(Tl) crystals. In fact, newer model liquid scintillation counters are available with personal computers that incorporate multichannel analyzers, radionuclide sample libraries, and spectroscopic packages that are modeled along those originally developed for gamma-ray spectrometry.

The only other differences between systems equipped with solid and liquid scintillators are that liquid scintillators require a light-tight shutter on the sample chamber and they perform optimally at lower temperatures (6 to 10°C). Early liquid scintillation counters were refrigerated to reduce dark noise in the EMs. With newer tubes this is unnecessary,

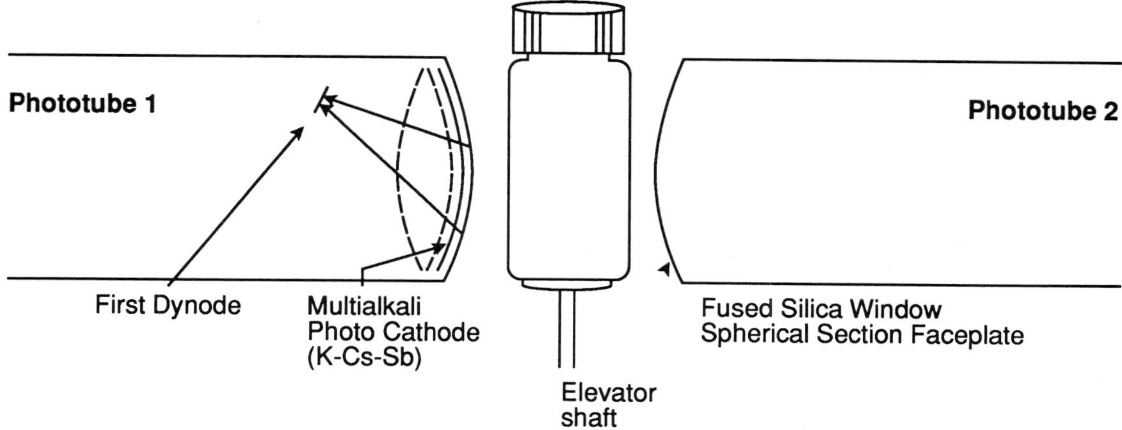

Figure 14. Schematic diagram of a standard counting vial and phototubes used for typical commercial liquid scintillation counter.

and most commercial systems operate at room temperature. However, refrigerated systems still offer lower background count rates and better stability of the scintillator formulation for many samples.

Photocathodes

The thin coating of semitransparent material applied to the inner surface of the EM tube is the photocathode. Light photons produced in the crystal strike the photocathode and eject loosely bound electrons from the valence band into the conduction band, where they wander to the surface and escape into the vacuum of the EM tube. The photon must be of sufficient energy to not only raise the electron from the valence band but to overcome the potential barrier that exists at the surface of the photocathode layer (1.5 to 2 eV). The photocathode usually consists of some alkali metal deposited on the glass window of the EM tube. Many modern EM tubes have a bialkali photocathode consisting of Sb-K_2-Cs, which has a high *quantum efficiency* in the spectral range of NaI(Tl) emissions. The quantum efficiency QE = the number of photoelectrons emitted/the number of incident photons. When the photocathode material is properly matched to the light wavelength produced in the scintillator, efficiencies of 20 to 30% are achieved (Fig. 16). Thus a 0.5-MeV gamma ray produces approximately 10^3 photons within the crystal, which results in the ejection of about 200 to 300 electrons from the photocathode. The photocathode must be thick enough to absorb the incident photon efficiently yet thin enough to minimize self-absorption of the ejected electrons. In bialkali tubes, the optimal photocathode thickness is about 200 nm. Good energy resolution also demands a uniform thickness in the photocathode, which may be difficult to achieve with large-diameter EM tubes.

The photocathode is sensitive to ambient temperature variations, which may affect its efficiency. Elevated temperatures also increase *thermionic* noise. Thermionic noise is spurious counts caused by electrons in the conduction band being ejected from the photocathode when they gain sufficient thermal energy to overcome the photocathode barrier potential. Ordinarily this noise is random and merely increases the *background* counting rate. With very low-activity samples in which the counting rate is only slightly above background, cooling the EM tube to 0°C may reduce this noise as well as the relative counting times required for statistical significance (see Chapter 4).

The window material of the EM tube is also important and must be matched to the light wavelength produced in the scintillation crystal. These materials are made of synthetic silica and various types of glass containing MgF_2, Al_2O_3, borosilicates, etc. Well-matched materials have a transmittance of 95% of incident light.

Table 4. Typical Parameters and Figure of Merit for a Commercial Liquid-Scintillation Counter

System characteristics	
Phototube	2 RCA 4501-V4
Tube face	Quartz, spherical
First dynode	Cu Be (Cs)
Light coupling	Air
Vial volume	15 cm^3
Vial material	Glass
Photophysical parameters	
Scintillation yield (S_E)	4%
Average photon energy ($h\bar{\nu}$)	3.2 eV
Number of primary photons	71
Light collection for each PM (G)	0.11
Spectral matching factor (m)	0.97
Quantum efficiency of PM (C)	0.32
Photoelectron collection efficiency (g)	0.8
System performance parameters	
Figure of merit η	0.4
Coincidence efficiency for ^{3}H	63%

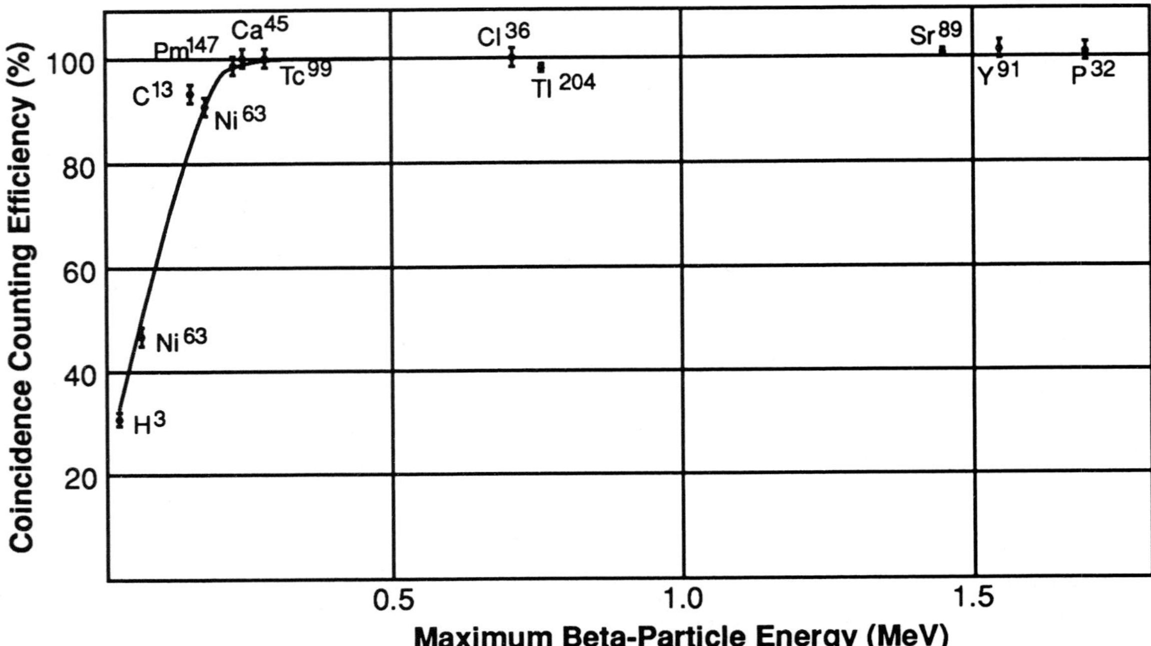

Figure 15. Liquid scintillation counting efficiency as a function of maximum beta-particle energy for pure beta-emitting radionuclides. Adapted from Goldstein.[23]

Electron Multiplier Tubes

There are several different design types of EM tube. The tube illustrated in Figure 9 is a "head-on" type, commonly used in nuclear medicine in which light enters the end of the evacuated glass tube to strike the photocathode layered on the inside of the input window.

Once ejected from the photocathode, the photoelectrons are accelerated toward the first dynode. Dynodes are metal plates covered with *negative electron affinity* (NEA) materials such as gallium phosphide that yield a high number of secondary electrons for each incident electron.[1] The first dynode is positively charged with respect to the photocathode. Electrons emitted from the photocathode are accelerated and gain sufficient energy to eject secondary electrons from the dynode. These secondary electrons are then accelerated toward the second dynode, where further multiplication occurs and so on through 10 to 14 dynodes. Ideally, the current amplification of a EM tube having n dynodes and an average secondary emission ratio δ per stage is δ^n. Conventional tubes with $\delta = 5$ and ten dynodes achieve current amplifications of 5^{10} or 10^7. Some modern tubes with high-NEA materials with $\delta = 50$ can achieve the same amplification with 4 or 5 dynodes.

A constant gain at each dynode is essential to maintaining proportionality between the input scintillation event and the output pulse, because a small variation at one dynode is amplified by each succeeding dynode, thus magnifying the error. Capacitors at the higher dynode stages help maintain the stability of charge on each dynode.

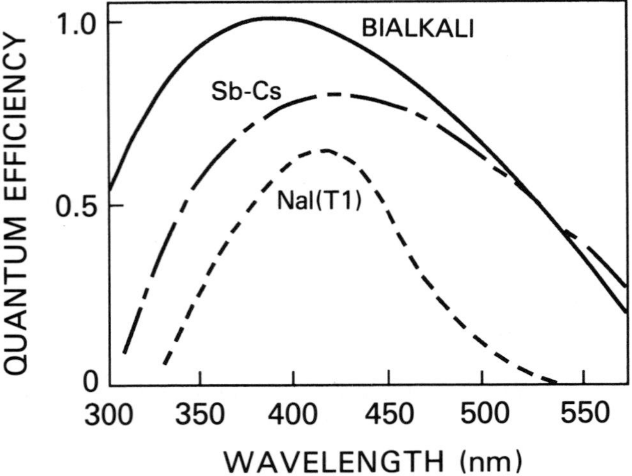

Figure 16. The quantum efficiency for two photocathode materials, K-Cs (Bialkali) and Sb-Cs. The emission spectrum of NaI(Tl) is shown for reference.

MAGNETIC SHIELDING

Because the electrons traveling from stage to stage within the EM tube have very low average energy (about 100 eV), their trajectories are sensitive to changing magnetic fields. Even the earth's magnetic field can effect tube output, depending on how the tube is oriented. To reduce such effects, PM tubes are shielded with a surrounding casing of nonmagnetic metal. Nevertheless, large changes in ambient magnetic fields, such as proximity to magnetic resonance (MR) magnets, may alter and distort the function of EM tubes.

High-Voltage Supply

The EM tube is almost always energized by a separate source to supply high voltage to the dynodes. Each dynode is charged with progressively higher voltage by a voltage divider circuit (Fig. 9). If 1000 V are applied across ten dynodes, the potential across each dynode is 100 V more than that across the preceding dynode. In this way, the electron direction is always toward the anode, and the amplification between dynodes is approximately equal per incident electron. To maintain proportionality between gamma energy and pulse output, the voltage supply must be very stable. Instability is called *drift* and may be caused by temperature changes or alterations in line voltage. If the drift is downward, the pulse output is low relative to gamma-energy input. If the drift is upward, the pulse output is erroneously high. If drift becomes too high, another effect may occur: electrons may be pulled off preceding dynodes in the absence of any photon emission (*dark current*). These electrons may be produced by thermionic electrons, ionization of residual gases in the EM tube, *ohmic leakage* caused by insufficient insulation at the base of the tube, and by *field emission* caused by operating at a voltage near the maximum rating value. Dark current can be demonstrated easily in a scintillation counter by increasing the high voltage until the scaler begins to register spontaneous counting rate in the absence of any radioactive source.

Preamplifiers

The output pulses from EM tubes are of low voltage, typically on the order of a few millivolts, and often have undesirable characteristics for subsequent electronic manipulation. Consequently, a preamplifier is inserted between the EM tube and the pulse-processing and analysis electronics that follow. The preamplifier has three essential functions: (1) to amplify the signal; (2) to match electrical impedance between the EM tube and the amplifier; and in some cases (3) to shape the signal for optimum handling by the amplifier. Shaping is usually accomplished by an R-C circuit that typically increases the pulse time constant. An essential feature of preamplifiers is linearity, ie, the signal output must be proportional to the input. Usually, this is not too difficult to accomplish with EM tubes, but it is more exacting when amplifying the weak signals of semiconductor detectors.

The pulse in Figure 17 has a rapid rise and long tail. The rise time is a reflection of (1) the decay time of the scintillation event within the crystal (usually about 0.2 μs) and (2) the *electron transit time*, the time required for the electrons to traverse the dynodes in the EM tube (10 to 100 ns). This time varies with the number and structure of the dynodes.[8] The pulse *rise time* generally requires 2 to 20 ns to complete, and the tail is much longer. If subsequent pulses fall within this tail, the voltage height will be increased and thus distorted. Pulse-shaping circuits, including R-C clipping and delay lines, help to eliminate tailing by producing pulses of 5 ns or less, thus greatly increasing the pulse pair resolution, ie, the number of pulses per second that can be separated and correctly discriminated (Fig. 18).

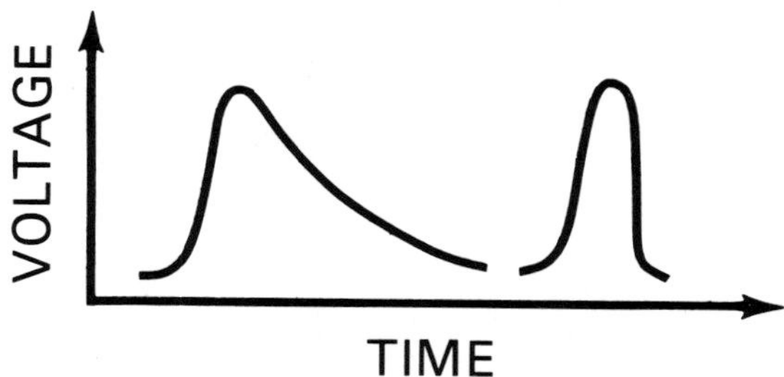

Figure 17. The output pulse from the EM tube has a long tail, which increases the probability of "pulse pileup" at high counting rates. The clipped pulse at right preserves the pulse-height information but eliminates the long tail.

Amplifiers

Boyd et al[9] have listed the characteristics of amplifiers:

1. Shape pulse to decrease resolving time.
2. Increase gain to drive pulse-height analyzers, scalers, etc.
3. Increase signal-to-noise ratio. Noise is any unwanted signal arising anywhere in the system. Sources include EM dark current, electrostatic frequencies, arcing of high voltage, and other radio frequency (RF) sources.
4. Stabilize signal gain to maintain proportionality between pulse height and photon energy deposition in the crystal.
5. Provide proper polarity of the output signal (usually positive).

Most modern amplifiers utilize transisters, which have the advantage of small size, short warm-up time, low heat generation, minimum drift, and low power requirements.

Pulse-Height Analyzers

The pulse height from a linear amplifier is proportional to the radiation energy deposited within the crystal. The implication is that, if a monoenergetic beam strikes the crystal and each photon is completely absorbed, all of the output pulses will be the same height. Perfect registry, however, is

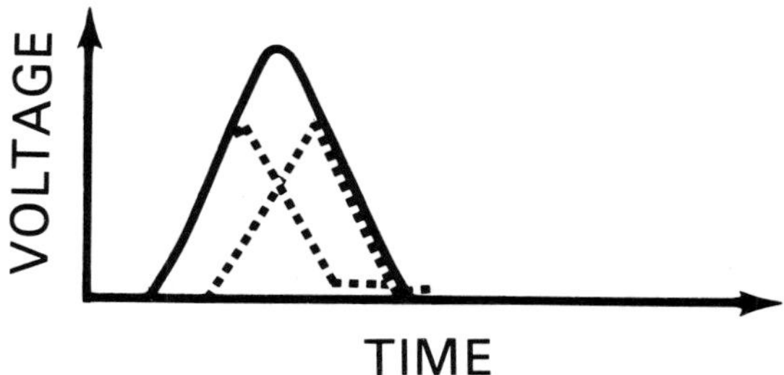

Figure 18. Pulse pileup occurs when two pulses (dashed lines) overlap. The resulting output pulse (solid line) is distorted. Depending on the discriminator settings, one or both pulses may be lost.

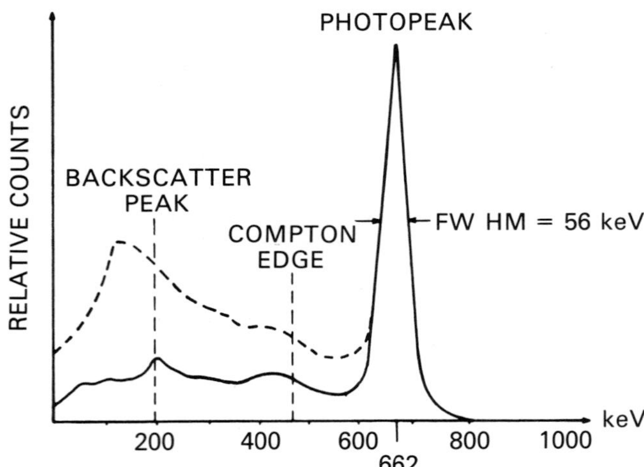

Figure 19. Pulse-height spectrum of ^{137}Cs, using a 5-in NaI(Tl) detector. The addition of a scattering medium (dotted line) affects primarily the lower end of the spectrum.

an elusive goal. Some loss of incident energy occurs through Compton scattering, in which scattered photons escape the crystal, and through the photoelectric effect, when characteristic x-rays, particularly at the edge of the crystal, escape. As a result, a distribution of pulse heights forms around the photopeak value, and the shape of this distribution depends on photon-to-photoelectric transfer variance; crystal size, composition, and intrinsic resolution; EM efficiency; and amplifier stability and linearity (Fig. 19). Pulse-height analyzers measure the frequency distribution of these pulse amplitudes. This distribution is known as the *pulse-height spectrum.*

The essential components of a single-channel analyzer (SCA) are two *pulse-height discriminators*, which may be set at E and $E + \Delta E$, respectively (Fig. 20). The upper- and lower-level discriminators consist of electronic circuits called *comparators*, which serve to compare the input pulse amplitude with their own voltage setting. They produce an output only when the input pulse exceeds their voltage setting. The discriminator output pulses are sent to an *anticoincidence circuit*, which operates in two modes. In the *integral* mode the upper level discriminator is turned off and the anticoincidence circuit passes all pulses that exceed the energy set by the lower level (threshold) discriminator. Thus all pulses of amplitude E or greater are passed. In the *differential* mode the upper level discriminator is turned on and only those pulses with energies between E and $E + \Delta E$ are passed. The output pulses from the SCA are then used to drive scalers, ratemeters, and other devices for count registration.

Most detection devices with SCAs have two controls for adjusting the discriminators, usually calibrated in keV. The lower-level discriminator is often called the *base level* or "threshold." In some cases, one determines the center of the window, while the other determines the window width as a percentage of the center window setting. For example, if ^{99m}Tc (E_γ = 140 keV) were being counted with a symmetric 20% window, the energy range selected would be 140 ± 14 keV, or 126 to 154 keV. In some situations, exclusion of some of the Compton scatter below the 140-keV photopeak is desirable. An "asymmetric window" can be selected merely by increasing the center-line adjustment to 150 keV. If the 20% window is retained, the new range is 150 ± 15 keV, or 135 to 165 keV. Notice that the same "percent window" now encompasses a wider energy range. Most modern detection devices have push-button selectors that designate the radionuclides most frequently counted. For special counting situations, however, it is important to have manual controls that override these automatic selectors.

Some applications of pulse-height analysis require multiple levels of discrimination. An example is gamma-ray spec-

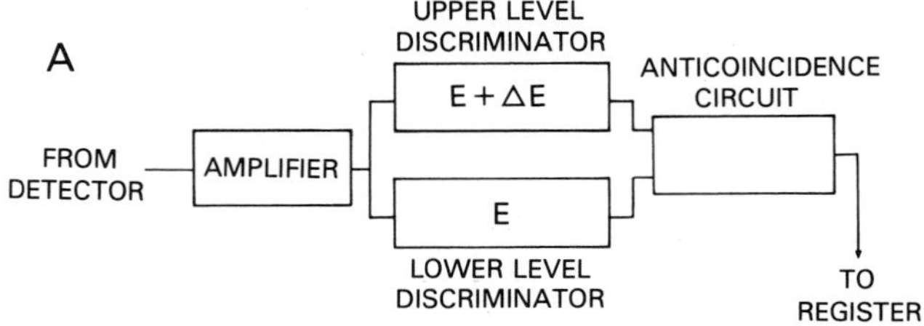

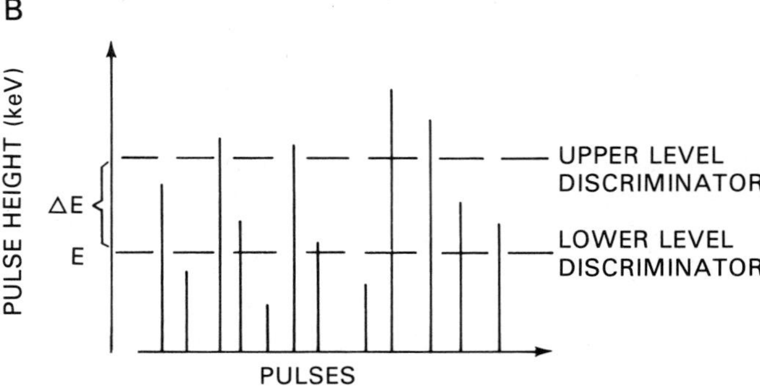

Figure 20. **(A).** Components of a single-channel PHA. **(B).** In the differential mode, the pulse-height analyzer passes only those pulses falling within the window (five counts). In the integral mode, the upper level discriminator is disabled and all pulses with energy greater than E are counted (nine counts).

troscopy (see Chapter 3). Rather than connect numerous SCAs, a *multichannel analyzer* (MCA) is employed. The heart of an MCA is a pulse-sorting device known as an *analog-to-digital converter* (ADC). Incoming pulses are separated according to amplitude and stored in a series of channels numbering from 128 to as many as 8192, each channel proportional to a preselected energy or amplitude range, ΔE. To accomplish this, the ADC uses either a series of comparators or a *ramp converter.*[10] The MCA uses a *digital storage* device that receives and sums pulses selected by the ADC as corresponding to various energy levels. This storage device contains X-Y locations, usually in a magnetic core in which the X location corresponds to $E + \Delta E$ and the Y location corresponds to the number of pulses falling within that window width. Once accumulated, the spectrum may be displayed by an X-Y plotter, cathode-ray tube, line printer, or other readout device.

From Figure 19, it is apparent that the monoenergetic gamma rays of ^{137}Cs (actually they come from the short-lived daughter radionuclide, ^{137m}Ba) result in a distribution of pulse heights. The width of the principal peak at half its height, or full-width-half-maximum (FWHM), characterizes the system's resolution, ie, the distribution of pulses around the true photon energy. This distribution determines the detector's ability to differentiate between gamma rays of different energies. Energy resolution is often expressed as a percentage of the peak energy of ^{137}Cs.

$$\% \text{ resolution} = \frac{^{137}\text{Cs FWHM (keV)}}{662} \times 100$$

Good NaI(Tl) detection systems have approximately 7 to 9% resolution. The value varies greatly with the size crystal, the type of EM tube, and the detection geometry. For example, for scintillation cameras with several EM tubes, light pipe, and capacitor circuitry, resolutions of about 15% can be expected.[8] For low-activity samples, very large NaI(Tl) systems are available (5- or 8-in diameter), but there is a tradeoff between higher efficiency and lower resolution.

Scalers

The scaler integrates the number of pulses accepted by the analyzer, either mechanically or, more commonly, electronically. Most scalers now read in decimal, using LEDs, although the primary circuitry usually operates in a binary system. Most counting systems are equipped with scaler timers, which measure both elapsed time and accumulated counts. The scaler timer permits the detector to count for a *preset time* or until a *present count* has been scaled.

Ratemeters

The ratemeter provides a direct and continuous measurement of the rate at which accepted pulses are processed, usually by means of a meter that fluctuates continuously with the changing count per unit time. *Analog* ratemeters operate by means of an R-C circuit in which the arriving pulses build up on a capacitor and are shunted through a resistor (Fig.

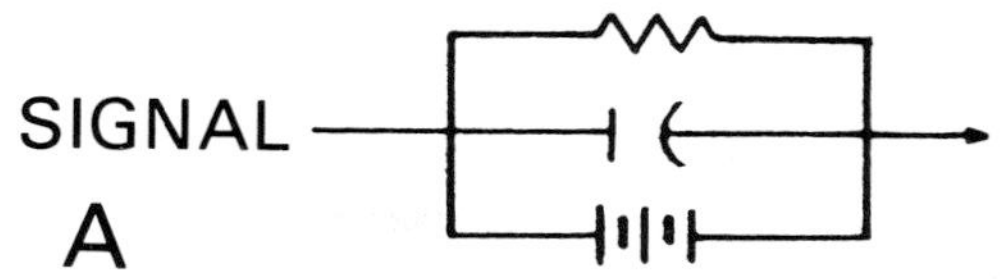

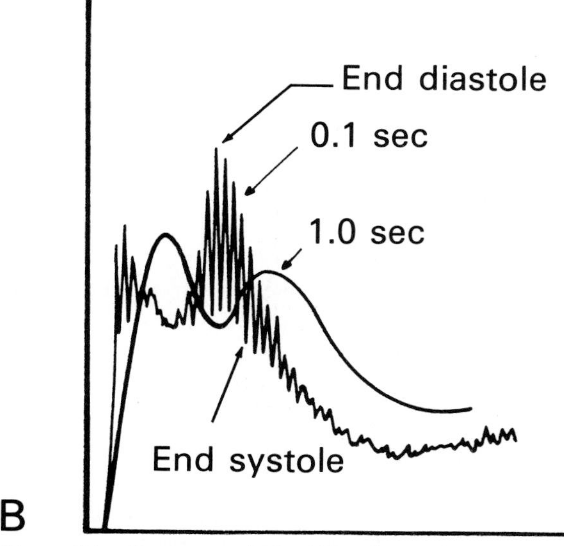

Figure 21. Ratemeter circuit (A) and recordings (B) of a radioactive bolus through the heart recorded by a strip-chart recorder with 0.1- and 1.0-second time constant. With 1.0-second time constant, individual heart beats are completely lost.

21A). The time to reach equilibrium is a function of the rate of the pulses and of the *R-C time constant* of the circuit. Most ratemeters have several time constants, which may be selected to reflect rapid fluctuations or to average the counts over greater time (long time constant). The effect is illustrated in Figure 21B, which represents the passage of a bolus of activity through the heart. With a time constant of 1 second, it is possible to discern the bolus entering and leaving the right and left chambers. The individual heart beats, however, which are seen easily with a 0.1-second time constant, cannot be resolved at the longer time constant.

Errors caused by time lag may be avoided using a *digital ratemeter.* A scaler is a type of digital ratemeter. After a preset time, the scaler indicates the counts accumulated during that period. A digital ratemeter is merely a constantly resetting scaler. The recycle frequency, however, is in reality a time constant. If long frequency intervals are selected, rapidly changing count rates may go undetected. Very short recycle times may themselves induce some counting error unless some buffering device is used.

The ratemeter output can be recorded in several ways, using a strip-chart recorder, magnetic tape, or magnetic disk. The strip-chart recorder, which reflects the changing rate on paper moving at a predetermined speed, has largely been replaced by computer printouts that represent digital re-

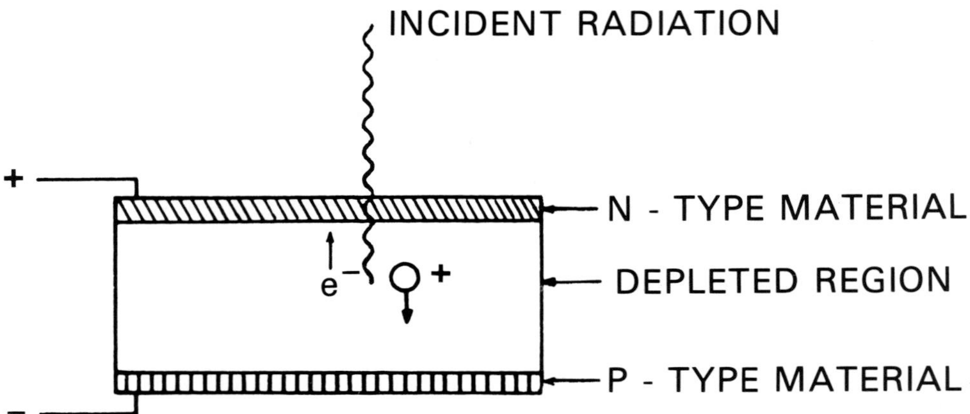

Figure 22. *p-n*-type semiconductor.

cordings wherein the "frame" rates are preselected and depend on the rate of change of counting events.

SEMICONDUCTOR DETECTORS

Solid-state detectors made of semiconducting materials are becoming increasingly important in radiation detection. Semiconductor detectors operate in a manner analogous to gas-filled detectors, except that they are 2000 to 5000 times more dense and are therefore much more efficient as radiation absorbers. Ordinarily, semiconducting substances such as silicon and germanium are poor electrical conductors. When they are subjected to ionizing radiation, however, the charges generated within the semiconductor material can be collected by applying a voltage potential across the detector crystal.

Semiconductors take many forms, but they generally consist of a *p-n junction*, made by creating two zones within the semiconductor material: a *p*-type material zone, which acts as an electron acceptor, and an *n*-type material zone, which acts as an electron donor (Fig. 22). If an electrical potential or bias, typically 500 to 4000 V, is applied across the detector, the electrical field draws electrons toward the *n* side and electron holes (in the valence band) toward the *p* side, thus forming an electrically neutral and insulating *depletion* region between the two. In this depleted region, no current flows. When radiation is absorbed within the depleted region (and only in this region), electron-hole pairs are formed. The electrons are raised from the valence band to the conduction band and drift toward the positive *n* side. The electron holes drift toward the *p* side. As a result, a small change in the bias develops proportional to the energy deposited in the depletion region. The physical principles thus contain elements analogous to both scintillation crystals and ionization chambers.

Semiconductor detectors have several advantages. The most important is that they have very high resolution and are thus capable of resolving energies only a few electron volts apart. The reason for this capability is that far more electrons are collected per MeV of energy absorbed than in ion chambers or scintillation detectors. Germanium requires only 2.9 eV and silicon 3.5 eV to form an electron-hole pair, while NaI(Tl) requires about 30 eV. Furthermore, the variability and inefficiency of the photocathode and EM tube are eliminated. Thus the energy resolution of semiconductors may be 20 times greater than that of NaI(Tl) crystals (Fig. 23). Semiconductors have a very short response time, so that pulse pair resolution is high. These semiconductors can be made so small that they can be inserted directly into the body, if desired.

Semiconductors also have several disadvantages. Because very low energy is required to produce a conduction electron,

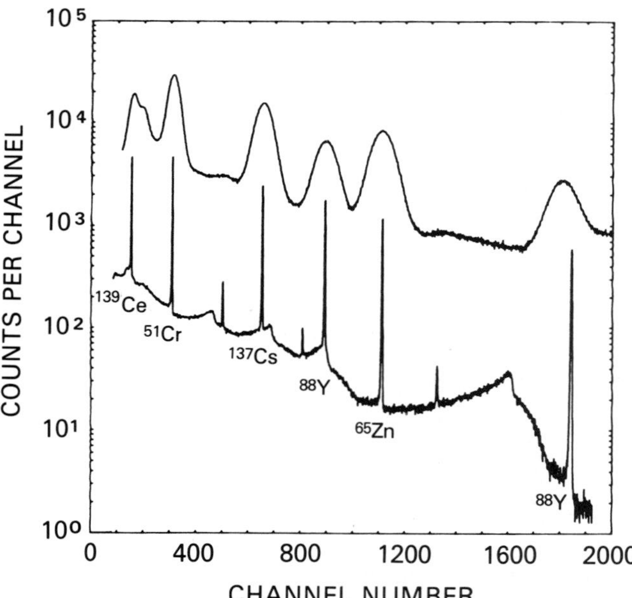

Figure 23. Gamma-ray spectra of a 5-mL mixed-radionuclide-solution source taken with the source within a 5-in NaI(Tl) well crystal (upper curve) and at the face of a 60-cm^3 Ge(Li) detector (lower curve). The counting time in each case was 2000 seconds. (From measurements made at the National Bureau of Standards.)

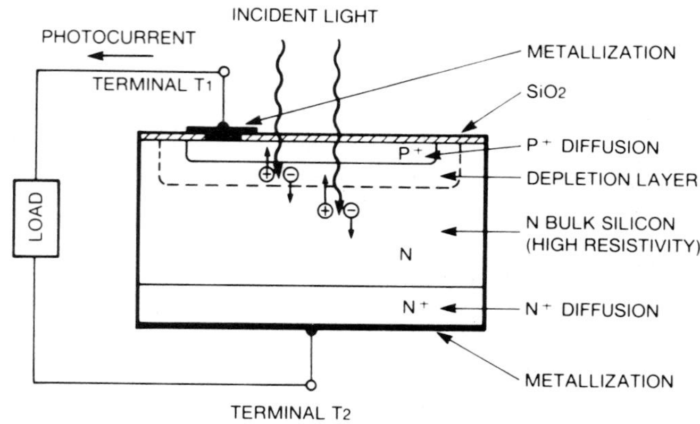

A

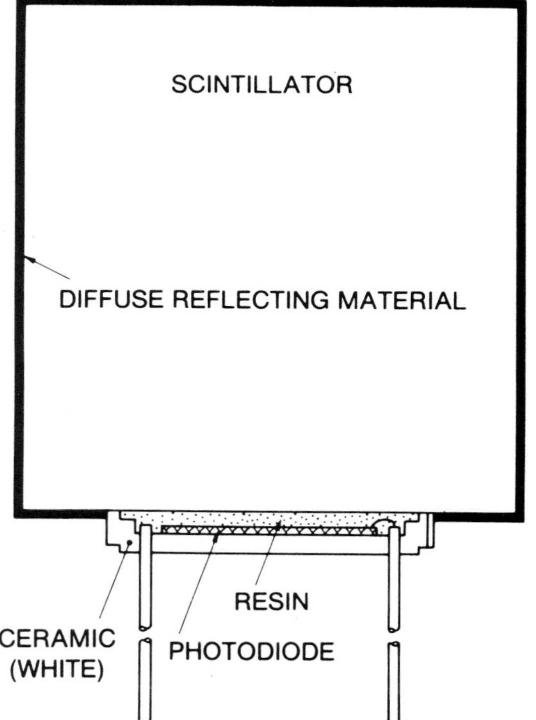

B

Figure 24. (A). Cross section of a photodiode. The *p*-type region on the light incident side (SiO_2) forms a *p-n* junction with the *n*-type silicon substrate, and this acts as a photoelectric converter. **(B).** Photodiode-scintillator coupling. Courtesy of Hamamatsu Corporation.

thermal noise may be high. Most applications require liquid nitrogen cooling to reduce this noise both in the detector and in the preamplifier. The bias voltage must be relatively high, which necessitates careful shielding, and the detectors are sensitive to atmospheric moisture. A major problem is encountered in producing detectors with sufficiently large volume to be efficient for gamma-ray detection; however, recent advances permit volumes up to 150 cm^3.

The *surface-barrier* detector is similar to *p-n* junction detectors with a very thin entrance window for the efficient detection of charged particles and weak x-rays. It is created by exposing a wafer on *n*-type germanium of silicon to air for a period of time to form a thin oxide layer. Oxygen is electronegative and therefore an electron acceptor, so a *p-n* junction is formed. The whole crystal is then covered with thin electroplating to form electrical contacts and to stop the oxidation process.

Photodiodes vs Electron Multipliers

Photodiodes operate in much the same way as semiconductor detectors, except that they produce a signal in response to visible or ultraviolet light rays, such as produced within scintillation detectors (Fig. 24A). Thus, if a photodiode is coupled optically to a scintillation crystal as in Figure 24B, electronic signals are produced in response to scintillation events within the crystal without the need for an EM tube.

When light strikes the photodiode, the electrons within the diode crystal structure become stimulated. Electrons are pulled up into the conduction band, leaving holes in their place in the valence band (see Fig. 10). These electron-hole pairs occur throughout the *p* layer, depletion layer, and *n*-layer materials, and in the depletion layer the electric field accelerates the electrons toward the *n* layer and the holes toward the *p* layer. The number of electron-hole pairs formed are directly proportional to the amount of incident light. This results in a positive charge in the *p* layer and a negative charge in the *n* layer. If an external circuit is connected between the *p* and *n* layers, electrons will flow away from the *n* layer and holes from the *p* layers toward the opposite electrode, respectively.

There are numerous advantages of photodiodes over EMTs, including their small size, low energy requirements, stability, fast response, and relative lower cost. The principle drawback is its lack of internal amplification, which has precluded its total replacement of EMTs.[14] This is especially true in applications such as PET where both energy and time resolution are demanded. In such cases high-speed, low-noise internal amplification is indispensible. Currently, large sensitive-area *avalanche photodiodes* are being developed for such applications.[15] The response time for these devices is on the order of several nanoseconds, with internal amplification in the region of 100 to 200, making them competitive with EMTs in PET applications.

REFERENCES

1. Knoll GF. *Radiation Detection and Measurement.* 2nd ed. New York: John Wiley & Sons, 1989.
2. Mann WB, Rytz A, Spernol A. *Radioactivity Measurements, Principles and Practice.* Oxford: Pergamon Press, 1991.
3. National Council on Radiation Protection. *A Handbook of Radioactivity Measurement Procedures.* Bethesda, MD: NCRP Publications, 1985. NCRP Report No. 58.
4. National Council on Radiation Protection. *Specification of Gamma Ray Brachytherapy Sources.* Washington, DC: National Council on Radiation Protection and Measurements, 1974:8. NCRP Report No. 41.
5. International Commission on Radiation Units. *Specification of High Activity Gamma-Ray Sources.* Washington DC: Interna-

tional Commission on Radiation Units and Measurements, 1971. ICRU Report No. 19.

6. Price WJ. *Nuclear Radiation Detection*. New York: McGraw-Hill, 1964:162.
7. Watt DE, Lawson RD, Clare DM. An experimental appraisal of the validity of neutron dosimetry theory in radiation protection. In: *Neutron Monitoring*. Vienna: International Atomic Energy Agency, 1967:27.
8. Murray RB. *IEEE Trans Nucl Sci* 1975;NS-22(1):54.
9. Boyd CM, Dalrymple GV, eds. *Basic Scientific Principles of Nuclear Medicine*. St Louis: C.V. Mosby, 1974.
10. Kowalski E. *Nuclear Counting Electronics*. New York: Springer-Verlag, 1970.
11. Nestor OH. Scintillator material growth. In: Haller EE et al, eds. *Nuclear Radiation Detector Material*. Elsever Science and North-Holland Publishing Companies, New York: Elsevier/North-Holland, 1983:77.
12. Ter-Pogossian MM, Phelps ME. Semiconductor detector systems. *Semin Nucl Med* 1973;3:343.
13. Thompson CJ, Yamamoto YL, Mer E. Positome II: a high efficiency positron imaging device for dynamic brain studies. *IEEE Trans Nucl Sci* 1979;NS-26:583.
14. Derenzo SE. Initial characterization of a BGO-photodiode detector for high resolution positron emission tomography. *IEEE Trans Nucl Sci* 1984;NS-31:620.
15. Lecomte R, et al. Performance characteristics of BGO-silicon avalanche photodiode detector for PET. *IEEE Trans Nucl Sci* 1985;NS-32:529.
16. Peng C-T. Liquid scintillation and Cerenkov counting. In: Coomber DI, ed. *Radiochemical Methods in Analysis*. New York: Plenum Press, 1975.
17. Horrocks DL. *Applications of Liquid Scintillation Counting*. New York: Academic Press, 1974.
18. Birks JB. *The Theory and Practice of Scintillation Counting*. Oxford: Pergamon Press, 1964.
19. Heath RL. Status of photon counting using solid scintillators. In: McQuarrie SA, Edis C, Wiebe LI, eds. *Advances in Scintillation Counting*. Edmonton: University of Alberta Press, 1983.
20. Coursey BM. *Use of NBS Mixed Radionuclide Gamma-ray Standards for Calibration of Ge(Li) Detectors Used in the Assay of Environmental Radioactivity*. Washington, DC: National Bureau of Standards, 1976. NBS Special Publication 456.
21. Coursey BM, Moghissi AA. Preparation of counting samples for liquid scintillation counting. In: Mann WB, Taylor JGV, eds. *Applications of Liquid Scintillation Counting in Radionuclide Metrology*. Sevres: Bureau International des Poids et Measures, 1980.
22. Coursey BM, Mann WB. Design considerations for the construction of high-efficiency liquid scintillation counting systems. In: *Application of Liquid Scintillation Counting in Radionuclide Metrology*. Sevres: BIPM Monographie 3, 1980.
23. Goldstein G. Absolute liquid scintillation counting of beta emitters. *Nucleonics* 1965;23:67.
24. Birks JB. *An Introduction to Liquid Scintillation Counting*. Buckinghamshire, U.K., Koch-Light Laboratories, 1975.
25. McDowell WJ. *Alpha Counting and Spectrometry Using Liquid Scintillation Methods*. Oak Ridge, TN: US Department of Energy; 1986. National Academy of Sciences-National Research Council Report NAS-NS-3116.

3 Counting Radioactivity

John C. Harbert, Bert M. Coursey

Radioactivity measurement techniques differ greatly, depending upon the type of radiation counted and the nature of the radioactive source. Beta- and gamma-ray detection are discussed separately; some principles common to both are considered first. Individual radionuclide disintegrations are random, but the rate of transformation can be described by the decay law:

$$\text{(1)} \qquad \frac{-dN}{dt} = N\lambda,$$

where N is the number of radioactive atoms present and λ is the decay constant, $\ln 2/T_{1/2}$. Equation 1 suggests two ways to quantify radioactivity in the sample. One can measure all disintegrations ($-dN/dt$) or, if the half-life is sufficiently long, one can measure the number of atoms (N) by gravimetric or spectrophotometric techniques. This is illustrated in Table 1, where the masses corresponding to 1 mCi are tabulated for several radioisotopes of iodine and technetium. One can see that milligram quantities of the long-lived ^{99}Tc can be used to synthesize Tc compounds which can then be characterized by various means such as x-ray diffraction. The corresponding masses for short-lived nuclides are exceedingly small however, and one must measure decay rates, $-dN/dt$.

COUNTING EFFICIENCY

The overall efficiency of any radiation counting system is defined as the ratio of the counting rate to the number of disintegrations per unit time:

$$\text{(2)} \qquad \varepsilon = \frac{R\ (\text{cpm})}{A\ (\text{dpm})}.$$

The factors that affect overall efficiency, ε_T, of a counting system are the geometry, absorption, scatter, intrinsic detector efficiency, and fidelity of count registration.

Overall detector efficiency can be expressed as

$$\text{(3)} \qquad \varepsilon_T = \varepsilon_1\, \varepsilon_2\, \varepsilon_3\, \varepsilon_4$$

where ε_1 is a factor accounting for absorbed and scattered radiation, ε_2 is the geometric efficiency, ε_3 is the intrinsic efficiency of the detector, and ε_4 is the fraction of pulses accepted by the pulse-height analyzer.

Geometry

The greatest factors affecting the efficiency of any counting system are the location, size, and shape of the sample in relation to the sensitive volume of the detector. The radiations from a radioactive source are emitted isotropically, ie, equally in every direction. For the case of a point source and detector with radius r located at some distance R from the source (Fig. 1a), the area exposed to the sphere of radiation flux emanating from the source is given by

$$\text{(4)} \qquad \varepsilon_2 = \frac{\pi r^2}{4\pi R^2} = \frac{\text{crystal area}}{\text{sphere area}}.$$

If the crystal measures 4 cm in diameter and is situated 10 cm from the source, the exposed area is only

$$\text{(5)} \qquad \varepsilon_2 = \frac{3.14 \times 2^2}{4 \times 3.14 \times 10^2} = \frac{12.56}{1256} = 1\%.$$

If the same crystal is moved twice this distance away, the geometric factor is less by

$$\text{(6)} \qquad \varepsilon_2 = \frac{12.56}{12.56 \times 20^2} = 0.25\%.$$

This example is a simple demonstration of the *inverse square law* which states that the counting rate decreases by $1/R^2$ as the detector moves away from a point source and increases by the same proportion as it is moved toward the source.

The inverse square law is only an approximation and does not hold for either large detectors or extended sources, such as activity within the human body. Thus, if R is reduced to zero and the source is placed against the detector (Fig. 1b), the counting rate does not become infinite; it reaches only about 50% of dN/dt. A closer approximation to the true geometric efficiency for cylindrical detectors is given by the factor $1/2\,(1 - \cos\theta)$, where θ is one-half the angle subtended by the crystal. In the case of Figure 1b where $\theta = 90°$ and $\cos\theta = 0$, the geometric factor becomes 0.5, which represents the actual condition.

Even higher detector efficiency is achieved by placing the source within the crystal as seen in Figure 1c, which is the geometry of a well counter. Now only the narrow angle subtended by the well opening allows radiations to escape. Figure 2 relates the response of a typical well counter (in percent of gamma rays detected) to the volume of sample measured. The loss of counts is due almost entirely to the

Table 1. Some Properties of Iodine and Technetium Radioisotopes

ISOTOPE	HALF-LIFE	ATOMIC MASS (g)	NUMBER OF ATOMS	MASS (g)
^{123}I	13.2 h	122.90	2.54×10^{12}	5.2×10^{-10}
^{125}I	59.6 d	124.90	2.75×10^{14}	5.7×10^{-8}
^{129}I	1.7×10^{7} y	128.90	2.86×10^{22}	6.1
^{99m}Tc	6.01 h	98.906	1.16×10^{12}	1.9×10^{-10}
^{99}Tc	2.11×10^{5} y	98.906	3.56×10^{20}	5.8×10^{-2}

Quantities of the nuclide corresponding to 1 mCi (3.7×10^{7} Bq).

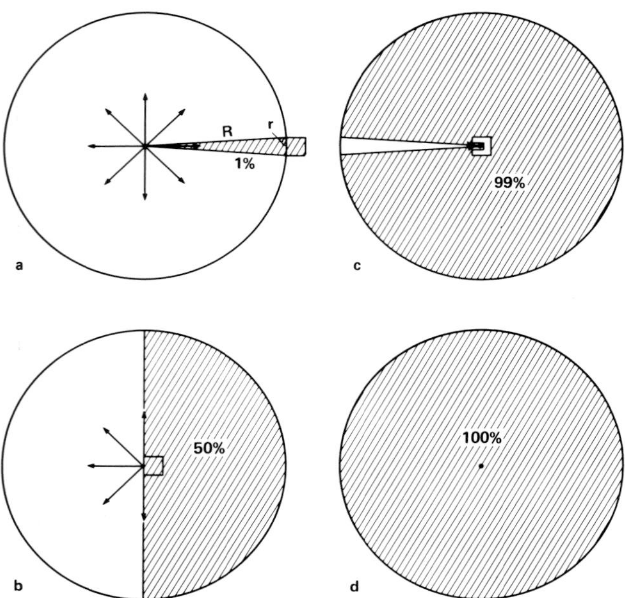

Figure 1. Four different counting geometries: **(a)** point source *R* cm from a cylindric crystal detector of radius *r*; **(b)** point source at the detector face; **(c)** point source inside well crystal; **(d)** 4π geometry as in liquid scintillation counting.

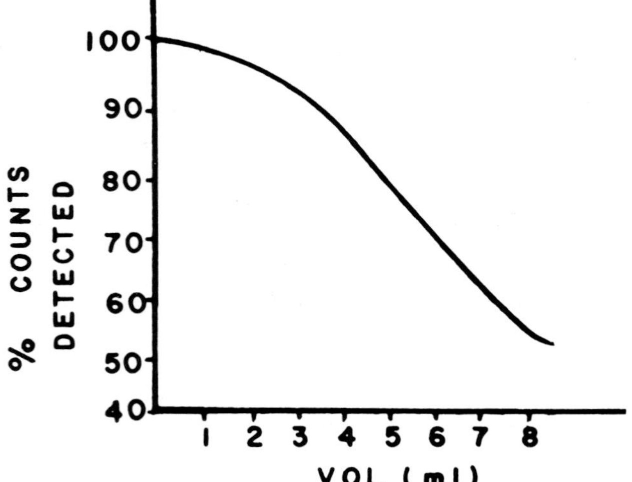

Figure 2. Changing counting rate as a function of source volume in a typical well counter.

decreasing angle subtended by the crystal and only slightly to the increased self-absorption due to increasing volume.

Virtually 100% geometric efficiency can be obtained by suspending the source completely within the detector (Fig. 1d). Such 4π geometry is most commonly encountered in liquid scintillation counting.

Absorption

Not all radiations emitted from the radioactive source and subtended by the detector reach the detector. Some are absorbed through interaction with the material of the source (*self-absorption*), in the medium between the source and the detector, and in the cladding of the detector itself. Self-absorption is more important with particulate radiation than with gamma radiation. Every beta emitter has a *saturation thickness* beyond which adding to the sample fails to increase the detected counts. Absorption outside the detector always decreases counting rate.

The usual method of correcting for external absorption is to count an aliquot of activity with and without the addition of absorber material while keeping all other factors of geometry equal. In general, the fraction of gamma rays that are emitted from a source and undergo absorption before reaching the detector decreases with increasing gamma-ray energy.

Scatter

Scattered photons in the source may either increase or decrease detection efficiency. Figure 3 shows a source of photons distributed within a scattering medium. Photons *e*, *g*, and *h* are Compton-scattered photons, which increase the counting rate. Photon *e* has been scattered off the wall of the collimator. Photon *g* has arisen outside the field of view of the collimator and is scattered into the detector. Photon *h* has undergone *multiple scattering* to reach the detector. Scattering reduces the photon energy but may increase the total counts observed.

Scattering of gamma photons increases with *Z* of the material and varies with the energy of the photon, as shown in Figure 4. One of the chief functions of pulse-height discrimination in gamma-ray detection systems is the elimination of scattered photons (particularly in imaging because of the degradation of image resolution). Figure 4 also plots the contribution of Compton scattering to the photopeak.

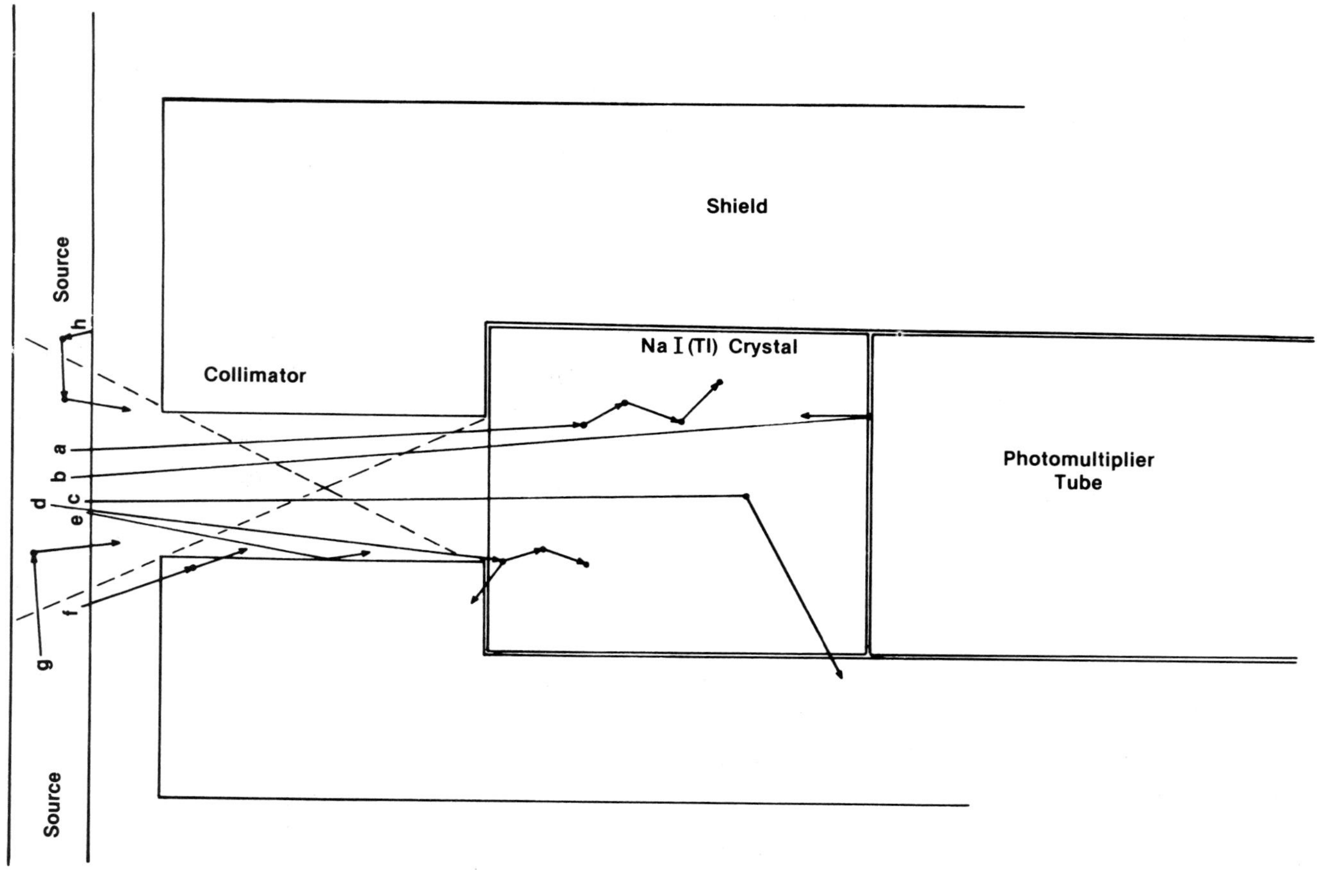

Figure 3. Extended gamma photon source and collimated NaI(Tl) detector. See text for description.

The reason for the decreasing Compton contribution with increasing energy is that the distance between photopeak and *Compton edge* increases. Most analyzer windows are set as a percentage of photopeak energy. Table 2 indicates angles of gamma-ray scattering that result in only 10% energy loss for several radionuclides. Gamma rays with 10% less than photopeak energy fall within a 20% analyzer window. Obviously, with lower-energy photons, a significant portion of the counts accepted result from scattered photons.

Scattered beta particles usually increase counting rate,

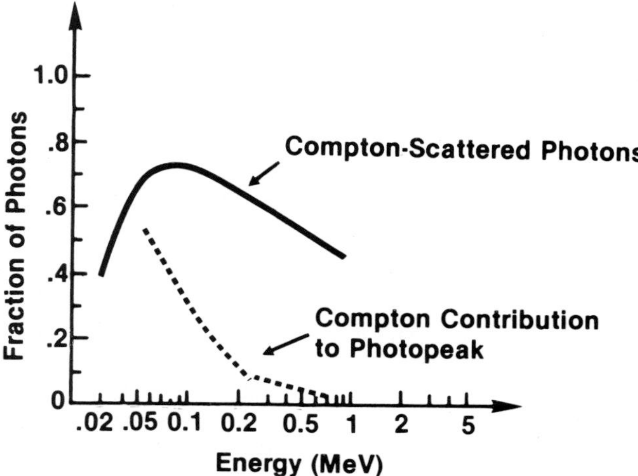

Figure 4. The fraction of gamma rays scattered in tissue medium (solid line) as a function of energy. The fraction appearing in the photopeak (broken line) is calculated for a 20% window and a NaI(Tl) crystal. (Modified from Reference 1.)

Table 2. The Angle of Scatter Resulting in 10% Loss of Energy for Several Radionuclides

RADIONUCLIDE	INCIDENT GAMMA-RAY ENERGY (keV)	SCATTERING ANGLE (°)	SCATTERED GAMMA-RAY ENERGY (keV)
^{125}I	35	152	32
^{133}Xe	81	68	73
^{99m}Tc	140	39	126
^{131}I	364	31	330
^{137m}Ba	662	22	600

From Hine GJ. Performance characteristics of nuclear instruments. In: Rhodes BA, ed. *Quality Control in Nuclear Medicine.* St Louis: C.V. Mosby, 1977.

especially with higher-energy particles, which scatter from the sample mount back into the detector volume (*backscatter*).

Detector Efficiency

The intrinsic efficiency of a detector ε_3 is defined as the ratio of the number of radiations (photons or particles) that interact in the detector to the total number of incident radiations. Intrinsic efficiency of most detectors is nearly 100% for alpha and beta particles because of their short path length. Intrinsic efficiency for gamma rays, however, depends upon the photon energy and the size, shape, and composition of the sensitive volume of the detector.

If each photon absorbed results in an output signal, the intrinsic efficiency may be represented as follows:

$$\varepsilon = 1 - \exp\left[-\mu(E)\,x\right], \tag{7}$$

where $-\mu(E)$ is the linear attenuation coefficient of the detector material for photon energy, E, and x is the detector thickness. The relationship between linear attenuation coefficient $-\mu(E)$ and photon energy is shown in Figure 5 for water, sodium iodide, and lead. Detector attenuation, and therefore intrinsic efficiency, decrease nearly logarithmically with increasing energy. For higher-energy photons, larger, denser crystals are usually employed. Germanium crystals are denser than NaI(Tl) crystals by 5.68:3.67 g/cm^3. Ge(Li) semiconductors, however, are restricted to thicknesses of less than about 5 cm because of limitations imposed by the depletion zone (see Chapter 2).

Most gas-filled detectors have efficiencies of less than 1% for the gamma-ray energies encountered in nuclear medicine. Some multiwire proportional counters have been filled with xenon gas under pressure for use as imaging devices, but they are suitable only for radionuclides that emit low-energy gamma and x-rays, such as ^{178}Ta, ^{133}Xe, and ^{201}Tl. One such "camera" containing xenon gas at 10 atm was described by Zimmerman et al.[2] Its intrinsic efficiency was 70% of that of an Anger camera with a 6-mm thick NaI(Tl) crystal for photons of 60 to 81 keV. With such detector systems, scatter with partial absorption of photons commonly gives rise to escape peaks (see "Gamma-Ray Spectrometry" in this chapter).

Use of a pulse-height analyzer and photopeak counting further reduces the intrinsic efficiency. In this case, only those photons that are completely absorbed in the crystal, the *photofraction*, and meet the energy requirements of the window enclosing the photopeak are counted. The photofraction of any radionuclide depends on the photon energy and the size and composition of the detector, as discussed earlier.

Instrument Deadtime

All radiation detectors have counting rate limitations imposed by the time required to transform the ionizing event into an electronic signal. In the case of Geiger-Müller (G–M) tubes, this time is relatively long (100 to 500 μs) because of the time required for the large positive gas ions to reach the outer wall cathode. In the case of modern scintillation detectors, this time is shorter (nanoseconds) because of short light decay times and fast electron multiplier (E–M) tubes. In both cases, the electronic signal is produced by the sharp drop in potential difference between electrodes once the electrons reach the anode. The signal strength, or *pulse height*, is proportional to the change in potential difference across the electrodes (Fig. 6B). During the *recovery time*, the potential difference between electrodes is restored. Several terms that refer to this process are defined as follows. The *deadtime* is the period following the first pulse during which the detector is insensitive to incoming ionizing events. The *resolving time* is the time required for the potential difference to increase sufficiently to produce a pulse that can "trigger" the counter. It is also the shortest time interval by which two pulses must be divided to be detected as separate pulses. The recovery time is the period required for regaining a potential difference sufficient to produce a full amplitude pulse. Ionizing events that enter the detector before the resolving time are lost because of *coincidence*. This loss is called *pulse pileup*, or *deadtime loss*. Ionizing events that occur during the recovery time result in lower pulse heights, or *baseline shift*. Such pulses are also lost if they fall below the lower-level discriminator of the pulse-height analyzer (PHA).

Counting systems are *paralyzable* (or extendable) if each event introduces a deadtime τ, whether or not the event is counted (dotted lines in Fig. 6B). In a nonparalyzable (or nonextendable) system, an event occurring during the deadtime has no effect on the recovery of potential difference. In such a system, the deadtime equals the resolving time.

Figure 7 demonstrates that, as counting rate increases, coincidence losses result in a variation between the observed counting rate r and the true counting rate R. At low counting rates, the values are identical. However, as true counting increases (dashed line), the observed counting rate declines, approaching zero in a paralyzable counting system and reaching $r_{\max} = 1/\tau$ in a nonparalyzable system. The shape of this curve depends upon the resolving time and the type of system. For a nonparalyzable system

$$\frac{R}{r} = \frac{1}{1 - R\tau}. \tag{8}$$

This equation is difficult to solve. Because $(1 - R\tau)$ is closely approximated by $(1 - r\tau)$ for the usual counting rates encountered in the laboratory, the above equation can be simplified to

$$R = \frac{r}{1 - r\tau}. \tag{9}$$

In the case of paralyzable systems, the dead periods are not all the same but dependent on the distribution of intervals between random events. For the paralyzable model

$$r = Re^{-R\tau}.$$

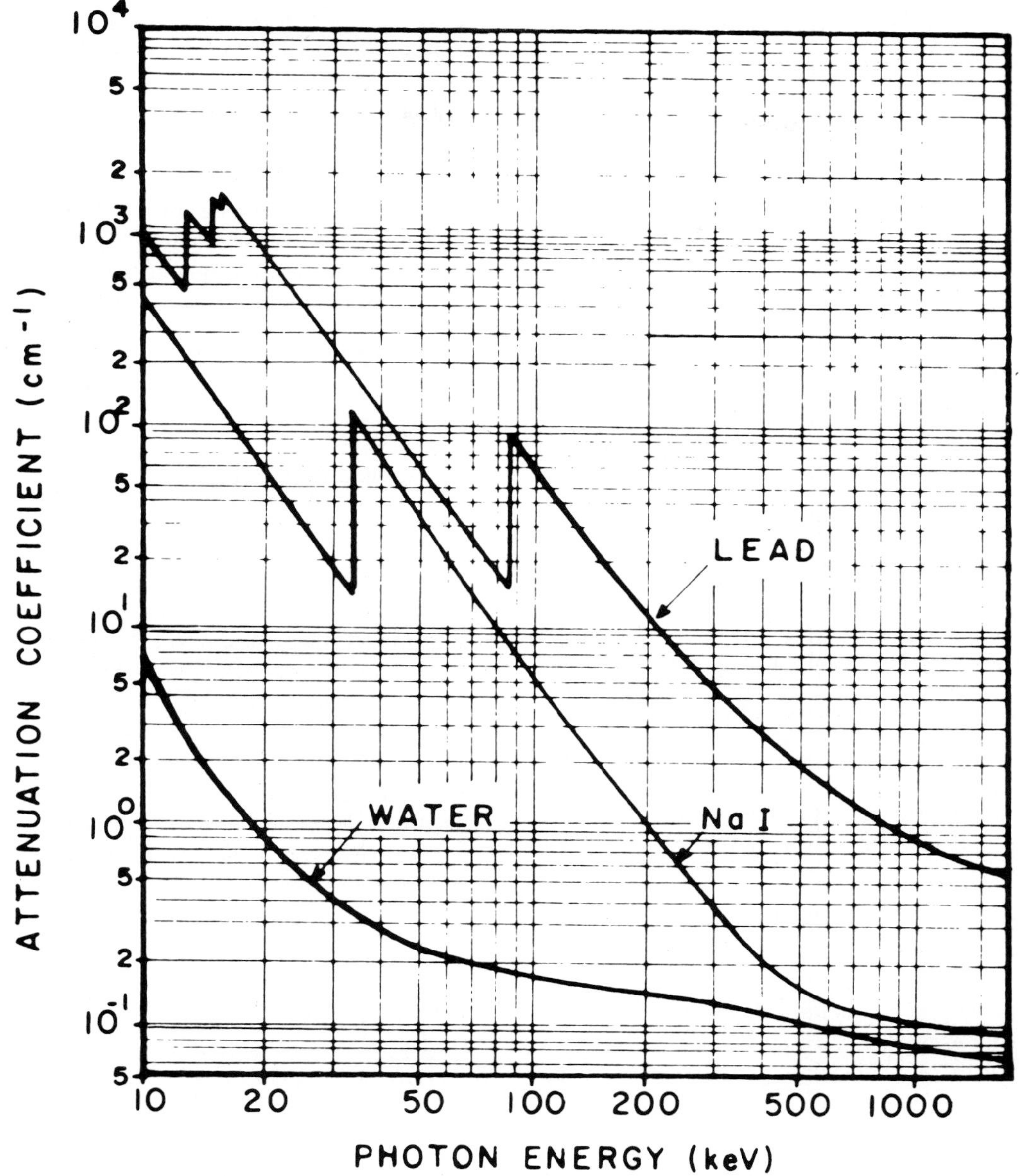

Figure 5. Linear attenuation coefficients for water, NaI, and lead as a function of photon energy.

This equation does not permit a direct solution of the true rate R. Instead, an iterative solution is required.

A deadtime τ is determined most often by the paired-source method, wherein the counting rates of two sources are counted separately as r_1 and r_2, and together as r_{12}. Then, for a nonparalyzable system for which negligible background is assumed,

$$\tau \cong \frac{r_1 + r_2 - r_{12}}{r_{12}^2 - r_1^2 - r_2^2}. \tag{10}$$

For a paralyzable system,

$$\tau \simeq \left(\frac{r_{12}}{2r_1r_2}\right) \ln \left(\frac{r_1 + r_2}{r_{12}}\right). \tag{11}$$

The sources are counted separately and simultaneously under constant conditions of geometry, scatter, and absorption. The activity of each source must be selected carefully so that neither source counted by itself induces appreciable coincidence loss, but when counted together the sources induce about 20% coincidence loss.

A second method, the *decaying source* technique, may be used if a short-lived radionuclide is available in sufficient quantity. Taking advantage of the known change in count rate through decay,

$$R = R_0\, e^{-\lambda t} \tag{12}$$

where R_0 is the true counting rate at the beginning of the determination.[3]

Some detectors have built-in coincidence correction cir-

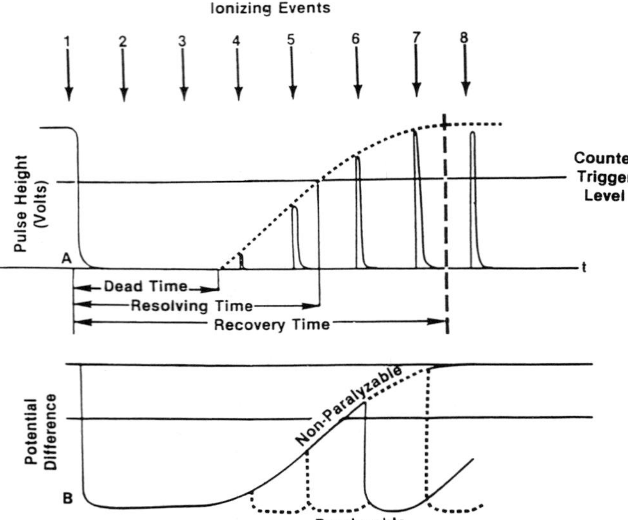

Figure 6. Output pulses from a radiation detector illustrating the effect of coincidence on pulse height in paralyzable and nonparalyzable systems. **(A)** The dotted line represents the return of potential difference across the electrodes following an initial pulse. During the deadtime, no pulse results from ionizing events 2 and 3. Pulses 4 to 7 would result in pulses of reduced amplitude. Only event 8, which occurs after the recovery time, will produce a full amplitude pulse. **(B)** The potential difference from the detector is represented here as a solid line. In a nonparalyzable system, event 6 would produce a second pulse of reduced amplitude. In a paralyzable system (broken line) only the first event would produce a pulse.

cuitry through storage buffers, but these buffers are effective only up to about 30% coincidence loss. While the usual solution to this problem is to avoid coincidence loss by limiting source activity, such a solution is not always possible, and coincidence errors must be corrected using Equation 9, or graphically using plotted counting rate response as in Figure 7. Knowledge of the counting rate response of each instrument used is therefore essential. If the instrument is equipped with a PHA, one must remember that any detected event can cause pulse pileup, whether it falls within the analyzer window or not. To determine the maximum counting rate to be encountered in any experimental situation, the integral mode should be used (see Chapter 2). The value of τ is determined by the counts from the total spectrum, not merely by those passing the analyzer window.

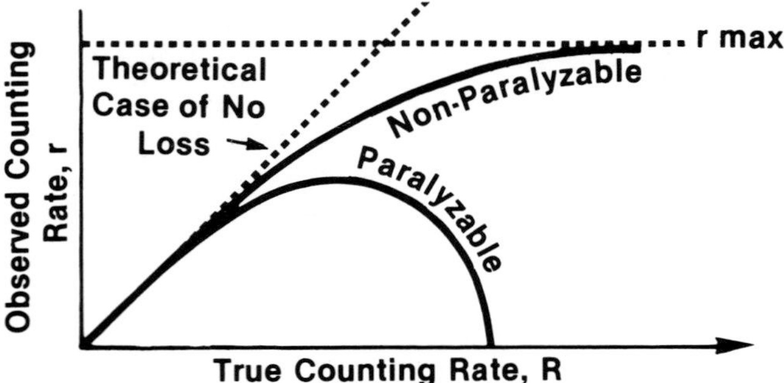

Figure 7. The relationship between true and observed counting rates in paralyzable and nonparalyzable counting systems.

Standards

The problem of determining absolute activity, which requires knowledge of the overall counting efficiency, is usually overcome by comparing the counting rate of the unknown source with that of a known standard of the same radionuclide:

$$\frac{\text{unknown activity } (\mu\text{Ci})}{\text{standard } (\mu\text{Ci})} = \frac{\text{cps unknown}}{\text{cps standard}}. \tag{13}$$

Therefore,

$$\text{unknown activity } (\mu\text{Ci}) = \text{standard } (\mu\text{Ci}) \times \frac{\text{cps unknown}}{\text{cps standard}}. \tag{14}$$

The only criterion for assuring the validity of this relationship is that the same conditions exist for counting both unknown and standard. Usually, this condition is easily fulfilled for samples contained in counting vials, but when the source is located inside the patient additional problems arise. Many standard reference materials for radionuclides used in nuclear medicine are available from the National Institute of Standards and Technology (formerly National Bureau of Standards).[5] These are listed in Table 3. Most of these materials are also available as standards from radiopharmaceutical manufacturers who maintain traceability to NIST.

Extraneous Counts

An important consideration in many radioactivity measurements, in most *in vivo* measurements, and in all low-level counting is the occurrence of extraneous counts, which may be defined as counts having any origin other than the radioactive atoms of interest. Two origins of extraneous counts are background counts and interfering radioactivity in the source.

BACKGROUND

Ambient background radiation derives principally from three sources (Table 4):

1. Primordial radionuclides
   The most important of these are uranium and thorium, found in many rocks and soil, and their daughters; ^{40}K; and ^{87}Rb, found in air and ground water.
2. Cosmic rays and cosmogenic radionuclides
   These include ^{14}C and radioberyllium. Cosmic rays derive from radiation of galactic particles upon the upper atmosphere and from the sun, especially during solar flares.
3. Man-made radionuclides
   The most notable of these are ^{90}Sr and ^{137}Cs from nuclear fallout.

Table 3. Radiopharmaceutical Standard Reference Materials from the National Institute of Standards and Technology[5]

RADIONUCLIDE	HALF-LIFE	APPROXIMATE ACTIVITY CONCENTRATION (Bq · g^{-1}) AT TIME OF DISPATCH	OVERALL UNCERTAINTY (%)	SRM NO. OF LAST ISSUE
^{51}Cr	27.702 d	4×10^6	0.7	4400LK
^{67}Ga	3.261 d	4×10^6	0.8	4416LK
^{195}Au	183 d	5×10^5	2.3	4421L
^{198}Au	2.696 d	4×10^6	1.7	4405LB
^{111}In	2.805 d	5×10^6	0.7	4417LJ
^{123}I	13.221 h	6×10^7	1.5	4414LC
^{125}I	59.6 d	1×10^6	1.0	4407LO
^{131}I	8.021 d	5×10^6	0.9	4401LP
^{59}Fe	44.51 d	8×10^5	1.5	4411LB
^{203}Pb	51.88 h	3×10^6	1.0	4420LB
^{203}Hg	46.60 d	1×10^6	1.0	4418L
^{99}Mo	65.92 h	1×10^7	1.0	4412LP
^{32}P	14.29 d	2×10^6	1.2	4406LK
^{75}Se	119.8 d	1×10^6	2.8	4409LD
^{85}Sr	64.854 d	1×10^6	1.4	4403LB
^{99m}Tc	6.007 h	1×10^9	0.9	4410HP
^{201}Tl	72.91 h	4×10^6	1.6	4404LL
^{113}Sn	115.08 d	1×10^6	3.1	4402LC
^{133}Xe	5.243 d	5×10^8 Bq total	1.0	4415LN
^{169}Yb	32.03 d	2×10^6	1.3	4419LC

Background radiation varies from location to location, depending upon altitude, building material, construction, and geographic location. Particularly variable background may occur in nuclear laboratories, because of stored radionuclides, ambient contamination, and often radioactive patients injected with radiopharmaceuticals. Measured background varies directly with the detector volume and inversely with detector shielding. Background corrections should always be applied unless the sample counting rate is greater than 100 times the background rate. In addition, background may arise from the detector instrumentation in the form of electronic "noise" pulses, which have already been discussed. Usually, background is allowed for by measuring a "dummy," or "blank" sample that is identical to the unknown source in all respects except for its absence of radioactivity.

INTERFERING RADIOACTIVITY

Both source and standard may contain interfering radioactivity. It may be added as a contaminant during sample processing; it may be generated during isotope production; or it may arise merely as a consequence of source geometry. If the interfering radionuclide in the unknown source is the same as the radioactive source, it cannot be distinguished by either chemical or physical techniques. An example is the variable blood activity encountered in organ imaging. If the

Table 4. Typical Environmental Radiation Field

RADIATION	ENERGY (MeV)	SOURCE	ABSORBED DOSE RATE IN FREE AIR (μrad/h)
α	1–9	Radon (atm)	2.7
β	0.1–200	Radon (atm)	
		K, U, Th, Sr (soil) Cosmic rays	3.4
γ	0.8–2.6	K, U, Th, Cs, Rn	5.9
η	0.1–100	Cosmic rays	0.1
ρ	10–2000	Cosmic rays	0.1
μ	100–30,000	Cosmic rays	2.3
			Total 14.5

Modified from NCRP Report No. 50.[4]

interfering nuclide is a different isotope of the same element, separating them by spectrometry may be possible. For example, the $^{122}Te(d,n)^{123}I$ reaction in a cyclotron produces various quantities of ^{130}I, ^{126}I, and ^{124}I, which are only partially discriminated by spectrometry. If the interfering radioactivity is a different element, it may be distinguished by chemical separation or by physical methods. The most common physical procedure is separation by half-life. For example, ^{197}Hg ($T_{1/2}$ = 2.7 days) contamination of ^{203}Hg ($T_{1/2}$ = 46.9 days) may be reduced by simple decay. Often, beta-emitting radionuclides, which have continuous energy spectra, can be discriminated only by physical separation methods.

COUNTING BETA PARTICLES

The measurement of beta-emitting nuclides presents some special problems not encountered with gamma-emitting nuclides. Beta particles are negatively charged and are emitted in a continuous energy distribution ranging from zero to the maximum energy characteristic of the particular nuclide, E_{max}. Because they are charged, beta particles readily interact with matter and are easily absorbed and scattered.

The most commonly used beta counters are liquid scintillation counters. Their principal advantage over solid-state detectors, GM tubes, and gas flow proportional counters is that the radioactive sample is intimately mixed with the liquid fluor, resulting in high geometric efficiency and good overall efficiency even for such low-energy beta emitters as ^{3}H and ^{35}S. Beta particles may also be counted with GM tubes fitted with thin mica windows. Gas flow proportional counters may be used to count weak-energy beta particles. In the latter instrument, the radioactive sample is placed directly into the sensitive volume of the detector, thus eliminating beta absorption in the detector window.

Samples are prepared by pipetting small amounts (0.1 mL) of a radioactive solution onto a sample counting planchette, usually stamped from copper or aluminum. The sample is then dried and often covered with Scotch tape to prevent loss. Liquid samples are almost never counted because of the changing absorption due to evaporation. It is essential to prepare the samples and standard in an identical manner so that the loss of efficiency due to self-absorption is the same. Also, both samples and standard must be counted on the same type of planchette so that backscatter will be the same. For example, ^{32}P mounted on a copper planchette has almost 30% higher counting rate than when counted on paper.

GAMMA-RAY SPECTROMETRY

Gamma-emitting nuclides are preferred to beta emitters in biologic tracer studies because

1. They are easier to detect and quantify in patients.
2. They are easier to detect within the environment, which improves radiation protection.
3. They can generally be administered in larger quantities per unit of absorbed dose to the patient.
4. The administered dose is more easily calibrated.

Most applications of gamma-ray detection in nuclear medicine involve the measurement of pulse height, particularly to identify or separate different radionuclides and to reject scattered radiation and thus improve resolution in radionuclide images. In most cases, spectrometry is performed with NaI(Tl) crystals for reasons already described. Consequently, the spectra illustrated here are those derived from NaI(Tl) systems.

Photon attenuation or absorption within the scintillation crystal occurs by the three processes of photon interaction described in Chapter 1:

1. In the photoelectric effect, all of the photon energy is transferred directly to an orbital electron, the photoelectron, which behaves as a beta particle, causing secondary ionization over a short path length. The chance that all of the original photon energy will be deposited within the crystal is high if the crystal is more than a few centimeters in thickness. Each ion pair formed ultimately results in the production of fluorescent light photons. However, the process occurs so quickly that the many individual photons appear as a single flash of light of brightness proportional to the incident photon energy.
2. Compton scattering results in only part of the photon energy being imparted to the orbital electron. The scattered photon may interact elsewhere in the crystal and undergo a photoelectric interaction or another Compton scattering. In either case, the processes occur so quickly that the total energy transfer is registered in a manner identical to the photoelectric effect. If the Compton-scattered photon passes out of the crystal, a lesser amount of light is produced and a lower pulse from the EM tube results (photon c, Fig. 3).
3. Pair production results in the conversion of 1.022 MeV of the photon energy into an electron and positron, with the remaining photon energy divided between the two particles as kinetic energy. The positron combines with an electron and annihilates to produce two 0.511-MeV photons. Either or both of these photons may interact in the crystal by the preceding two processes. If one or both of these annihilation photons escapes the crystal, the resultant pulse is 0.511 or 1.022 MeV lower than the photopeak. Such losses contribute to *escape peaks* superimposed upon the photopeak. The most probable of these occurrences, however, is total energy transfer.

In a perfect detection system, a monoenergetic gamma source such as ^{137}Cs should yield a single-line photopeak at 662 keV. The spectrum in Figure 8 using a 3- × 3-in NaI(Tl) crystal shows a spread of energies about the photopeak with a complex lower-energy component.

The distribution of energies of unscattered photons, ie,

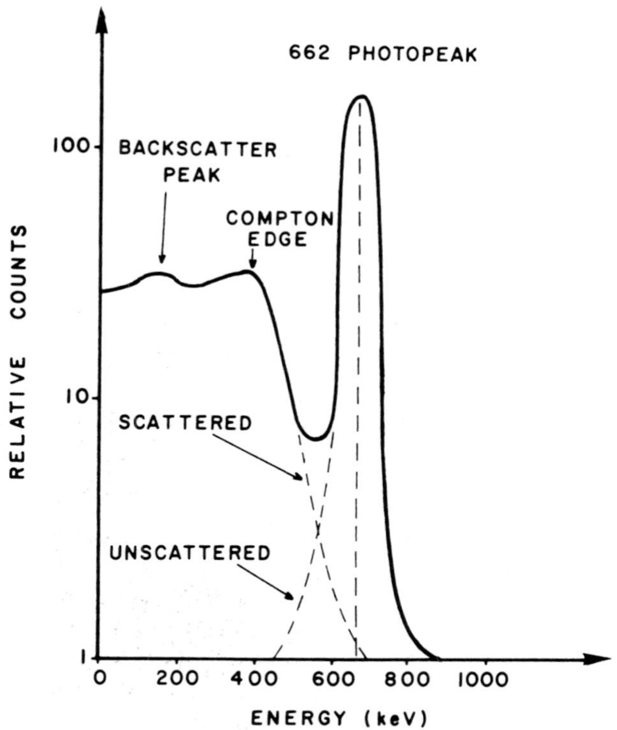

Figure 8. Pulse-height spectrum showing the distribution of unscattered and scattered photons forming the Compton trough, Compton edge, and backscatter peak.

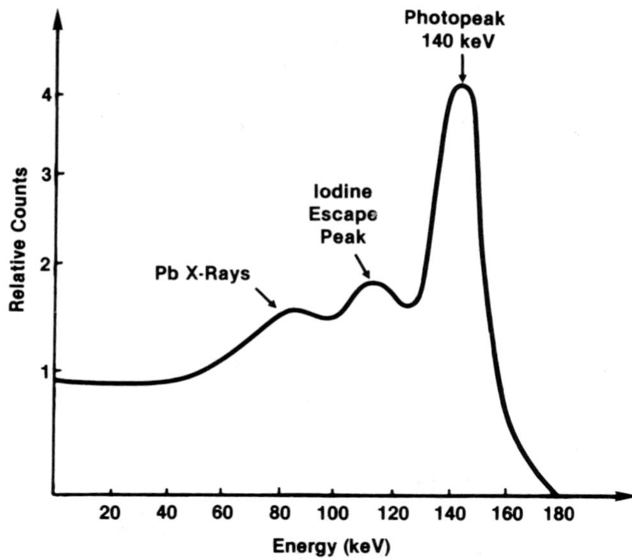

Figure 9. Iodine escape peak in ^{99m}Tc spectrum using a thin crystal.

photons completely absorbed within the crystal, stems from several variables operating within the scintillation detection system:

1. Variable amount of absorbed energy converted to heat rather than light photons.
2. Variable self-absorption of light within the crystal.
3. Variable photon absorption caused by nonuniform photocathode thickness.
4. Imperfect dynode amplification.
5. Fluctuating background or electronic noise.
6. Variable amplifier gain.

Most of these variables are random and additive. Therefore, the final spectrum has a photopeak with a more or less Gaussian distribution about a maximum. This spectrum is illustrated in Figure 8 by the dashed line extending down from the peak, which represents the theoretic distribution of unscattered photons.

Scattering, which makes up the lower energy portion of the spectrum, derives from several phenomena, as shown in Figure 3. The principal mechanism of photon absorption in NaI(Tl) above 100 keV is Compton scattering. There is a high probability that the Compton electron will be absorbed and a lesser probability that the Compton-scattered photon will be absorbed: a scattered photon that escapes from the crystal (photon c in Fig. 3) results in a pulse that falls into the *Compton plateau* between the *Compton edge* and the *backscatter peak* (Fig. 8).

Recall that the maximum energy is imparted to a Compton electron when the electron is scattered at 180° to the incident photon. The Compton edge is determined by the relation

$$\text{Compton edge (keV)} = \frac{E^2}{E + 256}, \tag{15}$$

where E is the photon energy. The backscatter peak occurs at the lower end of the Compton plateau and is caused by photons that pass completely through the crystal unabsorbed, strike the shielding or PM tube, and are scattered back 180° into the crystal, where they are absorbed (photon b, Fig. 3). These photons have an energy about equal to the photopeak minus the Compton edge. The backscatter peak can be calculated:

$$\text{Backscatter peak (keV)} = \frac{256\,E}{E + 256} \tag{16}$$

Other types of scattering that degrade the spectrum include

1. Iodine K escape
   Photon d in Figure 3 has undergone Compton scattering. The photoelectron from the K shell leaves an orbital vacancy, which is filled by an outer electron with the emissions of a K-characteristic x-ray. If this x-ray escapes the crystal, a pulse 28 keV lower than the photopeak results. This iodine K x-ray escape usually occurs at the edge of the crystal. The resultant iodine escape peak is apt to be seen only with thin crystals (Fig. 9).
2. Single and double escape peaks that result from pair production
   These have already been discussed. Following positron annihilation, one or both annihilation photons may es-

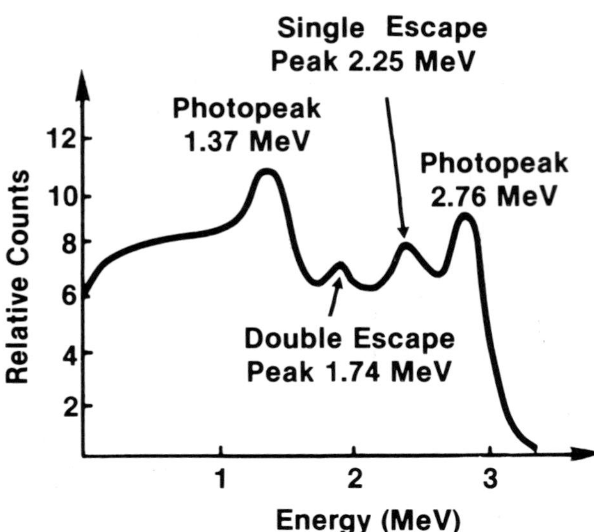

Figure 10. Spectrum of ^{24}Na showing the two photopeaks and single and double escape peaks below the 2.76-MeV photopeak.

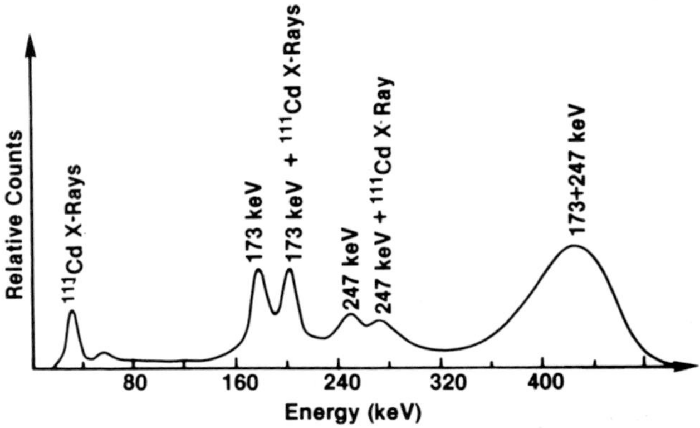

Figure 11. Pulse-height spectrum of ^{111}In taken from a NaI(Tl) well counter. Coincidence summing occurs with both x- and gamma rays. The probability of summing increases with the geometric efficiency.

cape the crystal, resulting in pulses 0.511 and 1.022 MeV below the photopeak (Fig. 10). These escape peaks also decrease with increasing crystal size.

3. Scattering within the source

   This is the most common origin of low energy pulses (photons g and h, Fig. 3). The scattered photon energy decreases with increasing angle of scatter and the number of scatter events before striking the crystal. It may be desirable to exclude these scattered photons by pulse-height discrimination.

4. Collimator scatter

   This is a source of two different kinds of scatter. The simplest type is represented by photon e in Figure 3, in which the incident photon undergoes Compton scattering and the degraded photon strikes the crystal producing a lower-energy pulse. The second is illustrated by photon f, which produces a Compton electron in the collimator with resultant production of a lead x-ray at 73 to 75 keV (Fig. 9).

Coincidence Summing

Many radionuclides emit more than one photon in the decay process, except in the case of metastable isotopes, such as ^{99m}Tc, that are characterized by having prolonged intervals between successive emissions leading to the ground state. Multiple emissions occur almost simultaneously. The direction of emission is random, so that the probability of two or more photons striking the detector simultaneously increases in proportion with geometric efficiency. When this occurs, the detector output registers a single pulse equal to the sum of the absorbed photon energies (Fig. 11). The result may be a dramatic alteration of the pulse-height spectrum. Coincidence sum peaks are encountered in the spectra derived from well counters much more frequently than in those derived from scintillation cameras. One means of identifying sum peaks is to observe the changing spectrum and record successive spectra as a source is raised out of a well counter.

Automated "Gamma Counters"

The most popular counting systems for counting large numbers of samples are NaI(Tl) "gamma counters." A typical gamma counter has an automated sample changer that can accommodate as many as 200 samples, a NaI(Tl) well crystal, and a personal computer (PC). The PC has a multichannel analyzer (MCA) board so that the entire pulse-height distribution for the gamma-ray emitter is accumulated for each sample. The counting efficiency for a typical well crystal as a function of gamma-ray energy is shown in Fig. 12. Only the photopeak efficiency is included in this curve. For a given radionuclide with multiple gamma and x rays, such as ^{111}In, the counting efficiency will be given by a complex summation which includes the photopeak efficiencies and branching ratios for the various radiations. Most often the efficiency is measured for a standard source of known activity. Efficiencies for several radionuclides in a commercial gamma counter are shown in Table 5.[6]

Effects of Counting Rate

Distortions of the pulse-height spectrum are also introduced by high counting rates. The effect is usually manifested by a broadening of the photopeak and by a shift of the photopeak toward lower energies (Fig. 13). These changes are caused by pulse pileup and baseline shift, respectively. Since the window does not change, both distortion and shift of the photopeak result in lost counts, which cause errors in counting determinations. Counting rates that result in 3 to 5% deadtime losses should be posted on all instruments being used for quantitative measurements. Samples exceeding these counting rates should be remeasured (along with their standards) after sufficient decay or dilution to reduce the

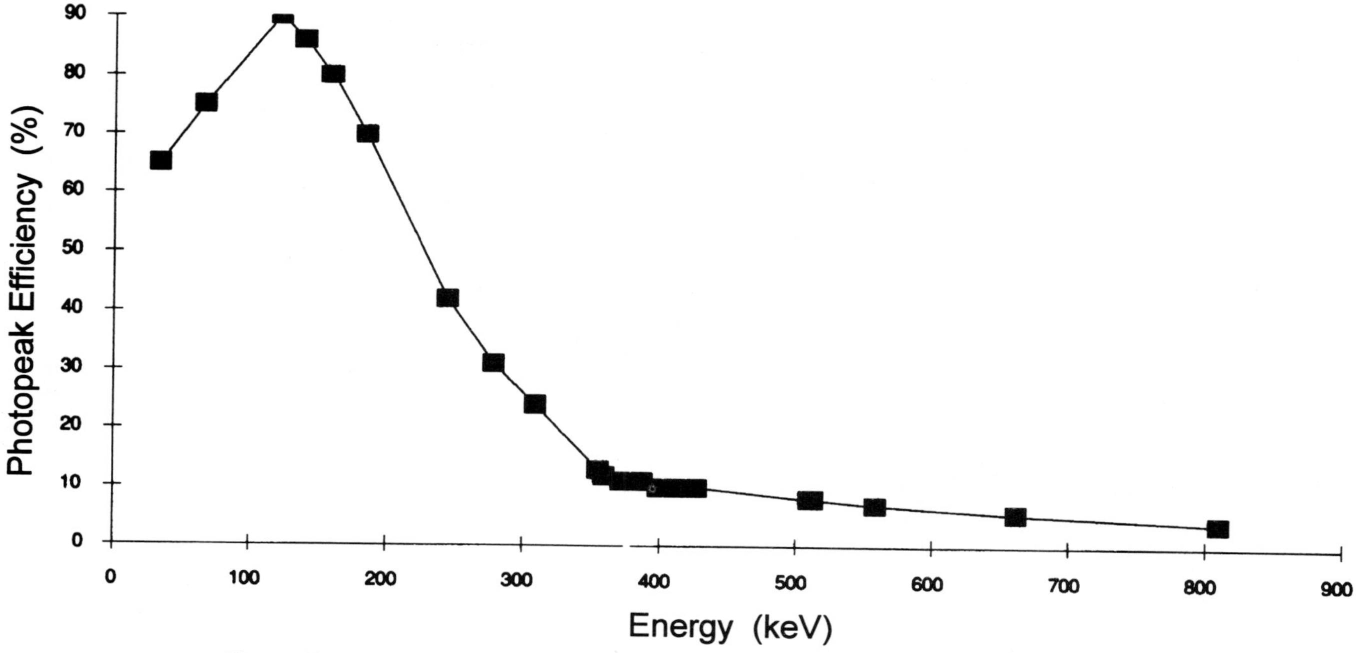

Figure 12. The photopeak efficiency curve for a NaI(Tl) well crystal. (From Reference 6.)

Table 5. Counting Efficiencies in an NaI(Tl) Well Crystal[6]

RADIONUCLIDE	ENERGY (keV)	EFFICIENCY (%)
^{76}As	559	7
^{195}Au	67	75
^{198}Au	412	10
^{133}Ba	356	13
^{77}Br	240	42
^{57}Co	122	90
^{58}Co	810	4
^{51}Cr	320	24
^{137}Cs	662	5.6
^{18}F	511	8
^{67}Ga	185	70
^{203}Hg	279	31
^{123}I	159	80
^{125}I	30	82
^{129}I	35	65
^{131}I	364	12
^{111}In	245	42
^{43}K	373	11
^{22}Na	511	8
^{203}Pb	279	31
^{125}Sb	428	10
^{85}Sr	514	8
^{87m}Sr	388	11
^{99m}Tc	140	86

counting rate. The counting rate of importance is the rate that includes the entire spectrum, not just the photopeak.

DUAL-ISOTOPE COUNTING

By means of pulse-height analysis and differential spectrometry two radionuclides can be easily counted simultaneously provided their photopeaks are reasonably well separated. Figure 14 shows the contributions of ^{131}I and ^{99m}Tc. When counted together, the activity (disintegrations per minute) of unknown samples containing both ^{131}I (A_I) and ^{99m}Tc (A_{Tc})

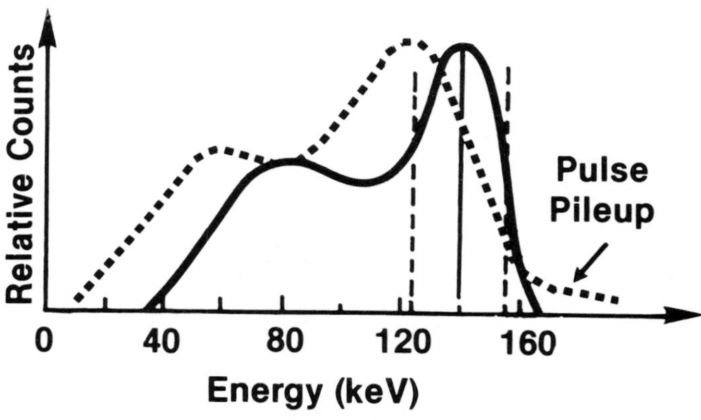

Figure 13. Spectrum of ^{99m}Tc at low (solid line) and high (broken line) counting rates. Pulse pileup causes *tailing* on the upper end of the spectrum while baseline shift causes lowering and broadening of the peak.

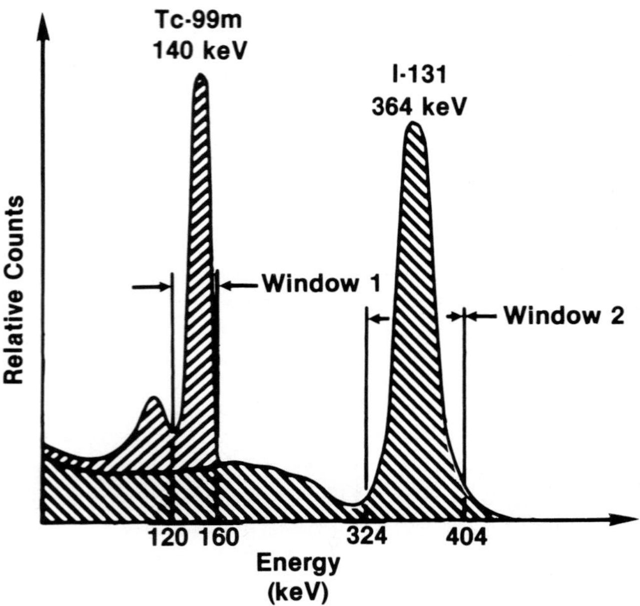

Figure 14. Appropriate window settings for counting ^{99m}Tc and ^{131}I with a linear amplifier. The contribution of ^{131}I-scattered radiation (crosstalk) within the ^{99m}Tc window is substantial and must be subtracted.

can be determined by counting separate ^{131}I and ^{99m}Tc standards and by using the relationships

$$A_I = \frac{n_1 f_2 - n_2 f_1}{C_1 f_2 - C_2 f_1} \tag{17}$$

and

$$A_{Tc} = \frac{n_1 C_2 - n_2 C_1}{C_1 f_2 - C_2 f_1}, \tag{18}$$

where

C_1 = cpm/dpm of I in lower window,
C_2 = cpm/dpm of I in upper window,
f_1 = cpm/dpm of Tc in lower window,
f_2 = cpm/dpm of Tc in upper window,
n_1 = counting rate in lower window,
n_2 = counting rate in upper window.

COINCIDENCE COUNTING

Many radionuclides decay with more than one emission. An example is ^{131}I, which decays with beta emission followed by prompt emission of one or more gamma rays (Appendix B). An effective means of reducing interfering background in low-activity samples is to arrange separate beta and gamma detectors so that both emissions are registered simultaneously. The output of these detectors is channeled through coincidence circuitry, which registers a count only if both detectors register counts simultaneously (Fig. 15). Extraneous counts that fail to activate both detectors are thus eliminated.

Radionuclides that emit cascades of gamma rays, such as ^{75}Se, ^{111}In, and ^{123m}Te, have been proposed for tomographic scanning.[7]

ABSORPTION-EDGE COUNTING

An ingenious method for measuring the concentration of specific atoms in biologic specimens makes use of the differential absorption of closely separated *K* x-rays that just straddle the *K*-shell absorption edge of the atoms to be measured. This technique is based upon the marked decrease in the attenuation coefficient at the absorption edge for gamma-ray transmission. As an example, Sorenson[8] has used the transmission of ^{139}Ce x-rays to measure iodine concentration in biologic samples. Cerium-139 decays to ^{139}La by electron capture with a 140-day half-life. The emissions of interest are the K_α x-rays from the lanthanum daughter, which neatly bracket the 33.2-keV absorption edge at 33.0 and 33.4 keV (Fig. 16). Samples containing iodine are exposed to a source of ^{139}Ce, and the transmission of the two x-rays is measured. The difference in x-rays detected is proportional to the concentration of iodine in the sample. The principle behind this technique is that the 33.0-keV x-ray is only slightly attenuated by iodine, but 33.4-keV x-ray is greatly attenuated.

The relative decrease in absorption of the two x-rays compared with known standards yields the iodine concentration in the unknown. Of course, separating two such closely placed x-ray energies is beyond the capabilities of all but the most sensitive spectrometers. By appropriate use of energy-

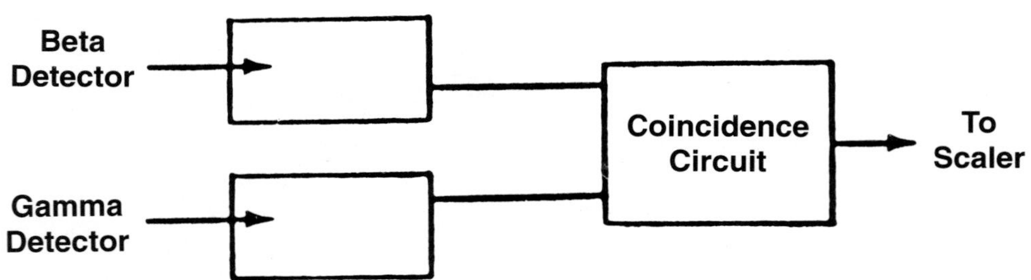

Figure 15. Schematic representation of coincidence counting for low-level detection of beta-emitting radionuclides.

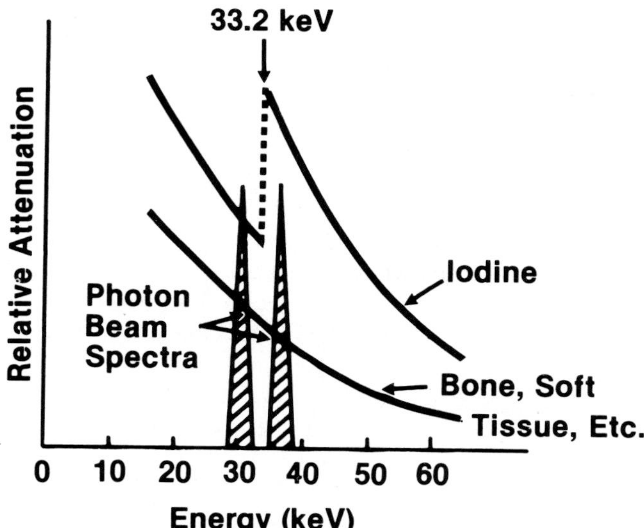

Figure 16. The photon beam from a ^{139}Ce source contains two photopeaks at 33.0 and 33.4 keV. The 33.4-keV photons are strongly attenuated by iodine in the absorbing medium because of the *K*-shell absorption edge at 33.2 keV. The 33.0-photopeak is attenuated much less by iodine.

selection filtration, however, the higher-energy x-ray can be largely eliminated from the source beam. Measuring the transmitted beams with and without filtration then allows calculation of the sample attenuation, even with coarse spectrometric systems employing NaI crystal detectors. The sensitivity of this technique for in vitro samples is approximately 5 μg/mL. The possibility of using this technique for in vivo measurement also exists.

LIQUID SCINTILLATION COUNTING

The basic instrumentation of liquid scintillation counters was discussed in the previous chapter. Preparation of samples prior to counting is somewhat more critical with liquid scintillation counting than with most other detector systems. Along with the usual considerations of sample mixing, container characteristics, and geometry, the chemical composition and optical characteristics of the counting medium must be controlled to avoid quenching, a phenomenon that results in reduced counting efficiency.

The amount of water in the sample must be matched to the solubility of the solvent. The content of inorganic salts, heavy metals, oxygen, as well as pH and temperature must all be controlled. These considerations are reviewed in detail by Bransome,[9] Crook et al,[10] and Peng et al.[11]

In general, it is not possible to solve every problem induced by sample preparation. The validity of the final count result, however, is most often secured by scrupulously avoiding any difference between treatment of the sample and that of the standard against which it is compared.

Instrument Settings

If one radionuclide is being counted, the instrument setting is simple: the lower discriminator is set near zero, just above the range of instrument noise. The upper discriminator is set at the point that gives the highest signal:background ratio (R_s/R_b). Since background is largely a function of window width, the ratio can be determined by serially counting background and a standard at various settings of the upper discriminator. A slightly better *figure of merit* (ε^2/B) can be achieved using the highest value of R_s^2/R_b.

Quench Correction

There are several means of reducing quenching. Oxygen quenching can be reduced by purging the sample with nitrogen, although this solution is generally impractical. More often, additional secondary solute is added to increase the competition for energy transfer from the solvent molecules. Other types of impurities may be reduced by precipitation, filtration, ion exchange, distillation, and other sample preparation measures. Color quenching can be reduced by bleaching agents, charcoal filtration, and sample combustion.

Even with all these precautions, however, some quenching occurs in all liquid scintillation samples. Therefore, the degree of quenching must be determined. Several methods of quench correction have been reviewed by Peng et al.[11]

Internal Standard

One of the simplest (and most time-consuming) methods is the addition of a known standard *S* to the unknown sample *U*. After measuring the sample activity R_u, a small amount of standard is added, a procedure known as "spiking" the sample, which gives a total activity $R_t = R_u + R_s$. Since the absolute activity of the standard A_s is known, the absolute activity of the sample A_u can be calculated:

$$A_u = A_s \frac{R_u}{R_t - R_u}. \tag{19}$$

To determine quenching due to the added standard, a chemically identical solution without radioactivity is added to a second unknown sample and the decrease in counting rate R_t noted. This factor is applied to the final calculation of A_u.

External Standard

In this method, a sealed gamma source (usually ^{137}Cs, ^{133}Ba, or ^{152}Eu) is used to irradiate the sample before R_u is determined. The secondary Compton and recoil electrons generated in the sample by the external gamma rays produce a broad pulse-height spectrum, which is recorded in an MCA. The spectrum for the external source shifts with quenching in a predictable way. For example, Horrocks[12] used the shift in the Compton edge for the 662-keV gamma ray from ^{137}Cs to define a quench parameter called the *H#*. This is illustrated in Figure 17. A series of standard samples is prepared with increasing quenching agent, and these are used to obtain a calibration curve of counting efficiency vs *H#*. For unknown

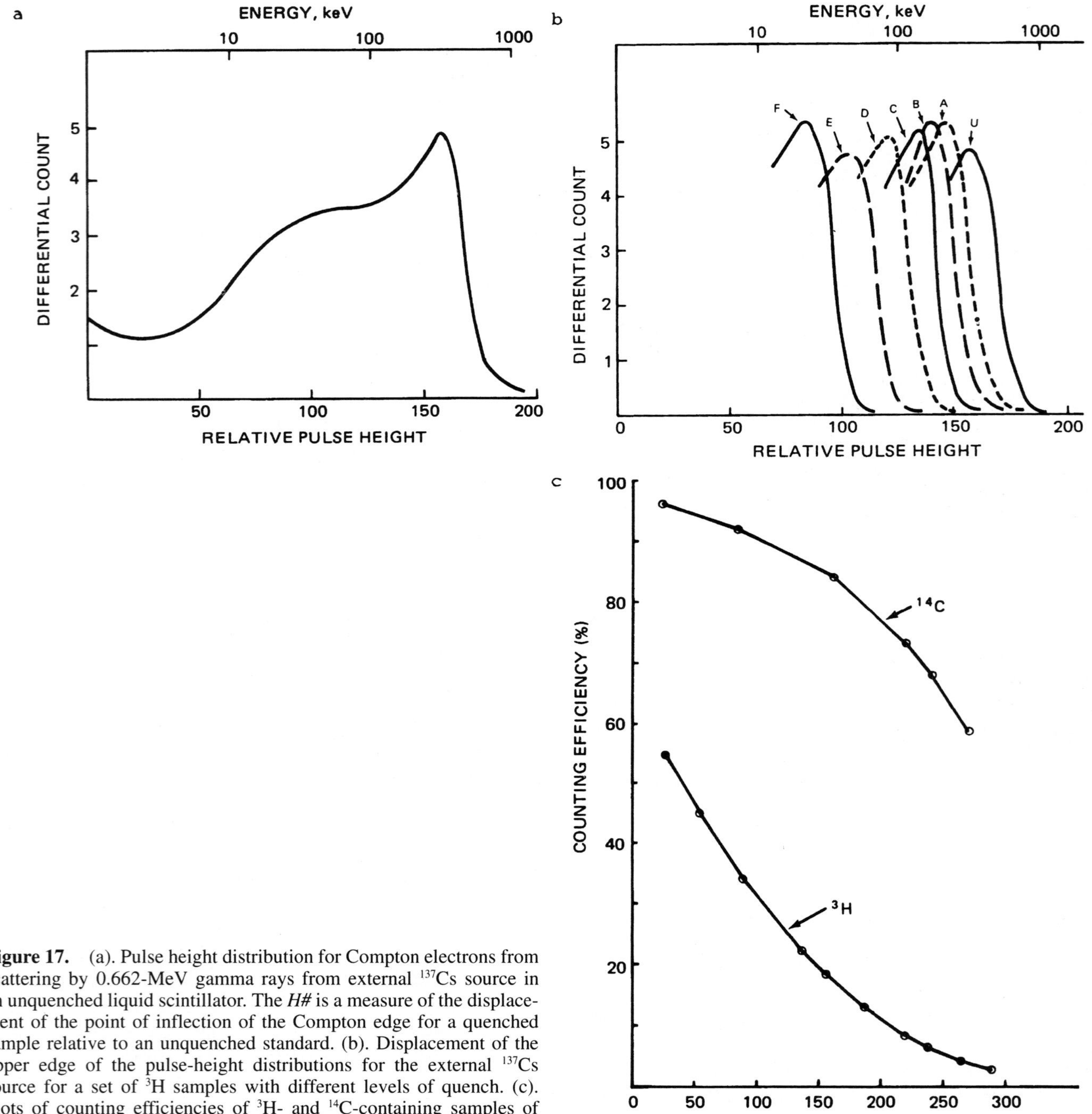

Figure 17. (a). Pulse height distribution for Compton electrons from scattering by 0.662-MeV gamma rays from external ^{137}Cs source in an unquenched liquid scintillator. The *H#* is a measure of the displacement of the point of inflection of the Compton edge for a quenched sample relative to an unquenched standard. (b). Displacement of the upper edge of the pulse-height distributions for the external ^{137}Cs source for a set of ^{3}H samples with different levels of quench. (c). Plots of counting efficiencies of ^{3}H- and ^{14}C-containing samples of different quench levels as a function of the *H#*. (From Reference 12.)

samples, *H#* is measured and the calibration curve is used to obtain the sample counting efficiency.

For the most careful work, the quenched set of standards must be prepared using the same scintillators, vials, and sample additives as the unknown samples. In practice, most users rely on a standard quench set of ^{14}C and ^{3}H samples from the manufacturer, and a built-in program computes quench curves, which are used to make an automatic quench correction.

Channels Ratio Method

Quenching shifts the observed spectrum of a radioactive sample to the left, ie, toward lower energies (Fig. 18). If the spectrum is divided into two adjacent or overlapping windows, quenching causes a shift in the counts in the two windows, and the ratio between them is proportional to the shift. A series of quenched standards is determined, and a curve of the ratio of counts between windows vs counting efficiency is plotted. The windows should be unequal, with

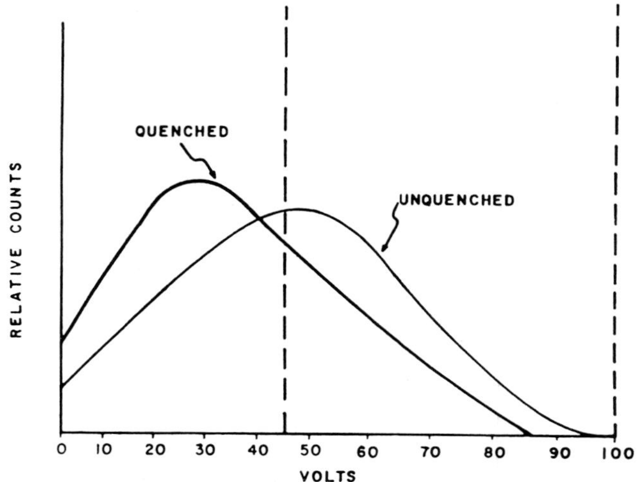

Figure 18. The channels ratio method for counting ^{14}C. The ratio of counts in the upper window (channel 45 to 100) to that in the lower window (channel 0 to 45) is measured for each sample. This ratio is plotted vs counting efficiency for a series of standards. The counting efficiency for an unknown sample may be interpolated from the calibration curve.

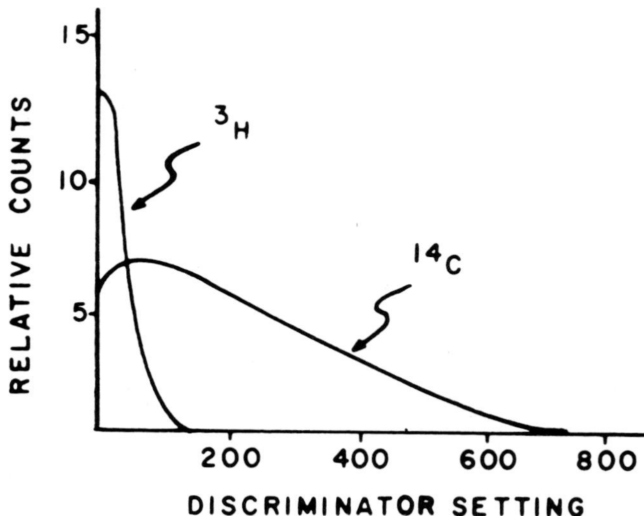

Figure 19. The effect of quench on pulse-height distribution for $^{3}H/^{14}C$ dual label samples. These spectra were acquired with a counting system employing a logarithmic amplifier. (From Reference 14.)

the narrower window viewing the lower energy range of the spectrum. This method is best employed with only moderately quenched samples with high counting rates. The statistical accuracy is too low for correcting low activity samples.

Background

As with all radiation detector systems, background is a constant concern in liquid scintillation counting. Besides all of the contributions to background to which scintillation crystal detectors are subject (cosmic radiation, ^{40}K in the counting equipment, EM thermal noise), liquid scintillation systems may contain another: *chemiluminescence*.[13]

This type of phosphorescence is of much longer duration than fluorescence and is caused by chemical reactions in the scintillation media. It is one of several mechanisms, such as heat production, of dissipating energy. When chemiluminescence occurs in the spectral range to which the photocathode is sensitive, it contributes to background. One common source of chemiluminescence is exposure to heat and light. Therefore, it is advisable to cool samples in a dark enclosure before counting. This type of chemiluminescence declines quickly. Other forms, however, are more subtle, eg, impurities in the solvents and chemical reactions with the counting vial caps. Often, these problems are detected only by serial counts over several hours or days as a means of observing the declining background counting rate. Another way of detecting the presence of chemiluminescence is to prepare a blank that contains all the elements of the assay system except the radionuclide.

Dual-Isotope Counting

Because of the low energies of many of the radiations being measured, the inefficient transfer of photons to the photocathode by quenching and self-absorption, and the broad inherent beta-emission spectrum, the ability of liquid scintillation spectrometry to separate two radionuclides is more limited than, for example, that of proportional counters. Nevertheless, if the energies of the two nuclides are sufficiently different, they can be distinguished when counted simultaneously. Fortunately, an energy difference does exist in the nuclide pairs most commonly used in biomedical research: ^{3}H and ^{14}C, ^{3}H and ^{35}S, ^{3}H and ^{32}P, and ^{14}C and ^{32}P. In cases such as ^{14}C and ^{35}S, which have similar spectra, the radionuclides must be chemically separated before counting.

Radionuclide	E_{max} (MeV)
^{3}H	0.018
^{14}C	0.155
^{35}S	0.167
^{36}Cl	0.714
^{32}P	1.710

Figure 19 shows the relative count rates for quenched and unquenched samples of ^{3}H and ^{14}C in a counter with a logarithmic amplifier. It is generally possible to select discriminator settings so that one radionuclide (in this case ^{3}H) is completely excluded from one channel; however, overlap of spectra will always occur in the lower channel, necessitating correction of the counts in the lower channel for the contribution of the more-energetic nuclide. Eliminating ^{3}H from the ^{14}C channel permits accurate determination of ^{14}C, but also greatly decreases the ^{14}C counting efficiency. It may be more useful to allow a small "spillover" of ^{3}H into the ^{14}C channel to increase the counting efficiency for ^{14}C. In this case simultaneous equations must be used to calculate the ^{3}H and ^{14}C activities.

Counting on Solid Supports

Solid supports include chromatographic strips, filter paper discs, and wipe test swabs. Radioactivity adhered to these supports is counted by immersing the entire support into the liquid scintillators. Frequently, a liquid scintillation system is more convenient to use than a gas-flow proportional counter for measuring these samples, especially with ^{3}H, which is not counted efficiently in a gas-flow system. The greatest problem involves geometry and absorption of the weak beta emissions by the support substance. Furlong[15] has offered several recommendations for solid support counting.

1. Use an internal standard whenever possible to check sample-to-sample variability. External standards have no meaning whatever for evaluating quenching under these conditions.
2. If the counting problem involves measuring a radioactive substrate and metabolic products, the assay conditions for the two should be identical.
3. The quenching characteristics of the support materials should be determined.

Solid Scintillator Systems

One of the chief disadvantages of liquid scintillation counting is the volume of radioactive waste generated from used scintillation samples. In early commercial counting systems vials of 20-mL volume were used and liter quantities of toluene-type scintillators containing ^{3}H and ^{14}C would accumulate rapidly for a few samples. With the increasing costs of disposal and heightened concern for the environmental impact of disposal of low-level radioactive wastes, manufacturers developed "minivials" in which as little as 1 mL scintillator is used. A more recent development is a solid scintillator described by Wunderly and Threadgill.[16] The product from Beckman Instruments is XtalScint, a solid scintillator in the form of a fine powder (3 to 8 μm) that is coated onto small vials and filters. In the case of the vial (Ready Cap), a sample, of the order of 200 μL, is placed in the vial and allowed to dry. The activity is in close proximity to the scintillating layer and the light output is sufficiently high to allow counting with good efficiency in a normal liquid-scintillation counter. Ready Filters are glass fiber filters coated on one side with XstalScint. There are two versions: a filter mat for automated cell harvesters and 25-mm filter circles for manual filtration experiments. These solid scintillator systems are in general less accurate than larger-volume liquid-scintillation vials because of the inhomogeneity in sample/scintillator contact and less-than-optimal light coupling. However, these factors may be offset by the ease of use and the reduction in hazardous radioactive wastes.

Cerenkov Counting

Cerenkov radiation is a particular form of light emission that beta particles give off as they travel through a liquid medium. Cerenkov radiation is emitted when the velocity of the particle exceeds the speed of light c in the medium, which is c/n where n is the refractive index of the medium. This light is mostly in the ultraviolet range but extends into the visible range and is responsible for the blue-white light surrounding the core in swimming pool reactors. The light is not propagated in all directions but is conical, with the path of the electron at the axis of the cone. The result is analogous to the shock wave caused by supersonic aircraft.

Cerenkov radiation is particularly useful since its detection does not require a scintillator and since it is not quenched by chemical impurities, although it is subject to color quenching. Water, solvents, and even strong acids can be used as counting media. They are only useful, however, for counting strong beta emitters. For water, beta particles must have energies greater than 0.263 MeV. With solvents of very high refractive indices, however, weaker-energy betas can be detected. For example, Ross[17] reported efficient detection of ^{14}C in α-bromonaphthalene. Because no scintillator is required, many samples such as urine (which has been decolorized), waste water, and tissue fluids can be counted directly without the addition of fluors. Color quenching may be corrected by internal standards, the channel ratio method, or external standards, provided the radiation is sufficiently energetic to produce Compton electrons.

Many of the energetic beta-particle emitters being used in radionuclide therapy (^{153}Sm, ^{186}Re, ^{188}Re, ^{166}Ho)[18–21] are suitable for analysis by Cerenkov counting. The Cerenkov counting efficiency for ^{90}Y as a function of sample volume[22] is shown in Figure 20.

IN VIVO MEASUREMENTS

When the radioactivity to be measured is located within the body, additional problems are encountered because of a variable amount of scattering from overlying and surrounding tissues. The most common means of quantifying in vivo activity is to construct a phantom of approximately the same size, dimensions, and elemental composition as the body or organ and to place a known amount of activity within the phantom to simulate the in vivo distribution. An example is the measurement of radioiodine uptake by the thyroid. The usual neck phantom is made of tissue-equivalent plastic with a hole drilled in the location of the trachea; through this hole, a standard quantity of radioiodine can be inserted to simulate the intrathyroidal radioiodine. This kind of comparison necessarily entails a significant error because, while the phantom may simulate the physical scatter and attenuation conditions for one neck, it is inadequate for

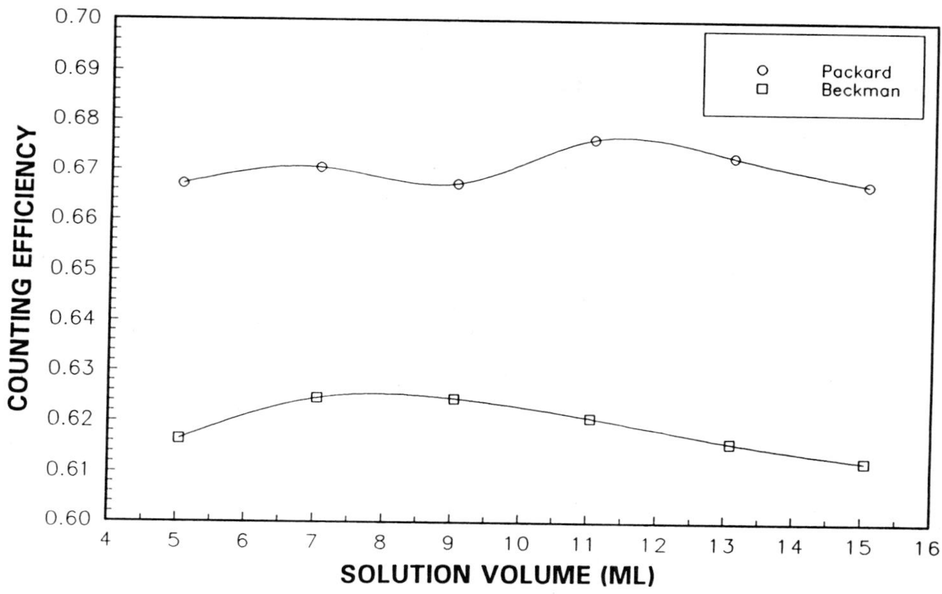

Figure 20. The Cerenkov counting efficiency as a function of sample volume for a high energy beta emitter ^{90}Y in conventional liquid-scintillation counters. (From Reference 22.)

another. Nevertheless, with the detector placed about 25 cm from the phantom, the percent error is acceptably small for meaningful clinical results, in which the normal range of uptake may vary from 6 to 30%—a fivefold variation.

The error caused by uncertainties due to different organ sizes and body habitus can be reduced by using pulse-height analysis to reduce the contribution due to scattered radiation. Another means of reducing error is to place the external detector at some distance from the organ of interest to reduce the error due to uncertainty of depth. For example, an error of 2 cm in depth at 10 cm from the detector produces a counting error of ±40%, while the same positional error at 20-cm distance from the crystal produces only about ±20% error.

To reproduce the scatter contributed by tissue surrounding and overlying the in vivo radioactive source, a variety of materials may be used that simulate the gamma-ray attenuation properties of soft tissue. These materials include water, presswood, lucite, and masonite. By carefully standardizing the counting geometry and instrument calibration, serial measurements in the same patient can be reproduced with a variability of about 10%. Variations between patients of different body habitus are much higher.

CONJUGATE VIEW METHODS

Several methods have been described for the quantification of organ radioactivity in vivo. Most of these utilize *conjugate* counting with a scintillation camera, with or without attenuation correction. Conjugate views are simply serial views (or simultaneous views using dual-headed imaging systems) of the organ region of interest in the anterior, *A*, and posterior, *P*, views (or both lateral views, depending of activity location). Deriving the *geometric mean* $(I_A I_P)^{1/2}$ or the *arithmetic mean* $(I_A + I_P)$ yields an estimate of the activity, *I*, approximately independent of source depth within the body. These quantitative methods have largely been applied to dosimetric problems, in which it is important to know the changing concentrations of organ activity with time, and in studies in which the activity within the body significantly changes depth during the course of a single study, such as in gastrointestinal transit studies. These considerations, including rigorous discussions of attenuation correction, buildup factors, etc, have been well-presented by Thomas et al,[23] Fleming,[24] and Myers et al.[25]

WHOLE BODY COUNTERS

The measurement of low levels of radioactivity, particularly when the radioactivity is widely distributed within the body, imposes special requirements on the construction and design of detectors. Whole body counters for measuring gamma-emitting radionuclides in the human body were originally conceived to measure radionuclide contaminations in radiation workers and accident victims, but have since been used for a variety of clinical applications.[26,27]

Physical Characteristics

Whole body counters have two types of detectors, liquid and solid. The liquid scintillation whole body counter, developed by Anderson,[28] consisted of a steel cylinder whose outer shell was filled with a mixture of toluene, *p*-terphenyl, and POPOP. The design is shown in Figure 21.[29] Various PM tubes are arranged around the cylinder, and the entire apparatus is enclosed in a shielded room to reduce background radiation. The advantage of the cylindric design is that it provides 4π geometry, so that sensitivity is largely

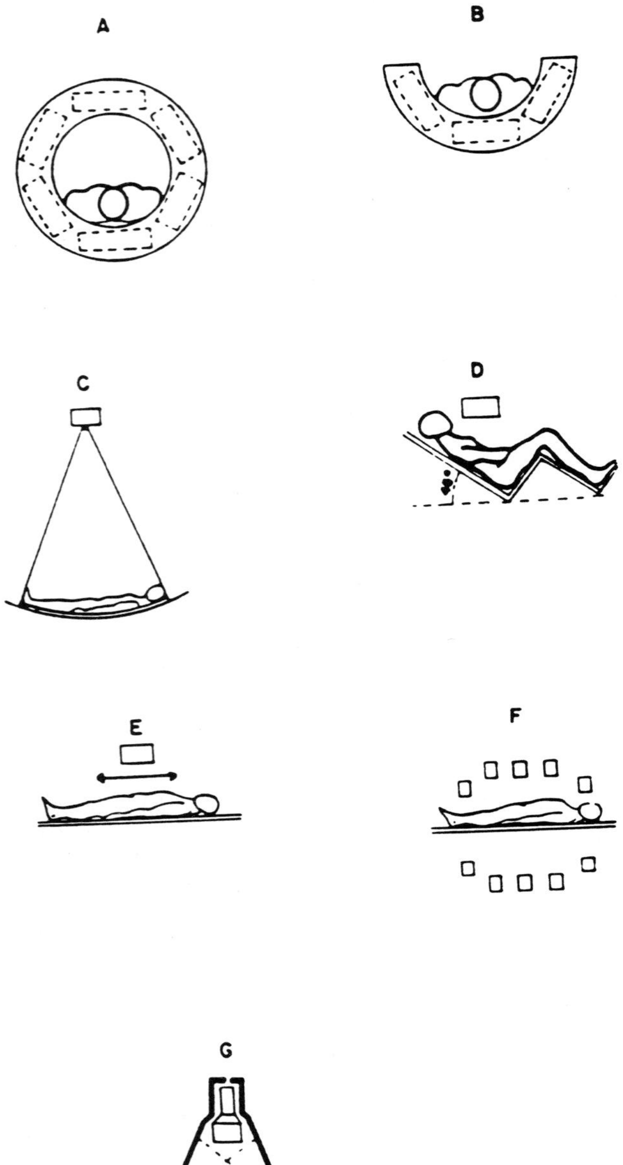

Figure 21. Commonly used detector geometries in whole body counters. (From Reference 29.)

independent of the spatial distribution of the radionuclide within the body.

Solid plastics in large volume have also been used.[30] A common 2π configuration is shown in Figure 21B. While these counters have high sensitivity, the spectrometric resolution is quite poor, and their use must be largely restricted to counting previously identified radionuclides. The sensitivity of sodium iodide crystals is less because of smaller detector volumes, but they have much greater energy resolution, thus allowing radionuclide identification by means of gamma-ray spectroscopy. Two basic characteristics of whole body counters that must be considered in all of their applications are (1) detector sensitivity and (2) uniformity of spatial response. Detector sensitivity depends essentially upon detector efficiency and the level of background radiation. The uniformity of response depends upon the spatial relationship between the detector and the radiation source. Sensitivity can most easily be increased by enlarging the sensitive volume of the detector and/or reducing background radiation. To this end, the early trend of whole body counter construction was toward larger detector crystals and more elaborate shielding. The latter was necessary because, as the detector volume increases, the sensitivity to background radiation also increases. Best results are achieved by a judicious combination of detector size and shield mass, composition, and arrangement. By this means, it is possible to achieve a level of detectability in fractions of nanocuries sufficient to detect natural body burdens of ^{40}K and radium, which vary between 10^{-2} and 10^{-4} dpm.

Geometry

The detector geometry varies as functions of both the type of detector used and the position of the subject relative to the detector, but the system must always be designed to assure measurement reproducibility with changes in radionuclide distribution. Several detector arrangements are shown in Figure 21.

The most commonly encountered systems make use of a stationary or moving couch geometry. The individual lies on a bed or couch viewed by one or more detectors (Fig. 21E through G). In the case of a single detector, it may be fixed or movable. Alternatively, the couch may move in relation to the detector.

An elaborate 54-detector system similar to that diagrammed in Figure 21F has been constructed at Brookhaven National Laboratory. It has a nearly invariant response to radionuclide distribution.[31] Other methods of improving uniformity include counting systems with rotational detectors and the substitution of Compton scatter for photopeak counting.[32]

Many shielding systems have been devised for the couch geometry. One of the simplest is the "shadow" shield (Fig. 21G).[33] In this counting system, the patient lies in a shielded trough. The detector overhead is also shielded, but open beneath. Either the trough or the detector moves longitudinally to scan the total length of the body. This system combines several desirable features, including favorable geometry, economy, and acceptable background levels for most counting problems.

To avoid the high cost of these elaborate special-purpose counters, many laboratories have adapted more conventional instruments for whole body counting. Short et al[34] described the use of a scintillation camera which, without its collimator, has a high sensitivity and uniform response at some distance. Rehani et al[35] have adopted a rectilinear scanner for the same purpose.

Clinical Applications

TOTAL BODY POTASSIUM

The fractional abundance of ^{40}K in natural potassium is *0.0118%*. From this relationship, it is possible to determine the total body potassium content by measuring the mass of ^{40}K. With well-designed and carefully calibrated whole body counters, an accuracy of ±5% can be achieved, but the technique is not simple.[29,36–38] Because of the low abundance of ^{40}K, its high-energy gamma emission (1.47 keV), and the ubiquity of potassium in the environment, elaborate detectors and shielding must be utilized. Organic scintillation detectors with 2π or 4π geometry have been used most often, although the couch arrangement with multiple detectors (Fig. 21F) also can be used.

The critical aspect in the direct measurement of ^{40}K is system calibration. Calibration is generally performed by administration of ^{42}K to a group of normal subjects with various heights and weights or by constructing phantoms containing known amounts of potassium and simulate the human distribution and approximate as closely as possible the geometry and gamma attenuation of the patient being counted. A range of normal individuals separated according to age and sex is measured and graphed according to height and weight.

Potassium is primarily an intracellular element and, because relatively little exists in fat, potassium content is proportional to "lean body mass."

$$\text{Lean Body Mass} \cong \text{Total Body Potassium (mEq)}/68.1$$
$$\text{Body Fat} = \text{Body Weight} - \text{Lean Body Mass}$$

The measurement of total potassium is useful in studies of obesity and diets designed for weight loss without loss of lean body mass.[36] It is also an indicator of the fraction of intracellular water and in nutritional studies provides an index of global synthesis.

Total body potassium can be estimated with less-sensitive counters by measuring total exchangeable potassium by the indicator dilution principle using ^{42}K. The use of the whole body counter obviates collecting excreta and confining patients to metabolic units. Potassium-42 is usually administered intravenously, and the total body activity is determined. The retained fraction is determined again at 24 or 48 hours. This fraction plus the ratio of serum ^{42}K to cold serum potassium is used to calculate exchangeable potassium, which in turn is an estimate of total body potassium. Use of the whole body counter is somewhat more reproducible than the dilution technique, which requires the determination of excreted ^{42}K to derive the retained dose.

INTESTINAL ABSORPTION OF IRON

Measurements of iron absorption are useful in several anemic and malabsorption diseases.[39–41] In the whole body counter technique, 0.5 to 5 μCi (~20 to 200 kBq) ^{59}Fe in the form of chloride, citrate, ascorbate, or hemoglobin-bound is administered orally. The absorbed fraction is determined by measuring total body activity 4 hours after ingestion and 14 days later. The advantage of whole body counting over other techniques is that measurements of excreta are avoided. It is especially useful for population studies in which it is important to avoid removing patients from their normal habitats and routines.

ABSORPTION OF B_{12}

The technique of measuring B_{12} absorption is similar to that described for iron. B_{12} labeled with ^{58}Co or ^{60}Co is administered orally in doses of 0.5 to 1.0 μCi (~20 to 40 kBq). Total body activity is measured after administration and 7 to 10 days later. The normal absorbed fraction is between 45 and 80% of the administered dose. In patients with pernicious anemia, the absorbed fraction is 0 to 17%. This technique has been used by Belcher et al[42] and Reizenstein et al,[43] among others.

STRONTIUM AND CALCIUM

Calcium turnover studies using ^{47}Ca and ^{85}Sr have been helpful in understanding bone metabolism. Calcium-47 is used more often when measures of intestinal absorption and body retention are of interest. These studies are performed in a manner similar to that described for B_{12} absorption, counting 7 to 10 days after administration of the tracer.[44,45]

Strontium-85 has been used for studying bone metabolism in cases of osteoporosis, osteomalacia, and bone metastases.[46] The use of this tracer is valid because of the similar compartmental distribution and a longer useful physical half-life (65 days) than ^{47}Ca. Strontium-85 has also been used as a tracer to quantify ^{89}Sr used in palliation of bone metastases.[47]

IN VIVO NEUTRON ACTIVATION ANALYSIS

Neutron activation analysis utilizes a source of neutrons to irradiate a distribution of target nuclei, which in the process of absorbing neutrons create unstable radionuclides that revert to a stable state by the emission of one or more gamma rays of characteristic energy. These energy levels identify the element, and the amount of radioactivity produced is proportional to its abundance. With properly designed sources and carefully planned irradiation and counting geometry, in vivo total-body neutron activation analysis (TBNAA) is possible. Thus, for example, total body calcium can be determined by irradiating the subject with neutrons using the $^{48}Ca(n,\gamma)^{49}Ca$ reaction. The induced ^{49}Ca has a half-life of 8.7 minutes and can be quantified by counting the subject in a whole body counter which has been calibrated using appropriate phantoms. This section will review the principals, techniques, and common applications of in vivo activation analysis.

Table 6. Measurement of Body Elements by In Vivo Neutron Activation Analysis[87]

STABLE ELEMENT	AMOUNT IN 70-KG STANDARD MAN (G)	PROPORTION BY WEIGHT IN 70-KG STANDARD MAN (%)	INDUCED NUCLIDE	NEUTRON REACTION	GAMMA RAY MEASURED (MeV)
Oxygen	42,000	60	^{16}N	n,p (fast)	Delayed (6–7)
Hydrogen	7,000	10	^{2}H	n,γ (thermal)	Prompt (2.2)
Nitrogen	2,100	3	^{13}N	n,2n (14 MeV)	Delayed (0.51)
				n,γ (thermal)	Prompt (10.8)
Calcium	1,050	1.5	^{49}Ca	n,γ (thermal)	Prompt (many); delayed (3.10)
Phosphorus	700	1	^{28}Al	n,α (fast)	Delayed (1.78)
			^{32}P	n,γ (thermal)	Prompt (0.08)
Sodium	105	0.15	^{24}Na	n,γ (thermal)	Prompt (many); delayed (2.75)
Chlorine	105	0.15	^{38}Cl	n,γ (thermal)	Prompt (many); delayed (1.6, 2.2)
			^{37}S	n,p (fast)	Delayed (3.10)
Magnesium	35	0.05	^{27}Mg	n,γ (thermal)	Delayed (0.84)
			^{24}Na	n,p (fast)	Delayed (2.75)
Iron*	4.2	0.006	^{56}Mn	n,p (fast)	Delayed (0.84)
Iodine*	0.01 (in thyroid)	0.03 (in thyroid)	^{128}I	n,γ (thermal)	Delayed (0.45)
Manganese*	Trace	Trace	^{56}Mn	n,γ (thermal)	Delayed (0.84)
Copper*	Trace	Trace	^{64}Cu	n,γ (thermal)	Delayed (0.51)
Cadmium*	Trace	Trace	^{114}Cd	n,γ (thermal)	Prompt (0.559)

*Partial-body activation.

Basic Principles

If a target is irradiated for some time t_1, the activity induced at the end of bombardment I_0, is given by

$$I_0 = \frac{WN\phi\sigma m}{A}[1 - \exp(-\lambda t_1)], \quad (20)$$

where

W = mass of element (g),
N = Avogadro's number = 6.0229×10^{23} atoms per gram atomic weight,
A = atomic weight,
ϕ = average neutron flux density (n/m^2),
σ = absorption cross section in barns (10^{-28} m^2),
m = fractional isotopic abundance,
λ = decay constant = $0.69315/T_{1/2}$.

The quantity in brackets is the *saturation factor* and depends on the length of bombardment and the half-life of the nuclide formed. When $t_1 = T_{1/2}$ of the induced radionuclide, this factor has a value of 0.5; when t_1 is large compared with $T_{1/2}$, it approaches unity. In practice, an irradiation time of about six half-lives induces a near maximum, ie, the *saturation activity.* Some body elements commonly measured and the activation techniques used are given in Tables 6 and 7.

INTERFERING NUCLEAR REACTIONS

Interfering nuclear reactions can occur when elements other than those being analyzed become radioactive and emit photons in the energy region being studied. There are two types of such interfering reactions. The first involves reactions that cause irradiation of two different elements to produce the same radionuclide being measured. For example, the reactions $^{23}Na(n,\gamma)^{24}Na$ and $^{24}Mg(n,p)^{24}Na$ both produce the same end product. The magnitude of this interfering reaction depends on the abundance of the target nuclei and the cross section (ie, probability) of the reaction. The second type of reaction occurs when secondary particles are produced within the target that can interact with other target nuclei to produce the same end product as the primary reaction. An example is the $^{16}O(p,\alpha)^{13}N$ reaction, which can occur as a secondary reaction to the $^{14}N(n,2n)^{13}N$ reaction using fast neutrons.

Neutron Sources

Several sources of neutrons are listed in Table 7. In early studies cyclotrons or neutron generators were used.[48–51] However, single point sources such as these impose requirements of special moderators and positioning to achieve uniform irradiation of a target as massive as the human body. More recently sealed sources, using, for example, the $^{238}Pu(\alpha,n)Be$ reaction, which generates neutrons with average energies of about 4 MeV, have been widely used.[52,53] Such sealed sources when configured in arrays above and below the patient have several advantages over accelerator-produced neutrons. The radiation dose to patients is reduced. The irradiation geometry is improved and the average neutron energy is more stable. The operation of α,n neutron sources is much simpler because they do not require expensive equipment and highly trained personnel required of particle accelerators. Finally,

Table 7. Characteristics of Neutron Sources Used for Total-Body Neutron Activation Analysis in Man and Elements Measured[87]

SOURCES AND REACTIONS	NEUTRON OUTPUT (n/s)	ENERGY (MeV)	IRRADIATION TIME (min)	PREMODERATOR THICKNESS (cm)	SSD* (m)	PATIENT POSITION	ELEMENTS MEASURED
1. Cyclotron	8×10^{10}	0.1–8 peak:3.5	5	1.5	2	Lying on side	CA, NA, N, Cd
$^{7}Li(p,n)^{7}Be$	5×10^{11}		10	Nil	3	Supine, motorized bed	
2. Cyclotron $^{9}Be(d,n)^{10}B$	5×10^{11}†	4–12 peak:8	1.3	0–few cm	3.7	Standing, turntable	Ca, Na, P
3. Cockcroft-Walton	1.5×10^{10}†	14	—	3	1.1	Lying in arc	Na, Ca, Cl
$^{3}T(d,n)^{4}He$	8×10^{10}	14	3	Various	1.0	Lying on side, motorized bed	
4. Cockcroft-Walton $^{3}T(d,n)^{4}He$	3×10^{10}	14	5	3.8	1.5	Standing, turntable	Ca, NA, Cl, P, N
5. $^{238}Pu(\alpha,n)Be$ $^{9}Be(\alpha,n)^{12}C$	1.4×10^{9}	2–8 Mean:4.5	5	2.9	0.3	Supine on bed	Ca, NA, Cl, P
^{241}Am-Be $^{9}Be(\alpha,n)^{12}C$	$2 \times (2 \times 10^{4})$‡	2–8 Mean:4.5	33	None	~0.2	Supine, motorized bed	H
6. Sealed tube neutron-generator $^{3}T(d,n)^{4}He$	$2 \times (3 \times 10^{10})$‡	14	1	4.0		Supine, motorized bed	Ca, Na, Cl, P, N

*SSD, Source-to-skin distance.
†Estimated value.
‡Two opposed sources.

such α,n neutron sources can be conveniently located within the hospital environment, making it much easier to conduct patient studies.

Most activation reactions occur with thermal neutrons (ie, energy ≅ 0.025 eV). However, in most cases fast neutrons are used for irradiation because of the poor penetration of thermal neutrons into the human body. The fast neutrons are thermalized in the body primarily by elastic scattering with body hydrogen.

A major contributor to the precision of activation analysis is the uniformity of neutron flux density throughout the target subject. Uniformity is often achieved by using *moderators* to prevent buildup of neutron flux densities at surface layers.[54] The use of bilateral irradiation geometry also helps assure uniformity. Neutron flux densities are measured by placing some type of neutron detector on or within the target.[55]

The radiation-absorbed dose to the patient in most tissue assay measurements is determined using tissue-equivalent ionization chambers. Absorbed doses range from about 0.001 to 0.02 Sv for common elements assayed.

Measuring Induced Activity

Once irradiation is complete, the induced activity is measured in a whole body counter (see preceding section), usually using an array of large NaI(Tl) detectors. Spectra similar to those shown in Figure 22 are obtained. The area beneath isotope peaks is measured to estimate induced activity. Using Equation 20, concentration of the unknown element is determined. Because the short half-lives of many of the radionuclides induced decay, corrections during counting must be made.

Detector configurations can be designed to count the entire body simultaneously[54] or to scan the body lengthwise. By either technique, the counter must be carefully calibrated with appropriate phantoms to relate counts from the unknown subject to a known amount of activity within a similar distribution of equivalent geometry and attenuation.

In *prompt gamma neutron activation analysis*, the excess energy released in binding neutrons is emitted as prompt gammas, ie, in less than 10^{-16} seconds. The principal difference here is that measurement of induced activity must take place simultaneously with neutron exposure.[56–63] Special collimation of neutron sources and shielding of NaI(Tl) detectors can overcome many detection problems associated with simultaneous activation and measurement.[64,65]

Clinical Applications

Total body calcium, particularly in osteoporosis and renal osteodystrophy studies, has been analyzed extensively using the $^{48}Ca(n,\gamma)^{49}Ca$ reaction. To obtain normative data on the relation of body calcium to sex, body habitus, and age, a noninvasive means of measuring calcium in normal subjects is important.[66–78] Measurement of calcium has also been useful in studying Paget's disease, thyroid and parathyroid disorders, Cushing's syndrome, acromegaly, rheumatoid arthritis, osteogenesis imperfecta, the effects of corticosteroid therapy, and vitamin D rickets. The influence of various dietary and therapeutic regimens on calcium levels in the body has also been investigated. Sodium, chlorine, and phosphorus can be measured simultaneously with calcium from the same spectra (Fig. 22).[62]

Other studies include

1. Estimates of nitrogen and potassium as indices of muscle

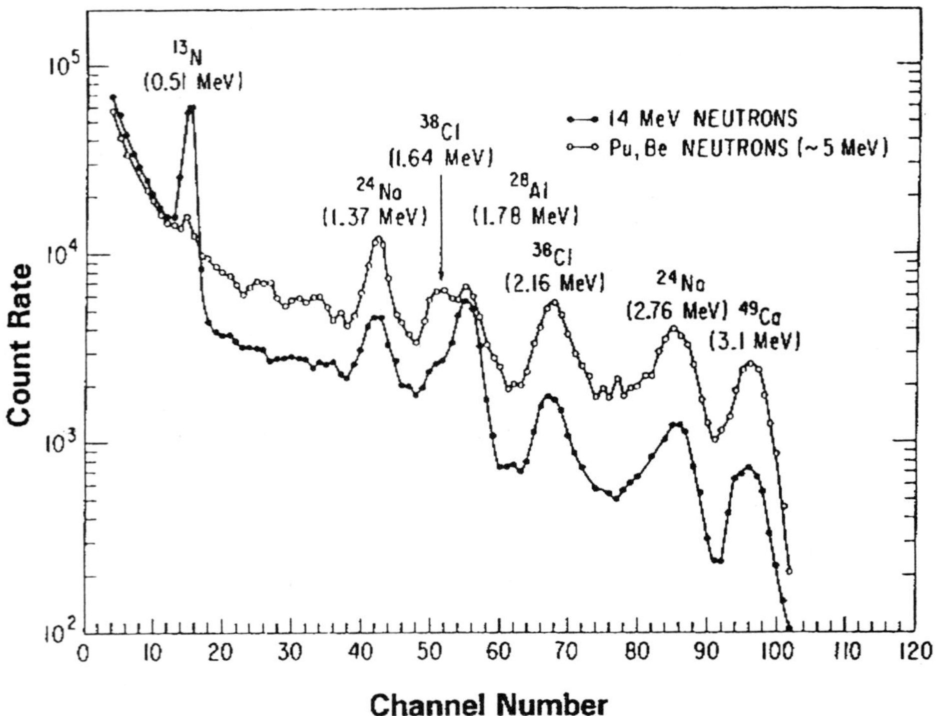

Figure 22. Gamma-ray spectra in human subject irradiated with 14-MeV neutrons and 5-MeV ^{238}Pu-Be neutrons. (From Reference 88.)

mass, body protein content, and the efficacy of nutrition regimens.[79–81]

2. Measures of body composition differences between normal subjects and patients with neoplastic diseases.[79,82,83]
3. The health consequences of internal accumulation of cadmium, which deposits chiefly in the liver and kidneys, addressed in both industrial workers[84,85] and smokers.[86]

REFERENCES

1. Anger HO. Radioisotope cameras. In: Hine CT, ed. *Instrumentation in Nuclear Medicine*. vol 1. New York: Academic Press, 1967.
2. Zimmerman RE, Fahey FH, Burns RE. High pressure, multiwire proportional chamber for cardiac imaging. *J Nucl Med* 1980; 21:91. Abstract.
3. Knoll GF. *Radiation Detection and Measurement*. 2nd ed. New York: John Wiley & Sons, 1988.
4. National Council on Radiation Protection. *Environmental Radiation Measurement*. Washington, DC: National Council on Radiation Protection, 1976. NCRP Report No. 50.
5. National Institute of Standards and Technology. *Radioactivity Standard Reference Materials*. Gaithersburg, MD: National Institute of Standards and Technology, 1993.
6. Wallac Oy. *Practical Considerations on the use of Radioactive Nuclides with 1470 Wizard Gamma Counter*. Turku, Finland: Pharmacia Wallac, 1993.
7. Chung V, Chak KC, Zacuto P, Hart HE. Multiple photo coincidence tomography. *Semin Nucl Med* 1980;10:345.
8. Sorenson JA. Absorption-edge transmission technique using ^{139}C for measurement of stable iodine concentration. *J Nucl Med* 1979;20:1286.
9. Bransome ED, ed. *The Current Status of Liquid Scintillation Counting*. New York: Grune & Stratton, 1970.
10. Crook MA, Johnson P, Scales B, eds. *Liquid Scintillation Counting*. vols 1 and 2. London: Heyden and Son, 1972.
11. Peng CT, Horrocks DL, Alpen EL, eds. *Liquid Scintillation Counting*. vols 1 and 2. New York: Academic Press, 1980.
12. Horrocks DL. *The H# Concept*. Fullerton, CA: Beckman Instruments, 1976.
13. Scales B. Questions regarding the occurrence of unwanted luminescence in liquid scintillation samples. In: Crook MA, Johnson P, Scales B, eds. *Liquid Scintillation Counting*. vols 1 and 2. London: Heyden and Son, 1972.
14. Kolb A. *Liquid Scintillation Counting: Recent Applications and Developments*. vol 1, New York: Academic Press, 1980.
15. Furlong NB. Liquid scintillation counting of samples on solid supports. In: Bransome ED, ed. *The Current Status of Liquid Scintillation Counting*. New York: Grune & Stratton, 1970.
16. Wunderly SW, Threadgill GJ: Solid scintillation counting: a new technique—theory and applications. In: Ross H, Noakes JE, Spaulding JD, eds. *Liquid Scintillation Counting and Organic Scintillators*. Chelsea, MI: Lewis Publishers, 1989; Chap. 16.
17. Ross HH. Cerenkov radiations: photon yield application to (^{14}C) assay. In: Bransome ED, ed. *The Current Status of Liquid Scintillation Counting*. New York: Grune & Stratton, 1970.
18. Coursey BM, Hoppes DD, Schima FJ, Unterweger MP. The standardization of samarium-153. *Appl Radiat Isot* 1987;38:31.
19. Coursey BM, Calhoun JM, Cessna J, et al. Assay of the eluent from the alumina-based tungsten-188-rhenium-188 generator. *Radioact Radiochem* 1990;V1/N4:38.
20. Coursey BM, Garcia-Torano E, Golas DB, et al. The standardization and decay scheme of rhenium-186. *Appl Radiat Isot* 1991;42:865.
21. Calhoun JM, Cessna J, Coursey BM, Hoppes DD, Schima FJ,

Unterweger, MP. The standardization and decay scheme of holmium-166. *Radioact Radiochem* 1991;V2/N4:38.
22. Coursey BM, Calhoun JM, Cessna J. Radioassays of Yttrium-90 for use in nuclear medicine, *Nucl Med Biol* in press.
23. Thomas SR, Maxon HR, Kereiakes JG, Saenger EL: Quantitative external counting techniques enabling improved diagnostic and therapeutic decisions in patients with well-differentiated thyroid cancer. *Radiology* 1977;122:731.
24. Fleming JS. A technique for the absolute measurement of activity using a gamma camera and computer. *Phys Med Biol* 1979;24:176.
23. Myers MJ, Lavender JP, de Oliveira JB, Maseri A. A simplified method of quantitating organ uptake using a gamma camera. *Br J Radiol* 1981;54:1062.
26. Van Dilla MA. Some applications of the Los Alamos human spectrometer. In: Mennely G, ed. *Radioactivity in Man*. Springfield, IL: Charles C Thomas, 1961.
27. Marinelli LD et al. Low-level gamma ray scintillation spectrometry: experimental requirements and biomedical applications. *Adv Biol Med Phys* 1962;8:81.
28. Anderson EC. The Los Alamos human counter. *Br J Radiol* 1957;7:27.
29. Kessler WV et al. A 4π liquid scintillation whole body counter. I-design operating characteristics and calibration. *Int J Appl Radiat Isot* 1968;19:287.
30. Forbes GB. A 4π plastic scintillation detector. *Int J Appl Radiat Isot* 1968;19:535.
31. Cohn SH, Dombrowski CS, Pate HR, Robertson JS. A whole body counter with an invariant response to radionuclide distribution and body size. *Phys Med Biol* 1969;14:645.
32. Cohn SH, Palmer HE. Recent advances in whole-body counting: a review. *J Nucl Med Biol* 1974;1:155.
33. Oliver R, Warner GT. A clinical whole body counter using shadow field principle. *Br J Radiol* 1966;36:806.
34. Short MD, Richards AR, Glass HI. The use of a gamma camera as a whole body counter. *Br J Radiol* 1972;45:289.
35. Rehani MM et al. A simple and inexpensive clinical whole body counter. *Nuklearmedizin* 1976;15:248.
36. Woodward KT et al. Correlations of total body potassium with body water. *Nature* 1956;178:97.
37. Forbes GB, Gallup J, Hursh JB. Estimation of total body potassium-40 content. *Science* 1961;133:101.
38. Forbes CB. Methods for determining composition of the human body with a note on the effect of diet and body composition. *Pediatrics* 1962;29:477.
39. Callender ST et al. The use of a single whole body counter for hematological investigations. *Br J Haematol* 1966;12: 276.
40. Deller DJ. Fe-59 absorption measurement by whole body counting: studies in alcoholic cirrhosis, hemochromatosis and pancreatitis. *Am J Dig Dis* 1956;10:249.
41. Pollack S, Balcerzac SP, Crosby WH. ^{59}Fe absorption in human subjects using total body counting technique. *Blood* 1966; 28:94.
42. Belcher EH, Anderson BB, Robinson CJ. The measurement of gastrointestinal absorption of Co-58 labeled vit. B_{12} by whole body counting. *Nucl Med* 1963;3:349.
43. Reizenstein PC, Conkite E, Cohn SH. Measurement of absorption of vitamin B_{12} by whole body gamma spectrometry. *Blood* 1961;18:95.
44. Caderquist E. Short term kinetic studies of ^{85}Sr and ^{47}Ca by whole body counting in malignant diseases of the skeleton. *Acta Radiol* 1964;2:42.
45. Sargent T, Linfoot JA, Isaac EL. Whole body counting of ^{47}Ca and ^{85}Sr in the study of bone diseases. In: *Clinical Uses of Whole Body Counting*. Vienna: International Atomic Energy Agency, 1966.
46. MacDonald NS. Recent uses of total-body counter facility in metabolic research and clinical diagnosis with radionuclides. In: *Whole Body Counting*. Vienna: International Atomic Energy Agency, 1962.
47. Blake GM, Zivanovic MA, Blaquiere RM, Fine DR, McEwan AJ, Ackery DM. Strontium-89 therapy: measurement of absorbed dose to skeletal metastases, *J Nucl Med* 1988;29:549.
48. Chamberlain MJ et al. Total body calcium by whole body neutron activation: new technique for study of bone disease. *Br Med J* 1968;2:581.
49. Chamberlain MJ et al. Use of cyclotron for whole body activation analysis: theoretical and practical considerations. *Int J Appl Radiat Isot* 1970;21:725.
50. Palmer HE et al. The feasibility of *in vivo* neutron activation analysis of total body calcium and other elements of body composition. *Phys Med Biol* 1968;13:269.
51. Nelp WB et al. Measurements of total body calcium (bone mass) *in vivo* with the use of total body neutron activation analysis. *J Lab Clin Med* 1970;76:151.
52. Cohn SH et al. Design and calibration on a "broad beam" ^{238}Pu,Be neutron source for total body neutron activation analysis. *J Nucl Med* 1972;13:487.
53. Cohn SH, Dombrowski CS. Measurements of total body calcium, sodium chloride, nitrogen and phosphorus in man by *in vivo* neutron activation analysis. *J Nucl Med* 1971;12:499.
54. Cohn SH, Fairchild RG, Shukla KK. Comparison of techniques for total body neutron activation analysis on calcium in man. Panel on *In Vivo* Neutron Activation Analysis. Vienna: International Atomic Energy Agency, STI/PUB/322, 1973.
55. Guey A. Estimation of total body calcium. Panel on *In Vivo* Neutron Activation Analysis. Vienna: International Atomic Energy Agency, STI/PUB/322, 1973.
56. Rundo J, Bunce LJ. Estimation of total hydrogen content of the human body. *Nature* 1966;210:1023.
57. Biggin HC, Chen NS, Ettinger KV, et al. *Radioanal Chem* 1974;19:207.
58. McLellan JS, Thomas BJ, Fremlin JH, Harvey TC. Cadmium—its *in vivo* detection in man. *Phys Med Biol* 1975;20:88.
59. Harvey TC et al. Measurement of liver cadmium in patients and industrial workers by neutron activation analysis. *Lancet* 1975;1:1209.
60. Thomas BJ, Harvey TC, Chettle DR et al. A transportable system for measurement of liver cadmium *in vivo*. *Phys Med Biol* 1979;23:432.
61. Evans CJ, Cummins P, Dutton J et al. Californium-252 facility for the *in vivo* measurement of organ cadmium. In: *Nuclear Activation Techniques in the Life Sciences*. Proc. Symp. 1978. Vienna: International Atomic Energy Agency, 1979;719.
62. Ellis KJ, Vartsky D, Cohn SH. A mobile prompt gamma neutron activation facility. In: *Nuclear Activation Techniques in the Life Sciences*. Proc. Symp 1978. Vienna: International Atomic Energy Agency, 1979;733.
63. Vartsky D, Ellis KJ, Chen NS, Cohn SH. A facility for *in vivo* measurement of kidney and liver cadmium by neutron capture prompt gamma analysis. *Phys Med Biol* 1977;22:1985.
64. Vartsky D, Ellis KJ, Cohn SH. *In vivo* measurement of body nitrogen by analysis of prompt gamma from neutron capture. *J Nucl Med* 1979;20:1158.
65. Mernagh JR, Harrison JE, McNeill KG. *In vivo* determination of nitrogen using Pu-Be sources. *Phys Med Biol* 1977;5:831.
66. Harrison JE et al. A bone calcium index based on partial body calcium measurements by *in vivo* activation analysis. *J Nucl Med* 1975;16:116.
67. Cohn SH, Vaswani AN, Zanzi I, Ellis KJ. Effect of aging on bone mass in adult women. *Am J Physiol* 1976;230:143.
68. Cohn SH, Vaswani AN, Aloia JF, et al. Changes in body chemi-

cal composition with age measured by total body neutron activation. *Metabolism* 1976;25:89.
69. Cohn SH, Abesamis C, Zanzi I, et al. Body elemental composition: comparison between black and white adults. *Am J Physiol* 1977;232:419.
70. Cohn SH, Abesamis C, Yasumura S, et al. Comparative skeletal mass and bone density in black and white women. *Metab Clin Exp* 1977;26:171.
71. Harrison JE, McNeill KG. Partial body calcium measurements by *in vivo* neutron activation analysis. *Am J Roentgenol* 1976;126:1308.
72. Harrison JE, Meema E, McNeill KG. A comparison of results from IVNAA of the trunk with results from X-ray densitometry of radium. In: Boddy K, ed. *Progress and Problems of In Vivo Activation Analysis*. Proc. 2nd Symp. East Kilbride, Scotland: Scottish Universities Research and Reactor Centre, 1976.
73. Harrison JE, McNeill KG, Hitchman AJ, Britt BA. Bone mineral measurements of the central skeleton by *in vivo* neutron activation analysis for routine investigation of osteopenia. *Invest Radiol* 1979;14:27.
74. McNeill KG, Harrison JE. Measurement of the axial skeleton for the diagnosis of osteoporosis by neutron activation analysis. *J Nucl Med* 1977;18:1136.
75. Maziere B, Kuntz D, Comar D, Ryckewaert A. *In vivo* analysis of bone calcium by local neutron activation of the hand: results in normal and osteoporotic subjects. *J Nucl Med* 1979;20:85.
76. Catto GRD, Macleod M. The investigation and treatment of renal bone disease. *Am J Med* 1978;61:64.
77. Meema HE, Harrison JE, McNeill KG, Oreopoulos DG. Correlations between peripheral and central skeletal mineral content in chronic renal failure patients and in osteoporosis. *Skelet Radiol* 1977;1:169.
78. Hoskins DJ, Chamberlain MJ. Calcium balance in chronic renal failure. *Q J Med* 1973;42:467.
79. Cohn SH, Sawitsky A, Vartsky D, et al. *In vivo* quantification of body composition in normal subjects and in cancer patients. *Nutr Cancer* 1980;2:67.
80. McNeill KG, Mernagh JR, Harrison JE, Jeejeebhoy KN. *In vivo* measurement of body protein based on the determination of nitrogen by prompt gamma neutron activation analysis. *Am J Clin Nutr* 1979;32:1955.
81. Burkinshaw L, Hill GL, Morgan DB. Assessment of the distribution of protein in the human body by *in vivo* neutron activation analysis. In: *Nuclear Activation Techniques in the Life Sciences*. Proc. Symp. 1978. Vienna: International Atomic Energy Agency, 1979;787.
82. Cohn SH, Gartenhaus C, Sawitsky A, et al. Compartmental body composition of cancer patients by measurement of total body nitrogen, potassium and water. *Metabolism* 1980;30:222.
83. Cohn SH, Vartsky D, Yasumura S, et al. Compartmental body composition based on total body nitrogen, potassium and calcium. *Am J Physiol* 1980;239:524.
84. Roels H et al. Critical concentrations of cadmium in renal cortex and urine. *Lancet* 1979;221.
85. Ellis KJ, Morgan WD, Zanai I, et al. Critical concentration of cadmium in human renal cortex (dose effect studies in cadmium smelter workers). *J Toxicol Environ Health* 1981;7:691.
86. Ellis KJ, Vartsky D, Zanzi I, et al. Cadmium: *in vivo* measurement in smokers and non smokers. *Science* 1979;205:323.
87. *In Vivo Neutron Activation Analysis*. Proc. Panel Vienna: International Atomic Energy Agency. STI/PUB/322, 1973.
88. Cohn SH, Fairchild RG, Shukla KK. Theoretical considerations in the selection of neutron sources for total body neutron activation analysis. *Phys Med Biol* 1973;18:648.

4 Statistical Methods

Robert P. Hirsch

In this chapter we will examine statistical methods in general as well as how these methods apply to the field of nuclear medicine. This is a task that is ambitious for an entire text, let alone for a single chapter. The field of statistics is immense, subsuming rather complicated logical processes as well as formidable mathematical methods. Much of this must be sacrificed to fit within this chapter. The traditional approach for a nuclear medicine text would be to concentrate on the mathematical methodology associated with the simplest statistical procedures. There are three problems with this traditional approach. First, the simplest statistical procedures are seldom appropriate to analyze real data, ie, data that are collected as part of actual clinical or research activities. Second, an ability to perform mathematical manipulations of data without understanding the basic logical processes is a dangerous level of knowledge. It is similar to knowing how to operate an automobile without knowing the rules of the road. Third, most mathematical manipulations in statistical analysis are, in practice, performed by computers rather than by hand. Thus, knowledge of those mathematical procedures is useful only to the extent that it helps us to understand the underlying logical processes. For most of us, the logical processes are lost in our struggle to follow the mathematics.

For these reasons, this chapter is not written using the usual approach to statistics. Rather, it emphasizes logical processes and interpretation of the results of statistical procedures rather than emphasizing the mathematical methods. Further, the statistical methods discussed in this chapter were selected based on the frequency with which they are encountered in the medical literature rather than on their simplicity.

Thus, we begin by examining some basic principles from a nonmathematical point of view. Next, we will learn how statistical methods are selected to analyze a particular set of data. Finally, we will consider how these issues relate to special types of data encountered in nuclear medicine. Still, this provides only an overview. If you wish to learn more about statistics, we recommend either a text that emphasizes concepts[1] or one that emphasizes mathematics,[2] depending on which approach you find more accessible.

BASIC PRINCIPLES

Let us begin by putting statistics in its place. Because of the great volume of information that has accumulated on statistics, it is easy to be swayed into believing that statistics has a corresponding position of great importance in the interpretation of clinical or research data. Not so. The great volume of information on statistics is a result of the fact that statistics is a mathematical field. Anything that we can express in mathematical language is more open to examination, derivation, and extrapolation than things that can be expressed only in literary language, that is, in words rather than in numbers. Of at least equal importance is the design of studies. The accumulated literature on issues of design is less than on issues of statistics only because of the difficulty of expressing design issues mathematically. Without good design, however, statistical issues are moot.[3]

Assuming that we have used an appropriate study design to collect our data, there are three ways statistics can help us to interpret those data: (1) to summarize a large volume of data (information) with a manageable few numbers; (2) to take the role of chance into account; and (3) to control for the effect of some types of information while examining relationships among other types of information. To examine the basic principles of statistics, we will consider how statistical methods help us to accomplish those three purposes.

Summarizing Data

To summarize data, we first need to think about how data can be organized. The way that we organize data is by constructing something called a *distribution*. A distribution of data is a description of how frequently (or with what probability) various data values occur. The description of the distribution can be mathematical or graphical. Figure 1 illustrates a graphical description of a hypothetical distribution.

To develop statistical procedures, statisticians rely on mathematical descriptions of distributions. The type of distribution that is used depends, in part, on the type of data that is being organized. There are three types of data that are important to us: *continuous, ordinal*, and *nominal*. Continuous data have a large number of possible values that are evenly spaced. Examples of continuous data include age and blood pressure. Ordinal data have a limited number of possible values that can be ordered but are not necessarily evenly spaced. Examples of ordinal data include stage of disease and number of persons in a family. Nominal data have a limited number of values that cannot be ordered. Examples of nominal data include gender and diagnosis.

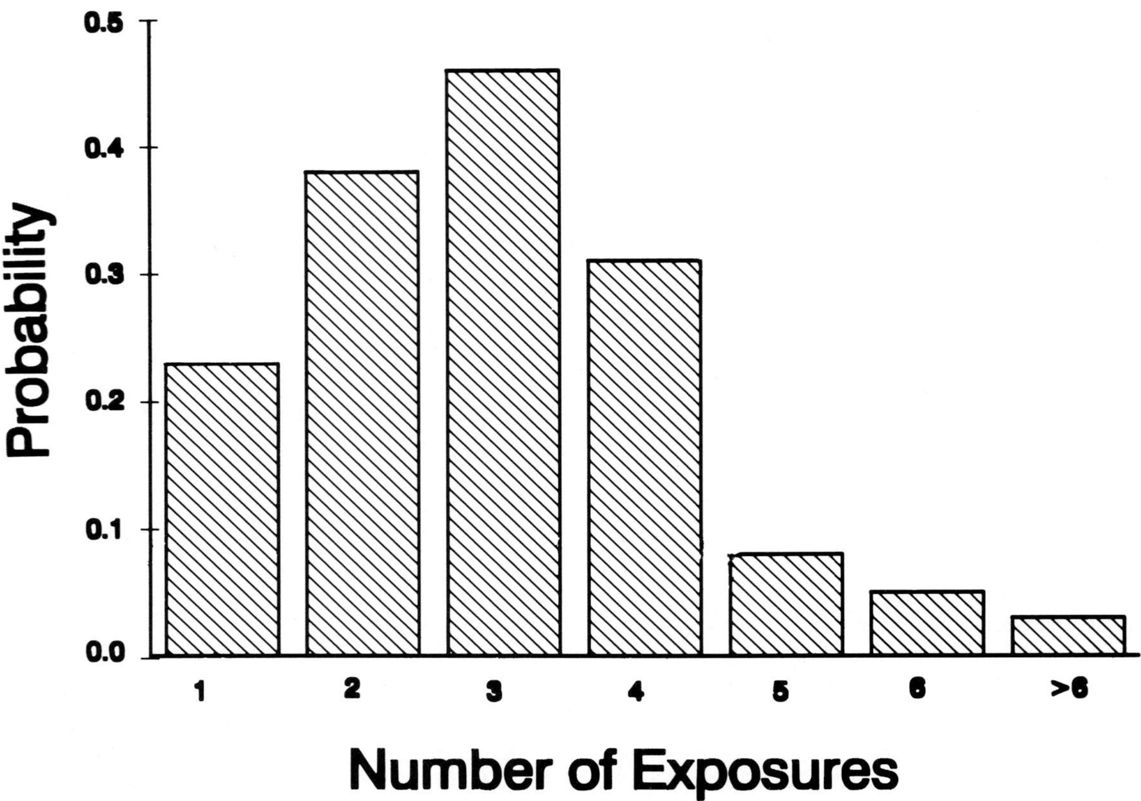

Figure 1. Graphical representation of a hypothetical distribution of the number of exposures required to achieve a particular clinical endpoint.

Also, any data with only two possible values are nominal data even if those two possible values can be ordered. For example, ages measured as young or old are nominal data.

There are only two groups or families of distributions on which nearly every statistical procedure is based. The most important of those is the *Gaussian distribution*. The Gaussian distribution is a symmetric bell-shaped distribution that can describe a collection of continuous data. Figure 2 illustrates a hypothetical Gaussian distribution.

The second most important distribution of data is the *binomial distribution*. It is, most often, asymmetric. The binomial distribution (or a related distribution) can be used to describe a collection of nominal data. This distribution is appropriate for data that have two possible categories. For data that have more than two possible categories, combinations of binomial distributions can be used to describe the data. This issue will be clarified in the next section when we discuss variables.

Analysis of ordinal data is a bit different from analysis of continuous or nominal data in that most statistical procedures for ordinal data do not rely on a particular type of distribution. We will discover the implications of this feature of ordinal data in the next section of this chapter.

Even though distributions of data allow us to organize large collections of information, knowing only the type of distribution is not enough to completely characterize the data. In fact, there are an infinite number of possible distributions of any particular type. What we need is some way to specify the distribution that corresponds to the set of data we wish to describe. A particular distribution is specified by its *parameters*. The parameters of a distribution are numbers that tell us which Gaussian distribution, for example, corresponds to our data.

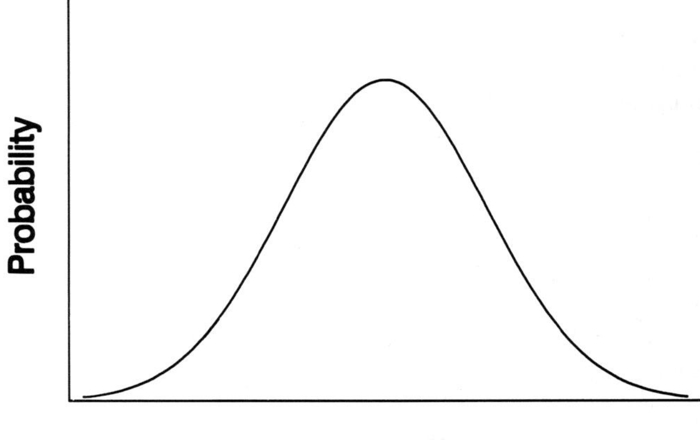

Figure 2. Graphical representation of a hypothetical distribution of the absorbed dose of a particular radionuclide in a certain target organ.

A Gaussian distribution has two parameters. One of those parameters tells us the location of the distribution along a continuum of values. The parameter of the Gaussian distribution that indicates the location of the distribution is the *mean*. The mean is the center of gravity of the distribution, that is, data in the distribution are balanced on either side of the mean. The mean is calculated as shown in Equation 1.

$$(1) \qquad \mu = \frac{\sum_{i=1}^{N} Y_i}{N},$$

where μ = the mean of the distribution; $\sum_{i=1}^{N}$ = the sum for all values between the first value and the Nth value; Y_i = the ith data value; N = the total number of data values.

The other parameter of the Gaussian distribution is a measure of dispersion. This parameter indicates how spread out the data values are around the mean. Dispersion can be expressed as the *variance* of the data (Equation 2) or as the *standard deviation*, which is the square root of the variance. The variance is the average squared deviation of each data value from the mean of the distribution. The reason for squaring the deviations is to prevent them from adding up to zero. Since the mean is the center of gravity of the distribution, there will always be an equal balance between deviations in a positive and a negative direction.

$$(2) \qquad \sigma^2 = \frac{\sum_{i=1}^{N} (Y_i - \mu)^2}{N},$$

where σ^2 = the variance of the distribution of data.

Thus, to summarize a collection of continuous data, assuming the data have a Gaussian distribution, we can specify everything we need to know about those data by calculating two parameters: the mean and the variance (or standard deviation). Even if the distribution of data does not appear to be a Gaussian distribution, the mean and the variance (or standard deviation) can still be useful in summarizing the data. Also, continuous data that do not have a Gaussian distribution usually have a distribution that can be transformed into a Gaussian distribution by a rather straightforward arithmetic manipulation of the data. For example, a common distribution in medicine is the *log normal distribution*. Data that have a log normal distribution will have a Gaussian distribution if the logarithm of each of the data values is used instead of the data values themselves.

When the data that we wish to summarize is nominal, usually we need to be concerned with calculating only one parameter. This is because a binomial distribution is completely specified by calculating its location. For each location of a binomial distribution, there is only one possible dispersion of values around that location. The location of a binomial distribution is the *probability* of the event addressed by the data. A probability is calculated by dividing the number of times the nominal event occurs by the number of times it is possible for the nominal event to occur (ie, the number of observations).

$$(3) \theta(\text{event}) = \frac{\text{Number of times event occurs}}{\text{Number of opportunities for event to occur}} = \frac{\text{Number of events}}{\text{Number of observations}},$$

where θ(event) = the probability of the event occurring.

Another way to summarize a collection of nominal data is with a *rate*. A rate tells us how fast events occur. A rate differs from a probability in that a probability is dimensionless while a rate has the dimension of 1/time.

$$(4) \qquad \mathit{rate}(\text{event}) = \frac{\text{Number of times event occurs over time}}{f(\text{time})},$$

where f(time) = some function of time.

An example of a rate commonly encountered in medicine is *incidence*. Incidence is the rate at which new cases of a disease occur. In nuclear medicine, rates are often used to measure radioactivity. Here, the event is a radionuclide disintegration. These events are counted over a period of time and summarized by calculating the number of disintegrations per unit time.

Rates are a little more complicated than are probabilities since they include the dimension of time. This dimension implies that the numeric value of a rate is dependent on the measure of time used. For instance, a disintegration rate of 200 counts per minute is the same as 3.33 counts per second. Thus, rates cannot be described by using a binomial distribution. Rather they are described by using a distribution that is closely related to the binomial distribution called the *Poisson distribution*.

The Poisson distribution can be derived from the binomial distribution by letting the number of events occurring (the numerator of a probability) become very small relative to the number of opportunities for an event to occur (the denominator of a probability). This is true in the case of radionuclide disintegrations since the observed number of disintegrations is very small relative to the number of radioactive particles available to disintegrate.

The Poisson distribution, like the binomial distribution, needs only a measure of location as the parameter specifying a particular distribution. The parameter of a Poisson distribution is the number of events. The usual symbol for this parameter is λ. This is the same as the numerator of a probability (see Equation 3). That the Poisson distribution is not concerned with the denominator is very convenient when we wish to summarize nominal data with a rate because that allows us to ignore the units of time in the denominator.

Thus, nominal data can be summarized either by using a probability or a rate as the parameter of the binomial or the Poisson distribution. Only one parameter (a measure of location) is needed to specify a distribution of nominal data. The Gaussian distribution, a distribution of continuous data, on the other hand, requires two parameters: a measure of location (the mean) and a measure of dispersion (the variance or the standard deviation).

Ordinal data is different from either continuous or nominal data in that there are no distributions that specifically describe ordinal data. Without a distribution, we have no parameters. As we will see in the next section, this is an important characteristic of ordinal data, but this lack of parameters makes it difficult for us to summarize collections of ordinal data. Generally, in summarizing ordinal data we use something that is similar to the mean: the *median*. The median is the physical center of a collection of data selected so that half of the data values are above and half are below the median. The median is not the parameter of a distribution, but it is a useful way to summarize ordinal data.

Taking Chance into Account

The second purpose of statistics is to provide us with a way to take chance into account. To understand how this is accomplished, we first need to understand why chance is an issue in the interpretation of a collection of data. We need to recognize that every collection of data we examine is only a subset of a larger group of data that is really of interest to us. The subset is called the *sample* and the larger group of data is called the *population*. From examination of the data in the sample, we wish to estimate the values of the parameters of the distribution of data in the population. We can interpret those estimates only if the sample can be thought of as a representative subset of the population. The way that we attempt to select a representative sample is by making a random choice of which of the data values in the population are selected to be in the sample. By a random choice, we imply that chance is the determinant of which data values are examined in the sample.

Thus, chance becomes an issue because it determines which of the data values in the population are included in the sample and, as a result, which of the data values are used to estimate the values of the parameters of the data distribution in the population. Those estimates are calculated from a sample's data in such a way that, on the average, the estimates are equal to the population's parameter. Equations 5 through 7 illustrate how a sample's data can be used to estimate the population's mean, variance, and probability of an event.

$$(5) \qquad \overline{Y} = \frac{\sum_{i=1}^{n} Y_i}{n},$$

where $\overline{Y}$ = the sample's estimate of the mean of the distribution of data in the population; n = the total number of data values in the sample.

$$(6) \qquad s^2 = \frac{\sum_{i=1}^{n} (Y_i - \overline{Y})^2}{n - 1},$$

where s^2 = the sample's estimate of the variance of the distribution of data in the population.

$$(7) \qquad p(\text{event}) = \frac{\text{Number of events in the sample}}{\text{Number of observations in sample}},$$

where p(event) = the sample's estimate of the probability of the event occurring.

For the most part, the equations illustrating the sample's estimates of the population's parameters (Equations 5 through 7) are the same as the equations for the population's parameters themselves (Equations 1 through 3). There are two notable exceptions. The first is the use of Greek letters for the population's parameters while Arabic letters are used for the sample's estimates. The other exception is specific to the variance of data in a Gaussian distribution. The denominator of the population's value is equal to N (the number of data values in the population) while the denominator of the sample's estimate of the variance of data is equal to $n - 1$. Subtracting one from the sample's size corrects for the bias that results from underrepresentation of extreme data values in the sample.

If we were to take many samples of a certain size (ie, each with the same number of data values), we would find many different estimates of the population's parameters. In practice, we do not really take many samples from the same population. Rather, we take only one sample. We need to think about this theoretical possibility, however, to understand how statistics can take into account the role of chance. Why this is so will be explained shortly.

If we were to organize estimates from all possible samples of a certain size as a distribution, we would find that the distribution would usually be a Gaussian distribution. This is especially true for estimates of location for the distribution of data. This tendency of the distribution of estimates from all possible samples of a given size to have a Gaussian distribution is an important principle in statistics. This principle is known as the *central limit theorem*. The central limit theorem not only tells us that distributions of estimates from all possible samples of a given size tend to be Gaussian distributions, but also that this tendency is greater for larger samples.

Since the distribution of all possible estimates tends to be a Gaussian distribution, we know that a particular distribution of estimates can be specified by two parameters: a mean and a variance (or standard deviation). The mean of the distribution of estimates from all possible samples is equal to the value of the population's parameter. The variance of the distribution of estimates from all possible samples is a function of the variance of the distribution of data and the size of the sample. The variance of the distribution of estimates of the mean from all possible samples of a given size is illustrated in Equation 8.

$$(8) \qquad \sigma_{\overline{Y}}^2 = \frac{\sigma^2}{n},$$

where $\sigma_{\overline{Y}}^2$ = the variance of the distribution of estimates of the mean from all possible samples with the size of n.

The square root of the variance of estimates is the standard deviation of the distribution of estimates. The standard deviation of the distribution of estimates from all possible samples, however, is usually called by a special name: the *standard error.*

Thus, there are two different types of distributions we have to think about to understand statistical procedures. One of those is the distribution of data. It is the parameters of the distribution of data for which we wish to make estimates from the sample. The other distribution is the distribution of estimates from all possible samples of a given size. This distribution is more difficult to consider because it is only theoretical. As we will see, however, this distribution of estimates is important to statistical procedures.

Now, we are ready to consider the role of chance. Because we assume that the particular sample we have taken has been selected at random from the population, chance determines which of the possible estimates of each population's parameter we have actually observed in our sample. On average, the samples' estimates are equal to the population's parameter, but any particular estimate can have any value. Because the estimates tend to have a Gaussian distribution, the probability of getting certain estimate values decreases the further the sample's estimate is from the mean of the distribution of all possible estimates. Further, we can use the (theoretical) distribution of all possible estimates from samples of a given size to calculate the probability of getting any particular estimate, or an estimate farther from the population's value. We can calculate that probability by determining the area of the distribution that is associated with that particular estimate or more extreme estimates.

To make calculation of probabilities from the distribution of estimates less tedious and to avoid the necessity of using calculus, we convert the distribution of estimates that is associated with our sample to a standard distribution. The probabilities for these standard distributions have been calculated for us. In fact, the probabilities associated with standard distributions are what we find in statistical tables. Most of the mathematical manipulations that are part of statistics are concerned with conversion of estimates to standard scales.

Thus, we can take into account the role of chance in determining the content of the sample selected from the population by calculating probabilities from the distribution of estimates from all possible samples of a given size. Those probabilities are determined by first converting the estimates to a standard scale. After that conversion, there are two ways we can choose to express the probability of obtaining a particular estimate. These are through the processes of *interval estimation* or *statistical inference.*

In the process of interval estimation, we recognize that the estimate of the population's parameter we have calculated from the sample's data is our single best guess of the value of the population's parameter. Even so, that estimate (called the *point estimate*) has a very low probability of being exactly equal to the population's parameter. The goal of interval estimation is to calculate an interval of values that has a high probability of including the population's parameter. That probability is usually chosen to be equal to 0.95. The interval of values that is calculated to have a 95% chance of including the population's value is called an *interval estimate* or a *confidence interval.**

One way to take chance into account is to calculate a confidence interval for a population's parameter. Another way is to test a hypothesis about the value of the population's parameter. In this process of statistical inference, we calculate the probability of obtaining the sample's estimate if the population's parameter were equal to some hypothesized value. The hypothesized value of the population's parameter is stated in the *null hypothesis.* This hypothesized value is a specific value for the parameter and usually reflects a *parsimonious* world in which nothing is related to anything else. For example, if the population's parameter were a difference between the means for two groups, the null hypothesis would state that the difference between those means in the population is equal to zero. This is a statement of parsimony because it says there is no distinction between the groups as far as the means are concerned.

All of the calculations that are performed in the process of statistical inference assume that the null hypothesis is true. Then, making that assumption, the probability of obtaining a sample with an estimate of the population's parameter that is at least as far away from the hypothesized value as the actual sample's estimate is calculated. That probability is known as the *P-value.* To calculate the *P*-value, we use the distribution of estimates from all possible samples of a given size. This is nearly the same distribution that was used in interval estimation. The only difference is that the location of the distribution used in inference is determined by the null hypothesis while the location of the distribution used in interval estimation is determined by the point estimate.

Thus, the *P*-value is the probability of obtaining an estimate from a sample that is at least as far from the value in the null hypothesis as the estimate in the sample actually obtained if the population's parameter is equal to the hypothesized value. If that sounds like a complicated probability to you, you are correct. The *P*-value is a complicated probability that is difficult to interpret quantitatively. Rather than attempt a quantitative interpretation, *P*-values are usually interpreted qualitatively, that is, if a *P*-value is equal to or less than a specified value, then we draw the conclusion that the null hypothesis probably does not correctly reflect the value of the population's parameter. That specified value is called *alpha.*

The value that we choose for alpha does two things for

*Some statisticians who adhere to an older philosophy of interval estimation might take offense at the statement that the interval estimate has a 95% chance of including the population's parameter. They would rather we say that 95% of the intervals so constructed will include the population's parameter. A more modern view is that these two statements are both correct.

Table 1. How the Relationship between the Truth of the Null Hypothesis in the Population and the Conclusion Drawn in Statistical Inference from Examination of the Data in a Sample Lead to Type I and Type II Errors

		CONCLUSION FROM SAMPLE	
		Null Hypothesis True	Null Hypothesis False
TRUTH IN POPULATION	Null Hypothesis True	Correct	Type I error
	Null Hypothesis False	Type II error	Correct

the process of inference. First, it defines the point at which a sample is considered too unusual, if the null hypothesis is true, to continue to believe that the null hypothesis is, indeed, true. Rather than believe that an unusual sample has been observed, we reject the null hypothesis as a reasonable statement of the nature of the population. How unusual should be considered too unusual? Generally, if a sample would be drawn 5% or less of the time from a population in which the null hypothesis were true, we consider that sample to be unusual enough for us to doubt that our sample was drawn from such a population. Thus, the conventual value of alpha is 0.05. If the *P*-value is equal or less than 0.05, we reject the null hypothesis as a reasonable reflection of the population.

The second thing that the chosen value of alpha does is to determine the probability that we will mistakenly conclude that the null hypothesis is false (ie, reject the null hypothesis) when, in fact, the sample was drawn from a population in which the null hypothesis correctly states the value of the parameter. This is one of two types of error that we could make in the process of statistical inference. This is called a *type I error*. To accept as true a null hypothesis that is, in fact, false is called a *type II error*. Those errors in statistical inference are summarized in Table 1.

If the null hypothesis is not a true reflection of the value of the parameter in the population, there is another hypothesis that is used in statistical inference to represent the value of the parameter. That hypothesis is called the *alternative hypothesis*. While the null hypothesis provides a specific value for the population's parameter, the alternative hypothesis provides an interval of values. The alternative hypothesis is accepted by default when the null hypothesis is rejected.

The most common type of alternative hypothesis includes in the interval all possible values for the population's parameter except that value specified in the null hypothesis. This is known as a *two-tailed* alternative hypothesis. Another type of alternative hypothesis, called a *one-tailed* alternative hypothesis, includes in its interval only those values that deviate in one direction from the value in the null hypothesis. One must have a strong argument that deviations from the value in the null hypothesis in the other direction cannot occur to use a one-tailed alternative hypothesis.

The chance of making a type I error (alpha) is specified by the researcher. The probability of making a type II error (beta), however, cannot be specified. The reason for this difference between alpha and beta is that alpha is the probability of making an error in inference under the condition that the null hypothesis is true and beta is the probability of making an error under the condition that the alternative hypothesis is true (ie, that the null hypothesis is false). Since the null hypothesis states a specific value for the population's parameter, we can determine the specific probability of making an error if the null hypothesis is assumed to be true. The alternative hypothesis, on the other hand, does not state a specific value for the population's parameter. Therefore, we cannot determine the specific value of beta.

Even though we do not know the value of beta, we know what influences it. Most often under the control of the researcher is the number of observations in the sample (called the *sample's size*). As the size of the sample increases, the value of beta decreases.

This inability to specify the probability of making a type II error (beta) causes us to be more cautious about making that sort of inferential error than about making a type I error. When we conclude that the null hypothesis is false, we know that the probability of making a mistake is equal to the specific value that we have chosen for alpha (see Table 1). If we were to conclude, however, that the null hypothesis is true, we would not know the probability of making a mistake because the probability of making a type II error is unknown. The solution to this problem is to avoid drawing the conclusion that the null hypothesis is true (referred to as "accepting the null hypothesis"). Rather, when the results of statistical inference do not lead to the conclusion that the null hypothesis is false (referred to as "rejecting the null hypothesis"), we refrain from drawing any conclusion about which hypothesis we believe is correct. This refusal to draw a specific conclusion in statistical inference is called "failing to reject" the null hypothesis. By failing to reject the null hypothesis instead of accepting that hypothesis, we avoid making a type II error since we avoid drawing a specific conclusion about the null hypothesis. Thus, the results of statistical inference can be rejection of the null hypothesis (concluding that the null hypothesis is false) or failure to reject the null hypothesis (deciding not to draw a conclusion about the validity of the null hypothesis).

We have seen that there are two ways statistical methods can help us to take into account the role of chance in determining which of all the possible samples that could have been collected from the population that we actually have examined. Interval estimation takes that role of chance into account by calculating an interval of values within which there is a high probability that the population's value is included. Statistical inference takes chance into account by allowing us to draw conclusions about the population's value with a specified probability of making a (type I) mistake. Now, let us see how statistical methods can help us control for some measurements while examining relationships among other measurements.

Controlling for Confounders

Often we are interested in removing the influence of some characteristics of individuals in a sample before we make comparisons among measurements made on those individuals. Suppose, for example, we wish to compare survival rates of persons with a particular type of tumor who receive different radiotherapy regimens. It is likely that we would be interested in comparing survival rates only after we have controlled for the influence on survival of such other characteristics as their ages and genders. These other characteristics are referred to as *confounders*.

Confounders can create an apparent relationship between an exposure (such as the radiotherapy dose) and an outcome (such as survival) if the confounder is associated with the exposure and it is a determinate of the outcome. For example, if younger persons tend to receive higher doses in radiotherapy, it might appear that higher doses are associated with better survival only because of that association rather than the fact that survival is greater due to higher doses. To control for this effect, we need to adjust the rates of survival for differences in patient ages. Certain statistical procedures, which will be discussed later, can make this sort of adjustment.

SELECTING STATISTICAL PROCEDURES

One of the more confusing aspects of statistical analysis is the choice among the many statistical procedures to analyze a particular set of data. Actually, this choice is less complicated than it seems at first if we follow the logical processes used by statisticians. Rather than think about data, statisticians think about *variables*. Variables represent data in the mathematics of statistical procedures. To select appropriate statistical procedures, we need to be able to identify variables and specify them by their type. The types of variables are defined by two characteristics: (1) the type of data they represent and (2) their function in the analysis.

Earlier, we considered three types of data: continuous, ordinal, and nominal. We use these same labels to specify variables that represent these data. For the most part, there is a one-to-one correspondence between data and a variable. One exception is in the number of nominal variables that are used to represent nominal data. A nominal variable can have only two possible values, but nominal data can have two or more possible values. When nominal data have more than two possible values, we need to represent those data with more than two nominal variables. More specifically, nominal data that has k possible values requires $k - 1$ nominal variables in statistical analysis. As an example, consider race as nominal data with four possible categories: Asian, black, white, and other. Those data require three nominal variables to specify those four values. For instance, we could have dichotomous (yes/no) variables representing the first three racial categories. We would not need a separate nominal variable for the fourth category since we would know that an individual was a member of that race if (s)he were not a member of the first three races.

To define a variable according to the type of data it represents, we first need to determine the type of data and then, if the data are nominal, we need to count the number of possible categories to ascertain how many nominal variables are needed to represent those data. Once we have defined the variables according to the type of data they represent, we need to define the variables further by their function in the statistical analysis.

Dependent and Independent Variables

There are two functions of variables in statistical analyses. The first function is to represent the data for which we are interested in making estimates or testing hypotheses. The variable that represents those data of primary interest in an analysis is called the *dependent variable*. In most statistical analyses, a set of data contains only one dependent variable. A set of data that contains one dependent variable is called a *univariate* data set. Data sets with more than one dependent variable (*multivariate* data sets) are common only in psychosocial areas of medical research.

The second function of variables is to specify the conditions under which we are interested in making estimates of or testing hypotheses about the dependent variable. The variables that specify those conditions are called *independent variables*. A set of data can contain no, one, or more than one independent variable. Data sets that contain no, one, and more than one independent variable are called *univariable*, *bivariable*, and *multivariable* data sets, respectively. Note that "-variable" refers to the number of variables in a data set regardless of their function. This is distinct from "-variate" which refers to the number of dependent variables.

To illustrate the functions of variables, let us reconsider the previous example of a study of survival of cancer patients relative to the dose they receive in radiotherapy, controlling for the effects of age and gender. The dependent variable in this example represents the survival rates. The remaining data (dose, age, and gender) are represented in the statistical analysis by independent variables. Thus, we are interested in examining the relationship between survival and dose under the condition that we have controlled for age and gender.

The most common independent variables are those that represent either continuous or nominal data. With continuous data, we are interested in how values of the dependent variable change along the continuum of independent variable values. For example, if survival is represented by the depen-

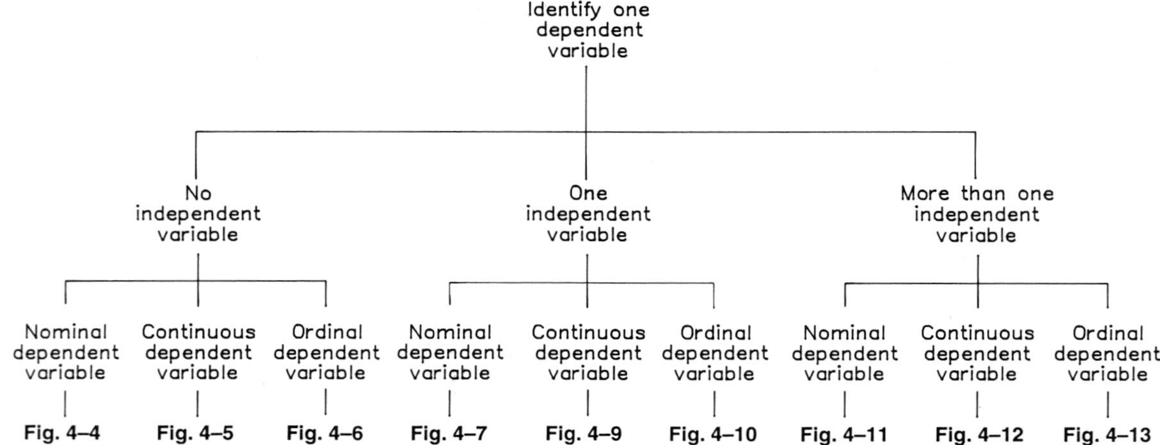

Figure 3. Flowchart illustrating the first logical steps involved in selecting a statistical procedure for a particular set of data. Identifying the dependent and independent variables and the type of data represented by the dependent variable leads to another flowchart that appears in the figure indicated at the end of each logical pathway.

dent variable and dose is represented by the independent variable, our interest is in examining how survival changes as dose changes.

On the other hand, a nominal independent variable has the effect of dividing dependent variable values into groups between which we wish to compare dependent variable values. For instance, if survival is represented by the dependent variable and gender is represented by the independent variable, we are interested in comparing the survival rates between the two genders.

Knowing how statisticians think about variables, let us see how a statistical test is selected for a particular set of data. The logical process of selecting a statistical procedure begins with the following steps:

1. Identify the dependent variable by determining what it is that you wish to make an estimate of or test a hypothesis about.
2. Count the number of independent variables. In most cases, the independent variables will be all the variables left after one dependent variable has been identified.
3. Determine the type of data represented by the dependent variable.

Those steps have been organized in a flowchart in Figure 3.

To look at some of the most commonly used statistical procedures in medicine, we will examine data sets of increasing complexity starting with data sets that contain only a dependent variable (univariable analyses), then data sets that contain a dependent variable and one independent variable (bivariable analyses), and, finally, we will look at procedures for one dependent variable and more than one independent variable (multivariable analyses).

Univariable Analyses

In univariable analyses, a data set contains only one variable: the dependent variable. In this case, estimation is more often of interest than is inference. The reason for this emphasis on estimation is the difficulty we have in imagining a valid null hypothesis to test when a data set contains no independent variables. To appreciate why this is so, recall that the null hypothesis must hypothesize that the dependent variable has a specific value in the population and that value reflects parsimony. When the data set contains an independent variable, we can hypothesize that there is no relationship between the dependent and independent variables. Without an independent variable, there is no specific value to reflect parsimony.

There is one circumstance, however, in which statistical inference is warranted even though we have a univariable data set. That is in the case of a study that contains *paired data*. In that sort of study, two measurements are made on the same individual under different circumstances. For example, suppose we were interested in comparing absorbed doses of a particular radionuclide in two different target organs. The way that we would make that comparison would be to measure the absorbed dose for those two organs in each patient and to calculate the difference between the absorbed doses. Those differences would be the data of interest that we would like to make estimates of or test hypotheses about. Thus, the data set would be represented by a single dependent variable (representing the differences in absorbed dose) and no independent variables. If we were to make statistical inferences on those data, a sensible null hypothesis would be that the mean of the differences between absorbed doses is equal to zero in the population.

Regardless of whether we are interested in estimation or inference, every univariable sample will be used to accomplish the first two purposes of statistical procedures: (1) to summarize measurements and (2) to take chance into account. The particular value we calculate to summarize measurements relies, in part, on the type of data represented by the dependent variable. Also, the calculations involved in taking chance into account are different for different types of data. Therefore, let us consider each type of data represented by the dependent variable separately.

First, we will investigate univariable samples that contain nominal data. As we learned before, there are two ways that we most often summarize a collection of nominal data in medicine. These are by calculating a probability or by calculating a rate. Thus, the first purpose of statistical procedures, to summarize measurements, is accomplished for univariable samples with a nominal dependent variable using either a probability or a rate.

To take chance into account, we need to determine the standard distribution of the samples' estimates that we will use. As we discussed earlier, this same standard distribution is used for either interval estimation or for inference. We also saw that the most commonly assumed distribution for probabilities is the binomial distribution and that the corresponding distribution for rates is the Poisson distribution. Unfortunately, these distributions are rather difficult to use. However, when the sample's size is large enough, the binomial and Poisson distributions are similar to a Gaussian distribution which is easier to use. Thus, we most often take chance into account for probabilities and rates using the Gaussian distribution. Because these distributions are only approximately the same as a Gaussian distribution, these procedures are called *normal approximations*. The particular standard distribution we use in normal approximations to the binomial and Poisson distributions is called the *standard normal distribution*. These statistical procedures are summarized in the flowchart in Figure 4.

Figure 4 gives us the names of the statistical procedures that we would use to analyze a univariable data set that includes a nominal dependent variable. We will not examine the actual calculations that are used in these procedures or in the procedures that are presented in any of the following flowcharts. The reason for this is that those calculations are, in practice, performed by computer programs rather than by hand. Thus, it is more important for us to understand the names of the procedures and how to interpret the results of analysis than it is to examine the underlying calculations.

The statistical procedures for a univariable sample with a continuous dependent variable are summarized in Figure 5.

When the dependent variable in a univariable data set represents continuous data, the point estimate that is most often used to summarize the data is the measure of location of the Gaussian distribution: the mean. Means estimated from samples tend to have a Gaussian distribution. We do not, however, use the standard normal distribution to take chance into account. Rather, we use the *Student's t distribution*. The Student's t distribution is similar to the standard normal distribution with the addition of a third parameter.

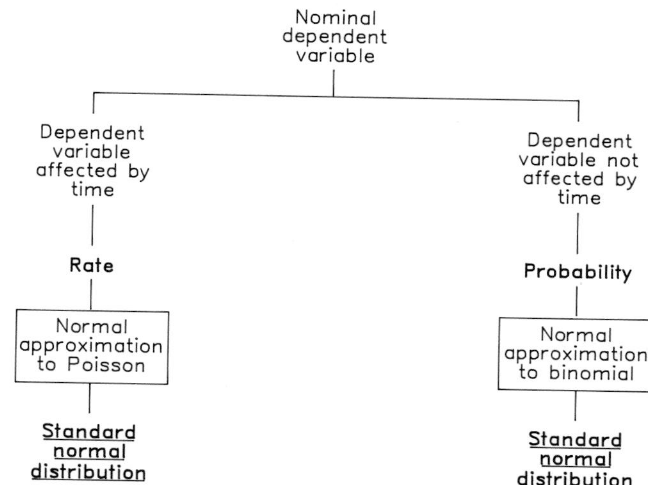

Figure 4. Flowchart illustrating the logical steps involved in selecting a point estimate (bold) and a standard distribution (bold and underlined) for analysis of a univariable sample with a nominal dependent variable. The common names of statistical procedures appear in boxes.

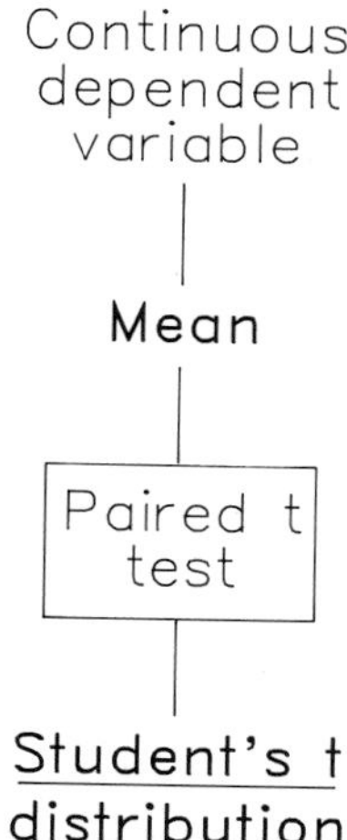

Figure 5. Flowchart illustrating the logical steps involved in selecting a point estimate (bold) and a standard distribution (bold and underlined) for analyzing a univariable sample with a continuous dependent variable. The common name of this statistical test is the paired t test.

That parameter is called *degrees of freedom*. The degrees of freedom take into account the role of chance in estimating the population's variance from the sample's observations when using the standard distribution.*

Data in medicine do not commonly occur on an ordinal scale, yet statistical procedures for ordinal dependent variables are not uncommonly used. The reason for this apparent

*We do not need to take into account the role of chance in estimation of the variance when the dependent variable is nominal since that variance can be equal to only one value for a particular probability or rate.

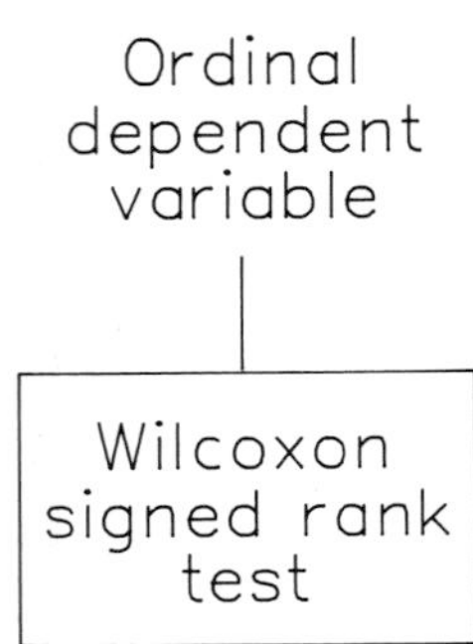

Figure 6. Flowchart illustrating the logical step involved in selecting a nonparametric procedure for analysis of a univariable sample with an ordinal dependent variable. The common name of this statistical test is the Wilcoxon signed rank test. Neither a point estimate nor a standard distribution are indicated since they are irrelevant to a nonparametric procedure.

contradiction is that statistical procedures for ordinal dependent variables are often used to analyze continuous data that have been converted to an ordinal scale. To perform this conversion of continuous data to an ordinal scale, the continuous data values are represented by their relative ranks rather than their actual numeric values.

Conversion of continuous data to an ordinal scale allows statistical analyses to be performed with fewer assumptions than are required for continuous data analyzed on a continuous scale. There are fewer assumptions required for the statistical procedures designed for ordinal data because estimates for ordinal data are not assumed to come from any particular type of distribution. Because we are not thinking about distributions for analysis of ordinal data, we do not think about parameters of distributions. This feature has led to the term "*nonparametric*" analyses for these procedures. Interest in nonparametric analyses is most often limited to statistical inference. Figure 6 illustrates the nonparametric procedure for a univariable data set.

Bivariable Analyses

In bivariable analyses, we have an independent, as well as a dependent, variable. This implies that there are certain conditions under which we are interested in making estimates of or testing hypotheses about dependent variable values in the population. As mentioned earlier, the types of data represented by an independent variable that are most commonly encountered in medicine are nominal and continuous data. Nominal and continuous independent variables specify different conditions under which values of the dependent variable change. Now, let us take a closer look at how those conditions are examined statistically.

Let us begin, as we did for univariable analyses, by thinking about a nominal dependent variable. Recall from that discussion that we summarize a collection of nominal data represented by the dependent variable either as a probability or as a rate. The same is true in bivariable analyses. If the independent variable represents nominal data, that nominal independent variable has the effect of separating the nominal data represented by the dependent variable into two groups. Thus, we can visualize analysis of a data set containing a nominal dependent variable and a nominal independent variable as a method to compare two probabilities or two rates between two groups.

The issue now is how to compare the two probabilities or rates between the two groups specified by the two values of the nominal independent variable. There are two possibilities. We could make that comparison by examining the difference between the probabilities or rates or by examining the ratio of the probabilities or rates. The interpretation of these two methods of comparison has an important distinction. That distinction is in whether or not the underlying probability or rate of the data represented by the dependent variable is reflected in the comparison. That underlying probability or rate is reflected in the difference but not in the ratio.

EXAMPLE

To understand the distinction between a comparison made by examining a difference and a comparison made by examining a ratio, let us look at an example. Suppose that we wish to compare the probabilities of surviving 5 years post-treatment (a nominal dependent variable)* between men and women (a nominal independent variable). Further suppose that the 5-year probability of survival is 0.10 for women and 0.05 for men. If we compare those probabilities as a difference, we would summarize that comparison by reporting that the difference between the probabilities is equal to 0.05. If, on the other hand, we compare those probabilities as a ratio, we would summarize that comparison by reporting that the ratio of the probabilities is equal to 2.00.

Now, to see how the difference between the probabilities reflects the underlying probability of survival, consider a comparison of survival between women and men for another treatment that is less efficacious. Specifically, imagine that the 5-year probabilities for survival are 0.01 for women and 0.005 for men with this less-efficacious treatment. The difference between the probabilities is equal to 0.005 and the ratio of the probabilities is equal to 2.00. Notice that the difference between the probabilities has decreased, just as the underlying probabilities of survival have decreased, with the less-efficacious treatment. The ratio of the probabilities, however, has remained the same, reflecting only the relationship between the probabilities without being affected by the distinction in overall survival between the two treatments.

Thus, we can compare probabilities or rates between two groups either as differences or ratios. Another important way in which nominal dependent variable values are compared between two groups in medicine is with a value known as

*Notice that this probability of survival addresses a particular period of time; namely, 5 years. In medicine, a probability that addresses a specified period of time is called a *risk*. On the other hand, a probability that addresses a point in time is called a *prevalence*.

the *odds ratio*. Odds are similar to probabilities in that they are dimensionless. They are different from probabilities in that the denominator of odds does not include the events that are included in the numerator of odds and probabilities. Equation 9 illustrates the calculation of the odds of an event.

$$(9)\quad \text{odds of event} = \frac{\text{number of events}}{(\text{number of observations}) - (\text{number of events})} = \frac{\text{number of events}}{\text{number of nonevents}}$$

Many people find that odds, by themselves, are more difficult to interpret than are probabilities or rates. In part, that is the reason we do not encounter odds as point estimates in univariable analysis of a nominal dependent variable. Further, we do not make comparisons between odds by using differences. Rather, we make those comparisons only by using ratios. The odds ratio is not difficult to interpret, especially when the underlying probabilities are small. In that circumstance, the odds ratio is very similar to the probability ratio. The advantages of using the odds ratio instead of the probability ratio are (1) the odds ratio can be used for case-control studies; (2) it is less sensitive to some kinds of bias; and (3) it has mathematical properties that make analysis easier. Thus, odds ratios are commonly encountered in medical research.

The interpretation of the point estimates from differences or ratios of probabilities or rates or from odds ratios is somewhat distinct. The methods of taking chance into account, however, are less distinct. This is especially true in statistical inference. The reason for this similarity in statistical inference is that the null hypotheses reflecting parsimony for each of those point estimates all occur under the same condition. That condition is when the probabilities, rates, or odds are equal in the two groups specified by values of the nominal independent variable. That occurs when a ratio is equal to one or when a difference is equal to zero. This similarity is the reason the flowchart for bivariable analysis of a nominal dependent variable (Fig. 7) does not show separate logical pathways for ratios and differences.

CHI-SQUARE DISTRIBUTION

To take chance into account when comparing probabilities, rates, or odds, we most often use a normal approximation method as we did when we had a univariable sample with a nominal dependent variable. Although the distribution for probabilities and odds that is being approximated by a Gaussian distribution in bivariable analysis is a combination of two binomial distributions, it has a special name: the *hypergeometric distribution*. The hypergeometric distribution can be approximated by the standard normal distribution or, more commonly, by a related distribution called the *chi-square distribution*. In bivariable analyses, the square root of the chi-square value is exactly equal to the standard normal value. Thus, use of either standard distribution leads to the same result.

When the independent variable represents continuous, rather than nominal, data, our interest is in how probabilities, rates, or odds change along a continuum of independent variable values rather than in comparing those estimates between two groups. Most of the commonly used methods of investigating a continuum of nominal dependent variable values are the same as the multivariable methods we will examine. There is one method, however, that is especially designed for the bivariable case in which the dependent variable represents nominal data. This method is called the *chi-square test for trend*. Actually, there are several methods that might be called a chi-square test for trend. The one that we will examine here is probably the most commonly used of the methods.

LINEAR MODEL

To describe how dependent variable values change as values of the independent variable change, we need to decide on some particular mathematical model. The most commonly used model in statistics is the *linear model*. The linear model is a mathematical description of a straight line. The linear model as it usually appears in the chi-square test for trend is illustrated in Equation 10.

$$(10)\qquad p_i = a + (b \cdot X_i)$$

where p_i = probability of event represented by the dependent variable corresponding to the ith value of the independent variable; X_i= the ith value of the independent variable; a = intercept; b = slope.

The linear model consists of two parameters that are estimated from the sample's observations. These are the *slope* and the *intercept* (see Fig. 8). The slope indicates the amount that values of the dependent variable change for each unit change in the value of the independent variable. The intercept indicates the value of the dependent variable that corresponds to the independent variable being equal to zero. In other words, the intercept is a specific estimate of the value of the dependent variable while the slope tells us how dependent variable values change along a continuum of independent variable values. Thus, it is the slope that provides the most information about the relationship between the dependent and independent variables and, therefore, is of greater interest in a linear model.

REGRESSION ANALYSIS

When the dependent variable represents continuous data, we might also have an interest in a linear model if the bivariable data set includes a continuous independent variable. With a continuous dependent variable, estimation of the slope and intercept is part of *regression analysis*. The linear model for a continuous dependent variable is illustrated in Equation 11.

$$(11)\qquad \hat{Y}_i = a + (b \cdot X_i),$$

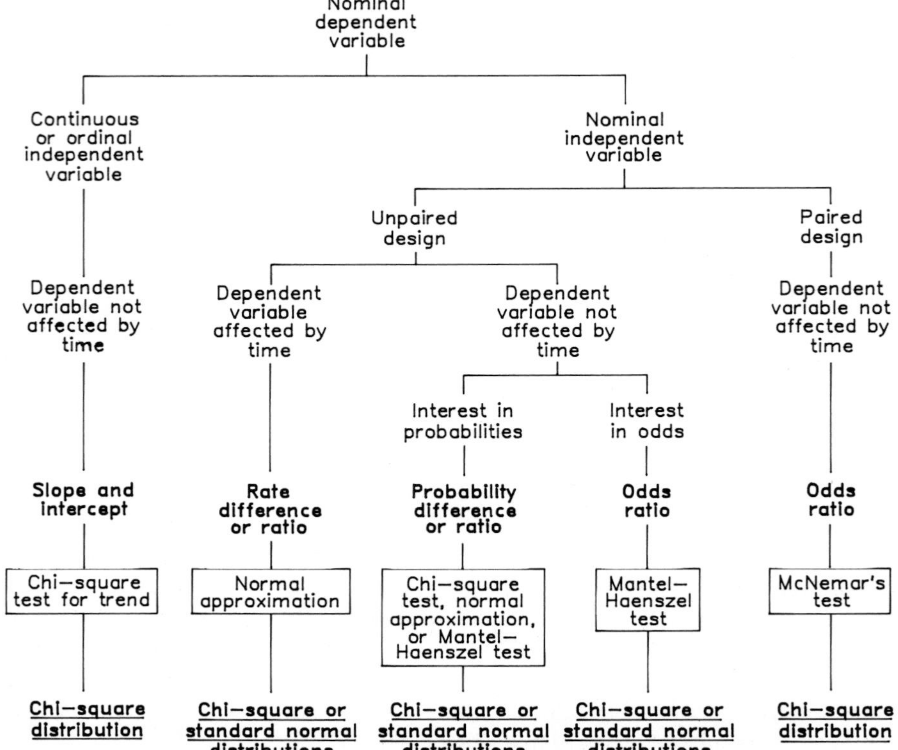

Figure 7. Flowchart illustrating the logical steps involved in selecting a point estimate (bold) and a standard distribution (bold and underlined) for analysis of a bivariable sample with a nominal dependent variable. The common names of statistical procedures appear in boxes.

where $\hat{Y}_i$ = estimated value of the continuous dependent variable corresponding to the *i*th value of the independent variable.

In regression analysis, the point estimates that we can calculate are the slope, the intercept, and the value of the dependent variable that corresponds to a particular value of the independent variable. To take chance into account, we can calculate confidence intervals for each of those point estimates. Also, we can test hypotheses about the slope, the intercept, or the entire linear model. The null hypothesis that addresses the entire linear model is called the *omnibus null hypothesis*.

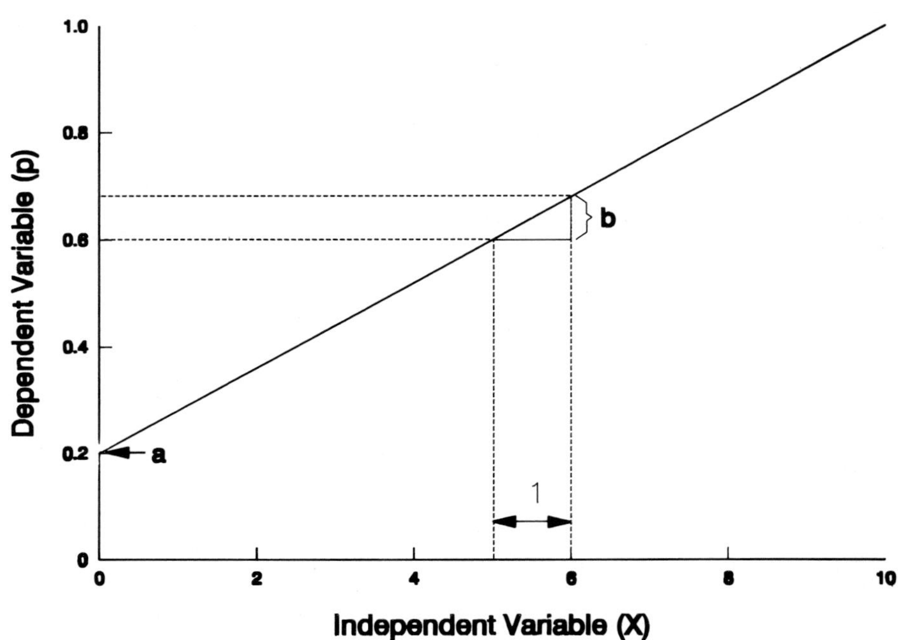

Figure 8. The straight line relationship assumed by a linear model in which the dependent variable represents nominal data. The information about the straight line contained in the slope (b) and the intercept (a) are indicated.

The omnibus null hypothesis states that knowledge of the value of the independent variable does not help us to estimate a value for the dependent variable. We test the omnibus null hypothesis by examining the *F ratio* which is a ratio of the explained variation to the unexplained variation in dependent variable values. If the null hypothesis is correct, the F ratio will, on the average, be equal to one. The distribution of F ratios from all possible samples of a given size is called the *F distribution*. The F distribution is closely related to the Student's t distribution, but differs from it in that the F distribution includes two (rather than one) parameters that are called degrees of freedom.

We also can test null hypotheses about the slope and the intercept. The usual null hypothesis for either the slope or the intercept is that the value of the parameter is equal to zero in the population. That null hypothesis can be tested using the Student's t distribution or the F distribution. In bivariable regression analysis, the test of the null hypothesis that the slope is equal to zero in the population is exactly the same as the test of the omnibus null hypothesis. This underlines the importance of the slope in telling us about the relationship between the dependent and independent variables.

CORRELATION ANALYSIS

Even though the slope is the more important parameter in regression analysis, it does not reliably tell us how strong the relationship is between a continuous dependent variable and a continuous independent variable. To examine the strength of the association between the variables, we need to consider a second way we can analyze a bivariable data set with two continuous variables: using *correlation analysis*. In correlation analysis, we estimate the *correlation coefficient*. The sample's estimate of the population's correlation coefficient is symbolized with the letter r.

The correlation coefficient has a range of possible values from -1 to $+1$. The extremes of that range indicate perfect relationships between the dependent and independent variables. Positive values tell us that dependent variable values increase as independent variable values increase. This is called a *direct relationship* between the variables. Negative values of the correlation coefficient tell us that dependent variable values decrease as independent variable values increase. This is known as an *inverse relationship* between the variables. A correlation coefficient equal to zero indicates that there is no relationship between the variables.

Correlation coefficients that have values between zero and positive one or values between minus one and zero indicate that the existence of an association between the dependent and independent variables that is somewhere in the continuum between a perfect association and no association. Exactly how strong the association is, however. is not so easy to interpret directly from the numeric value of the correlation coefficient. For instance, a correlation coefficient equal to 0.5 does not imply that the strength of the association is halfway between zero and positive one even though 0.5 is numerically halfway between those values. In fact, a correlation coefficient of 0.5 indicates that the strength of the association is one quarter of the way between no association and a perfect association. The method we use to make that interpretation is to square the value of the correlation coefficient. The square of the correlation coefficient is called the *coefficient of determination*, often called *R-squared*. The coefficient of determination tells us the proportion of the variation in the dependent variable that is associated with variation in the independent variable.

Correlation analysis is similar to regression analysis in that the relationship that is examined in both is a straight line relationship. These two methods of analyzing two continuous variables differ in the information they provide about that relationship. Regression analysis helps us estimate dependent variable values corresponding to values of the independent variable. Correlation analysis provides us with a number (the correlation coefficient or the coefficient of determination) that tells us how strong the relationship is between the two variables.

These two methods of analyzing two continuous variables also differ in the way the results of those analyses are influenced by the distribution of independent variable values in the sample.* The distribution of independent variable values does not influence the estimates made in regression analysis, but that distribution can have a substantial effect on the estimate of the correlation coefficient. Specifically, the more spread out the independent variable values are, the closer the estimate of the correlation coefficient will be to (either positive or negative) one.

NATURALISTIC AND PURPOSIVE SAMPLING

The sample's estimate of the correlation coefficient has relevance to the population if and only if the distribution of independent variable values in the sample is representative of the distribution of independent variable values in the population. As discussed previously for values of the dependent variable, the way that we accomplish representatives of independent variable values is by taking a random sample in which the independent variable values chosen to be included in the sample are selected by chance. This method of sampling is called *naturalistic sampling*. The alternative is to have the independent variable values to be included in the sample selected by the researcher. This is called *purposive sampling*.

This distinction between naturalistic and purposive sampling is an important point, so let us consider an example. Suppose we were interested in investigating the absorbed

*The reason that we focus on the distribution of independent variable values in the sample and not the distribution of both variables here is because we always assume, in every statistical procedure, that the distribution of dependent variable values in the sample is representative of their distribution in the population.

dose of a particular radionuclide in a specific target organ for persons with various body mass indices. Here the dependent variable would represent the absorbed dose and the independent variable would represent the body mass index of each person in the study. If persons were selected to be in the sample at random and without regard to their body mass index, the result would be a naturalistic sample. In this case, we could choose to use regression analysis to estimate the absorbed dose we would expect for a particular body mass index and/or we could choose to use correlation analysis to estimate the strength of the association between the absorbed dose and the body mass index. If, on the other hand, we selected a given number of persons with specific body mass indices to be in the sample, the distribution of body mass indices in that sample would reflect our choice rather than the distribution of body mass indices in the population. This would be a purposive sample and we would be limited to using regression analysis to analyze these data. Correlation analysis would not be appropriate in this case since the value of the correlation coefficient would reflect the number of persons with specific body mass indices that we chose to include in the sample as well as the strength of the association between absorbed dose and body mass index.

Therefore, it is important to determine whether the sample is naturalistic or purposive before attempting to interpret the correlation coefficient as an indicator of the strength of the association between two continuous variables. Probably the most frequently encountered situation in which this principle is overlooked is when a dose-response relationship is being investigated. Most often, the number of persons to receive specific doses is determined by the researcher. When that is true, the sample is purposive and correlation coefficients cannot be taken as estimates of the strength of the association in the population. This distinction is important enough to be included as a decision point in the flowchart for bivariable analysis of a continuous dependent variable (Fig. 9).

When we have a continuous dependent variable and a nominal independent variable, the nominal independent variable has the effect of dividing the dependent variable values into two groups. Then, our interest is usually in comparing the means of the dependent variable values between the groups. This is parallel to when the dependent variable is nominal. With means, however, we make this comparison only by examining the difference between the means, that is, we do not compare means as a ratio. The reason for this is that differences between estimates tend to meet the assumptions of statistical procedures much more often than do ratios. Comparing probabilities, rates, and odds as ratios is done for nominal dependent variables only because of the interpretability of ratios in that case. There is not a similar motivation to examine the ratio of means.

As we discovered in our discussion of univariable analyses, statistical procedures for ordinal dependent variables are used most often on continuous data converted to an ordinal scale to circumvent some of the assumptions inherent to procedures for continuous dependent variables. It should

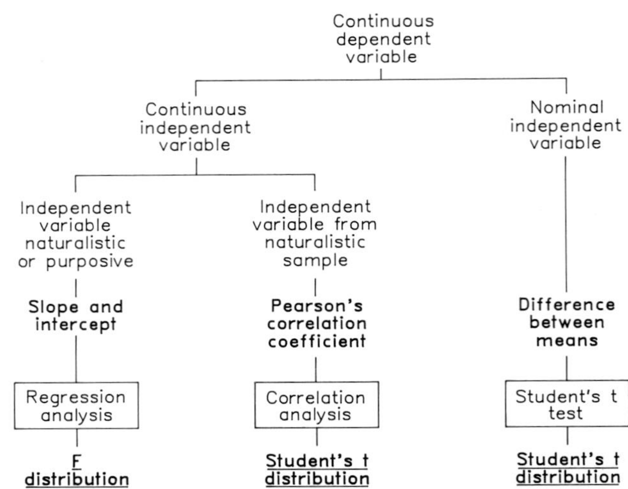

Figure 9. Flowchart illustrating the logical steps involved in selecting a point estimate (bold) and a standard distribution (bold and underlined) for analysis of a bivariable sample with a continuous dependent variable. The common names of statistical procedures appear in boxes.

not be surprising, therefore, to find procedures for ordinal dependent variables that are parallel to procedures for continuous dependent variables. Not all procedures for continuous dependent variables, however, can be performed on ordinal data. Specifically, it is not possible to perform regression analysis on ordinal data, because the distances between values of ordinal data are not known. Without that knowledge, we cannot estimate a slope and, therefore, we cannot estimate a linear model. As shown in Figure 10, however, we can

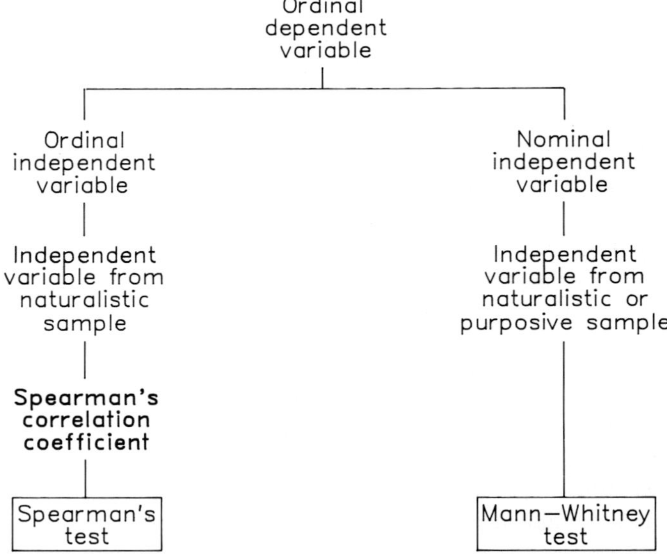

Figure 10. Flowchart illustrating the logical steps involved in selecting a nonparametric procedure for analysis of a bivariable sample with an ordinal dependent variable. The common names of statistical tests appear in boxes.

perform correlation analysis or compare two groups of ordinal dependent variable values.

Multivariable Analyses

For the most part, multivariable analyses are like bivariable analyses extended to accommodate more than one independent variable. For instance, a single nominal independent variable has the effect of dividing dependent variable values into two groups. More than one nominal independent variable has the effect of dividing dependent variable values into more than two groups. When the independent variable in bivariable analysis represents continuous data, we are interested in estimating values of the dependent variable that correspond to values along the continuum of independent variable values. When we have more than one continuous independent variable, we are interested in estimating dependent variable values that correspond to the combination of values of each of those independent variables.

There is, however, an important distinction between bivariable analyses and multivariable analyses. This distinction is that only multivariable procedures are able to accomplish the third purpose of statistics: to control for the effect of some independent variables while examining the relationship between the dependent variable and another independent variable.

To illustrate how multivariable analyses control for some variables while examining others, it is most convenient to consider multivariable regression analysis, although the same principle is applicable to all multivariable procedures. To begin, let us take a look at a linear model that includes, for example, three independent variables. Equation 12 illustrates such a linear model for a continuous dependent variable. Notice that Equation 12 is similar to the bivariable regression linear model in Equation 11 in that Equation 12 includes an intercept as well as a slope corresponding to each of the independent variables. When a linear model contains more than one independent variable, however, the slopes in that model are usually called *regression coefficients*.

$$(12) \qquad \hat{Y}_{ijk} = a + (b_1 \cdot X_{1i}) + (b_2 \cdot X_{2j}) + (b_3 \cdot X_{3k}),$$

where $\hat{Y}_{ijk}$ = estimated value of the continuous dependent variable corresponding to the *i*th value of the first independent variable, the *j*th value of the second independent variable, and the *k*th value of the third independent variable.

THE FULL AND REDUCED MODELS

If our set of data contained only three independent variables, then Equation 12 would constitute what is called the *full model*. This refers to the regression equation in which we estimate values of the dependent variable by considering all of the independent variables. To examine the contribution of any one of the independent variables to the estimation of dependent variable values, we compare the capacity of the full model to estimate dependent variable values to the capacity of a *reduced model* to estimate those values. The reduced model contains all of the independent variables except the one for which we are examining the contribution. Thus, the reduced model that is used to examine the contribution of the first independent variable in Equation 12 is one that includes the second and third independent variables but excludes the first independent variable. This reduced model is illustrated in Equation 13.*

$$(13) \qquad \hat{Y}_{ijk} = a' + (b_2' \cdot X_{2j}) + (b_3' \cdot X_{3k}).$$

In both Equations 12 and 13, variability in dependent variable values that is associated with the second and third independent variables is taken into account. Thus, the contribution of the first independent variable to estimate dependent variable values in the full model must be over and above the contributions of the second and third independent variables. The same is true for the contributions of the second and third independent variables. The reduced model for examination of the second independent variable includes the first and third independent variables and the reduced model for examination of the third independent variable includes the first and second independent variables. Therefore, each independent variable in a multivariable analysis is examined controlling for all the other independent variables.

In this way, multivariable analyses allow us to accomplish the third purpose of statistical methods: to control for the effect of some independent variables while examining the relationship between the dependent variable and another independent variable.

Nearly all multivariable statistical procedures that we use in medicine make comparisons between measurements after making adjustments for all the other characteristics that have been included in the same analysis. This is to our benefit when we wish to control for the effect of confounders since all we need to do is to include those confounders in the statistical analysis. This feature of multivariable statistical procedures, however, can lead to erroneous conclusions about relationships among measurements. For example, suppose we were interested in studying the biological effects of industrial exposure to ionizing radiation. Suppose that, in this industry, there is a strong association between levels of exposure to gamma and x-radiation and both types of ionizing radiation could lead to the biologic effect under study. If we were to include the doses of both gamma and x-radiation in the same statistical analysis, neither type of radiation might appear to have a dose-response relationship! The reason for this is that the analysis would control for x-radiation when evaluating gamma radiation and vice versa.

This characteristic of multivariable statistical methods results in something known as *multicollinearity*. If we wish to use multicollinearity to control for some measurements while examining others, then multicollinearity is a desirable

*Primes are used in Equation 13 to signify different numeric values for the intercept and regression coefficients in the reduced model compared to the full model.

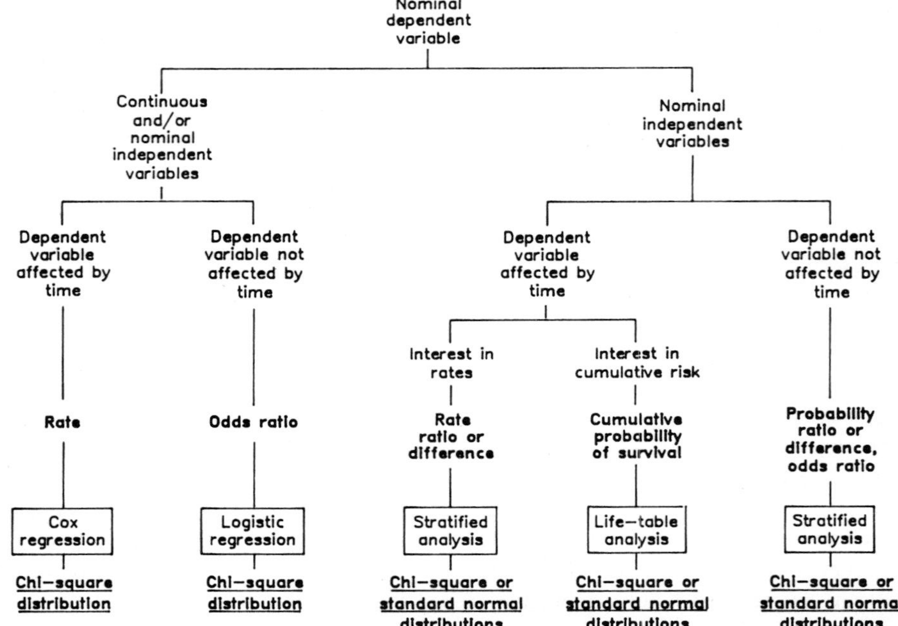

Figure 11. Flowchart illustrating the logical steps involved in selecting a point estimate (bold) and a standard distribution (bold and underlined) for analysis of a multivariable sample with a nominal dependent variable. The common names of statistical procedures appear in boxes.

feature. If, on the other hand, we interpret the results of multivariable statistical analysis of two or more associated measurements as if we had used bivariable statistical analysis, we are likely to be misled in our conclusions about the relationships among measurements. The most likely error in interpretation that we would make, in that circumstance, would be to erroneously conclude that there is no relationship between the associated independent variables and the dependent variable. Thus, it is well to keep this feature of multivariable analyses in mind when analyzing sets of data that contain independent variables that are associated with one another.

For the most part, multivariable analyses are like bivariable procedures that have been expanded to allow the inclusion of more than one independent variable. An exception is the way in which regression analysis is performed for a nominal dependent variable and more than one independent variable. There are two, commonly encountered regression methods for multivariable analysis of nominal dependent variables (Fig. 11). One of these, *logistic regression analysis*, is designed to analyze a nominal dependent variable that can be summarized using probabilities or odds. The other, *Cox proportional hazards regression*, is designed to analyze a nominal dependent variable that is summarized as a rate. Both of these regression methods use a mathematical *transformation* of the dependent variable values rather than a simple probability or rate as shown in Equation 10. The transformation allows the relationship between the dependent variable and the collection of independent variables to be *curvilinear* rather than linear. This is especially important when the dependent variable is summarized by using probabilities. A linear model for probabilities does nothing to avoid estimated probabilities being less than zero or greater than one; both of which are beyond the range of values that are possible for a probability.

When the independent variables represent nominal data, dependent variable values are separated into groups. In bivariable analyses of a nominal dependent variable, probabilities, rates, or odds are compared between two groups. In multivariable analysis of a nominal dependent variable, we also compare probabilities, rates, or odds between two groups even though we have more than one nominal independent variable. This method of analysis is called *stratified analysis*.

In stratified analysis, the two groups that we compare are specified by one of the nominal independent variables which we can call the independent variable of main interest. The remaining nominal independent variables specify subgroups (called *strata*) within which we examine the relationship between the dependent variable and the independent variable of main interest. The result of stratified analysis is a difference or ratio of probabilities or rates or an odds ratio that summarizes the association between the dependent variable and the independent variable of main interest controlling for the other nominal independent variables. Unlike other types of multivariable analyses, stratified analysis does not ordinarily provide corresponding estimates of the associations between the dependent and each of those other independent variables.

One type of stratified analysis is commonly encountered in reports of clinical trials. That type is *life-table analysis*. In life-table analysis, time since the beginning of treatment (or any exposure) is represented by nominal independent variables. These independent variables are then used to specify strata. In essence, life-table analysis allows for the confounding effects of different lengths of follow-up for various

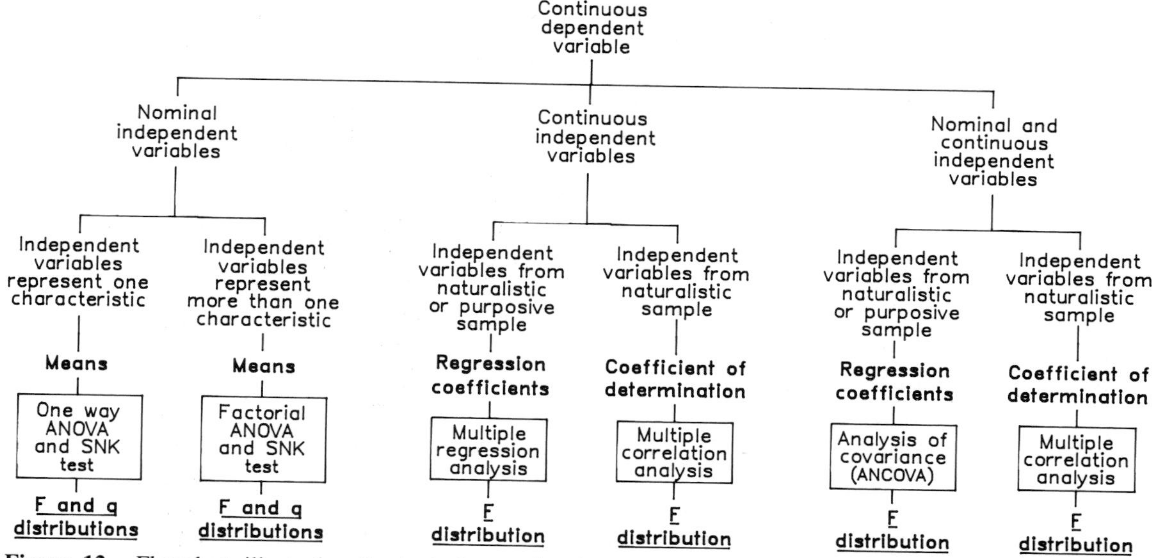

Figure 12. Flowchart illustrating the logical steps involved in selecting a point estimate (bold) and a standard distribution (bold and underlined) for analysis of a multivariable sample with a continuous dependent variable. The common names of statistical procedures appear in boxes.

patients in a study. This approach allows the frequencies of outcomes to be compared between groups with different lengths of follow-up by comparing probabilities rather than rates.

Techniques used in multivariable analysis of a continuous dependent variable are more similar to bivariable techniques than are methods for nominal dependent variables (Fig. 12). When the dependent and independent variables all represent continuous data, we can use *multiple correlation analysis* to measure the strength of the association between the continuous dependent variable and the entire collection of continuous independent variables if all of those independent variables are the result of naturalistic sampling. Otherwise, we can use *multiple regression analysis* to estimate values of the dependent variable from values of the independent variables.

ANALYSIS OF VARIANCE

When the independent variables represent nominal data, those independent variables have the effect of separating dependent variable values into groups. Since a multivariable data set contains more than one independent variable, more than two groups of dependent variable values are specified in multivariable analyses. Comparison of the means of the dependent variable values in each group is accomplished with a technique called *analysis of variance* or *ANOVA*.

Actually, there are several different types of analysis of variance that are appropriate for a continuous dependent variable and more than one nominal independent variable. Two of those types of analysis of variance are indicated in Figure 9: *one-way* and *factorial*. The distinction between those is how the nominal independent variables relate to each other.

One way in which nominal independent variables might relate is that they might all specify categories of the same characteristic. For instance, suppose we were interested in comparing absorbed doses of a particular radionuclide in a specific target organ (the dependent variable) among persons in four racial categories (Asian, black, white, and other). The three nominal independent variables that are required to represent those four categories are related in the sense that they specify different categories of the same characteristic: race. In statistical terminology, we say that they represent categories of a single *factor*.

Now suppose that we are interested in comparing absorbed doses among those four racial categories and between the two genders. The addition of gender to the data set increases the number of groups of dependent variable values that we wish to compare from four to eight. To specify those eight groups, however, we need to add only one nominal independent variable to our analysis. Specifically, we need a nominal independent variable that distinguishes between the two genders as well as the three nominal independent variables that specify the four racial categories. These independent variables are required to distinguish among the categories within only a single characteristic (or, in statistical terminology, within a single factor). Two characteristics are included in this set of data. Thus, the analysis of variance must address more than one factor.

When an analysis of variance consists of more than one factor, there are two different ways in which we can examine the relationships between values of the dependent variable and the categories specified by the nominal independent variables. One of those ways is to compare the means of the dependent variable values among the categories of one factor controlling for the confounding effects of the other factor(s). When we do this, we say that we are examining the *main effect* of the factor for which we are comparing dependent variable value means. Other than the fact that variation in dependent variable values associated with the other factors has been removed when comparing these means, examining the main effect of a factor is the same regardless of whether the analysis contains one or more than one factor.

The other way in which we can examine the relationships between values of the dependent variable and the categories specified by the nominal independent variables is unique to analyses that contain more than one factor. This way is to examine the consistency of the relationship among the means of the dependent variable values for categories of one factor between categories of another factor. For instance, we could compare mean absorbed doses for four racial categories to determine if the relationship of the means among the four racial categories is the same for the men as it is for women. If the relationship among the four racial categories differs between the two genders, we say that there is an *interaction* between race and gender.

When all the nominal independent variables distinguish among (more than two) categories of a single factor (such as when race was the only characteristic of interest), we call the method of analysis a *one-way ANOVA*. When the nominal independent variables specify categories of more than one factor (such as when both race and gender were characteristics of interest), we call the method of analysis a *factorial ANOVA*. These are just two of many different types of analysis of variance. Most of those other types are seldom used in medical research. One special type of ANOVA that is not uncommonly used, however, is a *repeated measures ANOVA*. A repeated measures ANOVA has one (or more) factor that consists of more than one value of the dependent variable measured for each individual. For instance, suppose that we are interested in comparing absorbed doses among the four racial categories and between the two genders as we imagined previously, but now we are also interested in comparing absorbed doses in two different target organs. In that case, target organ is known as a *repeated factor* since each person in the study contributes a dependent variable value for each category of the factor. This is similar to the paired data situation discussed in the section of this chapter that addresses univariable analyses.

Multivariable analyses provide us with two more distinctions from bivariable analyses. One concerns the level at which we examine the relationship between the dependent variable and the independent variables. In multivariable analysis we have a choice between two levels. One possibility is to examine the relationship between the dependent variable and the entire collection of independent variables. In regression analysis, this would imply that we are interested in whether or not all the independent variables taken as a group help to estimate dependent variable values. In analysis of variance, this level involves examination of the consistency of means of the dependent variable values among all categories specified by the nominal independent variables. Inference at this level, testing the relationship between the dependent variable and the entire collection of independent variables, addresses what is known as the *omnibus null hypothesis*.

The other way in which we can examine the relationship between the dependent variable and the independent variables in multivariable analysis is to examine how values of the dependent variable are associated with values of each individual independent variable. In regression analysis, that implies that we would be interested in testing a null hypothesis about the regression coefficient associated with a particular independent variable. The parallel in analysis of variance is comparing two means of dependent variable values. Examination of individual regression coefficients is a usual part of regression analysis. The pairwise comparison of means in analysis of variance, however, is performed using a separate statistical procedure. The most commonly used methods for pairwise comparisons of means is the *Student-Newman-Kuels test*.

ANALYSIS OF COVARIANCE

The other distinction between multivariable and bivariable analyses is that the collection of independent variables in multivariable analyses is not restricted to independent variables that all represent the same type of data. For instance, a data set might contain some nominal independent variables that specify groups of dependent variable values and also contain some continuous independent variables that specify continua along which we wish to examine dependent variable values. The general method of analysis of a continuous dependent variable, one or more nominal independent variables, and one or more continuous independent variables is called *analysis of covariance* or *ANCOVA*.

There are two ways to consider analysis of covariance. If our primary interest is in comparing dependent variable values among the groups specified by the nominal independent variables, we can consider analysis of covariance to be like an analysis of variance in which we control for the confounding effects of one or more continuous variables. For example, suppose that we are interested in comparing absorbed doses of a particular radionuclide among four racial categories as before, but we would like to make that comparison controlling for body mass (represented by a continuous independent variable). Inclusion of body mass as a *covariate* in an analysis of variance computer program would accomplish that comparison.

The other way to consider analysis of covariance is to imagine a regression analysis in which one or more of the independent variables represents nominal data. To understand this view of analysis of covariance, we first need to understand how nominal data can be represented in a regression equation. All of the independent variables in a regression equation must be quantitative. We represent nominal data in a regression equation by using *indicator variables*. Most commonly, indicator variables can be equal to either zero or one. The indicator variable is made equal to one when the nominal event occurs and equal to zero when that event does not occur. For example, if we were interested in examining the relationship between absorbed dose (the dependent variable) and body mass (a continuous independent variable) while taking gender into account, we could perform a regression analysis with gender represented by an indicator variable that was equal to, say, one for women and zero for men. Then, the regression equation would be as shown in Equation 14.

$$(14) \qquad \hat{Y}_{ij} = a + (b_1 \cdot X_i) + (b_2 \cdot I_j),$$

where I_j = the jth value of the indicator variable.

Since the indicator variable is equal to zero for men (in this example), Equation 14 is the same as the following bivariable regression equation when the relationship between absorbed dose (Y) and body mass (X) is examined for men:

$$(15) \qquad \hat{Y}_{i,\text{men}} = a + (b_1 \cdot X_i).$$

When women are considered, the indicator variable is equal to one. Thus, Equation 14 is the same as the following regression equation when the relationship between absorbed dose and body mass is examined for women:

$$(16) \qquad \hat{Y}_{i,\text{women}} = a + (b_1 \cdot X_i) + (b_2) = (a + b_2) + (b_1 \cdot X_i).$$

Equation 16 also is a bivariable regression equation that differs from the bivariable regression equation in Equation 15 in that the intercepts of the regression lines are different for women and men. Specifically, the intercepts of those two regression lines differ by the value of b_2.

We also can make the slopes of the regression lines for men and women differ. To do that, we have to create another variable known as an *interaction variable*. An interaction variable is created by multiplying an indicator variable by another variable. The other variable can be a continuous independent variable or another indicator variable. The following equation illustrates the addition of an interaction variable to Equation 14.

$$(17) \qquad \hat{Y}_{ij} = a + (b_1 \cdot X_i) + (b_2 \cdot I_j) + (b_3 \cdot X_i \cdot I_j).$$

The indicator variable for men is equal to zero and, therefore, the interaction variable is also equal to zero. Thus, the relationship between absorbed dose and body mass for men still is examined in Equation 15 as it was before the addition of the interaction variable. When women are considered, however, the indicator variable is equal to one. Thus, Equation 17 becomes equal to the following regression equation when the relationship between absorbed dose and body mass is examined for women:

$$(18) \qquad \hat{Y}_{i,\text{women}} = a + (b_1 \cdot X_i) + (b_2) + (b_3 \cdot X_i) = (a + b_2) + [(b_1 + b_3) \cdot X_i].$$

Now, the slopes of the regression lines for men and women differ by b_3, the regression coefficient for the interaction variable. This regression analysis view of analysis of covariance, therefore, allows us to compare regression equations examining the relationship between the dependent variable and the continuous independent variable(s) for various categories specified by the nominal independent variable(s). Differences in intercepts between nominal categories are expressed by the coefficients associated with the indicator variables and differences in slopes between nominal categories are expressed by the coefficients associated with the interaction variables.

While thinking about this regression view of analysis of covariance, you might wonder if it is possible to have a regression equation that includes only nominal independent variables. Not only is this possible, but the result of such a regression analysis is the same as analyses we have previously discussed. A regression analysis with one nominal independent variable is exactly the same as the Student's t test we discussed when considering bivariable analysis of a continuous dependent variable. A regression analysis with more than one nominal independent variable is the same as analysis of variance. In fact, every method that we use to analyze a continuous dependent variable can be expressed as a regression analysis. This uniformity of analytic approach for continuous dependent variables is called the *general linear model*.

In multivariable analysis of an ordinal dependent variable, procedures are, as much as possible, parallel to procedures for a continuous dependent variable. The ability to do this, however, is more limited in multivariable analysis than it was in either bivariable or univariable analyses. The reason for this is our inability to perform a regression analysis with an ordinal dependent variable. This inability to perform a regression analysis precludes a nonparametric equivalent to multiple regression analysis, multiple correlation analysis, and analysis of covariance. Thus, we are left only with a nonparametric parallel to analysis of variance.

KENDALL'S COEFFICIENT OF CONCORDANCE

In addition to a nonparametric equivalent to analysis of variance, Figure 13 shows us that we can perform a statistical procedure that has some similarity to correlation analysis. This procedure involves calculation of *Kendall's coefficient of concordance*. Although this is a multivariable procedure, Kendall's coefficient of concordance is more closely related to bivariable correlation analysis than it is to multivariable correlation analysis. It can be interpreted as the average bivariable (Spearman's) correlation coefficient for all possible pairs of variables without regard to whether the variables are the dependent or independent variables. Thus, Kendall's coefficient of concordance cannot be considered as a nonparametric substitute for the multiple correlation coefficient.

Kendall's coefficient of concordance is distinct from other multivariable analyses in another way: the absence of control

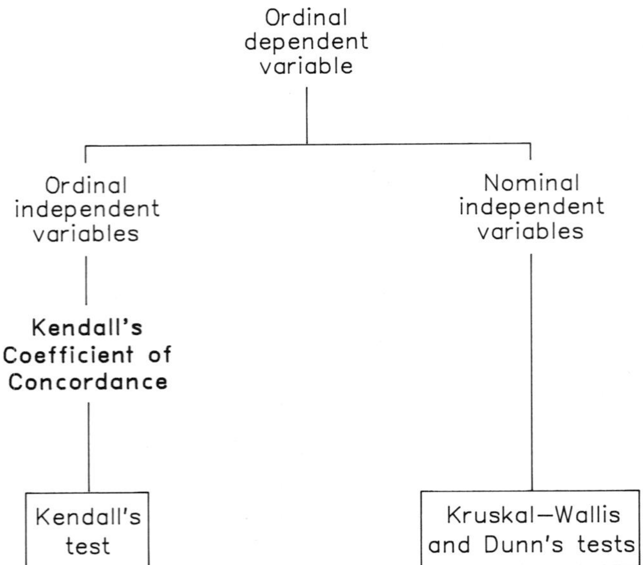

Figure 13. Flowchart illustrating the logical steps involved in selecting a nonparametric procedure for analysis of a multivariable sample with an ordinal dependent variable. The common names of statistical tests appear in boxes.

for the effect of other independent variables when examining the relationship between one independent variable and the dependent variable. In other words, this is a multivariable procedure in which multicollinearity is not functioning.

Special Concerns in Nuclear Medicine

Although any of the statistical procedures we have discussed in the previous sections can be useful in analysis of data in nuclear medicine, a special problem relates to counts when, for instance, there is an interest in the number of radionuclide disintegrations per unit of time. Since this information has a measure of time in the denominator, the number of disintegrations per unit time is a rate (see Equation 4).

As we discussed previously, rates have a Poisson distribution. The statistical procedures for rates that we have discussed so far are based on an approximation of the Gaussian distribution. To use these normal approximations, samples must be relatively large, because the Poisson distribution is a discrete distribution having a limited number of possible values while the Gaussian distribution is a continuous distribution having an unlimited number of possible values. To approximate a continuous distribution with information from a discrete distribution, there should be a large number of possible values. For nominal data, the number of possible values is determined by the size of the sample.

There are two advantages of using normal approximations for discrete distributions compared to using those discrete distributions themselves. The first advantage is that the calculations involved in a normal approximation are fewer than the calculations involved in using the actual discrete distribution. This is not really an important issue if we can rely on computers to perform these calculations for us.

The second advantage of using normal approximations is more an issue of aesthetics than an issue of difficulty. By definition, discrete distributions address frequencies of discrete data values. When calculating probabilities associated with discrete data values, each value has a finite probability of occurrence and values not specified in the distribution have a zero probability of occurrence. This is different from a continuous distribution, such as the Gaussian distribution, in which each specific data value has a probability of occurrence near zero and every data value is possible. The implication of this feature of discrete distributions is that it is often impossible to specify an interval of values that correspond to a particular percentage of the distribution. In interval estimation, this could result in an ability to calculate a 94% confidence interval or a 96% confidence interval, but not a 95% confidence interval. Likewise, it might be possible to conduct statistical inference with an alpha of 0.03, but impossible to use an alpha exactly equal to 0.05.

Even though normal approximations have these advantages compared to using the discrete distribution with which nominal dependent variables are actually associated, there are situations in which these discrete distributions are not well approximated by the Gaussian distribution. This is when the sample is too small. When a sample fails to meet the size requirement for a normal approximation, we are compelled to use a statistical method based on the actual discrete distribution. These methods are known as *exact methods* which must be used when the size requirement for a normal approximation is not satisfied. The use of exact methods, however, is not limited to situations in which a sample is too small to use a normal approximation.

Recall from our earlier discussion that the parameter of the Poisson distribution is the number of events. The population's value for the number of events is symbolized by the Greek letter lambda (λ). The sample's estimate of the number of events is symbolized by a. The probability of obtaining a sample with a events from a population with λ events is calculated using the following equation if we assume that the number of events in all possible samples has a Poisson distribution.

$$p(a) = \frac{\lambda^a \cdot e^{-\lambda}}{a!}, \tag{19}$$

where e = the base of the natural logarithm scale approximately equal to 2.718; $a! = a$ factorial, $a \cdot (a - 1) \cdot (a - 2) \cdot \ldots \cdot 1$.

Now, let us take a look at an example of using the Poisson distribution to calculate an exact interval estimate for a rate.

EXAMPLE

Suppose that we were to count 18 disintegrations during a period of 5 seconds. Let us calculate an exact 95%, two-tailed confidence interval for this rate of decay.

When we calculate an interval estimate, we assume that the sample's estimate is equal to the population's parameter.

Table 2.

NUMBER OF DISINTEGRATIONS	PROBABILITY OF OBSERVING THAT NUMBER	CUMULATIVE PROBABILITY FOR THAT NUMBER
0	0.00000002	0.00000001
1	0.00000027	0.00000029
2	0.00000247	0.00000276
3	0.00001480	0.00001756
4	0.00006662	0.00008418
5	0.00023982	0.00032399
6	0.00071945	0.00104345
7	0.00185002	0.00289347
8	0.00416254	0.00705601
9	0.00832509	0.01538110
10	0.01498516	0.03036626

The parameter of the Poisson distribution (λ) is equal to the number of persons with the event. Thus, we will assume that λ is equal to 18.

The procedure for calculation of a confidence interval using the Poisson distribution involves first calculating a confidence interval for the numerator of the rate and then converting the limits of the confidence interval to rates by dividing the limits by the period of time in the sample. To determine the limits of the confidence interval for the numerator, we calculate probabilities associated with each possible value using Equation 19. For instance, the probability of obtaining a sample in which we observe 18 disintegrations if λ is equal to 18 is calculated as follows:

$$p(a) = \frac{\lambda^a \cdot e^{-\lambda}}{a!} = \frac{18^{10} \cdot e^{-18}}{10!} = 0.01498516$$

First, let us determine the lower limit of the interval estimate. To do this, we calculate the probabilities associated with small numbers of disintegrations. For each of those numbers, we calculate the cumulative probability of obtaining a sample in which we observe that number or fewer disintegrations. Starting with zero disintegrations, we increase the number of disintegrations until we find the number associated with a cumulative probability close to 0.025. For a 95%, two-tailed interval estimate, this is the proportion of the distribution of estimates from all possible samples in the lower tail that we would like to exclude from the interval estimate. Table 2 summarizes those calculations.

From those calculations, we see that the cumulative probability that is closest to 0.025 is 0.03036626 associated with ten disintegrations. Thus, 10 is the lower limit of our interval estimate for the number of disintegrations.

Next, we need to determine the upper limit for the interval estimate. The approach to calculation of the upper limit is somewhat different from the approach to calculation of the lower limit. That difference is in the number of events at which we begin calculating cumulative probabilities. For the lower limit, we begin with zero events, because it is

Table 3.

NUMBER OF DISINTEGRATIONS	PROBABILITY OF OBSERVING THAT NUMBER	CUMULATIVE PROBABILITY FOR THAT NUMBER OR FEWER	CUMULATIVE PROBABILITY FOR THAT NUMBER OR MORE
11	0.02452117	0.05488742	0.96963374
12	0.03678175	0.09166918	0.94511258
13	0.05092858	0.14259776	0.90833082
14	0.06547960	0.20807736	0.85740224
15	0.07857552	0.28665289	0.79192264
16	0.08839747	0.37505035	0.71334711
17	0.09359732	0.46864767	0.62494965
18	0.09359732	0.56224499	0.53135233
19	0.08867114	0.65091613	0.43775501
20	0.07980403	0.73072016	0.34908387
21	0.06840345	0.79912361	0.26927984
22	0.05596646	0.85509007	0.20087639
23	0.04379984	0.89888991	0.14490993
24	0.03284988	0.93173979	0.10111009
25	0.02365191	0.95539170	0.06826021
26	0.01637440	0.97176610	0.04460830
27	0.01091627	0.98268237	0.02823390
28	0.00701760	0.98969997	0.01731763

impossible to observe fewer than zero events. There is no corresponding upper limit to the Poisson distribution. Thus, we need to calculate cumulative probabilities for each number of disintegrations or fewer (as we did in the previous table) and, from those cumulative probabilities, calculate the cumulative probabilities of observing each number of events or more. The following equation shows that calculation for 11 or more disintegrations if the population's parameter is equal to 18.

$$p(a \geq 11) = 1 - p(a \leq 11) + p(a = 11)$$

Table 3 summarizes those calculations beginning where the previous table ended.

For the number of disintegrations that we need for the upper limit of the 95%, two-tailed interval estimate we want to choose the number corresponding to a cumulative probability for that number or greater than 0.025. The closest cumulative probability is 0.02823390 corresponding to 27 disintegrations. Thus, our interval estimate for the number of disintegrations extends from 10 to 27. Instead of a 95% interval estimate this is a 94.14% [1 − (0.03036626 + 0.02823390) = 0.94139984] interval estimate.

Finally, we use the limits of the interval estimate for the number of disintegrations to calculate an interval estimate for the rate of disintegration by dividing each of those limits by the sampling period (5 seconds). From this calculation, we find that the 94.14%, two-tailed exact interval estimate for the rate of disintegration extends from 2.0 to 5.4 per second.

Exact methods can be used for inference or interval estimation in any univariable sample with a nominal dependent variable. Their use makes no assumptions about the size of the sample. They should be used for samples that contain too few observations for normal approximation procedures to be reliable. They also can be used for larger samples. The drawback to their use in larger samples is that the calculations required for exact procedures are more complicated and time consuming than for normal approximation procedures. Further, the results of exact methods are not much different from the results of normal approximation methods when the assumptions of the normal approximation are satisfied.

REFERENCES

1. Hirsch RP, Riegelman RK. *Statistical First Aid. Interpretation of Health Research Data.* Boston: Blackwell Scientific, 1992.
2. Armitage P, Berry G. *Statistical Methods in Medical Research.* 2nd ed. Boston: Blackwell Scientific, 1987.
3. Riegelman RK, Hirsch RP. *Studying a Study and Testing a Test. How to Read the Medical Literature.* 2nd ed. Boston: Little, Brown, 1989.

5 Single Photon Imaging

Michael V. Green, Jürgen Seidel

A general nuclear medicine imaging system performs five basic tasks: (1) photon detection; (2) data acquisition; (3) data processing; (4) image formation; and (5) display and analysis. In this chapter, the first four of these elements are considered as they relate to planar and SPECT (single photon emission computed tomography) imaging with the scintillation camera,[1–144] currently the most common imaging device in nuclear medicine. The last element, image formation, is treated elsewhere in this volume.

Image formation and detection, are intimately connected with the physical processes by which gamma radiation interacts with matter. Image acquisition and processing methods reflect design choices intended to yield images of the highest possible fidelity and these elements are discussed next. The chapter concludes with a discussion of both the physical and computational basis for SPECT imaging with the scintillation camera. We note at the outset that the following work treats a few basic, selected concepts from each of these areas in some detail rather than attempting a broader generalization. The topics selected for presentation, though few, are intended to reveal the essential operational features of the modern scintillation camera in its principal applications and to provide a common framework for understanding these systems regardless of manufacturer. More extensive and general treatments of these and related issues can be found elsewhere in the literature.[145–152]

PHOTON INTERACTIONS WITH MATTER

The modern scintillation camera is designed to create a high-fidelity, two-dimensional representation (or "projection") of three-dimensional radioactivity distributions in the body. Information about these internal distributions, and thus the compounds to which they are attached, is carried by photons liberated by radioactive decay of the tracer nuclide. Most radionuclides used in common clinical single-photon studies emit gamma-ray photons in the energy range between about 50 and 400 keV. In this energy range, two physical processes account for nearly all photon interactions with matter, the photoelectric effect and Compton scattering. In a photoelectric interaction, the photon is absorbed by an atom of the scintillation crystal material through which it is passing. The photon's energy is used to set free an atomic electron and provide it with kinetic energy which, eventually, will be dissipated in the crystal. In contrast, Compton scattering is conceptually like a billiard ball collision between a photon and an electron in the crystal. In such interactions, the incident photon can be regarded as bouncing off the electron and emerging with reduced energy at some angle with respect to its original direction. The portion of the primary photon energy transferred to the electron is dissipated in the crystal.

Given these interaction mechanisms, several possible fates await a photon emitted by a tracer within the body: the photon can simply escape the body without interaction, traveling along the original direction of emission, or it can interact by one of the two processes just noted. The total interaction probability (photoelectric or Compton processes) falls as the photon energy increases, so that the fraction of photons leaving the body without interaction rises with increasing photon energy. If all other factors could be ignored, tracers emitting high-energy photons would be preferred since only noninteracting photons can contribute unambiguously to knowledge of the internal source distribution.

The relative importance of the photoelectric and Compton processes for those photons that do interact in the body (or external instrument) depends on the physical properties of the medium through which the photon is passing and on photon energy. The probability of photoelectric interactions, while modest in low atomic number (Z) materials like the body, rises rapidly with increasing Z number and is very large in materials such as lead (Pb). For example, at a photon energy of 140 keV associated with ^{99m}Tc, the photoelectric mass absorption coefficient for Pb (2.2 cm^2/g) is more than three orders of magnitude greater than for water (0.001 cm^2/g).[153] The Compton effect, on the other hand, is weakly dependent on Z number and the Compton mass absorption coefficients for lead and water at 140 keV differ only slightly. As noted, the probability of either form of interaction decreases as the photon energy increases, but the probability of photoelectric events falls much more rapidly. As a result, at 140 keV in water, only a few percent of all interactions are photoelectric events and the remainder are Compton events. Compton scattering is thus the dominant form of photon interactions in the body in the photon energy range associated with most nuclear medicine tracer studies. On the other hand, where the intention is to intercept every photon in an image-forming or detection device, the photoelectric effect is made to dominate by using high Z-

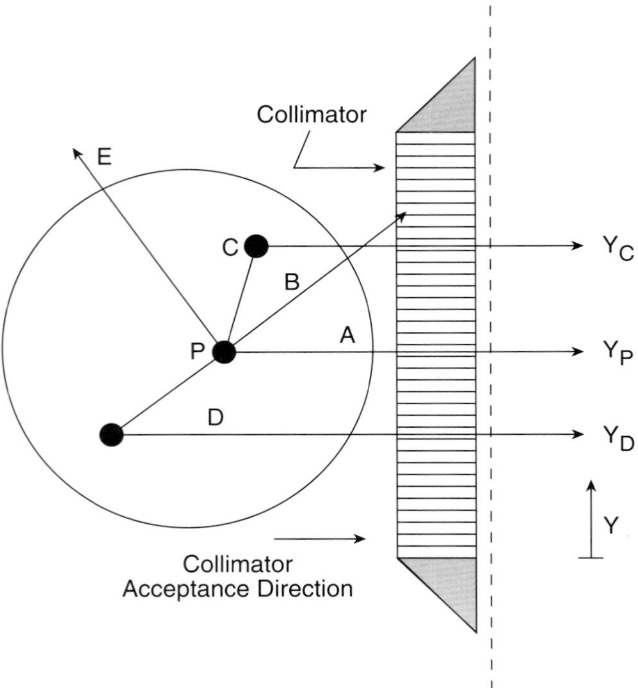

Figure 1. Some photon paths out of the body from a source *P*. Path A events represent "good" photons that emerge from the body without interaction and pass down the collimator holes. Path C and D events are Compton-scatter events and give rise to image "blur."

number materials of high physical density to maximize absorption.

The consequences of these two interaction processes on image formation are schematically illustrated in Figure 1. A point source of radioactivity is assumed to be located at point *P* in an object composed of low-density material such as the body. The paths followed by a few photons emitted from this source are shown. Photons following path A do not interact in the body and are emitted in a direction such that they will pass down one of the holes of the image-forming parallel-hole collimator and emerge at point Y_P. Photons following path B, on the other hand, also escape the body without interaction but are stopped by the collimator and do not contribute to the image. The collimator thus selects for passage only those photons traveling along the direction of path A and excludes all others. All noninteracting photons emitted from all possible source points in the body and traveling parallel to path A constitute the photon set from which the best possible two-dimensional projection image can be made. In general, formation of an ideal image is accomplished with a photon projection set consisting of noninteracting photons traveling in a specified direction or range of directions. For the parallel-hole collimator these paths are (ideally) parallel, while for other collimators the paths are not parallel. With the pinhole collimator, for example, the ideal projection set consists of all noninteracting photons paths lying within a cone whose apex is a single hole (Fig. 2B).

Unlike photons following ideal trajectories without interaction, photons following paths C and D in Figure 1 can also emerge from the body parallel to path A after a Compton interaction and thus can contribute potentially to image formation. However, their passage through the collimator to Y_C and Y_D do not coincide with the point of origin of the photons, Y_P. Thus, the complete set of these Compton-scattered photons can be regarded as forming a blurred image of the object. Inclusion of photons of this kind in an image will degrade image quality by reducing contrast and will make quantification of source activity inaccurate.

Each of the processes illustrated in Figure 1, though conceptually elementary, represents a problem that must be solved if a scintillation camera design is to be successful. We begin by considering how these processes affect the sensitivity and resolution of the image-forming process.

IMAGE FORMATION

Consider first, photons following path E in Figure 1. These photons escape detection by emerging from the body in a direction away from the detector. For a detector that occupies only a portion of the viewing space, as most detectors do, only a fraction of photons will be emitted in a direction that permits even potential detection. Furthermore, since gamma radiation cannot be focused like visible light, image formation is accomplished by photon rejection. In Figure 1, only photons traveling toward the collimator within the small acceptance angle of each individual collimator hole can contribute potentially to an image. All other photons traveling at angles outside this acceptance angle will either miss the collimator altogether or will be intercepted by the collimator material ("septa") and be absorbed. As a consequence, the number of photons emerging from the exit plane of a collimator ("image-forming device") is usually a very small fraction of the total number of photons emitted by the source. Typical values of this fraction are of the order of 10^{-4} to 10^{-5} so that less than 1 photon out of every 10,000 emitted are potentially detectable. This is a severe reduction of sensitivity which consequently sets very stringent limits on nuclear-imaging procedures. It is thus not surprising that collimators are designed to maximize sensitivity to the greatest possible degree subject to other necessary requirements. Since collimators should absorb all photons not traveling in the acceptance direction, they are made of materials that maximize total absorption by the photoelectric effect. The most common collimator material is Pb, a material that possesses a high atomic number and high density ($Z = 82$, $\rho = 11.35$ g/cm^3). For Pb parallel-hole collimators and typical photon energies, the thickness of material between holes ranges from a fraction of a millimeter to a few millimeters and is usually selected such that septal penetration is reduced to

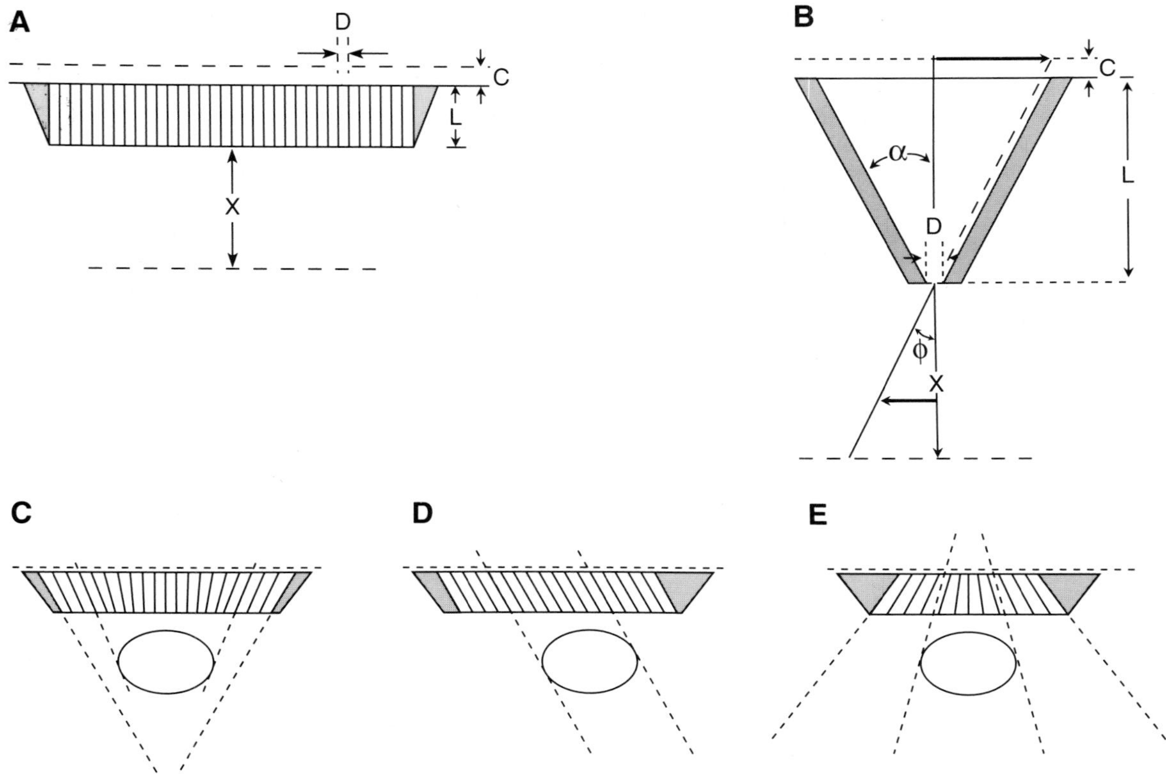

Figure 2. Parallel hole **(A)**, pinhole **(B)**, converging **(C)**, slant **(D)**, and diverging **(E)** collimators used with the scintillation camera. Variables indicated in A and B are defined in the text.

less than 5%. At 100 keV, half of the photons falling perpendicularly on a Pb sheet 0.16 mm thick will be absorbed in the material.

Once the collimator material is chosen, the geometric form into which this material is shaped becomes paramount in achieving a balance between collimator sensitivity, resolution, and image distortion.[25,146] Because this balance is crucial to the imaging process, we will consider two different types of collimators in some detail to illustrate how these tradeoffs can be made.

Parallel-Hole Collimation

The most common type of image formation utilizes the parallel, multihole collimator illustrated schematically in Figure 2A. The performance of this collimator depends on hole diameter (D), hole length (L), septal thickness (T), and the distance between collimator exit plane and the plane in which the image is actually detected (C). Performance also depends on object distance from the front of the collimator (X) and on the collimator material as characterized by its linear attenuation coefficient, μ. (The linear attenuation coefficient is the product of density and mass attenuation coefficient and is expressed in units of inverse centimeters.) The *resolution* of a collimator is its power to differentiate two points on a plane source. The geometric resolution (R) of a parallel-hole collimator is given by the relation[25]:

$$R = D\,\{1 + [(C + X)/L_{eff}]\}, \tag{1}$$

where $L_{eff} = L - 2/\mu$ and is the "effective" hole length, which includes the effects of septal penetration. As the linear attenuation coefficient increases, L_{eff} approaches the true hole length, L. The effect of a finite attenuation coefficient is thus to make the length of each collimator hole appear somewhat less than the true length.

The *sensitivity* (S) of this collimator is the fraction of photons emitted by a source in front of the collimator that emerge from the collimator exit plane. It is given by the relation[25]:

$$S = \{B\,D^2/[L_{eff}(D + T)]\}^2, \tag{2}$$

where B is a constant that depends on hole shape and arrangement.

These equations can be used to assess the relative changes in resolution and sensitivity that occur as the collimator design variables are changed. Imagine, for example, that we wish to image a 140-keV photon emitter. At this energy, C will be small compared to X, and D will probably be large compared to T, ie, septa are thin, so that Equations 1 and 2 reduce approximately to

(3) $$R \approx D + X\,(D/L_{\mathrm{eff}}).$$
(4) $$S \approx B^2\,(D/L_{\mathrm{eff}})^2.$$

According to Equation 3, the geometric resolution of a parallel-hole collimator under the assumed conditions increases, ie, becomes poorer, with growing source distance from the front of the collimator. When the source is against the collimator face, ie, $X = 0$, the geometric resolution of the collimator is equal to the hole diameter D (as it must be). As the source distance increases, the rate of increase of R is set by the slope, D/L_{eff}. When the effective hole length is much greater than the hole diameter, the rate of increase of R is small and resolution degrades slowly as one moves deeper into the object. Conversely, if the hole diameter and effective length are not very different, then the rate of resolution loss as one moves further from the collimator is larger and the resolution at the front of an object and the back of the object may be very different depending on object size. It is clear from Equation 3 that the highest geometric resolution collimator with the most uniform depth response would consist of holes of very small absolute diameter and very great length (absolutely small D, very large L_{eff}). If no other requirements needed to be met, a collimator with these properties would be "ideal" in the sense that it would form a very high resolution image on the subsequent element in the image-processing chain (the image detector). In addition to geometric resolution, however, the sensitivity of the collimator must also be considered. Unfortunately, according to Equation 4, the conditions that optimize the geometric resolution are exactly the same conditions that minimize the sensitivity of the collimator, ie, small D/large L_{eff}. Moreover, the sensitivity S varies as the *square* of this ratio, while the geometric resolution varies more slowly. Thus, small reductions in this ratio to improve geometric resolution will reduce sensitivity disproportionately and care must be taken to achieve a reasonable balance between these factors. Equation 4 also indicates that sensitivity can be increased by choosing a hole shape and a hole arrangement that maximizes the factor B. It has been shown that hexagonal holes arranged in a honeycomb pattern give the largest value of B (25) and most modern collimators are fabricated in this form.

Given these geometric dependencies, it is not surprising that several collimators with different hole lengths and/or diameters (and septal thicknesses) are usually supplied with each scintillation camera so that the collimator can be best matched to the imaging problem at hand. Common parallel-hole collimators for general imaging are often described as high or low sensitivity, high or low resolution, high or low energy, or "all-purpose." Each of these permutations represents some set of geometric factors selected to emphasize one or more performance variables for that collimator. For example, a high- and a low-resolution collimator intended to image 140-keV radiation emitted by ^{99m}Tc might differ in hole diameter by 50%. The high-resolution collimator would possess improved spatial resolution and depth response by virtue of the absolutely smaller hole diameter, but would be four times less sensitive than the low-resolution collimator. In applications where imaging time could be extended to compensate for such a sensitivity loss, the high-resolution collimator might be the collimator of choice. On the other hand, in applications where imaging time, target tracer activity, or both are minimal, lower-resolution collimation might have to be accepted in the interest of acquiring enough data to form a meaningful image. As suggested by this example, differences between real collimators spanning the typical range of performance characteristics do not often differ by more than a factor of 4.

We also note that Equation 4 does not contain the variable X so that the sensitivity of a parallel-hole collimator is independent of source distance, provided that the photon image of the source at the exit plane lies completely within the field of view of the collimator. When this condition is met and a source is moved around within the collimator field of view, photons emerge from the collimator exit plane at a constant rate, independent of source distance or lateral position within the field of view. Resolution, of course, deteriorates with increasing depth but is the same across the field of view if depth is constant.

Pinhole Collimation

Instead of forming an image by selecting photons traveling along parallel paths, image formation is achieved with the pinhole collimator (Fig. 2B) by selecting all photons traveling along lines passing through a single hole. This set of photon paths sweeps out a cone whose apex lies at the pinhole and whose angular width is determined by the angular width of the conical collimator. The geometric resolution (R) and sensitivity (S) of a pinhole collimator are given by the relations[146]:

(5) $$R = D_{\mathrm{eff}}\,[1 + (X/L)].$$
(6) $$S = D_{\mathrm{eff}}^2 \cos^3(\phi)/16X^2.$$

Here, D_{eff} is the effective diameter of the pinhole, X is the perpendicular distance from the pinhole to the plane containing the source, L is the collimator length, and ϕ is the angle between the pinhole axis and the source point location. Like the effective length of a hole in a parallel-hole collimator, D_{eff} depends on the physical diameter of the pinhole, the linear attenuation coefficient of the collimator material, and on the convergence angle of the collimator cone (α). The relationship between actual pinhole diameter and the effective diameter is more complex than for the parallel hole case but the effect is the same, ie, the pinhole appears larger than it actually is because of incomplete attenuation of radiation incident on the edges of the hole.

The equation describing the geometrical resolution of a pinhole collimator is similar in form to that describing the geometrical resolution of a parallel-hole collimator (Equation 1). The best geometric resolution that can be attained with a pinhole collimator is, according to this expression, equal to the effective pinhole diameter. Otherwise, the variation of R with source distance and hole 'length' is identical to that of the parallel hole case and the previous comments about the parallel-hole case also hold here. The expression for the geometric sensitivity of a pinhole collimator, however, is very different from the parallel-hole case. Pinhole sensitivity depends on the inverse square of the distance of the source from the pinhole and on the lateral position of the source within the field of view (due to the strong dependence on the angle ϕ). In contrast, the geometric sensitivity of a parallel-hole collimator is independent of both source distance and location across the field of view. A parallel-hole collimator, moreover, will project a life-size image of an object onto the image detector, in one-to-one correspondence with the real object. An object projected onto the exit plane of a pinhole collimator, however, will be reversed and will vary in size with the distance between object and pinhole. If the arrow shown in Figure 2B lies within the distance L of the pinhole, the length of this arrow when projected onto the collimator exit plane will be physically greater than the actual length of the arrow, ie, the arrow will appear magnified. The behavior of resolution and sensitivity expressed in Equations 5 and 6 and this magnification capability suggest that pinhole collimators can be very useful for imaging small, thin objects that can be placed close to the pinhole. Under these conditions, the otherwise poor sensitivity of a single hole can be increased by placing the object relatively near the hole (small X), along the central axis of the field of view (to minimize the effects of lateral sensitivity variation) and by imaging thin objects to minimize the strong sensitivity variation with source depth. In man, these requirements can be met for superficially located structures that are small, thin, and accessible, eg, the thyroid gland. In small animals such as rats, where these requirements hold for almost all internal body organs, pinhole imaging can be successfully employed to image structures as small as the individual chambers of the heart.[46]

While the pinhole collimator itself is capable of yielding a projection image with the resolution specified in Equation 5, we must also detect this projection image with a device usually of much lower resolution than attainable with the collimator. In practice, as with all collimator-camera combinations, the overall resolution of the image is determined by the combined resolution of camera and collimator. Here, the magnification effect of the pinhole for objects located within a distance L of the pinhole acts to improve the apparent resolution of the system. Since the *intrinsic* resolution (R_i) of a camera is independent of the collimator, an increasingly magnified projection image examined at a fixed (though poor) resolution will appear to exhibit increasingly finer detail, ie, will appear to portray objects at higher resolution. If the magnification M is given by the ratio L/X, then the overall resolution (R_o) of a pinhole image is given by the expression:

$$R_o = [R^2 + (R_i/M)^2]^{1/2}, \qquad (7)$$

where, as M increases, the image resolution approaches that of the projected pinhole image, as it should.

Other Collimators

Collimators have been designed that span the range of possibilities suggested by the two types described above. Several of these are also shown in Figure 2. In the multihole converging collimator (Fig. 2C), all of the holes "look" at a single point, the focal spot.[93,99,100] Though the field of view of a converging collimator is smaller than that of a parallel hole collimator of identical exit plane size, the converging collimator produces a magnified image of objects located between the collimator face and the focal point with relatively greater sensitivity. The diverging collimator shown in Figure 2E is used to produce a minified view of an object larger than the actual camera field of view. The resolution and sensitivity response functions for these two collimators are more complex than for the simple parallel-hole or pinhole collimators. The slant-hole collimator (Fig. 2D) can be placed flat against the body surface to obtain an oblique view of an internal organ.[33] A parallel-hole collimator used for this purpose would have to be rotated away from the body to obtain the same view and spatial resolution would be reduced. Further details about all of these collimator types can be found in References 25, 145, and 146.

Each of the collimators noted above, despite their differences, performs the task of selecting a set of image-forming photon trajectories emanating from a radioactive object and rejecting all others. Possibilities exist for creating magnified or minified images of such objects at high or low resolution, at high or low sensitivities, and with greater or lesser amounts of image distortion that might be introduced by a particular collimator design. The choice of collimator, therefore, depends strongly on the imaging situation if optimum images of a given object are to be obtained. Among the factors that must be considered in this choice are the amount of tracer nuclide likely to appear in the imaging target, the length of time available to image the target, the size and proximity of the target relative to other radioactive objects in the surrounding environment, and, ultimately, the kinds of measurements one wishes to make on the acquired image data. Each of these elements (and others) must be considered if the basic data selected by the image forming device are to optimally portray the spatial and temporal distribution of the administered radiopharmaceutical. If these choices have been carefully made, the next step in the imaging procedure is to detect this optimized image at the collimator exit plane. We consider this process of image detection with the scintillation camera in the next section.

IMAGE DETECTION

Early Scanners

The density of photon paths through the collimator exit plane defines a two-dimensional projection image of the distribution of photon origins as they exist in the object. In order to record this two-dimensional density function, an image detector is required that can accurately locate over the entire exit plane each point where a photon emerges from this plane. Prior to the development of the scintillation camera, images of internal radiotracer distributions were most often made with a single, mechanically driven detector moved slowly from point to point in a plane over the organ of interest. These *rectilinear* scanners, as they were known, consisted of a single, collimated sodium iodide detector coupled to a single photomultiplier tube. Collimators for these mechanical scanners were most often of the converging type (see Fig. 2C) with relatively short focal lengths. When imaging an organ, the detector was placed such that the focal point of the collimator scanned through the organ of interest at an appropriate depth. Because activity at the focal point of a converging collimator is seen by all collimator holes, the focal plane was scanned with the greatest sensitivity. Planes above and below the focal plane were seen with less sensitivity. This depth dependent sensitivity variation caused rectilinear scanners to produce images in which one plane of activity contributed more to the image than others, an early form of tomographic imaging. While these rectilinear scanners produced images of good diagnostic quality for very slowly changing activity distributions, imaging times were often very long because, effectively, only one point in the object could be examined at once. Because of the serial nature of this data acquisition process, dynamic imaging procedures with time scales of the order of seconds were unknown, and to some degree unthinkable, given the characteristics of the rectilinear scanner.

THE ANGER CAMERA

In the late 1950s and 1960s, Anger[6–8] described an imaging system that overcame nearly all of the limitations of the rectilinear scanner while simultaneously opening the way for high-speed, dynamic imaging. With the development of ^{99m}Tc-labeled radiopharmaceuticals in the 1960s and 1970s, agents that could be administered in high doses, the scintillation camera became the standard imaging system in diagnostic nuclear medicine, a position the camera occupies to this day. The scintillation camera has been dramatically improved technologically during the intervening years and has been adapted to SPECT imaging,[2–5] but the principles first outlined by Anger continue to provide the conceptual basis for all modern single-photon cameras. The reasons for the success of this device lie primarily in the approach that Anger took toward image detection.

A cutaway view of a stylized scintillation camera is shown in Figure 3. There are three essential elements to this system: (1) the image-forming collimator; (2) a disc or slab of scintillation material, most often sodium iodide (NaI) doped with small amounts of thallium (Tl); and (3) a bank of photomultiplier (electron multiplier) tubes (PMTs) packed together to cover the full area of the scintillator and optically coupled by

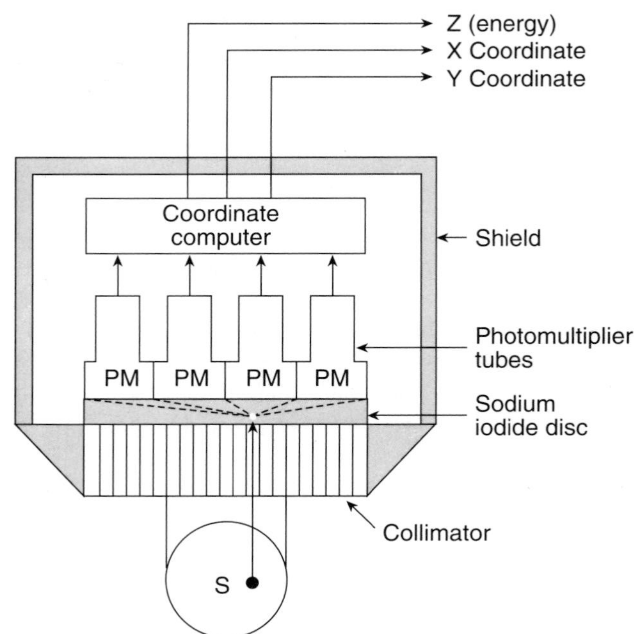

Figure 3. Cutaway view of an idealized scintillation camera.

"lightpipes" (not shown) to the rear surface of the scintillator crystal. The scintillator acts as the image detection element in this system.

The operation of the camera is conceptually straightforward. Photons passed by the image-forming device emerge from the collimator exit plane and are intercepted by the scintillator disc. Depending on photon energy, many of these photons are completely absorbed within the scintillator. When a photon is absorbed, a portion of the absorbed energy [NaI(Tl): $\approx 3\%$][157] is converted to fluorescent radiation that radiates away from the point of interaction inside the crystal. The number of these fluorescent photons is proportional to the amount of energy deposited in the crystal by the original photon: a "bright" flash of fluorescent radiation in the crystal corresponds to a large energy deposition while a "faint" flash corresponds to a small amount of deposited energy. The number of the fluorescent photons varies almost linearly with deposited energy but is never really very large even in the most efficient scintillators. Typical values range from less than a hundred to a few thousand fluorescent photons per event. These photons move away from the site of production and some will exit the crystal through the rear face where they can fall on the photocathodes of the coupled photomultiplier tubes. The purpose of these tubes is to collect for each individual event as many of the fluorescent photons as possible and for each tube to produce an amplified signal proportional to the number collected by that tube. By inspection of Figure 3, it is clear that the number of fluorescent photons falling on any given phototube will depend on the location of the gamma-ray interaction relative to that tube. If, for example, the gamma ray interacts near the center of a phototube (as illustrated in Fig. 3), the signal from this tube will be relatively large, since many photons will fall on its photocathode. Tubes farther away from the interaction site will produce progressively smaller signals, since they will "see" fewer and fewer of the emitted fluorescent photons. Because the entire set of photomultiplier signals will change continuously with changes in the position of the initial gamma-ray interaction, it would seem intuitively plausible that this set of signals could be used to compute the location of the primary interaction. Anger recognized that the *X-Y* location of any interaction point could be computed by taking the weighted average of these signals and in the original camera this computation was accomplished in analog form for each scintillation event. The image-forming component of the camera thus intercepts gamma rays passed by the image-forming device, converts this gamma-ray pattern into an equivalent pattern of fluorescent photon origins, and computes the location of these origins for each event as it occurs. In operation, the camera generates a stream of *X-Y* coordinates that locate the point of interaction of each gamma ray within the field of view and, by summing the outputs of all of the phototubes, produces an estimate of the total energy (*Z*) deposited in the crystal by that gamma-ray interaction.

Scintillators

In order to understand the relative importance of these various processes on the overall image-forming process, we consider each of these components in some detail. First, because the intent is to stop all photons emerging from the exit plane of a collimator, the scintillator material should maximize total photon absorption by the photoelectric effect subject, of course, to the added condition that the absorber also be a "good" scintillator (see Chapters 2 and 3 for further details). Although many scintillators have been discovered, crystals of sodium iodide doped with the element thallium are, by far, the most common scintillating material used in modern cameras. NaI(Tl) has a density of 3.7 g/cm^3 and a total mass absorption coefficient of 0.8 cm^2/g at 140 keV.[153] At this energy, the linear attenuation coefficient of this material is near 3 cm^{-1} and the half-value thickness (thickness required to absorb half the photons) is about 2.3 mm. Thus, more than 75% of 140-keV photons falling on a slab of NaI (Tl) scintillator will be absorbed in a crystal less than 5 mm thick.

The number of fluorescent photons emitted per kiloelectron volt of energy deposited in the crystal by an absorption event determines the quality of the scintillator. If all other factors could be ignored, a material exhibiting a high fluorescent photon yield would be preferred to a scintillator with lower yield. NaI(Tl) possesses one of the highest fluorescent photon yields of any known scintillator, making this material a good choice for image detection in the scintillation camera. This effect is important to the image detection process because the number of fluorescent photons produced in a given absorption event is a statistical variable. If, for example, two gamma rays are totally absorbed in the scintillator, the number of fluorescent photons produced in each interaction will generally not be the same even though the energy deposited in the crystal was the same. The actual number produced will vary somewhat around the mean number for that absorbed energy so that the energy deposited by the gamma ray will appear somewhat uncertain. The lower the conversion efficiency, the larger this uncertainty will be.

Photomultipliers

This effect is further exacerbated in the next step in image detection. Fluorescent photons radiate away from the point of gamma-ray interaction and fall on the photocathodes of the coupled PMTs in varying proportions depending on the distance from the point of interaction. For the phototube to produce a useful signal, the incoming fluorescent photons must be captured on the photocathode of the phototube and the fluorescent energy converted to a proportionate electron output inside the tube. This process can be accomplished efficiently only if the wavelength of the fluorescent light matches the wavelength at which the photocathode material most efficiently releases photoelectrons. In NaI(Tl), for example, the maximum number of fluorescent photons are emitted at a wavelength of 415 nm. Photocathodes with a spectral response far from this value would produce a small photoelectron yield, and hence a small output signal. In addition, like the number of fluorescent photons produced by gamma-ray absorption, the number of photoelectrons produced by fluorescent photon absorption is also a statistical variable. The smaller this number, the larger the relative uncertainty in photoelectron number. To take advantage of the high light output of NaI(Tl), and thus minimize the relative uncertainty in photoelectron number, phototubes with bialkali photocathodes are now used in almost all scintillation cameras. These materials are well matched to the 415-nm spectral output of NaI(Tl) and have their peak response at nearly the same wavelength.

The next step in the PMT signal-generating chain is to efficiently collect, and then multiply, all photoelectrons generated by the burst of fluorescent radiation falling on the photocathode. Collection of these photoelectrons at the first tube "dynode" is particularly important in determining the eventual magnitude of the amplified tube output. Because the number of photoelectrons produced by a typical gamma-ray absorption event is generally small, the loss of even a few of these photoelectrons at the first amplification stage can have a substantial effect on the magnitude of the tube output. The loss of a few electrons farther down the amplification chain, however, has less and less of an effect because the total number of electrons increases rapidly from one amplification stage to the next. Care must be taken, therefore, in the design of phototubes to insure that the relatively small number of photoelectrons that comprise the initial photoelectron signal input to the amplification chain are collected with the greatest possible efficiency. PMTs used in modern cameras have been optimized to achieve such high-collection efficiencies.

Gamma-Ray Energy (Z Signal) and Energy Resolution

Each of the effects just described contributes to uncertainties in locating a gamma-ray interaction within the camera's field of view and in determining the amount of energy deposited in the crystal by that interaction. The relationship between these physical processes and uncertainties can be visualized by considering how the set of simultaneous PMT outputs is used to compute event locations and energy deposition. From previous comments, the sum of all phototube signals for each event is an estimate of the total energy deposited in the crystal by the gamma-ray interaction. Through a chain of successive proportions, energy deposition is linearly related to the magnitude of this sum pulse or "Z" signal as it is often called. This sum pulse, however, has some variability due to the cumulative uncertainties noted for each step connecting the initial energy deposition in the crystal to the magnitude of the output pulse. Thus, even if a crystal is illuminated with purely monoenergetic gamma radiation and this radiation is totally absorbed, there will appear to be a range of gamma-ray energies distributed about a mean energy in a Gaussian-like fashion. The full width at half maximum (FWHM) of this distribution divided by the mean photopeak energy is called the relative energy resolution of the scintillator/PMT combination. For modern scintillation cameras, relative energy resolution is of the order of 10 to 15% at 140 keV.

Event Positioning

The effect of these perturbing physical processes on event location is somewhat more complex and, to understand this relationship, we need to understand how event positions are computed from the phototube output signals. As an illustration of the physical basis for this computational process, we show in Figure 4A an ideal, very long one-dimensional scintillation camera.

We first assume that all the phototubes are physically identical, uniformly spaced, and have identical electrical properties. If we now move a point source across the full camera field, the pattern of signal outputs S_i from the tubes will change as the source position changes. When the point source is at the left, for example, the output from the left-hand tubes will be large since most of the fluorescent radiation will fall on these tubes. As the source moves further to the right, the size of the signals from the left-hand tubes decreases while signal size increases for the right-hand tubes. This pattern of magnitudes is unique for each source position, so it should be possible to compute the source position from this pattern. Indeed, the pattern of signal responses for a given source position can be regarded as discrete samples of the fluorescent light output curve shown in Figure 4B taken in increments equal to the center-to-center tube spacing. Such a sampling provides the information necessary to locate the "centroid" of the light output curve being sampled. A centroid or center-of-gravity calculation has the form:

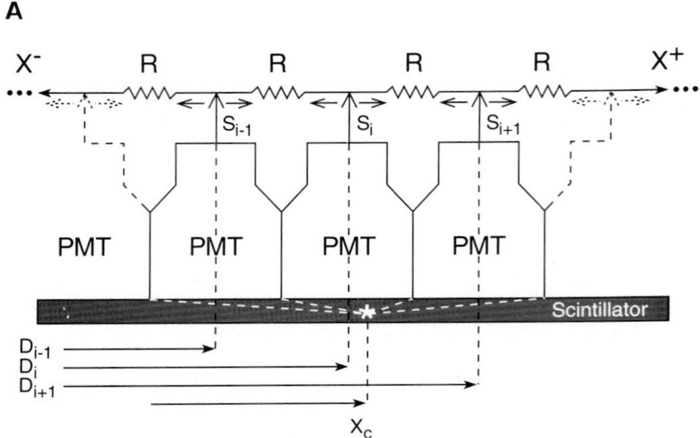

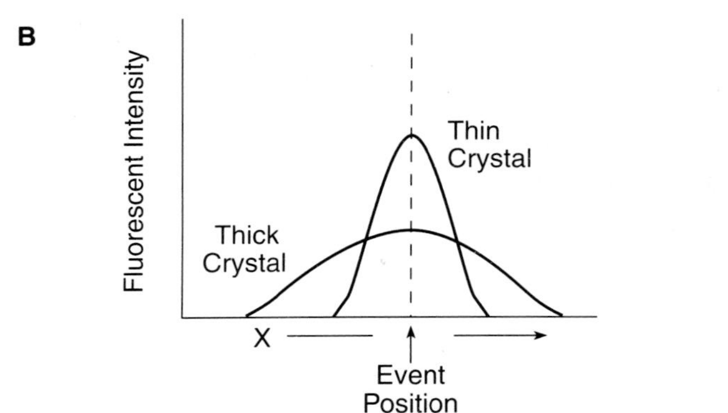

Figure 4. Idealized one-dimensional scintillation camera using resistive (R) division of the photomultiplier tube (PMT) signals, S_i, for event positioning **(A).** Fluorescent light output curves at the rear surface of a thick and a thin scintillator for a gamma-photon absorption **(B).**

$$X_c = \Sigma[S_i(D_i/W)]/\Sigma(S_i). \quad (8)$$

Here, X_c is the centroid value expressed as a fractional distance across the field of view, D_i is the distance from the origin of the X coordinate system to the center of tube i, W is the width of the camera's field of view, and S_i is the magnitude of the output signal from tube i. In this relation, the tube signals S_i serve to weight the tube distances D_i/W according to the magnitude of S_i. The larger the S_i, the larger will be the contribution of distance D_i/W to the centroid sum. Equivalently, the nearer the interaction point is to the tube center, the greater will be the size of S_i for that tube and the greater will be the weight applied to the corresponding distance D_i/W.

In order to calculate the centroid value, the sequence of operations indicated in Equation 8 must be carried out for each scintillation event, that is, for every light flash in the crystal, a signal pattern S_i is generated. Each S_i must then be multiplied by the corresponding distance factor D_i/W and summed with all other $S_i(D_i/W)$ products to yield the numerator in Equation 8. The individual signals S_i must also be simultaneously summed to yield the denominator in Equation 8. The final step is to compute the ratio of numerator to denominator and output this result as the X_c coordinate of the event. This entire computation must be performed on a time scale of microseconds (including a Y coordinate computation in a real camera) so that a practical method of performing this calculation is essential.

Anger performed the centroid calculation by passing the signal set for each event through an analog computing network. Several different physical processes have been used to perform this calculation and one of these is shown in Figure 4A. Here, the output of each tube is divided by a resistor chain whose total resistance to the left and to the right depends on the distance of the tube along the chain (or distance between the left and right edges of the camera's field of view). Output current from any tube i will be divided by this array such that $(W - D_i)/W$ of the current flows to the left and D_i/W flows to the right. The currents in each of these paths from all tubes are physically additive and yield two signals (usually) called X^+ and X^- to distinguish one from the other:

(9) (a) $X^- = \Sigma(S_i(W - D_i)/W)$
(b) $X^+ = \Sigma[S_i(D_i/W)]$

The most common method for computing the centroid is to use the sum and the difference of these signals:

(10) $X^+ - X^- = \Sigma[2\, S_i(D_i/W) - S_i]$ and
$X^+ + X^- = \Sigma(S_i)$.

The ratio of the difference to the sum gives

(11) $(X^+ - X^-)/(X^+ + X^-) = 2\{\Sigma[S_i(D_i/W)]/\Sigma(S_i)\} - 1$
$= 2\, X_c - 1$.

Thus, the ratio of the difference to the sum is proportional to the centroid position or solving explicitly,

(12) $X_c = (1/2)\, [(X^+ - X^-)/(X^+ + X^-)] + (1/2)$

This calculation, carried out by passively partitioning the tube outputs and using simple sum and division circuits, allows the position of scintillation events to be calculated at a very high rate. According to this expression, when the two signals are equal, $X^+ = X^-$, the X_c position equals 1/2, or halfway across the field of view (as it must be symmetry). On the other hand, when X^+ is much greater than X^-, X_c equals 1 (the far right edge of the camera). When the opposite is true, X_c is zero and the event occurred at the far left edge of the camera. This ratio technique thereby generates all possible positions along the X axis. The tube currents are also partitioned in the Y direction and the same calculation is made to compute Y_c. The final step is to sum the two denominators $(X^+ + X^-) + (Y^+ + Y^-)$ to obtain an estimate of the energy of the absorbed photon (Z). Each scintillation event, therefore, results in three simultaneously generated values: X_c and Y_c that locate the event and the Z pulse which is proportional to the absorbed photon energy for that event. The stream of these triplets emerging from the camera constitutes the information from which images of the target object are formed.

Spatial Resolution

This positioning scheme is not perfect and a number of factors conspire to introduce uncertainty into the computed X_c and Y_c values. The amount of uncertainty is known as the *intrinsic spatial resolution* of the camera, and it is of interest to determine the variables upon which intrinsic spatial resolution depends.

If we use Equation 8 to calculate the X_c values for our ideal camera, it is not difficult to show that the variance of this centroid value is given by

(13) $\mathrm{var}(X_c) \approx [1/(\Sigma S_i)]\ \{\Sigma[S_i(D_i/W)^2]/\Sigma S_i\} - X_c^2]$

and the resolution by

(14) $R \approx [\mathrm{var}(X_c)]^{1/2}$,

where $\mathrm{var}(X_c)$ is the square of the standard deviation of the estimated value of X_c and R is the camera resolution. We obtained Equation 13 by applying "error propagation"[154] to the centroid equation and by using the fact that the variance of an individual phototube signal is given by

(15) $\mathrm{var}(S_i) \approx S_i$.

According to Equation 13, the variance in X_c can be expressed as the product of two terms. The first term depends inversely on the sum of the phototube signals and will decrease as the signal sum increases. The signal sum can be increased in two ways. First, the energy of the incident photons could be increased thereby increasing the brightness of each scintillation and each S_i. Since the signal sum is proportional to the photon energy (E):

(16) $R \approx 1/E^{1/2}$

so that camera resolution improves with increasing photon energy.

The second way that the signal sum could be increased would be to improve the efficiency of the fluorescent light production/collection/conversion process. If the incident photon energy is fixed, improvement in the efficiency of any of the steps leading to the output S_i will increase the size of the S_i. Such improvements might include using a scintillator with a higher light conversion efficiency, a greater transmission efficiency to its own fluorescent light, a more efficient optical coupling of the scintillator to the phototubes, increased conversion efficiency of the photocathode material of the phototubes, and so on. Indeed, Equation 16 suggests a means of improving camera performance by improving each of these component elements.

The second term in Equation 13 also affects spatial resolution, but in a less obvious way. This term, however, can be used to predict the effects of increasing the phototube packing density and diminishing the crystal thickness. As crystal thickness decreases, the shape of the light output curve at the rear surface of the scintillator changes (Fig. 4B) and becomes more sharply peaked along the shortest path to the crystal surface. If we now simultaneously increase the number of phototubes per unit length, ie, more smaller tubes, we will sample this new, narrower light output curve completely but over a smaller absolute distance across the crystal. This is entirely equivalent to saying that the distances between the calculated centroid value and the tube centers that contribute to the centroid value are small. The consequences of this effect can be visualized by imagining what happens when crystal thickness approaches zero and the number of phototubes becomes infinitely large. As these conditions are approached, the light output curve will become more and more sharply peaked until only one infinitely narrow phototube is illuminated giving rise to a single PMT signal S_0. If this single constant S_0 is substituted appropriately into the second term of Equation 13, the second term becomes zero and the corresponding spatial resolution is perfect. Thus, spatial resolution can be improved by decreasing crystal thickness and increasing the phototube packing density. There are obvious limits to this strategy in the design of real cameras, however, since a camera with an infinitely thin crystal will also have zero sensitivity.

Camera Improvements

Early scintillation cameras were constructed with thick crystals, in part because radiopharmaceuticals available at the time emitted relatively high energy photons, eg, I-131 at 364 keV, and thick crystals were required to increase sensitivity. Early cameras were also fabricated with a small number of relatively large-diameter phototubes whose performance characteristics were substantially different (poorer) from those available today. When these factors were added to other inefficiencies in the signal processing chain, the net result was cameras with relatively poor performance.[6,8–14]

With the rapid proliferation of ^{99m}Tc-labeled radiopharmaceuticals in the 1970s and 1980s, however, camera manufacturers began to redesign their systems to capitalize on the high stopping power of NaI (Tl) for 140-keV radiation. At this energy, crystals could be made thinner and smaller. High-performance phototubes were used to improve the efficiency of the overall light collection/signal generation process. Other improvements were also introduced, including the use of threshold amplifiers on each of the PMTs. With such amplifiers, a minimum signal must be detected by a phototube before a signal is emitted. If the signal level does not exceed the preset threshold, the tube remains silent and does not emit a signal. The effect of this thresholding can be predicted by Equation 13. According to this equation, tubes far from the calculated centroid, X_c, can contribute a substantial amount to the variance sum even though the signals generated by these distant tubes are small. On the other hand, these distant tubes contribute little to the centroid calculation itself. Thus, elimination of the contribution of distant tubes that see little light will have little or no effect on the centroid calculation, but will reduce the variance and improve intrinsic spatial resolution. This and the other improvements noted above have, in fact, lead to very substantial improvements in spatial resolution.

Attempts to increase spatial resolution, however, can introduce new variables that adversely affect system performance. In the discussion above regarding event positioning, we assumed that the gain of a phototube, ie, the electron multiplication factor of the tube, was independent of the location of the scintillation event. Spatially dependent inhomogeneities in the photocathodes of phototubes or in the charge collection/amplification process, however, can cause tube gain to appear to depend on exactly where the light flash occurred. In thick crystals coupled to thick light pipes, scintillation events tend to occur relatively far from the photocathodes of each phototube so that the variation in light intensity across each tube is not very great and photocathode inhomogeneities are averaged out. In cameras with thin crystals and thin (or no) light pipes, the light distribution across a given phototube can vary appreciably and spatial inhomogeneity in the photocathode will give rise to gain variations that depend on source position. If this is so, the positioning equations noted earlier cannot be rigorously correct since they were derived by assuming a constant, position-independent gain response for each tube. Such behavior could give rise to nonlinearities in the positioning of scintillation events and, for the same reason, to apparent changes in uniformity by crowding events together at some locations in the field of view and spreading them out at others. These and other similar effects are addressed in modern scintillation cameras by applying several corrections to each event, corrections that compensate for distortions in linearity and uniformity. Since these corrections are responsible for the rather remarkable performance of contemporary cameras,[2–5,25,146] it is worthwhile examining these corrections in some detail.

Gain and Linearity Corrections

Consider first the Z energy signal output of a camera that has spatial variations in gain. Illumination of the full crystal of this camera causes different Z pulse values, even though the brightness of each light flash does not vary from one location to the next. The difference in regional gains gives rise to energy spectra at each image point compressed or expanded along the energy axis. If these spectra are summed to produce an energy spectrum for the full field of view, a photopeak in this summed spectrum will be artificially broader than the same photopeak observed at any single image point. As a result, the energy resolution of the system is degraded and the ability to reject scattered radiation becomes spatially dependent.

Corrections for spatial variations in gain are accomplished in a two-step process and require some specialized hardware.

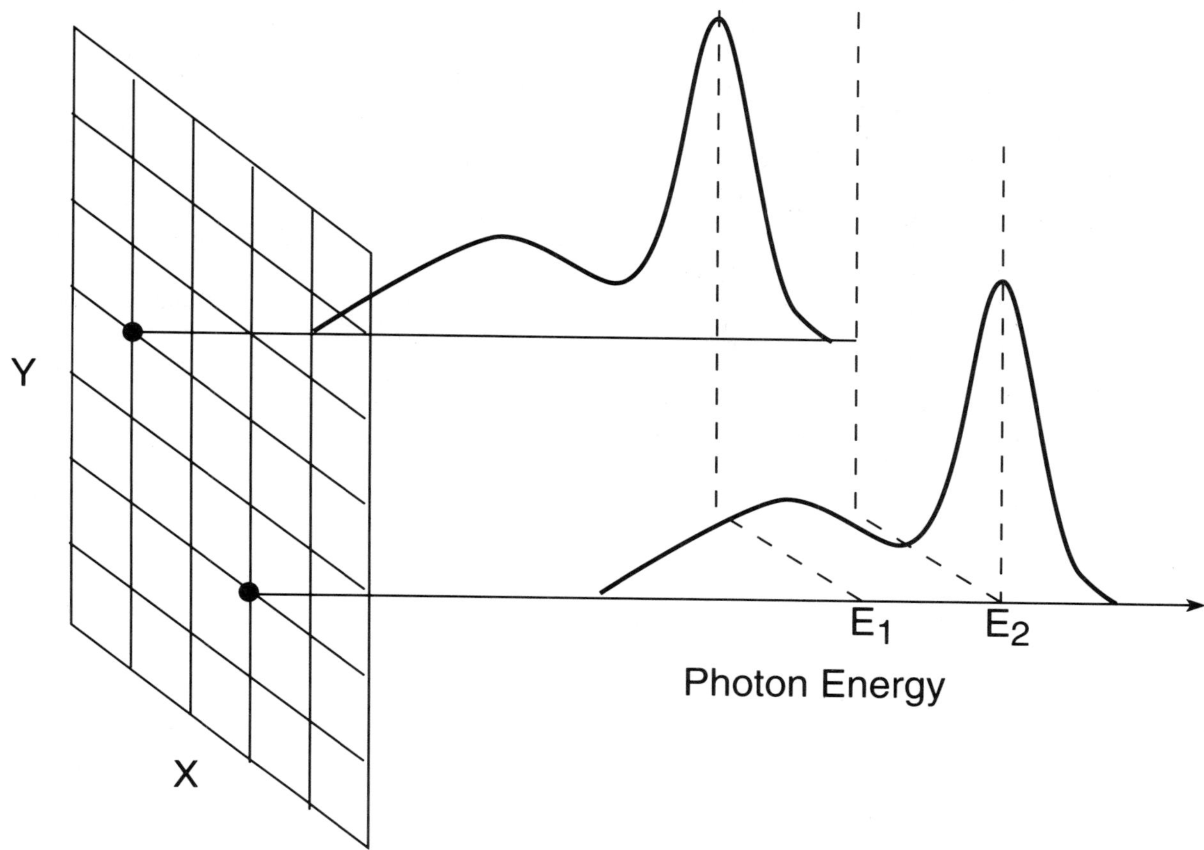

Figure 5. Schematic illustration of an energy acquisition in which the photon energy spectrum is recorded at each image point. Due to a gain difference at the two locations, the photopeak maxima do not occur at the same energy location along the energy axis. The observed locations, eg, E_1 and E_2, are used to calculate multiplicative corrections to remove this gain variation.

First, a uniform (flood) source of ^{99m}Tc or some other radionuclide is imaged for an extended period at a moderate count rate. Instead of simply recording the number of events, the energy spectrum is recorded at each image point. This is accomplished in practice by adding a third parameter to the acquisition, namely, the magnitude of the *Z* pulse associated with each event. This kind of "energy acquisition" is illustrated in Figure 5. If the gain of the camera were the same everywhere in the field of view, the location of the maximum of each photopeak along the energy axis would be identical. In reality, however, gain varies with position so that the location of the maximum of each photopeak is generally different (E_1 and E_2 in the figure). Since the intrinsic brightness of a total-absorption event does not change from one point in the crystal to the next, the observed variation in the location of a photopeak maximum must be due to a local gain variation in the camera. Thus, we may use the measured locations of the photopeak maxima to calculate gain corrections at each image point that normalizes gain across the field of view. These corrections are calculated by examining each energy spectrum in Figure 5 and locating the largest count value. The average channel number at which these maxima occur is computed for all points in the full field of view. Using this value as the normalizing factor, the ratio of this average to the channel number of each individual photopeak maximum location is computed and stored as a two-dimensional "lookup" table or gain correction "map" of the field of view. The dimensions of this map are *X* by *Y* and each *X,Y* value addresses the correction factor for that location. A photopeak maximum location exceeding the mean location gives rise to a correction factor less than unity, while photopeak maxima less than the mean photopeak location give rise to correction factors greater than unity.

In practice, gain corrections are applied "on the fly" for each detected event by first computing the *X,Y* location of the event. This coordinate pair is then used to address the lookup table at location *X,Y* and retrieve the correction factor for that location. The magnitude of the current *Z* pulse is then multiplied by this factor to obtain the gain-corrected *Z* pulse. If all image points are subjected to this method of correction, the entire field of view will appear to have uniform gain equal to the mean gain, and the energy location of every photopeak maximum will occur at the same point along the energy axis. As was noted earlier, summation of

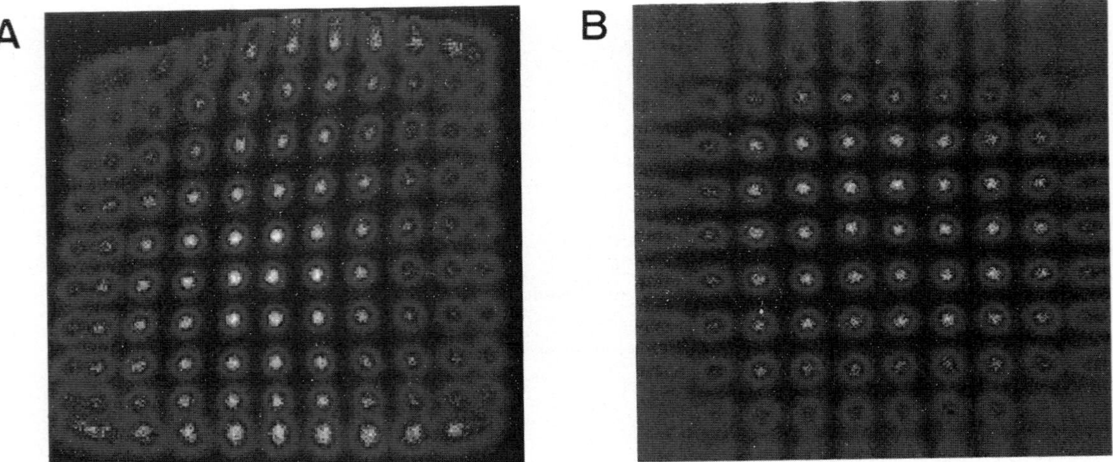

Figure 6. Orthogonal hole plate image before **(A)** and after **(B)** correction for spatial nonlinearities. (See Plate 1.)

uncorrected Z pulses in the output energy spectrum of a camera reduces the energy resolution of the system by combing individual spectra acquired at different gains. The scheme just described reduces this energy blurring by locally adjusting all of the gains to the same effective value. As a result, energy resolution (and scatter rejection) and spatial uniformity are improved.

The accuracy of event positioning, for reasons already noted, varies across the field of view of a typical scintillation camera. Correction of these positioning errors, like the gain correction, is a two-step process: first, a test image with known properties is acquired and, second, these data are used to compute a lookup table whose elements are the corrections that remove the observed X and Y positioning errors from all subsequently acquired images. A suitable test object for making these spatial linearity corrections is a Pb sheet drilled through with pinholes spaced at regular intervals in a square array. With the camera collimator removed, this orthogonal hole plate is placed over the crystal and illuminated by photons from a distant source, eg, several meters away, to provide a near parallel incident photon beam. An image of the hole pattern is thereby projected onto the crystal. In general, the image of the holes and the known regular pattern of the holes differs and it is from these differences that position corrections are computed. An image obtained with such an orthogonal hole plate is shown in Figure 6A. Although the hole array is regular, the image of the hole array shows spatial nonlinearities. In the upper left-hand corner of the image, the relationship between projected and imaged holes is markedly distorted. Deviations from straightness in the alignment of the holes are also evident over the remainder of the field of view. Such deviations are best appreciated by viewing this figure at a glancing angle and looking along a row or column of the projected dots. (These images, and those in Figure 19, were obtained with an experimental small-field-of-view scintillation camera that uses a single position-sensitive PMT for event location.[45,47])

Given the distortions shown in the figure, it is not difficult to imagine how a correction for these distortions might be performed. We could first identify the location of maximum brightness at each projected spot and assume that this maximum identifies the spot center. Since we know that each spot center is actually part of a regular array, we could determine the displacements of each spot center in both the X and Y directions that would force each spot center to lie on a regular array. If, during data acquisition, an event occurred at a spot center, we would simply apply the stored corrections to that coordinate point to map the event onto the regular array. While this strategy would work for events occurring at spot centers, most events occur between spot centers. Corrections for these intermediate events can be computed by noting that corrections for such events lie intermediate to the corrections computed for the four spot centers that bound each local quadrilateral; methods for calculating such corrections have been developed.[25,156] Within a given quadrilateral region, for example, the corrected position ($X_{corrected}$, $Y_{corrected}$) of an event can be obtained via "bilinear interpolation"[156]:

$$(17)\qquad \begin{aligned} X_{corrected} &= A*X + B*Y + C*X*Y + D \\ Y_{corrected} &= E*X + F*Y + G*X*Y + H, \end{aligned}$$

where the coefficients A, B, $C \ldots H$ are constant and X and Y are the measured coordinates of the event. The four coefficients in each equation can be found from the measured (or distorted) coordinates of the four vertices and the known locations of the four vertices in "corrected" space.

The results obtained with a correction scheme of this kind are illustrated in Figure 6B. The test image (Fig. 6A) was used to calculate corrections for each spatial location in the manner described above. This particular linearity correction method was selected because of the nature of the variations revealed in the test image. If these distortions were regular over the entire field of view, two simple global functions might be sufficient to calculate the "true" location of each event. In Figure 6A, however, the spatial nonlinearities are not regular and have both long- and short-range components that cannot be accurately modeled over the whole field of view by a few, simple continuous algebraic functions. The only way to achieve accuracy over the whole field is to subdivide the field of view into small regions within which spatial variations are relatively small, but in aggregate can reflect spatial variations over greater distances. Over most of the field of view (Fig. 6B) this strategy is effective, failing only at the edges of the field of view where uniformity and linearity distortions are large.

When all local corrections have been computed and stored as a lookup table, the measured X,Y coordinates of an event are used to address this table and recall the corrections for that coordinate set or the corrected coordinates directly. In the system used to create the images shown in Figure 6, this correction process occurs in real time as the event is acquired, which is the usual way such corrections are implemented in commercial imaging systems. These corrected coordinates are then used thereafter to represent the detected event. A number of subtleties are associated with spatial linearity corrections that must be considered in the real implementation of these techniques.[156]

Both of the correction techniques described above, for regional gain and spatial linearity, can be applied in real time using very fast computational techniques preceded by detailed system calibrations. These corrections presume, however, that the energy signals and position coordinates of detected events have the same meaning over time as when the calibrations were performed so that corrections made at some later date remain valid. Because, ultimately, changes in individual phototube gains will introduce variations into both regional position and energy calculations (and into certain scatter correction methods described later), methods must be devised to maintain individual phototube performance within narrow tolerances. A number of novel methods[25,146] have been developed to improve phototube gain stability. In one commercial scheme, for example, each phototube is periodically exposed to a pulse of light coming from a source of known and constant brightness. If the tube output voltage due to this pulse is outside a preset range, an automatic gain adjustment is activated and the gain of the tube altered so that the output pulse from the test flash returns to the specified range. Monitoring all phototubes in this way on a time scale short compared to other events (eg, such as the movement of the detector head during a SPECT study) insures that the signal inputs to the correction programs have the same physical meaning over time and under conditions nearly identical to those present during calibration. Despite these precautions it is customary to periodically recompute the gain and linearity lookup tables to account for long-term drifts in system performance. With modern systems, the gain and linearity maps are often recomputed, or checked, during preventative maintenance by company service personnel or, in some cases, by the user.

The effect of these corrections working together is perhaps best illustrated by improvements in uniformity.[9,13] In early cameras, exposure of the whole crystal to a broad, uniform beam of radiation gave rise to an image that was usually not uniform but varied in brightness from one region to the next. Initially, this effect was believed to arise from actual spatial variations in detection efficiency. Based on this belief, a variety of correction schemes were implemented by different camera manufacturers to give the appearance of uniform sensitivity over the full field of view. One such method was to acquire a high-count image of a uniform field and use this "field flood" image to compute a multiplicative correction factor at each image point. This factor was the ratio of the mean counts per point in the flood image divided by the counts at that image point. This correction factor array would then be applied to all subsequent images to normalize these images for apparent sensitivity variations. Application of this correction to another field flood image, for example, would produce a seemingly perfect correction of the observed nonuniformity. Eventually, however, it was recognized that apparent sensitivity variations were primarily the result of event mispositioning and gain variations, so that the premise underlying simple multiplicative correction schemes was incorrect. The lookup table methods noted above, however, correct explicitly for these effects, and uniformity is concomitantly improved.

Digital Cameras

The original Anger camera[6–8] was entirely analog in design, that is, all signals in the system took on continuously varying values and the position and energy of each event was calculated by manipulating these continuously varying voltages. Such complex analog systems, however, are subject to electronic drifts, gain changes in various subsystems, and baseline shifts that introduce sources of error into the computed quantities. Moreover, accurate correction of gain nonuniformities and position nonlinearities such as those described above are all but impossible to implement in analog form.

Most of these difficulties can be dealt with by replacing the analog components of an imaging system with digital elements that perform similar tasks. The advantages offered by this approach are appreciable so it is not surprising that modern scintillation cameras have become increasingly digital in character. In several recently described camera systems,[1,45,47] the position of a scintillation event is determined by digitizing the output of each PMT and using this set of digital signal representations to either compute[45] the location of the event using the centroid algorithm (Equation 8) or to consult a lookup table addressed by this signal set.[1] In this latter case, a given pattern of PMT signals is matched to a single, unique crystal location during system calibration with a test source. When this same pattern occurs during a subsequent data acquisition, the location of the calibration point in the field of view is retrieved from the lookup table and assigned to that event. In this scheme, spatial linearity distortions are automatically removed since the retrieved values are obtained from the "true" (undistorted) source positions measured during calibration. In a fully digital system, the remaining analog components are restricted to high-speed processing of incoming PMT signals in order to prepare these signals for digitization. Once digitized, the PMT signals are manipulated by algorithm or digital logic circuits to create the final corrected image.

SCATTER REJECTION

The various electronic and computed corrections described above depend only on the characteristics of the imaging device itself. Image quality, however, also depends on the nature of the object being imaged since "real" objects are sources of scattered as well as primary radiation. Inclusion of scattered radiation in an image, as illustrated in Figure 1, "blurs" the image and degrades image quality.

A substantial fraction of the scattered radiation incident on a camera crystal can be rejected through "pulse height analysis" of the *Z*-energy signal. As described previously, a Compton-scattering event results both in a change in direction of the incident photon and in a reduction in the energy of the scattered photon. Since the *Z* signal is a measure of photon energy and a Compton event always reduces the photon energy, an energy or *Z* threshold can be set below which events are considered scatter and rejected. The *Z* signal of an event is compared to a lower-level threshold previously established by imaging a source in air, a nearly scatter-free environment. An upper-level threshold is also established to reject high-energy background events or signals generated by higher-energy photons of the same radionuclide. The combination of lower and upper thresholds forms an energy "window" that defines the range of *Z*-signal magnitudes considered to be valid primary events. All events that do not possess *Z* signals falling within this window are rejected. The electronic device that performs this accept/reject test is called a pulse height analyzer (PHA). Under typical in vivo imaging conditions, pulse height analysis might reject 50% or more of the incoming signals as scattered events.

While pulse height analysis is effective in removing a large fraction of the scattered radiation incident on the detector, the energy resolution of a scintillation camera, even after correction for spatial gain variations, is of the order of 10 to 15%. As a result, photons scattered through relatively large angles can still possess sufficient energy to be detected within the established energy window. The nature of this effect is illustrated in Figure 7 where the energy of the scattered photon is plotted against scattering angle for several different initial photon energies. For an initial photon energy of 140 keV, a photon can undergo a scattering collision of more than 45° yet lose less than 14 keV in energy. For a camera operating with a typical 20% energy window (±14 keV), many of these events will fall within the window of acceptable pulse heights and contribute to the image. Thus, pulse height analysis, while effective for large-angle scatter (and higher initial photon energies), becomes ineffective at rejecting photons scattered through smaller angles (at lower initial photon energies). Unfortunately, the fraction of scattered photons that continues to satisfy the energy window conditions is quite large. The "scatter fraction," the ratio of scattered events to total events detected within the energy window, although highly variable, is typically of the order of 30%, a large fraction of the total.[62] Failure to discriminate against these scattered events reduces contrast and introduces serious inaccuracies in attempts to quantify organ activity. These inaccuracies can be very large as illustrated by an example later in this section where regional activity is overestimated by more than a *factor* of two in a simple phantom test object. This large and variable error should be contrasted with the quantitative capability of positron emission tomography (PET). Unlike single photon studies, effective scatter correction methods have been devised for PET and exact methods exist for attenuation correction. As a result, regional concentrations in similar test objects can be measured with PET to within a few percent of their true value, and physiological variables, eg, regional myocardial blood flow, often to within about 10 to 20% in vivo.[158]

Unlike PET attenuation corrections[78–95] that can be computed from transmission images, practical scatter correction methods in single photon studies have no such simple starting point. It is not surprising, therefore, that several methods of scatter correction are under study.[66–80] In the following discussion, we consider two of these methods to illustrate continuing efforts to improve image quality, the photopeak curve-fitting[66,68,69] and dual window[74] scatter rejection methods. Although correction of image data for scattered radiation is not now considered to be part of the usual group of instrumentation-based corrections, some of these methods of scatter correction require specialized hardware[67,71] and software. Thus, implementation of scatter correction methods in future systems may well have hardware implications so it is useful to include these methods under the general heading of instrument-based corrections.

Photopeak Curve-Fitting Scatter Rejection

With photopeak curve fitting, energy spectra are acquired at every image point (Fig. 5) within the field of view rather than just the number of events. It is then assumed that the shape of these individual energy spectra in the photopeak region (delineated by the vertical lines in Fig. 8A) can be represented as the sum of two (or sometimes more) mathematical functions. The first function is a Gaussian-shaped curve representing primary photons that have emerged from the object without interaction. The second function is selected to represent the energy-dependent distribution of scattered radiation thought to exist within the photopeak region. Functions selected for this purpose have included a straight line and sigmoid[68] and a complex function derived from the

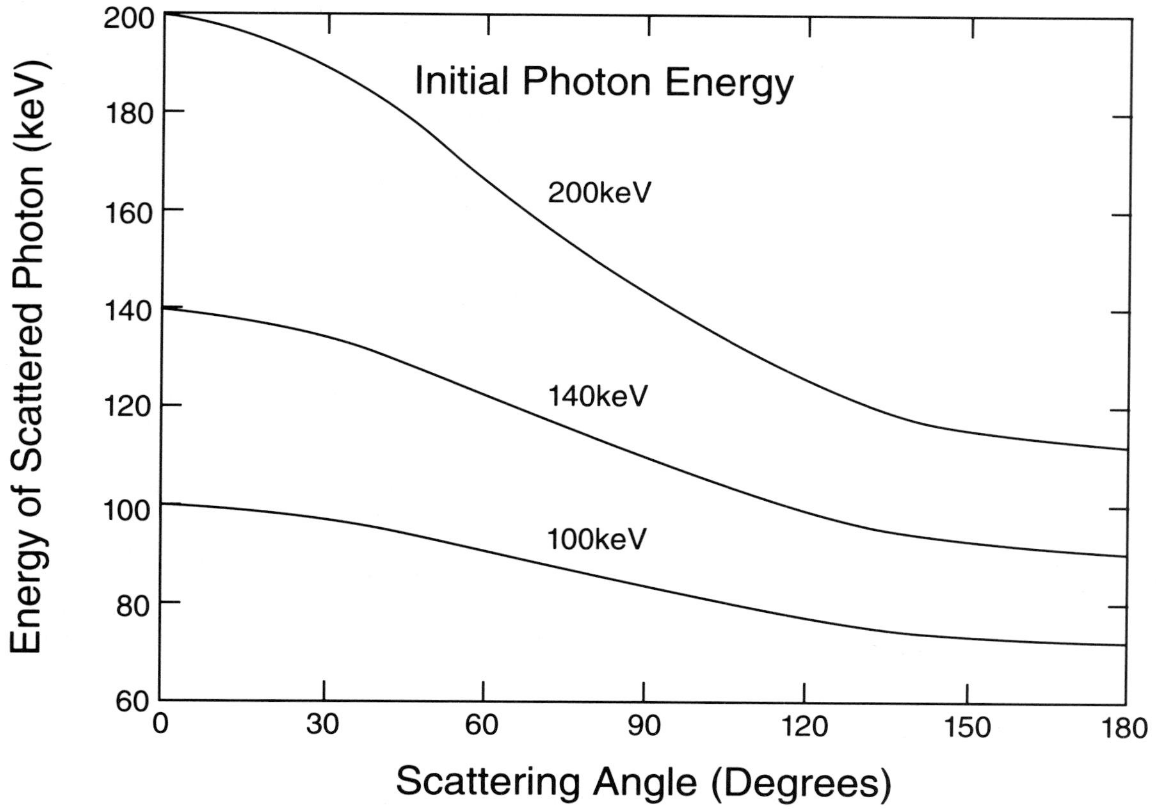

Figure 7. Energy of scattered photon vs scattering angle for several different initial photon energies.

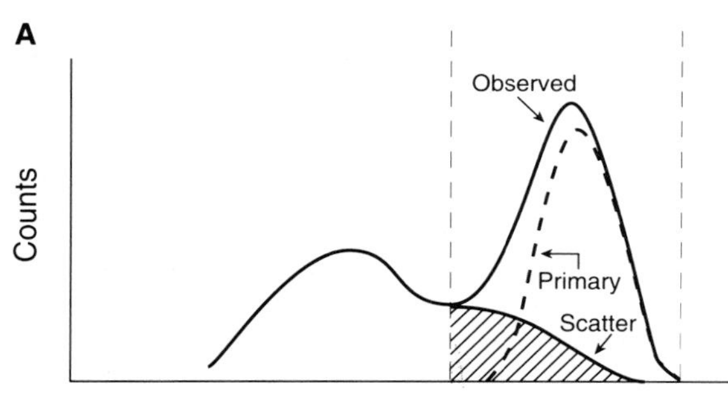

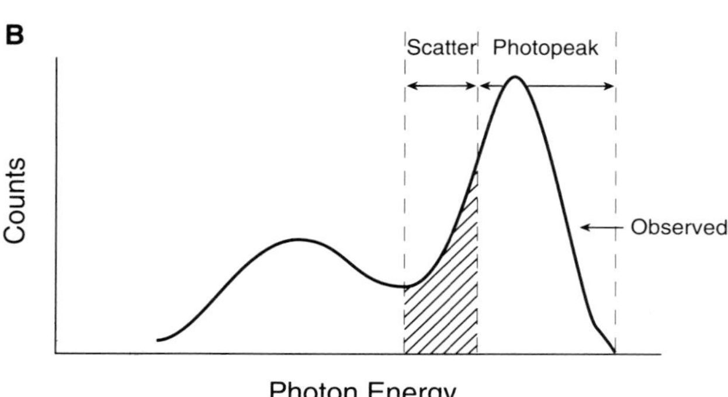

Figure 8. Schematic representation of photopeak curve-fitting (**A**) and dual-window (**B**) scatter rejection methods.

Klein-Nishina distribution.[69] Regardless of which of these approximations is used, the sum of the Gaussian and the chosen scatter function is fit to the observed curve in the photopeak region of each individual energy spectrum at each image point. This fitting operation, in turn, yields the parameters that define the Gaussian function and scatter function at every image point. Since, by hypothesis, the events represented by the Gaussian function are primary, unscattered photons, the area under this Gaussian is just the total number of unscattered events recorded at that image point. Thus, a new image is formed from the integral of the Gaussians obtained at each image point, an image from which the scatter component has putatively been removed.

In one implementation of this method,[68] the width and location of each Gaussian along the energy axis are predetermined from reference spectra acquired in air. These (relatively) scatter-free estimates of photopeak energy and width are then inserted into the curve-fitting routine applied at each image point. Inclusion of these a priori data is essential in order that the fitting operation yield valid estimates of the primary and scatter components. This approach also speeds the curve-fitting operation by reducing the number of free parameters in the fit.

The results of applying a method of this kind to a phantom test object are shown in Figure 9. The test object is a 20-cm diameter plastic cylinder viewed along the cylinder axis. Three smaller diameter water-filled cylinders are inside the

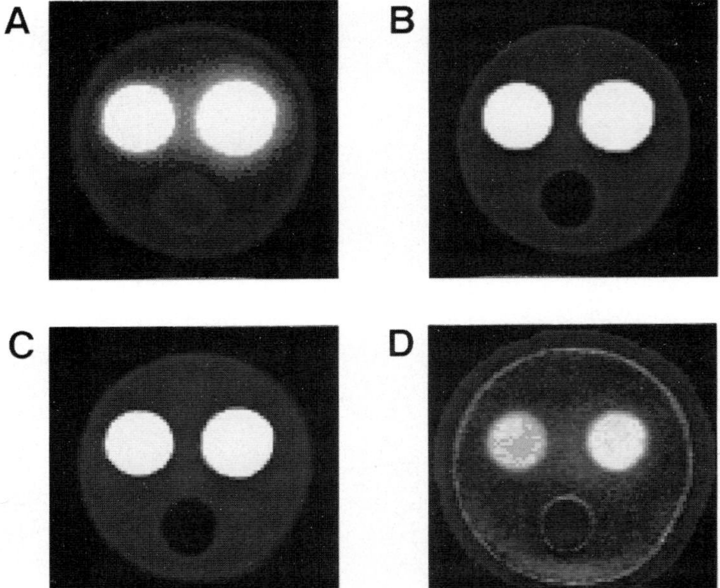

Figure 9. Planar, end-on images of a 20-cm diameter water-filled cylindrical "phantom" test object without scatter correction **(A),** with photopeak curve-fitting scatter correction **(B),** and with dual-window scatter correction ($K = 0.5$) **(C).** Panel D portrays spatial variations in the factor K assuming the photopeak correction method is exact. (See Plate 2.)

larger cylinder. These cylinders contain ^{99m}Tc at high (upper right), medium (upper left), and zero concentration (bottom middle). The void outside and around the smaller cylinders, but inside the large cylinder, is also filled with a water solution of ^{99m}Tc at a lower concentration to create general background activity. An image of this test object obtained with a 20% energy window is shown in panel A and represents the conventional appearance of this object without scatter correction. The image shown in panel B, on the other hand, is the image of the same phantom after scatter correction with the photopeak curve-fitting method as described above. In this example, the scatter component in the photopeak region has been modeled by the falling sigmoid across the photopeak region shown in Figure 8A. The applied fitting function is thus a Gaussian plus this sigmoid. The image in panel B is formed by integrating the counts under the computed Gaussian component at each image point. To the extent that the assumptions underlying this method are correct, this image should be free of scatter and accurately portray, within the limits set by the finite spatial resolution of the system, the correct ratios of activities between cylinders and the ratios of cylinder activities to surrounding activity.

To evaluate this method under more realistic conditions than permitted by the test object, an energy image was acquired in the anterior projection in a patient whose blood pool (red blood cells) was labeled with 20 mCi (740 MBq) of ^{99m}Tc. An image created in the usual way from this data set, ie, 20% energy window centered on the photopeak with no scatter correction, is shown in Figure 10A. The image obtained after scatter correction with the photopeak curve-fitting method is shown in Figure 10B.

Dual-Window Scatter Rejection

A second method of scatter correction uses more than one energy window to estimate scatter.[70,71] The method shown in Figure 8B employs a second energy window located immediately below and adjacent to a photopeak energy window. Since two energy windows are used (photopeak and scatter windows), this method is often referred to as the "dual-window" method.[74] During a dual-window acquisition, all Z pulses are compared against two energy windows rather than just one. Events with Z pulses falling within the limits set by the second PHA are routed into the second (scatter) image while events satisfying the photopeak energy requirements are sorted into the photopeak image. It is then assumed that the amount of scattered radiation detected in the photopeak region is a constant fraction, K, of the amount of scattered radiation detected in the scatter window. If this is so, then an image created from these scattered events (using a camera with a dual-energy window capability) can be scaled by K and simply subtracted from the image created from photopeak events. The result, if these assumptions are correct, should be an image free of scattered radiation. Images obtained with this method of correction are shown in Figure 9C for the same test object, and Figure 10C for the same patient study, used to evaluate the photopeak curve-fitting method. A constant multiplier of $K = 0.5$ was used to create these images.

Visual comparison of the scatter-corrected images in Figures 9 and 10 to the uncorrected images suggests, to a first approximation, that both correction methods improve image contrast. The uncorrected images (Figs. 9A and 10A) exhibit the characteristic lack of edge sharpness associated with

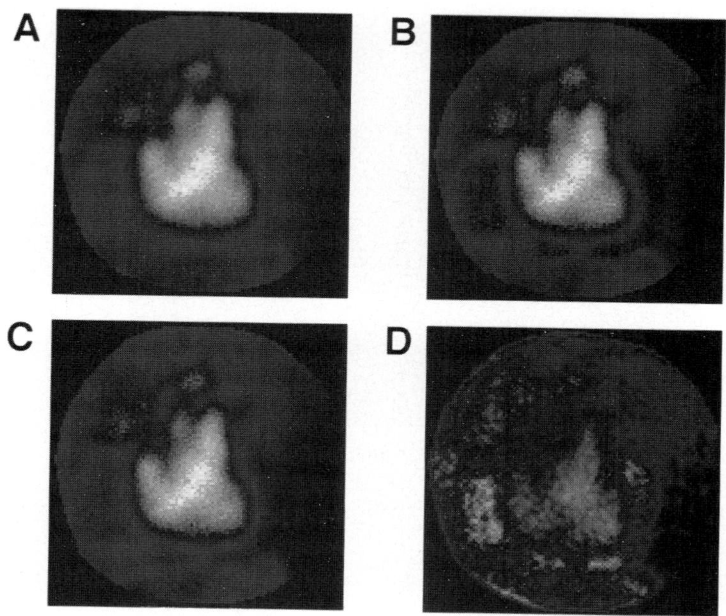

Figure 10. Anterior view of a patient's cardiac blood pool before scatter correction **(A),** after scatter correction with the photopeak curve-fitting method **(B)** and after correction with the dual-window method ($K = 0.05$), **(C).** Panel D portrays spatial variations in the factor K assuming the photopeak curve-fitting method is exact. (See Plate 3.)

scattered radiation and object borders appear "fuzzy." The corrected images, on the other hand, exhibit much sharper edges and, in the test object, more uniform distributions of activity within each of the regions of differing, but constant, tracer concentrations.

Visual inspection cannot, however, reveal subtle differences between the methods that might depend on the interplay between source activity and the distribution of scattering material in the object. To reveal such differences, K images were computed for both the test object and patient study (Fig. 9D and 10D). In these images, brightness is proportional to the ratio at each image point of photopeak scatter events calculated by the photopeak curve-fitting method to the total scatter counts within the low-energy scatter window of the dual-window method. If the photopeak curve-fitting method is assumed to give the true number of scatter events in the photopeak region, then this ratio is, in effect, an image of the scaling factor K at every image point. If K is truly constant, as required by the dual-window method, and the photopeak curve-fitting method is exact, then these images should be uniformly bright (or colored) everywhere. Inspection of these figures, however, indicates that regions exist within the phantom and patient images that are brighter or fainter than the average brightness. K, therefore, is not constant at least when compared to the photopeak curve-fitting method and varies with the distribution of source activity. In particular, K values tend to be larger in high-activity regions than in moderate-activity regions and to change rapidly at boundaries on one side of which is zero activity (bright rings around the cold rod and the outer boundary of the cylinder).

A second step toward ranking, these methods in order of their quantitative accuracy is illustrated in Figure 11. Here, count profiles (panel B) have been generated along the vertical path (Y) shown in panel A for the uncorrected (white curve), dual-window corrected (blue curve), and photopeak curve-fitting corrected (red curve) phantom images. As can be seen by inspection, the uncorrected profile variably overestimates the true activity level in the background region (dashed horizontal line). Immediately between the two hot rods this overestimate rises to almost 300% of the true activity. Activity also appears to be present within the region of zero activity.

In contrast, both scatter correction methods give count profiles that are much closer to the true, uniform activity distribution between the warm and hot cylinders and both give activity estimates near zero in the cold cylinder. In the region along the Y profile, therefore, both methods offer substantial improvements in quantitative accuracy compared to the profile without scatter correction. A more extensive quantitative comparison, however, indicates that the photopeak curve fitting method accurately estimates the true activity throughout the entire phantom whereas the dual-window method does not.

Both of the methods just described improve image quality to a greater or lesser degree. In addition to accuracy of correction, however, methods of this kind must also be relatively simple to implement and cannot extend appreciably the amount of patient imaging or processing time required to produce the scatter-corrected result. Methods of the dual- or multiple-window correction types[70,71] are simplest to implement and require only a camera with a dual- or multienergy-window acquisition capability. This feature is already available on most scintillation camera systems. The correc-

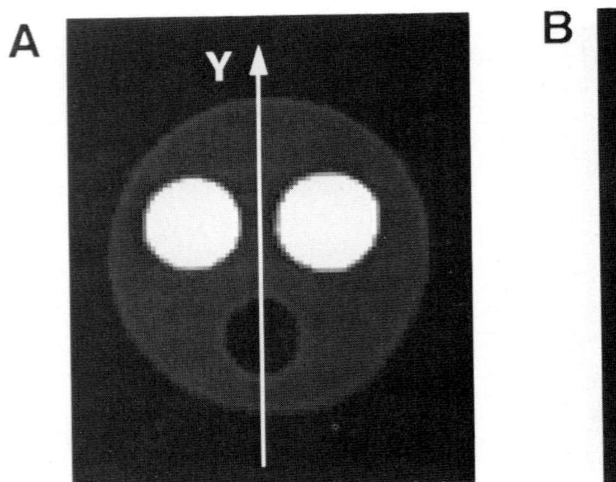

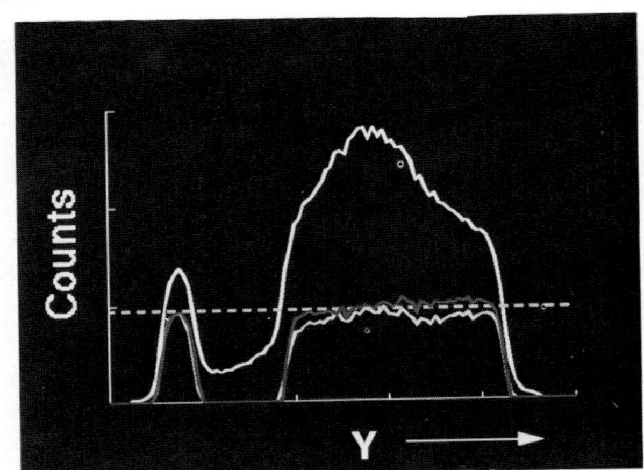

Figure 11. Image of the cylindrical phantom (**A**) showing the vertical path (*Y*) along which the count profiles shown in panel B were generated. Upper curve in panel B is without correction, lower curves are with photopeak curve-fitting scatter correction, and with dual-window scatter correction. Dashed horizontal line indicates true count level in warm background region. (See Plate 4.)

tion image, moreover, can be acquired simultaneously with the photopeak image so that no additional acquisition time or processing time beyond a simple multiplication and subtraction is required to achieve the final scatter-corrected result.

Photopeak curve-fitting methods,[68,69] in contrast, seemingly require specialized hardware such as a large memory array to hold the incoming point-by-point energy spectra, additional large amounts of memory to store sequences of such energy images when imaging dynamically, very high-speed hardware/software for efficient curve-fitting of the energy spectra in multiple images to minimize postacquisition processing time, and so forth. In fact, however, some of these elements already exist in modern camera systems so that implementation of the photopeak curve-fitting scheme may not be as difficult as first imagined. For example, the spatial gain correction method described in a previous section, and illustrated in Figure 5, utilizes the same three-dimensional energy spectra acquisition capability required by the photopeak curve-fitting method. In present-day cameras, this large array is usually used only during the gain correction calibration procedure, although nothing in principle prevents its use in routine imaging. The required memory for real-time acquisition of point-by-point energy spectra thus already exists in most systems. The other factors noted above that adversely affect the practical implementation of this method can be minimized but it is probable that this method will require some modifications in data acquisition that could impact on study length and postprocessing time. It should also be noted that there are a number of technical subtleties associated with these methods, particularly with photopeak curve-fitting methods that use any kind of a priori information. Drifts in phototube gain over time can, for example, shift the photopeak energy channel away from the photopeak location measured at the time of energy calibration. If this now incorrect reference channel number is used to position the Gaussian component, the resulting fit will be in error. Since the fit is in error, so too will be the estimate of primary radiation at that image point. Particular care may be required, therefore, in controlling for gain drifts and offsets with these methods since very small changes away from the reference or calibration values can have significant consequences.

At the present time, no single scatter correction method has been embraced as the final answer to the problem of scatter removal from scintigraphic images.[66–80] The methods alluded to above achieve this end, but with varying degrees of success and simplicity. Nonetheless, interest in this matter has increased and it is likely that some generally accepted form of scatter correction will emerge in the near future, possibly accompanied by commercial hardware developments intended to facilitate the process. Should such a method be combined with a practical scheme for attenuation correction, SPECT imaging studies could approach the accuracy of quantification previously achieved only with PET.

COUNT RATE AND DEAD TIME

A conventional single crystal scintillation camera records gamma-ray absorptions sequentially as they occur. Since a finite time is required to process each event, the possibility exists that events will be lost during this processing interval or "dead-time." Indeed, if increasing amounts of activity are placed in front of a camera and the count rate recorded at each increment, a plot of these data will yield a curve similar to that shown in Figure 12. At low count rates, the measured count rate increases nearly linearly with increasing activity. As the activity continues to increase, however, the measured rate begins to lag behind the increase in activity and the plot of measured count rate vs activity becomes increasingly flat. When the rate of gamma-ray interactions in the crystal

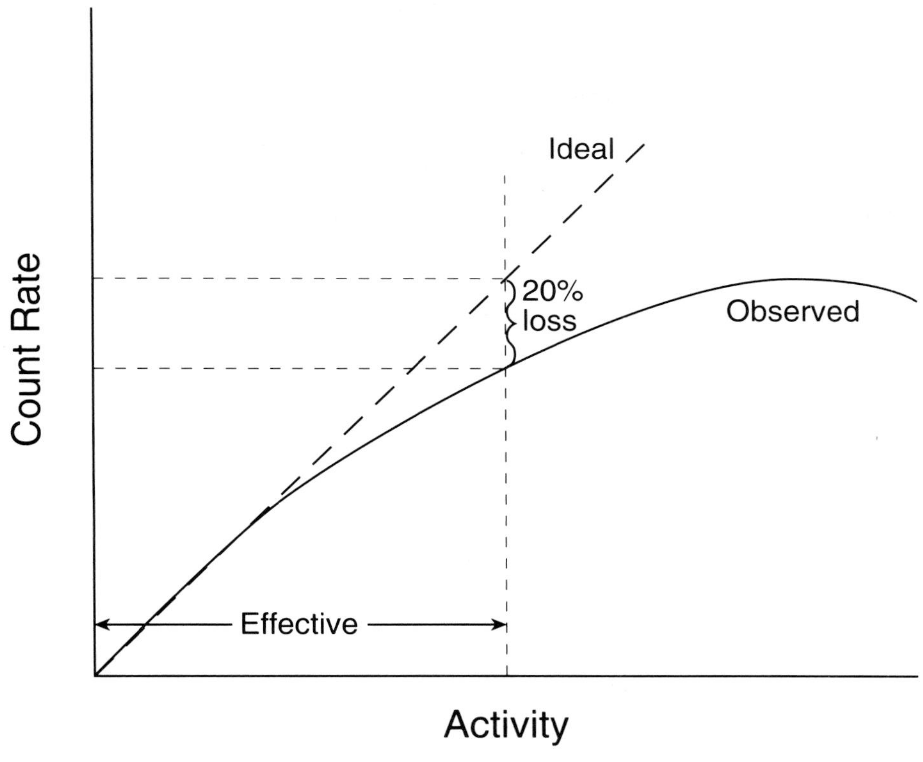

Figure 12. Count rate vs activity for an idealized scintillation camera.

increases even further, the measured count actually decreases and the camera is said to be "paralyzed." Furthermore, spatial resolution (or image quality) also usually deteriorates due to "pulse pile-up" at high count rates. Pile-up is a condition in which two or more events occur nearly simultaneously in the crystal and sum to a height acceptable to the pulse height analyzer. The resulting composite event is positioned at some average (fictitious) position that corresponds to neither true interaction site.

The relationship between count rate and activity can thus be divided roughly into three operating regimes.[25,146,157] At relatively low count rates, count rate and activity are nearly linearly related and in this operating region measured count rate directly reflects source activity and changes in source activity. As count rate increases further, the departure from linearity increases until count rate losses are large enough that further increases in activity are not warranted. Finally, in the paralyzable range, the camera is useless and further increases in activity are literally counterproductive. It follows from these observations that quantitative nuclear medicine studies generally should be performed with tracer doses adjusted so that the camera is always operating in or near the linear regime. Moreover, the breadth of this linear regime should be as great as possible so that linearity is preserved over the greatest possible activity range. A common measure of the boundary of this near-linear, or *effective*, range is the point at which count rate losses due to dead time are 20% of the true rate. In early cameras, this point was reached for measured count rates of less than 20,000 events per second. In modern cameras, the 20% boundary can occur at count rates as high as 100,000 (or more) per second depending on manufacturer.

In order to attain such high rates, a number of innovations have been introduced over the years that have progressively raised the 20% boundary to higher and higher levels.[22] These advances have occurred as a result of a careful consideration of the physical processes involved in photon detection and the use of efficient signal-processing circuits.

One technique to improve count rate performance is based on the observation that the spacing in time between consecutive interactions in a scintillation crystal is not constant and uniformly spaced. Instead, the spacing in time between events has a Poisson distribution. As a result, the camera appears to experience very high input event rates for short periods even though the mean event rate may be nominal. This effect, as might be expected, also increases with increasing count rate. Since this "burst" effect is a direct result of the random nature of radioactive decay, one solution to this problem would be to "derandomize" these events by quickly storing a short sequence of input pulses in analog storage buffers. By storing these pulses, subsequent analysis circuits downstream from these buffers are not subjected to high event rates that exceed their processing speeds. Instead, these stored pulses proceed down the processing chain at a rate dictated by the circuits rather than by the Poisson distribution of arrival times. Such techniques are very effective at improving camera count rate performance by large factors, particularly when multiple analog buffers are used to acquire events; circuits of this kind are often present in modern cameras.

Additional improvements in count rate performance can be traced more directly to electronic elements in camera systems. A pulse from a PMT quickly rises to a maximum and then slowly falls (exponentially) to zero. Rise times are typically a small fraction of a microsecond while decay times are many tens of microseconds. The peak magnitudes of these "raw" pulses are small so it is customary to integrate the PMT signal over time and to output this integrated value. On the other hand, if this integration process takes too long, the dead time of the system will be increased, potentially dramatically. As a result, modern systems usually employ some combination of pulse "clipping" and pulse integration that is a compromise between the requirements of large signal output and good count rate performance. As a result of these advances, including those described above, modern cameras exhibit dead times typically of the order of 5 microseconds or less.

QUALITY ASSURANCE

Each of the elements described in previous sections, collimation, spatial uniformity and linearity, scatter rejection, etc., together determine the fidelity of images output by a scintillation camera system. Camera manufacturers routinely provide a list of specifications for the performance of their systems and these specifications serve as useful benchmarks for the performance of a system over time. When a system is installed at a new location, acceptance tests should be performed to verify that both the hardware and software elements of the system meet these written specifications, specifications that probably played an important role in the camera selection process in the first place. Once a camera has been installed and accepted, it is essential that a continuous and rigorous program of quality control be instituted to insure that the camera continues to exhibit these same performance characteristics over time. Fortunately, intercomparison and acceptance testing of camera systems have been greatly facilitated by the development of a set of standards (National Electrical Manufacturers Association or NEMA standards) that specifies exactly how each of the system parameters is to be measured. This set of standards permits the performance of different cameras to be compared (since the testing procedures are the same across manufacturers). These standards also provide a useful guide for developing quality control programs to insure that these (or similar) standards are met over the useful life of the imaging system. Details of the NEMA testing protocol and guidelines for ongoing quality control procedures can be found in several publications.[23,25,146] We will describe here only the NEMA test for spatial uniformity and one of several possible quality control procedures for this parameter.

The NEMA test for intrinsic spatial uniformity requires that a detailed list of conditions be met: that two parameters, integral and differential uniformity, be measured, that such measurements be made over both the useful field of view (UFOV) and the central field of view (CFOV), that the full field count rate not exceed 20,000 events per second, that ^{99m}Tc be the photon source, that a 20% energy window be set around this photopeak, and that the crystal area outside the UFOV be masked with a Pb ring to prevent photons from interacting in this region. During image acquisition by computer, the acquired field flood image is digitized as a 64×64 array containing not less than 4000 (and preferably more than 10,000) counts at the central point in this array. The (point) photon source should be placed at least five UFOV diameters away from the camera during data acquisition. When the uniformity image is acquired under these conditions, and after digital filtering to suppress statistical fluctuations in regional count density, measurements of uniformity are performed and reported for both the UFOV and the CFOV. The definition of useful field-of-view is based on those pixels whose count content equals or exceeds half the central pixel value. For a camera with a circular field-of-view, these pixels define a disc having a certain diameter. If this diameter is multiplied by the factor 0.95, the disc with this new diameter centered on the center pixel is the UFOV. If this diameter is multiplied by the factor 0.75, the new disc centered on the center pixel defines the CFOV. Performance parameters calculated for the CFOV are often slightly better than for the UFOV since the UFOV includes a crystal annulus nearer to the crystal edge where distortions, and corrections for distortions, are usually larger.

Integral and differential spatial uniformity are designed to reflect two somewhat different aspects of spatial uniformity. Integral uniformity is, in a sense, a global measure of uniformity, while differential uniformity attempts to convey local or regional uniformity. Both parameters are expressed in percent and both are computed as the ratio of a difference between maximum and minimum values to the sum of those two values. For integral uniformity, the maximum and minimum values are just the largest and smallest count values, respectively, located anywhere within the UFOV (or CFOV). The difference between these values is the largest that occurs within the prescribed field so it is a worst-case measurement. By definition, no other deviations can be larger so that integral uniformity sets the maximum variation within the field of view. Differential linearity is also a worst-case estimator but for local, rather than global, variations in spatial uniformity. In this case, the computer-acquired uniform field flood image is inspected along each row and each column in six pixel increments. In each such increment, the maximum and minimum counts are identified and their difference-to-sum ratio is formed, as above. The largest of these differences along all rows and columns is the differential linearity. This parameter measures the largest uniformity variation that occurs on the specified length scale (6×1 pixels) anywhere in the field of view.

Like these tests for spatial uniformity, other NEMA tests also require specific types of test objects, imaging procedures, data analysis methods, and result calculation and expression. Moreover, these procedures must be carefully followed in all of their details or the resulting measurements can be substantially in error. For example, in the case of spatial uniformity measurements, failure to acquire a large number of counts per pixel could substantially skew the calculation of integral and differential linearity. Since the largest and smallest count values anywhere in the field flood image are being systematically sought in these measurements, there is already a built-in bias toward overestimation of these parameters. The reason for this is that the counts acquired at a given pixel are subject to statistical variations. If we systematically select only the largest and smallest count values from this image, the largest real differences in spatial uniformity are combined with the largest possible statistical variations in pixel counts. If these latter variations are large compared to the true variation, then these tests are really measuring how poorly the test was performed rather than spatial uniformity. It is not surprising, therefore, that the NEMA test for spatial uniformity also contains a specification for minimum count density. Similar detailed testing specifications also accompany the other NEMA tests.

While NEMA procedures are often used for acceptance testing of newly acquired scintillation cameras, these tests are generally too time consuming and laborious to perform on a routine basis. Instead, a number of simpler procedures have been devised over the years that can test the essential elements of machine performance quickly and with sufficient acuity to determine whether the system is performing near specifications. A number of these procedures are described elsewhere so only a brief description is included here.[25]

Quality control procedures for spatial uniformity and spatial linearity illustrate the type of testing procedures that can be easily and routinely used to insure adequate camera performance. Both kinds of measurements can be performed so as to measure either "extrinsic" or "intrinsic" performance. Extrinsic performance is measured with the collimator in place while intrinsic performance is measured without the collimator. Each of the approaches offers advantages. Extrinsic performance measurements are, in a sense, more complete than intrinsic measurements because damage to the collimator can also be detected. Although collimators are protected to some degree by metallic covers, penetration of these covers by sharp objects or deformation of a collimator by denting with blunt objects is not unknown. Such defects, moreover, might be interpreted as defects in organs imaged with such collimators so it is important to periodically perform extrinsic tests to insure that such damage has not been incurred. In the context of spatial uniformity measurements, a field flood source of size sufficient to cover the full field of view of the camera is placed in contact with the collimator. Such sources can come in two forms, liquid or solid. Solid sources, usually circular discs containing a long-lived isotope such as Co-57, are available commercially in a variety of diameters. Since these sources require no preparation, they are always available and ready to use. Moreover, by virtue of their long life, such sources provide a convenient means of following changes in system sensitivity over both short and long time scales.

Liquid uniformity sources, thin, large area circular cavities filled with a uniform solution of radioisotope, are usually prepared daily by injecting and thoroughly mixing a known quantity of ^{99m}Tc with water in the cavity. Such sources require some amount of time to prepare and increase the amount of time spent on quality control procedures. Moreover, some care must be taken to insure that the cavity thickness is uniform across the field of view and special filling techniques are often required. The primary differences between these two types of flood sources are practical and economic. Solid sources are relatively expensive and have to be replaced at roughly yearly intervals. Liquid uniformity phantoms and the ^{99m}Tc that goes into them are, in contrast, relatively inexpensive but do require an ongoing investment in preparation time. It is also likely that some increase in radiation exposure is associated with the filling and use of liquid sources. Considering these advantages and disadvantages, solid sources are probably the test object of choice if extrinsic spatial uniformity testing is to be performed on a daily or near-daily basis. If extrinsic testing is performed only occasionally, then liquid sources are more cost effective. Many of these complications or differences disappear, however, if intrinsic testing is selected as the routine method for assessing field uniformity. With the collimator removed, camera sensitivity increases by a very large factor so that relatively weak point (small volume) sources of ^{99m}Tc or any other isotope can be used to generate a relatively high count rate. The multimillicurie levels of activity associated with fillable liquid sources is thus avoided. A spatially uniform input distribution of gamma rays on the crystal surface is also easy to achieve with a small volume source simply by centering the source in the uncollimated field of view at five or six field diameters from the crystal surface. The deviation from true parallelism at these distance is modest and the input beam is essentially parallel.

Regardless of the test method used, the result is an image obtained when the number of photons falling on the crystal (or collimator) per unit area per second is nearly identical everywhere within the field of view. In a properly working camera, this image should also appear uniform. Visually detectable departures from uniformity can indicate any one of many potential problems. A dark hole in an image can, for example, indicate and locate a PMT that has failed. Streaks and other artifacts may indicate conditions ranging from a cracked crystal to electronic failure or malfunction of some other system component(s). The most common method of interpreting such images is by simple visual inspection, often accompanied by a comparison of the current uniformity image with images obtained previously. Alternatively, a more detailed, quantitative description of spatial uniformity can be obtained by computer analysis. For example, it is a relatively simple matter to implement a computer algorithm to examine a uniformity image in a manner analo-

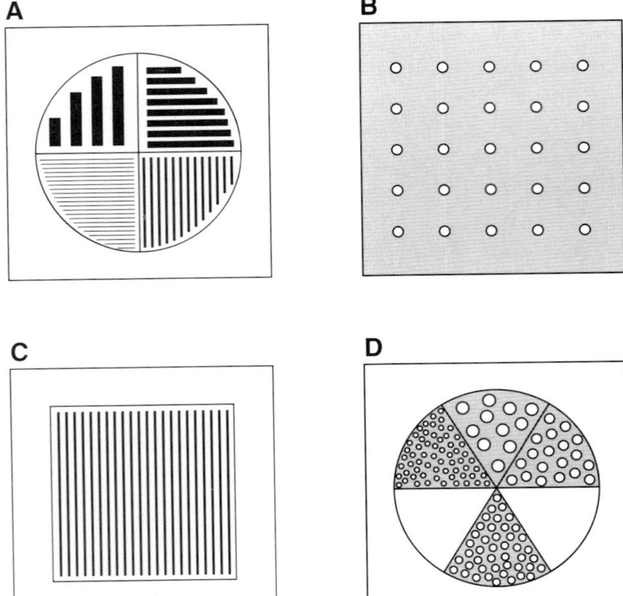

Figure 13. Pb test grids used to assess camera spatial resolution and spatial linearity: four quadrant **(A),** orthogonal hole **(B),** parallel bar **(C),** and pie slice **(D).** Blank pie slices are assumed to contain holes of sizes intermediate to those shown on either side.

gous to that prescribed in the NEMA standards if the data acquisition time and source strength have been properly chosen. In either case, visual or computer analysis, a significant qualitative or quantitative departure from previous, or specified, performance, should signal a service call to correct the problem.

While field uniformity is arguably the single most useful measurement of system status, changes in other essential system parameters cannot be reliably inferred from these images alone. Spatial resolution must also be periodically monitored and a number of test objects and procedures have been devised for this purpose. Like spatial uniformity, spatial resolution and linearity can be measured extrinsically or intrinsically using point or extended flood sources of radiation that uniformly illuminate the field of view. In addition to such a source, however, an additional test object is inserted between source and detector that projects a known, spatially varying pattern of photons onto the crystal (or collimator). A number of test patterns have been devised to measure various aspects of resolution and linearity including those illustrated schematically in Figure 13. The four-quadrant phantom (Fig. 13A), for example, consists of parallel Pb bars with equal width and equal between-bar spacing in a given quadrant but progressively smaller spacing and width from one quadrant to the next. By a judicious selection of bar width and spacing, it should be possible to just detect a pattern of bars in the quadrant with the smallest bar spacing. Failure to detect this pattern in the minimum spacing quadrant in subsequent studies would indicate a departure from system norms. Spatial resolution and linearity can also be evaluated with the orthogonal hole phantom (Fig. 13B). This phantom is a Pb plate drilled with small-diameter holes at regular intervals. If the collimator is removed and this plate placed over the crystal and illuminated by a distant point source of gamma radiation, the hole array will be projected onto the crystal. The apparent width of each projected hole is a measure of local intrinsic spatial resolution. The variation of the projected hole centers around the horizontal and vertical lines on which the hole center actually lies is a measure of intrinsic spatial linearity. An orthogonal hole plate of this kind was used to visualize (Fig. 6A) and correct (Fig. 6B) spatial nonlinearities found in an experimental scintillation camera. The two blank slices in the pie-slice grid (Fig. 13D) are imagined to be filled in with holes of appropriate intermediate sizes.

The choice of such test grids is somewhat arbitrary and is dictated largely by practical factors. The orthogonal hole phantom requires only a single data collection in order to sample the entire field of view while the four-quadrant phantom technically requires four data collections (each followed by a 90° rotation) to achieve full sampling. The construction of the four-quadrant phantom, moreover, does not allow linearity to be evaluated across the full field of view since each resolution pattern occupies only one fourth of the field of view. For qualitative quality control procedures, both methods can reveal comparable departures from normality. However, if resolution and linearity are to be quantified, the orthogonal hole phantom is probably superior since the regular hole pattern simplifies computer analysis.

Quality control procedures such as these are intended to reveal significant short-term deviations from normal system operation. While some deviations from normal operation occur because of a single, easily detectable catastrophic failure, daily operation of a camera will usually be accompanied by drifts in system performance with time, drifts that can only be detected with a continuous surveillance program specifically tailored to detect such variations. Such a program implies consistent and interpretable record keeping and a methodical approach to system testing. Only with such an approach can images obtained daily with these systems be regarded as reliably portraying the distribution of activity in the patient.

A CLINICAL APPLICATION

The previous sections of this chapter have been devoted to an exposition of a few of the basic operating principles underlying the scintillation camera in its conventional mode of operation. In clinical practice, however, the scintillation camera is often only one component in the data acquisition/processing chain that makes up a typical clinical imaging study. In this section, a clinical imaging procedure is described that is intended to illustrate how the camera and associated data-processing elements are combined in a relatively complex clinical procedure, gated blood pool imaging.[26–28,48–59] Specific cardiac disorders in which gated blood imaging is useful are detailed in Chapter 23.

Gated Blood Pool Imaging

Gated blood pool imaging, or radionuclide cineangiography, was developed to measure cardiac function and to visualize myocardial wall motion. Imaging of the heart is performed following equilibration of a suitable tracer throughout the blood pool. The procedure is based on the premise that, at equilibrium, global and regional count rates over the cardiac chambers are proportional to global and regional chamber volumes. If changes in these volumes can be accurately measured during a single cardiac cycle, then descriptors of cardiac performance such as left ventricular ejection fraction, peak filling rates, etc., can be computed. The cardiac cycle, however, is only about 1 second long in resting subjects and the number of photons released from the cardiac blood pool during a single beat is too small to form usable images of the cardiac chambers. If cardiac function is stable, however, the cyclic volume variations of the cardiac chambers from one beat to the next are nearly the same. If we were somehow able to superimpose image data collected from many cardiac cycles, we might be able to construct an average cardiac cycle with a sufficient number of photons not only to visualize cardiac performance, but to do so at a high temporal resolution (high frame rate).

To construct an average cardiac cycle, we must be able to temporally align the cardiac image data acquired during each beat to the same starting point in time, ie, to the same moment in each cardiac cycle. The most common fiducial or timing marker used for this purpose is the time of occurrence of the *R*-wave in the patient's externally monitored ECG signal, an event that signals the onset of ventricular systole in each beat. Various commercial devices are available that continuously examine this signal, detect some aspect of the *R*-wave (maximum positive rate of change, maximum value, etc.), and emit a logic pulse indicating that the *R*-wave has occurred and that the next cardiac cycle is about to begin. The first signal necessary for gated imaging is this *R*-wave logic pulse. The second and third required signals are the *X* and *Y* positions of each valid, ie, within the selected energy window, scintillation event detected within the camera's field of view. Finally, a fourth logic signal is generated at each "tick" of a clock, usually internal to the computer, that divides the time between *R*-waves into short increments. As indicated in Figure 14, these four signals are passed to a "word encoder" that writes each event into a unique computer word. This stream of encoded words is then passed to the computer where they are used to create an average cardiac cycle in real time, or passed to a storage device where they are recorded as a long, sequential "LIST" of events.

The word-encoding procedure is illustrated in Figure 15 for the case where each member of a valid *X*,*Y* coordinate pair has been digitized into one of 128 levels. To encode a 128-level *X*-signal into this word requires 7 bits ($2^7 = 128$) and the same number for *Y*. Thus, 14 bits of the 16-bit word are needed to encode the *X*,*Y* positions of a single scintillation event within the camera's field of view. In the figure, the values $X = 96$ and $Y = 90$ have been encoded in their binary representations by turning on (checked boxes) the appropriate combination of bits. The remaining two "extra" bits (15 and 16) can be used to encode the occurrence of an *R*-wave signal or the occurrence of a clock tick. To encode an *R*-wave marker, we simply create a computer word with the 16th bit "turned on" (set to 1) and leave all other bits off (zero). Similarly, whenever a clock tick occurs, we create a computer word with the 15th bit set to one, leaving the 16th and all other bits off. In this manner, we transform the four input signals into computer words, each identifiable by its format. Later, we can scan a list of these words and, knowing this "code," reconstruct exactly the sequence of events during the original data collection.

The average cardiac cycle can be created by processing these encoded words with one of two different algorithms (Fig. 16). The first of the methods, the "frame mode" method,

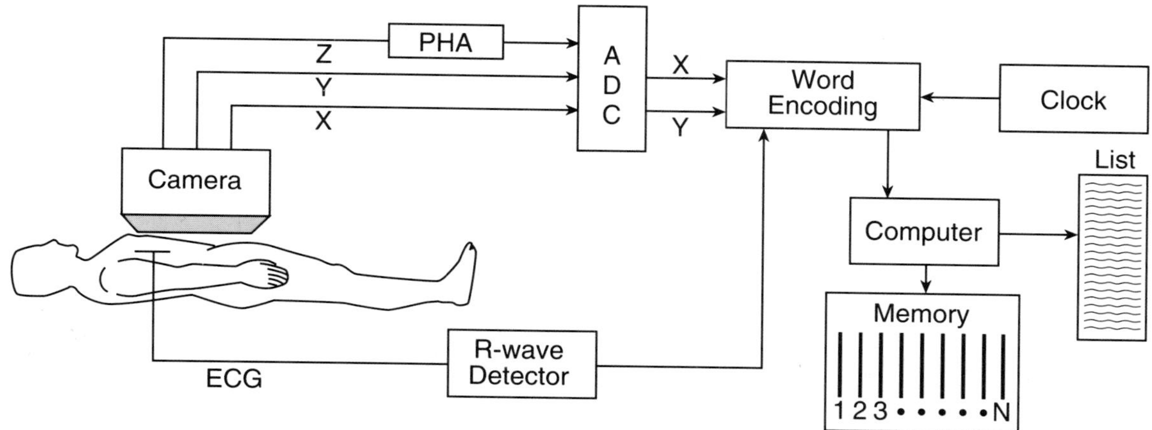

Figure 14. System elements required to perform gated blood pool imaging. PHA = pulse height analyzer; ADC = analog-to-digital converter.

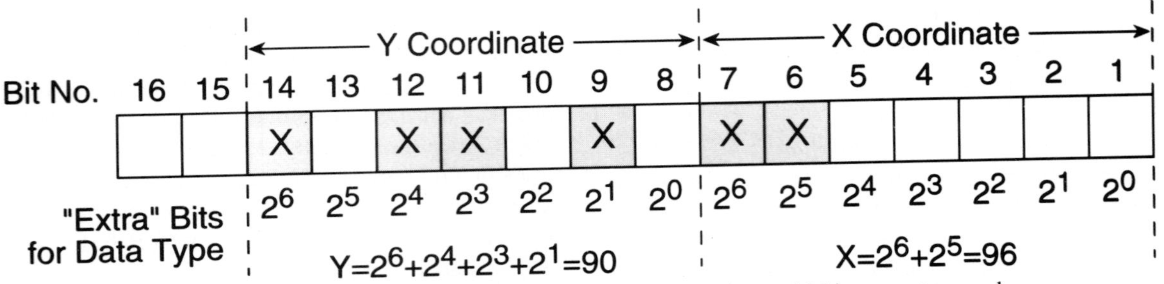

Figure 15. Encoding of timing and position information into a 16-bit computer word.

is the simpler method to implement in real time but is limited in many clinical applications because "bad" heart beats cannot be rejected from the acquired data nor can "backward-forward" framing be performed to eliminate data falloff at the end of the average cardiac cycle. The second method, though more difficult to implement in real time, is the "list mode" method. This method, in contrast to the first, permits rejection of bad beats and end-cycle corrections. We shall describe this method in some detail since the frame mode method is simply a subset of the list mode method.

After the encoding step, each encoded word is passed to the computer. Two temporary storage buffers (A and B in Fig. 16) are established in computer memory. The incoming stream of words is first written sequentially into one buffer until it is full, and then into the second buffer. While the second buffer is filling, the contents of the first buffer are analyzed and also written to some suitable storage device. When the second buffer is full, data are again directed into the first buffer and the second buffer is read out and analyzed. This process flip-flops back and forth until data collection is terminated. The reason for using two buffers in this manner is to prevent losing data during the read-out process.

At the end of data collection, the storage device will contain a single long list of computer words that encode in correct temporal order all of the position and timing data generated during the study. This long list can be examined

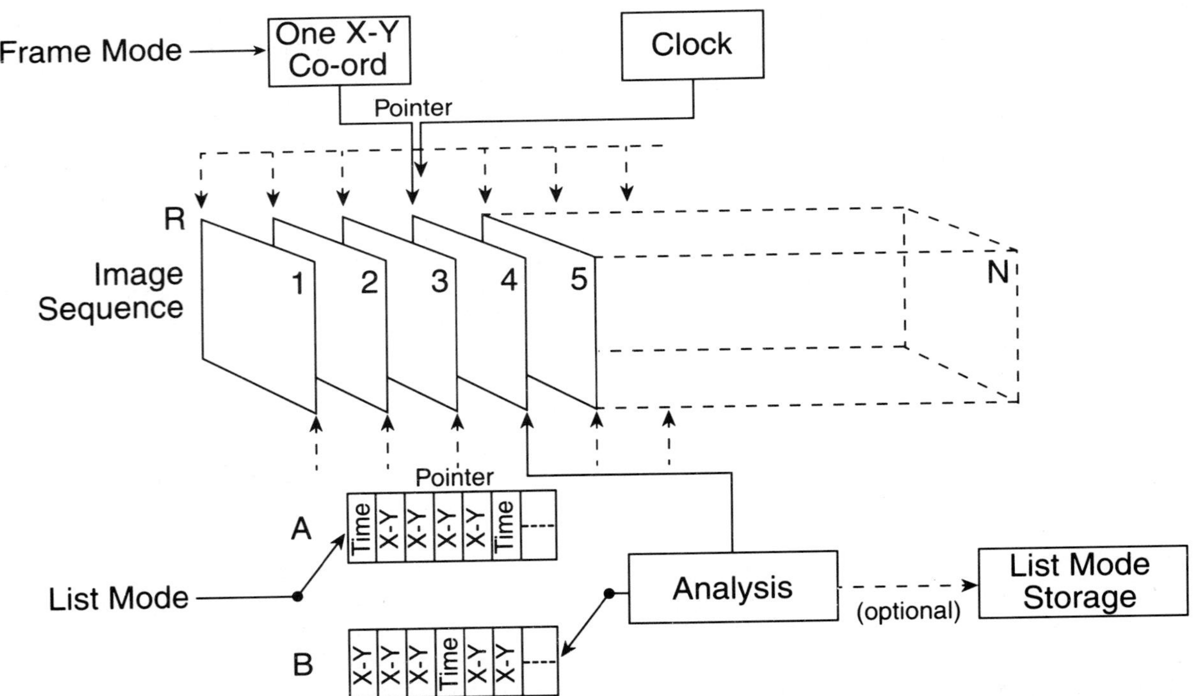

Figure 16. Frame mode and list mode methods of creating an average cardiac cycle.

retrospectively event by event to create the gated blood pool image sequence. This process can also be carried out in real-time during the "analysis" phase of data collection by using very large list mode storage buffers to store entire cardiac cycles,[60] but it is conceptually simpler to describe this task as an after-the-fact procedure.

The first step in this process is to establish in computer memory a set of images into which the acquired list mode data will be sorted. This set might consist of as many as 50 to 70 images, each 64 pixels square. Initially each pixel in each image contains zero counts. The stored list mode data are then examined beginning with the first computer word in the list and continuing through the list one word at a time. As each new word is encountered, it is decoded, as described above, to determine the kind of event represented by that word. The sorting algorithm uses this information to direct the flow of position data into the proper image in the image sequence. If a clock tick word is encountered, a tick counter is incremented by one count. If the clock ticks once every 10 milliseconds, 100 ticks will occur per second. Detection of an event representing an R-wave serves to reset this clock tick counter to zero. Detection of a position event (the 15th and 16th bits of a word being zero) initiates decoding of the first 7 bits of the word to define the X coordinate of the event and decoding of the second 7 bits to define the Y coordinate of the event. When the location of the event is known, the sorting algorithm looks at the tick counter. The contents of the tick counter at that moment determine the number of the image in the sequence into which that X,Y coordinate should be sorted. If, for example, the tick counter registers 37, the X,Y point in image 37 is incremented by one count. Since the tick counter measures time since the last R-wave, this event must have occurred 370 milliseconds after the R-wave at location X,Y in the field of view. Since the next R-wave resets the tick counter to zero, events occurring when the tick counter again registers 37 will be additively sorted into this same image. Thus, data from the same phase of all cardiac cycles will contribute to the same image in the sequence.

If this process is allowed to run to completion, an image sequence will be created that portrays the time variation of the cardiac chambers during a single, complete, average heartbeat. Since scintillation data are acquired during many heartbeats, the statistical reliability of this sequence can be high. Moreover, since the apparent temporal resolution of the sequence is set by the clock interval (10 milliseconds per image in the example), changes in cardiac chamber volumes can be examined reliably on short time scales. Both of these capabilities are significant in clinical practice.

As noted earlier, the list mode method allows the user to "look back" in time and discard image data that do not meet some specified condition prior to inclusion in the final image sequence. This look-back capability is particularly useful in rejecting image data that occurred during "bad" heartbeats such as premature ventricular contractions or other arrhythmias. To reject such data, the list is scanned and the distance in time between consecutive R-wave markers is calculated. This time interval, along with the number of that heart beat counted from the beginning of the study, is recorded in a new list. These data can be displayed as a frequency distribution function of cycle lengths to the user who can then select a range of beat lengths to be included in the final image sequence. The list is again scanned, this time checking whether the length of the current beat falls within the user specified window. If it does, the sorting algorithm described above is applied until all image data up to the next R-wave signal have been included in the sequence. If the cycle length is outside the selected window, then the image data between these two R-wave markers are simply skipped and the next cardiac cycle is examined in the same manner. This process is repeated beat-by-beat until all cycles recorded during the study have been examined. The result is an image sequence free of image data that occurred during cardiac cycles outside the specified range of beat lengths. It should also be noted that this same technique can be used to study cardiac function during "bad" beats by using the same method to reject "good" beats.[32]

Another advantage of the list mode method is the ability to portray more accurately events that occur late in the cardiac cycle such as atrial filling.[60] The look-back capability of the list mode method allows construction of a second cardiac image sequence framed backward in time from the R-wave. In a conventional frame mode acquisition, the number of heart beats contributing to the late images progressively declines and the resulting image sequence does not portray accurately late diastolic events. The same number of cardiac cycles, however, can be made to contribute to the late diastolic events if these data are framed backward in time from the R-wave. The decline in contributing cycles now will occur at the beginning of systole rather than during late diastole. If now the forward-framed sequence is merged with the backward-framed sequence, the combined image data will form a complete, undistorted cardiac cycle that portrays late as well as early cardiac events. If the merge point has been selected to occur during diastasis, when cardiac chamber variations are small, residual distortions due to heart rate variations are negligible and the events portrayed in the image sequence are quantitatively as well as qualitatively correct. The merge operation is performed to yield an average cardiac cycle whose length is equal to the mean cycle length.

Many subtleties are associated with the implementation of this and other methods for visualizing cardiac function.[29,31,40–42,44] This example does suggest, however, how the scintillation camera can be coupled to data acquisition/processing elements[61] to yield new or novel clinical procedures. Radionuclide cineangiography represented a solution to the problem of measuring a high-speed dynamic process with good statistical reliability, requirements that are usually mutually exclusive. As a result, much as been learned with this method about the response of the heart to disease, physical stress, therapeutic drugs, and other interventions.[48–59] Radionuclide cineangiography, however, is only one of several contemporary methods in which the computer and camera form an inseparable combination. SPECT is another and is treated in the next section.

SPECT IMAGING

The scintillation camera, as described so far, yields planar projection images of activity distributions in the body. In such projection images the third dimension is collapsed onto the plane and all knowledge of the distribution of activity with depth is lost. Moreover, image contrast in projection images is reduced by activity anterior and posterior to the labeled target object. Both of these deficiencies can be avoided to a substantial degree by acquiring many projection images at equally spaced intervals around the body which can then be manipulated mathematically to produce a tomographic image sequence that represents the three-dimensional activity distribution that gave rise to the projection set. This technique is known as single photon emission computed tomography (SPECT) and is increasingly important in nuclear medicine.[77–144] Although a number of different tomographic techniques have been devised in nuclear medicine over the years, SPECT today usually refers to transaxial tomography with one or more scintillation cameras rotating around the patient.[2–4] Other types of SPECT imaging systems have been introduced recently,[159–161] but we shall focus on the scintillation camera approach.

The conceptual basis for SPECT and other forms of transaxial tomography is illustrated in Figure 17A. Equally spaced projection images are obtained by physically rotating the camera in small angular steps around the patient. At each location the camera is allowed to dwell for a specified length of time sufficient to acquire a usable number of events to form an image. At the end of this interval the camera is stepped through the selected angular increment and another projection image acquired. This process is continued until the object has been viewed through 180 or 360°.[106,107] In a typical imaging situation with typical amounts of tracer, 30 to 120 projection images (180 or 360° acquisitions) might be acquired, with dwell times for each projection ranging from 10 to 60 seconds depending on count rate. A typical single camera SPECT study might thus require about 30 minutes of imaging time and contain millions of counts. These factors, however, are subject to large variations, depending on the exact imaging conditions.

Once the projection set is acquired, these image data can be manipulated to yield a sequence of tomographic images spaced along, and perpendicular to, the axis of rotation (in the plane of Fig. 17A). If a source of radioactivity located somewhere in the field of view of a camera is viewed in different projections, the location of the source in each image will generally be different (except if the source is located on

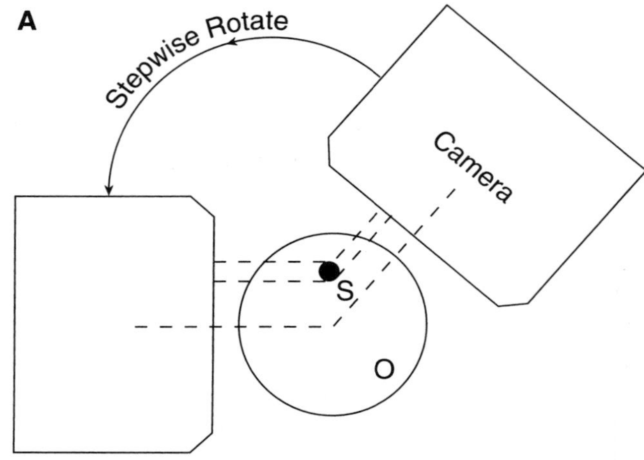

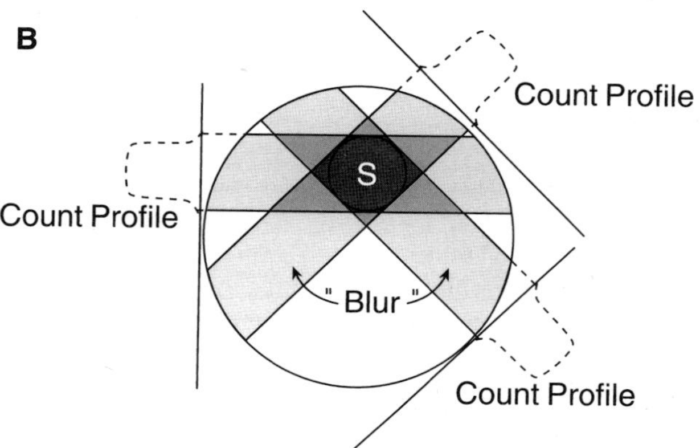

Figure 17. SPECT imaging of a source *S* in an object space *O* with a scintillation camera. Camera rotates around a fixed center from one position to the next, acquiring an image (projection) at each location **(A).** Additive backprojection of the acquired count profiles **(B)** in an attempt to reconstruct the source distribution.

the rotation axis). If we assume that the source is physically stationary in space and that the source is seen in each projection, then we might reconstruct the source distribution by simply "backprojecting" each source count profile through the image space as shown in Figure 17B. Since we do not know where the source is before reconstruction, we are forced to assume that the source is located with equal probability along the line of sight in each projection. Thus, when the source is backprojected, lines or bands of uniform probability density are generated across the image space. Wherever these lines or bands intersect, we allow them to add together, thereby reinforcing one another, forming a crude image of the source. It is clear, however, that such a simple backprojection scheme will not, by itself, accurately portray the true source distribution. Increasing the number of projections smooths the backprojection image but the source still appears extended in space beyond its actual size. The backprojection image, though not a true portrayal of the source distribution, does play an important role in reconstruction tomography.

To see why this is so, it is useful to find an expression that connects the intensity at a point in the backprojection image, $BP(x',y')$, with the true source distribution $S(x,y)$. If a circle with radius R is drawn around a source point x,y, the density of lines passing through this circle will be $N/(2\pi R)$, where N is the number of lines and $R = [(x' - x)^2 + (y' - y)^2]^{1/2}$. Since the same number of lines, N, will pass through *all* such concentric circles, the contribution of this source point to the backprojection image will be $S(x,y)(1/R)$. The total intensity at x',y' in the backprojection image is the sum of these products for all points in the source distribution. The sum of these products can be written as the integral:

$$BP(x', y') = \int S(x,y)\,[1/R]\,dx\,dy. \tag{18}$$

An integral whose arguments have this form is called the "convolution" of the two functions S and $1/R$ and can be written symbolically as

$$BP(x',y') = [S(x,y)]*[1/R], \tag{19}$$

where the asterisk indicates the product-integration operation. The backprojection image can thus be regarded as the convolution of the source distribution with the "blurring" function $1/R$. When cast in this light, the problem of reconstructing the source distribution from projections is equivalent to the problem of somehow solving this equation for $S(x,y)$ in terms of the other variables and recovering the true source distribution. The detailed mathematical methods necessary to carry out this task are contained in references 150 and 155 and we will simply outline the procedure and its outcome.

The convolution of two functions has a number of interesting mathematical properties. Specifically, the Fourier transform of the convolution of two functions is the product of the Fourier transforms of the functions themselves (the convolution theorem). If T is taken to symbolically represent the Fourier transform operation, then applying this rule to the BP convolution integral gives

$$\begin{aligned} T[BP(x',y')] &= T[(1/R)*S(x,y)] \\ &= T[1/R]\,T[S(x,y)]. \end{aligned} \tag{20}$$

Inspection of this relation indicates that through this operation we have managed to separate the source function S from the blurring function $1/R$. Since each function now appears as a transform in this relation, we have also succeeded in casting this problem into the spatial frequency domain rather than the spatial domain.

Solving for $T[S(x,y)]$ gives

$$T[S(x,y)] = T[BP(x',y')]/T[1/R]. \tag{21}$$

Further, it can be shown[150] that the Fourier transform of the function $1/R$ is just $1/K$ where "K" is the spatial frequency:

$$K = (K_x^2 + K_y^2)^{1/2}. \tag{22}$$

Substitution of $1/K$ for $T[1/R]$ in Equation 21 gives

$$T[S(x,y)] = K\,T[BP(x',y')]. \tag{23}$$

According to this expression, the Fourier transform of the source distribution can be obtained by multiplying the transform of the backprojection image by the linearly increasing "ramp" function, K. If all possible values of spatial frequency were contained in the transformed backprojection image, K would increase without bound. In imaging systems, however, there is always an upper limit to K. Imagine first, that the parallel lead bar pattern in Figure 13C is projected onto the crystal of a camera. When the bar width and spacing are large, the image of this pattern will vary regularly and periodically in brightness across the field of view and follow the variations in the real pattern. Suppose now that the spacing and width of the bars are slowly decreased, thereby increasing the rapidity (or frequency) of changes in brightness per unit distance across the field of view. At some point the image of this pattern and the real pattern will differ, a point where the spacing and width of the bars are comparable to the spatial resolution of the camera. Thus, there is some spatial frequency beyond which the camera will fail to portray the true input intensity distribution. In addition to this physical limit imposed wholly by the imaging device, we are also forced to sample the incoming image data in discrete spatial or digital increments. With too few increments information is lost and with too many, unnecessarily large images are created. According to the "sampling theorem,"[150] we can record without loss all information passed by the camera by sampling at a rate greater than the Nyquist rate, a rate that is twice the highest spatial frequency passed by the system. The practical consequence of these effects is that a ramp function for a real system, rather than increasing without bound, is truncated or "cutoff" at the Nyquist frequency for that system. The ramp increases linearly between zero and the cutoff frequency, K_c, and is zero for all higher frequencies (Fig. 18A). Since $T[T^{-1}(K)] = K$, where T^{-1} is the inverse Fourier transform, we may substitute this relation for K to obtain

$$T[S(x,y)] = T[T^{-1}(K)]\,T[BP(x',y')]. \tag{24}$$

By the convolution theorem, the term on the right is the product of two Fourier transforms and must be equal to the Fourier transform of their convolution:

$$T[S(x,y)] = T[T^{-1}(K)*BP(x',y')]. \tag{25}$$

If now the inverse Fourier transform of each side of this equation is taken, the source distribution becomes

$$S(x,y) = T^{-1}(K)*BP(x',y'). \tag{26}$$

According to this expression, the source distribution, $S(x,y)$ can be recovered by convolving the function $T^{-1}(K)$ with the backprojection image $BP(x',y')$. The inverse Fourier transform of the truncated ramp, K, is shown in Figure 18B. This method of reconstructing the source distribution (or removing the blur from the backprojection image) is known

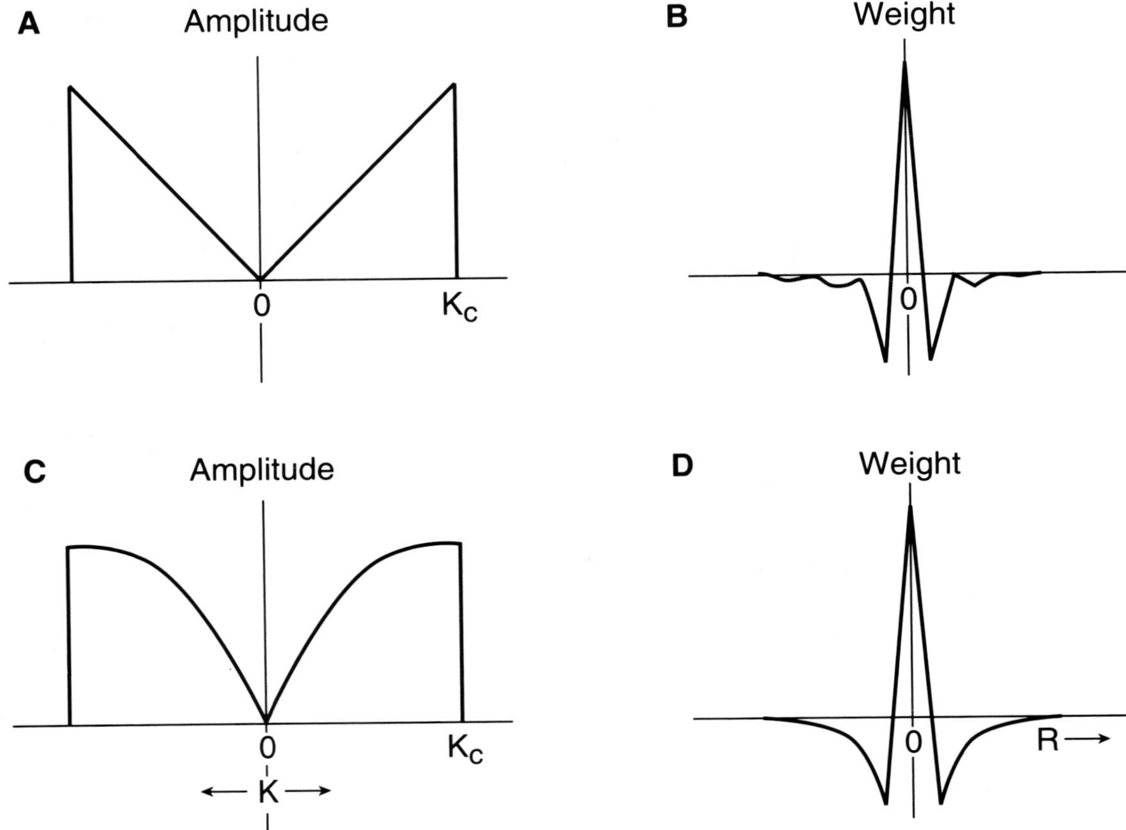

Figure 18. Frequency and spatial domain-equivalent filters used in SPECT. Truncated ramp filter **(A)** and its spatial equivalent **(B)** and modified ramp filter **(C)** and its spatial equivalent **(D).** K_c is the Nyquist frequency.

as the "convolution method" and is carried out in the spatial domain.

Equation 23 suggests another equivalent, but procedurally different, method of reconstructing $S(x,y)$. Instead of computating in the spatial domain, we could calculate in the frequency domain. In this case, we first take the Fourier transform of the backprojection image, multiply this image by the truncated ramp, and then take the inverse Fourier transform to obtain $S(x,y)$. This method is attractive for several reasons. First, unlike the convolution method, filtering is a simple multiplication in frequency space and not a matrix operation as in real space. In addition, efficient computational schemes have been devised to calculate Fourier transforms and their inverses and these two advantages can have great practical significance. This method of reconstructing $S(x,y)$ is known as the "filtered backprojection" or Fourier method and is probably the most commonly used method.

In the greatly simplified treatment above, many implicit assumptions were made about the nature of the projection data that are never realized in practice. We assumed, for example, an infinite number of projections with projection lines parallel and evenly spaced and image data free of counting "noise." This latter assumption is violated in real SPECT studies since data acquisition times and attainable count rates are finite. Although the total number of events acquired in a SPECT study can be large, perhaps in the millions, the counts along individual projection profiles of a single tomographic slice are small. As a result, counting noise is a substantial source of image degradation in SPECT imaging. In order to deal with counting noise (and other) effects, reconstruction is often performed with a modified ramp function similar to that shown in Figure 18C rather than the truncated ramp. The modified ramp is obtained by multiplying the truncated ramp point-by-point by a function that changes the shape of the ramp at higher frequencies. Instead of sharply terminating at the cutoff frequency like the truncated ramp, the modified ramp "rolls off" the high frequencies gradually as the cutoff frequency is approached. Since any of these functional forms are really just frequency weighting functions that accentuate or diminish the contribution of each spatial frequency to the final reconstructed image, the modified ramp increasingly reduces the contribution of the higher frequencies as one approaches the cutoff frequency. Conversely, the modified ramp accentuates the contribution of the lower frequencies and effectively acts as a "low-pass" filter in the frequency domain. The inverse Fourier transform, or spatial equivalent, of the modified ramp in Figure 18C is shown in Figure 18D. Although superficially similar to the inverse transform of the truncated ramp, transforms of modified ramp functions generally have a somewhat broader central peak and smaller, smoother oscillations near the horizontal axis. These are the features of

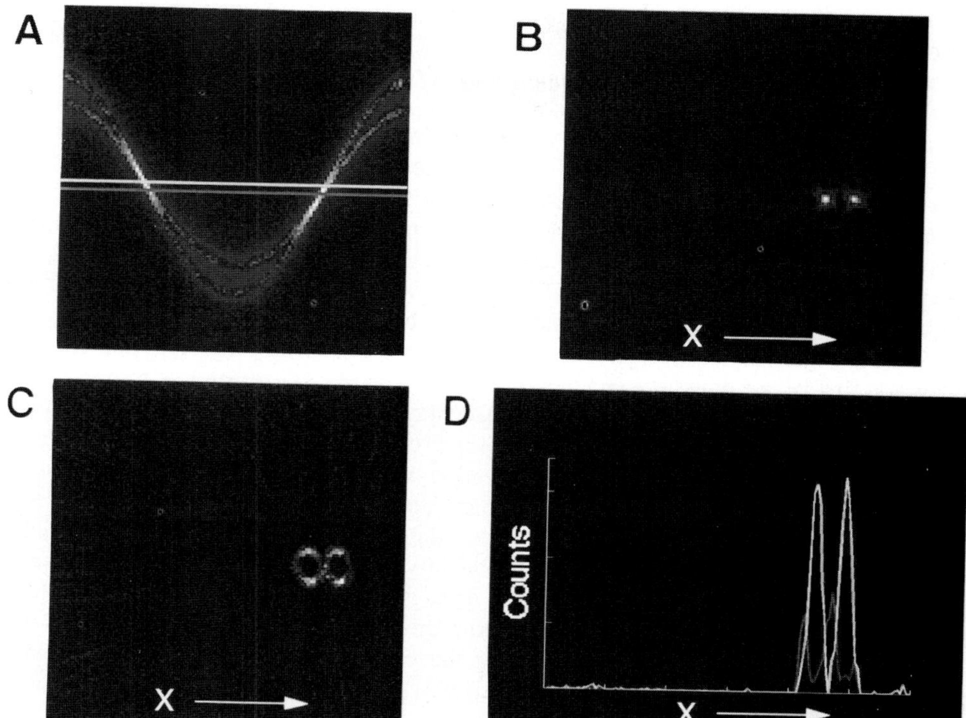

Figure 19. **(A)** 360° single-slice sinogram through two capillary tube sources parallel to the axis of rotation. **(B)** Transverse section image computed using the true center of rotation. **(C)** Transverse section image computed using the wrong center of rotation. **(D)** Comparison of count profiles through points in B and C. (See Plate 5.)

a filter in the spatial domain that combines, or averages, data over larger spatial regions in order to reduce the effects of local counting fluctuations (though at the cost of reduced spatial resolution). Many modifications to the truncated ramp function have been devised and evaluated for SPECT imaging, including the Wiener and Hanning modifications.[118,131,132,147] In modern SPECT systems, the user is often able to select, or create, a modified ramp that optimizes the tradeoff between resolution and image noise most appropriate for a particular kind of imaging study. We should point out, before leaving the subject of reconstruction, that a number of reconstruction methods have been devised that offer some advantages over the two treated here. Iterative methods that allow for incorporation of machine performance parameters and other physical effects into the reconstruction model have shown promise in improving the quantitative accuracy of SPECT images.[134–144]

In addition to counting noise[96,97] and problems associated with discrete sampling,[150] reconstruction of real objects is directly affected by the performance of the imaging system[101–108] and by the imaging environment.[79–95,98] Any violation of an assumption underlying the reconstruction algorithm will, to a greater or lesser degree, give rise to artifacts in the reconstructed images. We illustrated this effect by considering the consequences of inaccurately measuring the location of the camera's center of rotation.

The results of reconstructing a single, transverse slice through two capillary tubes parallel to the axis of rotation and filled with radioactivity are shown in Figure 19. In Figure 19A, the acquired projection data are portrayed as a "sinogram," a plot in which the ordinate is the distance along the camera's field of view and the abscissa is the projection angle. Although a 180° degree acquisition is all that is technically necessary for reconstruction, the acquisition shown in the figure was over 360°, giving two complete sinusoids, one for each source. These data were then combined to produce a single tomographic image set with improved counting statistics. The true center of rotation of this system is identified in A by the yellow horizontal line. When this correct location is used in the (convolution) reconstruction algorithm, the resulting transverse section image (Fig. 19B) contains, as expected, two in-focus dots corresponding to a cross section through the two capillary tubes.

In Figure 19C, however, these same sinogram data were reconstructed using the incorrect center of rotation identified by the red horizontal line in A. Instead of two sharply focused dots, this reconstruction shows two rings, each centered on a source. Count profiles through the two objects in Figures 19B and C are compared in panel D. By inspection, the apparent magnitudes of the sources in Figure 19C and their spatial distributions are markedly distorted compared to their appearance in Figure 19B. Thus, a relatively modest error (4 pixels out of 128 or about 3% in this case) in estimating the true location of the center of rotation gives rise to significant spatial artifacts and quantitative inaccuracies.

The reconstruction process also assumes that the object being imaged is motionless within the imaging field. If the object moves, or somehow gives the appearance of moving during the imaging interval, this assumption is violated and the collection of projection profiles of the object will not be consistent with the distribution of radioactivity in the object: the reconstruction will contain artifacts. Such artifacts can occur when a patient (or organ) moves during image acquisition or when there is an apparent inappropriate movement between the imaging field and the object. Apparent movements can occur in several ways. For example, when a camera rotates around a subject, the direction of the gravitational force vector relative to the camera and its support structure changes. When the camera is looking down on the patient from above, the camera may droop downward on the end of its support beam (if suspended this way). When the camera is viewing the subject from the side, however, the gravitational force may deflect the camera sideways, first in one direction, and then in the other when the camera is on the opposite side of the patient. An oscillation in the apparent location of the center of rotation will give rise to an inconsistent projection set and image artifacts. Improvements in the mechanical design of modern SPECT systems have substantially reduced this kind of center-of-rotation error. Nonetheless, the stability of the center of rotation must be carefully checked during acceptance testing and monitored periodically during the useful life of the system. Patient movement during the imaging procedure can also introduce similar artifacts in the reconstruction. Since SPECT studies are often lengthy, patient movement is of particular concern and a number of methods have been devised to detect and correct for such motions.[111–116]

The reconstruction process also assumes that the intrinsic "brightness" of the source remains constant throughout the imaging period. If a camera has a spatial variation in sensitivity, the same object will appear to change in brightness when viewed in different projections since it will appear at different locations in the camera's field of view. Apparent changes in brightness can occur due to differences in attenuation in different projections, and real changes can occur through radioactive decay or redistribution of source activity during the imaging period. All of these effects, whether from imperfections in the camera or from the imaging environment, can introduce subtle inaccuracies in the reconstructed images. As a result, quality control of SPECT imaging systems[149] and an understanding of these sources of error is essential if these images are to be correctly interpreted.

SUMMARY

In the previous sections, we have attempted to describe a few of the essential operational features of the scintillation camera as a planar imaging system and as a single photon tomograph. Although the scintillation camera has been refined continuously over the years into a high-performance device, the principles and the technology underlying the scintillation camera have continued to be applied in new and novel ways. The size of the imaging field has increased enormously to accommodate whole-body imaging, an important contemporary clinical application of the camera. Multiheaded scintillation camera systems[2–5] have been developed to increase the sensitivity and decrease the time required to perform cardiac, brain, and other SPECT studies. The Anger principle has been utilized for PET imaging[161] and in the design of dedicated SPECT brain imaging systems.[159,160] The cameras themselves have been improved substantially, and will continue to improve through increasing use of high-speed digital processing techniques that provide unprecedented control over all aspects of system performance.

As suggested in this chapter, a major goal of current research is to improve the quantitative accuracy of SPECT and other planar nuclear medicine studies.[62–95] While improvements in camera performance aid directly in this goal, the challenge remains to develop practical, efficient, and accurate methods of scatter rejection and radiation attenuation correction that can be employed routinely in clinical practice. Should these efforts to improve quantification be ultimately successful, the diagnostic power and utility of single photon studies will increase substantially. The ability to accurately estimate absolute tracer concentrations throughout the body with SPECT would allow clinicians to extract the greatest possible information from the acquired data, both for dignostic as well as therapeutic purposes, increasing, in turn, the value of nuclear medicine to the medical community. Although the exact form these advances might take in the future cannot be predicted, it is certain that such refinements will occur and that the scintillation camera, the centerpiece of single photon imaging, will continue to play a central and vital role in nuclear medicine.

REFERENCES

1. Milster TD, Aarsvold JN, Barrett HH, et al. A full-field modular gamma camera. *J Nucl Med* 1990;31:632.
2. Kimura K, Hashikawa K, Etani H, et al. A new apparatus for brain imaging: four head rotating gamma camera single-photon emission computed tomograph. *J Nucl Med* 1990; 31:603.
3. Kouris K, Clarke GA, Jarritt PH, et al. Physical performance evaluation of the Toshiba GCA-9300A triple-headed system. *J Nucl Med* 1993;34:1778.
4. Nakajima K, Taki J, Bunko H, et al. Dynamic acquisition with a three-headed SPECT system: application to technetium 99m-SQ30217 myocardial imaging. *J Nucl Med* 1991; 32:1273.
5. Fahey FH, Harkness BA, Keyes JW Jr, et al. Sensitivity, resolution and image quality with a multi-head SPECT camera. *J Nucl Med* 1992;33:1859.
6. Anger HO. Scintillation camera. *Rev Sci Instr* 1958;29:27.
7. Anger HO. Scintillation camera with multi-aperture collimators. *J Nucl Med* 1964;5:515.
8. Anger HO. Radioisotope cameras. In: Hine GJ, ed. *Instrumentation in Nuclear Medicine*, vol 1. New York: Academic Press, 1967.
9. Wicks R, Blau M. Effect of spatial distortion on Anger camera field-uniformity correction. *J Nucl Med* 1979;20:252.

10. Wicks R, Blau M. Effect of window fraction on the deadtime of Anger cameras. *J Nucl Med* 1977;18:732.
11. Adams R, Hine GJ, Zimmerman CD. Deadtime measurements in scintillation cameras under scatter conditions simulating quantative nuclear cardiography. *J Nucl Med* 1978;19:538.
12. Guldberg C, Rossing N. Comparing the performance of two gamma cameras under high counting rates: principles and practice. *J Nucl Med* 1978;19:545.
13. Lewis JT, Neff RA, Nishiyama H, et al. The effect of photon energy on tests of field uniformity in scintillation cameras. *J Nucl Med* 1978;19:553.
14. Lim CB, Hoffer PB, Rollo FD, et al. Performance evaluations of recent wide field scintillation gamma cameras. *J Nucl Med* 1978;19:942.
15. Lewellen TK, Williams DL, Murano R, et al. A field procedure for the quantitative assessment of nuclear imaging cameras. *J Nucl Med* 1978;19:954.
16. Chang W, Shuqiang L, Williams JJ, et al. New methods of examining gamma camera collimators. *J Nucl Med* 1988; 29:676.
17. Gillen GJ, Hilditch TE, Elliott AT. Nonisotropic point spread function as a result of collimator design and manufacturing defects. *J Nucl Med* 1988;29:1096.
18. Zasadny KR, Koral KF, Swailem FM. Dead time of an Anger camera in dual-energy-window-acquisition mode. *Med Phys* 1993;30:1115.
19. Bartkiewicz B, Huda W, McLellan Y. Impact of gamma camera parameters on imaging performance, evaluated by receiver operating characteristics (ROC) analysis. *Phys Med Biol* 1991;36:1065.
20. Gibson CJ. Gamma-camera linearity and resolution assessed using coarsely sampled line spread functions. *Phys Med Biol* 1992;37:371.
21. O'Connor MK, Oswald WM. The line resolution pattern: a new intrinsic resolution test pattern for nuclear medicine. *J Nucl Med* 1988;29:1856.
22. Lewellen TK, Bice AN, Pollard KR, et al. Evaluation of a clinical scintillation camera with pulse tail extrapolation electronics. *J Nucl Med* 1989;30:1554.
23. Geldenhuys EM, Lötter MG, Minnaar PC. A new approach to NEMA scintillation camera count rate curve determination. *J Nucl Med* 1988;29:538.
24. Busemann-Sokole E, Farrell TJ, Cradduck TD. Effect of scintillation camera non-uniformity on ejection fraction measurements. *J Nucl Med* 1985;26:1323.
25. Simmons GH, ed. *The Scintillation Camera.* New York: The Society of Nuclear Medicine, 1988.
26. Green MV, Ostrow HG, Douglas MA, et al. *Scintigraphic Cineangiography of the Heart.* Medinfo 74. Amsterdam: North Holland Publishing Co, 1974;827.
27. Green MV, Ostrow HG, Douglas MA, et al. High temporal resolution ECG-gated scintigraphic angiocardiography. *J Nucl Med* 1975;16:95.
28. Bacharach SL, Green MV, Borer JS, et al. A real-time system for multi-image gated cardiac studies. *J Nucl Med* 1977; 18:79.
29. Bacharach SL, Green MV, Borer JS, et al. Left ventricular peak ejection rate, filling rate and ejection fraction: frame rate requirements at rest and exercise. *J Nucl Med* 1979; 20:189.
30. Green MV, Ostrow HG, Douglas MA, et al. A comparison of simultaneous measurements of systolic function in the baboon by electromagnetic flowmeter and high frame rate ECG-gated blood pool scintigraphy. *Circulation* 1979;60:312.
31. Bachrach SL, Green MV, Borer JS, et al. Beat by beat validation of ECG gating. *J Nucl Med* 1980;21:307.
32. Bachrach SL, Green MV, Bonow RO, et al. Measurement of ventricular function by ECG gating during atrial fibrillation. *J Nucl Med* 1981;22:226.
33. Parker JA, Uren RF, Jones AG, et al. Radionuclide left ventriculography with the slant hole collimator. *J Nucl Med* 1977;18:848.
34. Strauss HW, Zaret BL, Hurley PJ, et al. A scintiphotographic method for measuring left ventricular ejection fraction in man without cardiac catherization. *Am J Cardiol* 1971;28:575.
35. Zaret BL, Strauss HW, Hurley PJ, et al. A noninvasive scintiphotographic method for detecting regional dysfunction in man. *N Engl J Med* 1971;284:1165.
36. Parker JA, Secker-Walker R, Hill R, et al. A new technique for calculation of left ventricular ejection fraction. *J Nucl Med* 1972;13:649.
37. Alpert NM, McKusick KA, Pohost GM, et al. Non-invasive nuclear kinecardiography. *J Nucl Med* 1974;15:1182.
38. Burow RD, Strauss HW, Singleton R, et al. Analysis of left ventricular function from multiple gated acquisition cardiac blood pool imaging: comparison to contrast angiography. *Circulation* 1977;56:1024.
39. Wagner RH, Halama JR, Henkin RE, et al. Errors in the determination of left ventricular functional parameters. *J Nucl Med* 1989;30:1870.
40. Simon TR, Walker BS, Matthiesen S, et al. A realistic dynamic cardiac phantom for evaluating radionuclide ventriculography: description and initial studies with the left ventricular chamber. *J Nucl Med* 1989;30:542.
41. Juni JE, Chen CC. Effects of gating modes on the analysis of left ventricular function in the presence of heart rate variation. *J Nucl Med* 1988;29:1272.
42. Bacharach SL, Bonow RO, Green MV. Comparison of fixed and variable temporal resolution methods for creating gated blood pool image sequences. *J Nucl Med* 1990;31:38.
43. Bacharach SL, Ostrow HG, Bonow RO, et al. ECG-gated pressure volume relationships utilizing scintigraphic image data. In: *Computers in Cardiology, Boston, MA.* Los Alamitos, CA: IEEE Computer Society Press, 1985;353.
44. Green MV, Bacharach SL, Borer JS, et al. A theoretical comparison of first pass and gated equilibrium methods of measuring systolic left ventricular function. *J Nucl Med* 1991; 32:1801.
45. Green MV, Andrich MP, Doudet D. Evaluation of cardiovascular function in small animals using a microcomputer-based scintigraphic imaging system. In: *Computers in Cardiology, Venice, Italy,* Los Alamitos, CA: IEEE Computer Society Press, 1991;233.
46. Pierluigi P, Fischman AJ, Ahmad M, et al. Cardiac bloodpool scintigraphy in rats and hamsters: comparison of five radiopharmaceuticals and three pinhole collimator apertures. *J Nucl Med* 1991;32:851.
47. Green MV, Markowitz A, Tedder TE, et al. SPECT imaging in small animals. *J Nucl Med* 1992;33:852.
48. Borer JS, Bacharach SL, Green MV, et al. Real-time radionuclide cineangiography in the non-invasive evaluation of global and regional left ventricular function at rest and during exercise in patients with coronary artery disease. *N Engl J Med* 1977;296:839.
49. Kent KM, Broer JS, Bacharach SL, et al. Effects of coronary artery bypass operation on global and regional left ventricular function during exercise. *N Engl J Med* 1978; 298:1434.
50. Borer JS, Bacharach SL, Green MV, et al. Effect of nitroglycerin on exercise-induced abnormalities of regional and global left ventricular function in coronary artery disease: assessment by radionuclide cineangiography in symptomatic and asymptomatic patients. *Circulation* 1978;57:314.
51. Gottdiener JS, Katin MJ, Borer JS, et al. Late cardiac effects

of therapeutic mediastinal irradiation. *N Engl J Med* 1983; 308:559.

52. Leon MB, Borer JS, Bacharach SL, et al. Detection of early cardiac dysfunction in patients with severe beta-thallassemia and chronic iron overload. *N Engl J Med* 1979;301:1143.
53. Bonow RO, Vitale SF, Bacharach SL. Effects of aging on asynchronous left ventricular regional function and global ventricular filling in normal human subjects. *J Am Coll Cardiol* 1988;11:50.
54. Rothendler JA, Schick EC, Leppo J, et al. Diagnosis of pericardial effusions from routine gated blood-pool imaging. *J Nucl Med* 1987;28:1419.
55. Bonaduce D, Morgano G, Petretta M, et al. Diastolic function in acute myocardial infarction: a radionucleide study. *J Nucl Med* 1988;29:1786.
56. Starling MR, Gross MD, Walsh RA, et al. Assessment of the radionuclide angiographic left ventricular maximum time-varying elastance calculation in man. *J Nucl Med* 1988; 29:1368.
57. Brown EJ Jr, Idoine J, Swinford RD, et al. Regional left ventricular filling: does it reflect diastolic abnormalities in continuous areas of myocardium? *J Nucl Med* 1989;30:165.
58. Marmor A, Sharir T, Shlomo IB, et al. Radionuclide ventriculography and central aorta pressure change in noninvasive assessment of myocardial performance. *J Nucl Med* 1989; 30:1657.
59. Verani MS, Sanders WE Jr, Noon GP. Functional assessment of the total artificial heart by blood-pool radionuclide angiography. *J Nucl Med* 1989;30:1405.
60. Bacharach SL, Green MV, Borer JS. Instrumentation and data processing in cardiovascular nuclear medicine: evaluation of ventricular function. *Semin Nucl Med* 1979;IX:257.
61. Rosenthal MS, Klein HA, Orenstein SR. Simultaneous acquisition of physiological data and nuclear medicine images. *J Nucl Med* 1988;29:1848.
62. Kojima A, Matsumoto M, Takahashi M, et al. Effect of energy resolution on scatter fraction in scintigraphic imaging: Monte Carlo study. *Med Phys* 1993;20:1107.
63. Singh M, Horne C. Use of a germanium detector to optimize scatter correction in SPECT. *J Nucl Med* 1987;28:1853.
64. Gagnon D, Laperrière L, Pouliot N, et al. Monte Carlo analysis of camera-induced spectral contamination for different primary energies. *Phys Med Biol* 1992;37:1725.
65. Wirth V. Effective energy resolution and scatter rejection in nuclear medicine. *Phys Med Biol* 1989;34:85.
66. Koral KF, Wang X, Rogers WL, et al. SPECT Compton-scattering correction by analysis of energy spectra. *J Nucl Med* 1988;29:195.
67. Koral KF, Buchbinder S, Clinthorne NH. Validation of a spectral-image acquisition system. *J Nucl Med* 1993;34: 113.
68. Seidel J, Green MV, Bacharach SL, et al. Correction for compton scatter by curve fitting the photopeak region of energy spectra acquired at every image point. *J Nucl Med* 1993;34:60.
69. Maor D, Berlad G, Chrem Y, et al. Klein-Nishina based energy factors for Compton free imaging (CFI). *J Nucl Med* 1991;32:1000.
70. King MA, Hademenos GJ, Glick SJ. A dual-photopeak window method for scatter correction. *J Nucl Med* 1992;33:605.
71. Ichihara T, Ogawa K, Motomura N, et al. Compton scatter compensation using the triple-energy window method for single-and dual-isotope SPECT. *J Nucl Med* 1993;34:2216.
72. Mas J, Hannequin P, Ben Younes R, et al. Scatter correction in planar imaging and SPECT by constrained factor analysis of dynamic structures (FADS). *Phys Med Biol* 1990;35:1451.
73. Msaki P, Axelsson B, Dahl CM, et al. Generalized scatter correction method in SPECT using point scatter distribution functions. *J Nucl Med* 1987;28:1861.
74. Gilardi MC, Bettinardi V, Todd-Pokropek A, et al. Assessment and comparison of three scatter correction techniques in single photon emission computed tomography. *J Nucl Med* 1988;29:1971.
75. DeVito RP, Hamill JJ, Treffert JD, et al. Energy-weighted acquisition of scintigraphic images using finite spatial filters. *J Nucl Med* 1989;30:2029.
76. DeVito RP, Hamill JJ, Determination of weighting functions for energy-weighted acquisition. *J Nucl Med* 1991;32:343.
77. Bowsher JE, Floyd CE Jr. Treatment of compton scattering in maximum-likelihood, expectation-maximization reconstructions of SPECT images. *J Nucl Med* 1991;32:1285.
78. Ljungberg M, Strand S-E. Scatter and attenuation correction in SPECT using density maps and Monte Carlo simulated scatter functions. *J Nucl Med* 1990;31:1560.
79. Galt JR, Cullom SJ, Garcia EV. SPECT quantification: a simplified method of attenuation and scatter correction for cardiac imaging. *J Nucl Med* 1992;33:2232.
80. Ljungberg M, Strand S-E. Attenuation and scatter correction in SPECT for sources in a nonhomogenous object: A Monte Carlo study. *J Nucl Med* 1991;32:1278.
81. Hansen CL, Siegel JA. Attenuation correction of thallium SPECT using differential attenuation of thallium photons. *J Nucl Med* 1992;33:1574.
82. Kemp BJ, Prato FS, Dean GW, et al. Correction for attenuation in technetium-99m-HMPAO SPECT brain imaging. *J Nucl Med* 1992;33:1875.
83. Cao ZJ, Tsui BMW. Performance characteristics of transmission imaging using a uniform sheet source with parallel-hole collimation. *Med Phys* 1992;19:1205.
84. van Elmbt L, Walrand S. Simultaneous correction of attenuation and distance-dependent resolution in SPECT: an analytical approach. *Phys Med Biol* 1993;38:1207.
85. Ljungberg M, Strand S-E. Attenuation correction in SPECT based on transmission studies and Monte Carlo simulations of build-up functions. *J Nucl Med* 1990;31:493.
86. Frey EC, Tsui BMW, Perry JR. Simultaneous acquisition of emission and transmission data for improved thallium-201 cardiac SPECT imaging using a technetium-99m transmission source. *J Nucl Med* 1992;33:2238.
87. Jaszczak RJ, Gilland DR, Hanson MW, et al. Fast transmission CT for determining attenuation maps using a collimated line source, rotatable air-copper-lead attenuators and fan-beam collimation. *J Nucl Med* 1993;34:1577.
88. Tan P, Bailey DL, Meikle SR et al. A scanning line source for simultaneous emission and transmission measurements in SPECT. *J Nucl Med* 1993;34:1752.
89. Lang TF, Hasegawa BH, Liew SC, et al. Description of a prototype emission-transmission computed tomography imaging system. *J Nucl Med* 1992;33:1881.
90. Tsui BMW, Gullberg GT, Edgerton ER, et al. Correction of nonuniform attenuation in cardiac SPECT imaging. *J Nucl Med* 1989;30:497.
91. Manglos SH, Thomas FD, Hellwig BJ. The effect of nonuniform attenuation compensation on myocardial SPECT defect analysis. *Phys Med Biol* 1993;38:897.
92. Manglos SH, Jaszczak RJ, Floyd CE, et al. Nonisotropic attenuation in SPECT: phantom tests of quantitative effects and compensation techniques. *J Nucl Med* 1987;28:1584.
93. Welch A, Webb S, Flower M. Improved cone-beam SPECT via an accurate correction for non-uniform photon attenuation. *Phys Med Biol* 1993;38:909.
94. Manglos SH, Bassano DA, Thomas FD. Cone-beam transmission computed tomography for nonuniform attenuation compensation of SPECT images. *J Nucl Med* 1991;32:1813.

95. Manglos SH, Bassano DA, Thomas FD. Imaging of the human torso using cone-beam transmission CT implemented on a rotating gamma camera. *J Nucl Med* 1992;33:150.
96. Madsen MT, Chang W, Hichwa RD. Spatial resolution and count density requirements in brain SPECT imaging. *Phys Med Biol* 1992;37:1625.
97. Gillen GJ. A simple method for the measurement of local statistical noise levels in SPECT. *Phys Med Biol* 1992; 37:1573.
98. Boulfelfel D, Rangayyan RM, Hahn LJ, et al. Use of the geometric mean of opposing planar projections in pre-reconstruction restoration of SPECT images. *Phys Med Biol* 1992; 37:1915.
99. Jaszczak RJ, Greer KL, Coleman RW. SPECT using a specially designed cone beam collimator. *J Nucl Med* 1988; 29:1398.
100. Li J, Jaszczak RJ, Greer KL, et al. Direct cone beam SPECT reconstruction with camera tile. *Phys Med Biol* 1993;38:241.
101. Malmain RE, Stanley PC, Guth WR. Collimator angulation error and its effect on SPECT. *J Nucl Med* 1990;31:655.
102. Cerqueira MD, Matsuoka D, Ritchie JL, et al. The influence of collimators on SPECT center of rotation measurements: artifact generation and acceptance testing. *J Nucl Med* 1988;29:1393.
103. Busemann-Sokole E. Measurement of collimator hole angulation and camera head tilt for slant and parallel hole collimators used in SPECT. *J Nucl Med* 1987;28:1592.
104. Bieszk JA, Hawman EG. Evaluation of SPECT angular sampling effects: continuous versus step-and-shoot acquisition. *J Nucl Med* 1987;28:1308.
105. Kojima A, Matsumoto M, Takahashi M, et al. Effect of spatial resolution on SPECT quantification values. *J Nucl Med* 1989;30:508.
106. Knesaurek K, King MA, Glick SJ, et al. Investigation of causes of geometric distortion in 180° and 360° angular sampling in SPECT. *J Nucl Med* 1989;30:1666.
107. Maublant JC, Peycelon P, Kwiatkowski F, et al. Comparison between 180° and 360° data collection in technetium-99m MIBI SPECT of the myocardium. *J Nucl Med* 1989;30: 295.
108. Maniawski PJ, Morgan HT, Wackers FJT. Orbit-related variation in spatial resolution as a source of artifactual defects in thallium-201 SPECT. *J Nucl Med* 1991;32:871.
109. Faber TL, Stokely EM, Templeton GH, et al. Quantification of three-dimensional left ventricular segmental wall motion and volumes from gated tomographic radionuclide ventriculograms. *J Nucl Med* 1989;30:638.
110. Nuyts J, Mortelmans L, Suetens P, et al. Model-based quantification of myocardial perfusion images from SPECT. *J Nucl Med* 1989;30:1992.
111. Botvinick EH, Zhu YY, O'Connell WJ, et al. A quantitative assessment of patient motion and its effect on myocardial perfusion SPECT images. *J Nucl Med* 1993;34:303.
112. Cooper JA, Neumann PH, McCandless BK. Effect of patient motion on tomographic myocardial perfusion imaging. *J Nucl Med* 1992;33:1566.
113. Chen Q-S, Franken PR, Defrise M, et al. Detection and correction of patient motion in SPECT imaging. *J Nucl Med Technol* 1993;21:198.
114. Geckle WJ, Frank TL, Links JM, et al. Correction for patient and organ movement in SPECT: application to exercise thallium-201 cardiac imaging. *J Nucl Med* 1988;29:441.
115. Cooper JA, Neumann PH, McCandless BK. Detection of patient motion during tomographic myocardial perfusion imaging. *J Nucl Med* 1993;34:1341.
116. Germano G, Chua T, Kavanagh PB, et al. Detection and correction of patient motion in dynamic and static myocardial SPECT using a multi-detector camera. *J Nucl Med* 1993; 34:1349.
117. Lowe VJ, Greer KL, Hanson MW, et al. Cardiac phantom evaluation of simultaneously acquired dual-isotope rest thallium-201/stress technetium-99m SPECT images. *J Nucl Med* 1993;34:1998.
118. Links JM, Jeremy RW, Dyer SM, et al. Wiener filtering improves quantification of regional myocardial perfusion with thallium-201 SPECT. *J Nucl Med* 1990;31:1230.
119. Gilland DR, Jaszczak RJ, Greer KL, et al. Quantitative SPECT reconstruction of iodine-123 data. *J Nucl Med* 1991;32:527.
120. Devous MD Sr, Lowe JL, Payne JK. Dual-isotope brain SPECT imaging with technetium and iodine-123: validation by phantom studies. *J Nucl Med* 1992;33:2030.
121. Kim H-J, Zeeberg BR, Loew MH, et al. Three-dimensional simulations of multidetector point-focusing SPECT imaging. *J Nucl Med* 1991;32:333.
122. Kim H-J, Zeeburg BR, Gahey FH, et al. Three-dimensional SPECT simulations of a complex three-dimensional mathematical brain model and measurements of the three-dimensional physical brain phantom. *J Nucl Med* 1991;32:1923.
123. Nakajima K, Shuke N, Taki J, et al. A simulation of dynamic SPECT using radiopharmaceuticals with rapid clearance. *J Nucl Med* 1992;33:1200.
124. Palmer J, Wollmer P. Pinhole emission computed tomography: method and experimental evaluation. *Phys Med Biol* 1990;35:339.
125. DePuey EG, Guertler-Krawczynska E, Robbins WL. Thallium-201 SPECT in coronary artery disease patients with left bundle branch block. *J Nucl Med* 1988;29:1479.
126. Neumann DR. Simultaneous dual-isotope SPECT imaging for the detection and characterization of parathyroid pathology. *J Nucl Med* 1992;33:131.
127. Faber TL, Akers MS, Peshock RM, et al. Three-dimensional motion and perfusion quantification in gated single-photon emission computed tomograms. *J Nucl Med* 1991;32:2311.
128. Front D, Israel O, Jerushalmi J, et al. Quantitative bone scintigraphy using SPECT. *J Nucl Med* 1989;30:240.
129. Groshar D, Frankel A, Iosilevsky G, et al. Quantitation of renal uptake of technetium-99m DMSA using SPECT. *J Nucl Med* 1989;30:246.
130. Leichner PK, Vriesendorp HM, Hawkins WG, et al. Quantitative SPECT for indium-111-labeled antibodies in the livers of beagle dogs. *J Nucl Med* 1991;32:1442.
131. Gilland DR, Tsui BMW, McCartney WH, et al. Determination of the optimum filter function for SPECT imaging. *J Nucl Med* 1988;29:643.
132. Suzuki S. Spatially limited filters for the two-dimensional convolution method of reconstruction, and their application to SPECT. *Phys Med Biol* 1992;37:37.
133. Kim H-J, Zeeburg BR, Reba RC. Evaluation of reconstruction algorithms in SPECT neuroimaging. I. Comparison of statistical noise in SPECT neuroimages with 'naive' and 'realistic' predictions. *Phys Med Biol* 1993;38:863.
134. Webb S. SPECT reconstruction by simulated annealing. *Phys Med Biol* 1989;34:259.
135. Gilland DR, Tsui BMW, Metz CE, et al. An evaluation of maximum likelihood-expectation maximization reconstruction for SPECT by ROC analysis. *J Nucl Med* 1992;33:451.
136. Liow J-S, Strother SC. The convergence of object dependent resolution in maximum likelihood based tomographic image reconstruction. *Phys Med Biol* 1993;38:55.
137. Lalush DS, Tsui BMW. A generalized Gibbs prior for maximum *a posteriori* reconstruction in SPECT. *Phys Med Biol* 1993;38:739.
138. Hawkins WG, Yang N-C, Leichner PK. Validation of the

circular harmonic transform (CHT) algorithm for quantitative SPECT. *J Nucl Med* 1991;32:141.

139. Formiconi AR, Pupi A, Passeri A. Compensation of spatial system response in SPECT with conjugate gradient reconstruction technique. *Phys Med Biol* 1989;34:69.
140. Wallis JW, Miller TR. Rapidly converging iterative reconstruction algorithms in single-photon emission computed tomography. *J Nucl Med* 1993;34:1793.
141. Xu X-L, Liow J-S, Strother SC. Iterative algebraic reconstruction algorithms for emission computed tomography: a unified framework and its application to positron emission tomography. *Med Phys* 1993;20:1675.
142. Liang Z. Compensation for attenuation, scatter, and detector response in SPECT reconstruction via iterative FBP methods. *Med Phys* 1993;20:1097.
143. Maze A, Le Cloirec J, Collorec R, et al. Iterative reconstruction methods for nonuniform attenuation distribution in SPECT. *J Nucl Med* 1993;34:1204.
144. Miller TR, Wallis JW. Fast maximum-likelihood reconstruction. *J Nucl Med* 1992;33:1710.
145. Sprawls P Jr. *Physical Principles of Medical Imaging*. Rockville, MD: Aspen Publications, 1987.
146. Williams LE, ed. *Nuclear Medical Physics*. vol 2. Boca Raton FL: CRC Press, 1987.
147. Williams LE, ed. *Nuclear Medical Physics*. vol. 3. Boca Raton, FL: CRC Press, 1987.
148. Hoffer PB, ed. *The Year Book of Nuclear Medicine*. Chicago, IL: Year Book Medical Publishers, 1986.
149. Williams ED, ed. *An Introduction to Emission Computed Tomography*, Report No. 44, London: Institute of Physical Sciences in Medicine, Report No. 44. 1985.
150. Parker JA. *Image Reconstruction in Radiology*. Boca Raton, FL: CRC Press, 1990.
151. Freedman GS, ed. *Tomographic Imaging in Nuclear Medicine*. New York: The Society of Nuclear Medicine, 1972.
152. Johns HE, Cunningham JR. *The Physics of Radiology*. 3rd ed. Springfield, IL: Charles C Thomas, 1969.
153. Hine GJ, Brownell GL, eds. *Radiation Dosimetry*. New York: Academic Press, 1956.
154. Bevington PR. *Data Reduction and Error Analysis for the Physical Sciences*. New York: McGraw-Hill, 1969.
155. Bracewell RN. *The Fourier Transform and its Applications*. 2nd ed, rev. New York: McGraw-Hill, 1965.
156. Jericevic Z, Wiese B, Bryan J, et al. *Methods in Cell Biology*. vol. 30. San Diego: Academic Press, 1989.
157. Knoll GF. *Radiation Detection and Measurement*. 2nd ed. New York: John Wiley & Sons, 1989.
158. Schelbert HR. Principles of positron emission tomography. In: *Cardiac Imaging*. Marcus ML, ed. Philadelphia: W.B. Saunders, 1991.
159. Zito F, Savi A, Fazio F. CERASPECT: a brain-dedicated SPECT system. Performance evaluation and comparison with the rotating gamma camera. *Phys Med Biol* 1993;38:1433.
160. Rowe RK, Aarsvold JN, Barrett HH, et al. A stationary hemispherical SPECT imager for three-dimensional brain imaging. *J Nucl Med* 1993;34:474.
161. Karp JS, Muehllehner G, Mankoff DA, et al. Continuous-slice PENN-PET: a positron tomograph with volume imaging capability. *J Nucl Med* 1990;31:617.

6 Positron Emission Tomography

Margaret E. Daube-Witherspoon, Peter Herscovitch

Positron emission tomography (PET) is a technique for imaging the concentration of positron-emitting radionuclides in the body by means of radiation detectors arrayed around the body. The data are presented in the form of gray-scale images of cross-sections through the body. The intensity of each point or pixel in the image is proportional to the amount of radioactivity at the corresponding position in the body. From these images one can derive quantitative images of useful physiological parameters, such as regional blood flow or metabolism.

From the 1950s until the early 1970s numerous articles reported of devices to image positron-emitting radioactivity.[1–6] However, it was not until the mid-1970s, when image reconstruction techniques developed for x-ray computed tomography were applied, that tomographic imaging of positron-emitting radiotracers began to advance. The first PET scanner which "... [incorporated] the fundamental features of modern PET devices"[7] was developed at Washington University in St. Louis in the mid-1970s.[8,9] Since that time, PET scanners have improved in spatial resolution and sampling, both in-plane and out-of-plane, and in the number of slices acquired simultaneously, through the use of smaller radiation detectors. There have also been improvements in quantitative accuracy through the use of sophisticated algorithms to correct for the various physical effects associated with the imaging process.

Initially, PET was used primarily to study the brain[10] and heart.[11,12] Subsequently, a wide variety of radiotracer techniques were developed to study these and other organs. For the brain, methods have been developed to assess regional cerebral blood flow and volume; glucose, oxygen, and protein metabolism; blood-brain barrier function; neuroreceptor-neurotransmitter systems; tissue pH; and concentrations of radiolabeled drugs in brain. PET brain studies have focused on normal brain function and the pathophysiology of neurologic and psychiatric disease.[13,14] For the heart, several PET methods now assess cardiac perfusion, glucose consumption, oxidative metabolism, and receptor function.[15,16] In addition, PET is used to study the lung and abdominal organs, and is finding increasing application in oncology.[17–19] Although most PET studies have emphasized organ physiology and pathophysiology, increasingly it is being applied to patient diagnosis and management.[20]

Conceptually, there are three components involved in PET: (1) tracer compounds of physiologic interest that are labeled with positron-emitting radionuclides; (2) PET scanners to visualize the concentration of positron-emitting radioactivity; and (3) mathematical models that describe the in vivo behavior of specific radiotracers used, so that physiologic processes under study can be quantified from tomographic measurements of regional radioactivity. This chapter focuses on PET imaging devices. Radiotracer compounds and mathematical modeling are discussed elsewhere in this volume.

PHYSICAL BASIS OF PET

Event Detection

Certain radionuclides, such as ^{18}F and ^{15}O, decay by positron emission from the nucleus. Positrons are "antimatter" particles to electrons; they have the same mass as electrons, but positive charge. After emission from the nucleus, positrons travel variable distances in tissue, up to a few millimeters, losing kinetic energy. When almost at rest, they interact with atomic electrons, resulting in the annihilation of both particles. Their combined mass is converted into two high-energy, 511-keV photons that travel in opposite directions away from the annihilation site at the speed of light (Fig. 1). (The 511-keV energy of each annihilation photon is equivalent to the rest mass of an electron or positron.) Positrons from a specific radionuclide are not monoenergetic. Rather, they are emitted with a range of energies from zero to a maximum value (E_{max}). The maximum positron energy varies considerably among radionuclides, from about 0.635 MeV for ^{18}F to 3.35 MeV for ^{82}Rb. The average energy of the positron is approximately 40% of E_{max}.[21] The greater the positron energy, the farther it travels from the nucleus before annihilation. The term *positron range* refers to the net distance away from the decay site that the positron travels before annihilating. The actual path the positron takes is tortuous, and path length is longer than the positron range.

In PET, what is detected is not the positron emitted by decay. Rather, detection of the photon pair that results from positron annihilation (one pair per radioactive decay event) is used to measure both the location and amount of radioactivity in the field of view. The annihilation photons are detected by two opposing radiation detectors connected by an electronic coincidence circuit (Fig. 2). This circuit records a decay event only when both detectors sense the almost

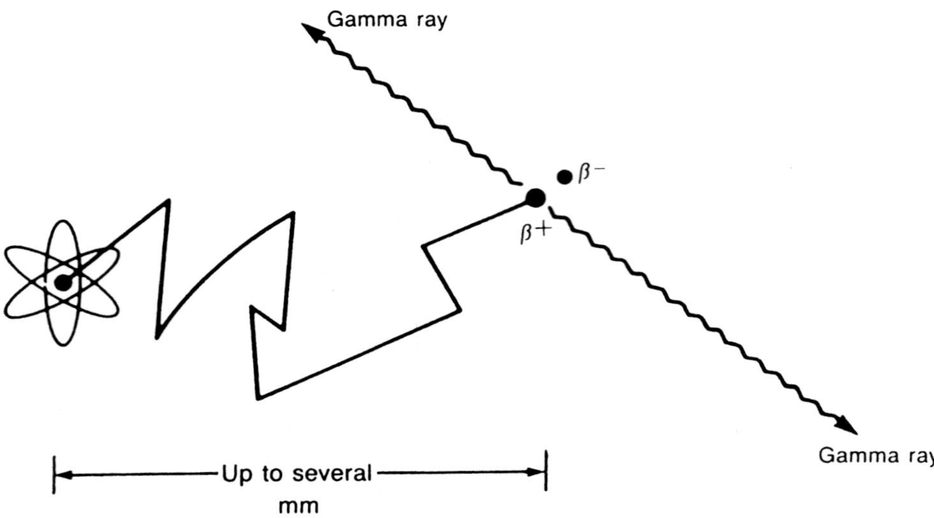

Figure 1. β^+ decay and positron annihilation. The positron created from the β^+ decay of the neutron-poor/proton-rich nucleus travels a short distance in tissue before annihilating both itself and an atomic electron (β^-), forming two 511-keV gamma rays. The gamma rays travel approximately 180° apart (from Bacharach[35]).

simultaneous arrival of both photons. A very short time window for photon arrival called the *coincidence resolving time* is allowed for registration of coincidence events. This time window is typically 5 to 20 nanoseconds and is limited primarily by the response time of the radiation detectors.

The coincidence requirement for photon detection localizes the site of the decay event between the detector pair. Unlike single-photon imaging, additional collimation of the photons, which reduces the efficiency of detection, is not needed to define their direction. This event localization by the coincidence requirement is sometimes referred to as "electronic" collimation. Except for time-of-flight PET imagers (discussed later in this chapter), which have specialized detectors and electronics, there is no information about the depth or location of the radioactive source within the volume between the two detectors.

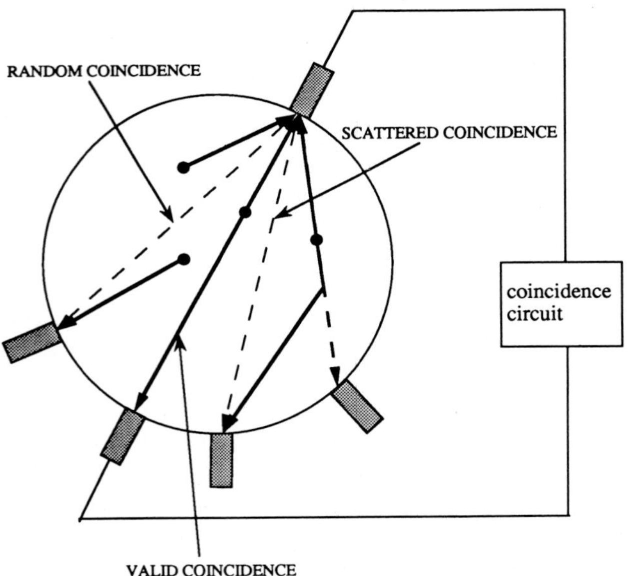

Figure 2. Coincidence detection. The two photons resulting from a positron emission and annihilation are detected by two radiation detectors that are connected by an electronic coincidence circuit. A decay event is recorded as a coincidence line between the detectors only when both photons are detected almost simultaneously. This coincidence requirement localizes the site of the annihilation to the volume of space between the detectors. A *random coincidence* is registered if two photons from two *different* positron annihilations are sensed by a detector pair within the coincidence resolving time. A *scattered coincidence* occurs when an annihilation photon traveling in tissue is deflected, so that its direction changes. This results in incorrect positioning of the measured coincidence line.

Formation of the PET Image

In most PET imagers several rings each consisting of many radiation detectors are used, with each detector paired with many detector elements on the opposite side of the ring in a fan-beam fashion. This configuration increases the number of coincidence lines detected, which in turn increases the scanner's sensitivity by sampling coincidence events from more areas at the same time. The number of coincidence events recorded by any pair of detectors is proportional to the amount of radioactivity between them. The coincidence data are sorted into parallel groups, each group representing a profile or one-dimensional projection of the radioactivity distribution in the tomographic slice viewed from a different angle (Fig. 3). These profiles are then combined to obtain a cross-sectional or *tomographic* image. In addition, in conventional two-dimensional (2-D) imaging, "cross slices" are derived from coincidences between detectors in different rings; events in these planes are placed halfway between the detector rings (Fig. 4).

Two-dimensional PET images are reconstructed from projection data usually by application of the same mathematical principles used in x-ray computed tomography.[22,23] The technique, referred to as *filtered back-projection*, consists of two steps: (1) radial filtering of the projection data and (2) back-projecting, or smearing, the filtered projection across the

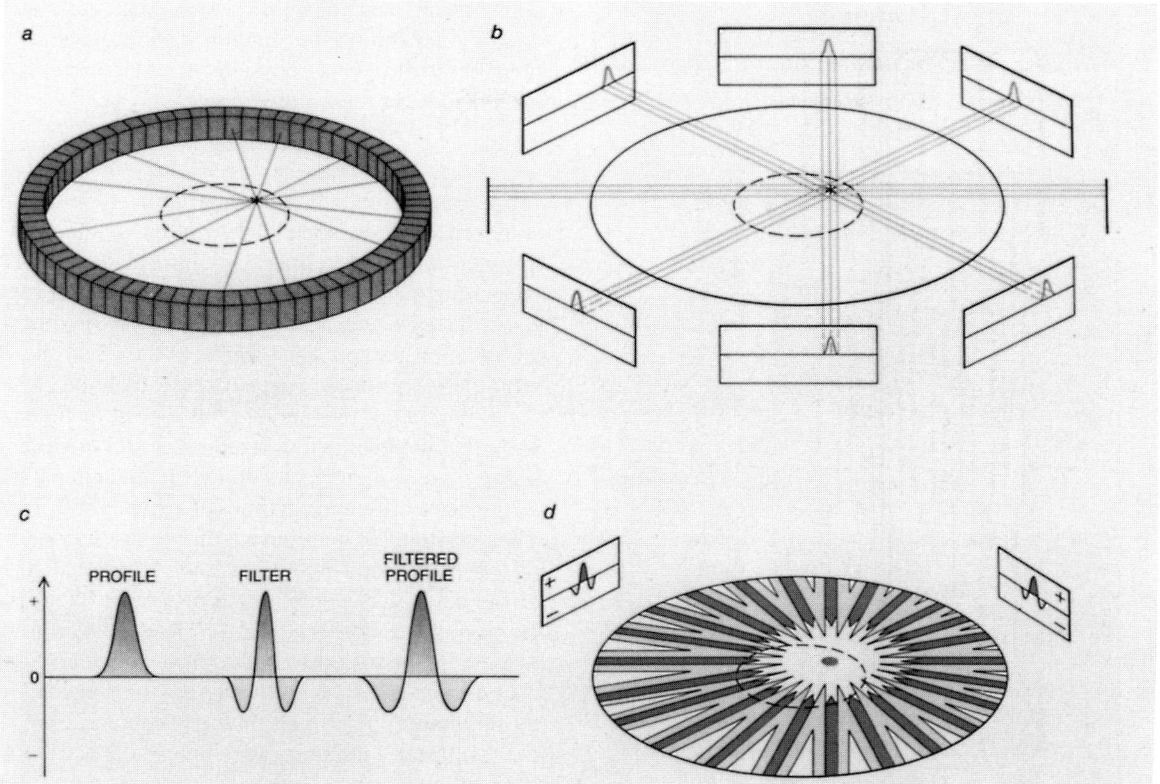

Figure 3. Formation of the PET image. The steps in PET image formation are depicted in these diagrams that illustrate the imaging of a small region of uniform radioactivity in a single tomographic plane. (a). Multiple coincidence lines are recorded by opposing detector pairs in the ring. Each line results from a positron emission and annihilation so that the number of coincidence lines recorded by any detector pair is proportional to the amount of radioactivity between them. (b). After imaging, the coincidence lines are sorted into parallel groups representing the profile or projection of the radioactivity distribution viewed from a different angle. (c). Each projection is mathematically processed by means of a special function called the *filter function* to remove unwanted contributions to pixels with no underlying radioactivity. (d). The modified projections are then combined by "back-projection" to reconstruct an image of the radioactivity distribution. Note that there are several other steps in reconstruction, eg, corrections for attenuation, deadtime, and random and scattered coincidence counts, as described in the text (from Ter-Pogossian et al[117]).

image plane (Fig. 3 and 5). In the back-projection step there is no information as to the location of the source contributing to a given coincidence line. Therefore, the counts in that line are distributed uniformly to all pixels that the coincidence line intersects. If the projection data are not filtered prior to back-projection, the image of each source has a star-pattern with a $1/r$-shaped intensity in the background because each count is applied not only to the area of activity (from which it was measured) but also to other pixels along that direction (see Fig. 5). Filtering produces negative projection values which, when back-projected, cancel out the positive counts in areas of no activity (see Figs. 3 and 5). The filter function can be varied, with more or less smoothing being applied during reconstruction. Filtering with a function that eliminates high spatial frequencies will decrease the noise in the image; however, it also results in poorer spatial resolution and can lead to poorer quantitative accuracy. The choice of reconstruction filter is determined by the purpose of the study and the quality of the acquired data. In general, it is preferable to do as little filtering during reconstruction as possible in order to preserve resolution and quantitative accuracy in the image.

The filtered back-projection algorithm makes a number of assumptions about the projection data that usually are not completely met. The data are assumed to be "perfect"; to satisfy this condition, the data must first be corrected for physical effects such as attenuation, nonuniform detector response, scatter, and random coincidences (discussed later in the chapter) prior to reconstruction. In addition, data are assumed to be measured from all possible coincidence lines passing through the object to be reconstructed, and the region of coincidence response is taken to be infinitely thin. The former is approximately true for 2-D reconstructions from most PET devices; the latter is never strictly met because the coincidences are localized only to the finite-sized volume between the detectors. Finally, the data are assumed to be noise-free. This condition is rarely met in PET.

In addition to filtered back-projection, there are other

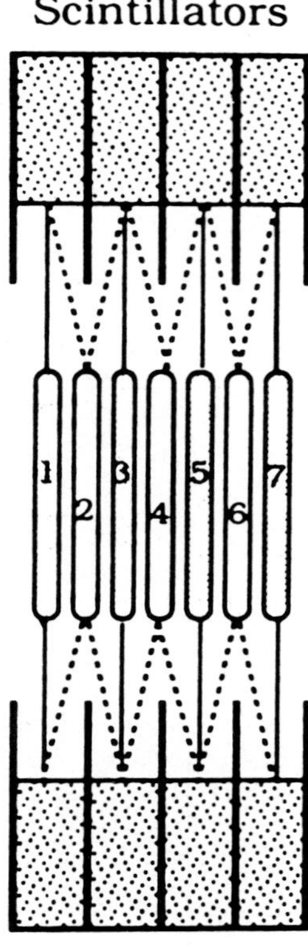

Figure 4. Straight and cross slices in 2-D imaging. A straight slice consists of coincident events between detectors in the same ring or axial position (indicated by the odd numbers). A cross slice is created from slightly oblique coincidences which are detected by detectors in different rings at different axial positions (indicated by the even numbers). The events in these cross slices are assigned to a fictitious slice parallel to the straight slices and positioned at an axial location which is the average of the two detected axial positions. In this figure, only cross slices arising from coincidences between detectors in adjacent rings are shown (from Kanno[118]).

reconstruction algorithms that are used much less frequently.[24–30] These methods, many of which require significant additional computation time, result in images with different bias and noise properties than those obtained by filtered back-projection. It is beyond the scope of this chapter to review these algorithms.

The intensity of any point in the PET image is proportional to the amount of radioactivity in the corresponding region of tissue.[31] To calibrate the PET system in order to obtain *absolute* radioactivity measurements, a cylinder containing a uniform solution of radioactivity is imaged. The radioactivity in an aliquot of the solution is then measured with a calibrated well counter, and the scanner calibration factor is calculated so that one can convert PET image counts (in units of counts per second per pixel) to units of radioactivity concentration (eg, nanocuries per cubic centimeter). The PET image can then be scaled and displayed to represent the absolute amount of radioactivity. It should be noted that the accuracy of this calibration depends upon the ability to correct for such effects as attenuation, scatter, random coincidences, and deadtime losses. The calibration procedure should mimic the imaging conditions encountered in practice as closely as possible in order to compensate for inaccuracies in these corrections.

Time-of-Flight Systems

Data from so-called "time-of-flight" systems do contain some information about the location of the activity along a given coincidence line. This information is obtained by measuring the difference in arrival times of the two photons. For a decay event near the edge of the field of view, one annihilation photon must travel farther than the other, and will, therefore, strike a detector later than the closer photon. Annihilation photons travel at the speed of light, so that an annihilation generated at a radius of 10 cm from the center of the field of view results in a difference in path lengths of 20 cm, for a difference in times of arrival of 667 picoseconds. Time-of-flight devices have a timing resolution on the order of 600 picoseconds[32] and can, therefore, localize the source of the coincident photons to a distance of approximately 9 cm from the center. The time difference can be used in image reconstruction to constrain the smearing of the counts during back-projection, thereby improving the signal-to-noise ratio in the image.[33] However, time-of-flight systems require the use of faster radiation detectors and electronics and are used infrequently.

PHYSICAL EFFECTS—LIMITATIONS TO IMAGE QUALITY AND QUANTIFICATION

Several factors limit quality and quantitative accuracy of PET images. Physical effects such as differences in detector pair efficiencies, attenuation, scatter, random coincidences, and scanner deadtime require correction prior to image reconstruction. Other factors inherent in the PET imaging process, such as image noise and spatial resolution, have a major impact on image quality and on the design or interpretation of PET studies. These issues are discussed below.

Spatial Resolution

The concept of spatial resolution is critical in understanding the limitations to both qualitative and quantitative PET imaging. One interpretation of resolution is that it is the minimum distance by which two points of radioactivity must be separated to be perceived independently in the reconstructed image. Structures that are closer than the spatial resolution of the scanner in any direction cannot be perfectly distinguished from adjacent structures and will receive a contribution from nearby areas. The resultant spreading or smearing reduces the quantitative accuracy in measurements of small objects and decreases image contrast.

Operationally, scanner resolution is measured separately for the transverse ("in-plane") and axial ("out-of-plane") directions. The in-plane spatial resolution is determined by imaging a thin point or line source of positron-emitting radioactivity (Fig. 6). Because of limited spatial resolution,

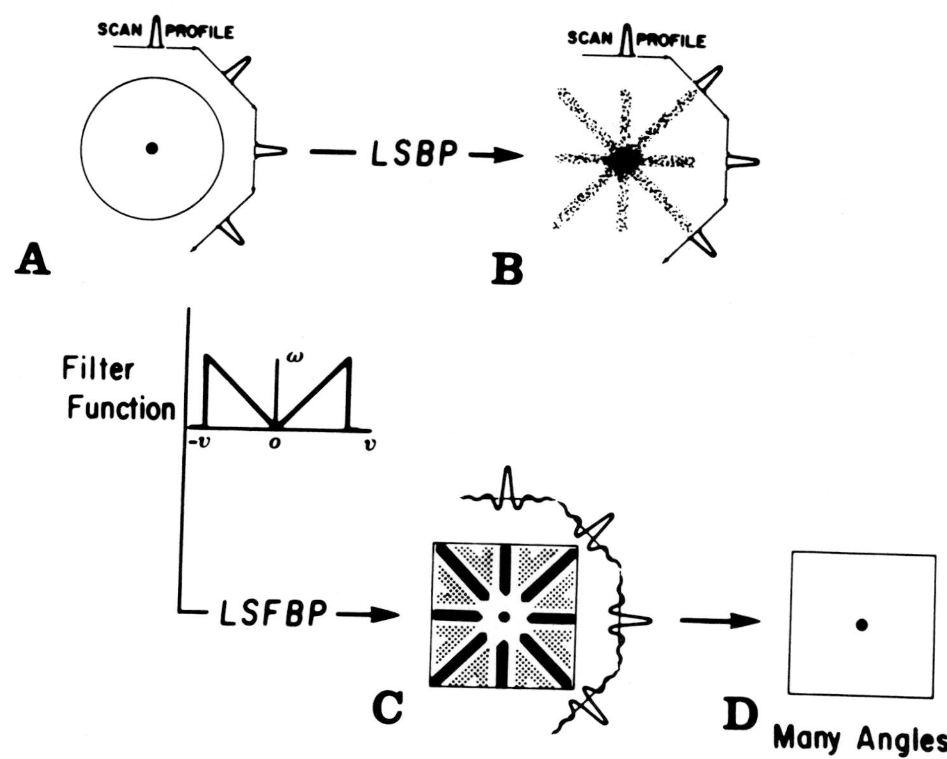

Figure 5. Effects of filtering in image reconstruction. (A). Projection data measured from different angles. (B). Results of linear superposition of back-projections (LSBP), where the projection data are not filtered prior to back-projection. Because the projection counts are back-projected evenly across the image, sources of activity also contribute to areas of no activity in a star-pattern with a $1/r$-shaped intensity. (C). Results of linear superposition of filtered back-projections (LSFBP). If the data are mathematically processed with a filter function prior to back-projection, the negative projection values cancel out the positive counts in areas of no activity, and the star artifact is eliminated. (D). The image produced when profiles at an adequate number of angles are acquired (from Hoffman et al[122]).

the dot-like image that would be expected appears blurred or spread out. Within a slice, the resulting radioactivity distribution, called the *line-spread function*, approximates a Gaussian or bell-shaped curve. The width of the line-spread function at one-half its maximum amplitude, termed the *full width at half maximum* (FWHM), is used to quantify resolution.[34] The FWHM is measured in two directions, along a line from the center of the gantry to the source ("radial resolution") and perpendicular to that line ("tangential resolution").

The in-plane resolution should be clearly distinguished from the pixel size in the image matrix. The pixel size is determined by the size of the reconstructed field of view and the number of elements in the image matrix (eg, 128 × 128 or 256 × 256). In general, the choice of pixel size in the image has no effect upon the spatial resolution in the PET image. However, if the pixel size selected is too large with respect to the scanner's in-plane resolution (ie, through the choice of too coarse an image matrix), then the resolution achieved in the patient image will be less than could have been obtained with a smaller pixel size. It is recommended that the pixel size be no more than one third FWHM.[35]

In addition to in-plane resolution, spatial resolution in the out-of-plane direction also affects quantification.[36] The *axial resolution* is the FWHM of the response measured in the axial direction with a stationary point source in the field of view and is analogous to transverse resolution. This parameter is meaningful only if the sampling (ie, detector spacing) in the axial direction does not exceed one third FWHM of the axial point spread function.[34] Most commercial PET systems, even those capable of 3-D acquisition, do not meet this criterion. An alternative parameter, the *slice profile width*, is measured by moving a point source of activity in small increments perpendicular to the tomographic plane and can be thought of as the effective thickness of a slice. It is determined primarily by the axial thickness of the detectors. The *slice separation*, or center-to-center distance between adjacent reconstructed slices (ie, including cross-slices, not just the detector ring separation), is the axial equivalent of the pixel size in conventional 2-D images.

PHYSICAL LIMITATIONS TO EVENT LOCALIZATION

Spatial resolution depends upon how accurately radioactivity in the field of view can be located. The physics of positron annihilation and scanner design both limit resolution. As discussed above, annihilation photons do not originate in the nucleus, the location of which one wishes to determine, but rather are produced only after the positron has traveled some distance from the nucleus. This distance is random and depends on positron energy and on tissue density. The effect of positron range on the spatial resolution for several positron-emitting radionuclides is listed in Table 1.

A second factor limiting the accuracy of event localization and, hence, spatial resolution is the noncolinearity of annihilation photons. Because positrons may have residual kinetic energy at the time of annihilation, the angle between the two photons deviates slightly (±0.6°) from 180°.[37] This results in a small misplacement of the coincidence line, and a slight

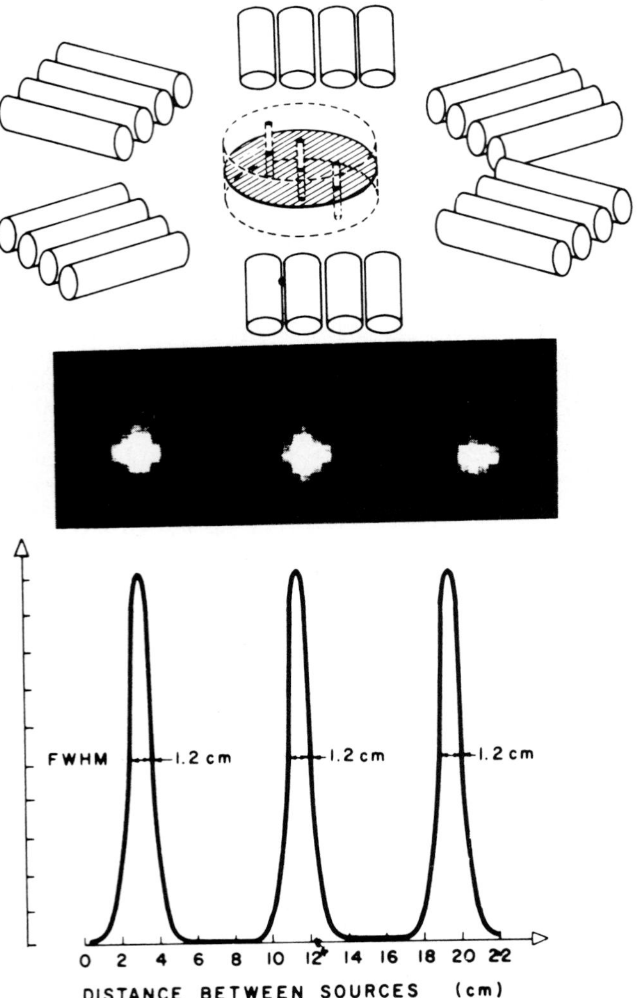

Figure 6. Measurement of transverse spatial resolution. This figure shows how PET resolution is defined and measured. Thin line sources of positron-emitting radioactivity perpendicular to the image plane are scanned (upper panel). Because of resolution limitations, the radioactivity in each source appears blurred or spread over a larger area (middle panel). Scanner resolution is defined by the amount of spreading that occurs. A plot of the image intensity (lower panel) shows that this spreading approximates a bell-shaped or Gaussian curve, called the *line spread function.* The width of the line spread function at one half its maximum amplitude (termed the full width at half maximum, FWHM) is the measure of resolution. Here, the resolution is 1.2 cm (from Ter-Pogossian et al[8]).

degradation of resolution by about 1 to 2 mm.[38,39] This degradation increases when the detectors are farther apart, as in a body scanner. The combined effects of positron range and noncolinearity define the theoretical best resolution achievable with PET, which is about 1 to 2 mm for a whole-body system with ^{18}F, the radionuclide with the shortest positron range.[40]

It is tomograph design, rather than the effects of positron range and noncolinearity, that limits the resolution achieved with current PET systems. Specifically, the detector size and shape determine how accurately the positions of coincidence lines are recorded; smaller crystals provide better resolution. The *intrinsic resolution*, or the resolution of a detector pair before image reconstruction, determines the best resolution achievable. It can be measured by moving a point source across the detector field of view. (The slice profile width, discussed earlier, is equivalent to the intrinsic resolution in the axial direction.) The reconstructed transverse resolution of commercial PET systems is currently 4 to 6 mm in the image plane,[41–45] although a single-ring device with a spatial resolution of 2.6 mm has been constructed.[46] Current tomographs have a transverse resolution and slice profile width that are approximately equivalent.[41–45]

NONUNIFORMITY OF SPATIAL RESOLUTION

Resolution in either the transverse or axial direction is not uniform across the scanner's field of view, and, therefore, its effect on image quality or quantitative accuracy can vary for different structures, depending on their positions and orientations. One reason why resolution varies is penetration of the photon into the crystal. Because annihilation photons are so energetic, they do not interact at the front surface of the detector, but can penetrate into the crystal before interacting. Fewer than 25% of all interactions occur in the front 3 mm of a bismuth germanate (BGO) crystal, a commonly used detector material in PET. The photon may even pass through one crystal before interacting in an adjacent crystal (event A in Fig. 7). It is also possible that a photon may interact by scattering in the detector, in which only a portion of the 511-keV energy is deposited and a secondary gamma ray is produced that may then escape the first crystal to interact in an adjacent one (event B in Fig. 7). In both instances, the coincidence line is mispositioned by an unknown amount. The distance in the detector that a given photon travels and the depth of interaction are usually not known, so it is not possible to correct the coincidence line to the actual path followed by the photon. The mispositioning is greater for off-center coincidence lines where the amount of entrance crystal seen by the photon is reduced by the oblique angle and where a scattered photon is more likely to escape into an adjacent crystal. For coincidence lines passing through the center, the probabilities of crystal penetration and of a scattered photon's escaping the entrance crystal are much reduced.

The shape and FWHM of the axial response function also changes with radial and axial position due to the size of the axial acceptance angle or window and the shadowing effects of the thin shielding placed between detector rings (discussed below). Slices with a large axial acceptance angle occur when coincidences between detectors in different rings or at different axial positions are included (eg, cross slices). In 2-D imaging, these coincidences are assigned to a slice parallel to the straight slices, positioned midway between the axial locations of the two detectors. This approximation breaks down for sources at large radial positions and for coincidence lines with large axial differences. These slices

Table 1. Effect of Positron Range on Spatial Resolution in PET

RADIONUCLIDE	E_{max} (MeV)*	FWHM (mm)†	PSF RANGE (mm)‡
F-18	0.635 (97%)	4.11	1.2
C-11	0.961 (99+%)	4.29	2.1
Ga-68	1.899 (90%)	5.01	5.4
Rb-82	3.35 (83%), 2.57 (13%)	7.72	12.4

*From Lederer.[120] E_{max} is the maximum energy of the positron. The numbers in parentheses are the percentage of β^+-decay. Rb-82 has two modes of β^+-decay with different values of E_{max}.

†System resolution degradation from positron range blurring for a PET resolution of 4.0 mm. The FWHM listed is the net resolution achieved (ie, for F-18, the resolution is blurred from 4.0 to 4.11 mm). Estimated from Equation 1 in Bacharach[35] where D is twice the average distance the positron travels.

‡Diameter of a circle containing 75% of all counts in the point spread function (PSF) resulting from positron range broadening alone. This PSF is very sharply peaked with long tails and is not well-approximated by a Gaussian function. The long tails of the function are the source of the resolution blurring in the system FWHM. From Derenzo.[121]

have a greater nonuniformity of axial resolution and slice profile width across the transverse field of view than slices in which only coincidences between detectors in the same detector ring are recorded[47] or where slices are created with a small axial acceptance window.[45]

For most PET scanners, the nonuniformity in resolution across a slice is small. The transverse resolution and the axial slice profile width typically degrade by 1.0 to 1.5 mm from the center out to 10 cm.[41,44] For radial distances beyond 10 cm, however, the effect can be quite large and will reduce the ability to resolve activity in small structures near the edge of the transverse field of view. The axial slice profile width also shows small differences between slices (<1 mm) with different axial acceptance windows out to 10 cm.[41,44]

PARTIAL VOLUME EFFECT

The effect of limited resolution is visually apparent as a blurring or lack of sharpness of the PET image. More important though is its impact on the accuracy of the radioactivity measurement[48,49] (Fig. 8). The radioactivity in a small region appears blurred or spread out over a larger area. The

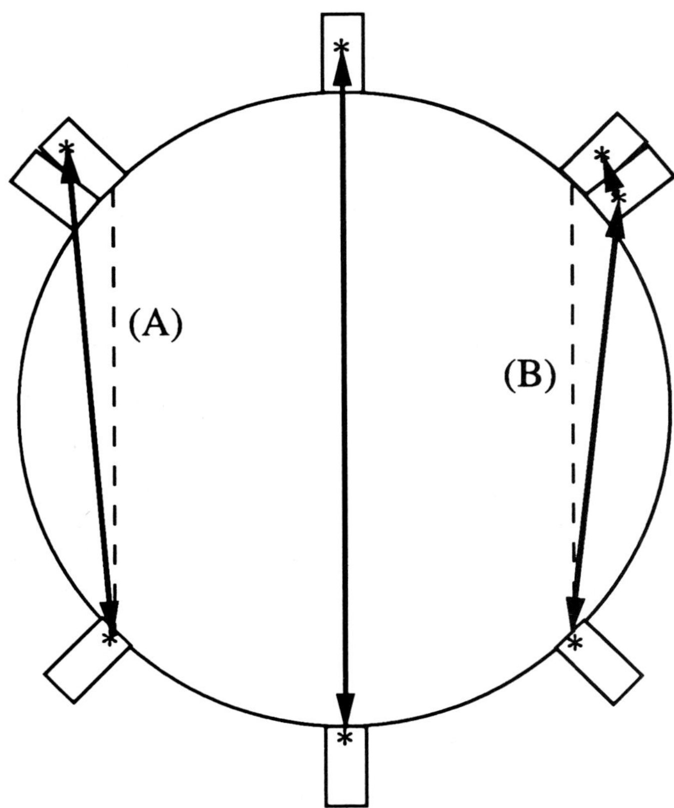

Figure 7. Degradation of transverse spatial resolution. Penetration of adjacent detectors before interaction (**A**) and multiple interactions of the photon in the detectors (**B**) lead to mispositioning of measured coincidence lines (denoted by dashed lines) because the depth of interaction of the photon in the crystal is not measured. This effect is most pronounced in circular gantry geometries, where the radial resolution degrades as the line source is moved off-center, while the tangential resolution remains more uniform across the transverse field of view.

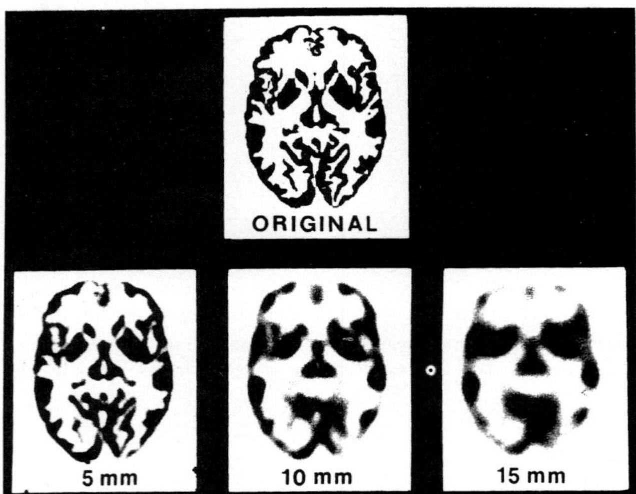

Figure 8. Effect of scanner resolution on a brain image. At the upper center is an original brain image. Subsequent images simulate the effect of scanning this image with tomographs of varying resolution, from 5 to 15 mm FWHM. The fine structure in the original image is lost as the resolution degrades (from Mazziotta et al[49]).

worse the resolution, the greater this effect. Thus, in the reconstructed image, a region of interest (ROI) contains only a portion of the radioactivity that was in the corresponding structure of interest. In addition, some of the radioactivity in surrounding areas appears to be spread into the ROI. As a result of this effect, termed *partial volume averaging*, a regional measurement contains a contribution both from the structure of interest and from surrounding structures. High radioactivity levels surrounded by lower values will be underestimated, while low radioactivity surrounded by high activity will be overestimated. These errors are less when the size of the structure of interest is large with respect to scanner resolution (Fig. 9). In a circular structure with a uniform radioactivity concentration and a diameter of twice the FWHM, the radioactivity will be accurately represented only at the center. However, statistical considerations limit how small an ROI can be used to obtain radioactivity measurements. Furthermore, the radioactivity in large structures, eg, thalamus, may not be uniform because of physiological heterogeneity. Generally in studies of the brain it is not possible to obtain measurements that reflect pure gray matter radioactivity, especially in cortical regions. In addition, partial volume averaging with cerebrospinal fluid in sulci or ventricles can underestimate tissue blood flow and metabolism, especially if there is cerebral atrophy.[50,51] Similarly, in myocardial perfusion studies, activity in the heart wall is blurred due to the thin size of the wall (10 to 20 mm) relative to a typical resolution (5 to 7 mm), while residual activity in the blood pool of the heart cavity is smeared into ROIs drawn on the heart muscle.[35] Partial volume averaging is also important when imaging tumors. The radioactivity in small tumors may be underestimated. If a tumor changes size, eg, during therapy or with further growth, the measured activity can change even if the measured physiological parameter (eg, glucose metabolic rate) per gram of tumor has not changed.

SAMPLING

Sampling refers to the spacing of the measured coincidence lines across the fields of view. The spatial resolution in an image is affected not only by the intrinsic resolution but also by the spacing of measured coincidence lines. Two parallel coincidences separated by a distance equal to the crystal size cannot be distinguished from each other if they strike the same detector pair. With smaller crystals, it is possible to distinguish between coincidence events that are closer together, that is, the sampling of the coincidence lines is finer. In scanners with multiple rings of small crystals, the transverse sampling is determined by the detector spacing within the ring; the axial sampling is determined by the distance between detector rings in the axial direction. Inadequate sampling, either radially, angularly, or axially, degrades resolution and potentially introduces artifacts into the image because of an effect termed "aliasing." In order to achieve artifact-free images with a resolution in the reconstructed image approaching the intrinsic resolution, the sampling distance in-plane must be less than one third of the intrinsic FWHM.[52]

Until recently, sampling in the axial direction has been coarser than that in-plane. The quantitative accuracy of the activity measurement in a given structure in those older systems (and even in some newer ones) depends upon the axial location of the structure within the slice (Fig. 10). Two ways to improve the axial sampling are (1) to acquire two (or more) scans, separated axially by one half of the center-to-center slice separation (or finer) or (2) to have an axial "wobble" motion[53] where the detector rings move back and forth axially during acquisition of measurements from twice as many slices. With the latter method, the distribution of radioactivity is assumed to remain relatively unchanged throughout the study. One drawback to these techniques is fewer counts in each individual image, if the total duration of the study is not increased. This technique has been used effectively when imaging ^{18}FDG to measure regional glucose metabolism.

There are also ways to improve the in-plane sampling. Many older systems and some new ones have the ability to move the detectors in-plane (eg, to "wobble," where the entire detector ring moves in a small circular motion about a point 1 to 2 cm off center).[54–57] This motion increases the density of coincidence lines that are registered and eliminates the image artifacts resulting from inadequate sampling.[52] Transverse resolution is improved with increased sampling, as is the uniformity of resolution across the field of view.

PATIENT MOTION

The spatial resolution achieved in patient images is often degraded by patient motion during the study. Patient motion

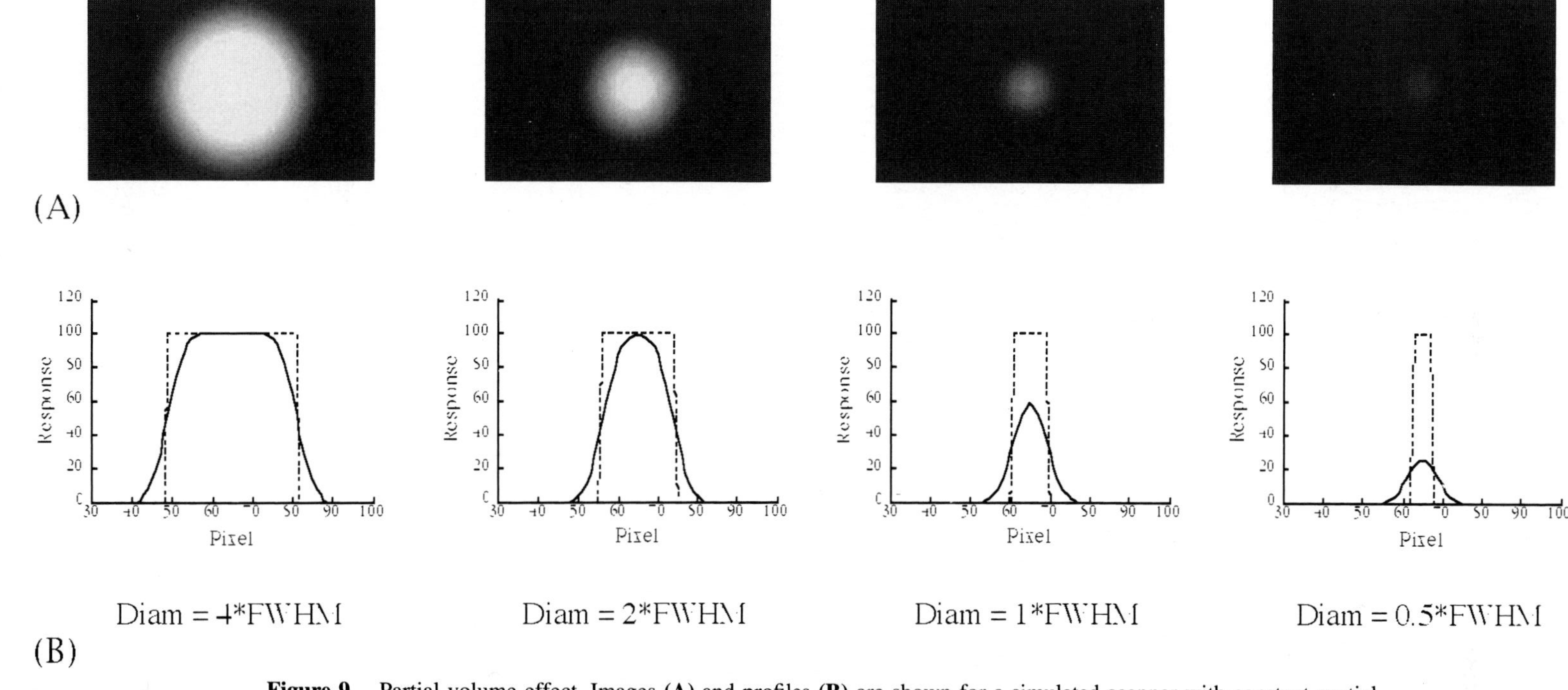

Figure 9. Partial volume effect. Images **(A)** and profiles **(B)** are shown for a simulated scanner with constant spatial resolution (FWHM) for object diameters of 4*FWHM, 2*FWHM, 1*FWHM, and 0.5*FWHM. The profiles are taken through the center of the object and are plotted as a percentage of the true value in the object. Similar results would be observed if the object size were held fixed and the FWHM varied from 0.25* object size to 2*object size. Note that, for the object with a diameter of 2*FWHM, an accurate value for the radioactivity concentration is recovered only at the center.

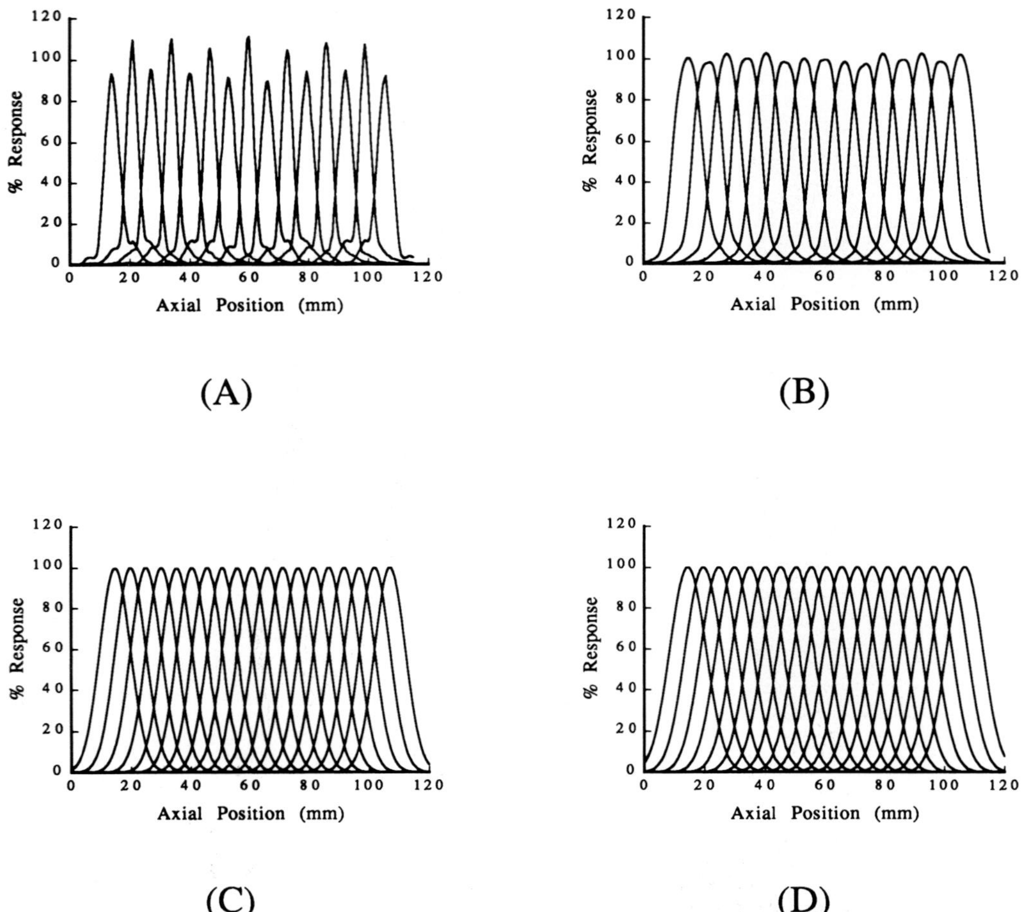

Figure 10. Axial slice sensitivity profiles for two scanners. The axial slice sensitivity profile provides an indication of the uniformity of response at various positions within a slice. To determine the axial slice sensitivity profile, the axial response functions obtained by measuring the count rate as a point source is moved axially in small increments, are normalized by the slice sensitivity. These normalized profiles are then plotted for all slices. (Top). Axial slice sensitivity profile for the Scanditronix/GE PC2048-15B brain scanner with 15 slices, a 6.5-mm slice separation, and a 4.5 to 5.8-mm slice profile width at the center, scaled to an average maximum response of 100%. Figure 10A is the measured response for an infinitely thin object. Figure 10B shows the calculated profiles for a 10-mm (in the axial direction) rectangular object, determined by convolving the slice profile widths by a 10-mm wide rectangular function. Note the large difference in the response at the center (peak) and edge (valley) of the slice. (Bottom). Axial slice sensitivity profile for the Positron Corporation Posicam 6.5 body scanner with 21 slices, a 5.125-mm slice separation, and a 11.9-mm slice profile width at the center, scaled as above. Figure 10C is the response for an infinitely thin object, and Figure 10D is after convolution with a 10-mm rectangular object. Because the axial sampling is finer than the slice profile width, the axial response is more uniform, and the peak-to-valley differences are much smaller for this system.

between transmission and emission scans can lead to a mismatch in the attenuation correction factors (see below), which results in inaccurate correction for attenuation of the emission data.[58,59] Motion can blur the images in a nonuniform manner and increase partial volume errors. Motion between studies obtained at rest and during performance of a task in a given subject can cause differences in activity to be misinterpreted as activation when, in fact, they are due to motion. The relative impact of this blurring becomes greater as system resolution improves.

Head motion during imaging can be reduced in several ways,[60,61] but cannot be eliminated entirely.[62,63] For this reason, several methods of detecting and correcting for motion have been developed. One technique utilized in brain imaging is based on radioactive fiducial markers that are used to align images of short duration, which are then summed.[64] Another method employs the brain images themselves to estimate the corrections necessary to attain maximum alignment of the serial images.[65] Separate real-time measurements of patient motion can be incorporated into data acquisition to permit a correction either in real time or postacquisition.[66]

Patient motion is less critical in cardiac and abdominal imaging. Cardiac and respiratory motions are the greater sources of blurring and quantification errors in these studies.[67] The effect of cardiac motion can be reduced by gating, ie, relating the acquisition periods to specific parts of the cardiac cycle. Eliminating the effects of respiratory motion is more difficult and is rarely performed.

Attenuation

Most annihilation photons interact with tissue, thus never reaching the detectors; in other words, they are *attenuated*. Attenuation substantially decreases the number of valid coincidence events sensed by each detector pair. There are two sources of photon loss, photoelectric absorption and Compton scatter. In both of these processes, the photon interacts with an atomic electron in tissue. In the photoelectric effect, the photon completely disappears, and its energy is used to eject an electron from the atom. Because of the relatively high energy of annihilation photons, few (<0.1%) are lost as the result of a photoelectric interaction of the 511-keV photon with tissue; Compton scattering is, instead, the main source of attenuation. In Compton scattering, the photon strikes a loosely bound orbital electron, and only part of the photon's energy is lost to the electron, which is ejected from the atom. The photon is deflected or scattered in a new direction, carrying with it a fraction of its original energy. The greater the energy lost in the interaction, the greater the angle that the photon is scattered. Depending upon the angle of scatter, an annihilation photon may not reach the detector to which it was originally traveling. It may hit another detector in the same or a different ring, or it may be completely deflected out of the field of view of the scanner. If it loses too much energy, it may be rejected as an invalid photon even if it reaches a detector. Because of the nature of coincidence detection, if either of the annihilation photons is lost through the photoelectric effect or scattering, the decay event will not be recorded by the appropriate detector pair. Fewer coincidence events will be registered, and the amount of radioactivity in the field of view will be underestimated.

Attenuation is important in both SPECT and PET because it results in a substantial decrease in the number of decay events detected. In fact, the impact of attenuation may be greater in PET than in SPECT, despite the higher probability of attenuation of the lower-energy photons in SPECT, because in PET the photon *pair* must traverse the entire tissue thickness unimpeded, whereas in SPECT the single photon is attenuated by a lesser amount of tissue. A critical feature that distinguishes PET from SPECT is that in PET the amount of attenuation for a given detector pair is independent of the depth in tissue where the decay occurred. This can be explained as follows (see Fig. 11). The probability (P_1) that a photon will escape the tissue, ie, not be attenuated, depends upon the amount and type of tissue it must pass through.

$$P_1 \propto e^{-\int_{L_1} \mu(x)dx} \tag{1}$$

where $\mu(x)$ is the attenuation coefficient determined by the type(s) of tissue and the photon's energy and L_1 is the path the photon travels. For 511-keV photons in water (tissue), $\mu = 0.096\ \text{cm}^{-1}$. The probability ($P_2$) of the second photon escaping unattenuated is

$$P_2 \propto e^{-\int_{L_2} \mu(x)dx} \tag{2}$$

where L_2 is that photon's path. The probability of a coincidence event where neither photon is attenuated (P_{coin}) is the product of P_1 and P_2

$$\begin{aligned} P_{\text{coin}} &= P_1 P_2 \\ &\propto e^{-\int_{L_1} \mu(x)dx}\, e^{-\int_{L_2} \mu(x)dx} \\ &\propto e^{-\int_{L} \mu(x)dx} \end{aligned} \tag{3}$$

where L is the path $L_1 + L_2$. For a constant attenuation coefficient $\mu = \mu_o$, Equation 3 reduces to

$$P_{\text{coin}} \propto e^{-\mu_o L} \tag{4}$$

and the probability of an unattenuated coincidence event depends only on the total path length L, not on the path lengths of the individual photons. It also follows from Equations 3 and 4 that the sensitivity of coincidence detection is independent of depth, unlike SPECT. A detector pair will register the same number of counts from a source located in its field of view regardless of where the source is positioned, because the attenuation of photon pairs depends only on the total amount of tissue between the detectors.

Attenuation is greater for coincidence lines passing through the center of an object because the annihilation photon pairs have a greater distance to travel in tissue. The loss due to attenuation is substantial; for example, detected counts decrease by a factor of 5 to 6 in the center of the head and up to a factor of 10 to 20 in the abdomen (Fig. 12). Therefore, a correction is required for this loss. There are two general methods of compensating for attenuation, (1) calculated and (2) measured.

The amount of attenuation in areas of reasonably homogeneous tissue (eg, the brain) can be estimated using an assumed value for the attenuation coefficient(s) of the tissue between each detector pair. One must also determine the outline/shape of the body. For the head, this can be obtained by fitting an ellipse or an irregular contour to the outline of the head in the slices of the emission images.[68–70] In this technique, it is assumed that μ is a constant within the outline; some algorithms take into account the higher attenuation of the skull by increasing the size of the contour slightly.[68]

Because the amount of attenuation is independent of source depth (ie, the annihilation site), a direct measurement of the attenuation can be made using an external source. Even for the head, an actual measurement of attenuation is more accurate than calculated methods[58,71] because of varying amounts of bone (both person-to-person and slice-to-slice), and the nonelliptical shape of the head, especially in lower slices. Measured attenuation correction is essential

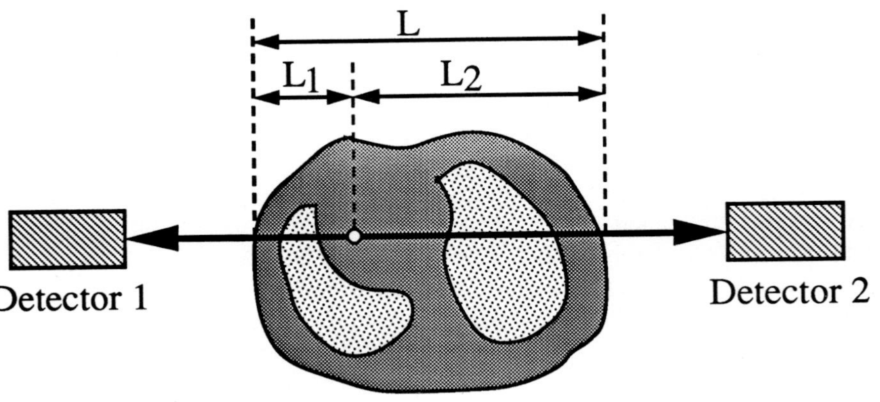

Figure 11. Attenuation. The probability that a single photon will escape the body, unattenuated, depends on the amount and type(s) of tissue it must traverse (paths L_1 and L_2). However, the probability that both photons in a coincidence pair will be unattenuated depends only on the total amount of tissue between the two detectors (path L).

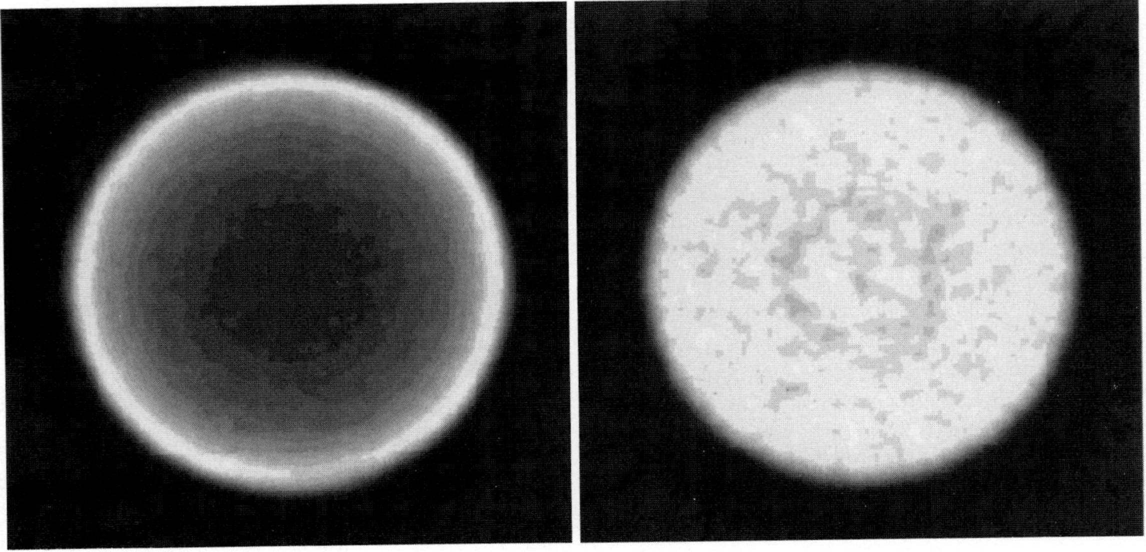

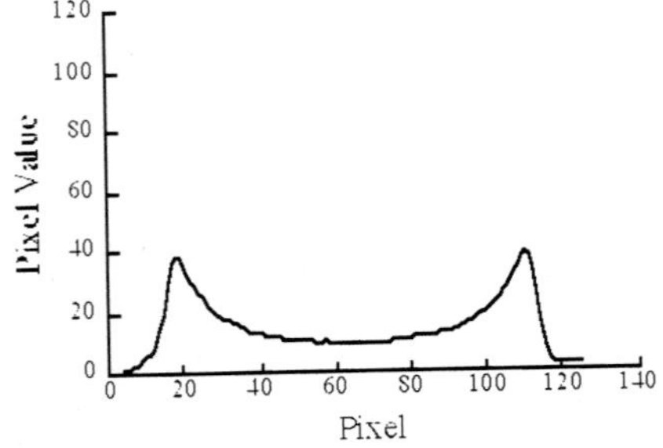

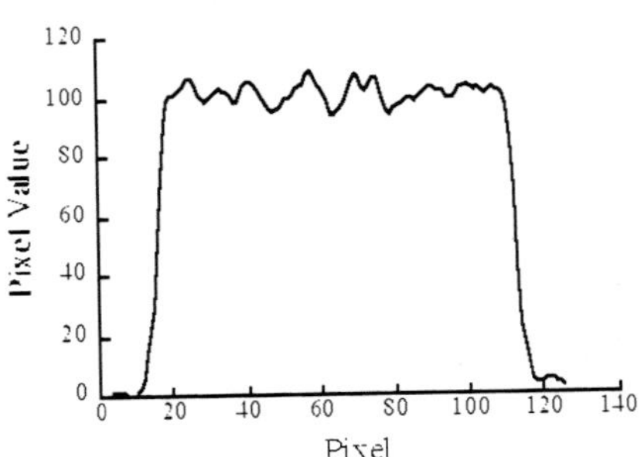

Figure 12. Effects of attenuation. The images shown are of a 16-cm cylindrical phantom, uniformly filled with radioactivity. The plots below are profiles taken through the center of the phantom. (Left). No correction for attenuation has been performed. Note that the count loss is greatest in the center and decreases toward the edge of the phantom, although no areas inside the phantom recover an accurate value for the radioactivity concentration. (Right). Correction for attenuation based upon a transmission scan has been performed. The cylinder now appears uniform, and the profile is flat.

for quantitative body imaging because of inhomogeneous attenuating tissues. To measure attenuation, a *transmission* scan is made prior to injecting radiotracer using an external source of positron-emitting radioactivity between the subject and the detector rings. A similar measurement with nothing in the field of view of the scanner, called a *blank scan*, is also made. The ratio of the two measurements gives the amount of photon attenuation between each detector pair and is used in the emission image reconstruction process to generate attenuation correction factors (ACF^{meas}).

$$\mathrm{ACF}_i^{\mathrm{meas}} = \frac{B_i}{T_i} = \frac{B_i}{B_i e^{-\int_{L_i} \mu(x)dx}} = e^{+\int_{L_i} \mu(x)dx} \qquad (5)$$

where B_i and T_i are the blank and transmission data, respectively, for coincidence line i, and L_i is the path through tissue for that coincidence line. Although it is not required for the attenuation correction of the emission data, it is common to reconstruct the transmission images, which represent the local attenuation coefficient of bone and tissue (Fig. 13). The transmission image can be used to verify patient position in the scanner prior to the injection of radiotracer.

In the past, ring transmission sources filled with positron-emitting radioactivity and placed within the gantry were used to perform the blank and transmission scans. More recently, however, one or more rod sources of long-lived ^{68}Ge/^{68}Ga activity which rotate around the subject have been used. Because the source location is known at all times, coincidence events that do not pass through the source can be rejected (Fig. 14). This has the effect of reducing the unwanted contribution from spurious events in the transmission data.[72,73] For a given source activity, the noise is much reduced with a rotating rod(s) configuration, as compared with a ring source geometry, because of this "masking" process. Therefore, the scan time or amount of activity in the transmission source can be significantly reduced.

Measured attenuation correction is accurate because it makes no assumptions about the shape or homogeneity of the attenuating tissue. However, it is subject to statistical noise arising from the blank and transmission scans which propagates into the emission images.[58,74] Noise in the transmission scan can be reduced by acquiring more counts, either by imaging longer or using a transmission source with higher activity. Noise can also be reduced by smoothing the blank and transmission data prior to generating the attenuation correction factors.[74] However, artifacts and errors in quantification can occur if there is a significant mismatch between the spatial resolutions of the emission and transmission data.[75,76] Another method to reduce noise in the attenuation correction factors is to segment the transmission image into areas of constant attenuation coefficient $\hat{\mu}(x)$ and then compute the line integral from the segmented image to obtain the correction factors from Equation 5.[77,78]

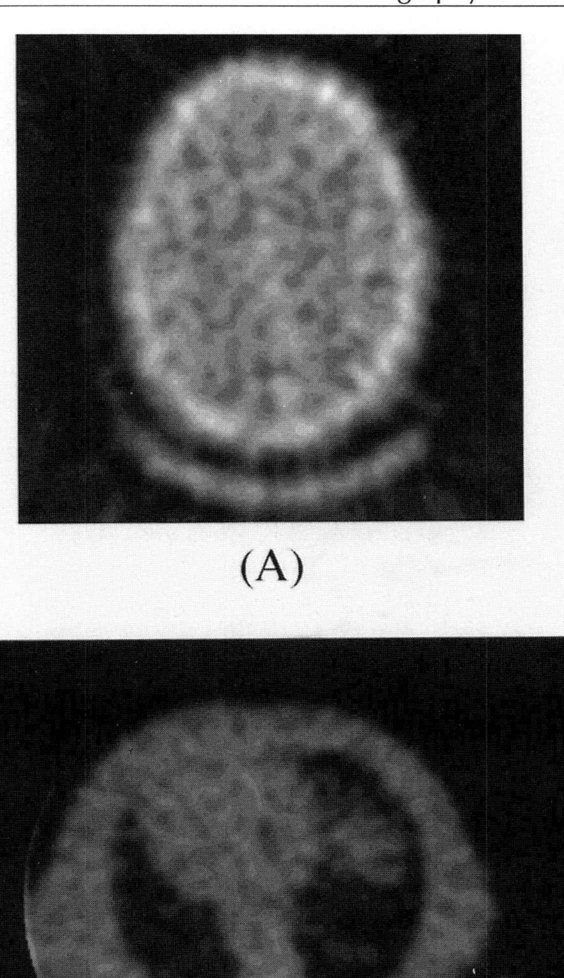

Figure 13. Transmission images. (A). Typical transmission image of the head, showing the different attenuation coefficients of brain tissue, skull, and the head support. (B). Transmission image of the chest, where the different attenuation coefficients of lung, tissue, and the patient bed are seen.

To reduce the time a patient needs to lie motionless, one can perform transmission scans *after* the tracer has been administered, immediately before or after the emission imaging[79,80] or simultaneously with emission imaging.[81] This technique is useful for longer-lived radionuclides with reasonably static tracer distributions, where a long period of time is necessary to reach a steady state before imaging or where the patient is likely to move during long studies. This typically occurs when ^{18}FDG is used to measure regional glucose metabolism, where there is a 30- to 45-minute period

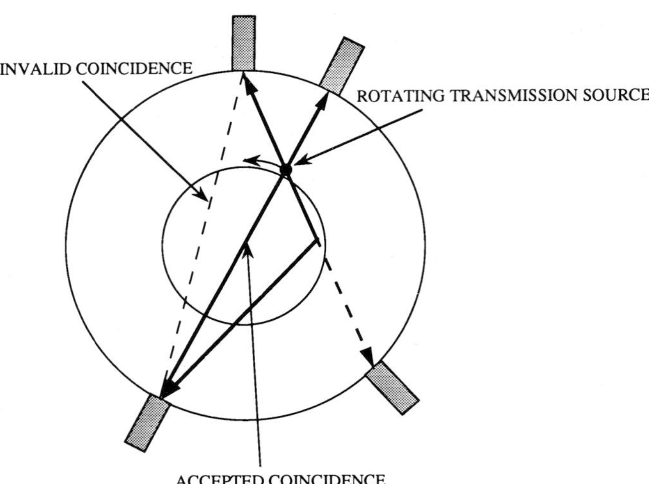

Figure 14. Rotating line source for transmission imaging. Only coincident photons that pass through the source at each position as it rotates around the subject are accepted as valid coincidence events. An event in which one photon scatters will be rejected as invalid if the resultant measured coincidence line does not pass through the transmission source.

between tracer administration and emission imaging. With a rotating transmission source, the emission events that do not pass through the source are eliminated from the transmission data by the windowing process. Thus, contamination of the transmission data by emission counts is restricted to the few emission coincidences coming from the patient that happen to occur along coincidence lines passing through the rotating transmission source (<10%). These accepted emission events must be subtracted in order to generate accurate attenuation correction factors.[79,80]

Count Rate Performance

There are two limitations to the activity level that can be accurately measured with a PET scanner, deadtime losses and random coincidences. *Deadtime loss* refers to the decreasing ability of the scanner to register counts as the count rate increases, because of the time required to handle each count. Deadtime causes a reduction in measured coincidences with increasing activity. *Random* or *"accidental" coincidences* occur when two photons from two *different* positron annihilations are sensed by a detector pair within the coincidence resolving time (see Fig. 2), so that a false or random coincidence count is registered. Random coincidences add counts uniformly to the image and lead to a loss of contrast and accuracy if they are not subtracted. Deadtime losses and random coincidences both affect the quantitative accuracy of the data and the statistical noise of the image.

DEADTIME LOSSES

Sources of deadtime losses in PET include the electronic circuitry used for energy and position discrimination of each photon that strikes a detector, the coincidence processing circuitry, the scintillation decay time of the crystal used in the radiation detectors, and, to a lesser extent, the transfer of data from the electronics to the computer. For systems in which there are more detectors than photomultiplier tubes (PMTs), electronic circuitry is needed to determine which crystal detected the photon. In these systems the major source of deadtime is in this processing circuitry.[44,82] At high count rates, in addition to count losses, accepted photons can also be mispositioned by this circuitry, with more events assigned to the detector elements near the center of the crystal array and fewer to the edges.[83–86] Event mispositioning degrades not only the in-plane resolution but also the axial resolution and slice profile width because of the misbinning (ie, erroneous assignment) of events between slices.[86] The in-plane resolution can worsen by 1 to 2 mm with high activity levels,[86] and the slice mispositioning errors can result in slice-to-slice quantification errors of 5 to 10%.[87]

The count loss due to deadtime can often be predicted for a given count rate[87] and a correction factor applied to the data to compensate for underestimation of counts. However, deadtime correction, no matter how accurate, does not compensate for the loss in statistical accuracy that occurs because fewer counts were actually collected. In addition, the patient will be exposed to increased radiation without a proportionate increase in detected counts.

RANDOM COINCIDENCES

Two factors affect the number of random coincidences measured, the coincidence resolving time (2τ) of the detector pairs and the amount of radioactivity in the field of view. The random coincidence count rate (R) for a detector pair is related to the coincidence resolving time by

$$R = 2\tau S_1 S_2 \qquad (6)$$

where S_1 and S_2 are the rates at which single photons strike the two detectors. Because the singles' rate for each detector is proportional to the amount of activity seen by the detector, it follows from Equation 6 that the random coincidence rate is proportional to the *square* of the activity. The true coincidence rate increases only linearly with activity, so the fraction of accepted coincidence counts that are actually random coincidences is then proportional to the amount of activity in the field of view.

Random coincidences can be reduced by using a shorter coincidence resolving time, but the timing uncertainty in the detectors and the signal processing circuitry, as well as the actual difference in times of arrival of the two photons at the detectors (0 to 2 nanoseconds), necessitate that a 10- to 20-nanosecond coincidence window be used. In systems where the time of flight of the two photons is measured, faster detectors and electronics are used, and the effective timing window can be reduced to 0.4 to 0.6 nanoseconds.[32,88] However, even for such small resolving times, the rate of random coincidences can be sufficiently high to require correction.[89]

Random coincidences are usually determined in one of two ways: (1) direct measurement by the delayed coincidence technique and (2) estimation from singles' count rates and the measured coincidence resolving time. The first method employs a second coincidence circuit in which one signal is delayed by several times the length of the coincidence window, so that only random coincidences are measured. The second method takes advantage of the relationship between coincidence resolving time and the two singles' rates (Equation 6) to estimate the random coincidence rate. In both methods, random coincidences are subtracted from measured coincidence data prior to image reconstruction. As with deadtime, the correction for random coincidences subtracts a reasonably accurate estimate of the false counts, but their contribution to image noise persists.[90]

DEADTIME LOSSES AND RANDOM COINCIDENCES—PRACTICAL CONSIDERATIONS

As discussed previously, deadtime losses and random coincidences can affect not only the accuracy of data during acquisition but also the statistical noise of the image. To help determine the optimum or maximum dose to be administered to the patient, one can measure, as a function of activity in the scanner field of view, the bias and coefficient of variation (standard deviation of pixel values as a percentage of the mean pixel value) in a large ROI from a decaying emission phantom study (see Fig. 15). Beyond a certain count rate, the corrections may break down. As illustrated in Figure 15B, there is no significant improvement in the coefficient of variation above a certain activity level. There may, in fact, be an *increase* in noise at very large injected activities, due to the high deadtime and random coincidence levels. Thus, for any given tomograph and radiopharmaceutical, the amount of radioactivity administered must be carefully selected to balance the competing effects of improved counting statistics with the "diminishing returns" of deadtime losses and random coincidences.

In practice, the injected dose should be limited to activities that result in less than 50% deadtime losses or that cause fewer than 50% of the measured coincidence events to be random coincidences. It is also preferable not to exceed the activity where the true count rate peaks due to instrument saturation.[34] Figure 16 demonstrates these effects as a function of activity in a 20-cm cylindrical phantom, initially filled uniformly with a high ^{11}C activity and imaged repeatedly as the activity decayed. Different system designs and source configurations perform differently at high count rates.

A useful parameter that expresses the combined degrading effects of deadtime losses, random coincidences, and scatter

(A)

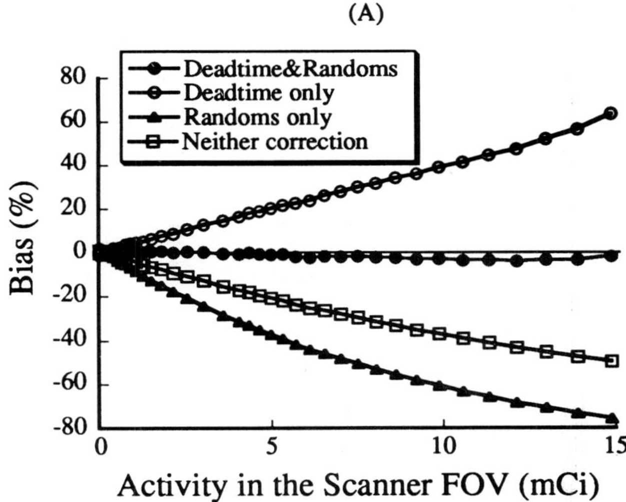

(B)

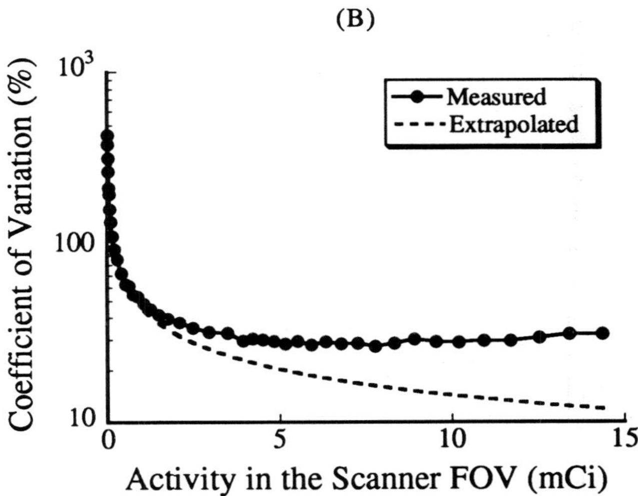

Figure 15. Bias and coefficient of variation in a uniform phantom as a function of activity. (A). The difference in mean value from values obtained with low levels of activity for a 16-cm circular ROI drawn on a 20-cm cylinder are shown as a function of activity in the field of view. Also shown are the results for cases where no randoms or deadtime correction has been performed. (B). The pixel-to-pixel coefficient of variation for the same ROI is shown as a function of activity in the field of view. The dashed line is the extrapolation from a fit of the low-activity data to $1/\sqrt{\text{activity}}$, the theoretical Poisson noise prediction that accounts for image noise only due to counting statistics.

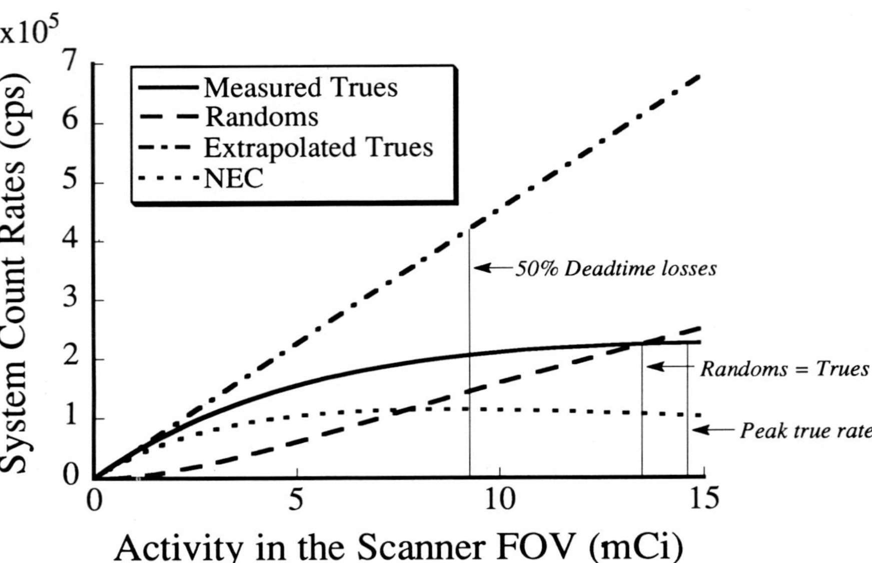

Figure 16. Count rate performance. The system count rates from a decaying 20-cm cylindrical phantom are plotted as function of activity concentration in the phantom. The measured true, random, extrapolated true, and NEC count rates are shown. The extrapolated true rates were determined from the measured true count rates at low activities and are the true rates one would obtain in the absence of deadtime losses. On this scanner and for this source configuration, the Scanditronix/GE PC2048-15B, the activity in the field of view where there are 50% deadtime losses is 9.2 mCi. The random and true coincidence rates are equal at 13.5 mCi, and the true count rate peaks at 14.8 mCi.

on the image noise is the *noise-equivalent count* (NEC) rate. This parameter is defined as

$$\text{NEC} = \frac{T}{1 + \frac{S}{T} + k\frac{R}{T}} \tag{7}$$

where *T*, *S*, and *R* are the true, scatter, and random coincidence rates, respectively, and *k* is a factor of 1 or 2, depending upon whether the random coincidences are calculated or measured.[91] The NEC rate is also plotted in Figure 16. As can be seen from Equation 7, the NEC rate is lower (worse) for cases of high randoms or scatter and is also degraded by deadtime losses.

Scatter

Another important source of image noise is Compton scatter which occurs when an annihilation photon traveling in tissue is deflected in a collision with an electron. This results in a change in direction of the photon as well as some loss in its energy. The greater the angle of scattering, the greater the energy loss. If scattered photons strike a detector and are of sufficient energy to be registered, the coincidence line will be incorrectly positioned (see Fig. 2). Therefore, not only is information lost from the affected "true" coincidence line, but also the accepted coincidence events that result from scattered photons will add a slowly varying background level to the image. This leads to an overestimation of radioactivity, which can be substantial in areas containing relatively less radioactivity, (eg, regions with low blood flow or metabolism or areas of nonspecific binding of receptor radioligands). Scattered photons reaching a detector originate not just in the plane of detector ring, but from the entire body. Photons can also be scattered back from the shielding into a detector. In addition, there is scatter from one detector into another. The amount of scatter in an image depends upon the distribution of radioactivity, the anatomy of the tissue scattering media, and scanner design.

There are both hardware and software strategies to reduce scatter. In two-dimensional imaging, thin lead or tungsten shields, or *septa*, are placed between detector rings to reduce scatter from out of the plane, while shielding between detector crystals decreases scatter from one crystal to another. Detector rings with larger diameters decrease scatter, because of the smaller solid angle for photon detection. Therefore, scatter is typically less in a whole body than a head unit. One can also reduce scatter by raising the energy threshold for accepted photons[92] because scattered photons have a lower energy than true events. Unfortunately, the energy resolution of PET detectors, 50 to 100 keV, is inadequate to eliminate most of the scatter. PET systems constructed with bismuth germanate (BGO) detectors usually operate with a minimum energy threshold of 300 to 380 keV,[44,93,94] while NaI(Tl) crystals have better energy resolution and use a higher energy threshold of 400 to 450 keV.[45] Compton scatter for 511-keV photons is primarily small-angle, that is, there is little energy loss; more than half of all scattered photons have energies above 450 keV, and almost 75% have energies above 350 keV. Therefore, most scattered coincidences are accepted by the electronics as valid events.

Regardless of tomograph design, it is necessary to perform a software correction for scatter, because it still can contribute as much as 10 to 20% of the counts in a conventional 2-D image. The amount of scatter depends upon the distribution of both source radioactivity and scattering/attenuating media. If the radiotracer distribution changes, the scatter distribution will also vary. Unlike random coincidences, scatter cannot be distinguished from true coincidences electronically, and there are no exact methods of estimating scatter as there are for random coincidences. Techniques have been developed to correct for scatter which vary in their complex-

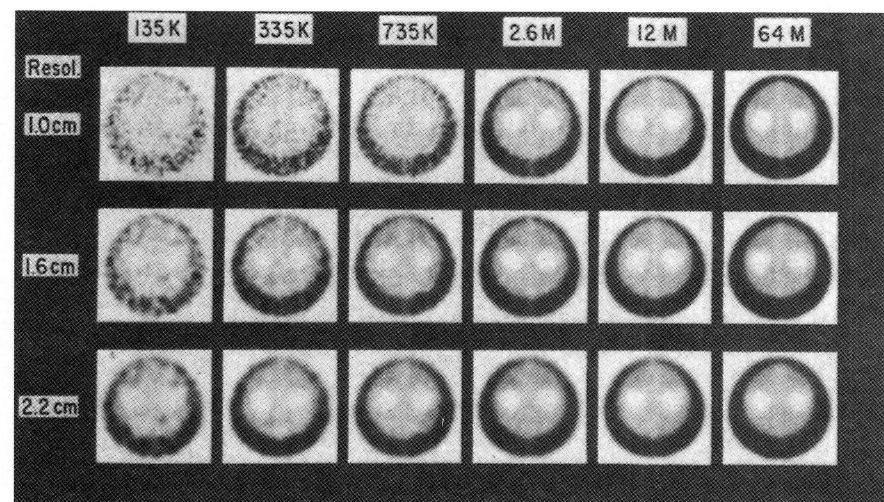

Figure 17. Effect of number of counts and spatial resolution on image noise. The images are of a cylindrical phantom containing chambers with relative radiotracer concentrations of 3 in the outer rim, 1 in the large inner portion, and 0 in the two small regions. Image noise, apparent as graininess, decreases with increasing counts (toward the right) and with decreasing resolution (down) (from Phelps et al[119]).

ity and effectiveness.[95–97] One method is a spatially varying deconvolution technique developed for the brain.[95] It assumes that the only source of scatter is activity from within the plane itself. This approximation is acceptable for the brain. Scatter correction techniques are reasonably accurate for the brain because the activity and tissue distributions are fairly uniform. Their accuracy in imaging situations where the activity distribution and/or attenuation distribution is nonuniform (eg, the chest) is less certain.

Image Noise

The PET image has inherent statistical noise because of the random nature of radioactive decay. The disintegration rate of a radioactive sample undergoes moment-to-moment variation that can be described by a Poisson statistical distribution.[98] The resultant uncertainty in the measurement of radioactivity, expressed as a fraction of the number of counts (N) recorded along a given coincidence line, is proportional to $1/\sqrt{N}$. Thus, counting noise decreases as the number of counts increases. Similarly, the statistical reliability of a PET image depends on the number of counts recorded. The situation is more complex, however, than the simple Poisson prediction because the estimate of radioactivity in any small ROI is obtained from an image reconstructed from multiple measurements of radioactivity distribution throughout the slice. Thus, the noise in any individual region of the image is affected by noise in other areas.[99–102] The resultant image noise is greater than would be predicted by Poisson statistics.[99] The statistical noise in an ROI is due not only to the uncertainty related to the number of counts contributing to that part of the image but also to the variances associated with the corrections for random and scattered coincidences, attenuation, detector nonuniformities, as well as the size and location of the ROI.[102] Excessive noise gives the PET image a "salt and pepper"-type appearance (Fig. 17) and decreases the ability to quantify radioactivity accurately. Within certain limitations, however, the more counts acquired, the better image quality and the higher statistical accuracy the images will have.

For a given radiotracer concentration in the field of view, the number of counts in the PET image depends upon the sensitivity of the scanner. Sensitivity is defined as the number of counts detected in a unit time per unit amount of radioactivity for a given distribution of activity. It is determined by system design features, such as detector material, size, and arrangement in the gantry; detector ring diameter; axial acceptance window (ie, the number of accepted coincidence lines between detectors with different axial locations); and the inter-ring septa. Sensitivity of a system varies inversely with the diameter of the detector rings. Systems with smaller ring diameters have greater sensitivity than those with larger detector separations because smaller detector rings subtend greater solid angles and "see" more emitted photons. It should be pointed out that PET scanners are, in general, rather inefficient. Because photon pairs are emitted in all directions, relatively few are actually detected because the detectors subtend only a small solid angle. Even if one disregards photon attenuation, only 1 to 3% of decay events are counted.[103]

PET sensitivity is typically measured with a standard 20-cm diameter cylindrical phantom, uniformly filled with known activity.[34] A small amount of activity is used to minimize the effects of random coincidences and deadtime losses. Correction is made for scatter so that the value reflects the sensitivity of the system to true coincidences, in units of (counts per second/microcuries per cubic centimeter). The sensitivity value depends on the source and attenuation distributions. Nonetheless, the use of a standard phantom for this measurement permits comparisons between different systems.

Image noise can be reduced by increasing the counts collected. This is achieved by increasing imaging time or the amount of radioactivity administered. Increasing imaging time is not always practicable for certain radiotracers, however, because of their short physical or physiological half-life or because it would not be compatible with the radiotracer strategy being used. For example, it may be necessary to acquire multiple, short frames to measure the time-activity curve of a radiotracer whose tissue concentration changes. Increasing imaging time is possible for radiotracers that achieve stable distributions in tissue, eg, ^{18}FDG in the brain or $^{13}NH_4^+$ in the heart, within the constraints of patient comfort and motion. Administering more radioactivity increases counts, but this approach is limited by radiation safety considerations and by increasing deadtime losses and random coincidence counts.

Detector Normalization

PET detectors do not all have the same efficiency. Accordingly, the efficiency for detecting coincidence lines can differ by factors of 4 to 5. Before image reconstruction, these differences in coincidence line response must be corrected. If left uncorrected, the resultant image will have obvious streak or fan artifacts, with more sensitive coincidence pairs appearing as hot stripes in the image and weaker ones exhibiting cold stripes. Correction factors should be measured periodically with a low-activity, uniform source (eg, a low-activity rotating line source). These correction factors can then be applied to emission data prior to image reconstruction.

SCANNER DESIGN

General Considerations

PET design involves complex, interacting factors.[40,96,104,105] These include the size, shape, and composition of the scintillation crystals; the arrangement of the crystals and photomultiplier tubes (PMTs) in the gantry; the design of coincidence electronic circuitry; and the mathematical methods for reconstruction and for the various corrections required for attenuation, deadtime, random coincidences, scatter, and detector nonuniformity. All of these features ultimately affect image quality and the ability to obtain accurate measurement of regional radioactivity.

Most PET systems have several rings of radiation detectors mounted in a gantry. A detector is typically a small scintillation crystal that emits light when an annihilation photon's energy is deposited in it. The relevant properties of several inorganic scintillation materials used in PET are summarized in Table 2.[106] Superior crystal materials have high stopping power for the energetic annihilation photons by means of high density and high atomic number, large light output, rapid decay of scintillation light, and no special packaging needs (eg, nonhygroscopic, room-temperature operation). BGO, used in most commercial scanners, has the advantage of high stopping power due to high density and effective atomic number. Other scintillation materials have been used for particular applications. In particular, BaF_2 has been used in time-of-flight scanners because of its fast decay time. The development of new detector materials for PET is an ongoing area of research.[107,108]

The radiation detector is coupled to a PMT which converts light pulses to electrical signals that are fed into the electronic coincidence circuitry. In most systems, several detectors are coupled to one PMT (Fig. 18). Because more than one crystal can contribute to a PMT signal, decoding electronics are required to determine which crystal actually detected the event. The crystal that detected the photon is determined by the relative signal intensities of the (fewer) PMTs in the detector "block." The detector block arrangement permits the use of very small crystals (smaller than the PMT) to improve resolution and sampling, while reducing the cost and complexity of the subsequent coincidence electronics.

Current commercially available systems[41–45] have from 18 to 32 rings, each containing several hundred detector elements. A tomographic slice is provided by each ring. In multiring systems "cross-slices" are also derived from coincidences between detectors in different rings. These planes are positioned halfway between detector rings. Therefore, $2n$-1 contiguous 2-D tomographic slices can be obtained simultaneously by n-ring systems.

An alternative design to the detector ring-based approach is that of the PENN-PET, designed by Muehllehner, et al.[45,109] This consists of a hexagonal array of large, single crystals of NaI(Tl) with an array of PMTs, which employ Anger logic to localize the event to 2-mm bins. There are effectively 128 slices in this system.

The transverse field of view and ring diameter are selected based on the type of imaging studies planned. A larger field of view and patient aperture are used in body imaging than in dedicated brain systems. Systems also have been designed specifically for imaging the brain or heart of laboratory animals, such as dogs or monkeys.[110] These have fewer rings with smaller diameters and can have higher sensitivity and resolution than standard tomographs at lower cost. The axial field of view has recently increased from 10 to 12 cm to 15 to 25 cm to image the entire brain or heart.

During imaging subjects rest on a special couch fitted with a head holder to restrain head movement (for brain studies) or Velcro straps to restrict body motion (for cardiac or abdominal studies). The gantry is equipped with several low-power lasers to aid in positioning. Some gantries can be tilted to obtain slices in desired anatomic planes, eg, parallel to the canthomeatal line. As the axial sampling of PET improves, this feature becomes less critical to accurate quantification and lesion detection, as the image data can be resliced to the desired orientation. Reslicing is already routinely done in cardiac PET to obtain short- and long-axis views of the heart from the transverse images. A dedicated computer is used to control the imaging process, collect coincidence count information, and reconstruct and display images.

Some PET systems can operate in a whole-body mode, in addition to transverse section imaging. During these acquisitions, longitudinal projection images of the body are ob-

Table 2. Physical Properties of Scintillators Used in PET

	NaI(T1)	BGO	GSO	BaF_2	CsF
Density (g/cc)	3.67	7.13	6.70	4.88	4.64
Effective atomic #	51	75	59	51	52
Index of refraction	1.85	2.15	.85	1.50	1.48
Relative emission intensity	100	15	25	10	5
Peak wavelength (nm)	410	480	440	310 (slow) 220 (fast)	390
Decay constant (ns)	230	300	56,600	430,620 (slow) 0.60,0.79 (fast)	5
Hygroscopic?	Yes	No	No	No	Yes

From Koeppe et al.[106]

tained by rearranging the acquired data from several axial locations.[111] These studies are useful for qualitative analysis of tracer uptake in the body, especially $^{18}F^-$ and ^{18}FDG uptake in studies of primary and metastatic cancers.

Three-Dimensional Imaging

A new approach to image formation is true three-dimensional (3-D) volume imaging,[45,112] accomplished by removing the inter-ring septa and permitting more cross-ring coincidences between detectors in different, possibly widely separated rings. Many more coincidence lines can be sampled, and system sensitivity increases substantially. This improves image quality, or alternatively, requires less radioactivity be administered. Removing the septa also increases the number of scattered coincidences accepted. Scatter accounts for up to 40 to 60% of the counts in a 3-D image taken without the septa. Accurate scatter correction becomes more important in these studies for both image contrast and quantification. Several techniques for scatter correction of 3-D data are under investigation. There are a number of other considerations involved in 3-D imaging; further work is required before this approach is routinely used.

An additional consideration to note is that the filtered back-projection algorithm is not appropriate for 3-D PET data because the measured data are not complete (ie, not all possible coincidences lines in 3-D space are sampled, especially those with large axial acceptance angles). For 3-D PET data, other algorithms are under investigation[112–115] and their qualitative and quantitative performance is being evaluated for different imaging situations.

PERFORMANCE EVALUATION AND QUALITY CONTROL

Formal procedures have been devised to test system performance characteristics.[34] These are performed when the instrument is accepted from the manufacturer to ensure that it meets specifications and must be repeated at regular intervals to verify that it continues to operate within those specifications. An understanding of the quantitative reliability of the image depends upon how carefully performance has been characterized. Specific questions involving quantification of radiotracer in small structures, in areas of low uptake or in

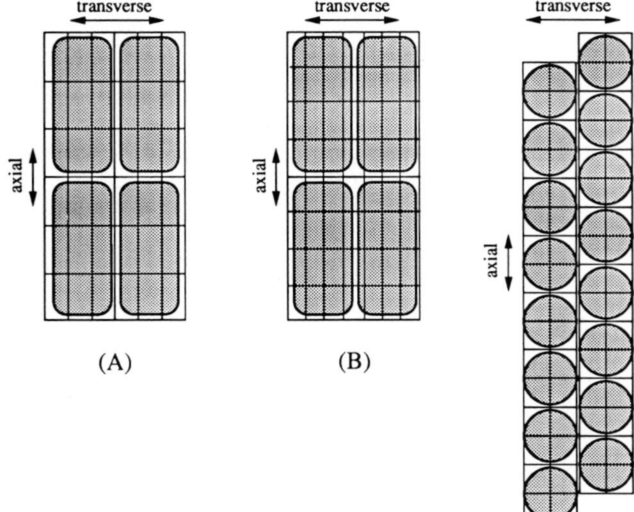

Figure 18. Detector block configurations. Schematics of detector blocks from three commercial PET systems are shown. The shaded areas represent PMTs, while the underlying unshaded areas are scintillator crystals. (A). GE Advance—The block is a 6 × 6 array of BGO with crystal dimensions of 4.0 mm (transverse) and 8.4 mm (axial). There are two Hamamatsu (R1548) dual-photomultipliers per block. (B). Siemens ECAT EXACT HR—The block is a 7 × 8 array of BGO with crystal dimensions of 2.8 mm (transverse) and 5.5 to 5.8 mm (axial). There are also two Hamamatsu dual-PMTs per block in this design. (C). Positron Corporation Posicam HZL-R—The block is a 2 × 16 array of BGO with crystal dimensions of 8.5 mm (transverse) and 9.8 mm (axial). There are eight Amperex (XP-1911) circular (3/4″ diameter) PMTs per block. Two adjacent blocks are shown. Each block extends across the entire axial field of view; adjacent blocks are staggered to increase the axial sampling. Figures are not drawn to scale.

the presence of high count rates, require more stringent performance and more extensive characterization than would be necessary for studies where images are interpreted only visually.[116] The accuracy and reliability of PET data in specific situations can be predicted by measuring performance characteristics. The extent of testing needed, whether for initial acceptance testing after purchase or for routine quality control, is dictated by the specific uses of the instrument. For example, if it is utilized primarily to generate images for visual interpretation, the accuracy of the corrections for deadtime losses or random coincidences may be less important than the spatial resolution of the system. While the use of phantoms to assess performance does not perfectly mimic actual imaging conditions, the information that is provided is, nonetheless, valuable.[34] One could imagine an unlimited number of specialized phantom measurements to simulate various imaging conditions. The commonly performed tests represent a compromise between having realistic measurement conditions and minimizing the time and effort associated with testing to optimize the practical information obtained about performance.

Almost all performance characteristics can be affected by changes in the system hardware or software. Parameters that are less likely to change over time include slice profile width, unless removable septa are not replaced at exactly the same location, and the accuracy of the attenuation correction, unless it is sensitive to the activity in the transmission source. Changes in any of the performance characteristics will be reflected in the image quality or quantitative accuracy of patient data, so it is important that these parameters be assessed periodically in addition to the daily quality control procedures.

REFERENCES

1. Brownell GL, Sweet WH. Localization of brain tumors with positron emitters. *Nucleonics* 1953;11:40–45.
2. Anger HO, Rosenthal DJ. Scintillation camera and positron camera. In: *Medical Radioisotope Scanning, Proceedings of a Seminar held in Vienna, Austria, February 25 to 27, 1959*. Vienna: International Atomic Energy Agency, 1959:59–82.
3. Rankowitz S, Robertson JS, Higgenbotham WA. Positron scanner for locating brain tumors. *IRE Int Conv Rec* 1962;10:49–56.
4. Burnham CA, Brownell GL. A multicrystal positron camera. *IEEE Trans Nucl Sci* 1972;NS-19:201–205.
5. Robertson JS, Marr RB, Rosenblum M, et al. 32-Crystal positron transverse section detector. In: Freedman GS, ed. *Tomographic Imaging in Nuclear Medicine*. New York: Society of Nuclear Medicine, 1973;142–153.
6. Brownell GL, Burnham CA. MGH positron camera. In: Freedman GS, ed. *Tomographic Imaging in Nuclear Medicine*. New York: Society of Nuclear Medicine, 1973;154–164.
7. Ter-Pogossian MM. The origins of positron emission tomography. *Semin Nucl Med* 1992;22:140–149.
8. Ter-Pogossian MM, Phelps ME, Hoffman EJ, et al. A positron-emission transaxial tomograph for nuclear imaging (PETT). *Radiology* 1975;11:89–98.
9. Phelps ME, Hoffman EJ, Mullani NA, et al. Application of annihilation coincidence detection to transaxial reconstruction tomography. *J Nucl Med* 1975;16:210–224.
10. Phelps ME, Mazziotta JC, Huang S-C. Study of cerebral function with positron computed tomography. *J Cereb Blood Flow Metab* 1982;2:113–162.
11. Schelbert HR, Henze E, Phelps ME. Emission tomography of the heart. *Semin Nucl Med* 1980;X:355–373.
12. Budinger TF, Yano Y, Huesman RH, et al. Positron emission tomography of the heart. *Physiologist* 1983;26:31–34.
13. Grafton ST, Mazziotta JC. Cerebral pathophysiology evaluated with positron emission tomography. In: Asbury AK, McKhann GM, McDonald WI, eds. *Diseases of the Nervous System: Clinical Neurobiology*. 2nd ed. Philadelphia: W.B. Saunders, 1992;1573–1588.
14. Volkow N, Fowler JS. Neuropsychiatric disorders: investigation of schizophrenia and substance abuse. *Semin Nucl Med* 1992;22:254–267.
15. Bergmann SR. Positron emission tomography of the heart. In: Gerson MC, ed. *Cardiac Nuclear Medicine*. 2nd ed. New York: McGraw-Hill, 1991;299–335.
16. Goldstein DS, Eisenhofer G, Dunn BB, et al. Positron emission tomographic imaging of cardiac sympathetic innervation using 6-[^{18}F]fluorodopamine: initial findings in humans. *J Am Coll Cardiol* 1993;22:1961–1971.
17. Shuster DP. Positron emission tomography: theory and its application to the study of lung disease. *Am Rev Respir Dis* 1989;139:818–840.
18. Strauss LG, Conti PS. The applications of PET in clinical oncology. *J Nucl Med* 1991;32:623–648.
19. Hawkins RA, Hoh C, Glaspy J, et al. The role of positron emission tomography in oncology and other whole-body applications. *Semin Nucl Med* 1992;XXII:268–284.
20. Hoffman JM, Hanson MW, Coleman RE. Clinical positron emission tomography imaging. *Radiol Clin N Am* 1993; 31:935–959.
21. Marinelli LD, Brinckeroff RF, Hine GJ. Average energy of beta-rays emitted by radioactive isotopes. *Rev Mod Phys* 1947;19:25–28.
22. Hounsfield GN, Ambrose J, Perry J, et al. Computerized transverse axial scanning. *Br J Radiol* 1973;46:1016–1022.
23. Brooks RA, Di Chiro G: Principles of computer assisted tomography (CAT) in radiographic and radioisotopic imaging. *Phys Med Biol* 1976;21:689–732.
24. Gordon R, Bender R, Herman GT. Algebraic reconstruction techniques (ART) for three-dimensional electron microscopy and x-ray photography. *J Theor Biol* 1970;29:471–481.
25. Goitein M. Three-dimensional density reconstruction from a series of two-dimensional projections. *Nucl Instrum Meth* 1972;101:509.
26. Gilbert P. Iterative methods for the three-dimensional reconstruction of an object from projections. *J Theor Biol* 1972; 36:105.
27. Herman GT, Lent A. Iterative reconstruction algorithms. *Comput Biol Med* 1976;6:273–294.
28. Lent A. A convergent algorithm for maximum entropy image restoration, with a medical x-ray application. In: Shaw R, ed. *Image Analysis and Evaluation*. Washington, DC: Society of Photographic Scientists and Engineers, 1977;249–257.
29. Shepp LA, Vardi Y. Maximum likelihood reconstruction for emission tomography. *IEEE Trans Med Imag* 1982;MI-1:113–132.
30. Lange K, Carson R. EM reconstruction algorithms for emission and transmission tomography. *J Comput Assist Tomogr* 1984;8:306–316.
31. Eichling JO, Higgins CS, Ter-Pogossian MM. Determination of radionuclide concentration with positron CT scanning. *J Nucl Med* 1977;18:845–847.

32. Ter-Pogossian MM, Ficke DC, Yamamoto M, et al. A positron emission tomograph utilizing photon time-of-flight information. *IEEE Trans Med Imag* 1982;MI-1:179–187.
33. Politte D. Image improvements in positron-emission tomography due to measuring differential time-of-flight and using maximum-likelihood estimation. *IEEE Trans Nucl Sci* 1990;37:737–742.
34. Karp JS, Daube-Witherspoon ME, Hoffman EJ, et al. Performance standards in positron emission tomography. *J Nucl Med* 1991;32:2342–2350.
35. Bacharach SL. The physics of positron emission tomography. In: Bergmann SR, Sobel BE, eds. *Positron Emission Tomography of the Heart*. Mount Kisco, NY: Futura Publishing, 1992;13–44.
36. Kessler RM, Ellis JR Jr., Eden M. Analysis of emission tomographic scan data: limitations imposed by resolution and background. *J Comput Assist Tomogr* 1984;8:514–522.
37. De Benedetti S, Cowan CE, Konneker WR, et al. On the angular distribution of two-photon annihilation radiation. *Phys Rev* 1950;77:205–212.
38. Muehllehner G. Resolution limit of positron cameras. *J Nucl Med* 1976;17:757.
39. Phelps ME, Hoffman EJ. Resolution limit of positron cameras. *J Nucl Med* 1976;17:757, 758.
40. Muehllehner G, Karp JS. Positron emission tomography imaging—technical consideration. *Semin Nucl Med* 1986; 16:35–50.
41. DeGrado TR, Turkington TG, Williams JJ, et al. Performance characteristics of a new generation PET scanner. *J Nucl Med* 1993;34:101P. Abstract.
42. Wienhard K, Dahlbom M, Eriksson L, et al. Performance evaluation of the high resolution PET scanner ECAT EXACT HR. *J Nucl Med* 1993;34:101P. Abstract.
43. Wienhard K, Eriksson L, Grootoonk S, et al. Performance evaluation of the positron scanner ECAT EXACT. *J Comput Assist Tomog* 1992;16:804–813.
44. Spinks TJ, Jones T, Bailey DL, et al. Physical performance of a positron tomograph for brain imaging with retractable septa. *Phys Med Biol* 1992;37:1637–1655.
45. Karp JS, Muehllehner G, Mankoff DA, et al. Continuous-slice PENN-PET: a positron tomograph with volume imaging capability. *J Nucl Med* 1990;31:617–627.
46. Derenzo SE, Huesman RH, Cahoon JL, et al. A positron tomograph with 600 BGO crystals and 2.6 mm resolution. *IEEE Trans Nucl Sci* 1988;35:659–664.
47. Hoffman EJ, Huang S-C, Plummer D, et al. Quantitation in positron emission computed tomography: Part 6. Effect of nonuniform resolution. *J Comput Assist Tomogr* 1982; 6:987–999.
48. Hoffman EJ, Huang S-C, Phelps ME. Quantitation in positron emission computed tomography: Part 1. Effect of object size. *J Comput Assist Tomogr* 1979;3:299–308.
49. Mazziotta JC, Phelps ME, Plummer D, et al. Quantitation in positron emission computed tomography: Part 5. Physical-anatomical effects. *J Comput Assist Tomogr* 1981; 5:734–743.
50. Herscovitch P, Auchus A, Gado M, et al. Correction of positron emission tomography data for cerebral atrophy. *J Cereb Blood Flow Metab* 1986;6:120–124.
51. Videen TO, Perlmutter JS, Mintun MA, et al. Regional correction of positron emission tomography data for the effects of cerebral atrophy. *J Cereb Blood Flow Metab* 1988;8:662–670.
52. Huang S-C, Hoffman EJ, Phelps ME, et al. Quantitation in positron emission computed tomography: Part 3. Effect of sampling. *J Comput Assist Tomogr* 1980;4:819–826.
53. Ficke DC, Beecher DE, Bergmann SR, et al. Performance characterization of a whole body PET system designed for dynamic cardiac imaging. In: *Proceedings of IEEE Nuclear Science Symposium and Medical Imaging Conference, Santa Fe, NM*. Piscataway, NJ: IEEE, 1991;1635–1638.
54. Bohm C, Eriksson L, Bergstrom M, et al. A computer assisted ringdetector positron camera system for reconstruction tomography of the brain. *IEEE Trans Nucl Sci* 1978;NS-25:624–637.
55. Brooks RA, Sank VJ, Talbert AJ, et al. Sampling requirements and detector motion for positron emission tomography. *IEEE Trans Nucl Sci* 1979;NS-26:2760–2763.
56. Mullani NA, Ter-Pogossian MM, Higgins CS, et al. Engineering aspects of PETT V. *IEEE Trans Nucl Sci* 1979;NS-26:2703–2706.
57. Colsher JG, Muehllehner G. Effects of wobbling motion on image quality in positron tomography. *IEEE Trans Nucl Sci* 1981;NS-28:90–93.
58. Huang S-C, Hoffman EJ, Phelps ME, et al. Quantitation in positron emission computed tomography: Part 2. Effects of inaccurate attenuation correction. *J Comput Assist Tomogr* 1979;3:804–814.
59. McCord ME, Bacharach SL, Bonow RO, et al. Misalignment between PET transmission and emission scans: its effect on myocardial imaging. *J Nucl Med* 1992;33:1209–1214.
60. Bergstrom M, Boethius J, Eriksson L, et al. Head fixation device for reproducible position alignment in transmission CT and positron emission tomography. *J Comput Assist Tomogr* 1981;5:136–141.
61. Fox PT, Perlmutter JS, Raichle ME. A stereotactic method of anatomical localization for positron emission tomography. *J Comput Assist Tomogr* 1985;9:141–153.
62. Phillips RL, London ED, Links JM, et al. Program for PET image alignment: effects on calculated differences in cerebral metabolic rates for glucose. *J Nucl Med* 1990;31:2052–2057.
63. Seitz RJ, Bohm C, Greitz T, et al. Accuracy and precision of the computerized brain atlas programme for localization and quantification in positron emission tomography. *J Cereb Blood Flow Metab* 1990;10:443–457.
64. Koeppe RA, Holthoff VA, Frey KA, et al. Compartmental analysis of [^{11}C]flumazenil kinetics for the estimation of ligand transport rate and receptor distribution using positron emission tomography. *J Cereb Blood Flow Metab* 1991; 11:735–744.
65. Minoshima S, Berger KL, Lee KS, et al. An automated method for rotational correction and centering of three-dimensional functional brain images. *J Nucl Med* 1992; 33:1579–1585.
66. Daube-Witherspoon ME, Yan YC, Green MV, et al. Correction for motion distortion in PET by dynamic monitoring of patient position. *J Nucl Med* 1990;31:816. Abstract.
67. Ter-Pogossian MM, Bergmann SR, Sobel BE. Influence of cardiac and respiratory motion on tomographic reconstructions of the heart: implications for quantitative nuclear cardiology. *J Comput Assist Tomogr* 1982;6:1148–1155.
68. Bergstrom M, Litton J, Eriksson L, et al. Determination of object contour from projections for attenuation correction in cranial positron emission tomography. *J Comput Assist Tomogr* 1982;6:365–372.
69. Tomitami T. An edge detection algorithm for attenuation correction in emission CT. *IEEE Trans Nucl Sci* 1987;NS-34:309–312.
70. Michel C, Bol A, De Volder AG, et al. Online brain attenuation correction in PET: towards a fully automated data handling in a clinical environment. *Eur J Nucl Med* 1989; 15:712–718.
71. Frackowiak RSJ, Lenzi G-L, Jones T, et al. Quantitative measurement of regional cerebral blood flow and oxygen metabolism in man using ^{15}O and positron emission tomography:

theory, procedure and normal values. *J Comput Assist Tomogr* 1980;4:727–736.

72. Carroll LR, Kretz P, Orcutt G. The orbiting rod source: improving performance in PET transmission correction scans. In: *Emission Computed Tomography: Current Trends*. New York: The Society of Nuclear Medicine, 1983;235–247.
73. Thompson CJ, Dagher A, Lunney DN, et al. A technique to reject scattered radiation in PET transmission scans. International workshop on physics and engineering of computerized multidimensional imaging and processing. *Proc SPIE* 1986;671:244–253.
74. Dahlbom M, Hoffman EJ. Problems in signal-to-noise ratio for attenuation correction in high resolution PET. *IEEE Trans Nucl Sci* 1987;34:288–293.
75. Palmer MR, Rogers JG, Bergstrom M, et al. Transmission profile filtering for positron emission tomography. *IEEE Trans Nucl Sci* 1986;NS-33:478–481.
76. Meikle SR, Dahlbom M, Cherry SR. Attenuation correction using count-limited transmission data in positron emission tomography. *J Nucl Med* 1993;34:143–150.
77. Huang SC, Carson R, Phelps M, et al. A boundary method for attenuation correction in positron emission tomography. *J Nucl Med* 1981;22:627–637.
78. Xu EZ, Mullani NA, Gould KL, et al. A segmented attenuation correction for PET. *J Nucl Med* 1991;32:161–165.
79. Carson RE, Daube-Witherspoon ME, Green MV. A method for postinjection PET transmission measurements. *J Nucl Med* 1988;29:1558–1567.
80. Daube-Witherspoon ME, Carson RE, Green MV. Post-injection transmission attenuation measurements for PET. *IEEE Trans Nucl Sci* 1988;35:757–761.
81. Thompson CJ, Ranger NT, Evans AC. Simultaneous transmission and emission scans in positron emission tomography. *IEEE Trans Nucl Sci* 1989;36:1011–1016.
82. Holte S, Eriksson L, Larsson JE, et al. A preliminary evaluation of a positron camera system using weighted decoding of individual crystals. *IEEE Trans Nucl Sci* 1988;35:730–734.
83. Karp JS, Muehllehner G. Performance of a positron-sensitive scintillation detector. *Phys Med Biol* 1985;30:643–655.
84. Mankoff DA, Muehllehner G, Karp JS. The effect of detector performance on high countrate PET imaging with a tomograph based on position-sensitive detectors. *IEEE Trans Nucl Sci* 1988;35:592–597.
85. Knoop BO, Jordan K, Spinks T. Evaluation of PET count rate performance. *Eur J Nucl Med* 1989;15:705–711.
86. Germano G, Hoffman EJ. A study of data loss and mispositioning due to pileup in 2-D detectors in PET. *IEEE Trans Nucl Sci* 1990;37:671–675.
87. Daube-Witherspoon ME, Carson RE. Unified deadtime correction model for PET. *IEEE Trans Med Imag* 1991; 10:267–275.
88. Holmes TJ, Ficke DC, Snyder DL. Modeling of accidental coincidences in both conventional and time-of-flight positron-emission tomography. *IEEE Trans Nucl Sci* 1984;NS-31:627–631.
89. Haynor DR, Harrison RL, Lewellen TK. A scheme for accidental coincidence correction in time-of-flight positron tomography. *IEEE Trans Nucl Sci* 1988;35:753–756.
90. Hoffman EJ, Huang S-C, Phelps ME, et al. Quantitation in positron emission computed tomography: Part 4. Effect of accidental coincidences. *J Comput Assist Tomogr* 1981; 5:391–400.
91. Strother SC, Casey ME, Hoffman EJ. Measuring PET scanner sensitivity: relating count rates to image signal-to-noise ratios using noise equivalent counts. *IEEE Trans Nucl Sci* 1990;37:783–788.
92. Mankoff D, Muehllehner G. Performance of positron imaging systems as a function of energy threshold and shielding depth. *IEEE Trans Med Imag* 1984;MI-3:18–24.
93. Kops ER, Herzog H, Schmid A, et al. Performance characteristics of an eight-ring whole body PET scanner. *J Comput Assist Tomogr* 1990;14:437–445.
94. Evans AC, Thompson CJ, Marrett S, et al. Performance evaluation of the PC-2048: a new 15-slice encoded-crystal PET scanner for neurological studies. *IEEE Trans Med Imag* 1991;10:90–98.
95. Bergstrom M, Eriksson L, Bohm C, et al. Correction for scattered radiation in a ring detector positron camera by integral transformation of the projections. *J Comput Assist Tomogr* 1983;7:42–50.
96. Hoffman EJ, Phelps ME. Positron emission tomography: principles and quantitation. In: Phelps ME, Mazziotta JC, Schelbert HR, eds. *Positron Emission Tomography and Autoradiography*. New York: Raven Press, 1986;237–286.
97. Bendriem B, Soussaline F, Campagnolo R, et al. A technique for the correction of scattered radiation in a PET system using time-of-flight information. *J Comput Assist Tomogr* 1986; 10:287–295.
98. Evans RD. *The Atomic Nucleus*. New York: McGraw-Hill, 1955.
99. Budinger TF, Derenzo SE, Greenberg WL, et al. Quantitative potentials of dynamic emission computed tomography. *J Nucl Med* 1978;19:309–315.
100. Alpert NM, Chesler DA, Correia JA, et al. Estimation of the local statistical noise in emission computed tomography. *IEEE Trans Med Imag* 1982;MI-1:142–146.
101. Huesman RH. A new fast algorithm for the evaluation of regions of interest and statistical uncertainty in computed tomography. *Phys Med Biol* 1984;29:543–552.
102. Carson RE, Yan Y, Daube-Witherspoon ME, et al. An approximation formula for the variance of PET region-of-interest values. *IEEE Trans Med Imag* 1993;12:240–250.
103. Bailey DL, Jones T, Spinks TJ, et al. Noise equivalent count measurements in a neuro-PET scanner with retractable septa. *IEEE Trans Med Imaging* 1991;10:256–260.
104. Brooks RA, Sank VJ, Friauf WS, et al. Design considerations for positron emission tomography. *IEEE Trans Biomed Eng*, 1981;28:158–177.
105. Council on Scientific Affairs. Instrumentation in positron emission tomography. *JAMA* 1988;259:1351–1356.
106. Koeppe RA, Hutchins GD. Instrumentation for positron emission tomography: tomographs and data processing and display systems. *Semin Nucl Med* 1992;22:162–181.
107. Derenzo SE, Moses WW, Cahoon JL, et al. Prospects for new inorganic scintillators. *IEEE Trans Nucl Sci* 1990; 37: 203–208.
108. Moses WW, Derenzo SE, Shlichta PJ. Scintillation properties of lead sulfate. *IEEE Trans Nucl Sci* 1992;39:1190–1194.
109. Muehllehner G, Karp JS, Mankoff DA, et al. Design and performance of a new positron tomograph. *IEEE Trans Nucl Sci* 1988;35:670–674.
110. Cherry SR, Dahlbom M, Hoffman EJ. 3D PET using a conventional multislice tomograph without septa. *J Comput Assist Tomogr* 1991;15:655–668.
111. Dahlbom M, Hoffman EJ, Hoh CK, et al. Whole-body positron emission tomography: Part 1. Methods and performance characteristics. *J Nucl Med* 1992;33:1191–1199.
112. Townsend DW, Geissbuhler A, Defrise M, et al. Fully three-dimensional reconstruction for a PET camera with retractable septa. *IEEE Trans Med Imag* 1991;10:505–512.
113. Kinahan PE, Rogers JG. Analytic three-dimensional image reconstruction using all detected events. *IEEE Trans Nucl Sci* 1989;36:964–968.
114. Daube-Witherspoon ME, Muehllehner G. Treatment of axial

data in three-dimensional PET. *J Nucl Med* 1987; 28:1717–1724.

115. Lewitt RM, Muehllehner G, Karp JS. 3D image reconstruction for PET by multi-slice rebinning and axial filtering. In: *Proceedings of IEEE 1991 Nuclear Science Symposium and Medical Imaging Conference, Santa Fe, New Mexico*. Piscataway, NJ: IEEE, 1991;2054–2061.
116. Guzzardi R, Bellina CR, Knoop B, et al. Methodologies for performance evaluation of positron emission tomographs. *J Nucl Biol Med* 1991;35:141–157.
117. Ter-Pogossian MM, Raichle ME, Sobel BE. Positron-emission tomography. *Sci Am* 1980;243(4):170–181.
118. Kanno I. PET instrumentation for quantitative tracing of radiopharmaceuticals. In: Diksic M, Reba RC, eds. *Radiopharmaceuticals and Brain Pathology Studied with PET and SPECT*. Boca Raton, FL: CRC Press, 1991;69–92.
119. Phelps ME, Hoffman EJ, Huang S-C, et al. Design considerations in positron computed tomography (PCT). *IEEE Trans Nucl Sci* 1979;NS-26:2746–2751.
120. Lederer CM, Shirley VS, eds. *Table of Isotopes*. 7th ed. New York: John Wiley & Sons, 1978.
121. Derenzo SE. Mathematical removal of positron range blurring in high resolution tomography. *IEEE Trans Nucl Sci* 1986; 33:565–569.
122. Phelps ME, Hoffman EJ, Gado M, et al. Computerized transaxial transmission reconstruction tomography. In: DeBlanc Jr. HJ, Sorenson JA, eds. *Noninvasive Brain Imaging: Computer Tomography and Radionuclides*. New York: Society of Nuclear Medicine, 1975;111–145.

7 Computer Systems

Stephen L. Bacharach

Computer systems are used in medicine to perform a wide range of operations, from the control of simple instruments to the reconstruction of tomographic images. Many devices that depend on computers are designed so that the user can operate them correctly without even knowing that they contain a computer. The operation of computers that control such instruments needs to be understood no more than the principles of solid-state electronics need be understood to play a transistor radio. Unfortunately, this is not the case for the computers used for image collection and analysis in nuclear medicine.

The computer systems used to collect and process images in nuclear medicine must be under more direct control by the user. There is often no standard method for acquiring, processing, analyzing, or displaying computer-acquired nuclear medicine images. Nuclear medicine is constantly evolving as new radiopharmaceuticals are developed, and new methods of data analysis devised. Even for well-established procedures there is often wide variation in opinion as to how best to acquire, analyze, and display the images. For these reasons it is essential that the nuclear medicine computer system be highly flexible. This in turn requires that the user have some understanding of those aspects of computer systems that affect the subjective quality and quantitative accuracy of the nuclear medicine images they produce. In the first section of this chapter, use of computer systems as instruments is discussed, and attention is given to the associated devices (*hardware*) essential to their operation. Only those aspects of computer systems likely to impact directly on their clinical use in nuclear medicine are discussed. The remaining sections discuss some of the basic elements of nuclear medicine *software*—the programs used to acquire and process data. Later chapters focus on ways in which this basic software can be used clinically.

OVERVIEW

Nuclear medicine computer systems are made up of several major components, each of which may be considered independently (Fig. 1). Although most systems contain many more devices than are shown in Figure 1, all systems must have at least the basic elements shown: a module for *data acquisition*, a module for *mass storage*, a module for *image display*, and the *computer* itself. The varous devices connected to the computer are referred to as "peripheral" devices. The computer controls the flow of information between itself and the peripheral devices, and performs necessary calculations on the data. For example computers may instruct the data acquisition peripheral to convert the data produced by the imaging device (usually an Anger scintillation camera) into digital form, ie, into numbers. The converted data might then be relayed to the computer memory (often called RAM for *random access memory*) and sorted into an image. Later the computer might send the image data to the display device, allowing the user to examine the image being formed, or the computer might send the image to the mass storage device—perhaps a magnetic disk drive—for permanent storage. The components necessary to perform each of these tasks (at least those important to the performance of good-quality nuclear medicine studies) are discussed in detail in the following sections.

DIGITIZING THE IMAGE

Digital computers operate only on numeric data. The signals produced by most gamma cameras, however, are not in numeric form. Rather, they are "analog" signals. An analog signal is one whose magnitude is related in some way to the actual information of interest (ie, the signal is the analog of that information). For example the column height in a mercury thermometer is the analog of temperature. Similarly the voltages produced by the x and y outputs of the scintillation camera are the analogs of the x and y positions describing where the gamma ray interacted in the camera crystal. Analog signals, like the height of the mercury column, are continuous signals—they can assume any possible value. Digital signals, on the other hand, can have only certain discrete values. For example, a digital thermometer with a three-digit display can produce only discrete readings of temperature, eg, 28.4 or 28.5 or 28.6, etc, degrees. It cannot produce intermediate values, eg, 28.467. One could make a digital thermometer with more digits displayed, for example a 5-digit thermometer, but still, it would be limited to discrete values, eg, 28.451 or 28.452, or 28.453, etc, and nothing in between. In the analog thermometer, on the other hand, the height of the column is not limited to only certain discrete values—it can take on all possible values. This is a fundamental difference between analog and digital signals. To convert the height of the mercury column to a discrete (ie, digital) value of temperature, we use an "analog-to-digital"

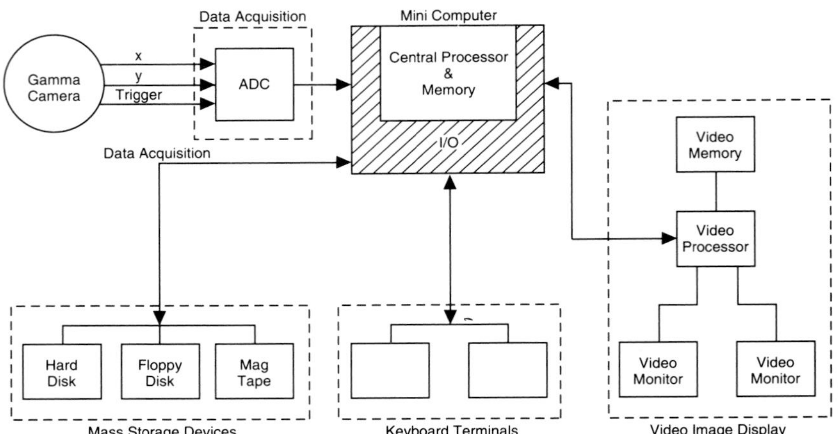

Figure 1. Components of a typical nuclear medicine computer system.

convertor (ADC). In the case of the mercury thermometer the ADC might consist simply of ruling off the glass tube into steps of, for example, tenths of degrees. Then the rule mark closest to the level of the mercury tells us the digital value of temperature. Our eye and brain would use the rule marks to do the analog (height) to digital (temperature in degrees) conversion. The digital resolution of this thermometer is determined by the number of rule markings per degree—one mark per 0.1° in this example. Similarly, the magnitude of the x and y voltage signals produced by all scintillation cameras are analog signals. The magnitude of their voltage is the analog of the position of the gamma ray that struck the camera crystal. These analog signals must be converted to digital form, ie, to a pair of numbers describing the position of the signal on the camera face, before the computer is able to use them. Again an analog-to-digital convertor is used (actually two—one for x and one for y), this time one that converts the magnitude (height) of the voltage to a number indicating position. Just as the number of divisions per degree determined the digital "resolution" of the thermometer, so the number of divisions per centimeter in x or y determines the digital resolution of the x and y ADCs of the gamma camera. A 40-cm field of view (FOV) gamma camera might utilize an electronic ADC which divides the gamma camera field of view into 64 rule marks along the 40-cm long horizontal direction (usually called x) and 64 rule marks in the vertical direction (usually called y). The squares formed by the intersections of these rule marks are called *pixels* (short for picture elements). In this example, the digital resolution of the ADC (not to be confused with the resolution of the gamma camera itself, discussed in Chapter 5) would be 64 pixels per 40 cm, or 1.6 pixels per centimeter. Sometimes digital resolution is expressed as the reciprocal of this value, ie, the number of centimeters or millimeters per pixel (0.625 cm per pixel in this example). However, expressing the digital resolution of the ADC as simply "64 by 64 pixels" or "4096 pixels" (the product of 64 × 64) is incorrect, as one must also know the number of centimeters these pixels span. For example, a 40-cm large-field-of-view (LFOV) gamma camera when divided into 64 by 64 pixels* corresponds to a much poorer digital resolution than if a 20-cm diameter small-field-of-view camera were divided up into the same 64 by 64 pixels. In the first case the distance between pixels would be 0.625 cm; in the latter case the pixels would be 0.3125 cm apart. In the former case one could measure positions (eg, the location at which a gamma ray interacted) only to within 0.625 cm, and in the latter to within 0.3125 cm. This has great practical importance when deciding on what digital resolution to use in acquiring a clinical image. A small-field-of-view gamma camera, such as might be used for cardiac imaging, requires many fewer pixels than an LFOV camera, to achieve the same spacing between pixels. Therefore certain applications that might require a 128 × 128 "matrix" of pixels on an LFOV camera may well require only a 64 × 64 "matrix" of pixels on a small FOV camera.

All nuclear medicine computers allow the user to define the digital resolution of the x and y ADCs by selecting the number of rule marks to be used over the camera field of view (although some computers force the two numbers to be the same). It is important then, that the clinician or technologist understand how properly to choose this number for a particular clinical application, with a particular gamma camera. The factors influencing this decision will be discussed later, in the context of the acquisition software.

There are many electronic methods of converting the analog x and y signals to digital form.[1] The user need not be concerned with the electronic details by which the ADC operates. However, the speed with which it performs the conversion *is* important to the user. There may be tens of thousands of photons striking the gamma camera each second. The ADC must be fast enough to convert each of the resulting pairs of signals before the next pair of signals

*For reasons related to the binary number system used by computers, the number of rule marks is nearly always specified in even powers of two, ie, 32, 64, 128, 256, 512, etc.

arrives. If a signal pair arrives while the ADCs are still converting a previous signal, the later signal pair may be missed, which contributes to the system count loss. Ideally, ADC deadtime (ie, the time it takes for the ADC to perform a conversion and be ready for the next *x*, *y* signal pair) should be shorter than the most closely spaced pulses that the gamma camera is capable of producing (typically a few microseconds).

THE COMPUTER

The computer can be thought of as the "brain" of the processing system. It consists of a "central processor unit" (CPU), memory, and means to communicate between itself and the outside world (ie, the peripheral devices attached to it). The CPU is in charge of performing all computations and making all decisions expected of the computer. While this may sound a complex task, the computer is able to understand only a small number (often 100 or fewer) of quite simple "instructions." These instructions are usually no more complex than, for example, "add one to the number stored in a specific memory location" or "skip the next instruction if the number stored in a specified memory location is zero." Each elementary instruction recognized by the CPU is represented by a number. A computer "program" is just a sequence of these elementary instructions, and therefore is simply a sequence of numbers (each representing one of the basic instructions) stored in the computer's memory. To perform the complex tasks required of a nuclear medicine computer many thousands of such simple instructions must be executed in the proper sequence. The computer's memory is used to temporarily store these thousands of instructions. The CPU goes from one memory location to the next, executing the instructions stored there.

The speed with which the CPU can execute its instructions affects the speed at which the system can perform its tasks. Typically the CPU can perform each of its elementary instructions in a millionth of a second or faster. Even so, many calculations, such as tomographic reconstructions and manipulations involving digital images, may require 10's or 100's of millions of instructions—and hence tens or hundreds of seconds to carry out. To decrease this time a faster CPU chip may be available, or one can purchase specialized hardware modules that speed certain computations. Two such devices are the *floating point processor* (often included in many computer systems), which greatly speeds the performance of noninteger arithmetic calculations, and the *array processor*, which greatly speeds certain operations performed on images, and speeds tomographic reconstruction.

Computer Memory

As will be seen later, the user of a nuclear medicine computer system often controls the way in which the computer's memory is utilized. It is therefore necessary to understand a little more about how this memory is organized.

Computer memory consists of many discrete locations for storing numbers. Each storage location is called a *word* of memory, and can be used to store any numeric data of interest. For example, we have already seen that memory can be used to store *programs*. Also, memory can be used to store data such as the digitized *x* and *y* coordinate values from the gamma camera ADC, or the numbers comprising a digital representation of an image.

A computer's memory, or RAM, is located on computer chips. Computer memory of this type is "volatile," ie, when power to the computer is turned off all numbers stored in the chips are lost. Cost and design constraints limit the number of words of memory in a computer. The size of each word, ie, the largest numeric value that each word can store, is also limited. The reason for this limit becomes obvious if the problem of storing numbers on a pad of paper is considered. If each number falls in the range of 0 to 99, only two digits are required to "store" each number by writing it on the paper. If numbers are allowed to be as large as 9999, four digits are required, which uses more storage space (room on the paper) than if only two digits are allowed. This example, however, is based on the decimal system of numbers with which we are all familiar. The computer does not use the decimal numbering system, but rather the binary numbering system. The digits of the binary system (called *bits*, for *b*inary dig*its*) are not the ten numbers from 0 to 9, but rather the two numbers 0 and 1. The ten numbers making up the digits of the decimal system lead to numbers written as powers of 10. For example, the decimal number 782 is seven in the 100's column, eight in the 10's column, and two in the 1's column. Similarly the two digits of a binary system lead to numbers written as powers of two—1, 2, 4, 8, 16, etc. Therefore, the number 1011 would be one in the 8 column, zero in the 4 column, 1 in the 2 column, and one in the 1 column, making a total (in decimal) of eleven. The reason computers use the binary system is that the computer's memory is made up of devices resembling switches. These switches can have not ten different states but only two—on and off. Therefore, the basic unit of memory can store not ten different numbers (0 to 9) as the decimal system requires, but rather only two—0 and 1. By convention, a single word of computer memory is 16 "bits" long, that is, it is a string of 16 binary digits. The largest number that can be stored in a word made up of 16 binary digits is $(2^{16} - 1)$, or 65,535 (just as the largest number that can be stored in a string of 3 decimal digits is $10^3 - 1$ or 999). If the words in the computer's memory were being used to store the number of counts detected at a particular location on the gamma camera crystal (one method of storing an "image"), then the maximum number of counts that could be stored at a particular location would also be 65,535—a limitation that must be always borne in mind. Because the number of words in memory is limited, storage of not one number but two numbers in each word is frequently desirable. Each half word of memory (8 bits) is called a *byte* of memory and can store a number only as large as 255

($2^8 - 1$). At first, it might seem that a half word should be able to store a number half as large as a full word. That this is not so can be understood from the previous example of writing a number on paper. With a word capable of holding four digits, a number as large as 9999 ($10^4 - 1$) can be stored, while with a half word capable of holding only two digits a number only as large as 99 ($10^2 - 1$) can be stored.

If data, such as a digitized image, can be stored in bytes instead of words, only half as much memory is needed, allowing, for example, twice as many images to be stored in the memory at once. The 255 maximum of each byte, however, means that only 255 counts can be stored at any pixel. This limitation often creates problems, some of which will be discussed further in the section on acquisition software below.

Creating an Image

Before describing the rest of the nuclear medicine system hardware, it is useful to see how the computer might use the ADC to create an image in its memory. The user must first decide on the desired digital acquisition resolution, eg, 128 pixels over the 40-cm camera field of view in *x* and in *y*. The computer instructs each of the two ADCs respectively to digitize the analog *x* and *y* data from the gamma camera at this resolution. The computer then sets aside room in its memory to hold a representation of the image. If, as in this example, a 128 × 128 image is desired, then 16384 words of memory are set aside (one word for each pixel, or half that amount if a byte image is desired). One can envision the image as a table or matrix of 128 rows by 128 columns each element of which is one word of memory. The computer first writes the number 0 in each of the words of the image (ie, it erases the values that might have been previously stored in each location). Data acquisition then begins. Each photon detected produces an *x* and *y* coordinate signal that is digitized by the two ADCs. The values of *x* and *y* produced by the two ADCs give the row and column locations at which the photon interacted in the gamma camera. The computer then adds the number one to the word in memory at that row and column. The value stored in each word, then, is the number of photons that interacted at the corresponding position on the camera face. Each time a photon interacts at that position, one more count is added to the memory location at the corresponding position in memory. At the end of the acquisition the value contained in each of the 128 rows and 128 columns of memory contains the number of counts that occurred at corresponding locations in the gamma camera. The "image" in the computer's memory is just a list of 16384 numbers, each number representing counts. Mentally, however, it is more convenient to think of the memory containing the image as arranged as the 128 rows of numbers by 128 columns of numbers.

Mass Storage Devices

Usually digitized images, programs, and other useful data are stored temporarily in memory, in either byte or word mode. Because memory size is limited (and expensive), and because the memory is erased when the power is turned off, RAM is unsuitable for long-term data storage. The most common device for image storage is a magnetic disk. There are two kinds of magnetic disks: *hard* and *flexible* (or *floppy*). A disk storage system consists of two parts: the disk itself (similar in shape to a phonograph record), on which data are stored, and the disk drive (analogous to a photograph player), which is the device used to read from, or record onto, the disk.

Hard disks are available in many capacities. Popular disk capacities for nuclear medicine computers range from hundreds to thousands of megabytes (a "mega"byte is a million bytes, and a thousand megabytes is known as a "giga"byte). To put these numbers into perspective, consider that many nuclear medicine images are produced by digitizing the field of view of the gamma camera into a 128 × 128 array of pixels. If the counts at each pixel are stored in one word of memory, then the image requires 16,384 words of memory. These 16,384 words of memory then must be transferred to the hard disk, for long-term storage. If the disk holds 100 megabytes (ie, 50 million words), then the number of 128 × 128 images that can be stored is given by

50,000,000 words of storage on disk/
(16,384 words per image)
= about 3050 images,

or in general:

number of images storable
=disk capacity in words (bytes)/
[size of image in words (bytes)].

The above calculation assumes that nothing besides images are being stored on the disk (which we will see later is an incorrect assumption).

Of course, when a SPECT study is performed, using, for example, 64 views, the raw data occupy 64 times 128 × 128 words per study (assuming a 128 × 128 acquisition matrix). If it is a ^{201}Tl stress/redistribution study, then each patient has two such studies. The number of stress/redistribution SPECT studies that could fit on the disk would then be 3050/(64 × 2) = about 24 patients. This only accounts for the raw data. If the reconstructed images are also stored (as presumably they would be), the number of patient studies that can be stored is limited still further. Clearly, large amounts of storage space may be required if one wishes to store studies for any length of time.

Images stored on hard disks typically require only tens of milliseconds to retrieve. Hard disks, then, allow rapid access to a large volume of data stored in a reasonably small space. The disk and disk drive are quite fragile; they are sensitive to shocks (mechanical and thermal) and to the presence of dust and particulate matter (eg, smoke). For this reason, the disk itself is most commonly an integral sealed unit consisting of the disk and the disk drive. In older computer systems the disk was removable from the drive, and was contained in a protective plastic container, called a *disk pack*, the whole of which could be inserted into the disk drive. These removable disk packs usually contained only tens of megabytes of storage, while the newer nonremovable disks routinely store many hundreds of megabytes, or even 1 or 2 gigabytes. When these older disk packs were filled with images, they could be removed from the disk drive and stored on a shelf, and a new disk pack inserted. Each 10-megabyte disk pack might cost from $50 to $100, while the older-style disk drives might cost $10,000 or $20,000. On the other hand, the newer, nonremovable disk and disk drives now cost only $2000 or $3000 for a *giga*byte of storage. The most popular of these new disk drives are called "SCSI" (pronounced "scuzzi," standing for Small Computer Systems Interface) disk drives, because their manufacturers have developed a standardized way of connecting the disk drive to the computer, making them compatible with many different computer types.

Floppy Disks

"Floppy" disk units (originally called by that name because the disk itself was flexible) also consist of two parts: a disk drive and the "diskette" on which the data are actually stored. The disks are removable. The original floppy disks (used now only on older machines) consisted of a 5.25-in diameter thin, flexible disk, enclosed in a protective paper or plastic wrapper. The whole disk and protective wrapper had some degree of flexibility, and could typically store a few tenths of a megabyte. The newer "floppy" disks (sometimes called micro disks, or microfloppy disks) are only about 3.5 in in diameter, and are enclosed in a plastic case that is not flexible. Newer-style microfloppy disks can typically hold around a megabyte (ie, about 30 128×128 word mode images), and cost about a dollar. Older style microfloppy disk drives exist which can only store about half this much information on a disk. The newer "high-density" or "double-density" drives can usually read data stored by either type of disk drive, but the old-style drives can only read data stored by another "single"-density drive.

Floppy disks are much slower than hard disks. It may take the computer many seconds to read an image from them. Both floppy disk drives and diskettes are considerably less expensive than hard disks. Floppy disks are much less subject to environmental and mechanical damage, but when handled carelessly can be rendered unreadable. Their small physical size makes them convenient for storing or mailing patient images from a single (small) study. A series of gated cardiac images (at 64×64 word mode, or 128×128 byte mode) obtained from one patient study might be stored on a single floppy disk.

Magnetic Tapes

Clearly, even the largest hard disk will eventually fill up. One can then either delete (ie, erase) older studies from the disk or use another storage medium to store the data for a longer term. The problem of long-term storage is important, for possible legal requirements and to be able to compare old studies to current ones. In many cases (eg, gated bloodpool movies or SPECT wall motion studies) film does not contain sufficient information to make such comparisons. As mentioned above, in older machines, hard disks could be removed from their drives and stored. This allowed for permanent (albeit bulky and expensive) storage. Alternatively, data can be stored on magnetic tape. The standard on many larger computer systems is still 1/2-in wide, nine-track tape. Reels of such tape range from about 6 to 12 in in diameter. The newest of these tape drives can only store a few hundred megabytes on a single 12-in reel of tape. It might typically take many minutes to write or read data from such a tape, at a cost of about $10 to $20 per tape (and up to tens of thousands of dollars for the tape drive itself, depending on its speed). Obviously, this is much slower than a disk. For archiving, however, it may often be a perfectly acceptable, if somewhat bulky, method of long-term storage. It has the advantage of being transportable. Any "high-density" nine-track tape drive can read nine-track tapes written by any other computer (providing a program is written to do the reading)—a compatibility that does not generally exist for removable disks.

Newer tape technologies exist that allow even more compact (but not necessarily faster) storage of data. Eight- or 4-mm tapes (similar to those used for video purposes and about the size of an audio tape cassette, or smaller) can be used to store digital data, with a tape often holding one or a few gigabytes. Unfortunately, each manufacturer's tape is usually physically unreadable by another manufacturer's tape drive. Also, at this writing, these tape drives are somewhat more error prone than the older nine-track drives (but technology is improving rapidly). Alternatively, 1/4-in tape cassettes, sometimes called "streamer" tapes, are available that can hold tens or even a few hundreds of megabytes in a 4- to 5- by 3-in cassette. Some of these newer technologies are not as fast as a modern nine-track tape drive, but often this is not a critical issue, as the data are being stored only for archival purposes.

Optical Disks

Tapes are not a wholly satisfactory solution to the archiving problem in nuclear medicine—in fact at this writing there *is* no really good solution to this problem. The faster nine-track tapes are very bulky, and the tape drives are very expensive. The smaller 8- and 4-mm units are less expensive and very compact, but often excruciatingly slow and prone to errors. When a physician is interpreting a study and wishes to compare the study with a previous one the patient may have had many months (or years) ago, speed becomes important. One still-evolving technology that may eventually aid in the solution to the archiving problem is the optical disk. These disks resemble audio "CDs." Drives selling for a few thousand dollars (at this writing) can write and read disks holding several hundred megabytes to around a gigabyte. They are quite fast (compared to tapes), although not nearly as fast as hard disks. Some units are able to write data onto a disk only once, and thereafter data can only be read from the disk. For archival purposes (in which you wish to keep the data indefinitely), this is not a significant drawback—in fact it may be an advantage as it prevents accidentally overwriting a disk. Such devices are called "Write Once Read Many" times, or WORM, drives. Other (slightly more costly) units can be used to write many times. A typical optical disk may cost a few hundred dollars, so one pays a significant price for the speed improvement over tape, and the optical disk can hold no more data (in fact, usually a factor of 2 less) than an 8- or 4-mm tape. "Juke boxes" are available, however, in which one can store a large number of optical disks for automatic insertion into the disk drive. Such devices are still quite expensive, however, and the technology of optical disks is still only a potential, not an actual, solution to the archiving problem. The technology is, however, evolving very rapidly.

Video Display

The video display system is the primary tool used by clinicians to observe and interact with images the computer acquires. Unlike film viewing, the computer permits a high degree of flexibility in image display.[2-4] The observer can alter the image appearance by altering contrast, brightness, and many other features that affect image perception. This flexibility is both advantageous and potentially troublesome. In theory one could adjust the way the display device portrays the image so as to optimize the diagnostic utility of the image. In practice, it is all too easy to adjust the display characteristics in ways that mislead the viewer, and potentially cause misinterpretation of the image. Clearly, it is critical that the clinician (and technologist) understand the way the display device functions, and some of the basic concepts of image perception.

There are many different designs of video display systems. Most consist of three elements (Fig. 2A): a video controller, a video memory, and a video monitor. The display controller is a small microcomputer (separate from, but communicating with, the nuclear medicine computer) that controls the basic operation of the display. This microprocessor has its own memory, sometimes called display memory or video memory. This memory is sometimes shared with the main nuclear medicine computer, and is used to store the images being displayed. The video controller and its memory may all be contained on a single circuit board that plugs into the nuclear medicine computer. Finally, the video monitor (similar to a TV set, without the channel selection or audio) is used to display the images.

The most important task the video processor performs is to translate the array of numbers representing the image into various intensities of light on the display. This translation from digitized image to display brightness is determined by a *look-up table* (LUT). The LUT, by controlling the way counts are displayed as brightness, controls the way the image is perceived. The user therefore can control the way the image is perceived by altering the LUT. Figure 2B illustrates how the LUT works. The LUT can be thought of as a table of brightness values. Each entry in the table contains a number that specifies the brightness that will appear on the screen. Consider a black and white video monitor. If the table entries are each 1 byte (ie, 8 bits) in size, then the maximum screen brightness (ie, the brightest white the monitor can display on the screen) will correspond to the maximum value that can be written in the table—255 in this case. A value of 128 would give only half of maximum brightness, and a value of 0 would appear completely dark on the screen. An 8-bit "wide" LUT, then, can produce 255 shades of gray.

How does the LUT translate the value of "counts" at a particular pixel in the image to an intensity on the screen? It is done simply by the order of the table. Any pixel containing zero counts has its brightness value contained in the first entry in the LUT. All pixels containing one count have their brightness displayed as whatever brightness value is listed in the second entry in the LUT, and so on. The example in Figure 2B illustrates how a value of six counts is translated ("looked up") by the table. Since there are six counts in the pixel, the microprocessor looks in the seventh location (remember 0 counts corresponds to the first location) of the LUT, which, in this example, contains the value of ten. Therefore 6 counts are displayed with a brightness value of "10," or 10/255ths of maximum brightness. If one wanted to display all the pixels containing 6 counts more brightly, one could insert a larger value into the corresponding entry of the LUT, for example, replacing the 10 with 100. In that case all pixels containing 6 counts would be displayed with a brightness of 100 (or 100/255 of maximum brightness).

Since every possible value of counts maps into one element in the LUT, the number of entries in the table is usually determined by the maximum value that can be stored in a pixel of video memory. In most display systems, the digital images are transferred from the main computer memory to video memory. Frequently, video memory is only 8 bits, ie, 1 byte, and so the maximum count value that can be stored in video memory is only 255. In this case, 256 LUT entries (255 + 1 entry for the value zero) would be required to map every possible value of count into a different brightness. In word-mode images (ie, 16-bit images), the maximum value of counts is 65535. The data would therefore have to be scaled to 255 maximum before transferring it to a display memory that could only hold 8 bits. Some newer displays have "deeper" video memories (ie, more bits), for example 10, 12, or 16 bits, permitting maximum counts of 1023, 4095, or 65533 counts per pixel to be stored. One would then need an equivalent number of entries in the LUT to map each count value into an intensity. These extra entries would at first not seem to be of much use, however, if the size of each entry in the LUT were still kept at 1 byte. The entry in each element of the table could only range from 0 to 255, and so only 255 shades of brightness could be displayed, even though the counts might vary from 0 to 4095. However, even with a LUT that is only 1 byte wide, having the extra

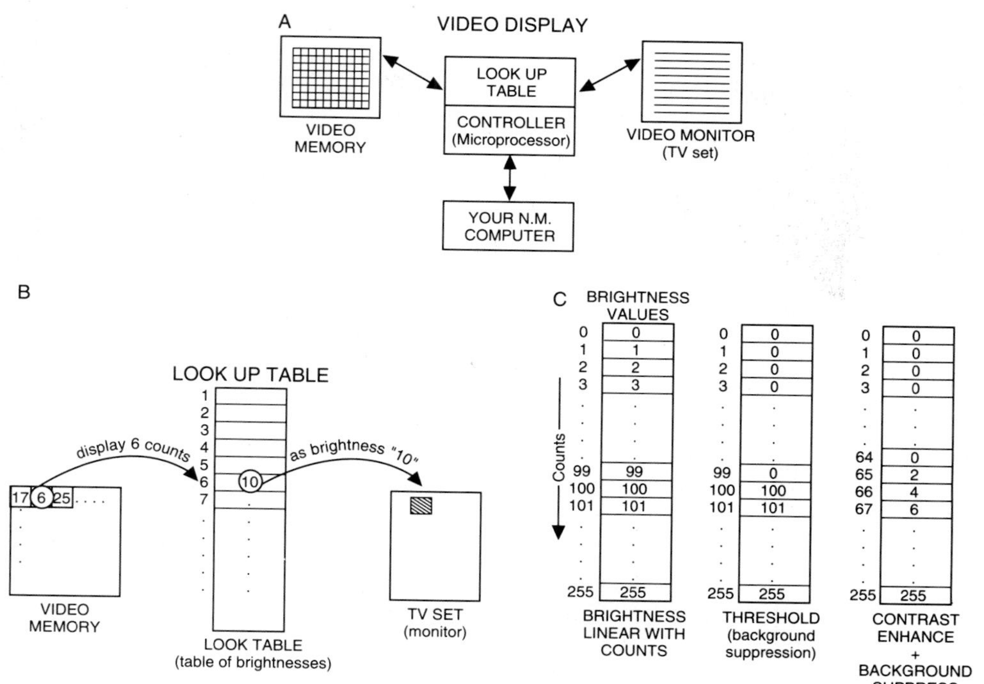

Figure 2. **(A).** Components of video display system. **(B).** Use of look-up table to convert counts to brightness. **(C).** Use of look-up table to change the way an image is perceived through thresholding and increased display contrast.

number of entries in the table permits a small range of the total 4095 counts to be displayed using the full 256 shades of gray, as will become clear in the next paragraph. One could of course increase the width of the LUT entries. However, the eye cannot really distinguish more than 256 shades of gray.

The LUT allows the user to dynamically adjust contrast, brightness, and other features that affect image perception, without actually changing image data. For example, the left panel of Figure 2C shows an LUT containing linearly increasing brightness values. Therefore, increasing counts are displayed with increasing brightnesses.* The middle panel of Figure 2C shows an LUT that results in *thresholding* of the image. All counts below 100 are displayed with 0 brightness, that is, they do not appear on the screen, while the remaining count values (100 to 255) are displayed as they were with the LUT to the left. The visual effects of this process can be seen in Figure 3A and B. Thresholding can be combined with display contrast enhancement, as is shown in the LUT on the far right of Figure 2C. Here the counts from 0 through 127 are displayed with 0 brightness, but the remaining counts increase 2 units of brightness for each additional count. Therefore, small changes in counts cause larger changes in brightness. Display *contrast* (defined as the change in brightness for a given change in counts) is thereby increased. The visual effects produced are shown in Figure 3C. Again, note that these effects (similar to those produced by thresholding, or background subtraction and scaling) are achieved by altering only the LUT, ie, without altering the data. Changes in the LUT are effected on most nuclear medicine systems by means of digital knobs or by moving "slider" bars with a cursor. Usually two knobs or cursors are available. Often one changes the lower level threshold value (below which all counts are displayed with zero brightness) and the other the upper threshold value, beyond which all counts are displayed either with maximum intensity or with zero intensity (at the users discretion). The user should also be able to easily load other progressions of numbers into the LUT, for example, exponentially increasing or logarithmically increasing values, in order to accentuate or depress the display of certain count ranges, or to be able to visualize simultaneously regions of both low and high counts.

Suppose an image contains a region with approximately 100 counts per pixel, and within that region there is a 40% hotter "hot spot" of 140 counts per pixel. Suppose a second region of the image has an average count per pixel of 10,000, and also contains a 40% hotter hot spot of 14,000. Although the 40% change in counts from 14,000 to 10,000 might be easily visible when the image is displayed in a linear manner, the same 40% count change from 140 to 100 would be imperceptible. Use of a logarithmic LUT offers a possible solution to this dilema. The logarithmic transformation is

*The eye, however, does not respond linearly to linearly increasing brightnesses. This can be compensated for either in the hardware which sends brightness signals to the video monitor or by adjusting the look-up table.

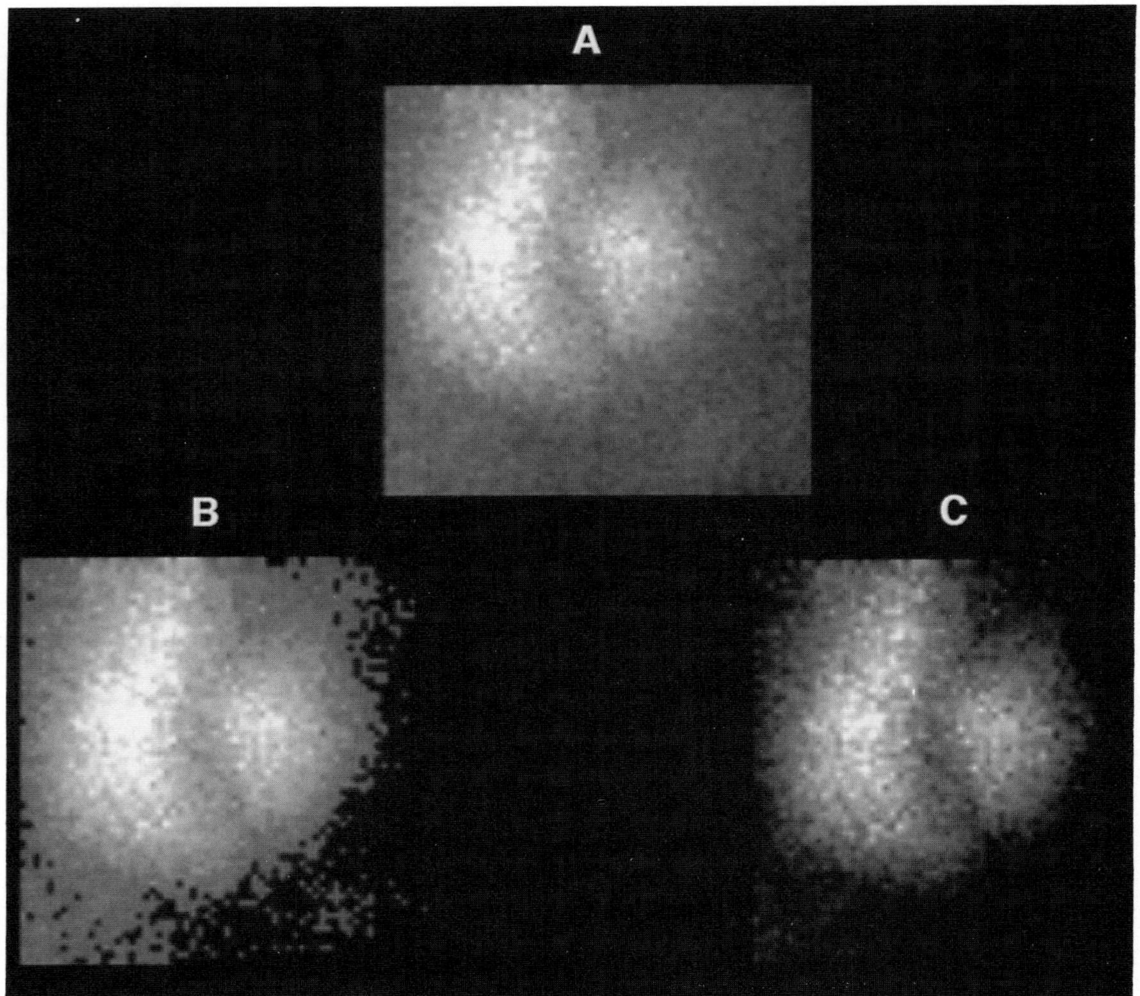

Figure 3. (A). Original cardiac end diastolic image from a gated blood pool study. **(B).** Same image as in A, but with LUT adjusted as in middle panel of Figure 2C so that all "background" pixels are displayed with zero intensity. **(C).** As in (B) but entire gray-scale range expanded between lowest nonzero pixel value and highest pixel value, as in LUT of Figure 2C, right panel. Note increased contrast.

illustrated in Table 1. When brightness is directly proportional to counts, the 40% count density change in the high region of the image produces a brightness change 100 times greater than that of the 40% change in the cold region. When the logarithm of counts at each pixel is displayed, the 40% change in the hot region results in exactly the same brightness difference as does the 40% change in the cold region. This equalization is obtained at a cost of (1) nonlinearity between absolute counts and brightness and (2) reduction in display contrast at the high count density region of the image. Again, the image transformations being discussed do not involve actually altering the individual pixel values, only altering the LUT which translates counts into brightnesses. Many other forms of display manipulation are possible by judicious use of the video LUT. One could emphasize high-count regions of the image by loading exponentially increasing values into the LUT, or even reverse the intensity values in an image (ie, make hot areas dark and cold areas bright) by loading the LUT with decreasing values.

Table 1. Linear and Logarithmic Transformations of Pixel Counts to Image Brightness

LINEAR		LOGARITHMIC	
Counts	*Brightness*	*Log Counts*	*Brightness*
14,000	1.0	4.15	1.0
10,000	0.7	4.0	0.96
140	0.01	2.15	0.52
100	0.007	2.0	0.48

Most display systems contain hardware that can be used to alter image size. This is called *video zoom*, and is illustrated in Figure 4. Note that video zoom increases only the size of the image, not its resolution. The principal use of

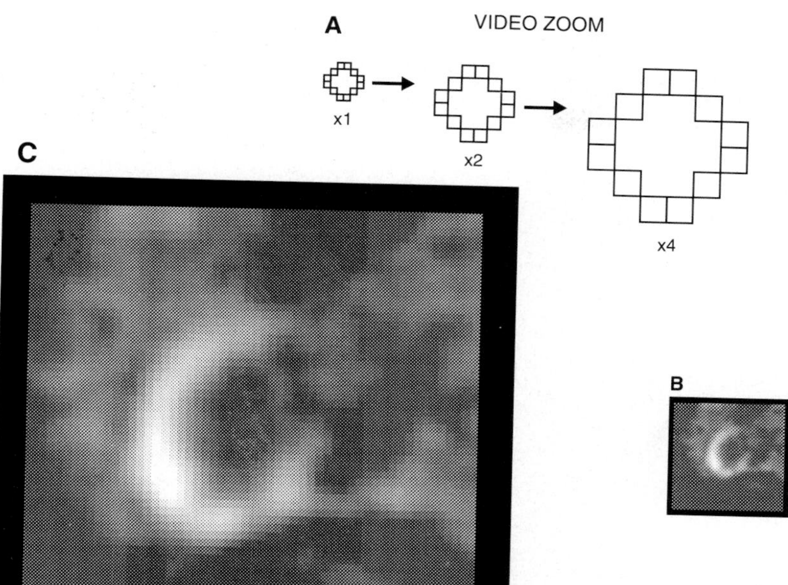

Figure 4. **(A).** Illustrating the concept of video zoom. **(B).** Original image (single transverse slice of cardiac Tl-201 image). **(C).** Same image, but zoomed by a factor of 6. Each pixel has been made larger, and individual pixels can now be seen.

video zoom is to adjust the image size to match the viewing distance. By increasing the size of each pixel, one can stand further from the screen, thus accomodating larger groups of viewers. However, if one does not stand sufficiently far from a hardware video-zoomed image, the individual pixels are too easily discerned, interfering with the brain's ability to perceive the image in its entirety. Viewing a zoomed image at too close a distance is analogous to viewing a greatly magnified photo in the newspaper at close range. When the photo is shown greatly magnified, the individual dots making up the image prevent the eye-brain "computer" from perceiving what object the collection of dots are meant to represent. Only by standing farther away from the image are the eye and brain able to integrate the individual dots into an entity, and thereby perceive the image as an object, rather than as a collection of dots. It is thought that, if a single pixel subtends somewhere between 0.1 and 0.5° of viewing angle to the eye, the brain is able to interpret the array of pixels as an object. At larger angles (ie, viewing the monitor at too close a distance), the individual pixels interfere with the brain's ability to integrate the structure into a recognizable object. Of course, standing *too* far from the screen results in a perceived loss of resolution, since several pixels will get blurred together by the eye. It is important to properly adjust the combination of viewing distance and zoom, to optimize the diagnostic information perceived from the image.

One way to make the display larger, yet maintain the same viewing distance, is by *interpolation*. Interpolation is used to create more pixels in the video display of an image than are actually present in the computer matrix. This is done by making a new image with "extra" pixels in between the pixels representing the original data. In the interpolatively zoomed image, the "extra" pixels are formed by averaging adjacent pixel values in the original data together. This is illustrated in Figure 5, in which noninterpolative and interpolative zooming are compared. Although interpolative zooming improves the image cosmetically (allowing you to view a zoomed image at closer distances), it does *not* increase the resolution of the image. Structures that were unable to be resolved by the gamma camera do not become visible simply by enlarging the image. The same features seen in Figure 5B can be perceived in Figure 5A by standing further from the image. Similarly, interpolatively zooming the image after its acquisition cannot compensate for failing to acquire the image with sufficient digital resolution in the first place. The intermediate pixels produced by the interpolation process are "phony" in that they do not represent real data. Interpolatively zoomed images require much more video memory than the original, since the intermediate pixel values must be stored (although some advanced video displays can perform interpolation "on the fly," and so need no additional memory). An interpolative factor of 2 zoom requires four times as much memory as the original image. Ideally, any calculations based on pixel values are performed only using the original image data, *not* by using the pixel values in the interpolated image. For this reason, the original image is often kept in the main computer memory, while the interpolatively zoomed image is kept in video memory. Regions of interest "drawn" by the user on interpolatively zoomed images should be translated by the computer back to the corresponding coordinates of the original image to give the proper quantitative values.

The hardware in video display systems in general only

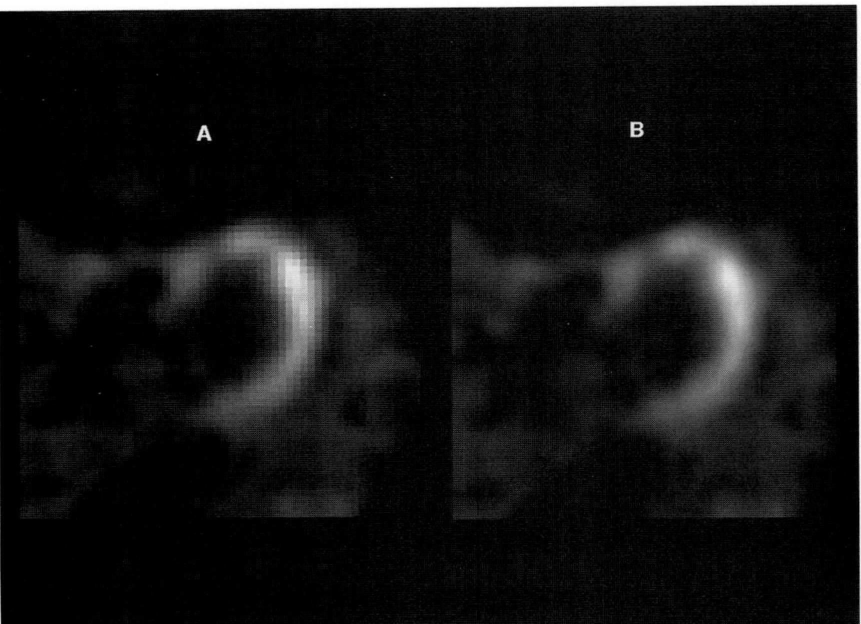

Figure 5. **(A).** Zoomed image (same image as in Figure 4), with no interpolation. **(B).** Same image with interpolation. Individual pixels are now same size as in Figure 4B (and hence are not discernable). Extra pixels are "fake" in the sense that they are simply a weighted average of neighboring original pixels.

supports the display of a certain number of pixels on the monitor. The monitor itself must be designed to handle that number of pixels (actually, it is the speed at which the video display device transmits its signals to the monitor that determines the ability of the monitor to be compatible with the rest of the display hardware). Typical pixel sizes might be 1024 pixels horizontally by 768 vertically. Some specialized display devices can display nearly four times this number of pixels. For comparison, a home TV set has only the equivalent of about 520 rows of pixels vertically. Another important parameter to assess when evaluating a video display system is the speed at which it refreshes the screen. That is, how many times per second is the video system able to completely "paint" the 1024 by 768 (or whatever) full screen? If this number is too low, the screen may appear to flicker, which can seriously degrade the visual image. For a 1024 by 768 display device, typically at least 60 Hz would be required, although it depends to some extent on how long the screen phosphors "glow" after a pixel has been displayed.

Color Displays

Video display systems also can be used to display different count ranges as different colors. To do so, not one but three LUTs are used, one for each of the three primary colors of the color TV monitor—red, green, and blue. Each count value is then translated into three intensities—one for each color. By varying the relative intensities of the three colors, any desired color can be achieved.

The eye can distinguish more colors than shades of gray scale. This is sometimes an advantage because it allows data to be displayed with increased "contrast" (ie, ability to visualize small differences in counts). It can also be a disadvantage in that the greatly contrasting borders between regions of different colors stand out as edges to the eye, edges as arbitrary as the values in the LUT used to produce them. Figure 6 illustrates the problem. The creation of artificial borders in color images can also be a significant source of image misinterpretation. Another disadvantage of color is that it is unnatural, that is, a particular color does not necessarily have any natural relevance or widely accepted meaning related to the function of the organ being imaged (Is green "hot" or "cold"? Is yellow a defect, or is red?). Despite these potential pitfalls, there are many valuable uses for color in medical imaging.

Several color scales have been devised to reduce the creation of artificial borders, yet keep the relationship between counts and color a "natural" one. The so-called "hot-body" spectrum is an example of such a color scale (Fig. 7). The scale is meant to represent increasing counts by the color an object (eg, iron) would attain as it is heated from "red hot" to "white hot." Another suitable use of color might be to display functional images in which many easily distinguishable colors could be used to represent the various functional values of the parameter of interest (eg, blood flow or metabolic rate). Such color scales are also frequently used in the display of positron emission tomograms (PET). The color-coded image gives the observer a better idea of the magnitudes of parameters such as the metabolic rates within each region of the image, while gray-scale images (or hot-body look-up tables) portray the morphology more faithfully. Comparison of two images from two different modalities (eg, MRI and PET) is often aided by using color. The MRI image might be portrayed in black and white, while the PET image is overlayed on top of the MRI image in color. Other

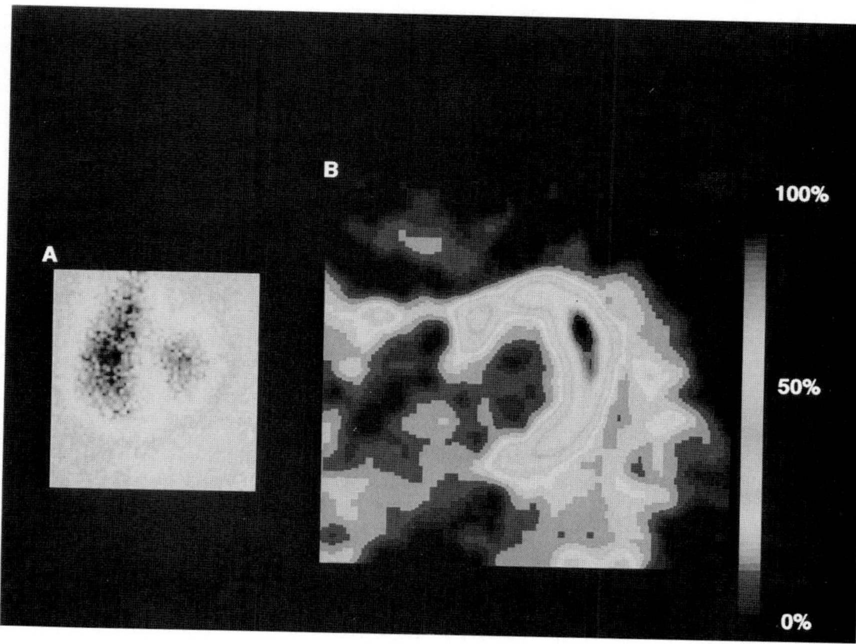

Figure 6. **(A).** Same image as Figure 3A, but with three (red, green, blue) LUTs rather than just one. Yellow seems to define the borders of the LV—or does it? **(B).** Same image as Figure 5B but in color. Here a color bar is shown to allow the user to translate colors into pixel values. The numbers to the right indicate percentage of maximum pixel value. (See Plate 6.)

potential uses of color displays are based on the fact that there are two attributes to a particular color (eg, red): its intensity and its frequency (ie, its "redness"). Theoretically, two quantities could then be represented by each pixel within a single image. The value of one quantity might be represented by the intensity of a color, while a second quantity might be represented by the frequency (ie, the "shade" of the color). Unfortunately, the human eye's perception of intensity is itself a function of color. How the eye and brain extract information from an image, especially a color image, remains only partially understood, and therefore the optimum way to display an image is correspondingly uncertain.

SOFTWARE

In modern nuclear medicine computer systems, the cost of writing and developing software (programs) is a major fraction of the system cost because of the time required to write and test ("debug") programs. The computer itself can

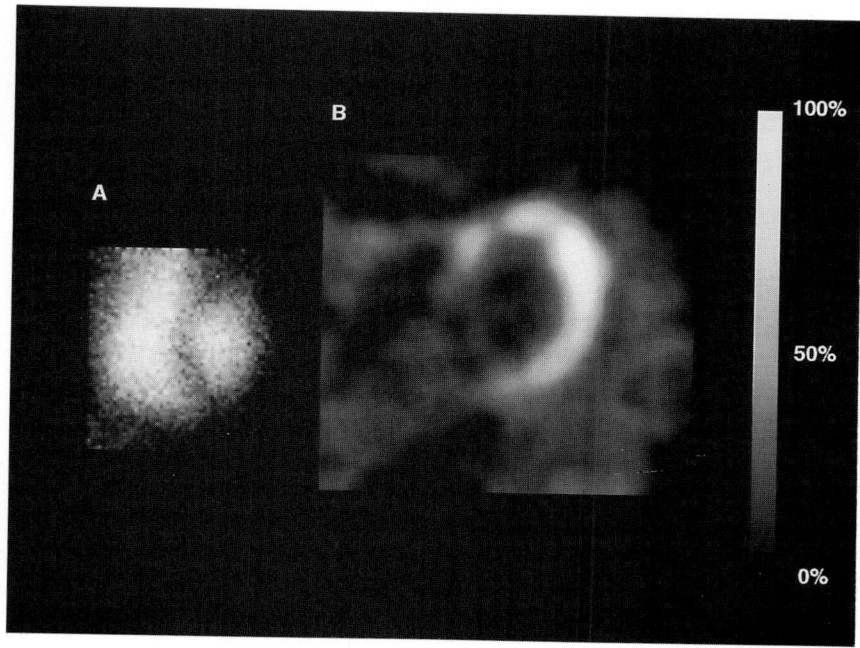

Figure 7. **(A).** Same image as Figure 3C, but using "hot-body" color spectrum. **(B).** Same image as Figure 5B but using hot-body spectrum. Artificial edges of Figure 6 are for the most part eliminated with this color LUT. (See Plate 7.)

only understand instructions written in "machine language", that is, the long sequences of numbers, each of which represents the very elemental instructions discussed previously.[5] Most humans, however, would have great difficulty dealing with this language (if for no other reason than it would be difficult to remember which number represented which instruction). Instead, most computers have programs that translate instructions given in a more "human" oriented language into the machine language understood by the computer. Many of these so called "high-level" languages exist—Fortran, Basic, C, Pascal to name a few—and every computer has translator programs available for one or more of these high-level languages. Only computer programmers need to use these programming languages on a nuclear medicine computer system. Instead, vendors have already written programs using these languages to provide most of the fundamental image manipulations the user will need. For example, the user must be able to add, subtract, and perform other operations with images. The user must be able to draw regions of interest to extract quantitative information from the image and perform a myriad of other basic operations essential to the analysis of image data. Although all these basic operations are presumably already "programmed" into the system, the physician or technologist often needs some way of automatically stringing these basic operations together. To do this, another language, called a "command" language or "macro" language, must be included in the computer system. Command languages allow the user to string together series of individual commands so that complex processing and acquisition protocols can be initiated with only one or a few keystrokes. Sophisticated computer systems may have command languages that permit loops and branching, which can be useful for increasing efficiency and speed of acquiring and processing clinical studies. Later chapters, as well as other texts[6] give detailed descriptions about how such manipulations can be used clinically.

Acquisition Software

STATIC ACQUISITIONS AND SELECTION OF MATRIX SIZE

A static image is a single image acquired for some predetermined length of time (or predetermined number of counts). In static acquisitions, one usually assumes that the distribution of radiopharmaceutical does not change during the time of the acquisition (or that whatever changes do occur are unimportant). In acquiring a static image the user must be able to determine that imaging last either a preset time, or until a preset number of counts have been acquired, or until "overflow" occurs, or combinations thereof. Overflow refers to the situation in which the number of counts at a pixel exceeds its capacity. For example, in a byte mode acquisition, each pixel can hold only 255 counts maximum. In this case, imaging would stop whenever any single pixel reached 255 counts. In word mode, a single pixel would have to reach 32767 or in some computers 65535 counts (the difference being that some computers use one of the 16 bits to indicate the sign of a number, ie, plus or minus, leaving only 15 bits for the actual number). What happens if "stop on overflow" is not selected? In that case, when a pixel overflows, the number stored in that pixel usually recycles back to 0. Permitting overflow is sometimes appropriate. For example, consider an image in which the organ of interest and a (hot) injection site or catheter are both within the field of view. Stopping on overflow might well stop acquisition before sufficient counts in the organ had been accumulated, due to overflow in the few pixels representing the injection site. Similarly, when performing a gated blood pool study with a hot spleen in the field of view, one does not usually wish the acquisition to terminate just because the counts in the spleen reached overflow.

The operator is expected to be knowledgeable enough to select the proper ADC digital resolution (ie, the number of pixels per millimeter) to be used for the image and either to specify the millimeters per pixel (or its inverse, pixels per millimeter), or, more commonly to specify the matrix size, eg, 64 × 64, 128 × 128, 256 × 256, etc, to be used for acquisition. For circular-field-of-view cameras the matrix is usually square (ie, equal in x and y), but for rectangular cameras (or for whole body-scanning cameras) the matrix size will in general be rectangular. Nearly always the digital acquisition resolution (ie, the number of millimeters per pixel) is chosen to be the same in both directions (eg, a 20-by 40-cm rectangular camera would then require a nonsquare matrix, such as 64 × 128). The appropriate digital acquisition resolution is the poorest digital acquisition resolution (ie, largest number of millimeters per pixel) that still is able to capture all the information inherent in the gamma camera/collimator, under the imaging conditions employed. A good rule of thumb is to first estimate the camera resolution expected from the camera collimator combination (including the effects of finite patient-to-collimator distance). Then use at least three pixels but no more than five pixels per FWHM of resolution expected in the image. For example, if the gamma-camera resolution of a liver image is expected to be about 10 mm FWHM (this should be the *real* resolution of the gamma camera plus collimator, at the actual collimator-to-liver distance, not the intrisic resolution of the camera), then one should use a minimum of 3 pixels/10 mm or 3.33 millimeters per pixel. For a 40-cm diameter FOV camera, this would mean using a matrix size of 128 × 128. Using fewer pixels than this would produce an image that would fail to capture all the information produced by the camera. Using more pixels (eg, 512 × 512) takes up much more disk space and does *not* improve image resolution. The resolution of the final image is set by the camera, collimator, and camera-patient distance. The digital acquisition resolution of the ADC cannot improve upon this. The ADC resolution, if improperly set at too coarse a matrix, can *reduce* the resolution of the image, but setting it at too fine a matrix only costs space and does not improve image resolution.

Table 2 summarizes typical storage requirements and the

Table 2. Image Matrix Characteristics

MATRIX SIZE	NO. PIXELS	MAX. COUNTS PER PIXEL	MEMORY REQUIRED (WORDS)	ADC DIGITAL RESOLUTION (mm/PIXEL)	
				37 cm FOV	*25 cm FOV*
32 × 32	1024	255 (byte mode)	512	11.60	7.80
		65535 (word mode)	1024		
64 × 64	4096	255	2048	5.78	3.90
		65535	4096		
128 × 128	16,384	255	8192	2.89	1.95
		65535	16384		
256 × 256	65,536	255	32768	1.45	.98
		65535	65536		

digital acquisition resolutions that can be achieved for several acquisition matrices and camera sizes.

ANALOG ZOOM

Frequently, the matrix sizes listed in Table 2 do not permit optimum digital resolution. For example, a gated cardiac image with a high-resolution collimator may require a larger matrix than 64 × 64 to avoid compromising image resolution. Computer memory, however, may be insufficient to accomodate the fourfold larger 128 × 128 matrix. In such cases, the *analog zoom* feature on the ADCs of most computers can be used to select a small part of the camera field of view (eg, the cardiac chambers) and to digitize only that portion of the image rather than the entire field of view. This feature improves digital acquisition resolution without changing matrix size. The price paid is a reduction in the camera's apparent field of view, an acceptable price if the organ of interest is small. The analog zoom is usually specified as a factor by which each axis of the image is magnified. For example, assume at no zoom (zoom factor of 1.0) a 64 × 64 matrix may just encompass the 40-cm field of view of the camera, as in Figure 8A. The digital resolution is 40 cm/64 pixels = 6.25 mm per pixel (therefore, at best, we could capture the resolution of a 19-mm FWHM image, using our 3 to 5 pixels per FWHM rule of thumb). At a zoom factor of 1.5, the X and Y axes of the image are each magnified by a factor of 1.5 (Fig. 8B). The new digital resolution is 40 cm/(1.5 × 64) = 4.1 mm per pixel. The digital acquisition resolution is now 50% higher and is equivalent to digitizing the entire camera field of view with a 96 × 96 matrix. Similarly, a 64 × 64 matrix at a zoom factor of 2.0 is equivalent to the digital acquisition resolution of a 128 × 128 matrix but requires only one fourth the memory because only one quarter of the camera field of view is digitized and stored.

Dynamic Frame Mode Acquisition

Many nuclear medicine studies require monitoring the changes in activity in an organ with time. One method for following changing patterns of activity is to acquire the data in *dynamic frame mode*.* In this mode, the user first specifies (1) the matrix size desired, (2) either the duration of each image or the number of images to be acquired each second, and (3) the total duration of the study. Specification of the number of images per second is usually referred to as the *framing rate*. For example, if the study duration is 60 seconds at a framing rate of 2 frames per second, 120 images will be created, each of 0.5-second duration. Alternatively, the computer might ask the user to specify the duration of each frame (0.5 seconds in this case) and the maximum number of frames required. Preferably, the acquisition software would allow the user to specify the parameters of the dynamic study in either way.

The memory in most nuclear medicine computers is not usually large enough to hold the total number of dynamic images specified for a dynamic frame mode acquisition. Instead the images are usually stored on disk immediately after they are created. One possible way to implement a dynamic acquisition would be to acquire each image as described for a static acquisition, transfer that image to disk, and then begin acquiring the next image. This would in general be unacceptable, due to the time lost waiting before acquiring the second image while the first was being written to disk. To illustrate the general method by which this problem is circumvented, consider a 64 × 64 (word mode) matrix size at a framing rate of four images per second (0.25 seconds per image). The computer sets aside space in memory for *two* 64 × 64 matrices. For the first 0.25 second, data are stored (framed) in the first matrix. During the next 0.25 seconds, data are stored in the second matrix. Simultaneously, the computer begins transferring the first matrix from memory to disk and then resets each element of the first matrix to zero. At the end of the second 0.25-second interval,

*The word "frame" is "computerese" for matrix or image matrix. It is sometimes used as a verb—"to frame data" meaning to sort data into an image matrix.

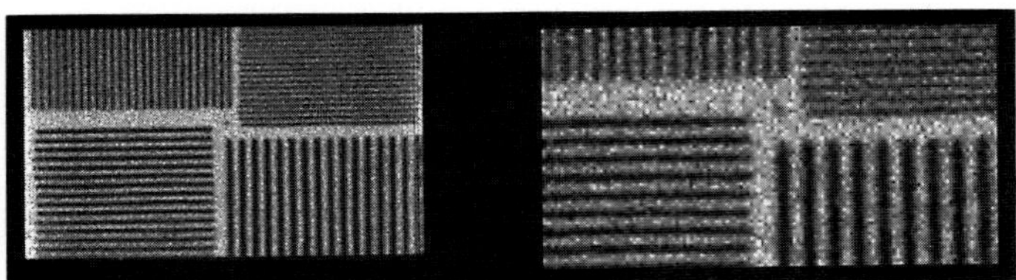

Figure 8. **(A).** Bar phantom with analog zoom = 1. **(B).** Same bar phantom with analog zoom = 1.5. The ADC analog zoomed image not only is enlarged (at the expense of a smaller field of view), but also has a larger number of pixels per square centimeter (2.25 times as many pixels per square centimeter).

data are stored in the first matrix again, while the second are being written to disk.

Several practical considerations are apparent. First, the computer must have sufficient memory to hold *two* images in memory at the same time. This occasionally sets an upper limit on the matrix size allowable for dynamic acquisition. Second, images cannot be acquired any more rapidly than they can be written to disk, which usually sets an upper limit on the possible framing rate. Since a 64 × 64 image contains only one fourth as many pixels of data as a 128 × 128 image, the former can be written to disk four times faster than a 128 × 128 image, and usually the maximum framing rate is about four times faster. Likewise, byte mode images can support twice the framing rate as word mode images. Typical dynamic framing rates achievable by some modern computers using hard disks are on the order of tens of 128 × 128 (byte mode) images per second. Dynamic frame mode studies are often acquired in byte mode rather than word mode when the framing interval is short because for a short acquisition the chance of exceeding 255 counts in any pixel is small.

The dynamic frame mode acquisition program must allow the frame rates to be adjusted over the course of a study. For example, in many studies, the activity is changing rapidly immediately following the injection (requiring high frame rates early in the study), but after a minute or two the activity within the organ may change much more slowly (requiring only slow frame rates). In this case the computer should be able to acquire data at several different frame rates during the course of the study. For example, one might select one frame per second for the first 40 seconds of the study, then switch to 10 seconds per frame for the next 60 seconds, and finally change to 1 minute per frame for the slowly changing portion of the study. The computer software must provide an easy way to enter such sequences.

Usually, dynamic frame mode acquisitions are the simplest, most straightforward solution to the problem of dynamic acquisition. Several factors must be considered, however, when dynamic frame mode acquisitions are performed:

1. A large number of images are often required for high framing rate studies (eg, bolus studies, such as first-transit cardiac ventricular function studies).
2. The temporal resolution (framing rate) required must be known in advance.
3. The framing rate is limited by the disk-writing speed, especially for large-matrix sizes.
4. In some circumstances, much more data must be stored on the disk than are actually used in analyzing the image, that is, if high frame rate studies are acquired, it may well be that during the short duration of each image many pixels contain few (or no) counts.

In most clinical studies, these factors are inconsequential. In a few special cases, however, they become serious limitations, especially when the required framing rate can be determined only from the data alone. When it is not known in advance how fast the injected radionuclide will be taken up by, or cleared from, the organ of interest, *list mode* acquisition may be preferable.

LIST MODE ACQUISITION

In *list mode* acquisition, the computer simply records in sequence the position (X,Y) of each photon detected by the camera. Later, when the study is complete, this sequential "list" of data is sorted into frames whose matrix size and rate can then, after the fact, be specified. To retain timing information, the list also contains timing marks so that the time of each photon occurrence may be determined. These timing marks might typically be recorded once every millisecond (ie, 1000 per second).

Two potential disadvantages of list mode acquisition are apparent. First, the list of x,y coordinates must be stored on disk. If a 1-million count study is to be acquired, 1 million words (plus 1000 words per second for timing marks) must be stored. Second, at the conclusion of the study, the data are not yet ready for visual inspection but must be "framed" (ie, sorted) into images. This sorting or framing proceeds exactly as in a dynamic frame mode acquisition except that the data come from the disk instead of from the gamma camera. The necessity for retrospective framing adds a few extra minutes of processing to the study. The patient need not be present during this time, however, and neither the framing rate nor matrix size is limited except by the time resolution inherent in the timing marks. If the initial framing rate and matrix size selected are inappropriate, the study need not be repeated. Instead, the data are simply reframed from the disk at the newly selected temporal or spatial resolution. When an acceptable set of framed images is produced, the list mode data can then be discarded and that space on the disk reused. Acquiring studies directly in dynamic frame mode often requires less disk space than if the study were acquired in list mode. High counting rate studies, at modest or slow frame rates in particular, are usually handled more efficiently in dynamic frame mode. Under certain conditions,

Table 3. A Comparison of List and Frame Mode Acquisition

	LIST MODE	DYNAMIC FRAME MODE
Disk usage	Equals total counts Independent of matrix size Independent of framing rate	Independent of total counts Increases with increasing matrix size Increases with increasing framing rate
Matrix size	Unlimited	Limited by maximum disk writing speed
Frame rate	Unlimited	Limited by maximum disk writing speed
Maximum counting rate	Limited by disk writing speed	Unlimited (except by system deadtime)

however, the reverse is true. For example, consider a first-pass cardiac dynamic study of 20-second duration with a peak counting rate of 60,000 cps, a 64×64 matrix size, and a framing rate of 25 frames per second. List mode acquisition would require a disk space for less than $20 \times 61{,}000$ words per second (including timing marks) = 1.22×10^6 words. The disk space required is independent of matrix size or framing rate. For dynamic frame mode acquisition, the disk space consumed critically depends on framing rate and matrix size. For the above example:

$$\begin{aligned} &20 \text{ seconds} \times 25 \text{ frames per second} \\ &\quad \times 4096 \text{ words per frame} \\ &\quad = 2.0 \times 10^6 \text{ words} \end{aligned}$$

In this case then using a list mode acquisition conserves disk space (although, after the studies were framed, the storage space requirements would be the same for the same framing rate parameters). List mode is also more flexible because framing rate and matrix size can be altered after the study. Table 3 summarizes the advantages and disadvantages of frame and list mode acquisition. Note that in list mode acquisition the maximum counting rate must be less than the maximum speed at which the disk is capable of storing data (typically 100,000 to 200,000 words per second). Dynamic frame mode is not limited by counting rate, but instead the product of framing rate and matrix size must not exceed the maximum rate at which data can be written to disk. There are other circumstances in which list mode acquisition may be of value—in particular in certain kinds of gated cardiac studies.

Gated Cardiac Acquisitions

Many physiologic events occur very quickly and require high framing rates to capture the information. At high framing rates, however, the frame duration may be so short that too few counts are available in each image to permit adequate analysis to be performed. If the physiologic process is cyclic, or can be reproducibly repeated, this limitation can be overcome by performing a *gated study.*[7] In a gated study, some physiologic parameter must be used to demarcate the repetition cycle. For example, in attempting to produce a series of images that span the cardiac cycle, the electrocardiographic *R* wave can be used as a gate to demarcate the cycle. Gated studies can be acquired in either frame or list mode. In cardiac gated studies, the heart cycle is defined by the *R* wave to *R* wave interval. This interval is then divided into as many frames as are necessary to provide the desired temporal resolution. For example, 16 images are usually adequate for visual determinations of cardiac wall motion. If the average *R-R* interval is 800 milliseconds, then 16 images per *R-R* would correspond to a framing rate of 50 milliseconds per frame or 20 frames per second. The computer then establishes in its memory 16 separate matrices of the desired size (eg, 64×64), into which counts are sorted sequentially. At the first *R* wave, marking the beginning of a new cycle, data are sorted into the first matrix. After 50 milliseconds have elapsed, data are acquired into the second matrix in memory, and so on, until the next *R* wave. At each subsequent *R* wave, data are once again sorted into the first matrix. Usually, several hundred cycles are required to obtain adequate statistics in the composite, 16-image cycle. Following (or during) acquisition, the frames can be displayed sequentially and looped, giving the cine effect of a beating heart. Many parameters can be measured from such studies. Implicit in the method of gating is the assumption that all cycles are equivalent. This assumption may not be valid, however, for patients whose *R-R* interval is highly variable. Nonetheless, gated cardiac imaging has proved to be of great value and is widely used. Other cyclic phenomena (eg, the respiratory cycle) have also been studied using the concept of "gating" but have not proven as useful as in the case of cardiac imaging.

There are many other important considerations involved in performing gated cardiac studies, and there are many variants on the basic concept of gating described above.[7,8]

IMAGE PROCESSING

One advantage of acquiring images in digital format is that they can be further processed to (1) alter visual appearance, possibly enhancing clinical interpretation, and (2) derive quantitative information from the images. Image processing is a complete field in itself, and as such is beyond the scope of this chapter. However, most commercially available nuclear medicine computer systems include some elementary image processing software. In this section, a few of these basic image processing operations are described. First some common manipulations used primarily to alter the appearance of the image are discussed, then a few of the techniques used to extract quantitative information from the images are presented. Later chapters will discuss in more detail some of the image-processing methodologies that have been found to be useful in specific clinical applications. For a more complete review of image processing and analysis in general, the reader is referred to other texts.[6,8,9]

Altering Visual Perception

Commercial nuclear medicine computer systems provide many methods of altering the data that represent the image. Such methods are often used to alter the appearance of the image, but, unlike the LUT methods discussed above, altering the image data implies actually changing the value stored at each pixel. A few of the more common manipulations are described below.

THRESHOLDING

An image can be *thresholded* by setting to zero counts all pixels with counts below a certain selected value, called the *lower-level threshold*. This produces exactly the same visual effect as depicted in Figures 2C and 3B, except the actual data, rather than the LUT, are changed. Notice in Figure 3B that the appearance of image pixels above the threshold is not altered; the display contrast of the image is not changed. Thresholding can be used to focus the observer's attention on a particular portion of the image above the threshold. Often an image of an organ that has been thresholded gives the appearance of having a well-defined edge, the location of which depends upon the value selected for the threshold. While a fixed-threshold method of edge detection may be of use occasionally, it can also mislead the observer into falsely thinking the edge so obtained has anatomical significance.

It is also possible to set both upper- and lower-level thresholds, so that pixels either exceeding the upper level or below the lower level are set to zero. This is called *windowing* the image. Again, the same visual effect could be achieved by setting LUT values above and below preset high and low values to zero.

BACKGROUND SUBTRACTION

When an image of an organ is viewed, it is often desirable to eliminate or reduce the counts from overlaying or underlaying tissue. In a xenon lung ventilation image, for example, background activity from the muscle and fat tissues of the surrounding chest wall is superimposed upon the actual lung activity. A commonly employed, but simplistic, scheme for compensating for such background activity is based on the assumption that the background is constant everywhere within the image. This value is therefore subtracted from each pixel in the image. Unlike thresholding, background subtraction can alter the displayed image contrast (for a linear LUT). The effect is similar to that shown in Figures 2C and 3C, except again the actual data are changed, rather than just the LUT.

To better understand the effect that background subtraction has on the image it is necessary to distinguish between "image contrast" and the previously defined "display contrast." Recall that display contrast is the change in displayed brightness for a given change in image counts. Display contrast can be altered simply by changing the values in the LUT (or even by changing the controls on the video monitor). Image contrast, on the other hand, refers to the inherent differences in counts between one region of the image and another. For example, when imaging a liver tumor, a radiopharmaceutical might be evaluated on the basis of how much of the agent localized in the tumor compared to how much appeared in normal liver tissue. The image contrast of the resulting image could be defined as the fractional difference in counts between tumor and normal tissue. Consider the following example. Imagine a liver image in which a tumor in the liver contained 150 counts per pixel, while the counts over normal liver averaged 100 counts per pixel. The image contrast between the normal and tumor liver tissue could be defined as the fractional difference in counts between these two regions:

$$= (\text{tumor-normal})/\text{normal}$$
$$= (150 - 100)/100$$
$$= 0.50,$$

That is, there is only a 50% difference in counts between the normal and tumor tissue. This counts difference is completely independent of how the user chooses to *display* the image (ie, of how the LUT is adjusted). It is primarily dependent on the biodistribution of the radiopharmaceutical. However, it may be known (or suspected) that some of the counts in the image are due to the presence of activity uptake in overlying (and underlying) abdominal fat. This "background" activity might be suspected to be uniform over the liver, and perhaps could be estimated by examining regions of the image adjacent to the liver. If the background activity was estimated to be 50 counts per pixel on the average, then this background value could be subtracted from each pixel in the image. By subtracting this background value from the image, one would (hopefully) obtain a more accurate portrayal of the actual activity distribution in the normal liver and the tumor. The resulting contrast in the background subtracted image would now be

$$(100 - 50)/50 = 1.0$$

The fractional change in counts (ie, the image contrast between normal and tumor tissue) is now 100%, rather than the previous 50%. This background subtraction may also change the display contrast. More importantly, however, it changes the numerical values of relative counts between the two regions—numerical values which may be used to more accurately assess the true changes in concentrations of the radiopharmaceutical in the normal and abnormal tissues. Of

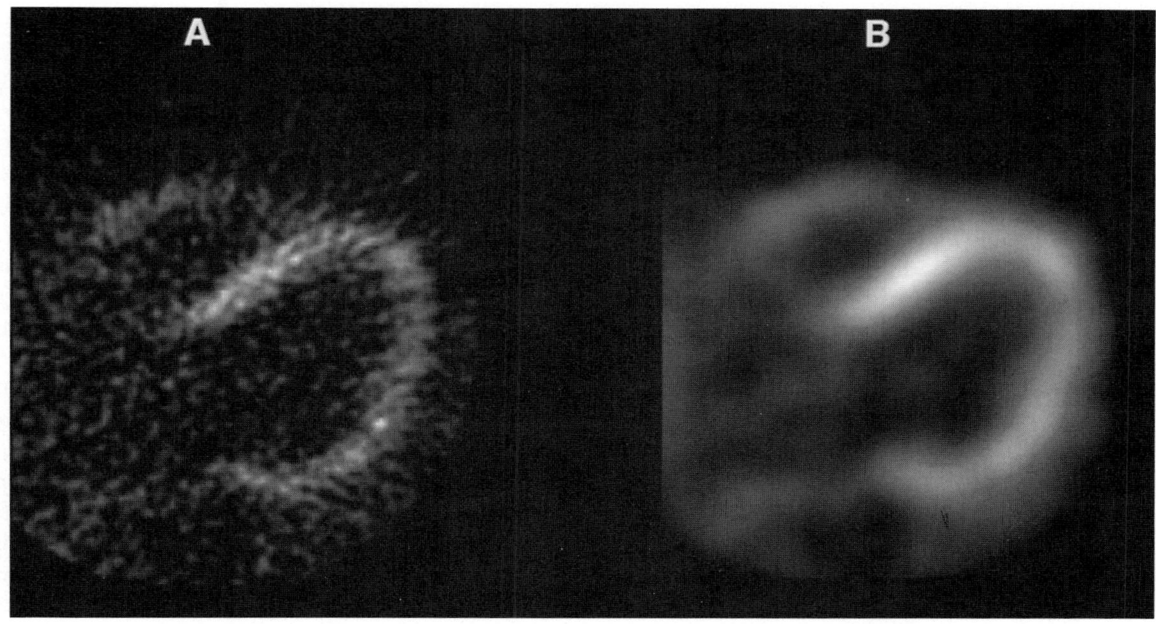

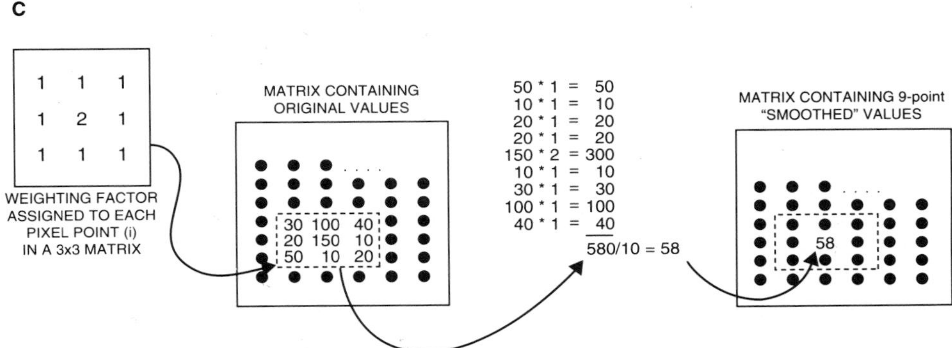

Figure 9. **(A).** Unsmoothed image (128 × 128, 1.7 mm per pixel PET cardiac N^{13} ammonia perfusion image). **(B).** Same image after nine-point FWHM gaussian weighted smooth. Note that resolution of this camera (Posicam PC6.5) is approximately 7 mm FWHM. Therefore, a nine-point smooth is quite "heavy" smoothing, resulting in considerable loss of resolution. **(C).** An example of weighted averaging. For simplicity, a 3 pixel wide "smooth" is shown.

course, if the estimate of background is incorrect, so too will be the values of counts in the various tissues.

SMOOTHING

All images have statistical fluctuations owing to limited counts. If the fluctuations are large, the ability of the clinician to interpret the image is impaired. The best means for improving such an image is to collect more counts. When this is not practical, however, several mathematical operations are available that may improve the appearance of the image, by altering the value stored in each pixel. One class of such operations are called *smoothing* operations and they have both advantageous and deleterious effects on the perceived image quality and on the relationship between counts and activity at each pixel.

A common method of smoothing an image is illustrated in Figure 9. This method involves averaging the counts from a group of neighboring pixels and replacing the center pixel in the group with this average value. The averaging can be performed either by treating all pixel values equally or by counting pixels far from the center pixel less heavily than the closer pixels when computing the average (called *weighted smoothing*). The number of pixels used in the average may vary. In Figure 9B, a nine pixel FWHM smooth with gaussian weighting is shown. This technique therefore is referred to as *gaussian nine-point FWHM weighted smoothing*. There is a potential problem in specifying the degree of smoothing in terms of number of pixels averaged together (eg, nine-point smoothing). Consider a certain FOV gamma camera digitized into either a 128 × 128 or 256 × 256 matrix. A nine-point smooth in the 128 × 128 image will produce twice the smoothing as in the 256 × 256 image, because 9 pixels represents twice the distance in the 128 × 128 image as in the 256 × 256 image. Therefore, if one wishes to specify the degree of smoothing in terms of pixels, one must also always specify the pixel size.

Smoothing reduces statistical noise by averaging. The averaging process, however, results in loss of resolution—edges become blurred. It is possible to estimate the effect smoothing will have on image resolution. If, for example, a certain number of pixels (and therefore a certain number of mm) are used in the smoothing, with a gaussian weighting of N mm FWHM, and if the initial resolution is M mm FWHM, then the resolution in the smoothed image will be approximately

$$\text{Smoothed resolution} = (N^2 + M^2)^{0.5}.$$

For example, in Figure 9, the resolution of the original image (Fig. 9A) is 7 mm FWHM, and each pixel is 1.7 mm. In Figure 9B, a 9-pixel FWHM gaussian smooth has been performed, corresponding to a $9 \times 1.7 = 15.3$ mm FWHM smooth. The resulting resolution, using the above formula is therefore $(7^2 + 15.3^2)^{0.5} = 16.8$ mm FWHM—a considerable loss of resolution.

Several factors are important when deciding whether to smooth an image in this way. First, smoothing by averaging should be used primarily for visual purposes (to aid in qualitative image interpretation or in drawing a region of interest). Usually, computations are best performed on the original data. Second, spatial smoothing by averaging should be applied only when counting fluctuations are the principal factor affecting visual perception. Applying this type of smoothing operation to an image that has high counts per pixel does not significantly improve visual smoothness but does decrease resolution (eg, blurring true changes in counts such as those occurring at organ edges or at borders between hot and cold regions). Some spatial smoothing operations attempt to minimize the problem of blurring true edges by adjusting the "amount" of smoothing at different regions within the image—smoothing heavily where statistics are the principal cause of the observed counting fluctuations, smoothing less heavily in regions where changes in counts are not explicable on a statistical basis. Such smoothing operations are called "nonstationary" because the degree of smoothing varies over the image. Many nonstationary smoothing algorithms have been suggested for use in nuclear medicine. There are also schemes that average pixel values together in a way that actually improves resolution, but at the expense of worsened statistical fluctuations. These methods use weighting factors that have both positive and negative values. The reader is referred to texts on image processing for more detailed descriptions of these methods.[6,8,9] It should be remembered that quantitative information present in the image is not necessarily preserved following application of nonstationary smoothing procedures, and so such operations should be used with care.

The aforementioned smoothing procedures are all *spatial* in nature, ie, the averaging procedures are performed in the X and Y directions of a single image. In a set of dynamic images, one may also average together pixel values that are neighbors in time, rather than in space. Such "temporal" smoothing has many advantages over spatial smoothing. The same techniques used for spatial smoothing apply to temporal smoothing, except that only one dimension, time, is used. To understand temporal smoothing, consider the 10th image in a series of 20 dynamically acquired images. The 5-point temporally smoothed value of the nth pixel in this image would be created by averaging its counts with the nth pixel counts in images 8 and 9 and in images 11 and 12. This averaging procedure may be weighted or not, and may be stationary or nonstationary in time, just as with spatial imaging. If temporal imaging is combined with spatial imaging, the two spatial dimensions of smoothing (eg, 9 points—a square of 3 by 3 pixels in x and y) are combined with the one additional temporal dimension (eg, 5 points in time). In this case, the resulting pixel value is influenced by the content in 45 temporally and spatially neighboring pixels. Temporal smoothing has the advantage of not necessarily blurring spatial resolution, since only temporally adjacent, not spatially adjacent, data are averaged together. Of course, in certain types of dynamic studies (eg, gated cardiac studies) successive time points represent anatomical structures that are moving. In this case, temporal smoothing can also cause spatial blurring of the moving structure.

Quantifying Images

In many nuclear medicine images, the counts at each pixel are closely related to a physiologic property of interest, and so the counts at each pixel in an organ may give information about the *function* of that organ. For example, in a microsphere lung perfusion image the counts at any pixel need only be divided by the total counts to estimate fractional blood flow to the lung region corresponding to that pixel. The image resulting from this simple calculation is a *functional image* because the resultant value at each pixel no longer represents counts, but rather the value of a functional parameter, in this case fractional blood flow. Often, the functional information about an organ cannot be obtained from a single image, but rather can be obtained only by observing how the counts in the image change with time. Consider, for example, an end diastolic (ED) image and an end systolic (ES) image, both obtained from a gated cardiac blood pool scan. To evaluate the relative volume of blood ejected from each region within the ventricles (the *regional stroke volume*), a functional image could be created by subtracting the ES image from the ED image. The intensity of each pixel in this image would then be related to the change in blood volume that occurred at that region. A bright pixel would correspond to a region with a high stroke volume (a large difference between ES and ED counts), and a dark pixel to a region with a low stroke volume (Fig. 10). This "difference image" might be referred to as a functional image of stroke volume (or more accurately, stroke counts). Alternatively, one could divide the stroke counts image by the

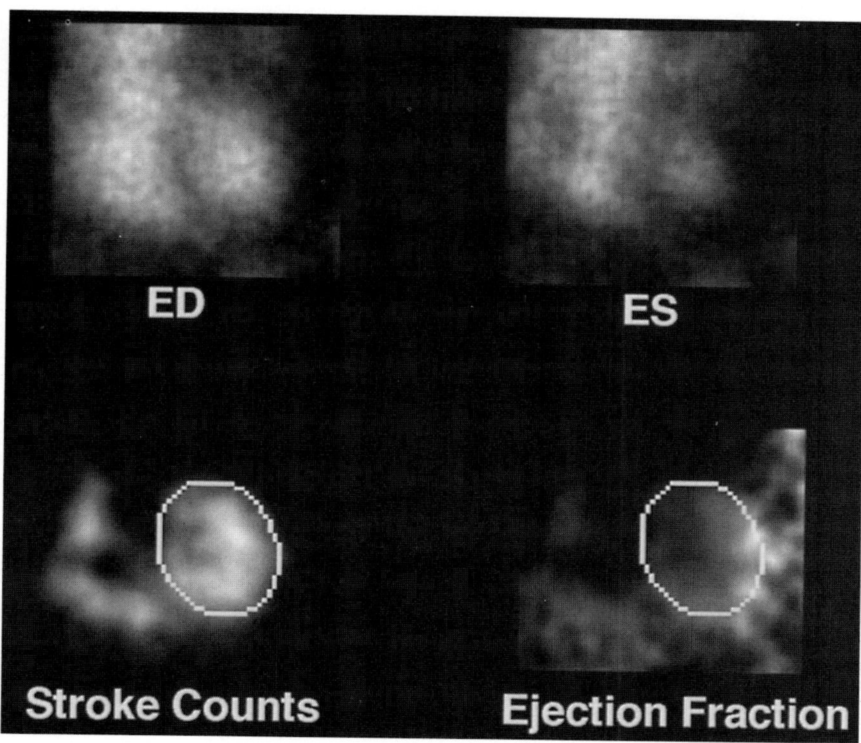

Figure 10. Upper panels: End diastolic and end systolic images from series of gated blood pool images. Lower left: stroke counts image. Lower right: ejection fraction (EF) image. In both lower panels negative values are displayed as zero, but nonzero values are maintained in the pixel data. Left ventricular region of interest shown superimposed. Note large values of EF outside the heart in the lower right panel, caused by noise.

ED image to get an image in which each pixel is given by the ED counts at that pixel minus the ES counts at the pixel, divided by the ED counts. The resultant value is (apart from background corrections) the pixel by pixel value of ejection fraction (Fig. 10, lower right):

$$\text{EF of } i\text{th pixel} = \text{EF}_i = (\text{ED}_i - \text{ES}_i)/\text{ED}_i.$$

Care is needed in performing such arithmetic operations with images. Most nuclear medicine computer systems store images only in word or byte mode, ie, as integer numbers. Fractional numbers are rounded or truncated to either the nearest or next lower integer value. In two of the examples above, calculating either fractional blood flow to each pixel or regional EF, the resulting pixel value will often be less than 1, causing each pixel value to be truncated to zero following the division. The resultant image would then be blank. This is avoided by first scaling (ie, multiplying) the image by a suitable factor so that the resulting counts at each pixel lie, for example, between 0 and 100. For such numeric manipulations, word mode data often are more convenient than byte mode data. Even with word mode data, care must be taken to insure that the values resulting from the numerical calculations do not exceed the capacity of the 16 bits available to store the resultant image. In addition, arithmetic operations often result in negative values. In the ejection fraction or stroke counts functional image described above, it is possible that for some pixels the ES counts will be greater than the ED counts, giving a negative value of stroke counts or EF. In some computer systems, these negative numbers are simply set to zero. Doing this, however, biases any numerical data obtained from the resultant image, since statistical fluctuations will cause regions that do not change with time to fluctuate around zero in the difference image. A region of interest (ROI), ie, a group of pixels identified to the computer as a single entity, usually by "drawing" an enclosing line around them with a mouse on the computer screen, drawn about such a nonvarying region should yield zero average "stroke counts." However, if all the negatives have been set to zero, then an ROI will erroneously yield a positive, rather than zero, value of stroke counts. Also, it must be remembered that often the physical meaning of the functional image may be valid only in the region encompassing the organ of interest. For example, in the EF image of Figure 10, values of EF at regions outside the heart can be evaluated, but there is no physiologic meaning to such calculations.

TIME-ACTIVITY CURVES

Often, information about the functioning of an organ requires observation of how activity (and hence counts) changes in a pixel, or group of pixels, over time. To observe such changes, a series of images must be acquired (ie, a dynamic acquisition). From the series of sequential frames produced by the dynamic acquisition, a curve, called a *time-activity curve* (TAC), can be generated. This curve is produced by plotting the number of counts (or count rate, or mean count rate) within an ROI on the y axis, against time on the x axis. The ROI identifies to the computer which pixels are to be used in creating the TAC.

on the x axis. The ROI identifies to the computer which pixels are to be used in creating the TAC.

TACs can be analyzed either subjectively by visual inspection or objectively by quantifying some parameter of interest from the TAC. For example, TACs could be obtained from a series of renal images after injection of Tc-DTPA. It has been suggested that certain features of such curves may be of clinical significance, eg, the rate of uptake (measured perhaps by the time to reach the peak of the curve) or the rate of clearance (measured perhaps by the time to fall from peak activity to half the peak). Obviously different pharmaceuticals and different organs produce different curves, requiring different analysis schemes. Often it is desired to analyze curves not just from one or a few regions of the organ of interest, but rather from every pixel or from many small groups of pixels. While this is possible, presenting the resulting data in a meaningful way is difficult. Simply presenting the clinician with a list of hundreds of values for "time to peak activity" at each pixel in the organ, for example, is clearly of limited value. Functional images are one obvious solution to this problem. TACs are created for each pixel within an image, and each TAC is analyzed to produce some index of function (eg, time to peak, time to half max, etc). A new image is then created in which each pixel's value (and therefore intensity) is proportional to the value of the functional parameter (eg, time to peak activity) obtained from the TAC at that pixel. Thus functional images permit visual presentation of a large number of numeric results. Color is often used in the display of such functional images, since it is easier to distinguish a large number of different pixel values if they are encoded in color. Since the image is not an image depicting morphology, the distracting artificial boundaries often produced when using color displays are not as important. Later chapters in this book discuss clinical situations in which functional images have proven valuable.

ACTIVITY PROFILES

Most nuclear medicine computer systems allow the user to interactively display a profile of pixel values across an image. A pixel value profile is the sequence of values corresponding to pixels that lie on a chosen line across the image. In a usual two-dimensional image, the line defining the profile can be taken in any orientation within the image plane. The profile may consist of a line one pixel wide or a wider strip up to the entire width of the image. The profile then is displayed as a graph of counts per pixel (averaged over the line width) on one axis and pixel number on the other axis. Such profiles are useful for subjective evaluation of uniformity in objects (eg, in a uniformity flood field image).

IMAGE ORIENTATION AND POSITIONING

The computer system must permit easy reorientation of images in space. Orientation parameters should include both rotation of the image by user-chosen angles about user-specified centers of rotation as well as image shifting and flipping (mirroring) about arbitrary axes. In addition, it should be possible to zoom the image (and save the resultant zoomed image) by any fractional factor to allow two images with initially unequal pixel spacing to be compared. For SPECT applications, as will be discussed in later chapters, many of these operations must be carried out in three dimensions. All of the above-mentioned operations can be performed in a manner to produce minimal distortions in the underlying quantitative pixel values, but of course many of the operations rely on interpolations that often produce the same effects as pixel averaging (ie, smoothing).

FOURIER ANALYSIS OF CYCLIC DATA

Any cyclic curve can be represented mathematically by a sum of sinusoid and cosinusoid curves of various amplitudes and frequencies, known as a *Fourier series*. The principles are familiar in music: any complex tone (eg, a note played on a piano) can be identically reproduced by adding together the proper number of pure tones (called harmonics) of varying pitch (frequency) and intensity (amplitude). Fourier series are useful in analyzing the cyclic data produced from gated cardiac studies. As an example, consider a TAC produced from a left ventricular ROI. This TAC is a cyclic function of time and can be written as a Fourier series:

$$\begin{aligned}\text{TAC} &= A_1 \sin(ft) + A_2 \sin(2ft) + A_3 \sin(3ft) + \ldots \\ &+ B_1 \cos(ft) + B_2 \cos(2ft) + B_3 \cos(3ft) + \ldots \\ &= \Sigma A_n \sin(n\,\text{ft}) + B_n \cos(n\,\text{ft})\end{aligned}$$

where A_n and B_n are the amplitudes, or intensities, of each frequency, t is time; and f is frequency (cycles per second). Each term of a certain frequency is called a *harmonic*. The *fundamental frequency* f, or first harmonic, is given by $2\pi/p$ where p is the period of the cardiac cycle in seconds. Note that the summation implies that, in principle, an infinite number of harmonics is required to reproduce a curve exactly. In practice, because the left ventricular TAC often closely resembles a cosine wave that falls and rises in the time of one heart beat, fewer terms (harmonics) are needed to describe the TAC. In Figure 11 (top), a left ventricular TAC is shown. In Figure 11A is the Fourier series that describes this TAC if only the first harmonic is used. This curve has the same general shape as the TAC but is missing much detail (eg, the rapid filling, the diastasis period, atrial contraction, etc). In Figures 11B, C, and D, two, three, and four harmonics are added, producing a curve successively closer to the original. If the number of harmonics were increased still further, the Fourier series would eventually reproduce the original identically (including the statistical fluctuations). By omitting the high-frequency harmonics (eg, using only the first four harmonics, as in Fig. 11D), a much smoother curve is produced. This is one use of Fourier

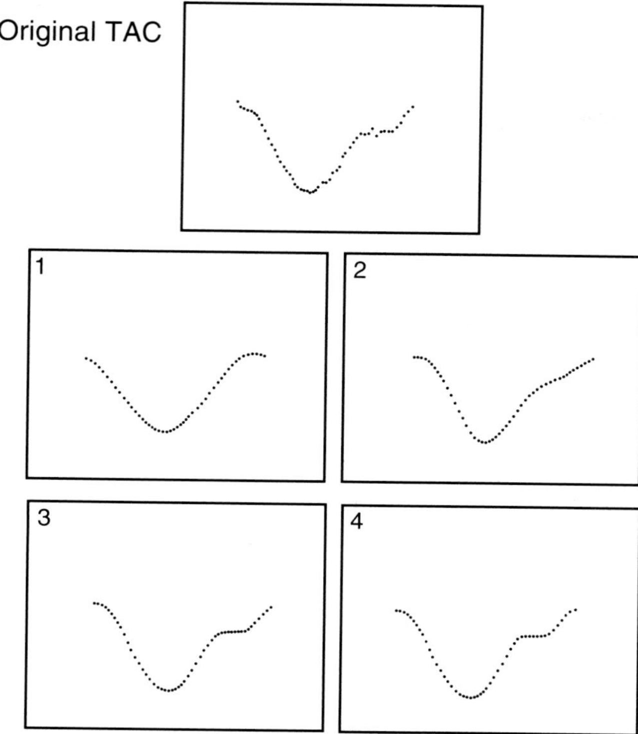

Figure 11. Top: Time activity curve (TAC) obtained from a left ventricular region of interest in a high-count gated blood pool study. (1 to 4). Approximations to this TAC using 1, 2, 3, and 4 harmonics respectively.

series—to smooth, or *Fourier filter*, TACs by omitting high-frequency harmonics. Fourier series are also used in cardiac *phase analysis*, in which the TAC is assumed to be described adequately by one harmonic.

Fourier analysis can be used to filter images, not just TACs. For example, by describing each single-pixel TAC in a gated cardiac image sequence by its Fourier series, and omitting all high harmonics, each image in the sequence becomes effectively temporally smoothed. There are a great many other ways Fourier analysis can be used in medical imaging, ranging from reconstruction of tomographic images to improving image resolution. The reader is referred to other texts for more details.[6,8,10]

REFERENCES

1. Bacharach SL, De Graaf CN. Data acquisition and processing in *in vivo* nuclear medicine. In: Van Rijk PP, ed. *Nuclear Techniques in Diagnostic Medicine*. Dordrecht: Martinus Nijhoff, 1986;163–188.
2. Todd-Pokropek AE, Pizer SM. Displays in scintigraphy. In: *Medical Radionuclide Imaging*. Vol. 1. Vienna: IAEA, 1977.
3. Cornsweet TN. *Visual Perception*. New York: Academic Press, 1970.
4. James AE, Anderson JH, Higgins CB. *Digital Image Processing in Radiology*. Baltimore: Williams & Wilkins, 1985.
5. Lieberman DE, ed. *Computer Methods: The Fundamentals of Digital Nuclear Medicine*. St. Louis: C.V. Mosby, 1977.
6. Goris ML, Briandet PA. *A Clinical and Mathematical Introduction to Computer Processing of Scintigraphic Images*. New York: Raven Press, 1983.
7. Bacharach SL, Green MV, Borer JS. Instrumentation and data processing in cardiovascular nuclear medicine: evaluation of ventricular function. *Semin Nucl Med* 1979;IX:257–274.
8. Collins SM, Skorton DJ. *Cardiac Imaging and Image Processing*. New York: McGraw-Hill, 1986.
9. Pratt WK. *Digital Image Processing*. New York: John Wiley & Sons, 1991.
10. Parker JA. *Image Reconstruction in Radiology*. Boca Raton, FL: CRC Press, 1990.

8 Mathematical Modeling and Compartmental Analysis

Richard E. Carson

Progress in nuclear medicine depends heavily upon the development and application of new radiopharmaceuticals and the imaging of their biodistribution and kinetics with modern instrumentation. Clever design and synthesis of more sensitive and specific radiopharmaceuticals is the necessary first step. Each tracer is targeted to measure a physiological parameter of interest such as blood flow, metabolism, receptor content, etc, in one or more organs or regions. State-of-the-art instrumentation, eg, positron emission tomography (PET) and single photon emission computed tomography (SPECT) scanners and cameras, can produce high-quality three-dimensional images after injection of tracer into a patient, normal volunteer, or research animal. At a minimum, these images provide a qualitative measure of the radioactivity distribution. At best, with an appropriate reconstruction algorithm and with proper corrections for the physical effects in emission tomography (eg, attenuation, scatter), quantitatively accurate measurements of regional radioactivity concentration can be obtained. These images of tracer distribution, both qualitative and quantitative, can be usefully applied to answer clinical and scientific questions.

With the additional use of tracer kinetic modeling techniques, however, there is the potential for a substantial improvement in the kind and quality of information that can be extracted from these biological data. The purpose of a mathematical model is to define the relationships between the measurable data and the physiological parameters that affect the uptake and metabolism of the tracer.

In this chapter, the concepts of mathematical modeling as applied to nuclear medicine modalities are presented. Many of these concepts can be applied to radioactivity measurements from small animals made by tissue sampling or quantitative autoradiography. The primary focus in this chapter will be on methods applicable to data that can be acquired with quantitative imaging technology, particularly PET. The advantages and disadvantages of various modeling approaches are presented. Then, classes of models are introduced, followed by a detailed description of compartment modeling and of the process of model development and application. Finally, the factors to be considered in choosing and using various model-based methods are presented.

OVERVIEW OF MODELING

Nuclear medicine imaging modalities produce relative or absolute radioactivity measurements throughout a target structure or organ. A single static image may be collected at a single specific time postinjection or the full time course of radioactivity can be measured, depending on the characteristics of the radiopharmaceutical and the instrumentation. Data from multiple studies under different biological conditions may also be obtained. If the appropriate tracer is selected and suitable imaging conditions are used, the activity values measured in a region of interest (ROI) in the image should be most heavily influenced by the physiological characteristic of interest, be it blood flow, receptor concentration, etc. A model attempts to describe in an exact fashion this relationship between the measurements and the parameters of interest. In other words, an appropriate tracer kinetic model can account for all the biological factors that contribute to the tissue radioactivity signal.

The concentration of radioactivity in a given tissue region at a particular time postinjection primarily depends upon two factors. First, and of most interest, is the local tissue physiology, eg, the blood flow or metabolism in that region. Second is the input function, ie, the time course of tracer radioactivity concentration in the blood or plasma, which defines the availability of tracer to the target organ. A model is a mathematical description (ie, one or more equations) of the relationship between tissue concentration and these controlling factors. A full model can predict the time course of radioactivity concentration in a tissue region from knowledge of the local physiological variables and the input function. A simpler model might predict only certain aspects of the tissue concentration curve, such as the initial slope, the area under the curve, or the relative activity concentration between the target organ and a reference region.

The development of a model is not a simple task. The studies that are necessary to develop and validate a model can be quite complex. There are no absolute rules defining the essential components of a model. A successful model-based method must account for the limitations imposed by instrumentation, statistics, and patient logistics. To determine the ultimate form of a useful model, many factors must be considered and compromises must be made. The complexity of a "100%-accurate" model may make it impractical to use or may produce statistically unreliable results. A "less-accurate" model may be more useful.

A model can predict the tissue radioactivity measurements given knowledge of the underlying physiology. This does not appear to be useful, since it requires knowledge of exactly the information that we seek to determine. However, the model can be made useful by inverting its equations. In this way, measurements of tissue and blood concentration can be used to estimate regional physiological parameters on a regional or even pixel-by-pixel basis. There are many ways to invert the model equations and solve for these parameters. Such techniques are called model-based methods. They may be very complex, requiring multiple scans and blood samples and using iterative parameter estimation techniques. Alternatively, a model-based method may be a simple clinically oriented procedure. With the knowledge of the behavior of the tracer provided by the model, straightforward study conditions (tracer administration scheme, scanning and blood data collection, and data processing) can be defined to measure one or more physiological parameters.

This chapter provides an overview of the wide assortment of ways to develop useful models and to use the models to obtain absolute or relative values of physiological parameters.

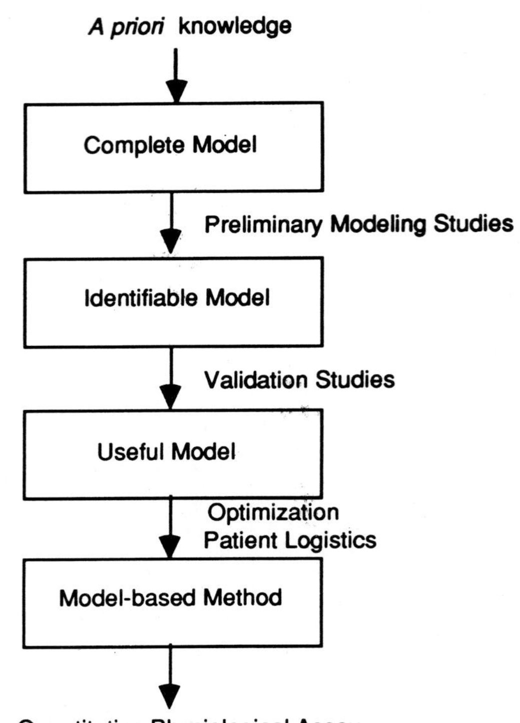

Figure 1. Steps in developing a model. A priori knowledge of the expected biochemical behavior of the tracer is used to specify a complete model. Preliminary modeling studies will define an identifiable model, appropriate for the measurable data. Validation studies are used to refine the model, verify its assumptions, and test the accuracy of its estimates. After optimization procedures, error analysis, and accounting for patient logistic considerations, a model-based method can be developed that is both practical and produces reliable, accurate physiological measurements.

The Modeling Process

Once a radioactive tracer has been selected for evaluation, there are a number of steps involved in developing a useful model and a model-based method. Figure 1 gives an overview of this process. Based on a priori knowledge of the expected in vivo behavior of the tracer, a complete model can be specified. Such a model is usually overly complex and will have many more parameters than can be determined from nuclear medicine data due to statistical noise. Based on preliminary modeling studies, a simpler model whose parameters can be determined (identified) can be developed. Then, validation studies can be performed to refine the model and verify that its assumptions are correct and that its estimates of physiological parameters are accurate. Finally, based on the understanding of the tracer provided by these modeling studies, a simpler protocol can be defined and applied for routine patient use. This method may involve limited or no blood measurements and simple data analysis procedures. Under many conditions, such a protocol may produce physiological estimates of comparable precision and accuracy as those determined from the more complex modeling studies.

Many factors affect the ultimate form of a useful model. In addition to the biological characteristics of the tracer, the characteristics of the instrumentation to be used to measure tissue radioactivity are important. It is essential to understand the accuracy of the reconstruction algorithm and its corrections as well as the noise level in the measurements, which depends on the injected dose, camera sensitivity, reconstruction parameters, and imaging time. It may be of little use to develop a sophisticated model if there are significant inaccuracies in the radioactivity measurements due to improper corrections for attenuation or scatter. The noise level in the data also affects the number of parameters that may be estimated. Noise also is the primary determinant of the precision (variability) in the estimated parameters.

TRACERS AND MODELS

In this chapter, labeled compounds are referred to as tracer, radiotracer, or radiopharmaceutical. The term tracer implies that the injected compound, including both labeled and unlabelled molecules, is present in the tissue at negligible mass concentrations, so that little or no change in the saturation of relevant enzymes or receptors occurs. For this discussion, we assume that tracer levels are appropriate, except where explicitly noted.

Characteristics of Radiotracers

Before discussing models, it is important to consider the basic characteristics of radioactive tracers (see Chapter 11 for a more complete discussion). A tracer is designed to provide information about a particular physiological function of interest, such as blood flow, blood volume, a metabolic process, a synthetic process, a transport step, a binding process, etc. However, since any given tracer will likely have many biochemical fates following injection, great care and judgment are required to choose an appropriate compound. Ideally, the only factor controlling the uptake and distribution of the tracer will be the physiological process under study. Realistically, other factors always affect a tracer's distribution and kinetics. For example, for a receptor-binding radiotracer, regional radioactivity concentration data are affected by regional blood flow, plasma protein binding, capillary permeability, nonspecific tissue binding, receptor association and dissociation rates, free receptor concentration, tracer clearance from blood (controlled by whole body uptake), tracer metabolism (throughout the body), and regional uptake of any radioactive metabolites. One hopes the net effect of extraneous factors will be minor.

A tracer may either be a direct radiolabeled version of a naturally occurring compound, an analog of a natural compound, or a unique compound, perhaps a radiolabeled drug. An analog is a compound whose chemical properties are slightly different from the natural compound to which it is related. For example, ^{11}C-glucose is identical to glucose except for the replacement of a ^{12}C atom with ^{11}C. Analogs of glucose are deoxyglucose[1] and fluorodeoxyglucose (FDG),[2–4] which are chemically different from glucose. Often, because the naturally occurring compound has a very complex biochemical fate, a model describing the tissue radioactivity curve of a directly labeled compound may also need to be quite complex. A carefully designed analog can dramatically simplify the modeling and improve the sensitivity of the model to the parameter of interest. Deoxyglucose and FDG are good examples. Deoxyglucose and glucose enter cells by the same transport enzyme and are both phosphorylated by the enzyme hexokinase. However, deoxyglucose is not a substrate for the next enzyme in the glycolytic pathway, so deoxyglucose-6-phosphate accumulates in tissue. In this way, the tissue signal directly reflects the rate of metabolism, since there is little clearance of metabolized tracer. One important disadvantage of using an analog is that the measured kinetic parameters are those of the analog itself, not of the natural compound of interest. To correct for this, the relationship between the native compound and the radioactive analog must be determined. For deoxyglucose and FDG, this relationship is summarized by the *lumped constant*.[1,5] To make the analog approach widely applicable, it is necessary to test whether this constant changes over a wide range of pathological conditions.[5–9]

Ideally, the parameter of interest is the primary determinant of the uptake and retention of a tracer, ie, the tissue uptake after an appropriate period is directly (ie, linearly) proportional to this parameter. This is the case for radioactive microspheres.[10] Many other compounds are substantially trapped in tissue shortly after uptake and are called chemical microspheres.[11,12] For this class of compounds, a single scan at an appropriate time postinjection will give information about the parameter of interest. For other tracers, which both enter and exit tissue, imaging at multiple time points postinjection may be necessary to extract useful physiological information.

It is obvious that another important attribute of a tracer is that there be sufficient uptake in the organ of interest, ie, the radioactivity concentration must provide sufficient counting statistics in an image of reasonable length after injection of an allowable dose. Thus, the size of the structure of interest and the characteristics of the imaging equipment can also affect the choice of tracer.

Types of Models

There are a wide variety of approaches to extract meaningful physiological data from tissue radioactivity measurements made with nuclear medicine techniques. All modeling approaches share some basic assumptions, in particular the principle of conservation of mass. Several sources present comprehensive modeling alternatives.[13–18] Some approaches are termed *stochastic* or *noncompartmental*, and require few assumptions concerning the underlying physiology of the tracer's uptake and metabolism.[19] These methods permit measurements of certain physiological parameters, such as mean transit time and volume of distribution, without explicit descriptions of all of the specific pools or compartments that a tracer molecule may enter.

Alternatively, there are *distrubuted* models that try to achieve a precise description of the fate of the radiotracer. These models not only specify the possible physical locations and biochemical forms of the tracer, but also include concentration gradients that exist within different physiological domains. In particular, distributed models for exchange of tracer between capillary and tissue have been extensively developed.[20–26] Since this is a necessary step in the uptake of any tracer into tissue, a precise model for trans-capillary delivery of tracer is important. Distributed models are also used to account for processes, such as diffusion, where concentration gradients are present.[27]

A class of models whose complexity lies between stochastic and distributed are the *compartmental* models. These models define some of the details of the underlying physiology, but do not include concentration gradients present in distributed models. The development and application of these models is the principal topic of this chapter. A common application of compartmental modeling is the mathematical description of the distribution of a tracer throughout the body.[28,29] Here different body organs or groups of organs are assigned to individual compartments, and the model defines the kinetics into and out of each compartment. This type of model is useful when the primary measurable data are the concentration of the tracer in blood and urine. If there are many measurements with good accuracy, fairly complex models with many compartments and parameters can be used.

In nuclear medicine, compartmental modeling is applied in a different manner. Here, one or more measurements of radioactivity levels in a specific organ, region, or even pixel are made. If the tracer enters and leaves the organ via the blood, the tracer kinetics in other body regions need not be considered to evaluate the physiological traits of the organ of interest. In this way, each region or pixel can be analyzed independently. Generally, there must be some knowledge of the time course of blood activity. Since each region can be evaluated separately, the models can be relatively simple, and can therefore be usefully applied to determine regional physiological parameters from nuclear medicine data.

COMPARTMENTAL MODELING

Compartmental modeling is the most commonly used method for describing the uptake and clearance of radioactive tracers in tissue.[28,30,31] These models specify that all molecules of tracer delivered to the system (ie, injected) will at any given time exist in one of many compartments. Each compartment defines one possible state of the tracer, specifically its physical location (eg, intravascular space, extracellular space, intracellular space, synapse) and its chemical state (ie, its current metabolic form or its binding state to different tissue elements, such as plasma proteins, receptors, etc). Usually, a single compartment represents a number of these states lumped together. Compartments are typically numbered for mathematical notation.

The compartmental model also describes the possible transformations that can occur to the tracer, allowing it to "move" between compartments. For example, a molecule of tracer in the vascular space may enter the extracellular space, or a molecule of receptor-binding tracer that is free in the synapse may become bound to its receptor. The model defines the chance or probability that any tracer molecule will "move" to a different compartment within a specified time. This fractional rate of change of the tracer concentration in one compartment is called a *rate constant*, usually expressed as "k", and has units of inverse minute (or another time unit). The inverse minute unit reflects the fraction per minute, ie, the proportion of tracer molecules in a given compartment that will move to another compartment in 1 minute. To distinguish the various rate constants in a given model, subscripts are used to define the source and destination compartment numbers. In much of the compartmental modeling literature, k_{12}, for example, reflects the rate of tracer movement to compartment 1 from compartment 2. This nomenclature is especially convenient for large models and is motivated by the nature of matrix algebra notation. In nuclear medicine applications, the number of compartments is often small (1 to 3), as is the number of rate constants (1 to 5), so it is typical to use a notation with one subscript (eg, k_3) where the source and destination compartments associated with each constant are explicitly defined.

The physiological interpretation of the source and destination compartments defines the meaning of the rate constants for movement of tracer between them. For example, the rate constant describing tracer movement from a receptor-bound compartment to the unbound compartment reflects the receptor dissociation rate. For a freely diffusible inert tracer, the rate constant between arterial blood and a tissue compartment defines local blood flow. By determining these rate constants (or some algebraic combination of them), quantitative estimates of local physiological parameters can be obtained. The underlying goal of all modeling methods is the estimation of one or more of these rate constants from tissue radioactivity measurements.

Examples of Compartmental Models

Figure 2 shows examples of compartmental model configurations. In many authors' depictions of models, a rectangular box is drawn for each compartment, with arrows labeled with the rate constants placed between the boxes. In most whole-body compartmental models, the blood is usually counted as a compartment. Measurements from blood are often the primary set of data used to estimate the model rate constants. In the nuclear medicine applications described here, we are most interested in the model constants associated with the tissue regions that are being imaged. Typically, measurements are made from the blood to define the "input function" to the first tissue compartment (see Input Functions and Convolution). In this presentation, we will treat these blood input measurements as known values, not as concentration values to be predicted by the model. Thus, blood will not be counted as a compartment.

Figure 2A shows the simplest model having one tissue compartment with irreversible uptake of tracer. This irreversible uptake is shown by the presence of a rate constant K_1 for tracer moving from the blood to compartment 1, but with no rate constant for exit of tracer back to blood. Such a model is appropriate for radioactive microspheres[10] or for a tracer that is irreversibly trapped in tissue. This model is often used as an approximation when tissue trapping is nearly irreversible.[11] Figure 2B shows a one-tissue compartment model, appropriate for a tracer that exhibits reversible tissue uptake. This is a common model for inert tracers used to measure local blood flow.[13] Here, the rate at which the tracer exits the tissue compartment and returns to the blood is denoted k_2. Figure 2C shows a model with two tissue compartments. This model may be appropriate for a tracer that enters tissue from blood, and then is either metabolized to a form that is trapped in the tissue (at a rate k_3) or returns to blood (at a rate k_2), such as deoxyglucose.[1] Compartment 1 represents the unmetabolized tracer and compartment 2 the metabolized tracer. Figure 2D shows a three-tissue com-

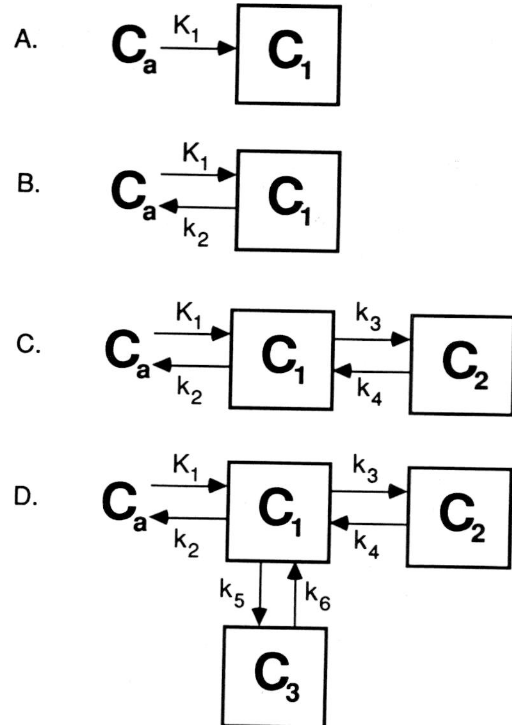

Figure 2. Examples of compartmental models. C_a is the concentration of tracer in arterial blood; C_1, C_2, and C_3 are the tracer concentrations in compartments 1 to 3; and K_1 k_2, etc, are the rate constants that define the fractional rate of tracer movement between compartments. **(A).** The simplest compartmental model having one tissue compartment with irreversible uptake of tracer, eg, microspheres. **(B).** A model with one tissue compartment appropriate for a tracer that exhibits reversible tissue uptake, eg, diffusible blood flow tracer. **(C).** A model with two tissue compartments, eg, FDG. **(D).** A three-tissue compartment model for a receptor-binding ligand where the three compartments represent (1) free tracer; (2) tracer specifically bound to receptor; and (3) tracer nonspecifically bound to other tissue elements.

partment model for a receptor-binding ligand where the three compartments represent free tracer; tracer specifically bound to receptor; and tracer nonspecifically bound to other tissue elements.[32]

Compartmental Modeling Assumptions

The successful application of simple compartmental models to a complex biological system requires that many assumptions be true. These assumptions are typically not completely valid, so that successful use of these models depends upon whether errors in these assumptions produce acceptable errors in model measurements (see Error Analysis). Compartmental models, by their nature, assume that each compartment is well mixed, ie, there are no concentration gradients within a single compartment. Therefore, all tracer molecules in a given compartment have equal probability of exchange into other compartments. This well-mixed assumption has the great advantage of producing relatively simple mathematical relationships. However, it limits the ability of compartmental models to provide an accurate description of some biological structures. For example, a compartmental model cannot include the change of activity concentration in a capillary from arterial to venous ends, or the heterogeneous distribution of receptors in a patch of tissue. Often, in nuclear medicine applications, the "well-mixed" assumption is also violated by the nature of the imaging process. Due to low resolution, even single-pixel data from reconstructed images represent a mixture of underlying tissue types. When larger ROIs are used to reduce the statistical uncertainty of the measurements, heterogeneity in the measurements increases.

A primary assumption of most compartmental models is that the underlying physiological processes are in steady state. Mathematically, this means that the rate constants of the system do not change with time during a study, resulting in a model consisting of linear differential equations (see Model Implementation). If these rate constants reflect local blood flow or the rate of a metabolic or binding process, then the rate at which these processes occur should remain constant during a study. Since the rates of many biological processes are regulated by substrate and product concentrations, maintaining processes in steady state usually requires constant concentrations of these compounds. In practice, this requirement is never precisely met. However, these assumptions are adequately met so long as any changes in the underlying rates of flow, metabolism, receptor binding, etc, are small with respect to the time scale of the data being analyzed. Note that the concentrations of the injected radiopharmaceuticals may change dramatically during a study; however, this does not violate the steady-state assumption as long as the radioactive species exists at a negligible (tracer) concentration with respect to the nonradioactive natural biological substrates (see Biochemical Reactions and Receptor-ligand Binding). For studies using injections of radiopharmaceuticals with low specific activity, saturation of receptors or enzymes can be significant, and nonlinear modeling techniques are required.

To generate the equations of a model, the magnitude of tracer movement from compartment A to compartment B per unit of time must be defined. This is called the *flux* (J_{AB}). If tracer concentration is expressed in units of nanocuries per milliliter, then flux has units of nanocuries per milliliter per minute (or another appropriate time unit). The assumptions of well-mixed compartments and physiological processes in steady state lead to the mathematical relationship that the flux J_{AB} is a linear multiple of the amount, or concentration, of tracer in the source compartment A (C_A), ie,

$$J_{AB} = k\, C_A \tag{1}$$

where k is a rate constant with inverse minute units, which is independent of the concentration in any compartment. This simple equation is the basis of the differential equations that describe compartmental models (see Model Implementation).

Interpretation of Model Rate Constants

The physiological interpretation of the rate constant (such as k in Equation 1) depends upon the definition of the source and destination compartments. A single compartment of a model may often lump a number of physiological entities, eg, tracer in extracellular and intracellular spaces or tracer that is free in tissue and nonspecifically bound. This section discusses the physiological meaning of model rate constants.

BLOOD FLOW AND EXTRACTION

The first step in most in vivo models is the delivery of tracer to the target region from the circulation. The flux of tracer into the first tissue compartment from the blood is governed by the local blood flow and the rate of extraction of the tracer from the intracapillary blood into the tissue. Conventional fluid flow describes the volume of liquid passing a given point per unit of time and has units of milliliters per minute. A more useful physiological measure is *perfusion flow*, the volume of blood passing in and out of a given volume (or weight) of tissue per unit of time, which has units of milliliters per minute per milliliter of tissue or milliliters per minute per gram of tissue. In the physiological literature, the term blood flow usually means perfusion flow.

Determining blood flow and extraction information from model parameters begins with the Fick Principle (see, for example, Lassen and Perl[15]). The net flux (J) of tracer into or out of a tissue element equals the difference between the influx (J_{in}) and outflux (J_{out}), ie,

$$J = J_{in} - J_{out} = F\,C_a - F\,C_v \tag{2}$$

where the influx is the product of the blood flow (F) and the arterial concentration (C_a), and the outflux is the product of the blood flow and the venous concentration (C_v). The unidirectional (or first-pass) *extraction fraction* E is the fraction of tracer that exits the blood and enters the tissue on one capillary pass, or

$$E = \frac{C_a - C_v}{C_a} \tag{3}$$

A tracer with low extraction has a small arterial-venous difference on first-pass. Equation 2 can then be rewritten as

$$J = (F \cdot E)\,C_a = k\,C_a \tag{4}$$

Equation 4 describes the unidirectional delivery of tracer from blood to tissue. The rate constant k defining this uptake process is thus the product of blood flow and unidirectional extraction fraction. The interpretation of the extraction fraction was further developed by Kety,[13] Renkin,[33] and Crone[34] by considering the capillary as a cylinder to produce the following relationship:

$$E = 1 - exp(-PS/F) \tag{5}$$

where P is the permeability of the tracer across the capillary surface (centimeters per minute), S is the capillary surface area per gram of tissue (square centimeters per gram), and F is the blood flow (milliliters per minute per gram). For highly permeable tracers, the product PS is much greater than the flow F, the exponential term in Equation 5 is small, and the extraction fraction is nearly 1.0; thus the rate constant for delivery is approximately equal to flow. Such tracers are therefore useful to measure regional blood flow and not useful to measure permeability, ie, they are flow limited. For tracers with permeability much lower than flow, the relationship in Equation 5 can be approximated as

$$E \cong \frac{PS}{F} \tag{6}$$

and the rate constant k ($F \cdot E$) becomes PS. Such tracers are useful to measure permeability and not useful to measure flow. Most tracers lie between these two extremes, so that the rate constant for delivery from arterial blood to tissue is affected by both blood flow and permeability. These relationships are directly applicable to tracers that enter and leave tissue by passive diffusion. For tracers transported into and out of tissue by facilitated or active transport, the PS product is mathematically equivalent to the transport rate, which depends upon the concentration and reaction rate of the transport enzymes (see Biochemical Reactions).

The interpretation of a delivery rate constant k as the product of flow and extraction fraction may depend upon whether the blood activity concentration C_a is measured in whole blood or in plasma. If there is very rapid equilibration between plasma and red blood cells, then whole blood and plasma concentrations will be identical. However, if equilibrium is slow with respect to tracer uptake rates into tissue, or if there is trapping or metabolism of the tracer in red blood cells, then the plasma concentration should be used. In the extreme of no uptake of tracer into red cells, then the delivery rate constant k is the product of extraction fraction and plasma flow, where plasma flow is related to whole blood flow based on the hematocrit.

DIFFUSIBLE TRACERS AND VOLUME OF DISTRIBUTION

One of the simplest classes of tracers are those that enter tissue from blood and then later return to blood. The net flux of tracer into a tissue compartment can be expressed as follows:

$$J = K_1 C_a - k_2\,C \tag{7}$$

K_1 is the rate of entry of tracer from blood to tissue and is equal to the product of extraction fraction and blood flow, and C_a is the concentration of tracer in arterial blood. The rate constant k_2 describes the rate of return of tracer from tissue to blood, where C is the concentration of tracer in tissue. The physiological interpretation of k_2 can best be defined by introducing the concept of the volume of distribution. Suppose the concentration of tracer in the blood remained constant. Ultimately, the concentration of a diffusible tracer in the tissue compartment would also become constant and equilibrium would be achieved. The ratio of the tissue concentration to the blood concentration at equilibrium is called the *volume of distribution* (or alternatively the *partition coefficient*). It is termed a volume because it can be thought of as the volume of blood that contains the same quantity of radioactivity as 1 mL (or 1 g) of tissue. Once the blood and tissue tracer concentrations have reached constant levels, ie, equilibrium, the net flux J into the tissue compartment is 0, so the volume of distribution V_D can be expressed as

$$V_D = \frac{C}{C_a} = \frac{K_1}{k_2} \tag{8}$$

where the last equality is derived by setting the flux J in Equation 7 to 0. Therefore, the physiological definition for the rate constant k_2 is the ratio of K_1 to V_D.

BIOCHEMICAL REACTIONS

Often, two compartments of a model represent the substrate and product of a chemical reaction. In that case, the rate constant describing the "exchange" between these compartments is indicative of the reaction rate. For enzyme-catalyzed reactions,[35] the flux from substrate to product compartments is the *reaction velocity* v:

$$v = \frac{v_m C}{K_m + C} \tag{9}$$

where v_m is the maximum rate of the reaction, C is the concentration of substrate, and K_m is the concentration of substrate that produces half-maximum velocity. This is the classic Michaelis-Menten relationship. It shows that the velocity is not a linear function of the substrate concentration, as in Equation 1. However, when using tracer concentrations of a radioactive species and if the concentrations of the native substrates are in steady state (see Compartmental Modeling Assumptions), the linear form of Equation 1 still holds. In the presence of a native substrate with concentration C, and the radioactive analog with concentration C^*, the reaction rate for the generation of radioactive product v^* is as follows:

$$v^* = \frac{v_m^* C^*}{K_m^* \,(1 + C/K_m + C^*/K_m^*)} \tag{10}$$

v_m^* and K_m^* are the maximum velocity and half-maximum substrate concentration for the radioactive analog. If the radioactive species has high specific activity (the concentration ratio of labeled to unlabeled compound in the injectate) so that its total concentration (labeled and unlabeled) is small compared to the native substrate, ie, $C^*/K_m^* \ll C/K_m$, then Equation 10 reduces to

$$v^* = \left(\frac{v_m^*}{K_m^*(1 + C/K_m)}\right) C^* = k\, C^* \tag{11}$$

The term in large brackets in Equation 11 is composed of terms that are assumed to be constant throughout a tracer experiment. Therefore, when using radiopharmaceuticals at tracer concentrations, enzyme-catalyzed reactions can be described with a linear relationship as the product of a rate constant k and the radioactive substrate concentration C^*.

RECEPTOR-LIGAND BINDING

For radiotracers that bind to receptors in the tissue (eg, see Eckleman[36]), the rate of binding, ie, the rate of passage of tracer from the free compartment to the bound compartment, can also be described by the linear form of Equation 1 under tracer concentration assumptions. For many receptor systems, the binding rate is proportional to the product of the concentrations of free ligand and free receptor. This classical bimolecular association can be described mathematically as

$$v = k_{on}(B_{\max} - B)F \tag{12}$$

where k_{on} is the bimolecular association rate (per nanomolar per minute) $B_{\max}$ is the total concentration of receptors (nanomolar), B is the concentration of receptors currently bound (either by the injected ligand or by endogenous ligand), and F is the concentration of free ligand. When a radioactive species is added and competes with endogenous ligand for receptor binding, the radiopharmaceutical binding velocity is

$$v^* = k_{\text{on}}^* \,(B_{\max} - B - B^*)\, F^* \tag{13}$$

where k_{on}^* is the association rate of the radiopharmaceutical. If the radioactive compound has high specific activity, then $B^* \ll B$, and Equation 13 becomes

$$v^* = (k_{\text{on}}^*\, B'_{\max})\, F^* = k\, F^* \tag{14}$$

where $B'_{\max}$ is the free receptor concentration ($B_{\max} - B$). Thus, using a high specific activity receptor-binding ligand, measurement of the reaction rate constant k provides information about the product of k_{on} and $B'_{\max}$, but cannot separate these parameters. Note that this description of receptor-binding radioligands is mathematically identical to that for enzyme-catalyzed reactions, although the conventional nomenclature is different.

MODEL IMPLEMENTATION

This section presents an overview of the mathematics associated with compartmental modeling. This includes the mathematical formulation of these models into differential equations, the solutions to a few simple models, and a summary of parameter estimation techniques used to determine model rate constants from measured data. Here we concentrate on applications where we have made measurements in an organ or region of interest which we wish to use to ascertain estimates of the underlying physiological rates of this region.

Mathematics of Compartmental Models

This section describes the process of converting a compartmental model into its mathematical form and its solution. For a more complete discussion of these topics, consult basic texts on differential equations[37] as well as specialized texts on mathematical modeling of biologic systems.[16,28]

First we start with a particular model configuration such as those in Figure 2. The compartments are numbered 1, 2, etc, and the radioactivity concentration in each compartment is designated C_1, C_2, etc. Radioactivity measurements in tissue are typically of a form such as counts per milliliter or nanocuries per gram. The volume or weight unit in the denominator reflects the full tissue volume. However, the tracer may exist only in portions of the tissue, eg, just the extracellular space. In this case, the concentration of the tracer within its distribution space will be higher than its apparent concentration per gram of tissue. The compartmental model equations are written in terms of C_1, C_2, etc, which are in units of radioactivity per volume (or weight) of tissue. When these concentration values are used to define reaction rates, which are based on the true local concentration, the interpretation of the relevant rate constant includes a correction for the fraction of total tissue volume in which the tracer distributes.

DIFFERENTIAL EQUATIONS

The net flux into each compartment can be defined as the sum of all the inflows minus the sum of all the outflows. Each of these components is symbolized by an arrow into or out of the compartment, and the magnitude of each flux is the product of the rate constant and the concentration in the source compartment. The net flux into a compartment has units of concentration per unit time and is equal to the rate of change of the compartment concentration, or dC/dt. Consider the simple one-compartment model in Figure 2B. The differential equation describing the rate of change of the tissue concentration C_1 is

$$\text{(15)} \qquad \frac{dC_1}{dt} = K_1C_a(t) - k_2C_1(t)$$

Here, $C_a(t)$ is the time course of tracer in the arterial blood, also called the input function. K_1 is the rate constant for entry of tracer from blood to tissue, and k_2 is the rate constant for return of tracer to blood. The capitalization of the rate constant K_1 is not a typographical error. K_1 is capitalized to designate the fact that it has units different from other rate constants. The blood radiotracer measurements are typically made per milliliter of blood or plasma. In the earlier nonimaging studies in animals, tissue concentration measurements were made per gram of tissue. Thus C_1 had units of nanocuries per gram, and C_a had units of nanocuries per milliliter. Therefore, K_1 must have units of milliliters blood per minute per gram tissue (usually written as mL/min/g). The other rate constants have inverse minute units. Modern nuclear medicine imaging devices actually acquire tissue radioactivity measurements per milliliter of tissue. Thus, to present results in comparable units to earlier work, corrections for the density of tissue must be applied to convert nanocuries per milliliter to nanocuries per gram.

Before solving Equation 15 for a general input function $C_a(t)$, first consider the case of an ideal bolus input, ie, the tracer passes through the tissue capillaries in one brief instant at time $t = 0$, and there is no recirculation. If C_a is the magnitude of this bolus, the model solution for the time-concentration curve for compartment 1 is as follows:

$$\text{(16)} \qquad C_1(t) = C_a\, K_1\, exp(-k_2t\,).$$

Thus, at time zero, the tissue activity jumps from 0 to a level K_1C_a and then drops toward zero exponentially with a rate k_2 or a half-life of $0.693/k_2$.

Now consider the two compartment model in Figure 2C. For this model there will be two differential equations, one per compartment:

$$\text{(17)} \qquad \frac{dC_1}{dt} = K_1C_a(t) - k_2C_1(t) - k_3C_1(t) + k_4C_2(t)$$

$$\text{(18)} \qquad \frac{dC_2}{dt} = k_3C_1(t) - k_4C_2(t)$$

Note that there is a term on the right sides of Equations 17 and 18 for each of the connections between compartments in Figure 2C. An outflux term in Equation 17 [eg, $-k_3C_1(t)$] has a corresponding influx term in Equation 18 [$+k_3C_1(t)$]. The solution to these coupled differential equations, again for the case of an ideal bolus input, is as follows:

$$\text{(19)} \qquad C_1(t) = C_a[A_{11}exp(-\alpha_1t\,) + A_{12}\, exp(-\alpha_2t)]$$

$$\text{(20)} \qquad C_2(t) = C_a\, A_{22}[exp(-\alpha_1t\,) - exp(-\alpha_2t)]$$

where A_{11}, A_{12}, A_{21}, A_{22}, α_1, and α_2 are algebraic functions of the rate constants K_1, k_2, k_3, and k_4^4. Here, the time course of each compartment is the sum of two exponentials. One special case of interest is when the tracer is irreversibly bound in tissue so that the rate of return of tracer from compartment 2 to compartment 1, k_4, is zero. In this case, the solutions become

$$\text{(21)} \qquad C_1(t) = C_a\, K_1exp[-(k_2 + k_3)t]$$

$$\text{(22)} \qquad C_2(t) = C_a\frac{K_1k_3}{k_2 + k_3}\{1 - exp[-(k_2 + k_3)t]\}$$

Note that, in most cases, the measured tissue activity will be the total in both compartments, so that the model prediction will be the sum $C_1(t) + C_2(t)$.

These solutions for tissue concentration are linearly proportional to the magnitude of the input, C_a. Doubling the magnitude of the input (injecting more) will double the resultant tissue concentration. The equations are nonlinear with respect to many of the model rate constants, since they appear in the exponents.

Input Functions and Convolution

In the previous section, mathematical solutions were presented for simple models under the condition of an ideal bolus, ie, the tracer appears for one brief capillary transit with no recirculation. In reality, the input to the tissue is the continuous blood time-activity curve. The equations above are linear with respect to the input function C_a. This permits a direct extension of these bolus equations to be applied to solve the case of a continuous input function. Figure 3 illustrates this concept. The relationships depicted in Figure 3 can be expressed mathematically as follows. Suppose, as in Figure 3E, there is a bolus input of magnitude A at time $t = T_1$, and a second bolus of magnitude B at $t = T_2$. The resulting tissue activity curve is

$$(23) \quad C_1(t) = K_1\, A\, exp[-k_2(t - T_1)] \qquad \text{for } T_1 \leq t < T_2.$$

$$(24) \quad C_1(t) = K_1\, A\, exp[-k_2(t - T_1)] + K_1\, B\, exp[-k_2(t - T_2)] \qquad \text{for } t \geq T_2.$$

In other words, the tissue response is a sum of the individual responses to each bolus input. The responses are scaled in magnitude and shifted in time to match each bolus. Suppose now there is a series of bolus administrations at times T_i, $i = 1, \ldots$, each of magnitude $C_a(T_i)$. The total tissue response can be written as the summation:

$$(25) \qquad C_1(t) = \sum_i C_a(T_i) K_1\, exp[-k_2(t - T_i)]$$

where the exponentials are considered to have zero value for negative arguments (ie, $t < T_i$). If we now consider the continuous input function $C_a(t)$ as an infinite series of individual boluses, the summation becomes an integral:

$$(26) \qquad C_1(t) = \int_0^t C_a(s)\, K_1\, exp[-k_2(t - s)]\, ds$$

Here s is the integration variable. This is called a *convolution integral*, which is often written as

$$(27) \qquad C_1(t) = C_a(t) \otimes K_1\, exp(-k_2 t)$$

with the symbol $\otimes$ denoting convolution. This analysis corresponds to the one-compartment model of Figure 2B and extends the bolus solution (Equation 16) to the case of a general input function (Equation 27). However, convolution applies to any compartmental model whose solution is linear in its input function. Let $h_i(t)$ be the impulse response function for compartment i, ie, the time course of tissue response from a bolus input of magnitude 1 [$K_1\, exp(-k_2 t)$ for the one-compartment model]. Then the tissue activity resulting from a general input function is written as

$$(28) \qquad C_i(t) = C_a(t) \otimes h_i(t)$$

Thus, for linear compartmental models, the tissue time-activity curve is the convolution of the input function with the impulse response function. The latter is a sum of exponentials, typically one exponential per compartment. A number of approaches have been used to implement and solve Equation 28 on a computer if the arterial input function is determined from serial samples. One approach is to fit the measured input function data to a suitable model[38] and then solve the convolution integral by standard mathematical methods. Alternatively, a continuous input function can be approximated by linear interpolation between the sample data values, and then Equation 28 can be solved by analytical integration over each time period between blood samples.

Figure 4 shows the effects that variations in the input function can produce on the resulting tissue response. Figure 4A shows three input functions. The solid line is a measured arterial input function. The other two input curves were simulated based on the measured data so that the area under all curves is a constant. The tissue concentration curves produced in response to each input function are shown in Figure 4B. In all cases, the tissue response is calculated based on the one-compartment model, Equation 27, using the same parameters ($K_1 = 0.1$ mL/min/mL and $k_2 = 0.1$ min^{-1}). The difference in shape between the input functions produces comparable differences in the tissue concentration curves. These differences in shape do not reflect differences in the local physiological parameters of the tissue, since here these rate constants were the same in all cases. Therefore, the main point of Figure 4 is that a time-activity curve in a tissue region cannot be interpreted without knowledge of the input function.

The linear compartmental models discussed to this point have the great advantage of providing exact mathematical solutions, predicting the tissue response in the form of Equation 28. In some cases, the flux between compartments cannot be described mathematically as the product of a rate constant times the concentration of tracer in the source compartment ($J = kC$). For example, in modeling receptor-binding ligands, the linear flux assumption holds if the radiopharmaceutical is administered at trace levels and does not produce detectable saturation of the receptor sites (Equation 14). If such a ligand is administered in low specific activity so that it produces a change in receptor occupancy, the differential equations governing the model are no longer linear. This can be seen in Equation 13 where the flux from the free to the bound compartments v^* cannot be described as a constant multiplied by F^*, since the bound concentration B^* also appears in the relationship. Solving the equations for this and most other nonlinear cases requires techniques of numerical integration of differential equations.[39,40] The basic means of estimating numerically the activity in each compartment is to take small time intervals and use the differential equation to determine how much each compartment's concentration should change over each interval. The simplest method can be derived from the definition of the derivative, ie, for a very small time interval, Δt,

$$(29) \qquad \frac{dC}{dt} \cong \frac{C(t + \Delta t) - C(t)}{\Delta t}$$

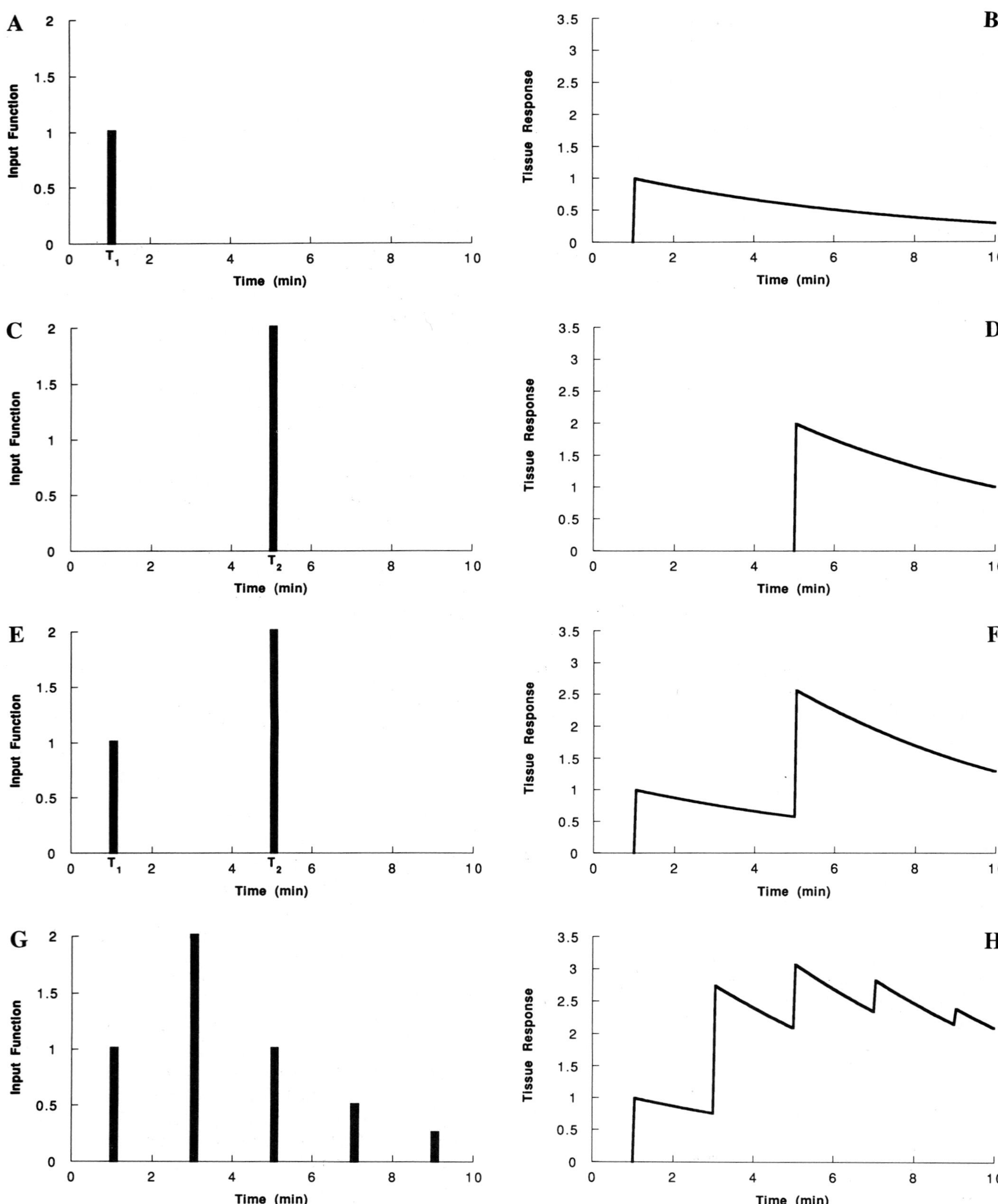

Figure 3. Convolution. A, C, E, and G show the input functions that produce the tissue responses in B, D, F, and H, respectively. **(A).** An ideal bolus input at 1 minute. **(B).** The corresponding tissue response to the one-compartment model of Figure 2B, ie, exponential clearance following Equation 16. **(C).** A single bolus of twice the magnitude in A at $t = 5$ minutes. **(D).** The tissue response to C is altered (from that in B) in a corresponding manner. **(E).** Combination of inputs in A and C. **(F).** The tissue response to E, which is the sum of the tissue responses from each bolus administered separately (B + D). This demonstrates the linearity of the model equations. **(G).** A cascade of bolus inputs with different magnitudes. **(H).** The tissue activity response to G composed of the sum of the responses to each bolus.

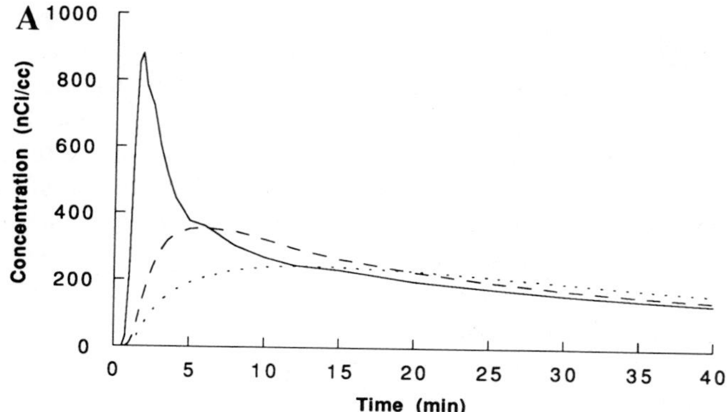

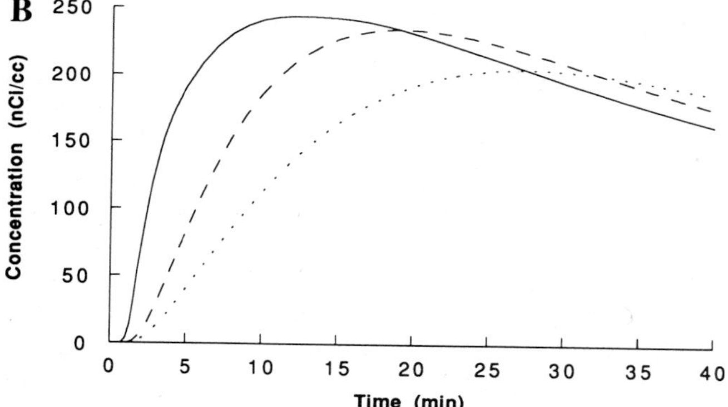

Figure 4. Effects of input functions on tissue curves. **(A).** Three input functions. The solid line is a measured arterial input function following a bolus injection of ^{18}F-fluorodeoxyglucose. The dashed and dotted lines represent other input functions derived from the first curve, so that the area under these curves is the same, ie, same injected activity. **(B).** The tissue response curves from the three input functions in **A.** In all cases the same model and rate constants were used (see text for details).

This can be inverted to solve for the tissue concentration at time $t + \Delta t$,

$$C(t + \Delta t) \cong C(t) + \frac{dC}{dt}\Delta t \tag{30}$$

If the interval size is chosen properly, the approximation of Equation 30 will introduce only small errors in the estimation of $C(t + \Delta t)$. The most commonly used method for numerical integration is called Runge-Kutta. This approach provides increased accuracy with longer intervals by averaging estimates of the derivative dC/dt at the beginning, middle, and end of each interval.

In implementing models, it is important that the model formulation match the nature of nuclear medicine imaging data. The models presented above predict the tissue concentration at an instant in time. Image values represent the average tissue activity collected over each scan interval. The instantaneous model value can be used to determine the integrated image value. For example, for the one-compartment model (Equations 15 and 27), the integrated value from time T_1 to T_2 is as follows:

$$\int_{T_1}^{T_2} C_1(t)dt = \frac{K_1 \int_{T_1}^{T_2} C_a(t)dt - [C_1(T_2) - C_1(T_1)]}{k_2} \tag{31}$$

Another practical issue is radioactive decay. This can be handled either by explicit decay correction of both the tissue and blood data or by incorporating decay into the model formulation. The latter approach can be accomplished by adding an additional rate constant corresponding to the decay rate (0.693/half-life) to each compartment. This method is slightly more accurate than explicit decay correction for short-lived tracers, since decay correction does not account for biologic change in tracer concentration within one scan interval.

Parameter Estimation

The previous sections presented the mathematical techniques necessary to solve the model equations. Thus, with knowledge of the input function $C_a(t)$, the model configuration, and its rate constants, the tissue concentration curve can be predicted mathematically. This section provides an overview of the inverse problem, that is, given measurements of the tissue activity and the input function and a proposed model configuration, one can estimate the underlying rate constants. Many references are available on the topic of parameter estimation.[41–43]

There are many ways of estimating model parameters. The choices available and the success of any given method depends upon the form of the model and the sampling and statistical quality of the measured data. If only a single measurement of tissue radioactivity is made, only a single parameter can be determined. Collection of multiple time points permits the estimation of some or all of the parameters of a model. Since measured data always have some associated noise, the estimates of model parameters from such data will also be noisy. It is often the goal of a statistical estimation method to minimize the variability of the resulting parameter estimates. Note also that the values of the parameters affect the statistical quality of the results. For example, blood flow estimates produced by a particular method may be reliable for high-flow regions but unreliable for low-flow regions.

When many tissue measurements are collected after radionuclide administration, the most commonly used method of parameter estimation is called *least-squares estimation.* Qualitatively, the goal of this technique is to find values for the model rate constants that, when inserted into the model equations, produce the best fit to the tissue measurements. Quantitatively, the goal is to minimize an optimization function, specifically the sum of the squared differences between the measured tissue concentration data and the model prediction, ie,

$$\sum_{i=1}^{N} [C_i - C(T_i)]^2 \tag{32}$$

where there are N tissue measurements, C_i, $i = 1, \ldots, N$, at times T_i, and $C(T_i)$ is the model prediction of tissue activity at each of these times. This particular form is used because of the nature of the noise in the measured data. Parameter estimates produced by minimizing the sum of squared differences have minimum variability if the noise in each measurement is statistically independent, additive, Gaussian, and of equal magnitude. Additive and independent statistical noise is usually a good assumption for imaging data; however, sometimes the variance of the measurements will not be constant throughout multiple-scan acquisitions, particularly for short-lived isotopes such as ^{15}O or ^{11}C. In this case, the least-squares function can be modified to accommodate variable noise levels as follows:

$$\sum_{i=1}^{N} w_i[C_i - C(T_i)]^2 \tag{33}$$

where w_i is a weight assigned to data point i. This method is called *weighted least-squares estimation*, and the optimum weight for each sample is the inverse of the variance of the data.[42] For simple count data, the variance of the data can be estimated from the count data itself based on its Poisson distribution.[44] For reconstructed data, many algorithms have been proposed to calculate or approximate the noise in pixel or region-of-interest data.[45–50]

It is important to recognize that there are many potential error sources in the modeling process, excluding random noise, that cause inconsistencies between the model and measured data (see Sources of Error in Modeling Approaches). These nonrandom errors are called *deterministic*. When fitting data to a model, the parameter estimation procedure is naive in that it assumes that the specified model is absolutely correct. Therefore, if there are deterministic errors in the model or the input function, the estimation algorithm can produce unsuitable results. It may be appropriate in some situations to adjust the weights of some data points (eg, early time points where errors in the model due to intravascular activity are most significant) to reduce the sensitivity of the model to the presence of deterministic errors.

Once an optimization function (Equations 32 and 33) has been defined, there are many algorithms available to determine the values of the model parameters that minimize it.[40,42] Unfortunately, in most cases with compartmental models, there are no direct solutions for the parameters. This is true because, although the models themselves are linear (ie, all fluxes between compartments are linear multiples of the concentration in the source compartment), the solutions to these models are functions that are nonlinear in at least one of the model parameters. For example, Equation 27, the solution to the one-compartment model (Fig. 2B) is linear with respect to the parameter K_1 but is nonlinear with respect to the parameter k_2. To solve for the parameters, iterative algorithms are required. First, an initial guess is made for the parameter values. Then the algorithm repeatedly modifies the parameters at each step reducing the optimization function. Convergence is reached when changes to the parameters from one iteration to the next become exceedingly small. Great care is required in the use of iterative algorithms because incorrect solutions can be obtained, particularly if the initial guess is not appropriate.

Figure 5 provides an example of the process of parameter estimation applied to time-activity data collected after a bolus injection of fluorodeoxyglucose (FDG).[51] Figure 5A shows the measured plasma input function. Figure 5B shows a plot of region-of-interest values (occipital cortex) taken from reconstructed PET images. The solid line through the data points is the best fit obtained by minimizing the weighted sum of squared differences between the data and the two-compartment model (Figure 2C). Figure 5C shows a plot of the weighted residuals vs time. The *residual* is the difference between each data point and the model prediction. When weighted least-squares is used, the residuals are scaled by the square root of each weight, w_i, so that the sum-of-squares optimization function equals the sum of squared residuals. Ideally the residuals would be random, have zero mean, and uniform variance. If a good estimate of the noise level in the data is known, the weighted residuals should have a standard deviation of approximately 1. Thus, when plotting the residuals vs time or concentration, the residuals would appear as a uniform band centered on zero. The residuals in Figure 5C reasonably satisfy these expectations.

Many parameter estimation algorithms provide estimates of the uncertainties of the parameter estimates called *standard errors*. These values can be used as estimates of the minimum random uncertainty in the estimate. The algorithm determines these standard errors based on the structure of the model, the parameter estimates, and the magnitude of the residual sum of squares. Usually, however, this measure is an underestimate of the true uncertainty of the parameters, since there are usually many sources of errors that are not explicitly included.

It is also useful to calculate functions of the rate constants that provide different physiological information. For example, in the one-compartment model (Fig. 2B), a parameter estimation problem may be posed to estimate the rate constants K_1 and k_2. From these parameters, the distribution volume ($V = K_1/k_2$) can be calculated. To determine the uncertainty in the distribution volume estimate, information about the individual standard errors in K_1 and k_2 is required along with the correlation between them. The parameter estimates will be correlated, since both values are determined simultaneously from the same noisy data. The coefficient of variation (*CV*, the ratio of the standard error to the parameter

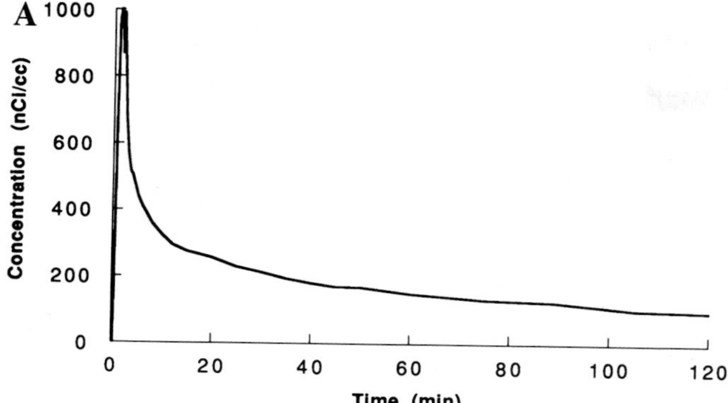

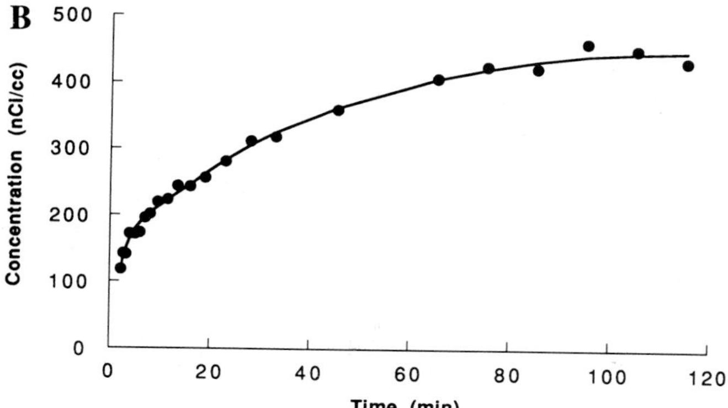

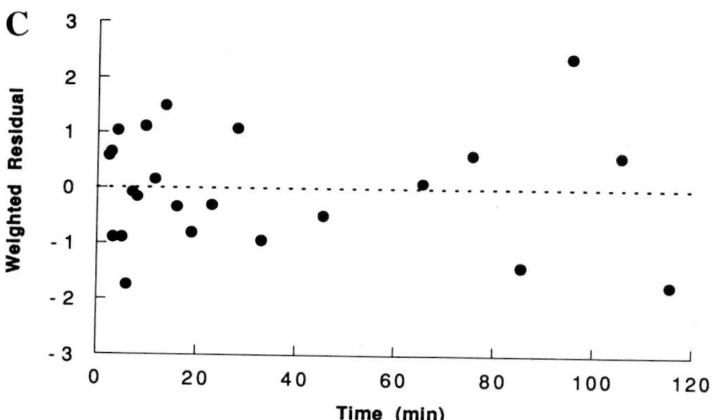

Figure 5. Examples of parameter estimation results from PET data after bolus injection of FDG. **(A).** Measured plasma time-activity curve. **(B).** Tissue time-activity curve from region-of-interest in occipital cortex. Symbols are measured data points. Solid line is fitted function for the two-compartment model (Fig. 2C) based on weighted least-squares parameter estimation. **(C).** Plot of weighted residuals vs time.

value) of the distribution volume can be calculated by propagation of errors calculations:

$$CV^2(V) = CV^2(K_1) + CV^2(k_2) - 2\,\rho_{12}\,CV(K_1)\,CV(k_2) \tag{34}$$

where ρ_{12} is the estimated correlation coefficient between the parameter estimates K_1 and k_2.

In some cases, estimated model rate constants have large uncertainties. However, algebraic functions of these rate constants may have less variability (due to the correlation between estimated model parameters) and may provide more useful physiological measures. For example, in a complete receptor model, the free receptor concentration B'_{max} appears in the rate constant describing the movement of tracer from a free to a bound compartment. Therefore, receptor information can be obtained from this rate constant or from functions that include this rate constant. The total volume of distribution, which can be derived from the model rate constants, has been found to be a particularly useful and reliable measure for receptor quantification.[52–54]

Least squares is the best optimization criterion for estimating parameters when a large number of assumptions are met. If any of these assumptions are not true, then better estimates may be obtained by other methods (see Error Analysis). A better estimate is one that may be more accurate (less biased) or more precise (less variable). In addition, iterative least-squares algorithms may be a computationally intensive procedure, particularly if it must be carried out individually for every pixel in an imaging volume. Often, iterative least-squares procedures are used only when being applied to a small number of regions of interest. However, it is often more useful if the data analysis procedure produces functional images where each pixel already represents a physiological parameter of interest. To do this, rapid computation schemes are required. Rapid implementations of iterative least-squares procedures have been developed for the simplest nonlinear models with just one nonlinear parameter, eg, the one-compartment model with solution in Equation 27. These techniques have been applied to the measurement of cerebral blood flow[55,56] and total volume of distribution of receptors.[53,57] In addition, a number of methods have been derived that allow direct noniterative calculation of the parameter estimates by reformulating the problem in terms of integrals of the tissue and blood data.[58–65] These methods do not minimize the sum-of-squares optimization function, but in many cases have been shown to have comparable statistical quality to the least-squares techniques and often have less sensitivity to deterministic errors in the model. Another interesting approach for parameter estimation from nonlinear models uses the methods of linear programming based on the knowledge that all the exponential clearance terms (eg, α_i in Equations 19 and 20) are positive.[66]

As shown above, the measured tissue activity is the convolution of the input function with the underlying impulse-response function (Equation 28). This impulse-response function has a much simpler mathematical form (usually a sum of exponentials) and is therefore more easily analyzed. Some investigators have used the approach of deconvolution, whereby an estimate of the impulse response function is determined from measurements of the tissue response and the input function.[67] However, because the process of deconvolution greatly amplifies noise in the tissue measurements and is often mathematically unstable, great care is required in the application of these techniques.

DEVELOPMENT OF MATHEMATICAL MODELS

The primary factor affecting the form of a model is the nature of the tracer itself. Usually, a priori information can be used to predict all of the relevant metabolic paths of the tracer in tissue, ie, a complete model. However, technical and statistical limitations of the available data will prevent the use of such a comprehensive model, which includes all steps in the physiological uptake, metabolism, and clearance of a tracer.

Figure 1 shows the process of development and application of a model in nuclear medicine.[68,69] This section presents the steps of starting with a complete model and then generating an *identifiable* model and ultimately a *useful* model. An identifiable model is one that can be applied to kinetic regional data and used to extract estimates of model parameters. Such a model is a simplified version of a comprehensive description of the interactions of a radiotracer in tissue. However, this model may not be workable if its parameter estimates are too variable or inaccurate. A useful model may be derived by further simplification of the identifiable model. The useful model provides reproducible and accurate estimates of model parameters. Validation studies are necessary to demonstrate these characteristics.

Model Identifiability

The first step in defining a model is to determine identifiability, which means that the parameters of a model can be uniquely determined from measurable data. There is an extensive literature on this topic,[16,19,70–76] including studies with particular attention to nuclear medicine applications.[77–79] In some cases, the structure of the model itself does not permit the unique definition of parameter values, even with noise-free data. One example of this is the case of high specific-activity studies with receptor-binding ligands. Here the association rate k_{on} and the free receptor concentration B'_{max} appear together as a product in the model differential equations (Equation 14) and can therefore not be separated.[32,80] A more significant problem in many applications is that of numerical identifiability. Here, parameter estimation can be successfully performed with low-noise data, but, with realistic noise levels, the uncertainties in the resulting parameter estimates are large. In addition, small deterministic errors in the model or in tissue radioactivity quantification can produce large changes in the parameter estimates. Thus, while an identifiable model is essential, it is not necessarily a useful model.

The process of model selection is as follows. Tissue measurements after injection of the radiopharmaceutical are collected. Then, a number of possible model configurations are proposed. Parameter estimation procedures are performed with the measured data using each model. The goodness-of-fit of each model to the data is assessed from the residual sum of squares (Equation 33) using statistical tests such as the F-test, the Akaike information criterion,[81] or the Schwarz criterion[82] to determine which model is most appropriate. In general, the use of a more complex model with additional parameters will produce a better fit to the data and a smaller residual sum of squares. However, this will be the case even if the additional parameters added by the more complex model are only providing a better fit to the noise in the data and have no relationship to the underlying true tissue model. The statistical tests used for model comparison determine whether the residual sum of squares has been reduced using the more complex model by an amount that is significantly greater than that expected by random chance.

Another useful approach for model comparison is the examination of the pattern of residuals as in Figure 5C.[42] If the residuals from a fit of one model configuration do not appear as randomly distributed around zero, then a more complex model may be appropriate. However, given all the error sources (see Sources of Error in Modeling Approaches), no model will ever be perfect. It will therefore often be the case that an overly complex model will still provide a statistically significant improvement in the fit compared to a simple model. The modeler must have a good understanding of the degree of accuracy in the data to avoid an unduly complicated model.

To simplify models, pairs of compartments can be collapsed together. Two compartments can be collapsed into one by assuming that the rate constants "connecting" them are large enough so that the two compartments remain in constant equilibrium. When this occurs, the physiological interpretation of the remaining rate constants in the reduced model must be changed. In this way, a set of "nested" models can be defined. Figure 2 shows some examples of nested models. Here a simple model with a few rate constants can be considered to be a special case of a more complex model with more parameters. For example, the model in Figure 2B is a simplified version of Figure 2C which is itself a simplified version of Figure 2D.

It is good practice to test a set of nested models to determine which one best characterizes a set of measured data.[53] An example of this process is shown in Figure 6 for the opiate receptor antagonist ^{18}F-cyclofoxy.[54,83–85] Figure 6A shows a typical time-activity curve measured in the thalamus with PET after bolus injection. The dots are measured data points. The solid line is the best weighted least-squares fit using a model with two tissue compartments (Fig. 2C). The dashed line is the best fit using a model with one tissue compartment (Fig. 2B). Both models also included an additional parameter to account for radioactivity present in the tissue vascular space, so five and three parameters were estimated, respectively. The plots of weighted residuals vs time from these fits are shown in Figures 6B (one compartment) and C (two compartment). The one-compartment results show a deterministic pattern of residuals. The residual points are not randomly distributed about zero, but instead show runs

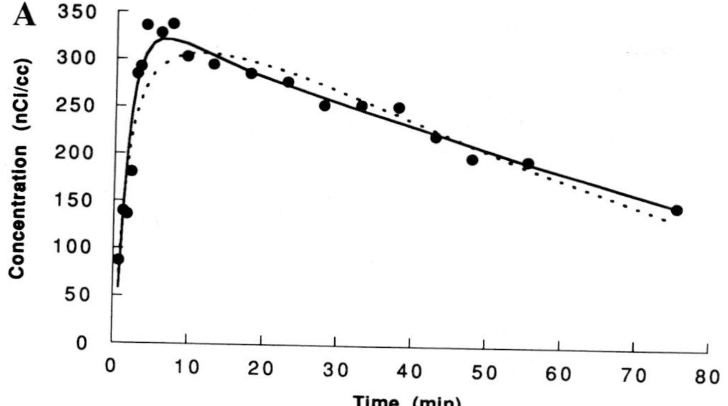

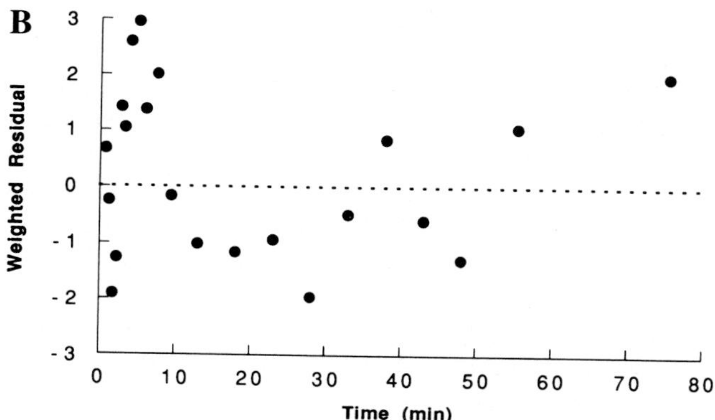

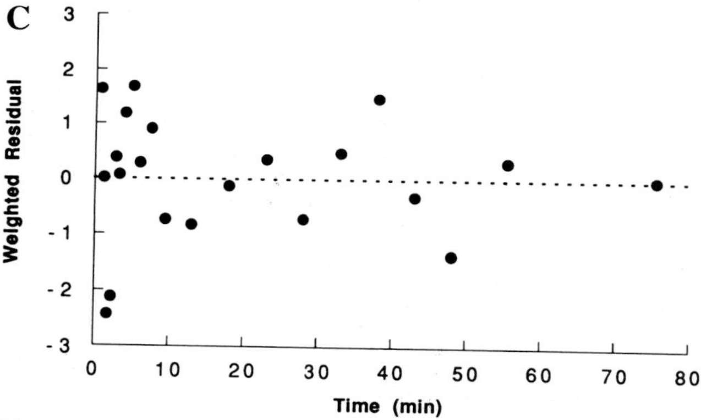

Figure 6. Comparison of model fits. **(A).** PET tissue concentration data from the thalamus acquired after bolus injection of the opiate antagonist ^{18}F-cyclofoxy. Symbols are measured data points. Solid line is weighted least-squares fit using a model with two compartments and five parameters (K_1, k_2, k_3, k_4, and vascular fraction). Dashed line is best fit using a model with one compartment and three parameters (K_1, k_2, and vascular fraction). **(B).** Plot of weighted residuals vs time for the three-parameter model. **(C).** Plot of weighted residuals vs time for the five-parameter model. The residuals for the three-parameter model show a nonrandom pattern that is reduced with the five-parameter model.

of sequential values that are all positive or all negative. The residual pattern is more random when using the two-compartment model. In this case, the more complex model was found to have produced a statistically significant reduction in the residual sum of squares. However, this improvement was not large and was not found uniformly for all patients or for all brain regions.

The absolute magnitude of the residual noise can also be useful in determining if a particular model configuration is appropriate. If the model is exactly correct and the magnitude of data noise is known, the weighted sum of squares (Equation 33) will be approximately equal to $N - n_p$, where N is the number of data points and n_p is the number of model parameters being estimated. If the actual sum of squares from data fits are close to this value, the modeler gains more confidence that the chosen model configuration is appropriate.

Model Constraints

A typical situation in nuclear medicine modeling problems is that a simple model with few parameters is often not adequate to describe the tissue concentration curve. However, a more complex model that does adequately describe the data frequently produces parameter estimates that have large uncertainties (standard errors). Specifically, a simple one-compartment, two-parameter model is often insufficient, whereas a two-compartment, four-parameter model is better by various statistically significant measures. A number of authors have dealt with this conflict by applying constraints. These entail specifying exact values for certain parameters or defining relationships between the parameters that must be met. In either case, the effect is to reduce the number of parameters that must be determined from the model. If the constraints are accurate (or reasonably so), then the sensitivity of the model to the remaining parameters is increased and the uncertainty in their estimation is reduced. Often the constraint equations use a priori values for physiological constants based on the presumed interpretation of the model parameters in terms of Michaelis-Menten parameters.[86–88] Alternatively, some parameters may be constrained based on measurements made in other regions. For example, a common approach for receptor-binding tracers is to first analyze a reference region known to have little or no specific binding to determine parameters associated with the magnitude of nonspecific binding. Then, regions with specific binding are analyzed with nonspecific-binding rate constants constrained to equal those estimated in the reference region.[80,89] Alternatively, additional studies can be performed to aid the estimation process by constraining parameters to be common to the analysis of both studies. For receptor-binding tracers, a study with an inactive enantiomer can be used to determine parameters of nonspecific binding.[90,91] In addition, paired studies with high-and low-specific-activity injections and/or displacement can be performed and analyzed simultaneously with some parameters shared in the models for the two studies.[92,93]

Validation of Physiological Measures

In the process of developing and selecting a suitable model formulation and methodology, it is important to perform validation studies that prove that the parameter estimates produced by a model are correct. These studies determine the precision and accuracy of model estimates, verify the legitimacy of the model assumptions, and help choose between various approaches. Such an evaluation invariably must be done in animals because of constraints on experimental design, scan duration, and radiation dosimetry in humans. Practical limits on animals studies include limitations on total blood sampling for input function measurements and the effects of anesthesia.

Although much of the work of model development and and validation is performed using small or large animals, it is important to realize that there are considerable differences between nuclear medicine image data and autoradiographic or tissue-sampling measurements, as well as the species differences among rodents, large animals, and humans, which may limit the applicability of the information obtained in the animal experiments. For example, measurement of tissue concentration data at multiple time points in rodents requires several animals. Nuclear medicine studies allow acquisition of multiple time points in a single study, avoiding interindividual variability. However, the spatial resolution and statistical reliability of image data are substantially worse than measurements from tissue samples in rats. Therefore, kinetic parameters that can be reliably determined from rat data may not be numerically identifiable from human imaging data. Therefore, many validation studies should be repeated wherever practical with human subjects.

The simplest test of a model is reproducibility, ie, what is the variability of the model parameters under identical conditions, either on the same day or different days[94]? Repeating studies on the same day generally produces smaller differences in imaging data results, since there is less variation in subject positioning and scanner calibration. Measurements of population variability of model estimates provide information concerning the most useful model configurations. Clearly, model parameters with large coefficients of variation are not generally useful. Also, models should provide physiologically reasonable values. Although in vivo measurements can certainly produce results different from in vitro tests, it is up to the investigator to demonstrate the accuracy of a model that produces parameter estimates inconsistent with previous results in the literature.

The next steps in validation of a model are intervention studies. Here, one or more of the physiological parameters that affect tracer uptake are altered, and the model is tested to verify that the model parameters change in the proper direction and by an appropriate magnitude in response to a variety of biologic stimuli. For example, brain blood flow can be altered by changing arterial pCO_2, or free receptor concentration can be reduced by administration of a cold ligand. It is also useful to test whether the parameters of interest do *not* change in response to a perturbation in a different factor, eg, does an estimate of receptor number remain unchanged when blood flow is increased?[95] Alternatively, changing the form of the input function should ideally have no effect of the model parameters.[54] Model assumptions, eg, parameters whose values have been constrained, should be tested. At a minimum, computer simulations of the effects of errors in various assumptions upon model results can be performed (see Error Analysis). The limitation of these simulations is that they are only as good as the models on which they are based. Therefore, experimental validation of model assumptions should be performed where possible.

Finally, the absolute accuracy of model parameters can be tested by direct comparison with a "gold standard." To test the accuracy of regional measurements, such a validation study can only be carried out with animals. While this validation step is appealing, is often difficult to achieve. There is often no gold standard available for the measurement of interest. Even if such a standard is available, the comparison requires careful matching of imaging data with tissue sample data. If the regions being compared are small, the effects of inaccurate registration and scanner resolution can make evaluation of the model's accuracy difficult at best. Even without a gold standard, other validations of the model can be performed. For example, model predictions of concentrations in separate compartments can be compared to biochemical measurements of tissue samples.[96] Also, microdialysis provides a method to assess extracellular tracer concentration directly for comparison to model predictions.[97]

MODEL-BASED METHODS

To this point, the design, development, and validation of a tracer kinetic model have been presented. Ideally, the modeling effort generates a complete, validated model that describes the relationship between tissue measurements and the underlying regional physiological parameters. With this knowledge, we can design a method of data acquisition and processing suitable for human studies. This section concerns this final step in the modeling process shown in Figure 1: the adaptation of such a useful model to produce a practical patient protocol.[68,98] It is often the case that the original modeling studies are complex and may not be suitable for human subjects, particularly certain patient populations. For example, arterial blood sampling may not be feasible, or a long data acquisition period may not be practical, or the statistical quality of data in humans may limit the number of parameters that can be reliably estimated. From the understanding of the characteristics of the tracer and with knowledge of the limitations imposed by instrumentation and logistical considerations, a model-based method can be developed that can achieve a useful level of physiological accuracy and reliability.

Many questions must be considered in converting a model into a model-based method. To what extent are the extra complexities of a full modeling study necessary or useful? What are the best tradeoffs to maintain an adequate signal-to-noise ratio in the data? Can an appropriate input function be measured less invasively than from arterial samples, eg, from direct image measurements, from venous samples, or from a reference region? What is a practical data collection period that is compatible with the time availability on the scanner, the statistical requirements of the collected images, and the characteristics of the patients? Which parameters are of prime importance? Can parameter estimates be calculated on a pixel-by-pixel basis to generate functional images or must iterative nonlinear methods be applied to region-of-interest data? What reasonable assumptions can be incorporated into the model to reduce the number of parameters to a workable set that can be determined with reasonable precision? Is the method overly sensitive to measurement errors or to inaccuracies in model assumptions, particularly in patient groups? If the method is simplified too much, could differences between patients and controls be exaggerated or hidden because physiological factors included in the original model are now excluded?

This section presents some approaches that have been used to produce model-based methods. These methods are generally simpler than the parameter estimation studies, use additional assumptions, and typically allow production of functional images of the physiological estimates. In addition, sources of error in model approaches are discussed along with error analysis methodology. Finally, the tradeoffs between using model-based techniques and simple empirical methods are examined.

Graphical Analysis

One increasingly common method applied to tracer kinetic data is that of graphical analysis.[86,99–104] The basic concept of this method is that, after appropriate mathematical transformation, the measured data can be converted into a straight-line plot whose slope and/or intercept has physiological meaning. This approach has advantages, since it is simple to verify visually the linearity of the data and it is easy to determine the slope and intercept by noniterative linear regression methods. It is also generally easy to determine these values on a pixel-by-pixel basis, thus producing a functional image of the parameter.[105] For many models, the simplified equations of graphical analysis do not apply for all times postinjection, eg, at early times when the blood activity is changing rapidly and some tissue compartments have not yet reached equilibrium with the blood. Therefore, care must be taken in selecting the time period for determining the slope and intercept. However, it is also true that avoiding the time periods where the kinetics are rapid also makes the methods less sensitive to errors introduced by oversimplifications in the model, particularly those dealing with tracer exchange between capillary, extracellular space, and intracellular space.

The most widely used graphical analysis technique is the Patlak plot.[99–101] This approach is appropriate when there is an irreversible or nearly irreversible trapping step in the model. Conceptually, the transformations of the Patlak plot convert a bolus injection experiment to a constant infusion. A simple example of this model is the two-compartment model (Fig. 2C), in which the rate constant for return of tracer from compartment 2 to compartment 1, k_4, is zero or is small, ie, irreversible trapping. In this case, the model solution (from Equations 21, 22, and 28) for the total tissue tracer concentration $C(t)$ for an arbitrary input function $C_a(t)$ is

$$(35) \qquad C(t) = C_a(t) \otimes \left(\frac{K_1k_2}{k_2 + k_3} exp[-(k_2 + k_3)t] + \frac{K_1k_3}{k_2 + k_3}\right)$$

If the arterial input function were held constant, the solution to Equation 35 would be

$$(36) \qquad C(t) = C_a \left(\frac{K_1k_2}{(k_2 + k_3)^2} (1 - exp[-(k_2 + k_3)t] + \frac{K_1k_3}{k_2 + k_3} t\right)$$

After an appropriate time, t^*, after which the exponential term in Equation 36 is sufficiently small, the ratio of tissue to blood activity becomes

$$(37) \qquad \frac{C(t)}{C_a} = \frac{K_1k_2}{(k_2 + k_3)^2} + \frac{K_1k_3}{k_2 + k_3} t$$

which is a linear equation. The slope of this equation, K, is

$$(38) \qquad K = \frac{K_1k_3}{k_2 + k_3}$$

This is the net uptake rate of tracer into the irreversibly bound compartment 2. It is the product of two terms: K_1, the rate of entry into the tissue from the blood, and $k_3/(k_2 + k_3)$, the fraction of the tracer that enters the tissue that reaches the irreversible compartment.

For the case in which the input function is not a constant, the Patlak transformation is as follows:

$$(39) \qquad \frac{C(t)}{C_a(t)} = V_0 + K \left(\frac{\int_0^t C_a(s)\, ds}{C_a(t)}\right)$$

The term in large brackets is often called *stretched time* or normalized time, since it has units of time and it distorts time based on the nature of the input function. If the ratio of tissue to blood activity, which is called the apparent volume of distribution, is plotted vs stretched time, under the appropriate conditions, a linear plot is obtained with slope K and intercept V_0 (the initial volume of distribution). Note that, in the case of a constant arterial input, stretched time becomes exactly equal to true time.

Figure 7 provides an example of the use of Patlak plot as applied to brain PET data after the injection of FDG.[51] In this study, subjects were studied on two occasions, approximately 1 week apart. For one scan, the subjects underwent a hyperinsulinemic euglycemic clamp, whereby high levels of insulin were infused, and simultaneously blood glucose levels were maintained at a constant level, thus ensuring the steady-state assumption of the tracer kinetic model. On the second occasion, a sham clamp was performed, ie, a control study. Figure 7A shows the measured plasma input functions for the two studies in one individual. The high insulin levels in the clamp study caused a dramatic increase in the rate of FDG clearance from plasma. Figure 7B shows the tissue curves for an average of gray matter regions. There is clearly a dramatic difference in the two curves. The Patlak transformation of Equation 39 was applied to this data and is shown in Figure 7C with a plot of the apparent volume of distribution vs stretched time. The two plots nearly overlay each other, demonstrating that most of the difference between the two tissue time-activity curves of Figure 7B can be accounted for by the differences in the input function, not by differences in the tissue kinetic parameters. Note that the hyperinsulinemic study covers a longer period in stretched time than the control study.

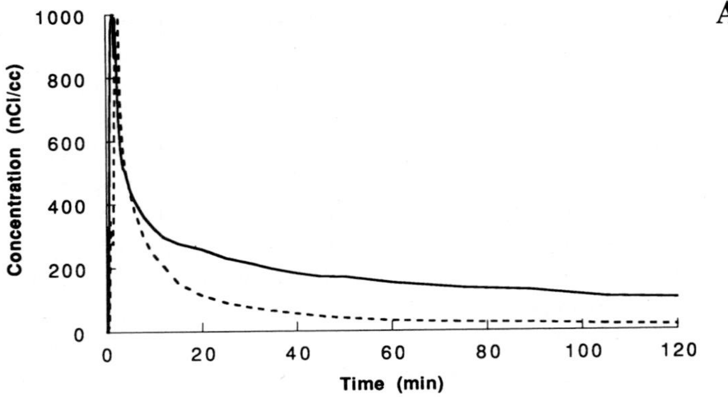

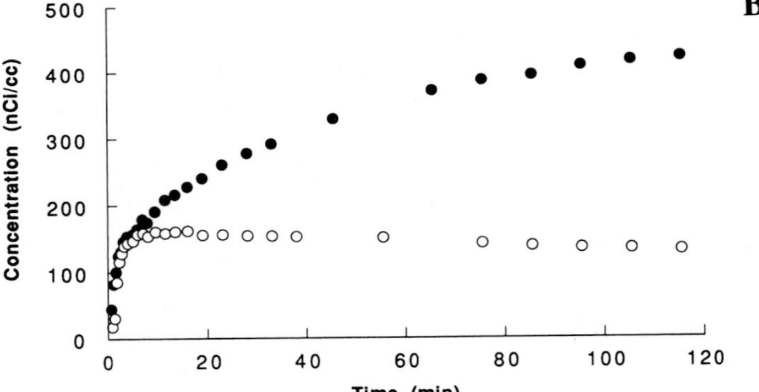

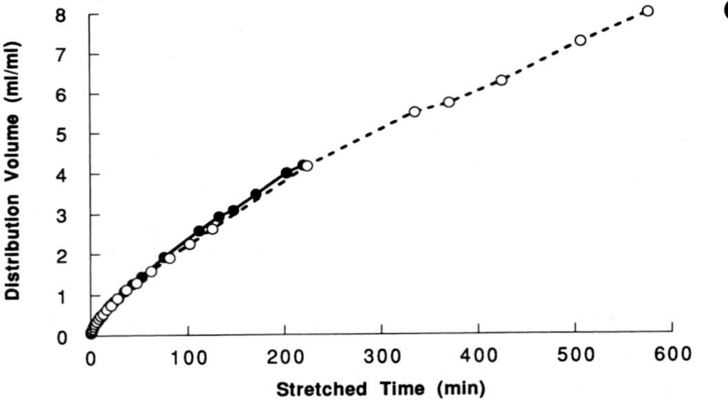

Figure 7. Example of graphical analysis (Patlak plot) from FDG PET data. The study involved a control scan one day and a hyperinsulinemic euglycemic clamp on another day. **(A).** Plasma input functions. Solid line is the control study and the dashed line is the clamp study. The high insulin levels produce substantially more rapid plasma clearance of FDG. **(B).** Average tissue time concentration curves in cortical gray matter. Filled and open symbols are imaging data values from the control and clamp studies, respectively. **(C).** Patlak plots from the control (filled symbols and solid line) and clamp (open symbols and dashed line) studies computed from the data in A and B using Equation 39. Despite the large differences in plasma and tissue data between the two studies due to the different insulin levels, the tissue kinetics in both cases as shown by graphical analysis are very similar, ie, there is at most a small effect of insulin on gray matter metabolism of FDG.

Single-Scan Techniques

A common approach to produce simplified model-based methods is the use of single-scan techniques. Here, based on a good understanding of the relationship between tissue radioactivity and the underlying physiological parameters, tissue radioactivity information is acquired during one scan interval. This single measurement permits the estimation of a single unknown physiological parameter. Since most models have multiple rate constants, some corrections must be applied to account for these other unknowns. Careful design of a single-scan technique ensures that variation in these nuisance parameters produces only minor errors in the parameter of interest.

For the measurement of cerebral blood flow with ^{15}O-H_2O or comparable diffusible tracers, two approaches have been taken to produce single-scan methods. Some of the earliest studies used continuous inhalation of ^{15}O-CO_2,[106] which is rapidly converted to ^{15}O-H_2O in the lungs. By achieving constant radioactivity levels, the derivative in the differential equation of uptake of the tracer (Equation 15 with additional terms for radioactive decay) can be set to zero, and K_1 can be determined from an algebraic formula in terms of tissue and blood radioactivity. A different approach uses a bolus injection followed by a single short scan.[107,108] This autoradiographic method uses the explicit solution of the model (Equation 27) to determine K_1 from the integrated tissue radioactivity and a measured input function. Both of these methods treat the estimated K_1 values as equal to blood flow, assuming a large permeability-surface area product for the tracer (Equation 5). Both methods also require the use of an assumed value for the tracer distribution volume V in order to specify k_2 as K_1/V. Because only one tissue measurement is made, only one unknown parameter can be determined. The short scan of the autoradiographic method was designed in part to minimize the sensitivity of this method to errors in the assumed value of the distribution volume.

Another example of single-scan, model-based techniques is the autoradiographic method for measurement of glucose metabolism, which was developed in rats with ^{14}C-deoxyglucose[1] and extended to PET using ^{18}F-2-fluoro-2-deoxy-D-glucose.[2–4] These methods take advantage of the fact that most of the radioactivity in the tissue approximately 45 minutes postinjection has been phosphorylated, so that the total tissue radioactivity can be used to estimate the net flux into tissue of deoxyglucose, K. This is the same rate constant as determined from the slope of the Patlak plot. Effectively, these methods estimate the slope of a Patlak plot by using the measured tissue value as one data point and by using population values of the model rate constants to estimate the y-intercept of the straight line. A number of other formulations of this approach have been developed,[109–111] each with different sensitivities to errors in the assumed rate constants. Finally, since FDG is an analog of glucose, the metabolic rate of glucose is estimated from the measured net flux of FDG using the measured plasma glucose level and an assumed scaling factor, the lumped constant.[1,5–9]

Another single-scan technique has been developed for quantification of receptors using infusion to produce true equilibrium.[54,112,113] By administering tracer as a combination of bolus plus continuous infusion, constant radioactivity levels can be reached in blood and in all regions of interest. The total tissue volume of distribution can be determined from the ratio of tissue activity to metabolite-corrected plasma activity. This value will include free, nonspecifically bound, and specifically bound tracer. Estimates of the nonspecific component, eg, from a region with low receptor binding, measurements with an inactive enantiomer, or made after displacement with excess cold ligand, can be subtracted to estimate the binding potential, B_{max}/K_D.[114] (K_D is the dissociation equilibrium constant.) Multiple infusions at different specific activities can be used to determine B_{max}.[84,115]

Sources of Error in Modeling Approaches

In making the choices necessary to implement a tracer method, it is important to be aware of the many sources of error that affect the precision and accuracy of these physiological measurements.[98] A good understanding of what effects are more or less significant to a given tracer and to the particular biologic question of interest is essential in designing a sensitive, reliable technique that is not overly complex. Here we do not consider random statistical noise in the data, but rather nonrandom deterministic errors. Table 1 lists sources of errors in modeling methods. These factors are discussed in this section.

Table 1. Sources of Error in Modeling

- Tissue radioactivity measurements
  - Resolution—partial volume effect
  - Attenuation and accuracy of attenuation correction
  - Scatter and accuracy of scatter correction
  - Randoms and accuracy of random correction
  - Deadtime and accuracy of deadtime correction
  - Detector normalization
  - Reconstruction algorithm and filter
  - Object size and radioactivity distribution within object
  - Local radioactivity contrast
  - Region size and data sampling strategy
  - Region-of-interest placement accuracy (including errors due to registration with anatomical images)
  - Subject or organ motion
- Models
  - Model oversimplifications (eg, lumping compartments)
  - Intravascular radioactivity
  - Heterogeneity in regional data
  - Incorrect values for assumed model parameters
  - Change in physiological parameters during imaging period
  - Associated blood measurements (eg, blood glucose concentration)
  - Tomograph—blood counting calibration
  - Use of venous blood instead of arterial blood for the input function
  - The measurement of the input function
    - Speed of sampling
    - Sample timing
    - Sample counting
    - Pipetting/weighing
    - Counting corrections
    - Data handling
    - Metabolite correction
    - Plasma protein binding measurements
  - Difference between organ and peripheral input function
    - Delay
    - Dispersion
  - Parameter estimation uncertainties

The measurement of regional radioactivity from imaging devices is a primary source of error (see Chapters 5 and 6). Although the quantitative accuracy of imaging methodology continues to improve, there are still many sources of inaccuracies. Quantitative SPECT depends upon accurate corrections for attenuation, varying resolution with depth, and scatter. PET imaging is quantitatively more accurate, but the accuracy of scatter corrections is limited, particularly for whole-body imaging and for 3-D septaless acquisition. A key effect corrupting all nuclear medicine imaging modalities is finite resolution, ie, the partial volume effect.[116] The magnitude of bias in concentration measurements depends on the size of the underlying structure, the distribution of radiotracer within and around the structure, the resolution of the imaging device, the reconstruction algorithm, and the strategy for extracting regional concentration values. Definition of the regions of interest using registered anatomical scans (MRI or CT) is important, as long as registration errors are minimized.

The partial volume effect produces heterogeneity, that

is, the tissue response measured from even a single pixel represents a weighted average of the tissue in the surrounding region, and is thus a combination of different kinetic responses. This can have minimal to large effects on model results depending on the magnitude of heterogeneity and how the parameter of interest affects the tissue concentration measurements. This effect has been studied in great detail for a number of methods.[117–122] Since finite resolution is unavoidable in real imaging data, ideally application of modeling techniques will not introduce artifactual changes in the data. In other words, suppose a heterogeneous region was composed of two tissue types. Ideally, the kinetic estimates from that area would be weighted averages of the appropriate values for each tissue type, weighted by the fraction of the region occupied by each tissue type. If the parameter is estimated in a linear fashion from the data, this will be the case.

Another source of error in model applications is the presence of intravascular radioactivity in the tissue measurements.[123–128] Some fraction of the measured counts originate from radioactivity in the blood within the tissue. Since the radioactivity time course in blood differs from that in tissue, errors in model measurements occur unless this effect is properly handled. Often, the fraction of tissue volume occupied by blood can be measured in a separate tracer experiment. Alternatively, this vascular fraction is added as a parameter to account for this effect. Obviously, these errors are most important in regions with large blood volumes or in regions near the heart chambers or large blood vessels. Typically, errors due to vascular radioactivity are more significant when data collected immediately after injection are included in the analysis. However, these early data are often most sensitive to the parameter of interest, such as in the case of blood flow tracers where the rate constant for movement of tracer from blood into tissue is of prime importance. Various strategies involving selection of time intervals for analysis or optimum region-of-interest placement have been proposed to handle these effects.[126,129]

A key to successful quantitative methods is the accurate measurement of the input function. Typically, the blood time-activity curve is measured in a peripheral blood vessel (usually radial artery) unless the heart chambers can be imaged directly.[130–132] When individual blood samples are drawn by hand, they must be taken at a sufficiently rapid rate to characterize the curve accurately. Careful attention is required for accurate sample timing, centrifugation, pipetting or weighing, radioactivity counting, counting corrections (background, decay, dead time, etc), and data handling. Some investigators have developed devices for automatic withdrawal and measurement of whole blood radioactivity.[133] These devices provide consistent data, but they may have increased statistical noise depending upon their counting geometry. Timing and dispersion differences between the brain and the peripheral artery require correction, particularly for studies of short duration with sharp bolus

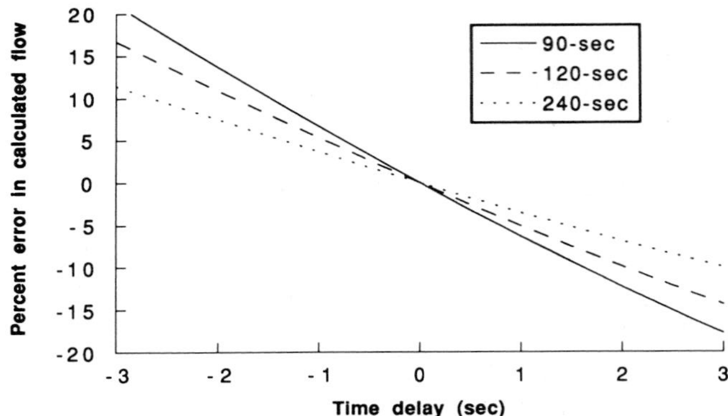

Figure 8. Example of error analysis—the effect of errors in time delay corrections between the brain and peripheral artery on measurement of cerebral blood flow with $^{15}O\text{-}H_2O$. A positive time delay means that the tissue data have been shifted forward in time with respect to the arterial input function. The three curves show the percent error in estimated flow, based on data collection periods of 90, 120, and 240 seconds. See text for additional details.

inputs.[134–137] A number of studies have been undertaken to assess the effects of statistical noise in the input function on estimated parameters and to develop appropriate estimation methodology.[138–141] If there are radioactive metabolites of the tracer in blood, it is important to determine the percentage of blood radioactivity that corresponds to the original tracer as well as the extent to which these metabolites pass into tissue. Since metabolite determinations are often complex, particularly for short-lived tracers, metabolite measurements are made at only a small number of postinjection time points. Appropriate interpolation or modeling schemes are necessary to generate a continuous estimate of the metabolite fraction throughout the study.[142]

Error Analysis

Error analysis is a useful tool in developing an appropriate model-based method. A thorough error analysis is a critical step in assessing the utility of a given method. Papers dedicated solely to error analysis are commonly found in the literature.[117,118,126,143–152] These analyses usually proceed as follows: (1) Choose a particular source of error. (2) Select values for the model parameters and use the model equations to simulate tissue data including this error effect, usually covering a range of effect magnitudes. (3) Then, analyze these simulated measurements with one or more methods, compare the derived parameter estimates to their original values, and determine the magnitude of error that is produced.

Figure 8 provides an example of the results of an error analysis. Cerebral blood flow measurements with the tracer $^{15}O\text{-}H_2O$ are altered in the presence of errors in correction for the time delay between the measured arterial input function and the actual input to the brain. Using an actual measured input function, tissue time activity data were simulated over a 4-minute period using the model of Equation 27, with a flow value of 0.5 mL/min/g and a distribution volume of 0.8 mL/g. CBF (K_1) was then calculated by direct estimation of the two model parameters for total time intervals of 90, 120, and 240 seconds. In each case, the tissue data were shifted with respect to the arterial input function by -3 to $+3$ seconds (a positive shift means that the tissue data have been shifted later in time with respect to the blood data). The figure shows the percent error as a function of time delay. Positive time shifts produce underestimates in blood flow. This error is larger for shorter total acquisition times. This analysis suggests that the effect of time shift errors can be reduced by using longer data acquisition periods. Even then, errors as large as 10% occur with time shifts of 3 seconds, so care should be taken to measure or estimate time delays between tissue and blood data.[136,153]

A careful analysis of all the relevant error sources can be used to optimize methodology or to choose one approach over another. For example, various studies have been performed to choose opimum total imaging times and scan schedules.[125,154–156] Unfortunately, it is difficult to determine the total error of a method based on the independent error analyses of a number of measurements or assumptions. First, error analyses are only as good as their ability to simulate the biologic reality. That includes recognizing and analyzing all potential error sources and making appropriate choices for the magnitude of each error term. Even then, many error sources are not independent, ie, errors in one term affect other terms. Thus actual errors may be larger or smaller than those predicted from independent error analyses. Therefore, it is best if the ultimate choice of a method can be made by analyzing many studies with a variety of techniques and choosing the approach that has the best reproducibility, the minimum population variability, or the maximum statistical power to extract a particular physiological signal.

Selection of Model-based Methods

This chapter has presented an overview of modeling methods, from the most complex dynamic data acquisition with iterative parameter estimation to simplified methods including Patlak plots or single-scan techniques. Choosing the best approach is not simple, and other options are available when selecting a tracer method. In some studies, investigators normalize the physiological measurements. Instead of using the absolute values provided by a method, these results are scaled in some manner by a reference value, such as the average value in the entire organ or in a particular reference structure. This procedure may significantly reduce intersubject variation introduced by instrumentation, reconstruction, and application of the model, as well as variability due to global flow, metabolism, etc. In some cases where the model equations are linear (or nearly so) with respect to the parameter of interest, investigators can avoid measuring the input function and use normalized tissue concentration measurements as equivalent to a normalized model-based method.[107,157,158] Interpretation of results from normalized methods must be performed with care, however, since changes in ratios may be caused by changes in the numerator, denominator, or both.

An alternative to using a model-based method is to use a simple empirical approach. Such approaches make no explicit attempt to estimate the physiological parameter(s) of interest. Instead, an index based on tissue measurements is used and presumed to reflect the underlying physiology. Empirical indices include absolute radioactivity values, radioactivity values corrected for dose and/or subject weight, and ratios of radioactivity values between target and reference regions (normalized values).

How can an investigator determine the best approach when using a tracer? Many tradeoffs must be considered in designing a study, and there are no simple answers.[98] As an example, consider the use of a receptor-binding radiotracer for measurements in the brain with PET. Suppose the tracer binds reversibly, ie, its dissociation rate from the receptor is sufficiently fast to approach equilibrium during the study period. Possible model-based quantification approaches include the following: (1) complete modeling study with iterative parameter estimation; (2) use of a simplified model with estimation of the volume of distribution[53]; and (3) use of a linearization formula to derive the volume of distribution from the later portion of the data.[103] Empirical alternatives to model-based methods include the following: (1) ratio of tissue region of interest to (metabolite-corrected) blood during the apparent equilibrium phase or (2) ratio of tissue region of interest to reference region with few receptors during the apparent equilibrium phase.

Although the empirical approaches are the simplest, they can provide misleading results. For tracers that can reversibly bind with receptors, indices derived from ratios of tissue concentration to reference regions or to plasma levels can be significantly distorted due to lack of true equilibrium.[54] This effect is demonstrated in Figure 9 with a "bolus plus infusion" protocol in the baboon using the opiate antagonist ^{18}F-cyclofoxy (see Single-Scan Techniques). In one study, the infusion was interrupted at 70 minutes postinjection. The purpose of this interruption was to demonstrate with measured data the sensitivity of ratio measures, in particular the ratio of tissue to metabolite-corrected plasma (the apparent volume of distribution), to the plasma clearance rate. Radioactivity in the plasma (Fig. 9A) and tissue regions (Fig. 9B) reached steady levels by 20 and 30 minutes, respectively. At 70 minutes postinjection, the infusion was discontinued, and plasma and tissue concentrations dropped. Figure 9C shows the apparent volume of distribution plotted against time. Discontinuing the infusion caused a dramatic increase in the receptor-rich thalamus with smaller increases in frontal cortex and cerebellum. The magnitude of this effect depends upon the relative magnitudes of the rate of tracer clearance from plasma and the receptor dissociation rate. The change in Figure 9C is due solely to the change in clearance of radiotracer from plasma and demonstrates that this ratio

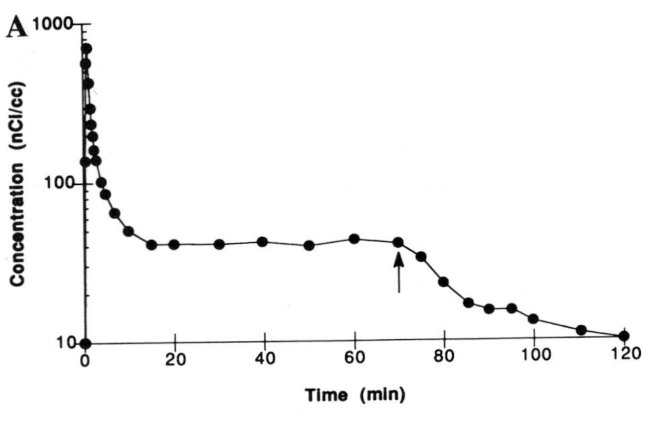

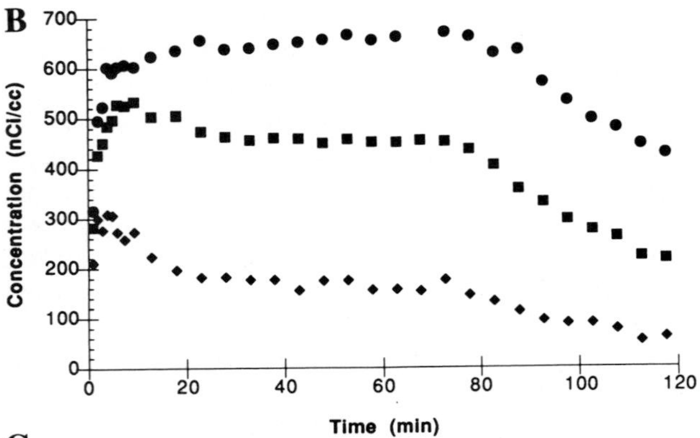

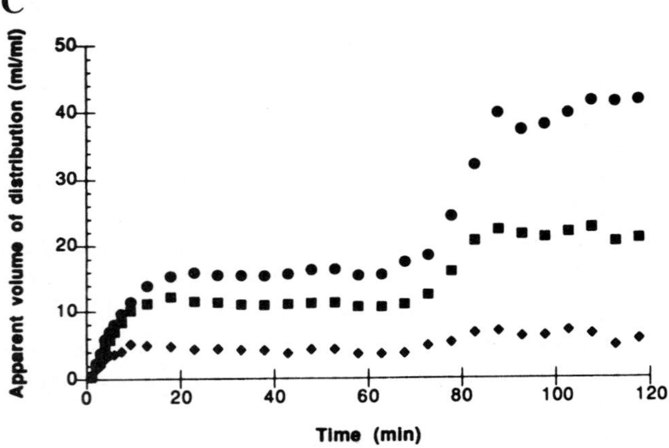

Figure 9. Effect of transient equilibrium on tissue concentration and apparent volume of distribution (ratio of tissue to metabolite-corrected plasma) as demonstrated by a discontinued-infusion study. **(A).** Total plasma radioactivity. ^{18}F-cyclofoxy was administered according to a bolus/infusion protocol, but the infusion was discontinued at 70 minutes (arrow). **(B).** Tissue time-activity data for thalamus (●), frontal cortex (■), and cerebellum (◆). **(C).** Apparent volume of distribution as a function of time for regions in B. There is a dramatic increase in apparent distribution volume due to increased plasma clearance beginning at 70 minutes. See text for additional details.

measure can be significantly affected by the plasma clearance rate.

Another choice to be made with this type of study is how to administer the tracer, ie, as a bolus or as a continuous infusion to reach equilibrium.[54,112] Use of infusions has advantages and disadvantages. Data analysis is greatly simplified, since the volume of distribution can be obtained directly from the ratio of tissue radioactivity to metabolite-corrected blood. Scans need only be collected during the equilibrium period, providing more patient comfort. Scans can be acquired and analyzed at different axial positions, since measurement of a full time course of tracer activity is not required. Fewer measurements in blood are required. Also, the technique is model independent and only relies on equilibrium conditions. However, if true equilibrium is not obtained, errors that could have been eliminated by a more complex modeling procedure will occur. Due to normal variation in plasma clearance rates of the tracer, deviations from equilibrium add variability to the results. The time interval corresponding to true equilibrium must be carefully assessed and ideally verified in each subject. There are also increased logistical requirements due to a long infusion of radioactivity compared to a simple bolus injection. Furthermore, it is necessary to assess whether bolus or infusion approaches provide better statistical quality to the physiological measurements.

SIGNAL-TO-NOISE CONSIDERATIONS

Does the use of model-based methods improve the signal-to-noise characteristics of data? In other words, can small biologic signals be detected more easily by using modeling methodology? Use of appropriate quantification methodology can reduce intersubject variability by accounting for factors affecting the raw concentration measurements that are unrelated to the physiological measure of interest. If intersubject variability is decreased, the power of the study to detect group differences is increased. However, if this extraneous variability is small, then use of a model-based method may produce little improvement in the signal-to-noise ratio. In fact, since there are a large number of potential sources of error in applying modeling techniques (Table 1), errors in these corrections or in the implementation of these procedures can actually increase variability over simpler, empirical methods. The net effect of applying a model on measurement variability thus depends upon the magnitude of physiological variation in the patient groups that can be removed by the model vs the accuracy of the model and the reliability of the additional measurements that it requires.

MODEL-BASED VS EMPIRICAL METHODS

Model-based methods have one important advantage over empirical approaches. With model-based results, it is easier to justify the conclusion that any significant findings are in fact due to real differences in the biologic function of interest and not due to extraneous physiological factors. When empirical methods detect significant differences, these other physiological factors may contribute substantially to the measured differences. Thus, interpretation of the results is less straightforward. This is particularly true when there are known differences in physiology between subject groups in a study. For example, if plasma tracer clearance differs between patients and control subjects, substantial errors may be made if tissue radioactivity values are directly interpreted as reflecting the relevant physiological process. On these grounds, model-based methods, which usually require a more complicated study procedure, are superior to empirical approaches. It is important, however, to remember that model-based methods rely on many assumptions, which can produce misleading results when applied inappropriately. For example, in ischemic tissue, the FDG rate constants and the lumped constant differ from normal.[6,159,160] If appropriate lumped constant and rate constant values are not used in single-scan FDG studies, the results may be as misleading as an empirical index.

REFERENCES

1. Sokoloff L, Reivich M, Kennedy C, Des Rosiers MH, Patlak CS, Pettigrew KD, Sakurada O, Shinohara M. The [^{14}C]deoxyglucose method for the measurement of local cerebral glucose utilization; theory, procedure, and normal values in the conscious and anesthetized albino rat. *J Neurochem* 1977; 28:897–916.
2. Reivich M, Kuhl D, Wolf A, Greenberg J, Phelps M, Ido T, Casella V, Fowler J, Hoffman E, Alavi A, Som P, Sokoloff L. The [^{18}F]fluorodeoxyglucose method for the measurement of local cerebral glucose utilization in man. *Circ Res* 1979; 44:127–137.
3. Phelps ME, Huang SC, Hoffman EJ, Selin C, Sokoloff L, Kuhl DE. Tomographic measurement of local cerebral glucose metabolic rate in humans with (F-18) 2-fluoro-2-deoxy-D-glucose: validation of method. *Ann Neurol* 1979;6:371–388.
4. Huang SC, Phelps ME, Hoffman EJ, Sideris K, Selin CJ, Kuhl DE. Non-invasive determination of local cerebral metabolic rate of glucose in man. *Am J Physiol* 1980;238: E69–E82.
5. Reivich M, Alavi A, Wolf A, Fowler J, Russell J, Arnett C, MacGregor RR, Shiue CY, Atkins H, Anand A, Dann R, Greenberg JH. Glucose metabolic rate kinetic model parameter determination in humans: the lumped constants and rate constants for [^{18}F]fluorodeoxyglucose and [^{11}C]deoxyglucose. *J Cereb Blood Flow Metab* 1985;5:179–192.
6. Gjedde A, Wienhard K, Heiss WD, Kloster G, Diemer NH, Herholz K, Pawlik G. Comparative regional analysis of 2-fluorodeoxyglucose and methylglucose uptake in brain of four stroke patients. With special reference to the regional estimation of the lumped constant. *J Cereb Blood Flow Metab* 1985;5:163–178.
7. Spence A, Graham M, Muzi M, Abbott G, Krohn K, Kapoor R, Woods S. Deoxyglucose lumped constant estimated in a transplanted rat astrocytic glioma by the hexose utilization index. *J Cereb Blood Flow Metab* 1990;10:190–198.
8. Dienel GA, Cruz NF, Mori K, Holden JE, Sokoloff L. Direct measurement of the lambda of the lumped constant of the deoxyglucose method in rat brain: determination of lambda and lumped constant from tissue glucose concentration or equilibrium brain/plasma distribution ratio for methylglucose. *J Cereb Blood Flow Metab* 1991;11:25–34.
9. Holden JE, Mori K, Dienel GA, Cruz NF, Nelson T, Sokoloff L. Modeling the dependence of hexose distribution volumes in brain on plasma glucose concentration: implications for estimation of the local 2-deoxyglucose lumped constant. *J Cereb Blood Flow Metab* 1991;11:171–182.
10. Heymann M, Payne B, Hoffman J, Rudolph A. Blood flow measurements with radionuclide-labeled particles. *Prog Cardiovasc Dis* 1977;20:55–79.
11. Phelps ME, Huang S-C, Hoffman EJ, Selin C, Kuhl DE. Cerebral extraction of N-13 ammonia: its dependence on cerebral blood flow and capillary permeability—surface area product. *Stroke* 1981;12:607–619.
12. Neirinckx R, Canning L, Piper I, Nowotnik D, Pickett R, Holmes R, Volkert W, Forster A, Weisner P, Marriott J, Chaplin S. Tc-99m d,1-HM-PAO: a new radiopharmaceutical for SPECT imaging of regional cerebral blood perfusion. *J Nucl Med* 1987;28:191–202.
13. Kety SS. The theory and applications of the exchange of inert gas at the lungs and tissues. *Pharmacol Rev* 1951;3: 1–41.
14. Zierler KL. Circulation times and the theory of indicator-dilution methods for determining blood flow and volume. In: *Handbook of Physiology.* Baltimore: Waverly Press, 1962, 585–615.
15. Lassen NA, Peri W. *Tracer Kinetic Methods in Medical Physiology.* New York: Raven Press, 1979.
16. Carson ER, Cobelli C, Finkelstein L. *The Mathematical Modeling of Metabolic and Endocrine Systems.* New York: John Wiley & Sons, 1983.
17. Lambrecht R, Rescigno A, ed. *Tracer Kinetics and Physiological Modeling.* Berlin: Springer-Verlag, 1983.
18. Peters A. A unified approach to quantification by kinetic analysis in nuclear medicine. *J Nucl Med* 1993;34:706–713.
19. DiStefano JJ. Non-compartmental vs. compartmental analysis: some basis for choice. *Am J Physiol* 1982;243:R1–R6.
20. Johnson J, Wilson T. A model for capillary exchange. *Am J Physiol* 1966;210:1299–1303.
21. Bassingthwaighte JB. A concurrent flow model for extraction during transcapillary passage. *Circ Res* 1974;35:483–503.
22. Bassingthwaighte JB, Holloway GA. Estimation of blood flow with radioactive tracers. *Semin Nucl Med* 1976;6:141–161.
23. Goresky CA, Ziegler WH, Bach GG. Capillary exchange modeling: brain-limited and flow-limited distribution. *Circ Res* 1970;27:739–764.
24. Rose CP, Goresky CA. Constraints on the uptake of labeled palmitate by the heart. *Circ Res* 1977;41:534–545.
25. Larson KB, Markham J, Raichle ME. Comparison of distributed and compartmental models for analysis of cerebral blood flow measurements. *J Cereb Blood Flow Metab* 1985; 5(suppl 1):649, 650.
26. Larson KB, Markham J, Raichle ME. Tracer-kinetic models for measuring cerebral blood flow using externally detected radiotracers. *J Cereb Blood Flow Metab* 1987;7:443–463.
27. van Osdol W,Sung C, Dedrick R, Weinstein J. A distributed pharmacokinetic model of two-step imaging and treatment protocols using streptavidin-conjugated monoclonal antibodies and radiolabeled biotin. *J Nucl Med* 1993;34:1552–1564.
28. Jacquez JA. *Compartmental Analysis in Biology and Medicine.* Amsterdam: Elsevier/North-Holland, 1972.
29. Wagner JG. *Fundamentals of Clinical Pharmacokinetics.* Hamilton, IL: Drug Intelligence, 1975.
30. Anderson D. *Compartmental Modeling and Tracer Kinetics.* Berlin: Springer-Verlag, 1983.
31. Robertson J, ed. *Compartmental Distribution of Radiotracers.* Boca Raton, FL: CRC Press, 1983.
32. Huang SC, Barrio JR, Phelps ME. Neuroreceptor assay with positron emission tomography. *J Cereb Blood Flow Metab* 1986;6:515–521.

33. Renkin EM. Transport of potassium-42 from blood to tissue in isolated mammalian skeletal muscles. *Am J Physiol* 1959;197:1205–1210.
34. Crone C. Permeability of capillaries in various organs as determined by use of the indicator diffusion method. *Acta Physiol Scand* 1964;58:292–305.
35. Lehninger A. *Biochemistry*. New York: Worth, 1975.
36. Eckelman W, ed. *Receptor-Binding Radiotracers*. Boca Raton, FL: CRC Press, 1982.
37. Braun M. *Differential Equations and their Applications*. New York: Springer-Verlag, 1975.
38. Feng D, Huang S, Wang X. Models for computer simulation studies of input functions for tracer kinetic modeling with positron emission tomography. *Int J Biomed Comput* 1993; 32:95–110.
39. Gear C. *Numerical Initial Value Problems in Ordinary Differential Equations*. Englewood Cliffs, NJ: Prentice Hall, 1971.
40. Press W, Flannery B, Teukolsy S, Vetterling W. *Numerical Recipes: The Art of Scientific Computing*. Cambridge: Cambridge University Press, 1986.
41. Bard Y. *Nonlinear Parameter Estimation*. Academic Press, New York, 1974.
42. Beck JV, Arnold KJ. *Parameter Estimation in Engineering and Science*. New York: John Wiley & Sons, 1977.
43. Carson RE. Parameter estimation in positron emission tomography. In: Phelps ME, Mazziotta JC, Schelbert HR, eds. *Positron Emission Tomography and Autoradiography*. New York: Raven Press, 1986, 347–390.
44. Sorenson JA, Phelps ME. *Physics in Nuclear Medicine*. Orlando: Grune & Stratton, 1987.
45. Budinger TF, Derenzo SE, Greenberg WL, Gullberg GT, Huesman RH. Quantitative potentials of dynamic emission computed tomography. *J Nucl Med* 1978;19:309–315.
46. Alpert NM, Chesler DA, Correia JA, Ackerman RH, Chang JY, Finklestein S, Davis SM, Brownell GL, Taveras JM. Estimation of the local statistical noise in emission computed tomography. *IEEE Trans Med Imag* 1982;1:142–146.
47. Huesman RH. A new fast algorithm for the evaluation of regions of interest and statistical uncertainty in computed tomography. *Phys Med Biol* 1984;29:543–552.
48. Alpert NM, Barker WC, Gelman A, Weise S, Senda M, Correia JA. The precision of positron emission tomography: theory and measurement. *J Cereb Blood Flow Metab* 1991;11:A26–A30.
49. Haynor DR, Harrison RL, Lewellen TK. The use of importance sampling techniques to improve the efficiency of photon tracking in emission tomography simulations. *Med Phys* 1991;18:990–1001.
50. Carson RE, Yan Y, Daube-Witherspoon ME, Freedman N, Bacharach SL, Herscovitch P. An approximation formula for the variance of PET region-of-interest values. *IEEE Trans Med Imag* 1993;12:240–250.
51. Eastman R, Carson R, Gordon M, Berg G, Lillioja S, Larson S, Roth J. Brain glucose metabolism in non-insulin dependent diabetes mellitus: a study in Pima Indians using positron emission tomography during hyperinsulinemia with euglycemic glucose clamp. *J Clin Endocrinol Metab* 1990;71: 1602–1610.
52. Salmon E, Brooks DJ, Leenders KL, Turton DR, Hume SP, Cremer JE, Jones T, Frackowiak RSJ. A two-compartment description and kinetic procedure for measuring regional cerebral [^{11}C]nomifensine uptake using positron emission tomography. *J Cereb Blood Flow Metab* 1990;10: 307–316.
53. Koeppe RA, Holthoff VA, Frey KA, Kilbourn MR, Kuhl DE. Compartmental analysis of [^{11}C]flumazenil kinetic for the estimation of ligand transport rate and receptor distribution using positron emission tomography. *J Cereb Blood Flow Metab* 1991;11:735–744.
54. Carson RE, Channing MA, Blasberg RG, Dunn BB, Cohen RM, Rice KC, Herscovitch P. Comparison of bolus and infusion methods for receptor quantitation: application to [^{18}F]-cyclofoxy and positron emission tomography. *J Cereb Blood Flow Metab* 1993;13:24–42.
55. Holden JE, Gatley SJ, Hichwa RD, Ip WR, Shaughnessy WJ, Nickles RJ, Polcyn RE. Cerebral blood flow using PET measurements of fluoromethane kinetics. *J Nucl Med* 1981; 22:1084–1088.
56. Koeppe RA, Holden JE, Ip WR. Performance comparison of parameter estimation techniques for the quantitation of local cerebral blood flow by dynamic positron computed tomography. *J Cereb Blood Flow Metab* 1985;5:224–234.
57. Frey KA, Holthoff VA, Koeppe RA, Jewett DM, Kilbourn MR, Kuhl DE. Parametric in vivo imaging of benzodiazepine receptor distribution in human brain. *Ann Neurol* 1991; 30:663–672.
58. Huang S, Carson R, Phelps M. Measurement of local blood flow and distribution volume with short-lived isotopes: a general input technique. *J Cereb Blood Flow Metab* 1982; 2:99–108.
59. Huang S-C, Carson RE, Hoffman EJ, Carson J, MacDonald N, Barrio JR, Phelps ME. Quantitative measurement of local cerebral blood flow in humans by positron computed tomography and ^{15}O-water. *J Cereb Blood Flow Metab* 1983;3: 141–153.
60. Alpert NM, Eriksson L, Chang JY, Bergstrom M, Litton JE, Correia JA, Bohm C, Ackerman RH, Taveras JM. Strategy for the measurement of regional cerebral blood flow using short-lived tracers and emission tomography. *J Cereb Blood Flow Metab* 1984;4:28–34.
61. Blomqvist G. On the construction of functional maps in positron emission tomography. *J Cereb Blood Flow Metab* 1984;4:629–632.
62. Carson RE, Huang SC, Green MV. Weighted integration method for local cerebral blood flow measurements with positron emission tomography. *J Cereb Blood Flow Metab* 1986;6:245–258.
63. Blomqvist G, Pauli S, Farde L, Eriksson L, Persson A, Halldin C. Maps of receptor binding parameters in human brain—a kinetic analysis of PET measurements. *Eur J Nucl Med* 1990;16:257–265.
64. Yokoi T, Kanno I, Iida H, Miura S, Uemura K. A new approach of weighted integration technique based on accumulated images using dynamic PET and $H_2{}^{15}O$. *J Cereb Blood Flow Metab* 1991;11:492–501.
65. Carson RE. PET parameter estimation using linear integration methods: Bias and variability considerations, In: *Quantification of Brain Function. Tracer Kinetics and Image Analysis in Brain PET*, Eds. K Uemura, NA Lassen, T Jones, and I Kanno, Elsevier Science Publishers B.V., Amsterdam, 1993, pp. 499–507.
66. Cunningham VJ, Jones T. Spectral-analysis of dynamic PET studies. *J Cereb Blood Flow Metab* 1993;13:15–23.
67. Howman-Giles R, Moase A, Gaskin K, Uren R. Hepatobiliary scintigraphy in a pediatric population: determination of hepatic extraction fraction by deconvolution analysis. *J Nucl Med* 1993;34:214–221.
68. Huang SC, Phelps ME. Principles of tracer kinetic modeling in positron emission tomography and autoradiography. In: Phelps M, Mazziotta J, Schelbert H, eds. *Positron Emission Tomography and Autoradiography: Principles and Applications for the Brain and Heart*. New York: Raven Press, 1986; 287–346.
69. Carson RE. The development and application of mathematical

models in nuclear medicine. *J Nucl Med* 1991;32:2206–2208. Editorial.

70. Berman M, Schoenfeld R. Invariants in experimental data on linear kinetics and the formulation of models. *J Appl Physiol* 1956;27:1361–1370.
71. Berman M. The formulation of testing models. *Ann NY Acad Sci* 1963;108:192–194.
72. Carson ER, Jones EA. Use of kinetic analysis and mathematical modeling in the study of metabolic pathway *in vivo. N Engl J Med* 1979;300:1016–1027.
73. Carson ER, Cobelli C, Finkelstein L. Modeling and identification of metabolic systems. *Am J Physiol* 1981;240:R120–R129.
74. Cobelli C, Ruggerin A. Evaluation of alternative model structures of metabolic systems: two case studies on model identification and validation. *Med Biol Eng Comput* 1982;20:444–450.
75. DiStefano J, Landaw E. Multiexponential, multicompartmental, and noncompartmental modeling. I. Methodological limitations and physiological interpretations. *Am J Physiol* 1984;246:R651–R664.
76. Landaw EW, DiStefano JJ. Multiexponential, multicompartmental and noncompartmental modeling. II. Data analysis and statistical considerations. *Am J Physiol* 1984;246:R665–R677.
77. Vera D, Krohn K, Scheibe P, Stadalnik R. Identifiability analysis of an in vivo receptor-binding radiopharmacokinetic system. *IEEE Trans Biomed Eng* 1985;32:312–322.
78. Delforge J, Syrota A, Mazoyer BM. Experimental design optimisation: theory and application to estimation of receptor model parameters using dynamic positron emission tomography. *Phys Med Biol* 1989;34:419–435.
79. Delforge J, Syrota A, Mazoyer Bm. Identifiability analysis and parameter identification of an in vivo ligand-receptor model from PET data. *IEEE Trans Biomed Eng* 1990; 37:653–661.
80. Wong DR, Gjedde A, Wagner HM. Quantification of neuroreceptors in the living human brain. I. Irreversible binding of ligands. *J Cereb Blood Flow Metab* 1986;6:137–146.
81. Akaike H. An information criterion (AIC). *Math Sci* 1976;14:5–9.
82. Schwarz G. Estimating the dimension of a model. *Ann Stat* 1978;6:461–464.
83. Pert CB, Danks JA, Channing MA, Eckelman WC, Larson SM, Bennett JM, Burke TRJ, Rice KC: 3-[^{18}F] Acetylcyclofoxy: a useful probe for the visualization of opiate receptors in living animals. *FEBS Lett* 1984;177:281–286.
84. Kawai R, Carson RE, Dunn B, Newman AH, Rice KC, Blasberg RG. Regional brain measurement of B_{max} and K_D with the opiate antagonist cyclofoxy: equilibrium studies in the conscious rate. *J Cereb Blood Flow Metab* 1991;11:529–544.
85. Theodore WH, Carson RE, Andreason P, Zametkin A, Blasberg R, Leiderman DB, Rice K, Newman A, Channing M, Dunn B, Simpson N, Herscovitch P. PET imaging of opiate receptor binding in human epilepsy using [^{18}F]cyclofoxy. *Epilepsy Res* 1992;13:129–139.
86. Gjedde A, Reith J, Dyve S, Leger G, Guttman M, Diksic M, Evans A, Kuwabara H. Dopa decarboxylase activity of the living human brain. *Proc Natl Acad Sci USA* 1991;88: 2721–2725.
87. Kuwabara H, Evans AC, Gjedde A. Michaelis-Menten constraints improved cerebral glucose metabolism and regional lumped constant measurements with [^{18}F]fluorodeoxyglucose. *J Cereb Blood Flow Metab* 1990;10:180–189.
88. Kuwabara H, Cumming P, Reith J, Leger G, Diksic M, Evans AC, Gjedde A. Human striatal L-dopa decarboxylase activity estimated in vivo using 6-[^{18}F]fluoro-dopa and positron emission tomography: error analysis and application to normal subjects. *J Cereb Blood Flow Metab* 1993;13:43–56.
89. Frost JJ, Douglass DH, Mayberg HS, Dannals RF, Links JM, Wilson AA, Ravert HT, Crozier WC, Wagner HN. Multicompartmental analysis of [^{11}C]-carfentanil binding to opiate receptors in humans measured by positron emission tomography. *J Cereb Blood Flow Metab* 1989;9:398–409.
90. Farde L, Eriksson L, Blomquist G, Halldin C. Kinetic analysis of central [^{11}C]raclopride binding to D_2-dopamine receptors studied by PET: a comparison to the equilibrium analysis. *J Cereb Blood Flow Metab* 1989;9:696–708.
91. Carson RE, Blasberg RG, Channing MA, Yolles PS, Dunn BB, Newman AH, Rice KC, Herscovitch P. A kinetic study of the active and inactive enantiomers of ^{18}F-cyclofoxy with PET. *J Cereb Blood Flow Metab* 1989;9(suppl):16.
92. Delforge J, Syrota A, Bottlaender M, Varastet M, Loc'h C, Bendrieum B, Crouzel C, Brouillet E, Maziere M. Modeling analysis of [^{11}-C]flumazenil kinetics studied by PET: application to a critical study of the equilibrium approaches. *J Cereb Blood Flow Metab* 1993;13:454–468.
93. Price J, Mayberg H, Dannals R, Wilson A, Ravert H, Sadzot B, Rattner Z, Kimball A, Feldman M, Frost J. Measurement of benzodiazepine receptor number and affinity in humans using tracer kinetic modeling, positron emission tomography, and [^{11}C]flumazenil. *J Cereb Blood Flow Metab* 1993;13: 656–667.
94. Dewey SL, Smith GS, Logan J, Brodie JD, Yu DW, Ferrieri RA, King PT, MacGregor RR, Martin TP, Wolf AP, et al. GABAergic inhibition of endogenous dopamine release measured in vivo with ^{11}C-raclopride and positron emission tomography. *J Neurosci* 1992;12:3773–3780.
95. Holthoff VA, Koeppe RA, Frey KA, Paradise AH, Kuhl DE. Differentiation of radioligand delivery and binding in the brain: validation of a two-compartment model for [^{11}C]flumazenil. *J Cereb Blood Flow Metab* 1991;11:745–752.
96. Nelson T, Lucignani G, Goochee J, Crane AM, Sokoloff L. Invalidity of criticisms of the deoxyglucose method based on alleged glucose-6-phosphatase activity in brain. *J Neurochem* 1986;46:905–919.
97. Benveniste H. Brain microdialysis. *J Neurochem* 1989; 52:1667–1679.
98. Carson RE. Precision and accuracy considerations of physiological quantitation in PET. *J Cereb Blood Flow Metab* 1991;11:A45–50.
99. Gjedde A. High- and low-affinity transport of D-glucose from blood to brain. *J Neurochem* 1981;36:1463–1471.
100. Patlak CS, Blasberg RG, Fenstermacher JD. Graphical evaluation of blood-to-brain transfer constants from multiple-time uptake data. *J Cereb Blood Flow Metab* 1983;3:1–7.
101. Patlak CS, Blasberg RG. Graphical evaluation of blood-to-brain transfer constants from multiple-time uptake data. Generalizations. *J Cereb Blood Flow Metab* 1985;5:584–590.
102. Martin W, Palmer M, Patlak C, Calne D. Nigrostriatal function in humans studied with positron emission tomography. *Ann Neurol* 1989;20:535–542.
103. Logan J, Fowler JS, Volkow ND, Wolf AP, Dewey SL, Schyler DJ, MacGregor RR, Hitzemann R, Bendriem B, Gatley SJ, Christman D. Graphical analysis of reversible radioligand binding from time-activity measurements applied to [N-^{11}C-methyl]-(−)-cocaine: PET studies in human subjects. *J Cereb Blood Flow Metab* 1990;10:740–747.
104. Yokoi T, Iida H, Itoh H, Kanno I. A new graphic plot analysis for cerebral blood flow and partition coefficient with iodine-123-iodoamphetamine and dynamic SPECT validation studies using oxygen-15-water and PET. *J Nucl Med* 1993;34: 498–505.
105. Choi Y, Hawkins RA, Huang SC, Gambhir SS, Brunken RC,

Phelps ME, Schelbert HR. Parametric images of myocardial metabolic rate of glucose generated from dynamic cardiac PET and 2-[^{18}F]fluoro-2-deoxy-D-glucose studies. *J Nucl Med* 1991;32:733–738.

106. Frackowiak RSJ, Lenzi G-L, Jones T, Heather JD. Quantitative measurement of regional cerebral blood flow and oxygen metabolism in man using ^{15}O and positron emission tomography: theory, procedure and normal values. *J Comput Assist Tomogr* 1980;4:727–736.
107. Herscovitch P, Markham J, Raichle ME. Brain blood flow measured with intravenous $H_2{}^{15}O$. I. Theory and error analysis. *J Nucl Med* 1983;24:782–789.
108. Raichle ME, Martin WRW, Herscovitch P, Mintun MA, Markham J. Brain blood flow measured with intravenous $H_2{}^{15}O$. II. Implementation and validation. *J Nucl Med* 1983;24:790–798.
109. Brooks RA. Alternative formula for glucose utilization using labeled deoxyglucose. *J Nucl Med* 1982;23:538, 539.
110. Hutchins GD, Holden JE, Koeppe RA, Halama JR, Gatley SJ, Nickels RJ. Alternative approach to single-scan estimation of cerebral glucose metabolic rate using glucose analogs, with particular application to ischemia. *J Cereb Blood Flow Metab* 1984;4:35–40.
111. Wilson PD, Huang SC, Hawkins RA. Single-scan Bayes estimation of cerebral glucose metabolic rate: comparison with non-Bayes single-scan methods using FDG PET scans in stroke. *J Cereb Blood Flow Metab* 1988;8:418–425.
112. Frey KA, Ehrenkaufer RLE, Beaucage S, Agranoff BW. Quantitative in vivo receptor binding. I. Theory and application to the muscarinic cholinergic receptor. *J Neurosci* 1985;5:421–428.
113. Laruelle M, Abi-Dargham A, Rattner Z, Al-Tikriti M, Zea-Ponce Y, Zoghbi S, Charney D, Price J, Frost J, Hoffer P, Baldwin R, Innis R. Single photon emission tomography measurement of benzodiazepine receptor number and affinity in primate brain: a constant infusion paradigm with [^{123}I]iomazenil. *Eur J Pharmacol* 1993;230:119–123.
114. Mintun MA, Raichle ME, Kilbourn MR, Wooton GF, Welch MJ. A quantative model for the in vivo assessment of drug binding sites with positron emission tomography. *Ann Neurol* 1984;15:217–227.
115. Carson RE, Doudet DJ, Channing MA, Dunn BB, Der MG, Newman AH, Rice KC, Cohen RM, Blasberg RG, Herscovitch P. Equilibrium measurement of B_{max} and K_D of the opiate antagonist ^{18}F-cyclofoxy with PET: pixel-by-pixel analysis. *J Cereb Blood Flow Metab* 1991;11(suppl):618.
116. Hoffman EJ, Huang S-C, Phelps ME. Quantitation in positron emission computed tomography: 1. Effect of object size. *J Comput Assist Tomogr* 1979;3:299–308.
117. Herscovitch P, Raichle ME. Effect of tissue heterogeneity on the measurement of cerebral blood flow with the equilibrium $C^{15}O_2$ inhalation technique. *J Cereb Blood Flow Metab* 1983;3:407–415.
118. Herscovitch P, Raichle ME. Effect of tissue heterogeneity on the measurement of regional cerebral oxygen extraction and metabolic rate with positron emission tomography. *J Cereb Blood Flow Metab* 1985;5(suppl 1):671, 672.
119. Herholz K, Patlak CS. The influence of tissue heterogeneity on results of fitting nonlinear model equations to regional tracer uptake curves: with an application to compartmental models used in positron emission tomography. *J Cereb Blood Flow Metab* 1987;7:214–229.
120. Huang SC, Mahoney DK, Phelps ME. Quantitation in positron emission tomography: 8. Effects of nonlinear parameter estimation on functional images. *J Comput Assist Tomogr* 1987;11:314–325.
121. Schmidt K, Mies G, Sokoloff L. Model of kinetic behavior of deoxyglucose in heterogeneous tissues in brain: a reinterpretation of the significance of parameters fitted to homogeneous tissue models. *J Cereb Blood Flow Metab* 1991;11:10–24.
122. Schmidt K, Lucignani G, Moresco R, Rizzo G, Gilardi M, Messa C, Colombo F, Fazio F, Sokoloff L. Errors introduced by tissue heterogeneity in estimation of local cerebral glucose utilization with current kinetic models of the [^{18}F]fluorodeoxyglucose method. *J Cereb Blood Flow Metab* 1992;12:823–834.
123. Lammertsma AA, Jones T. Correction for the presence of intravascular oxygen-15 in the steady state technique for measuring regional oxygen extraction ratio in the brain: 1. Description of the method. *J Cereb Blood Flow Metab* 1983;13:416–424.
124. Evans AC, Diksic M, Yamamoto YL, Kato A, Dagher A, Redies C, Hakim A. Effect of vascular activity in the determination of rate constants for the uptake of ^{18}F-labeled 2-fluoro-2-deoxy-D-glucose: error analysis and normal values in older subjects. *J Cereb Blood Flow Metab* 1986;6:724–738.
125. Hawkins RA, Phelps ME, Huang SC. Effects of temporal sampling, glucose metabolic rates, and disruptions of the blood-brain barrier on the FDG model with and without a vascular compartment: studies in human brain tumors with PET. *J Cereb Blood Flow Metab* 1986;6:170–183.
126. KoeppeRA, Hutchins GD, Rothley JM, Hichwa RD. Examination of assumptions for local cerebral blood flow studies in PET. *J Nucl Med* 1987;28:1695–1703.
127. Iida H, Kanno I, Takahashi A, Miura S, Murakami M, Takahashi K, Ono Y, Shishido F, Inugami A, Tomura N, et al. Measurement of absolute myocardial blood flow with $H_2{}^{15}O$ and dynamic positron-emission tomography. Strategy for quantification in relation to the partial-volume effect. *Circulation* 1988;78:104–115.
128. Herrero P, Markham J, Shelton ME, Weinheimer CJ, Bergmann SR. Noninvasive quantification of regional myocardial perfusion with rubidium-82 and positron emission tomography. Exploration of a mathematical model. *Circulation* 1990;82:1377–1386.
129. Hutchins GD, Caraher JM, Raylman RR. A region of interest strategy for minimizing resolution distortions in quantitative myocardial PET studies. *J Nucl Med* 1992;33:1243–1250.
130. Weinberg I, Huang S, Hoffman E, Araujo L, Nienaber C, Grover-McKay M, Dahlbom M, Schelbert H. Validation of PET-acquired input functions for cardiac studies. *J Nucl Med* 1988;29:241–247.
131. Iida H, Rhodes CG, de Silva R, Araujo LI, Bloomfield PM, Lammertsma AA, Jones T. Use of the left ventricular time-activity curve as a noninvasive input function in dynamic oxygen-15-water positron emission tomography. *J Nucl Med* 1992;33:1669–1677.
132. Germano G, Chen BC, Huang SC, Gambhir SS, Hoffman EJ, Phelps ME. Use of the abdominal aorta for arterial input function determination in hepatic and renal PET studies. *J Nucl Med* 1992;33:613–620.
133. Eriksson L, Kanno I: Blood sampling devices and measurements. *Med Prog Technol* 1991;17:249–257.
134. Dhawan V, Conti J, Mernyk M, Jarden JO, Rottenberg DA. Accuracy of PET RCBF measurements: effect of time shift between blood and brain radioactivity curves. *Phys Med Biol* 1986;31:507–514.
135. Dhawan V, Jarden JO, Strother S, Rottenberg DA. Effect of blood curve smearing on the accuracy of parameter estimates for [82-Rb] PET studies of blood-brain barrier permeability. *Phys Med Biol* 1988;33:61–74.
136. Iida H, Kanno I, Miura S, Murakami M, Takahashi K, Uemura K. Evaluation of regional differences of tracer appearance

time in cerebral tissues using [^{15}O]water and dynamic positron emission tomography. *J Cereb Blood Flow Metab* 1988;8: 285–288.

137. Meyer E. Simultaneous correction for tracer arrival delay and dispersion in CBF measurements by the $H_2{}^{15}O$ autoradiographic method and dynamic PET. *J Nucl Med* 1989;30: 1069–1078.
138. Huesman RH, Mazoyer BM. Kinetic data analysis with a noisy input function. *Phys Med Biol* 1987;32:1569–1579.
139. Chen KW, Huang SC, Yu DC. The effects of measurement errors in plasma radioactivity curve on parameter estimation in positron emission tomography. *Phys Med Biol* 1991;36: 1183–1200.
140. Markham J, Schuster DP. Effects of nonideal input functions on PET measurements of pulmonary blood flow. *J Appl Physiol* 1992;72:2495–2500.
141. Feng D, Wang X. A computer simulation study on the effects of input function measurement noise in tracer kinetic modeling with positron emission tomography. *Comput Biol Med* 1993;23:57–68.
142. Huang SC, Barrio JR, Yu DC, Chen B, Grafton S, Melega WP, Hoffman JM, Satyamurthy N. Modelling approach for separating blood time-activity curves in positron emission tomographic studies. *Phys Med Biol* 1991;36:749–761.
143. Huang S-C, Phelps ME, Hoffman EJ, Kuhl DE. A theoretical study of quantitative flow measurements with constant infusion of short-lived isotopes. *Phys Med Biol* 1979;24: 1151–1161.
144. Huang S-C, Phelps ME, Hoffman EJ, Kuhl DE. Error sensitivity of fluorodeoxyglucose method for measurement of cerebral metabolic rate of glucose. *J Cereb Blood Flow Metab* 1981;1:391–401.
145. Lammertsma AA, Jones T, Frackowiak RSJ, Lenzi G-L. A theoretical study of the steady-state model for measuring regional cerebral blood flow and oxygen utilization using oxygen-15. *J Comput Assist Tomogr* 1981;5:544–550.
146. Lammertsma AA, Heather JD, Jones T, Frackowiak RSJ, Lenzi G-L. A statistical study of the steady state technique for measuring regional cerebral blood flow and oxygen utilization using ^{15}O. *J Comput Assist Tomogr* 1982;6:566–573.
147. Brownell G, Kearfott K, Kairentoi A, Elmaleh D, Alpert N, Correia J, Wechsle L, Ackerman R. Quantitation of regional cerebral glucose metabolism. *J Comput Assist Tomogr* 1983; 7:919–924.
148. Wienhard K, Pawlik G, Herholz K, Wagner R, Heiss W-D. Estimation of local cerebral glucose utilization by positron emission tomography of [^{18}F]2-fluoro-2-deoxy-D-glucose: a critical appraisal of optimization procedures. *J Cereb Blood Flow Metab* 1985;5:115–125.
149. Huang S-C, Feng D, Phelps ME. Model dependency and estimation reliability in measurement of cerebral oxygen utilization rate with oxygen-15 and dynamic positron emission tomography. *J Cereb Blood Flow Metab* 1986;6:105–119.
150. Iida H, Kanno I, Miura S, Murakami M, Takahashi K, Uemura K. Error analysis of a quantitative cerebral blood flow measurement using $H_2{}^{15}O$ autoradiography and positron emission tomography, with respect to the dispersion of the input function. *J Cereb Blood Flow Metab* 1986;6:536–545.
151. Jagust WJ, Budinger TF, Huesman RH, Friedland RP, Mazoyer BM, Knittel BL. Methodologic factors affecting PET measurements of cerebral glucose metabolism. *J Nucl Med* 1986;27:1358–1361.
152. Senda M, Buxton RB, Alpert NM, Correia JA, Mackay BC, Weise SB, Ackerman RH. The ^{15}O steady-state method: correction for variation in arterial concentration. *J Cereb Blood Flow Metab* 1988;8:681–690.
153. Lammertsma AA, Cunningham VJ, Deiber MP, Heather JD, Bloomfield PM, Nutt J, Frackowiak RSJ, Jones T. Combination of dynamic and integral methods for generating reproducible functional CBF images. *J Cereb Blood Flow Metab* 1990;10:675–686.
154. Mazoyer BM, Huesman RH, Budinger TF, Knittel BL. Dynamic PET data analysis. *J Comput Assist Tomogr* 1986;10: 645–653.
155. Jovkar S, Evans AC, Diksic M, Nakai H, Yamamoto YL. Minimisation of parameter estimation errors in dynamic PET: choice of scanning schedules. *Phys Med Biol* 1989;34: 895–908.
156. Kanno I, Iida H, Miura S, Murakami M. Optimal scan time of oxygen-15-labeled water injection method for measurement of cerebral blood flow. *J Nucl Med* 1991;32:1931–1934.
157. Fox PT, Mintun MA, Raichle ME, Herscovitch P. A noninvasive approach to quantitative functional brain mapping with $H_2{}^{15}O$ and positron emission tomography. *J Cereb Blood Flow Metab* 1984;4:329–333.
158. Mazziotta JC, Huang SC, Phelps ME, Carson RE, MacDonald NS, Mahoney K. A noninvasive positron computed tomography technique using oxygen-15-labeled water for the evaluation of neurobehavioral task batteries. *J Cereb Blood Flow Metab* 1985;5:70–78.
159. Hawkins RA, Phelps ME, Huang S-C, Kuhl DE. Effect of ischemia on quantification of local cerebral glucose metabolic rate in man. *J Cereb Blood Flow Metab* 1981;1:37–51.
160. Nakai H, Yamamoto Y, Diksic M, Matsuda M, Takar E, Meyer E, Redies C. Time-dependent changes of lumped and rate constant in the deoxyglucose method in experimental cerebral ischemia. *J Cereb Blood Flow Metab* 1987;7:640–648.

9 Production of Radionuclides

John C. Harbert

Nearly all naturally occurring radionuclides found in sufficient abundance for use in tracer studies have long half-lives, which make them unsuitable for medical use. All medically important radionuclides are produced in nuclear reactors or particle accelerators of various types. This chapter examines the radionuclides most frequently used in nuclear medicine and identifies their modes of production and general details of processing.

REACTOR-PRODUCED RADIONUCLIDES

A nuclear reactor consists essentially of a tightly contained enclosure with a central core of fissionable fuel, usually ^{238}U and ^{235}U, the latter enriched significantly above its natural abundance of 0.7%. Uranium-235 undergoes spontaneous fission ($T_{1/2} \sim 7 \times 10^8$ years), which yields two smaller, more stable fission fragments and two or three neutrons per fission event. Some of these fission neutrons stimulate additional fission events. For example, if each nucleus undergoing fission produces two neutrons capable of stimulating two additional events, the sequence of the fission events would increase in geometric proportion, or 2:4:8:16:32:64:128 . . . leading to a *chain reaction.* The relationship between the number of fissions in one generation and the number of fissions in the immediately preceding generation is called the *multiplication factor.* When this factor is greater than unity, the speed of the chain reaction increases and the reaction is called *supercritical.* When the factor is less than unity, the reaction eventually ceases and is said to be *subcritical.* The reaction is *sustained*, or *critical*, when the factor equals unity exactly.

The average number of neutrons produced per fission is approximately 2.4. To sustain criticality, an equilibrium must be established between the rate of neutron production and the rate of dissipation by either escape or absorption. The size, shape, and composition of the reactor core are all important in achieving and sustaining a chain reaction. If the ^{235}U is contained within a small sphere, most of the neutrons escape the system without producing a critical reaction. As the radius of the sphere increases, neutron escape increases as r^2, but absorption increases as r^3. Combining the appropriate radius with a sufficient quantity of fuel achieves a critical radius and critical mass. In the case of pure ^{235}U, the critical radius is about 8.7 cm and the critical mass is about 5.2 kg.

In a nuclear reactor, the speed of the reaction is governed by control rods made of a material with a high *cross section* for neutrons, such as boron or cadmium; the rods are raised or lowered to speed or slow the nuclear reaction (Fig. 1). The *moderator* also slows the neutrons, thereby increasing the probability of neutron absorption by ^{235}U nuclei. The moderator is distributed throughout the fuel and consists of such light atoms as hydrogen, deuterium, or carbon. These nuclei have low cross sections for neutron absorption, but cause elastic collisions, which slow them to a *thermal neutron* state (about 0.3 eV). This energy state is most efficient in inducing fission. Some reactors, eg, the "swimming pool" reactor, are moderated by water that circulates between the elements and serves as a coolant. Deuterium is an even more efficient moderator.

Usually, the target to be irradiated is inserted into the reactor core by a pneumatic conduction system, which is enclosed within a suitable container called a *thimble*. This system is best used to produce radionuclides of relatively short half-lives. Nuclides with longer half-lives may be extracted from fixed targets attached to the control rods or may be processed from spent fuel rods.

Principal Nuclear Reactions

Several nuclear reactions can occur in the course of neutron activation. The most common production mode is the (n,γ) reaction, known also as the *neutron capture reaction*:

$$^{A}_{Z}X\ (n,\gamma)^{A+1}_{Z}X.$$

In this reaction, the target nucleus $^{A}_{Z}X$ captures a neutron, forming an excited nucleus $^{A+1}_{Z}X^*$, which undergoes deexcitation by emission of a *prompt* gamma ray. The resulting nucleus is usually radioactive and most often decays by beta emission because of neutron excess. Because the product is an isotope of the target atom, the product is not carrier-free. Only a tiny fraction of the target nuclei are activated ($1:10^6$ to $1:10^9$), so that specific activity is quite low. Szillard and Chalmers described a process to separate the formed radioisotope based on the fact that the recoil energy generated by nuclear emission of a photon after neutron capture is often sufficient to break chemical bonds in the target material.[1] An appreciable number of the activated nuclei then exist in a chemical form different from that of the target atoms, and

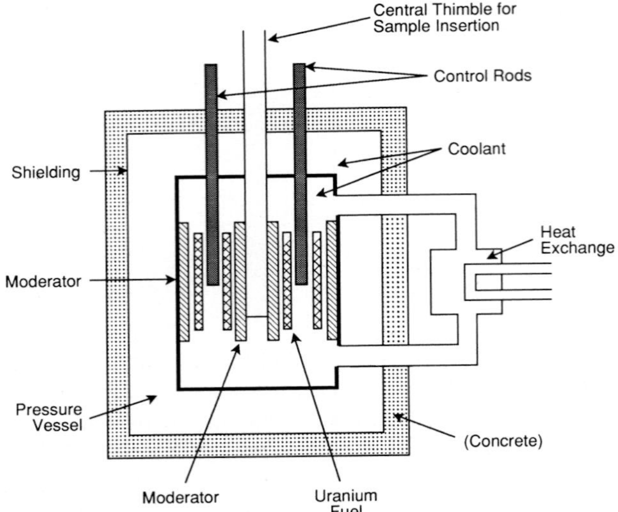

Figure 1. Essential features of a nuclear reactor.

this difference allows chemical separation. An example is the separation of trivalent ^{51}Cr after neutron bombardment of hexavalent potassium chromate. Specific activities of 30 mCi/mg are easily obtainable.

Carrier-free products result when the activated nucleus is a short-lived intermediate, as in the production of ^{131}I from ^{130}Te:

$$^{130}_{52}\text{Te}\ (n,\gamma)\ ^{131}_{52}\text{Te}\ (\beta^-,\ T_{1/2} = 25\ \text{minutes})\ ^{131}_{53}\text{I}$$

Both ^{99m}Tc and ^{113m}In are obtained from parent nuclides produced by (n,γ) reactions. The relatively long half-lives of the parents ^{99}Mo (66.6 hours) and ^{113}Sn (115 days) make these nuclides ideal for use in generator systems.

(n,p) and (n,α) Reactions

In these reactions, the incident neutrons have energies in the 2- to 6-MeV range, resulting in the emission of charged particles. In (n,p) reactions, the atomic number of the product nuclide decreases by one while the mass remains the same:

$$^{A}_{Z}X(n,p)^{A}_{Z-1}X$$

For (n,α) reactions, the atomic number decreases by two and atomic mass decreases by three:

$$^{A}_{Z}X\ (n,\alpha)\ ^{A-3}_{Z-2}X$$

The products in these cases are separated easily from the target by chemical means and are thus carrier-free radionuclides. Some examples of these reactions are listed in Table 1.

BUILDUP OF RADIOACTIVITY

The buildup of radioactivity produced in a thin target when irradiated by a source of particles is given by the equation:

$$dN/dt = n\phi\sigma - \lambda N,$$

where N is the number of atoms undergoing the reaction, n is the number of target nuclei capable of undergoing the reaction, ϕ is the flux density of particles per square centimeter per second, σ is the cross section for the particular reaction in barns, 10^{-24} cm^2 (10^{-28} m^2 in SI units), and λ is the decay constant of the radionuclide formed. In this equation, $n\phi\sigma$ equals the number of transformations per second, and $-\lambda N$ describes the radioactive decay occurring during irradiation. After irradiation continues for some finite time t, the number of radioactive nuclei N^* formed is found by integration:

$$N_t^* = \frac{n\phi\sigma}{\lambda}(1 - e^{-\lambda t})$$

The amount of activity formed is calculated using the relations between mass in grams; the atomic weight A; and Avogadro's number, 6.02×10^{23} atoms/mol:

$$\text{Activity} = \frac{6.02 \times 10^{23}\ \phi\sigma}{A}(1 - e^{\lambda t})\text{dps/g}$$

(or Bq/g)

Dividing by 3.7×10^{10} dps/Ci

$$\text{Activity} = \frac{1.62 \times 10^{13}\ \phi\sigma}{A}(1 - e^{-\lambda t})\ \text{Ci/g}$$

This equation gives the *specific activity* at any time t.

The buildup of activity is illustrated in Figure 2. The curve approaches a limit where the rate of production equals

Table 1. Some Reactor-Produced Radionuclides

PRINCIPLE PRODUCTION		
Radionuclide	*Decay Modes*	*Reaction*
^{14}C	β^-	^{14}N (n, p) ^{14}C
^{24}Na	β^-, γ	^{23}Na (n, γ) ^{24}Na
^{32}P	β^-	^{31}P (n, γ) ^{32}P ^{32}S (n, p) ^{32}P ^{34}S (n, γ) ^{35}S
^{35}S	β^-	^{35}Cl (n, p) ^{35}S
^{42}K	β^-, γ	^{41}K (n, γ) ^{42}K
^{47}Ca	β^-, γ	^{46}Ca (n, γ) ^{47}Ca
^{51}Cr	EC, γ	^{50}Cr (n, γ) ^{51}Cr
^{59}Fe	β^-, γ	^{58}Fe (n, γ) ^{59}Fe
^{75}Se	EC, γ	^{74}Se (n, γ) ^{75}Se
^{99}Mo	β^-, γ	^{98}Mo (n, γ) ^{99}Mo
^{113}Sn	EC, γ	^{112}Sn (n, γ) ^{113}Sn
^{125}I	EC, γ	^{124}Xe (n, γ) ^{125}Xe$\rightarrow$^{125}I
^{131}I	β^-, γ	^{130}Te (n, γ) ^{131}Te$\rightarrow$^{131}I

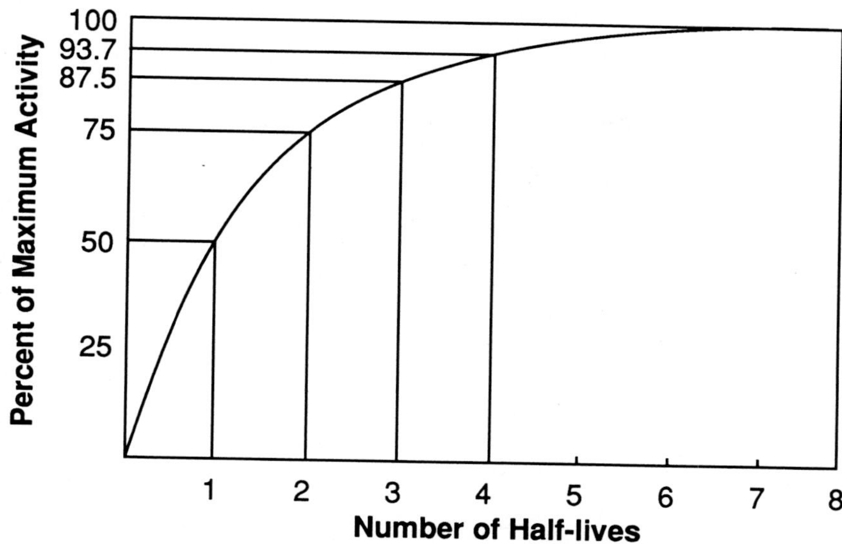

Figure 2. Buildup of activity as a function of time (in half-lives) of bombardment.

the rate of disintegration. The point at which activity reaches a maximum is known as the *saturation specific activity.* When t is *long* with respect to $T_{1/2}$:

$$\text{Maximum activity} = \frac{1.62 \times 10^{13}\ \phi\sigma}{A}\ \text{Ci/g}$$

Figure 2 shows that maximum activity is reached after approximately five half-lives. In fact, irradiation longer than 3 to 4 half-lives is inefficient. The rate of production is

$$R = \frac{6.02 \times 10^{23}\ \phi\sigma}{A}\ \text{activations/g}\cdot\text{s}$$
$$= \frac{1.62 \times 10^{13}\ \phi\sigma}{A}\ \text{Ci/g}\cdot\text{s}$$

This equation assumes no attenuation of flux by the target. Of course, this does not hold for thick targets, nor for bombardment with charged particles, in which particle flux decreases as the particles pass through the target material of thickness X, i.e., $\Delta\phi/\Delta X$ is high. The activation cross section also decreases because of loss of particle energy. Lapp and Andrews discuss these considerations in more detail.[2]

The reaction cross sections noted in these equations are the *activation cross sections.* The cross section values listed in nuclide charts are the *isotopic cross sections* for specific reactions and specific nuclides. For example, consider the production of ^{113}Sn by the ^{112}Sn (n,γ) ^{113}Sn reaction. The cross section for this reaction is 0.9 barns,[3] and the isotopic abundance of metallic tin is 95%. In a 1-g tin target:

$$N = \frac{6.02 \times 10^{23} \times 0.95}{112}$$

In a flux of 10^{12} neutrons/cm^2/s the maximum activity produced per gram would be

$$= \frac{N\ \phi\sigma}{A\ (3.7 \times 10^{10})}$$
$$= \frac{6.02 \times 10^{23} \times 0.95 \times 10^{12} \times 0.9 \times 10^{-24}}{112 \times 3.7 \times 10^{10}}$$
$$= 0.123\ \text{Ci}$$
$$= 4.55 \times 10^{9}\ \text{Bq}$$

The maximum activity obtainable in these reactions is a linear function of the concentration of the nuclei undergoing reaction. Targets should be packed as densely as possible and, when the natural abundance of the reacting nuclide is low, isotopic enrichment may be necessary to increase specific activity. For example, the production of ^{45}Ca from the ^{44}Ca (n,γ) ^{45}Ca reaction is facilitated greatly by using ^{44}Ca that is enriched tenfold above its 2.06% natural abundance. Nevertheless, the final specific activity is low.

NUCLEAR FISSION

Fission of ^{235}U or ^{239}Pu gives rise to a great variety of nuclides, whose masses range from 72 to 162, with the majority between 95 and 135. Some fission products useful to medicine are ^{99}Mo, ^{131}I, and ^{133}Xe. While fission products may be recovered from spent fuel rods, the usual method is by processing targets of enriched ^{235}U inserted directly into the reactor core. The separation of radionuclides obtained by fission is difficult because many radionuclides are formed, and usually several isotopes of the same element are formed. Thus, separation of ^{131}I from stable ^{127}I and long-lived ^{129}I ($T_{1/2} = 1.6 \times 10^{7}$ years) is nearly impossible. On the other

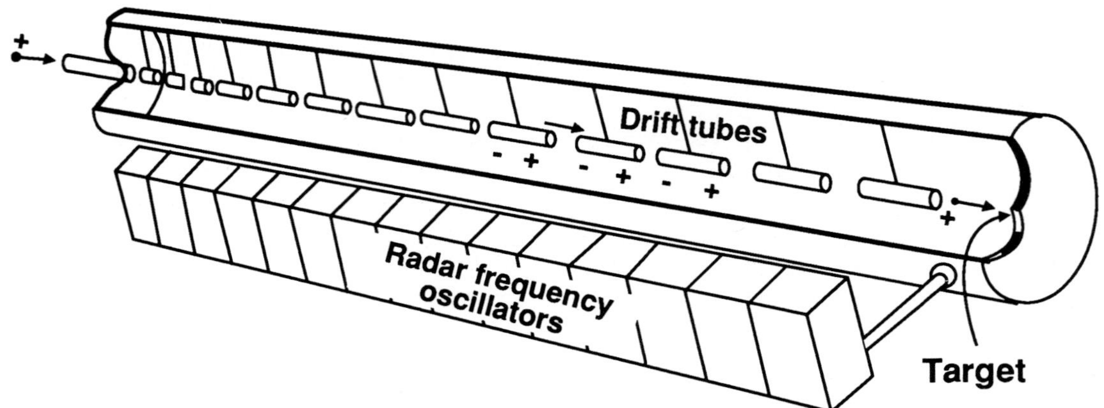

Figure 3. Schematic diagram of a linear accelerator.

hand, ^{99}Mo used in the preparation of ^{99}Mo- ^{99m}Tc generators can be recovered in high-specific activities.

PARTICLE ACCELERATORS

Charged particle accelerators may be divided into two groups based on the acceleration path: linear and circular. Particle acceleration in both groups is accomplished by electrostatic attraction between the charged particle and an oppositely charged drift tube, separated by an electronically insulated gap. In a *linear accelerator*, or LINAC, segmented drift tubes of increasing length are aligned linearly, up to 1 mile in length in some cases (Fig. 3). High-frequency alternating voltage is applied to each tube segment, so that adjacent segments are oppositely charged. Charged particles injected into the tube are accelerated in the segment gaps, owing to the temporary opposite charge in the succeeding tube. The velocity, or kinetic energy, of the accelerated particle is directly related to the electrostatic charge applied and to the number of gaps in the assembly. Energies of up to 800 MeV for protons and in the GeV range for electrons have been achieved at national laboratory facilities. The type of particle accelerated and the energies generated are selected carefully according to the nuclear reaction desired and the target material used.

In a *circular accelerator*, or *cyclotron*, the accelerated particles are held in a tight spiral by the application of a magnetic field perpendicular to the particle's direction. Initially, charged particles to be accelerated are injected into the center of a space between two hollow D-shaped copper electrodes (Fig. 4). Opposite alternating electric charges are placed on the "Ds" and oscillated at frequencies of about 10^7 Hz.

The charged particle is accelerated into the oppositely charged D, is bent by the magnetic field, and returns to the gap in time to be accelerated across the gap and into the other D, which is now oppositely charged. The velocity, or energy, of the particle increases each time the particle passes

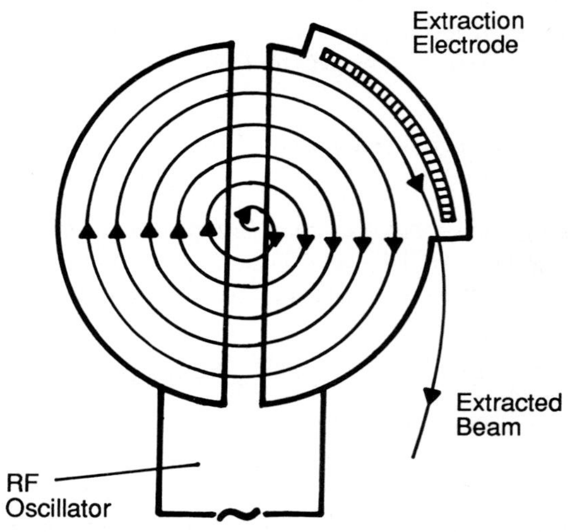

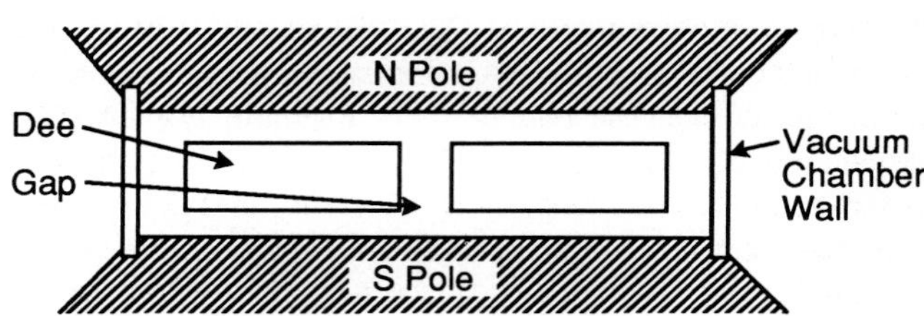

Figure 4. Schematic drawings of a cyclotron viewed from above (top) and the side (bottom).

through the gap, and the radius of the particle's path increases due to centrifugal force. Proton energies approaching 30 MeV are achieved with an orbit radius of less than 40 cm.

Cyclotrons capable of accelerating protons, deuterons, alpha particles, and ^{3}He ions to energies between 8 and 50 MeV are available commercially and are the principal machines used for radionuclide production.

PRINCIPAL NUCLEAR REACTIONS

Charged particle nuclear reactions change the number of protons in the nuclei of the target atoms and therefore change the element. For example, cyclotron production of ^{67}Ga from isotopically enriched ^{68}Zn utilizes the following nuclear reaction: ^{68}Zn $(p,2n)$ ^{67}Ga. Occasionally, the product of the nuclear reaction is the radioactive parent of the desired nuclide. For example, ^{201}Tl ($T_{1/2}$ = 73.5 hours) is the daughter of ^{201}Pb ($T_{1/2}$ = 9.4 hours) formed by the $^{203}Tl(p,3n)$ ^{201}Pb reaction using isotopically enriched ^{203}Tl as the target. Just as chemical reactions either absorb energy (must be heated) or release energy (heat is released), nuclear reactions either absorb or release energy. This energy is expressed as a Q value and can be calculated from the difference in the sum of the masses of the reactants and products. For example:

$$^{68}Zn + p \rightarrow {}^{67}Ga + 2n + Q$$
$$67.9248 + 1.0073 = 66.9282 + 2.0173 - 0.0134$$
$$Q = -0.0134 \text{ amu} \times 931.4 \text{ MeV/amu} = -12.48 \text{ MeV}$$

The energy Q must be supplied by the projectile causing the nuclear reaction. For a positively charged particle (p^+, d^+, $^{3}He^{++}$, $^{4}He^{++}$) to penetrate the nucleus of a target atom, sufficient energy must be supplied to overcome the potential barrier due to coulombic repulsion of like charges. Therefore, to effect a charged particle reaction, positively charged projectiles must be accelerated to energies sufficient to overcome the potential barrier of the positively charged nucleus even though the nuclear reaction itself may be exoergic. In general, (p,n) reactions are formed in the 10- to 15-MeV range, $(p,2n)$ in the 15- to 25-MeV range, $(p,3n)$ in the 20- to 35-MeV range, etc. To determine Q values experimentally, a stack of thin foils is placed in the charged particle beam and irradiated for a known time at known beam current. Following irradiation, each foil is assayed for the various radionuclides produced by the reactions (x,n), $(x,2n)$, $(x,3n)$, etc. All data from the foils are plotted for activity produced vs energy produced for the various reactions. The resulting curves for each reaction are called *excitation functions* and describe the production yield in μCi/μA-hr over an energy range.

The beam current can be determined accurately by integrating the current produced in an evacuated aluminum Faraday cup or from the radioactivity induced in high-purity metallic disks placed in the beam during the bombardment. The disks are made of such a metal as copper or silver, for which the excitation function (μCi/μA-hr) has been thoroughly studied and is well known.

For the production of any radionuclide, several nuclear reactions are possible. The best method is chosen by the energy and charged particles available, physical and chemical properties of the target material, competing nuclear reactions and the radionuclidic purity desired, total activity required (ie, mCi or Ci), and economic considerations.[4] An example is the production of ^{123}I ($T_{1/2}$ = 13 hr), for which more than a dozen nuclear reactions are possible, each with its own set of problems and advantages. With few exceptions, the radiopharmaceutical industry uses proton reactions in the 15- to 30-MeV range for production of radionuclides. Some typical reactions for accelerator-produced radionuclides are shown in Table 2.

PRODUCTION YIELDS

Production rates for charged particle nuclear reactions follow the same rules as described earlier in this chapter and can be calculated from reaction cross section values. The concept of flux, however, as presented for nuclear reactors is not practical for cyclotron production. Instead, the beam of charged particles generated per second is measured as *beam current* in microamperes. The area over which the beam is spread depends upon the beam profile and target configuration. Radionuclide production is optimized by delivering as much beam current as the target can withstand at the optimum particle energy. The limiting factor is usually the rate at which heat can be removed from the target to prevent it from melting. The amount of heat generated in the target is the product of the particle energy and the beam current; therefore, as particle energy is increased, the beam current must be decreased to produce the same heat load.

Usually, production yields are reported as mCi/μA-hr (1-μA bombardment for 1 hour) at a given particle energy and target size and thickness.

CYCLOTRON TARGETS

A *cyclotron target* is a deposit of a chemical element on a target base or holder of high thermal conductivity. Ideally, the target material is a monoisotopic element having a low vapor pressure and high melting point. The target base is usually composed of copper, nickel, silver, or aluminum, with machined holes for water cooling. An internal target intercepts the beam as it circulates within the cyclotron and must be designed to dissipate large quantities of heat. These high-power targets are usually metallic elements electroplated or vapor deposited on a copper base for high thermal conductivity.

The cyclotron beam may be deflected from its circular orbit inside the Ds and extracted into an evacuated beam tube external to the tank. Targets placed in this beam are called *external targets*. With external targets, space and con-

Table 2. Some Accelerator-Produced Radionuclides

RADIONUCLIDE	PRINCIPAL DECAY MODE	NUCLEAR REACTION
^{11}C	β^+	^{11}B (*p,n*) ^{11}C ^{10}B (*d,n*) ^{11}C ^{14}N (*p,α*) ^{11}C
^{13}N	β^+	^{12}C (*d,n*) ^{13}N ^{16}O (*p,α*) ^{13}N
^{15}O	β^+	^{14}N (*d,n*) ^{15}O ^{16}O (*p,pn*) ^{15}O
^{18}F	β^+, EC	^{18}O (*p,n*) ^{18}F ^{20}Ne (*d,α*) ^{18}F
^{43}K	β^-, γ	^{40}Ar (*α,p*) ^{43}K
^{52}Fe	β^+, EC	^{50}Cr (*α,2n*) ^{52}Fe
^{57}Co	EC	^{56}Fe (*p,γ*) ^{57}Co
^{67}Ga	EC	^{66}Zn (*d,n*) ^{67}Ga ^{68}Zn (*p,2n*) ^{67}Ga
^{75}Br	β^+, EC	^{74}Se (*d,n*) ^{75}Br ^{74}Se (*p,γ*) ^{75}Br
^{81m}Kr	γ	^{79}Br (*α,2n*) $^{81}Rb \xrightarrow[T_{1/2} = 4.7\text{ h}]{\text{EC, }\beta^+} 81\text{ m}_{Kr}$
^{111}In	EC	^{111}Cd (*p,n*) ^{111}In ^{112}Cd (*p,2n*) ^{111}In
^{123}I	EC	^{122}Te (*d,n*) ^{123}I ^{123}Te (*p,n*) ^{123}I ^{124}Te (*p,2n*) ^{123}I ^{127}I (*p,5n*) $^{123}Xe \xrightarrow[T_{1/2} = 2.1\text{ h}]{\text{EC, }\beta^+} {}^{123}I$
^{201}Tl	EC	^{200}Hg (*d,n*) ^{201}Tl ^{201}Hg (*d,2n*) ^{201}Tl ^{203}Tl (*p,3n*) $^{201}Pb \xrightarrow[T_{1/2} = 9.4\text{ h}]{\text{EC, }\beta^+} {}^{201}Tl$

figuration requirements are not severe, and greater flexibility is possible. Foils, pressed powder, and gaseous targets, though not practical as internal targets, are possible as external targets.

Because the radionuclide produced in charged particle reactions differs chemically from the target material, separation yields a carrier-free product. High beam current internal targets are quite radioactive (ie, often more than 1000 R/hour), owing in part to short-lived radionuclides induced in the target base; thus they must be chemically processed in a hot cell or with other heavily shielded containment, using remote manipulation. Usually, the target material is an expensive isotopically enriched stable isotope and must be recovered chemically after separation of the desired product. The monetary investment of materials, equipment, and personnel required for target preparation, processing, and recovery coupled with generally lower yields results in higher costs for cyclotron-produced radionuclides than for reactor-produced products.

Examples

GALLIUM-67

Gallium-67 is commercially prepared using the ^{68}Zn (*p*,2*n*) ^{67}Ga reaction. Isotopically enriched ^{68}Zn is electroplated on a copper internal target base. Naturally occurring zinc (18.5% ^{68}Zn) can be used; however, the ^{67}Ga yield is reduced accordingly, and the content of 9.5-hour ^{66}Ga is increased. The target is bombarded at an incident proton energy of 26 MeV for 10 to 20 hours, producing several curies of ^{67}Ga.

IODINE-123

Several nuclear reactions are capable of forming ^{123}I. Unfortunately, all of them have some disadvantages that translate to high cost: low yield, poor radionuclidic purity, or high energy requirements. The ^{127}I (*p*,5*n*) $^{123}Xe \rightarrow {}^{123}I$ reaction produces large quantities of relatively pure ^{123}I, with varying, but generally low, percentages of ^{125}I as radionuclidic impurity. This reaction requires 60 to 70 MeV protons, and cyclotrons having this energy are few and expensive to build. A good compromise is the ^{124}Xe(*p, pn*) $^{123}Xe \rightarrow {}^{123}I$ reaction, currently used to produce commercial ^{123}I.

FLUORINE-18

Fluorine-18 is one of several relatively short-lived positron-emitting radionuclides that can be produced from gaseous external targets. Other such radionuclides include ^{15}O, ^{13}N, and ^{11}C.

One useful nuclear reaction for production of ^{18}F

is $^{20}Ne(d,\alpha)^{18}F$, which uses naturally occurring neon gas with $\geq 0.1\%$ fluorine carrier contained in an external gas target. Deuterons between 2 and 14 MeV used to bombard the target produce approximately 350 mCi in 1 hour. At the end of bombardment, the gas in the target is released and conducted through a suitable system of tubing and valves to a reaction vessel for subsequent chemical processing.

In the preparation of ^{18}F-2-deoxy-2-fluoro-D-glucose (^{18}F FDG), the anhydrous ^{18}F as F_2 is bubbled through a cooled solution of 3,4,6 tri-*O*-acetyl D-glucal in freon-11 to form glycopyranosyl fluoride.[5] After the freon evaporates, the residue is dissolved in petroleum ether and passed over a silica gel column to remove impurities. The mixture is evaporated to dryness, suspended in dilute hydrochloric acid, and refluxed to hydrolyze the product to ^{18}F FDG.

Similar on-line systems have been developed for processing ^{15}O, ^{13}N, and ^{11}C.

REFERENCES

1. Szillard L, Chalmers TA. Chemical separation of radioactive element from its bombarded isotope in the Fermi effect. *Nature* 1934;134:462.
2. Lapp RE, Andrews HL. *Nuclear Radiation Physics*. 4th ed. Englewood Cliffs, NJ: Prentice Hall, 1934.
3. Lederer CM, Shirly VS, et al. *Table of Isotopes*. 7th ed. New York: John Wiley & Sons, 1978.
4. Tilbury RS, Laughlin JS. Cyclotron production of radioactive isotopes for medical uses. *Semin Nucl Med* 1974;4:245.
5. Barrio JR, et al. Remote, semiautomated production of ^{18}F-labeled 2-deoxy-2-fluoro-D-glucose. *J Nucl Med* 1981;22:372.

10 Radionuclide Generator Systems

F.F. (Russ) Knapp, Jr.

Radionuclide generators provide a ready source of medically useful radionuclides, while eliminating the two major impediments to the use of short-lived products: cost of production and uncertainty of transportation. In successful generator systems, the long-lived parent radionuclide can be shipped to the nuclear medicine laboratory in a suitable separation system from which the short-lived daughter can be extracted as needed during the functional life of the generator.

The evolution of radionuclide generators can be traced back to the 1920s, when Failla separated ^{222}Rn from ^{226}Ra.[1] This concept fluorished, and since then numerous successful generator systems have been developed (Tables 1 and 2).[2-4]

To be useful, generator systems must have certain essential properties[5]:

1. They should yield a daughter with high radiochemical and radionuclidic purity in an injectable solvent.
2. They must be safe and easily operated.
3. They must yield sterile and pyrogen-free products.
4. The products must be convenient for on-sight radiopharmaceutical preparation.
5. They must be capable of multiple separations.
6. The daughter half-life should be less than about 24 hours.

Otherwise, the radionuclide may be better obtained directly from a commercial source.

PARENT-DAUGHTER RELATIONSHIPS

In any generator system, the parent-daughter relationship can be described by

$$\frac{dN_1}{dt} = -N_1\lambda_1 \tag{1}$$

and

$$\frac{dN_2}{dt} = N_1\lambda_1 - N_2\lambda_2, \tag{2}$$

where N_1 = the number of atoms of the parent nuclide, N_2 = the number of atoms of the daughter nuclide, λ_1 = the disintegration constant of the parent, λ_2 = the disintegration constant of the daughter. $N_1\lambda_1$ represents the rate at which daughter atoms are formed, and $N_2\lambda_2$ represents the rate of their disappearance. These relationships are illustrated in Figure 1.

Figure 2 shows the changing relationships of parent and daughter nuclides in the ^{99}Mo-^{99m}Tc generator. When the half-life of the daughter is short compared with that of the parent, as in this case, approximately 50% of the equilibrium activity is reached within one daughter half-life, 75% at the end of two half-lives, and >99% after six half-lives.

The curves in Figure 2 reflect the branching scheme of ^{99}Mo, where only about 87% of ^{99}Mo disintegrations give rise to the metastable ^{99m}Tc.

CLINICALLY USEFUL GENERATOR SYSTEMS

The usual means of separating the daughter from the parent nuclide takes advantage of different oxidation states of the two radionuclides. The most common system employs a chromatographic column in which the parent is adsorbed onto some binder substance, such as an ion exchange resin, alumina, or other inorganic exchanger. The daughter, with a different chemical form and weaker affinity for the binder, is then washed off the column by a suitable eluting solution.

Figure 3 illustrates an "open" separation system consisting of a shielded column fitted with a porous fitted disc. Above this column, the chromatographic ion-exchange medium is placed and sealed with a retaining ring filter.

When generators are designed for commercial use, they are usually "closed" ie, the top and bottom are sealed to prevent contaminants from entering the column. Such seals can often be merely the insertion of Millipore filters into the outlet line. Bacteriostatic agents such as benzyl alcohol or phenol may be used in the eluting solution, provided they do not interfere with either binding of the parent nuclide or the stability of radiopharmaceuticals for which the daughter radionuclide is intended.

^{99}Mo-^{99m}Tc Generator

The ^{99}Mo-^{99m}Tc generator system, originally described by Richards,[6] has been by far the most widely used and in many respects remains the best example. Molybdenum-99 is obtained either in the carrier-free state separated from ^{235}U fission products from a reactor or by the ^{98}Mo (n,γ) reaction.

Most commercial ^{99}Mo-^{99m}Tc generators have used column chromatography, in which ^{99}Mo is adsorbed onto alumina and eluted with normal saline. The amount of alumina required

Table 1. Principal Characteristics of Currently and Potentially Useful Radionuclide Generators

DAUGHTER	$T_{1/2}$ (h)	DECAY MODE	PRINCIPAL EMISSION* keV (%)	PARENT	$T_{1/2}$	SELECTED REFERENCES
^{99m}Tc	6	IT	140 (89)	^{99}Mo	2.7 d	6, 38, 39
^{113m}In	1.7	IT	392 (64)	^{113}Sn	118 d	58
^{87m}Sr	2.8	IT	388 (82)	^{87}Y	3.3 d	56
^{103m}Rh	0.95	IT	Multiple	^{103}Ru	39.3 d	40
^{68}Ga	1.13	β+	836 (88)	^{68}Ge	271 d	48, 51
^{52m}Mn	0.35	β+	1173 (96)	^{52}Fe	8.2 h	52, 53
^{132}I	2.3	β−	Multiple	^{132}Te	78 h	49, 50
^{188}Re	17	β−	728 (25) 795 (71)	^{188}W	69 d	13, 14, 41, 42
^{90}Y	64	β−	935 (100)	^{90}Sr	28.8 y	12
^{194}Ir	19	β−	745	^{194}Os	6 y	43
^{212}Bi	1	α,β−	α = 6050 (25 d) β-multiple	^{212}Pb	10.6 h	44

*β− and β+ are average energies.
Source: MIRD Decay Schemes.

depends upon the specific activity of the ^{99}Mo to be bound. Since the extraction efficiency of ^{99m}Tc is inversely proportional to the square root of the alumina thickness, the mass of alumina employed in the generator should be at a minimum. This presents essentially no problem when carrier-free fission ^{99}Mo is used. Current radiochemical extraction techniques can render ^{99}Mo virtually free of such other fission contaminants as ^{131}I, ^{140}La, ^{103}Ru, and ^{132}Te.

With reactor-produced ^{99}Mo, radionuclidic contaminants are low, but the mass of residual ^{98}Mo reduces specific activity. One approach that permits the use of low specific activity ^{99}Mo is the preparation of a molybdenum-zirconium gel which is then packed into a column.[7]

Most commercial ^{99}Mo-^{99m}Tc generators have a useful shelf-life of about 1 week, between two and three half-lives of the ^{99}Mo. This shelf-life is practically determined by the activity concentrations required for most imaging agent "kits." In some cases higher concentrations can be obtained by *fractional elution*. In this case only the middle fraction of a total elution is used for labeling, since this fraction contains the highest ^{99m}Tc concentration.

After an elution, ^{99m}Tc begins to grow in again by decay of ^{99}Mo (Fig. 2). The daughter can be removed at any time, but the yield or amount of ^{99m}Tc available from decay depends on the time elapsed since the previous elution. Practical elution cycles for the ^{99}Mo-^{99m}Tc generator are about 24 hours. Typical commercial generators contain 2 to 16 Ci (90 to 600 GBq) of ^{99}Mo.

The chemistry of ^{99m}Tc radiopharmaceuticals is discussed in detail in Chapter 11. Quality control procedures prescribed for ^{99}Mo-^{99m}Tc generators are similar to those required of most radionuclide generators. A test of ^{99}Mo breakthrough is essential. This is simple in the case of ^{99m}Tc-^{99}Mo solutions, because the 740-keV gamma emission (14%) of ^{99}Mo is easily detected through calibrated shields that effectively absorb all of the 140-keV gamma rays of ^{99m}Tc. The current maximum legal limit of breakthrough in the United States is 0.15 μCi ^{99}Mo per millicurie ^{99m}Tc per administered dose.

Table 2. Some Ultrashort-Lived Radionuclide Generators

DAUGHTER	$T_{1/2}$	DECAY MODE	PRINCIPAL EMISSION keV (%)	PARENT	$T_{1/2}$	SELECTED REFERENCES
^{81m}Kr	13 s	IT	190 (67)	^{81}Rb	4.6 h	23–25
^{109m}Ag	39.6 s	IT	88 (3.6)	^{109}Cd	1.24 y	47
^{191m}Ir	4.9 s	IT	129 (25)	^{191}Os	15.4 d	28–30
^{137m}Ba	2.55 min	IT	662 (90)	^{137}Cs	30 y	54, 55
^{195m}Au	30.5 s	IT	260 (68)	^{195m}Hg	41.6 h	31, 32, 45
^{82}Rb	1.3 min	β+	1523* (83)	^{82}Sr	25 d	18–22
^{62}Cu	9.7 min	β+	Multiple	^{62}Zn	9.26 h	35–37
^{178}Ta	9.25 min	EC	55 (67) 64 (18)	^{178}W	21.5 d	

*Average energy.

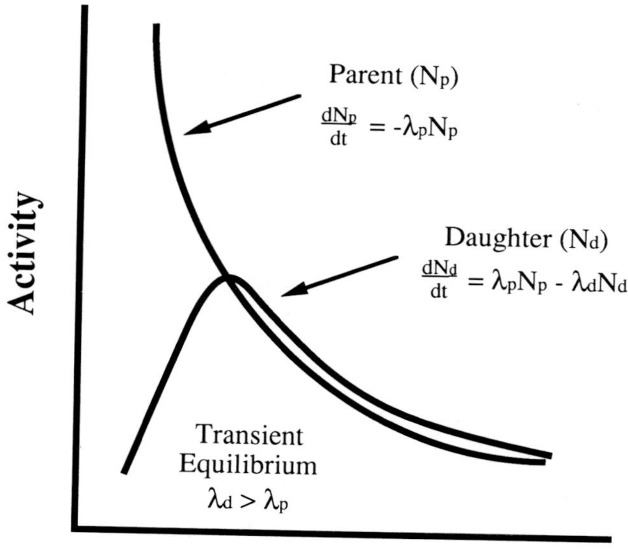

Figure 1. Parent and daughter activities as a function of time when a transient equilibrium exists ($\lambda_2 > \lambda_1$).

Aluminum breakthrough must also be tested because aluminum interferes with the radiolabeling of some radiopharmaceuticals.

^{113}Sn-^{113m}In Generator

Tin-113 decays to ^{113m}In. The metastable ^{113m}In decays with a half-life of 1.7 hour to stable ^{113}In. The 393-keV gamma emission is generally too high for efficient scintillation camera imaging, but suitable for rectilinear scanners. This generator is seldom used clinically today. However, the 118-day half-life of ^{113}Sn makes this system a convenient laboratory source of radionuclides since generator replacement is necessitated only once or twice annually.

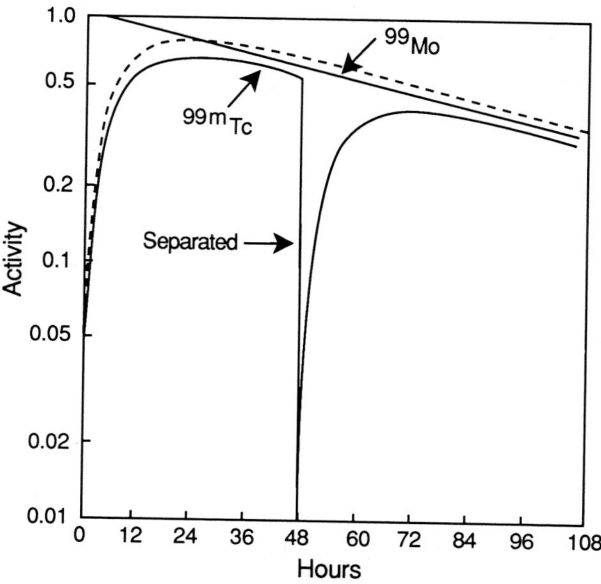

Figure 2. The buildup and transient equilibrium of ^{99m}Tc in a ^{99}Mo-^{99m}Tc generator. The dotted line indicates the hypothetical ^{99m}Tc activity if ^{99}Mo decayed 100% to ^{99m}Tc, instead of only 87% of disintegrations.

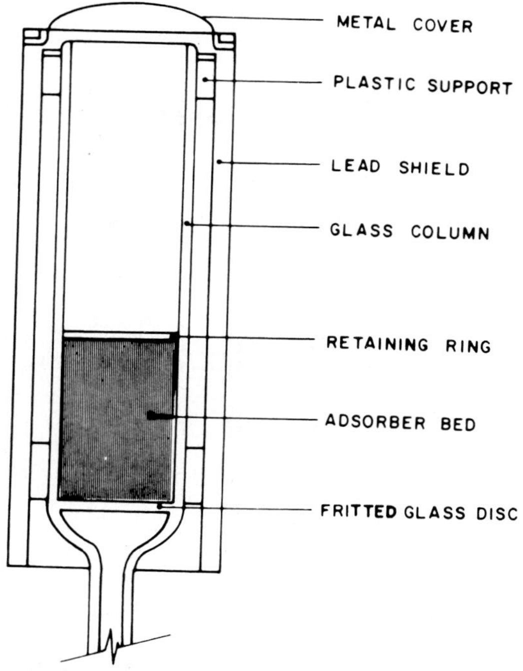

Figure 3. A typical chromatographic column used in open generator systems.

The ^{113}Sn is bound either to hydrous zirconium oxide or to silica gel and is eluted with HCl solution at pH 1.2 to 1.6. Breakthrough of ^{113}Sn must be checked scrupulously at the beginning of each new generator and periodically during its shelf life. This quality control check can be made by allowing the eluate to decay for 48 hours, after which all of the eluted ^{113m}In will have decayed. Any detectable ^{113m}In can then be assumed to be in equilibrium with breakthrough ^{113}Sn.

^{90}Sr-^{90}Y Generator

Yttrium-90 is the daughter of ^{90}Sr and is used increasingly for such therapeutic applications as radiolabeled antibodies (See Chapter 51). While most ^{90}Y is obtained from commercial sources, it can be produced in local radiopharmacies using a chromatographic generator system. Chinol and Hnatowich have described a generator in which ^{90}Sr is loaded onto Dowex 50 cation exchange resin as the solid support.[12] They describe elution with 0.03 *M* EDTA with an average elution efficiency of 98% and ^{90}Sr breakthrough averaging 0.002%.

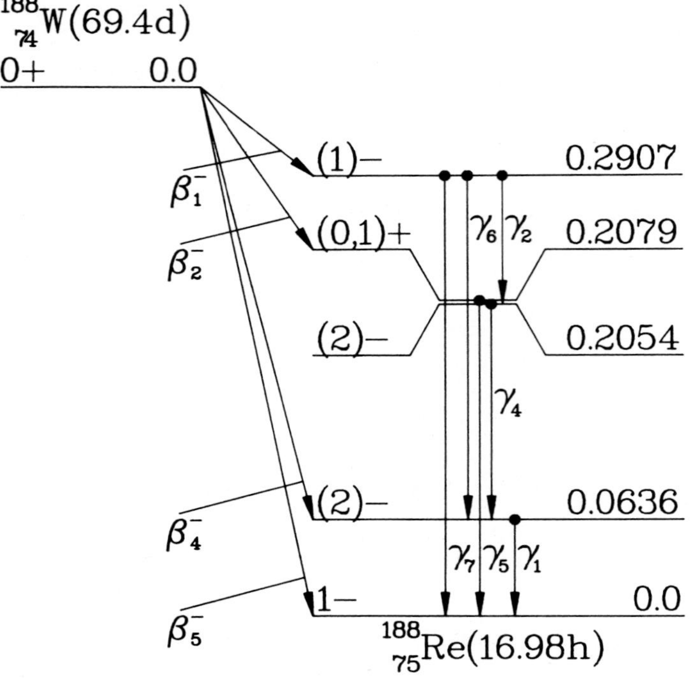

Figure 4. The decay scheme of ^{188}W.

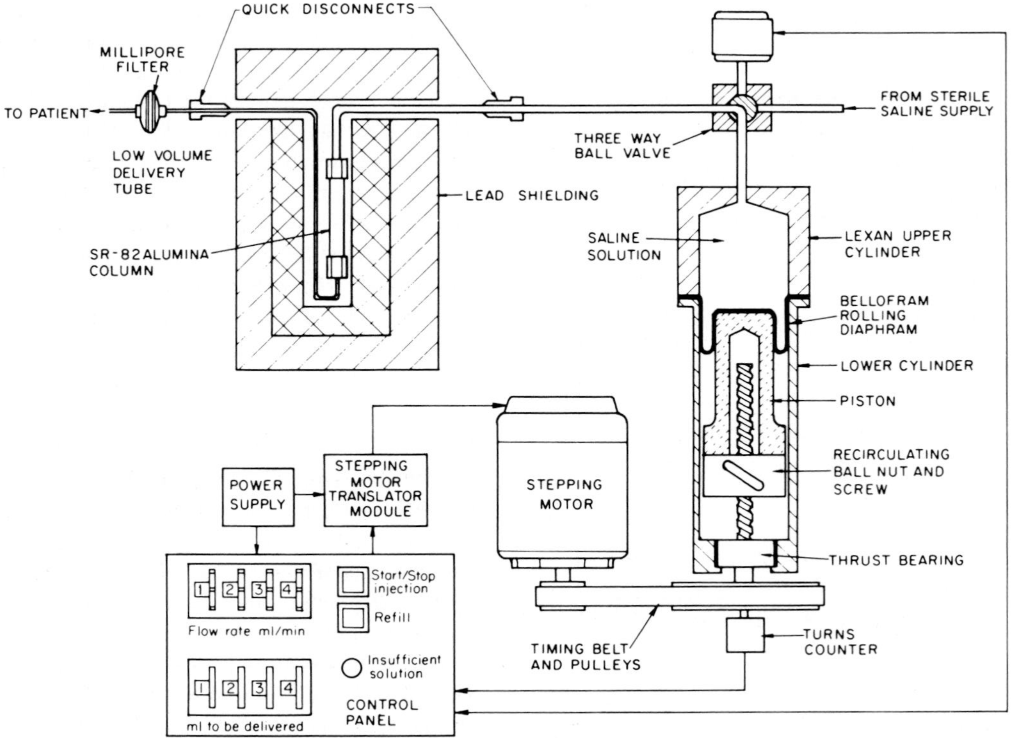

Figure 5. Rubidium-82 closed generator system. (From Reference 57.)

^{188}W-^{188}Re *Generator*

Another promising candidate for antibody labeling for radioimmunotherapy is ^{188}Re, the daughter of ^{188}W (Fig. 4).[13,14] Rhenium-188 decays with β^- emissions along with 15% 155-keV gamma emissions, which are useful to localize the radionuclide in dosimetry and biodistribution studies.

Reactor-produced ^{188}W is loaded as acidified sodium tungstate onto BioRad alumina, from which ^{188}Re can be eluted as sodium perrhenate with 99% efficiency.[14] Prototype generators as large as 225 mCi have been evaluated with consistently high yields for several months.[2]

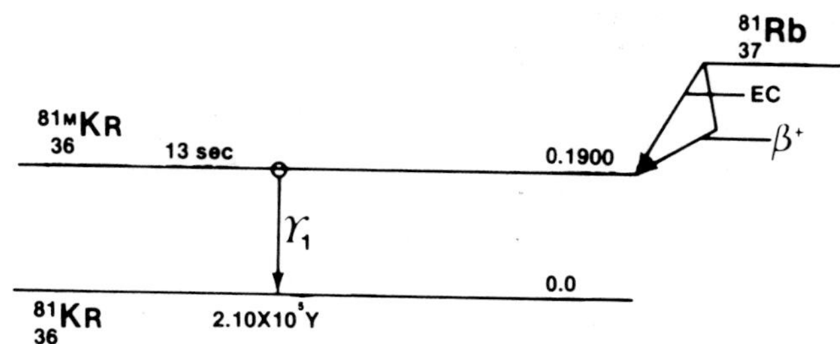

Figure 6. Principal decay characteristics of ^{81}Rb and ^{81m}Kr.

ULTRASHORT-LIVED GENERATORS

The attraction of radionuclides with very short half-lives is that they deliver low radiation-absorbed dose, studies can be repeated at short intervals without interfering background, and from a radiation safety point of view spills and waste do not create the problems of longer-lived nuclides. A substantial limitation to wider use of short-lived radionuclides is the problem of decay during preparation and delivery.

The first ultrashort-lived radiotracers were used to measure velocity and relative volume of blood circulating through various organs. Bender and Blau[15] used ^{137m}Ba and Yano and Anger demonstrated the use of generator-produced ^{109m}Ag and ^{191m}Ir for these studies.[16]

A list of potentially useful generator-produced ultrashort-lived radionuclides is given in Table 2. Only radionuclide daughters with half-lives of less than 10 minutes are classified as ultrashort lived. Not all radionuclides listed here can be used with currently available imaging systems, because many emit high-energy photons, eg, ^{28}Al (1.78 MeV). Others are impractical for widespread use because of such short half-lived parents as ^{62}Zn (9.26 hours) and ^{81}Rb (4.58 hours). Both require generator production or delivery on the same day. Nevertheless, useful applications have been found.

Yano's first automated ultrashort-lived radionuclide generator system was designed to elute ^{191m}Ir from its ^{191}Os parent, but it was also used, with minor changes, to separate other ultrashort-lived radionuclides.[17] The system was automated to provide a continuous flow of sterile eluant solution. The resin column, inside a 5-cm thick lead shield, was connected to a 20-mL syringe, which was automatically filled from an eluant reservoir and forced through the generator by an electric motor drive and automatic two-way valve. A second reservoir contained sterile water to dilute the highly saline eluant before reaching the patient's vein. This generator system made it possible to deliver the radionuclide daughter by direct intravenous infusion at the time intervals desired, before appreciable radionuclide decay. A Millipore filter at the end of the system ensured eluate sterility.

^{82}Sr-^{82}Rb *Generator*

The long half-life of ^{82}Sr (25 days) makes the ^{82}Sr-^{82}Rb generator an attractive source of a short-lived positron-emitting radionuclide. This generator is now available commercially for use with PET studies of myocardium.[18–20] It is especially valuable for facilities that do not have in-house cyclotrons.[21,22]

The chemistry of separation and binding of $^{82}SrCl_2$ to hydrous SnO_2 as the solid support is relatively straightforward. There is negligible ^{82}Sr breakthrough when the column is eluted with isotonic saline at physiologic pH.

The generator is shown in Figure 5. Its use in cardiovascular nuclear medicine requires a system for rapid elution and on-line injection of the eluate; every 5 to 10 minutes, 30 to 60 mCi (1 to 2 GBq) of ^{82}Rb can be injected automatically in 7 to 8 mL of eluant. The syringe plunger is bidirectionally actuated by a low-friction, recirculating ball screw jack that is coupled to a stepping motor through a reduction gear. The speed of the motor driving the syringe plunger and infusion rate are regulated automatically by a radiation monitor in line with the infusion tubing to deliver a predetermined dose. The entire system is self-contained on a mobile cart.

^{81}Rb-^{81m}Kr *Generator*

Krypton-81m has a 13-second half-life and decays by isomeric transition to ^{81}Kr, emitting 190-keV gamma rays in 67% of disintegrations (Fig. 6). The development of the ^{81}Rb-^{81m}Kr generator was described by Jones and Clark and by Yano et al.[23–25] Generators are available for both perfusion studies[26,46] and for pulmonary function studies.[27]

A variety of exchangers have been used in generator prototypes. The most widely used adsorbent is strongly basic Dowex 50 × 8. Krypton-81m is extracted from this generator by passage of filtered medical-grade air through the column. Since the daughter is a gas, ^{81}Rb breakthrough is inconsequential when eluted with air. The presence of other rubidium isotopes, such as ^{82m}Rb, on the column is also of no consequence since they do not decay to a gas. Furthermore, the 13-second half-life of the daughter makes leakage to the environment almost trivial. In fact, waste gas collection systems are eliminated in pulmonary ventilation studies. A significant drawback is the short, 4.7-hour half-life of the parent, which requires daily production (or delivery) of the generator system.

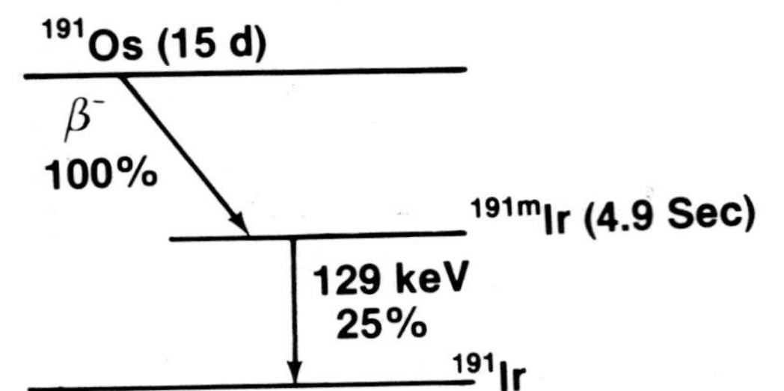

Figure 7. Principal decay characteristics of ^{191}Os and ^{191m}Ir.

^{191}Os-^{191m}Ir Generator

Iridium-191m has many characteristics of an ideal ultrashort-lived radionuclide. It has a half-life of only 4.9 seconds and decays by isomeric transition to stable ^{191}Ir (Fig. 7). The parent ^{191}Os has a 15-day half-life, necessitating infrequent production. The 25% of the 129-keV gamma rays that are not internally converted provides an efficient means of external detection. Osmium-191 can be produced by the ^{190}Os (n,γ) ^{191}Os reaction of 98%-enriched ^{191}Os.

The first ^{191}Os-^{191m}Ir generator was reported by Yano and Anger.[16] Recent modifications incorporate Os (VI) as osmyl chloride bound to silica gel impregnated with tridodecyl-methylammonium chloride. This mixture is slurried into the generator column with pH 1 saline. Equilibration of the generator at room temperature for 24 hours before elution is evidently important to insure proper generator performance. Elution with acidic (HCl) saline at pH 1 provides yields of 21 to 33%.[28,29] An activated carbon "scavenger" column is used in tandem with the generator column to remove ^{191}Os breakthrough before the eluant is rapidly buffered with 1 *M* succinate solution to pH 9. A 0.22-μm Millipore filter is attached at the end of the elution line prior to intravenous administration.

Studies by Franken et al[30] describe the advantages of using ^{191m}Ir for rapid sequential radionuclide angiography. An important aspect of the use of this generator and other generators providing ultra short-lived daughter nuclides is the rapid in-growth period. With ^{191m}Ir, for example, complete return to equilibrium is reached in less than 1 minute, at which time the generator can again be eluted. The portability of these systems in conjunction with portable scintillation cameras allows their use in critical care units.

The generator prototype used to obtain ^{191m}Ir for Franken's studies consists of a specially activated carbon adsorbent with the ^{191}Os bound as an Os(VI) species. The ^{191m}Ir is eluted with pH 2 saline containing 0.025% potassium iodide with the 2 mL bolus buffered with Tris to pH 7.2 just prior to flushing into the intravenous line. The generator system has a consistently high ^{191m}Ir yield (~18% per bolus) and low parent breakthrough (<2×10^{-4}% per bolus) over a useful shelf life of at least 3 weeks.

^{195m}Hg-^{195m}Au Generator

Panek et al developed a reliable ^{195m}Hg-^{195m}Au generator (Fig. 8 and 9).[31] The ^{195m}Hg ($T_{1/2}$ = 41.6 hours) is prepared from a metallic gold target by the $(p,3n)$ reaction and loaded on a ZnS-coated silica gel column. The ^{195m}Au ($T_{1/2}$ = 30.6 seconds; γ = 262 keV) is eluted with thiosulfate solution. This generator is intended for cardiac and blood pool studies.[32] It can be eluted using either a bolus or a continuous infusion technique. The yield from a 7.5 G GBq (200 mCi) generator approaches 30% at flow rates of 12 mL/minute. Mercury breakthrough in the most recent generator models is 2 to 3×10^{-3}%/mL. This results in an elution of about 1 μCi of ^{195m}Hg per millicurie of ^{195m}Au, which is small enough to permit 10 to 12 successive cardiac studies while imposing an acceptable radiation burden to the kidneys.

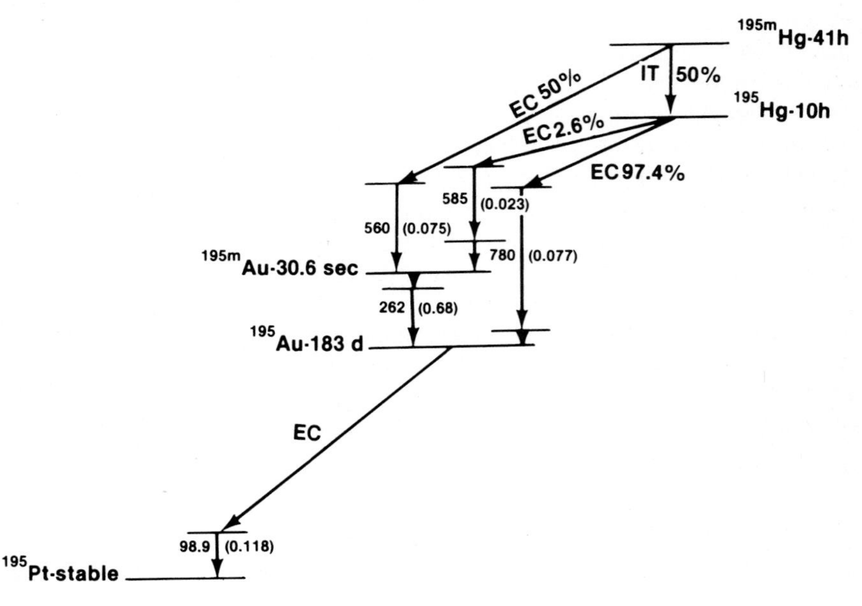

Figure 8. Principal decay characteristics of ^{195m}Hg and ^{195m}Au.

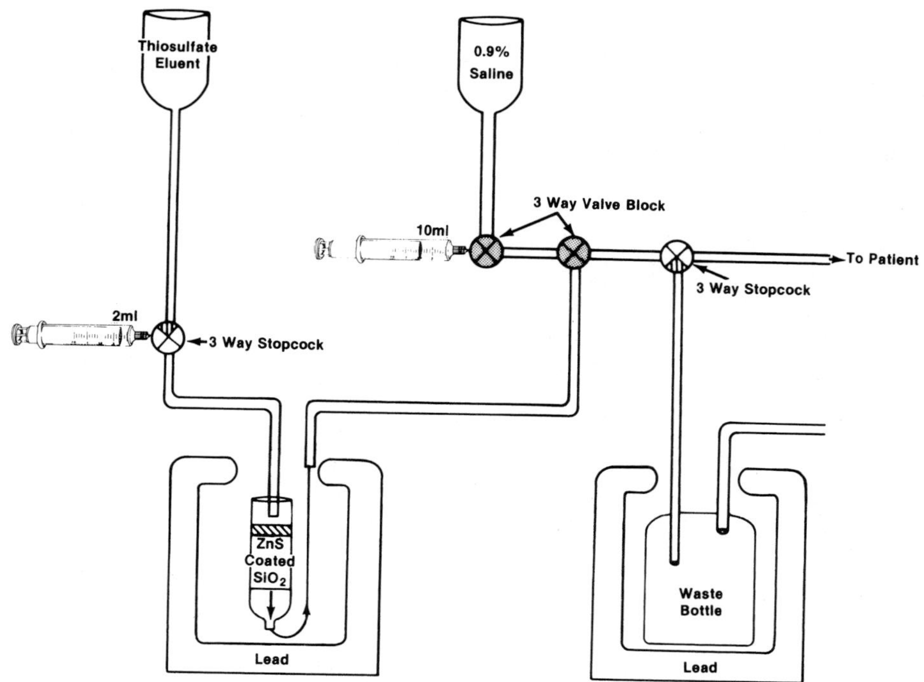

Figure 9. Prototype generator system for ^{195m}Au.

^{62}Zn-^{62}Cu Generator

The ^{62}Zn-^{62}Cu generator was first described by Robinson et al.[35] The parent ^{62}Zn is loaded on a Dowex 1 × 8 anion exchange resin column in the chloride form, from which the daughter ^{62}Cu is eluted with 2 *M* HCl (Fig. 10). Initial clinical interest has been focused on ^{62}Cu(II)-labeled pyruvaldehyde bis(N^4-methylthiosemicarbazone), ^{62}Cu-PTSM, a lipophilic agent used for PET organ perfusion imaging.[36,37]

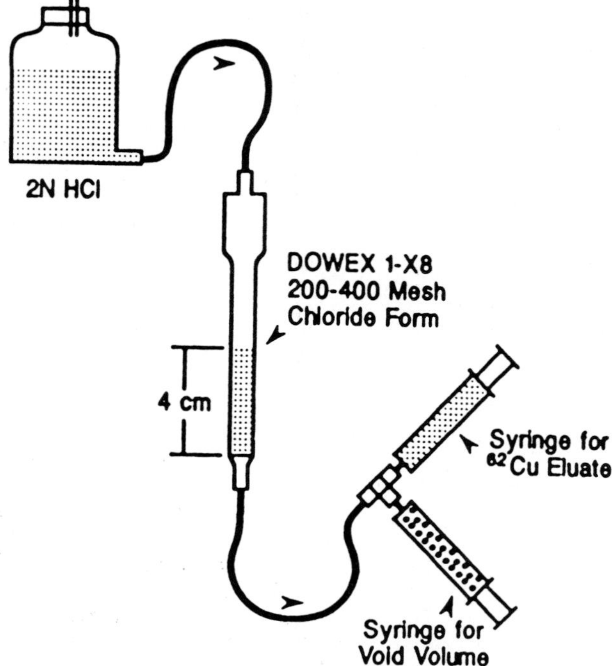

Figure 10. A prototype ^{62}Zn-^{62}Cu generator.

In the preparation of ^{62}Cu-PTSM the acidic generator eluate is neutralized with 3 *N* sodium acetate buffer, which is added to the PTSM ligand in ethanol. The reaction mixture is then added to a C_{18}-SepPak® solid-phase extraction cartridge, and the lipophilic ^{62}Cu-PTSM is obtained by elution with ethanol. The ethanol eluant is diluted with saline prior to filtration through a sterile 0.22-μm Millipore filter before intravenous injection. The complete elution, synthesis, and purification procedure can be complete in 1 to 6 minutes with a final yield of about 50%.

The greatest drawback of this generator system is the short, 9.26-hour half-life of the parent ^{62}Cu.

This brief review has focused on some of the important factors concerning the use of radionuclide generator systems for nuclear medicine. With the emergence of PET as an important clinical modality and the wider use of radionuclide therapy, generator systems will become increasingly important sources of radionuclides.

REFERENCES

1. Failla G. The development of filtered radium implants. *Am J Roentgenol* 1926;16:507.
2. Knapp FF, Callahan AP, Mirzadeh S, Brihaye C, Guillaume M. The development of radionuclide generators. In: Schubiger PA, Westera G, eds. *Progress in Radiopharmacy.* Dordrecht: Kluwer Academic, 1992;67–88.
3. Knapp FF Jr, Butler TA, eds. *Radionuclide Generators: New Systems for Nuclear Medicine Applications.* American Chemi-

cal Society Advances in Chemistry Series No. 241. Washington DC: American Chemical Society, 1984.

4. Lambrecht RM. Radionuclide generators. *Radiochim Acta* 1983;34:9–24.
5. Colombetti LG. Radionuclide generator systems. In: *Textbook of Nuclear Medicine*. vol. 1. Ricker A, Harbert JC, eds, Philadelphia: Lea & Febiger, 1984.
6. Richards P. Nuclide generators. In: *Radioactive Pharmaceuticals*. Symposium No. 6, Conf 651111. Oak Ridge, TN: US Atomic Energy Commission, 1966;155.
7. Evans JV, Moore PW, Shying ME, Sodeau JM. A new generator for technetium-99m. In: *Proceedings of the 3rd World Congress of Nuclear Medicine and Biology, August 29–September 2, Paris, France*. vol. 2, Raynuad C, ed. Elmsford, NY: Pergamon Press, 1982;1592–1595.
8. Perrier C, Segré E. Chemical properties of element 43. *J Chem Physiol*. 1937;5:712.
9. Hallaba E, El-Asrag HA. On the sublimation of ^{99m}Tc from irradiated molybdenum trioxide. *Isotopenpraxis* 1975;8:290.
10. Colombetti LG. Performance of ^{99m}Tc generating systems. In: *Quality Control in Nuclear Medicine*. Rhodes BA, ed. St. Louis: C.V. Mosby, 1977.
11. Gerlit JB. *Some Chemical Properties of Technetium*. vol. 7. New York: Int. Conf. Peaceful Uses Atom. Energy 1956;145.
12. Chinol M, Hnatowich DJ. Generator-produced yttrium-90 for radioimmunotherapy. *J Nucl Med* 1987;28:1465–1470.
13. Griffiths GL, Knapp FF Jr, Callahan AP, Chang C-H, Hansen HJ, Goldenberg DM. Direct radiolabeling of monoclonal antibodies with generator-produced rhenium-188 for radioimmunotherapy. *Can Res* 1991b,51:4592–4602.
14. Callahan AP, Rice DE, Knapp FF Jr. Rhenium-188 for therapeutic applications from an alumina based tungsten-188/rhenium-188 radionuclide generator. *NucCompact-Eur/Am Commun Nucl Med* 1989;20:3–6.
15. Bender MA, Blau M. The autofluoroscope. *Nucleonics* 1963; 21:52.
16. Yano Y, Anger HO. Ultrashort-lived radioisotopes for visualizing blood vessels and organs. *J Nucl Med* 1968;9:2.
17. Yano Y, Anger HO. Visualization of heart and kidneys in animals with ultrashort-lived ^{82}Rb and the positron scintillation camera. *J Nucl Med* 1968;9:412.
18. Yano Y, Budinger TF, Cahoon JL, Huesman RH. An automated microprocessor-controlled Rb-82 generator for positron emission tomography studies. In: Knapp FF Jr, Butler TA, eds. *Radionuclide Generators—New Systems for Nuclear Medicine Applications*. ACS Symposium Series No. 242, Washington DC: American Chemical Society, 1984;97–122.
19. Gennaro GP, Neirinckx RD, Bergner B, Muller WR, Waranis A, Haney TA, Barker SL, Loberg MD, Yarnais A. A radionuclide generator and infusion system for pharmaceutical quality rubidium-82. In: *Radionuclide Generators—New Systems for Nuclear Medicine Applications*. Knapp FF Jr, Butler TA, eds. ACS Symposium Series No. 242, Washington DC: American Chemical Society 1984;135–150.
20. Brihaye C, Guillaume M, Cogneau M. Distribution coefficients of Sr and Rb ions on various adsorbents in view to achieving a Sr-Rb generator for medical use. *Radiochem Radioanal Lett* 1981;48:157–164.
21. Gould KL, Goldstein RA, Mullani NA. Economic analysis of clinical positron emission tomography of the heart with rubidium-82. *J Nucl Med* 30:707–717.
22. Gould KL, Goldstein RA, Mullani NA. Non-invasive assessment of coronary stenoses by myocardial perfusion imaging during pharmacologic coronary vasodilation. VIII. Clinical feasibility of positron cardiac imaging without a cyclotron using generator-produced rubidium-82. *J Am Coll Cardiol* 1986;7:775–789.
23. Jones T, Clark JC. A cyclotron produced ^{81}Rb-^{81m}Kr generator and its uses in gamma camera studies. *Br J Radiol* 1969;42:237.
24. Jones T et al. ^{81m}Kr generator and its uses in cardiopulmonary studies with the scintillation camera. *J Nucl Med* 1970;11:118.
25. Yano Y, McRae J, Anger HO. Lung function studies using short-lived ^{81m}Kr and the scintillation camera. *J Nucl Med* 1970;11:674.
26. Guillaume M, Brihaye C. Generators for short-lived gamma and positron emitting radionuclides: current status and prospects. *Nucl Med Biol* 1986;13:89–100.
27. Guillaume M, Czichosz R, Richard P, Fagard E. Krypton-81m generator for ventilation and perfusion (Monograph in English). *Bull Soc R Liège*, 1983;LII:213–281.
28. Issachar D, Abrashkin S, Weiniger J, Zemach D, Lubin E, Hellman C, Trumper D. Osmium-191/iridium-191m generator based on silica gel impregnated with tridodecylmethylammonium chloride. *J Nucl Med* 1989;30:538–541.
29. Hellman C, Zafrir N, Shimoni A, Issachar D, Trumper J, Abrashkin S, Lubin E. Evaluation of ventricular function with first-pass iridium-191m radionuclide angiography. *J Nucl Med* 1989;30:450–457.
30. Franken PR, Dobbeleir A, Ham HR, Brihaye C, Guillaume M, Knapp FF Jr, Vandevivere J. Ultrashort-lived iridium-191m from a new carbon-based generator system for left ventricular first-pass angiocardiography. *J Nucl Med* 1989;30:1025–1031.
31. Panek KJ, Lindeyer J, van der Vlught NC. A new generator system for production of short-living Au-195m radioisotope. *J Nucl Med* 1982;23:P108.
32. Mena I, Narahara KA, de Jong R, Maublaut J. Gold-195m, and ultra-short-lived generator-produced radionuclide: clinical application in sequential first-pass ventriculography. *J Nucl Med* 1983;24:139.
33. Neirinckx RD, Trumper J, LeBlanc A, Johnson PC. Evaluation of adsorbents for the Ta-178 generator. In: Knapp FF Jr, Butler TA, eds. *Radionuclide Generators—New Systems for Nuclear Medicine Applications*. ACS Symposium Series No. 242, Washington DC: American Chemical Society, 1984;151–168.
34. Lacy JL, Ball ME, Verani MS, Wiles HB, Babich JW, LeBlanc AD, Stabin M, Bolomey L, Roberts R. An improved tungsten-178/tantalum-178. *J Nucl Med* 1988b;29:1526–1538.
35. Robinson GD Jr, Zielinsky FW, Lee AW. The zinc-62/copper-62 generator. A convenient source of copper-62 for radiopharmaceuticals. *Int J Appl Rad Isot* 1980;31:111–116.
36. Green MA, Klippenstein DL. Copper(II)bis-(thiosemicarbazone) complexes as potential tracers for evaluation of cerebral and myocardial blood flow with PET. *J Nucl Med* 1988; 29:1549–1559.
37. Green MA, Mathias JC, Welch MJ, McGuire AH, Perry D, Fernandex-Rubio F, Perlmutter JS, Raichle ME, Bergmann SR. Copper-62-labeled pyruvaldehyde bis (N^4-methylthiosemicarbaxonato) copper(II): synthesis and evaluation as a positron emission tomography tracer for cerebral and myocardial perfusion. *J Nucl Med* 1990;31:1989–1996.
38. Eckelman WC, Coursey BM, eds. Technetium-99m: generators, chemistry and preparation of radiopharmaceuticals. *Int J Appl Radiat Isot* 1982;33:793.
39. Boyd RE. Technetium generator: status and prospects. In: *Seminar on Radionuclide Generator Technology*. IAEA-SR-131, paper 21, 1986.
40. Lambrecht RM, Sajjad M. Accelerator-derived radionuclide generators. *Radiochim Acta* 1988;43:171–179.
41. Kodina G, Tulskaya T, Gureev E, Brodskaya G, Gapurova O, Drosdovsky B. Production and investigationof rhenium-188 generator. In: Nicolini M, Bandoli G, eds. *Technetium and Rhenium in Chemistry and Nuclear Medicine*. Verona: Cortina International, 1990;635–641.
42. Ehrhardt G, Ketring AP, Turpin TA, Razavi MS, Vanderheyden

J-L, Fritzberg AR. An improved tungsten-188 generator for radiotherapeutic applications. *J Nucl Med* 1987;28:656, 657.

43. Mirzadeh S, Callahan AP, Knapp FF Jr. Iridium-194—a new candidate for radioimmunotherapy (RAIT) from an osmium-194 generator system. *J Nucl Med* 1991;32:1089. Abstract.
44. Atcher RW, Friedman AM, Hines JJ. An improved generator for the production of ^{21}Pb and ^{212}Bi from ^{224}Ra. *Appl Radiat Isot* 1988;39:283–286.
45. Bett R, Cunningham JG, Sims HE, Willis HE, Dymond DS, Flatman W, Stone DL, Elliot AT. Development of the ^{195m}Hg/^{195m}Au generator for first-pass radionuclide angiography of the heart. *Int J Appl Radiat Isot* 1983;34:959–963.
46. Phillip MS, Ramsey CI, Ma JM, Lamb JF. A Krypton-81m perfusion generator. In: Knapp FF Jr, Butler TA, eds. *Radionuclide Generators—New Systems for Nuclear Medicine Applications.* ACS Symposium Series No. 242, Washington DC: American Chemical Society, 1984;67–76.
47. Steinkruger FJ, Wanek PM, Moody DC. *Cadmium-109/Silver-109m Biomedical Generator.* International Atomic Energy Agency. Seminar on Radionuclide Generator Technology. Vienna, October 13–17, 1986. Symposium, IAEA-SR-131/08, 1986.
48. Loc'h C, Mazière B, Comar D. A new genertor for ionic gallium-68. *J Nucl Med* 1980;21:171–173.
49. Stang LG et al. Production of iodine-132. *Nucleonics* 1954; 12:22.
50. Tucker WD et al. Practical methods of milking Y^{90}, Tc^{99m} and I^{132} from their respective parents. *Trans Am Nucl Soc* 1960;3:451.
51. Neirinckx RD, Davis MA. Development of a generator for ionic gallium-68. *J Nucl Med* 1979;20:681.
52. Ku TH, Richards P, Stang LG, et al. Generator production of manganese-52m for positron tomography. *J Nucl Med* 1979;20:682.
53. Atcher RW, Friedman AM. Manganese-52m, a new short-lived generator produced radionuclide: a potential tracer for positron tomography. *J Nucl Med* 1980;21:569.
54. Vernejoul P, Valeyre J, Kellershohn C. Dosimetry and technique for the use of ^{137m}Ba in cardiac hemodynamics. *C R Acad Sci* 1967;264:10.
55. Castronovo FP, Reba RC, Wagner HN. System for sustained intravenous infusion of a sterile solution of ^{137m}Ba-ethylenediaminetetraacetic acid (EDTA). *J Nucl Med* 1969;10:242.
56. Meckelnburg RL. Clinical value of generator produced ^{87m}strontium. *J Nucl Med* 1964;5:929.
57. Yano Y, Cahoon JL, Budinger TF. A precision flow-controlled Rb82 generator for bolus or constant infusion studies of the heart and brain. *J Nucl Med* 1981;22:1006.
58. Colombetti LG, Goodwin DA, Hinkley RL. Preparation and testing of a sterile ^{113}Sn-^{113n}In generator. *Am J Roentg Rad Ther Nucl Med* 1969;CVI:745.

11 Radiopharmaceutical Chemistry

William C. Eckelman, Joseph Steigman, Chang H. Paik

INTRODUCTION

Definitions and Scope

Radiopharmaceutical chemistry is the study of those aspects of chemistry, radiochemistry, biochemistry, pharmacology, physiology, and molecular biology that relate to the development of radiolabeled compounds suitable for tracing physiological processes. One of the success stories of the peaceful use of the atom is the discovery and development of radiopharmaceuticals for use as noninvasive diagnostic agents that are capable of probing a system on the molecular level. Molecular imaging with high specific activity radiopharmaceuticals affords the opportunity to translate the laboratory discoveries to the study in humans in health and disease.

Diagnostic radiopharmaceuticals are generally labeled with single photon-emitting radionuclides although many important uses for positron-emitting radionuclides are being developed. The ability to incorporate readily available radionuclides with optimum decay characteristics into tracer molecules has been the foremost consideration in developing diagnostic radiopharmaceuticals. In this respect, ^{99m}Tc is the ideal choice. The radioisotopes of iodine have played a pioneering role in radiopharmaceutical chemistry since their early use in thyroid metabolism studies and the in vitro techniques of radioimmunoassay. Because none of the iodine isotopes have the ideal nuclear properties and availability of ^{99m}Tc, earlier iodinated imaging agents have mostly been replaced by ^{99m}Tc-labeled radiopharmaceuticals. Only in radiolabeling specific biochemicals does iodine, especially ^{123}I, play an important role because of the greater structural disruption caused by incorporating technetium. This chapter contains a detailed discussion of the complex chemistry of technetium and iodine, along with examples of clinically useful radiopharmaceuticals. Other radionuclides with important diagnostic applications, including short-lived cyclotron products, are also reviewed with an emphasis on their radiochemistry and quality assurance.

History of the Discovery of Radioactivity[1]

In the course of investigating fluorescence from potassium uranyl sulfate, Becquerel discovered that the emissions that blackened a photographic plate were present whether or not the crystals were exposed to light or to the newly discovered x-rays. In 1898, Pierre and Marie Sklodowska Curie concluded that the emissions from the uranium salts were an atomic phenomenon and introduced the name "radioactivity." The field of radiochemistry was born in the attempts to isolate characteristic radioactivity from various ores. The early radioactive species identified were isotopes of uranium, thorium, polonium, and radon. As the various emissions from the radioactive elements were identified, these emissions were used in turn to produce artificial radioactivity. In January of 1934, Irene Curie and Frederick Joliet produced radioactive species by bombarding aluminum and boron with alpha particles from polonium. Nuclear fission was discovered by Otto Hahn and F. Strassmann 4 years later and both of these discoveries led to the production of an increasing number of new radionuclides.

History of Applications to Clinical Research

Martin D. Kamen in the three editions of his book entitled *Isotopic Tracers in Biology* chronicled the rapid progress in applying the newly discovered radionuclides to uses in clinical research.[2] Some of the important "firsts" were the determination of the speed of diffusion and peripheral circulation using ^{24}Na by Blumgart and Weiss in 1927 and thyroid metabolism by Hamilton and Stone in 1937. Uptake, retention, and excretion of radiolabeled phosphate (^{32}P) and radiolabeled iodide (^{131}I) provided valuable information about the selectivity of proposed therapeutic regimens. Radioisotopes were also valuable in applications in hematology. Red cell survival, iron physiology, and blood volume were some of the important contributions. In the early 1940s, ^{32}P followed by ^{35}S and ^{131}I was used to label antigens and antibodies. In the process of studying the behavior of ^{131}I insulin, Berson and Yalow developed the sensitive assay system for blood components known as radioimmunoassay.[3]

RADIOPHARMACEUTICAL CHEMISTRY OF TECHNETIUM

Discovery of Tc and ^{99m}Tc

Perhaps the most successful peaceful use of the atom has been the development of ^{99m}Tc radiopharmaceuticals as noninvasive diagnostic agents. The element technetium was identified by Perrier and Segre in 1937.[4] Two years later, ^{99m}Tc was discovered.[5] Only a few years after that, the molybdenum-technetium pair was separated in the midst of analyzing fission products at Brookhaven National Laboratory.[6]

This new radioisotope, eluted from a molybdenum generator in the form of pertechnetate, was soon tested as a diagnostic agent.[7]

At present there are 17 known isotopes of technetium, all radioactive, and 6 nuclear isomers. Of these, the short-lived nuclear isomer ^{99m}Tc ($T_{1/2}$ = 6.03 hours) is used in nuclear medicine, and the much longer-lived ^{99}Tc ($T_{1/2} = 2.1 \times 10^5$ years), which is available from uranium fission, is used to establish the general chemistry of the element at conventional chemical concentrations.[8] The radiation characteristics of ^{99m}Tc are excellent for external imaging. Its half-life is 6.03 hours, it emits gamma-ray photons, but no beta particles and only low energy or low-frequency Auger electrons. The predominant photon energy—140 KeV—is almost totally absorbed in the thin thallium-doped sodium iodide single-crystal slabs used in most scintillation cameras.[9] Although other generator systems offer some real advantages over the ^{99}Mo-^{99m}Tc generator,[10] its use is increasing. Three shorter-lived isotopes, ^{92}Tc ($T_{1/2}$ = 4.44 minutes), ^{93}Tc ($T_{1/2}$ = 165 minutes), and ^{94m}Tc ($T_{1/2}$ = 52 minutes), which are positron emitters, may find use in positron emission tomography.[11]

The first injection of Na $^{99m}TcO_4$ into a human was made in 1961,[7] following the development of the so-called Brookhaven generator.[6,12] Its use in diagnostic medicine expanded rapidly. Two important advances led to the rapid proliferation of ^{99m}Tc in nuclear medicine: the further development of a generator that could be eluted with isotonic saline[13] and the development of a single vial kit containing both stannous ion (as the reducing agent) and the chelating agent.[14] These so-called "instant kits" produce a high-yield radiopharmaceutical in one step upon the addition of pertechnetate. In 1970 more than 2000 daily diagnostic procedures based on ^{99m}Tc were carried out in the United States alone.[15] Today, more than 85% of the diagnostic nuclear medicine procedures use ^{99m}Tc radiopharmaceuticals.[15] The history of the development of commercial ^{99m}Tc radiopharmaceutical is given in Table 1.

Technetium is a second-row transition metal. It is in group VIIa of the periodic table,[43] below manganese and above rhenium. Its neighbors are molybdenum, #42, and ruthenium #44. The second- and third-row transition metals show much greater complexities in their chemical behavior than the first-row elements. Their spin-orbital coupling constants are much larger, as are ligand field splittings, leading to more electron pairing, with resulting low magnetic moments (except for d-3 states). The highest oxidation states are more stable than those of their first-row congeners, and the chemistry of the lower oxidation states becomes quite complicated, often exhibiting metal-metal bonding. Technetium itself can assume any oxidation state from +7 to 0. It resembles manganese to a limited extent, and rhenium to a much greater extent. In its compounds it exhibits coordination numbers from 4 to 9, and their crystal structures show great variety.[44,45] In water, and, of necessity our major interest is in its aqueous chemistry, many of its compounds hydrolyze, polymerize, and become colloidal. In this treatment, we shall draw upon the chemistry of rhenium compounds, which often resemble their technetium analogs, and occasionally on the chemistry of isoelectronic molybdenum compounds.

The lanthanide contraction causes the ionic radii of Tc and of Re to be very similar, and many of their compounds are isomorphous. The Tc-O distance in the tetrahedral TcO_4 anion is 1.711Å, and that of Re-O in ReO_4 is 1.717Å.[46] Perrhenate is reported to form very weak complexes with rare earth ions,[47] much weaker than those of chloride ion. The only reported pertechnetate complex is one with uranyl nitrate, determined qualitatively by extraction.

Pertechnetate is much like other oxo-anions such as perchlorate, ClO_4^-, in its solution behavior. Pertechnic acid, $HTcO_4$, is described as a strong acid in aqueous acid-base titrations. A recent estimate of its acid strength in water by osmotic coefficient measurement (which agrees with Raman spectra) shows it, like $HReO_4$ and $HClO_4$, to be completely dissociated even in 6 *M* solutions.[48]

It is a widely accepted principle in inorganic chemistry that salts of large anions and large cations are insoluble in water, and dissolve in various organic solvents. This is true of anions such as ClO_4^-, ReO_4^-, and even I^-, which tend to precipitate with large quaternary ammonium, phosphonium, or arsonium cations. The precipitates can then be extracted into water-immiscible solvents such as benzene.[49,50] This is also true of both millimolar and nanomolar pertechnetate solutions. In addition, strongly basic anion-exchange resins in the chloride form will extract pertechnetate from water at all levels of concentration.[51,52] The resins are cross-linked quaternary ammonium compounds. Probably the type of interaction between quaternary ammonium salts and water, which is called "water-structure enforced ion-pairing," is responsible for the high selectivity of the resins toward pertechnetate.[53]

Methods of Analysis of ^{99m}Tc

Methods of analysis for total technetium are of limited direct interest in nuclear medicine because the central analytical problem in that area is the determination of the quantity of ^{99m}Tc in a particular chemical form rather than a determination of the total technetium present in a sample. Usually physical methods (with perhaps some preliminary chemical separations) suffice for determining total technetium. These methods include liquid scintillation counting,[54] neutron activation analysis,[55-57] atomic absorption,[58] x-ray fluorescence,[59] and mass spectrometry.[60]

The pertechnetate ion in water shows strong absorption in the UV at 244 and 287 nm (ϵ = 5690 and 2170 M^{-1} cm^{-1}, respectively).*[61] In addition, a strong infrared band at 901 cm^{-1}, characteristic of the Tc=O bond, has been used.[62]

A number of spectrophotometric methods for measuring technetium have been developed over the years. In most of these, strongly colored complexes or chelates of technetium

*Molar Absorptivity as defined in *Anal. Chem.* 1982, 54:157.

Table 1. Development of ^{99m}Tc Radiopharmaceuticals that Proceeded to Routine Clinical Use

YEAR	^{99m}Tc RADIOPHARMACEUTICAL	INVESTIGATORS
1960	Pertechnetate	Shellabarger, Richards[16]
1964	Sulfur colloid by the hydrogen sulfide method	Atkins, Richards, and Schiffer[17]
1964	Albumin by the iron ascorbate method	McAfee et al[18]
1965	Aerosols	Taplin and Poe[19]
1966	Sulfur colloid by thiosulfate method	Stern, McAfee, and Subramanian[20]
1966	Iron ascorbate	Harper, Lathrop, and Gottschalk[21]
1966	Macroaggregated albumin (MAA)	Gwyther and Field[22]
1968	DTPA by the iron ascorbate method	Richards and Atkins[23]
1970	DTPA by the stannous ion instant kit[24]	Eckelman and Richards[14]
1971	Albumin by the stannous ion instant kit	Eckelman, Meinken, and Richards[25]
1971	Red blood cells by the stannous ion method	Eckelman, Richards, Hauser, and Atkins[26]
1971	Polyphosphate by the stannous ion instant kit	Subramanian and McAfee[27]
1971	Microsphere	Rhodes et al[28]
1973	Diphosphonate by the stannous ion instant kit	Yano, McRae, and Van Dyke[29]
1974	Dimercaptosuccinate	Lin, Khentigan, and Winchell[30]
1975	Methylene diphosphonate	Subramanian et al[31]
1976	Iminodiacetic acid (HIDA) by the stannous ion instant kit leading to disofenin,[33] lidofenin, and mebrofenin[34]	Loberg et al[32]
1980	Hydroxymethylene diphosphonate	Bevan et al[35]
1984	Propylene amine oxime leading to exametazine[36]	Volkert et al[37]
1984	Isonitriles leading to sestamibi	Holman et al[38]
1986	Tetrapeptides leading to mertiatide	Taylor et al[39]
1986	Boron adducts of dioximes leading to teboroxime	Treher et al[40]
1986	Technegas	Burch et al[41]
1988	Bicisate (^{99m}Tc ECD)	Walovitch et al[42]

are formed, with high molar extinction coefficients. The chemistry is known in only a few of these. The first is the thiocyanate method of determination originated by Crouthamel[63] and chemically characterized by Trop et al.[64] In short, the standard analysis for technetium in strongly acidic thiocyanate solutions probably involves the early formation of the Tc(V) complex, which is rapidly reduced by excess thiocyanate to a mixture of the Tc(III) and Tc(IV) complexes, absorbing at 400 and 510 nm, respectively. The second example is concerned with the use of thioglycolic acid, $HSCH_2COOH$, as an analytical reagent for technetium. The sulfhydryl group is the reductant in a test developed by Miller and Thomason.[65] They found that at pH 8 a green complex (λ_{max} 655 nm, $E = 1800$) was formed, but that in acid solution there was only general absorption in the range 350 to 500 nm. DePamphilis et al., attempting to synthesize a technetium complex of thioglycolic acid found a product that was derived from an impurity in a commercial preparation. This impurity was mercaptothioacetic acid, $HSCH_2COSH$, which made up 15% of the starting material, and which reacted preferentially relative to the thioglycolic acid itself, forming $TcO(SCH_2COS)_2$.[66]

Sources of ^{99m}Tc

Pertechnetate-99m is obtained in three ways: from a generator, as "instant technetium" by extraction, or as Tc_2O_7 by high-temperature evaporation. In all three cases it is produced by the decay of ^{99}Mo. The latter is either a fission product or is made by neutron bombardment of highly purified molybdenum metal in a reactor.

^{99}Mo decays mostly to the ^{99m}Tc metastable nuclide, and to a lesser extent (13%) directly to the long-lived ^{99}Tc nuclide.[1,67] There is therefore a modification of the equation that describes the growth and decay of ^{99m}Tc from ^{99}Mo. For a simple parent-daughter pair, in which the half-life of the parent is longer than that of the daughter, the pair will eventually enter a state of transient equilibrium. The number of daughter nuclei, (N_2) is related to N_1, the number of parent nuclei at the same time, t, in the following equation:

$$N_2 = \frac{\lambda_1}{\lambda_2 - \lambda_1} N_1^0(e^{-\lambda_1 t} - e^{-\lambda_2 t}) + N_2^0 e^{-\lambda_2 t}$$

where N_1^0 and N_2^0, respectively, are the number of parent and daughter atoms present at $t = 0$ and where λ_1 and λ_2 are the decay constants for the parent and daughter, respectively. This general equation can be simplified at transient equilibrium to

$$\frac{N_2}{N_1} = \frac{\lambda_1}{\lambda_2 - \lambda_1}$$

if one takes N_2^0, the number of daughter atoms initially present, as zero. The condition for transient equilibrium is that

$e^{-\lambda_2 t}$ is negligible compared to $e^{-\lambda_1 t}$. The accuracy of this assumption is a matter of personal decision but the second term represents a 1.2% contribution at 42 hours. For the molybdenum-technetium system, the general equation becomes

$$N_2 = 0.87 \frac{\lambda_1}{\lambda_2 - \lambda_1} N_1^0 (e^{-\lambda_1 t} - e^{-\lambda_2 t})$$

Expressed in terms of disintegration rates or activities, it becomes

$$A_2 = 0.87\, A_1^0 \frac{\lambda_2}{\lambda_2 - \lambda_1} (e^{-\lambda_1 t} - e^{-\lambda_2 t})$$

If ^{99}Mo decayed only to ^{99m}Tc, the ratio of activities of daughter to parent at transient equilibrium would be 1.10. However, because 13% of the ^{99}Mo nuclides decay directly to the ^{99}Tc ground state, the equation take the form:

$$\frac{A_2}{A_1} = 0.87 \frac{\lambda_2}{\lambda_2 - \lambda_1}$$

At transient equilibrium, the ^{99m}Tc radioactivity is 96.25% of that of ^{99}Mo. Long-lived ^{99}Tc atoms will be present in the generators from the decay of ^{99}Mo as well as from the decay of ^{99m}Tc. The chemical consequences of the appearance of ^{99}Tc in the generator from both these decay processes (but mainly from the decay of ^{99m}Tc) are discussed in the section on reduced ^{99m}Tc compounds.

The technetium produced in solution or on a column by the decay of molybdenum-99(VI) is largely in the oxidation state VII corresponding to the following equation, with no breaking of chemical bonds.

```
       O                    O               O
       ||       beta-      +||              ||
 -O — Mo — O- → -O — Tc — O- → -O — Tc  =O
       ||       decay       ||              ||
       O                    O               O
```

THE BROOKHAVEN GENERATOR

The Brookhaven generator[6,68] consists of a column of about 5 grams of activated alumina, which has been acidified and treated with a sodium molybdate solution containing molybdenum-99. If the latter is a fission product, the specific activity will be very high, (>10^4 Ci/g), with very little carrier molybdate. If the molybdenum-99 is a reactor product, there will be many milligrams of carrier molybdate on the column.

In weakly acid solution the molybdate anion polymerizes, forming the $Mo_7O_{24}^{6-}$ homopolymer.[43] If aluminum ions are present, a stable heteropolymer, $Al(Mo_6O_{24})^{9-}$, is formed.[43,69,70] While the structure of the molybdate polymer on activated alumina is not necessarily the same as that formed in aqueous acid, it can be concluded that aluminum ions on the activated alumina surface will bind some octahedral polymeric variety of MoO_3 groups, probably by the displacement of hydroxy groups coordinated to aluminum ions.[71] The nature, properties, and preparation of activated alumina have been described elsewhere in some detail.[72]

Problems of chemical and radiochemical purity arise in the use of generators. Aluminum salt displacement from the column must be limited to less than 20 μg/mL of eluate for reactor material, and to half of that for fission-derived molybdate. Aluminum must be analyzed colorimetrically, by reaction with methyl orange. Molybdenum-99 breakthrough is limited to less than 0.15 μCi/mCi (0.15kBq/MBq) of ^{99m}Tc at the time of use. Other gamma-emitting radioactive products in fission-based generators are limited to less than 0.5 μCi/mCi of ^{99m}Tc at the time of injection. ^{89}Sr, a beta-emitter, is limited to 6×10^{-4} μCi per millicurie of ^{99m}Tc whereas ^{90}Sr is limited to 6×10^{-5} μCi Sr per millicurie of ^{99m}Tc at the time of injection. ^{103}Ru and ^{131}I are also common contaminants, limited to 0.05 μCi/mCi of ^{99m}Tc.[73]

There is a problem that sometimes arises in generators: a yield of pertechnetate less than expected. A large and sometimes preponderant fraction of the expected pertechnetate remains on the column after elution. Two groups of investigators have concluded that the effect is due mainly to the chemical reduction of pertechnetate caused by the radiolysis of water by the molybdenum-99 beta particles. This reduction, however, is seen only in the presence of alumina.[74,75] The radiolysis of water produces solvated electrons, H atoms, OH radicals, HO_2 (from dissolved oxygen), H_2O_2, and H_2.[76] An encounter between a pertechnetate ion and a solvated electron will produce technetate, TcO_4^{2-}.[77,78] In the absence of alumina, reduced technetium species are not observed in irradiated pertechnetate solutions.[74,75] However, in the presence of alumina, if the TcO_4^{2-} ion is formed on or near the alumina surface, it will be strongly adsorbed at an anionic site like any other polyvalent anion, and it will probably not encounter another technetate anion because of its high dilution, so that a disproportionation reaction between distant neighbors is unlikely. Oxygen reduces the adsorption of technetium by the columns.

If the ^{99}Mo is a fission product, the loss of ^{99m}Tc activity by adsorption is unimportant, except with very high activities of molybdenum.[79] On the other hand, if the ^{99}Mo is a reactor product the retention of ^{99m}Tc by the column increases with increasing carrier molybdenum content.[68] This is now attributed to the semiconductor properties of molybdic oxide, MoO_3 (or its polymerized form).[80] This interpretation means that the phenomenon of pertechnetate reduction is inherent in the carrier molybdate columns.[81] Various remedies have been employed to correct this condition. In one form or another they involve adding oxidizing agents to the column[13,81] or adding scavengers of solvated electrons.[82]

The chemical condition of the eluate is important for labeling efficiency, especially when the pertechnetate is used with "instant" kits containing small amounts of stannous ion as the reducing agent. It is interesting to note that, although oxidants are needed in the column, their presence in the eluate causes low yields. Oxidants include not only peroxide but excess ^{99}Tc also.

Srivastava et al.[83] found that at low concentrations of stannous ion reduction in DTPA kits was stoichiometric, but reduction in pyrophosphate kits was not, based on a four-electron change in each. At <20 μg of tin(II), no improvement in the yield was seen after 4 hours of mixing and the reduction was substantially less than that calculated on the basis of the ^{99}Tc-to-tin(II) ratio. Various kits for the preparation of ^{99m}TcMAA gave very different labeling yields as a function of added ^{99}Tc, presumably because of different amounts of "usable" stannous ion. In many modern "instant" kits, the amount of total stannous ion is small so that limitations on the ^{99}Tc content are recommended, eg, for RBC[84] and exametazine (HMPAO).[85]

For large generators (>2 Ci), Salehi and Guignard[86] found that discarding the small volume of saline that remained in the dead volume below the column bed improved the binding efficiencies for radiolabeling platelets and lymphocytes with ^{99m}Tc. This experimental solution to low labeling yields did not address the mechanistic questions. The cause of the low labeling yield could be attributed to the presence of decayed ^{99m}Tc and ^{99}Tc, peroxide due to radiolysis, or disulfide compounds extracted from the rubber or plastic components.

Excess ^{99}Tc above the usual amount of stannous ion can be produced on Curie-level generators.[87] For a 7-Ci (260 GBq) generator, ^{99}Tc was present at 10^{-7} to 10^{-6} M as measured using ion exchange HPLC with UV detection. The experimental values are higher than the theoretical values for ^{99}Tc by as much as 35%.

Peroxide is the second possible oxidizing agent that could reduce the radiochemical yield. Molinski[88] determined the yield of peroxide to be 0.33 ng/mCi/hour and found microgram quantities of peroxide per milliliter eluate. This is generally too small to oxidize a substantial percentage of the stannous ion.

Reducing agents that place ^{99m}Tc in an inert complex also can reduce yields of ^{99m}Tc radiopharmaceuticals. Molinski[88] reported that the presence of organic impurities reduced the elution yield, but it is possible that they also interfere with the labeling yield. Boyd and Sorby[89] claimed that the vinyl bag containing the saline in the so-called wet generators (those that remain in contact with the saline) is a source of organic material. They increased the elution yields by purifying the saline eluent with charcoal, but did not comment on the effect of the purified eluate on radiochemical yields. In addition to plasticizers, they found cyclohexanone and propan-1-ol. Deutsch[87] also found compounds with strong UV absorption being eluted from one commercial generator. The low radiochemical yield is more prevalent for the initial elutions of the generator and more severe for the "wet" generators.[87] The final reducing agent suggested as a source of low radiochemical yields is the ill-defined group of rubber formation accelerators, which usually contains disulfide compounds. Hamilton found that microgram per milliliter of sulfhydryl compounds could be extracted from rubber by solutions of iodinated contrast media.[90] The exact cause of the low radiochemical purity on eluting the "Monday morning" generator is still unknown.

INSTANT TECHNETIUM

A second source of pertechnetate-99m is commonly called "instant technetium." A solution of Na_2MoO_4 containing ^{99}Mo is made strongly alkaline with NaOH (>2.5 M) and is then extracted with a solvent such as methyl ethyl ketone. The ketone is normally quite soluble in water at room temperature, but it is salted out by various concentrated electrolyte solutions. In strong alkali the molybdate remains in the aqueous phase, and sodium pertechnetate is extracted almost completely into the ketone. The organic solvent is then evaporated and the sodium pertechnetate is dissolved in saline solution.[91] If this procedure is used on a large scale, it is necessary to add an oxidizing agent (eg, air or H_2O_2) to the aqueous solution to maintain the technetium in the heptavalent state. An additional problem arises from the inevitable reactions of ketones in strong alkali, yielding substituted mesityl oxides and other condensation products and possible pyrogens.[92] These are said to exert a deleterious effect on some labeling formulations.[93]

SUBLIMATION GENERATOR

A third source of pertechnetate-99m is a sublimation generator. Heating Mo/Tc mixtures causes sublimation of Tc_2O_7 which is much more volatile than MoO_3. Such a generator has been reported to yield more than 50% of the theoretical activity from active MoO_3. This technique has few clinical applications, having been used primarily by central radiopharmacy operations in Australia.[67]

Protein Binding of Pertechnetate

Pertechnetate-99m in saline solution is injected intravenously into patients in a number of diagnostic procedures. Its condition in blood is not known. However, it is almost certainly bound to various proteins. Hays and Green reported that about 80% of $^{99m}TcO_4^-$ was bound to serum proteins at 37°C in a phosphate buffer at pH 7.4. Equilibrium dialysis was used to determine this; a lower value was obtained using gel chromatography.[94] The binding increased with decreasing temperature and increasing acidity. There was little difference between binding to normal serum and to 2.5 g% HSA solution. The binding was assumed to be weak, since prolonged electrophoresis or prolonged dialysis resulted in the complete release of the pertechnetate from the protein(s).[95]

Several investigators provide reliable estimations of association constants[96,97] of between 1 and 6×10^3 M^{-1} and binding to protein between 64 and 80% at different temperatures, pH, and TcO_4^- concentrations.[98–101]

Tc(VII) Sulfur Colloid

Apart from pertechnetate itself, the only other Tc(VII) compound is technetium heptasulfide, Tc_2S_7. At a no carrier-added level, an undefined insoluble colloid is formed which measures perfusion in liver and spleen. There are three reported methods of making the preparation, which is called technetium sulfur colloid.

1. $^{99m}TcO_4^-$ + H_2S in acid solution
2. $^{99m}TcO_4^-$ + Sb_2S_3 colloid in acid
3. $^{99m}TcO_4^-$ + $Na_2S_2O_3$ in acid

Historically, the first formulation of TcS-colloid was based on the reaction of $^{99m}TcO_4^-$ with H_2S in HCl solution.[102] A technetium-containing colloidal dispersion of very small particle size was produced, probably with some colloidal sulfur. The latter, if present, was formed by air oxidation of H_2S. The need to eliminate H_2S completely before injection led to technical complications.

The reaction of no-carrier-added TcO_4^- with previously prepared colloidal Sb_2S_3 was introduced in 1965.[103] It is probably a surface reaction in which sulfide ions of the antimony compound are exchanged with oxide ions of the pertechnetate. This means that the final particle size will be determined by the size of the Sb_2S_3 colloid which can be made as small as several millimicrons in diameter. This is a well-studied colloidal system,[104] very much like As_2S_3.[105] There is, for example, an analytical procedure for various metals in which an exchange of oxygen atoms is carried out on cellulose-containing metallic sulfides such as Ag_2S, CdS, and As_2S_3. Pertechnetate is one of the anions that undergoes sulfide formation on such treated papers in acid solution.[106,107]

The major commercial source of colloidal technetium preparations is TcS-colloid formed from pertechnetate-99m in an acidified solution of sodium thiosulfate.[17,20] The reaction involves Tc(VII) for the most part. While thiosulfates are known to reduce pertechnetate to a limited extent under some conditions, a ^{99m}Tc(IV) compound added to a radiopharmaceutical preparation was not incorporated into the colloid.[108] Because high radiochemical yields are obtained with ^{99m}Tc-S-colloid, reduction must not be a serious problem.

An investigation of the distribution of Tc activity as a function of particle size in a standard sulfur colloid preparation showed that, for particle sizes greater than 0.1 μm diameter, the percent of sulfur in the filtrate was not too different from that of technetium. However, for particles smaller than 0.1 μm, there was a 15% yield of the technetium, and almost no sulfur.[109] This means that Tc colloid was forming more rapidly than the sulfur colloid, and the sulfur colloid was formed at least in part on the Tc colloid, which serves as a nucleus. At the same time some sulfur nuclei probably formed independently, ie, homogeneously. The classical work of Zaiser and LaMer showed that homogeneous nucleation of the sulfur colloid takes place at room temperature in 0.001 to 0.002 *M* $Na_2S_2O_3$ and up to 0.002 *M* HCl.[110] When sulfur was generated in the thiosulfate-HCl solution studied by them, it was initially in homogeneous solution. As its concentration increased, it became supersaturated and at a certain degree of supersaturation it suddenly formed nuclei that grew as more sulfur was homogeneously generated. The condition of radiopharmaceutical preparations are not drastically different from those of Zaiser and LaMer. In fact, the yield of polythionite (determined by difference) was 8 to 10% of total reacted sulfur for both the LaMer sols and the standard preparation.

In one set of radiopharmaceutical preparations, a solution with 10^{-12} *M* TcO_4^- in place of the 10^{-9} *M* concentrations in the standard preparation, the distribution of radioactivity as a function of particle size was about the same in the two solutions. This suggested that other metal sulfides were acting as nuclei in the more dilute solution, and perhaps in the standard solution as well. Analyses showed the presence of Ag, Cu, Sb, Sn, and W in $Na_2S_2O_3.5H_2O$ (reagent grade). More metal salts of this type undoubtedly are present in HCl and in gelatin. If these metals form sulfides more quickly than technetium, they may carry the latter by sulfide-oxide exchange.

In summary, Tc colloid is formed rapidly from acidified thiosulfate solutions at 100°C, directly and by reaction with other metal or metalloid sulfides (the latter arising from impurities in the reagents). Sulfur is formed independently by homogeneous nucleation and by condensation from supersaturated solution on the Tc colloid nuclei. The sulfur can be dissolved by heating the colloidal dispersion in mild alkaline solution, reforming thiosulfate from the sulfite which is present and leaving extremely small colloidal particles carrying the technetium.

Reducing Agents for Tc(VII)

With the advent of the ^{99}Mo/^{99m}Tc generator system in the 1960s,[6] "instant" kits,[14] and innovations in chelation, use of ^{99m}Tc-labeled compounds has expanded. However, the chemical form of ^{99m}Tc eluted from the generator is pertechnetate, TcO_4^-, which is Tc(VII), the most stable chemical state of technetium in aqueous solution.

Pertechnetate does not bind to chelating agents nor does it coprecipitate with particles necessary for bone, renal, or pulmonary imaging procedures. Consequently, a less-stable reduced state of technetium, capable of participating in chemical reactions, must be formed. The only exception to this is ^{99m}Tc sulfur colloid, which is considered to contain Tc(VII).

Reduced states of technetium can be achieved by treatment with such reducing agents as stannous ion, the combination of ferric chloride and ascorbic acid, ferrous ion, sodium borohydride, concentrated hydrochloric acid, sodium dithionite, hypophosphorus acid, and hydrazine. The sulfhydryl group and the aldehyde group have been used as reducing agents, but both require heat and time to produce reasonable yields, which makes them somewhat less convenient. Pertechnetate can also be reduced electrolytically, ie, electrons can be supplied by a voltage applied to inert electrodes. With zirconium and tin electrodes, metallic reducing species probably are responsible for the reduction. In the reduced state, the technetium binds readily to chelating agents, thereby forming such compounds as ^{99m}Tc diethylenetriaminepentaacetic acid (DTPA), ^{99m}Tc hydroxyethylidene diphosphonate (HEDP), and ^{99m}Tc glucoheptonate, which are commonly used in diagnostic imaging. Reduced technetium also coprecipitates with colloids to produce such compounds as ^{99m}Tc stannous oxide or ^{99m}Tc microaggregates and with particles to produce ^{99m}Tc stannous macroaggregated albumin (MAA).

Many of the first ^{99m}Tc chelates were formed using ferric chloride and ascorbic acid as the reducing agent. Although these agents produced a suitable radiopharmaceutical, the need to use special equipment, such as a pH meter, and to prepare sterile buffers prevented their routine use in most nuclear medicine laboratories. The introduction of stannous ion as a reducing agent permitted pertechnetate to be added to the reaction vial with no pH adjustment or addition of other substances. Pertechnetate is reduced at pH 4 to 7 and then bound by the chelating agent. On a practical level, this use of stannous ion was a key development; most current radiopharmaceutical kits employ the stannous reduction technique. For blood cells, which are sensitive to changes in pH, stannous ion is also ideal.

The disadvantage of using a stannous or ferrous salt as the reducing agent is that at neutral pH it reacts readily with water to form colloids or large particles. These colloids and particles coprecipitate with reduced technetium and, in fact, this property has been used purposely to prepare imaging agents for liver and lung, respectively. If the desired product is a ^{99m}Tc chelate, however, these radiolabeled particles are unwanted radiochemical impurities. To avoid this side reaction, the metallic salt is kept soluble at neutral pH by binding it to a chelating agent, most often the same compound to be labeled with ^{99m}Tc. For instance, in the preparation of ^{99m}Tc DTPA, an excess of DTPA is added to the kit to bind all of the stannous ion present.

$SnCl_2.2H_2O$

This reagent is the most widely used reductant for pertechnetate in radiopharmaceutical practice. Because it is present in kits in large excess relative to pertechnetate, it maintains a reducing presence in solutions prior to injection. It is difficult to obtain as a pure compound, free of tin (IV). Commercial grades of $SnCl_2 \cdot 2H_2O$ may contain more than 5% of Sn(IV)[111] and there is some evidence that autooxidation occurs in the solid state.[112] Solid $SnSO_4$[112] and solid Sn(II)acetate[113] are much more stable than the chloride, and can be maintained in a pure state.

Tobias investigated the equilibria of stannous perchlorate in 3 *M* sodium perchlorate solutions at various acidities.[114] He found that Sn^{2+} ions existed in these solutions, that they hydrolyzed even in acid, that they hydrolyzed to cyclic complexes—$Sn_3(OH)_4^{2+}$ or $Sn_3O(OH)_2^{2+}$, and that they formed soluble $Sn(OH)_3^-$ in alkali. The main ions in solution before precipitation of the hydroxide are $Sn(OH)^{1+}$, $Sn_2(OH)_2^{2+}$, and the predominant species, $Sn_3(OH)_4^{2+}$. The addition of chloride ions to stannous perchlorate-perchloric acid solutions produced additional complexes. Formation constants at 25°C were determined for $Sn(OH)^+$, for a mixed chlorohydroxy tin complex, and for $SnCl^+$, $SnCl_2$, and $SnCl_3^-$.[115] The successive formation constants for the latter three complexes were approximately 14, 3.6, and 0.97 M^{-1}.

Another determination of these constants showed essentially the same values.[116]A basic salt was isolated from chloride-containing solutions below pH 4.5. Its composition is $Sn_4(OH)_6Cl_2$.[117] Above pH 4.5 mixtures of various solids were obtained. Above pH 5.5 colloidal tin species are formed before the hydroxide precipitates. The latter is not a true hydroxide, but is an amorphous hydrous oxide whose composition is $Sn_5O_3(OH)_4$ (formed at pH 10 from $SnSO_4$ solutions).[118]

We conclude that in radiopharmaceutical preparations (which are always made in saline solution) there will be very few Sn^{2+} ions, probably some chloro complexes, some polymers [in the absence of ligands which can complex Sn(II)] and some colloidal tin aggregates. Hence, to describe the real reducing agent as Sn^{2+} is incorrect, and to describe it as $SnCl_2$ or $SnCl_3^-$ in saline solutions may be only partly correct.

With respect to technetium compounds, there is little evidence of widespread tin-technetium mixed-metal complexes. A Tc-Sn mixed complex is reported by Deutsch et al in which the critical bond is an oxygen bridge between Tc and Sn.[119] This compound, a dimethylglyoxime complex, has been characterized by its x-ray diffraction pattern. A second reported complex, a Sn(II)-Tc(III)-Tc(IV)-phosphate complex of unknown composition, was indirectly shown to exist by Steigman et al.[120] Hydroxyethylidene diphosphonate (HEDP) has been reported to form mixed-metal complexes with Sn(II) and reduced technetium.[121,122] The latter claim was based on low-performance polyamide chromatography. However, recent investigation of the system employing HPLC spectophotometry and double-isotope labeling showed that there was no detectable tin in the four to five main HEDP complexes and only 1 of 13 minor complexes contained the tin isotope.[123]

On the other hand, no mixed-metal complex was found in the Tc-HIDA complexes,[124] in the Tc-pyrophosphate complex,[121] or in the Tc-gluconate complex.[125] In the latter two cases, $SnCl_2$ reduction and another method of reduction in the presence of the appropriate ligand yielded identical spectra of the technetium complexes.

HYDROCHLORIC ACID

Hydrochloric acid has not been used in a clinically useful radiopharmaceutical because of the difficulty of handling concentrated acid. It interests researchers, however, because it provides one example of different oxidation states being produced at carrier-free levels of ^{99m}Tc and at millimolar carrier levels of ^{99}Tc. Hydrochloric acid was first reported to reduce ^{99}Tc by Gerlit, who showed that quantitative reduction could be achieved at 20°C in concentrated HCl in 1 hour or at 75°C in 9 *N* HCl in 1/2 hours.[126] The exact oxidation state was not identified, but reduction was indicated by decreased extraction by diethyldithiocarbamate in $CHCl_3$. Busey identified the oxidation state as Tc(V) by titration with $SnCl_2$.[127] He showed that at room temperature >80% yield of Tc(V) could be achieved immediately. The reduction to $TcCl_6^{2-}$ was slow.

Ossicini et al developed a chromatographic method of separating the oxychlorocomplexes of Tc(IV), Tc(V), and Tc(VII) using HCl.[128]

Because oxidation states per se cannot be separated by chromatography there is the possibility of various complex oxychlorocompounds having the same R_f value but different oxidation states. With development of this chromatographic system using 0.6 *N* HCl on Whatman No. 3 MM paper, differences were noted between the rates of reduction for ^{99m}Tc and ^{99}Tc. Because 13% of ^{99}Mo decays to ^{99}Tc directly and ^{99}Tc is the decay product of ^{99m}Tc, the actual concentration of Tc in any study using "^{99m}Tc" is usually unknown. With ^{99}Tc, Ossicini et al showed an immediate reduction to ^{99}Tc(V) in concentrated HCl.[128] At 100°C in concentrated HCl, ^{99}Tc(IV) is observed. At 1/2 hour, approximately 50% ^{99}Tc(V) remained. The ^{99}Tc(V) decreased to 30% after 1 hour. In HBr at room temperature, ^{99}Tc(VII) produced ^{99}Tc(V), but when heated at 100°C, it produced ^{99}Tc(IV).

Williams and Deegan varied the concentration of ^{99}Tc from 10 mg/mL to trace concentrations.[129] They found Tc(V) at higher concentrations but Tc(IV) at 0.05 mg/mL and at trace levels. Thus Tc is reduced to a lower oxidation state at trace levels, violating the generally accepted second-order kinetic rate dependence. The reducing agent Cl^- was held constant (11 N HCl) in these studies.

Cifka has shown an HCl concentration dependence on the reduction of ^{99m}Tc pertechnetate to Tc(IV). Above 5 *N* HCl at 100°C, the reduction was quantitative.[130] De Liverant and Wolf have confirmed this, using ^{99m}Tc eluted from a commercial generator.[131] Cifka also observed Tc(IV) at 22°C in concentrated HCl, whereas De Liverant and Wolf found only 20% Tc(V) under the same conditions. Earlier, Eckelman et al observed that DTPA could bind up to 45% of the ^{99m}Tc reduced by HCl but only 9% of the ^{99}Tc at 4×10^{-2} *M* in concentrated HCl, again implying that trace and millimolar concentrations of Tc are chemically different.[132] Based on Cifka's work with trace impurities and on the fact that the lower oxidation state is observed at lower concentrations, the parameters of the reduction of Tc with HCl need further study.

The reduction of millimolar concentrations of Tc(VII) to Tc(IV) can be achieved by using stronger reducing agents. Concentrated HCl in the presence of KI can reduce Tc(VII) to Tc(IV) quantitatively. Thomas et al showed that at 25°C concentrated HCl produces Tc(V) rapidly at carrier Tc levels but reduction to Tc(IV) is slow.[133] With concentrated HBr at 25°C, Tc(IV) is rapidly produced. At 0°C, HBr produces Tc(V). With HI, Tc(V) can be produced only at isopropanol-dry ice bath temperatures. The HCl system has been suggested as the reducing system of choice to produce $TcOCl_4^-$.

HCl occupies a special place in the group of reagents that have been used to reduce pertechnetate. Concentrated HCl produces two starting materials that have been used in substitution reactions with various ligands, salts of the $TcOCl_4^{1-}$ anion for Tc(V) compounds and salts of the $TcCl_6^{2-}$ anion for Tc(IV) compounds. The corresponding bromo compounds are often preferred because of their higher reactivity. Pertechnetate reacts with HCl at room temperature. A transient yellow color develops which is believed to be a Tc(VII)chloro-addition product, fac $TcO_3Cl_3^{2-}$,[134] by analogy with a Re(VII) chloro-addition product whose cesium salt was isolated.[135] The yellow product was temporarily stabilized in concentrated choline chloride solution (in HCl), its spectrum was recorded, and it formed a Tc(VII) complex with dipyridyl.[135,136] In concentrated HCl, this transient yellow species is rapidly transformed to the green Tc(V) complex, $TcOCl_4^{1-}$, and chlorine. On heating in concentrated HCl, the $TcOCl_4^{1-}$ is further reduced to the Tc(IV) complex anion, $TcCl_6^{2-}$.

OTHER REDUCING AGENTS

Sodium Borohydride. $NaBH_4$ was introduced into nuclear medicine by Subramanian and McAfee.[136] It is a commonly used reducing agent in organic synthesis. It is regarded by organic chemists as "mild" in its reducing action compared to $LiAlH_4$.[137]

Sodium Dithionite. $Na_2S_2O_4$ is an extremely powerful reducing agent, particularly in alkaline solution.[43] In acid solution, it decomposes to thiosulfate and bisulfite and its reducing ability is attributed to the sulfoxylate ion radical formed by dissociation. It can reduce many metallic salts to lower oxidation states or to the metal. It was found to be an effective reagent in the pH range 11 to 13 for reducing TcO_4^{1-} to $[TcO(SCH_2CH_2S)_2]^{1-}$ in the presence of ethanedithiol.[138]

Hypophosphorous Acid. Hypophosphorous acid, H_3PO_2, is an extremely powerful reducing agent in both acid and alkaline solution.[139,140] Hypophosphorous acid has been used as a reductant in concentrated HCl for the synthesis of quaternary ammonium salts of the $TcOCl_4^{1-}$ anion.[141]

Hydrazine. Hydrazine, NH_2NH_2, is both an oxidizing and a reducing agent. In alkaline solution it is a powerful reductant.

Ascorbic Acid. Ascorbic acid, $C_6H_8O_6$, has been used alone or with a ferrous or ferric salt as a reducing agent in radiopharmaceuticals. One of the early methods of labeling albumin with technetium was based on a Fe(III)-ascorbate reduction of pertechnetate in the presence of air.[142] It is possible that the labeling was accompanied by some breakdown of the protein, an effect that was quite evident in the reactions of albumin with Cu(II)-ascorbate.[143] Free sulfhydryl groups may have been formed in both cases.

Sulfhydryl (and Related) Compounds. The standard reduction potentials of sulfhydryl compounds such as cysteine are difficult to measure. The reactions at electrode surfaces are sluggish and electrode poisoning (such as that caused by H_2S) has been found. The difficulties in such measurements are described in detail in Clark's monograph.[144] The generalized reaction is

$$R\text{-}S\text{-}S\text{-}R + 2H^+ + 2e = 2RSH$$

Thiourea, $(NH_2)_2C = S$, and its oxidized product, formamidine disulfide, have been studied in acid.

The mechanism of reduction by thiols such as cysteine is complicated. The reaction between Ce(IV) and cysteine in acid solution proceeds by way of the formation of thiol free radicals (RS·) in a one-electron-transfer reaction, but may produce further oxidized free radicals such as RSO· and RSO_2.[145]

Sulfur Dioxide. Sulfur dioxide has been used to reduce pertechnetate. Sulfite (as sulfurous acid), SO_2, or bisulfite can react with one-electron-transfer oxidants such as Fe(III) to give SO_3^{1-} (actually the dimer dithionate, $S_2O_6^{2-}$) as well as sulfate, and with two-electron-transfer oxidants such as halogens to give sulfate alone.[146,147]

Formamidine Sulfinic Acid. Formamidine sulfinic acid, also known as aminoimino-methanesulfinic acid and thiourea dioxide, has been used as a substitute for stannous salts in the preparation of a number of ^{99m}Tc-tagged radiopharmaceuticals.[148]

Hydroxylamine. Hydroxylamine, NH_2OH, which is better known as a ligand in various metal-ion complexes, can act as either an oxidant or a reductant. Qualitatively, its reactions as a reductant are complicated.[149]

Tertiary Organic Phosphines and Arsines. These compounds, such as triphenyl phosphine or mixed aryl-alkyl tertiary phosphines and arsines, have served as both ligands and reducing agents. A relatively simple reduction scheme involves the reaction of pertechnetate with a tertiary phosphine. The phosphine-oxide R_3PO is formed, and a phosphine complex, often a Tc(III) complex, is the main product. The reduction of Tc(IV) hexahalo complexes by phosphines and arsines to form Tc(III) complexes (because phosphines are two-electron reductants) suggests that individual halogen atoms are probably transferred to one phosphine molecule before or during the attachment of another to the technetium.

NATURE OF THE REDUCED TECHNETIUM COMPLEXES

There is an unspoken assumption in the search for reducing agents to replace $SnCl_2$ because, in the presence of a particular ligand, the same technetium complex will be formed regardless of the reductant. While this may be true in general, several exceptions to this assumption have been described.[150–160]

A less well-defined but nevertheless definite example of different products arising from the use of different reducing agents of pertechnetate-99m was found in the labeling of human serum albumin. An early method of labeling albumin with ^{99m}Tc was based on the reaction of pertechnetate with ascorbic acid containing ferric chloride in neutral solution, adding albumin, adjusting the pH to 2, and then raising it to pH 5 to 6.[18] In this procedure, it was later established that blocking the one free sulfhydryl group on the albumin very markedly reduced the yield of Tc-labeled albumin. Two blocking agents were used: N-ethylmaleimide and (very dilute) mercuric chloride.[160]

These examples show that more attention must be paid to the products of reaction of pertechnetate with reducing agents, and that more study of the mechanisms is also required.

Tc(V) Compounds

Until recently the opinion was widely held that the aqueous chemistry of technetium was largely limited to compounds of Tc(VII) and Tc(IV), and that Tc(V) compounds would be unstable in water.[161] This opinion was held in spite of the existence of a large number of stable octahedral complexes of Re(V) that had multiple bonds between the metal and oxygen or nitrogen atoms.[162] Chronologically, the first established case of the existence of a Tc(V) compound in water came from a study of Tc(V) citrate.[163] This was soon followed by a study of the Tc(V)-gluconate and -glucoheptonate complexes prepared by $SnCl_2$ reduction of pertechnetate.[164] These are examples of a large number of actual and potential polyhydroxy compounds that also serve as sources of other Tc(V) complexes by displacement of part or all of the polyhydroxy ligand.[165] This and related researchers were based on chemical investigations of already established useful radiopharmaceutical products, and were carried out on aqueous solutions of the complexes.

A different approach consists of the production (mostly in nonaqueous solutions and often by substitution reactions) of the Tc(V) complexes $TcOCl_4^-$ and $TcOBr_4^-$ of crystalline solids whose stoichiometries, coordination, and structures could be definitively characterized. This is true of the dithiol complexes described below. Because numerous Tc(V) complexes emerged from the Tc(V) dithiol studies, the sulfur chemistry of Tc(V) will be discussed before the oxygen and nitrogen chemistry.

SULFHYDRYL COMPOUNDS

Sulfur, which is less electronegative than oxygen or nitrogen, has very different bonding properties. It has low-lying empty 3d orbitals that are available for electron donation by other atoms, and its coordination number can be as high as 6.[166] Johannsen and co-workers investigated the formation of complexes of technetium with cysteine, cystine derivatives, and penicillamine.[167] The Tc(V) complexes were formed either by reduction of pertechnetate by the mercaptan or by substitution reactions of $TcOCl_4^-$ (in solution) or of Tc(V) citrate [prepared by adding 1 mol of Sn(II) for each mol of $^{99}TcO_4^-$ in a citrate buffer].

The fairly complete characterization of a number of technetium complexes, including the study of the properties of Tc(V) chelates of bidentate thiol ligands, has broadened perspectives and furnished at least the beginning of a generalized approach to the structural chemistry of Tc(V) complexes (unfortunately, not all studied in water). Two notes appeared simultaneously in 1978. In one, pertechnetate was reported to have reacted with an impurity in thioglycolic acid and was reduced to the oxotechnetium bis (thiomercaptoacetate) anion, which was isolated as the tetra-*n*-butylammonium salt: $n\text{-}Bu_4N[TcO(SCH_2COS)_2]$.[66] In the other work, pertechnetate was reduced by $NaBH_4$ in ethanol in the presence of 1,2- or 1,3-dithiols and the products were isolated as the tetraphenylarsonium salts, eg, $Ph_4As\text{-}[TcO(SCH_2CH_2S)_2]$.[168]

In both reported Tc(V) dithiol complexes, the four sulfur atoms of the five-membered rings are nearly co-planar. The technetium atom is about 0.8 Å above that plane, and the oxygen atom lies above it. The Tc-O distance is 1.6 to 1.7 Å. The structures are thus approximately square pyramidal with the oxygen at the apex. The IR and Raman spectra of the 1,2-ethylenedithiol complex show absorption at 940 cm^{-1}; in the case of the other compound, it is at 950 cm^{-1}. These bands are assigned to the Tc=O stretching frequency by comparison with many Re(V) oxo compounds.[162]

MIXED SULFUR-OXYGEN AND SULFUR-NITROGEN COMPOUNDS

The structure of tetraphenylarsonium bis (2-mercapto-ethanolato) oxotechnetate, $[Ph_4As][TcO(SCH_2CH_2O)_2]$ is an almost square-based pyramid very much like those found in the dithiol complexes.[169] There is some distortion in the five-membered rings because of the difference in Tc-O and Tc-S bond lengths. The distortion causes the formation of a trapezoid in the plane. The Tc=O distance is 0.72 Å, a little less than those found in the dithiol complexes. The IR spectrum shows a strong band at 948 cm^{-1}, assigned to the Tc=O stretch.

It can be concluded that the substitution of one oxygen for one sulfur atom in dithiol ligands produces only a small structural change. However, there is a loss of stability. This complex will react in solution with two equivalents of 1,2-ethanedithiol to form $[TcO(SCH_2CH_2S)_2]$. It appears to do so by way of an intermediate species which may be a dimer: $[(TcO)_2(SCH_2CH_2S)_3]$.[170]

When dissimilar chelating atoms are present in a ligand, it can be expected that *cis* and *trans* isomers of the complex will form, and this may present a problem in the preparation of a pure compound. The solid compound that was actually isolated in the cited work[170] was the *cis* isomer. The *trans* isomer was not physically separated, but was detected in the NMR spectrum of the initial reaction mixture. *Cis* and *trans* isomers were also found in the formation of the unsymmetrical mercaptothioacetate complex.[170]

A series of bisimidobisthiolate complexes of Tc(V) were prepared in which the core was $TcON_2S_2$.[171] The amide groups were deprotonated in the formation of the complexes. The technetium was 5-coordinate in these compounds; the structural characteristics resembled those of the mercapto-ethanol Tc(V) compounds. Thus, in the simplest of these, based on ethylene bis (2-mercaptoacetamide),[172] the basal plane was a distorted square pyramid with some ring angle distortion, the Tc=O distance was 1.679 Å, and the technetium atom was 0.771 Å above the plane.

Another type of mixed S-N compound of technetium is found in the diaminodithiol (DADT) compounds. When technetium is coordinated to these ligands, the resulting complexes are neutral, quite stable, and exhibit a lipophilicity that depends on the overall structure of the ligand.[173] While a large part of the work was performed with ^{99m}Tc,[174] a particular ligand, (N-piperidinylethyl) hexamethyl diaminodithiol, was reacted with $^{99}TcO_4^-$, reduced in basic solution by sodium hydrosulfite, and compared (by HPLC and paper chromatography) with the ^{99m}Tc complex. There were two complexes in each system: ^{99}Tc NEP-DADT syn- and anti-isomers in which the N-piperidinylethyl side chain was located either syn or anti to the Tc=O core. In synthesizing the complexes, one of the two secondary amine groups lost a proton, whereas the other did not. When this was coupled to the loss of two protons from the two sulfhydryl groups, the net charge on the complex was reduced to zero.[175]

In summary Tc(V) forms complexes with various dithiols in which the coordination number of the metal is five in crystals, and in which there is no group *trans* to the Tc=O bond. With dithiols, Tc(V) can form four-, five-, and six-membered rings. If a nitrogen atom is substituted for one of the sulfur atoms, as in *N,N*-ethylene bis (2-mercaptoacetamide), only a five-membered ring has been found. The attempts to form a six-membered ring by the inclusion of an additional CH_2 group were unsuccessful.[176] The short Tc=O distance is characterized by an IR stretching frequency in the 900 to 1000 cm^{-1} region. This band offers a convenient means of identifying the Tc=O moiety in Tc(V) compounds.

There is also a *trans* effect associated with M=O bonds (where M represents a metal), already noted in Re(V) compounds.[163] Groups that are *trans* to the oxide ion (in a hypothetical or actual 6-coordinate compound) are rendered labile, in both a kinetic and an equilibrium sense. In the solid state the complexes discussed thus far are five-coordinate. In solution, it is possible that there is weak solvation in the position *trans* to the Tc=O bond. Only a qualitative statement can be made about the *trans* effect in octahedral substitution. More quantitative knowledge in this area has come from the study of square planar complexes.[177] The magnitude of the *trans* effect depends on the nature of the ligands.

OXYGEN COMPOUNDS

The first demonstration of the existence of a Tc(V)-oxygen-linked complex in aqueous solution was reported by Steigman et al in a study of the reaction of pertechnetate-99 with excess $SnCl_2$ in a citrate buffer at pH 7.[163] The first reported study of a gluconate complex of technetium maintained that the reduction of pertechnetate by $SnCl_2$ in the presence of a gluconate salt produced a Tc(IV)-gluconate complex.[178] The oxidation state of the technetium was determined by an iodometric titration of the solution, with the implicit assumption that the iodine reacted only with excess Sn(II). Both the analytical method and the chemical conclusions were questioned because of the possibility of oxidation of some reduced form of the technetium by the iodine reagent.[179]

Another study of the reduction of pertechnetate by $SnCl_2$ in the presence of various polyhydroxy compounds including sodium gluconate and sodium glucoheptonate concluded that there was a large family of Tc(V) compounds formed in dilute alkali.[178] The oxidation state of the technetium in these complexes was established as Tc(V) by the polarographic analysis of excess (unreacted) Sn(II), by spectrophotometric titrations,[178] and by coulometry at fixed potential.[180] The gluconate-technetium ratio was critical in determining the electron number n (the number of electrons taken up by the pertechnetate). In alkaline solution the value of n was 2.0 down to ratio 17. At pH 5, n was almost 2.4 when the ratio was 110.

POLYHYDRIC ALCOHOLS

In the polyhydric alcohol series starting with ethylene glycol and finishing with perseitol, $C_7H_9(OH)_7$, pale pink-violet solutions were formed in their presence when pertechnetate-99 was reacted with excess $SnCl_2$ at pH 12. Tc(V) could form alkoxide-based chelates with five-membered rings, but not with six-membered rings. The early members of the series—complexes of Tc(V) with ethylene glycol and glycerol—disproportionated rapidly when their alkaline solutions were acidified to form TcO_2. Complexes formed with longer-chain polyols such as mannitol showed virtually no change in spectrum on acidification. These complexes, like those of the polyhydroxy acids described below, are not very stable in water, and require a fairly large excess of ligand for stabilization.

Tc-GLUCOHEPTONATE

It is assumed that two glucoheptonate ligands react with the technetium at the carboxylate and the alpha-carbon alkoxide groups. However, if this were correct, any alpha-hydroxycarboxylic acid should form similar complexes. Yet lactic and glycolic acids do not form Tc(V) complexes, and glyceric acid, which does, disproportionates raidly in acid solution, unlike Tc(V) glucoheptonate, which merely undergoes a reversible spectral shift. The projected structure for Tc(V) glucoheptonate does not explain the source of the greater stability of the longer-chain Tc(V) polyhydroxy carboxylic acid complexes in this regard.[181] It appears, then, that the polyhydroxy carboxylic acids form the same alkoxide-based chelate found for the Tc(V) polyhydric alcohols.

NITROGEN-CONTAINING LIGANDS

An early paper by Spitsyn and collaborators described a dioxo Tc(V) tetrapyridine complex which was characterized by its IR spectrum.[182] In addition, the reduction of pertechnetate-99m by $SnCl_2$ in alkali in the presence of cyclamo-macrocyclic nitrogen compounds produced technetium complexes.[183] One ligand in particular, 1,4,8,11-tetraazatetradecan, with four nitrogen atoms in a ring, did form a Tc(V) complex. It was free of tin. It was cationic and had the same electrophoretic mobility as Co(II) cyclam pseudohalide complexes with a +1 charge, about half the mobility of Ni(II) cyclam complexes with a +2 charge, and about one third of the mobility of Co(III) complexes with a +3 charge. The authors also prepared a Tc-ethylenediamine complex in solution. The same group published the crystal structure of a Tc(V) cyclam perchlorate,[184] which confirmed the conclusions drawn from the earlier chemical work performed on aqueous solutions of the ^{99m}Tc complex. Other Tc(V) complexes with nitrogen bases have been prepared and studied. They include the ethylenediamine complex,[185] pyridine, imidazole, and picoline complexes,[186] and a series of aliphatic amino, heterocyclic, and amino acid ligands that form cationic Tc(V) complexes.[187] All tetramines that have been studied show the *trans*-dioxo structure in their Tc complexes. In terms of stability in solution, the cyclam type of structure appears to be most stable. The ethylenediamine complex decomposes in water unless excess ligand is present. This is also true of the complexes of monodentate ligands.

Diamine complexes of Tc(V) have been prepared with 1,2-propylenediamine[186] and 1,3-propylenediamine;[186] which means that Tc(V) can form both five-membered and six-membered rings with two nitrogen atoms.

Zuckman and collaborators have suggested that dioxo complexes of Tc(V) and Re(V) are formed when the ligands are uncharged and are poor donors, such as the nitrogen bases mentioned above. When the ligands are negatively charged and operate as strong donors, such as oxygen, sulfur, and halogen anions, five-coordinate complexes with a Tc=O core are formed,[184] that is, formation of a dioxo core is a means of reducing the effective central charge of the technetium, but this is also effectively done by the above anions.

However, the existence of another type of nitrogen-based ligand complicated this picture. This is the amine-oxime class of reagents. In the reactions with Tc(V), two amino nitrogen atoms are deprotonated on complex formation and the two nitrogen atoms of the oxime groups complete the formation of the complex.[188,189] The OH groups of the two oximes lose a proton, and form a hydrogen bond between them. In spite of coordination to four nitrogen atoms, the Tc(V) forms a TcO^{3+} core rather than the expected *trans*-TcO_2^+ core. This emerged after the earlier radiochemical studies with ^{99m}Tc and 3,3-(1,3-propanediyldiimino) bis (3-methyl-2-butanone oxime) (known as PnAO).[190]

These radiochemical studies by Troutner and collaborators showed that the complex was neutral and lipophilic.[191] Crystals of the Tc-PnAO were then prepared with ^{99}Tc and analyzed.[190] There was a planar arrangement with the four nitrogen atoms, a shortened oximate-O-oximate-O distance compatible with a single hydrogen bond, and a Tc-O distance—1.679 Å—comparable with other Tc=O distances and occupying the apical position. More recently, after the discovery that the ^{99m}Tc PnAO complex penetrated the intact blood brain barrier (but was washed out too rapidly for use with a slowly rotating gamma camera), a number of other ligands of this type were synthesized and structures and various properties of their Tc complexes were examined.[192] The Tc=O distance is a little on the long side (1.676 Å) when compared with those of other complexes (1.61 to 1.67 Å). The IR stretches for Tc=O range from 908 to 923 cm^{-1}. The average $Tc\text{-}N_{(amide)}$ bond is 1.913 Å; typical $TcN_{(amine)}$ distances are 2.088 to 2.259 Å. The authors concluded that the two deprotonated N atoms show sp^2 rather than sp^3 hybridized character. This, together with the deprotonation of the amine groups makes the TcO^{3+} core more stable than a *trans* TcO_2^+ species, which in any event may be geometrically difficult to form, given the steric crowding of the Tc=O by methyl groups on the carbon atoms adjacent to the amide nitrogens.

A further investigation by the same group shifted the inquiry from the effects of substituent charge on the backbone to a study of the effects of changing the lengths of the hydrocarbon backbone itself.[193] The backbone groups were ethylene, propylene, butylene, and pentylene. The prototype is the original $Pn(AO)_2$, commonly called PnAO.[194] This work turned up both monoxo (Tc=O) and dioxo (O=Tc=O) cores.

The longer backbone group and larger ring size caused a charge from TcO^{3+} (with a Tc=O stretch at 930 cm^{-1}) to a TcO_2^+ core. The electronic nature of the groups *cis* to the oxo groups is the primary factor in deciding whether TcO_3^+ or TcO_2^+ will form. Anions will help to stabilize the TcO^{3+} core by reducing the effects of the central charge. Thus, an amide will lose a proton, forming an amido anion and will show sp^2 character, and (from the decrease in the Tc-N distance) will show multiple bond formation-factors that stabilize TcO^{3+}. However, with the longer backbone, steric constraints become very important and too great a Tc-N distance will result in TcO_2^+ formation, the N atoms will retain sp^3 character with their hydrogen, and they will behave like hard, neutral donor atoms. The increased ring size introduces too much strain for the deprotonation of the amino group, forcing long Tc-N distances.

Overall, more stabilization is obtained through deprotonation and sp^2 hybridization of amine nitrogens, and through formation of Tc-N multiple bonds (as with Tc(V) PnAO) than is achieved by formation of the *trans*-dioxo species TcO_2^+.

ARSINE COMPOUNDS

A Tc(III) arsine complex, $[Tc(diars)_2Cl_2]ClO_4$ in which diars stands for *o*-phenylenebis(diarsine) was oxidized in alcohol solution by means of Cl_2.[194] This produced an eight-coordinate Tc(V) complex: $[Tc(diars)_2Cl_4]$ PF_6. The new compound possessed dodecahedral coordination. These were tested as potential myocardial imaging agents when labeled with ^{99m}Tc.

EDTA COMPLEX

A seven-coordinate oxo technetium(V) complex with EDTA was prepared as the barium salt by Deutsch and collaborators. It was synthesized by reacting H_4EDTA with $TcOCl_4^{1-}$ in anhydrous dimethyl sulfoxide, yielding the $Tc(O)EDTA^{1-}$ anion as the acid.[195]

A NEW TYPE OF Tc(V) CORE

It is possible to classify T(V) compounds by the core containing Tc and another atom. The cores would include TcO^{3+}, TcO_2^{1+}, Tc-O-Tc(dimer), and $Tc{=}N^{2+}$(nitrido). Compounds containing a new Tc-imino core were recently reported.[196,197] The complexes contain the core $(Tc^V{=}NR)^{3+}$ in which NR represents an amino group. The core $(TcNR)^{3+}$ is formally analogous to TcO^{3+}. In one method of synthesis, the salt (Bu_4N) $(TcOX_4)$ (X = Cl,Br) is reacted with excess RNCO in toluene, producing $Bu_4N(TcNRX_4)$. In turn the latter is a good starting material for new Tc=NR complexes. A second synthesis was made by reacting an aromatic amine with $Bu_4NTcOCl_4$ in the presence of phosphine. If the latter was triphenyl phosphine (PPh_3), the resulting product was $[Tc^V(NC_6H_4Z)(Cl_3)(PPh_3)_2]$. If the phosphine was $R_2P\text{-}CH_2\text{-}CH_2\text{-}PR_2$, the product was a Tc(IV) complex.

DISPLACEMENT REACTIONS AND MIXED-LIGAND COMPLEXES OF Tc(V)

Displacement reactions have been used in the synthesis of many Re(V) and of some Tc(V) complexes. One group of compounds, $TcOCl_4^-$ and $TcOBr_4^-$ salts, has been used in a number of syntheses that were described earlier. The solid salts (usually quaternary ammonium or arsonium compounds) have been characterized structurally and show the pyramidal structure of oxotechnetium(V) compound. Perhaps the simplest synthesis is that reported by Bandoli et al.[195] As Ph_4AsTcO_4 was precipitated from aqueous solution, reduced with concentrated HCl, and recrystallized from a methylene chloride, pentane mixture. Displacement reactions with these anions cannot be used in water because of rapid solvolysis and disproportionation.[198] The displacements are usually carried out in methanol or ethanol.

Steigman[198A] and collaborators introduced the use of Tc(V) polyhydroxy compounds, including the gluconate, as intermediates in the preparation of more stable Tc(V) compounds in water by displacement reactions. Equal moles of pertechnetate and $SnCl_2$ were reacted in alkali in the presence of excess sodium gluconate to form the Tc(V) complex, and after pH adjustment a second ligand, such as cysteine, was added to the solution.[181] This procedure was used by Spies et al in preparing a large number of Tc(V) complexes (mostly dithiols).[199] Probably any labile complex of Tc(V) can be used in this way.

Tc(IV) Compounds

Complexes of ^{99}Tc(IV) of radiopharmaceutical interest have been produced in the following ways: by the reaction of pertechnetate with a reducing agent in the presence of a ligand, by the coulometric reduction of pertechnetate in the presence of a ligand, by ligand displacement reactions on hexahalide complexes of Tc (IV), and by reaction between a ligand and precipitated $TcO_2 \cdot xH_2O$ after dissolution of the oxide in acid.

HALIDE COMPLEXES

Three of the four hexahalide complexes of Tc (IV) have been used in syntheses of various Tc (IV) compounds by displacement. The hexafluoride anion, TcF_6^{2-}, is different from the other hexahalide complexes in that it resists hydrolysis and undergoes substitution reactions with difficulty. It has been prepared by reacting salts of $TcCl_6^{2-}$ or $TcBr_6^{2-}$ with KHF_2 in a melt.[200,201] K_2TcCl_6 can be prepared by prolonged heating of $KTcO_4$ in concentrated HCl.[202]

K_2TcBr_6 has been made by repeatedly evaporating K_2TcCl_6 with concentrated HBr[203] or by the direct action of cold concentrated HBr on a pertechnetate salt.[204] Salts of the TCl_6^{2-} anion have been prepared by repeatedly digesting a hexabromo salt with concentrated HI.[204]

The hexahalotechnetates, particularly the chloro and bromo compounds, have been used in displacement reactions with various ligands in the synthesis of many Tc (IV) complexes. These preparations have been most successful when they were carried out in nonaqueous solvents. If they are run in water there may be hydrolysis accompanying the displacement reaction with attendant complications (TcO_2 formation, mixed complex formation, etc).

In any solvent there is the possibility of other complications: oxidation (by air) to a higher oxidation state or reduction by the ligand to a lower oxidation state. There should be some independent verification of the valence of the technetium in the complex. It cannot be assumed that the final oxidation state of the technetium in a compound is the (IV) state because one started with a Tc (IV) hexahalogenate.

OXIDE OF Tc(IV)

Hydrated TcO_2 ($TcO_2 \cdot xH_2O$) has also been used in the synthesis of Tc (IV) compounds. The oxide has been prepared by the electrolytic reduction of pertechnetate in alkaline solution,[205] by the reduction of pertechnetate using zinc in HCl[206] by the action of hydrazine on pertechnetate, or by the hydrolysis of K_2TcCl_6 and K_2TcBr_6.[206] However, there are no standardized and universally accepted methods of synthesizing $TcO_2 \cdot xH_2O$. Thus, Nelson et al reported that the reduction of pertechnetate by zinc in HCl to hydrated TcO_2 was quantitative.[206] However, Schwochau and Herr maintained that in this reduction some 20% of the technetium was reduced to metal.[207] They preferred to prepare the oxide by hydrolysis of the hexachloro complex. On the other hand, Colton and Tomkins reported that a purer product was obtained from the hydrolysis of the hexaiodo compound because too much cationic impurity was incorporated in the product of hexachloro-technetate hydrolysis.[208] The condition of $TcO_2 \cdot xH_2O$ in aqueous solution was investigated by Gorski and Koch.[209] This material was prepared by the hydrazine reduction of pertechnetate, and was subsequently dissolved or dispersed in dilute perchloric acid. The concentration of technetium was not given. They measured its electrical mobility through a column of sea sand, in perchloric acid solutions whose pH ranged from 1 to 2.5. From this it was concluded that hydrolysis was taking place in two steps involving 0, 1+, and 2+ species.

Noll et al studied the electrophoresis of $TcO_2 \cdot xH_2O$ dissolved initially in 1 *M* $HClO_4$.[210] Their apparatus was somewhat more conventional than that of Gorski and Koch, and they used small glass spheres in place of sea sand. They were unable to reproduce the results reported by Gorski and Koch. They concluded that the reported hydrolytic equilibria did not exist, at least on the basis of electrophoretic and pH-titrimetric measurements. Dialysis measurements showed that there was colloidal matter present in solution until acidities of the order of 1 *M* or higher in $HClO_4$ were reached. Sundrehagen also failed to reproduce Gorski and Koch's results.[211]

There is possible confirmation of the hydrolysis mechanism of Gorski and Koch in the work of Owunwanne et al.[212] These workers studied the exchange reactions between TcO_2 in $HClO_4$ and Sr $(ClO_4)_2$ on a cation-exchange resin. They postulated a 2+ charge on the Tc species between pH 1.1 to 2.0. A solvent extraction method of determining the nature of TcO_2 in aqueous solution was developed by Guennec and Guillaumont.[213] However, the percent of extracted ^{99m}Tc (IV) (extracted as a complex) was small.

SOLUBILITY OF $TcO_2 \cdot xH_2O$

Any knowledge of the behavior of TcO_2 in aqueous solutions must ultimately depend on well-established determinations of its solubility in water, in dilute acid, and alkaline solutions. An extensive research on the solubility of TcO_2 in various aqueous solutions was undertaken by Meyer et al at the Oak Ridge National Laboratory.[214] They prepared the oxide either by the electroreduction of pertechnetate on platinum or by the reduction of pertechnetate by hydrazine. They also precipitated TcO_2 from pertechnetate-hydrazine mixtures onto purified sand. Solubilities were determined by measuring the beta activity of ^{99}Tc in solutions that had been in contact with the solid oxide and had been recirculated or stirred. Oxygen was removed from these solutions by displacement with argon gas. Nevertheless, pertechnetate was found in varying amounts in all samples. In the pH interval 4 to 10 the solubility of TcO_2 ranged from 8.8×10^{-8} to 9.4×10^{-7} *M*, but most values fell between 1×10^{-8} and 2×10^{-8} *M*. At pH zero, solubilities from 10^{-7} to 10^{-4} *M* were found, depending on the oxide source.

Meyer et al assumed that in the pH interval from 4 to 10 the dissolved Tc (IV) was uncharged, but that the increase in solubility in more acid solutions was probably due to the formation of cationic species (eg, $[TcO(OH)]^{1+}$). However, there is another possible explanation: radiocolloid formation. Early in the history of radiochemistry a number of radioactive nuclides in aqueous solution exhibited colloidal behavior (filterability, lowered diffusion coefficients, anomalous adsorption on solid surfaces) at concentrations far below those predicted from solubility product constants for the onset of precipitation and hence of colloid formation.[215,216] The phenomenon has been attributed to adsorption on colloidal impurities in the water, as well as to the formation of true colloids. This led to a critical reexamination of the solubility product determinations of water-insoluble salts and hydroxides by Haissinsky.[217,218] He found that different solubility determinations of insoluble halides, carbonates, sulfates, and other salts were in fair agreement. However, in the case of insoluble sulfides and hydroxides there were very large differences in reported solubilities for even the same sample of a given compound, depending (perhaps) on age, history, prior treatments, etc. Measured solubilities differed from one another by orders of magnitude for the same compound. This led to his conclusion that one is dealing with polydispersed systems containing ions both simple and complex, and colloidal micelles of various dimensions in a slow state of evolution. The ordinary principles of solubility and solubility product are not applicable.[217] This may well apply to TcO_2 in water, especially in mildly acid solution.

THIOSEMICARBAZONE COMPLEX OF Tc(IV)

A complex of technetium was formed by the reduction of pertechnetate with stannous chloride in the presence of potassium kethoxal-bis-(thiosemicarbazone) (KTS).[219] The complex was extracted into various organic solvents, suggesting strongly that it carried no charge. It had an absorption maximum at 450 nm, as did a solution in which a $TcCl_6^{2-}$ salt had been reacted with the thiosemicarbazone. There appear to be a number of products formed.

COMPLEXES WITH PHOSPHORUS (V) LIGANDS

Pyrophosphate. The reduction of pertechnetate by excess $SnCl_2$ in 0.2 *M* sodium pyrophosphate solution at pH 7 could not be analyzed for unreacted Sn(II) by polarography, because the Sn(II) oxidation wave at −0.24 V vs the standard calomel electrode was severely distorted in the presence of pertechnetate.[163] At the same time, iodometric titrations were found to be unreliable in this system. Coulometry at fixed potential produced a pink color, which was followed by a pale blue. The pink compound was a Tc(IV) complex (n = 3, A_{max} = 520 nm, $\epsilon = 500\ M^{-1}\ cm^{-1}$). The coulometrically produced pale blue solution initially had Tc(III) (n = 4) and was unstable; slowly liberating a gas. Excess $SnCl_2$ added to TcO_4^- in sodium pyrophosphate at pH 7 produced a faint blue color that deepened on standing. The final (limiting) spectrum, after 100 hours at room temperature, was the same as that of the coulometrically produced product after rereduction. This was interpreted as the absence of any mixed-metal complex of $SnCl_2$ and technetium. The velocity constant was $490 \pm 74\ LM^{-1}\ h^{-1}$ at room temperature. The reaction was probably a slow dimerization reaction. In a more concentrated pyrophosphate solution (1 *M* $K_4P_2O_7$), the coulometrically reduced technetium, yellowish in color, had an average electron number of 4.6 [a mixture of Tc(III) and Tc(II)]. The product prepared with excess $SnCl_2$ in that medium was colorless, with no detectable light absorption in either the visible or near-UV region.

Methylene Diphosphonate (MDP). HPLC was used to characterize both carrier-added and no-carrier-added technetium-MDP formulations.[220] The purpose of this investigation was the examination of the bone-imaging properties of various separated fractions. The Tc-MDP complexes were prepared by the reduction of pertechnetate by $NaBH_4$ at pH 2, 6, 8, 9, 10, and 12. Both aerobic and anaerobic solutions were studied. On the acid side both types gave yellow solutions. At pH 8 the anaerobic solution was green, and the aerobic solution turned yellow on standing. At pH 9 the anaerobic specimen was greenish-blue, and the aerobic specimen slowly turned orange-red. At pH 10 both turned pink on standing. At pH 12 both were colorless. These obviously complicated changes, which were both time and pH dependent, appear to have little connection with the brown compound obtained by displacement.[221] The HPLC separations were conducted on an anion-exchange column with 0.85 *M* sodium acetate as the eluant. Depending on the pH, two to five peaks were observed (more in alkali than in acid). With the carrier-added solution there was visible but limited interconversion by changing pH. The no-carrier-added samples showed two peaks in acid and four in alkali, and much more interconvertibility of peaks by changing pH than the other specimens. The conclusion was drawn that "increasing the formulation pH favors production of complexes with short retention times, which within the modes of anion exchange chromatography corresponds to complexes of low negative charge density."[220] This appears to mean that a higher charge density in a complex anion means a longer retention time—or a greater selectivity coefficient—with respect to anion-exchange columns. The conclusion is incorrect; if anything, the reverse is true.[222]

Hydroxyethylidene Diphosphonate. The oxidation state of technetium which had been reduced from TcO_4^- by excess $SnCl_2$ in 0.2 *M* Na_2EHDP at pH 5 was determined by a polarographic analysis of unreacted Sn(II).[121] Two maxima were observed, one at $-0.12V$ and the other at $+0.080V$ (vs standard calomel). The concentrations of tin were equivalent to a four-electron and a three-electron change, respectively. The waves were poorly defined.

Russell and Cash performed pulse polarography on pertechnetate in acid, neutral, and alkaline solutions of EHDP.[223] They reported the formation of Tc (III) in the acid solution, and the formation of Tc (V) in neutral and alkaline solution.

A fast-scan cyclic voltammetric study of the reduction of pertechnetate in EHDP at pH 3.5 and 7 gave somewhat different results.[224] There was an initial reversible 1-electron reduction, followed by the formation of Tc (V) in a complicated fashion. This product may have undergone further reaction with ligand or solvent molecules. There was an additional reduction step in a second reduction peak. It was hypothesized that this step (at pH 7) formed Tc(IV). The time scale for this operation was in milliseconds. The usual polarographic studies require seconds, and slower reduction reactions following the rapid ones may well have been observed in the usual studies.

Amperometric titrations of pertechnetate in acid EHDP solution with $SnCl_2$ showed a three-electron change, forming Tc (IV).[225] Excess $SnCl_2$ was back-titrated with I_2, and gave the same result.[226] This latter titration (without potentiometry) had been carried out by Hambright et al, who drew the same conclusion.[178] However, this is not a definitive finding, since the same data would have been obtained if a lower oxidation state [such as Tc (III)] had been oxidized to Tc (IV), along with a smaller titer of unreacted $SnCl_2$.[163] A specific analysis for unreacted $SnCl_2$ would have been preferable.

Muenze reacted a $TcBr_6^{2-}$ salt with EHDP, and isolated a solid whose composition was $[K_2TcO\ (OH)]^{3+}\ [EHDP]^{3-}$.[227] While this seems to establish that the product is a Tc (IV) complex of EHDP, its preparation by displacement in water rather than in a nonaqueous solvent raises the possibility of complications from the independently occurring hydrolysis of the $TcBr_6^{2-}$ anion.

Van den Brand et al examined reaction mixtures containing pertechnetate, $SnCl_2$ and EHDP at pH 7 in water by gel chromatography.[228] They used the cross-linked polyacrylamide gel Bio-Gel P-4 rather than Sephadex because of the possibility that Sephadex would decompose Tc-EHDP complexes.[178] As it turned out, the complexes decomposed on Bio-Gel. It was necessary to add Na_2EHDP to the saline eluant to avoid this decomposition. They assumed that the gel functioned by steric exclusion and, accordingly, they calibrated the column with a variety of inorganic and organic compounds of different molecular weights preliminary to the estimation of the molecular weights of any Tc-EHDP complexes. Technetium-99 was at 10^{-6} *M*, and ^{99m}Tc at 10^{-11} to 10^{-12} *M*. The technetium elution curves were unsymmetrical in shape, suggesting that a number of compounds were being eluted close to one another. They concluded that there were five components with ^{99}Tc, four with ^{99m}Tc, and two with ^{113}Sn.

The application of HPLC techniques to the analysis of Tc-HEDP complexes was undertaken by Pinkerton et al[229] using millimolar pertechnetate reduced by $NaBH_4$ and tagged with ^{99m}Tc. The column consisted of a strongly basic anion-exchange resin, Aminex A-27. The eluant was 0.85 *M* sodium acetate maintained at pH 8.4, and monitored by radiation detection and UV scanning. A large number of components were found, including several that were produced at atmospheric pressure.

Pinkerton and later associates continued this work. With the same sodium acetate eluant they found 13 fractions produced by $NaBH_4$ reduction.[230] They also found that reduction by $SnCl_2$ produced at least 15 fractions of which 7 were also found in $NaBH_4$ reductions.[123] The work was based on UV spectra and on chromatographic retention times. It made possible the testing of a number of the separated fractions in radiopharmaceutical preparations and is undoubtedly valuable in an applied sense.

Tc (III) Compounds

AMINOCARBOXYLATE COMPLEXES

The reduction of pertechnetate-99 by excess $SnCl_2$ in the presence of DTPA produced a Tc(III) complex. This conclusion was based on a polarographic analysis of unreacted Sn(II). The complex was not otherwise characterized.[163] The chemistry of Tc(III) aminocarboxylate complexes involves Tc dimer formation, as Linder has demonstrated, but the Tc(III)-O-Tc(III) compounds have not been investigated as thoroughly as the mixed-valence Tc(III)-O-Tc(IV) entities.[231] The ^{99m}Tc DTPA complex is used to measure glomerular filtration rate.

Russell and Speiser studied the electrochemistry of a number of aminocarboxylate complexes of technetium by polarography.[232] The ligands included DTPA, EDTA, ADA [*N*-(2-acetamido) iminodiacetate], and HIDA [*N*-(2,6-dimethylphenylcarbamoylmethyl) iminodiacetic acid]. In acid solution Tc(III) was formed in all cases. The electron number gradually increased with increasing pH. Coulometry in a 3 m*M* TcO_4^- solution at pH 6 with 0.1 *M* DTPA produced a brown color (presumably TcO_2), but cutting the pertechnetate concentration in half again produced Tc(III). Amperometric titrations with $SnCl_2$ were carried out on the various solutions with a dropping mercury electrode. The Sn(II) anodic wave was reported to give results concordant with the cathodic Tc wave. In acid solution, values between Tc(III) and Tc(IV) were found for DTPA, EDTA, and ADA. In alkaline solutions of all the ligands, three-electron reductions to Tc(IV) were found, as well as in neutral DTPA and EDTA solutions. The amperometric titrations in acid solution gave the same nonintegral oxidation states at the end points that had been reported by Steigman et al in the direct titration of pertechnetate by $SnCl_2$ in a pH 4 solution of DTPA.[163,178] The more relevant information for radiopharmaceutical purposes would have been the oxidation state obtained with an excess of $SnCl_2$. The results obtained in alkali should be accepted with caution because of the instability of various DTPA and EDTA complexes in basic solution.[233,234]

PHOSPHINE AND ARSINE COMPLEXES

A large body of chemical information about mixed phosphine and arsine complexes of Tc(III) has been accumulated in the course of a search for cationic Tc complexes that might be useful in heart imaging. These are of the type *trans*-$[TcD_2X_2]^+$, in which D represents a chelating diphosphine ligand, and X represents a halogen. Libson et al systematically investigated the synthesis of nine of these complexes, varying the nature of the phosphine or arsine ligand and of the halogen, and characterized the resulting compounds by a variety of techniques, including structural and electrochemical methods.[235] The halogen and halogen-like ligands included Cl, Br, and SCN. The organic ligands included DPPE (1,2 bis-diphenylphosphino) ethane and several variants, DMPE [bis (1,2-dimethylphosphino)] ethane, and DIARS [*o*-phenylene bis (dimethylarsine)]. The favored preparations involved the reduction of pertechnetate or TcX_6^{2-} by excess phosphine or arsine ligand. Structural analysis showed that in the DPPE complex the technetium was central and octahedral, coordinated with four equatorial phosphorus atoms and two *trans*-axial halogen atoms.

The electrochemistry of these compounds was carried out by cyclic voltammetry in dimethylformamide with gold, platinum, and glassy carbon electrodes. It was concluded that complexes with Cl or Br were robust (ie, difficult to displace). The E° values of the various complexes depended on the nature of both ligands. The Br complexes were stronger oxidants than the Cl compounds. Aryl substituents on phosphorus gave stronger oxidants than alkyl residues. Both the Tc(III)-(II) and the Tc(II)-(I) equilibria were reversible in this medium. There was no indication of a Tc(IV)-(III) wave.

A second paper dealt with the redox chemistry of the Tc(III) $D_2X_2^+$ cations [and the Tc(I)D_3^+ cations].[236] Spectroelectrochemistry was added to the usual electrochemical measurements. The Tc $D_2X_2^+$ complexes in DMF showed two reversible changes, corresponding to two one-electron reversible reactions forming Tc(II) and Tc(I). Conventional pulse polarography was also performed in aqueous solution for $TcD_2X_2^{+/0}$ [ie, Tc(III) cation and Tc(II) neutral product]. The supporting electrolyte was 0.5 *M* KNO_3. The E° value in this solution was −0.122 V (vs NHE) for the DMPE chloride and −0.016 V for the dibromo complex. These values were much more positive, by several hundred millivolts, than the values expected from the measurements in DMF. In the case of the DEPE complexes, the differences were about 350 mV more positive than the values in DMF. The differences were attributed to the insolubility in water of the reduced form, which would make it easier to reduce the Tc(III) complex. Such a facilitated reduction could be expected to take place in biological media as well.

Even assuming that the reduction of the Tc(III) complex and the reoxidation of the Tc(II) insoluble form together are reversible in the time frame of normal pulse polarography, it does not follow that in the high dilution encountered in ^{99m}Tc solutions and in the biological media (ie, blood) the same considerations, ie, reversible equilibrium influenced by the insolubility of one reactant, will apply. In the first pass the concentration of the Tc(III) complex is about 10^{-8} *M*. In subsequent passes it will be much less. The neutral Tc(II) complex may be soluble at those levels of concentration, which would make the reduction process more difficult. There is the possibility that the insoluble Tc(II) complex would be solubilized by proteins or cholate salts or similar solubilizing agents. In addition, the mechanisms of reduction by biological molecules (presumably those carrying sulfhydryl groups) are often complicated. In particular it is quite possible that the reduction by a thiol group, producing a thiol radical, may not be reversible. If this is the case, the insolubility of the Tc(II) complex in water will not contribute to rendering the reduction of the Tc(III) complex easier. A direct demonstration of such a reduction is needed.

OXIME COMPLEXES

Unlike most of the technetium chemical literature, in which similar work had already been carried out on rhenium compounds, there is very little on the reactions of rhenium compounds with oximes, except for analytical determinations. A number of spectrophotometric analytical procedures based on the reduction of perrhenate, usually by acid $SnCl_2$ in the presence of oximes, are in the literature, but there are few investigations of composition, oxidation state, etc. Meloche et al, working with α-furildioxime, reported that Re (IV) did not react with the oxime unless $SnCl_2$ was added, and that an electrolytic reduction of perrhenate in the presence of the oxime was ineffective, as were a number of reducing agents other than $SnCl_2$.[237] Narayanan and Umland examined the stoichiometry of the reaction between $SnCl_2$ and reduced perrhenate in the presence of dimethylglyoxime.[238] They concluded that in 1:1 methanol-acetic acid solution there were three DMG moieties per rhenium, but that in aqueous HCl the stoichiometry was 2:1.

There have been several assays for technetium based on oxime complexation.[239,240] The first more complete investigation of the reaction between reduced technetium and dimethylglyoxime in the presence of $SnCl_2$ was reported by Deutsch et al.[119] These workers had obtained two crystalline compounds by reacting $SnCl_2$ in HCl with pertechnetate in 95% ethanol saturated with dimethylglyoxime. The technetium was seven coordinate, and the tin had octahedral coordination. The tin was believed to be in the (IV) state, and the technetium was thought to be Tc(V). In effect, the tin served to cap the trigonal prismatic structure around the technetium. This capping explains the findings of Meloche et al that $SnCl_2$ was unique among the reducing agents in the formation of a reduced perrhenate complex with α-furil.[237]

The same Tc complex was re-investigated by Linder et al[241] as part of a more general inquiry into technetium dioxime complexes capped with various derivatives of boric acid. They found that they could prepare the same complex reported by Deutsch et al but in good (50%) yield simply by adding *two* equivalents of $SnCl_2$ to a refluxing HCl-alcohol solution of DMG and NH_4TcO_4. The complex is diamagnetic, as previously reported, and is neutral. These workers concluded, however, that it was not a Tc(V) complex, but rather a Tc(III) compound. The mass spectral analysis (FAB spectrum) showed a strong molecular ion with a major peak at a mass to charge ratio (m/c) of 685. This corresponds to a Tc(III) compound with four protons for charge balance. If it were a Tc(V) compound it would require only two protons for charge balance, with m/c = 683. This was not seen. While it is possible that the Tc(V) compound was readily reduced in the mass spectrometer, chemical reaction pointed to a Tc(III) complex. In the absence of reducing agents, the complex is readily changed to other Tc(III) oxime species, including TcCl $(DMG)_3$ and TcCl $(DMG)_3$ BR (BR stands for boronic aryl or alkyl acids). Finally, if the Tc(III) complex TcCl $(DMG)_3$ is treated with $SnCl_4$ in ethanol, the original compound, Tc $(DMG)_3$ μ-OH $SnCl_3$, is quantitatively reformed.

Research at the Squibb Institute for Medical Research has produced a class of neutral technetium (III) compounds derived from tris-oxime complexes, and capped with boronic acids. The compounds, whose ^{99m}Tc analogs show brain and heart uptake, are called BATOs (for boronic acid adducts of technetium dioxime complexes.)[242] The compounds included [bis[1,2-cyclohexanedione dioximato (1-)-*O*]-[1,2-cyclohexanedione dioximato (2-)-0] borato (2-*N,N′,N″,N‴,N⁗,N*‴″]-chlorotechnetium (SQ 32014) and bis[1,2-cyclohexandione dioximato (1-)-0]-[1,2-cyclohexane-dionedioximato(2-)-*O*]methyl)borato (2-)-(*N, N′,N″,N‴,N⁗,N*‴″)-chlorotechnetium (SQ 30,217), in both of which the dioxime was cyclohexanedione dioxime. The complexes were characterized by x-ray crystallography, conductivity, elemental analysis, HPLC, infra-red, NMR, and UV-visible spectra, lipophilicity, and a wide variety of mass spectra. In the cyclohexanedione complexes, the technetium was coordinated to three N-bonded dioxime molecules, and to one Cl atom in an axial position. The technetium has a monocapped distorted trigonal prismatic geometry. At one end of the molecule the dioxime groups are held together by a proton bridge in which two H atoms are shared by three O atoms. The other end of the molecule is held together by a methylboron cap through the remaining three O atoms of the oxime groups. The dimethylglyoximate complex, which was also exhaustively characterized, is quite similar in structure to the other two, with a seven-coordinate Tc(III) atom capped with boron at one end, and holding two proton bridges at the other end.[243]

The BATO complexes are robust, that is, they are resistant to oxidation, reduction, or metal exchange. However, the axial chloride can be replaced in water by a hydroxy group. The rates of exchange of four complexes were determined in three solutions of different pH (all, however, near 7) and at two temperatures (both near room temperature).[244] The exchange rate is measured in minutes to slightly more than 1 hour for the half-times, suggesting that the interchange does not take place immediately on injection. The hydroxy compound in general resembles the parent chloro compound, except for decreased lipophilicity.

Tc(I) Compounds, Isonitriles

The first reported isonitrile complex of technetium was the hexakis (tert-butyl isocyanide) technetium (I) hexafluorophosphate, which was synthesized from hexakis (thiourea-S) technetium (III) chloride by reaction with tert-butylisocyanide in methanol under reflux.[245] A later synthesis of isonitrile complexes was based on the reduction of pertechnetate-99 by alkaline sodium dithionite in the presence of the ligand in an ethanol-water mixture.[246] This facile synthesis of Tc(I) complexes from pertechnetate was extended to the tert-butyl, methyl, cyclohexyl, and phenyl isocyanide compounds. All (as the hexafluorophosphates) were characterized by elemental analysis, electronic, infrared, and proton magnetic resonance, conductance, cyclic voltametry, and field desorption mass spectrometry. The various compounds were stable in air and water, were soluble in polar organic solvents, and showed the conductance expected of 1:1 electrolytes in acetonitrile solution. The alkyl complexes exhibited a reversible one-electron oxidation at 0.82 to 0.88 V vs SCE in acetonitrile. That of the aryl complex was at 1.18 V vs SCE. The direct synthesis from pertechnetate also made it possible to prepare the complexes at the 10^{-8} to 10^{-9} *M* level with ^{99m}Tc.

Another method of synthesis of the hexakis isonitrile complexes of Tc(I) was reported by Kennedy and Pinkerton.[247] This involved the prior synthesis by electrolytic or chemical reduction of formate, acetate, or pivalate complexes of technetium, whose oxidized form was reacted with the hexakis isocyanide reagents.

The Tc(I) oxidation state is achieved with isonitriles because of the nature of the ligand. In the formal sense, the carbon atoms are divalent. If the metal ion has filled d-orbitals that can overlap with low, empty, antibonding orbitals of the attached ligand atom, a back-donating bond can reduce the negative charge on the metal. Back donation increases as the positive charge on the complex decreases. In this sense, isocyanides will behave like carbon monoxide, in that low oxidation states of metals will be stabilized.[248]

^{99m}Tc Radiopharmaceuticals for Diagnosis

OXIDATION STATES OF ^{99m}Tc RADIOPHARMACEUTICALS

Although efforts to characterize Tc compounds have been considerable,[43] most have been carried out in nonaqueous solutions and therefore are not directly applicable to clinical ^{99m}Tc radiopharmaceuticals. On the other hand, some recent work on Tc compounds in aqueous solution has involved thiol compounds that are not used routinely.[249] Efforts in both cases, however, have led to the discovery of important chemical information.

Most ^{99m}Tc radiopharmaceuticals in clinical use are treated with stannous ion and therefore studies with this reducing agent are relevant to the understanding of clinical ^{99m}Tc radiopharmaceuticals. While it is desirable to know the exact oxidation state of technetium in clinically used radiopharmaceuticals, present methodology makes the determination of nanomolar concentrations difficult. Experiments with millimolar concentrations of ^{99}Tc have indicated that it is reduced by stannous ion to the V state, and then slowly to Tc(IV) at pH 7 in citrate buffer. In HCl also, ^{99}Tc is reduced by stannous ion to the IV state. With a DTPA buffer at pH 4, the ^{99}Tc(III) state prevails.[163] It is not known, however, whether these millimolar determinations can be extrapolated to the nanomolar concentrations used in diagnostic imaging procedures.

Investigators also have attempted to define the reduced oxidation state of ^{99m}Tc in the DTPA chelate.[132] It is known that millimolar concentrations of $^{99}TcO_4^-$, for which in vitro analysis can be made, form ^{99}Tc(IV) in the presence of the following reducing agents: (1) stannous ion, (2) ferric chloride and ascorbic acid, (3) ferrous ion, and (4) concentrated HCl-HI and ^{99}Tc(V) with concentrated HCl. In each case, and for concentrations ranging from millimolar ^{99}Tc to tracer ^{99m}Tc, binding efficiency of the reduced technetium to DTPA is greater than 85% for those reducing agents producing Tc(IV). When the same measurements are performed with concentrated HCl alone as the reducing agent, only 10% of ^{99}Tc, but 45% of ^{99m}Tc, is bound to DTPA. Differences in the efficiency of compound formation almost certainly reflect a difference in oxidation state produced by concentrated HCl. When the same binding trend is evident for ^{99m}Tc and ^{99}Tc, the same oxidation state that occurs with ^{99}Tc is assumed for ^{99m}Tc. Although in the absence of DTPA Tc(IV) is produced with the first four reducing agents, any conclusions regarding the oxidation state of stannous-reduced technetium labeled to DTPA are unwarranted in view of the changes in the stannous-stannic electrochemical potential caused by the addition of DTPA.

Efforts to extrapolate from millimolar to nanomolar chemistry by observing the biological behavior of the resulting radiopharmaceuticals have shown that ^{99m}Tc HEDP and ^{99m}Tc glucoheptonate (GHA) have the same biologic distributions as the ^{99}Tc compounds and therefore are probably in the same oxidation state, namely, Tc(IV).[178] On the other hand, Steigman has shown that a stable complex is formed with gluconate in the Tc(V) oxidation state at high pH.[250] He has also shown, using millimolar concentrations of ^{99}Tc, that a mixture of Tc(III) and Tc(IV) pyrophosphate exists. Finally, TcHIDA, a hepatobiliary agent, has been shown to be in the Tc(III) oxidation state when millimolar concentrations of ^{99}Tc are used.[251] Using HPLC, the following radiopharmaceuticals have been shown to have the same oxidation state for the ^{99m}Tc compound as found for the ^{99}Tc compound: teboroxime, the Tc-Isonitriles including sestamibi, and the Tc amine-oximes including exametazine.

PROTEIN LABELING WITH REDUCED Tc

Methods to Radiolabel Proteins. Most iodinated radiopharmaceuticals used in nuclear medicine have eventually been replaced by ones labeled with ^{99m}Tc. The inferior nuclear properties of ^{131}I and the chemical instability of the iodine-carbon bond are usually given as the reasons for this. In the case of ^{131}I labeling of antibodies, the logic is complicated by its therapeutic properties. Therefore, this comparison is valid only for radiolabeled antibodies used for diagnosis. Soon after the discovery of ^{131}I in a tellurium target bombarded in the Berkeley cyclotron, Hamilton and Soley[252] used this radionuclide in its simplest chemical form, iodide, to study iodine metabolism. In the following years various molecules were radioiodinated; the ability to radioiodinate proteins at high specific activity was a major factor in the development of the insulin radioimmunoassay by Berson and Yalow.[253] Antibodies were also first radiolabeled with ^{131}I.[254] As early as 1957, Pressman et al were able to localize tumors by scanning using radiolabeled antibodies. With the development of the ^{99}Mo-^{99m}Tc generator system in the late 1950s, there has been a continuous effort to first label proteins and later to label antibodies with ^{99m}Tc. The effort to radiolabel antibodies with ^{99m}Tc is the topic of this review.

Since ^{99m}Tc-labeled antibodies will be used for diagnosis, the ideal radiolabeled antibody is the one for which the ^{99m}Tc "traces" the distribution of the antibody. However, the clinical importance of antibody radiolabeled with ^{99m}Tc is still not well documented. Nuclear medicine is competing with other imaging modalities that are capable of much higher information density. Although the use of ^{99m}Tc-labeled antibodies will increase the specificity of the nuclear medicine study, no studies have been published showing that the sensitivity is comparable to CT or NMR imaging in establishing the size, shape, and position of a tumor. In general, nuclear medicine's strength lies in the ability to map either perfusion or biochemical changes. The contrast agents used to enhance CT or NMR imaging are at relatively high concentrations and therefore are not suited for measuring tissue perfusion changes and especially not well suited for measuring biochemical processes.

In general, CT and NMR imaging have higher resolution than the planar scintillation camera or SPECT. If the general location of the tumor or the metastases can be specified, CT or NMR imaging should be superior in detecting small tumors. High tumor to nontumor ratios and high count ratios are necessary to detect even 1-cm^2 tumors at depths of 1 to 5 cm using the planar Anger camera.[255] In the very important case where the metastases are extensive and a whole body survey is indicated, the radiodiagnostic technique has an advantage. Larson et al[256] have also suggested staging and monitoring therapeutic response as important goals of cancer diagnosis with radionuclides. SPECT offers some improvement in resolution, especially when overlying structures are involved, but the need for information density is increased. Most SPECT studies to date are carried out with 5 to 10% of the injected dose in the target organ whereas antibody concentrations rarely reach the level of 0.1% dose localized in the tumor.[257]

Based on nuclear properties, it would appear that ^{123}I is equal to ^{99m}Tc. Given that ^{123}I is easier to manipulate chemically than ^{99m}Tc, the former should be the radionuclide of choice for labeling antibodies. However, pure ^{123}I is only produced at a high-energy cyclotron whereas ^{99m}Tc is available from a generator system and therefore ^{123}I is not competitive with ^{99m}Tc. Even with the rather complicated chemistry needed to label antibodies with ^{99m}Tc, the overall advantage still lies far to the side of technetium.

Direct labeling, ie, using the amino acids of the antibody to complex the metal, may result in a labile chemical bond because of the stereochemistry of the functional groups in the tertiary structure of the antibody. Only when the protein is known to bind the metal with high affinity is direct labeling useful. Even in those cases, the protein is usually labeled by injecting a soluble salt that exchanges with the protein. The injection of ^{67}Ga-citrate and ^{111}In-chloride are examples of direct labeling of proteins (eg, transferrin) in vivo. On the other hand, ^{99m}Tc has been directly labeled to proteins and particularly to antibodies,[258–260] but the stability and inertness of the bond are in question. Although the investigators utilized different buffer systems, pH, and incubation times, a common feature is the use of stannous ion as a reducing agent. The advantage of direct labeling is the experimental simplicity. However, in at least one case, the resulting antibody complex with ^{99m}Tc has been reported to be unstable. This necessitated the use of an elaborate molecular permeation chromatographic system to purify the ^{99m}Tc labeled antibodies. This is consistent with the observation of Eckelman et al,[25] who had published in 1971 that albumin binding of ^{99m}Tc is so weak that multiple chromatographic purifications resulted in further radiochemical impurities as a result of dissociation. The competitive binding of ^{99m}Tc by stannous oxide also was a source of radiochemical impurities. Since then, other reviews have documented the same instabilities. Steigman et al[160] suggested that the mechanism of binding was related to sulfhydryl groups, but Hnatowich's group[261] recently proposed the importance of a helix structure. Paik et al[262] suggested that ^{99m}Tc is bound by both a high-affinity, low-capacity site and by a low-affinity, high-capacity site. Their study suggests that the high affinity site is indeed related to the presence of sulfhydryl groups. However, the extent of high-affinity site binding is not quantitative and depends on the antibody fragment used. For IgG and $F(ab')_2$ that contain disulfide bridges between the heavy chains, high titers of reduced disulfide groups are detected in the presence of stannous ion. For Fab that does not have a disulfide bridge between heavy chains, very few sulfhydryl groups could be detected. This trend parallels the percentage binding of ^{99m}Tc when binding to the low-affinity site is prevented by the presence of excess DTPA. For IgG, about 24% of the ^{99m}Tc binds to high-affinity sites whereas for $F(ab')_2$ only 16% of the ^{99m}Tc is bound to the high-affinity sites. Very little ^{99m}Tc is bound to Fab with high affinity. These results are useful in interpreting other data. For instance, Rhodes et al[259] probably increase the high-affinity binding by long incubation of antibodies with stannous ion. Khaw et al[263] probably have a small percentage of directly bound antibody because they use Fab fragments, whereas Lanteigne et al[261] show binding via DTPA and directly to IgG. The best solution to the problem of low-affinity binding of ^{99m}Tc has been put forth by Paik et al.[262] They suggest that all radiolabeling with ^{99m}Tc or with ^{111}In should be done in the presence of excess DTPA. Even though that may decrease the radiochemical yield, it guarantees an inert chemical bond either directly to the protein through the high-affinity sites for ^{99m}Tc or through the bifunctional chelate for Tc and In.

The early indirect labeling methods have mostly involved the use of DTPA conjugated to the protein. The DTPA is considered a bifunctional chelate in that it binds to the protein and to the ^{99m}Tc. Other chelating agents, derivatives of dimercaptoacetamide (DADS),[264] derivatives of bis-*N*-methylthiosemicarbazone,[265] metallothionein,[266] thiolactone diaminedithiol,[267] hydrazinonicotinic acid,[268] and diaminetetrathiol[269] have been conjugated to antibodies for ^{99m}Tc labeling.

Because both the direct labeling methods, which apparently depend on free sulfhydryl groups for binding ^{99m}Tc, and the bifunctional chelate approach, which depends on a competition between weak and strong direct binding and binding by the covalently bound chelating agent, do not achieve high radiochemical purity, investigators have turned to prelabeling the ligand and then reacting this ^{99m}Tc chelate with the antibody. Fritzberg et al[270] have prelabeled the DADS ligand and then bound the ligand to the antibody via an activated ester. Likewise Franz et al[271] have prelabeled a *N*-propylamine derivative of cyclam with ^{99m}Tc and then reacted that chelate with an activated antibody. Recently BATO derivatives[272] were used for a preformed ^{99m}Tc chelate approach to label antibody. This method assumes that the ^{99m}Tc is bound to the chelating agent and therefore a single radiochemical should be produced. On the other hand, the development of an "instant kit" will be difficult with this approach.

Direct Labeling of Proteins. In 1988, we presented three approaches to radiolabeling antibodies with ^{99m}Tc[273]: (1) direct labeling, (2) indirect labeling via a chelating group attached to the antibody, and (3) indirect labeling by attaching a ^{99m}Tc chelate to the antibody. Among the three, direct labeling was thought to give the least reliable label whereas labeling by attaching a ^{99m}Tc chelate was thought to represent a true tracer of the antibody. Since the last presentation more attention has been paid to direct labeling because of the possibilities of a "instant kit" formulation.

Direct protein labeling can occur by at least two chemical processes or a combination of these processes. The ^{99m}Tc can be bound to (1) a colloid that is coated with antibody or (2) the sulfhydryl groups in the antibody and this concentration can be increased by reducing agents.

In the direct labeling procedure, stannous ion has been used most often to label proteins with ^{99m}Tc. In one of the first attempts,[274] excess stannous ion was adsorbed to ion-exchange resin in the presence of albumin and pertechnetate to radiolabel the protein. At that time the analytical techniques could not differentiate between labeled protein and labeled colloid coated with protein. Later, Eckelman et al[25] developed a number of techniques for radiolabeling albumin with ^{99m}Tc. In the course of this investigation, it became clear that tin colloid was being formed and this colloid was a competitive binder for the ^{99m}Tc. The use of Sephadex G25 allowed the separation of tin colloid from albumin, but gave no indication if the albumin was, in fact, colloid coated with albumin. Using radiolabeled stannous ion, tin was found in the albumin peak in inverse relation to the amount of stannous ion added. Albumin could also be labeled at low pH (2.5) where tin colloid is unlikely to form. They concluded that very high concentrations of albumin (50 mg/mL) were necessary to produce high radiochemical yields. Because colloid was often present, the presence of ^{99m}Tc-labeled protein bound to small colloids could not be ruled out.

The question of the oxidation state of technetium in protein complexes has been discussed extensively with no clear-cut answer emerging. An argument based on the oxidation state achieved in the absence of protein with a certain reducing system is not sound because a different oxidation state could be more stable in the presence of proteins. Because the exact site of binding to protein is not known, the question is all the more difficult. The use of Fe(II) or Sn(II) alone as the reducing agent suggests that Tc(IV) is present.[275]

However, these arguments are based on the expected oxidation state for a protein-free system and the possibility still exists that the Tc(IV) is oxidized to Tc(V) and bound in that state by the protein. ^{99m}Tc albumin was prepared by Williams and Deegan by mixing pertechnetate with dilute HCl and evaporating the mixture to dryness.[129] The yield of labeled albumin was 30% using this reagent. With the addition of ascorbic acid to albumin at pH 2.5, Williams and Deegan obtained a 90% apparent yield. The minimal reaction of albumin with technetium reduced by concentrated HCl with no ascorbate present is consistent with the observation of Eckelman et al[132] that this source of reduced technetium [probably Tc(V)] binds to DTPA with a <10% yield on the carrier level but with about a 40% yield on the no-carrier-added level (probably Tc(IV)). If it is Tc(IV) that binds efficiently to DTPA and concentrated HCl produces Tc(IV) on the carrier-free level, then the fact that Williams and Deegan obtained low protein-labeling yields with ^{99m}Tc reduced with concentrated HCl indicates that Tc(V) not Tc(IV) is involved in protein binding. The higher yields with addition of ascorbate also supports that hypothesis because it is thought to stabilize Tc(V). A colloidal mechanism of binding also should not be eliminated, in view of the presence of colloid in a number of preparations and the slow blood clearance of small zirconyl colloids as reported by Kyker et al[276] even with nonmetallic reducing agents. Lebowitz et al[277] have labeled gelatin with technetium using sodium borohydride as the reducing agent, but Johnson and Gollan observed colloids using only pertechnenate and sodium borohydride. The resulting radiopharmaceutical was taken up by the liver.[278] Metallic colloids are not possible with this reducing agent, but molybdenum blue eluted from a low specific activity ^{99}Mo generator may be the colloidal carrier for the technetium.

The second possibility is the binding of technetium to sulfhydryl groups produced by the reduction of disulfide bonds. This is especially true for antibodies of the IgG type that contain from four to six interchain disulfide bonds and numerous intrachain disulfide bonds.[279] Steigman et al[160] are the first to suggest that sulfhydryl groups were responsible for the direct binding of ^{99m}Tc. Paik et al[262] substantiated this hypothesis by carrying out a number of competitive experiments and by titrating the SH groups using Ellman's reagent.

The amount of stannous chloride is important in direct labeling because too little results in incomplete reduction and too much results in colloid formation when the labeling is performed in acetate buffer which is not a good chelate. The available sulfhydryl groups were determined after 30-minute incubation of stannous chloride with antibody. The stannous chloride was present in eight-fold excess over the protein. The following results were obtained (expressed as sulfhydryl groups/antibody)— IgG: 5.5 ± 0.7; F(ab')2: 4.2 ± 0.6; Fab: 0.9 ± 0.15. The presence of both high- and low-affinity sites on the protein was defined by competition studies using DTPA. The high-affinity sites were determined as those from which ^{99m}Tc could not be removed by DTPA even at large molar excesses. The percentage bound to protein was determined at various ratios of DTPA to protein.

These results are obtained only under conditions of direct competition between DTPA and antibody. If the protein is labeled first, then DTPA is effective only at high pH. One hypothesis is that the high-affinity binding to IgG involves a Tc(V) species whereas the binding to DTPA involves a Tc(III) or Tc(IV) species. Competitive experiments indicate that the distribution of ^{99m}Tc between the competing ligands is determined by the forward rate constants but not by the equilibrium constants for these reaction conditions. This approach has been refined by others to maximize the percentage of free sulfhydryl groups. Paik et al[280] estimate that about ten times molar excess of DTPA is required to prevent ^{99m}Tc complexation with low-affinity sites. However, the presence of free DTPA reduces drastically the percent ^{99m}Tc bound to antibody.

One possible solution for this low yield is to reequilibrate the mixture of low- and high-affinity sites in the presence of DTPA at high pH. This apparently increases the percent Tc on the high-affinity sites. Distribution studies in mice show similarities between the antibodies labeled by different techniques at the high-affinity sites.

The generally lower percent ID per gram values in the tumor for the antibody containing both strongly and weakly bound ^{99m}Tc indicates that a soluble chelate rather than pertechnetate may be the major radiochemical impurity.

Hnatowich's group has determined the expected ratio of ^{99m}Tc binding to the chelating agent in the bifunctional chelate compared to direct binding to the antibody. Using 50 μg/mL DTPA as the molar equivalent to 20 mg/mL IgG, various binding conditions were tested. Without protein present, DTPA complexed reduced ^{99m}Tc efficiently, but not quantitatively.

In a subsequent paper, they determined the appropriate tin-to-DTPA ratio. The labeling of conjugated protein via the bifunctional chelate is about 80%. The distribution in normal mice at 1 hour is similar for ^{111}In-DTPA-IgG and ^{99m}Tc-DTPA-IgG.

If the source of ^{99m}Tc is ^{99m}Tc-EDTA at 100 μg/mL, then the requirement for chelator concentration is less. Using 150,000 as the molecular weight of IgG there is 33 nmol/mL of IgG. If the molecular weight of the free amine is used, 268, then 3 μg of DADT is 13 nmol/mL and 8 μg of DADT is 34 nmol/mL. These molar values do not agree with the molar ratios stated by Liang et al.[281] However, it appears that the chelation to DADT is more effective when Tc-EDTA is used than when the chelator is labeled directly.

It has been more than 10 years since Rhodes developed the direct labeling method by pretinning the antibody by overnight incubation with stannous chloride.[282] This procedure is the basis for the many "direct labeling" methods being pursued today. In Rhodes' current method 0.67 mL of a solution containing 5 m*M* $SnCl_2$, 40 m*M* potassium phthalate, and 13.4 m*M* sodium potassium tartrate at pH 5.6 is added to 1 mL of 1 mg/mL antibody and incubated for 21 hours at room temperature.[283] The pretinned antibody can be stored frozen at −70°C. Pertechnetate is added and incubated for 1 hour at room temperature before using. The radiochemical purity was determined using a TSK G3000SW column eluted with phosphate buffer. A transchelation challenge test used either 3 m*M* EDTA, 100 μg of pretinned antibody in phosphate buffer, 100 μg of pretinned antibody in 1% human serum albumin, or phosphate buffer. Equal volumes were mixed and incubated at room temperature for 1 hour or more before HPLC analysis. HPLC analysis of technetium-labeled IgG mixed with one of the four challenge solutions showed that the technetium remains bound to the IgG. If the antibody has not been pretinned, the exchange with the challenge agent is rapid. The antibody must be rigorously purified before radiolabeling or low molecular weight components will be radiolabeled. Others have shown that the presence of citrate, for example, can reduce the radiochemical purity of labeled proteins.[284]

Reno and Bottino[285] refined and expanded on Rhodes' approach by suggesting a series of reducing agents (dithiothreitol, sodium borohydride, sodium phosphorothioate, dithioerythritol, 2-mercaptoethanol, cysteine, *N*-acetyl cysteine, and glutathione), weak chelating agents for ^{99m}Tc (tartrate, glucoheptonate), and stabilizers for the formed sulfhydryl groups (zinc ion). They show that untreated antibody binds only 24% of added ^{99m}Tc, whereas DTT-treated antibody binds 85%. Zn-stabilized antibody has a longer shelf life than reduced but unprotected antibody. Pak et al[286] in a recent patent used a reducing agent such as dithiothreitol along with stannous chloride and a water-soluble ligand. Saccharic acid, glucoheptonic acid, and tartaric or another polyhydroxy carboxylic acid capable of complexing technetium were proposed as stabilizing agents.

In most cases, the direct labeling technique is a combination of the approach to increase the number of sulfhydryl groups in an antibody with a reducing agent and the use of a ligand capable of solubilizing Tc(V) yet still undergo rapid metal exchange with the antibody. Steigman et al had proposed Tc(V) gluconate as the ideal exchange ligand some years ago after studying a series of polyalcohols and polyhydroxy carboxylic acids.[163,180,287] A competition was set up between the chelating agent and a Sephadex gel column which is a composed of cross-linked dextrans. The column was eluted with a 55-m*M* solution of the chelating agent. Ethylene glycol, glycerol, erythritol, 1,6-hexanediol,inositol, *D*-mannose, and fructose-O-dextrose (sucrose) did not form stable or inert enough complexes with Tc to compete effectively with the binding on the column. No Tc was eluted using these chelating agents. In a series of three- and four-carbon polyols, stereochemistry played a major part in the ability to bind technetium. Xylitol bound Tc, but ribitol did not. Of the four carbon compounds, mannitol, sorbitol, and galactitol all were capable of eluting 60 to 70% of the reduced technetium from Sephadex. The hydroxy acids, lactic and glyceric, produced minimal complex whereas of the five-, six-, and seven-carbon homologs, xylonic acid eluted 22%, D-gluconic acid eluted 82%, and L-galactonic acid did not elute Tc, but glucoheptonate eluted 94% of the Tc. The chelating agents suggested by Pak et al are hydroxydiacids. Nevertheless, they serve the same purpose by being strong-enough chelating agents to prevent the formation of hydrolyzed technetium but weak enough to transfer the technetium to the protein.

A recent variation on this theme was presented by Bremer et al[288] who used propylenetetraphosphonate as the solubilizing ligand. They also preincubated the protein with a reducing agent such as 2-mercaptoethanol or 2-aminoethanethiol to increase the sulfhydryl concentration. Their formulation is (1) 2.0 mg antibody in phosphate (preincubated with reducing agent) and (2) 0.12 mg $SnCl_2$-$2H_2O$ in 2.9 mg 1,1,3,3-propanetetraphosphonic acid, tetrasodium salt $4H_2O$.

Hansen et al recently published a similar procedure whereby the freshly prepared Fab fragment is mixed with their reducing agent for 24 hours before adding pertechnetate.[289] No additional details are available.

Feitsma et al[290] have published a direct method using a Tc nitride intermediate. The undefined species is produced by heating a mixture of dimethylformamide, HCl, and pertechnetate in normal saline. The technetium complex is extracted in chloroform, the chloroform is evaporated, and the protein solution is added. Blok et al showed that the yields with various proteins were higher with this method than with the pretinning procedure.[291] Competition studies with primary amines indicate that the technetium is binding to amines in the protein. Baldas et al described a procedure that may give a similar technetium intermediate.[292] They prepared a well-characterized Tc-nitrido compound by refluxing a solution of pertechnetate, azide, and HCl. They suggest that a $TcNCl_4$ group is binding to sulfhydryl groups created by partial reduction of the disulfide bridges.

DeFulvio and Thakur[293] have recently titrated free sulfhydryl groups using ninhydrin. Using molar ratios of between 1000 to 5000 of dithiothreitol (DTT), dierythritol (DTE), or 2-mercaptoethanol (2-ME) to IgG, they observed less than 2% reduction of the available 35 disulfide groups in IgG. Stannous chloride at molar ratios of 500 to 2500 reduced up to 1.8% of the available disulfide groups. The highest percentage reduction was obtained with molar ratios of 3500 to 17,500 of ascorbic acid. All reducing agents were mixed with IgG for 30 minutes. Radiolabeling with ^{99m}Tc led to various yields with a maximum of 96% for an ascorbic acid ratio of 3500. Incubation of the radiolabeled protein with 500 molar excess of DTPA or with HSA did not result in transchelation. Blocking the sulfhydryl groups with iodoacetate or cysteine decreased ^{99m}Tc binding. This is the most comprehensive report relating reducing agents to number of sulfhydryl groups produced and radiochemical yield.

There have been few comparisons in vivo of different methods of radiolabeling.[294] The direct method of radiolabeling used was that of Rhodes.[295] The indirect method was that of Abrams using the hydrazino nicotinamide chelator.[296] In this case, direct labeling reduced the immunoreactivity to a greater extent than indirect labeling. Electrophoresis showed that direct labeling led to lower molecular weight species. The in vivo distribution shows the direct method produces more radioactivity in the kidney and less in the liver compared to the indirect method. However, there was no difference in clearance in patients using radiolabeled fragments.[297] This is probably due in part to the greater renal clearance of the fragments and therefore increased difficulty in observing increased renal radioactivity.

The competition studies carried out by Rhodes, Thakur, and Hansen may not be conclusive because of the pH used and the chelating agent. Fritzberg found that the DADS compounds (4,5-dimercaptoacetamidopentanoic acid) were more competitive for Tc bound to antibodies than was DTPA.[298] His results show that 1 m*M* DTPA was not effective in removing directly bound Tc from labeled antibodies after 18- to 24-hour incubation at 37°C but that the DADS compound at 1 m*M* removed 54% of the protein bound Tc. Incidentally, the efficiency of a chelating agent that is known to bind Tc(V) rather than Tc(IV) supports the hypothesis that protein bound Tc is probably Tc(V). The solubilizing agents as well as the most efficient competitors for directly bound ^{99m}Tc are all known to bind Tc(V) in the absence of protein, yet many of the direct labeling methods use reducing agents that produce Tc(IV) in the absence of protein. There is no immediate solution to this dichotomy, but Tc(V) is favored. Since these DADS compounds have high affinity for the Tc, Fritzberg has stated that "while these donor atoms form highly stable complexes when optimal five-membered chelate rings of sufficient number result in small molecule ligands, the likelihood of finding four or more donor atoms in a preferred arrangement in the protein is low."[299] Another interesting difference in labeling conditions is that antibodies treated with reducing agents are labeled at room temperature, whereas diamidedithiols and triamidemonothiol such as MAG_3 cannot be labeled at room temperature and at the pH (6 to 7) used for the direct labeling of antibodies. Although amino acid sequences are known for many antibodies, there are no crystal structures indicating the three-dimensional stereochemistry and so this statement cannot be verified at present, but the implications are clear. In vivo Paik et al showed that the directly labeled antibody cleared the body more rapidly as if a percentage of the ^{99m}Tc was bound to low molecular weight compounds.[262,280] Buraggi et al[300] have reported rapid blood clearance and Burchiel et al have observed renal uptake.

Another approach to binding ^{99m}Tc directly to antibodies is to increase the sulfhydryl groups using 2-iminothiolane.[301] A molar ratio of 50 of 2-iminothiolane to IgG mixed for 30 minutes led to a 94% radiochemical yield with ^{99m}Tc using 1.4 μg tin(II). Using DTPA in a molar excess of 764 did not decrease the yield after 2.5 hours. Challenge experiments with cysteine led to 50% transchelation after 4 hours. Serum did not remove ^{99m}Tc. Goedemans et al quote earlier work on Pb protein labeling as the basis for their approach.[301] IgG has sufficient exposed lysine groups such that six to nine attached sulfhydryl groups are introduced. Joiris et al[302] studied the same reaction for directly labeling antibodies. They state that this procedure is superior to the use of a disulfide reducing agent because the latter produces fragments, eg, Fab is produced from $F(ab')_2$ whereas the former, ie, 1-iminothiolane, does not produce such fragmentation.

The direct labeling of proteins in general and antibodies in particular is progressing with a number of these approaches being used in clinical trials. There is no doubt that the ^{99m}Tc is bound to the antibody. Nevertheless, identification of the binding site, the oxidation state of Tc, and the stability of the site(s) needs to be pursued. With the low percentage of the injected dose in the tumor and the photon-poor nature of nuclear medicine imaging, the search for these answers is of utmost importance.

Indirect Methods. An indirect method involves the use of a bifunctional chelating agent. The bifunctional chelating agent is either radiolabeled with ^{99m}Tc before or after the chelating agent is conjugated to antibodies. The advantage of this indirect approach is that one can select a bifunctional chelating agent with a known chelate structure and a well-defined ^{99m}Tc chelation chemistry. One example is an analogue of diamidodithiol or diaminodithiol. Because of the high stability of its ^{99m}Tc complex and good in vivo clearance, a diamidodithiol and diaminodithiol derivative has been most actively pursued as a bifunctional chelating agent. However, the use of the thiol and amino ligands requires caution because they are very reactive nucleophiles that can deactivate an organic functional groups such as an activated ester which must be activated for the conjugation of the chelating agent to antibody. The thiol ligand also can react with disulfide bridges of antibodies to generate thiol groups into antibody, thereby producing the direct binding of ^{99m}Tc to the sulfhydryl groups of antibody. Because of these reasons, it is important to protect the reactive thiol and amino groups but also be able to remove these groups under a mild condition when needed for complexation with ^{99m}Tc.

There are two indirect approaches, the preformed ^{99m}Tc chelate approach and the chelator-antibody approach. A general procedure for the preformed chelate approach involves the removal of the protecting group, ^{99m}Tc complexation of the bifunctional chelator, the purification of this preformed chelate, the activation of a carboxy group to an activated ester, and the conjugation of the preformed chelate to antibody. The advantage of the preformed chelate approach is that ^{99m}Tc is complexed exclusively to the chelator moiety of antibody through well-defined chemical steps. A weakness of this method is that highly trained personnel are required to perform these experiments successfully and the overall labeling yield is generally low. For the chelator-antibody approach, a chelator is conjugated to antibody before the ^{99m}Tc labeling is performed. The advantage of this approach is that the labeling experiment is simple. However, one has to be certain that the sulfhydryl group of the chelator is protected when the bifunctional chelator is conjugated to antibody but can be deprotected under a gentle condition before the radiolabeling of the conjugate is performed. One has to be able to perform a control experiment to prove that the deprotected sulfhydryl group of the chelator does not reduce the disulfide bridges of antibody, thereby causing a direct binding of ^{99m}Tc to antibody.

The Preformed Chelate Approach. Derivatives of diamido dithiol, triamido, monothiol, cyclam, and BATO have been used for a preformed chelate approach to label antibodies. The advantage of this approach is that one can ensure that ^{99m}Tc is bound to the chelator moiety and not to amino acid residues of antibody. The disadvantage is that this approach involves several additional experimental steps to obtain the ^{99m}Tc-labeled antibody after the chelator is labeled with ^{99m}Tc.

Diamidodithio Bifunctional Chelate.[298,299] Fritzberg has compared the use of direct labeling a bifunctional chelate and a preformed chelate to determine relative radiochemical purity and stability. He used the 2,5-dimercaptoacetamidopropanoate as the ligand. The core ligand (TcDADS) has been suggested as a ^{99m}Tc substitute for Hippuran. In the case of the bifunctional chelate, the ligand was conjugated to antibody using an activated ester. The Ab-ligand complex was then radiolabeled by ligand exchange. For the prelabeled ligand, the diamidodithio ligand was radiolabeled first, the carboxylic acid of the diamidodithio ligand was activated to the ester, and then the prelabeled ligand was reacted with the Ab. The relative stabilities were tested by incubation of each radiolabeled antibody type with either DTPA or excess diamidodithio ligand.

It is clear from this experiment that the prelabeled ligand forms the most stable bond. Esterification of the preformed Tc complex went in about 70% yield. Conjugation yields using 2.5 mg/mL $F(ab')_2$ at pH 9 were between 50 and 70%.

A diamidodithio derivative, 4,5-bis(benzoylthioacetamido)pentanoic acid has been most actively investigated by Fritzberg et al.[298] An important parameter determining the radiolabeling condition has been the removal of the benzoyl group. Because the debenzoylation requires high pH or heating, the ^{99m}Tc labeling was performed under the same conditions as the hydrolysis of the benzoyl group using sodium dithionite as a reducing agent or exchange labeling with ^{99m}Tc gluconate. The carboxy group of ^{99m}Tc chelate was converted to the activated ester from the reaction with 500-fold molar excess 2,3,5,6-tetrafluorophenol in the presence of an equal molar excess of 1-(3-dimethylaminopropyl)-3-ethylcarbodiimide as a coupling agent at 75°C for 30 minutes. The esterification yield was reported to be 70%. The activated ester of ^{99m}Tc 4,5-bis(thioacetamido)pentanoic acid was purified and conjugated to antibody at pH 9.0 with a 50 to 70% conjugation yield. Recently, Fritzberg's group[303] protected the mercapto group with an ethoxyethyl group. This protecting group was removed at pH 3 as ^{99m}Tc is complexed to the thio group. Under this condition the ethoxyethyl group on the sulfur which was not complexed with ^{99m}Tc and the tetrafluorophenyl ester were reported to be stable. Using this ethoxy ethyl protecting group, antibody was labeled with ^{99m}Tc with an overall yield of 70%.

Boronic Acid Adduct of Technetium Dioximes (BATO). Linder et al[272] have modified the boronic acid moiety of BATO to generate an isothiocyanato functional group and also to increase hydrophilicity so that BATO complex can be reacted with antibody in aqueous medium. To achieve this goal they synthesized 2-carboxy 4-isothiocyanatophenyl boronic acid (CPITC). ^{99m}TcCl (dioxime) 3CPITC complexes were prepared with a 30% yield. The isothiocyanato functional group of the CPITC complex was then conjugated to amino groups of antibody with a yield of 30%.

Cyclam-Based Bifunctional Chelate. Franz et al[271] have used a derivative of the well-characterized cyclam to avoid direct antibody binding. Cyclam was derivatized at the 1-nitrogen with a 3-aminopropyl derivative. The cyclam derivative was reacted with 2-imino thiolate to introduce a sulfhydryl functional group. This was reacted with activated IgG to form the bifunctional chelate. The relationship of activated antibody and number of chelates incorporated is given.

These experiments show one of the problems with using prelabeled ligands. Only 4% of the ^{99m}Tc becomes bound to the IgG. A more-efficient coupling reaction is needed. If the ligand is labeled with ^{99m}Tc in the presence of the activated coupling group, then optimal radiolabeling conditions may not be available. On the other hand, if the Tc complex is activated toward conjugation after formation, another procedural step is required. This balance must be dealt with to obtain maximum efficiency.

The Antibody Chelator Conjugate. This approach involves the conjugation of the bifunctional chelator to antibody prior to radiolabeling with ^{99m}Tc. This approach has been pursued with the assumption that ^{99m}Tc would bind solely to the chelator moieties if the chelator forms a more stable complex with ^{99m}Tc than the amino acid residues of the antibody. DTPA was first tried. Although DTPA is not an ideal chelator for ^{99m}Tc, this early study revealed two sites of binding, a high-affinity, low-capacity site and a low-affinity, high-capacity site for binding ^{99m}Tc. The high-affinity site was qualitatively related to the sulfhydryl group generated by the reduction of the disulfide bridges of the antibody. The amino residues corresponding to the low-affinity site are not yet well defined. The ^{99m}Tc labeling of the low-affinity site was reported to be prevented by the presence of free DTPA, glucoheptonate, tartrate, and glucarate. The ^{99m}Tc binding to the high-affinity sulfhydryl-containing site is difficult to prevent. It is, therefore, important to prove before the labeling of chelator antibody conjugate with ^{99m}Tc that the free chelator binds all of the reduced ^{99m}Tc when antibody is present. This competition experiment is especially important for sulfhydryl-containing bifunctional chelating agents because these agents can reduce the disulfide bridges of antibody to sulhydryl groups that can bind ^{99m}Tc. The following chelating agents were used for the chelator-antibody approach.

Thiolactone Diaminedithiol. A thiolactone diaminodithiol derivative was synthesized by Baidoo et al.[267] The carbonyl group of this bifunctional chelating agent was then conjugated to amino groups of the antibody. The conjugation reaction was more efficient at pH 8 than at pH 7. However, the conjugation reaction was very slow even at pH 8 such that the yield of the chelator conjugation was 6% at the reaction time of 24 hours with the protein at 2 mg/mL. It was reported that the rate of the ^{99m}Tc labeling to the chelator-antibody conjugate was dependent on the concentration of the chelator molecules. The labeling yield was 85% at 10 minutes when the chelator-antibody (1 mg) with three chelator molecules per antibody was transchelated with ^{99m}Tc glucoheptonate at pH 7. There was no report on what percent of the label was due to direct ^{99m}Tc binding to sulfhydryl groups of antibody generated by the exposure of the antibody to the sulfhydryl groups of the chelating agent.

Diaminotetrathiol. Najafi et al have recently synthesized tetrakis (2-mercaptoethyl) ethylenediamine.[269] This agent was reacted with antibody at a 1:1 molar ratio. The authors believed that one mercapto group of this agent reacted with a disulfide of antibody to couple the agent to antibody through a disulfide bond that generates a sulfhydryl group to antibody. Although the ^{99m}Tc labeling yield of this chelator-antibody conjugate was reported to be 95%, it was not known what percent of the total activity was bound directly to the sulfhydryl groups of antibody. The authors reported that 50% of the antibody-bound activity was liberated as ^{99m}Tc N_2S_4 when treated with 2-mercaptoethanol or cysteine. This might indicate that only 50% of the total bound activity was bound to the chelator moiety.

Metallothionein. The metal-binding protein metallothionein was conjugated to antibody using succinimidyl 4-(*N*-maleimido)cyclohexane 1-carboxylate by Brown et al.[266] The metallothionein antibody (1.3×10^{-5} *M*) with two metallothionein molecules per antibody was labeled by incubating with ^{99m}Tc glucoheptonate at room temperature for 60 minutes. The labeling yield to the conjugate was 70 to 95%. Since metallothionein also can reduce the disulfide bridges of antibody to sulfhydryl groups, it is not certain how many percent of the total ^{99m}Tc activity is bound to the metallothionein moiety.

Hydrazinonicotinic Acid. Schwartz et al[268] synthesized *N*-hydroxysuccinimide ester of 6-hydrazinonicotinic acid. The carbonyl group of the active ester was then conjugated to amino groups of antibody. The hydrazino-modified antibody was then labeled with ^{99m}Tc via an exchange labeling using ^{99m}Tc glucoheptonate in citrate buffer at pH 5.2 to 6.2 at room temperature for 1 hour. The radiolabel was reported to be stable (92% retained with antibody) in the presence of 10 m*M* L-cysteine in PBS, pH 7.4, at 37°C for 24 hours. The precise nature of the bonding between ^{99m}Tc and the hydrazino moiety has not been established. This ^{99m}Tc complex might contain a Tc=N bond based on the crystal structure of a technetium-hydralazine complex.

Bis-thiosemicarbazone Bifunctional Chelates. Yokoyama's group has developed the neutral ^{99m}Tc chelate KTS (keto-bis-thiosemicarbazone) for use in bifunctional chelates.[304] Various derivatives have been prepared including the *p*-carbonylethylphenyl-glycol derivative (CE-DTS) that has been conjugated to antibody by activating the acid group using the phosphorylazide method. Stannous ascorbate was used as the reducing agent and ^{99m}Tc ascorbate as the transfer agent. As in most of these studies the optimal pH is between

4.5 and 6.2. The labeling experiments were carried out to determine what percent of the ^{99m}Tc binds to the chelating agent and what percent binds directly to the antibody. At ratios of chelating agent to antibody that preserve the immunologic activity (ie, 1:1 molar ratio), about 15 to 20% of the ^{99m}Tc is directly bound to the protein. In vitro and in vivo stability of the derivatized antibody is high.

The ideal nuclear properties of ^{99m}Tc warrant further definition of the role of diagnostic radiolabeled antibodies and of the chemistry of technetium. To date, the labeling of antibodies with ^{99m}Tc using an "instant kit" has not resulted in a product with high radiochemical purity. High purity is obtained using the prelabeled ligands, but this necessitates a multistep kit. However, in light of the large number of variables involved in each experiment with radiolabeled monoclonal antibodies, it seems prudent to use only preformed ligands, not only with ^{99m}Tc, but with all metallic radionuclides, until such time that an ideal combination of radionuclide and antibody can be identified. The use of directly labeled antibodies or antibodies labeled nominally via bifunctional chelates has added an unnecessary complication to the already complicated experiment involving the search for the ideal diagnostic or therapeutic antibody.

DIRECT LABELING OF CHELATING AGENTS

Technetium chelates are used to varying degrees in the study of three organ systems: the kidneys, liver, and bone. For the kidneys, Arnold documents 12 different chelating agents that have been combined with ^{99m}Tc.[305] These include (1) EDTA,[306] (2) DTPA,[14,307] (3) mannitol,[27] (4) mannitol with gelatin,[277] (5) penicillamine-acetazolamide,[308,309] (6) caseidin,[310] (7) citrate,[311] (8) tetracycline,[312] (9) inulin,[277] (10) dimercaptosuccinic acid (DMSA),[30] (11) glucoheptonate, and (12) gluconate.[313] More recently, other compounds, mostly thiol derivatives, have been proposed: penicillamine,[314] cysteine,[315] acetylcysteine,[316] glutathione,[317] and Unithiol.[318] These are discussed in a recent review.[249]

Few of these compounds are used clinically to determine size, shape, and position of the kidneys because of the advent of computed tomography and ultrasound. The most common clinical agents for kidney studies are ^{99m}Tc DTPA, ^{99m}Tc glucoheptonate, and ^{99m}Tc DMSA. Four other important ^{99m}Tc chelates also have been prepared: cyclam,[319] DADS [*N,N'*-bis(mercaptoacetamido)-ethylenediamine],[320] and KTS [kethoxalbis(thiosemicarbazone)].[265,321] Technetium-99m cyclam is important, not so much as a kidney agent per se, but as a positively charged chelate for bifunctional derivatives. Technetium-99m DADS is important because it is secreted by the renal tubules. A carboxylic derivative ^{99m}Tc-CO_2-DADS has higher renal excretion but can exist as a mixture of four isomers.[322] Only one of these has high renal excretion. It has been replaced by TcMAG3 which was fewer stereoisomers.[323] Technetium-99m KTS is a neutral, lipophilic chelate useful for labeling structures that must cross cell membranes.

Hepatic and hepatobiliary ^{99m}Tc chelates have been proposed as possible replacements for ^{131}I rose bengal, the advantage being the increased photon yield. They are as follows: (1) penicillamine,[324] (2) pyridoxylideneglutamate (PG), a Schiff base,[325] (3) dihydrothiotic acid,[326] (4) tetracycline,[312] (5) mercaptoisobutyric acid,[327] (6) 6-mercaptopurine,[328] and (7) HIDA, a lidocaine derivative containing iminodiacetic acid.[32,329] A convenient method has been developed to prepare various HIDA derivatives with substituents in the benzene ring.[330] Briefly, substituted anilines are reacted with the anhydride of nitrilotriacetic acid to produce chelating agents for ^{99m}Tc. Several structure-distribution studies have been carried out.[331–336]

The third group of technetium chelates, those used for bone imaging, were developed in 1971.[27] Prior to that, only the less-desirable fluorine or strontium nuclides were available. Tripolyphosphate was the first of these.[337] Shortly thereafter, ^{99m}Tc polyphosphate was introduced. The slow blood clearance and varying chain length, described by Subramanian et al[338] led to further investigation and subsequent synthesis of today's conventional skeletal imaging agents: pyrophosphate,[337] diphosphonate (HEDP)[29] methylene diphosphonate (MDP),[31] and hydroxymethylene diphosphonate (HMDP).[35,339] These compounds have been compared to other diphosphonate and imidodiphosphonate derivatives in terms of bone uptake and blood.[340–342]

The final group of chelates includes the new radiopharmaceuticals for heart and brain. In the heart, ^{201}Tl-as the thallous cation is most often used. However, ^{99m}Tc cations, such as hexakis (2-methoxy-2-methylpropyl) isonitrile [also known as Sestamibi[38] and RP-30] and neutral ^{99m}Tc complexes such as [bis[1,2-cyclohexanedionedioximato(1″)-O]-1, 2-cyclohexane-dione-dioximato(2-cyclohexane-dione-dioximato(2)-O]methylborato(2)-*N,N′,N″,N‴,N⁗,N*‴″]-chlorotechnetium (one of a class of boron adducts of technetium dioximes [BATOs] also know as teboroxime, SQ 30,217, or CDO-MeB)[343–345] are being tested to determine their suitability as myocardial perfusion agents. Although these two radiopharmaceuticals are both indicated for use as myocardial perfusion agents, their biological properties differ substantially. Cardiolite is a positively charged, lipid-soluble ^{99m}Tc complex that appears to be bound in the mitochondria of myocytes by virtue of the transmembrane potential.[346] Cardiolite is taken up by the myocardium and retained with a half-life of greater than 12 hours, whereas ^{99m}Tc-labeled teboroxime is taken up rapidly and released rapidly.[347] With Cardiotec, the imaging must be completed within the first 10 minutes after injection. This latter compound is more characteristic of xenon than of thallium and can be used to obtain rapid repeat studies. Cardiotec is a neutral compound that is more highly extracted than thallium and significantly higher than Cardiolite and should therefore be more sensitive to small changes in flow, especially during a stress test. Both ^{99m}Tc radiopharmaceuticals do not "redistribute" to the extent that ^{201}Tl does and therefore two injections are required to obtain a stress and a rest study. There have been recent efforts to view the net efflux of teboroxime from the heart as "redistri-

Table 2. Recently Approved Radiopharmaceuticals

TRADE NAMES	GENERIC NAME
CardioTec	Teboroxime
Cardiolite	Sestamibi
Technescan MAG_3	Mertiatide
Ceretec	Exametazime (HMPAO)
I.V. Persantine (for ^{201}Tl)	Dipyridamole, USP
Cardiogen-82	Rubidium-82 Generator

bution"[348,349] and obtain both stress and rest information from a single injection. A recent review of cardiac imaging with Sestambi and Teboroxime by Leppo et al, which crowns an excellent series of ten articles on these two heart agents, appears in the October 1991 edition of the *Journal of Nuclear Medicine*.[350] Both heart agents were approved at the end of 1990 and are rapidly expanding the type of information obtained in diagnostic myocardial perfusion studies.

^{133}Xe is approved by the US FDA for the measurement of cerebral perfusion. ^{123}I labeled *N*-isopropylamphetamine[351] (Spectamine) in 1989 became the second commercially available agent that crosses the intact blood-brain barrier. The distribution immediately after injection is flow related, but the immediate uptake and later distribution are dependent on amine uptake processes. Recently, several neutral ^{99m}Tc-labeled compounds were proposed for measuring cerebral blood flow in disease states in which the blood-brain barrier is intact. The series of propyleneamineoximes are interesting cerebral perfusion agents.[37] Whereas ^{99m}Tc PNAO (propyleneamine oxime) is taken up efficiently and released from the cerebrum rapidly, a derivative, ^{99m}Tc, D,L-hexamethylpropylene-amine oxime (HMPAO) is taken up and retained. The mechanism of retention is thought to be binding to glutathione in the brain, although this is far from proven.[352] Because the available rotating SPECT instrumentation is relatively insensitive, the latter compound is being studied in the clinic after approval by the FDA in 1989. However, with the proliferation of multihead SPECT machines, those compounds with fast pharmacokinetics may be more useful because repeat studies can be carried out with minimal delay. The analogy with myocardial imaging agents is important. Finally, there is an ester derivative of the diamino, disulfide chelation system (*N,N'*-1,2-ethylenediyl-bis-L-cysteine diethylester, Neurolite, and Tc-ECD) that is taken up in the human brain.[353] This compound depends on the slow hydrolysis of the ester groups in the blood and the rapid hydrolysis of ester groups in the brain to give high cerebral uptake and retention of the more hydrophilic metabolite. It appears that a series of first-generation ^{99m}Tc compounds has been developed to measure perfusion in the brain; these hold great promise for establishing the usefulness of nuclear medicine studies of cerebral perfusion in diseases that do not disrupt the blood-brain barrier. Dementia and stroke are the two most frequently mentioned abnormalities. Table 2 contains the trade names (in the first column), and the USAN names

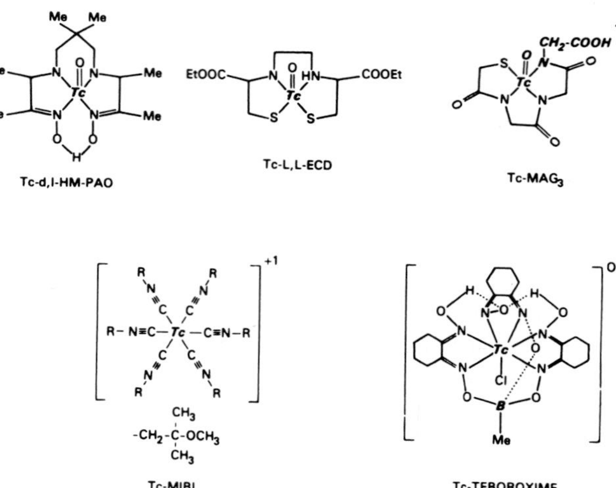

Figure 1. Structure of Tc–d, I–HMPAO (exametazime), Tc–L, L–ECD, Tc–MAG_3 (mertiatide), Tc–MIBI (Sestamibi), and Tc teboroxime (teboroxime).

(in the second column), for the recently FDA-approved radiopharmaceuticals. The chemical structures are given in Figure 1. The preparation conditions for these new radiopharmaceuticals are given in Table 3. In general, the preparation is more complicated than that needed for the previously established kits, but still falls under the general concept of "instant kits."

In Vitro Radiochemical Purity. Of the chelating agents studied, ^{99m}TcSn DTPA is one that appears to be radiochemically pure.[354] By definition, this implies that only the chemical form stated is present in the compound. In contrast, most of the other chelating agents mentioned seem to have a low affinity (are weak chelates) for Tc; in these instances, the risk of radiochemical impurity (species other than those desired) is high.

The ^{99m}Tc chelates suggested for renal scintigraphy are mostly weak chelates and may give confusing results if studied on certain chromatographic systems. One source of error, previously mentioned, can result from interaction with the solid phase of the system because chelating moieties in the solid support compete for the ^{99m}Tc.

Among the agents suggested for hepatobiliary imaging,

Table 3. Preparation Conditions

RADIOPHARMACEUTICAL	PROTOCOL FOR PREPARATION
CardioTec	Heat for 15 min at 100°C
Cardiolite	Heat for 10 min at 100°C
Ceretec	Generator within 24 hr; use within 30 min
MAG_3	Add 2 ml of air; heat for 10 min at 100°C
Cardiogen	Use with infusion system

^{99m}Tc pyridoxyleneglutamate,[325,355,356] ^{99m}Tc penicillamine, and ^{99m}Tc IDA compounds have been shown to be radiochemically pure.

Technetium HIDA has been chromatographed in two systems and shown to be a pure radiochemical.[32,329] There have been reports that various Tc-IDA compounds, eg, *N*-(2,6-diisopropylacetanilide) iminodiacetic acid and *N*-(*p*-isopropylacetanilide) iminodiacetic acid, showed two components on HPLC when prepared at low pH. Only a single peak was evident at neutral pH.

Of the bone-imaging agents, ^{99m}Tc HEDP appears to be a strong chelate and has been chromatographed on Sephadex G25 eluted with saline.[357,358] Technetium pyrophosphate on the other hand, dissociates on Sephasex G25 and on Whatman paper when saline is used. This artifact was described earlier and is remedied by eluting with a pyrophosphate solution; the change produces a single peak in both systems, which indicates a radiochemically pure product. Technetium polyphosphate also elutes from Sephadex G25 with saline, but presents an additional radiochemical purity analysis problem. Although one radioactive peak has been obtained in the chromatography of ^{99m}Tc polyphosphate, the variations in phosphate chain length raise uncertainties concerning the identity of the localizing species.[359] It is hoped that the use of high performance liquid chromatography (HPLC) will clarify many of these and other questions concerning the radiochemical purity of chelates labeled with technetium.

The chemistry of ^{99m}Tc HMPAO and ^{99m}Tc ECD has been reviewed recently by Nowotnik.[360] ^{99m}Tc HMPAO can be prepared as the D,L mixture or the meso compound. Only the D,L pair is taken up and retained in the brain. In vitro the D,L pair is unstable, giving a number of more polar radiopharmaceuticals in relatively short time. This has led to various restrictions on its use in the routine clinic.[361] ^{99m}Tc ECD is stable in solution.

HPLC is state of the art for analysis of radiopharmaceuticals. Wieland edited a series of papers dealing with the technique and applications of HPLC to radiopharmaceutical research.[362] Various contributors covered not only the basic technique but applications to the development of organic and metal chelate radiopharmaceuticals. Recently, Boothe and Emran[363] reviewed the current methods for a series of SPECT and PET radiopharmaceuticals (Table 4). Pike et al in the same textbook give similar information on various PET radiopharmaceuticals.[364]

Table 4. Application of HPLC to the Analysis of Radiopharmaceuticals

APPLICATION TO TECHNETIUM RADIOPHARMACEUTICALS
Pertechnetate
Ethylene-1-hydroxy-1,1-diphosphonate (EHDP)
Methylene-1,1-diphosphonate (MDP)
Dimethylaminomethylene diphosphonate (DMAD)
N-Benzyl-*N*-methyl-piperazinyl-bis-(aminoethanethiol) (BPA-BAT)
HMPAO
Hepatobiliary iminodiacetic acids (HIDAs)
APPLICATION TO MONOCLONAL ANTIBODIES
^{111}In IgG 1a murine anti-CEA
^{125}I B72.3
^{125}I Fab 96.5
APPLICATION TO RECEPTOR-BASED RADIOPHARMACEUTICALS
11-beta-methoxy-[16-alpha ^{123}I]-iodoestradiol
N-[Methyl ^{11}C]-nomifensine
d-[^{11}C]-octopamine
3-*N*-[^{11}C]-Methylspiperone
^{123}I SCH 23982
3-(2′[^{18}F])-Fluoroethylspiperone
^{18}F benzamide analogs
3-Quinuclidinyl 4-iodo-[^{123}I]-benzilate
OTHER RADIOLABELED BIOCHEMICALS
6-[^{18}F]-fluoro-DOPA
^{11}C Amino acids
N-3-[^{18}F]-fluoropropylputrescine
[^{18}F] FDG

In Vivo Radiochemical Purity. ***Renal Agents.*** Information about the chemical forms of ^{99m}Tc renal imaging agents is sparse. Chromatography of plasma and urine samples after injection of Tc-Sn-DTPA indicates that at 1 hour after administration the Tc-Sn-DTPA is 90% radiochemically pure in the plasma and 98% radiochemically pure in the urine.

These chelates for kidney imaging fall into three categories: those that are filtered, those that are secreted, and those that exhibit a mixed behavior of filtration, secretion, and binding in the kidneys. Technetium-99m DADS is largely secreted by the tubules. Although the mechanism is not certain, the secretion rate appears to be faster than DTPA and can be blocked by probenecid, which suggests that tubular secretion plays a dominant role in renal clearance of the chelate.[365]

Most of the chelates with mixed functions, such as Tc-ascorbate, Tc-glucoheptonate, and Tc-DMSA, have not been characterized chemically. Partly because the starting radiotracer is not a single component, researchers have been reluctant to investigate the chemical form in blood and urine. Renal extraction efficiencies were determined by McAfee et al for a series of kidney agents.[366] Ortho-iodohippurate had the highest extraction efficiency. The ^{99m}Tc complexes of DTPA and glucoheptonate have extraction efficiencies of 27 to 29%. Technetium-99m DMSA and Hg-197 chlormerodrin had lower extraction values of 8 and 14%, respectively.

An interesting aspect of the mixed-function renal imaging agents is the effect of stannous ion on retention in the renal cortex. In the DMSA kit, the absolute amount of stannous ion is important in accelerating the formation of the kidney localizing component. Both chromatographic and biologic differences were observed when ^{99m}Tc DMSA was prepared with stannous ion, electrochemically or with sodium borohydride.[367]

A number of possible mechanisms were outlined but a causal relationship could not be extracted from the data.[368]

Steigman et al unified these concepts by showing that stannous ion increased the renal retention of ^{99m}Tc for several chelating agents.[250] In general, for DTPA, pyrophosphate, and HEDP preparations, the kidney-to-background ratio was higher for the electrolytic kit than for the stannous ion kit. However, with stannous-reduced ^{99m}Tc gluconate, ^{99m}Tc was retained longer in the kidney. The effect of stannous ion on renal physiology was demonstrated by injecting a stannous gluconate complex within 5 minutes of the electrolytic ^{99m}Tc gluconate. The image showed the same high kidney retention observed with the $^{99m}Tc(Sn)$gluconate preparations. This can be explained by a change in membrane permeability.

Bone Agents. Some information concerning the in vivo fate of the skeletal imaging agents is also available. Krishnamurthy et al, in comparing ^{99m}Tc pyrophosphate with diphosphonate, established the early binding properties of these compounds.[369–371] At 1 hour post-administration, approximately 80% of the serum ^{99m}Tc activity was bound to serum proteins, most of which was associated with the globulin fraction. Red blood cell binding was also found. In another investigation, Bowen and Garnett determined that, 1 hour following the intravenous administration of ^{99m}Tc PYP, greater than 50% of the plasma activity was due to free ^{99m}Tc polyphosphate;[372] this contrasts with the plasma clearance data obtained with ^{99m}Tc PYP, which indicated that less than 33% of the total plasma activity was free ^{99m}Tc pyrophosphate. Interestingly, the major urinary constituent after the administration of either ^{99m}Tc PYP or ^{99m}Tc PPi was ^{99m}Tc PYP. This finding suggests that ^{99m}Tc PYP was present in the ^{99m}Tc PPi.

Schumichen et al compared various methods of analyzing protein-bound ^{99m}Tc-labeled bone-imaging agents.[373] Using the ammonium sulfate precipitation method, the investigators found that bone-imaging agents had varying amounts of ^{99m}Tc bound to plasma proteins. For example, ^{99m}Tc HEDP had 8.6 and 24.5% of the ^{99m}Tc bound to protein at 10 minutes and 5 hours, respectively after a patient's injection. The comparable percentages were 13.3 to 48% for ^{99m}Tc MDP, 18.2 to 79.3% for ^{99m}Tc pyrophosphate, and 49.6 to 90.0% for ^{99m}Tc tripolyphosphate. These are percentages of the radioactivity left in the blood at the time of sampling and are not related to the injected dose. When these human-plasma samples were injected in rats, the concentration of radioactivity in the bone at 1 hour was compared with the protein-bound concentration in the original sample. There was a good correlation between the nonprotein-bound ^{99m}Tc in human plasma and the bone uptake in rats for all ^{99m}Tc bone-imaging agents. Similar correlations were obtained when activity in the blood and urine of the rats was compared with the nonprotein-bound plasma fraction of ^{99m}Tc from humans.

In 1971, Subramanian and McAfee published the first studies using a ^{99m}Tc bone-imaging agent.[27] Since that time, criteria for ^{99m}Tc uptake in bone have been determined almost entirely by organ distribution studies. In fact, the first phosphate, sodium tripolyphosphate, was not a pure ligand, and it prompted further studies on the effect of chain length on bone localization. For polyphosphates, bone uptake was found to be inversely proportional to the chain length, ie, pyrophosphate gives the highest bone uptake. The initial organ distribution studies focused on blood clearance, which did little to define the bone-localizing species. In this respect, ^{99m}Tc MDP appears to be one of the quickest bone-imaging agents in clearing the blood and is the most widely used, clinically. More recent organ distribution studies have focused less on blood clearance than on bone uptake. In two articles, Bevan et al studied in vivo binding of technetium skeletal imaging agents.[35] Technetium-99m MDP and Tc-99m HMDP appear to clear the blood rapidly. On the other hand, ^{99m}Tc HEDP has lower bone uptake but a higher ratio between areas of bone with different metabolic rates.

Buja et al have shown that the uptake of ^{99}Tc HEDP is positively related to serum calcium levels.[374] Other proposed uptake mechanisms, such as high-affinity binding to organic matrix,[375,376] to tissue phosphatases,[377,378] or to various proteins of damaged tissue,[379] may play minor roles in ^{99m}Tc localization in the bone.

Autoradiographic studies confirm that the growing face of the apatite crystal is the point of uptake of ^{99m}Tc bone-imaging agents.[380] The chemical state of ^{99m}Tc at the bone surface has not been determined. Christensen and Krogsgaard dissolved bone with EDTA and found that the ^{99m}Tc-labeled chemical form could not be distinguished from ^{99m}Tc MDP.[381] Earlier theories had proposed that ^{99m}Tc would be displaced on the bone surface by calcium to produce TcO_2.[382] Pinkerton et al have shown that ^{99m}Tc HEDP prepared with sodium borohydride contains many components before injection,[229] and Steigman et al have suggested the possibility of polymeric species.[164] Therefore, in vivo radiochemical purity is uncertain until pure starting material is used.

The localization mechanism of ^{99m}Tc phosphorus radiotracers in myocardial infarcts and in other soft-tissue abnormalities is probably due to microcalcification. Of the bone tracers, ^{99m}Tc PYP is the most widely used in clinical evaluation of myocardial infarcts.[383] The reasons for the discrepancies between the relative uptakes of ^{99m}Tc PYP and ^{99m}Tc MDP in damaged myocardial tissue and the relative uptakes of these complexes in bone are not known.

Hepatobiliary Agents.[384] The hepatocytes in the liver clear hepatobiliary agents from plasma by an active transport process. Most current ^{99m}Tc hepatobiliary agents are cleared by the same general anionic mechanism operative for bilirubin. Therefore, in hyperbilirubinemia, there is competitive inhibition for transport of the ^{99m}Tc agents. All hepatobiliary agents appear to have certain chemical characteristics that distinguish them from substances excreted by the kidney. The molecular weight of hepatobiliary agents is usually between 300 and 1000 d; the molecules contain at least two planar, lipophilic structures and a polar group. These hepatobiliary agents usually are protein bound, although neither ^{99m}Tc PG nor ^{99m}Tc HIDA are extensively protein bound in plasma.[385]

To optimize these chemical properties, many ^{99m}Tc agents have been prepared and evaluated. As early as 1974, hepatobiliary ^{99m}Tc chelates were proposed as possible replacements for ^{131}I rose bengal.[32] The early ^{99m}Tc hepatobiliary agents were excreted by both kidney and liver. The first improvements focused on decreasing the kidney component; later, efforts to accelerate clearnce were made. Loberg proposed a pharmacokinetic model that describes the competition between hepatobiliary and renal clearance.[386]

Either an increase in hepatobiliary clearance or a decrease in renal clearance increases hepatobiliary specificity. When liver function is impaired, however, renal clearance becomes relatively more significant.[385] This effect is observed even when the ^{99m}Tc HIDA derivative is one in which elimination by the hepatobiliary pathway is both efficient and rapid in normal patients and animals. Therefore, in addition to simply finding chelates that are rapidly cleared by the liver, chelates that more successfully compete with bilirubin are being sought so that these agents may be used in patients with high serum bilirubin.[384] For this reason, the most suitable chelates probably have a high affinity for anionic receptors or hepatocytes, compared to bilirubin, as well as normally rapid clearance rates.

Several analogs of ^{99m}Tc HIDA are sufficiently lipophilic and characterized by the other properties outlined by Firnau to be excreted by the hepatobiliary system.[387] Further refinements in the structure have been proposed to increase the blood and liver clearance.

Regarding the in vivo behavior of ^{99m}Tc hepatobiliary chelates, Loberg et al have shown that the ^{99m}Tc activity in the bile has the same chromatographic behavior and distributes in rats in the same manner as the original compound.[385] The search continues for derivatives that are cleared from the blood and liver at a faster rate.

Heart and Brain Agents. The in vivo chemistry of the newer ^{99m}Tc radiopharmaceuticals is critical because of the attempts to quantify the functional study and to understand the mechanism of localization. As a result the HPLC procedure developed for the in vitro assay is applied to an organic extract of plasma to determine the in vivo fate of the radiopharmaceutical. In the case of ^{99m}Tc HMPAO, the same decomposition that occurs in vitro also occurs in vivo; this is the method of retention in the brain. The parent compound rapidly converts to hydrophilic species.[388] The injection of the hydrophilic species prepared in vitro does not result in brain uptake. The theory is that the lipophilic species crosses the blood-brain barrier and then the ^{99m}Tc is retained as the hydrophilic compound.

The in vivo stability of ^{99m}Tc ECD is also low, with the hydrolysis of the diester thought to be the main route of metabolism. The L,L-ECD shows the best brain retention. The ^{99m}Tc L,L-ECD is hydrolyzed rapidly to the monacid in brain, lung, kidney, liver, and blood. The retention is presumably due to the hydrolysis in brain, but the higher retention in baboon and human brain compared to rat brain cannot be explained by the rate of conversion.[353]

The in vivo behavior of the recently developed myocardial imaging agents was review by Nunn.[389] Both sestamibi and teboroxime clear the blood rapidly. Recent studies show that teboroxime is slowly degraded in the blood by hydrolysis of the axial chloride.

^{99m}Tc MAG3 is stable in vivo, but highly protein bound. It clears the blood in proportion to renal plasma flow.[390]

DIRECT LABELING OF COLLOIDS AND PARTICLES

Numerous radiolabeled colloids for use in hepatic scintigraphy have been reported. The one most commonly used is ^{99m}Tc sulfur colloid prepared from the acid decomposition of sodium thiosulfate in the presence of a variety of stabilizing agents. Among these are gelatin (the most popular), albumin, poylvinylpyrrolidine, and polyhydric alcohol.[21,391–393] Stabilizer-free preparations also have been proposed as well as compounds with carrier rhenium and antimony.[102,394,395] Other types of colloids include stannous oxide,[396] technetium oxide,[397] and microaggregated albumin.[398]

Several ^{99m}Tc labeled particles can be used for lung scanning. Methods and types of preparations include macroaggregation of ^{99m}Tc-labeled albumin, the conversion of Tc sulfur colloids into HSA macroaggregates,[399] coprecipitation of ^{99m}Tc with iron hydroxide,[400] macroaggregation of albumin in the presence of colloid,[401] and incorporation of ^{99m}Tc sulfur colloid or reduced technetium into microspheres.[28] Macroaggregates are the most commonly used.

In Vitro Radiochemical Purity. The work of Cifka and Vesely is notable for having shown that premixing pertechnetate with sodium thiosulfate produces a nonpertechnetate radiochemical impurity.[108] In routine silica gel thin layer chromatography (TLC) systems, this impurity was not identified because it remained at the origin and therefore was indistinguishable from ^{99m}Tc sulfur colloid. On Whatman No. 3 paper with 0.3 N HCl, however, the impurity did manifest itself. Differences in chromatographic behavior of technetium sulfur colloid preparations are known,[402] but they have not been related to biological behavior.

Determination of the particle size of colloids is important because the size appears to be related to the distribution. Methods of determining particle size differ, depending on whether the colloids are radioactive or nonradioactive. Traditionally, colloid chemists have used electron microscopy to determine particle size because it provides a direct measurement.[403] Steigman, however, has shown that Tc-labeled sulfur colloid has a different particle size distribution from that of cold sulfur colloid. Electron microscopy therefore may not be useful for measuring these particles.[404]

The major difference between ^{99m}Tc colloid and sulfur colloid is in the size range <100 nm, where a larger percentage of ^{99m}Tc colloid particles fall.[109] Warbick et al, assuming no differences between labeled and nonlabeled colloid particle size distribution, compared several sizing methods (Table

Table 5. Colloid Size

MATERIAL	DIAMETER (nm)
Tc-phytate	In vivo
^{99m}Tc-antimony sulfide	4–14
^{113}m-colloid	10–20
^{198}Au colloid	10
^{99m}Tc-Sn-phosphate	In vivo
^{99m}Tc-liposomes (neutral)	33
^{99m}Tc-minimicroaggregates (HSA)	90
^{99m}Tc-sulfur colloid (thiosulfate)	200–500

From Spencer, RP: Reticuloendothelial compounds. In: Spencer RP, ed. *Radiopharmaceuticals: Structure-Activity Relationships.* New York, Grune & Stratton, 1981. Reprinted by permission of the publisher.

5).[405] Technetium-99m sulfur colloid prepared with perrhenate carrier showed at least three major size components: 22% particle <100 nm; 39% between 200 and 400 nm; and 24%/400 nm. Davis et al also showed that such cellulose membrane filters as Millipore do not filter particles according to size because of the filter thickness and irregular path.[406] For the Tc sulfur colloid analyzed by Warbick et al electron microscopy revealed the presence of aggregates as the cause of the bimodal distribution observed with Nucleopore filters.

Warbick et al chose electron microscopy because it allows direct observation of the particles and chemical components. Technetium-99m antimony sulfur colloid was determined to have a smaller particle size (average = 10 nm) than thiosulfate-prepared sulfur colloid. The presence of aggregates makes data of antimony colloid difficult to interpret. Billinghurst and Jette used gel filtration to measure particle size because of the general unavailability of electron microscopes and the evaporation of sulfur that occurs with that technique.[407] They proposed gel filtration for colloidal particles below 100-nm diameter because larger particles are above the maximum operating range. In addition, based on the relationship between percentage radioactivity and number of particles, they proposed that the surface area, not the volume, is the relevant variable. Only certain particle size ranges can be analyzed on these columns, and the elution time is long.

Pedersen and Kristensen have compared several techniques, including filtration, photon correlation spectroscopy, and light microscopy.[408] They confirmed by these methods that several ^{99m}Tc colloid preparations change with time, especially the ^{99m}Tc colloids. They reemphasize that the Nucleopore filtration technique measures the distribution of radioactivity in particles of different sizes, whereas photon correlation spectroscopy (Nanosizer) measures particle size. For example, for rhenium-sulfur gelatin, the mean particle size by Nanosizer measurement was 420 ± 40 nm, whereas only 30% of the ^{99m}Tc radioactivity was retained on a 400-nm filter, 33% on a 200-nm filter, and 36% on a 100-nm filter. The lower level of size detection for the spectroscopic method can also create inconsistencies.

In some preparations of ^{99m}Tc sulfur colloid, the colloid adheres to the walls of the glass vial in which it has been prepared. If the total vial is assayed, an aliquot removed may not represent the true fraction removed. It is therefore necessary to assay the dose in the syringe. Unless the syringe containing colloid is flushed with the patient's blood, a substantial fraction of the dose remains in the syringe.

Microspheres are particles formed by extrusion of albumin into hot oil, as opposed to macroaggregates, which are formed by heating albumin in water.[409] After sieving, they are uniformly sized and can be readily labeled. Microspheres have also been prepared from gelatin and amylose by modification of the albumin methods.[410] Other microspheres of various compositions are available for diagnostic and therapeutic purposes.[411]

It is important that labeled particles be of nearly uniform size and that a small proportion of unbound radionuclide exist. Microspheres are supplied presieved and have a narrow size range. Unbound radionuclides may be determined by washing or incubating with the fluid to be used, filtering the mixture of spheres and fluid through a 0.45-μm filter to retain the spheres, and determining the activity of the filtrate. The U.S. Pharmacopeia (USP) specifies that no less than 90% of ^{99m}Tc-macroaggregated albumin (MAA) have diameters between 10 and 90 μm, and none may have a diameter greater than 150 μm.[73] On some occasions, the spheres may break under rough handling. For a general reference to albumin microspheres, the reader is referred to Reference 412.

In Vivo Radiochemical Purity. The chemical form of ^{99m}Tc following the intravenous administration of either radiolabeled particles or colloids is not known. Radiochemical impurities are easily demonstrated by chromatography, but their relationship to the biologic behavior of the compound is not well understood.

In further support of Steigman's contention that the particle size of the ^{99m}Tc particles differs from the sulfur colloid itself, two groups have studied the distribution of sulfur colloid doubly labeled with ^{99m}Tc and ^{35}S and found 86% of the ^{99m}Tc in the liver at 4 minutes but only 11% of ^{35}S at the same length of time. With longer heating time, only 29% of the ^{99m}Tc concentrated in the liver, while a much greater percentage concentrated in the lung. Clearance rates were also different. Technetium-99m remained in the liver (87% at 36 hours), but the ^{35}S cleared more rapidly (4% at 36 hours). Frier et al observed similar pharmacokinetics.[413] When they used ^{99}Tc in equimolar amounts, they observed high liver uptake with both ^{99m}Tc and ^{35}S. They suggest that sulfur colloid is broken down by serum whereas Tc colloid is not. Although this may occur in sera, accelerated breakdown also occurs in the liver, as shown in the first case. Both groups removed soluble sulfur by dialysis. The ^{35}S can be incorporated in either of the nonequivalent sulfur atoms in thiosulfate.[414]

Many experiments have been carried out to determine the effect of size, number of particles, surface charge, and stabilizer on the distribution. Most of these have been designed to increase the concentration of colloid in the bone marrow. Atkins et al studied the distribution of sulfur colloid produced by H_2S and by thiosulfate.[415] Increasing either the number of colloid particles or the gelatin concentration increased the marrow uptake. Pretreatment of animals with either gelatin or nonradioactive colloid also decreased liver uptake and increased bone marrow uptake. At large doses, relatively more H_2S-produced colloid than thiosulfate-produced colloid goes to the marrow. Quantitative studies of the effect of particle size and number by Cohen et al and by Caro and Ciscato revealed that the clearance halftime could be described by the Michaelis-Menten equation for enzyme reactions.[416,417]

The colloid disappears from the blood by an exponential function, is adsorbed on the surface of Kupffer's cells, and then is bound irreversibly. Caro and Ciscato used gold colloid stablized by PVP or gelatin.[416,417] The hepatic clearance time was not affected by the mean size of the particles that were at least in the range of 2.5 to 30 nm. The overall rate constant is greater for PVP-protected colloids than for gelatin-protected colloids. The gelatin-protected particles have a greater affinity for the cell sites, but their entry into the cell is slower. Smaller particles seem to be cleared from the blood faster,[276,418] but a kinetic analysis using the methods of Caro and Ciscato has not been applied; therefore, the surface charge and the rate of binding and internalization still may be determining factors.

McAfee et al compared several colloids to determine relative bone marrow uptake.[366] No significant increase in uptake was observed among different colloids such as antimony sulfur colloid, stannous oxide colloid, microaggregated albumin, and small albumin microspheres. McAfee et al showed that mini microaggregated albumin had the highest marrow concentration in dogs, and this was confirmed by comparative imaging.

Several factors must be kept in mind during discussion of colloid distribution as a function of physicochemical properties. The measurement of size can be misleading because the radioactive particles may not have the same size distribution as the nonradioactive particles, and the extrapolation from one physical measurement to another is beset with difficulties. Emphasis on particle size may be incorrect, based on the work of Caro and Ciscato and Myers.[417,419] Also, the difference in relative distribution between the liver and bone marrow might best be explained by a difference in mechanism of sequestration. Martindale et al conclude that small colloids, such as ^{99m}Tc antimony sulfur colloid, concentrate in the subendothelial dendritic phagocytes of the bone marrow. The actual route to these cells may be by micropinocytosis across the endothelial lining of the sinusoid, through the junctions between adjoining endothelial cells. Only occasionally was the radiocolloid found in the endothelial cells lining the bone-marrow sinusoids. Thus small colloids are better suited to localization in the bone marrow.[420]

DIRECT LABELING OF CELLS AND BLOOD ELEMENTS

The two blood components, erythrocytes (RBCs), and albumin (HSA), have received the most attention in radiolabeling with ^{99m}Tc.[421] Although in vitro labeling of RBC appears to be superior to in vivo labeling (injecting tin intravenously, followed 20 minutes later by injecting ^{99m}Tc pertechnetate), many laboratories still use the latter because of technical ease. In vitro methods, especially those using the pretinning kit developed byBrookhaven National Laboratory,[422] appear to produce quantitative retention of radioactivity.[423] The problem with the in vivo labeling technique, as described by Pavel and Zimmer,[424] is the low labeling yield in some patients.[425] Gottchalk et al have suggested that the two techniques can be combined as follows: stannous pyrophosphate is injected as in the in vivo technique, but, instead of injecting pertechnetate 15 minutes later, blood is withdrawn and labeled in vitro.[426] This permits determination of the labeling yield before reinjection.

Attempts have also been made to label leukocytes,[427] lymphocytes,[428] and platelets,[429,439] although little success has been achieved with these blood cells. Many tumor cells have been labeled with technetium, including murine fibrosarcoma, human carcinoma of the breast, lung, and colon, and malignant melanoma.[431] Thymocyte labeling with ^{99m}Tc also has been reported.[432]

Because of the frequency of thromboembolic disorders, great interest has surrounded labeled fibrinogen and urokinase for thrombus localization.[433–435] Streptokinase, although not found in humans, has been studied for the same reasons,[436] as has plasmin.[437] For these and all other blood products and cells mentioned, the labeling procedure is based on the stannous chloride method developed for RBCs and HSA.

The majority of the labeling methods using ^{111}In are reviewed in the Clinical Chapter (see Chapter 35) by Dr. John McAfee.[438,439]

In Vitro Radiochemical Purity. The best method of determining labeling yield of cells is by centrifugation, which readily separates unbound radioactivity from the labeled cells. It does not separate ^{99m}Tc-labeled colloids or particles, because they sediment also.

For blood protein components, the most widely employed means of separation is by gel filtration with Sephadex G25 using saline solution.[25] Radiochemical impurities do exist. Early investigators erroneously assumed that pertechnetate is the only possible impurity. This led to much confusion when the in vivo stability of Tc-HSA was determined. In the production of ^{99m}Tc HSA by the iron ascorbate reduction method, impurities include not only pertechnetate, but also Tc-ascorbate, which is excreted rapidly and therefore overestimates plasma volume.

With development of the highly efficient tin reduction

method for preparing ^{99m}Tc HSA, not only is the production of ascorbate avoided, but the probability of a pertechnetate impurity is remote. Those labeling procedures that use stannous chelate and HSA at neutral pH, however, may result in the formation of small colloids with slow blood clearance. The clearance of Tc-HSA and small colloid is similar, so that the clinical observation is not affected.

The binding of ^{99m}Tc to blood clot agents is variable. Persson et al demonstrated that, even under optimal reaction conditions, ^{99m}Tc streptokinase was only 70 to 80% radiochemically pure.[440] With fibrinogen, 85% labeling occurred following electrolysis using zirconium electrodes.[429] Duffy and Duffy obtained the same yield using stannous chloride and streptokinase at pH 1 to 2.[441] However, upon increasing the pH to 7, approximately 15 to 20% of the ^{99m}Tc was released. Streptokinase also can be labeled by using stannous pyrophosphate as the reducing agent, yielding between 50 and 60% for a 2-hour labeling time at neutral pH. The radiochemical purity of radiolabeled streptokinase was determined on TLC, Sephadex column chromatography, and polyacrylamide gel electrophoresis. The commercially available streptokinase contains gelatin which is also labeled. To obtain radiochemically pure streptokinase, pure streptokinase must be used. The product is labeled at neutral pH and must be purified on a Sephadex column eluted with saline.

In Vivo Radiochemical Purity. Demonstrating radiochemical purity of labeled blood products is a minor task compared with the problem of proving that the radiolabeled product truly represents its natural blood counterpart.

For RBCs, red cell volume determinations have indirectly confirmed 95% radiochemical purity as much as 1 hour after injection.[442] Similar studies with ^{99m}Tc HSA remain in doubt because they are not accompanied by in vitro radiochemical purity data.

Two problems complicate labeling of cells other than RBCs. First, conclusively determining the chemical form of technetium in vivo is difficult. The second problem pertains to cell fragility. Labeling such cells as leukocytes, platelets, and thymocytes necessitates an evaluation of cell viability following the labeling procedure. Although such viability tests as trypan blue staining or determinations of cellular ability to incorporate thymidine and amino acids can indicate that the function tested is intact, the in vivo distribution does not represent that of native cells. A possible explanation is that the cell membrane is compromised during the labeling process, which changes the cell characteristics and behavior.

Nevertheless, even large quantities of radiochemical impurities may not frustrate the clinical objective. Acceptable thrombus visualization has been achieved with as little as 18% of ^{99m}Tc fibrinogen migrating electrophoretically with the clotting fractions.[429]

NEW DIRECTIONS IN ^{99m}Tc RADIOPHARMACEUTICALS

Future progress in nuclear medicine appears to rest upon more specific approaches to compound localization, mechanisms that depend upon the use of radiolabeled biologically active compounds or synthetic drugs. In spite of the potential suggested by this type of application, major difficulties are encountered in directly radiolabeling the functional groups of such compounds as hormones, enzymes, and drugs. First, the native functional group(s) may be essential to interaction with the active biological site responsible for compound localization; second, the affinity binding the radionuclide to the molecule may be insufficient to produce a stable chelate.

The importance of both of these factors is exemplified by radiolabeled bleomycin. Bleomycin is a mixture of closely related antibiotics that have been used successfully to treat a variety of malignancies. Chemically, this antibiotic acts as a chelating agent and binds a number of divalent and trivalent cations with varying affinities.[443] Although chelates of indium, gallium, and copper have not demonstrated the necessary in vivo and in vitro stability, cobalt-labeled bleomycin is more stable.[444] A technetium-labeled bleomycin would be more useful. While inspection of the bleomycin structure indicates that the disaccharide moiety is the most likely chelating group, it is unfortunately a low-affinity site for ^{99m}Tc.[445] The sugar moiety has a high affinity for ^{99m}Tc at pH 10 to 12, but a weak affinity at neutral pH. Therefore, the use of the native functional groups of bleomycin to bind technetium results in a weak chelate with poor stability.

The biologic activity of a drug may also change with the addition of a radiolabel. For example, the chelation of copper to bleomycin destroys its ability to cleave strands of DNA.[446] When labeled with cobalt, the antibacterial activity of bleomycin is deleteriously affected and becomes negligible when tested against the usually responsive *Bacillus subtilis* ATC 6633.[447] In this instance, cobalt appears to alter the biologic effectiveness of the bleomycin because of its bond to the functional groups responsible for maintaining the antibiotic integrity of this drug.

Another approach for labeling biochemicals (for which there have been many precedents) is derivatization. Drug derivatives have been prepared to increase absorption, eliminate bitterness and odor, diminish gastric upset, increase or decrease metabolism, and improve stability of the parent compound both in vivo and in vitro. Derivatives might also be developed that will accept a radiolabel without altering biologic activity.

Increasingly, specific site-directed synthetic derivatives are being developed. These are molecules that concentrate within the body by virtue of their physiologic action. Examples are (1) steroid hormones, (2) peptide hormones, (3) adrenergic substances, (4) vitamins, and (5) certain synthetic drugs. The ideal properties for any site-directed derivative were outlined by Paul Ehrlich approximately 80 years ago and more recently have been enumerated by Sinkula and Yalkowsky as follows[448]: (1) Exclusive and complete transport to the diseased tissue or target organ, including high binding affinity and interaction with these cell systems and tissues; (2) absence of binding by the derivative to protein or tissue not specifically diseased; (3) absence of degradation or metabolism of the derivative prior to contact with the diseased bioenvironment; (4) lack of toxicity for normal tissue in the body; (5) complete elimination from the body of the nonlocalized pharmaceutical.

Because these criteria are so stringent, the "ideal" site-directed drug derivative has yet to be synthesized. Even with radioiodide, perhaps the best example of a physiological site-directed radiopharmaceutical, the normal 24-hour thyroid uptake is only 15 to 25% of the administered dose. Localization also occurs in the stomach and salivary glands, with most of the dose excreted in the urine.

Regarding the use of radiopharmaceuticals, certain other factors must be considered. One factor is the time frame during which a radiopharmaceutical must maintain its integrity. During evaluation of pharmacokinetics, no absolute criteria exist, but rather a medical tracer needs to remain stable in vivo only for the duration of the study. For example, if a blood pool label reflects the vascular pool size accurately for only 30 minutes after injection, then it fulfills the criteria for a stable in vivo derivative, and its use is valid during that period of time.

In the reduced oxidation states, technetium usually requires an octahedral coordination structure, ie, up to six coordination sites in a target molecule are bound directly to the radionuclide. This structure can prevent the biologic molecule's expected interaction with the active site responsible for localization. Technetium-99m probably is not bound directly to many molecules with affinities able to withstand in vivo dilution or ligand substitution. As a result, the radiolabeled tracer in many cases may not reflect the biologic behavior of the parent molecule. In addition, the ready oxidation of certain reduced weak chelates interferes with studies of radiochemical purity and in vivo metabolism. To avoid the problems encountered with direct labeling of a biologically active molecule, derivatives are formed by covalent bonding of a chelating agent to a molecule known to act on a specific organ or to follow a specific pathway.

Labeling derivatives of biologically active compounds for use as tracers is a recent procedure. For reasons already elucidated, technetium appears to be the most logical of the radioactive metals for development of agents with widespread applicability. To bind such "positively charged" metal ions as ^{99m}Tc requires a relatively large chelating agent. The chelate, however, adds a large polar group to the molecule, altering its biologic activity.

Since the discovery of ^{99m}Tc in the late 1930s and its introduction into nuclear medicine via the ^{99}Mo/^{99m}Tc in the 1950s, ^{99m}Tc has been the radionuclide of choice in radiopharmaceutical development. From the "instant kits" that were measuring a combination of function and anatomy in the early years of ^{99m}Tc to the recent perfusion agents for the heart and brain, ^{99m}Tc has been amazingly resilient. In the past year, we have seen substantial progress in the attempt to link ^{99m}Tc to biochemicals. Chen and Janda[449] have prepared a Tc complex of a ribonucleoside. In this case, the Tc complex inhibits ribonuclease U2 activity at about 10% of the present gold standard, uridine vanadate. However, it is stable in aqueous solution and has the possibility of containing a high-affinity isomer in the diastereomer mixture.

DiZio et al[450] have radiolabeled a progestin derivative with ^{99m}Tc. This is yet another example of a ^{99m}Tc-labeled biochemical. The best ^{99m}Tc compound in this series has a relative binding affinity for the progestin receptor of 47% compared to R5020. The high nonspecific binding in vivo is still a major hurdle with the ^{99m}Tc chelates adding about 2 log units to the partition coefficient of the parent compound.

Piwnica-Worms et al[451] have investigated the behavior of ^{99m}Tc sestamibi on the subcellular level and discovered another application for the myocardial perfusion agent. Through careful evaluation of its subcellular distribution, these authors have found that radiolabeled sestamibi binds to P-glycoprotein and may be useful in monitoring the development of drug resistance.

Finally, Mäcke et al[452] have labeled Sandostatin, a somatostatin analog, with ^{99m}Tc using a diaminodiimino complex (PnAO) attached to the amino group of the N-terminal phenylalanine amino acid. The unlabeled derivative had a pKi of 9.94 compared to 9.45 for actreotide. However, the ^{99m}Tc-labeled compound showed high nonspecific binding in vitro. In general, the addition of a neutral ^{99m}Tc chelate to a biochemical has caused an increase in the lipophilicity that has interfered with specific binding.

PITFALLS

Factors that can affect the integrity of technetium radiopharmaceuticals adversely and deteriorate the quality of the scan image are due primarily to (1) improper preparation of nonradioactive components; (2) improper technique in the introduction of pertechnetate; and (3) differences in patient biophysiology. In the first case, oxidation of stannous chloride ($Sn\ 2^+$) to $Sn\ 4^+$, inadequate binding of the stannous ion to the chelating agent, or binding of stannous ion to a degradation product of the chelating agent fails either to reduce technetium or to introduce a competitive binder involving the degradation product. Should any of these problems occur during the manufacturing of stannous pyrophosphate or MAA particles, for example, the desired product will not be obtained.

Improper technique in the addition of pertechnetate to stannous-labeled chelating agents also degrades image quality. Careless contamination with O_2 during the addition of pertechnetate can prevent technetium reduction and ruin the ^{99m}Tc bone-scanning agent.

Metabolic variations among patients receiving technetium-labeled compounds affect tracer distribution. For example, both prospective and retrospective evaluations of ^{99m}Tc diphosphonate following bone scans with excess soft tissue activity have demonstrated no chromatographic irregularities in the administered compound or in analyzed samples of the patient's urine and blood. Local variations in tissue metabolism probably are responsible for distributional variations. Several of these so-called iatrogenic effects on radionuclide distribution have been reviewed.[453–457] Any of these factors can produce ineffective agents, and all have been responsible for suboptimal scintigraphs. Although the incidence of these problems is low, nuclear medicine laboratories should be capable of differentiating between these sources of error, particularly now that university and community hospitals are preparing, at least in part, their own technetium radiopharmaceuticals.

The most significant factor in successful ^{99m}Tc chromatography is a complete understanding of each system's function and limitations. For the determination of pertechnetate, there are no distinct advantages to either the column or the TLC systems. Each system has certain attributes that become apparent after extensive use. As new radiopharmaceuticals are developed, the chromatographic system must be validated with pure radiopharmaceutical. A case in point is the use of the silica gel:acetone system for analyzing ^{99m}Tc HIDA compounds. Because of the increased lipophilicity, ^{99m}Tc HIDA is not retained at the origin as is ^{99m}Tc DTPA; rather, it spreads over the entire strip in a broad peak. With 75% $CHCl_3$ and 25% acetone as the solvent, the ^{99m}Tc HIDA is retained at the origin in a sharp peak and TcO_4^- migrates with the solvent front. As in most areas of quality control, baseline reference determinations of the radiopharmaceutical are imperative.

With these concepts, a rational approach to ^{99m}Tc compound chromatography can be adopted. If the presence of pertechnetate is suspected from a bone scan, eg, gastrointestinal visualization, then the systems should be used exclusively for the detection of pertechnetate; should be used to determine the presence of reduced but unchelated technetium.

UNSATISFACTORY IMAGES AND THEIR CAUSES

Unexpected distribution of a radiopharmaceutical may be attributed to the radiopharmaceutical or to an altered physiological or pathologic process in the patient. As mentioned in the last section, unsatisfactory ^{99m}Tc radiopharmaceuticals can easily result from adding oxygen (air bubbles) along with pertechnetate to the kit. The oxidation produces pertechnetate, which results in thyroid and stomach localization. More subtle changes in distribution are observed when the nonradioactive kit is prepared in such a fashion that stannous oxide colloid is produced in a chelate kit. When some colloid is formed, soft tissue background or liver uptake occurs. This same effect is observed when too little chelating agent is used or when the kit is diluted excessively.

Many reports have been published in which an abnormal physiologic state of the patient was believed to cause the poor image.[453–457]

RADIOCHEMICAL PURITY

Most radiopharmaceuticals cannot be studied by ultraviolet or infrared spectroscopy, nuclear magnetic resonance, or elemental analysis because they are carrier free. Accordingly, chromatography has become the major analytic tool for determining their radiochemical purity. The term radiochemical purity, however, is much abused. The strict definition is the percentage of the radionuclide in question in the desired chemical form. The common mistake is to use a chromatographic system that can separate only one radiochemical impurity, usually pertechnetate, and then to report the radiochemical purity on that basis. Certainly, pertechnetate is the most obvious impurity in ^{99m}Tc radiopharmaceuticals, but as early as 1967, another impurity, commonly called reduced unbound ^{99m}Tc or reduced hydrolyzed ^{99m}Tc, had been identified. The exact nature of this species is not known; it may be a combination of impurities. Nevertheless, it is an impurity to be recognized.

Chromatographic Techniques. The most common method of separating radiochemical impurities in ^{99m}Tc radiopharmaceuticals is chromatography. Paper chromatography and TLC are simple methods of separation with closely related techniques for sample application, development, detection, etc. Column chromatography, which is a more complicated technique, offers a wider variety of solid supports (adsorption, gel filtration, and permeation for molecular size, ion exchange, etc) and is more adaptable to large-scale separations and to quantification of the species present. Recently, HPLC has been used for less-polar ^{99m}Tc chelates. This sensitive technique promises to make the definition of radiochemical purity more restrictive. With TLC and paper chromatography, only unchelated ^{99m}Tc species have been identified as radiochemical impurities, but with HPLC various chelated species are identified.

Paper and Thin-Layer Chromatography. These two chromatographic techniques, used primarily to determine the presence of pertechnetate in radiopharmaceuticals, can be completed within 1 hour, are simple to perform, and do not require expensive equipment. The procedure in each case consists of the application of microliter amounts of the radiochemical to a plate coated with a thin layer of absorbent, or to the paper chromatogram, at a point approximately 1 inch from the end that is to be immersed in the eluting solution. This point is called the origin and is marked at the lateral surface of the strip or plate for identification. The chromatogram then is immersed in the preferred solvent and the chromatographic tank is tightly covered. The solution level must be clearly below the point at which the radioactive sample is spotted. The solution ascends the strip by capillary action, carrying each radiochemical component according to its partition between the solid support material, eg, the paper or silica gel, and the solution. When the solution has traveled the desired distance, the solvent front is marked, and the plate or strip is removed from the container and allowed to dry.

The distance traveled by each radioactive component of the solution under analysis is the most important factor in these determinations. This distance, termed the R_f value, is defined as the ratio of the distance traveled by a given radiochemical component compared to the solvent front. It depends upon such conditions as temperature, quality of the support material, and preequilibration of the solution; because of these variables, R_f values are not always reproducible. For this reason, the suspected radiochemical impurity (eg, pertechnetate) should be chromatographed simultaneously with the product being evaluated and in the same container as this product.

The radioactivity associated with the various components now can be determined by counting cut-up portions of the chromatogram, or by counting on a radiochromatogram scanner, which gives the distribution of the radioactivity as a function of distance in a polygraph-like printout. Since glass-backed, thin-layer strips must be scraped before counting the sectioned pieces, which thus lengthens the procedure, fiber-backed or aluminum-backed, thin layer plates are preferred when cutting is necessary.

One main source of error in the chromatographic analysis of ^{99m}Tc radiochemical purity derives from the ease of oxidation of certain reduced states of technetium. For this reason, compounds should not be dried on the TLC plate or paper strip before elution in either chromatographic system. In the event that this is done inadvertently, oxidation may ensue with subsequent formation of pertechnetate not originally present in the radiopharmaceutical. In addition, nonspecific adsorption of the compound, as has been reported with ^{99m}TcSn HSA, may occur, owing to the small number of highly active sites on the chromatography strip or plate.[458] This phenomenon also has been observed in the preparation of high-specific activity iodinated hormones used for radioimmunoassay.[459]

Column Chromatography. Column chromatography is more sophisticated chromatographic system than TLC. Larger samples of radiochemical (0.1 mL to 5% of the column volume) can be used, which is an advantage when analyzing for oxidation-sensitive compounds produced with ^{99m}Tc. Each type of solid support, however, must be carefully prepared to obtain satisfactory performance, and the appropriate product manual must be consulted. Here, instead of measuring an R_f value, an elution volume is quantitated. Elution volume is defined as the volume of eluate require to elute the particular compound from the column. This volume also depends upon experimental conditions and must be calibrated using verified samples of the expected impurities.

Column chromatography requires more expensive equipment than do paper and TLC methods; fraction collectors and automatic gamma counters are needed. It is also more time consuming because of the large number of fractions that must be collected and counted. Finally, an attentive, competent technician is mandatory.

With these added complexities, however, determinations of radiochemical purity rather than pertechnetate contamination can be obtained. Short columns (10 cm) have been useful for relatively rapid determination of a certain impurity, whereas longer columns (greater than 30 cm) generally have been reserved for radiochemical purity determinations.

Another source of error may result from interaction between the solid phase of the chromatography system and the radiopharmaceutical. In this case, the solid support itself competes for the ^{99m}Tc because of its own chelating ability. For example, the polysaccharide Sephadex can compete favorably for certain weak chelates, eg, ^{99m}Tc gluconate and ^{99m}Tc mannitol.[163,460] Therefore, a ^{99m}Tc radiopharmaceutical analyzed on such a chromatographic system might appear to contain a radiochemical impurity (a reduced form of technetium) that is not bound to the chelating agent. This shortcoming has been demonstrated for a number of weak chelates analyzed with Sephadex column chromatography. To avoid this artifact, the inert solid phase polyacrylamide, Bio Gel P-10, with which there is no competitive adsorption of ^{99m}Tc to the base support, may be used. Alternatively, the Sephadex column can be eluted with the same concentration of chelating agent that is used in the preparation of the radiopharmaceutical.[461,462] Both options provide reasonable assurance that the determination of radiochemical purity is accurate.

This same phenomenon also may occur with paper chromatographic systems. When radiochemically pure ^{99m}Tc pyrophosphate (PYP) is eluted with saline, most of the reduced ^{99m}Tc appears to be unbound; however, if the paper is eluted with a pyrophosphate solution, the chelate is found to be radiochemically pure.[463] With the dilutional effect of the saline solvent and the rapid dissociation constant of polyphosphate (TcPPi), the chelate can release the ^{99m}Tc to another chelating compound. This property must be considered when evaluating radiochemical purity determinations with these systems.

Chelate stability on Sephadex and paper does not imply in vivo stability of the compound, but serves merely as an index of the competition (at the specific concentrations used) between the respective groups and the chelating agent.

HPLC. HPLC brings both improved column efficiency and high mobile-phase velocities to the separation procedures. Improved column efficiency is brought about by increased surface area per column length, which results from the use of decreased particle size (5 to 10 μm). The decreased particle size increases resistance to mobile-phase flow, however. This is overcome by using high pressure, usually on the order of 1000 psi. The most popular column packing consists of nonpolar chemically bonded phases. These columns are the "reverse" of the usual polar solid supports, such as silica gel and alumina. The reversed-phase columns are better suited for separating the nonpolar molecules that characterize many biochemicals and drugs. The columns are eluted with such polar mobile phases as mixtures of water and methanol, tetrahydrofuran, or acetonitrile. As in classical liquid chromatography, the retention time t_R is measured relative to the retention time of a nonadsorbed component t_0 to determine the capacity factor $k' = t_R - t_0/t_0$. The relative retention of two components α is given by the equation:

$$\alpha = k'_2/k'_1$$

Pertechnetate Generator Chromatography

The most important factor in the preparation of ^{99m}Tc radiopharmaceuticals is the radiochemical purity of pertechnetate eluted from the generator.

Two primary paper chromatography systems, based on the original work of Shukla, have been suggested to identify the various technetium species present in the generator eluate.[464] These systems contrast with the majority of chromatographic systems, in which the sole purpose has been to identify pertechnetate in ^{99m}Tc chelate and colloid preparations. Here, technetium species IV, V, and VII, which act as impurities with paper chromatography (in 0.3 *M* HCl or 90% methanol solutions), can be identified.

Although these systems are capable of identifying the Tc(IV), Tc(V), and Tc(VII), only the Tc(V) state can be eluted with TcO_4^- directly from the alumina column in the generator.[74] This species does not bind to DTPA and can be implicated in certain instances of nonbonding by the effluent of the Mo-99 generator product.[132]

Pertechnetate Impurity Chromatography

Following the determinations for reduced ^{99m}Tc species in generator pertechnetate, of major concern after the formation of ^{99m}Tc compounds is reoxidation of the reduced state of TcO_4^-. This can be rapidly determined by several chromatographic systems. No information, however, is provided regarding the radiochemical purity of the reduced compound. Usually, nonradioactive kits for the various compounds are prepared properly; as a result, impurities that form most likely result from pertechnetate formed by oxidation of the reduced technetium in one's own laboratory. These systems are designed to adsorb all nonpertechnetate compounds at the origin in TLC or on the support in column chromatography. Only the presence or absence of TcO_4^- is evaluated.

Radiochemical Purity Chromatography

To assure that a ^{99m}Tc radiopharmaceutical contains only the desired reduced species, at least two chromatographic systems must be used. Both systems used to assay for radiochemical purity should demonstrate a single band of radioactivity and possess a partition coefficient such that the compound is not freely eluted nor strongly adsorbed. Because of the complexity of these techniques, they are utilized primarily as research tools. Since pertechnetate is the most frequent impurity formed by ^{99m}Tc chelate degradation, the previously described chromatographic systems usually suffice.

Paper chromatography has been used for many years, whereas gel chromatography (Sephadex) was adopted in 1967. Richards and Atkins demonstrated the special advantage of the gel system, which strongly adsorbs reduced unchelated technetium.[23] Furthermore, ^{99m}Tc HSA was shown not to be radiochemically pure, as was originally suggested by paper systems[142]; it only appeared so because of the limitations inherent in these earlier techniques. Since its introduction, gel chromatography has been widely used in combination with paper chromatographic systems to determine radiochemical purity.[25,465]

Other systems also are capable of separating radiochemical impurities and, by necessity, new systems will be developed with the ever-increasing number of chelating agents. These systems often can be adapted from methods used to purify nonradioactive chelates.[466] For example, a system is needed to separate DTPA from Tc-DTPA, compounds with obvious differences. Separations may be possible with compounds that show slow dissociation on HPLC.

The more polar ^{99m}Tc chelates have been difficult to analyze on HPLC because of their poor retention. Russell and Majerik used a weak basic anion-exchange column eluted with buffer-separated pertechnetate from such polar chelates as DTPA, EHDP, and glucoheptonate, but since these chelates are not retained they appeared to be radiochemically pure.[354] Wong et al also studied a number of ^{99m}Tc chelates on HPLC using a μ Bondagel column eluted with buffer and a Bondapak C-18 column eluted with buffer acetonitrile.[467] There was good separation between Tc-HIDA or Tc-HSA and pertechnetate, but minimal separation between polar chelates (DTPA, MDP, and pyrophosphate) and pertechnetate.

Nonpolar chelates such as Tc-HIDA are more easily retained, especially on reversed-phase columns, as first shown by Loberg and Fields.[124] They were able to separate SnHIDA, HIDA, and Tc-HIDA on HPLC, using a Bondapak C-18 column eluted with acetonitrile and buffer. In a subsequent study, Fields et al were able to separate a number of chelate-containing ^{99m}Tc HIDA radiochemical impurites when analogs were used with pKa values for the imino nitrogen of greater than seven.[468]

Fritzberg and Lewis also have discovered radiochemical impurities other than pertechnetate and reduced-hydrolyzed Tc in ^{99m}Tc HIDA derivatives that have large substituents in the ortho position.[358] These impurities convert to the major component as a function of either time or increased pH. Pinkerton et al were the first to develop an HPLC system to separate bone-imaging agents.[229] Using an anion exchange column eluted with buffer, they found as many as seven components in Tc-HEDP, in addition to pertechnetate and reduced hydrolyzed technetium. This result was observed using ^{99}Tc whereas with ^{99m}Tc only one major peak was found. Srivastava et al, however, found multiple peaks for ^{99m}Tc MDP using reversed-phase HPLC.[469]

RADIOPHARMACEUTICAL CHEMISTRY OF IODINE

Radionuclides of Iodine

The radionuclides of iodine having the best nuclear properties for gamma-ray detecting systems are ^{123}I, ^{125}I, and ^{131}I. Both ^{125}I and ^{131}I are reactor produced and therefore less expensive and more readily available than the cyclotron product, ^{123}I. The radiation-absorbed dose to the patient from both ^{131}I and ^{125}I is high, however. Iodine-123 is a superior radionuclide for imaging systems, with a 159-keV gamma ray and low radiation-absorbed dose. This gamma ray has a half thickness in water of 4.7 cm and therefore affords satisfactory tissue penetration, yet its energy is low enough to be collimated easily. This radionuclide, though, can be produced only in a cyclotron and currently cannot easily be made free of ^{124}I and/or ^{125}I. High-energy protons or helium particles form the purest ^{123}I, but accelerators that produce them are not readily available.[470] The most frequently used reaction to produce ^{123}I of high purity is the $^{127}I(p,5n)^{123}I$ reaction or the ^{124}Xe (p, x) ^{123}I.[470A]

Iodine-124 is an undersirable radionuclide impurity because of its long half-life (4.2 days) and its positron and high-energy photons (511, 603, and 723 keV). A 1% concentration of ^{124}I at time of production usually results in 5% contamination at an imaging time 24 hours later. The ^{124}I degrades resolution because a significant fraction of the high-energy gamma rays are detected as scattered radiation in the 159-keV energy window. With a low-energy collimator, the scatter contribution is about 28%. With a high-resolution, medium-energy collimator, the contribution is 10%. With a high-energy collimator, only 3% is scattered radiation, but the sensitivity is greatly reduced. The need for high radionuclidic purity is obvious.[471]

Chemistry of Iodine

Of the halogens, iodine is most likely to support a positive charge and thus is the least reactive toward electrophilic addition or substitution. The chemical properties of iodine stem from the decreasing ionization potential, larger atomic radii, larger van der Waals forces, and increased polarizability that are found as the atomic number in the group VII congeners increases. Also, iodine forms the weakest bonds to carbon and the other first-row elements. Despite its anticipated stability, the I^+ ion does not exist alone but usually forms a complex with a nucleophilic species, such as water or pyridine.

Target Molecules for Electrophilic Substitution by Iodine

In electrophilic substitution, the most reactive aromatic compound is phenol, followed by aniline, methoxybenzene, and imidazole. The anion seems to be the reactive species, so close attention must be paid to the pKa and pH values of the reaction. Imidazole and pyrazole are iodinated in the 4-position and, therefore, fused ring compounds such as benzimidazole are not easily iodinated. Iso-oxazole, oxazole, and thiozole are less reactive than imidazole. In other heterocyclic compounds, the order of iodination at a specific reaction site is 2-thiophen = 3-furan < 3-benzofuran = 2-benzothiophen < 3-benzothiophen = 2-benzofuran ≪ 2-thiophen ≪ 2-furan. For benzothiophen and indole the 3-position is preferred, although in the heterocyclic alone (thiophen and pyrole), the 2-position is more reactive. The 2-position is most reactive in furan and benzofuran.[472]

Pyridine is not easily iodinated at a carbon atom, but rather, it forms charge transfer complexes with the halogen at nitrogen. Aliphatic unsaturated compounds can be iodinated, but the carbon-iodine bond is much less stable than the bond in aromatic compounds, although the mode of deiodination differs in each case.

The most popular iodinating agents used to produce electrophilic addition or substitution in activated aromatic rings are (1) iodine[473]; (2) iodine monochloride[474]; (3) chloramine-T[475]; (4) lactoperoxidase[476]; (5) electrolysis[477]; and (6) prelabeled ligands.[478]

Iodination Using Iodine

The reaction mechanism for the electrophilic aromatic substitution has been studied extensively. Reactions with phenols and imidazole generally show an isotope effect, indicating that the rate-determining step involves removal of hydrogen from the intermediate. In this case, the rate of catalysis seems to be determined by the type of base used. Where no isotope effect is observed, as in the iodination of dimethylaminobenzenesulfonic acid, the rate of reaction appears to be related to the basicity of the catalyst. This observation suggests that the formation of a complex iodinating agent may be involved in a rate-determining step.

Papers by Grovenstein et al showed a definite effect of iodide on the rate of iodination.[479] This effect is consistent with I_2 as the reactive species. These same authors observed that, as the iodide concentration decreased, the kinetic isotope effect also decreased, and the first step involving the attack of the iodine became rate determining. At high concentrations of iodide, the removal of hydrogen became the rate-determining step.

In radioiodination, half of the radioisotope is converted to the iodide chemical form after the reaction of the positive iodinating species. This process limits the theoretical yield.

Iodination Using Iodine Monochloride

McFarland showed, that compared to I_2 solutions, ICI increases the iodination efficiency because all iodine atoms can be incorporated.[474] Radioiodide is mixed with ICI and then added to the target molecule. Since carrier ICI is added, the specific activity of the product is lower than that obtained with chloramine-T. Lambrecht et al have proposed a recoil method for preparing carrier-free $^{*}ICI$,[480] but because of the complicated techniques involved it is not in common use.

The mechanism of ICI iodination has been studied by Berliner.[481] He suggested that either H_2OI^+ or ICI might be the electrophile in the rate-determining step. Batts and Gold, by studying the reverse reaction, ie, deiodination, showed that the chloride concentration affected the rate of reaction, and that ICI must therefore be the electrophile.[482] The deiodination was also acid catalyzed and the iodine released could be trapped by either chloride or dimedone. A substantial catalysis by chloride was observed, but the deiodination rate approached zero as the pH approached 7.

Iodination Using Chloramine-T

Chloramine-T, the sodium salt of *N*-chloro-*p*-toluenesulfonamide, has been used as an oxidant since its discovery by Chattaway in 1905. It is widely used at present because it has advantages over a standard iodine solution. Chloramine-T is unstable when exposed to light, but a 0.05 *M* solution in water decreases in oxidizing power by only 0.02%/month when stored in the dark.

The free acid and $RNCI_2$ exist at pH 1; at pH 2.6, the concentrations of $RNCI^-$ and RNCIH are equal, and at pH 4, only RNCI exists. The rate of reaction for the hydrolysis at pH 3.7 and 25°C is 10.10 L/mol/s, and the reverse reaction is 2.5 L/mol/s.

In addition to being a powerful oxidizing agent, chloramine-T can act also as a chlorinating agent in electrophilic substitution of aromatic molecules. Huguchi and Hussain describe the active species as the *N,N*-dichloro *p*-toluenesulfonamide (dichloramine-T).[483]

When phenol is used as the target molecule and the chloramine-T-to-phenol ratio is 10, chlorophenol is found in the reaction mixture after 3 minutes in a yield of 10 to 19%, in the pH range of 9.6 to 6.5. In the presence of radioiodide, the average yield of iodophenol based on radioiodide is 50% whereas the average yield of chlorophenol based on phenol is approximately 10%. In attempts to produce iodinated molecules with maximum specific activity, equimolar amounts of chloramine-T, iodide, and target molecule can produce mixed chloroiodo compounds that are difficult to separate and identify from the desired radioiodine compounds.

The use of chloramine-T has been discouraged because of these possible side reactions. Nevertheless, use of appropriate molar ratios can produce satisfactory products even with the most sensitive target molecules. Freychet et al have reported that equimolar amounts of either chloramine-T or chloramine-T added in small aliquots produces radiolabeled insulin that retains its biological activity.[484] Eckelman et al found that bleomycin can be radiolabeled by the chloramine-T method and that this sensitive molecule retained its antibacterial activity after iodination.[447]

To use chloramine-T, the target molecule must contain a tyrosine or imidazole moiety. The major advantages of iodination using chloramine-T are the simplicity and high reactivity that allow rapid preparation of products with high specific activity.

Iodination Using Lactoperoxidase

Iodide can be enzymatically oxidized to active iodine.[476] Immunoglobulin and bovine serum albumin were iodinated at low specific activity. Later, Thorell and Johansson improved the method to prepare high-specific activity, iodinated polypeptides, and proteins.[485] This method is claimed to be less destructive to the target molecule but involves the usual problems encountered when dealing with enzymes, such as purification, determination of enzymatic activity, and separation from the reaction mixture. It is advantageous, however, in that carrier-free iodide, which yields products with high specific activity, can be used.

Iodination Using Electrolysis

Although the reaction conditions needed for the electrolytic oxidation of iodide are generally mild, carrier iodine is needed, and the reaction volumes are usually larger than needed for other methods.[477] Miller and Watkins proposed a method of electrolytic iodination in acetonitrile that is effective for molecules as unreactive to electrophilic substitution as ethyl benzoate.[486] This reaction apparently proceeds through a nitrogen iodine intermediate.

Iodination Using Prelabeled Ligands

Bolton and Hunter proposed iodinated 3-(4-hydroxyphenyl)-propionic acid *N*-hydroxysuccinimide ester as an indirect iodinating reagent that avoids many of the problems of direct iodination.[478] In this indirect method of iodination, the active ester is iodinated and purified from oxidizing and reducing agents before being mixed with the target molecule. In this way, the impurities inherent in other iodination methods, eg, chloramine-T and metabisulfate, do not come into contact with the target molecule. The reaction results in the formation of an amide bond with lysine groups of the target molecule. This method permits iodination of molecules that do not contain tyrosine or whose biologic activity might be lowered by alteration at the tyrosine rather than at the lysine moiety. The specific activity obtained is usually lower than that obtained with chloramine-T. The Bolton-Hunter reagent is the most popular, although two other prelabeled ligands, iodoaniline, which is converted to a reactive diazonium ion, and methyl-3,5-diiodo-*p*-hydrox-ybenzimilate have been offered as equally effective reagents.[487,488] This indirect iodination method has been practiced for some time in preparing iodinated tracers for use in radioimmunoassay. Iodinated histamine-, tyramine-, and tyrosine-methyl ester can be reacted with carboxymethyl groups to produce iodinated derivatives.[489] A recent review compares other prelabeled ligands.[489A]

Exchange Labeling

IODINATION OF AROMATIC RINGS BY REPLACEMENT OF OTHER SUBSTITUENTS

A large number of metal derivatives have been prepared to lend specificity and reactivity to iodination of deactivated rings. Various leaving groups have been studied both at the carrier iodine level and the carrier-free level. Iododeboronation,[490] iododesilylation,[491] and iododestannylation[492] are among the more popular for carrier-free reactions. These methods were recently compared in an attempt to incorporate short-lived ^{122}I ($T_{1/2}$ = 3.6 minutes) into aromatic rings.[493] Because of the short half-life of ^{122}I, the relative reactivities were important. Likewise, it will be important to radiolabel the receptor-binding radiotracers by efficient methods with ^{123}I so that the procedures can become a clinical reality. Of the five metal groups substituted on benzene, $SnMe_3$ and $HgCl_2$ were clearly the most reactive either in ethanol or acetic acid solvent. The oxidizing agent used to carry out the electrophilic substitution was dichloramine-T (DCT). The regioselectivity of these reagents is important for receptor-binding radiotracers because of the structure-distribution sensitivity. It also permits the facile iodination of nonactivated aromatic compounds and, in fact, the aromatic compound must be deactivated to prevent competitive deprotonation reactions.

NUCLEOPHILIC IODINATION

Nucleophilic iodination of aromatic rings is usually carried out using either a diazonium ion prepared in situ or a triazene derivative. The mechanism of decomposition of these derivatives has been discussed at great length in the literature.[494,495] The reaction mechanism rivals electrophilic iodination in terms of complexity and no simple theory has emerged. Szele and Zollinger[496] have presented an explanation for the effect of solvents on competitive heterolytic and homolytic dediazoniation. In most of the earlier studies in acidic aqueous solution, heterolytic dissociation to give an aryl cation and molecular nitrogen was the mechanism of choice. However, in other solvents such as 2,2,2-trifluoroethanol (TFE) at least two intermediates must be involved: the phenyl cation and a tight ion-pair between the phenyl cation and nitrogen. Solvent effects on heterolytic dediazonation are small; the difference between the slowest and fastest is only a factor of 10. Radical reactions are also prominent with abstraction of a hydrogen atom to give the original aryl compound. The radical reaction is more dependent on the solvent. The formation of a radical pair and N_2 is favored by the nucleophilicity of the anion present. However, the anion must be a good homolytic leaving group. Szele and Zollinger call this "the concept of a nucleofugic homolytic leaving group."

IODINE REPLACEMENT BY IODINE (IPSO REACTION)

One of the most popular methods of introducing radioidine into aromatic structures is by halogen exchange. Stockin[497] has outlined three methods: the melt method, low-pH halogen exchange reactions, and excitation labeling. These methods do not, in general, produce radioligands with specific activities high enough to be used for receptor-binding radiotracers.

BROMINE REPLACEMENT BY IODINE

Stocklin in his review[497] also mentions Br for I exchange analogous to the ipso reaction. Recently, Wieland's group had adapted the original ammonium sulfate method[498] to produce higher specific activity ligands starting with the bromoderivative.[499] The method of choice for replacement of either iodine or bromine by ^{123}I is the copper exchange method developed by Mertens.[500]

Purification

In the past, high-specific activities were attained by using one or more iodine molecules per target molecule. Heavily iodinated species are present even at low molar ratios,[501] and chlorocompounds might be present with chloramine-T. Discouraged with these findings, most investigators iodinate low molecular weight compounds at high target-to-iodide ratios and then separate the iodinated target molecule by HPLC to attain maximum specific activity. When carrier-free radioiodine is used and one iodine atom per molecule is assumed, the maximum specific activity is 2,200 Ci/mmol for ^{125}I, 16,000 Ci/mmol for ^{131}I, and 23,600 Ci/mmol for ^{123}I. This specific activity is not reached for ^{131}I prepared from natural tellurium, because ^{127}I and ^{129}I are also produced.[502] Depending on the irradiation time and the time after irradiation, various specific activities can be obtained.[503] Iodine-131 with higher specific activity is obtained by uranium fission. Using enriched tellurium, maximum specific activity is produced by the $^{130}Te(n,\gamma)^{131}I$ reaction, and this is now the method of choice.

Radiopharmaceuticals

An early review enumerates the iodinated radiopharmaceuticals that have been tested.[504] Labeled dyes, macromolecules, steroids, heterocyclics, and other labeled compounds have been studied as tracers of the parent molecule. Few have been used routinely.

An interesting iodinated radiopharmaceutical is 6-iodomethyl 19-norcholest 5(10)-en-3-ol,[505] which is used for imaging the adrenal cortex. The original method of preparing 19-iodocholesterol produced apparently as much as 30% of 6-iodomethyl 19-norcholesterol, and this "impurity" is now thought to be the adrenal concentrating species. The latter compound has higher adrenal uptake and less in vivo deiodination and is now the agent of choice. Iodine-131 must be used because the gamma camera images are taken several days after injection to allow clearance of nonadrenal activity.

Most of the modern-day iodinated compounds are designed as receptor-binding radiotracers. A recent chapter describes the in vitro and in vivo chemistry of this class of compounds.[506]

Iodine-125 is used most often as a label for in vitro radioimmunoassays and radioreceptor assays. Its long half-life, high specific activity, and low energy make it ideal for this application.

RESEARCH USES OF SPECT AND PET

Introduction

The early radiopharmaceuticals, mostly labeled with single photon-emitting radiotracers, were designed to measure physiology. One of the first, radioactive iodine, was used to study thyroid metabolism.[419] That certain radioisotopes of iodine could be used for therapy is also important to the development of nuclear medicine. Selenium-labeled amino acids, another class of physiologic tracers, were used primarily for pancreas studies.[507] Other compounds, such as $^{197/203}$Hg-labeled chlormerodrin, were adapted from pharmaceuticals that produced a physiologic effect.[508] At that time mercury compounds were used as diuretics and the use of radioactive mercury provided pharmacokinetic data by external imaging. A list of well-established compounds of the 1950s to the present shows a wide range of abilities to measure changes in physiological processes.

In spite of this unique attribute, diagnostic radiopharmaceuticals were often used to detect changes in size, shape, or position of an organ. With the arrival of computerized tomography (CT) and iodinated contrast media and, more recently, the use of paramagnetic contrast media with nuclear magnetic resonance imaging, attempts to use radiopharmaceuticals to detect anatomical changes suffered. Procedures that were mainly anatomical, such as liver imaging with colloids and brain imaging to detect a disrupted blood-brain barrier, have become less important.

Nuclear medicine procedures that measure physiology, such as myocardial perfusion imaging, have increased. PET studies are clearly aimed at physiologic determinations. On the other hand, attempts to use iodinated contrast media with CT to measure perfusion or a biochemical process have not been successful.[509] Iodinated contrast media have not been used in the diagnosis of biochemical changes since their development in the 1920s because of the high concentration of iodinated compound required to affect the image.[510] Magnetic resonance contrast media that change the relaxation times of the proton are now being developed to better define anatomical changes and functional changes in major organ systems by analogy with the early nuclear medicine studies.[511]

Both single photon emitting (SPE) and positron emitting (PE) radiotracers are available for measuring perfusion in the heart and the brain with a normal blood-brain barrier. The increased sensitivity of PET allows for the use of both diffusible and microsphere analogs, whereas SPE radiotracers are microsphere analogs. The recent introduction of more sensitive multihead ring SPECT[512] has optimized the use of SPE-diffusible tracers, especially in the heart, eg, for the ^{99m}Tc-labeled compound teboroxime.[513] The ^{82}Sr/^{82}Rb generator allows myocardial perfusion to be measured with PET without the expense of a cyclotron.[514] Rapid repeat studies are possible with ^{82}Rb because of its 75s-physical half-life. Although not approved by the FDA, ^{18}F-2-fluoro-2-deoxy glucose (FDG) and ^{15}O-H_2O have been used extensively in research studies. Glucose metabolism, as measured by FDG, is a measure of tumor aggressiveness[515] and focal epilepsy.[516]

The Correlation of Cognitive and Physiological Factors with Cerebral Blood Flow

Activation studies have been carried out with both PET and SPECT radiotracers to map normal cerebral function and as a baseline for studies of disease. The major SPECT radioligands are ^{133}Xe, ^{123}I-*N*-isopropyl iodoamphetamine, ^{99m}Tc HMPAO, and ^{99m}Tc ECD. Xe has the advantage of quantification and repeat studies within the hour, whereas the others are more difficult to quantify and have long cerebral half-lives. ^{133}Xe is approved by the FDA. ^{123}I-labeled *N*-isopropylamphetamine (spectamine) became the second commercially available agent that crosses the intact blood-brain barrier. The distribution immediately after injection is flow related, but the immediate uptake and later distribution are dependent on amine uptake processes. Two neutral ^{99m}Tc compounds have also been proposed for cerebral perfusion studies. These both cross the normal blood-brain barrier. ^{99m}Tc-labeled D,L-hexamethylpropylamine oxime (HMPAO) is highly extracted and retained in the brain.[360] Two-minute half-life ^{15}O-H_2O is the PET agent most often used because of its relative ease of preparation and the ability to carry out a series of studies in a single session. Recently, ^{15}O-butanol has been used in the clinic because of its linear response at high blood flow rates.[517]

A growing body of literature attests to the sensitivity of PET and SPECT for measuring the neurophysiological concomitants of a subject's mental state and behavior, sensory input, motor outputs, and cognitive activity. As a consequence of this unique capability, these tools are currently the most powerful in the armamentarium for investigating the normal human cerebral functional landscape, the physiological responses of the human brain to the challenges of daily activities, and its functional characteristics under pathological conditions.[518–523,533–535]

The Development of Radioligands for the Diagnosis of Diseases Involving Perfusion Changes or Biochemical Changes

The most recent development in nuclear medicine has centered on radioligands that measure a specific biochemical pathway. The development of PET for biochemical studies is based on the advantages of quantification, sensitivity, and resolution when compared to SPECT. From a biological point of view, it is considered advantageous to label with ^{11}C, ^{13}N, ^{15}O, or ^{18}F rather than ^{123}I or ^{99m}Tc. However, these advantages have been addressed by those who continued to work on SPE radiotracers. Consequently there are now numerous ^{123}I-labeled receptor binding radiotracers.[506] Most of the effort to map biochemical reactions with both SPECT and PET, outside of the seminal work on ^{18}F-FDG[524] and later on ^{18}F-6-fluoroDOPA,[525] has been directed toward receptor-binding radiotracers. There are three steps in the development of a biochemical probe. The first is to develop a diagnostic agent that binds preferentially to a chosen enzyme or receptor or takes part in a single biochemical step. Single-step reactions such as receptor or enzyme binding are preferred because interpretation of the data by external imaging is more straightforward. This latter approach has been designated metabolic trapping.[526] We now have several receptor binding radiotracers labeled with either SPE or PE radionuclides that do just that, bind to the receptor, that is, they fulfill the first criterion of a biochemical probe.[527,528] The second step is to determine the sensitivity of the diagnostic agent to a change in the biochemistry. Although many excellent pharmacokinetic analyses have been published,[529] use of collected data at one time point after injection where the distribution reflects the biochemical change and not flow or transport is simplest.[530] The third step is to find a biochemical change as a function of a specific disease that matches the determined sensitivity. It would be preferable to start the research with the disease state well defined, but in practice the determination of the sensitivity in disease states cannot be predicted.

The Selection of Drug Candidates Based on Pharmacokinetics in Man

To date, most new drugs have been developed on the basis of animal studies using ^{14}C- and ^{3}H-labeled forms of the drug. In addition, a surrogate marker of the biochemical action is measured in animals. For example, an angiotensin-converting enzyme blocker such as Captopril is chosen on the relative biodistribution of the drug and the strength and duration of reduced blood pressure in animals. There is no simple method to carry out these studies in man. In the early development of the receptor concept, investigators were faced with the same challenge until high specific activity ligands led to the direct measurement of a ligand on the molecular basis. Likewise, the development of SPECT and PET techniques to measure the pharmacokinetics in vivo in man by noninvasive imaging will lead to better understanding of the drug of choice.

There are at least three basic measurements that SPECT and PET can bring to the development of a new pharmaceutical in man: (1) the effect of the new drug on regional blood flow; (2) the relative binding of the new drug at the site of interaction; and (3) the duration of binding at the site of action. SPECT and PET perfusion agents have been discussed in detail in the previous sections. In this application, the perfusion to a specific region would be measured as a function of dose and time after injection or oral absorption. The duration of action can also be measured using a single radioligand and a series of nonradioactive compounds. An example of this approach is the use of the radioligand to measure the unbound sites after administration of the drug. Assuming that there is a low capacity site involved in the mode of action of the drug, the half-life of the drug at this site can be determined by titrating the unbound sites using the radiolabeled ligand. Once again this avoids the time-consuming necessity of radiolabeling every drug candidate and proving that the drug is a "true tracer." Examples of this use appear in the literature.[531,532]

SPECT and PET are rapidly expanding their sphere of influence from diagnosis, which is the primary focus to date, to cerebral mapping and drug testing. The power of these noninvasive techniques lies in their unique abilities to "map" biochemical changes with high sensitivity.

REFERENCES

1. Friedlander G, Kennedy JW, Miller JM. *Nuclear and Radiochemistry* 2nd ed. 1964, New York: John Wiley & Sons Inc; 1964;70.
2. Kamen MD. *Isotopic Tracers in Biology. Applications to Clinical Research* 3rd ed. Kamen M, ed. New York: Academic Press; 1957:246.
3. Berson SA, Yalow RS. Quantitative aspects of the reaction between insulin and insulin binding antibody. *J Clin Invest* 1959;38:1996.
4. Perrier C, Segre E. Radioactive isotopes of element 43. *Nature* 1937;140:193.
5. Segre E, Seaborg GT. Discovery of technetium. *Phys Rev* 1938:54.
6. Richards P. A survey of the production at Brookhaven National Laboratory of radioisotopes for Medical research. Trans. 5th Nuclear Congress, 7th Int. Electronic Nuclear Symposium. Rome, 1960;2:223–244.
7. Harper PV, Andros G, Lathrop K. Preliminary observations on the use of six-hour ^{99m}Tc as a tracer in biology and medicine. *Argonne Can Res Hospital* 1962;18:176.
8. *Handbook of Chemistry and Physics*. Vol. 59th ed. Boca Raton, FL: CRC Press Inc; 1979:B296–297.
9. Dillman LT, Vonder Loge FC. Radionuclide decay schemes and nuclear parameters for use in radiation-dose estimation. *MIRD Pamphlet*. 1975;10:119.
10. Wagner HN Jr. Present and future applications of radiopharmaceuticals from generator-produced radioisotopes. *Int Atomic Energy Agency* 1971:163.
11. Lederer CM, Shirley VS. *Table of Isotopes*. 7th ed. Lederer CM and Shirley VS, New York: John Wiley & Sons, Inc.; 1978.
12. Tucker D, et al. American Nuclear Society Annual Meeting, Los Angeles, CA. *Trans Am Nucl Soc* 1958;1(June):160.
13. Richards P, Tucker WD, Srivastava SC. Introduction; technetium-99m: an historical perspective. *Int J Appl Rad Isot* 1982;33(10):793–799.
14. Eckelman WC, Richards P. Instant ^{99m}Tc-DTPA. *J Nucl Med* 1970;11:761.
15. *The Nuclear Medicine Market*. New York, NY: Frost and Sullivan; 1988.
16. Shellabarger C, Richards P. Bulletin of the Medical Department. 1960, Brookhaven National Laboratory, Upton, NY.
17. Atkins HL, Richards P, Schiffer L. Scanning of liver, spleen, and bone marrow with colloidal 99m-technetium. *Nucl Appl* 1966;2:27.
18. McAfee JG, et al. ^{99m}Tc labeled serum albumin for scintillation scanning of the placenta. *J Nucl Med* 1964;5:936.
19. Taplin GV, Poe ND. A dual lung-scanning technic for evaluation of pulmonary function. *Radiology* 1965;85:365–368.
20. Stern H, McAfee JG, et al. Preparation, distribution, and utilization of technetium-99m-sulfur colloid. *J Nucl Med* 1966;7(9):665–675.
21. Harper P, Lathrop KA, Gottschalk A. Pharmacodynamics of Technetium-99m in Radioactive Pharmaceuticals. USAEC Technical Information Service, 1966:355.
22. Gwyther MM, Field EO. Aggregated ^{99m}Tc-labeled albumin for lung scintic scanning. *Int J Appl Rad Isot* 1966; 17(8):485–486.
23. Richards P, Atkins HL. Proc 7th Annual Meeting Japanese Society of Nuclear Medicine. *Jpn J Nucl Med* 1968;7:165.
24. Eckelman WC, Richards P. Instant ^{99m}Tc compounds. *Nucl Med* 1971;10:245–251.
25. Eckelman WC, Meinken G, Richards P. ^{99m}Tc human serum albumin. *J Nucl Med* 1971;11:707–710.

26. Eckelman WC, et al. Technetium-labeled red blood cells. *J Nucl Med* 1971;12(1):22–24.
27. Subramanian G, McAfee JG. A new complex of ^{99m}Tc for skeletal imaging. *Radiology* 1971;99(1):192–196.
28. Rhodes BA, Stern HS, Buchanan JA, et al. Lung scanning with ^{99m}Tc microspheres. *Radiology* 1971;99:613–621.
29. Yano Y, McRae J, Van Dyke DC, et al. Technetium-99m-labeled stannous ethane-1-hydroxy-1-diphosphonate: a new bone scanning agent. *J Nucl Med* 1973;14(2):73–78.
30. Lin TH, Khentigan A, Winchell HS. A ^{99m}Tc chelate substitute for organ radiomercurial renal agents. *J Nucl Med* 1974; 15(1):34–35.
31. Subramanian G, et al. Technetium-99m-methylene diphosphonate—a superior agent for skeletal imaging: comparison with other technetium complexes. *J Nucl Med* 1975; 16(8):744–755.
32. Loberg MD, Cooper M, Harvey E, et al. Development of new radiopharmaceuticals based on N-substitution of iminodiacetic acid. *J Nucl Med* 1976;17(7):633–638.
33. Winston BW, et al. Experimental and clinical trials of new ^{99m}Tc hepatobiliary agents. *Radiology* 1978;128:793.
34. Nunn AD, Loberg MD, Conley RA. A structure-distribution relationship approach leading to the development of Tc-99m mebrofenin; an improved cholescintigraphic agent. *J Nucl Med* 1983;24(5):423–430.
35. Bevan JA, et al. Tc-99m HMDP (hydroxymethylenediphosphonate): a radiopharmaceutical for skeletal and acute myocardial infarct imaging. I. Synthesis and distribution in animals. *J Nucl Med* 1980;21:961.
36. Neirinckx RD, et al.: Technetium-99m d,l-HM-PAO: a new radiopharmaceutical for SPECT imaging of regional cerebral blood perfusion. *J Nucl Med* 1987;28(2):191–202.
37. Volkert WA, Hoffman TJ, Seger TM, et al. ^{99m}Tc-propylene amine oxime (Tc-99m-PnAO): a potential brain radiopharmaceutical. *Eur J Nucl Med* 1984;9(11):511–516.
38. Holman BL, Jones AG, Lister-James J, et al. A new Tc-99m-labeled myocardial imaging agent, hexakis (t-butylisonitrile)-technetium (I) (Tc-99m TBI). Initial experience in the human. *J Nucl Med* 1984;25(12):1350–1355.
39. Taylor A, et al. Comparison of iodine-131-OIH and technetium-99m-MAG$_3$ renal imaging in volunteers. *J Nucl Med* 1986;27:795–803.
40. Treher EN, et al. New technetium radiopharmaceuticals: boronic acid adducts of vicinal dioxime complexes. *J Label Comp Radiopharm* 1986;23:118.
41. Burch WM, Sullivan PJ, McLaren CJ. Technegas–a new ventilation agent for lung scanning. *Nucl Med Comm* 1986; 7:865–871.
42. Walovitch RC, et al. Pharmacological characterization of Tc-99m ECD in non-human primates as a new agent for brain perfusion imaging. *J Nucl Med* 1988;29:788.
43. Cotton FA, Wilkinson G. *Advanced Inorganic Chemistry.* 3rd ed. New York: Wiley-Interscience; 1988:812–817.
44. Jones AG, Davison A. The chemistry of technetium I, II, III and IV. *Int J Appl Radiat Isot* 1982;33:867.
45. Davison A, Jones AG. The chemistry of technetium (V). *Int J Appl Radiat Isot* 1982;33:875.
46. Krebs B, Hasse KD. Refinements of the crystal structures of potassium pertechnetate, potassium perrhenate, and osmium tetroxide. The bond lengths in tetrahedral oxo-anions and oxides of d° transition metals. *Acta Crystallogr Sect B* 1976;32:1334.
47. Mayfield HG, Bull WE. Perrhenato complexes of bivalent cations. *Inorg Chim Acta* 1969;3:676.
48. Boyd GE. Osomotic and activity coefficients of aqueous pertechnetic acid and perrhenic acid solutions at 25°C. *Inorg Chem* 1978;17:1808.
49. Tribalat S, Beyden J. Isolation of technetium. *Anal Chim Acta* 1953;8:22.
50. Boyd GE, Larsen QV. Solvent extraction of septivalent technetium. *J Phys Chem* 1960;64:988.
51. Atteberry RW, Boyd GE. Separation of seventh group anions by ion-exchange chromatography. *J Am Chem Soc* 1950; 72:4805.
52. Boyd GE, Larsen QV, Motta EE. Isolation of milligram quantities of long-lived technetium from neutron irradiated molybdenum. *J Am Chem Soc* 1960;82:809.
53. Diamond RM. The aqueous solution behavior of large univalent ions. A new type of ion-pairing. *J Phys Chem* 1963;67:2513.
54. Rucker TL, Mullins WT. Radioanalysis of technetium-99 at the Oak Ridge Gaseous diffusion Plant, in *Radioelem. Anal. Prog. Probl.* Lyons WS, ed. Ann Arbor, MI: Ann Arbor, Science; 1980:95.
55. Foti SC, Delucchi E, Akamian V. Determination of picogram amounts of ^{99}Tc by neutron activation analysis. *Anal Chim Acta* 1972;60:261.
56. Foti SC, Delucchi E, Akamian V. Determination of picogram amounts of technetium in environmental samples by neutron activation analysis. *Anal Chim Acta* 1972;60:269.
57. Bate LC. Determination of technetium-99 in mixed fission products by neutron activation analysis. In: *Radioelem. Anal.: Prog. Probl Proc. Conf. Anal. Chem. Energy Technol.* Ann Arbor, MI: Ann Arbor Science; 1980.
58. Hareland WA, Ebersole ER, Ramachandran TP. Determination of technetium by atomic absorption spectrophotometry. *Anal Chem.* 1972;44:520.
59. Lux F, Ammentorp-Schmidt F, Opavsky W. X-ray fluorescence determination of Tc and Mo in solutions. *Z Anorg Allgem Chem* 1965;341:172.
60. Andersen TJ, Walker RL. Determination of picogram amounts of technetium-99 by resin bead mass spectrometric isotope dilution. *Anal Chem* 1980;52:709.
61. Mullen P, Schwochau K, Jorgensen CK. Vacuo ultraviolet spectra of permanganate, pertechnetate, and perrhenate. *Chem Phys Lett* 1969;3:49.
62. Magee RJ, Al-Kayssi M. Determination of rhenium and technetium by infrared spectroscopy. *Anal Chim Acta* 1962; 27:469.
63. Crouthamel CE. Thiocyanate spectrophotometric determination of technetium. *Anal Chem* 1957;29:1756.
64. Trop HS, Davison A, Jones AG, et al. Synthesis and physical properties of hexakis (isothiocyanato) technetate (III) and -(IV) complexes. Structure of the $[Tc(NCS)_6]^{3-}$ ion. *Inorg Chem* 1980;19:1105.
65. Miller FJ, Thomason PF. Spectrophotometric determination of technetium (VII) with thioglycolic acid. *Anal Chem* 1960;32:1429.
66. DePamphilis BV, Jones AG, Davis MA. Preparation and crystal structure of oxotechnetium bis (thiomercaptoacetate) and its relationship to radiopharmaceuticals labeled with ^{99m}Tc. *J Am Chem Soc* 1978;78:5570–5571.
67. Boyd RE. Technetium-99m generators—the available options. *Int J Appl Radiat Isot* 1982;33:801–809.
68. Tucker WD, Greene MW, Weiss AJ, et al. 1958, Brookhaven National Laboratory, Upton, NY.
69. Lebedva LI, Kyong K. Interaction between Phosphorous (V), Molybdenum (VI) and Aluminum(III) in Weak Acid Solutions. Vestnik Leningrad Univ., 1968;23:127.
70. Duca A, Budiu T. Determination of the instability constant of the phospho-12-molybdic acid by means of the paper chromatographic method. *Rev Roum Chim* 1966;11: 585.
71. Millman WS, Crispin M, Cirillo WS, et al. Studies of the

hydrogen held by solids. XXIL. The surface chemistry of reduced molybdena-alumina catalysts. *J Catal* 1979;60:404.
72. Wefers K, Bell GM. Oxides and hydroxides of alumina. Technical Paper. Alcoa Res. Lab., 1972;19:51.
73. The United States Pharmacopoeial Convention, Inc. in The United States Pharmacopoeial Convention, Inc. 1975. Rockville, MD 20852.
74. Cifka J, Vesely P. Some factors influencing the elution of technetium-99m generators. *Radiochim Acta* 1971;16:30.
75. Abrashkin S, Heller-Grossman L, Schafferman A, et al. Technetium-99m generators: the influence of the radiation dose on the elution yield. *Int J Appl Radiat Isot* 1978;29:395.
76. Draganic IG, Draganic ZD. *The radiation chemistry of water.* New York: Academic Press, 1971.
77. Pikaev AE, Kryuchkov SV, Kuzina AF, et al. Pulsed radiolysis of neutral aqueous solutions of potassium pertechnetate. *Dokl Akad Nauk SSSR.* (English Transl.) 1977;236:1155.
78. Deutsch E, Heineman WR, Hurst R, et al. Production, detection and characterization of transient hexavalent technetium in aqueous alkaline media by pulse radiolysis and very fast scan cyclic voltammetry. *J Chem Soc Chem Commun* 1978:1038.
79. Boyd RE. Recent developments with generators of ^{99m}Tc, in *Radiopharmaceuticals and Labelled Compounds.* Vienna: IAEA; 1973:3–26.
80. Steigman J. Chemistry of the alumina column. *Int J Appl Radiat Isot* 1982;33:829.
81. Levin VI, Kozyreva-Alexandrova LS, Sokolova TN, et al. A new technetium-99m generator of higher activity. *Int J Appl Radiat Isot* 1979;30:450.
82. Charlton JC, Lyons D. German Patent #2,238, 503, 1973, Feb. 22.
83. Srivastava SC, Meinken G, Smith TD, et al. Problems associated with stannous ^{99m}Tc radiopharmaceuticals. *Int J Appl Radiat Isot* 1977;28:83.
84. Smith TD, Richards P. A simple kit for the preparation of ^{99m}Tc labeled red blood cells. *J Nucl Med* 1976;17:126.
85. Bayne VJ, Forster AM, Tyrrell DA. Use of sodium iodide to overcome the eluate age restriction for Ceretec reconstitution. *Nucl Med* 1989;10:29–33.
86. Salehi N, Guignard PA. Milking techniques of 99m generators and labeling efficiencies. *Int J Appl Radiat Isot* 1985;36:417.
87. Deutsch E, Heineman WR, Zodda J, et al. Preparation of "no-carrier-added" technetium-99m complexes: determination of the total technetium content of generator eluents. *Int J Appl Radiat Isot* 1982;33:843–848.
88. Mokinski VJ. A review of ^{99m}Tc generator technology. *Int J Appl Radiat Isot* 1982;33:811.
89. Boyd RE, Sorby PJ. Improved elution efficiency of ^{99m}Tc generators following purification of the eluting saline. *Int J Appl Radiat Isot* 1984;35:993.
90. Hamilton G. Contamination of contrast agent by MBT in rubber seals. *J Can Med Assoc* 1987;136:1020.
91. Kuzina AF, Tagil TS, Zamosanikova NN, et al. Extraction of technetium-99 with acetone. *Proc Acad Sci USSR Chem Sec* 1962;142/147:569.
92. Gemmill WJ, King PA, Molinski VJ. Production of a solution containing radioactive technetium. U.S. Patent No. 3436354, 1969.
93. Tachimori S, Nakamura H, Amano H. Preparation of technetium-99m by direct absorption from organic solution. *J Nucl Sci Technol* 1971;8:357.
94. Hayes MT, Green FA. Binding of $^{99m}TcO_4$ by human serum and tissues. *J Nucl Med* 1971;12:365.
95. Hayes MT, Green FA. In vitro studies of technetium-99m-labeled pertechnetate binding by human serum and tissues. *J Nucl Med* 1973;14:149.
96. Scatchard G. The attraction of proteins for small molecules and ions. *Ann NY Acad Sci* 1949;51:660.
97. Kominami G, Yokoyama A, Tanaka H. The pertechnetate ion binding to human serum albumin—the competition with other anions. *Radioisotopes (Tokyo).* 1977;26:525.
98. Kominami G, Yokoyama A, Kikumoto S, et al. Pertechnetate binding to human serum and tissues. *J Nucl Med* 1973;14:149.
99. Scatchard G, Coleman JS, Shen AL. Physical chemistry of protein solutions. VII. The binding of some small anions to serum albumin. *J Am Chem Soc* 1957;79:12.
100. Johannsen B, Berger R, Schumacher K. The binding of technetium compounds by human serum albumin. *Radiochem Radioanal Lett* 1980;42:177.
101. Dewanjee MK, Brueggemann P, Wahner HW. Affinity constants of technetium-99-pertechnetate and technetium-chelates with human serum albumin. Radiopharmaceuticals II. International Symp., New York: Society of Nuclear Medicine. 1979:435.
102. Harper PV, Lathrop KA, Richards P. ^{99m}Tc as a radiocolloid. *J Nucl Med* 1964;5:382.
103. Garzon OL, Placos MC, Radicella R. Technetium-99m labeled colloid. *Int J Appl Radiat Isot* 1965;16:613.
104. Pauli WO, Kolbl LW, Laub A. The synthesis of highly purified sulfur sols. II. The antimony sulfide sol. *Kolloid-Z* 1937;80:175.
105. Pauli WO, Laub A. The synthesis of highly purified sulfur sols. I. The arsenious sulfide sol. *Kolloid-Z* 1937;78:295.
106. Schuessler HD, Herrmann G. Rapid exchange of metal ions on metal sulfide cellulose. *Radiochim Acta* 1970;13:65.
107. Zuber G, Liser KH. Selective separation of technetium. *Radiochim Acta* 1974;21:60.
108. Cifka J, Vesely P. Non-pertechnetate radiochemical impurity in sulfur colloid labeled with technetium-99m. Chemical study of the labeling process. In: *Radiopharmaceutical and Labelled Compounds.* Vienna: IAEA; 1973:53.
109. Steigman J, Solomon NA, Hwang LL-Y. Technetium sulfur-colloid. *Int J Appl Radiat Isot* 1986;37:223.
110. Zaiser EM, LaMer VK. The Kinetics of the formation and growth of monodispersed sulfur hydrosols. *J Colloid Sci* 1948;3:571.
111. Donaldson JD, Moser W. Pure tin(II) sulfate. *J Chem Soc* 1960:4000.
112. Abel E. Is autooxidation catalyzed by chloride ion? *Monatshefte* 1954;85:949.
113. Donaldson JD, Moser W, Simpson WB. Tin(II) acetates. *J Chem Soc* 1964;suppl:5942.
114. Tobias RS. Studies on the hydrolysis of metal ions. 21. The hydrolysis of tin(II) ion, Sn^{2+}. *Acta Chem Scand* 1958;12:198.
115. Vanderzee CE, Rhodes DE. Thermodynamic data on the stannous chloride complexes from electromotive force measurements. *J Am Chem Soc* 1952;74:3552.
116. Gobom S. The hydrolysis of the tin(II) ion. *Acta Chem Scand* 1976;30(Ser. A):745.
117. Donaldson JD, Moser W, Simpson WB. Basic tin(II) chloride. *J Chem Soc* 1963:1727.
118. Donaldson JD, Moser W. Hydrous tin oxide. *J Chem Soc* 1961:835.
119. Deutsch E, Elder RC, Large BA, et al. Structural characterization of a bridged technetium-99-tin-dimethylglyoxime complex: implications for the chemistry of technetium-99-labeled radiopharmaceuticals prepared by the tin(II) reduction of pertechnetate. *Proc Natl Acad Sci USA* 1976;73:4287.
120. Steigman J, Meinken G, Richards P. The reduction of pertechnetate-99 by stannous chloride II. The stoichiometry of the reaction in aqueous solutions of several phosphorus(V) compounds. *Int J Appl Radiat Isot* 1978;29:653.
121. Tofe AJ, Francis MD. Optimization of the ratio of stannous

tin: ethane-1-hydroxy-1, 1-diphosphonate for bone scanning with ^{99m}Tc-pertechnetate. *J Nucl Med* 1974;15:69.

122. Van den Brand J. Technetium (tin) ethane-1-hydroxy-1,1-diphosphonate complexes; preparation, composition and biodistribution. Netherlands Energy Research Foundation, 1981, October. ECN-98(ZG Petten (NH1), The Netherlands): 1755.
123. Mikelsons MV, Pinkerton TC. Liquid chromatography of tin-reduced technetium hydroxyethylidene diphosphonate complexes for on-line spectral characterization and double isotope labeling. *Anal Chem* 1986;58:1007–1013.
124. Loberg MD, Fields AT. Chemical structure of technetium-99m-labeled N-(2,6-dimethylphenylcarbamoylmethyl)-iminodiacetic acid (^{99m}Tc-HIDA). *Int J Appl Radiat Isot* 1978;29:167.
125. Steigman J, Hwang LL-Y, Solomon NA. Unpublished.
126. Gerlit JB. Some chemical properties of technetium. In: *Peaceful Uses of Atomic Energy.* Geneva: In Proc. Intern. Conf; 1965.
127. Busey RM. Chemistry of technetium in hydrochloric acid solution. U.S. Atomic Energy Commission. Document ORNL-2782;13:1959.
128. Ossicini L, Saracino F, Lederer M. The solution, chemistry and chromatographic behavior of technetium in aqueous HCl and HBr. *J Chromatogr* 1964;16:524.
129. Williams MJ, Deegan T. Processes involved in the binding of technetium-99m to human serum albumin. *Int J Appl Radiat Isot* 1971;22:767.
130. Cifka J. Lower-oxidation-state technetium-99m in the generator product: Its determination and occurence. *Int J Appl Radiat Isot* 1982;33:849.
131. De Liverant J, Wolf W. Studies on the reduction of ^{99m}Tc-TcO^{4-} by hydrochloric acid. *Int J Appl Radiat Isot* 1982;33:857.
132. Eckelman WC, Meinken G, Richard P, et al. The chemical state of ^{99m}Tc in biomedical products. II. The chelation of reduced technetium with DTPA. *J Nucl Med* 1972;13:577.
133. Thomas RW, et al. Technetium radiopharmaceuticals development. II. Preparation, characterization and synthetic utility of the oxotetrahalotechnetate (V) species. *Inorg Chem* 1980;19:2840.
134. Davison A, Jones AG, Abrams MJ. New 2,2-bipyridine and 1,10-phenanthroline oxohalide complexes of technetium (VII) and (V). *Inorg Chem* 1981;20:4300.
135. Grove DE, Johnson NP, Wilkinson G. Trioxotrichlororhenate (VII) ion. *Inorg Chem* 1969;8:1196.
136. Subramanian G, McAfee JG. Use of sodium borohydride in labeling biologically useful compounds with ^{99m}Tc. *J Nucl Med* 1969;10:443.
137. Brown HC, Krishnamurthy S. Forty years of hydride reductions. *Tetrahedron.* 1979:567.
138. Jones AG, Orvig C, Trop HS, et al. A survey of reducing agents for the synthesis of tetraphenylarsonium oxotechnetiumbis (ethanedithioloate) from [^{99}Tc] pertechnetate in aqueous solution. *J Nucl Med* 1979;21:279.
139. Latimer WM. *Oxidation Potentials.* 2nd ed. New York: Prentice Hall; 1952:109.
140. Van Wazer JR: *Phosphorus and its Compounds.* New York: John Wiley & Sons; 1966;351.
141. Cotton FA, Davison A, Day VW. Preparation and structural characterization of salts of oxotetrachlorotechnetate (V). *Inorg Chem* 1979;18:3024.
142. Stern HS, McAfee JG, Zolle I. Technetium-99m-albumin. In: Andrews GA, Kniseley RM, Wagner HN Jr, eds. *Radioactive Pharmaceuticals.* U.S. Atomic Energy Commission Conf. 651111; 1966:352.
143. Marx G, Chevion M. Site-specific modification of albumin by free radicals. Reaction with copper (II) and ascorbate. *J Biochem* 1986;236:397.
144. Clark WM. *Oxidation-Reduction Potentials of Organic Systems.* 1960, Baltimore MD: Williams & Wilkins Co; 1960: 471.
145. Gilbert BC, Norman ROC, Placucci G, et al. Electron spin resonance studies. XLV. Reactions of the methyl radical with some aliphatic compounds in aqueous solution. *J Am Chem Soc* 1975;892.
146. Higginson WCE, Marshall JW. Equivalence changes in oxidation-reduction reactions in solution: some aspects of the oxidation of sulfurous acid. *J Am Chem Soc* 1957:447.
147. Halpern J, Taube H. The transfer of oxygen atoms in oxidation-reduction reactions. III. The reaction of halogenates with sulfite in aqueous solution. *J Am Chem Soc* 1952; 74:375.
148. Fritzberg AR, Lyster DM, Dolphin DH. Evaluation of formamidine sulfinic acid and other reducing agents for use in the preparation of Tc-99m labelled radiopharmaceuticals. *J Nucl Med* 1977;18:553.
149. Nazer AFM, Wells CF. Kinetics and mechanism of the oxidation of hydroxylamine by aquovanadium (V) ions in aqueous perchlorate media. *J Chem Soc* 1971;93:5892.
150. Armstrong RA, Taube H. Chemistry of trans-aquonitrosyltetraammine technetium (I) and related studies. *Inorg Chem* 1976;15:1904.
151. Hieber W, Nast R, Gehring G. Reductive nitrosylation of tetraoxometallates with NH_2OH in strong alkali. *J Inorg Allg Chem* 1948;169:256.
152. Bhakacharyya R, Roy PS. Reductive nitrosylation of tetraoxometallates. II. Generation of [Re(NO)] moiety: a novel and virtually single step synthesis of $[Re(NO)(NCS)_3H_2O_7^-$ and its 2,2′-bipyridyl and 1,10-phenanthrolein derivatives directly from perrhenate in aqueous and aerobic media. *Transition Metal Chem* 1982;7:285.
153. Baldas J, Pojer PM. The use of formamidinesulfinic acid in the preparation of Tc-99m-labeled radiopharmaceuticals—a cautionary note. Aust. Radiat. Lab [Tech. Rep.], 1980. ARL/TR, ARL/TR015: p. 8.
154. Pojer PM, Baldas J. Technetium-99m-labeled *N,-N*-diethyldithio carbamate-a nonpolar complex with slow hepatic clearance. *Aust Radiat Lab.* 1980. ARL/TR, ARL/TR 025:6.
155. Baldas J, Pojer PM. The use of formamidine sulfinic acid in the preparation of Tc-99m-labeled radiopharmaceuticals—a cautionary note. *Int J Nucl Med Bio* 1981;8:110.
156. Baldas J, et al. The influence of reducing agents on the composition of technetium-99 complexes: implications for ^{99m}Tc-radiopharmaceutical preparation. *Eur J Nucl Med* 1982;7:187.
157. Baldas J, et al. Preparation and crystal structure of carbonyltris (diethyldithiocarbamato) technetium (III): an unexpected source of corrdinated carbon monoxide. *J Chem Soc Dalton Trans* 1982:451.
158. Baldas J, et al. Synthesis and structure of bis (diethyldithiocarbamato) nitridotechnetium (V): a technetium-nitrogen triple bond. *J Chem Soc Dalton Trans* 1981:1798.
159. Baldas J, et al. Studies of technetium complexes. VI. The preparation, characterization and electron spin resonance spectra of salts of tetrachloro- and tetrabromo-nitridotechnetate (VI). *J Chem Soc Dalton Trans* 1984:1798.
160. Steigman I, Williams HP, Solomon NA. The importance of the protein sulfhydryl group in HSA labelling with technetium-99m. *J Nucl Med* 1975;16:573.
161. Peacock RD. In "Comprehensive Inorganic Chemistry", 1966 (quoted in DePamphilis BV, Jones AG, Davis MA et al, *J Am Chem* 100:5570–5571, 1978) ed. J.H.E. J.C. Bailar R.S. Nyholm, A.F. Trotman-Dickinson. Vol. 3. 1973, Pergamon Press, Elsevier Publishing Co., N.Y.: Oxford. 877–903.

162. Rouschias G. Recent advances in the chemistry of rhenium. *Chem Rev* 1974;74:531–566.
163. Steigman J, Meinken G, Richards P. Reduction of pertechnetate-99 by stannous chloride. I. Stochiometry of the reaction in hydrochloric acid, in a citrate buffer, and in a DTPA buffer. *Int J Appl Radiat Isot* 1975;26:601–609.
164. Steigman J, Hwang L, Srivastava S. Complexes of reduced technetium-99 with polyhydric compounds. *J Labelled Compd Radiopharm* 1977;13:160.
165. Steigman J, et al. Cysteine and albumin complexes of technetium-99 and technetium-99m. *J Labelled Compd Radiopharm* 1977;13:162.
166. Kuhn CG, Isied SS. Some Aspects of the reactivity of metal ion-sulfur bonds. *Prog Inorg Chem* 1980;27:153.
167. Johannsen B, et al. Chemical and biological characterization of different technetium complexes of cysteine and cysteine derivative. *J Nucl Med* 1978;19:816.
168. Smith JE, et al. A thiol complex of technetium pertinent to radiopharmaceutical use of ^{99m}Tc. *J Am Chem Soc* 1978; 78:5571–5572.
169. Jones AG, DePamphilis BV, Davison A. Preparation and crystal structure of tetraphenylarsonium bis (2-mercaptoethanolato) oxotechnetate. *Inorg Chem* 1981;20:1617.
170. DePamphilis BV, Jones AG, Davison A. Ligand-exchange reactivity patterns of oxotechnetium (V) complexes. *Inorg Chem* 1983;22:2292.
171. DePamphilis BV, et al. A new class of Oxotechnetium (V) chelate complexes containing a $TcON_2S_2$ core. *Inorg Chem* 1981;20:1629.
172. Jones AG, et al. Chemical and in vivo studies of the anion oxo [*N,N'*-ethylenebis (2-mercaptoacetimido)] technetate(V). *J Nucl Med* 1982;23(9):801–809.
173. Burns HD, Manspeaker H, Miller REA. Preparation and biodistribution of neutral, lipid-soluble Tc-99m complexes of bis (2-mercaptoethylamine) ligands. *J Nucl Med* 1979;20:654.
174. Lever SZ, Burns HD, Kervitsky TM, et al. Design preparation and biodistribution of a technetium-99 triaminodithiol complex to assess regional cerebral blood flow. *J Nucl Med* 1985;26:1287.
175. Epps LA, Burns HD, Lever SZ, et al. Brain imaging agents: synthesis and characterization of (N-piperidinylethyl) hexamethyl diaminodithiolate oxotechnetium (V) complexes. *J Appl Radiat Isot* 1987;38:661.
176. Davison A, Jones AG, Orvig C, et al. A series of oxotechnetium (+5) chelate complexes containing a $TcOS_2N_2$ core. *J Nucl Med* 1981;22:59.
177. Basolo F, Pearson RG. The trans effect in metal complexes in progress. *Inorg Chem* 1962;4:381.
178. Hambright P, McRae J, Valk PE, et al. Chemistry of technetium radiopharmaceuticals. I. Exploration of the tissue distribution and oxidation state consequences of technetium (IV) in Tc-Sn-gluconate and Tc-Sn-EHDP using carrier ^{99}Tc. *J Nucl Med* 1975;16:478.
179. Steigman J. Chemical state of technetium in vivo (letter No. 2). *J Nucl Med* 1976;17:423.
180. Hwang L.L.-Y, et al. Complexes of technetium with polyhydric ligands. *Int J Appl Radiat Isot* 1985;36:475–480.
181. deKievet W. Technetium radiopharmaceuticals: Chemical characterization and tissue distribution of Tc-glucoheptonate using Tc-99m and carrier Tc-99. *J Nucl Med* 1981;22:703.
182. Kuzina AF, Oblova AA, Spitsyn VI. Complexes of technetium IV and V with amines. *Russ J Inorg Chem* (Engl. Transl.) 1972;17:1377.
183. Simon J, et al. Radiochemical characterization of technetium-cyclam. *Radiochem Radioanal Lett* 1981;47:111.
184. Zuckman SA, Freeman GM, Troutner DE, et al. Preparation and X-ray structure of trans-dioxo (1,4,8,11-tetraazacyclotetradecane) technetium (V) perchlorate hydrate. *Inorg Chem* 1981;20:2386.
185. Kastner ME, Lindsay MJ, Clarke MJ. Synthesis and structure of trans-$[O_2(en)_2Tc^V]^+$. *Inorg Chem* 1982;21:2037.
186. Kastner ME, et al. Synthesis and structure of trans-$[O_2(TBP)_4Tc]$ + (TBP = 4 tertbutylpyridine) and related complexes. *Inorg Chem* 1984;23:4683.
187. Seifert S, Muenze R, Johannsen B. Cationic technetium complexes with nitrogen-containing ligands: a new group of technetium compounds. *Radiochem Radioanal Lett* 1982; 54:153.
188. Siripaisarnpipat S, Schlemper EO. Preparation, spectra and crystal structures of two rhodium (III) complexes with short intramolecular hydrogen bonds. *Inorg Chem* 1984;23: 330–334.
189. Vassian EG, Murmann RK. Aromatization of an aliphatic amine oxime nickel (II) complex by molecular oxygen. *Inorg Chem* 1967;6:2043–2046.
190. Fair CK, et al. Oxo [3,3′-(1,3-propanediylidimino) bis (3-methyl-2-butane oximato)(3-)-*N*,1*N′*,*N′*,*N‴*) technetium V], [Tc O $(C_{13}H_{25}\text{-}N_4O_2)$]. *Acta Crystallogr Crystal Struct Commun* 1984;C40(Sec. C):1544–1546.
191. Troutner DE, et al. A neutral lipophilic complex of ^{99m}Tc with a multidentate amine oxime. *Int J Appl Radiat Isot* 1984;35:467–470.
192. Jurisson S, et al. Synthesis, characterization and X-ray structural determinations of technetium (V)-oxo-tetradentate amine oxime complexes. *Inorg Chem* 1986;25:543–549.
193. Jurisson S, et al. Effect of ring size on properties of technetium amine complexes. X-ray structures of TcO_2 (Pent $(AO)_2$) which contains an unusual eight-membered chelate ring and of $TcOEn(AO)_2$. *Inorg Chem* 1987;26:3576.
194. Glavan KA, Whittle R, Johnson SF, et al. Oxidative addition from a six-coordinate to an eight-coordinate complex, single-crystal structure of $[Tc(diars)_2Cl_2]$ ClO_4 and $[Tc(diars)_2Cl_4]PF_6$. *J Am Chem Soc* 1980;102:2103.
195. Bandoli G, Mazzi U, Roncari E, et al. Crystal structures of technetium compounds. *Coordination Chem Rev* 1982; 44:210.
196. Dilworth JR, Thompson RM, Archer CM, et al. Synthesis of some novel Tc imido complexes. In: Bandoli G, Nicolini M, Mazzi U, eds. *Technetium and Rhenium in Chemistry and Nuclear Medicine 3*, New York: Raven Press, 1990.
197. Nicholson T, Davison A, Jones A. The characterization of technetium organohydrazide chelate complexes. The synthesis of a technetium phenylimido complex. The X-ray crystal structure of $[TcO9SC_6H_2Pr^i_3)_2(PhNNCON_2HPh)]$. *Inorg Chim Acta* 1990;168:227.
198. Jezowska-Trzebiatowska B, Hanuza J, Baluka M. Force constants and vibration frequencies of the rhenium-oxygen bonds in the infrared region (200-4000 cm^{-1}). *Spectrochim Acta* 1971;27(Part A):1753.
198A. Steigman J, Hwang L, Solomon NA, Kan T. Cysteine and albumin complexes of technetium-99 and technetium-99m. *J Labelled Compd Radiopharm* 1977, 13:162.
199. Spies H, Johannsen B, Muenze R. Synthesis of bis (1,2-dithiolato-oxotechnetate (V) complexes. *Z Chem* 1980; 20:222.
200. Schwochau K, Herr W. Preparation, properties and crystal structure of potassium hexafluorotechnetate (IV). *Angew Chem Int Ed* 1963;2:97.
201. Colton R, Peacoc RD. An outline of technetium chemistry. *Q Rev (London)* 1963;16:299.
202. Gmelin TC. *Technetium*, Supplement Volume 2, in Gmelin Handbook of Inorganic Chemistry, System Number 69. New York: Springer; 1983:100.
203. Dilziel J, Gill NS, Nyholm RS, et al. Technetium. I. The

preparation and properties of potassium hexahalotechnetates. *J Chem Soc* 1958:4012.

204. Schwochau K. Zur chemie des technetiums. *Angew Chem* 1964;76:9.
205. Rogers LB. Electroseparation of technetium from rhenium and molybdenum. *J Am Chem Soc* 1949;71:1507.
206. Nelson CM, Boyd GE, Smith WT Jr. Magnetochemistry of technetium and rhenium. *J Am Chem Soc* 1954;76:348.
207. Schwochau K, Herr W. Chemistry of technetium complexes. I. Preparation and properties of cyanotechnetate (IV). *Z Anorg Allgem Chem* 1962;318:198.
208. Colton R, Tomkins IB. Halides and oxide halides of technetium. *Aust J Chem* 1968;21:1981.
209. Gorski B, Koch H. Chemistry of technetium in aqueous solution. I. State of tetravalent technetium in aqueous solution. *J Inorg Nucl Chem* 1969;31:3566.
210. Noll B, Seifert S, Muenze R. Zur Bildung des Tc(IV)-DTPA(1:1) Komplexes. Zentralinst Kernforsch. Rossendorf. Dresden (Ber.), 1975:145.
211. Sundrehagen E. Polymer formation and hydrolyzation of tetravalent technetium-99. *Int J Appl Radiat Isot* 1979; 30:739.
212. Owunwanne A, Marinsky J, Blau M. Charge and nature of technetium species produced in the reduction of pertechnetate by stannous ion. *J Nucl Med* 1977;18:1099.
213. Guennec JY, Guillaumont R. Behavior of technetium (IV) in a noncomplexing medium at tracer concentrations. *Radiochem Radioanal Lett* 1973;1:33.
214. Meyer RE, Arnold WD, Case FI. Valence effects on solubility and sorption: the solubility of Tc(IV) oxide. ORNL-6199, 1986, March. NUREG/CR-4309.
215. Schweitzer GK, Jackson M. Radiocolloids—a historical review. *J Chem Ed* 1952:513.
216. Haissinsky M. *Nuclear Chemistry and its Applications*. Reading, Ma: Addison-Wesley;1964:606–611.
217. Haissinsky M. Method of preparation of sources of radium. *E J Chim Phys* 1934;31:43.
218. Haissinsky M. The solubility of very slightly soluble electrolytes. *Acta Physicochem* 1935;3:517.
219. Yokoyama A, Terauchi Y, Horiuchi K. Technetium-99m-kethoxal-bis (thiosemicarbazone), an uncharged complex with a tetravalent ^{99m}Tc state, and its excretion into the bile. *J Nucl Med* 1976;17(9):816–819.
220. Tanabe S, et al. Effect of pH on the formation of Tc(NaBH4)-MDP radiopharmaceutical analogs. *Int J Appl Radiat Isot* 1983;34:1577.
221. Libson K, Deutsch E, Barnett BL. Structural characterization of a Tc-99 diphosphonate complex. Implications for the chemistry of technetium-99m skeletal imaging agents. *J Am Chem Soc* 1980;102:2476.
222. Steigman J, Eckelman WC. *Chemistry of Technetium in Medicine*. Washington, DC: National Academy of Science; 1992:74–78.
223. Russell CD, Cash AG. Complexes of technetium with pyrophosphate, etidronate and medronate. *J Nucl Med* 1979; 20:532.
224. Pinkerton TC, Heineman WR. The electrochemical reduction of pertechnetate in aqueous hydroxyethylidene diphosphonate media. *J Electronal Chem* 1983;158:323.
225. Russell CD, Cash AG. Oxidation state of technetium in bone-scanning agents as determined at carrier concentration by amperometric titration. *Int J Appl Radiat Isot* 1979; 30:485.
226. Korteland J, Dekker BG, DeLigny CL. The valence state of technetium-99 in its complexes with bleomycin, 1-hydroxyethylidene-1, 1-diphosphonate and human serum albumin. *Int J Appl Radiat Isot* 1980;31:315.
227. Muenze R. Compounds of technetium (IV) with hydroxyethylidenediphosphonic acid. *J Labelled Compd Radiopharm* 1978;15:215.
228. Van den Brand JAGM, et al. Gel chromatographic separation and identification of the technetium (tin)-EHDP complexes using the radiotracers phosphorus-32, technetium-99m, and tin-113. *Int J Appl Radiat Isot* 1981;32:44.
229. Pinkerton TC, Heineman WR, Deutsch E. Separation of technetium hydroxyethylidene diphosphonate complexes by anion-exchange high performance liquid chromatography. *Anal Chem* 1980;52:1106–1110.
230. Wilson GM, Pinkerton TC. Determination of charge and size of technetium diphosphonate complexes by anion-exchange liquid chromatography. *Anal Chem* 1985;57:246–253.
231. Linder KE. *Aminocarboxylate Complexes of Technetium.* Cambridge, MA: M.I.T., 1986.
232. Russell CD, Speiser AG. Iminodiacetate complexes of technetium: an electrochemical study. *Int J Appl Radiat Isot* 1982;33:903.
233. Volkert WA, Troutner DE, Holmes RA. Labeling of amine ligands with technetium-99m in aqueous solutions by ligand exchange. *Int J Appl Radiat Isot* 1982;33:891.
234. Wilkins RG, Yelen RE. Kinetics of monomer-dimer interconversion of iron (III) ethylenediaminetetraacetate and related chelates. *Inorg Chem* 1969;8:1470.
235. Libson K, Barnett BL, Deutsch E. Synthesis, characterization and electrochemical properties of tertiary diphosphine complexes of technetium: single-crystal structure of the prototype complex trans-[Tc(DPPE)$_2$Br$_2$] BF_4^-. *Inorg Chem* 1983; 22:1695.
236. Ichimura A, et al. Technetium electrochemistry. 21. Electrochemical and spectroelectrochemical studies of the Bis (tertiary phosphine) (D) complexes trans [$Tc^{III}D_2X_2$] + (X = Cl, Br) and [$Tc^{I}D_3$]$^+$. *Inorg Chem* 1984;23:1272.
237. Meloche VW, Martin RL, Webb WH. Spectrophotometric determination of rhenium with alpha-furildioxime. *Anal Chem* 1957;29:527.
238. Narayanan A, Umland F. Spectrophotometric investigation of rhenium-dimethylglyoxime complex in solution. *Mikrochim Acta* 1972:527.
239. Jasim F, Magee RJ, Wilson CL. New reagents for the detection of technetium. *Talanta* 1959;2:93.
240. Kuzina AF. Photometric determination of technetium with furil dioxime in hydrochloric acid solution. *Zh Analit Khim* (Engl. Trans.) 1962;17:487.
241. Linder KE, et al. A re-assessment of the oxidation state of Tc(DMG)$_3$ (u-OH)SnCl$_3$: evidence for Tc(III). Proc. 7th Int. Symp. on Radiopharm. Chem., Gronigen, The Netherlands, 1988.
242. Nunn AD, Feld T, Treher EN. Boronic acid adducts of technetium oxime complexes (BATOs) a new class of neutral complexes with myocardial imaging capabilities. United States Patent #4,705,849, 1987.
243. Linder K, et al. A new technetium agent, SQ 32, 097, which can be used to assess cerebral blood flow. *J Nucl Med* 1987;28:592.
244. Hirth W, et al. Chloro-Hydroxy substitution on technetium dioxime complexes: chemical and biological comparison of TcCl (Dioxime)$_3$ BR and Tc(OH)(Dioxime)$_3$ BR. Proc. 7th Int. Symp. Radiopharm. Chem. Gronigen, The Netherlands, 1988. 47.
245. Abrams MT, Davison A, Brodack JW, et al. The preparation of technetium (III) compounds in aqueous media. *J Labelled Compd Radiopharm* 1982;14:1596.
246. Abrams MJ, Davison A, Jones AG, et al. Synthesis and characterization of hexakis (alkyl isocyanide) and hexakis (aryl isocyanide) complexes of technetium (I). *Inorg Chem* 1983;22:2798–2800.

247. Kennedy CM, Pinkerton TC. Technetium carboxylate complexes. III. A new synthetic route to hexakis (isonitrile) technetium (I) salts. *Appl Radiat Isot* 1988;39:1179.
248. Ugi I: *Isonitrile Chemistry.* New York, NY: Academic Press; 218:1971.
249. Johannson B, Spies H. Chemie und radiopharmakologie von technetium komplexen. Academie der Wissenschaften der DDR. Dresden, DDR, 1981.
250. Steigman J. Scintiphotos in rabbits made with Tc-99m preparations reduced by electrolysis and by $SnCl_2$: concise communication. *J Nucl Med* 1979;20:766.
251. Loberg MD. Abstracts of the Eighth Northeast Regional Meeting of the American Chemical Society. Boston, MA, June 25, 1978. 1978, June.
252. Hamilton JG, Soley MH. Studies in iodine metabolism by the use of a new radioactive isotope of iodine. *Am J Physiol* 1939;127:557.
253. Berson S, et al. ^{131}I metabolism in human subject: demonstration of insulin binding globulin in the circulation of insulin treated subjects. *J Clin Invest* 1956;35:170.
254. Pressman D, Eisen HN. The zone of localization of antibodies. V. An attempt to saturate antibody-binding sites in mouse kidney. *J Immunol* 1950;64:273.
255. Rockoff SD, Goodenough DJ, McIntire KR. Theoretical limitations in the immunodiagnostic imaging of cancer with computed tomography and nuclear scanning. *Cancer Res* 1980;40:3054.
256. Larson SM, Carrasquillo JA, Reynolds JC. Radioimmunodetection and radioimmunotherapy. *Cancer Invest* 1984;2:363.
257. Keenan AM, Harbert JC, Larson SM. Monoclonal antibodies in nuclear medicine. *J Nucl Med* 1985;26:531.
258. Pettit WA, et al. Improved protein labeling with stannous tanrate reduction of pertechnetate. *J Nucl Med* 1980;21:59.
259. Rhodes BA, et al. ^{99m}Tc labeling and acceptance testing of radiolabeled antibodies. In: *Tumor Imaging*, Burchiel SW, Rhodes BA, New York: Masson; 1982:111.
260. Sundrehagen E. Formation of ^{99m}Tc immunoglobulin G complexes free from radionuclides, quality controlled by radioimmunoelectrophoresis. *Eur J Nucl Med* 1982;7:549.
261. Lanteigne D, Hnatowich DJ. The labeling of DTPA coupled proteins with ^{99m}Tc. *Int J Appl Radiat Isot* 1984;35:617.
262. Paik CH, et al. The labeling of high affinity sites of antibodies with ^{99m}Tc. *Int J Nucl Med Biol* 1985;12:3.
263. Khaw BA, et al. ^{99m}Tc labeling of antibodies to cardiac myosin Fab and to human fibrinogen. *J Nucl Med* 1982;23:1011.
264. Kasina S, Vanderheyden JL, Fritzberg AR. Application of diamide dimercaptide N_2S_2 bifunctional chelating agents for ^{99m}Tc labeling of proteins. Proc. 6th Int Symp. Radiopharmaceutical Chemistry, Boston, 1986. (29 June–3 July):269.
265. Arano Y, et al. Synthesis and evaluation of a new bifunctional chelating agent for ^{99m}Tc labeling proteins: p-carboxyethylphenyl-glyoxal-di(N-methylthiosemicarbazone). *Int J Nucl Med Bio* 1985;12:425.
266. Brown BA, Dearborn CB, Drozynsk CA, et al. Pharmacokinetics of ^{99m}Tc-metallothionein-B72.3 and its $F(ab')_2$ fragment. *Cancer Res. (Suppl.)* 1990;50:835.
267. Baidoo KE, Scheffel U, Lever SZ. ^{99m}Tc labeling of proteins: initial evaluation of a novel diamine dithiol bifunctional chelating agent. *Cancer Res (Suppl.)* 1990;1(50):799s–803s.
268. Schwartz DA, Abrams MJ, Hauser M, et al. Preparation of hydrazino-modified proteins and their use for the synthesis of ^{99m}Tc-protein conjugates. *Bioconj Chem* 1991;2(5):333–336.
269. Najafi A, Alauddin MM, Siegel ME, et al. Synthesis and preliminary evaluation of a new chelate N_2S_4 for use in labeling proteins with metallic radionuclides. *Int J Radiat Appl Instrum B* 1991;18(2):179–185.
270. Fritzberg AR. Advances in 99mTc-labeling of antibodies. *J Nucl Med* 1987;26:7.
271. Franz J, et al. The production of technetium-99m-labeled conjugated antibodies using a cyclam-based bifunctional chelating agent. *J Nucl Med Bio* 1987;14(6):569–572.
272. Linder KE, Wen MD, Nowotnik DP, et al. Technetium labeling of monoclonal antibodies with functionalized BATO's: 2.$TcCl(DMG)_3$ CPITC labeling of B72.3 and NP-4 whole antibodies and NP-4 $F(ab')_2$. *Bioconj Chem* 1991;2(6): 407–414.
273. Eckelman WC, Paik CH, Steigman J. Three approaches to radiolabeling antibodies. *J Nucl Med Bio* 1989;16:171.
274. Dreyer R, Muenze R. Markierung von Serumalbumin mit 99m Technetium. *Wiss Z Karl-Marx-Univ Leipzig Math-Naturwiss R* 1969;18:629.
275. Lin MS. In *Radiopharmaceuticals. Labeling proteins with ^{99m}Tc.* Subramanian G, Rhodes BA, and Cooper JF, eds. 1975; New York: Soc. Nucl. Med. 36.
276. Kyker GC, Rafter JJ. Colloidal properties of the lanthanides. In: *Radioactive Pharmaceuticals.* United States Atomic Energy Commission, 1966;503.
277. Lebowitz E, Atkins HL, Hauser W, et al. ^{99m}Tc-gelatin: a "compound" with high renal specificity. *Int J Appl Radiat Isot* 1971;22(12):786–789.
278. Johnson AE, Gollan F. ^{99m}Tc-technetium dioxide for liver scanning. *J Nucl Med* 1971;11:564.
279. Gorevic PD. In: Srivastava S, ed. *Radiolabeled Monoclonal Antibodies for Imaging and Therapy. Immunochemistry of Hybridomas.* New York: Plenum-Press; 1988:3–21.
280. Paik CH, Eckelman WC, Reba RC. Transchelation of ^{99m}Tc from low affinity sites to high affinity sites of antibody. *Nucl Med Bio* 1986;13:359.
281. Liang FH, Virzi F, Hnatowich DJ. Serum stability and nonspecific binding of technetium-99m labeled diamino dithiol for protein labeling. *Nucl Med Bio* 1987;14:555–562.
282. Rhodes BA, et al. A kit for direct labeling of antibody and antibody fragments with Tc-99m. *J Nucl Med* 1980;21:54.
283. Hawkins EB, Pant KD, Rhodes BA. Resistance of direct Tc-99m-protein bond to transchelation. *Antibody Immuno Conj Radiopharm* 1990;3:17–25.
284. Pszona A, Sakowicz A. The influence of citrate ions on the radiochemical purity of 99mTc-human serum albumin. *Int J Appl Radiat Isot* 1981;32:349–350.
285. Reno JM, Bottino BJ. Radiolabeled proteins, especially antibodies, and their preparation and use as diagnostic and therapeutic agents. Euro Pat. Appl. EP 237150 A2, 1987.
286. Pak KY, et al. Method for labeling antibodies with isotopic technetium or rhenium, their use in immunotherapy and scintigraphy, and kits for performing the method. International Patent WO 8807382, 1988.
287. Steigman J, Richards P. Chemistry of technetium as applied to radiopharmaceuticals. In: Subramanian G et al, ed. *Radiopharmaceuticals.* New York: Soc. Nucl. Med; 1975;23–35.
288. Bremer KH, et al. Preparation of a technetium-99m-labeled organ-specific substance. European Pat. Appl. EP 271806 A2, 1988.
289. Hansen HJ, et al. Preclinical evaluation of an "instant" ^{99m}Tc-labeling kit for antibody labeling. *Cancer Res (Suppl.)* 1990;50:794.
290. Feitsma RIJ, Blok D, Wasser MNJM, et al. A new method for technetium-99m-labeling of proteins with an application to clot detection with an antifibrin monoclonal antibody. *Nucl Med Comm* 1987;8:771–777.
291. Blok D, Feitsma RIJ, Wasser MNJM, et al. A new method for protein labeling with technetium-99m. *Nucl Med Bio* 1989;16:11–16.
292. Baldas J, Bonnyman J. Substitution reactions of $^{99m}TcNCl_4$.

A route to a new class of ^{99m}Tc radiopharmaceuticals. *Int J Appl Radiat Isot* 1985;36:133–139.

293. Thakur ML, et al. Technetium-99m labeled monoclonal antibodies: evaluation of reducing agents. *Int J Radiat Appl Instrum B* 1991;18(2):227–33.
294. Hnatowich DJ, et al. Directly and Indirectly technetium-99m-labeled antibodies-a comparison of in vitro and animal in vivo properties. *J Nucl Med* 1993;34:109–119.
295. Rhodes BA, Zamora PO, Newell KD, et al. Technetium-99m-labeling of murine monoclonal antibody fragments. *J Nucl Med* 1986;27:685–693.
296. Abrams MJ, et al. Technetium-99m-human polyclonal IgG radiolabeled via the hydrazino nicotinamide derivative for imaging focal sites of infection of rats. *J Nucl Med* 1990;31:2022–2028.
297. Hnatowich KJ, Mardirossian G, Roy S, et al. Pharmacokinetics of the FO23C4 anti-CEA antibody fragment labeled with technetium-99m and indium-111: a comparison in patients. *Nucl Med Comm* 1993:52–63.
298. Fritzberg AR, Abrams PG, Beaumier PL, et al. Specific and stable labeling of antibodies with technetium-99m with a diamide dithiolate chelating agent. *Proc Nat Acad Sci USA* 1988;85:4025–4029.
299. Fritzberg AR, et al. Approaches to radiolabeling of antibodies for diagnosis and therapy of cancer. *Pharm Res* 1988; 5:325–334.
300. Buraggi GL, et al. Rapid blood clearance. In: Donato L, Britton K, eds. *Immunoscintigraphy.* New York: Gordon and Breach; 1984;215–245.
301. Goedemans WT, et al. A new, single method for labeling of proteins with ^{99m}Tc by derivatization with 1-imino-4-mercaptobutyl groups. In: Nicolini M, Bandoli G, Mazzi U, eds. *Technetium and Rhenium in Chemistry and Nuclear Medicine*. New York, NY: Cortina International-Verona, Raven Press; 1990; 595–598.
302. Joiris E, Bastin B, Thornback JR. A new method of labeling of monoclonal antibodies and their fragments with technetium-99m. *Nucl Med Bio* 1991;18:353.
303. Kasina S, RaO TN, Srinivasan A, et al. Development and biologic evaluation of a kit for performed chelate technetium-99m radiolabeling of an antibody Fab fragment using a diamide dimercaptide chelating agent. *J Nucl Med* 1992; 32(7):1445–1451.
304. Arano Y, et al. Technetium-99m-labeled monoclonal antibody with preserved immunoreactivity and high in vivo stability. *J Nucl Med* 1987;28(6):1027–1033.
305. Arnold RW, et al. Comparison of ^{99m}Tc complexes for renal imaging. *J Nucl Med* 1975;16(5):357–367.
306. Fleay RF. ^{99m}Tc-Labeled EDTA for renal scanning. *Aust Radiol* 1968;12(3):265–267.
307. Hauser W, Atkins HL, Nelson KG, et al. Technetium-99m DTPA: a new radiopharmaceutical for brain and kidney scanning. *Radiology* 1970;94(3):679–684.
308. Halpern SE, Tubis M, Golden M, et al. ^{99m}TcPAC, a new renal scanning agent. II. Evaluation in humans. *J Nucl Med* 1972;13(10):723–728.
309. Halpern SE, Tubis M, Ensow SJ, et al. ^{99m}Tc-penicillamine-acetazolamide complex, a new renal scanning agent. *J Nucl Med* 1972;13(1):45–50.
310. Winchell HS, Lin M, Shipley B, et al. Localization of polypeptide caseidin in the renal cortex: a new radioisotope carrier for renal studies. *J Nucl Med* 1971;12(10): 678–682.
311. Kountz SL, Yeh SH, Wood J, et al. Technetium-99m(V)-citrate complex for estimation of glomerular filtration rate. *Nature* 1967;215(108):1397–1399.
312. Fliegel CP, Dewanjee MK, Holman LB. ^{99m}Tc tetracycline as a kidney and gallbladder imaging agent. *Radiology* 1974; 110(2):407–412.
313. Charamaza O, Budikova M. Herstellungsmethode eines ^{99m}Tc-zinn-komplexes fur die nierenszintigraphie. *J Nucl Med* 1969;8:301.
314. Lichte H, Hor G. Nierenszintigraphie mit Tc-99m penicillamine. *Fortschr Geb Rontgenstr Nuklearmed* 1975;122:119.
315. Ikeda I, Inoue O, Uchida J, et al. New renal scanning agents of Tc-99m compounds. *World Congress Nucl Med*, Tokyo, 1974.
316. Subramanian G, et al. Tc-99m-Sn-acetylcysteine: a new renal scanning agent. *Eur J Nucl Med* 1976;1(4):243–245.
317. Johannson B, Syhre P, Spies H. Analytische untersuchungen zer markierung von cystein und glutathion mit technetium-99m. Jahresbericht des Zentralinstitutes fur Kernforschung Rossendorf, *Zfk* 1976;312:53.
318. Oginski M, Rembelska M. Tc-99m-unithiol complex, a new pharmaceutical for kidney scintigraphy. *J Nucl Med* 1976;15(6):282–286.
319. Troutner DE, Simon J, Ketring AR, et al. Complexing of Tc-99m with cyclam: concise communication. *J Nucl Med* 1980;21(5):443–448.
320. Davison A, Sohn M, Orvig C. A tetradentate ligand designed specifically to coordinate technetium. *J Nucl Med* 1979; 20:641.
321. Yokoyama A, Saji H, Tanaka H, et al. Preparation of chemically characterized ^{99m}Tc-penicillamine complex. *J Nucl Med* 1976;17:810.
322. Verbruggen A, et al. Synthesis and renal excretion characteristics of the four stereoisomers present in ^{99m}Tc bis(mercaptoacetyl)-2,2-diaminopropanoate (Tc99m-CO_2-DADS). *J Nucl Med* 1985;26:19.
323. Fritzberg AR, et al. Synthesis and biological evaluation of technetium-99m-MAG_3 as a hippuran replacement. *J Nucl Med* 1986;27(1):111–116.
324. Tubis M, et al. 99m Tc-penicillamine, a new cholescintigraphic agent. *J Nucl Med* 1972;13(8):652–654.
325. Baker RJ, Bellen JC, Ronai PM. Technetium 99m-pyridoxylideneglutamate: a new hepatobiliary radiopharmaceutical. *J Nucl Med* 1975;16:720.
326. Dugal P, et al. A quantitative test for gallbladder function. *J Nucl Med* 1972;13:428.
327. Lin TH, Khentigan A, Winchell HS. A ^{99m}Tc-labelled replacement for ^{131}I-rose bengal in liver and biliary tract studies. *J Nucl Med* 1974;15(7):613–615.
328. Hunt FC, Maddalena DJ, Yeates MG. Technetium-99m-6 mercaptopurine, a new radiopharmaceutical for cholescintigraphy. In: *Recent Advances in Nuclear Medicine*. Proceedings of First World Congress for Nuclear Medicine, Tokyo, 1974.
329. Callery PS, Faith B, Loberg MD, et al. Tissue distribution of technetium-99m and carbon-14 labeled N-(2,6-dimethylphenylcarbamylmethyl) imino-diacetic acid. *J Med Chem* 1976;19(7):962–964.
330. Burns HD, Sowa DT, Marzilli LG. Improved synthesis of N(2,6-dimethylphenylcarbamolymethyl) iminodiacetic acid and analogs. *J Pharm Sci* 1978;67(10):1434–1436.
331. Wistow BW, Subramanian G, Van Heertum RL, et al. An evaluation of 99mTc-labeled hepatobiliary agents. *J Nucl Med* 1977;18(5):455–461.
332. Burns HD, Worley P, Wagner HN Jr, et al. Design of technetium radiopharmaceuticals. In: Heindel N, ed. *Chemistry of Radiopharmaceuticals*. New York: Masson; 1978.
333. Van Wyke AJ, Fourie PJ, Van Zyl WH, et al. Synthesis of five new ^{99m}Tc-HIDA isomers and comparison with ^{99m}Tc-HIDA. *Eur J Nucl Med* 1979;4(6):445–448.
334. Molter M, Kloss G. Studies of pharmacokinetics of various Tc-99m-IDA derivatives. Trends in Neurosciences. *Third Int Symp Radiopharm* 1980;19:9.

335. Nunn AD. Preliminary structure-distribution relationships of ^{99m}Tc hepatobiliary agents. I. Protein binding of HIDA's. *Third Intern Symp Radiopharm* 1980;18:12.
336. Nunn AD, Loberg MD. Hepatobiliary agents: Structure-Activity Relationships. In: Spencer RP, ed. *Radiopharmaceuticals.* New York: Grune & Stratton; 1981;539.
337. Perez R, Kohen Y, Henry R, et al. A new radiopharmaceutical for ^{99m}Tc bone scanning. *J Nucl Med* 1972;13:788.
338. Subramanian G, McAfee JG, Bell EG, et al. ^{99m}Tc-labeled polyphosphate as a skeletal imaging agent. *Radiology* 1972;102(3):701–704.
339. Bevan JA, Tofe AJ, Benedict JJ. Tc-99m HMDP (Hydroxymethylene diphosphonate): a radiopharmaceutical for skeletal and acute myocardial infarct imaging. II. comparison of Tc-99m hydroxymethylene diphosphonate (HMDP) with other technetium-labeled bone-imaging agents in a canine model. *J Nucl Med* 1980;21(10):967–970.
340. Subramanian G, McAfee JG, Blair RJ, et al. Technetium-99m labelled stannous imidodiphosphate, a new radiodiagnostic agent for bone scanning: comparison with other ^{99m}Tc complexes. *J Nucl Med* 1975;16(12):1137–1143.
341. Jones AG, Francis MD, Davis MA. Bone scanning: radionuclide reaction mechanisms. *Sem Nucl Med* 1976;6(1):3–18.
342. Davis MA, Jones AL. Comparison of ^{99m}Tc labeled phosphate and phosphonate agents for skeletal imaging. *Sem Nucl Med* 1976;6(1):19–31.
343. Johnson LL, Seldin DW, Muschel M, et al. Comparison of planar SQ 30,217 and TI-201 myocardial imaging with coronary anatomy. *Circulation* 1987;76(abstract):217.
344. Seldin DW, Johnson LL, Blood DK, et al. Myocardial perfusion imaging with technetium-99m SQ 30,217: comparison with thallium-201 and coronary anatomy. *J Nucl Med* 1989;30:312–319.
345. Meerdink DJ, Thuber M, Savage S, et al. Comparative myocardial extraction of two technetium labeled boron oxime derivatives (SQ 30,217, SQ 32,014) and thallium. *J Nucl Med* 1988;29:972.
346. Piwnica-Worms D, Kronauge JF, Chiu ML. Uptake and retention of hexakis (2-methoxy isobutyl isonitrile)technetium (I) in cultured chick myocardial cells. Mitochondrial and plasma membrane potential dependence. *Circulation* 1990;82:1826.
347. Narra RK, Nunn AD, Kuczynski BL, et al. A neutral ^{99m}Tc complex for myocardial imaging. *J Nucl Med* 1989; 30:1830–1837.
348. Kim AS, Akers MS, Faber TS, et al. Dynamic myocardial perfusion imaging with Tc-99m-teboroxime in patients; comparison with thallium-201 and arteriography. *Circulation* 1990;82(abstract):321 or 111.
349. Gewirtz H. Differential myocardial washout of technetium-99m teboroxime: mechanism and significance. *J Nucl Med* 1992;32:2009–2011.
350. Leppo JA, DePuey EG, Johnson LL. A review of cardiac imaging with sestamibi and teboroxime. *J Nucl Med* 1991;32:2012–2022.
351. Winchell HS, Horst WD, Braun L, et al. N-Isopropyl-[^{123}I]iodoamphetamine: single pass brain uptake and washout, binding to brain synaptosomes, and localization in dog and monkey brain. *J Nucl Med* 1980;21:947–952.
352. Neirinckx RD, Burke JF, Harrison RC, et al. The retention mechanism of ^{99m}Tc-HMPAO; intracellular reaction with glutahione. *J Cereb Blood Flow Metab* 1988;8:4–12.
353. Vallabhajosula S, Zimmerman RE, Picard M, et al. Technetium-99m ECD: a new brain imaging agent: in vivo kinetics and biodistribution studies in normal human subjects. *J Nucl Med* 1989;30:599–604.
354. Russell CD, Majerik J. Determination of pertechnetate in radiopharmaceuticals by high pressure liquid, thin layer and paper chromatography. *Int J Appl Radiat Isot* 1978; 29:109.
355. Kubota H, et al. Technetium-99m-pyridoxylideneglutamate: a new agent for gallbladder imaging. Comparison with ^{131}I-rose bengal. *J Nucl Med* 1976;17:36.
356. Kato M, Hazue M. Tc-99m(sn) pyridoxylideaminates: preparation and biologic evaluation. *J Nucl Med* 1978;19:397.
357. Castronovo CF Jr, Callahan RJ. A new bone scanning agent: Tc labeled 1-hydroxy-ethylidene-1,1-disodium phosphonate. *J Nucl Med* 1972;13:823.
358. Fritzberg AR, Lewis D. HPLC analysis of Tc-99m iminodiacetate hepatobiliary agents and a question of multiple peaks: concise communication. *J Nucl Med* 1980;21:1180.
359. King AG, Christy B, Hupf HB, et al. Polyphosphates: a chemical analysis of average chain length and the relationship to bone deposition in rats. *J Nucl Med* 1973;14:695.
360. Nowotnik DP. Technetium-based brain perfusion agents. In: Nunn A, ed. *Radiopharmaceuticals: Chemistry and Pharmacology.* New York: Marcel Dekker, Inc; 1992:37–95.
361. Volkert WA, et al. The behavior of neutral amine oxime chelates labelled at tracer level. *Int J Nucl Med Biol* 1984;11:243.
362. Wieland DM, Tobes MC, Mangner TJ. *Analytical and Chromatographic Techniques in Radiopharmaceutical Chemistry.* New York, NY: Springer-Verlag; 1986.
363. Boothe TE, Emran AM. The role of high performance liquid chromatography in radiochemical/radiopharmaceutical synthesis and quality assurance. In: Emran AM, ed. *New Trends in Radiopharmaceutical Synthesis, Quality Assurance, and Regulatory Control*, New York, NY: Plenum Press; 1991;409.
364. Pike VW, et al. Radiopharmaceutical Production for PET: Quality Assurance, Practice, Experiences and Issues. In: Emran AM, ed. *New Trends in Radiopharmaceutical Synthesis, Quality Assurance, and Regulatory Control.* New York: Plenum Press; 1991;433.
365. Fritzberg AR, Klingensmith WC, Whitney WP, et al. Chemical and biological studies of Tc-99m N,N-bis(mercaptoacetamido)-ethylenediamine: a potential replacement for I-131 iodohippurate. *J Nucl Med* 1981;22:258.
366. McAfee JG, Subramanian G, Aburano T, et al. A new formulation of Tc-99m minimicroaggregated albumin for marrow imaging: comparison with other colloids. In-111 and Fe-59. *J Nucl Med* 1982;23:21.
367. Ikeda I, Inoue O, Kurata K. Preparation of various Tc-99m dimercaptosuccinate complexes and their evaluation as radiotracers. *J Nucl Med* 1977;18:1222.
368. Fritzberg AR, Lyster DM, Dolphin DH. Tc-glutathione: role of reducing agent on renal retention. *Int J Nucl Med Biol* 1978;5:87.
369. Krishnamurthy GT, Tubis M, Endow JS, et al. Clinical comparison of the kinetics of ^{99m}Tc-labeled polyphosphate and diphosphonate. *J Nucl Med* 1974;15:848.
370. Krishnamurthy GT, et al. Comparison of ^{99m}Tc-polyphosphate and 18-F. I. Kinetics. *J Nucl Med* 1974;15:832.
371. Krishnamurthy GT, Hoebotter RL, Walsh CE. Kinetics of Tc-labeled pyrophosphate and polyphosphate in man. *J Nucl Med* 1975;16:109.
372. Bowen BM, Garnett ES. Analysis of the relationship between Tc-Sn-polyphosphate and ^{99m}Tc-Sn-pyrophosphate. *J Nucl Med* 1974;15:652.
373. Schumichen C, Koch K, Kraus A, et al. Binding of technetium-99m to plasma proteins: Influence on the distribution of Tc-99m phosphate agents. *J Nucl Med* 1980;21:1080.
374. Buja LM, Tofe AJ, Kulkarni PV, et al. Sites and mechanisms of localization of technetium-99m phosphorus radiopharmaceuticals in acute myocardial infarcts and other tissues. *J Clin Invest* 1977;60:724.
375. Rosenthall L, Kaye M. Technetium-99m pyrophosphate ki-

netics and imaging in metabolic bone disease. *J Nucl Med* 1975;16:33.
376. Kaye M, Silverton S, Rosenthall L. Technetium-99m-pyrophosphates. Studies in vivo and in vitro. *J Nucl Med* 1975;16:40.
377. Schmitt GH, Holmes RA, Isitman AT. A proposed mechanism for ^{99m}Tc-labeled polyphosphate and diphosphonate uptake by human breast tissue. *Radiology* 1974;112:733.
378. Zimmer AM, Isitman AT, Holmes RA. Enzymatic inhibition of diphosphonate: a proposed mechanism of tissue uptake. *J Nucl Med* 1975;16:352.
379. Dewanjee MK, Kahn PC. Mechanism of localization of ^{99m}Tc-labeled pyrophosphate and tetracycline in infarcted myocardium. *J Nucl Med* 1976;17:639.
380. Francis MD, Ferguson DL, Tofe AJ, et al. Comparative evaluation of three diphosphonates: in vitro absorption (C-14 labeled) and in vivo osteogenic uptake (Tc-99m complexed). *J Nucl Med* 1980;21:1185.
381. Christensen SB, Krogsgaard OW. Localization of Tc-99m MDP in epiphyseal growth plates of rats. *J Nucl Med* 1981;22:237.
382. Van Langevelde A, Driessen OMJ, Pauwels LKJ, et al. Aspects of ^{99m}technetium binding from an ethane-1-hydroxy-1,1-diphosphonate-^{99m}Tc complex to bone. *Eur J Nucl Med* 1977;2:47.
383. Lyons KP, Olson HG, Aronow WS. Pyrophosphate myocardial imaging. *Sem Nucl Med* 1980;10:168.
384. Loberg MD, Ryan JW, Porter DW. Hepatic clearance mechanisms of Tc-99m-N-(acetanilido)-iminodiacetic acid derivatives (letter to the editor). *J Nucl Med* 1980;21:1111.
385. Loberg MD, Porter DW. Review and current status of hepatobiliary imaging aspects. In: *Radiopharmaceuticals II.* New York: Society of Nuclear Medicine; 1979;519.
386. Loberg MD. Radiotracer distribution by active transport. In: Colombetti L, ed. *Principles of Radiopharmacology.* Boca Raton, FL: CRC Press; 1979;43.
387. Firnau G: Why do Tc-99m chelates work for cholescintigraphy? *Eur J Nucl Med* 1976;1:137.
388. Andersen AR, et al. Assessment of the arterial input curve for [^{99m}Tc]-d,l,HM-PAO by rapid octanol extraction. *J Cereb Blood Flow Metab* 1988;8:23.
389. Nunn A. Single photon radiopharmaceuticals for imaging myocardial perfusion. In: Nunn A, ed. *Radiopharmaceuticals, Chemistry and Pharmacology.* New York: Marcel Dekker, Inc; 1992;97.
390. Verbruggen AM, DeRoo. Renal Radiopharmaceuticals. In: Nunn A, ed. *Radiopharmaceuticals, Chemistry and Pharmacology.* New York: Marcel Dekker, Inc; 1992:365.
391. Larson JM, Bennett LR. Human serum albumin as a stabilizer for ^{99m}Tc-sulfur suspension. *J Nucl Med.* 1969;10:294.
392. Ege GN, Richards LP. Introducing PVP as a stabilizer in the preparation of technetium sulphur colloid. *Br J Radiol* 1969;42:552.
393. Hunter WW Jr. Stabilization of particulate suspensions with nonantigenic polyhydric alcohols: application to ^{99m}Tc-sulfur colloid. *J Nucl Med* 1969;10:607.
394. Webber MM, Victery W, Cragin MD. Stabilizer reaction-free ^{99m}Tc-sulfur suspension for liver, spleen, and bone-marrow scanning. *Radiology* 1969;92:170.
395. Larson SM, Nelp WR. Radiopharmacology of a simplified technetium-99m-colloid preparation for photo scanning. *J Nucl Med* 1966;7:817.
396. Maas R, Alvarez J, Arriaga C. On a new tracer for liver scanning. *Int J Appl Radiat Isot* 1967;18:653.
397. Johnson AE, Gollan F. ^{99m}Tc-technetium dioxide for liver scanning. *J Nucl Med* 1970;11:564.
398. Yamada H, Johnson DE, Griswold ML. Radioalbumin macroaggregates for reticuloendothelial organ scanning and function assessment. *J Nucl Med* 1969;10:453.
399. Cragin MD, Weber MM, Victery WK. Technique for the rapid preparation lung scan particles using Tc-sulfur and human serum albumin. *J Nucl Med* 1969;10:621.
400. Yano Y, McRae I, Honbo DS, et al. ^{99m}Tc-ferric hydroxide macroaggregates for pulmonary scintiphotography. *J Nucl Med.* 1969;10:683.
401. Lin MS, Winchell HS. Macroaggregation of an albumin-stabilized technetium-tin (11) colloid. *J Nucl Med* 1972; 13:928.
402. Kristensen K, Pedersen B. Letter: Lung retention of ^{99m}Tc-sulfur colloid. *J Nucl Med* 1975;16:439.
403. Enustun BV, Turkevich J. Coagulation of colloidal gold. *J Am Chem Soc* 1963;85:3317.
404. Steigman J, Eckelman WC. Tc Chemistry as Applied to Medicine. National Research Council, Technical Information Center, U.S.D.O.E., Washington, DC, 1992.
405. Warbick A, Ege GN, Henkelman RM, et al. An evaluation of radiocolloid sizing technique. *J Nucl Med* 1977;18:827.
406. Davis MA, Jones AG, Trindale H. A rapid and accurate method for sizing radiocolloids. *J Nucl Med* 1974;15:923.
407. Billinghurst MW, Jette D. Colloidal particle size determination by gel filtration. *J Nucl Med* 1979;20:133.
408. Pedersen B, Kristensen K. Evaluation of methods for sizing of colloidal radiopharmaceuticals. *Eur J Nucl Med* 1981;6:521.
409. Rhodes BA, et al. Radioactive albumin microspheres for studies of the pulmonary circulation. *Radiology* 1969;92:1453.
410. Subramanian LG, Bell EG, McAfee IG. Preparation and labeling of gelatin, amylose and human serum albumin microspheres for in vivo use in nuclear medicine. *J Nucl Med* 1969;10:373.
411. Tubis M. Hospital preparation and dispensing of radiopharmaceuticals. In: Tubis M, Wolf N, ed. *Radiopharmacy.* New York: Wiley Interscience; 1976.
412. Rhodes BA, Bolles TE. Albumin microspheres: current methods of preparation and use. In: Subramanian G et al, ed. *Radiopharmaceuticals.* New York: Society of Nuclear Medicine; 1974.
413. Frier M, Griffiths P, Ramsey A. The biological fate of sulfur colloid. *Eur J Nucl Med* 1981;6:371.
414. Szvmendera J, et al. Chemical and electron microscope observations of a safe PVP-stabilized colloid for liver and spleen scanning. *J Nucl Med* 1971;12:212.
415. Atkins HL, Cardinale KG, Eckelman WC, et al. Evaluation of ^{99m}Tc-DTPA prepared by three different methods. *Radiology* 1971;98:674.
416. Cohen Y, Ingrand J, Caro R. Kinetics of the disappearance of gelatin protected radiogold-colloids from the bloodstream. *Int J Appl Radiat Isot* 1968;19:703.
417. Caro RA, Ciscato VA. Kinetics of the phagocytosis of radiogold colloids by the reticuloendothelial system in the rat. *Int J Appl Radiat Isot* 1970;21:405.
418. Dobson EL, Goffman JW, Jones HB, et al. Studies with colloids containing radioisotopes of yttrium, zirconium, columbium, and lanthanum in bone marrow, liver, and spleen. *J Lab Clin Med* 1949;34:306.
419. Myers WG. Radioisotopes of iodine. In: Andrews GA, Kniseley RM, Wagner HN Jr, *Radioactive Pharmaceuticals.* Springfield, VA: U.S. Atomic Energy Commission; 1966:217.
420. Martindale AA, Papadimitrion JM, Turner JH. Technetium 99m antimony colloid for bone-marrow imaging. *J Nucl Med* 1980;21:1035.
421. Eckelman WC. Technical considerations in labeling of blood elements. *Semi Nucl Med* 1975;5:3.
422. Smith TD, Richards P. A simple kit for the rapid preparation of ^{99m}Tc red blood cells. *J Nucl Med* 1974;15:534.

423. Hegge FN, Hamilton GW, Larson SM, et al. Cardiac chamber imaging: a comparison of red blood cells labeled with Tc-99m in vitro and in vivo. *J Nucl Med* 1978;19:129.
424. Pavel DG, Zimmer AM. In vivo labeling of red cells with Tc pertechnetate. *J Nucl Med* 1978;19:972.
425. Leitl GP, et al. Interference with Tc-99m labeling of red blood cells (RBCs). *J Nucl Med* 1980;21:44.
426. Glottchalk A, Armas R, Thakur M. Reply to spleen scanning with Tc-99m-labeled red blood cells (RBC). *J Nucl Med* 1980;21:1000.
427. Dugan MA, et al. New radiopharmaceuticals for thrombosis localization. *J Nucl Med* 1972;13:782.
428. Barth RF, Singla O, Gillespie GY. Use of ^{99m}Tc as a radisotonic label to study the migratory patterns of normal and neoplastic cells. *J Nucl Med* 1974;15:656.
429. Harwig SSL, Harwig JF, Coleman RE, et al. In vivo behavior of ^{99m}Tc-fibrinogen and its potential as a thrombus-imaging agent. *J Nucl Med* 1976;17:40.
430. Uchida T, Yasunaga K, Kariyone S, et al. Survival and sequestration of ^{51}Cr- and $^{99m}TcO_4^-$-labeled platelets. *J Nucl Med* 1974;15:801.
431. Gillespie GY, Barth RE, Goburty A. Labeling of mammalian nucleated cells with ^{99m}Tc. *J Nucl Med* 1973;14:706.
432. Barth RF, Singla OJ. Organ distribution of ^{99m}Tc and ^{51}Cr labeled thymocytes. *J Nucl Med* 1975;16:633.
433. Wong DW, Mishkin FS. Technetium 99m-human fibrinogen. *J Nucl Med* 1975;16:343.
434. Jonckheer MH, Abramovici J, Jeghers O, et al. The interpretation of phlebograms using fibrinogen labeled with ^{99m}Tc. *Eur J Nucl Med* 1978;3:233.
435. Millar WT, Smith JF. Localization of deep-venous thrombosis using technetium 99m-labeled urokinase. *Lancet* 1974;2:695.
436. Dugan MA, et al. Localization of deep vein thrombosis using radioactive streptokinase. *J Nucl Med* 1973;14:233.
437. Deacon JM, et al. Technetium 99m-plasmin: a new test for the detection of deep vein thrombosis. *Br J Radiol* 1980;53:673.
438. McAfee JG, Kopecky RT, Frymoyer PA. Nuclear medicine comes of age: its present and future roles in diagnosis. *Radiology.* 1990; March 174 (3 pt 1):609–620.
439. Thakur ML. Radiolabeled blood cells: perspectives and directions. *Int J Rad Appl Instrum B* 1990;17(1):41–47.
440. Persson RBR, Kempi V. Labeling and testing of ^{99m}Tc-streptokinase for the diagnosis of deep vein thrombosis. *J Nucl Med* 1975;16:474.
441. Duffy MF, Duffy GJ. Studies on the labeling of streptokinase with ^{99m}Tc for use as a radiopharmaceutical in the detection of deep vein thrombosis: concise communication. *J Nucl Med* 1977;18:483.
442. Korubin V, Maisey M, McIntyre P. Evaluation of technetium-labeled red cells for determination of red cell volume in man. *J Nucl Med* 1972;13:760.
443. Renault H, et al. Chelation de cations radioactifs par un polypeptide: la bleomycine, in *Radiopharm Labeled Compounds* 1973;7:232–235.
444. Reba RC, Eckelman WC, Poulose KP, et al. Tumor-specific radiopharmaceuticals: radiolabeled bleomycin. In: *Radiopharmaceuticals*. Subramanian M. et al, eds. New York: Society of Nuclear Medicine; 1974.
445. Richards P, Steigman J. Chemistry of technetium as applied to radiopharmaceuticals. In: *Radiopharmaceuticals*. Subramanian, G. et al, eds. New York: Society of Nuclear Medicine; 1975.
446. Asakura H, Hori M, Umezawa H: Characterization of bleomycin action on DNA. *J Antibiot* 1975;28(7):537–542.
447. Eckelman WC, Kubota H, Siegel BA, et al. Iodinated bleomycin: an unsatisfactory radiopharmaceutical for tumor localization. *J Nucl Med* 1976;17(5):385–388.
448. Sinkula AA, Yalkowski SH. Rationale for design of biologically reversible drug derivatives: prodrugs. *J Pharm Sci* 1975;64(2):181–210.
449. Chen YCJ, Janda KD. A new approach toward the inhibition of ribonucleases: a water-stable ribonucleoside-technetium chelate. *J Am Chem Soc* 1992;114:1488–1489.
450. DiZio JP, et al. Technetium- and rhenium-labeled progestins: synthesis, receptor binding and in vivo distribution of a beta-substituted progestin labeled with technetium-99 and rhenium-186. *J Nucl Med* 1992;33(4):558–569.
451. Piwnica-Worms D, et al. Functional imaging of multidrug-resistant P-glycoprotein with an organotechnetium complex. *Cancer Res* 1993;53(5):977–984.
452. Macke HR, et al. New octreotide derivatives for in vivo targeting of somatostatin receptor-positive tumors for single photon emission computed tomography (SPECT) and positron emission tomography (PET). *Horm Metab Res Suppl.* 1993;27:12–17.
453. Lentle BC, Schmidt R, Nonjaim AA. Iatrogenic alterations in the biodistribution of radiotracers. *J Nucl Med* 1978; 19:743.
454. Hladik WB, Nigg KK, Rhodes BA. Drug-induced changes in the biologic distribution of radiopharmaceuticals. *Sem Nucl Med* 1982;12:184.
455. Hodges R. Iatrogenic alterations in the biodistribution of radiotracers as a result of drug therapy: theoretical considerations. In: Hladik WB, Saha GP, Study KT, eds. *Essentials of Nuclear Medicine Science*. Baltimore MD: Williams & Wilkins; 1987; 165.
456. HladikWB, et al. Iatrogenic alterations in the biodistribution of radiotracers as a result of drug therapy: theoretical considerations. In: Hladik WB, Saha GP, Study KT, eds. *Essentials of Nuclear Medicine Science*. Baltimore, MD: Williams & Wilkins: 1987;189.
457. Lentle BC, Styles CB. Iatrogenic alterations in the biodistribution of radiotracers as a result of radiation therapy, surgery, and other invasive medical procedures. In: Hladik WB, Saha GP, Study KT, eds. *Essentials of Nuclear Medicine Science*. Baltimore, MD: Williams & Wilkins; 1987;220.
458. Lin MS, Kruse SL, Goodwin DA, et al. Albumin loading effect: a pitfall in saline paper analysis of ^{99m}Tc-albumin. *J Nucl Med* 1974;15:1018.
459. Yalow RS, Berson SA. Immunoassay of plasma insulin. In: Glick D, ed. *Methods of Biochemical Analysis*. New York: Interscience; 1964.
460. Valk PE, Dilts CA, McRae J. A possible artifact in gel chromatography of some ^{99m}Tc-chelates. *J Nucl Med* 1973; 14:235.
461. Steigman I, Williams HP. Letter: Gel chromatography in the analysis of ^{99m}Tc-radiopharmaceuticals. *J Nucl Med* 1974; 15:318.
462. Schneider PB. A simple "electrolytic" preparation of a ^{99m}Tc (Sn) citrate renal scanning agent. *J Nucl Med* 1973;14:843.
463. Eckelman WC, et al. ^{99m}Tc-pyrophosphate for bone imaging. *J Nucl Med* 1974;15:279.
464. Shukla SK. Ion exchange paper chromatography of Tc (IV), Tc (V), and Tc (VII) in hydrochloric acid. *J Chromatogr* 1966;21:92.
465. Persson RBR, Liden K. ^{99m}Tc-labeled human serum albumin: a study of the labeling procedure. *Int J Appl Radiat Isot* 1969;20:241.
466. Zweig G, Sherma J. *Handbook of Chromatography*. Boca Raton, FL: CRC Press; 1, 2:1972.
467. Wong SH, Hosain P, Zeichner SJ, et al. Quality control studies of ^{99m}Tc-labeled radiopharmaceuticals by high performance liquid chromatography. *Int J Appl Radiat Isot* 1981;32:185.
468. Fields AT, Porter DW, Callery PS, et al. Synthesis and radiola-

beling of technetium radiopharmaceuticals based on N-substituted iminodiacetic acid. *J Label Compd Radiopharm* 1978;15:387.

469. Srivastava SC, et al. Characterization of ^{99m}Tc bone agents (MDP, EHDP) by reverse phase and ion exchange high performance liquid chromatography. *J Nucl Med* 1981;22:69.
470. Lambrecht RM, Wolf AP. Cyclotron and short-lived halogen isotopes for radiopharmaceutical applications. In: *Radiopharmaceuticals and Labeled Compounds*. Vienna: IAEA; 1973;275.

470A. Qaim SM, Tarkanyi F, Stöcklin G, Sajjad M, Lambrecht RM. Excitation functions of (p, 2n) and (p, pn) reactions on highly enriched ^{124}Xe with special reference to the production of ^{123}I. *J Label Compd Radiopharm* 1991;30:103–104.

471. Wellman HN, et al. Properties, production and clinical uses of radioisotopes of iodine. *Crit Rev Clin Radiol Nucl Med* 1975;6:81.
472. De La Mare PBD. *Electrophilic Halogenation*. New York: Cambridge University Press; 1976.
473. Clayton JC, Hems BA. The synthesis of 263. thyroxine and related substances. VI. The preparation of some derivatives of DL-thyroxine. *J Chem Soc* 1950:840.
474. MacFarland AS. Efficient trace-labeling of proteins with iodine. *Nature* 1958;182:53.
475. Hunter WM, Greenwood FC. Preparation of iodine-131 labeled human growth hormones of high specific activity. *Nature* 1962;194:495.
476. Marchalonis JJ. An enzymic method for the trace iodination of immunoglobulins and other proteins. *Biochemistry* 1969;113:299.
477. Katz I, Bonorris G. Electrolytic iodination of proteins with ^{125}I and ^{131}I. *J Lab Clin Med* 1968;72:966.
478. Bolton AE, Hunter WM. The labeling of proteins to high specific radioactivities by conjugation to a ^{125}I-containing acylating agent. *J Biochem* 1973;133:529.
479. Grovenstein E Jr., Aprahamian NS, Bryan CS, et al. Aromatic halogenation. IV. Kinetics and mechanism of iodination of phenol and 2,6 dibromophenol. *J Am Chem Soc* 1973; 75:4261.
480. Lambrecht RM, et al. Preparation of high purity carrier free ^{123}I-iodine monochloride as iodination reagent for synthesis of radiopharmaceuticals. *J Nucl Med* 1972;13:266.
481. Berliner E. Kinetics of aromatic halogenation. V The iodination of 2,4 dichlorophenol and anisole with iodine monochloride. *J Am Chem Soc* 1958;80:856.
482. Batts BD, Gold V. The kinetics of aromatic protio- and deuterio-deiodination. *J Chem Soc* 1964;5753.
483. Huguchi T, Hussain A. Mechanism of chlorination of cresol by chloramine-T. Mediation by dichloramine-T. *J Chem Soc* 1967;549.
484. Freychet P, Roth J, Neville DM Jr. Monoiodoinsulin: demonstration of its biological activity and binding to fat cells and liver membranes. *Biochem Biophys Res Commun* 1971; 43:400.
485. Thorell JI, Johansson BG. Enzymatic iodination of polypeptides with ^{125}I to high specific activity. *Biochim Biophys Acta* 1971;251:363.
486. Miller L, Watkins BF. Scope and mechanism of aromatic iodination with electrochemically generated iodine (I). *J Am Chem Soc* 1976;98:1515.
487. Hayes CE, Goldstein IS. Radioiodination of sulfhydryl-sensitive proteins. *Anal Biochem* 1975;67:580.
488. Wood FT, Wu MM, Cerhart JC. The radioactive labeling of proteins with an iodinated amidination reagent. *Anal Biochem* 1975;69:339.
489. Hunter W. Preparation and assessment of radioactive tracers. *Br Med Bull* 1974;30:18.

489A. Wilbur DS. Radiohalogenation of proteins: an overview of radionuclides, labeling methods, and reagents for conjugate labeling. *Bioconjugate Chem* 1992;3:433–470.

490. Kabalka GW, Gooch EE. Synthesis of organic iodides via reaction of organoboranes with sodium iodide. *J Org Chem* 1981;46:2582.
491. Stock LM, Spector AR. Rates and relative rates of chloro- and iododesilylation. Evidence for a four center transition state. *J Org Chem* 1963;28:3272.
492. Hanson RN, Seitz DE, Botarro JC. E-17 ^{125}I iodovinylestradiol: an estrogen-receptor-seeking radiopharmaceutical. *J Nucl Med* 1982;23:431.
493. Moerlein SM, Mathis CA, Yano V. Comparative evaluation of electrophilic aromatic demetallation techniques for labeling radiopharmaceuticals with iodine-122. *Intern J Appl Radiat Isot* 1987;38:85.
494. Zollinger H. *Diazo and Azo Chemistry, Aliphatic and Aromatic Compounds*. New York: Interscience; 1961.
495. Patai S. *The Chemistry of Diazonium and Diazo Groups*. Part 1 and Part 2. New York: Interscience; 1979.
496. Szele J, Zollinger H. Dediazonation of arenediazonium ions in homogeneous solution. Solvent effects in competitive heterolytic and homolytic dediazonations. *Helv Chim Acta* 1978;61:1721.
497. Stockin G. Bromine-77 and iodine-123 radiopharmaceuticals. *Intern J Appl Radiat Isot* 1977;28:131.
498. Mangner TJ, Wu J, Wieland DM. Solid-phase exchange radioiodination of aryl iodides. Facilitation by ammonium sulfate. *J Org Chem* 1982;47:1484.
499. Gildersleeve DL, et al. Synthesis of a high specific activity ^{125}I-labeled analog of PK 11195. Potential agent for SPECT imaging of the peripheral benzodiazenine binding site. *J Nucl Med Bio* 1989;16:423.
500. Mertens J, Gysemans M. Cu^{1+} assisted nucleophilic exchange radiohalogenation: applications and mechanistic approach. In: Emran AM, ed. *New Trends in Radiopharmaceutical Synthesis, Quality Assurance, and Regulatory Control*, New York, NY: Plenum Press, 1991:53–66.
501. Rosa U, Pennisi GE, Scarsellati GA. Factors affecting protein iodination. In: Donato L, Milhard G, Sirchis J, eds. *Labeled Proteins in Tracer Studies*, Brussels: Euratom; 1966.
502. Bale WF, Helmkamp RW, Davis TP, et al. High specific activity labeling of proteins with ^{131}I by the iodide monochloride method. *Proc Soc Exp Biol Med* 1966;122:407.
503. Bale WF, Contreras MA, Grady ED. Factors influencing localization of labeled antibodies in tumor. *Cancer Res* 1980;40:2965.
504. Wolf AP, et al. Synthesis of radiopharmaceuticals and labeled compounds using short-lived isotopes. In: *Radiopharmaceuticals and Labeled Compounds*. Vienna: IAEA; 1973:345.
505. Kojima M, Maeda M. Homoallylic rearrangement of 19-iodocholesterok. *J Chem Soc Commun*. 1975;47.
506. Eckelman WC. The testing of putative receptor binding radiotracers in vivo. In: Diksic M, Reba RC, eds. *Radiopharmaceuticals and Brain Pathology Studied with PET and SPECT*. Boca Raton, FL: CRC Press, Inc.; 1991;41.
507. Blau M, Manske RF. The pancreas specificity of 75Se-selenomethionine. *J Nucl Med* 1961;2:102.
508. Wagner HN Jr., Rhodes BA. The Radiopharmaceutical. In: Wagner HN, ed. *Principles of Nuclear Medicine*. Philadelphia, PA: WB Saunders Co; 1968:286.
509. Axel L. Cerebral blood flow determination by rapid-sequence computed tomography. *Radiology* 1980;137:679–686.
510. Hoey GB, Smith KR. Chemistry of X-ray contrast media in Radiocontrast Agents. In: Sovak M, ed. *Handbook of Experimental Pharmacology*. New York, NY: Springer-Verlag; 1984:23–126.

511. Partain CL, et al. *Magnetic Resonance Imaging*. 2nd ed. Partain CL, et al. eds. Philadelphia, PA: WB Saunders Co; 1989.
512. Budinger T. Editorial: Advances in emission tomography: quo vadis? *J Nucl Med* 1990;31:628.
513. Hendel RC, et al. Diagnostic value of a new myocardial perfusion agent, teboroxime (SQ 30,217), utilizing a rapid planar imaging protocol: preliminary results. *J Am Coll Cardiol* 1990;16:855–861.
514. Bonow RO, et al. Cardiac positron emission tomography. A report for health professionals from the committee on advanced cardiac imaging and technology of the Council on Chemical Cardiology. *Circulation* 1991;84:12447.
515. Di Chiro G, Brook RA. PET-FDG of untreated and treated cerebral gliomas. *J Nucl Med* 1988;29:421.
516. Engel J, et al. Local cerebral metabolism during partial seizures. *Neurology* 1983;33:400.
517. Berridge MS, Sassidy EH, Terris AH. A routine, automated synthesis of oxygen-15-labeled butanol for position tomography. *J Nucl Med* 1990;31:1727.
518. Wise R, et al. Language activation studies with positron emission tomography. *Ciba Found Symp* 1991;163:218–228.
519. Heiss WD, et al. PET correlates of normal and impaired memory functions. *Cerebrovasc Brain Metab* 1992;4(1):1–27.
520. Steinmetz H, Seitz RJ. Functional anatomy of language processing: neuroimaging and the problem of individual variability. *Neuropsychologia* 1991;29(12):1149–1161.
521. Volkow ND, et al. Metabolic studies of drugs of abuse. *NIDA Res Monogr* 1991;105:47–53.
522. Ring HA, et al. The use of cerebral activation procedures with single photon emission tomography. *Eur J Nucl Med* 1991;18(2):133–141.
523. Reba RC, Diksic M. *Radiopharmaceuticals and Brain Pathology Studied with PET and SPECT.* Boca Raton, FL: CRC Press; 1991.
524. Phelps ME, Huang SC, Hoffman EJ, et al. Tomographic measurement of local cerebral glucose metabolic rate in humans with (F-18) 2-fluoro-2-deoxy-glucose: validation of a method. *Ann Neurol* 1979;6:371.
525. Martin WRW: Dopa Metabolism in Quantitative Imaging. In: Frost JJ, Wagner HN Jr, eds. *Neuroreceptors, Neurotransmitters*. New York, NY: Raven Press; 1990;167.
526. Fowler JS, Wolf AP. 2-Deoxy-2-[18-F]fluoro-D-glucose for metabolic studies. *Intern J Appl Radiat Isot* 1986;37:663.
527. Eckelman WC. Radiopharmaceuticals and brain pathology studied with PET and SPECT. In: Diksic M, Reba RC, eds. *The testing of Putative Receptor Binding Radiotracers in Vivo*. Boca Raton, FL: CRC Press; 1990:41–68.
528. Kilbourn M. Radiotracers for PET studies of neurotransmitter binding sites: design considerations. In: In vivo Imaging of Neurotransmitter Functions in Brain, Heart and Tumors. *Am College Nucl Phys*. Washington DC, 1991;47.
529. Gjedde A, Wong DF. Modeling neuroreceptor binding of radioligands in vivo in quantitative imaging. In: Frost JJ, Wagner HN Jr, eds. *Neuroreceptors, Neurotransmitters, and Enzymes*. New York, NY: Raven Press, Ltd; 1990;51.
530. Eckelman WC. The status of radiopharmaceutical research. *Nucl Med Bio*. 1991;18:iii–vi.
531. Johnston CI, et al. Comparative studies of tissue inhibition by angiotensin converting enzyme inhibitors. *J Hypertension* 1989;6(suppl 5):11.
532. Hwang D-R, Eckelman WC, Mathis CJ, Petrillo EW Jr, Lloyd J, Welch MJ. Positron-labeled Angiotensin-Converting Enzyme (ACE) inhibitor: fluorine-18-fluorocaptopril. Probing the ACE activity in vivo by positron emission tomography. *J Nucl Med* 1991;32:1730–1737.
533. Frackowiak RS, Rriston KJ. Functional neuroanatomy of the human brain: positron emission tomography—a new neuroanatomical technique. *J Anat* 1994;184:211–225.
534. Raichle ME. Circulatory and metabolic corrrelates of brain function in normal humans. In: Mountcastle VB, Plum F, eds. *Handbook of Physiology. The Nervous System*. Bethesda, MD: American Physiological Society, pp 643–674.
535. Herscovitch P. Functional mapping of the human brain. In: Wagner HN Jr, ed. *Principles of Nuclear Medicine*, 2nd ed. 1995; Philadelphia, PA: Saunders WB. In Press.

12 Radiation Absorbed Dose Calculations

Ted W. Fowler, Lisa Langlois Coronado

DEFINITIONS AND SCOPE

Internal dosimetry is used to estimate radiation absorbed doses from medical procedures involving radionuclides. Internal dosimetry is defined as the assessment of radiation dose received from a radionuclide *inside the body.* Internal doses are *calculated* using biologic and radiologic (physical) parameters. Unlike external dosimetry, which is often based on measurements with a radiation survey instrument, internal dosimetry is based on calculated values because of the difficulty of obtaining actual measurements of radiation flux or deposited energy inside body organs. This chapter describes the methodology typically used in nuclear medicine to calculate doses to body organs from radiopharmaceuticals.

Absorbed dose is defined as the amount of energy deposited per unit of mass of tissue. Mathematically, this relationship is expressed as[1]

$$\overline{D} = \frac{d\overline{\epsilon}}{dm}$$

where $\overline{D}$ = mean absorbed dose and $d\overline{\epsilon}$ = mean energy imparted by ionizing radiation to matter of mass, dm.

The unit of radiation absorbed dose is the gray (Gy), which is the deposition of 1 J/kg of material. The gray has replaced the rad, which is defined as the deposition of 100 ergs per gram of material; 1 Gy equals 100 rad. Radiation absorbed dose can be calculated using several different methods, the two most common being the Marinelli and MIRD equations. The absorbed dose calculations developed by the Medical Internal Radiation Dose (MIRD) Committee of the Society of Nuclear Medicine is described in this chapter. Robertson has described how the Marinelli equations can be converted to the MIRD equations and users of Marinelli equations should consult this reference.[2] The MIRD radiation absorbed dose equations, utilizing absorbed fractions, is the methodology required by the Food and Drug Administration (FDA)[3] to meet FDA limits. This methodology is also used by the International Commission on Radiological Protection (ICRP).[4]

BODY DISTRIBUTION

Once radioactive material enters the body, it selectively localizes in certain organs of the body, called *source organs.* Organs irradiated by source organs are called *target organs.* The source organ and the target organ can be the same organ (ie, an organ can irradiate itself; this is referred to as the self-dose). Both the radionuclide and the chemical form of the compound affect the distribution of radioactive material inside the body. In most cases, the compound form governs the distribution. For example, ^{99m}Tc-methylene diphosphonate localizes in bone; ^{99m}Tc-sulfur colloid localizes in the reticuloendothelial system, and ^{99m}Tc-albumin macroaggregates localize in the lung. Furthermore, some radiopharmaceuticals contain contaminants that contribute to the absorbed dose to body organs. For example, ^{201}Tl is not radionuclidically pure; typical contaminants ^{200}Tl, ^{202}Tl, ^{203}Pb, and ^{210}Pb are assumed to be present for the purpose of estimating the ^{201}Tl absorbed dose. Radionuclide contaminants of commonly used radiopharmaceuticals are listed in Reference 5.

If the labeling efficiency in vivo is not 100%, the absorbed dose from the free compound must be considered in calculating the total absorbed dose. For example, erythrocytes can be labeled with ^{99m}Tc-pertechnetate. If there is incomplete labeling (eg, less than 100%), the dose from the pertechnetate has to be considered in calculating the total absorbed dose from the administered ^{99m}Tc.

REFERENCE MAN AND MATHEMATICAL PHANTOMS FOR DOSIMETRY

The estimation of absorbed dose from internal radiation sources requires us to specify certain information regarding the exposed individual. The ICRP Task Group on Reference Man specifies the characteristics of man needed for dosimetry purposes.[6] Snyder et al formulated a mathematical description of an adult human that incorporates much of the reference man data.[7] The Reference Man phantom is shown in Figure 1 and Reference 8 includes a detailed description of the phantom. Table 1 includes masses of body organs for both reference man and for the phantom. Simplified equations for the phantom organs were used to provide formulas that could be readily calculated on a digital computer[9] to provide estimates of photon absorbed fractions for various target/source organ configurations. Since no individual will have the exact characteristics of reference man and the phantom, doses calculated using these parameters should be considered as best estimates in absence of specific patient information.

In addition to the adult human phantom, a series of phantoms, developed at Oak Ridge National Laboratory, repre-

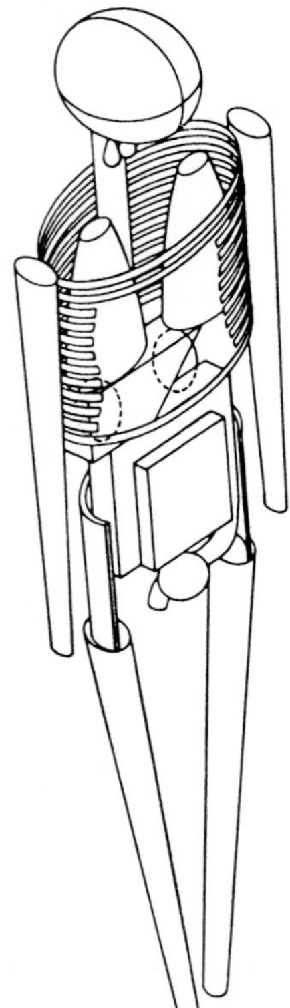

Figure 1. Reference man phantom showing some internal organs. (From Cloutier.[10])

sents individuals of various ages from newborns to adults. These phantoms and the specific absorbed fractions developed from them have been widely used to estimate the radiation absorbed dose for radiation workers, nuclear medicine patients, and members of the general public. The pediatric phantoms include newborn, 1-year old, 10-year old, and 15-year-old models.[11]

The 15-year old model has been used to represent the adult female and has been designated reference woman.[6] Recently, the Radiopharmaceutical Internal Dose Information Center, a unit funded by the Department of Energy and the Food and Drug Administration to improve radiation dose estimates, has incorporated the anatomical changes that occur during pregnancy into the 15-year-old model to represent the pregnant woman. Complete models for 3, 6, and 9 months of pregnancy have been developed and can be used to estimate the absorbed dose to various organs of the pregnant female as well as to the developing fetus.[12,13]

Table 1. Masses of Body Organs of Reference Man and of Anthropomorphic Phantom

BODY ORGANS	MASS (g) *Reference Man*	MASS (g) *Phantom*
Adrenals	14	15.5
Bladder		
Wall	45	45.1
Contents	200	200
Gastrointestinal tract		
Stomach		
Wall	150	150
Contents	250	247
Small intestine		
Wall	640	640*
Contents	400	400*
Upper large intestine		
Wall	210	209
Contents	220	200
Lower large intestine		
Wall	160	160
Contents	135	137
Kidneys (both)	310	284
Liver	1,800	1,810
Lungs (both, including blood)	1,000	999
Other tissue	48,000	48,500 (2800 g suggested for muscle; 12,500 g for separable adipose tissue)
Ovaries (both)	11	8.27
Pancreas	100	60.3
Salivary glands	85	Not represented
Skeleton	10,000	10,500
Cortical bone	4,000	4,000
Trabecular bone	1,000	1,000
Red marrow	1,500	1,500
Yellow marrow	1,500	1,500
Cartilage	1,100	1,100
Other constituents	900	1,400
Spleen	180	174
Testes	35	37.1
Thyroid	20	19.6
Uterus	80	65.4
Total body	70,000	69,900

*Small intestine wall and contents not separated in phantom.

From Cloutier.[10]

ABSORBED DOSE CALCULATIONS

General MIRD Equation

The complete MIRD equations for calculating absorbed dose are described by Loevinger and Berman.[14] Loevinger et al have further explained the MIRD schema in a comprehensive manner and have provided many examples of absorbed dose calculations in the MIRD Primer for Absorbed Dose Calculations.[15] Other references also contain useful information pertinent to the use of the MIRD equations in nuclear medicine.[16–20] This chapter briefly describes the *simplified* MIRD equation. Table 2 lists the symbols, quantities, and units used in the MIRD schema*. The general equation is as follows:

$$\overline{D}(T \leftarrow S) = \tilde{A}_S \cdot S(T \leftarrow S)$$

*Because the published MIRD tables use the traditional units rather than the International System of Units (ie, SI units), traditional units will be emphasized in this chapter and in the example absorbed dose calculations.

Table 2. Principal Symbols, Quantities, and Units Used in MIRD Schema

SYMBOL	QUANTITY	TRADITIONAL UNITS	SI UNITS
$\overline{D}$	Mean absorbed dose	rad	Gy
A_S	Activity in source organ S	μCi	Bq
$\tilde{A}_s$	Cumulated activity in source organ	μCi-h	Bq-s
$S(T \leftarrow S)$	S factor (mean absorbed dose to target organ, T, per unit cumulated activity in source organ, S)	rad/μCi-h	Gy/Bq-s
λ_R	Radiological decay constant	h^{-1}	s^{-1}
$T_{1/2\ rad}$	Radioactive half-life	h	s
λ_B	Biologic removal constant	h^{-1}	s^{-1}
$T_{1/2\ bio}$	Biologic half-life	h	s
λ_E	Effective removal constant	h^{-1}	s^{-1}
$T_{1/2\ eff}$	Effective half-life	h	s
α	Fractional distribution	1	1
τ	Residence time	h	s
Δ	Equilibrium dose constant (mean energy emitted per unit cumulated activity)	g-rad/μCi-h	kg-Gy/Bq-s
ϕ	Absorbed fraction	1	1
M_T	Mass of target organ T	g	kg
$\overline{E}$	Mean energy per particle or photon	MeV	J
n	Mean number of particles or photons per nuclear disintegration	1	1
Φ	Specific absorbed fraction	g^{-1}	kg^{-1}

The bar over the D indicates a mean value and the tilde over A_S denotes a time integral. $\overline{D}$ $(T \leftarrow S)$ = mean absorbed dose to a target organ, T, from a radionuclide uniformly distributed in a source organ, S (rad or gray). $\tilde{A}_S$ = cumulated activity in the source organ or the number of disintegrations in the source organ (microcurie-hour or becquerel-second). $S(T \leftarrow S)$ = mean absorbed dose to a target organ per unit cumulated activity in the source organ; also known as the S factor (rad per microcurie-hour or gray per becquerel-second).

Cumulated Activity

The time integral of activity, known as the cumulated activity ($\tilde{A}_S$), is calculated using metabolic data. The determination of $\tilde{A}_S$ is usually the most difficult part of the internal dose calculation. The metabolic data needed for this calculation may be obtained from animal studies or human clinical studies. To calculate $\tilde{A}_S$, the time course of activity in the source organ must be characterized and integrated. Mathematically, the simplest situation is a one-compartment model where the activity enters the compartment instantaneously and is removed by radioactive decay and a single biological clearance constant. The differential equation describing source organ activity, A_S, in a one-compartment model is

$$\frac{dA_S(t)}{dt} = -(\lambda_R + \lambda_B)\, A_S$$

where $A_S(t)$ = activity in source organ as a function of time; λ_R = radiological decay constant = $0.693/T_{1/2rad}$; λ_B = biological removal constant = $0.693/T_{1/2bio}$; and $T_{1/2bio}$ = biological half-life.

The total removal of activity from the source organ by physical (radiological) and biologic processes is described by a single term called the effective removal constant.

$$\lambda_E = \lambda_R + \lambda_B$$

where λ_E = effective removal constant = $0.693/T_{1/2eff}$ and $T_{1/2eff}$ = effective half-life.

$$T_{1/2eff} = \frac{T_{1/2rad}\, T_{1/2bio}}{T_{1/2rad} + T_{1/2bio}}$$

The effective half-life can be no greater than the smaller of the physical (radiological) or biologic half-lives.

The solution of the differential equation describing source organ activity as a function of time in a one-compartment model with a single biological removal constant is

$$A_S(t) = A_S(0)e^{-\lambda_E t}$$

$A_S(0)$ is the initial activity in the source organ which is defined as the fraction of the total activity administered into the body that accumulates in the source organ S. Figure 2

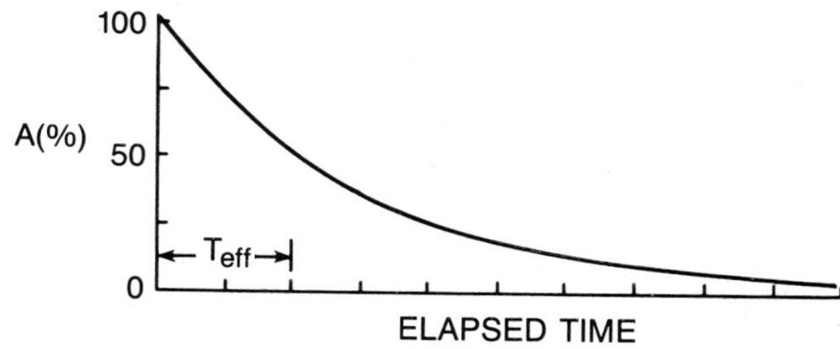

Figure 2. Amount of activity in compartment with respect to time. (From Cloutier.[10])

shows the activity in the compartment as a function of time with 50% of the activity being removed from the compartment after one effective half-life ($T_{1/2\text{eff}}$).

Unfortunately, the change in activity with time in most biological systems cannot be described with the above simple equation having one compartment[10] and a single biological removal half-life. A typical equation describing the activity in a source organ is as follows:

$$A_S(t) = A_S(0) \sum_j \alpha_{Sj} e^{-\lambda_{Ej} t}$$

where α = fractional distribution function. For a given source organ,

$$\sum_j \alpha_{Sj} = 1$$

where j = biological compartment; α_{Sj} = fractional distribution function for the jth biologic compartment in a source organ; and λ_{Ej} = effective removal constant for the jth biologic compartment in a source organ.

The cumulated activity, $\tilde{A}_S$, is represented by the area under the activity curve shown in Figure 2 and is the total number of disintegrations over time t. Mathematically, $\tilde{A}_S$ is calculated as follows:

$$\tilde{A}_S(0 - t) = \int_0^t A_S(t)\, dt$$

$$\tilde{A}_S(0 - t) = \int_0^t A_S(0)\, e^{-\lambda_E t}\, dt$$

$$\tilde{A}_S(0 - t) = \frac{A_S(0)}{-\lambda_E} e^{-\lambda_E t} \Big|_0^t$$

$$\tilde{A}_S(0 - t) = \frac{A_S(0)}{-\lambda_E} (e^{-\lambda_E t} - 1)$$

$$\tilde{A}_S(0 - t) = \frac{A_S(0)}{\lambda_E} (1 - e^{-\lambda_E t})$$

where $e^{-\lambda_E t}$ = fraction of activity remaining at time t and $1 - e^{-\lambda_E t}$ = fraction of total disintegrations to time t.

Example calculation, for $t = T_{1/2\text{eff}}$

$$e^{-\lambda_E T_{1/2eff}} = e^{\frac{-0.693}{T_{1/2eff}} T_{1/2eff}} = e^{-0.693} = 0.5$$

When t = ∞ (infinity),

$$\tilde{A}_S(0 - \infty) = \frac{A_S(0)}{\lambda_E}$$

$$\tilde{A}_S(0 - \infty) = A_S(0) \frac{1}{0.693} T_{1/2\text{eff}}$$

$$\tilde{A}_S(0 - \infty) = A_S(0)\ 1.44\ T_{1/2\text{eff}}$$

The above equation is valid when t is much greater than the effective half-life, ie, when t is at least ten effective half-lives.

$$\tilde{A}_S(\mu\text{Ci-hour}) = A_S(0)\ (\mu\text{Ci})\ 1.44\ T_{1/2\text{eff}}(\text{hour})$$

where $\tilde{A}_S$ = cumulated activity in source organ; $A_S(0)$ = initial activity in source organ = product of the administered activity (or intake of activity) times the fraction of activity that reaches the source organ; and $T_{1/2\text{eff}}$ = effective half-life in source organ.

Sometimes $\tilde{A}_S$ is defined using a term called residence time, τ_S. Residence time is the average time that activity remains in a source organ.

$$\tau_S = \frac{\tilde{A}_S}{A_S(0)} = 1.44\ T_{1/2\text{eff}} = \frac{1}{\lambda_E}$$

The MIRD Primer for Absorbed Dose Calculations[15] describes residence time in detail and how it is used in simple and complex dose calculations. Several other references also contain useful information pertinent to the use of kinetic models in the calculation of cumulated activity ($\tilde{A}_S$). In MIRD Pamphlet 12, Berman describes the kinetic model differential equations and solutions needed for absorbed dose calculations.[21] Robertson presents a summary discussion of kinetic analysis and general solutions of the differential and integral equations for a two-compartment closed system.[18] Biologic removal constants and the radiological decay constant can be substituted into Robertson's equations[18] and $\tilde{A}_S$ can be calculated for a two-compartment closed system without having to do the differential and integral mathematical calculations. Several references contain useful information pertinent to the kinetic analysis necessary to calculate the radiation absorbed dose to the urinary bladder wall.[22–24]

S Factors

The S factor is the absorbed dose to target organ T per disintegration of a radionuclide in source organ S and is defined as follows: $S(T \leftarrow S)$ = mean absorbed dose to a target organ per unit cumulated activity in source organ (rad per microcurie-hour or gray per becquerel-second).

$$S(T \leftarrow S) = \sum_i \Delta_i \frac{\phi_i(T \leftarrow S)}{M_T}$$

where i subscripts refer to a certain type of radiation; Δ_i = equilibrium absorbed-dose constant = mean energy emitted per unit cumulated activity for radiation i (gram-rad per microcuries-hour or kilogram-gray per becquerel-second). This is also the mean energy emitted per nuclear decay or disintegration. $\phi_i(T \leftarrow S)$ = absorbed fraction = fraction of the energy of the ith radiation from the radionuclide in the source organ that is imparted to the target organ (eg, this is the absorbed fraction of energy emitted from source S that is absorbed in target organ T); M_T = mass of the target organ (gram or kilogram). Note that M_T is the mass of the target organ, not the mass of the source organ. The absorbed dose is calculated to the target (ie, energy absorbed per unit mass of the target).

The S factor equation is also written as follows:

$$S(T \leftarrow S) = \sum_n \Delta_n \frac{\phi_n(T \leftarrow S)}{M_T} + \sum_p \Delta_p \frac{\phi_p(T \leftarrow S)}{M_T}$$

The subscripts n and p in the S factor equation denote nonpenetrating and penetrating emissions.

The term *nonpenetrating* is applied to those radiations for which only an insignificant amount of energy is absorbed outside a source volume (electromagnetic radiation of energy less or equal to 10 keV, and all particulate radiation).

The term *penetrating* is applied to those radiations for which a significant amount of energy may be absorbed outside a source volume (electromagnetic radiation having energy greater than 10 keV).

S factors have been tabulated for many source-target organs in the MIRD anthrophomorphic phantom in MIRD pamphlet No. 11[25] and in other publications such as Reference 8.

Equilibrium Dose Constant

Δ_i is also called the equilibrium (absorbed) dose constant because, for a uniform distribution of a radionuclide in an infinite, homogeneous absorbing material, the energy absorbed per gram is in equilibrium with the energy emitted per gram. Also, the equilibrium dose constant gives the dose rate in rad per hour for a concentration of 1 μCi/g on the assumption that all the emitted energy is locally absorbed.

$$\Delta_i = 2.13 n_i \overline{E}_i$$

where Δ_i = energy emitted per disintegration (gram-rad per microcurie-hour); n_i is the mean number of particles or photons per nuclear transformation; $\overline{E}_i$ is the mean energy (megaelectron volts); 2.13 is a unit conversion constant (gram-rad per microcurie-hour) (megaelectron volt per disintegration) and is the product of the following terms:

$$(1.602 \times 10^{-6}\ \text{erg/MeV})(10^{-2}\ \text{g-rad/erg})\ (3.7 \times 10^{4}\ \text{dis/}\mu\text{Ci-second})(3.6 \times 10^{3}\ \text{second/h})$$

Values of Δ_i are calculated from decay scheme information. The disintegration of a radionuclide is assumed to give rise to radiations of types $i = 1,2,3 \ldots$ each with a mean number n_i of particles (or photons) per disintegration, and a mean energy $\overline{E}_i$ MeV per particle (or photon).

Δ_i values for a number of radionuclides have been tabulated by Dillman in MIRD Pamphlets 4,[26] 6,[27] and 10.[28] A compilation by Kocher[29] contains Δ_i values for many of the radionuclides of interest in nuclear medicine.

The total energy emitted per disintegration is the sum of all radiations i emitted:

$$\Delta = \sum_i \Delta_i = 2.13 \sum_i n_i E_i$$

Decay scheme data and Δ_i values for fluorine-18 are shown in Appendix B. One hundred percent of the fluorine-18 disintegrations result in the emission of a 0.2498 Mev positron (positive beta particle) from the F-18 nucleus. The Δ_i value for the positron is calculated as

$$\Delta_i = (2.13)(1.00\ \beta^+/\text{dis.})(0.2498\ \text{Mev}/\beta^+) = 0.532\ \text{g-rad}/\mu\text{Ci-h}$$

Each positron ultimately combines with an electron in an interaction that results in the annihilation of both particles and their rest mass appears as two 0.51-Mev photons. The Δ_i value for the annihilation radiation is calculated as

$$\Delta_i = (2.13)(2.00\ \gamma/\text{dis.})(0.511\ \text{MeV}/\gamma) = 2.18\ \text{g-rad}/\mu\text{Ci-h}$$

Absorbed Fraction

The absorbed fraction depends on the type of radiation with the following general rules applying:

$$S \neq T \quad \phi = 0 \text{ for nonpenetrating radiation}$$
$$S = T \quad \phi = 1 \text{ for nonpenetrating radiation}$$
$$S = T \quad \phi < 1 \text{ for penetrating radiation}$$

$$0 \leq \phi_i(T \leftarrow S) \leq 1$$

For gamma emissions, the absorbed fraction depends on the gamma ray energy, size, and shape of the organs, and on the geometric configuration between source and target organs. The absorbed fraction as a function of gamma energy for a uniform distribution of activity is presented in MIRD Pamphlet 5[30] for organs within a heterogeneous phantom. Absorbed fractions for uniformly distributed photon sources are also presented in MIRD Pamphlets 3[31] and 8.[32] The data for small volumes are specifically helpful for dose calculations involving sizes of organs in children.

Specific Absorbed Fraction

Dividing the absorbed fraction, ϕ_i, by the mass of the target organ, M_T, yields the specific absorbed fraction. Tables providing values for Φ_i are presented in ICRP Publication 23.[6]

$$\Phi_i(T \leftarrow S) = \frac{\phi_i(T \leftarrow S)}{M_T}$$

$$0 \leq \Phi_i \leq \frac{1}{M_T}$$

Reciprocity Principal

The reciprocity principal is used in absorbed-dose calculations to relate the doses in different source regions. The reciprocal dose theorem states that two sources containing the same total amount of radioactivity deliver to each other the same average dose, irrespective of size, shape, or distance.[33] The reciprocity principal is applied to the specific absorbed fraction and the S factor in MIRD Pamphlet 1.[14] The specific absorbed fraction is independent of which region is designated source and which target, or in symbols

$$\Phi_i(T \leftarrow S) = \Phi_i(S \leftarrow T) \equiv \Phi_i(S \longleftrightarrow T)\text{g}^{-1}$$

The dose reciprocity theorem is useful when tables of Φ are not available for all source-target organ pairs. If $\Phi_i(S \leftarrow T)$ is known, then $\Phi_i(T \leftarrow S)$ can be obtained from the dose reciprocity theorem using the preceding equation. Also, the mean absorbed dose per microcurie-hour (or per disintegration) is independent of which region is designated source and which target,[14] or in symbols

$$S(T \leftarrow S) = S(S \leftarrow T)$$

Remainder of the Body

A common problem encountered during absorbed dose calculations involves the situation where only part of the administered activity is accounted for in source organs where S factors have been tabulated. The problem is obtaining the S factor for the "remainder" of the body. If one uses the S factor for the total body, S(target organ ← total body), to calculate the dose from the remainder of the body cumulated activity ($\tilde{A}_{\text{remainder}}$), doses to target organs that have been considered as source organs will be overestimated. When the S factor for the total body is used, it is assumed that the activity is uniformly distributed in the total body. This is not the case when the remainder of the body is considered as a source organ. To avoid accounting for activity in source organs twice, a value of S can be calculated to be used with the cumulated activity in the remainder of the body using the methodology of Roedler and Kaul.[34] The general equation for the S factor of target organ T from the remainder of the body RB is

$$S(T \leftarrow RB) = \frac{M_{TB}\, S(T \leftarrow TB) - \sum_{S} M_S\, S(T \leftarrow S)}{M_{TB} - \sum_{S} M_S}$$

where S represents the source organs, TB is total body, and

$$M_{TB} - \sum_{S} M_S = \text{mass of } RB$$

Summary

$$\bar{D}\,(T \leftarrow S) = \tilde{A}_S \cdot S(T \leftarrow S)$$

Ordinarily there will be many source organs, S, contributing dose to the target organ, T, and we must add together all these contributions. Expressed as an equation, this takes the form:

$$\bar{D}(T) = \sum_{S} \bar{D}(T \leftarrow S)$$

where the summation sign now indicates addition of contributions from all source organs S.

EXAMPLES OF DOSE CALCULATIONS

Since the absorbed dose to a target organ or tissue from the administration of a radiopharmaceutical is expressed as

$$\bar{D}(T \leftarrow S) = \tilde{A}_S \cdot S(T \leftarrow S)$$

the uncertainties in the calculated estimate reflect the uncertainties associated with the two quantities, the cumulated activity and the S factor. The uncertainty in the S factor is considered to be slight since this value is derived from well-analyzed and established physical data, eg, the radiation type, energy emitted per nuclear transformation and mass of the target organ. The major uncertainty associated with the cumulated activity, $\tilde{A}$, arises from the quantitative description of the biologic parameters, eg, uptake, retention, and excretion of the compound. Consequently, the estimated absorbed dose to different organs can deviate considerably from the actual absorbed dose in patients by a factor of perhaps two or three. The deviation is less for substances labeled with short-lived radionuclides such as ^{99m}Tc.[35]

In order to estimate radiation absorbed dose to a reference man phantom, which should approximate the dose to a patient undergoing administration of a radiopharmaceutical, information concerning the radionuclide, chemical form, biokinetic model, and administered activity is needed.

Example 1

Consider an example in which 3 mCi (111 MBq) of ^{99m}Tc as a colloid is administered to a patient. Assume the administered activity, A_0, is instantaneously distributed in the body, and that 60% is located in the liver, 30% is located in the spleen, and 10% is located in the red bone marrow. If no further distribution of the ^{99m}Tc occurs and no biologic removal from the three source organs takes place, the average absorbed dose to the liver can be calculated as follows:

$$\bar{D}_{LI} = \bar{D}(LI \leftarrow LI) + \bar{D}(LI \leftarrow SP) + \bar{D}(LI \leftarrow RBM)$$

where LI is the liver, SP is the spleen, and RBM is the red bone marrow.

$$\bar{D}_{LI} = \tilde{A}_{LI}S(LI \leftarrow LI) + \tilde{A}_{SP}S(LI \leftarrow SP) + \tilde{A}_{RBM}S(LI \leftarrow RBM)$$

In this case, since there is no biological elimination, $T_{1/2\text{eff}} = T_{1/2\text{rad}}$. Calculation of the cumulated activity for each source organ is as follows:

$$A_0 = 3\text{mCi} = 3000\ \mu\text{Ci}$$
$$\tilde{A}_s = f \cdot A_0 \cdot 1.44 \cdot T_{1/2\text{eff}}$$

$$\begin{aligned}
\tilde{A}_{LI} &= (0.60)(3000\ \mu\text{Ci})(1.44)(6.02\ \text{hours}) \\
&= 1.56 \times 10^4\ \mu\text{Ci-hour} \\
\tilde{A}_{SP} &= (0.30)(3000\ \mu\text{Ci})(1.44)(6.02\ \text{hours}) \\
&= 7.8 \times 10^3\ \mu\text{Ci-hour} \\
\tilde{A}_{RBM} &= (0.10)(3000\ \mu\text{Ci})(1.44)(6.02\ \text{hours}) \\
&= 2.6 \times 10^3\ \mu\text{Ci-hour}
\end{aligned}$$

Using the appropriate S factor listed in Table 3, the dose contribution from each source organ is as follows:

$$\begin{aligned}
&\bar{D}(LI \leftarrow LI) \\
&\quad = (1.56 \times 10^4\ \mu\text{Ci-hour})(4.6 \times 10^{-5}\ \text{rad}/\mu\text{Ci-hour}) \\
&\quad = 0.718\ \text{rad}\ (7.18\ \text{mGy}) \\
&\bar{D}(LI \leftarrow SP) \\
&\quad = (7.8 \times 10^3\ \mu\text{Ci-hour})(9.8 \times 10^{-7}\ \text{rad}/\mu\text{Ci-hour}) \\
&\quad = 0.0076\ \text{rad}\ (0.076\ \text{mGy}) \\
&\bar{D}(LI \leftarrow RBM) \\
&\quad = (2.6 \times 10^3\ \mu\text{Ci-hour})(9.2 \times 10^{-7}\ \text{rad}/\mu\text{Ci-hour}) \\
&\quad = 0.0024\ \text{rad}\ (0.024\ \text{mGy})
\end{aligned}$$

Table 3. *S* Factors (rad/μCi-h) for ^{99m}Tc*

	SOURCE ORGANS					
TARGET ORGANS	*Adrenals*	*Kidneys*	*Liver*	*Red Bone Marrow*	*Spleen*	*Total Body*
Adrenals	3.1 E-03	1.1 E-05	4.5 E-06	2.3 E-06	6.3 E-06	2.3 E-06
Bladder wall	1.3 E-07	2.8 E-07	1.6 E-07	9.9 E-07	1.2 E-07	2.3 E-06
Bone (total)	2.0 E-06	1.4 E-06	1.1 E-06	4.0 E-06	1.1 E-06	2.5 E-06
GI (stomach wall)	2.9 E-06	3.6 E-06	1.9 E-06	9.5 E-07	1.0 E-05	2.2 E-06
GI (SI)	8.3 E-07	2.9 E-06	1.6 E-06	2.6 E-06	1.4 E-06	2.5 E-06
GI (ULI wall)	9.3 E-07	2.9 E-06	2.5 E-06	2.1 E-06	1.4 E-06	2.4 E-06
GI (LLI wall)	2.2 E-07	7.2 E-07	2.3 E-07	2.9 E-06	6.1 E-07	2.3 E-06
Kidneys	1.1 E-05	1.9 E-04	3.9 E-06	2.2 E-06	9.1 E-06	2.2 E-06
Liver	4.9 E-06	3.9 E-06	4.6 E-05	9.2 E-07	9.8 E-07	2.2 E-06
Lungs	2.4 E-06	8.5 E-07	2.5 E-06	1.2 E-06	2.3 E-06	2.0 E-06
Red bone marrow	3.6 E-06	3.8 E-06	1.6 E-06	3.1 E-05	1.7 E-06	2.9 E-06
Muscle	1.4 E-06	1.3 E-06	1.1 E-06	1.2 E-06	1.4 E-06	1.9 E-06
Ovaries	6.1 E-07	1.1 E-06	4.5 E-07	3.2 E-06	4.0 E-07	2.4 E-06
Pancreas	9.0 E-06	6.6 E-06	4.2 E-06	1.7 E-06	1.9 E-05	2.4 E-06
Skin	5.1 E-07	5.3 E-07	4.9 E-07	5.9 E-07	4.7 E-07	1.3 E-06
Spleen	6.3 E-06	8.6 E-06	9.2 E-07	9.2 E-07	3.3 E-04	2.2 E-06
Testes	3.2 E-08	8.8 E-08	6.2 E-08	4.5 E-07	4.8 E-08	1.7 E-06
Thyroid	1.3 E-07	4.8 E-08	1.5 E-07	6.8 E-07	8.7 E-08	1.5 E-06
Uterus	1.1 E-06	9.4 E-07	3.9 E-07	2.2 E-06	4.0 E-07	2.6 E-06
Total body	2.2 E-06	2.2 E-06	2.2 E-06	2.2 E-06	2.2 E-06	2.0 E-06

Based on MIRD Pamphlet 11.[25]

*To convert from rad/μCi-h to Gy/Bq-s or rad/μCi-h to mGy/MBq-s, multiply the value in the table by 7.51×10^{-11} or 7.51×10^{-2}, respectively.

Thus, the total dose to the liver, the summation of the contribution from each source organ, is 0.728 rad (7.28 mGy). Note that approximately 98% of the total dose to the liver is contributed from the activity contained within the liver (ie, the organ self-dose).

Example 2

A more complex dose problem is encountered when the administered radiopharmaceutical is concentrated or readily excreted through the urinary excretion pathway. In these instances, the excretory organs (ie, kidneys, spleen, and urinary bladder wall) may have the highest radiation absorbed dose. Calculation of the dose to the urinary bladder wall from the activity contained within the bladder contents is more complex. In this example, a dynamic bladder model with a uniform void frequency is used.

Consider an example in which a patient is administered 1 mCi (37 MBq) of an ^{18}F compound for a PET study. Imaging requires a total of 2.0 hours, after which time the patient voids (ie, urinates). Assume the administered activity is instantaneously distributed in the body with 50%, having a $T_{1/2bio}$ of 1.5 hours, cleared through the urinary excretion system; the remaining 50% of the administered activity is distributed to various organs of the body from which there is no biologic elimination.

Calculation of the cumulated activity in the urinary bladder contents of the patient, $\tilde{A}_{BC}$, during the first 2 hours following administration of the ^{18}F compound is as follows:

$$\frac{dA_{BC}}{dt} = A_{Body}\lambda_B - A_{BC}\lambda_R$$

This equation reflects the change of radioactivity in the bladder contents and is valid until the patient voids. Note that A_{Body} is the activity in the body that is cleared through the urinary excretion system with a biological removal constant of λ_B.

Substituting in the equation,

$$A_{Body}(t) = A_{Body}(0)e^{-\lambda_E t}$$

for A_{Body} and solving the differential yields the following result:

$$A_{BC}(t) = A_{Body}(0)\,[e^{-\lambda_R t} - e^{-\lambda_E t}]$$

To solve for the cumulated activity, the following integration must be performed:

$$\tilde{A}_{BC}\ (0\text{ to }2\text{ hours}) = \int_0^2 A_{BC}(t)\,dt$$

Substituting the equation for $A_{BC}(t)$ into the right side of the equation yields

$$\tilde{A}_{BC}(0 \text{ to } 2 \text{ hours}) = \int_0^2 A_{Body}(0)\,[e^{-\lambda_R t} - e^{-\lambda_E t}]\,dt$$

Integrating this equation yields

$$\tilde{A}_{BC}(0 \text{ to } 2 \text{ hours}) = A_{Body}(0)\left[\frac{1 - e^{-\lambda_R(2)}}{\lambda_R} - \frac{1 - e^{-\lambda_E(2)}}{\lambda_E}\right]$$

Substituting in the parameters,

$T_{1/2rad} = 1.83$ hour; $\lambda_R = 0.379$ hour^{-1}; $\lambda_E = 0.841$ hour^{-1}

The calculation yields

$$\tilde{A}_{BC}(0 \text{ to } 2 \text{ hours}) = A_{Body}(0)(0.434 \text{ hour})$$

Since only 50% of the administered activity is cleared through the urinary bladder, for a 1-mCi injection, the initial activity in the body cleared through the urinary bladder is

$$A_{Body}(0) = f \cdot (A_0) = (0.50)(1000\ \mu\text{Ci}) = 500\ \mu\text{Ci}$$

Thus, the cumulated activity in the bladder for the first 2 hours following administration is

$$\tilde{A}_{BC}(0 \text{ to } 2 \text{ hour}) = (500\ \mu\text{Ci})(0.434) = 217\ \mu\text{Ci-hour}$$

The S factor for ^{18}F with the bladder contents as the source organ and the bladder wall as the target is 1.8×10^{-3} rad/μCi-hour.[25] Thus, the radiation absorbed dose to the bladder wall from the radioactivity contained in the bladder contents for the first 2 hours would then be

$$\overline{D}(BW \leftarrow BC) = \tilde{A}_{(BC)} \cdot S(BW \leftarrow BC) = 0.391 \text{ rad } (3.91 \text{ mGy})$$

where BW is the bladder wall and BC is the bladder contents.

If the bladder voids at constant intervals of 2 hours, the number of disintegrations during each succeeding bladder filling is equal to the product of the disintegrations that occurred during the first bladder filling times the factor

$$e^{-\lambda_E(t)}$$

where t is the elapsed time in hours since the administration of the ^{18}F compound. This term accounts for the activity remaining in the body that is available for excretion after radiological decay and biologic elimination have occurred through previous voids. Hence,

$$\tilde{A}_{BC}(0 \text{ to } 2 \text{ hours}) = e^{-\lambda_E(0)} A_{Body}(0)\left[\frac{1 - e^{-\lambda_R(2)}}{\lambda_R} - \frac{1 - e^{-\lambda_E(2)}}{\lambda_E}\right] dt$$

The expression in brackets will be the same for each interval since the bladder voiding time is considered to be constant at 2 hours. As shown previously, this expression reduces to a value of 0.434 hours when the parameters are substituted into the expression.

To determine the *total* dose to the urinary bladder wall (ie, from time 0 to infinity) the calculations are continued in a similar manner with the results as follows:

$$\begin{aligned}
\tilde{A}_{BC}(0 \text{ to } 2 \text{ hours}) &= A_{Body}(0) \cdot 0.434 \text{ hours}\\
\tilde{A}_{BC}(2 \text{ to } 4 \text{ hours}) &= e^{-\lambda_E(2)}\, \tilde{A}_{BC}(0 \text{ to } 2 \text{ hours})\\
\tilde{A}_{BC}(4 \text{ to } 6 \text{ hours}) &= e^{-\lambda_E(4)}\, \tilde{A}_{BC}(0 \text{ to } 2 \text{ hours})\\
\tilde{A}_{BC}(6 \text{ to } 8 \text{ hours}) &= e^{-\lambda_E(6)}\, \tilde{A}_{BC}(0 \text{ to } 2 \text{ hours})
\end{aligned}$$

Substituting in the parameters yields the following results:

$$\begin{aligned}
\tilde{A}_{BC}(0 \text{ to } 2 \text{ hours}) &= A_{Body}(0) \cdot 0.434 \text{ hours}\\
\tilde{A}_{BC}(2 \text{ to } 4 \text{ hours}) &= A_{Body}(0) \cdot 0.081 \text{ hours}\\
\tilde{A}_{BC}(4 \text{ to } 6 \text{ hours}) &= A_{Body}(0) \cdot 0.015 \text{ hours}\\
\tilde{A}_{BC}(6 \text{ to } 8 \text{ hours}) &= A_{Body}(0) \cdot 0.0028 \text{ hours}
\end{aligned}$$

At this point, it can be reasonably assumed that successive voids would yield negligible contributions to the bladder wall dose. Consequently, the *total* cumulated activity in the bladder is

$$\tilde{A}_{BC} = (500\ \mu\text{Ci}) \cdot (0.434 + 0.081 + 0.015 + 0.0028 \text{ hours})$$

This yields an average dose to the urinary bladder wall of

$$\overline{D}_{BW} = (266.4\ \mu\text{Ci-hour})(1.8 \times 10^{-3} \text{ rad}/\mu\text{Ci-hour}) = 0.48 \text{ rad } (4.8 \text{ mGy})$$

Note that almost 82% of the absorbed dose was delivered to the bladder wall within the first 2 hours following administration (ie, during the first void interval).

EXTRAPOLATION OF ANIMAL DATA

As discussed, the biological parameters of absorption, distribution, metabolism, and excretion of radiolabeled compounds are often the most difficult to quantify. Before a new radiolabeled drug can be administered to humans, radiation dose to various organs of the body must be estimated. The estimates are usually based on biodistribution studies in some animal species. The data collected from laboratory animals on the distribution of an internally administered radionuclide may be presented by scientists in a variety of ways, not all of which are easy to comprehend. To improve the reader's comprehension and the value of the raw data, two rules should be followed when conducting animal biodistribution studies: (1) account for 100% of the administered radioactivity and (2) report data as fraction of administered activity per organ.[36]

Since the interpretation of data gathered is not straightforward, researchers have proposed different schemes for extrapolating data. Tissue concentrations in man can be extrapolated from those in animals directly or on the basis of percentage distribution. Each extrapolation may lead to substantial variations in the dose estimate. If concentrations (percent dose per gram) are used, then the data must be normalized by multiplying by the ratio of the organ weights or the whole-body weights.

Regardless of the extrapolation method chosen, a biodistribution animal study must be designed to meet several key criteria[37]:

1. The choice of animal must be appropriate to the study. For example, rats do not have a gallbladder; hence, they would not be useful in characterizing the dosimetry of hepatobiliary agents.
2. A sufficient number of animals must be studied to adequately characterize the variability of dose distribution. A minimum of three animals per time point is recommended.
3. All of the administered radioactivity must be accounted for. Both retention (in all major internal organs) and excretion (from all major routes) should be tabulated. Unless a compound is known to have only urinary excretion, both urine and feces should be collected throughout the study.
4. A sufficient number of measurements must be taken to characterize both early and late clearance phases. Initially, the length of the study should be based upon the physical half-life of the radionuclide.

SOFTWARE USED FOR DOSE CALCULATIONS

Mirdose

The Radiopharmaceutical Internal Dose Information Center of the Oak Ridge Associated Universities* has created a software package that allows the user to calculate internal radiation dose estimates using the MIRD schema. The program, known as "MIRDOSE," or the revised "MIRDOSE2," is written for IBM PC microcomputers in BASIC language.[38] MIRDOSE2 is interactive, and allows the user to choose from 24 source and 25 target organs in any combination for an adult or pediatric subject. Alternatively, the user may merely request a printed table of S factors.

In order to use MIRDOSE2, the user must have a working knowledge of the MIRD schema and the biologic parameters for the radiolabeled compound of interest. If the urinary bladder is chosen as a source organ, the program enables the user to enter a constant void interval (in hours) or to enter the residence time for the urinary bladder. Dose estimates are then printed for all target organs chosen, in both traditional and SI units, with the source organs responsible for the first and second highest contributions listed automatically for each target organ.

The SAAM Software System

A digital computer program, written in FORTRAN, was developed at the National Institutes of Health* to assist individuals in analyzing and testing mathematical models for biologic systems, in particular, kinetic models. The program, entitled SAAM[39,40] (Simulation, Analysis And Modeling), enables biomedical models to be solved in a batch or conversational mode; models solved in the conversational mode require the use of CONSAM.[41–43] CONSAM is an interactive version of the SAAM modeling program that allows the user to create, test, revise, and develop mathematical models for simulation and data fitting.

The current SAAM user community is estimated to be 2000 users, distributed at 500 sites around the world. A majority of users are in the fields of pharmacokinetics, lipid and lipoprotein metabolism, intermediary metabolism, and trace element and mineral metabolism.

*Radiopharmaceutical Internal Dose Information Center, Oak Ridge Associated Universities, P.O. Box 117, Oak Ridge, TN 37831-0117. Telephone: (615) 576-3448.

*For copies of the manuals or SAAM/CONSAM programs, contact Loren A. Zech, M.D., National Institutes of Health/NCI, Laboratory of Mathematical Biology, Building 10, Room 4B-56, Bethesda, MD 20892; telephone: (301) 496-8914.

CONCLUSION

Radiation absorbed dose estimates for patients undergoing the administration of radiopharmaceuticals can be easily *calculated* using the MIRD equations; however, it should be recognized that the accuracy of the dose estimates is highly dependent upon the biologic data used in the equations. Improved biologic data on the distribution and retention of radiopharmaceuticals in both normal and diseased patients is greatly needed. At present, in the absence of human biologic data, distribution and retention information obtained from animal studies is extrapolated and used for calculating absorbed doses for patients.

The proceedings of several symposia on radiopharmaceutical dosimetry contain the most current biologic information available on a variety of radiopharmaceuticals.[34,35,44,45] As new biological data are obtained, absorbed dose estimates can be revised to more accurately calculate the true absorbed dose to patients. Consequently, a cooperative effort between nuclear medicine departments and internal dosimetrists is required to collect much needed human biologic data. Use of this biologic data will ensure proper risk assessment and the continued safe use of radiopharmaceuticals in medicine.

REFERENCES

1. ICRU Report No. 33. Radiation Quantities and Units. Washington, DC, International Commission on Radiation Units and Measurements, 1980.
2. Robertson JS. Reconciliation of marinelli and MIRD radiation absorbed dose formulas. *Health Physics* 1981;40:565–568.
3. Code of Federal Regulations, Title 21—Food and Drugs, Part 361—Prescription Drugs for Human Use Generally Recognized as Safe and Effective and Not Misbranded: Drugs Used in Research (10 CFR 361). Washington, DC: Office of the Federal Register, 1987.
4. ICRP Publication 30 Part 1. *Limits for Intakes of Radionuclides by Workers*. Vol 2, Nos. 3, 4. The International Commission on Radiological Protection, New York: Pergamon Press, 1979.
5. ICRP Publication 53. *Radiation Dose to Patients from Radiopharmaceuticals*. Vol 18, Nos. 1–4. The International Commission on Radiological Protection, New York: Pergamon Press, 1988;4.
6. ICRP Publication 23. *Report of the Task Group on Reference*

Man. The International Commission on Radiological Protection, New York: Pergamon Press, 1975.
7. Snyder WS et al. Estimates of absorbed fractions for monoenergetic photon sources uniformly distributed in various organs of a heterogeneous phantom. NM/MIRD Pamphlet No. 3. *J Nucl Med* 1969;10:suppl 3.
8. Snyder WS et al. *A Tabulation of Dose Equivalent per Microcurie-Day for Source and Target Organs of an Adult for Various Radionuclides*. ORNL-5000. Springfield, VA: National Technical Information Service, 1974.
9. Poston JW. Reference man: a system for internal dose calculations. In: Till JE, Meyer RH, eds. *Radiological Assessment, A Textbook on Environmental Dose Analysis*. NUREG/CR-3332, ORNL-5968. US Nuclear Regulatory Commission, Springfield, VA: National Technical Information Service, 1983.
10. Cloutier RJ, Watson EE, Coffey JL. Radiopharmaceutical dose calculation, in Harbert J, da Rocha AFG, eds. *Textbook of Nuclear Medicine*. Vol 1. Philadelphia: Lea & Febiger, 1984;267–282.
11. Cristy M. *Mathematical Phantoms Representing Children of Various Ages for Use in Estimates of Internal Dose*. ORNL/NUREG/TM-367. Oak Ridge, TN: Oak Ridge National Laboratory, 1980.
12. Sikov MR, Traub RJ, Hui TE, et al. *Contribution of Maternal Radionuclide Burdens to Prenatal Radiation Doses*. NUREG/CR-5631, PNL-7445 (Rev 1). US Nuclear Regulatory Commission, Springfield, VA: National Technical Information Service, 1992.
13. Stabin M, Watson EE, Eckerman K, et al. *Calculation of Absorbed Dose for the Adult Female at Three, Six and Nine Months of Pregnancy*. Paper presented at the 36th Annual Health Physics Society, Washington, DC, 1991.
14. Loevinger R, Berman M. *A Revised Schema for Calculating the Absorbed Dose from Biologically Distributed Radionuclides*. NM/MIRD Pamphlet No. 1, Revised. New York: The Society of Nuclear Medicine, 1976.
15. Loevinger R, Budinger T, Watson E. *MIRD Primer for Absorbed Dose Calculations*. New York: The Society of Nuclear Medicine, 1988.
16. ICRU Report No. 32. *Methods of Assessment of Absorbed Dose in Clinical Use of Radionuclides*. Washington, DC: International Commission on Radiation Units and Measurements, 1979.
17. NCRP Report No. 70. *Nuclear Medicine—Factors Influencing the Choice and Use of Radionuclides in Diagnosis and Therapy*. Bethesda, MD: National Council on Radiation Protection and Measurements, 1982.
18. Robertson J. Radiation absorbed dose calculations in diagnostic nuclear medicine. *Int J Appl Rad Isot* 1982;33:981.
19. NCRP Report No. 83. *The Experimental Basis for Absorbed Dose Calculations in Medical Uses of Radionuclides*. Bethesda, MD: National Council on Radiation Protection and Measurements, 1985.
20. NCRP Report No. 84. *General Concepts for the Dosimetry of Internally Deposited Radionuclides*. Bethesda MD: National Council on Radiation Protection and Measurements, 1985.
21. Berman M. *Kinetic Models for Absorbed Dose Calculations*. NM/MIRD Pamphlet No. 12. New York: The Society of Nuclear Medicine, 1976.
22. Thomas S et al. *A Dynamic Urinary Bladder Model for Radiation Dose Calculations*. Oak Ridge, TN: Oak Ridge Associated Universities, 1991.
23. Smith T et al. Dosimetry of renal radiopharmaceuticals: the importance of bladder radioactivity and a simple aid for its estimation. *Br J Radiol*, 1981;54:961–965.
24. Smith T et al. Bladder wall dose from administered radiopharmaceuticals: the effects of variations in urine flow rate, voiding interval and initial bladder content. *Rad Prot Dosimetry* 1982; 2(3):183–189.
25. Snyder WS et al. *"S", Absorbed Dose per Unit Cumulated Activity for Selected Radionuclides and Organs*. NM/MIRD Pamphlet No. 11. New York: The Society of Nuclear Medicine, 1975.
26. Dillman LT. *Radionuclide decay schemes and nuclear parameters for use in radiation—dose estimation. J Nucl Med*. NM/MIRD Pamphlet No. 4, 1969;10(suppl 2).
27. Dillman LT. *Radionuclide decay schemes and nuclear parameters for use in radiation—dose estimation. J Nucl Med*. NM/MIRD Pamphlet No. 6, 1970;11(suppl 4).
28. Dillman LT, Von der Lage FC. *Radionuclide Decay Schemes and Nuclear Parameters for Use in Radiation—Dose Estimation*. NM/MIRD Pamphlet No. 10. New York: The Society of Nuclear Medicine, 1975.
29. Kocher DC. *Radioactive Decay Data Tables*. A Handbook of Decay Data for Application to Radiation Dosimetry and Radiological Assessments, US Department of Energy Technical Information Center, DOE/TIC-11026, Springfield VA: National Technical Information Service, 1981.
30. Snyder WS et al. Estimates of absorbed fractions for monoenergetic photon sources uniformly distributed in various organs of a heterogeneous phantom. *J Nucl Med* NM/MIRD Pamphlet No. 5, 1969;10(suppl 3).
31. Brownell GL et al. Absorbed fractions for photon dosimetry. *J Nucl Med*, NM/MIRD Pamphlet No. 3, 1968;9(suppl 1).
32. Ellett WH, Humes RM. Absorbed fractions for small volumes containing photon-emitting radioactivity. *J Nucl Med*. NM/MIRD Pamphlet No. 8, 1971;12(suppl 5).
33. Loevinger R et al. Discrete radioisotope sources. In: Hine G, Brownell G, eds. *Radiation Dosimetry*. New York: Academic Press, 1956;693–765.
34. Roedler HD, Kaul A. Dose to target organs from remaining body activity: results of the formally exact and approximate solution. In: *Radiopharmaceutical Dosimetry Symposium*. HEW Publication (FDA) 76-8044, 1976.
35. Roedler HD. Accuracy of internal dose calculations with special consideration of radiopharmaceutical biokinetics. In: *Third International Radiopharmaceutical Dosimetry Symposium*. HEW Publication (FDA) 81-8166, 1981.
36. Lathrop KA. Collection and presentation of animal data relating to internally distributed radionuclides. In: *Third International Radiopharmaceutical Dosimetry Symposium*. HEW Publication (FDA) 81-8166, 1981;198–203.
37. Stabin M. *Radiation Dosimetry and Predictive Value of Preclinical Models*. Lecture presented at the National Institutes of Health, Bethesda, MD, 1991.
38. Watson E, Stabin M, Bolch W. "MIRDOSE", Oak Ridge, TN: Oak Ridge Associated Universities, 1984.
39. Berman M, Shahn E, Weiss MF. The routine fitting of kinetic data to models: a mathematical formalism for digital computers. *Biophysics J* 1962;2:275–287.
40. Berman M, Weiss MF. *SAAM Manual*. HEW Publication (NIH) 78-810, 1978.
41. Foster DM, Boston RC. The use of computers in compartmental analysis: the SAAM and CONSAM programs. In: Robertson J, ed. *Compartmental Distribution of Radiotracers*. Boca Raton, FL: CRC Press, 1983.

42. Boston RC, Greif PC, Berman M. CONSAM (conversational version of the SAAM modeling program). In: Berman et al, eds, *Lipoprotein Kinetics and Modeling*. New York: Academic Press, 1982.
43. Boston RC, Greif PC, Berman M. Conversational SAAM—an interactive program for kinetic analysis of biological systems. *Computer Prog Biomed* 1981;13:111–119.
44. Cloutier RJ, Edwards CL, Snyder WS, eds. *Medical Radionuclides: Radiation Dose and Effects*. CONF-691212, USAEC Symposium Series 20. Springfield, VA: National Technical Information Service, 1970.
45. Schlafke-Stelson AT, Watson EE, eds. *Fourth International Radiopharmaceutical Dosimetry Symposium*. CONF-851113, Springfield, VA: National Technical Information Service, 1986.

13 Radiation Effects in Nuclear Medicine

John D. Boice, Jr.

HISTORICAL BACKGROUND

The age of radiation began in 1895 when Roentgen announced the discovery of "a new kind of ray" that could penetrate the human body and reveal broken bones. The first radiograph was taken in January 1896, the same year that Becquerel discovered the natural radioactivity of uranium. In 1901, the first harmful effect of radiation was reported: a nasty skin burn was attributed to a vial of radium, obtained from Madame Curie, and carried in Becquerel's vest pocket. The first radiation-induced skin cancer was reported in 1902 on the hand of a roentgenologist. In the 1920s, bone cancer was linked to ingesting large quantities of radium in women who painted dials on watches and clocks. In the 1930s, Thorotrast, a colloid solution of thorium dioxide, was commonly used as a diagnostic contrast agent, particularly for cerebral angiography. Thorotrast remains in the body, and has resulted in liver cancer and leukemia. Artificial radioactivity was discovered in 1934 by Irène and Frédéric Joliot. Artificial radioactive tracers of biological importance were then produced by E.O. Lawrence, who invented the cyclotron in the 1930s. The "father of nuclear medicine," George Charles de Hevesy—a Hungarian chemist, obtained ^{32}P from Lawrence for use in metabolic studies. Therapeutic nuclear medicine began shortly thereafter when ^{32}P was used by John Lawrence to treat leukemia. Iodine-131 was synthesized in 1938 by Seaborg and Livingood, the same year that ^{99m}Tc was isolated by Segrè and Seaborg. The first reports of excess leukemia among radiologists appeared in the 1940s, and excess cancers attributable to medical radiation were reported in analytic studies in the 1950s. The studies of Japanese bomb survivors began in 1950, and have formed the basis of radiation protection guidelines ever since.[1–5,55]

BASIC CONCEPTS

Energy emitted from a source is generally referred to as radiation. Examples include heat or light from the sun, microwaves from an oven, x-rays from an x-ray tube, or gamma rays from radioactive elements. Radiation that can remove electrons from atoms is called *ionizing* and includes electromagnetic rays such as x- and gamma rays and energetic particles such as protons, fission nuclei, and alpha and beta particles. Neutrons, unlike these other particles, have no charge and cannot ionize directly. Instead they impart energy to protons through elastic collisions, and the protons cause subsequent ionizations. Another way in which energy can be released in tissue is by *excitation* where electrons are merely raised to a higher energy level within an atom but are not removed. The total amount of energy absorbed in matter as a result of radiation interactions is called the dose, which is measured in gray (Gy): 1 Gy = 1 J/kg. Until recently the standard unit for dose was the rad (1 rad = 100 ergs/g), but the conversion is simple: 1 Gy = 100 rad = 100 cGy. An acute whole-body dose of about 5 Gy (500 rad) is lethal about half of the time in humans; yet this dose ionizes only about 1 of every 40 million molecules. Permanent damage thus can be produced after a relatively small amount of energy is absorbed.

Radiation is absorbed randomly by atoms and molecules in cells and can alter molecular structure. These alterations can be amplified by biologic processes to result in observable effects. The biologic effects, however, depend not only on the total absorbed dose but also on the linear energy transfer (LET), or ionization density, of the type of radiation. LET is a measure of the energy loss per unit distance traveled and depends on the velocity, charge, and mass of a particle or on x- or gamma-ray energy. High-LET radiations such as alpha particles (helium nuclei) release energy in short tracks of dense ionizations. Low-LET, or sparsely ionizing, radiations such as gamma rays produce ionizing events that are not close together. Depending on the biologic endpoint, the effect per gray may differ widely as a function of LET but is usually greater for high-LET radiation.

The relative biologic effectiveness (RBE) of radiation characterizes its ability to produce a specific disorder (eg, cell death, cancer, or chromosome aberration) compared to a standard, usually x- or gamma rays. An RBE of 20 for alpha particles at 10 cGy, for example, would imply that the biologic effect from 10 cGy of alpha particles is the same as that from 200 cGy of gamma rays. The unit of biologic dose equivalence used in radiologic protection is the sievert (Sv), which has replaced the rem (1 Sv = 100 rem). The sievert represents the absorbed dose in grays multiplied by a quality factor (specific to the type of radiation) and other possible modifying factors. The sievert has also been applied to assess the effects of mixed field exposures. For example, the dose equivalence of an exposure to 10 cGy of gamma

Table 1. Radiation Effects on Some Key Cellular Molecules

MOLECULE	RADIATION EFFECT	POSSIBLE CELLULAR EFFECT
DNA	Disruption of linear arrangement of bases by base substitution, deletion, or addition; cross linking; single-strand break; double-strand break	Temporary or permanent inhibition of DNA synthesis; synthesis of incorrect DNA; inhibition or prevention of mitosis; synthesis of incorrect protein
Enzymes	Alteration in tertiary structure of molecule because of disruption of chemical bonds	Inhibition of enzymatic activity with resultant changes in cellular metabolism
Structural lipids composing cell membranes	Disruption of molecular bonds	Increased permeability to K^+, Na^+, etc., with resultant alteration in normal intracellular/extracellular environment

From Mossman.[76]

rays plus 10 cGy of alpha particles, with gamma rays as the standard and an RBE of 20 for alpha particles, would be 2.1 Sv (210 rem).

Mechanisms of Cellular Damage

Cellular damage depends on the type of radiation, the amount of energy deposited per volume of tissue, the rate at which the energy is deposited, the way in which the energy is distributed throughout the tissue of interest, and the amount of fractionation or splitting of the dose.[1]

Chemical changes in cells are brought about in two ways, either directly or indirectly. Radiation energy can be deposited directly within cellular molecules to alter biologic function, or it can interact with nearby molecules, usually water, to produce highly reactive ions and free radicals that then damage the biologically important macromolecules (indirect action). Ionizing events that occur in water, the most common substance in the body, can create highly reactive ions and free radicals such as H^+, $OH^\bullet$, and OH^-. The radiolysis of water occurs within microseconds and the ionization products, including H_2O_2, can interact with both the base and sugar components of DNA, as well as other cellular molecules, to bring about change (Table 1).

The physical properties of radiation have been used to describe how the transfer of energy at the cellular level might cause biological damage.[1] Essentially, it is postulated that sublesions are produced within cells at a rate proportional to the energy deposited, and a biologic effect results if two sublesions occur close enough in both time and space. The double-strand DNA molecule, essential for cellular replication, is thought to be the critical target for radiation-induced damage. For high-LET radiation, such as neutrons or alpha particles, the concentration of transferred energy is such that both sublesions are usually produced by one track or "hit," implying a biologic response proportional to dose, ie, a linear response.

For sparsely ionizing low-LET radiation, ionizations and any consequent sublesions will usually be distributed uniformly throughout the cell. The occurrence of two sublesions close together would be rare, with probability approximately proportional to the square of the dose, D^2, that is, two hits are required and a quadratic response would be expected. Low-LET radiation, however, is thought to have a high-LET component at the end of each track whose biologic effect should be proportional to dose.

For low-LET radiation, a general equation for biologic effect is

$$I = c + aD + bD^2$$

where I is the incidence of the effect, c is the spontaneous rate, D is the radiation dose, and a and b are positive constants. This model appears to fit a wide range of studies on the induction of chromosome aberrations, point mutations, and other radiation effects on single cells, and some carcinogenic studies in animals. In the past, this linear-quadratic model has been used to derive risk estimates from human studies for most cancers, except for the breast and thyroid, for which a linear relationship is used.[6] Recently, analyses of atomic bomb survivor data found little reason to reject linearity for most cancers except leukemia.[1]

A further modification can be made to account for the possible competing effects of cell killing or inactivation at high doses which can prevent cell division or function[1]:

$$I = (c + aD + bD^2)exp(-pD - qD^2)$$

where the exponential term, which predominates at high doses, corresponds to a decrease in incidence after some maximal value is reached. For low-LET radiation, the linear term predominates at very low doses, the quadratic at higher doses, and the exponential at very high doses. Cellular and tissue effects of very high doses are discussed more fully in later sections.

When exposures are protracted or separated in time, the contributions of D^2 become less and less important for both cancer induction and cell killing. It is generally found in experimental settings that lengthening the time over which a dose is delivered reduces the amount of cellular damage and cancer induction from low-LET radiations.[7,8] To estimate risks for persons exposed at low dose rates, various committees have recommended that a dose rate effectiveness factor (DREF) of between 2 and 10 should be used to scale down risk coefficients obtained from studies of acute exposure.[2] Except for leukemia, a DREF was not incorporated in risk

Table 2. Average Annual Effective Dose of Ionizing Radiation to US Citizens[1]

SOURCE	DOSE (mSv)
Natural sources	
Radon	2.0 (mainly lung)
Cosmic, terrestrial, internal	1.0
Medical	
x-ray diagnosis	0.39
Nuclear medicine	0.14
Consumer products	~0.1
Occupational	<0.01
Miscellaneous environmental sources	<0.001
Nuclear fuel cycle	<0.001
Total	1.6 (excluding radon)

1 mSv = 0.1 rem.

models employed by the BEIR V committee, although a preference for a value of about 2 was expressed.[1]

In experimental studies the induction of cancer by exposure to high-LET radiation has generally appeared to follow a linear dose response. Moreover, protraction and fractionation of dose from high-LET radiation tend not to decrease cancer risk but rather, especially at higher dose levels, to increase it somewhat because of a reduction in the competing effect of cell killing.[8] Recent studies suggest that this enhancement of risk at lower dose rates may also be at levels where cellular killing is minimal.

Sources of Exposure (Table 2)

Background radiation from natural sources contributes the most to population exposure, about 2.9 mSv/y (0.29 rem).[1,2] These sources include cosmic rays (0.27 mSv/y), which vary by altitude; terrestrial radiations (0.28 mSv/y), which vary according to the distribution in soil of radioactive elements such as uranium; internally deposited radionuclides (0.39 mSv/y) such as ^{40}K; and radon (2.0 mSv/y confined mainly to lung). The greatest source of man-made radiation is from medical procedures (0.53 mSv/y), with exposures increasing directly with patient age. Nuclear medicine procedures are estimated to contribute 0.14 mSv/y. Occupation, nuclear power, fallout from testing nuclear weapons, and consumer products make only a minor contribution (0.11 mSv/y). The average per capita dose from all sources of radiation, excluding radon, is thus about 1.6 mSv (0.160 rem) per year. Some individuals in the population, however, can experience much higher exposures such as cancer patients treated with radiation (Table 3).

CARCINOGENIC EFFECTS

In the 1950s, concern about excessive exposure to ionizing radiation centered mainly on the possibility of genetic effects, ie, changes in the germ cells of parents that would be passed on to their children. Large-scale studies of the children of the atomic bomb survivors in Japan, however, have revealed no apparent genetic alterations,[9] while the survivors themselves have developed various cancers in excess of expectation. On the basis of Japanese survivor studies, continuous lifetime exposure of 100,000 persons to 1 mSv/y has been estimated to induce about 65 leukemias, and 495 fatal cancers of other sites.[1] If true, then 3 to 5% of all cancers might be attributable to all sources of radiation exposure (1.6 mSv/y), excluding indoor radon which has been suggested as an important cause of lung cancer.[10] Estimates of lifetime cancer risks are presented in Table 4 for acute whole-body exposures of 1 Gy. While radiation has clearly been found to cause cancer and other harmful effects in man, there remain substantial uncertainties as to the level of risk from low doses and dose rates. At doses under about 10 cGy, the risks appear too low to be detected and extrapolations from high-dose studies are performed to estimate possible risks.

The activation of cellular protooncogenes, the so-called cancer genes found in normal cells that can exhibit transforming activity, and the inactivation of cellular tumor suppressor genes have been proposed as possible mechanisms by which radiation causes cancer.[1,11,12] Recently, ultraviolet light was found to cause human squamous cell cancer of the skin by inducing mutations at pyrimidine dimers in skin-cell p53 genes which prevent the gene from suppressing tumor growth.[13] Lung cancer tissue from underground uranium miners has also been shown to contain a rather unique mutational spectrum in the p53 tumor suppressor gene that might be characteristic of high levels of radon exposure.[14,15] Cancer apparently results after the accumulation of mutations in several oncogenes and suppressor genes. It is provocative to speculate that radiation, as well as other environmental carcinogens, may induce characteristic mutations in certain genes that are responsible for the initiation or progression of cancers.

RADIONUCLIDES IN MEDICINE

Therapeutic ^{131}I

Radioactive iodine has been commonly used in nuclear medicine since the 1940s for diagnostic and therapeutic purposes. Despite widespread patient exposure, few cancers have been convincingly linked to ^{131}I. Leukemia was not excessive in two large series of patients treated with ^{131}I for hyperthyroidism in the United States and Sweden.[16–18] Excess cancer of organs such as the bladder that concentrate iodine[19] and of the breast[20] have been reported in some studies, but not confirmed in larger series.[17] A modest increase in stomach and kidney cancer was suggested in one study.[21] Thyroid cancer has not been correlated with ^{131}I therapy, possibly because of the cellular destruction and loss of thyroid function that follows a dose of 60 to 100 Gy to the thyroid.[22]

Patients with thyroid cancer treated with ^{131}I experience relatively large exposures, on the order of 50 to 100 cGy to bone marrow and other organs. Exposures for metastatic

Table 3. Radiation Exposure in Man

SOURCE	POPULATION EXPOSED	DURATION OF EXPOSURE	EXPOSURE CONDITIONS	RADIATION EFFECTS
Medical radiodiagnosis (including nuclear medicine)	200 million/y	Intermittent throughout life	Low dose to part of body (~1 cGy)	Mutations? Cancer? In utero effects?
Natural background radiation	Entire population	Throughout life	Low dose to whole body (0.1 cGy/y)	Mutations? Cancer? In utero effects?
Radiotherapy	600,000/y	2 mo	High dose to part of body (>1,000 cGy)	Tumor control; normal tissue effects
Radiation accidents; military activities	Tens of thousands may be exposed	Seconds to days	High dose to whole body (doses vary widely)	Normal tissue dysfunction; death

From Mossman.[76]

disease can be much higher. Among 258 persons treated with high-dose ^{131}I for inoperable thyroid cancer, 4 leukemias were observed vs 0.08 expected based on general population rates; an excess of bladder cancer was also suggested.[23] In a recent Swedish study, slight excesses of leukemia (4 vs 1.6) and cancers of the kidney and salivary glands were reported among 834 patients with thyroid cancer treated with an average of 123 mCi (4551 MBq) of ^{131}I.[24]

Diagnostic ^{131}I

Among 35,074 Swedish patients given diagnostic doses of ^{131}I, primarily for scans, no increase in the incidence of any cancer was observed.[21] The dose to the thyroid was 50 cGy so that a substantial excess of thyroid cancer might have been expected based on data from other studies of brief exposures to x- or gamma rays.[25] The absence of an effect supports the notion that internal ^{131}I beta particles may be less carcinogenic than external x- or gamma rays, perhaps due to the protracted nature of the exposure (half-life = 8 days) or to the distribution of dose within the gland from ^{131}I.

Table 4. Estimates of Lifetime Cancer Risks Based on UNSCEAR and BEIR[1]

CANCER	CANCER DEATHS (PER 10^4 PERSONS PER GRAY)
Leukemia	85
Lung	100
Breast	20
Thyroid	10
Bone	5
Subtotal	220
Remainder	
GI Tract	150
Ovary	15
Bladder	30
Multiple myeloma	15
Skin	2
Other	63
Subtotal	280
Total	500

From Upton.[77]

^{224}Ra

In the 1940s ^{224}Ra was used to treat bone tuberculosis and ankylosing spondylitis in Germany. The half-time of ^{224}Ra is just a few days and most of the energy from alpha-particle emissions is deposited on bone surfaces, resulting in high rates of osteosarcoma.[26] Interestingly, protracted exposure to radium alpha particles appeared more carcinogenic than brief exposures. This "protraction enhancement" from alpha-emitting radiation might be related to less killing of premalignant cells, exposing more cells, increasing the stimulus for cell division, and/or preventing repair of local damage.

Radium dial painters who ingested large quantities of ^{226}Ra and ^{228}Ra experienced a bone cancer risk that was ten times lower than these German patients.[27] Different distributions of the release of energy in the bone has been suggested as the reason for this difference in risk. ^{224}Ra has a short half-life (3.62 days) and releases its energy on bone surfaces where the "critical" cells for osteosarcoma induction, the endosteal cells, are located. In contrast, ^{226}Ra is a bone-volume seeker with a very long half-life (1600 years), and distributes its energy more uniformly throughout the bone, the dose to the bone matrix being essentially irrelevant to cancer risk. For the same average bone dose, the risk from ^{224}Ra will always be greater than that from ^{226}Ra because more radiation will reach the endosteal cells.

^{32}P

^{32}P has been used to treat polycythemia vera (PV), a blood disease characterized by overproduction of red cells, and excess leukemias have arisen.[28] In a randomized clinical trial it was found that 9 of 156 (6%) patients treated with ^{32}P developed leukemia in contrast to 1 of 134 (1%) treated by phlebotomy.[29] Patients treated with chlorambucil were at highest risk (11%).

Thorotrast

Thorotrast, a colloidal solution of thorium dioxide, was used between 1928 and 1955 as a contrast agent during radiographic procedures, particularly cerebral angiography. Thorium remained in body tissue essentially for life and results in continuous alpha-particle exposure at a low-dose rate. The annual dose from a typical injection of 25 mL of Thorotrast was 25 cGy to liver and 16 cGy to bone marrow. Surveys in Denmark, Germany, Japan, and Portugal show substantial excesses of liver cancer, including angiosarcoma and cholangiocarcinoma, and acute myeloid leukemia.[10,30] Hemangioendothelioma of the liver appears uniquely related to Thorotrast. Excess lung cancer has been reported in some series, suggesting a possible effect of exhaled thoron (^{220}Rn).[31]

The nonuniform deposition of thorium in the liver likely resulted in very high local doses, which may be the important determinant of cancer risk.[32] The chemical nature of thorium, a heavy metal, also may be related to risk as might the combination of necrosis and liver regeneration. On the other hand, radiant energy expended in necrotic tissue probably contributed little to carcinogenesis. Although Thorotrast has not been used for about 40 years, its legacy remains. Thorotrast appears to be one of the most carcinogenic exposures known to man, with cumulative lifetime incidences of cancer estimated to be as high as 60%.

OCCUPATIONAL EXPOSURE

Radiologists

Skin cancer on the hand of a radiologist in 1902 was the first malignancy attributed to radiation.[1,33] In the 1940s, radiologists were first reported to be at high risk for leukemia, possibly due to chronic occupational exposures. Leukemia, aplastic anemia, and skin cancer were excessive among radiologists who practiced during the early part of this century before radiation protection guidelines were in use, but these risks appear to have disappeared among more recent radiologists. Multiple myeloma was increased among US radiologists practicing in later years, but not among English or Chinese radiologists. Cancers of the pancreas and lung were increased among the pioneering radiologists in the United Kingdom, but not in the United States or China. Suggested increases of breast, thyroid, and bone cancers were correlated with radiation work in China only.[34] Neither leukemia nor cancer was reported to be in excess among US Army x-ray technologists, who likely received much lower total doses. A new survey of 145,000 x-ray technologists in the United States may in the future be able to evaluate risks more precisely,[33] although breast cancer appears unrelated to radiation work in this series.[33A]

The absence of radiation dose estimates is a serious limitation of these studies. Cumulative doses were likely between 1 and 8 Gy during the early part of this century, and it is possible that radiologists who developed cancer were those who scorned safety measures and received even greater doses. It was not uncommon for x-ray workers to be given time off from work because of severe depression of white blood cell counts. Radiologists also receive more personal (nonoccupational) exposures to diagnostic and therapeutic radiation than other specialists.

Radium Dial and Clock Painters

Women who painted watch dials and clocks with radium prior to 1930 would lick their brushes and ingest large quantities of radium. They subsequently developed bone sarcomas and head carcinomas at a high rates.[27,35] The average dose to bone from ^{226}Ra and ^{228}Ra was 1700 cGy. Cancers in mastoid air cells or paranasal sinuses (head carcinomas) likely were caused by radon gas emitted as a decay product of radium. No excess of leukemia was observed among US or English radium luminizers.[36] Early reports linking breast cancer with radium or external gamma-ray exposures were not confirmed. Multiple myeloma was increased in the US study, but correlated with duration of employment (a surrogate for gamma-ray exposure) rather than radium intake. Liver cancer was not increased. The British study reported only 1 osteosarcoma, but the systemic intake of radium was much lower than for the United States.

Other Radiation Workers

Except for studies of underground miners who are at high risk of lung cancer,[10,37] studies of radiation workers in the nuclear industry are generally inconsistent.[1,38] Workers at US nuclear facilities were at significantly low risk of leukemia,[39] whereas workers in the United Kingdom were at significantly high risk.[40] Compared to the general population, both groups were at significantly low risk for dying of cancer overall. Multiple myeloma was recently found to be no longer significantly increased among Hanford workers in the United States. Early reports of excess cancer among naval nuclear shipyard workers have not been confirmed. Workers exposed to plutonium, thought at one time to be extremely toxic, have not been found to be at increased cancer risk.[41]

ENVIRONMENTAL EXPOSURES TO RADIONUCLIDES

Environmental exposures due to natural background radiation or to man-made contamination have not been convincingly linked to increases in cancer risk.[1,38] Indoor radon levels in some homes are quite high and should be reduced, but epidemiologic surveys have not convincingly linked lung cancer with indoor radon exposures.[42,43,43A] Although exposures in underground mines have been clearly linked to lung cancer, the relevance of such studies to indoor radon situations has been questioned because miners were also exposed to cigarette smoke, silica dust, diesel and blast fumes, arsenic, and other carcinogenic or lung irritants that could potentiate the effect of radon exposures.[44] Analytic studies of populations residing in areas of high background radiation, due to thorium-containing sands, have also failed to detect evidence of excess cancers, although chromosomal damage in circulating lymphocytes has been found.[45]

Children living near nuclear reactor installations in the United Kingdom,[46] but not in the United States[47] or other countries, have been reported to be at increased risk of developing leukemia. Although environmental contamination from reactor releases appears to be ruled out as a probable cause for the small clusters of leukemia seen in the United Kingdom, paternal occupational exposures to radiation prior to conception[48] and viral exposures[49] have been suggested as possible alternative causes. Paternal exposure to radiation, however, no longer appears a viable hypothesis to explain the small clusters of childhood leukemia.[50] Childhood leukemia has not been associated with fallout from the Chernobyl reactor accident,[51] nor has thyroid nodularity.[52] Such studies, however, may be too early to detect any radiation effects from the Chernobyl accident, and there are problems with accurately assessing radiation doses experienced by the surrounding populations.

MEDICAL X-RAY EXPOSURES

The possible contribution of diagnostic radiology to the overall cancer burden in our society appears small in comparison with other causes, and only a few studies have reported increased risks.[1,2,38] Women with tuberculosis who received frequent (well over 50) x-ray fluoroscopy examinations of the chest in the 1940s, for example, were found to be at increased risk of breast cancer, but not lung cancer or leukemia. Exposures after the age of 40 carried no detectable increase in breast cancer risk which was encouraging in light of recommendations for mammographic x-ray screening programs to detect early breast cancers among asymptomatic women at these and older ages.[53] Prenatal x-ray has been linked to increases in childhood cancer,[8] although the absence of a similar effect in atomic bomb survivors exposed in utero[54] and in all prospective studies[55] suggests that the fetus may not be overly sensitive to the carcinogenic action of radiation. General diagnostic radiation has not been convincingly linked to adult leukemia.[56]

Studies of patients treated with radiation have provided quantitative information on risk because of the ability to estimate accurately dose to organs (Table 5). British patients treated with radiation for ankylosing spondylitics were at high risk for developing leukemia and other cancers, especially lung cancer. Women irradiated for benign breast conditions were at high risk for subsequent breast cancer. Children given radiotherapy for benign head and neck conditions develop thyroid cancer at a high rate. Women treated for excessive uterine bleeding are at increased risk of leukemia and other pelvic tumors. Radiotherapy for peptic ulcer resulted in stomach cancer in later life.[1,2,33,55,57]

Table 5. Populations Studied for Cancer Development after Radiation Exposure[1,2,33,55]

EXPOSED POPULATION	EXCESS CANCERS
Military	
Japanese A-bomb survivors	Leukemia, lung, breast, thyroid, stomach, other
Marshall Islanders (fallout)	Thyroid
Radionuclides in medicine	
Spondylitis and bone TB (^{224}Ra)	Bone
Polycythemia vera (^{32}P)	Leukemia
Thorotrast (^{232}Th)	Liver, leukemia
Occupation	
Radium dial painters (^{226}Ra)	Bone
Underground miners (^{222}Rn)	Lung
Pioneering radiologists	Leukemia, skin
Diagnostic radiography	
Tuberculosis patients (fluoroscopy)	Breast
Prenatal x-ray	Leukemia
Radiotherapy	
Ankylosing spondylitis	Leukemia, lung, stomach, other
Benign breast disease	Breast
Tinea capitis	Thyroid, brain, skin
Thymus enlargement	Thyroid
Cervical cancer	Leukemia, bladder, rectum, other
Childhood cancer	Bone, thyroid

Radiotherapy for cervical cancer has been linked to small increases in leukemia; the relatively low risk observed, however, was attributed to the predominance of cell killing over transformation that occurs at therapeutic doses. Breast cancer patients treated with radiotherapy were at increased risk of leukemia, especially if systemic chemotherapy was also administered.[58] A small risk of contralateral breast cancer exists after radiotherapy for breast cancer but only among patients irradiated under age 45.[59] Patients with Hodgkin's disease are at increased risk of cancers of the breast, lung, and other tumors following radiotherapy. Children given radiotherapy develop second cancers of the bone, thyroid, brain, and other tumors in excess of expectation.[55]

EXPOSURES FROM ATOMIC AND THERMONUCLEAR WEAPONS

Japanese Atomic Bomb Survivors

The atomic bomb survivor studies provide an important human experience from which estimates of radiation risk can be derived.[1,60] The population is large, over 100,000, and not selected because of disease or occupation. Leukemia has one of the highest relative risk (RR) coefficients and one of the shortest times to onset, with the minimum latency of about 2 years. At 1 Gy whole body exposure, a RR of 6.21 is estimated, whereas it is 1.41 for all other cancers combined. No diagnoses of chronic lymphocytic leukemia have been made. The risk of CML was high, and the wave-like response over time was quite evident. The dose response for breast cancer incidence was linear; all major types of lung cancer have occurred in excess; significant excesses of papillary and follicular carcinoma of the thyroid, but not medullary or anaplastic cancer have been reported. Recent incidence data provide little evidence for a thyroid cancer excess following exposures in adult life.[60A] Increased deaths were reported for cancers of the esophagus, stomach, colon, lung, breast, ovary, and urinary bladder. Multiple myeloma but not malignant lymphoma was excessive. No excesses were seen for cancers of the rectum, gallbladder, pancreas, liver, uterus, bone, oral cavity and pharynx, nasal passages, or larynx. The minimal latent period for radiogenic cancers other than leukemia was about 10 years. Relative and absolute risks differed significantly by age at exposure, with younger survivors having somewhat higher risks.

Weapons Testing

Natives of four inhabited atolls east of Bikini Island were accidentally exposed to nuclear fallout in 1954.[1,59] Most of the exposure was to radioactive iodines and external gamma rays. Thyroid nodularity and cancer have occurred in excess. Most beta-particle energy from ^{131}I is supposedly deposited in the colloid of the large follicles without reaching the critical follicular cells, and the low dose rate would tend to minimize risk. In contrast, the shorter-lived and more energetic isotopes (^{132}I, ^{133}I, and ^{135}I) contributed two to three times the dose of ^{131}I, and more uniformly exposed the thyroid at a higher dose rate. A study of 7000 Marshall Islanders from 14 atolls revealed a linear relationship between thyroid nodules and proximity to Bikini.[61]

Among children exposed to fallout from nuclear weapons tests at the Nevada Test Site in the 1950s, there was little to no suggestion of increased thyroid neoplasm.[62] Assuming that ^{131}I was concentrated in milk and subsequently drunk by children, the thyroid dose was estimated to be between 30 to 240 cGy (mean, 120 cGy). An excess of 73 to 100 thyroid nodules at these doses would have been expected based on radiation risk estimates from studies of x-irradiation in childhood. A weak association between estimated bone marrow dose and leukemia, however, was reported.[63] Childhood leukemia was not convincingly linked to fallout from Soviet nuclear weapons tests.[64]

GENETIC EFFECTS

The perception of radiation hazards has shifted dramatically during the past 40 years from concern over possible genetic effects on future generations to somatic effects on the individual exposed[1,5,8] The genetic effects of radiation were first demonstrated by Muller in 1927 in experiments with the fruit fly *Drosophila*. Doses of tens of grays were used because insects are more resistant to radiation than mammals. The dose response was linear and the estimate of doubling dose, ie, the dose required to double the natural or spontaneous level of mutations in the next generation, was 5 cGy, a very low level. Further, spreading the dose over time did not result in a reduction in mutations, suggesting that radiation damage to the germ cells was permanent and cumulative.

Fortunately the genetic material of mammals was found to be much more robust than that of the fruit fly, most likely because of effective repair mechanisms that correct cellular damage caused by radiation. After World War II, the "mega-mice" experiments of Russell and colleagues modified our understanding of genetic effects.[1,5,8] The doubling dose was determined to be much higher than previously thought, spreading dose over time substantially reduced the genetic effect (approaching zero for the females), males were more sensitive than females, different genetic effects could have doubling doses that differed widely, radiation damage was not cumulative, and the number of mutations decreased significantly if the time between radiation and conception was increased.

The experimental studies provided clear evidence that radiation can cause changes in the genes and chromosomes of reproductive cells that are passed on to succeeding generations. However, despite extensive evaluations of the children of the atomic bomb survivors over the past 45 years, not a single inherited mutational change has been attributed to parental exposure.[9] Over 31,000 children born to exposed parents and 41,000 children of unexposed parents were compared with regard to 8 indicators of genetic damage, including stillbirths and congenital malformations, total mortality, cancer incidence, chromosome abnormalities, sex-chromosome aneuploidy, changes in blood proteins, sex ratio among children of exposed mothers, and growth and development. No significant differences in any of these measures were found, leading to the conclusion that humans must be much less sensitive to the genetic effects of radiation than previously thought based on animal experiments.[9] However, it should not be assumed that no heritable effects result from gonadal exposures, just that the dose to cause a detectable effect must be high. It is currently estimated that, for acute exposures in humans, about 2 Gy would be required to double the rate of mutations in the next generation. For chronic exposures the estimate of doubling dose is about 4 Gy.

The studies of atomic bomb survivors and laboratory experiments thus provide guidance for practical genetic counseling following exposure to radiopharmaceuticals.[5] If substantial gonadal exposures occur, any planned conception should be delayed for about 6 months to minimize the possible genetic impact. Tables published by the ICRP and others can be used to estimate radiation dose to germ cells for practically all nuclear medicine procedures.[65,66] For example, 13.6 mCi (505 MBq) of ^{131}I administered to treat hyperthyroidism would result in an ovarian dose of 2.1 cGy and a testicular dose of 0.8 cGy, assuming a 45% thyroid uptake. Such computations indicate that nuclear medicine procedures must contribute only a negligible portion of the *genetically significant dose* (GSD) to the population. The GSD is an index of presumed genetic impact of radiation that adjusts for the reproductive potential of the people exposed, eg, exposure of the ovaries of women past childbearing age would not result in any genetic effects in future generations. The GSD for all medical exposures, primarily radiograph procedures, was estimated to be 0.02 cSv in 1970. For comparison, the annual GSD from natural background radiation is 0.08 cSv, or 4 times as much.[5]

IN UTERO EFFECTS

An embryo or fetus exposed to excessive amounts of radiation can suffer death, malformation, growth retardation, or functional impairment, with the injury dependent upon gestational age and dose.[1,67,68] Prior to implantation in the uterine wall (0 to 12 days after inception), the developing embryo is highly susceptible to the lethal effects of toxic agents, and the pregnancy usually terminates with reabsorption of the embryo or continues without harm. After implantation, the fetus becomes increasingly sensitive to the induction of birth defects throughout the period of major organ development (2 to 10 weeks). As the pregnancy progresses, most organ systems become less susceptible to injury, although the central nervous system, ocular tissue, and the hematopoietic system continue to develop throughout gestation and remain vulnerable. During the second and third trimesters, radiotherapy does not generally produce congenital anomalies or fetal death. However, high-dose exposures during this period can result in growth retardation and developmental anomalies. No instance of cancer after in utero exposure to radiotherapy or chemotherapy has been reported, whereas low doses of diagnostic radiography have been associated with childhood cancer.

Radiotherapy

Observations of pregnant women who underwent radiotherapy in the 1920s established ionizing radiation as the first known environmental agent to cause congenital malformations in man. In most cases, fetal doses were estimated to be over 250 cGy, and many of the women were unaware of their pregnancy when treated with radiation. Very high fetal doses, ie, those well over 300 to 500 cGy, might be expected to cause death and subsequent abortion or stillbirth anytime during pregnancy, but especially prior to 14 weeks of gestation. Not all fetal exposures to radiotherapy, however, result in detectable abnormalities in the offspring.[69]

Radioactive Iodine

Direct evidence of the effects of radioisotopes on the human embryo and fetus is fragmentary.[67,68] However, therapeutic doses of ^{131}I administered to pregnant women can destroy the fetal thyroid and cause hypothyroidism and cretinism. Lower doses associated with fallout from a nuclear weapons test on Bikini island resulted in benign thyroid nodules in two of three men who were exposed in utero. In one of those men who was exposed at 22 weeks, the thyroid was probably functional, and radioiodine could have been transferred effectively from the mother.

Atomic Bomb Exposure

Small head size and mental retardation were found related to both radiation dose and gestational age among children exposed in utero to the atomic bombings in 1945.[1,67,68] The probability of mental retardation was estimated to be as high as 40% after 100 cGy if exposure occurred during the 8th to 15th week of gestation, a time of rapid proliferation of neurons and of neuroblast migration to the cerebral cortex. Prenatal radiation exposure also increased the frequency of chromosomal aberrations, caused minor abnormalities of the lens of the eye, and reduced stature. However, in utero exposure to the atomic bombs has not been associated with skeletal abnormalities, sterility, or childhood cancer.

Carcinogenesis

Radiotherapy during pregnancy has not been linked to childhood cancer, whereas lower diagnostic exposures anytime during gestation have. The causal nature of the association between diagnostic x-rays and childhood cancer is frequently questioned, in large part because of the absence of an effect among atomic bomb survivors exposed in utero. The most popular noncausal interpretation ascribes possible confounding influences to unknown selection factors—factors related to both an increased rate of prenatal x-ray exposure and to an increased tendency for a malignant condition to develop. However, no study has been able to identify any such factors. It is prudent, then, to assume that the developing fetus is susceptible to radiation carcinogenesis, but not necessarily more susceptible than the newborn child or infant.[55]

Nuclear Medicine Considerations

Since most nuclear medicine procedures result in only small doses to the embryo or developing fetus (Table 6),[65,66] the probability of causing any deleterious effect is accordingly low. The degree of placental permeability to specific radiopharmaceuticals is the most important determinant of radiation dose to the developing fetus. In general, the placenta is impermeable to large protein molecules, colloidal suspensions, and small molecules attached to protein carriers, while it is completely permeable to small molecules of sugars, amino acids, and inorganic radionuclides such as phosphorus, cesium, thallium, and strontium. Radioiodine is potentially the most dangerous radiopharmaceutical because of its ability to cross the placental barrier and concentrate in fetal thyroid tissue. Other radiopharmaceuticals that readily cross the placental barrier include ^{75}Se selenomethionine, radioactive noble gases, ionic ^{47}Ca, ^{85}Sr, and ^{201}Tl. Many newer radiopharmaceuticals such as ^{99m}Tc pertechnetate consist of large macromolecules that cannot easily pass through the placenta, and thus result in negligible fetal doses.

It is uncommon for an elective or nonurgent procedure to

Table 6. Doses to Embryo from Various Radiopharmaceuticals[65,66]

RADIOPHARMACEUTICAL	ADMINISTERED ACTIVITY mCi (MBq)*	DOSE TO EMBRYO (cGy)
^{99m}Tc—sodium pertechnetate	10 (370)	0.37
^{99m}Tc polyphosphate	10 (370)	0.36
^{99m}Tc DTPA	10 (370)	0.30
^{99m}Tc sulfur colloid	2 (74)	0.06
^{67}Ga citrate	2 (74)	0.06
^{75}Se methionine	0.25 (9)	2.40
^{131}I—sodium iodide (15% uptake)	0.10 (4)	0.01

1 mCi = 37 MBq.

be performed on a woman known to be pregnant. However, because of the anxiety and possible legal action associated with any fetal exposure, it has been recommended that all women of childbearing age be handled in the following manner. (1) Record the date of the last menstrual period and determine whether pregnancy is possible. (2) If pregnant, or if an unsuspected pregnancy is possible, determine the stage of gestation and estimate possible fetal dose. (3) Communicate this information to the woman or a responsible family member and obtain an informed consent to place in the patient's record.[68]

Despite procedures as above to minimize the possibility of fetal exposure, there will always be instances of clinical urgency, such as accidents or cancer, that result in radiation to a developing fetus, or it may happen that a woman with an unsuspected pregnancy is administered a radiopharmaceutical. The physician is then faced with providing guidance as to whether a therapeutic abortion should be considered. Such a decision is complex and would consider the stage of fetal development, the dose received, and the desires of the pregnant woman.[5,68] Some physicians have relied on the "Danish Rule" which suggests that therapeutic abortions are advised when the fetal dose exceeds 10 cGy.[70] This recommendation is clearly flexible and would vary with personal circumstances. For example, a pregnant woman who had been unable to become pregnant for many years may be willing to accept the small risk of giving birth to a deformed child. Because about 5% of all births carry an observable abnormality, relatively low radiation doses of 10 cGy would be expected to increase this proportion by only a tiny amount. The equation changes, however, as the fetal dose increases as well as the personal circumstances of the mother-to-be. Because a fetal dose of 10 cGy is rarely encountered in nuclear medicine procedures, the application of the "Danish Rule" would be a rare occurrence.

HIGH-DOSE EFFECTS

The effects of internally deposited radionuclides are qualitatively similar to those caused by external sources of radiation (Table 7). Cellular and tissue effects, however, depend on several factors, among which are (1) the physical-chemical form of the radionuclides; (2) the amount administered; (3) the route of administration; (4) the tissue distribution and rate of excretion; (5) the half-life of the isotopes; (6) the type and energy of emitted radiation, LET, and RBE; and (7) the radiosensitivity of irradiated cells in tissue.[71]

Cells

Very high doses of radiation can destroy tissue by either killing cells in interphase or, more commonly, by killing progenitor cells at mitosis, which results in an eventual depletion of mature cells. Most undifferentiated cells with high mitotic activity, eg, hematopoietic stem cells, can be killed with relatively low dose exposures (Table 8). Most mature or highly differentiated cells, eg, muscle cells, are radioresistant and substantial doses are required to cause a loss of function. A useful rule of thumb first put forth in 1906 by Bergonie and Tribondeau is that the radiosensitivity of cells is directly related to their mitotic activity and inversely related to their degree of differentiation. The lymphocyte, which is highly radiosensitive, is one of the few exceptions to this rule.

Cell survival is also a function of the cell cycle stage at which exposure occurs. Irradiation causes most damage during mitosis and least damaging during G_1 and the middle of S. In general, low doses can cause cell cycle delay, moderate doses can cause deaths of some daughter cells, and high doses can cause interphase death.

The direct action of radiation to kill or cause mammalian cells to lose reproductive capacity can be described mathematically as

$$S = N/N_0 = exp\ (-k\ D)$$

where N is the number of cells alive after dose D, N_0 is the initial number of cells, and k is a constant related to radiosensitivity. If only one radiation hit is required to kill a cell, then a typical exponential curve would be seen, ie, a straight line on a semilog plot. However, when more than one hit (or target) is required to kill a cell, a shoulder is seen at low doses, indicating that damage can be accumulated

Table 7. Biologic Effects of Radiation

LEVEL OF ORGANIZATION	TYPE OF DAMAGE	IMPORTANT EFFECTS	RELATIVE DOSAGE
Cell	Chromosomal aberrations; mutations	Cell death; inhibition of cell division; transformation to malignant state	Low
Tissue	Hypoplasia, transformation of cells to malignant state	Disruption in tissue function; death, induction of cancer	Low-medium
Whole body	Transformation of tissue to malignant state	Cancer	Low-medium
	Disruption of hemopoietic, gastrointestinal, central nervous systems	Death	High

From Mossman.[76]

before the lethal effect is evident. A special quantity is the D_0 (or D_{37}) dose, which is the dose that kills 63% of the cell population; for most mammalian cells this is between 100 and 200 cGy.

Tissue

As might be expected, the relative sensitivity of a tissue is determined largely by the radiosensitivity of its cells.[71] Tissue response is also influenced by cell turnover rate, various cellular interactions, and capacity to repopulate. Many of the acute effects of radiation in tissues are mediated through the death of cells when they attempt to divide. The incidence of cell death is dose dependent, and cells that have retained their capacity to divide contribute to postirradiation recovery of the tissues. Hemopoietic tissues are extremely sensitive to irradiation, whereas muscle and nerve tissue can withstand massive doses.

Whole-Body Effects

The acute radiation syndrome (ARS) can occur following total-body exposures exceeding 100 cGy.[2,72] Medical management of radiation accidents, including Chernobyl, and studies of atomic bomb survivors have shown that loss of tissue function can produce clinical symptoms that differ according to dose, severity, and duration (Table 9). The ARS is generally divided into three or four clinical syndromes: hematopoietic, gastrointestinal, cardiovascular, and neurological, although there can be considerable overlap. During the first 48 hours after whole-body irradiation, a prodromal phase of symptoms can arise that are gastrointestinal (eg, anorexia, nausea, vomiting, diarrhea) and neuromuscular (eg, fatigue, apathy, sweating) in nature. The dose estimated to induce vomiting in 50% of individuals is about 2 Gy.

The hematopoietic syndrome relates to damage of stem cells in the bone marrow and lymphatic organs and usually occurs when doses exceed 200 cGy. Hemorrhage and infection due to granulocytopenia and thrombocytopenia is the usual cause of death, which could occur within 3 weeks. The gastrointestinal syndrome usually occurs when doses exceed 700 cGy. Loss of intestinal stem cells occurs, the intestinal/vascular barrier is broken, and sepsis results. Death can occur within 3 days. The central nervous syndrome is characterized by the immediate onset of severe neurological changes with convulsions and death within 2 days following massive exposures of over 10,000 cGy.

Without medical attention, the dose that would kill 50%

Table 8. Relative Radiosensitivities of Mammalian Cells

RELATIVE RADIOSENSITIVITY (CLASS)	CELL TYPES	GENERAL CHARACTERISTICS
High (I)	Hemopoietic stem cells, spermatogonia, intestinal crypt cells, oogonia, epidermal cells, lymphocytes	Short lived; undifferentiated; divide regularly
Fairly high (II)	Precursor cells of hemopoietic series, spermatocytes, oocytes	Divide limited number of times; differentiate to some degree
Medium (III)	Endothelial cells, fibroblasts, mesenchymal cells	Divide irregularly; lifespan highly variable
Fairly low (IV)	Epithelial cells of liver, kidney, salivary gland, basal and parenchymal cells of thyroid and adrenal gland, tracheobronchial basal cells of lung	Long lived; do not divide often; variable degree of differentiation
Low (V)	Neurons, erythrocytes, muscle cells, sperm	Do not divide; highly differentiated

From Casarret.[71]

Table 9. Expected Symptoms (%) following High-Dose Whole-Body Irradiation

SYMPTOM	MIDLINE TISSUE DOSE (cGy) *50–99* (%)	*100–199* (%)	*200–349* (%)	*350–549* (%)	*550–750* (%)
Anorexia	15–50	50–90	90–100	100	100
Nausea	5–30	30–70	70–90	90–100	100
Vomiting	15–20	20–50	50–80	80–100	100
Diarrhea			10	10	10
Fatigue/weakness		25–60	60–90	90–100	100
Headache				50	80
Diziness/disorientation					100
Bleeding		10	10–50	50–100	100
Fever		10–60	10–80	80–100	100
Infection		10–50	10–80	80–100	100
Death		<5	5–50	50–99	100

Modified from Mettler.[72]

of a population within 60 days ($LD_{50/60}$) would be about 250 cGy. For healthy persons receiving good medical support the $LD_{50/60}$ would be about 500 cGy. If marrow transplantation were possible, the $LD_{50/60}$ might rise to 900 cGy.

Nuclear Medicine Consideration

In general, large amounts of internal emitters are required to produce radiation sickness in man. Hematologic injury has been reported, however, after the therapeutic use of radioactive colloids.[2,72] A patient incorrectly treated with colloidal ^{198}Au (7400 MBq injected into the peritoneal cavity) resulted in 440 cGy to bone marrow and death occurred within 3 months from cerebral hemorrhage due to thrombocytopenia. Single or multiple doses of ^{32}P are given to treat polycythemia vera; and the activity for treatment 4 to 6 mCi (140 to 220 MBq) delivers a cumulative dose to the marrow of about 140 cGy. Severe pancytopenia has been reported following administered ^{32}P activities of 57 mCi (2100 MBq). Treatment of chondrosarcoma by ^{35}S is limited by hemotoxicity which can occur at 55 mCi (200 MBq/kg). The use of radioiodine to treat metastatic thyroid cancer is also limited generally by the dose to bone marrow. Because thyroid tissue is relatively radioresistant to direct cytocidal actions of radiation, massive doses of radiation are usually needed to produce thyroid ablation. Administered activities in excess of 20 mCi (740 MBq) of ^{131}I are usually required to ablate the thyroid, and result in a marrow dose of about 5 cGy. Doses in excess of 300 mCi (11,000 MBq) of ^{131}I, however, are usually required to cause bone marrow depression.

RADIATION HORMESIS (ADAPTIVE RESPONSE)

Radiation exposures at sufficiently high doses can produce harmful effects, eg, increased cancer rates in man. It is generally assumed that even very low doses are detrimental, but that the effects of low doses are so small that they cannot be observed directly against the much higher "natural" occurrence of cancer or genetic effects from other causes. Recently, however, more attention has been given to the intriguing possibility that low-level exposures might be good for you.[55,73–75] Radiation hormesis and adaptive response are terms being used to describe this phenomena. A comprehensive summary of the literature on adaptive response to radiation in cells and organisms has recently been published.[55] Perhaps the most plausible mechanism for adaptive response relates to the induction of enhanced DNA repair processes after relatively low dose exposures.[55,75] Other purported mechanisms include increased production of free radical scavengers or of immune cells. In all cases it is suggested that the DNA damage from low-level radiation is somehow compensated for by an adaptive response. Some, but not all, laboratory studies find that animals exposed to low doses outlive unexposed animals. Recent cellular studies find that a conditioning dose of about 1 cGy can reduce or completely suppress the number of radiation-induced mutations and chromosome breaks caused by subsequent higher doses. Human data are inconclusive as to whether very low doses are beneficial (in a similar way that they are inconclusive as to whether very low doses are harmful). There is at present no consensus as to whether adaptive response can play a beneficial role in human health, but there does seem to be more of a willingness to at least consider the possibility.

REFERENCES

1. NAS. *Health Effects of Exposure to Low Levels of Ionizing Radiation* (*BEIR V*). Washington, DC: National Academy Press, 1990.
2. UNSCEAR. *Sources, Effects, and Risks of Ionizing Radiation.* Publ E.88.IX.7. New York: United Nations, 1988.
3. Wagner NH, Ketchum LE. *Living with Radiation.* Baltimore: The Johns Hopkins University Press, 1989.

4. Stannard JN. *Radioactivity and Health. A History*. Springfield, VA: National Technical Information Service, 1988.
5. Hall EJ. *Radiation and Life*. 2nd ed. New York: Pergamon Press, 1984.
6. National Institutes of Health. *Report of the National Institutes of Health Ad Hoc Working Group to Develop Radioepidemiological Tables*. Washington, DC: Public Health Service, NIH Publ. No. 85-2748, US DHHS, 1985.
7. National Council on Radiation Protection and Measurements. *Influence of Dose and Its Distribution in Time on Dose-Response Relationships for Low-LET Radiations*. Report No. 64. Washington, DC: NCRP, 1980.
8. UNSCEAR. *Genetic and Somatic Effects of Ionizing Radiation*. Publ E.86.IX.9. New York: United Nations, 1986.
9. Neel JV, Schull WJ, eds. *The Children of Atomic Bomb Survivors. A Genetic Study*. Washington, DC: National Academy Press, 1991, 1–518.
10. NAS. *Health Risks of Radon and Other Internally Deposited Alpha-emitters (BEIR IV Report)*. Washington, DC: National Academy Press, 1988.
11. Weichselbaum RR, Beckett MA, Diamond AA. An important step in radiation carcinogenesis may be inactivation of cellular genes. *Int J Radiat Oncol Biol Phy* 1989;16:277–282.
12. Elkind MM, Benjamin SA, Sinclair WK, et al. Oncogenic mechanisms in radiation-induced cancer. *Cancer Res* 1991; 51:2740–2747.
13. Brash DE, Rudolph JA, Simon JA, et al. A role for sunlight in skin cancer: UV-induced p53 mutations in squamous cell carcinoma. *Proc Natl Acad Sci USA* 1991;88:10124–10128.
14. Taylor JA, Watson MA, Deverux TR, et al. p53 mutation hotspot in radon-associated lung cancer. Lancet 1994;343:86–87.
15. VähäKangas KH, Samet JM, Metcalf RA, et al. Mutations of p53 and *ras* genes in radon-associated lung cancer from uranium miners. *Lancet* 1992;339:576–580.
16. Hall P, Boice JD Jr, Berg G, et al. Leukaemia incidence after iodine-131 exposure. *Lancet* 1992;340:1–4.
17. Holm L-E, Hall P, Wiklund KE, et al. Cancer risk after iodine-131 therapy for hyperthyroidism. *J Natl Cancer Inst* 1991; 83:1072–1077.
18. Saenger EL, Thoma GE, Tompkins EA. Incidence of leukemia following treatment of hyperthyroidism. Preliminary report of the cooperative thyrotoxicosis therapy follow-up study. *JAMA* 1968;205:855–862.
19. Hoffman D. Effects of I-131 therapy in the United States. In: Boice JD Jr, Fraumeni JF Jr, eds. *Radiation Carcinogenesis: Epidemiology and Biological Significance*. New York: Raven Press, 1984;273–280.
20. Goldman MB, Maloof F, Monson RR, et al. Radioactive iodine therapy and breast cancer: A follow-up study of hyperthyroid women. *Am J Epidemiol* 1988;127:969–980.
21. Holm L-E, Wiklund KE, Lundell GE, et al. Cancer risk in population examined with diagnostic doses of 131-I. *J Natl Cancer Inst* 1989;81:302–306.
22. Hall P, Berg G, Bjelkengren G, et al. Cancer mortality after iodine-131 therapy for hyperthyroidism. *Int J Cancer* 1992; 50:886–890.
23. Edmonds CJ, Smith T. The long-term hazards of the treatment of thyroid cancer with radioiodine. *Br J Radiol* 1986;59:45–51.
24. Hall P, Holm L-E, Lundell G, et al. Cancer risks in thyroid cancer patients. *Br J Cancer* 1991;64:159–163.
25. Ron E, Modan B, Preston D, et al. Thyroid neoplasia following low-dose radiation in childhood. *Radiat Res* 1989;120: 516–531.
26. Spiess H, Mays CW, Chmelevsky D. Malignancies in patients injected with radium 224. In: Taylor DM, Mays CW, Gerber GB, Thomas RG, eds. *Risks from Radium and Thorotrast*. BIR Report 21. London: British Institute of Radiology, 1989; 7–12.
27. Rowland RE, Stehney AF, Lucas HF Jr. Dose-response relationships for female radium dial workers. *Radiat Res* 1978;76:368–383.
28. Modan B, Lilienfeld AM. Leukaemogenic effects of ionizing-irradiation treatment in polycythemia. *Lancet* 1964;2:439–441.
29. Berk PD, Goldberg JD, Silverstein MN, et al. Increased incidence of acute leukemia in polycythemia vera associated with chlorambucil therapy. *N Engl J Med* 1981;304:441–447.
30. Taylor DM, Mays CW, Gerber GB, Thomas RG, eds. *Risks from Radium and Thorotrast*. BIR Report 21. London, British Institute of Radiology, 1989.
31. Andersson M, Storm HA. Cancer incidence among Danish Thorotrast patients. *J Natl Cancer Inst* 1992;1318–1325.
32. Guilmette RA, Mays DM, eds. Total body evaluation of a Thorotrast patient. *Health Phys* 1992;63:1–100.
33. Boice JD Jr, Mandel JS, Doody MM, et al. A health survey of radiologic technologists. *Cancer* 1992;69:586–598.
33A. Boice JD Jr, Mandel JS, Doody MM. Breast cancer among radiological technologists. *JAMA* (in press)
34. Wang J-X, Inskip PD, Boice JD Jr, et al. Cancer incidence among medical diagnostic X-ray workers in China; 1950 to 1985. *Int J Cancer* 1990;45:889–895.
35. Stebbings JH, Lucas H, Stehney A. Mortality from cancers of major sites in female radium dial workers. *Am J Ind Med* 1984;5:435–459.
36. Baverstock KF, Papworth DG. The UK radium luminiser survey. In: Taylor DM, Mays CW, Gerber GB, Thomas RG, eds. *Risks from Radium and Thorotrast*. BIR Report 21. London: British Institute of Radiology, 1989, 72–76.
37. Lubin JH, Boice JD Jr, Edling C, et al. *Lung Cancer Following Radon Exposure Among Underground Miners: A Joint Analysis of 11 Studies*. NIH Publ No. 94-3644. Washington DC: US Govt Printing Office, 1994.
38. Boice JD Jr. Radiation carcinogenesis—human epidemiology. In: Mossman KL, Mills WA, eds. *The Biological Basis of Radiation Protection Practice*. Baltimore: Williams & Wilkins, 1992;89–120.
39. Gilbert ES, Fry SA, Wiggs LD, et al. Analyses of combined mortality data on workers at the Hanford Site, Oak Ridge National Laboratory, and Rocky Flats Nuclear Weapons Plant. *Radiat Res* 1989;120:19–35.
40. Kendall GM, Muirhead CR, MacGibbon BH, et al. Mortality and occupational exposure to radiation: first analysis of the National Registry of Radiation Workers. *Br Med J* 1992; 304:220–225.
41. Voelz GL, Lawrence JNP. A 42-year medical follow-up of Manhattan's project plutonium workers. *Health Phys* 1991; 61:181–190.
42. Alavanja MCR, Brownson RC, Lubin JH, et al. Residential radon exposure and lung cancer among nonsmoking women. *J Natl Cancer Inst* 1994;86:1829–1837.
43. Blot WJ, Xu Z-Y, Boice JD Jr, et al. Indoor radon and lung cancer in China. *J Natl Cancer Inst* 1990;82:1025–1030.
43A. Lubin JH. Invited commentary: lung cancer and exposure to residential radon. *Am J Epidemiol* 1994;140:323–332.
44. Abelson PH. Mineral dusts and radon in uranium mines. *Science* 1991;254:777.
45. Wang Z, Boice JD Jr, Wei L, et al. Thyroid nodularity and chromosome aberrations among women in areas of high background radiation in China. *J Natl Cancer Inst* 1990; 82:478–485.
46. Forman D, Cook-Monzaffari P, Darby S, et al. Cancer near nuclear installations. *Nature* 1987;329:499–505.
47. Jablon S, Hrubec Z, Boice JD Jr, et al. Cancer in populations

living near nuclear facilities. A survey of mortality nationwide and incidence in two states. *JAMA* 1991;265:1403–1408.

48. Gardner MJ, Snee MP, Hall AJ, et al. Results of case-control study of leukaemia and lymphoma among young people near Sellafield nuclear plant in West Cumbria. *Br Med J* 1990;300:423–429.
49. Kinlen L. Evidence for an infective cause for childhood leukaemia: comparison of a Scottish New Town with nuclear reprocessing sites in Britain. *Lancet* 1988;2:1323–1327.
50. Doll R, Evans HJ, Darby SC. Paternal exposure not to blame. Nature 1994;367:678–680.
51. Parkin DM, Cardis E, Masuger E, et al. Childhood leukaemia following the Chernobyl accident. The European Childhood Leukaemia-Lymphoma Incidence Study (ECLIS). *Eur J Cancer* 1993;29A:87–95.
52. Mettler FA Jr, Williamson MR, Royal HD, et al. Thyroid nodules in the population living around Chernobyl. *JAMA* 1992; 268:616–619.
53. Boice JD Jr, Preston D, Davis FG, Monson RR. Frequent chest X-ray fluoroscopy and breast cancer incidence among tuberculosis patients in Massachusetts. *Radiat Res* 1991; 125:214–222.
54. Jablon S, Kato H. Childhood cancer in relation to prenatal exposure to atomic-bomb radiation. *Lancet* 1970;2:1000–1003.
55. UNSCEAR. *Sources and Effects of Ionizing Radiation*. Publ E.94.IX.11. New York: United Nations, 1994.
56. Boice JD Jr, Morin MM, Glass AG, et al. Diagnostic x-ray procedures and risk of leukemia, lymphoma, and multiple myeloma. *JAMA* 1991;265:1290–1294.
57. Griem ML, Kleinerman RA, Boice JD Jr, et al. Cancer following radiotherapy for peptic ulcer. *J Natl Cancer Inst* 1994;86:842–849.
58. Curtis RE, Boice JD Jr, Stovall M, et al. Risk of leukemia after chemotherapy and radiation treatment for breast cancer. *N Engl J Med* 1992;326:1745–1751.
59. Boice JD Jr, Harvey E, Blettner M, et al. Contralateral breast cancer following radiotherapy for breast cancer. *N Engl J Med* 1992;326:781–785.
60. Shimizu Y, Kato H, Schull WJ. Studies of the mortality of A-bomb survivors. 9. Mortality; 1950–1985: Part 2. Cancer mortality based on the recently revised doses (DS86). *Radiat Res* 1990;121:120–141.

60A. Thompson DE, Mabuchi K, Ron E, et al. Cancer incidence in atomic bomb survivors. Part II: solid tumors, 1958–1987. *Radiat Res* 1994;137:S17–S67.

61. Hamilton TE, van Belle G, LoGerfo JP. Thyroid neoplasia in Marshall Islanders exposed to nuclear fallout. *JAMA* 1987; 258:629–635.
62. Rallison ML, Lotz TM, Bishop M, et al. Cohort study of thyroid disease near the Nevada Test Site: a preliminary report. *Health Phys* 1990;59:739–746.
63. Stevens W, Thomas DC, Lyon JL, et al. Leukemia in Utah and radioactive fallout from the Neveda test site. A case-control study. *JAMA* 1990;264:585–591.
64. Darby SC, Olsen JH, Doll R, et al. Trends in childhood leukaemia in the Nordic countries in relation to fallout from atmospheric nuclear weapons testing. *Br Med J* 1992;304: 1005–1009.
65. International Commission on Radiological Protection. Radiation dose to patients from radiopharmaceuticals (ICRP Publ 53). *Ann ICRP* 1987;18:1–377.
66. Kereiakes JG, Rosenstein M. *Handbook of Radiation Doses in Nuclear Medicine and Diagnostic X-Ray*. Boca Raton, FL: CRC Press, 1980.
67. Boice JD Jr. Fetal risk to radiotherapy and chemotherapy exposure in utero. *Cancer Bull* 1986;38:293–300.
68. Brent RL. The effects of embryonic and fetal exposure to ionizing radiation: counseling the patient and worker about risks. In: Mossman KL, Mills WA, eds. *The Biological Basis of Radiation Protection Practice*. Baltimore: Williams & Wilkins, 1992;23–62.
69. Mulvihill JJ, Harvey ER, Boice JD Jr, et al. Normal findings 52 years after in utero radiation exposure. *Lancet* 1991; 338:1202, 1203.
70. Hammer-Jacobsen E. Therapeutic abortion on account of x-ray. *Dan Med Bull* 1959;6:113.
71. Casarett GW. *Radiation Histopathology*. Boca Raton, FL: CRC Press, 1980.
72. Mettler FA Jr. Effects of whole-body irradiation. In: Mettler FA Jr, Kelsey CA, Ricks RC, eds. *Medical Management of Radiation Accidents*. Boca Raton, FL: CRC Press, 1990;79–88.
73. Macklis RM, Beresford B. Radiation hormesis. *J Nucl Med* 1991;32:350–359.
74. Sagan LA. On radiation, paradigms, and hormesis. *Science* 1989;245:574.
75. Wolff S. Is radiation all bad? The search for adaptation. *Radiat Res* 1992;131:117–123.
76. Mossman KL. Radiation effects in nuclear medicine. In: Harbert JC, DaRocha A, eds. *Textbook of Nuclear Medicine*. Vol 1. Philadelphia: Lea & Febiger, 1984;283–302.
77. Upton AC. Cancer risk estimates for external radiation exposure (BEIR V). In: Mossman KL, Mills WA, eds. *The Biological Basis of Radiation Protection Practice*. Baltimore: Williams & Wilkins, 1992;121–137.

14 Quantitative Radioassays

Gyorgy Csako

HISTORY OF RADIOASSAYS

The use of radionuclides in quantitative analytical assays for biological substances began in 1940, when Rittenberg and Foster[1,2] reported the technique of isotope dilution for measuring amino acids and fatty acids. In this technique, a component in a mixture is quantitatively measured by recovering a known fraction, instead of the entire amount of the component. In 1946, Keston et al[3] introduced the double-isotope dilution derivative technique for measuring amino acids. Later, this technique was used to measure such biologically active substances as hormones and drugs. Radioassays were also introduced to measure enzyme activity (radioenzymometry) and the concentration of substrates, enzyme inhibitors, and activators in radioenzymatic assays.[4–7]

In the 1950s variants of the (radio)isotope dilution assay (RIDA) that do not require chemical purification were discovered. In 1956, Berson and Yalow[8] reported that (1) after long-term therapy with heterologous (beef/pork) insulin, diabetics developed antiinsulin antibodies and (2) by incubating antiinsulin antibody with labeled and unlabeled insulin, the ratio of antibody-bound and free radiolabeled insulin was inversely related to the concentration of unlabeled insulin. Recognition of the competition between unlabeled and radiolabeled insulin for limited numbers of binding sites on antiinsulin antibody led them to develop the first radioimmunoassay (RIA)[9,10] that measured insulin with high analytical sensitivity and specificity, thus obviating the need for bioassays. Concomitantly, other American researchers were developing similar RIAs for insulin,[11] glucagon,[12] and growth hormone.[13]

In the early 1960s, Ekins[14] and Murphy and Pattee[15] described competitive protein binding (CPB) assays based on thyroxin-binding globulin as binder for thyroxin; Barakat and Ekins[16] and Rothenberg[17] reported similar assays based on transcobalamin and intrinsic factor, respectively, as binders for vitamin B_{12}; and Murphy et al[18,19] published transcortin-based CPB for steroids.

In 1965, Rothenberg[20] used enzymes as saturable reagents in the radioenzymatic saturation analysis (RESA), which is essentially a competitive binding assay. The first competitive radioreceptor assays (RRAs) based on "cytosol" (but truly nuclear) proteins as binders were described by Baulieu et al[21] in 1967 and by Korenman[22] in 1968 for estrogens. In 1970, RRAs based on membrane proteins as binders were reported by Lefkowitz et al[23,24] for ACTH. In 1982, Potocnjak et al[25] published their "4i" (*i*nhibition of *i*diotype-anti *i*diotype *i*nteraction) assay. The 4i assay was the first competitive RIA where radiolabeled antiidiotypic antibody is substituted for radiolabeled antigen and competes with the antigen to be measured for limited numbers of binding sites on the antigen-specific antibody. The technique of double radioisotope-labeled ("dual") binding assay was introduced as a double RIA by Morgan in 1966.[26]

The concept of "sandwich" assays based on solid-phase bound antigens and the use of radiolabeled antibodies (radioallergosorbent test, RAST) was introduced by Wide et al.[27] This technique also represented the first noncompetitive binding radioassay. In 1968 Miles and Hales[28] used radiolabeled antibodies in another type of noncompetitive quantitative binding radioassay which they called immunoradiometric assay, IRMA. Soon the first two-site (sandwich) IRMA assays were reported by Haberman[29] and by Addison and Hales.[30] Recently, a receptor-antibody sandwich assay (RASA) was reported by Corti et al.[31]

In 1969, Rowe[32] used radiolabeled antibody to increase the analytical sensitivity of radial immunodiffusion (RID). The greatly increased sensitivity obtained by this approach demonstrated the advantage of radiolabeled reagents for quantitative precipitation and agglutination reactions.

In 1975, the discovery by Kohler and Milstein[33] of the hybridoma technology (in vitro production of specific monoclonal antibodies) represented a major contribution to the advancement of radioimmunobinding assays, particularly two/three-site IRMAs.

Obviously, many other contributions, too numerous to list here, have ensured the success of binding radioassays. Improvements in radioiodination, innovations in solid-phase technology and other methods of separating bound and free radiolabeled substances, the elaboration of theoretical and practical ways for data reduction, and assay automation are only some examples.

CLASSIFICATION AND NOMENCLATURE OF RADIOASSAYS

In vitro radioassays can be conveniently classified into two major types: (1) those that are based on specific binding of radiolabeled substance(s) (binding assays) and (2) those that

Table 1. Classification of radioassays

A. Binding assays
   I. "Limited reagent" (competitive or saturation analysis)
      1. Labeled ligand
         • Radioimmunoassay (RIA)
         • Radiotransinassay (RTA) (previously: Competitive protein binding [assay]); (CPB[A])
         • Radioreceptor assay (RRA)
      2. Labeled antibody
         • "Indirect immunoradiometric assay (IRMA)" or "indirect one [single]-site IRMA" (unoccupied sites measured on labeled antibody [="free fraction"])
      3. Labeled antiidiotypic antibody
         • Inhibition of idiotype-antiidiotype
         • interaction ("4i-assay")
      4. Radioenzymatic saturation analysis (RESA)
   II. "Reagent-excess" (noncompetitive)
      1. Labeled antibody
         • Radioallergo (antigen)sorbent test (RAST) ("sandwich assay")
         • One [single]-site IRMA (occupied sites measured on labeled antibody [=bound fraction])
         • Two/three-site IRMA ("sandwich" assay)
         • Receptor-antibody sandwich (radio)assay (RAS[R]A)
         • Radioactive quantitative precipitation/agglutination
           –Radioimmunoprecipitation assay (RIPA)
           –Radioactive (single) radial immunodiffusion (RID)
      2. Labeled antiidiotypic antibody
         • (Radio)idiometric assay (RIMA)
      3. Radioenzymometric assay (REMA)
      4. Radioenzymatic assay (REA)
         • Enzymatic single-isotope derivative methods
         • Measurement of enzyme activators and inhibitors
   III. "Dual" (double [radio] label) assays
      1. RIA/RIA
      2. RTA/RTA
      3. RIA/IRMA
      4. IRMA/immunoenzymometric assay (IEMA)
B. Nonbinding assays
   I. Isotope dilution
      1. Simple isotope dilution
      2. Reverse isotope dilution
      3. Inverse isotope dilution
      4. Derivative dilution
      5. Dual isotope dilution
   II. Indirect equilibrium dialysis

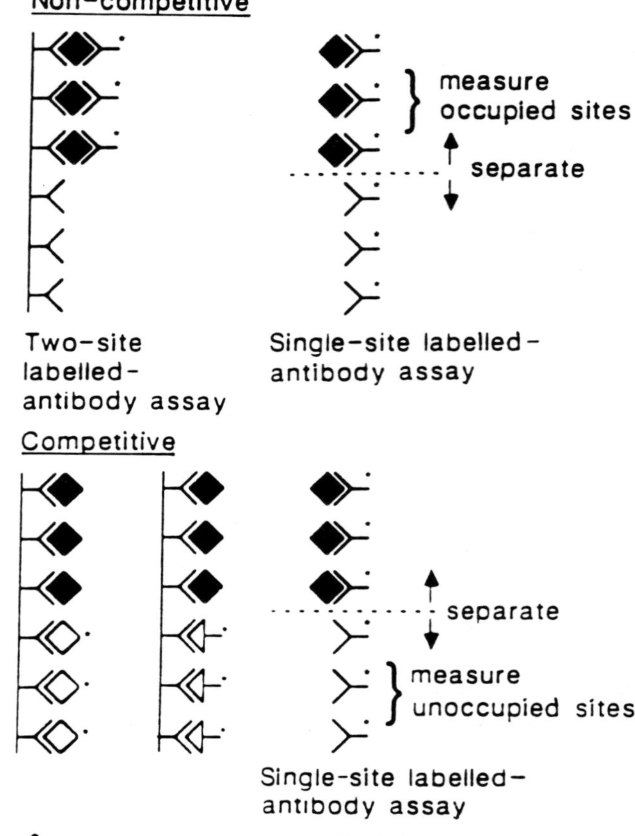

Figure 1. Alternative methods of measuring antibody binding site occupancy. Labeled antibody methods can be competitive or noncompetitive, depending on whether bound or unbound fraction is measured. Reactants may be introduced in any order, although assay sensitivity may thereby be affected, and optimal reactant concentrations may differ. (Reprinted with permission from Ekins.[37])

are not (nonbinding assays) (Table 1). For completeness, the table includes *all* clinically relevant quantitative radioassays.

The essential components of all binding assays include a ligand and its specific binder. The ligand, usually the substance measured, refers to any substance that is specifically bound by an appropriate binder and the binder refers to any substance that will specifically bind a ligand. Based on these definitions, binding assays encompass a heterogeneous group of analytical techniques in which the "binding reagents" include antibodies, "specific" binding proteins, and enzymes. The recent discovery of *abzymes* or *catalytic antibodies*, ie, antibodies that bind to and stabilize transition-state intermediates, and hence exhibit intrinsic enzymic activity,[34–36] highlights the similarities between various binding reactions.

In competitive binding, or *saturation assays*, the unoccupied binder sites are measured and the key reagents are available only in a limited quantity (Fig. 1), which is why these are also called "*limited reagent*" assays.[38]

The methods introduced by Ekins,[14,16] Rothenberg,[17] and Murphy[15,18,19] are widely referred to as competitive protein binding (CPB) assays, as Murphy[39] initially proposed it. These assays are, however, more appropriately called *radiotransin assays* (RTAs), as suggested later by Murphy,[40,41] because they utilize specific transport (binding) proteins ("transins") from body fluids to bind the ligands they measure.

There is no established name for the special version of

competitive RIA where radiolabeled antiidiotypic antibody is substituted for labeled antigen. The technique was termed 4i (*i*nhibition of *i*diotype-anti *i*diotype *i*nteraction) assay in the first report[25] using this approach. Although 4i is apparently a competitive binding assay, it was described by the authors[25] as an IRMA, apparently referring to the use of radiolabeled antibody.

In noncompetitive binding assays, the occupied sites of the binder are measured and all key reagents are provided in excess over the analyte of interest, hence the term "reagent-excess" assays.[38] Excess reagents include the immobilized antigen (allergen) and radiolabeled antibody in RAST and related assays, the radiolabeled antibody and solid-phase bound antigen ("immunosorbant") in the original IRMA, and the solid-phase bound and radiolabeled antibodies in two/three-site IRMAs (Fig. 1). The receptor-antibody sandwich assay (RASA) was described with the use of enzyme (peroxidase)-labeled antibody[31] and the idiometric assay with the use of nonradioactive (europium)-labeled alpha-type antiidiotypic antibody.[42,43] However, the assay principles are obviously applicable to radiolabeled reagent, and then the term RASRA (RA, radioassay) for the former and radioidiometric assay (RIMA) for the latter would be appropriate.

Depending on whether there is an extra separation step between the addition of key reactants, both competitive and noncompetitive binding radioassays can be of the "one-step" or "two-step" type. While the former is shorter in assay time and simpler in design, the latter has the advantage that, by adding an extra separation step, potentially interfering components are removed from the sample prior to addition of the tracer.

The nomenclature of nonbinding radioassays (Table 1) is more straightforward than that of the binding assays, and the designations used are descriptive of the analytical concepts involved in these methods. Different radioisotope dilution techniques have been reviewed recently.[44] The double-isotope derivative assays are highly sensitive, specific, and accurate; hence they are considered reference methods.[45] However, their complexity and expense generally preclude routine use. Indirect equilibrium dialysis techniques are used for measuring free (nonprotein bound) hormones and drugs.

THE BINDING REACTION

All binding assays are based on a reversible interaction between two molecules: a bindee (ligand, analyte, antigen, or substrate) and the respective binder, usually an antibody, transport protein (transin), receptor, or enzyme.* Some binding reactions may be stereospecific, eg, catecholamine binding to receptors. In contrast to classical chemical reactions, where two molecules are united by covalent bonds, binding reactions involve weak, noncovalent bonds and usually no alteration of the reacting molecules. Electrostatic forces have been implicated in a variety of biologically important intermolecular interactions. Primary (coulombic or ionic interactions, Lifschitz-van der Waals forces, and hydrogen bonds) and secondary (Lifschitz-van der Waals forces and hydrogen bonds comprising "hydrophobic interaction") bonds are involved in protein antigen-antibody reactions.[46–48] Transport proteins also exhibit multiple forms of interactions with ligands. Because of difficulties in isolating intact receptors, the nature of ligand-receptor interactions is relatively less established. Several types of interactions are thought, however, to contribute. Hydrophobic interactions may be the dominating force in steroid interactions with nuclear receptor proteins and in peptide interactions with membrane receptors. Hydrogen and ionic binding may also provide specificity in the reaction of some peptides with hormone receptors.

In the end, it is apparent that binding reactions involve relatively weak forces that act at short ranges. However, if there is a "good fit" between the ligand and binder, these weak forces combine to form a strong attraction that keeps the two reactants in close proximity.[49]

The forward rate of association between antigen and antibody is fairly high in hapten-antibody systems; equilibration in 0.2 to 0.3 μmol/L solutions of hapten-antibody is achieved within 50 to 100 milliseconds after the addition of hapten.[50] Nevertheless, prolonged incubations are often needed for maximum sensitivity in protein antigen-antibody systems. In haptenic systems, greater tracer binding may be obtained at 12 and 24 hours than at 1 and 4 hours.[51] The likely explanation is that very dilute solutions (often below the 0.1 μmol/L range) of antibody and radioligand are used in the assays and that the antigen-antibody reaction is bimolecular in nature.[51] Because of the heterogeneity of polyclonal antibodies, redistribution of antigen between high- and low-affinity antibodies may also necessitate long incubation times.[51]

Binding Reactions in Solid-Phase

The commercial success of binding assays was greatly enhanced by the introduction of insoluble reagents that are immobilized either by physical adsorption (coating) or chemical coupling onto solid support. Such supports may be the inside surface of plastic tubes or microtiter plate wells, glass beads, latex or iron ("magnetic") particles, agarose spheres, or cellulose membranes. Not surprisingly, however, this new technology raised questions about the physicochemical aspects of binding at surfaces. Recent studies revealed some unique features of antigen-antibody reactions at solid-liquid interfaces. In general, the water surrounding protein molecules is more highly ordered near the surface of the solid phase, which favors the Lipshitz-van der Waals forces (dipole-dipole interactions) and coulombic bonding, and,

*The binding reaction occurring between complementary oligonucleotide and/or polynucleotide chains via hydrogen bonding is an essential component of molecular biology technology. By incorporating radiolabeled nucleotides, quantitative assays exist based on this binding reaction, but, because of their unique application, will not be further discussed in this chapter.

hence, facilitates the formation of antigen-antibody complexes. Studying antibody binding to solid phase-bound antigens, Sternberg and Nygren[53] reported that, due to limitations in mass transport or steric interactions, the immune complexes dissociate so slowly that the antigen-antibody reactions are practically irreversible at solid-liquid interfaces. The increased stability of immune complexes may be due to lateral interactions between bound antibodies. However, in contrast to cell surface reactions, antigen-antibody reactions at solid-liquid interfaces often are diffusion limited due to depletion of reactants close to the surface. Even when the reactions are not limited by diffusion, both the intrinsic forward and reverse reactions are slower at solid-liquid surface than in solution. Nygren and Sternberg[53] observed greater antibody affinity to haptens immobilized on a carrier protein than in solution. Lastly, the binding reaction occurring on coated surfaces is known to be unusually sensitive to the protein concentration of reaction mixtures.

As a whole, it is widely believed that many immune complexes form more efficiently in solution than at solid-liquid interfaces. Consequently, detection limits of immunoassays may be lowered by allowing the formation of immune complexes in solution before capturing them on solid surface for separation.[54]

Modulation of the Binding Reaction

Understanding the dynamics of interactions between antigen-antibody binding reactions[46–48] provides clues for their manipulations. Such dynamics may be classified into three major categories: (1) reaction environment (pH, ionic strength, surface tension, addition of polymers, dehydrating and chaotropic agents); (2) reaction temperature; and (3) reaction time.

THE LAW OF MASS ACTION

In the simplest form, the binding reaction is a univalent, reversible, saturable, bimolecular interaction that, in analogy to the Michaelis-Menten equation for enzyme-substrate reaction, can be described as

(1) $$[L] + [B] \underset{k_d}{\overset{k_a}{\rightleftharpoons}} [LB]$$

where $[L]$ denotes the concentration of free ligand; $[B]$ is the concentration of free binder sites; $[LB]$ is the concentration of the ligand-binder complex formed; k_a is the rate constant for the forward (association) reaction; and k_d is the rate constant for the reverse (dissociation) reaction.

The rate constants represent the fraction of molecules available for reaction within a unit of time in each direction. While the rate constants are independent of the concentrations, the absolute rates of change, ie, the total number of molecules reacting within a unit of time, gradually decrease during the binding reaction. When the absolute rates of association and dissociation are equal, no more changes occur in concentrations of the two reactants and their complex, and the reaction are said to be in equilibrium. If certain conditions are met (see below), the first-order *law of mass action* governs the rate of reaction and the equilibrium state. According to this law, the rate of a (chemical) reaction is proportional to the concentrations of the reactants. Further, the ratios of the concentration of the ligand-binder complex and the concentration of the two reactants, ligand and binder, are constant and equal the ratios of the rate constants at equilibrium:

(2) $$K_a = \frac{[LB]}{[L]\,[B]} = \frac{k_a}{k_d} = \frac{1}{K_d}$$

and

(3) $$K_d = \frac{[L]\,[B]}{[LB]} = \frac{k_d}{k_a} = \frac{1}{K_a}$$

The units for the affinity constant K_a are in liter/mol, whereas units for the dissociation constant K_d are in mol/liter. Since the concentration of total binding sites $[n]$ equals $[B]$ + $[LB]$, Equation 3 may be rewritten as

(4) $$K_d = \frac{([n] - [LB])\,[L]}{[LB]}$$

which rearranges to

(5) $$\frac{[LB]}{[n]} = \frac{[L]}{K_d + [L]}$$

where the ratio $[LB]/[n]$ represents the fraction of total binding sites occupied by ligand. At one-half maximum occupancy of binding sites $[LB]/[n] = 0.5$ and $K_d = [L]$, implying that the concentration of ligand required for half-maximal occupancy of binding sites is equal to K_d or $1/K_a$. This concept is analogous to the estimation of the Michaelis' constant for enzymes. Michaelis' constant is equal numerically to the reciprocal of substrate concentration at 50% saturation of the enzyme. Thus, if saturation curves for the binder are prepared by adding progressively increasing amounts of either radiolabeled ligand or a mixture of radiolabeled and unlabeled ligand, and assuming the two behave identically, the concentration of free (or bound) ligand at 50% saturation may be used to determine an average association constant for the binding reaction. To differentiate from the association constant determined by Scatchard plot (see below), the term *intrinsic association constant* is proposed for the association constant based on 50% binder saturation.

Scatchard Plot

Redefining $[LB]$ as bound ligand or B, and $[L]$ as free ligand, or F, and recalling that $[n] = [B] + [LB]$, Equation 2 can be rewritten in form of the Scatchard equation:[55]

(6) $$B/F = K_a\,([n] - [LB])$$

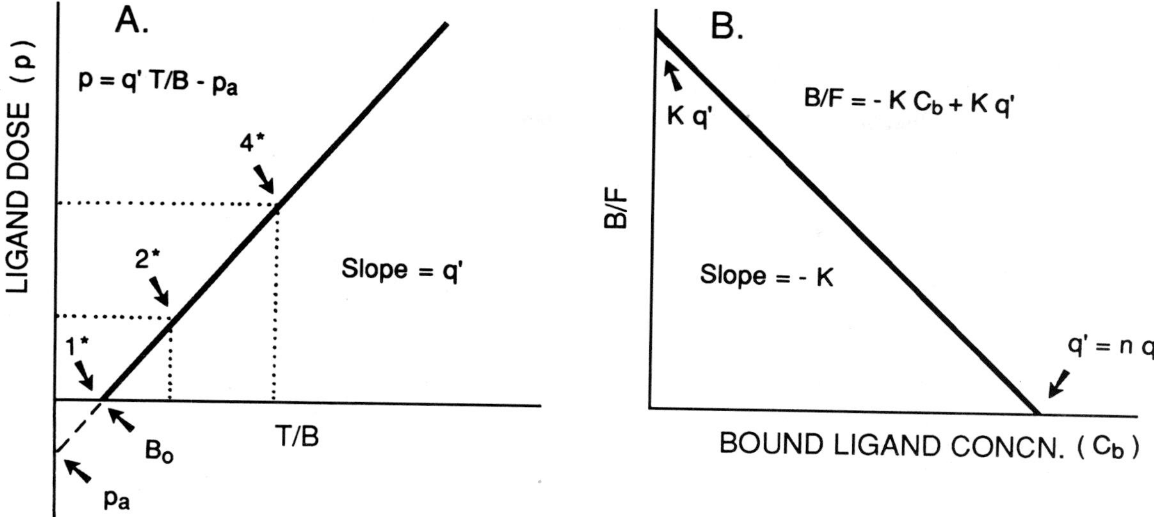

Figure 2. Determination of the affinity (equilibrium) constant and binding-site concentration by means of the Scatchard plot in RIA. (For details see text.)

If the reaction follows first-order kinetics, plotting the bound concentration against *B/F* yields a straight line (Fig. 2B). In RIAs the bound concentration, C_b, is the sum of the unlabeled (p) and labeled (p^*) ligand concentration ($C_b = p + p^*$); therefore, it is necessary to know the tracer concentration. This information usually is not provided by the manufacturer, but can be readily obtained when data are collected for the standard curve (Fig. 2A). In addition to the usual set of standards (all containing one aliquot of the tracer), two additional tubes are included, one containing two aliquots (2*) and the other four aliquots (4*) of tagged ligand. No unlabeled ligand is added to either tube. Both tubes (2* and 4*) are run as though they were unknowns, which they are. Then, a standard curve is prepared by plotting the ligand dose (p) as a function of *T/B* (total counts/bound counts) (Fig. 2A). The slope of the linear least squares regression line is the measure of the concentration of binding sites (q'). From the regression line, the ligand concentrations for two (2*) and four (4*) aliquots of tracer can also be read off. As 4* represents three aliquots of p^* in addition to the one normally used in the assay, the corresponding ligand concentration will be three times greater than that of 2*. With determination of the tracer concentration, it is now possible to calculate C_b, the concentration of the bound antigen for each standard [$C_b = (p + p^*)\ B/T$].

In the Scatchard plot (Fig. 2B), the slope is equal to $-K$, the affinity constant, and the x-axis intercept gives the concentration of binding sites, $q' = nq$. In this equation, n is the number of binding sites per molecule and q is the concentration of antibody or other binder. For monomeric (bivalent) antibodies $n = 2$ and $q' = 2q$. For a more detailed discussion of this technique see Chase.[56]

The main value of the Scatchard plot is that two critical parameters of the binding reaction, the affinity constant, K_a, and the concentration of total binding sites [n] can be directly determined. Nevertheless, the best way to analyze ligand-binding data is still debated.[57,58]

Radiolabeled Ligand

In the traditional formulation of competitive binding assays, radiolabeled ligand competes with unlabeled ligand for limited numbers of binding sites on the specific binder. Assuming identical behavior of labeled and unlabeled ligand, their respective forward and reverse rate constants are also identical, and at equilibrium the reaction can be described as

$$\frac{[L]}{[L^*]} + [B] \underset{k_d}{\overset{k_a}{\rightleftharpoons}} [LB] + [L^*B] \qquad (7)$$

where [L^*] represents the concentration of radiolabeled ligand. If other conditions also are met (see below), the law of mass action can then be applied for this situation in the same way as for unlabeled ligand alone (see Equation 1).

Conditions for the Law of Mass Action

As stated earlier, application of the mass action law assumes that certain conditions are met:

1. Full equilibrium is reached in the reaction.
2. The reaction is entirely reversible.
3. Both ligand and binder are present in only one chemical species.
4. Both ligand and binder are univalent, ie, one ligand molecule can react with one binder molecule and no other combinations exist.
5. No allosteric or cooperative (eg, ligand-ligand, site-site) interactions that could modify the reactivity of either reactant occur. This implies that ligand and binder react according to the first-order mass action law.

6. The bound and free ligand fractions are completely separated from each other.
7. The ratio of bound to free ligand or the ratio of bound to total ligand can be precisely measured, and the measurements are not influenced by factors like nonspecific binding.

Many of these requirements cannot be fully satisfied in routinely used binding assays. For instance, in traditional formulation of competitive binding reactions the labeled ligand is, at best, slightly different, but, at worst, can be completely different chemically from the unlabeled ligand, thus disobeying the requirement for a homogeneous ligand. Regarding antibodies as binders, only monoclonal antibodies satisfy the requirement for homogeneity because polyclonal antisera raised in animals yield antibodies with a spectrum of affinities and specificities. Full equilibrium, too, is seldom reached in most assays and, in fact, some assay protocols require sequential addition of reagents. Perfect separation of free from bound ligand without affecting the equilibrium is another often-violated requirement. Although these are only selected examples of the limitations found in binding assays, they explain why the law of mass action is so often unsatisfactory as a curve-fitting model. Nevertheless, the assay conditions are sometimes close enough to the ideal model to allow the use of experimental data in the equations shown above. Although it is theoretically desirable to develop binding assays that strictly follow the law of mass action, satisfying this law is neither the ultimate nor the sole measure of the practical value of a binding assay.

Multivalent Binding Reaction

In contrast to the simple univalent reaction described above, many reactions involve multivalent binding. These multivalent binding reactions have been analyzed for antigen-antibody interactions. The respective equations are, however, complex[59–64] and the applications often require computers.

LIGANDS

In general, ligands with molecular weights of less than about 5000 possess a well-defined chemical structure and can be purified into a single compound. Larger molecular size often is associated with heterogeneity due to minor structural and/or compositional differences among molecules of the same chemical species (eg, isohormones[65]). The expectations regarding the purity of different forms of ligands vary mainly with their intended use in the particular binding assay.

UNKNOWNS

Because of the high specificity of antibodies, usually there is little or no requirement for prior separation of the unknown components in immunoassays. Assuming 1:5 to 1:20 final dilutions in these assays, the use of unfractionated serum or plasma is generally suitable. There are, however, some exceptions. For instance, plasma from insulin-treated diabetics often contains antibodies to the injected heterologous insulin. In these cases, removal or destruction of interfering antibodies is necessary prior to assay for insulin.

Because of the relatively low specificity of transins, samples for RTAs routinely require pretreatment. Since the unknown ligands in these assays are nonprotein in nature and the samples commonly contain their respective binding proteins, samples are deproteinized prior to analysis.

Prior isolation of the ligand may also be required for an RTA. For instance, serum thyroxin binding globulin (TBG) binds both thyroxin (T4) and triiodothyronine (T3). Since the circulating concentration of T4 is approximately 50-fold higher than that of T3, T3 must first be separated from T4 for measurement with RTA.

Because of the comparatively low analytical specificity and sensitivity of RRAs, unknown ligands (hormones, antibodies to hormone receptors, and drugs) often require partial purification and concentration before analysis. Prepurification techniques remove cross-reacting metabolites and precursors and such interfering substances as antihormone antibodies, hormone or drug-binding substances, and proteases. The techniques employed include gel filtration, electrophoresis, ion exchange, and affinity chromatography.

TRACERS

When ligands are used as tracers, they should be very pure. The assay results ultimately depend on radioactivity measurements and high concentrations of radiolabeled impurities may thus invalidate the assay.

STANDARDS

When a ligand is used as the calibration standard, less-purified forms may be quite acceptable. Dilutions of whole serum or plasma may be appropriate as calibration standards. Because the identical behavior of standards and unknowns in a given assay system is critical, special consideration should be given to possible differences in their matrix. Heterologous ligands may serve as standards if they are sufficiently similar to the unknowns immunochemically. For instance, heterologous insulin standards and tracers were successfully employed to measure insulin from a number of mammalian species in RIAs. See further discussion of standards below.

LIGAND FOR ASSAY VALIDATION AND PERFORMANCE CHARACTERISTICS

Recovery and cross-reactivity studies require highly purified ligands. Other performance characteristics of the assay system (eg, imprecision) usually are established with impure ligand contained in a matrix that is similar if not identical to that of routine assay conditions.

IMMUNOGENS

For immunization, partially purified ligands may be satisfactory, but such ligands as steroids and glycoprotein hormones require high purity to generate sufficiently specific antisera. The hybridoma technology[33] is particularly well suited for antibody production by partially purified or unpurified ligands as immunogens. Full identity of the immunogen with the ligand of interest is desirable but not necessarily required for a usable binding assay. As long as the epitope(s) critical for the binding assay are present on the immunogen, antibodies with the appropriate specificities can be produced for interaction with the ligand to be measured.

Source of Ligands

For use as tracers or standards, ligands may be extracted from biologic materials, chemically synthesized, or produced by recombinant DNA techniques. Examples of synthetic ligands include various drugs, nonprotein hormones, and small peptide hormones such as G-17 gastrin. Chemical synthesis usually is less available for ligands of high molecular weight and hence they need to be either extracted from natural sources or, if possible, produced by recombinant DNA technology (eg, recombinant thyrotropin, TSH).

Stability and Storage of Ligands

The stability of ligands may be compromised by the presence of impurities, particularly in the case of samples (unknown ligands). However, even highly purified ligands can undergo degradation during storage, and some ligands are better preserved in a less-purified form. For example, the integrity of certain apolipoproteins and lipoproteins is difficult to preserve in a purified form. Another example is pure alpha-fetoprotein that tends to aggregate when stored in solution at −20°C.[66]

The integrity of protein ligands in solution is best preserved by rapid freezing to about −80°C, thus avoiding supercooling effects, followed by storage below −30°C. At higher temperatures and, in particular, around the eutectic point (which is the lowest melting point of a solution), most of the water is in the form of pure ice crystals that may concentrate small molecules, peptides, and proteins in liquid zones. This phenomenon causes changes in ionic strength and pH that may degrade ligands. For instance, the pH in a neutral phosphate buffer may decrease locally by several points when it is frozen to −30°C. The commonly used −20°C storage temperature is above the eutectic freezing point of physiologic saline (−23°C) and is, therefore, suboptimal for long-term storage.[67]

Stability and storage problems may also arise with nonprotein ligands, particularly in unpurified samples. For instance, steroids are stable in serum and plasma but not in whole blood. Red blood cells alter plasma concentrations of active steroids; they degrade estradiol to estrone and cortisol to cortisone and adsorb testosterone. Thus, prompt separation (within 30 minutes) of red blood cells in the specimen is necessary. Repeat freezing-thawing of plasma, serum, or urine causes hydrolysis of steroid conjugates and yields falsely high values for unconjugated steroids.

Standards

Standards are used to generate accurate and uniform test results in different runs, days, laboratories, and even countries.[68,69] Based on the specific goal to be reached, standards may be classified into such categories as calibration standard, working standard, in-house standard, and national and international reference standards. International reference standards such as the first international reference preparation (IRP) and the second international standard (IS) are established by the Expert Committee on Biological Standardization of the World Health Organization. They are based on international collaborative studies and contain a specified amount or activity of ligands. The activity of ligands for which the structure is not available in strict physicochemical terms is expressed in international units, IU. A general problem for complex ligands such as glycoprotein hormones is that their standardization is based on biologic activity, yet these materials are being utilized based on their mass as standards in immunoassays. Besides, storage may have a differential effect on biologic activity and antigenicity of these materials.

The basic requirement for all standards is that their behavior be indistinguishable from that of unknowns in the assay procedures. For quantitatively valid results, even in heterologous RIA the calibration standards should be superimposable on the dilution curve of unknowns.[70] Additional requirements include (1) sufficient quantity for assuring long-term standardization (in-house standards for months to years, whereas national and IRS standards possibly for a decade or longer); (2) sufficient stability and estimates of possible storage effects; (3) lack of interfering substances; (4) quantitative recovery with minimal vial-to-vial and batch-to-batch variation; and possibly (5) availability in a purified form. Sometimes, highly purified standards are not practical due to possible loss of biologic activity upon purification and/or storage.

Because recombinant DNA-derived proteins can be produced with great homogeneity and high purity in almost unlimited quantity, it is expected that they may obviate many of the current problems associated with standardization of protein hormones.

The choice of matrix for the preparation of standards is largely empirical. Standards may be stored in buffers with or without such added proteins as serum albumin, gelatin, or sera. The addition of proteins minimizes the adsorption of ligands to glassware, and simulates the matrix in which the unknown ligand will be presented for the assay to avoid the so-called "matrix effect." The infectious hazard should be minimal when using standards.

Antigens and Immunogens

Since most routinely used binding assays are immunoassays, the most commonly used ligands are either antigens or haptens. The *antigen* is defined as a substance that combines with its specific antibody or specifically sensitized T-lymphocytes. When injected into a suitable animal, the antigen acts as an *immunogen* and stimulates the production of specific antibodies or the generation of specifically sensitized T-lymphocytes. Hence, all immunogens are antigens but the reverse is not necessarily true.

Most immunogenic substances are either macromolecules or cell components. Immunogenicity depends on foreignness, chemical nature, molecular size, composition, and molecular complexity. In general, only substances that are recognized as nonself induce immune responses. Large proteins, polypeptides, and polysaccharides are immunogenic, whereas lipids and nucleic acids usually are not or only poorly immunogenic.*

Proteins with a molecular weight greater than 100,000 are the most potent immunogens. Immunogenicity is still strong for molecules greater than 10,000, whereas it is generally weak between 5000 and 10,000. This is why the immunogenicity of insulin, with a molecular weight of about 5800, was an unexpected finding in the original work of Berson and Yalow.[8] The minimum peptide length for immunogenicity is about 8 to 15 amino acids with molecular weights between 1000 and 2500.[71] These short peptides are, however, poorly immunogenic by themselves and frequently produce antisera of low titer and affinity not usable in binding radioassays. The smallest peptide hormone that has been shown to be immunogenic by itself is vasopressin with a molecular weight of 1080.[72]

Antigenic Determinants or Epitopes

Only a restricted portion of the antigen binds to antibody. This small portion of the antigen that fits the *antibody combining site* or *paratope* is called the *antigenic determinant* or *epitope*. The entire antigenic determinant is usually no greater than four amino acids or four or five sugar molecules. Thus, large antigens may carry a number of antigenic determinants. For instance, a single-chain protein consisting of 100 amino acids may contain up to 20 nonoverlapping, linearly continuous epitopes. With the formation of secondary structure, eg, helices, the entire molecule assumes a three-dimensional conformation. The assembly of other chemical macromolecules is based on similar principles. The development of higher-ordered structures has two major implications for antigenicity: (1) of the many antigenic determinants present in the primary structure (up to 20 in the above example) most will be "buried" and only a few will be exposed and actually available for reaction on the surface of large antigens in their native state and (2) since the primary requirement for forming an epitope is *spatial contiguity*, amino acids present in distinct regions of the same polypeptide chain or in different polypeptide chains can form *discontinuous epitopes*, which are not present in the primary structure.

These two observations explain (1) the finding of "unexpected" immunoreactivity by monoclonal antibodies of denatured macromolecules but not of those in the native state;[71] (2) the occasional loss of immunoreactivity with isolation and purification procedures that disrupt the tertiary and quaternary structure and, hence, the discontinuous epitopes of some macromolecules; and (3) that genetically manufactured peptides, by not assembling into the proper tertiary structure, may not express the same (discontinuous) epitopes as their native counterparts.[71] Fortunately, problems related to the use of synthetically produced peptides as antigens are uncommon.[73,74]

The importance of higher-ordered structures in defining discontinuous epitopes on proteins is well documented for the naturally occurring peptide hormone, insulin. It was observed that pork, dog, and sperm whale insulins have identical amino acid sequences (primary structure) but are immunologically distinguishable by some antisera.[75,76] The likely explanation is that the secondary and tertiary structure and the formation of some unique discontinuous epitopes is determined at the time the two polypeptide chains of insulin are synthesized in the proinsulin molecule. Indeed, the composition of the connecting (C-) peptides are different in pork and dog proinsulins.[77] Note that even solid-phase adsorption of proteins, eg, to tubes or microtiter plates, may produce conformational changes in their tertiary structure, leading to altered epitope expression.[71]

Haptens

Haptens are small, sometimes called incomplete, antigens that are not immunogenic by themselves but can be rendered immunogenic when coupled with high molecular weight molecules, the *carriers*. Haptens are somewhat analogous to antigenic determinants. Being antigenic means that haptens react with specific antibodies or specifically sensitized T-lymphocytes. As discussed above, peptides with molecular weights between 1000 and 5000 usually are poorly immunogenic. They are, therefore, functionally haptens and require conjugation with carrier proteins to generate potent antisera required for radioassays. The molecular weight of *true* haptens (with no immunogenicity at all) is below 1000 with a minimum molecular weight of approximately 150. Steroids and most drugs are true haptens.

Conjugation of Haptens to Carrier Proteins

In order to obtain a good antibody response, haptens known to be strong stimulators are conjugated with relatively weakly immunogenic carriers, whereas haptens known to

*By usual definition, proteins consist of at least 50 amino acids; fewer amino acid residues joined by amide bonds in a single chain are called polypeptides or peptides.

be weak stimulators are combined with strongly immunogenic carriers.

The binding of haptens to carrier proteins via covalent bonds requires bifunctional reagents, ie, compounds that can react at both ends. Common conjugation techniques include the mixed anhydride, carbodiimide, benzidine, and glutaraldehyde (Schiff's base) reactions.[78-81] The ideal site of attachment on the hapten molecule is selected on the basis of Landsteiner's principle[82] which states that antisera tend to be specific for that part of the hapten molecule farthest removed from the point of conjugation, ie, the penultimate [distal] portion of the antigen. This implies that those groups that are most unique for a given hapten and the reactivity of which will most likely discriminate them from other similar substances such as precursors, metabolites, and analogs should not be used for conjugation and, if possible, should be positioned distant from the actual point of attachment. The importance of the Landsteiner's principle has been particularly well documented for ring structures such as steroids and diphenylhydantoin.[83,84]

Binding Activity vs Biologic Activity and/or Chemical Identity

The use of biologically active ligands as antigens raises an important question about the biologic relevance of the results obtained and the chemical identity of the ligand measured by immunoassays. Ideally, there is a good agreement between bioactivity, immunoactivity, and chemical identity. However, even in properly validated immunoassays only immunologic but not biologic or chemical identity is required between unknowns and standards. At the beginning of RIA technology Berson and Yalow pointed out that specific recognition by antibody of part of a molecule does not necessarily guarantee a coincidence with those parts that are responsible for biologic activity. Since then numerous examples have been reported where the immunoactivity and bioactivity or chemical nature of a ligand in question disagree: confirming an inherent limitation of ligand immunoassays. There are three major situations in which this limitation may lead to erroneous results:

1. Antigenically and chemically similar but biologically inactive ligands. This is by far the most common problem for binding assays and most often occurs with large antigens that express multiple epitopes. The antibody may cross-react with functionally deficient isohormones, precursors, and degradation products. Proper selection of antibody specificity can reduce or eliminate this problem that usually results in an overestimate of the biologically active fraction. The measurement of biologically deficient or inactive substances is, however, not always a disadvantage. For instance, immunoassays for enzymes such as creatine kinase BB or MB are claimed to have a distinct advantage over catalytic methods in that they measure the actual protein concentration of the enzyme based on the presence of antigenic determinants rather than enzymic activity. In fact, these assays appear to have greater analytical sensitivity and specificity than catalytic methods.
2. Antigenically related but chemically and biologically different ligands. These ligands have no functional and chemical relationship, ie, they are biologically and chemically different, but, because of identity or similarity in some of their epitopes, they are immunologically cross-reactive. Obviously, the impact of this phenomenon on ligand immunoassays is the greatest when the cross-reactive substances occur in the same species; as is the case with human growth hormone (GH) and human chorionic somatomammotropin, (CS).[85,86] Although GH is of pituitary and CS is of placental origin and the two share no known biologic function, they may cross-react in immunoassays for growth hormone. In fact, CS was discovered by studying why serum dilutions from pregnant women did not follow linearity in immunoassays for GH.[85,86] On a theoretical basis, antibodies with too narrow binding specificity, such as monoclonals or affinity-purified polyclonals, may, paradoxically, lead to an increased rate of cross-reactivity between functionally and chemically different large antigens. This could occur because these antibodies are capable of recognizing a single epitope that, purely by chance, may be present on unrelated molecules. In other words, by not recognizing the biologically relevant portion of the antigen, antibodies with exquisite binding specificity may paradoxically reduce assay specificity for biologically active antigens. To avoid this problem, presenting as an overestimate of the antigen in question, proper selection of antibody specificity, pooling of monoclonal antibodies with different epitope specificities into a single reagent, or simultaneous use of several monoclonal antibodies in a sandwich assay format are suggested.[87,88] The noncompetitive IRMA format compensates well for possible narrowness of specificity but can only be applied to large antigens containing multiple epitopes.
3. Antigenically unrelated but chemically and biologically similar ligands. In these situations the high specificity of antibodies is again responsible for the discrepant results between immunoactivity and bioactivity when the antigens are only slightly different chemically. For instance, protein hormones bearing similar biological and chemical properties may produce little or no reaction in the immunoassay designed for another species. In RIAs for human thyrotropin, thyrotropins from dogs, cattle, rats, and rabbits, all with similar biological properties, failed to cross-react.[89,90] Likewise, in an RIA for lysine-vasopressin, arginine-vasopressin did not react.[91] The two types of vasopressin have similar biological properties and differ only in a single amino acid. Thus, if the goal is to establish uniqueness of a ligand, antibody specificities like the ones described for thyrotropin and vasopressin are appropriate or desirable. If, however, the goal is to establish biological activity irrespective of the source of ligand,

antibodies with specificity directed against epitopes that are possibly shared between functionally similar antigens are necessary for the binding reaction.

Ligand measurements based on binding reactions should be interpreted with caution. By proper design, the relationship between binding ability and biologic activity and/or chemical identity can be maximized in these assays for the ligand of interest. However, because of the inherent limitations of binding assays, in vitro or in vivo bioassays are still needed in selected cases to assay biologically active ligands. Extensive discussions of the relationship between immunoactivity, binding activity to receptors, and bioactivity have been published previously.[38,65,70,92–94]

BINDERS

Practically all currently used binders are proteins, including antibodies, circulating transport proteins (transins), and cell receptors. In RIAs, IRMAs, 4i assay, and RIMA, the binders are antibodies with an average molecular weight of 155,000; in RTAs, mainly glycoproteins with a molecular weight of less than 100,000; and in RRAs, a heterogenous group of proteins, eg, membrane-bound receptors or soluble muclear receptors with molecular weights ranging from 50,000 to 300,000. Alternative protein binders include lectins,[95] avidin[96,97] (68,000) or streptavidin[98] (60,000), and "nature's universal antibodies" staphylococcal protein A (42,000)[99–101] and streptococcal protein G (30,000).[102,103] The protein composition is, however, not a theoretical requirement; chelators and, as mentioned earlier, oligo- and polynucleotides could also serve as binders.

Saturability

All binding reagents are expected to show *saturability*, ie, to contain a finite number of binding sites. Competitive binding (limited reagent) methods also are called "saturation analysis" because they rely on the fact that the distribution of ligands between bound and free fractions depends on the ligand initially present, provided the binder is "saturable" and is held strictly constant.[38] Noncompetitive (reagent excess) assays, in turn, are based on excess amounts of binder.

Not surprisingly, the requirement for a saturable binder that is held constant in a competitive binding assay presents a special problem for those receptor assays in which intact cells act as binders. Regulation of receptor number by homologous hormone on cells may change the sensitivity of the system.[104–106] However, this phenomenon per se does not necessarily represent a disadvantage; in fact, in some cases it has been successfully exploited to increase assay sensitivity.[105,106]

During the development of binding radioassays it was recognized early that two additional characteristics of the binding reaction are critical for analytical performance of an assay: affinity (and related avidity) and specificity (and related cross-reactivity).

Affinity

The *affinity* is the thermodynamic expression of the binding energy contained in the ligand-binder complex. The affinity of a binder (for a given ligand) is quantitatively expressed by the affinity or equilibrium constant K_a of the binding reaction ($K_a = k_a/k_d$—see Equation 2). The minimum affinity constant required for a usable binding assay is between 10^6 and 10^7 L/mol. If K_a is less than 1×10^6 L/mol, the amount of binder required to obtain substantial ligand binding will be unreasonably large. Currently, the alternative binder avidin or streptavidin is the highest affinity binder with $K_a = 10^{15}$ L/mol in its interaction with biotin. This high affinity makes the binding reaction practically irreversible.

In general, the affinity constant for competitive binding assays should be within the same order of magnitude as the concentration of ligand to be measured. With RIAs this goal is achieved by selecting high-affinity polyclonal antibodies. In the case of RTAs for hormones, the assay sensitivity is within the capability of transins because circulating concentrations of both thyroxin and cortisol are about 10^{-7} mol/L, ie, much higher than those of many other hormones of interest. The receptor affinity for most hormones, when described by the dissociation constant ($K_d = 1/K_a$), falls approximately in the range of circulating hormone concentrations (ie, 10^{-9} to 10^{-12} mol/L). The therapeutic concentration of drugs usually is 10^{-4} to 10^{-8} mol/L, making them readily amenable to measurement with RRA. Monoclonal antibodies with relatively low binding affinity are primarily used in noncompetitive binding assays where binding affinity is not as critical for analytical sensitivity. The *minimum detectable concentration* in competitive binding assays approaches the reciprocal of the affinity constant, ie, close to $1/K_a$.

In competitive binding immunoassays, the higher the K_a value (1) the more sensitive the assay analytically; (2) the faster the development of equilibrium; and (3) the higher the concentration of the binder-ligand complex formed. On the other hand, because of differences in binding reaction forces, the rate of association usually is most rapid for receptors and transins (minutes to hours), and much slower for antibodies (hours to days).[49] These rates largely determine the speed at which competitive binding assays can be performed.

It is important to recognize that the affinity constant of polyclonal antibodies represents an average of a pool of antibodies with a range of affinities (and specificities). Monoclonal antibodies constitute the most homogeneous binders. Transins are usually a single binding substance. Receptors may have a single noninteracting binding site, a single interacting binding site, or more than one noninteracting binding site.[94] Fortunately, this receptor heterogeneity rarely leads to notable differences in assay results.[94]

When conditions for the law of mass action are met, K_a

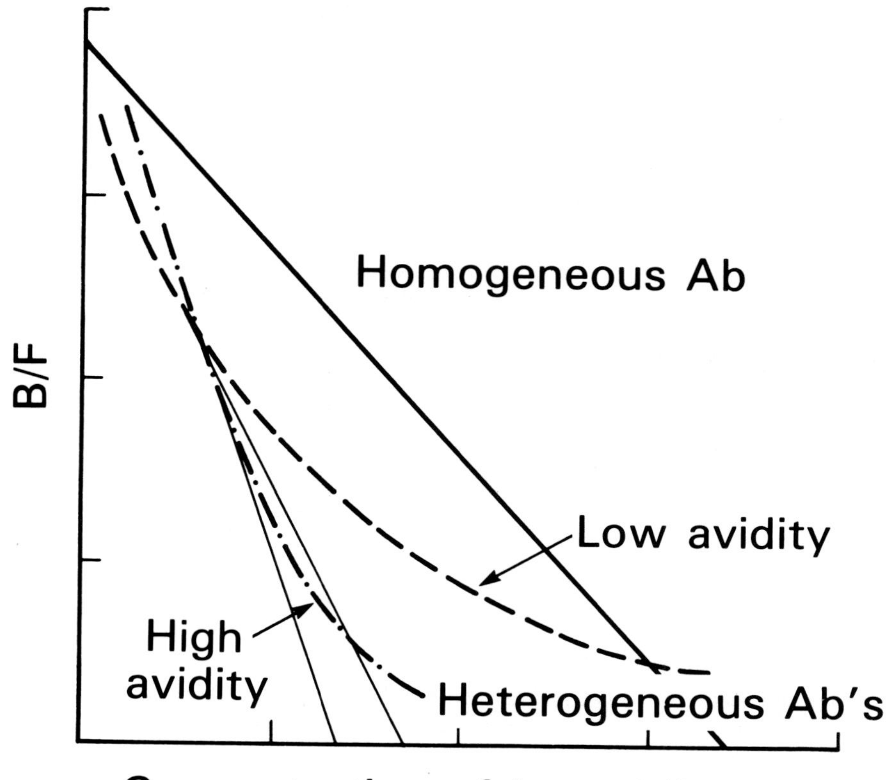

Figure 3. Scatchard plots of monoclonal (homogeneous) and various polyclonal (heterogeneous) antibodies.

can be determined from the Scatchard plot[55] (see Equation 6 and Fig. 3). A straight line in the Scatchard plot indicates homogeneous binding sites, whereas downward curved lines signify binding site heterogeneity. However, curved lines can have other causes as well.[107,108] Downward concavity of the Scatchard plot may indicate negative cooperativity, while upward concavity is consistent with positive cooperativity between the binding sites. Nonlinear curves showing positive curvature in RIAs may also result from imperfect experimental conditions. These include conditions when (1) nonspecific binding (NSB) is corrected for the free fraction; (2) labeled ligand affinity is less than unlabeled ligand affinity, eg, due to "aging" tracer; (3) the free and bound fractions are incompletely separated; and (4) RIA is performed under nonequilibrium conditions.

In the case of antibodies, the determination of affinity is most precise when the binding reaction is univalent, ie, when monovalent Fab fragments of monoclonal antibodies react with monovalent antigens. In turn, the determination of K_a is the least reliable when polyclonal antibodies react with multivalent antigens. Under these conditions, secondary reactions such as complement binding[109,110] and Fc-Fc interactions[111] may modify the primary antigen-antibody reaction.

In routine applications where divalent antibody (usually IgG) preparations are compared for their relative binding potential to the same univalent antigen, measurement of the *intrinsic association constant* is recommended.[71] This constant is the reciprocal of the free antigen concentration at half saturation of the antibody, ie, when half the antibody-combining sites are occupied by antigen (see Equation 5).[71] It has the same units as K_a.

Avidity

Since most current immunoassays involve intact monoclonal or polyclonal antibodies and multivalent antigens, the term *avidity* is used to describe the sum of total interactions between the two binding reactants. Thus, avidity is a broader term and may carry greater bond energy than affinity, which only reflects the interaction between individual antibody combining sites and antigenic determinants. In a way, affinity may be considered as the property of the substance bound (antigen) and avidity as the property of the binder (antibody). In the simplest case, assuming identical affinities for the individual binding sites of IgG and IgM, the IgM molecule (a pentamer with ten binding sites) will have much greater avidity for multivalent antigens than an IgG molecule with only two binding sites. It is, however, even more important that a typical IgG molecule binds at least 10,000 times more strongly to a multivalent antigen if both binding sites are involved than if only one site is engaged. The avidity also is augmented when several antibodies bind simultaneously to different epitopes on the same antigen molecule.

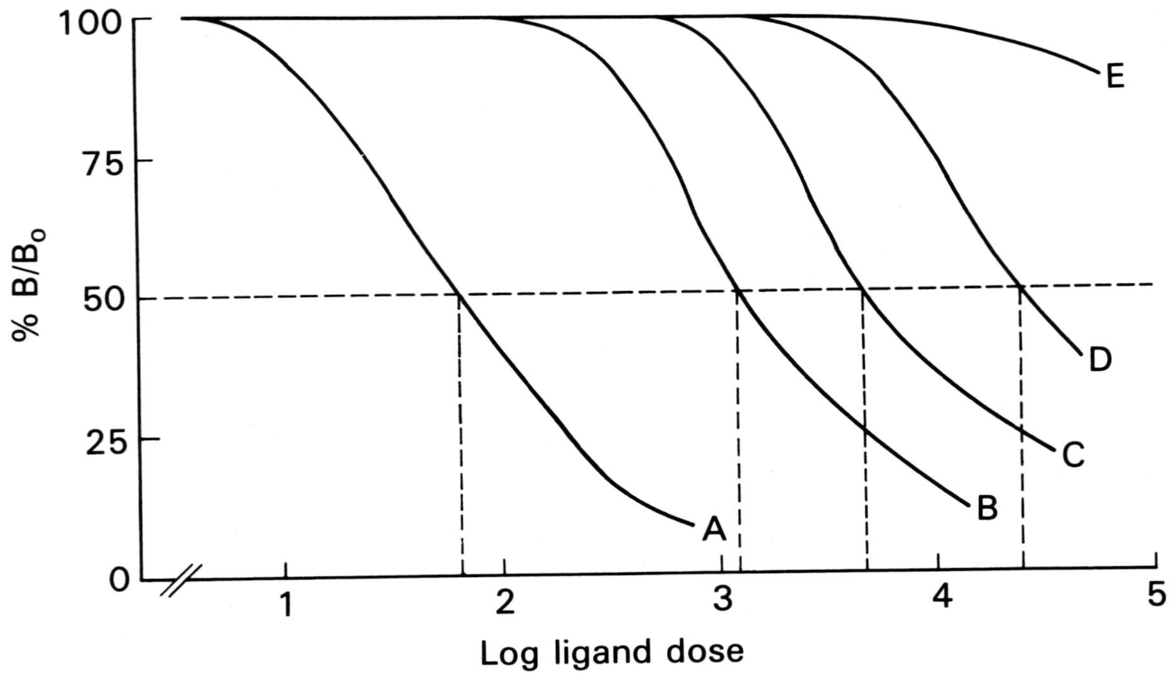

Figure 4. Determination of cross-reactivity in competitive binding radioassays. **(A)**. Standard dose-response curve for the ligand of interest. **(B, C, and D)**. Dose-response curves for cross-reactive substances with decreasing potency (approximately 8, 1, and 0.5% cross-reactivity, respectively). **(E)**. Dose-response curve for a substance with barely detectable cross-reactive potency. Degree of cross reactivity (%) is defined by the ratio of the dose of ligand of interest to the dose of cross-reacting substance, both causing the same degree (eg, 50% B/B_0) of tracer displacement.

Specificity

While affinity (or avidity) is a critical factor in determining the analytical sensitivity of a binding assay, the diagnostic usefulness of binding assays greatly depends on the *specificity.* Specificity can be defined as the uniqueness of interaction between a given binder and a given ligand, conferred by the intrinsic spatial configuration of the binding site(s) and the "goodness of fit" of the reactive site(s) of the ligand. Specificity is probably never confined to a single substance. According to Murphy and Lehotay,[49] the binding reaction is specific when "the degree of complementarity required for tight binding is so great that only a few closely related analogs can fit well enough to bind strongly." Indeed, some binding reactions, such as catecholamine binding to membrane receptors, exhibit *stereospecificity* as well. Binding of peptide/protein hormones by receptors shows, however, no stereospecificity.[94] Antibodies and transins may also be stereospecific binders. Not surprisingly, monoclonal antibodies exhibit more stereospecificity than do polyclonals. For instance, surveying four currently available immunoassays for free thyroxin, the two assays with polyclonal antithyroxin antibodies both were described to have a 100% cross-reactivity with D-thyroxin, whereas two assays with mouse monoclonal antithyroxin antibodies had only 30 and 60% cross-reactivity with D-thyroxin. As to transins, thyroxin-binding prealbumin (TBPA, transthyretin) binds L-thyroxin but has negligible affinity for D-thyroxin. In turn, thyroxin-binding globulin (TBG, thyropexin) shows no stereospecificity for the binding of thyroxin.

Cross-Reactivity

Specificity can also be defined as the reciprocal of *cross-reactivity* of the binder with other ligands, particularly with those similar in structure to the ligand in question. In competitive binding assays, cross-reactivity testing usually is performed by setting up serial dilutions of related or suspected ligands as unknowns in parallel with similar dilutions of the original ligand in the standard assay.[112] The results are then plotted as dose-response curves (Fig. 4). Ligands are commonly compared at 50% displacement of the labeled ligand (ie, reduction of the binding of the labeled ligand to 50% of the initial value, B_0 or b_0), and the degree of cross-reactivity is calculated as follows:

$$\text{Cross-reactivity (\%)} = \frac{\text{Concentration (dose) of original ligand causing 50\% displacement}}{\text{Concentration (dose) of cross-reacting ligand causing 50\% displacement}} \times 100$$

Cross-reactivity testing at other B_0 values (often between 70 and 90%) can also be carried out, but with nonparallel response curves the results depend on the % B_0.[113]

Table 2. Comparison of Polyclonal and Monoclonal Antibodies

	POLYCLONAL	MONOCLONAL
Antibody production		
Purity of immunogen	High purity desirable and/or required	May be produced with partially or unpurified immunogen
Technique involved	Easy and simple	More difficult (requires special skills and facilities)
Antibody yield	Limited both in time and quantity	Virtually unlimited
Characteristics of antibody		
Composition	Heterogeneous	Homogeneous
Specificity	Relatively low (antibodies react with a variety of epitopes)	Very high (all antibodies react with the same epitope)
Affinity	Usually high (affinity constant is the average of different antibodies)	Relatively low* (affinity constant is the same for all antibodies)
Stability	Good	Variable (may be sensitive to storage, iodination, variations in pH, temperature)
Ability to agglutinate/ precipitate	Often good (because of reaction with different epitopes present on large antigens)	Rarely present (because of recognition of unique epitopes, agglutinates/precipitates only if epitope is repeated on the antigen)

*High-affinity monoclonal antibodies can now be produced by special techniques.

Source of Binders

Since the most commonly used binding assays are immunoassays, the most widely used binders are antibodies. Polyclonal antibodies are obtained by immunizing animals or, rarely, by harvesting accidentally formed antibodies such as the human anti-bovine/pork insulin antibodies used initially by Berson and Yalow.[114] Although the affinity and specificity of polyclonal antibodies varies with time and the animal of origin, a single batch of high-titered polyclonal antibodies may be sufficient for thousands or millions of determinations. For example, a batch of sheep antiserum that can be used at a working dilution of 1:10^6 will enable the performance of 10^9 to 10^{10} individual RIAs.[38] Avian antibodies have potentially two advantages over those from mammalian species: (1) they can be harvested in large quantities from the yolks of eggs and (2) they may exhibit fewer nonspecific interactions (complement binding) than mammalian antibodies.[115]

Since the discovery of the hybridoma technology,[33] monoclonal antibodies, primarily from the mouse, are being used with increasing frequency in immunoassays (Table 2). Monoclonals provide a homogeneous and continuous supply of reagent. Recently, other new possibilities became available for the production of specific antibodies as binding reagents. Using recombinant DNA technology, antibodies or antibody fragments have been produced by bacteria such as *Escherichia coli*[116–119] and yeasts such as *Saccharomyces cerevisiae*.[119,120] Undoubtedly, this technology has the potential to provide well-characterized, homogeneous, and even "custom-designed" binding reagents in an essentially unlimited supply.

Transins are available from such diverse sources as mammalian serum, eg, human TBG for thyroxin, equine transcortin for steroids,[121] rat vitamin D-binding protein for vitamin D, bovine milk beta-lactoglobulin for folate, and hog gastric intrinsic factor for vitamin B_{12}. Plasma as a source of transins is generally used diluted about 1:10.

Isolated "cytosol" (but, truly, nuclear) binding proteins are the source of receptors for steroid and thyroid hormones, the vitamin D group, and such drugs as cyclosporine, FK-506, and rapamycin,[122,123] whereas crude or purified plasma membranes and single-cell suspensions prepared from mammalian tissues, blood, or cell culture lines serve as binders for protein/peptide hormones, the neurotransmitter γ-aminobutyric acid,[124] and several drugs such as digoxin and neuroleptics. Receptors may also be produced by chemical synthesis[31] and recombinant DNA technology.[125,126]

Initially, radioreceptor binding studies were performed with typical target tissues for the hormones. However, it is now well established that nontarget tissues may also carry specific binding sites for different ligands, and hence can be used for RRAs.[94] Interestingly, intact cells have also been exploited for the measurement of vitamin D that binds to a "cytosol" receptor protein.[127] In this "cytoreceptor" method, the 1,25-$(OH)_2$-vitamin D fraction of a plasma specimen is incubated with intact rat bone cells containing 1,25-$(OH)_2$-vitamin D_3 receptors. The cell membrane (1) decreases the entry of interfering vitamin D metabolites into the cell for binding to the "cytosol" receptor and thus reduces the usual degree of sample pre-purification and (2) separates the bound from the free ligand.

Immunoglobulin Structure

Antibodies are immunoglobulins with specific binding activity. The prototype of an antibody molecule usually is represented by IgG (Fig. 5). IgG consists of four polypeptide chains—two identical heavy (H)-chains each containing

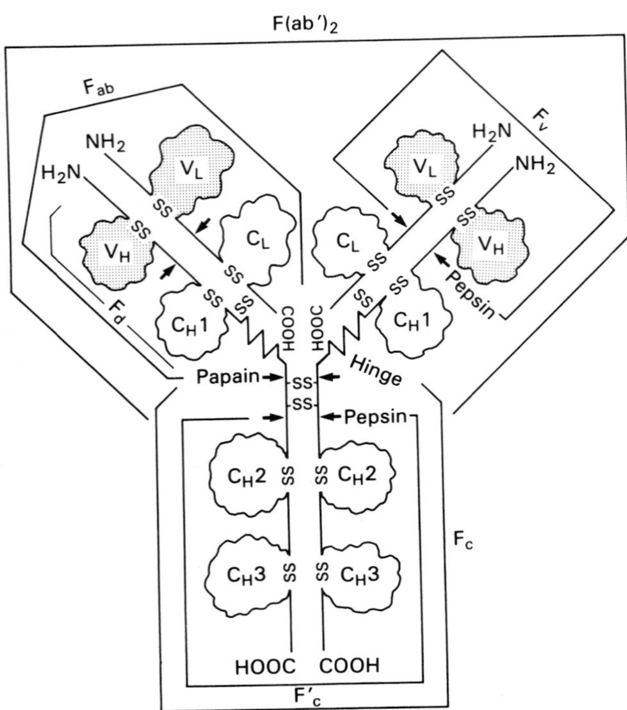

Figure 5. Schematic structure of immunoglobulin G molecule. Relative positions of interchain and intrachain disulfide bonds, intrachain loops and domains, and probable cleaving sites by papain and pepsin with the resultant fragments are shown. See text for description.

about 450 amino acids (molecular weight 55,000) and two identical light (L)-chains each containing about 220 amino acids (molecular weight 23,000). The four chains are held together by a combination of covalent bonds and noncovalent interactions. There are interchain disulfide (-S-S-) bonds between the two H-chains and between pairs of H-chains and L-chains. The mid-portion of the H-chains (*hinge region*) is unusually rich in proline and hydrophilic amino acid residues, conferring a certain degree of flexibility. This allows the molecule to assume its well-known Y-shaped structure and to bind simultaneously to two similar epitopes on the same antigen or on different antigens (cross-linking).

Each intrachain "loop" is composed of 50 to 70 amino acids. The loops and adjacent amino acids constitute the immunoglobulin *domains*. The variable regions have a single domain (designated V_H and V_L for H- and L-chains, respectively). The L-chains have one constant region domain (designated C_L), but the H-chains have three constant region domains in the case of IgG, IgA, and IgD, designated C_H1, C_H2, and C_H3 and an additional domain, C_H4, in the case of IgM and IgE. The hinge region is located between the C_H2 and C_H3 domains; this is the most common site of proteolysis. It is the variable domains of the H- and L-chains folded in close proximity that form a cleft or pouch (antigen-binding site or *paratope*) where the epitope with a sterically complementary configuration will fit. In each V-domain only about 20 to 30 amino acid residues contribute to the formation of paratopes. In fact, the amino acid sequence variability is restricted to three small hypervariable regions in the V_L domain, and to three, or may be four, hypervariable regions in the V_H domain. Only 4 to 8 amino acids in each paired hypervariable region (H- and L-chains) form the antigen-binding site and are responsible for its specificity and affinity. Because of the unique genetic mechanisms involved in the assembly of variable domains, it is estimated that humans are able to make as many as a 100 million different antibody molecules.

The incubation of purified IgG with papain splits the molecule in the hinge region above the disulfide bonds into two monovalent Fab (*a*ntigen *b*inding) and one Fc (*c*rystallizable) fragments (Fig. 5). Limited proteolysis with pepsin below the disulfide bonds produces a bivalent $F(ab')_2$ and an Fc′ fragment. Digestion with pepsin under proper conditions also disrupts a site between the variable and constant regions. The V_H and V_L domains remain noncovalently associated and yield the *Fv* (*v*ariable) fragment which is fully capable of antigen-binding. The part of H-chain that contains the Fab fragment is called *Fd*. The antigen-binding portion of the antibody molecule is called the *V*-module; a term often used in the context of genetic engineering of antibodies.

Humoral Immune Response

For triggering an immune response, the immunogen first must be recognized as nonself by immunocompetent cells (*immune recognition*). It is thought that for each possible antigenic specificity there is a clone of immunocytes bearing multiple copies of the receptor specific for that antigen. In B-lymphocytes these specific receptors are surface-bound immunoglobulins, particularly IgD and monomeric IgM molecules. In T-lymphocytes, the specific receptors are composed of two transmembrane polypeptide chains, termed α and β, with similar molecular weights (40,000 to 45,000). According to the involvement of T-cells in immune recognition, antigens may be T dependent or T independent.[128] *T-dependent antigens* contain a large number of epitopes with little repetition of a given type. In turn, most T-independent antigens are polysaccharides or lipopolysaccharides consisting of repeating sequences of a limited number of sugars. The antibody response to *T-independent antigens* occurs by direct stimulation of B-cells with antigen, either by binding to two receptors (one is a membrane-bound antigen-specific immunoglobulin, the other is a mitogen receptor) or by simultaneous binding to and cross-linking of antigen-specific membrane bound immunoglobulin receptors. The antibody response by B-cells to *T-dependent antigens* requires initial close contact with macrophages and other antigen-presenting cells (eg, Langerhans cells of the epidermis and the dendritic cells of the lymphoid tissues) and helper T-cells. While macrophages "process" the antigen for presentation to resting helper T-cells, other antigen-presenting cells do not.

Upon proper stimulation, each B-cell clone makes antibodies with a unique antigen binding site. First, the antibody

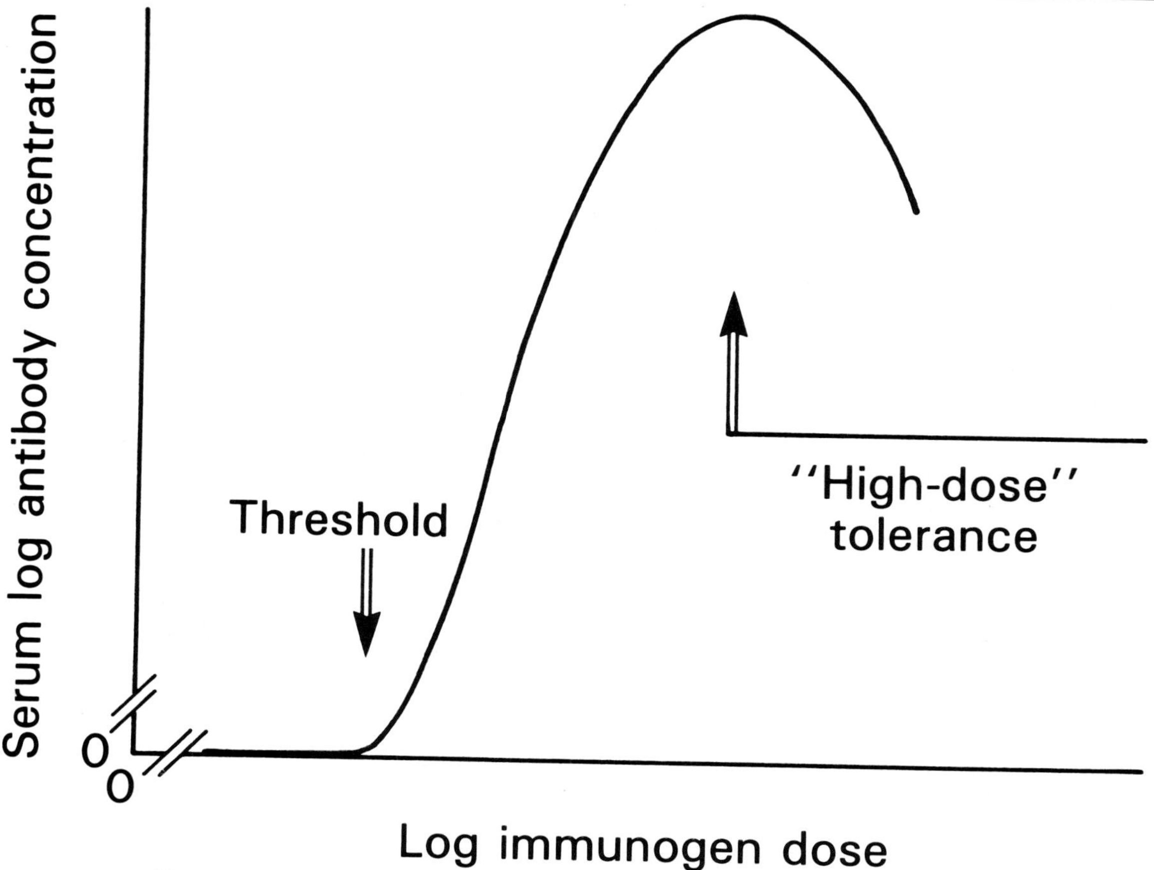

Figure 6. Dependence of serum antibody concentration on the dose of immunogen.

molecules are inserted into the cell membrane, where they serve as receptors for the respective antigen. When antigen binds to these surface receptors, the B-cells are triggered to multiply and differentiate into plasma cells that secrete large amounts of soluble antibody with the same antigen specificity into the circulation. The immune response is a complex and self-limiting phenomenon that also involves the production of a variety of soluble factors such as interleukins, interferons, and B-cell growth factors; feedback mechanisms such as suppressor T-cells and antibody feedback; the formation of memory cells (only for T-dependent antigens); and, possibly, the development of immune tolerance. All plasma cells initially synthesize IgM antibodies, but, in the case of T-dependent antigens, many eventually switch to making other classes of antibody, such as IgG or IgA ("*class switching*".) In this process, the initial L-chain type and antigen specificity are maintained but binding affinity may increase.

Polyclonal Antibodies

Traditionally, antibodies were raised by planned immunization of animals and humans, and only rarely obtained by harvesting antibodies formed incidentally, eg, human anti-pork/bovine insulin antibodies. Despite several years of experience in raising antibodies to a great variety of antigens and haptens, the production of a satisfactory antiserum is an imprecise art rather than a science. There is extensive literature on various practical aspects of immunization, but no general agreement as to (1) the dose and purity of immunogen; (2) the use and type of adjuvants; (3) the choice of animals; (4) the route of immunization; and (5) the immunization and bleeding schedule. Only a few general concepts can be summarized here and the best approach to produce a high-quality antiserum to a given substance remains largely empirical.

1. Both the *dose* and *purity of an immunogen* can affect the success of antibody production. Below a threshold dose there is no antibody production (Fig. 6). At higher doses, the serum antibody response increases almost linearly with the immunizing dose up to a peak serum antibody concentration, followed by a similar rate of decline with further increases in the dose of the immunogen (*high-dose* or *zone tolerance*). Excessively high doses of the immunogen also reduce the avidity of the antibodies formed.[129] Although the immunogen dose may depend on the animal species chosen, a suitable primary dose of peptide/protein antigens for mice, guinea pigs, and rabbits is in the order of 10 to 100 μg in complete Freund's adjuvant (CFA). Highly purified immunogens are not always required for the production of a good antiserum.

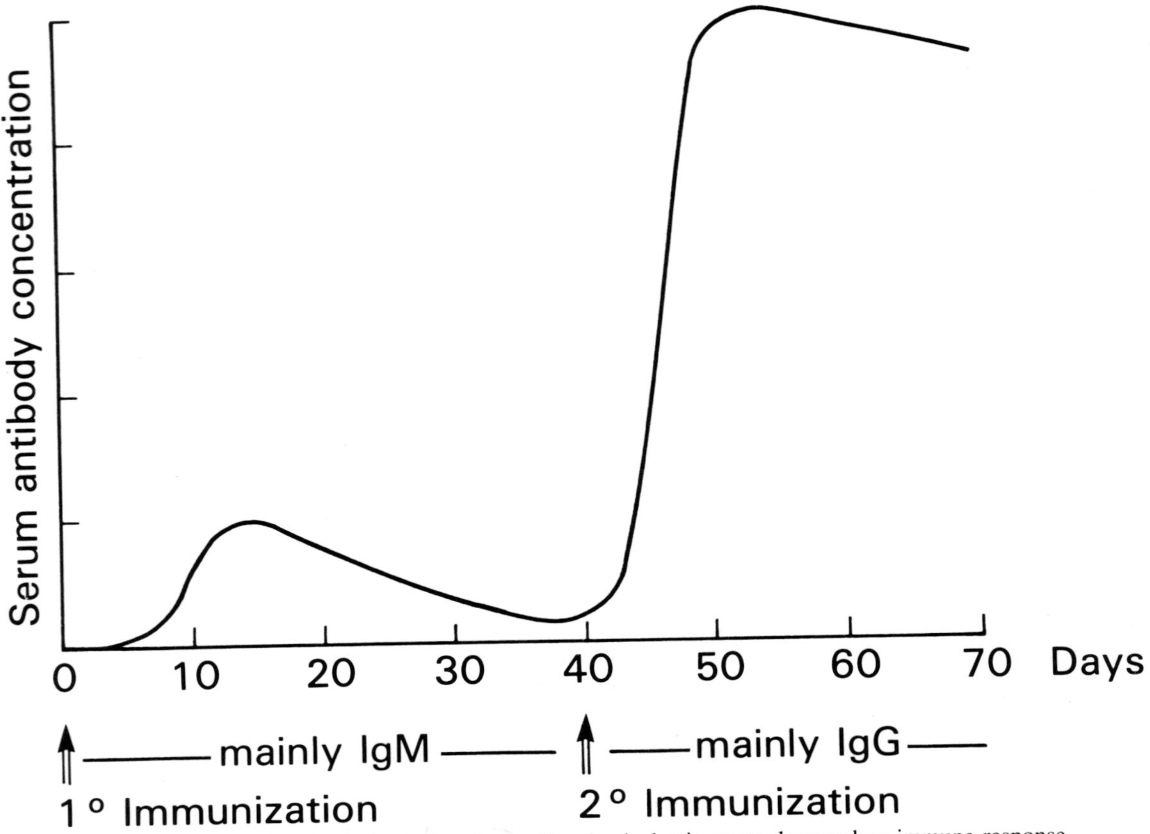

Figure 7. Serum antibody formation during the classical primary and secondary immune response.

In the early 1970s, in fact, it was suggested that impurities in a semipurified antigen may act as adjuvants to stimulate antibody production. Since then, this has been debated by many investigators. Nevertheless, immunization with several unrelated antigens can be performed simultaneously. Interestingly, no relationship appears to exist between the concentration and specificity of antibodies directed toward the various antigens.[70]

2. Immunological adjuvants nonspecifically potentiate the specific immune response.[130] They include a variety of unrelated substances such as CFA (heat-killed and dried *Mycobacterium tuberculosis* in a water-in-oil emulsion), incomplete Freund's adjuvant (without mycobacteria), emulsified lanolin, aluminum hydroxide, gelatin, bacterial cell wall isolates, and many others. The most popular adjuvant is CFA. The effect of adjuvants involves one or more of the following mechanisms:[131] (a) prolongation of the release of immunogen from the depot site; (b) induction of inflammation; and (c) activation of macrophages. Although most adjuvants exhibit undesirable side effects, their use remains critical for successful antibody production. Latex particles and liposomes may replace the rather toxic CFA in the future.[132]
3. The choice of animal may depend on the degree of foreignness of the immunogen to a given species, the amount of antiserum necessary, and practical issues such as cost and ease of housing, handling, and bleeding. Rabbits are popular, but guinea pigs, inbred strains of mice, goat, sheep, donkey, horse, and chicken also are commonly used. Newborn mammals are unresponsive and old animals show reduced responsiveness to immunication, as do those in poor health and/or nutritional condition. Because antibody responses often vary among different individuals of a given species, it is advisable to immunize several animals with the same antigen. Obviously, it is easier to find good responders to a given antigen in a group of genetically diverse animals than in a group of inbred animals, which, in turn, are expected to show more uniformity in their response.
4. The route of administration primarily depends on the composition of immunizing material. Depot preparations require subcutaneous or intramuscular administrations. Injections into the footpads are now discouraged because of animal discomfort. Multisite (30 to 50) intradermal injections[133] may result in skin ulcerations and appear to have no clear advantage in stimulating antibody response over the use of subcutaneous injections at only a few sites.[134]
5. The immunization and bleeding schedule vary with the properties of immunogen, the use and type of adjuvant,

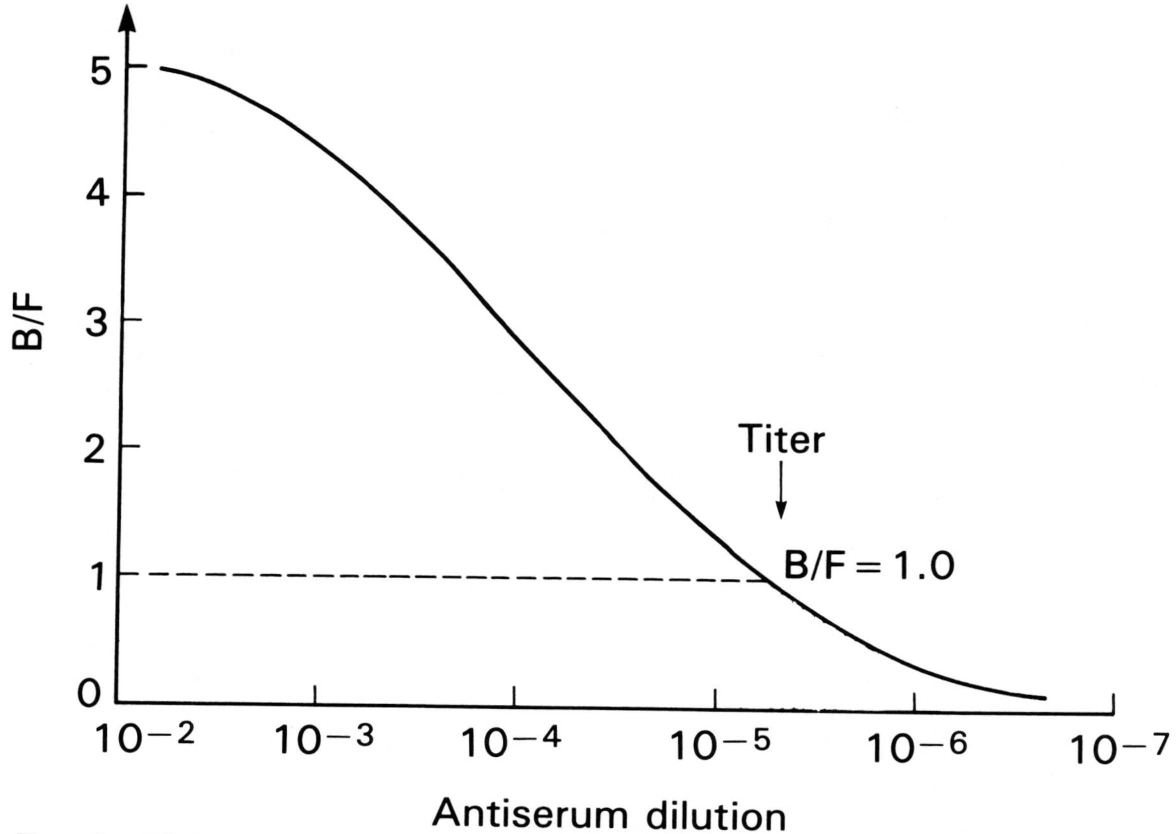

Figure 8. Dilution curve of antiserum with a fixed amount of labeled antigen. Antibody titer is defined by 50% tracer binding ($B/F = 1.0$). The dilution that gives $B/F = 0.5$ to 1.0 usually is the most appropriate working antibody titer for RIA.

the choice of animal, and the route of administration. Characteristic primary and secondary immune responses are shown in Figure 7. Compared to the primary response, (1) the secondary response occurs after a very short lag phase; (2) the antibody production rises more rapidly; (3) antibody concentration peaks much higher and faster; (4) peak antibody concentrations decline more slowly; and (5) instead of IgM, mostly IgG antibodies are formed and antibody affinity often is greater. Second and subsequent booster injections also require smaller immunogen doses. After booster injections, the animal continues to produce antibodies over a period of weeks to months. Consequently, blood as a source of antiserum may be collected for months to years from large animals receiving booster injections. In case of frequent bleeds, iron supplementation should be considered to prevent the development of anemia. With repeat injections at 2- to 3-week intervals, the serum antibody concentration reaches a plateau after three to five doses of the immunogen. Sometimes, immunogen boosters decrease serum antibody concentration, in which case immunization should be stopped for 3 to 6 months, after which reimmunization often enhances antibody response.

Antibody Titer and Concentration

The *antibody titer* is the capacity of an antiserum to bind a given antigen and can be conveniently defined by tracer-binding studies (Fig. 8). Serial dilutions of antiserum are incubated with a fixed amount of radiolabeled tracer antigen and the percent bound is plotted against the antiserum dilution. The antibody titer is then the dilution of antiserum that binds 50% of the tracer. As a measure of antigen-binding capacity, the titer is proportional to the product of both antibody concentration and affinity.

The antibody titer varies with the amount of tracer used in the analysis. For interlaboratory comparison, therefore, the titer should always be reported with the amount of tracer specified. For RIAs, working antiserum dilutions (which are often used synonymously with titer) of $1{:}10^5$ to $1{:}10^6$ are expected, and most investigators like to use at least a $1{:}10^3$ dilution.

To measure *antibody concentration*, the Heidelberger-Kendall quantitative precipitation technique[135] or such newer quantitative techniques as nephelometry[136] are employed. The serum concentration of specific antibodies obtained by optimum immunization is in the range of 0.1 to 2 mg of antibody per milliliter. This only represents 0.5 to 10% of the total serum immunoglobulin concentration. It is also interesting to note that even a 2 mg/mL antibody concentration corresponds to only 12 μmol/L antibody or 24 μmol/L total binding site concentration if all antibody is of the IgG type.

Monoclonal Antibodies

The hybridoma technology for the production of specific monoclonal antibodies was developed by Köhler and Milstein[33] in 1975. In this technique, animals (typically mice) are hyperimmunized, bled, screened for antibody titer, and those giving the greatest response are selected. The purity of immunogen often is of little concern. The B-lymphocytes of the best responding animals are isolated from the spleen and fused with properly selected immortal myeloma cells. The fused cells (hybridomas) are then tested for their ability to produce specific antibodies. Those secreting the best antibodies are cloned and grown either in the peritoneal cavity of mice or in a culture medium in the presence of feeder cells such as peritoneal macrophages.

Using in vivo expansion techniques, the ascitic fluid formed contains 5 to 15 mg/mL of the monoclonal antibody 7 to 10 days after implantation of hybridoma cells.[137] As the now popular single taps produce 5 to 15 mL of fluid per mouse, the total monoclonal antibody yield is 50 to 100 mg per mouse.

Since 1978, hybridomas secreting murine monoclonal antibodies have also been produced following in vitro immunization.[138] This technique allows theoretically unlimited production of specific monoclonal antibodies under highly controlled and reproducible conditions and with much reduced contamination. One disadvantage is that it mostly yields IgM monoclonal antibodies.[138–140]

Although most monoclonal antibodies for immunoassays are now produced using murine neoplastic cell lines, other animals may also be employed.[141] Heterohybridoma monoclonal antibodies can also be generated. For this purpose antibody-producing "mortal" cells of other animals are fused with neoplastic murine cells.[142,143] This technique is commonly associated with low efficiency and low antibody yield, but the resultant antibody may be of high affinity.[142]

Modified Antibodies

Antibodies as reagents have been modified by chemical treatment and proteolysis for decades. During the last few years, a number of alternative techniques became available, resulting in new opportunities for the production of modified antibodies.[144]

1. Antibody fragments. To reduce the potential for complement binding, Fc-Fc interaction, and cross-reactions in general, $F(ab')_2$ and Fab fragments of specific antibodies have been employed in a number of binding assays. When monovalent binders are required, Fab or Fv fragments can be produced by either proteolysis or recombinant DNA technology.
2. Somatic variants. Hybridoma cell-lines may undergo spontaneous somatic mutation and isotype switching in culture medium. C-region mutations may result in monoclonal antibodies with increased affinity.[145] A novel variant is the heterodimer immunoglobulin molecule composed of two different H-L pairs ($L_1H_1H_2L_2$) and expressing two different *V*-module specificities.[146,147]
3. Recombinant antibodies. The genes responsible for specific antibodies can now be cloned, amplified, and introduced by appropriate vectors or electroporation into mammalian neoplastic or hybridoma cells as *tranfectomas*, or into bacteria and yeasts. Although transfectomas have the best potential to produce properly assembled antibodies, the yield obtained with these cells is relatively low and the technique is expensive. The recovery of intact antibody molecules is poor from bacteria, but *E. coli* was successfully used to produce Fab and Fv fragments.[116–119] Complete recombinant antibody molecules have been synthesized with a yeast expression system.[119,120]

RADIOLABELING

The quality of tracer is a critical element of binding radioassays and improvements in radiolabeling techniques have been essential for the success of these assays. To optimize analytical sensitivity of an assay, highly pure substances should be used for labeling. ^{125}I is now the label of choice in more than 90% of all clinical binding radioassays. In such dual assays as vitamin B_{12}/folate and free thyroxin/thyrotropin, ^{57}Co also is used. ^{59}Fe may be used for serum iron determination and ^{3}H or ^{14}C is used for steroid and drug assays.

High specific activity of the radiotracer improves the precision and analytical sensitivity of binding assays and reduces sample counting time or the amount of tracer needed. Beyond a certain point, however, these reductions are of no practical benefit.[38] The dependence of analytical sensitivity on specific activity means that analytes occurring in relatively high concentrations in the sample (eg, nonpeptide hormones and drugs) can be measured with tracers of relatively low specific activity as with tritiated steroids. Sometimes, even ^{14}C-labeled tracers with low specific activity may be suitable for a steroid or drug assay. In turn, peptide/protein hormones occurring in comparatively low concentrations in the sample require tracers with high specific activity. Since the attainable specific activity with tritium (or ^{14}C) is low for peptides/proteins, the label of choice is ^{125}I. For good assay performance, specific activity in the range of 1.11 to 1.85 TBq/mmol (30 to 50 Ci/mmol) is needed for steroids, though tritiated steroids are commercially available with specific activities as high as 7.40 TBq/mmol (200 Ci/mmol).[150] However, 10 to 50 times higher specific activity is needed routinely for the measurement of peptide/protein hormones. For instance, if insulin (MW 5800) is labeled with ^{125}I at a level of 0.8 iodine atom per molecle and the isotopic abundance* is 100%, the resultant specific activity is approximately 11.1 MBq/mg protein (300 mCi/mg protein) or 64.38 TBq/mmol of insulin (1740 Ci/mmol).[150]

The high specific activity, particularly in association with high fractional decay rate, may affect stability, especially with radioiodinated peptides/proteins when two or more atoms of radioiodine are present in each molecule. Disintegration of the first radioiodine atom disrupts covalent bonds, producing radioactively labeled fragments that may exhibit altered immunological and chemical properties. Free radioiodide also is formed. This phenomenon of radiation self-damage has been designated by Yalow[151] as "decay catastrophe." The ensuing radiolysis reduces assay precision because of the increasing background of unreactive labeled materials. Decay catastrophe is avoided by limiting iodination to 0.8 to 1.0 atom of radioiodine per molecule. Some suggest even lower ratios such as 0.5 to 0.8 iodine per molecule. Nevertheless, Ekins[38] calculated that, even if the entire population of radioiodinated (^{125}I) molecules is doubly labeled, the generation of labeled protein fragments arising as a direct result of decay catastrophe would only be in the order of 1% per day. Thus, using a freshly purified preparation "catastrophic" degradation of molecules, even with prolonged incubations, would be an unlikely cause of altered assay performance.

It is also of importance that the labeling ratios represent only an average of all possible combinations between radioiodine and host molecule. When Monte Carlo simulation was used to calculate the theoretical distribution of iodine atoms in labeled insulin preparations at an average of 0.8 radioiodine atom per molecule, about half of the radioactivity was estimated to be in a form other than monoiodoinsulin.[152] Thus, if monoiodoinsulin (or any monoiodinated tracer) is required, additional separation techniques such as ion-exchange chromatography, starch gel electrophoresis, or high-performance liquid chromatography should be performed following radioiodination.

In addition to analytical sensitivity and radiation self-damage, the choice of label affects several other aspects of the assay. The long half-life of ^{3}H and ^{14}C represents only limited advantage in practice. Tritiated or ^{14}C-labeled compounds require expensive counting devices, the use of scintillation cocktails that are expensive both to purchase and discard, solubility in scintillation cocktails, and long counting times. Because of their relatively low specific activity, tritiated products require repurifications at regular intervals that are more expensive and cumbersome than those for ^{125}I-labeled substances. These limitations prompted the introduction of indirect labeling of steroids and other compounds, that traditionally were directly labeled with tritium (or ^{14}C), with γ-emitting radionuclides such as ^{75}Se and ^{125}I.

Radioiodination may considerably alter the binding of antigens if tyrosyl and/or histidyl residues (see below) form part of the epitope. The same problem may occur in RRAs when the binding site of peptide/protein hormones or other ligands to receptors is altered by iodination. Even a single atom of iodine may occasionally reduce the affinity of tracer for a particular antibody or cell receptor. The overall impact is loss of assay sensitivity.[153] Low radioiodination ratios reduce this problem.

*The relative amount (% by weight) of a particular isotope of an element compared to the total of all its isotopes.

Radioiodination

Iodine is easily incorporated into most peptides/proteins. The reactive species is cationic iodine (I^+) that is generated by oxidation of the relatively unreactive iodide ion (I^-) (normally supplied in the form of $Na^{125}I$). Iodine primarily is substituted for hydrogen into the aromatic side chain of tyrosyl residues, and, less efficiently, into histidyl residues of peptides/proteins. Direct and indirect iodination techniques are discussed in detail in Chapter 11.

Purification and Repurification of Labeled Materials

Purification of tracers is required immediately after labeling and at intervals thereafter. Radioiodinated peptides/proteins are customarily purified by gel filtration, ion-exchange chromatography, by adsorption onto specific solid-phase bound antibodies or cellular receptors, by adsorption onto silica, and by starch gel electrophoresis, etc.[154,155] Purified labeled peptides/proteins are then eluted from gel filtration and ion-exchange columns by appropriate buffers, from antibodies by reduction in pH, or from adsorbents by the use of acidified alcohol or acetone.[38] In some instances, high-performance liquid chromatography is used for further purification and/or assessment of the purity of the labeled material.[156]

Storage and Stability of Radiolabeled Materials

After purification, the radiolabeled substance is pooled, diluted with appropriate buffer, and then refrigerated. Aqueous solutions of tritiated compounds, in general, should not be stored frozen because molecular clustering may accelerate the rate of self-radiolysis. Under routine storage conditions most tritiated steroids are stable over at least a 6-month period.

Although the half-life of ^{3}H is very long, the shelf life of tritiated products is limited by the loss of ^{3}H and the appearance of antigenically altered molecules, both reducing assay sensitivity. In one study with three iodinated protein hormones, the specific binding decreased at a mean rate of 0.8%/d (range, 0 to 1.6%) during a follow-up period of 8 weeks.[157] In another study, the rate of release of ^{125}I from different iodinated protein hormones ranged from 0.6 to 4.5%/week, irrespective of the storage temperature.[158] In RIAs, 5 to 10% impurities of radioiodinated antigens generally reduce the assay sensitivity to the point that only antigens occurring in high concentrations can be measured. Greater than 10% impurities require repurification.

Quality Assessment of Radiolabeled Materials

There are several ways to assess the quality of a tracer.

1. Specific activity. Specific activity usually refers to the amount of radioactivity per amount of both labeled and unlabeled material present in the tracer. Thus, specific activity is a function of both the type of radionuclide and the degree of substitution. Recall that the specific activity of each radionuclide is inversely proportional to its half-life; the shorter the half-life, the higher the specific activity achievable.
2. Radiochemical purity. Based on physicochemical properties, the tracer can be analyzed for purity by techniques such as chromatography, electrophoresis, and adsorption. For radioiodinated proteins a simple technique is to determine the percentage of radioactivity that remains soluble in trichloroacetic acid.[150] This test primarily detects deiodination. The extent of maximum binding (B_0) and nonspecific binding (NSB) in competitive binding assays are also related to radiochemical purity of the tracer. Although these parameters provide indirect evidence of damage to the labeled material, they do not directly measure the most critical attribute, specific binding activity.
3. Binding activity/immunoreactivity. For an RIA, this may be first checked by determining the amount of tracer that is bound by a known amount of antibody added in excess. Large amounts of tracer that fail to bind to the antibody indicate impaired immunoreactivity. In practice, the test is carried out by determining the percentage of bound tracer (B_0-NSB/T-NSB) using the dilution of antibody routinely employed in the assay.[150] A better indicator of tracer quality is to run an actual assay standard curve. Higher-quality tracers result in higher assay sensitivity.[150] Finally, since receptors have a high built-in specificity and binding to these receptors is closely related to biologic activity, the most stringent test for integrity of a tracer is its ability to perform in an RRA.[150]

PHASE SEPARATION TECHNIQUES

With rare exceptions,[159–165] binding radioassays require complete separation of the free (F) and bound (B) fractions prior to estimating their radioactive content. Alternatively, the total radioactivity (T) may be counted in place of either F or B. Since errors occurring in phase separation have a profound effect on assay precision and may bias the assay, proper selection of the separation method also is critical for good assay performance.

Although a large variety of phase separation techniques are available today, simplicity and applicability to automation has made the use of immobilized reagents the most popular. Of these, solid phase-coupled antigen or antibody techniques, often referred to only as solid-phase techniques, are the most widely employed in clinical laboratories.

All separation methods require that the dissociation constant be small compared to the association constant. In practice, however, this is not always the case, and some loss of assay sensitivity commonly occurs during phase separation. In systems displaying high dissociation rates, the effect may be particularly evident with solid adsorbent methods and lead to *ligand stripping*. In this phenomenon, the free ligand fraction is increased and the bound fraction is decreased by disruption of the ligand-binder complex.

In many RIAs, RTAs, and solubilized receptor-based RRAs, blanks must be included for the determination of *nonspecific binding* (NSB) of labeled ligands to other reactants and to the vessels themselves. NSB is then used to correct results. NSB may be caused by (1) inadequate separation of F and B fractions; (2) labeled contaminants in tracer; (3) nonspecific adsorption of tracer to assay vessel; and (4) entrapment of free fraction in precipitate.

Phase separation techniques can be classified as follows:

1. Electrophoresis, chromatoelectrophoresis, radioimmunoelectrophoresis. Separation of F and B fractions is based on differences in ionic charge and size resulting in differential migration in an electrical field. The separation is enhanced in chromatoelectrophoresis by means of a support medium with high affinity for the free ligand. The term radioimmunoelectrophoresis refers to either of these early separation techniques.[10,166] These methods are not generally used today because they are too labor intensive for large numbers of samples.
2. Dialysis and Filtration. Both techniques are based on size difference between free ligand and ligand-binder complex.[167] Dialysis is also tedious when many assays are run.
3. Gel filtration (permeation) chromatography. The use of such gels as Sephadex relies predominantly on steric exclusion of large protein-bound material from the solution contained in the interstices of gel particles, while entry of the smaller-sized free ligand is permitted.[167] Consequently, the complexes that are larger than the largest pores of the swollen gel pass through in the first elution. Because the equilibrium is undisturbed by this procedure, the time of exposure of the reaction mixture to the gel particles is not critical, making the technique particularly valuable in systems characterized by high dissociation rates.[38] Gel filtration is time consuming and labor intensive. It is now rarely used in routine assays, but remains a research tool.
4. Centrifugation. Because of size differences, antigen-antibody complexes can be sometimes separated from free antigen by high-speed centrifugation. These separations are, however, usually incomplete. On the other hand, complexes of the ligand with cells and subcellular fragments as natural insoluble binding reagents are efficiently separated from the free fraction by this technique. Centrifugation also is commonly used in combination with other separation techniques such as solid-phase adsorption (eg, charcoal), particle-bound binding reagents (eg, microbead-coupled antibodies), nonspecific precipitation with ethanol, and second antibody-based immunoprecipitation.

5. Solid phase adsorption. In contrast to immune reactions, these techniques are nonspecific because they are based on simple physicochemical interaction between substances in solution and the surface of the "adsorbing" material. The intensity of adsorption depends on concentration of the adsorbent, charge of the ligand, temperature, incubation time, pH, ionic strength, and composition of the reaction mixture. Because the adsorbent ultimately may bind both free and bound ligand, the conditions of the reaction must be carefully controlled to permit selective adsorption of the free ligand and to leave the ligand-binder complexes in solution. For instance, if too much protein is present, adsorption of the free ligand to charcoal may be inhibited, whereas too low a protein concentration allows adsorption of the ligand-binder complex as well.[168] Adsorption techniques are well suited for the separation of *F* and *B* fractions when the ligand in question is of low molecular weight, less than 10,000, and the ligand-binder complex is relatively large.
6. Chemical precipitation. Unlike immune reactions, these phase separation techniques are based on precipitation of the antigen-antibody complex from solution by salting out[11] with Na_2SO_4 or $(NH_4)_2SO_4$, by dehydration with polyethylene glycol (PEG),[169] or by solvent (eg, ethanol, dioxane) partition. Normal animal serum or γ-globulin may be added as a carrier or coprecipitant to increase the size of the precipitate.
7. Double-antibody (immunoprecipitation) and related techniques. Despite higher cost and longer incubation time, double-antibody techniques quickly became popular in routine immunoassays. In these methods, a second antibody is raised against the γ-globulin of the animal species that produced the first antibody. In the original postimmunoprecipitation technique,[170] the second antibody, by binding to the antigen-antibody complex, forms a larger complex that often can be centrifuged out of solution directly. Serum from the animal against which the second antibody is directed is often added to provide a bulkier precipitate. The second antibody is used in much higher concentrations, and frequently produced in a larger animal species such as goat, than is the primary antibody. After sedimenting the immune complexes by centrifugation, great care should be taken to avoid disturbing the precipitate. The supernatant can be either aspirated or decanted. Radioactivity can be determined in the bound precipitate or in the free fraction by taking either the entire supernatant or an aliquot of the supernatant. In addition to the original postimmunoprecipitation technique, there are several modifications such as pre-precipitation of the first antibody with the second antibody,[171] combination of postimmunoprecipitation with PEG,[172] and the double-antibody solid phase (DASP) method.[173] Protein A or protein G may be used in place of the second antibody;[174] further, biotin-avidin[175] (or streptavidin) and fluorescein isothiocyanate (FITC)-anti-FITC[176] systems may be used as "universal" separators in modifications of the DASP method.
8. Solid phase-coupled antigen or first antibody. Although antigen may be the solid phase-coupled reagent in both competitive and noncompetitive assays, most commonly the antibody is bound to solid phase in both types of assays. The solid-phase material may be composed of inert materials such as plastic (polystyrene, polypropylene), glass, dextran polymer (eg, Sephadex), agarose, paraamino cellulose, polyacrylamide gel, or polymeric[177,178] antibody. The immobilized reagent may be located on the inner surface of tubes and microtiter wells, or on the surface of micro- and macrobeads, discs, and magnetizable particles. The antigen usually is immobilized by simple adsorption to the solid phase,[27,179] whereas the antibody may be physically adsorbed[179,180] (eg, plastic tubes, microtiter wells) or conjugated by covalent bonds using one of the numerous coupling methods.[179]

Besides simplicity and wide applicability, the separation with solid phase-bound reagents is rapid, irreversible, and associated with low NSB. Solid phase-bound reagents allow the performance of assay in two stages. When the reaction is carried out in the concomitant presence of both sample and tracer, the assay is called "one step." When the tracer is added only after unbound components of the sample are removed, the assay is called "two step." While one-step assays are technically simpler and faster, two-step assays are subjected to fewer interferences. This is because the first step eliminates interfering and degradative components of the sample that may cause incubation damage.

Pseudohomogeneous and Homogeneous Binding Radioassays

Since 1979, a few competitive binding radioassays (RIA and RRA methods) that require little or no separation of bound from free ligand have also been described.[159–165,181] Assays with a requirement for limited separation can be considered pseudohomogeneous, whereas those requiring no separation are true homogeneous assays (Table 3). In contrast to heterogenous assay systems, these newer assay designs are technically simpler, less time consuming, and more readily amenable to automation. While pseudohomogeneous techniques remain largely limited to the original reports, the true homogeneous assay now appears to be gaining popularity, particularly in the microtiter format.

COUNTING TECHNIQUES

For discussion see Chapter 3.

DATA REDUCTION

In each binding assay, a set of standards is run in parallel with the unknown samples. The counting data for the stan-

Table 3. Classification of Radiolabeled Binding Assays According to Requirement for Phase Separation of Free and Bound Fractions[a]

ASSAY DESIGN	YEAR REPORTED	REF.
Heterogeneous (complete separation)		
RIA	1956–1961	8–13
RTA (CPB)	1960–1964	14–19
RESA[b]	1965	20
"Dual" ([radio]label) assay	1966	
RAST	1967	27
RRA	1967–1970	21–24
One [single]-site IRMA	1968	28
Radioactive RID	1969	32
Two-site ("sandwich") IRMA	1970–1971	29, 30
"4i assay"	1982	25
RASA[c]	1987	31
Idiometric assay[d]	1990	39
Pseudohomogeneous ("limited" separation)		
Internal sample attenuator counting (ISAC)	1979–1981	167, 168
Ligand differentiation immunoassay (LIDIA)	1983	169
BioMAT™ (microparticulate solid-phase)	1987	170
Homogeneous (no separation)		
Scintillation proximity assay (SPA)	1979–1992	171–173

[a]Tests are listed in order of first report(s).

[b]Requires separation of radiolabeled substrate [as free] and radiolabeled product [as bound].

[c]No radiolabeled version is known yet. Reported method is based on peroxidase-labeled antibody.

[d]No radiolabeled version is known yet. Reported method is based on europium-labeled alphatype antiidiotypic antibody.

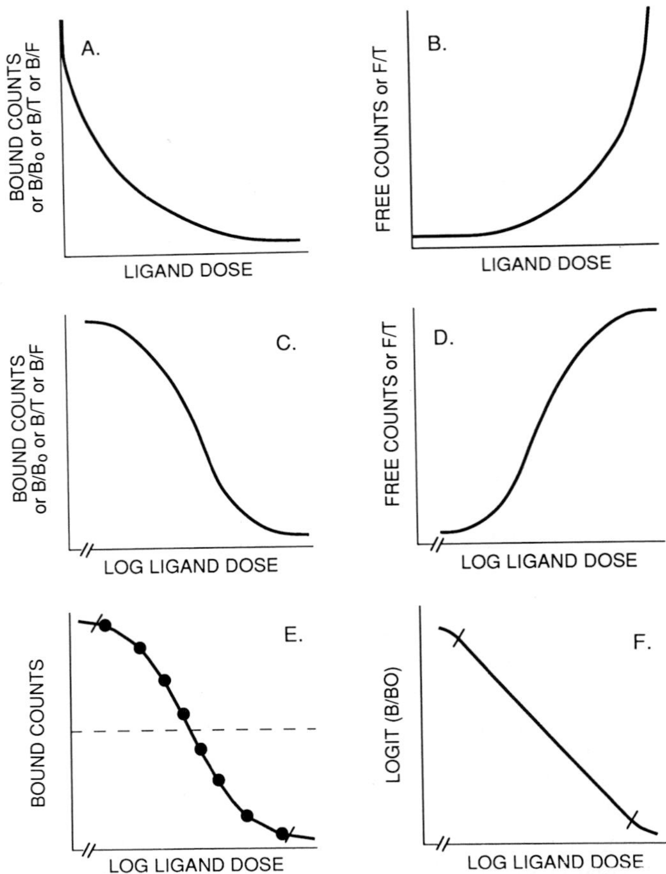

Figure 9. Examples of possible dose-response curves for competitive binding radioassays. Percent bound can be plotted with or without subtraction of NSB. Logit % bound ($B/B_0 \times 100$) = ln $\%B/(100 - \%B)$ with correction for NSB in the calculation. Curve E = four-parameter logistic curve fitting (NSB to be subtracted from B and B_0). B = bound counts, B_0 = zero standard counts (maximum binding), F = free counts, T = total counts, NSB = nonspecific binding (minimum binding).

dards are plotted to obtain a standard curve which is then used to determine the concentration of the unknowns. Theoretically, either the bound (B) or free (F) fraction can be measured. In practice, the type of phase separation technique largely determines the mode of quantification. For instance, with solid phase-bound reagent techniques, measuring the B fraction works best.

The doses (concentrations) of standards usually are plotted on the x-axis, whereas counts or transformations of the counts (metamers) are plotted on the y-axis. Depending on the derivation of response variable, either direct or inverse relationship between the dose and response may be obtained. Further, the relationship between the dose and response may be linear or nonlinear. Several mathematical transformations, eg, log and logit functions, are available for linearization of counting data. Basic data reduction techniques are illustrated in Figures 9 and 10.

In general, a data reduction method should be straightforward, yet capable of providing adequate statistical description of the assay. Some data reduction techniques can be easily carried out manually, but thorough statistical analyses require computers and appropriate software. Many commercial counters have data processing capability or are readily interfaceable with computers for carrying out this function.

Theoretically, the data reduction method should be based on the law of mass action in all binding radioassays. Classical liquid-phase RIAs are largely governed by this law. There are some programs available for the use of mass action law as a data reduction technique, but they are not routinely used. One major reason is the difficulty in describing the binding site of polyclonal antibodies (that carry several binding components) in the form of a single K_a value. Another problem is that, instead of equilibrium, many assays use the *sequential saturation* (quasiequilibrium) approach. In these systems, the antibody is allowed to react with the antigen before the addition of labeled antigen. Since the dissociation generally occurs at a slower rate than the association, this approach may increase assay sensitivity if the contact time with the tracer is sufficiently short. However, given enough time, the reaction eventually reaches equilibrium. Nevertheless, in their intended design, quasiequilibrium conditions

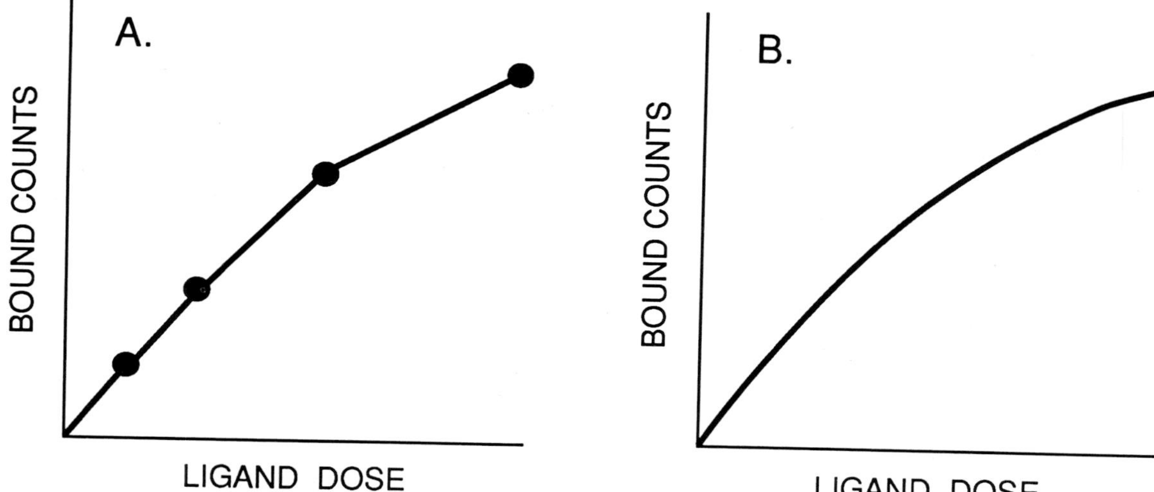

Figure 10. Examples of possible dose-response curves for noncompetitive binding radioassays. **(A)**. Point-to-point. **(B)**. Fitted curve (parabolic regression).

do not fulfill requirements of the mass action law. Likewise, since antigen-antibody reactions at solid surfaces dissociate only very slowly,[52,53] equilibrium is seldom reached within the time periods used for incubations in solid-phase based immunoassays.

Noncompetitive assays use a fundamentally different approach. In the typical format (two-site IRMA), two antibodies that react with different epitopes on the ligand are required. The binding of each antibody to the ligand also is governed by the mass action law, but at relatively low concentration of the ligand and in excess of antibodies,[38] binding of the tracer antibody will be directly proportional to the amount of ligand present.

Thus, most data reduction methods are either approximations of the law of mass action (semiempirical) or are empirical.[182,183] Numerous data reduction techniques have been published.[56,107,184–202] The existence of so many data reduction methods by itself implies that there is no single technique applicable to all binding radioassays. In case of commercial binding assays, the choice of transformation of counts to concentration usually is stated in the product insert. Critical examination of the plotted calibration curve is, however, necessary to visually verify the "goodness of fit." Even better, there are many curve-fit routines today that attempt to fit the curve several times and automatically select the best fit. Each of these attempts is referred to as an *iteration*. If no good fit is possible, some programs will alert the operator for further investigation.

An important issue in RIA data reduction is that the random errors are not homogeneous along the standard curve, but vary systematically. The variance is greater at the extremes than in the middle; this is called *heteroscedasticity*. When heteroscedasticity is present, it is desirable to perform a weighted regression analysis.

Of the many curve-fit methods, the *logit-log plot* continues to enjoy widespread popularity (Fig. 11). This technique linearizes sigmoid dose-response curves. The logistic function (logit) is defined as

$$\text{logit}(y) = \ln(y/1 - y) \quad (8)$$

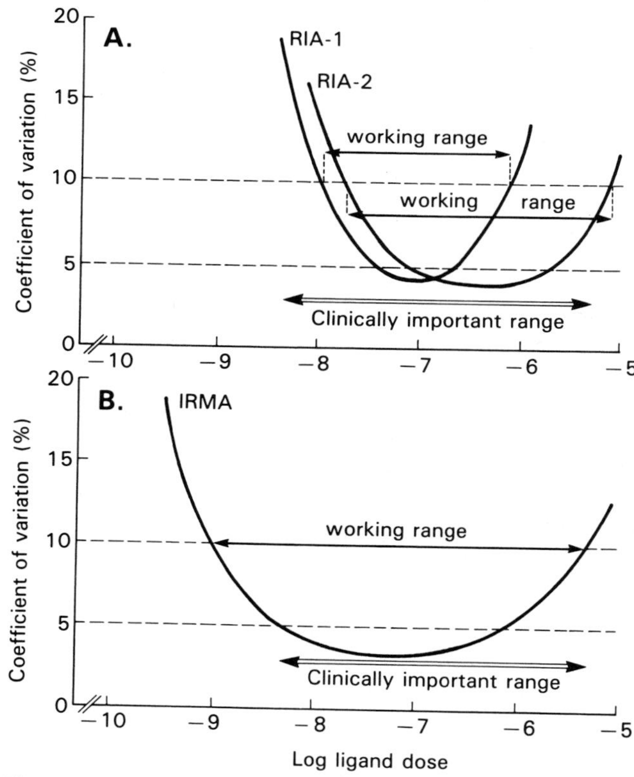

Figure 11. Typical precision profiles of RIAs and IRMA. Working ranges are arbitrarily defined at a CV of 10%. Note the much wider working range for IRMA and the relationship to clinical utility.

where y represents a measurable quantity of a response dependent on a variable dose (x). When logit(y) is plotted against log(x), a linear dose-response curve is obtained. In case of competitive binding assays, the percentage bound (B/B_0) is plotted against the log of dose:

$$\text{(9)} \qquad \text{logit}(B/B_0) = \log_e[(B/B_0)/(1 - B/B_0)]$$

This may be symbolized as

$$\text{(10)} \qquad \text{logit}(y) = \log_e\left(\frac{1}{1 - y}\right)$$

where

$$\text{(11)} \qquad y = \frac{B - \text{NSB}}{B_0 - \text{NSB}}$$

and where B represents bound activity, B_0 represents counts bound in the absence of unlabeled antigen, and NSB represents the nonspecific binding, ie, counts bound in the absence of antibody or receptor, ("assay blank"). The logit-log technique approximates the law of mass action and hence qualifies as a semiempirical approach for RIA data reduction. The *four-parameter logistic curve fitting* method represents the more general case of the two-parameter logit-log method. It also has some theoretical relationship to the mass action law. Although this technique requires nonlinear curve fitting, it may be the most effective method for RIA data reduction.

Noncompetitive (sandwich) assays are generally less demanding for curve-fit routines. Among the available options, empirical approaches represent the current state-of-the-art. Since an ideal data reduction approach for IRMAs remains to be identified, the choice of technique is largely personal. Simple point-to-point fit often is satisfactory.

Commercially available computer programs have been reviewed recently.[203]

Assay Parameters Used in Data Reduction

MAXIMUM OR INITIAL BINDING (%B_0)

This is the percent binding of tracer with zero or no standard in RIA (or other competitive binding assay). In RIA, the B_0 should be between 30 and 70% of the total activity. A change greater than 5% in this parameter over a period of time suggests possible problems in antibody affinity, incubation time, or separation method.

MINIMUM OR NONSPECIFIC BINDING (NSB)

NSB is the percent binding of tracer in the presence of an infinite dose of the standard. Experimentally, NSB is determined by omitting the antibody in an RIA. In an IRMA, the response at zero standard dose and NSB are the same.

Ideally, NSB should be about 1% of the total tracer added. Modern counters can automatically subtract NSB values as the detection data for either RIA or IRMA are accumulated.

LEAST DETECTABLE DOSE (LDD, OR ANALYTICAL SENSITIVITY)

LDD is usually defined as the ligand concentration read from the standard curve at a response plus (for IRMA) or minus (for RIA) two standard deviations from the mean of the zero standard.[204] The LDD depends on the sample matrix (note possible differences between standards and unknowns), on the shape and precision of the standard curve near zero, and on the method of data reduction. As stated before, in competitive binding radioassays such as RIAs, the analytical sensitivity approximates the reciprocal of the affinity constant of the binder (antibody), ie, about $1/K_a$. Thus, $1/K_a$ is an alternative way to define assay sensitivity.

QUALITY CONTROL

Regular monitoring of assay performance and the use of appropriate controls are integral parts of good laboratory practice. Participation in external proficiency testing also is essential for intermethod and interlaboratory comparisons. Quality-control techniques with respect to binding radioassays have been repeatedly reviewed.[187,189,199,205–207]

A short summary of some specific issues of quality control in binding radioassays follows.

1. Midrange slope of standard curve. This is used for monitoring interassay precision of RIAs. The slope of the standard curve is an indication of assay "sensitivity" in the sense that it determines the minimum detectable difference between two concentrations of antigen. The steeper the slope, the more sensitive the assay, all other variables being equal. This concept of sensitivity was introduced by Yalow and Berson,[208] who defined it as the slope of the dose-response curve relating B/F to ligand concentration. Flattening of the slope suggests binder degradation.[209] This meaning of sensitivity should not be mistaken for analytical sensitivity, which primarily refers to the least detectable dose (LDD).
2. Slope, intercept, correlation coefficient (R) of standard curve. These parameters should remain constant during the life of an RIA kit. Lack of stability indicates breakdown of assay components. The R^2 value (goodness of fit) should be greater than 0.95 for a good assay.[209]
3. Imprecision. This is monitored by calculating the coefficient of variation (CV) of replicates. The midrange CV is particularly useful for monitoring the performance of RIA. It should be less than 3%.[209]
4. Precision profile. This is the plot of the CV vs ligand concentration[38,210] (Fig. 11). The precision profile allows the operator to observe the precision of the assay throughout the range of the standard curve. Further, working (reporting) ranges can be established based on assay precision. Ideally, the working (reporting) range completely overlaps the concentration range expected for clinical use of an assay. From the precision profile, the analytical

Table 4. Comparison of the Three Major Types of Competitive Binding Radioassays

PROPERTY	RIA	RTA	RRA
Binding reagent			
Availability	Inducible	Easy to limited	Limited
Reproducible source	Variable to very high	High	Variable to high
"Titer"	Potentially very high	Low	Low
Stability	Usually good	Usually good	Variable
Affinity for ligand	Low to very high	Relatively low	Very high
Specificity	Potentially very high	High	Very high
Assay			
Link to bioactivity	Variable	High	Very high
Rapidity of reaction	Slow for equilibrium	Relatively fast for equilibrium	Fast for equilibrium
Validation	Relatively difficult (potentially many cross-reacting substances)	Relatively easy	Relatively easy

sensitivity is the ligand concentration read from the graph at the lower end of the precision profile curve at an acceptable precision level. The analytical sensitivity established by this method is more realistic in terms of overall confidence in the reported numerical result than LDD. Unfortunately, there may be a large difference between the LDD and a minimal acceptable level based on the precision profile and a predetermined CV value. An important mathematical limitation of the use of precision profile to establish sensitivity is that, even as assays increase in analytical sensitivity, the value will still tend toward infinity as the mean concentration moves toward zero. This is because CV is defined as standard deviation divided by mean concentration.

5. Parallelism. This ultimately represents a measure of specificity, since it is used to determine if there are any substances in the unknown specimen that cause immunochemical interferences.[209] In parallelism testing, serial dilutions of the unknown are compared with the standard curve. Nonparallelism indicates the presence of cross-reactive components in the unknown and precludes quantification of the ligand in question.

COMMON BINDING RADIOASSAYS

The relative advantages and disadvantages of the three most common types of competitive binding radioassays are summarized in Table 4. A critical issue is the sensitivity of competitive binding assays.[211] This is determined by the relative proportion of binder and tracer in the assay system. To increase sensitivity, a higher dilution of binder is usually chosen, whereas lesser dilution often increases the range of values covered by the assay curve. Too high initial binding (B_0) indicates excess binder in the system. In this case, addition of unlabeled ligand would be bound to unoccupied binding sites rather than acting to displace tracer. In turn, too-low initial binding (B_0) results in an assay in which the assay curve is too shallow and the results are less accurate. Guidelines assessing the quality of RIA systems have been published.[211a]

Radioimmunoassays (RIAs)

In the case of RIAs, the requirement for first-order kinetics implies that the antibody-binding sites are independent of each other and that the antigen and antibody-binding sites react in a one-to-one ratio. There has been a long debate on how to optimize assay conditions, ie, sensitivity and precision in RIAs.[38] For maximum assay performance, Berson and Yalow[211] first proposed that (1) the amount of labeled antigen should be vanishingly low and (2) the amount of antibody employed should bind 50% of the labeled antigen. Later they proposed 33% tracer binding as being optimum.[208] Subsequently, these general rules have been widely adopted by the majority of investigators in setting up RIAs. Largely on a theoretical basis, Ekins and co-workers[38,59] proposed a somewhat different approach that formally considers the errors in the measurement of assay response variable for the optimization of RIAs. Because of the more complex mathematical calculations involved, the conclusions emerging from Ekins' approach are less readily summarized than those of Berson and Yalow.[208,211] Under many circumstances, the two approaches correspond closely, but sometimes they differ significantly. Without complete resolution of the controversy, the approach advocated by Ekins and co-workers[38,59] now appears to be accurate with empirical validation.

Besides the classical *equilibrium saturation* RIA that can be carried out either in liquid phase or solid phase, *nonequilibrium* (*disequilibrium*) RIAs also are used. In *sequential saturation* RIA, first the unlabeled antigen of the sample is allowed to react with the antibody, then the labeled antigen is added to bind to the remaining antibody-binding sites. This technique reduces the effective measuring range, but often increases the sensitivity of assays based on low-affinity binders. In *displacement* RIA, the components are used in the reverse order: first labeled antigen is allowed to react with antibody, after which unlabeled antigen is added to displace the labeled antigen from binding sites. This approach may be advantageous when the affinity of labeled antigen is lower than that of unlabeled antigen.

Based on the number of separation steps, one- and two-step RIAs can be distinguished. Equilibrium RIAs are of the former, whereas some nonequilibrium RIAs are of the latter assay design. Sequential saturation two-step RIAs also are called *immunoextraction techniques* because during the first incubation step they "extract" the antigen from standards, unknowns, and controls, followed by "back-titration" of unoccupied binding sites by the labeled antigen in the second step. These assays really represent a unique category of binding assays with features of both RIA and IRMA.

According to a recent study, one-step methods, in general, provide a better performance profile: lower detection limit and more specific antigen recognition.[212] The quantity of reagents needed (both specific binding reagent and tracer) is three to four times less for one- than two-step methods. On the other hand, higher amounts of reagents employed in two-step techniques result in a higher measuring signal, which is important where concentration of the unknown antigen is low.[212]

Along with debate on the physiological role of free (non-protein bound) hormones[213,214] marches controversy about their measurement, particularly with RIAs.[215–219] Most of the technical controversy surrounds the use of so-called analog tracers, radiolabeled derivatives of the parent hormone.[215–219] These analogs are claimed, but not always proven, to exhibit negligible or no binding to serum transport proteins, the presence of which otherwise interferes with the distribution of analog tracers in one-step RIAs for free hormones.

Radiotransin Assays (RTAs)

The binding proteins used in RTAs are usually of lower affinity and are less specific than the antibodies employed in RIAs. This leads to lower analytical sensitivity, ie, higher LDD, and requires pretreatment of samples to remove endogenous binding proteins. The recent availability of highly specific antibodies for analytes traditionally measured in RTAs greatly reduces their appeal and they may soon be replaced altogether by RIAs.[220]

Radioreceptor Assays (RRAs)

RRAs are also similar in concept to RIAs. Because of their unique specificities, the receptors employed in RRAs can measure biologically active hormones and drugs that cannot be easily assayed by other techniques. Soluble intracellular receptors are used essentially the same way as RTAs, while the use of intact cells and plasma membrane preparations as binders requires certain assay modifications. By using the Scatchard plot,[55–58,200] quantitative assay of receptors also is possible for diagnostic use.[222,223]

Obvious disadvantages of RRAs include high cost, pH sensitivity, and assay complexity. However, since RRAs provide information not attainable by immunoassays, they will probably remain essential tools for both research and clinical diagnosis. In fact, progress in recombinant DNA and other evolving technologies opens the door to new opportunities for novel RRAs with improved sensitivity and specificity.[94]

Immunoradiometric Assays (IRMAs)

In single-site IRMA, the binding reaction can be represented as follows:

$$[Ag] + [Ab^*] \underset{k_d}{\overset{k_a}{\rightleftharpoons}} [AgAb^*] + [Ab^*] \tag{12}$$

where $[Ag]$ = free antigen concentration; $[Ab^*]$ = labeled antibody concentration; $[AgAb^*]$ = concentration of the complex formed; K_a = association constant; and K_d = dissociation constant. The basic difference from RIA is that one of the key reagents, the radiolabeled antibody, is provided in excess.[38] Because of excess antibody, there is no competition for binding sites in IRMA and the entire amount of antigen theoretically may be antibody bound. In RIA, free antigen is separated from bound antigen, whereas in single-site IRMA free labeled antibody is separated from the bound labeled antibody by binding the latter to excess immobilized antigen.[28] Since the bound fraction containing all the antigen is counted in IRMA, counts are directly related to antigen concentration.

At the present, "sandwich" IRMAs are most commonly used in two- or even in a three-site format (Fig. 12). Technically, all IRMAs can be of the one- or two-step assay design, depending on the number of phase separation steps. When polyclonal antibodies are used in sandwich IRMAs, there are usually two incubation and two washing steps because of the potential competition between the two antibody reagents. The use of two or three monoclonal antibodies recognizing different antigenic determinants on the antigen to be measured is especially advantageous in performing a one-incubation step sandwich IRMA.

IRMAs, particularly in the sandwich format and coupled with solid-phase technology, represented a major improvement in binding radioassays. IRMAs have several advantages over RIAs. The use of labeled antibodies obviated potential problems arising from iodination of labile antigens. Besides, antibodies regularly have amino acids available for labeling, they are fairly stable proteins, and can be labeled with high specific activity without damaging their binding activity. The use of two or three antibodies in the sandwich format greatly increases assay specificity. The specificity of IRMAs is further enhanced by the availability of homogeneous monoclonal antibodies that recognize a single epitope. Sandwich IRMAs may also have greater analytical sensitivity than RIAs (Fig. 13).[37] The working range of sandwich IRMAs often is 5- to 300-fold wider than that of RIAs with superior (1 to 2%) CVs at the response midcurve (Fig. 11). The nonspecific matrix effects are minimal and highly consistent in IRMAs. The incubation or equilibrium time decreases because of the presence of excess antibody. The IRMA techniques also allow for less precision in antibody addition. IRMAs have only one critical pipetting step—the addition of the unknown. In double-antibody RIAs, in turn, the pipetting of unknown, antibody, and tracer are all equally

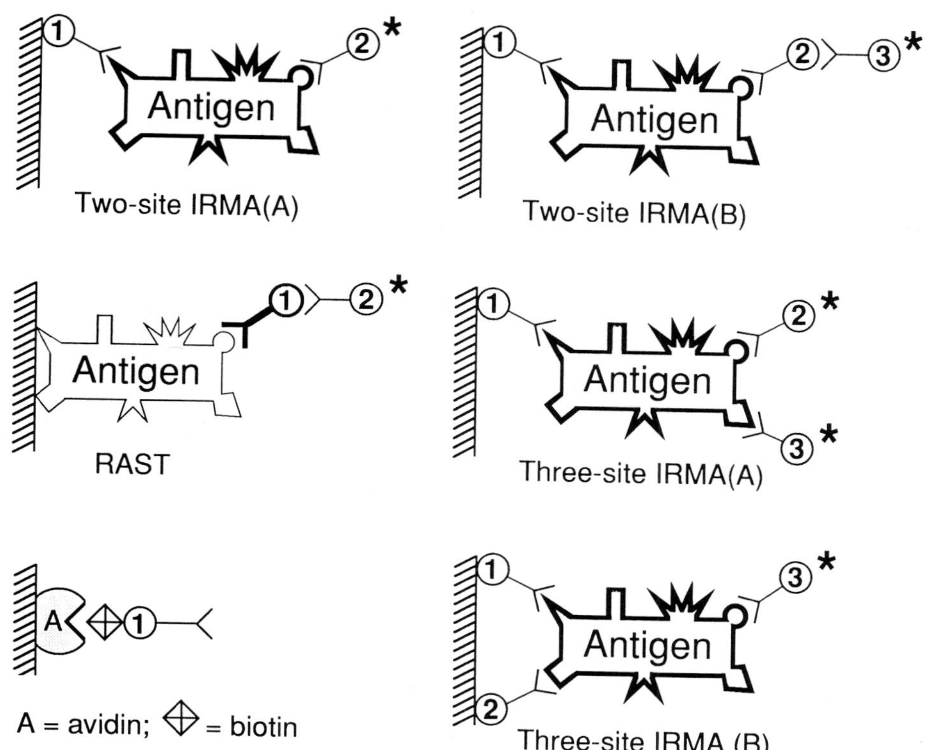

Figure 12. Types of solid phase "sandwich" immunoassays and the avidin-biotin reaction as a separation method (one of the antibodies is covalently coupled to biotin, ie, biotinylated).

important to assay precision. Overall, IRMAs represent a more robust system than RIAs.[224] The major limitation of sandwich IRMAs is that they require large antigens expressing multiple epitopes.

Dual Label Radioassays

In the first dual radioassay in 1966, human insulin and growth hormone were labeled with ^{131}I and ^{125}I, respectively.[26] In a later application,[225] triiodothyronine and thyroxin were measured simultaneously by using ^{125}I and ^{131}I. Other applications used ^{57}Co and ^{125}I for such clinically related analytes as T4 and TSH,[226,227] LH and FSH, and vitamin B_{12} and folate. Two radionuclides in dual assays are discriminated by appropriate adjustment of the spectrometer windows. Some spillover (usually up to 3%) from the higher-energy radionuclide into the lower-energy channel affects assay precision,[228] but does not necessarily limit practical application.

INTERFERENCES

A number of factors may affect binding radioassay performance and the validity of results. These include matrix effects exemplified by differences between serum and plasma, blood and urine or other body fluids, serum and tissue extracts, or the presence of such additives as citrate, oxalate, EDTA, heparin in whole blood, or plasma samples. Since the information regarding these issues usually is available before testing, these problems are relatively easy to resolve by selecting either proper techniques for specimen collection or appropriate assay conditions. Some components in samples that are not known before testing and are recognized as interferences only after the assay has been completed are discussed below.

Contamination with Radionuclides

Radionuclides may contaminate patient specimens due to administration of radiopharmaceuticals. Although most commonly ^{99m}Tc is administered, ^{67}Ga, ^{201}Tl, ^{131}I, ^{111}In, ^{57}Co, ^{51}Cr, and ^{32}P are occasional contaminants. Such contaminations can cause falsely increased, falsely decreased results, or have no effect at all, depending on the separation technique.[229,230]

Prior screening of specimens by γ-counting and inclusion of nonspecific binding tubes in the assay whenever possible help to identify radioactive contamination.[229] After allowing sufficient time for radioactive decay of the contaminant (if possible), the specimen may be reassayed to measure the analyte in question.[229]

Bridging Phenomenon in Hapten RIA

Many haptens cannot be radiolabeled directly but require a chemical bridge to small carrier molecules.[231,232] The carrier molecules either already carry a radiolabel or are readily accessible to radiolabeling. Since the production of good antisera also requires conjugation of haptens to carrier molecules (to make them immunogenic), there is a possibility that the two condensation processes involve the same chemical

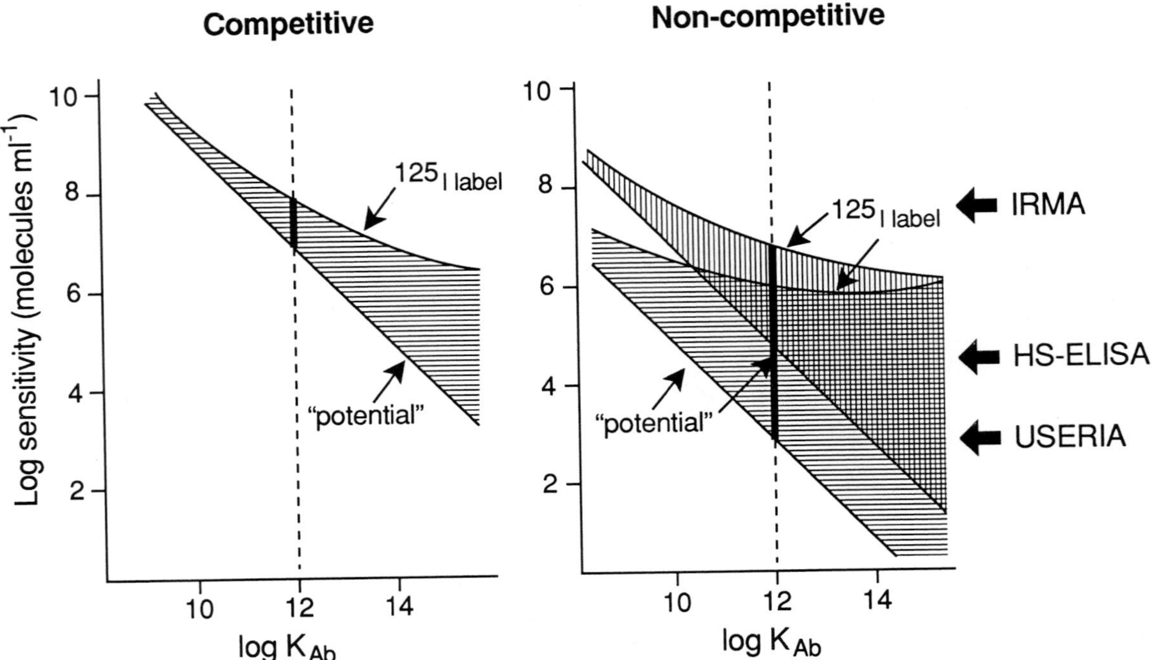

Figure 13. Predicted assay sensitivities (molecules per milliliter) plotted against antibody affinity (*L/M*). "Potential sensitivity" curves assume a label of infinite specific activity, implying zero error in label measurement per se. For competitive assays, other errors are assumed to cause a 1% CV in assay response. For "noncompetitive" assays, nonspecific binding of labeled antibody of 1% (upper curves) and 0.01% (lower curves) is assumed. Sensitivities using ^{125}I are also plotted, sensitivity loss being due to "counting" errors. In practice, highest antibody affinity constants normally approximate 10^{12} *L/M*, albeit antibody affinities seldom exceed 10^{11} *L/M*. Higher sensitivities are attainable using monoclonals in a noncompetitive mode than by using higher affinity antibodies in a competitive assay. Greater sensitivites require labels of specific activity higher than ^{125}I. Sensitivity of noncompetitive assays using ^{125}I (IRMA) and enzymes (yielding fluorescent (HS-ELISA) or radioactive products (USERIA) are shown. (Reprinted with permission from Ekins.[37])

bridge.[233,234] Antibodies that recognize this common bridge may be produced by immunization. The presence of such antibodies in the assay system results in a much higher binding affinity for the tracer than for the unlabeled analyte. The characteristic of this phenomenon is that the standard curves are long and shallow, requiring large concentrations of native analyte to inhibit binding of radiolabeled analyte to the antibody.

Induced and Heterophile Antibodies to Immunoglobulins

Human antibodies to animal immunoglobulins that interfere with immunoassays may arise in several ways.[235–245] The injection of both therapeutic and diagnostic animal antibodies represent growing opportunities for immunizing humans against animal immunoglobulins.[239,243] Human anti-mouse antibodies are now commonly referred to by the acronym HAMA. Interfering antibodies also may result from ingestion of bovine milk and meat from different animals and from handling animals. Passive transfer of maternal antibodies to the fetus can also interfere with neonatal serum testing.[241]

In some individuals, the etiology of circulating anti-animal immunoglobulin antibodies called *heterophile antibodies* is not as obvious. In contrast to antibodies induced by unintentional immunization, heterophile antibodies are characterized by substantial nonspecificity, developing in response to no clear immunogen.[235,238,240] They often are associated with autoimmune diseases or are sheep erythrocyte agglutinins associated with infectious mononucleosis.

Depending on assay design and the location of the epitope recognized by the interfering antibody, both falsely low and falsely high results have been documented. Competitive binding assays are less commonly affected by heterophile antibodies than IRMA assays.[235] RIAs exhibiting antibody interference use a large amount of patient serum and long incubation times in combination with high titers of interfering antibodies in the patient's serum.[235] Positive interference occurs with solid-phase RIA and its postulated mechanism is the blocking of antigenic sites by binding to the interfering antibody.[235] Negative interference is seen in double-antibody RIA techniques and may be due to formation of an antibody complex prior to the addition of the second antibody, thereby causing enhanced precipitation.[235]

The most common and usually greatest interferences are, however, seen in two (three)-site IRMAs.[236–245] The interfering antibodies, by linking the labeled and immobilized antibodies, simulate the analyte and hence result in its variable overestimation (Fig. 18). In one study, as many as 15% of

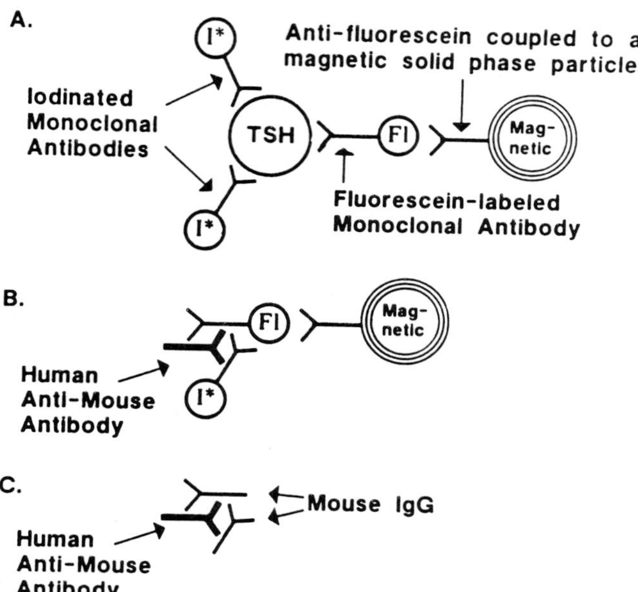

Figure 14. Probable mechanism for false serum TSH elevations in an IRMA using mouse monoclonal antibodies, and prevention by addition of mouse serum or Ig. **(A)**. Assay design. Patient serum is reacted with ^{125}I (I*) and fluorescein (Fl)-labeled anti-TSH monoclonal antibodies, forming a radiolabeled sandwich. After incubation with antifluorescein coupled to a magnetic solid-phase particle, radiolabeled sandwiches containing TSH are sedimented in a magnetic field. **(B)**. Positive interference. Human antimouse Ig antibodies bind to each of the labeled mouse monoclonal antibodies in the assay kit, creating a sandwich linking the [^{125}I]mouse Ig to a fluorescein-labeled mouse Ig which is bound to the magnetic particle, imitating the sandwich that is formed with TSH. **(C)**. Prevention of interference. Mouse Igs added as serum or purified Ig bind to the human antimouse antibodies, preventing the formation of artifactually labeled sandwiches that are not detected by the assay. Ig, immunoglobulin. (Reprinted with permission from Kahn et al.[238])

human serum specimens assayed disclosed some overestimate in a two-site IRMA with mouse monoclonal antibodies.[232] When a specially designed murine monoclonal antibody assay was used, the presence of interfering antibodies was detected in 40% of normal human sera.[236]

Interfering antibodies can be recognized in several ways: (1) clinically inappropriate assay result; (2) antibody neutralization test;[235] (3) nonlinear dilution curve of analyte;[238] and (4) reduction (RIA or IRMA) or increase (RIA) in the apparent assay result after the addition of blocking normal animal serum or immunoglobulin.[235,238,239]

Interfering antibodies or their effect can be eliminated by a number of techniques. Some block the effect of interfering antibodies (Fig. 14); others either eliminate the likely combining sites (epitopes of Fc) from assay antibodies (Fab or F(ab′)$_2$ fragments), or remove the interfering antibodies altogether from the specimen prior to assay.[235,237–245] Theoretically, removal of interfering antibodies from the specimen is an ideal solution, but it is difficult to apply to large numbers of specimens. It is also of interest that addition of blocking immunoglobulins to the assay may not always completely eliminate the interference.[240,244]

Rheumatoid Factor (RF)

Rheumatoid factors are autoantibodies that bind multiple epitopes on the Fc fragment of IgG, and hence readily cause interference with two-site IRMAs.[240] Although IgM-RF is known to be the cause of interference, most cases may be due to IgG-RF, which is not measured in the usual sheep cell or latex RF assays for IgM.[240] This suggests that the real incidence of interferences due to IgG-RF may be grossly underestimated.[240] Because of the well-defined reactivity of RFs with Fc, the addition of blocking immunoglobulins, the use of Fab or F(ab′)$_2$ antibody fragments or chimeric antibodies in the assay, and removal of immunoglobulins from the specimens in question all are expected to eliminate antibody interferences due to RF.

Autoantibodies to Hormones

Autoantibodies to thyroid hormones (T3 and T4)[246] and TSH[247] have been reported. According to some estimates the prevalence of antithyroid hormone antibodies may reach 40% in patients with Hashimoto's thyroiditis and Graves disease.[246] Interestingly, autoantibody to TSH may be an antiidiotypic antibody to TSH receptor antibody.[247] The laboratory significance of such antihormone antibodies is that they all are capable of interfering with immunoassays. Depending on the assays design, both falsely low and falsely high assay results may be obtained (Fig. 15).[246] Antithyroid hormone antibodies can be detected by assays specifically designed for this purpose.[246] Otherwise, these autoantibodies should be suspected in case of assay results that are inappropriate for the clinical status of patients and/or incompatible with other test results, or in patients with Hashimoto's thyroiditis or Graves disease. Proper assay selection (eg, two-step free hormone assay in case of antithyroid hormone antibodies) or removal of interfering antibodies from the specimen will eliminate this problem.

High-Dose "Hook Effect"

The high-dose "hook effect" in sandwich immunoassays is so named because the dose response curve at unusually high doses of the analyte begins to decline and thereby forms a "hook" (Fig. 16). The high-dose hook effect is particularly common in one-step sandwich assays in which both antibodies to the analyte are added at the same time (rather than sequentially) with no "wash" step to remove unbound analyte.[248,250] When the hook occurs at concentrations far beyond those usually encountered in clinical practice, there is little risk of falsely low test results. However, for some tests, such as those determining such tumor marker concentrations as alpha-fetoprotein and prostate-specific antigen, where homeostatic mechanisms are not involved, the range encountered may be broad enough to include the region of the hook.

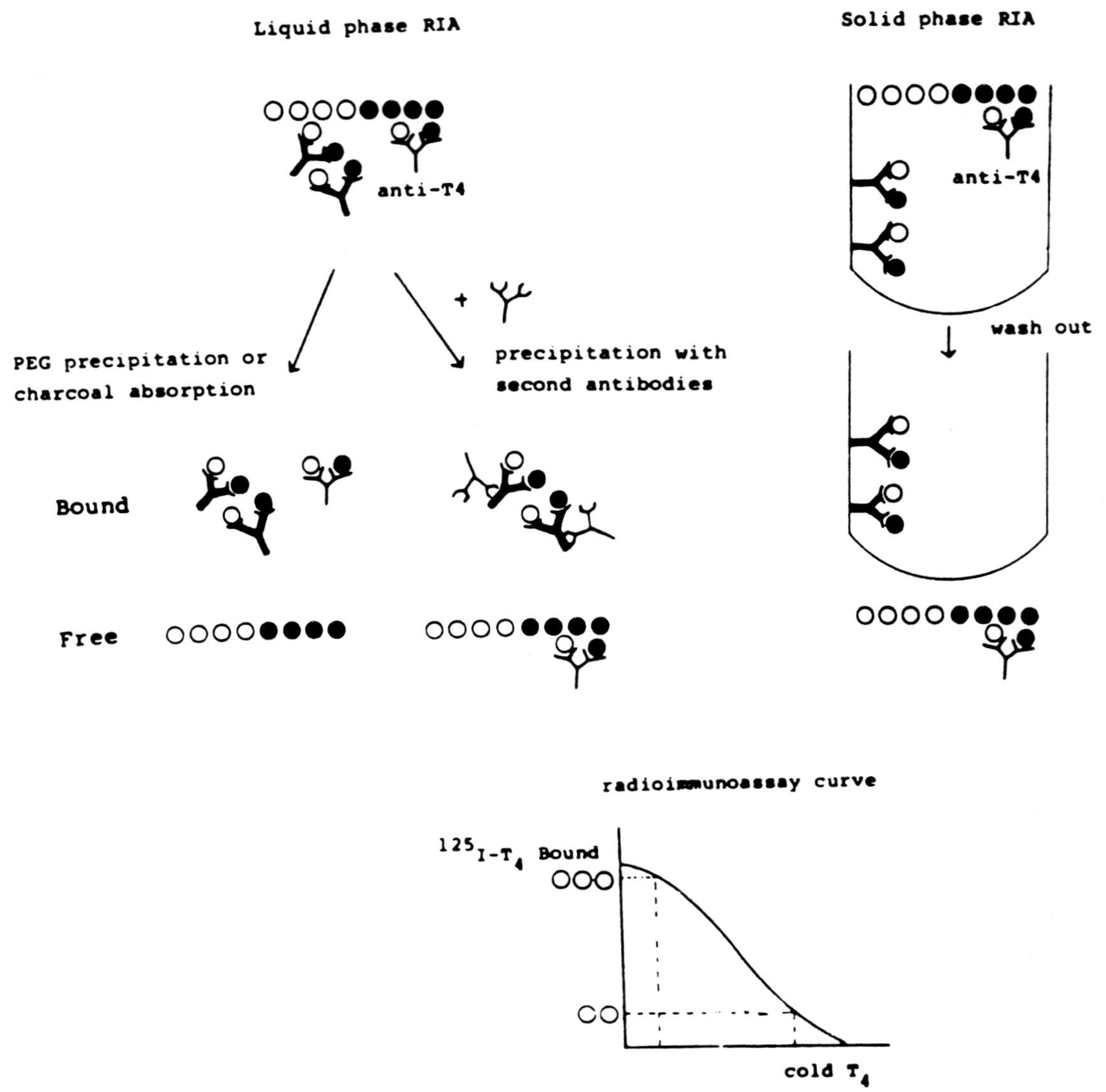

Figure 15. Schematic representation of how antithyroxine autoantibodies in patient's serum interfere with liquid phase (single- or double-antibody methods) and solid-phase RIA. In the presence of T4 autoantibodies, the bound ^{125}I-T4 is increased giving a falsely low value in single-antibody methods, whereas a falsely high result occurs in liquid-phase radioimmunoassays using second antibodies or in solid-phase radioimmunoassays. Similar patterns occur in the presence of T3 autoantibodies in radioimmunoassays for T3. The open circles represent ^{125}I-T4, and the solid circles represent "cold" T4; PEG = polyethylene glycol. (Reprinted with permission from Sakata et al.[246])

Extremely high concentrations of such hormones as HCG and TSH[249] may also occur and produce a hook effect.

In case of monoclonal antibody-based one-step sandwich assays, the high-dose hook effect is generally explained by the large excess of analyte which prevents simultaneous binding of solid- and liquid-phase antibodies to a single antigen molecule.[250] In case of polyclonal antibody-based two-step sandwich assays, additional causes of the high-dose hook effect may include low-affinity solid phase antibodies, inadequate washing after the first step, and "labile kinetics" during the second step if limiting amounts of labeled antibody are present or if incubation times are too long.[251,252]

An assay result that is inappropriate for the patient's clinical status and other laboratory results should suggest the possibility of high-dose hook effect when a sandwich assay is involved in the measurement. Two-step modifications, in general, reduce the possibility of the hook effect.[250] Some suggest routinely analyzing two widely different dilutions of specimens for analytes (eg, tumor markers) that are most commonly involved in producing high-dose hook effect.

TRENDS IN BINDING RADIOASSAYS

During the last decade two major trends appeared in the field of immunoassays: the rapidly increasing use of monoclonal

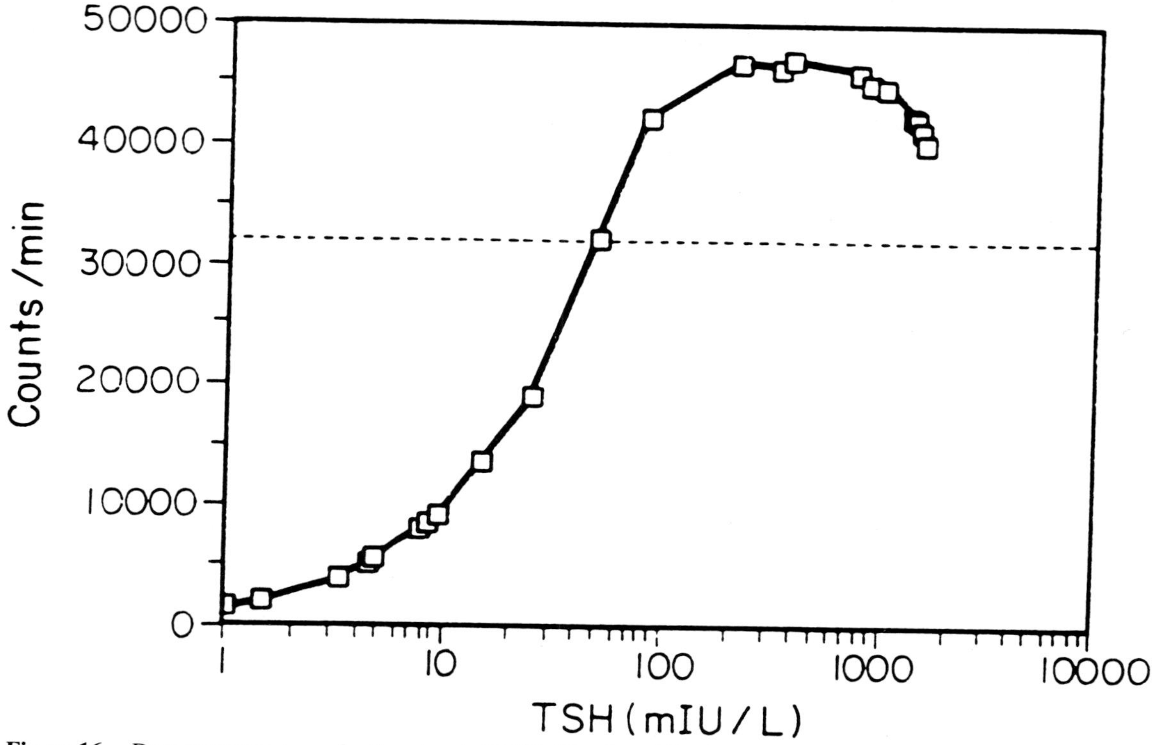

Figure 16. Dose-response curve for thyrotropin IRMA. The dotted line indicates the response for the highest standard (50 mIU/L). (Reprinted with permission from Zweig and Csako.[249])

antibodies and the growing use of nonisotopic labels.[253] The availability of monoclonal antibodies led to increasing use of highly specific sandwich assays for large antigens expressing multiple epitopes. New concepts such as the combined use of receptor and antibody (RASA)[31] and antiidiotypic antibodies for either competitive (4i assay)[25] or noncompetitive immunoassays (RIMA)[42] have also opened new ways for improving assays. The growing use of recombinant DNA products (binders, tracers, standards) is another intriguing area of development. The practical implementation of homogeneous binding radioassays exemplified by the scintillation proximity assay (SPA),[163–165] creates a novel opportunity, particularly in combination with the microtiter plate format, for the development of inexpensive and automated binding assays. After a gradual decline in the utilization of radiolabels for new assays during the 1980s, the current trend is stabilization at the level of about one fourth of all new immunoassays.[253] Radiolabeled immunoassays are still cheaper than nonisotopic assays to perform in most situations. It is particularly difficult to replace radiolabels in RRAs, which are essential tests in both endocrinology and drug research. The future of immunoassays in nuclear medicine has been questioned.[268] Nevertheless, because of their simplicity, high analytical sensitivity, and low cost, it appears likely that, for a select group of analytes that are more esoteric and generate a relatively low volume, binding radioassays remain the choice in the future for both diagnostic and research purpose.

Acknowledgments. This chapter is dedicated to the memory of my parents Margit and Janos Csako.

REFERENCES

1. Rittenberg D, Foster GL. A new procedure for quantitative analysis by isotope dilution, with application to the determination of amino acids and fatty acids. *J Biol Chem* 1940;133:737–752.
2. Graff S, Rittenberg D, Foster GL. The glutamic acid of malignant tumors. *J Biol Chem* 1940;133:745–752.
3. Keston AS, Udenfriend S, Cannan RK. Micro-analysis of mixtures (amino acids) in the form of isotopic derivatives. *J Am Chem Soc* 1946;68:1390 (correction on p. 2753).
4. Avivi P, Simpson SS, Tait JF, Whitehead JK. The use of ^{3}H and ^{14}C labelled acetic anhydride as analytical reagents in microbiochemistry. In: Johnston JE, Faires RA, Millett RJ, eds. *Proceedings of 2nd Radioisotope Conference*. Vol 1. New York: Academic Press, 1954;313–323.
5. Whitehead JK, Beale D. The determination of thyroxine levels in human plasma. *Clin Chim Acta* 1959;4:710–720.
6. Oldham KG. Radiotracer techniques for enzyme assays and enzymatic assays. In: Evans EA, Muramatsu M, eds. *Radiotracer Techniques and Applications*. Vol 2. New York: Marcel Dekker, 1977;823–891.
7. Reed DJ. Methodology of radiotracer enzyme assays. *Adv Tracer Methodol* 1968;4:145–175.
8. Berson SA, Yalow RS, Bauman A, et al. Insulin-I^{131} metabolism in human subjects: demonstration of insulin binding globulin in the circulation of insulin treated subjects. *J Clin Invest* 1956;35:170–190.
9. Yalow RS, Berson SA. Assay of plasma insulin in human subjects by immunological methods. *Nature* 1959; 184:1648, 1649.
10. Yalow RS, Berson SA. Immunoassay of endogenous plasma insulin in man. *J Clin Invest* 1960;39:1157–1175.
11. Grodsky GM, Peng CT. Extractable insulin measured by

immuno-chemical assay: effect of tolbutamide. *Proc Soc Exp Biol Med* 1959;101:100–103.
12. Unger RH, Eisentraut AM, McCall MS, et al. Glucagon antibodies and their use for immunoassay for glucagon. *Proc Soc Exp Biol Med* 1959;102:621–623.
13. Utiger RD, Parker ML, Daughaday WH. Studies on human growth hormone. I. A radio-immunoassay for human growth hormone. *J Clin Invest* 1962;41:254–261.
14. Ekins RP. The estimation of thyroxine in human plasma by an electrophoretic technique. *Clin Chim Acta* 1960; 5:453–459.
15. Murphy BEP, Pattee CJ. Determination of thyroxine utilizing the property of protein-binding. *J Clin Endocrinol Metab* 1964;24:187–196.
16. Barakat RM, Ekins RP. Assay of vitamin B_{12} in blood. *Lancet* 1961;2:25, 26.
17. Rothenberg SP. Assay of serum vitamin B_{12} concentration using Co^{57}-B_{12} and intrinsic factor. *Proc Soc Exp Biol Med* 1961;108:45–48.
18. Murphy BP, Engelberg W, Pattee CJ. A simple method for the determination of plasma corticoids. *J Clin Endocrinol Metab* 1963;23:293–300.
19. Murphy BEP, Hood AB, Pattee CJ. A simple method for the serial determination of plasma corticoids. *Can Med Assoc J* 1964;90:775–780.
20. Rothenberg SP. A radio-enzymatic assay for folic acid. *Nature* 1965;206:1154–1156.
21. Baulieu EE, Ablerge A, Jung I. Recepteurs hormonaux. Liaison specifique de l'oestradiol a des proteines uterines. *CR Acad Sci (D)* 1967;265:354–357.
22. Korenman SG. Radio-ligand binding assay of specific estrogens using a soluble uterine macromolecule. *J Clin Endocrinol Metab* 1968;28:127–130.
23. Lefkowitz RJ, Roth J, Pricer W, Pastan I. ACTH receptors in the adrenal: specific binding of ^{125}I-ACTH and its relation to adenyl cyclase. *Proc Natl Acad Sci USA* 1970;65: 745–752.
24. Lefkowitz RJ, Roth J, Pastan I. Radioreceptor assay of adrenocorticotropic hormone: a new approach to assay polypeptide hormones in plasma. *Science* 1970;170:633–635.
25. Potocnjak P, Zavala F, Nussenzweig R, Nussenzweig V. Inhibition of idiotype-anti-idiotype interaction for detection of a parasite antigen: a new immunoassay. *Science* 1982; 215:1637–1639.
26. Morgan CR. Immunoassay of human insulin and growth hormone simultaneously using ^{131}I and ^{125}I tracers. *Proc Soc Exp Biol Med* 1966;123:230–233.
27. Wide L, Bennich H, Johansson SGO. Diagnosis of allergy by an in-vitro test for allergen antibodies. *Lancet* 1967; 2:1105–1107.
28. Miles LEM, Hales CN. Labelled antibodies and immunological assay systems. *Nature* 1968;219:186–189.
29. Habermann E. Ein neues Prinzip zur quantitativen Bestimmung hochmolekular Antigene (Verknupfungstest) und seine Anwendung auf Tetanustoxin, Serumalbumin und Ovalbumin. *Z Klin Chem Klin Biochem* 1970;8:51–55.
30. Addison GM, Hales CN. Two site assay of human growth hormone. *Horm Metab Res* 1971;3:59, 60.
31. Corti A, Cavenaghi L, Giani E, Cassani G. A receptor-antibody sandwich assay for teicoplanin. *Clin Chem* 1987; 33:1615–1618.
32. Rowe DS. Radioactive single radial diffusion: a method for increasing the sensitivity of immunochemical quantification of proteins in agar gel. *Bull WHO* 1969;40:613–616.
33. Köhler G, Milstein C. Continuous cultures of fused cells secreting antibody of predefined specificity. *Nature* 1975;256:495–497.
34. Tramontano A, Janda KD, Lerner RA. Catalytic antibodies. *Science* 1986;234:1566–1570.
35. Pollack SJ, Jacobs JW, Schultz PG. Selective chemical catalysis by an antibody. *Science* 1986;234:1570–1573.
36. Lerner RA, Tramontano DS. Antibodies as enzymes. *Trends Biochem Sci* 1987;12:427–430.
37. Ekins R. A shadow over immunoassay. *Nature* 1989; 340:256–258.
38. Ekins R. General principles of hormone assay. In: Loraine JA, Bell ET, eds. *Hormone Assays and their Clinical Application*, 4th ed. Edinburgh: Churchill Livingstone, 1976; 1–72.
39. Murphy BEP. Application of the property of protein binding to the assay of minute quantities of hormones and other substances. *Nature* 1964;201:679–682.
40. Murphy BEP. Nuclear in vitro procedures. I. Competitive protein-binding radioassays. *Hospital Pract* 1972;7:65–68.
41. Murphy BEP. Non-chromatographic radiotransinassay for cortisol: application to human adult serum, umbilical cord serum, and amniotic fluid. *J Clin Endocrinol Metab* 1975; 41:1050–1057.
42. Barnard G, Kohen F. Idiometric assay: noncompetitive immunoassay for small molecules typified by the measurement of estradiol in serum. *Clin Chem* 1990;36:1945–1950.
43. Jerne NK, Rolan J, Cazenave P-A. Recurrent idiotypes and internal images. *EMBO J* 1982;1:243–247.
44. Knoche HW. *Radioisotopic Methods for Biological and Medical Research.* New York: Oxford University Press, 1991.
45. Dorfman RI, ed. *Methods in Hormone Research.* vol 1. ed. 2. New York: Academic Press, 1968.
46. Van Oss CJ, Good RJ, Chaudhury MK. Nature of the antigen-antibody interaction. Primary and secondary bonds: optimal conditions for association and dissociation. *J Chromatog* 1986;376:111–119.
47. Getzoff ED, Tainer JA, Lerner RA. The chemistry and mechanism of antibody binding to protein antigens. *Adv Immunol* 1988;43:1–98.
48. Davies DR, Padlan EA: Antigen-antibody complexes. *Annu Rev Biochem* 1990;59:439–473.
49. Murphy BEP, Lehotay DC. Competitive protein-binding assays (including radioimmunoassays). In: Evan EA, Muramatsu M, eds. *Radiotracer Techniques and Applications.* vol 2. New York: Marcel Dekker, 1977;969–1003.
50. Day LA, Sturtevant JM, Singer SJ. The kinetics of the reactions between antibodies to the 2,4-dinitrophenyl group and specific haptens. *Ann NY Acad Sci* 1963;103: 611–625.
51. Parker CW. Nature of immunological responses and antigen-antibody interaction. In: Odell WD, Daughaday WH, eds. *Principles of Competitive Protein Binding Assays.* Philadelphia: Lippincott, 1971;25–48.
52. Stenberg M, Nygren H. Kinetics of antigen-antibody reactions at solid-liquid interfaces. *J Immunol Math* 1988; 113:3–15.
53. Nygren H, Stenberg AM. Immunochemistry at interfaces. *Immunology* 1989;66:321–327.
54. Ishikawa E, Hashida S, Tanaka K, Kohno T. Methodological advances in enzymology: development and application of ultrasensitive enzyme immunoassays for antigens and antibodies. *Clin Chim Acta* 1989;185:223–230.
55. Scatchard G. The attractions of proteins for small molecules. *Ann NY Acad Sci* 1949;51:660–672.
56. Chase GD. Some concepts of RIA theory, data reduction, and quality control. III. The Scatchard plot and the equilibrium model. *Ligand Q* 1979;2:30–33.

57. Klotz IM. Numbers of receptor sites from Scatchard graphs: facts and fantasies. *Science* 1982;217:1247–1249.
58. Munson PJ, Rodbard D. Number of receptor sites from Scatchard and Klotz graphs: a constructive critique. *Science* 1983;220:979–981.
59. Ekins RP, Newman GB, O'Riordan JLH. Theoretical aspects of saturation and radioimmunoassay. In: Hayes RL, Goswitz FA, Murphy BEP, eds. *Radioisotopes in Medicine: In Vitro Studies*. Oak Ridge, TN: US Atomic Energy Commission, 1968;59–100.
60. Berson SA, Yalow RS. Quantitative aspects of the reaction between insulin and insulin-binding antibody. *J Clin Invest* 1959;38:1996–2016.
61. Baulieu EE, Raynaud JP. A "proportion graph" method for measuring binding systems. *Eur J Biochem* 1970; 13:293–304.
62. Keller N, Sendelbeck LR, Richardson UI, et al. Protein binding of corticosteroids in undiluted rat plasma. *Endocrinology* 1966;79:884–906.
63. Malan PG, Cox MG, Long EMR, Ekins RP. Curve fitting to radioimmunoassay standard curves: spline and multiple binding-site models. *Ann Clin Biochem* 1978;15:132–134.
64. Cantor CR, Schimmel PR. *Biophysical Chemistry. Part III The Behavior of Biological Macromolecules*. San Francisco: WH Freeman, 1980.
65. Chappel S. Biological to immunological ratios: reevaluation of a concept [Editorial]. *J Clin Endocrinol Metab* 1990; 70:1494, 1495.
66. Young JL, Meldrum WL, Willey KP. Centralized production of radioiodinated proteins: the provision of ^{125}I-alphafetoprotein. In: Hunter WM, Corrie JET, eds. *Immunoassays for Clinical Chemistry.* 2nd ed. Edinburgh: Churchill Livingstone, 1983;295–300.
67. Fishbein WN, Winkert JW. Parameters of freezing damage to enzymes. *Adv Chem Ser* 1979;180:55–82.
68. Bangham DR. 1982 update on standardization and standards. In: Hunter WM, Corrie JET, eds. *Immunoassays for Clinical Chemistry.* 2nd ed. Edinburgh, Churchill Livingstone, 1983:27–44.
69. Seth J. Standardisation and quality assurance. In: Price CP, Newman DJ, eds. *Principles and Practice of Immunoassay.* New York: Stockton Press, 1991;154–189.
70. Yalow RS. Radioimmunoassay of hormones. In: Wilson JD, Foster DW, eds. *Williams Textbook of Endocrinology.* 8th ed. Philadelphia: W.B. Saunders, 1992;1635–1645.
71. Burrin J, Newman D. Production and assessment of antibodies. In: Price CP, Newman DJ, eds. *Principles and Practice of Immunoassay.* New York, Stockton Press, 1991;19–52.
72. Roth J, Glick SM, Klein LA, Petersen MJ. Specific antibody to vasopressin in man. *J Clin Endocrinol Metab* 1966; 26:671–675.
73. Scheidtmann KH. Immunological detection of proteins of known sequence. In: Creighton TE, ed. *Protein Structure: A Practical Approach.* Oxford: IRL Press, 1989;93–116.
74. Argos P. Prediction of protein structure from gene and amino acid sequences. In: Creighton TE, eds. *Protein Structure: A Practical Approach.* Oxford: IRL Press, 1989;169–190.
75. Berson SA, Yalow RS. Immunochemical distinction between insulins with identical amino acid sequences from different mamalian species (pork and sperm whale insulins) *Nature* 1961;191:1392, 1393.
76. Berson SA, Yalow RS. Insulin in blood and insulin antibodies. *Am J Med* 1966;40:676–690.
77. Peterson JD, Nehrlich S, Oyer PE, Steiner DF. Determination of the amino acid sequence of the monkey, sheep, and dog proinsulin C-peptides by a semi-micro Edman degradation procedure. *J Biol Chem* 1972;247:4866–4871.
78. Kurzer F, Douraghi-Zadeh K. Advances in the chemistry of carbodiimides. *Chem Rev* 1967;67:107–152.
79. Kohen F, Bauminger S, Lindner HR. Preparation of antigenic steroid-protein conjugates. In: Cameron EHD, Hillier SG, Griffiths K, eds. *Fifth Tenovus Workshop: Steroid Immunoassay.* Cardifff: Alpha Omega, 1975;11–32.
80. Erlanger BF. The preparation of antigenic hapten-carrier conjugates: a survey. *Meth Enzymol* 1980;80:85–104.
81. Makela O, Seppala IJT. Haptens and carriers. In: Weir DM, ed. *Handbook of Experimental Immunology.* Vol 1. Oxford: Blackwell Scientific, 1986;3.1–3.31.
82. Landsteiner K. *The Specificity of Serological Reactions.* Boston: Harvard University Press, 1945.
83. Tigelaar RE, Rapport RL II, Inman JK, Kupferberg HJ. A radioimmunoassay for diphenylhydantoin. *Clin Chim Acta* 1973;43:231–241.
84. Cook CE, Kepler JA, Christensen DH. Antiserum to diphenylhydantoin: preparation and characterization. *Res Comm Chem Path Pharmacol* 1973;5:767–774.
85. Greenwood FC, Hunter WM, Klopper A. Assay of human growth hormone in pregnancy at parturition and in lactation: detection of a growth-hormone-like substance from the placenta. *Br Med J* 1964;1:22–24.
86. Glick SM, Roth J, Yalow RS, Berson SA. Regulation of growth hormone secretion. *Recent Progr Horm Res* 1965;21:241–283.
87. Pekary AE, Turner LF, Hershman JM. New immunoenzymatic assay for human thyrotropin compared with two radioimmunoassays. *Clin Chem* 1986;32:511–514.
88. Lindmo T, Bormer O, Ugelstad J, Nustad K. Immunometric assay by flow cytometry using mixtures of particle types of different affinity. *J Immunol Methods* 1990;126: 183–189.
89. Utiger RD, Odell WD, Condliffe PG. Immunologic studies of purified human and bovine thyrotropin. *Endocrinology* 1963;73:359–365.
90. Odell WD, Wilber JF, Utiger RD. Studies of thyrotropin physiology by means of radioimmunoassay. *Recent Progr Horm Res* 1967;23:47–85.
91. Skowsky WR, Fisher DA. The use of thyroglobulin to induce antigenicity to small molecules. *J Lab Clin Med* 1972; 80:134–144.
92. Jaakkola T, Ding Y-Q, Kellokumpu-Lehtinen P, et al. The ratios of serum bioactive/immunoreactive luteinizing hormone and follicle-stimulating hormone in various clinical conditions with increased and decreased gonadotropin secretion: reevaluation by a highly sensitive immunometric assay. *J Clin Endocrinol Metab* 1990;70:1489–1493.
93. Pastan I, Roth J, Macchia V. Binding of hormone to tissue: the first step in polypeptide hormone action. *Proc Natl Acad Sci USA* 1966;56:1802–1809.
94. Gorden P, Weintraub BD. Radioreceptor and other functional hormone assays. In: Wilson JD, Foster DW, eds. *Williams Textbook of Endocrinology.* 8th ed. Philadelphia: WB Saunders, 1992;1647–1661.
95. Thompson S, Stappenbeck R, Turner GA. A multiwell lectin-binding assay using *Lotus tetragonolobus* for measuring different glycosylated forms of haptoglobin. *Clin Chim Acta* 1989;189:277–284.
96. Green NM. Avidin. *Adv Protein Chem* 1975;29:85–133.
97. Bayer EA, Wilchek M. The use of the avidin-biotin complex as a tool in molecular biology. *Meth Biochem Anal* 1980;26:1–45.
98. Chaiet L, Wolf FJ. The properties of streptavidin, a biotin-binding protein produced by *Streptomycetes. Arch Biochem Biophys* 1964;106:1–5.

99. Kronvall G et al. Phylogenetic insight into evolution of mammalian Fc fragment of a G globulin using staphylococcal protein A. *J Immunol* 1970;104:140–147.
100. Goding JW. Use of staphylococcal protein A as an immunological reagent. *J Immunol Methods* 1978;20:241–253.
101. Surolia A, Pain D, Khan MI. Protein A: nature's universal antibody. *Trends Biochem Sci* 1982;7:74–76.
102. Bjork L, Kronvall G. Purification and some properties of streptococcal protein G, a novel IgG-binding reagent. *J Immunol* 1984;133:969–974.
103. Sjobring U, Bjorck L, Kastern W. Streptococcal protein G. *J Biol Chem* 1991;266:399–405.
104. Barazzone P, Lesniak MA, Gorden P, et al. Binding, internalization, and lysosomal association of ^{125}I-human growth hormone in cultured human lymphocytes: a quantitative morphological and biochemical study. *J Cell Biol* 1980; 87:360–369.
105. Eastman RC, Lesniak MA, Roth J, et al. Regulation of receptor by homologous hormone enhances sensitivity and broadens scope of radioreceptor assay for human growth hormone. *J Clin Endocrinol Metab* 1979;49:262–267.
106. Rosenfeld RG, Hintz RL. Modulation of homologous receptor concentrations: a sensitive radioassay for human growth hormone in acromegalic, newborn, and stimulated plasma. *J Endocrinol Metab* 1980;50:62–69.
107. Smith SW, Feldkamp CS. Qualitative features of Scatchard plots: positive curvature. *Ligand Q* 1979;2:37–40.
108. Bremner WS, Chase GD. Some concepts of RIA theory, data reduction, and quality control IV. Binding mechanisms and nonlinear Scatchard plots. *Ligand Q* 1980;3:21–27.
109. Bormer OP. Interference of complement with the binding of carcinoembryonic antigen to solid-phase monoclonal antibodies. *J Immunol Methods* 1989;121:85–93.
110. Larsson A, Sjoquist J. Binding of complement components C1q, C3, C4 and C5 to a model immune complex in ELISA. *J Immunol Methods* 1989;119:103–109.
111. Moller NPH, Steensgaards J. Fc-mediated immune precipitation. II. Analysis of precipitating immune complexes by rate-zonal ultracentrifugation. *Immunology* 1979;38:641–648.
112. Abraham GE. Solid-phase radioimmunoassay of estradiol-17β. *J Clin Endocrinol Metab* 1969;29:866–870.
113. Landon J. Discussion on antibodies. In: Hunter WM, Corrie JET, eds. *Immunoassays for Clinical Chemistry.* 2nd ed. Edinburgh: Churchill Livingstone, 1983;480.
114. Berson SA, Yalow RS. Recent studies on insulin-binding antibodies. *Ann NY Acad Sci* 1959;82:338–344.
115. Bauwens RM, Kint JA, Devos MP, et al. Production, purification and characterization of antibodies to 1.25-dihydroxyvitamin D raised in chicken egg yolk. *Clin Chim Acta* 1987;170:37–44.
116. Wetzel R. Active immunoglobulin fragments synthesised in *E. coli*—from Fab to Scantibodies. *Prot Eng* 1988;2:169, 170.
117. Skerra A, Pluckthun A. Assembly of a functional Fv fragment in *E. coli. Science* 1988;240:1038–1040.
118. Better M, Horwitz AH. Expression of engineered antibodies and antibody fragments in microorganisms. *Meth Enzymol* 1989;178:476–496.
119. Morrison S, Oi VT. Genetically engineered antibody molecules. *Adv Immunol* 1989;44:65–92.
120. Wood CR, Boss MA, Kenten JH, et al. The synthesis and in vivo assembly of functional antibodies in yeast. *Nature* 1985;314:446–449.
121. Murphy BEP, Barta A. One-tube radiotransinassay for determination of cortisol at ambient temperature. *Clin Chem* 1987;33:1137–1140.
122. Soldin SJ. Drug receptor assays: quo vadis? *Ann Clin Biochem* 1992;29:132–136.
123. Schreiber S. Chemistry and biology of the immunophilins and their immunosuppressive ligands. *Science* 1991; 250:283–287.
124. Mousah H, Jacqmin P, Lesne M. The quantification of gamma aminobutyric acid in the cerebrospinal fluid by a radioreceptor-assay. *Clin Chim Acta* 1987;170: 151–160.
125. Kobika BK, Kobika TS, Daniel H, et al. Chimeric α_2, β_2-adrenergic receptors: delineation of domains involved in effector coupling and ligand binding specificity. *Science* 1988;240:1310–1316.
126. Filetti S, Foti D, Costante G, Rapoport B. Recombinant human thyrotropin (TSH) receptor in a radioreceptor assay for the measurement of TSH receptor autoantibodies. *J Clin Endocrinol Metab* 1991;72:1096–1101.
127. Manolagas SC, Deftos LJ. Cytoreceptor assay for 1,25-dihydroxyvitamin D_3: a novel radiometric method based on binding of the hormone to intracellular receptors in vitro. *Lancet* 1980;2:401, 402.
128. Moller G, ed. T cell-dependent and independent B-cell activation. *Immunol Rev* 1987;99:5–299.
129. Dresser DW. Immunization of experimental animals. In: Weir DM, ed. *Handbook of Experimental Immunology.* Vol. 1. Oxford: Blackwell Scientific, 1986;8.1–8.21.
130. Bomford R. Adjuvants. In: Spier RE, Griffiths JB, eds. *Animal Cell Biotechnology.* vol 2. New York: Academic Press, 1985;235–250.
131. Allison AC, Byers NE. An adjuvant formulation that selectively elicits the formation of antibodies of protective isotypes and of cell-mediated immunity. *J Immunol Methods* 1986;95:157–186.
132. Gregoriadis G. Immunological adjuvants: a role for liposomes. *Immunol Today* 1990;11:89–97.
133. Lynch SS, Shirley A. Production of specific antisera to follicle-stimulating hormone and other hormones. *J Endocrinol* 1975;65:127–132.
134. Corrie JET. Production of anti-hapten sera in rabbits. In: Hunter WM, Corrie JET, eds. *Immunoassays for Clinical Chemistry.* Edinburgh: Churchill Livingstone, 1983;469–472.
135. Heidelberger M, Kendall FE. A quantitative theory of the precipitin reaction. *J Exp Med* 1935;62:697–720.
136. Deverill I. Turbidimetric and nephelometric techniques. In: Reeves WG, ed. *Research Monographs in Immunology.* Vol 6. Amsterdam, Elsevier, 1984;27–49.
137. Tung AS. Production of large amounts of antibodies, nonspecific immunoglobulins, and other serum proteins in ascitic fluid of individual mice and guinea pigs. *Meth Enzymol* 1983;93:12–23.
138. Van Ness J, Laemmli UK, Pettijohn DE. Immunization in vitro and production of monoclonal antibodies specific to insoluble and weakly immunogenic proteins. *Proc Natl Acad Sci USA* 1984;81:7897–7901.
139. Borrebaeck CAK, ed. *In Vitro Immunization in Hybridoma Technology. Progress in Biotechnology 5.* Amsterdam: Elsevier, 1988.
140. Borrebaeck CAK. In vitro immunization for production of murine and human monoclonal antibodies: present status. *Trends Biotech* 1986;4:147–153.
141. Bazin H, Xhutdebise L-M, Burtonboy G, et al. Rat monoclonal antibodies. I. Rapid purification from in vitro culture supernatants. *J Immunol Methods* 1984;66:261–269.
142. Groves DJ, Morris BA, Tan K, et al. Production of an ovine monoclonal antibody to testosterone by an interspecies fusion. *Hybridoma* 1987;6:71–76.
143. Flynn JN, Harkiss GD, Hopkins J. Generation of a

sheep × mouse heterohybridoma cell line (1C6.3a6T.1DT) and evaluation of its use in the production of ovine monoclonal antibodies. *J Immunol Methods* 1989;121: 237–246.
144. Seabrook R, Atkinson T. Modified antibodies. In: Price CP, Newman DJ, eds. *Principles and Practice of Immunoassay.* New York: Stockton Press, 1991;53–77.
145. French DL, Laskov R, Scharff MD. The role of somatic hypermutation in the generation of antibody diversity. *Science* 1989;244:1152–1157.
146. Milstein C, Cuello AC. Hybrid hybridomas and the production of bi-specific monoclonal antibodies. *Immunol Today* 1984;5:299–304.
147. Suresh MR, Cuello AC, Milstein C. Bispecific monoclonal antibodies from hybridomas. *Meth Enzymol* 1986; 121:210–228.
148. Sun LK, Curtis P, Rekowicz-Szulcynska E, et al. Chimeric antibody with human constant regions and mouse variable region directed against carcinoma-associated antigen 17-1A. *Proc Natl Acad Sci USA* 1987;84:214–218.
149. Reichmann L, Clark M, Waldmann H, Winter G. Reshaping human antibodies for therapy. *Nature* 1988;332:323–327.
150. Jacobs LS. Principles and practice of competitive binding assays. In: Sonnenwirth AC, Jarett L, eds. *Gradwohl's Clinical Laboratory Methods and Diagnosis.* 8th ed. St. Louis: CV Mosby, 1980;69–94.
151. Yalow RS. Preparation and stability of iodine labeled compounds, part 3. In: Margoulies M, ed. *Protein and Polypeptide Hormones.* Ser 161, Amsterdam: Excerpta Medica, 1968;605–607.
152. Schneider BS, Straus E, Yalow RS. Some considerations in the preparation of radioiodoinsulin for radioimmunoassay and receptor assay. *Diabetes* 1976;25:260–267.
153. Ekins RP, Newman GB. The optimisation of precision and sensitivity in the radioimmunoassay method, part 2. In: Margoulies M, ed. *Protein and Polypeptide Hormones.* Ser. 161, Amsterdam: Excerpta Medica, 1968;329–331.
154. Hunter WM. Preparation and assessment of radioactive tracers. *Br Med Bull* 1974;30:18–23.
155. Jaffe BM, Behrman HR, eds. *Methods of Hormone Radioimmunoassay.* 2nd ed. New York: Academic Pres, 1979.
156. Frank BH, Peavy DE, Hooker CS, Duckworth WC. Receptor binding properties of monoiodotyrosyl insulin isomers purified by high performance liquid chromatography. *Diabetes* 1983;32:705–711.
157. Butt WR, Lynch SS, Reay P, et al. Comparison of iodination methods. In: Hunter WM, Corrie JET, eds. *Immunoassays for Clinical Chemistry.* 2nd ed. Edinburgh: Churchill Livingstone, 1983;286–288.
158. Brown NS. Discussion on labelling of protein antigens. In: Hunter WM, Corrie JET, eds. *Immunoassays for Clinical Chemistry.* 2nd ed. Edinburgh: Churchill Livingstone, 1983;307–315.
159. Thorell JI. Internal sample attenuator. A new method for counting of bound and free activity in radioimmunoassay without physical separation of phases [Abstract]. *J Nucl Med* 1977;18:623.
160. Thorell JI. Internal sample attenuator counting (ISAC): a new technique for separating and measuring bound and free activity in radioimmunoassays. *Clin Chem* 1981;27:1969–1973.
161. Barnard GJR, Matson CM, Makawiti DW, et al. A novel liquid phase separation system for automated immunoassay. In: Hunter WM, Corrie JET, eds. *Immunoassays for Clinical Chemistry.* 2nd ed. Edinburgh: Churchill Livingstone, 1983;231–241.
162. Baldwin J, Hargreaves WR. BioMAT™: a rapid, self-washing immunoassay system with a microparticulate solid phase. *Clin Chem* 1987;33:1566, 1567. Abstract.
163. Hart HE, Greenwald ED. Scintillation proximity assay (SPA)—a new method of immunoassay. *Mol Immunol* 1979;16:265–267.
164. Wood TP, Towers P, Swann K, et al. Radioligand binding technology which eliminates the requirement for separation of free and bound radiolabel. *Br J Pharmacol* (Proceedings Supplement) 1990;100:492P. Abstract.
165. Poggeler B, Huether G. Versatile one-tube scintillation proximity homogeneous radioimmunoassay of melatonin. *Clin Chem* 1992;38:314, 315.
166. Hunter WM, Greenwood FC. A radio-immunoelectrophoretic assay for human growth hormone. *Biochem J* 1964;91:43–56.
167. Westphal U. *Steroid-Protein Interactions.* vol 4. New York: Springer-Verlag, 1971.
168. Skelley DS, Brown LP, Besch PK. Radioimmunoassay. *Clin Chem* 1973;19:146–186.
169. Desbuquois B, Auerbach GD. Use of polyethylene glycol to separate free and antibody-bound peptide hormones in radioimmunoassays. *J Clin Endocrinol Metab* 1971;33: 732–738.
170. Morgan CR, Lazarow A. Immunoassay of insulin using a two-antibody system. *Proc Soc Exp Biol Med* 1962; 110:29–32.
171. Hales CN, Randle PJ. Immunoassay of insulin with insulin-antibody precipitate. *Biochem J* 1963;88:137–146.
172. Edwards R. The development and use of PEG assisted second antibody precipitation as a separation technique in radioimmunoassays. In: Hunter WM, Corrie JET, eds. *Immunoassays for Clinical Chemistry.* 2nd ed. Edinburgh: Churchill Livingstone, 1983;139–146.
173. den Hollander FC, Schuurs AHWM. Solid phase antibody systems. In: Kirkham KE, Hunter WM, eds. *Radioimmunoassay Methods.* Edinburgh: Churchill Livingstone, 1971; 419–443.
174. Jonsson S, Kronvall G. The use of protein-A-containing *Staphylococcus aureus* as a solid phase anti-IgG reagent in radioimmunoassays as exemplified in the quantitation of α-fetoprotein in normal human adult serum. *Eur J Immunol* 1974;4:29–33.
175. Zahradnik R, Brennan G, Hutchison JS, Odell WD. Immunoradiometric assay of corticotropin with use of avidin-biotin separation. *Clin Chem* 1989;35:804–807.
176. Kang J, Kaladas P, Chang C, et al. A highly sensitive immunoenzymometric assay involving "common-capture" particles and membrane filtration. *Clin Chem* 1986;32: 1682–1686.
177. Donini S, Donini P. Radioimmunoassay employing polymerised antisera. *Acta Endocrinol* 1969;(suppl) 142:225–228.
178. Auditore-Hargreaves K, Houghton RL, Monji N, et al. Phase-separation immunoassays. *Clin Chem* 1987;33: 1509–1516.
179. Wood WG, Gadow A. Immobilisation of antibodies and antigens on macro solid phases: a comparison between adsorptive and covalent binding. Part 1 of a critical study of macro solid phases for use in immunoassay systems. *J Clin Chem Clin Biochem* 1983;21:789–797.
180. Catt K, Tregear GW. Solid phase radioimmunoassay in antibody-coated tubes. *Science* 1967;158:1570–1572.
181. Eriksson H, Mattiasson B, Thorell JI. Combination of solid-phase second antibody and internal sample attenuator counting techniques. Radioimmunoassay of thyroid stimulating hormone. *J Immunol Methods* 1984;71:117–225.
182. Grotjan HE, Keel BA. Immunoassay data reduction: Part 1. Basic concepts. In *Service Training and Continuing Educa-*

tion: EndocrinologyandMetabolism. 10(5). Washington, DC: American Association for Clinical Chemistry, 1991;5–20.

183. Grotjan HE, Keel BA. Immunoassay data reduction: Part 2. Approaches to fitting the standard curve. In *Service Training and Continuing Education: Endocrinology and Metabolism.* 10(6). Washington, DC: American Association for Clinical Chemistry, 1991;5–22.
184. Rodbard D, Feldman Y, Jaffe ML, Miles LEM. Kinetics of two-site immunoradiometric ("sandwich") assays. II. Studies on the nature of the "high-dose hook effect". *Immunochemistry* 1978;15:77–82.
185. Chard T. *An Introduction to Radioimmunoassay and Related Techniques*. New York: North-Holland, 1981.
186a. Cernosek SF. Data reduction in radioimmunoassays. Part 1 Introduction. *Ligand Rev* 1979;1:22–24.
186b. Cernosek SF. Data reduction in radioimmunoassays. Part 2 Linearization of dose-response data. ibid. 1979;1:34–37.
186c. Cernosek SF. Data reduction in radioimmunoassays. Part 3 Weighted regression analysis. ibid. 1980;2:7–11.
186d. Cernosek SF. Data reduction in radioimmunoassays. Part 4 Empirical curve fitting methods. ibid. 1980;2:56–60.
187. Chase GD. Some concepts of RIA theory, data reduction and quality control I. Basic approaches to data reduction. *Ligand Q* 1979;2:25–28; II. The "ideal" RIA. *Ligand Q* 1979;2:29–32.
188. Rodbard D, Lewald JE. Computer analysis of radioligand assay and radioimmunoassay data. *Acta Endocrinol* 1970;(suppl)147:79–103.
189. Rodbard D. Statistical quality control and routine data processing for radioimmunoassays and immunoradiometric assays. *Clin Chem* 1974;20:1255–1270.
190. Rodbard D, Hutt DM. Statstical analysis of radioimmunoassays and immunoradiometric (labelled antibody) assays. A generalized weighted, iterative, least squares method for logistic fitting. In: Int Atomic Energy Agency, ed. *Radioimmunoassay and Related Procedures in Medicine*. Vol 1. Vienna: IAEA, 1974;165–192.
191. Rodbard D et al. Statistical characterization of the random errors in the radioimmunoassay dose-response variable. *Clin Chem* 1976;22:350–358.
192. Rodbard D. Data processing for radioimmunoassays: an overview. In: Natelson S, Pesce AJ, Dietz AA. *Clinical Immunochemistry: Chemical and Cellular Bases and Application in Disease*. Washington, DC: American Association for Clinical Chemistry, 1978;477–494.
193. Rodbard D, Munson PJ, Delean A. Improved curve-fitting, parallelism testing, characterization of sensitivity and specificity, validation, and optimization for radioliand assays. In: International Atomic Energy Agency. *Radioimmunoassay and Related Procedures in Medicine*. Vienna: IAEA, 1977;469–514.
194. Munson PJ, Rodbard D. LIGAND: a versatile computerized approach for characterization of ligand-binding systems. *Anal Biochem* 1980;107:220–239.
195. DeLean A, Munson PJ, Rodbard D. Simultaneous analysis of families of sigmoidal curves: application to bioassay, radioligand assay, and physiological dose-response curves. *Am J Physiol* 1978;235:E97–E102.
196. Grotjan HE Jr, Steinberger E. Radioimmunoassay and bioassay data processing using a logistic curve fitting routine adapted to a desk computer. *Comput Biol Med* 1977; 7:159–163.
197. Guardabasso V, Rodbard D, Munson PJ. A model-free approach to estimation of relative potency in dose-response curve analysis. *Am J Physiol* 1987;252:E357–E364.
198. Guardabasso V, Rodbard D, Munson PJ. A versatile method for simultaneous analysis of families of curves. *FASEB J* 1988;2:209–215.
199. Dudley RA, Edwards P, Ekins RP, et al. Guidelines for immunoassay data proceeding. *Clin Chem* 1985;31:1264–1271.
200. Thakur A. Statistical methods for serum hormone assays. In: Keel BA, Webster BW, eds. *Handbook of the Laboratory Diagnosis and Treatment of Infertility.* Boca Raton, FL: CRC Press, 1990;271–290.
201. Finney DJ. *Statistical Methods in Biological Assay.* 3rd ed. New York: Macmillan, 1978.
202. Rodbard D, Munson PJ, Thakun AK. Quantitative characterization of hormone receptors. *Cancer* 1980;46(suppl): 2907–2918.
203. Cernosek SF Jr. Data reduction radioimmunoassay: computerized data reduction. *J Clin Immunoassay* 1985;8:203–212.
204. Rodbard D. Statistical estimation of the minimal detectable concentration ("sensitivity") for radioligand assays. *Anal Biochem* 1978;90:1–12.
205. Eckert GH, Carey RN. Application of statistical quality control rules to quality control in radioimmunoassay. *J Clin Immunoassay* 1985;8:107–114.
206. Carey RN, Tyvoll JL, Plaut DS, et al. Performance characteristics of some statistical quality control rules for radioimmunoassay. *J Clin Immunoassay* 1985;8:245–251.
207. Burrin JM. Quality assurance of hormone analyses. *Ann Clin Biochem* 1988;25:340–345.
208. Yalow RS, Berson SA. General principles of radioimmunoassay. In: Hayes RL, Goswitz FS, Murphy BEP, eds. *Radioisotopes in Medicine: In Vitro Studies*. Oak Ridge, TN: USAEC Div Technical Inf, 1968;7–39.
209. Hill A. Radioassay. In: Early PJ, Sodee DB, eds. *Principles and Practice of Nuclear Medicine*. St Louis: CV Mosby, 1985;856–924.
210. Ekins R. The "precision" profile: its use in RIA assessment and design. *Ligand Q* 1981;4:33–44.
211. Berson SA, Yalow RS. Immunoassay of protein hormones. In Pincus G, Thimann KU, Astwood EB, eds. *The Hormones: Physiology, Chemistry, and Applications*. New York: Academic Press, 1964;557–630.
211a. National Committee for Clinical Laboratory Standards. *Assessing the Quality of Radioimmunoassay Systems; Approved Guideline*. NCCLS Publication. LA1-A. Villanova, PA: NCCLS;1985.
212. Keilacker H, Besch W, Woltanski K-P, et al. Mathematical modelling of competitive labelled-ligand assay systems. Theoretical re-evaluation of optimum assay conditions and precision data for some experimentally established radioimmunoassay systems. *Eur J Clin Chem Clin Biochem* 1991;29:555–563.
213. Pardridge WM. Plasma protein-mediated transport of steroid and thyroid hormones. *Am J Physiol* 1987;252:E157–E164.
214. Ekins R. Measurement of free hormones in blood. *Endocrine Rev* 1990;11:5–46.
215. Ekins R. Validity of analog free thyroxin immunoassays. *Clin Chem* 1987;33:2137–2151.
216. Midgley JEM, Moon CR, Wilkins TA. Validity of analog free thyroxin immunoassays. Part II. *Clin Chem* 1987; 33:2145–2152.
217. Ekins R. Hirsutism: free and bound testosterone. *Ann Clin Biochem* 1990;27:9193.
218. Midgley JEM. Continuation of misrepresentations of analogue free hormone assays. *Ann Clin Biochem* 1990; 27:388, 389.
219. Csako G, Zweig MH, Ruddel, et al. Direct and indirect techniques for free thryoxin compared in patients with non-

thyroidal illness. III. Analysis of interference variables by stepwise regression. *Clin Chem* 1990;36:645–650.
220. O'Sullivan JJ, Leeming RJ, Lynch SS, Pollock A. Radioimmunoassay that measures serum vitamin B_{12}. *J Clin Pathol* 1992;45:328–331.
221. Chrousos GP. Radioreceptor assay of steroids and assay of receptors. In: *15th Training Course: Hormonal Assay Techniques*. Bethesda, MD: Endocrine Society, 1989;241.
222. Allegra JC et al. Estrogen receptor status: an important variable in predicting response to endocrine therapy in metastatic breast cancer. *Eur J Cancer* 1980;16:323–331.
223. Romic-Stojkovic R, Gamulin S. Relationship of cytoplasmic and nuclear estrogen receptors and progesterone receptors in human breast cancer. *Cancer Res* 1980;40:4821–4825.
224. Jackson TM, Marshall NJ, Ekins RP. Optimization of immunoradiometric (labelled antibody) assays. In: Hunter WM, Corrie JET, eds. *Immunoassays for Clinical Chemistry*. 2nd ed. Edinburgh: Churchill Livingstone, 1983;557–575.
225. Haynes SP, Goldie DJ. Simultaneous radioimmunoassay of thyroid hormones in unextracted serum. *Ann Clin Biochem* 1977;14:12–15.
226. Desai RK, Deppe WM, Norman RJ, et al. The SimulTRAC™ FT_4/TSH assay evaluated as first-line thyroid-function test. *Clin Chem* 1988;34:1488–1491.
227. Csako G, Zweig MH, Glickman J, et al. Direct and indirect techniques for free thyroxin compared in patients with nonthyroidal illness. I. Effect of free fatty acids. *Clin Chem* 1989;35:102–109.
228. Edwards R. Radiolabelled immunoassay. In: Price CP, Newman DJ, eds. *Principles and Practice of Immunoassay*. New York: Stockton Press, 1991;856–924.
229. Nickoloff EL. Radioisotopes as interfering substances in radioimmunoassays. *Ligand Q* 1979;2:22–24.
230. Carmel R. Artifactual radioassay results due to serum contamination by intravenous radioisotope administration. *Am J Clin Pathol* 1978;70:364–367.
231. Bolton AE, Hunter WM. The labelling of proteins to high specific radioactivities by conjugation to a ^{125}I-containing acylating agent. *Biochem J* 1973;133:529–538.
232. Midgley AR, Niswender GD, Gay VL, Reichert LJ Jr. Use of antibodies for characterization of gonadotropins and steroids. *Recent Progr Horm Res* 1971;27:235–301.
233. Nordblom GD, Counsell RE, England BG. Ligand specificity and bridging phenomena in hapten radioimmunoassays. *Ligand Q* 1979;2:34–36.
234. Corrie JET. ^{125}Iodinated tracers for steroid radioimmunoassay: the problem of bridge recognition. In: Hunter WM, Corrie JET, eds. *Immunoassays for Clinical Chemistry*. 2nd ed. Edinburgh: Churchill Livingstone, 1983;353–357.
235. Hunter WM, Budd PS. Circulating antibodies to ovine and bovine immunoglobulin in healthy subjects: a hazard for immunoassays. *Lancet* 1980;2:1136, 1137.
236. Boscato LM, Stuart MC. Incidence and specificity of interference in two-site immunoassays. *Clin Chem* 1986; 32:1491–1495.
237. Boscato LM, Stuart MC. Heterophilic antibodies: a problem for all immunoassays. *Clin Chem* 1988;34:27–33.
238. Kahn BB, Weintraub BD, Csako G, Zweig MH. Factitious elevation of thyrotropin in a new ultrasensitive assay: implications for the use of monoclonal antibodies in "sandwich" immunoassay. *J Clin Endocrinol Metab* 1988;66:526–533.
239. Zweig MH, Csako G, Reynolds JC, Carrasquillo JA. Interference by iatrogenically induced anti-mouse IgG antibodies in a two site immunometric assay for thyrotropin. *Arch Pathol Lab Med* 1991;115:164–168.
240. Levinson SS. Antibody multispecificity in immunoassay interference. *Clin Biochem* 1992;25:77–87.
241. Gendrel D, Feinstein MC, Grenier J, et al. Falsely elevated serum thyrotropin (TSH) in newborn infants; transfer from mothers to infants of a factor interfering in the TSH radioimmunoassay. *J Clin Endocrinol Metab* 1981;52:62–67.
242. Csako G, Weintraub BD, Zweig MH. The potency of immunoglobulin G fragments for inhibition of interference caused by anti-immunoglobulin antibodies in a monoclonal immunoradiometric assay for thyrotropin. *Clin Chem* 1988; 34:1481–1483.
243. Primus FJ, Kelley EA, Hansen HJ, Goldenberg DM. Sandwich-type immunoassay of carcinoembryonic antigen in patients receiving murine monoclonal antibodies for diagnosis and therapy. *Clin Chem* 1988;34:261–264.
244. Zweig MH, Csako G, Spero M. Escape from blockade of interfering heterophile antibodies in a two-site immunoradiometric assay for thyrotropin. *Clin Chem* 1988; 34:2589–2591.
245. Newman ES, Moskie LA, Duggal RN, Goldenberg DM, Hansen HJ: Murine monoclonal antibody adsorbed onto vinylidene fluoride floccules to eliminate antibody interference in "sandwich-type immunoassays. *Clin Chem* 1989; 35:1743–1746.
246. Sakata S, Nakamura S, Miura K. Autoantibodies against thyroid hormones or iodothyronine. Implications in diagnosis, thyroid function, treatment, and pathogenesis. *Ann Intern Med* 1985;103:579–589.
247. Eto S, Fujihara T, Ohnami S, Suzuki H. Autoantibody to bovine TSH in Hashimoto's thyroiditis. *Lancet* 1984;i:520.
248. Garrett PE. The hook: who's got it? when does it matter? what can you do about it? *J Clin Immunoassay* 1986; 9:170, 171.
249. Zweig MH, Csako G. High-dose hook effect in a two-site IRMA for measuring thyrotropin. *Ann Clin Biochem* 1990;27:494, 495.
250. Alfthan H, Stenman U. Falsely low results obtained with the Hybritech Tandem^R-PSA assay. *Clin Chem* 1988;34:2152.
251. Ryall RG, Story CJ, Turner DR. Reappraisal of the causes of the "hook effect" in two-site immunoradiometric assays. *Anal Biochem* 1982;127:308–315.
252. Chi K-F, Scanlon MD, Henkel R, et al. Detection of human plasma-associated hepatitis B surface antigens by monoclonal antibodies: the same monoclonal antibody can be used as both capture and tracer antibody. *Diagn Clin Immunol* 1987;5:91–99.
253. Gosling JP. A decade of development in immunoassay methodology. *Clin Chem* 1990;36:1408–1427.
254. Whitherspoon L. Immunoassay: is there a future role for nuclear medicine? *J Nucl Med* 1983;24:952–996.

15 Radiomicrobiology

Salman H. Siddiqi

The principle of radiomicrobiology is based on the metabolic activity of living cells or microorganisms in a nutritionally enriched support medium with one or more substrates in the medium labeled with a radionuclide. During metabolism, the labeled substrate is converted to radiolabeled by-products. These products are generally extracellular in gaseous form, although some are assimilated into the cell as well. Quantitative monitoring of radioactivity in these products provides information about

1. Multiplication and rate of growth of the cell population
2. Active metabolism and utilization of substrates by viable microorganisms without multiplication
3. Killing or inhibitory effects of antimicrobials on microorganisms
4. Enhancement effects on growth
5. Identification of microorganisms
6. Assimilation of specific substrates by microorganisms to define metabolic pathways

Radiomicrobiology is thus divided into two parts: (1) the radiometric detection of growth by $^{14}CO_2$ monitoring and (2) substrate assimilation by incorporation of radioactivity into cell materials such as RNA and DNA. We will concentrate on radiometric systems for the detection of $^{14}CO_2$ as an index of microbial growth since they are most commonly used.

RADIOMETRIC DETECTION

Among various means of monitoring metabolism of radiolabeled substrates, the most sensitive and convenient is the radiometric method in which evolved $^{14}CO_2$ is monitored. Other by-products with β-emitting radionuclides such as $^{14}CH_4$ and C^3H_4 are not produced as commonly as $^{14}CO_2$ and thus are not used in clinical microbiology. In the radiometric system, one or more substrates in a well-balanced nutritional medium are labeled with ^{14}C. These substrates are decarboxylated during metabolism (respiration) of microorganisms and the $^{14}CO_2$ produced is measured quantitatively by various means. The measurement of metabolic rates during the early phase of bacterial growth, while growth is still linear with respect to time, can be used to define bacterial growth or its inhibition. This technique is extremely sensitive and can detect very small quantities of $^{14}CO_2$ so that growth can be detected at an early stage which results in significant time savings.

Methods of Detection

There are two common methods for quantifying $^{14}CO_2$ generation: trapping in an alkaline solution and then counting by liquid scintillation counting and counting ^{14}C directly in an ion chamber (Fig. 1).

SCINTILLATION COUNTING

Although this technique had been used in different forms for a long time, Buddemeyer and co-workers developed a simple variation using a biphasic scintillation vial system.[1] This system consists of a sterile glass vial containing the growth medium. The vial is surrounded by an alkali impregnated-paper cylinder which is then placed in a plastic scintillation vial (Fig. 2).[1–3] The assembly is sealed with a cap. When microorganisms are inoculated into the medium in the inner vial and incubated, $^{14}CO_2$ is liberated and trapped on the alkali paper. Scintillation cocktail is then added and the trapped $^{14}CO_2$ is counted in a liquid scintillation counter. The system can be automated by connecting the digital output of the scintillation counting system through a computer with software capable of analyzing the data. The amount of $^{14}CO_2$ and its generation rate are directly proportional to the amount of growth occurring in the medium.

Various modifications have been developed that increase the counting efficiency from the original 7% to 70 to 80%, while at the same time reducing variability.[2–4] Schort et al developed a small enclosed radiorespirator apparatus in which a cell suspension was filtered through a membrane filter. The filter was then soaked with medium containing ^{14}C-labeled substrate and placed in a two-compartment apparatus, sealed with a cork.[5] Evolved $^{14}CO_2$ was collected in the side compartment on an alkali-impregnated filter paper and then counted with a scintillation counter. The apparatus was used for detecting bacteremia. Boonkitticharoen et al made further improvements in the system to handle larger volumes of growth medium with increased counting efficiency.[4]

One of the many advantages of the biphasic vial system is that $^{14}CO_2$ can be measured continuously and cumulatively. Moreover, it is very sensitive.[1,2] However, due to numerous

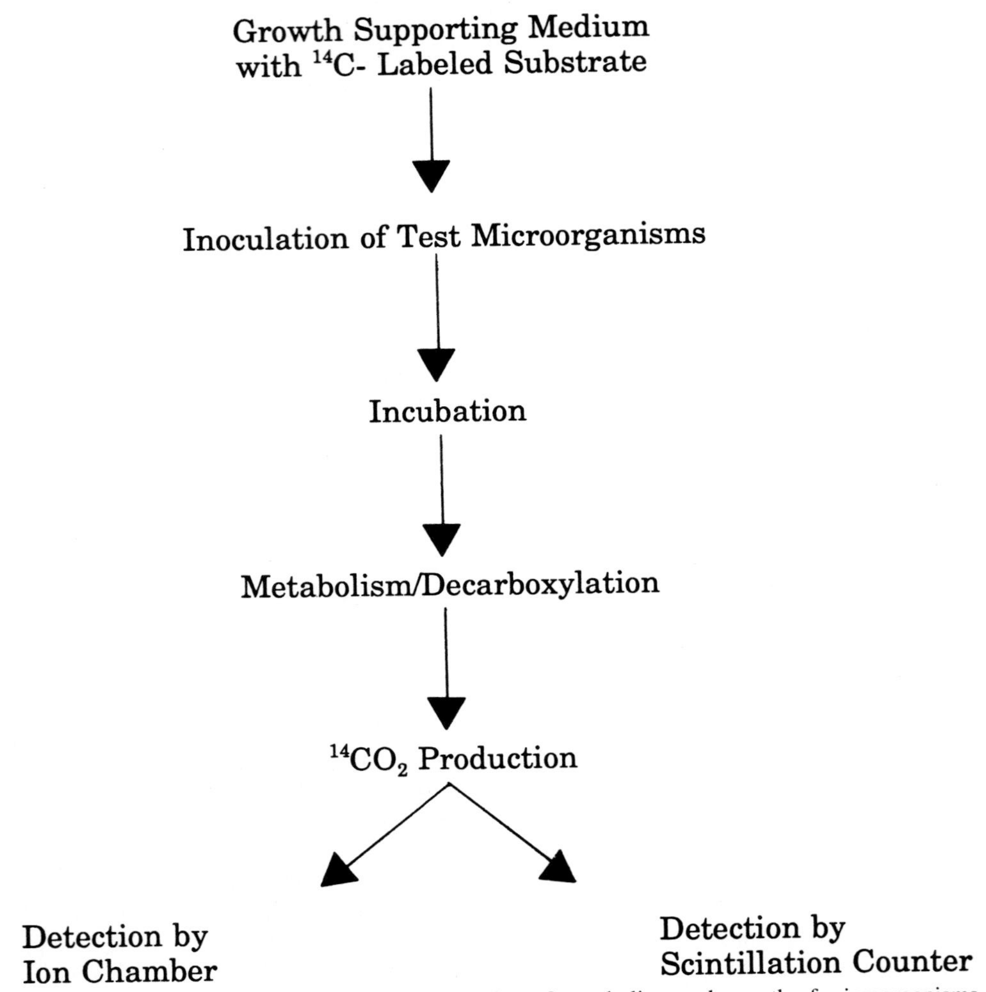

Figure 1. Basic outline for radiometric monitoring of metabolism and growth of microorganisms.

limitations, this approach has not been adopted for routine clinical microbiological investigations.

ION CHAMBER MONITORING

Initially, $^{14}CO_2$ production by coliform bacteria was monitored by Levin using a Geiger Counter.[6–8] However, the method was cumbersome and time consuming. Later, an ion chamber was developed by Deland and Wagner to monitor $^{14}CO_2$.[9] This approach was more practical and could be automated, although there are some disadvantages. Unlike the Buddemeyer system, the monitoring of $^{14}CO_2$ is not cumulative; at each measurement, $^{14}CO_2$ is evacuated from the medium vial and after the counting of radioactivity it is eliminated from the counting system. Thus, counting efficiency is lower than the Buddemeyer system. However, there are several advantages; it is simple to use, it has various options of culture gas (aerobic, anaerobic), and accomodates various volumes of media. Because of these advantages the method has been automated and commercialized.

Instrumentation and Automation

Deland and Wagner first reported a prototype ion chamber device to detect $^{14}CO_2$ produced by bacteria in blood cultures.[9,10] This led to further innovations and ultimately the BACTEC System (Johnston Laboratories, Cockeysville, MD) was developed commercially for blood cultures. Culture vials with different sizes (20 to 50 mL), containing various volumes of media (4 to 30 mL) can be used. The vials are sealed with a rubber septum to contain the $^{14}CO_2$ produced during incubation. The basic principle of the BACTEC system is illustrated in Figures 3 and 4. The most important component in this instrument is the sampling and air flow system. A gas tank, containing 5 to 10% CO_2 balanced air for aerobic or nitrogen for anaerobic bacteria is attached to the instrument. The head assembly contains a set of needles, one for drawing the gas sample from the culture vial and the other for supplying fresh gas each time the vial is sampled. A heating coil decontaminates the needles between testings. Once a vial is placed under the needle

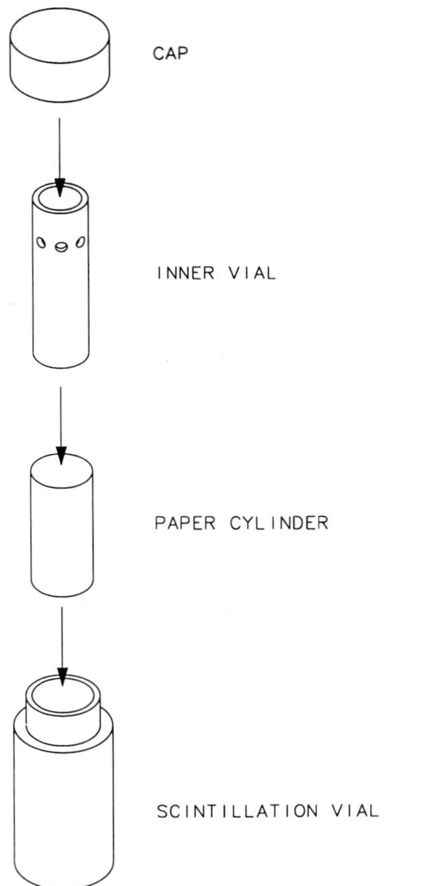

Figure 2. Monitoring $^{14}CO_2$ production by the scintillation counting method. Components of the Buddemeyer biphasic scintillation vial. See text for description.

assembly, the needles are depressed, penetrating the rubber septum of the vial, and the headspace gas from the vial is aspirated and transferred to the ion chamber to measure the evolved radioactivity. Concurrently, the other needle introduces fresh culture gas from the gas supply. After counting, the ion chamber is flushed with air to eliminate the sample. The entire cycle takes from 60 to 80 seconds per sample.

The $^{14}CO_2$ radioactivity measurement is converted to growth index or "GI" units ranging from 0 to 999. The instrument is calibrated in such a way that 100 GI units corresponds to an activity of 0.025 μCi (.92 Bq). This radiometric system is widely used in clinical microbiology for culturing clinical specimens for bacteria, yeasts, and molds. Methods have been developed for antimicrobial susceptibility testing, speciation of bacteria, and various research applications.

Data Handling

In radiometric systems, the culture vials can be tested periodically for $^{14}CO_2$ ranging from daily to weekly. The increase in the growth index between testings indicates the number of microorganisms present and their rate of growth. The way the data are plotted depends upon the parameters to be investigated.

DIFFERENTIAL PLOTTING

Because $^{14}CO_2$ does not accumulate with successive sampling the data can be plotted showing the GI values at each testing vs time. This is the most common method to demonstrate changes in metabolic rates over the time course of an experiment. When compared with controls, these curves are used to compare the differential metabolism of various substrates, or to study growth inhibition or enhancement by test substrates (Fig. 5).

CUMULATIVE PLOTTING

This represents the cumulative $^{14}CO_2$ produced with time, thus illustrating the total difference between the two test parameters, eg, the differential metabolism of two substrates (Fig. 6). If the inhibitory effect of an antimicrobial is to be determined quantitatively, one way of plotting is the cumulative percentage, taking the control as 100% and calculating the growth values in the antimicrobial containing medium as a percent of the control (Fig. 7).

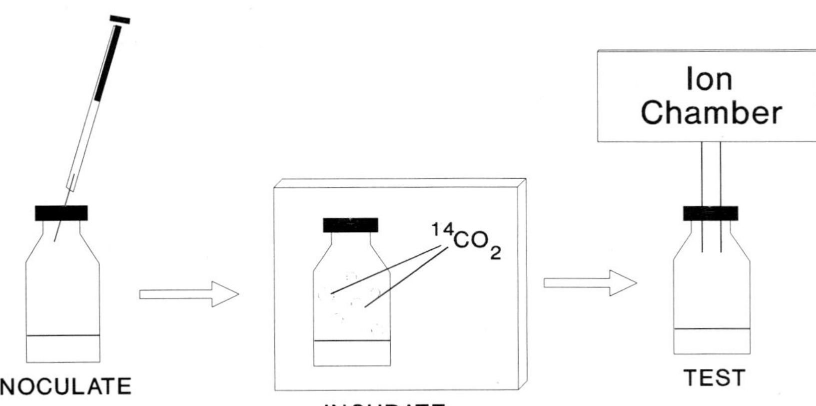

Figure 3. Monitoring of $^{14}CO_2$ by ion chamber method. Basic principle of BACTEC system.

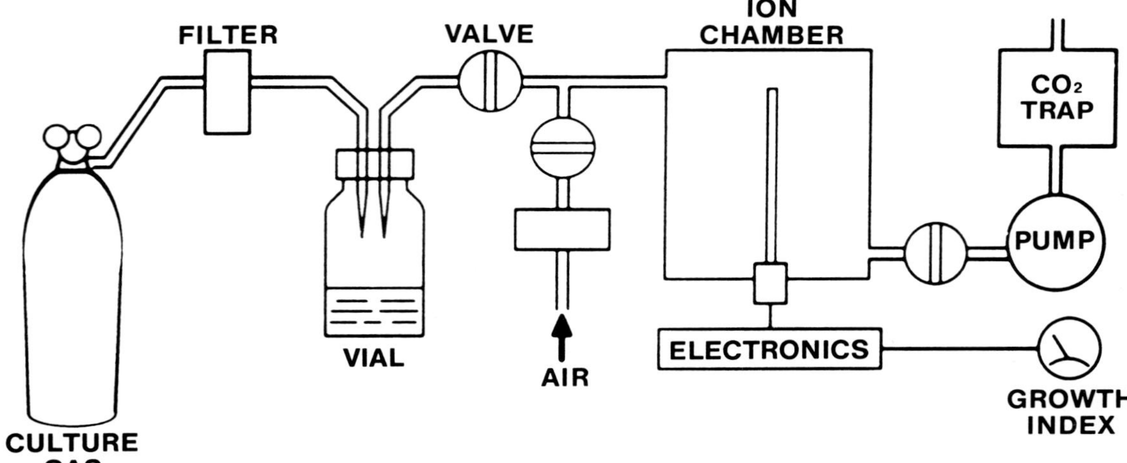

Figure 4. Schematic diagram of the BACTEC system.

SEMILOG PLOTTING

This method represents the data in linear form and is used for growth studies where the number of bacteria are to be evaluated or generation time is to be determined. This method is useful when an increase in the number of bacteria is to be enumerated at different intervals, either by total counts or by counts of colony forming units (CFU).

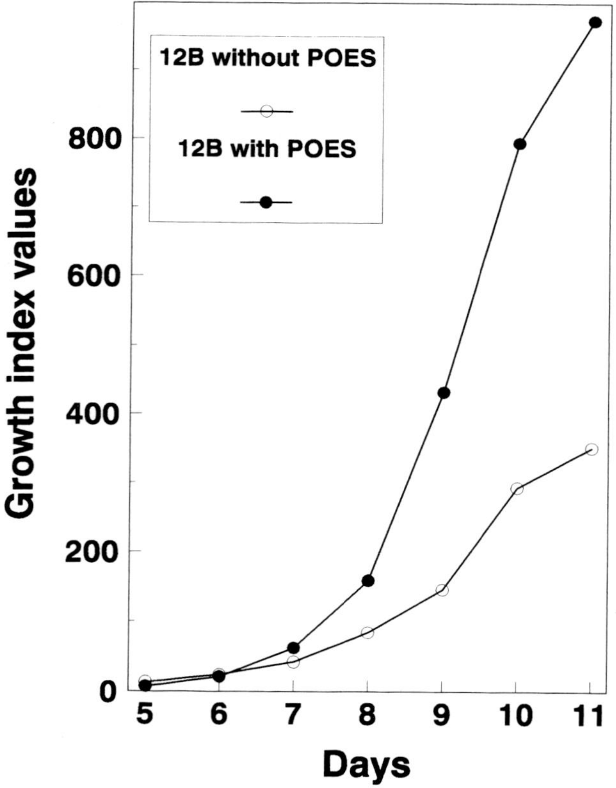

Figure 5. Enhancement effect of polyoxylethylene stearate on growth of *M. bovis* in radiometric 12B medium.

FACTORS AFFECTING RADIOMETRIC DETECTION

Radiolabeled Substrate

Selection of an appropriate radiolabeled substrate is the most important step in radiomicrobiological investigations. There are three main factors to be considered in the selection of radiolabeled substrates. First, it should be readily metabolized by the test organisms. Second, it should be decarboxylated with maximum production of $^{14}CO_2$ if $^{14}CO_2$ generation is monitored or it should be well incorporated into the organism in case of assimilation studies. Third, the substrate should be stable and not break down by autoradiolytic dissociation during storage, incubation, or testing of the medium.

The number and position of carbon radiolabeling in a substrate may also vary, the selection of which depends upon the metabolic pathway of the test organism. For example, glucose is generally used as uniformly labeled U-^{14}C-glucose while, for palmitic acid, the carbon at the first position is labeled 1-^{14}C-palmitic acid.

Since concentration of ^{14}C-labeled substrate is to some extent proportional to $^{14}CO_2$ production, optimum concentration of substrate results in earliest detection of growth. On the other hand, excessive concentrations of a substrate may have an inhibitory effect on bacterial growth. The problem of radioactive waste disposal also mandates using as little radioactive material as practicable.

It is important to have some balance between the nutrients present in the medium and the radiolabeled substrate. Since the amount of ^{14}C-labeled substrate is small compared to unlabeled (cold) substrates present in the medium, the metabolism of the ^{14}C-substrate is sometimes reduced in the competitive environment and growth detection time increases. For example, the presence of cold glycerol in NC-5 medium markedly inhibits the assimilation and oxidation of U-^{14}C-glycerol by *Mycobacterium lepraemurium*.[11] On the other

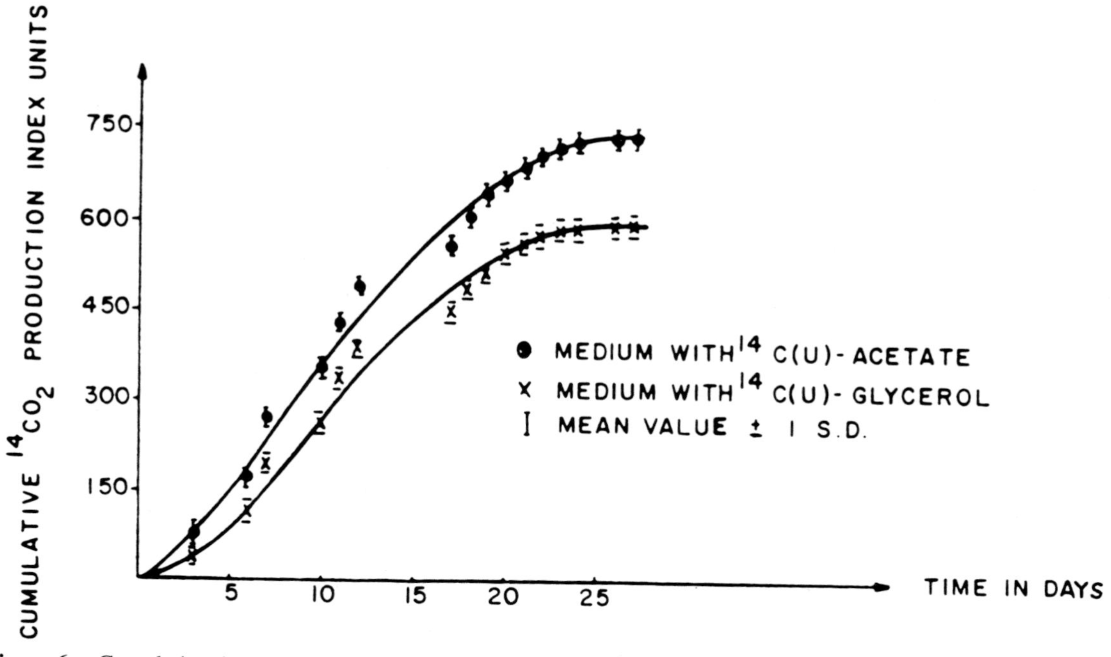

Figure 6. Cumulative data plotting. Metabolism of U-^{14}C acetate and U-^{14}C glycerol by *M. lepraemurium*. Cumulative plotting of the same data presented in Figure 5 provides an overall comparison of the substrates, medium with acetate performing better than glycerol. Reproduced with permission from Reference 103.

hand, in the Middlebrook 7H12 (BACTEC 12B) medium, bovine serum albumin (BSA) is added, which contains several fatty acids. These may compete with ^{14}C-palmitic acid. However, BSA is required for mycobacterial growth and thus, cannot be eliminated. Other enrichments such as glucose and oleic acid, which are generally used for mycobacterial culture media, are eliminated to reduce competition. For growth of *M. tuberculosis* glycerol is not used as a growth substrate in the presence of glutamate or glucose because of catabolic repression which arises from reduction in the cyclic AMP in the presence of glucose.[12] Thus, it is essential to investigate ingredients in the medium that may compete with the radiolabeled substrate.

Among various substrates, U-^{14}C glucose is the most com-

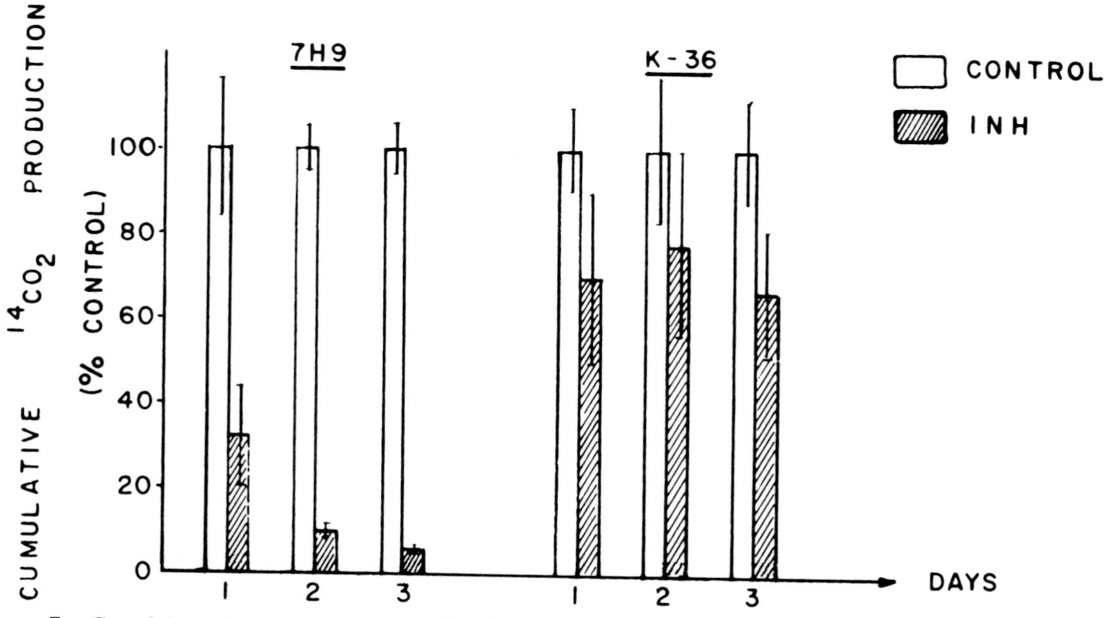

Figure 7. Comparison of the effects of 1.0 μg isoniazid on the metabolism of ^{14}C-formate by *M. tuberculosis* in 7H9 medium and K-36 buffer. Control vials do not contain INH. Reproduced with permission from Reference 103.

monly used for detecting clinical pathogens. A variety of other substrates have been used in radiometric detection of bacteria, such as uniformly labeled glutamic acid, aspartic acid, arginine, and formate.[13] Sometimes more than one radiolabeled substrate is used to increase detection sensitivity. Mycobacteria do not produce CO_2 from most substrates, and substrates such as glucose cannot be used for the detection. Camargo et al studied several 1-^{14}C fatty acids to establish metabolism and assimilation kinetics of mycobacteria.[14,15] They also studied oxidation patterns of 1-^{14}C fatty acids and U-^{14}C amino acids by drug susceptible and drug-resistant mycobacteria and reported that complex amino acids such as proline, phenylalanine, and tyrosine were not oxidized by the test mycobacteria, while butyric acid, octanoic acid, glycine, and alanine were oxidized.[16] The differential oxidation of these substrates by the test species of mycobacteria indicated the feasibility of using this approach to differentiate different species of mycobacteria.

Nature of Medium

The choice of media should be based on commonly available selections known to optimally support growth of the microorganisms under study. A simple medium is generally preferred because complex media are likely to contain substances that compete with radiolabeled substrates. In most studies performed with common clinical pathogens, glucose-free trypticase soy broth or thioglycolate broth is used. Depending upon the type of microorganisms to be investigated, the medium may be aerobic, anaerobic, or hypertonic. Agitation of liquid cultures helps growth of most aerobic bacteria when isolated from blood specimens.[17] Generally, liquid medium is preferred for radiometric studies, but solid medium may also be used.

pH of Medium

Most culture media have a pH of 7.0 to 7.2. At this pH, the solubility of $^{14}CO_2$ in the culture medium vial is high and release of $^{14}CO_2$ into the headspace of the culture medium vial is limited to surface exchange. Lowering the pH reduces CO_2 solubility in the medium and enhances its release into the headspace; this may be inhibitory for some bacterial growth.

In most culture systems, 2.5 to 10.0% CO_2 is added to air as the culture gas to ensure optimum bacterial growth. The absorption of CO_2 into the medium also reduces the pH gradually. Growth and metabolism by bacteria often result in decreased pH, especially if the medium is not buffered well. In the case of mycobacteria, there is no significant acid production, and thus the pH of the medium is not altered by growth. Generally, pH 6.8 is used for mycobacterial media, but in some special cases, eg, *M. paratuberculosis*, lower pH (5.9) is desirable for optimum growth.

Incubation Temperature

Optimum incubation temperature is critical for maximum generation of $^{14}CO_2$. Common clinical pathogens are usually incubated at 35 to 36°C while peak $^{14}CO_2$ production by *M. tuberculosis* occurs at 36 to 38°. The $^{14}CO_2$ production from U-^{14}C acetate by *M. lepraemurium* at 30°C is almost 60% higher than at 37°C.[14] Similarly, *M. marinum* or *M. chelonae* subspecies *chelonae* grow poorly or fail to grow on initial isolation at 37°C, while at 30°C the organisms grow very well. *M. xenopi* on the other hand grows best at a temperature higher than 37°C.

Stress Environments

When microorganisms are placed in stressed environments, there is a tendency to overcome the adverse conditions for a short while, resulting in increased metabolism and $^{14}CO_2$ production. This initial high $^{14}CO_2$ production is followed progressively by decreased metabolism, and ultimately death of the organism if the stress environment persists. The metabolism of lauric acid by *M. tuberculosis* in water and K-36 buffer is an example. Both media provide stress environment for metabolism, but water is more hostile than the buffer. In water, there is a higher $^{14}CO_2$ output followed by an abrupt fall in production. In K-36 buffer the initial $^{14}CO_2$ production is lower, but metabolism is maintained longer.[15] This indicates that in some instances, even if the medium does not provide good nutritional environment or does not support growth, there is a possibility of detecting metabolism with $^{14}CO_2$ production without having active multiplication.

Inoculum Size

The inoculum size is directly proportional to the quantity of growth, and hence the quantity of $^{14}CO_2$ production. With fewer organisms inoculated into a culture vial, it takes a longer time to detect growth radiometrically. Inoculum size also effects the peak of growth curves if daily $^{14}CO_2$ production is plotted against time. Figure 8 illustrates the effect of inoculum size on growth curves of *M. tuberculosis*.

For common clinical pathogens, inoculum size is not critical because they grow rapidly and growth is detected in a short period of time. For example, as few as ten organisms inoculated into a radiometric medium can be detected easily within 2 to 4 hours.[5,10] On the other hand, inoculum size is more critical for slow-growing bacteria such as *M. tuberculosis*, with which growth may be detected from 24 hours to several weeks depending on the inoculum size. In case of viable but non-culturable microorganisms, the detection of metabolism and $^{14}CO_2$ production is possible only with large inoculum sizes. For *M. lepraemurium* detection of metabolism was not possible with an inoculum less than 10^9 organisms per vial.[11]

Quality of Inoculum

The detection time of bacterial growth also depends upon the inoculum quality. When an actively growing culture in its logarithmic phase is inoculated, it grows faster and produces $^{14}CO_2$ earlier than a culture in a stationery phase or of low viability. Sometimes clumping of bacteria affects the growth rate and $^{14}CO_2$ production. For such bacteria as *M. tuberculo-*

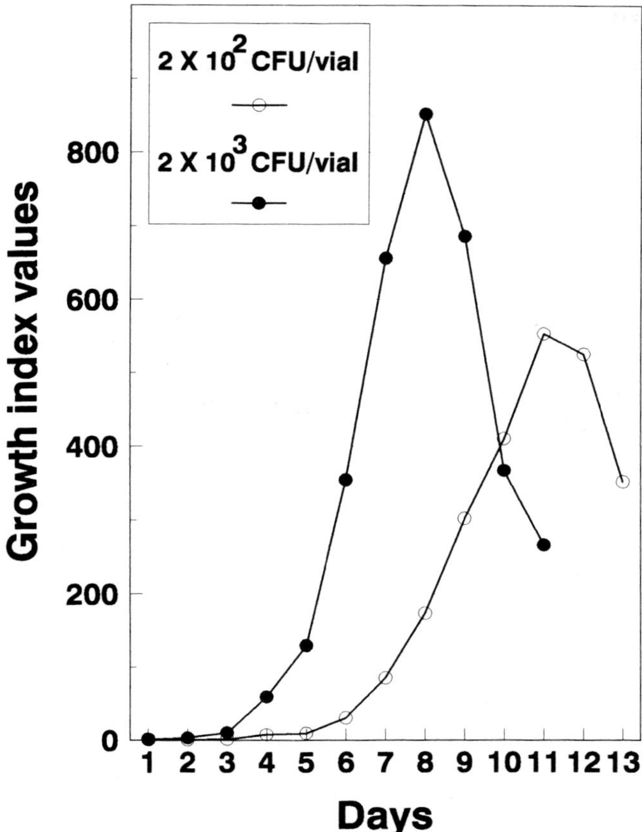

Figure 8. Effect of inoculum size on growth and $^{14}Co_2$ production of *M. tuberculosis* in radiometric 12B medium. Increase in the inoculum also increases the $^{14}CO_2$ output, resulting in earlier detection and an earlier, higher peak.

sis, a well-dispersed suspension is essential for metabolic or drug susceptibility studies. Sample preparation may also affect the quality of inoculum. In the case of sputum for mycobacterial culture, it is necessary to digest and decontaminate the specimen, usually with strong alkali or acid. This results in damaging the cell and mycobacteria may take longer to initiate growth, the delay depending upon the harshness of specimen processing.

Type of Bacteria

Bacteria have different rates of growth and metabolism. Most bacteria are detected faster than fungi and mycobacteria. Even among mycobacteria, *M. tuberculosis* and *M. bovis* are the slowest to detect because of their slow growth.

APPLICATIONS

Levin and co-workers were among the first investigators who reported the use of radionuclides to detect microorganisms. They measured $^{14}CO_2$ produced by *Escherichia coli* from the metabolism of ^{14}C-lactose and ^{14}C-formate.[8,18,19] In succeeding years, methodology was improved and various applications of radiomicrobiology were reported in such fields as space projects, diagnostic microbiology, and enzyme assays.[20–22] Radiometric procedures have been especially useful in clinical microbiology.[23,24]

Blood Culture

The use of radiometric techniques to diagnose bacteremia was one of the earliest and most important applications in clinical microbiology. Initial studies with a semiautomated instrument were carried out by Deland and Wagner in 1970. Using ^{14}C-glucose, 18 common pathogenic bacteria were tested with seeded blood specimens. All the organisms tested metabolized the radiolabeled glucose and produced sufficient $^{14}CO_2$ to be detected within a few hours.[10,25] Waters found the system was capable of detecting as few as 1 colony forming unit (CFU).[26] Later, the instrument and techniques were improved to detect most types of pathogenic bacteria in blood,[24,27–34] including fastidious bacteria and bacteria from antimocribial-containing specimens.[30,31,35–39] The radiometric technique has also been reported to detect mycoplasma and fungi from blood, body fluids, and other clinical specimens such as bone marrow, peritoneal fluid, etc.[29,40–46]

Nonradiometric methods based on total CO_2 production, oxygen consumption, pH, or pressure change are being developed and are now commercially available. These methods are replacing radiometric techniques because they reduce the problem of handling radioactive waste in clinical laboratories.

Culture for Mycobacteria and Other Microorganisms

Mycobacteria are difficult to grow in culture medium and require long incubation periods. Camargo and co-workers were among the first to apply radiometry in mycobacteriology through the metabolism of U-^{14}C-glycerol by *M. lepraemurium*.[11,14] Later, Cummings et al reported that metabolism of U-^{14}C-acetate and U-^{14}C-glycerol by *M. tuberculosis* could be detected as early as 18 hours.[47] Although several attempts were made to detect growth of mycobacteria by using various radiolabeled substrates and monitoring $^{14}CO_2$ production using either the biphasic vial technique or the ion chamber, Middlebrook et al reported the first practical application with a suitable radiometric medium to detect growth of *M. tuberculosis*.[11,48–50] In the initial studies, Middlebrook evaluated two radiolabeled substrates, 1-^{14}C formic acid and 1-^{14}C palmitic acid. Further studies lead to the development of Middlebrook 7H12 medium, which supports growth of almost all mycobacteria and increases the sensitivity in detecting culture-positive clinical specimens, with a significant time saving from 3 to 4 weeks to 10 to 12 days.[22,51–53]

Siddiqi developed Middlebrook 7H13, which is effective for isolating mycobacteria from blood without requiring prior processing of the specimen.[54,55] Radiometric techniques are also employed for isolating leptospira and protozoa[56,57] and for the detection of viral infections in tissue cultures. The infected cells cause a significant reduction of $^{14}CO_2$

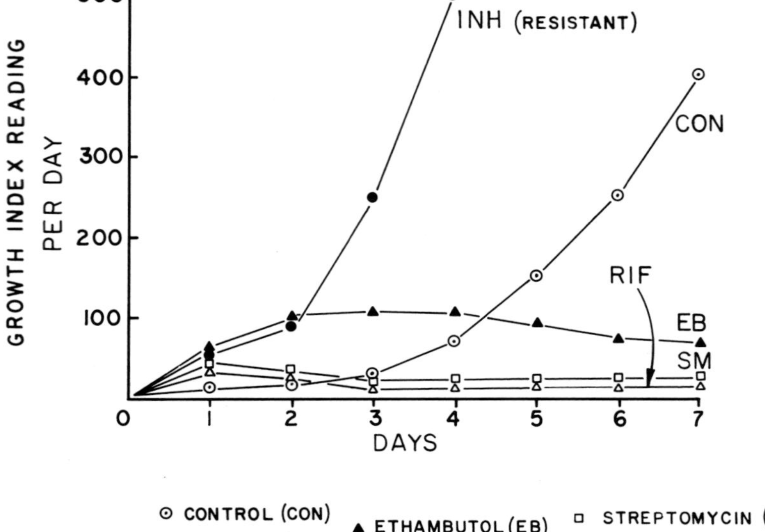

Figure 9. Radiometric drug susceptibility test pattern of an INH-resistant *M. tuberculosis*. Increase or decrease in the daily $^{14}CO_2$ output depends upon the degree of inhibitory effect of antimicrobial added to the medium.

production from 1-^{14}C–glucose compared to control cells cultures.[58]

Antimicrobial Susceptibility Testing

If a bactericidal or bacteriostatic substance is added to growth medium, growth and $^{14}CO_2$ production are inhibited. The extent of the effect on $^{14}CO_2$ production depends upon the degree of inhibition of the test agent added to the medium (Fig. 9). Heim and co-workers reported radiometric susceptibility testing of *E. coli*, *Staphylococcus aureus*, and *Proteus* against various concentrations of several antimicrobials.[59] The first clinical application of radiometric antimicrobial susceptibility testing of bacteria was reported by DeBlanc et al.[60] The antimicrobial concentration that reduced $^{14}CO_2$ production by at least 50% was considered the inhibitory concentration. A good correlation was found between the inhibitory concentrations by radiometric method and conventional susceptibility testing using tube dilution methods. Susceptibility testing of bacteria by radiometric methods, however, has not been used widely except for mycobacteria.[61–66]

Radiometric procedures may also be applied for testing serum bactericidal activity following the drug susceptibility principle. A 4-hour radiometric test to predict the bacteriostatic end-point for Gram-positive and -negative bacteria using a mixture of U-^{14}C-glucose, [guanidine-^{14}C]-arginine, and U-^{14}C-glycine has been successful.[67,68] More than 60% inhibition at 1:8 dilution was used to predict the outcome of the tube dilution test. Similar testing can be applied for fungi[69] and protozoa.[56] Radiometric susceptibility testing of noncultivable bacteria such as *M. leprae* has also been reported.[70,71]

Speciation of Bacteria

Before the introduction of rapid automated techniques for speciation, bacteria were identified by their characteristic patterns of sugar fermentation. Such differentiation tests required days to a week for speciation. Radiometric techniques are now applied to speciate bacteria on the basis of differential metabolism of various ^{14}C-substrates.[72–75]

Type-specific antibodies added to medium can inhibit growth of specific bacteria in much the same way that antimicrobials do. This technique has been used to identify Salmonella and group A streptococci and has been shown to be useful in detection of β-hemolytic streptococci in throat swabs.[76,77] Radiometric serum antimicrobial level determinations have also been reported for gentamicin and other antimicrobials.[78,79]

The most commonly used radiometric identification test is the NAP test developed by Siddiqi and Laszlo.[75,80] The addition of NAP (ρ-nitro-α-acetyl-amino β-hydroxy propiophenone) to 12B medium inhibits growth of the *M. tuberculosis* complex, while there is no significant inhibition of other mycobacteria. Inhibition of $^{14}CO_2$ production can usually be detected in 4 to 5 days. A radiometric inhibition test using hydroxylamine hydrochloride or azaguanine has also been reported for differentiating of the *M. tuberculosis* complex.[52,81] Inhibition by thiophene carboxylic acid hydrazide (TCH) may be used to differentiate between *M. tuberculosis* and *M. bovis*.[81]

Sterility Testing

Chen et al reported radiometric sterility testing of radiopharmaceuticals.[82] The sterility test has also been applied to frozen blood, commercial food products, and rapid detection of contaminated tissue specimens for burn patients.[83,84]

Growth Studies

Radiometry provides information about the growth kinetics of microorganisms in the presence of a test substances. Such information helps in the development of new media and improvement of existing media. It also determines whether a substrate is utilized or not and, in case of more than one substrates, which one is best utilized and by which metabolic pathway.

Enhancement effects of various additives on growth or metabolism of microorganisms can also be studied by radiometric techniques. Siddiqi et al reported that polyoxyethylene stearate significantly enhanced growth of the *M. tuberculosis* complex in 12B medium (Fig. 5).[85]

Water Microbiology

As early as 1956, Levin used radiometric techniques to detect coliform organisms in water and sewage using 1-^{14}C lactose.[6] Amino acid metabolism and bacterial products in aquatic systems have been evaluated by simultaneous incubation of water samples with both ^{3}H-methyl thymidine and ^{14}C-labeled amino acids.[86]

Phagocytosis Monitoring

In recent years, radiometric techniques have been used to monitoror phagocytosis of bacteria by human polymorphonuclear leukocytes. This can be done by measuring the uptake of ^{14}C-substrates by bacteria or by using a radiometric culture media to monitor the viability of bacteria before and after phagocytosis.[87–89]

Vitamin Assays

Vitamin levels in food and body fluids can be estimated by radiometric methods. The procedure is based on the selection of a microorganism that grows only in the presence of the test vitamin. A suitable ^{14}C-labeled substrate is added to the medium, which is readily decarboxylated by the vitamin-dependent strain. Standard curves are generated by adding known concentrations of the test vitamin to the vitamin-free medium. The production of $^{14}CO_2$ is plotted against the vitamin concentrations. An unknown sample is then added to the vitamin-deficient medium and the production of $^{14}CO_2$ is monitored. The concentration of vitamin present in the medium is estimated by comparing with the standard curve.

Chen et al measured vitamin B_{12} levels in human serum using *Lactobacillus leichmannii* in a medium containing [guanido-^{14}C]-arginine.[90] They also measured folate levels in plasma, red blood cells, and food using *L. casei* and 1-^{14}C-gluconate.[91] Niacin levels in food and plasma samples can be measured by using *L. plantarum* and U-^{14}C L-malic acid.[92] Similarly, vitamin B_6 can be measured with *Kloectera brevis* using 1-^{14}C-L-valine or methionine.[93–96]

Tissue Culture and Cancer Research

The use of radiometry in tissue cultures aids in monitoring cell activity during culture. The effect of various substrates on the metabolism of the tissue can also be determined.[97] The most important application of this technique is the screening of anticancer drugs to estimate chemotherapy sensitivity.[98] Tissue cell lines in a culture medium containing a suitable radiolabeled substrate, usually ^{14}C-glucose, are used to predict the responsiveness of an individual patient's tumor to various chemotherapeutic agents.[96,99]

ASSIMILATION STUDIES

Assimilation studies are carried out to investigate bacterial metabolism and the fate of particular substrates. The breakdown products of a radiolabeled substrate as well as the quantity of radioactivity incorporated within the cell are evaluated to better understand metabolic pathways.

Substrate assimilation studies may also be combined with oxidation and $^{14}CO_2$ monitoring. Generally, microorganisms are removed from the medium by filtration through 0.2- to 0.45-μm pore size filter. The filter is washed, dried, and then dissolved in ethyl acetate, scintillation fluid is added, and the radioactivity is counted, indicating the radiolabel assimilated within the cell. Radioactive counts of the filtrate, along with the washings, are also obtained to measure unutilized substrate.

As an extension of assimilation studies, radiochromatographic analysis of the metabolic products can be carried out. The radiochromatogram of the medium that contains live bacteria is compared with the radiochromatogram of the filtrate and the control vial in order to estimate assimilation of the substrate.

Radiolabeling of Bacteria

Sometimes bacteria are directly radiolabeled to investigate the fate of those bacteria during various processes such as adhesion to a surface or to study the efficiency of centrifugation or a cleaning procedure. Often gamma-emitting radionucleotides or radioisotopes are used for labeling. Indium 111 oxine, ^{14}C, and ^{125}I have been used in such studies.[100–102]

REFERENCES

1. Buddemeyer EW. Liquid scintillation vial for cumulative and continuous radiometric measurement of in-vitro metabolism. *Applied Microbiol* 1974;28:177.
2. Ganatra RD, Buddemeyer EU, Deodhar MN, et al. Modifications in biphasic liquid-scintillation vial system for radiometry. *J Nucl Med* 1980;21:480.
3. Buddemeyer E, Hutchinson R, Cooper M. Automatic quantitative radiometric assay of bacterial metabolism. *Clin Chem* 976;22:1459.
4. Boonkitticharoen V, Ehrhardt JC, Kirchner PT. Radiometric assay of bacterial growth: analysis of factors determining system performance and optimization of assay technique. *J Nucl Med* 1987;28:209.

5. Schort JR, Hess WC, Levin GV. Methods for radiorespirometric detection of bacteria in pure culture and in blood. *Appl Microbiol* 1973;26:867.
6. Levin GV, Harrison VR, Hess WC. Preliminary report on a one-hour presumptive test for coliform organisms. *J Am Water Works Assoc* 1956;48:75.
7. Levin GV, Harrison VR, Hess WC, Guerney HC. A radioisotope technique for rapid detection of coliform organisms. *Am J Public Health* 1956;46:1405.
8. Levin GV, Strauss VI, Hess WC. Rapid coliform organisms determination with ^{14}C. *J Water Pollu Contr Fed* 1961; 33:1021.
9. DeLand FH, Wagner HN Jr. Early detection of bacterial growth with carbon-14 labeled glucose. *Radiology* 1969; 92:154.
10. DeLand FH, Wagner HN Jr. Automated radiometric detection of bacterial growth in blood cultures. *J Lab Clin Med* 1970;75:529.
11. Camargo EE, Larson SM, Tepper BS, Wagner HN Jr. Radiometric measurement of metabolic activity of *M. lepraemurium. Appl Microbiol* 1974;28:452.
12. Ratledge C. Lipids: Cell composition, fatty acid biosynthesis. In: Ratledge C, Stanford J, Grang JM, eds. *Biology of the Mycobacteria*. Vol 1. New York: Academic Press, 1982; 186–271.
13. Bopp H, Ellner PD. Evaluation of substrates for radiometric detection of bacteria in blood cultures. *J Clin Microbiol* 1988;26:919.
14. Camargo EE, Kertcher JA, Larson SM, et al. Radiometric measurement of differential metabolism of fatty acids by *Mycobacterium lepraemurium, Int J Lepr* 1979;47:126.
15. Camargo EE, Kertcher JA, Larson SM, et al. Radiometric measurement of differential metabolism of fatty acid by mycobacteria. *Int J Lepr* 1982;50:200.
16. Camargo EE, Wagner HN Jr. Radiometric studies on the oxidation of [1-^{14}C] fatty acids and [U-^{14}C] L-amino acids by mycobacteria. *Int J Rad App Instrum* 1987;14:43.
17. Weinstein MP, Mirrett S, Reimer LG, Reller LB. Effect of agitation and terminal subcultures on yield and speed of detection of the oxoid signal blood culture system versus the BACTEC radiometric system. *J Clin Microbiol* 1989;27:427.
18. Scott RM, Seiz D, Shaughnessy HJ. Rapid carbon-14 test for coliform bacteria in water. *Am J Public Health*, 1964;54:827.
19. Scott RM, Seiz D, Shaughnessy HJ. Rapid carbon-14 test for sewage bacteria. *Am J Public Health* 1964;54:834.
20. Corkill JE. Effect of media, working practice, and automation on the rapid detection of bacteremia. *J Clin Pathol*, 1985; 38:336.
21. Levin GV, Heim AH, Glendenning JR, Thompson MF. "Gulliver"—a quest for life on Mars. *Science* 1962;138:114.
22. Roberts GD, Goodman NL, Heifets L, et al. Evaluation of the BACTEC radiometric method for recovery of mycobacteria and drug susceptibility testing of *Mycobacterium tuberculosis* from acid-fast smear-positive specimens. *J Clin Microbiol* 1983;18:689.
23. Strand CL, Jones MS, Daniel WD. Comparison of a radiometric and a conventional blood culture system: efficiency of recovery, speed of recovery, cost and technical time. *Lab Med* 1981;11:41.
24. Thiemke WA, Wicher K. Laboratory experience with a radiometric method for detecting bacteremia. *J Clin Microb* 1975; 1:302.
25. DeLand FH. Metabolic inhibition as an index of bacterial susceptibility to drugs. *Antimicrob Agents Chemother* 1972; 2:405.
26. Waters JR. Sensitivity of the $^{14}CO_2$ radiometric method for bacterial detection. *Appl Microbiol* 1972;23:198.
27. Bannatyne RM, Harnett N. Radiometric detection of bacteremia in neonates. *Appl Microbiol* 1974;27:1067.
28. Brannon P, Kiehn TE. Clinical comparison of lysis-centrifugation and radiometric resin systems for blood culture. *Clin Microbiol* 1986;24:886.
29. Holley J, Moss A. A prospective evaluation of blood culture versus standard plate techniques for diagnosing peritonitis in continuous ambulatory peritoneal dialysis. *Am J Kidney Dis* 1989;13:184.
30. LaScolea LJ, Dryja D, Sullivan TD, et al. Diagnosis of bacteremia in children by quantitative direct plating and a radiometric procedure. *J Clin Microbiol* 1981;13:478.
31. LaScolea LJ Jr, Sullivan TD, Dryja D, Neter E. Advantages of BACTEC Hypertonic culture medium for detection of *Haemophilus influenzae* bacteremia in children. *J Clin Microbiol* 1983;17:1177.
32. Renner ED, Gatheridge LA, Washington JA. Evaluation of radiometric system for detecting bacteremia. *Appl Microbiol*, 1973;26:368.
33. Rosner R. Comparison of macroscopic, microscopic and radiometric examinations of clinical blood cultures in hypertonic media. *Appl Microbiol* 1974;28:644.
34. Washington JA, Yu PKW. Radiometric method for detection of bacteremia. *Appl Microbiol* 1971;22:100.
35. Beckwith DG, Conyers WC, Etowski DC. Anaerobic radiometric detection of facultative gram-positive cocci in blood. *J Clin Microbiol* 1982;1:212.
36. Crist AE Jr, Amsterdam D, Neter E. Superiority of hypertonic culture medium for detection of *Haemophilus influenzae* by the BACTEC Procedure. *J Clin Microbiol* 1982;15:528.
37. Gross KC, Houghton MP, Roberts RB. Evaluation of blood culture media for isolation of pyridoxal dependent *Streptococcus mitior* (*mitis*). *Am J Clin Pathol* 1981;75:743.
38. Martinez OV, Malinin TI. Effect of osmotic stabilizers on radiometric detection of cell wall-damaged bacteria. *J Clin Microbiol* 1979;10:657.
39. Strand CL. Evaluation of the antimicrobial removal device when used with the BACTEC blood culture system. *Am J Clin Path*, 1982;78:853.
40. Body BA, Pfaller MA, Durrer J, et al. Comparison of the lysis centrifugation and radiometric blood culture systems for recovery of yeast. *Eur J Clin Microbiol Infect Dis* 1988;7:417.
41. Eng RHK, Bishburg E, Smith SM, et al. Bacteremia and fungemia in patients with acquired immune deficiency syndrome. *Am J Clin Path*, 1986;86:105.
42. Hopfer RL, Orengo A, Chestnut S, Wenglar M. Radiometric detection of yeasts in blood cultures of cancer patients. *J Clin Microbiol* 1980;12:329.
43. Prevost E, Bannister E. Detection of yeast septicemia by biphasic and radiometric methods. *J Clin Microbiol* 1981; 13:655.
44. Smaron MF, Boonlayangoor S, Zierdt CH. Detection of *Mycoplasma hominis* septicemia by radiometric blood culture. *J Clin Microbiol* 1985;21:298.
45. Bishburg E, Eng RHK, Smith SM, Kapila R. Yield of bone marrow culture in the diagnosis of infectious diseases in patients with acquired immunodeficiency syndrome. *J Clin Microbiol* 1986;24:312.
46. Doyle PW, Crichton EP, Mathias RG, Werb R. Clinical and microbiological evaluation of four culture methods for the diagnosis of peritonitis in patients on continuous ambulatory peritoneal dialysis. *J Clin Microbiol* 1989;27:1206.
47. Cummings DM, Ristroph D, Camargo EE, et al. Radiometric detection of the metabolic activity of *Mycobacterium tuberculosis. J Nucl Med* 1975;16:1189.
48. Camargo EE, Larson SM, Tepper BS, Wagner HN Jr. A

radiometric method for predicting effectiveness of chemotherapeutic agents in murine leprosy. *Int J Lepr* 1975;43:234.
49. Kertcher JA, Chen MF, Charache P, et al. Rapid radiometric susceptibility testing of *Mycobacterium tuberculosis. Am Rev Resp Dis* 1978;117:631.
50. Middlebrook G, Reggiardo Z, Tigertt WD. Automatable radiometric detection of growth of *Mycobacterium tuberculosis* in selective media. *Am Rev Respir Dis* 1977;115:1066.
51. Kirihara M, Hillier SL, Coyle MB. Improved detection times for *Mycobacterium avium* complex and *Mycobacterium tuberculosis* with the BACTEC Radiometric system. *J Clin Microbiol* 1985;22:841.
52. Park CH, Hixon DL, Ferguson CB, et al. Rapid recovery of mycobacteria from clinical specimens using automated radiometric technic. *Am J Clin Pathol* 1984;81:341.
53. Stager CE, Libonati JP, Siddiqi SH, et al. Role of solid media when used in conjunction with the BACTEC system for mycobacterial isolation and identification. *J Clin Microbiol* 1991;29:154.
54. Siddiqi SH, Hwangbo CC. A new medium (Middlebrook 7H13) for recovery of mycobacteria from blood specimens. *Abs Ann Mtg Am Soc for Microbiol* (ABS U78-ASM), 1988.
55. Strand CL, Epstein G, Verzosa S, et al. Evaluation of a new blood culture medium for mycobacteria. *Am J Clin Pathol* 1989;91:316.
56. Inge PM, Farthing MJ. A radiometric assay for antigiardial drugs. *Trans R Soc Trop Med Hyg* 1987;81:345.
57. Manca N, Veradi R, Colombrita D, et al. Radiometric method for the rapid detection of leptospira organisms. *J Clin Microbiol* 1986;23:401.
58. D'Antonio N, Tsan MF, Charache P, et al. Simple radiometric techniques for rapid detection of herpes simplex virus type 1 in Wi-38 cell culture. *J Nucl Med* 1976;17:503.
59. Heim AH, Curtin JA, Levin GV. Determination of antimicrobial activity by a radioisotope method. *Proc Antimicrob Agents Ann Conf* 1960;123.
60. DeBlanc HJ, Charache P, Wagner HN Jr. Automated radiometric measurement of antibiotic effect on bacterial growth. *Antimicrob Agents Chemother* 1972;2:360.
61. Snider DE, Good RC, Kilburn JO, et al. Rapid drug susceptibility testing for *Mycobacterium tuberculosis. Am Rev Respir Dis* 1981;123:402.
62. Siddiqi SH, Libonati JP, Middlebrook G. Evaluation of a rapid radiometric method for drug susceptibility testing of *Mycobacterium tuberculosis. J Clin Microbiol* 1981;13:908.
63. Siddiqi SH, Hawkins JE, Laszlo A. Interlaboratory drug susceptibility testing of *Mycobacterium tuberculosis* by a radiometric procedure and two conventional methods. *J Clin Microbiol*, 1985;22:919.
64. Hoffner SE, Kallenius G, Beezer AE, Svenson SB. Studies on the mechanisms of the synergistic effects of ethambutol and other antibacterial drugs on *Mycobacterium avium* complex. *Acta Leprol* 1989;7:195.
65. Lee C, Heifets LB. Determination of minimal inhibitory concentrations of antituberculosis drugs by radiometric and conventional methods. *Am Rev Respir Dis* 1987;136:349.
66. Lindholm-Levy P, Heifets L. Clofazimine and other riminocompounds: minimal inhibitory and minimal bactericidal concentrations at different pHs for *Mycobacterium avium* complex. *Tubercle* 1988;69:179.
67. Beckwith DG, Guidon PT Jr. Development of a five-hour radiometric serum antibacterial assay for gram-positive cocci. *J Nucl Med* 1981;22:274.
68. Kansu E, Akalin E, Civelek C, et al. Serum bactericidal and opsonic activities in chronic lymphocytic leukemia and multiple myeloma. *Am J Hematol* 1968;23:191.
69. Merz WG, Fay D, Thumar B, Dixon D. Susceptibility testing of filamentous fungi to amphotericin B by a rapid radiometric method. *J Clin Microbiol* 1985;19:54.
70. Franzblau SG. Oxidation of palmitic acid by *Mycobacterium leprae* in an axenic medium. *J Clin Microbiol* 1988;25:18.
71. Franzblau SG. Drug susceptibility testing of *Mycobacterium leprae* in the BACTEC 460 system. *Antimicrob Agents Chemother* 1989;33:2115.
72. Strauss RR, Holderback J, Friedman H. Comparison of a radiometric procedure with conventional methods for identification of *Neisseria. J Clin Microbiol* 1978;7:419.
73. Damato J, Collins MT, McClatchy JK. Urease testing of mycobacteria with BACTEC radiometric instrumentation. *J Clin Microbiol* 1982;15:478.
74. Damato J, Collins MT. Radiometric studies with gas-liquid and thin-layer chromatography for rapid demonstration of hemin dependence and characterization of *M. haemophilum. J Clin Microbiol* 1984;20:515.
75. Siddiqi SH, Hwangbo C, Silcox V, et al. Rapid radiometric methods to detect and differentiate *Mycobacterium tuberculosis/M. bovis* from other mycobacterial species. *Am Rev Respir Dis* 1984;130:634.
76. Larson SM, Charache P, Chen MF, Wagner HN Jr. Inhibition of the metabolism of Streptococcus and Salmonella by type specific antisera. *Appl Microbiol* 1974;27:351.
77. Larson SM, Chen MF, Charache P, Wagner HN Jr. A radiometric identification of streptococcus Group A in throat cultures. *J Nucl Med* 1975;16:1085.
78. Manos JP, Jacobs PF. Evaluation of the BACTEC serum gentamicin assay. *Antimicrob Agents Chemother* 1979; 16:631.
79. Hopfer RL, Groschel D. Radiometric determination of the concentration of amphotericin B in body fluids. *Antimicrob Agents Chemother* 1977;12:733.
80. Laszlo A, Siddiqi SH. Evaluation of a rapid radiometric differentiation test for the *Mycobacterium tuberculosis* complex by selective inhibition with ρ-nitro-α-acetylamino-β-hydroxypropiophenone. *J Clin Microbiol* 1984;19:694.
81. Gross WM, Hawkins JE. Radiometric selective inhibition tests for differentiation of *Mycobacterium tuberculosis, M. bovis*, and other mycobacteria. *J Clin Microbiol* 1985;21:565.
82. Chen MF, Rhodes BA, Larson SM, Wagner HN Jr. Sterility testing of radiopharmaceuticals. *J Nucl Med* 1974;15:1142.
83. Szymanski SO, Carrington EJ. Evaluation of a large scale frozen blood program. *Transfusion* 1977;17:431.
84. Martinez OV, Malinin TI, Ward CG. The use of a radiometric technic for the rapid detection of contaminated tissue specimens from burned patients. *Am J Clin Pathol* 1980;74:319.
85. Siddiqi SH, Libonati JP, Carter ME, et al. Enhancement of mycobacterial growth in Middlebrook 7H12 medium by polyoxyethylene stearate. *Curr Microbiol* 1988;17:105.
86. Jonas BJ, Tuttle JH, Stoner DL, Ducklow HW. Dual-label radioisotope method for simultaneously measuring bacterial production and metabolism in natural waters. *Appl Environ Microbiol* 1988;54:791.
87. Jones GS, Herold J, Amirault J, Andersen BR. Killing of *Mycobacterium tuberculosis* by neutrophils: a non-oxidative process. *J Infect Dis* 1990;162:700.
88. McGregor SJ, Brook JH, Briggs JD, Junor BJ. Bactericidal activity of peritoneal macrophages from continuous ambulatory dialysis patients. *Nephrol Dial Transplant* 1987;2:104.
89. Meylan PR, Richman DD, Kornbluth RS. Characterization and growth in human macrophages of *Mycobacterium avium* complex strains isolated from the blood of patients with acquired immunodeficiency syndrome. *Infect Immun* 1990; 58:564.
90. Chen MF, McIntyre PA, Wagner HN Jr. A radiometric micro-

biologic method for vitamin B_{12} assay. *J Nucl Med* 1977;18:388.

91. Chen MF, McIntyre PA, Kertcher JA. Measurement of folates in human plasma and erythrocytes by a radiometric microbiologic method. *J Nucl Med* 1978;19:906.
92. Kertcher JA, Guilarte TR, Chen MF, et al. A radiometric microbiologic assay for the biologically active forms of niacin. *J Nucl Med* 1979;20:419.
93. Guilarte TR, Shane B, McIntyre PA. Radiometric microbiologic assay of vitamin B^6: Application to food analysis. *J Nutr* 1981;111:1869.
94. Guilarte TR. A radiometric microbiological assay for pantothenic acid in biological fluids. *Ann Biochem* 1989;178:63.
95. Guilarte TR. Radiometric microbiological assay of B vitamins. *J Nutr Biochem* 1991;2:334.
96. Osterdahl BG, Johansson E. Comparison of radiometric and microbiological assays for the determination of folate in fortified gruel and porridge. *Int J Vitam Nutr Res* 1989;59:147.
97. Fajer AB. Changes in glucose metabolism in premeiotic and meiotic ovaries of the hamster. *J Repro Fertil* 1983;69:101.
98. Arteaga CL, Forseth BJ, Clark GM, et al. A radiometric method for evaluation of chemotherapy sensitivity: Results of screening a panel of human breast cancer cell lines. *Cancer Res* 1987;47:6248.
99. Von Hoff DD, Foreseth BJ, Turner JN, et al. Selection of chemotherapy for patient treatment utilizing a radiometric versus a cloning system. *Intl J Cell Cloning* 1986;4:16.
100. Bettin K, Allen MO, Gerding DN, et al. In-111 *Pseudomonas aeruginosa*: a simple method of labeling live bacteria with gamma-emitting radioisotope. *Eur J Nucl Med* 1986;12:277.
101. Brassart D, Woltz A, Golliard M, Neeser JR. In-vitro inhibition of adhesion of *Candida albicans*: clinical isolates to human buccal epithelial cells by FUC alpha 1-2 gal beta-bearing complex carbohydrates. *Infect Immun* 1991;59:1605.
102. Seon WK. Comparison of ultrasonic and mechanical cleaning of primary root canals using a novel radiometric method. *Pediatric Dent* 1991;13:136.
103. Camargo E. Radiomicrobiology. In: Harbert JC, Da Rocha AFG eds. *Textbook of Nuclear Medicine—Basic Sciences.* Philadelphia: Lea & Febiger, 1984, chap 15.

16 Radiation Safety Practices in the Nuclear Medicine Laboratory

William J. Walker, Lynn Evans Jenkins

Radiation is an essential part of nuclear medicine and, therefore, radiation safety must be an integral part of all nuclear medicine programs. The basics of radiation safety programs have changed little since the inception of nuclear medicine in the 1950s and the same basic principles still apply. However, in modern nuclear medicine radiation safety programs there are additional facets that must be considered, many of which result from regulatory requirements.

Radiation safety in the nuclear medicine laboratory is best addressed in a formal, written program that clearly states procedures, policies, and responsibilities. A well-written program is a valuable tool for management held responsible by regulatory agencies for safe operation and regulatory compliance. In private practice nuclear medicine clinics, management is the physician or physicians themselves and an authorized user named in the US Nuclear Regulatory Commission (NRC) or state license acts as a radiation safety officer (RSO). At hospitals and medical research facilities engaged in nuclear medicine, management is represented by an appointed radiation safety committee (RSC) in addition to an RSO. The RSO assists in the performance of the Committee's duties and serves as its secretary. The Committee is composed of a chairperson and one authorized user from each type of activity authorized by the license, the RSO, a representative of the nursing service, and a representative of management who is neither an authorized user nor an RSO.

The RSC oversees the radiation safety program for the facility management, ensuring that licensed materials are used safely by reviewing training programs, equipment, facilities, supplies, and procedures. The Committee ensures that licensed materials are used in compliance with NRC regulations and the facility's license and that the use of the licensed materials is consistent with the philosophy of maintaining personnel radiation exposures as low as reasonably achievable (ALARA). A well-run committee performs frequent reviews of the program to identify problems and implement their solutions. Most RSCs are required to meet at least quarterly and be attended by a quorum consisting of at least half of the membership including the RSO and the management representative. In private practice, the functions of the RSC are performed by the RSO.

Traditionally, regulatory agencies required radiation safety programs to be designed primarily to protect the occupationally exposed workers in nuclear medicine departments, the physicians and technologists, and of the general public. The protection of patients was considered a part of the practice of medicine and as such was at the sole discretion of the physician. Protection of patients has received much greater attention in the past few years and now holds a prominent place in formal radiation safety programs.

Some controversy exists within the scientific community over what constitutes a safe level of exposure to radiation and there is no level that is generally accepted by authorities as being "absolutely safe." For this reason the occupational dose limit should be considered a regulatory upper limit rather than an operational guide post. Good practice should result in doses to workers being maintained at the lowest possible levels consistent with doing the job. This philosophy is reflected in the ALARA principle. The principle is now a part of the NRC regulation under 10 CFR Part 20, paragraph 20.1101(b).[2] The term ALARA means as low as is reasonably achievable taking into account the state of technology, and the economics of improvements in relation to benefits to the public health and safety, and other societal and socioeconomic considerations, and in relation to the utilization of atomic energy in the public interest.

REGULATORY BASIS FOR RADIATION SAFETY IN NUCLEAR MEDICINE

All nuclear medicine clinics and departments or operations within the United States must be licensed by either the NRC or by an agreement state. Agreement states are states that have entered into an agreement under the Atomic Energy Act with the NRC to provide a regulatory program comparable to that administered by the NRC. Agreement state programs are similar or identical to those required by the NRC. The NRC does not regulate naturally occurring radioactive materials nor does it regulate radiation-producing machines. These, however, are all regulated by individual states.

RADIATION UNITS

Exposure, Absorbed Dose, and Dose Equivalent

The development of well-defined units of radioactivity and of energy deposition by ionizing radiation in matter was essential for the establishment of clear standards for the use of radionuclides. A number of national and international organizations are actively continuing this process. One of these organizations, the International Commission on Radiation Units and Measurements (ICRU), originally defined four special radiation units: the roentgen (R) to be used only as a measure of exposure, the rad (D) to be used as a measure of radiation absorbed dose, the rem (H) to be used as a measure of dose equivalent, and the curie (Ci) to be used as a measure of activity. These units have now been replaced with radiation units in the International System of Units (SI), which are given in Appendix A. New SI units include the gray (Gy = 1 J kg^{-1} = 100 rad), the sievert (Sv = 1 J kg^{-1} = 100 rem), and the becquerel (Bq = 1 d sec^{-1} = 2.703×10^{-11} Ci). However, a quantity termed the air kerma may be used to specify the exposure. The unit of the kerma is the gray (Gy).

The roentgen was first defined in 1928 as a measure of the energy deposition of x-rays in air. The restriction to x-rays has since been dropped, and the definition of R was expanded to include all photons with energy below 3 MeV. *Exposure* is defined as the total electrical charge of all ions of one sign produced in a unit mass of air. The roentgen is defined as 2.58×10^{-4} coulombs/kg in dry air at standard temperature and pressure. This amount is equivalent to 87 ergs/g of air at standard temperature and pressure. An air kerma of about 8.7 mGy is equivalent to an exposure of 1 R.

The rad was designed to fill the need for a unit of energy deposition that was not restricted to air and would be applicable to radiations other than photons. It is a measure of *radiation absorbed dose,* which is defined as the energy imparted to a unit mass of matter. The rad is specifically defined as the deposition of 100 ergs/g to the volume of interest. This is equal to 62.4×10^6 MeV/gram and 0.01 Gy. As a general rule of thumb, 1 rad is approximately equal to the dose to soft tissue resulting from exposure to 1 R of intermediate-energy x-rays or gamma rays.

The rem was developed in response to a considerable body of evidence that indicated that the biologic effects of exposure to different types or distribution patterns of radiation were often different for the same radiation absorbed dose. The *dose equivalent* is defined as the absorbed dose times two other factors: the *quality factor, Q,* a defined unit related to linear energy transfer used to express differences in biologic effectiveness of various ionizing radiations, and the *distribution factor, N,* which is used to correct for differences in the distribution of internally deposited radionclides on the observed biologic effects. The distribution factor and all other factors used in weighing the absorbed dose are

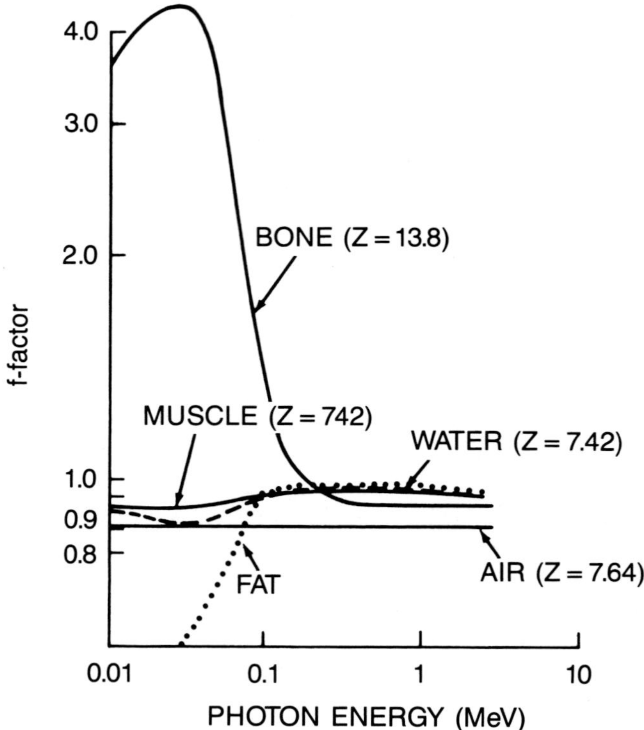

Figure 1. The f-factor for conversion between roentgens and rads in air, water, and different constituents of the body, plotted as a function of photon energy.

currently assigned the value of 1. Thus the dose equivalent, *H,* is the product of *D* and *Q,* or

$$H = DQ$$

The unit of dose equivalent is assigned the special name *sievert* (Sv) where 1 Sv = 100 rem (see Appendix A).

From a practical sense estimating the dose equivalent is simplified because most radiation sources used in most nuclear medicine applications are photon emitters with energies between 100 keV and 3 MeV. To make an adequate estimate of dose from exposure measurements, one must have a clear understanding of the relationship of these terms and the relative response of the instrumentation used to measure the exposure within those photon energies. By definition an exposure of 1 R yields an absorbed dose of 0.869 rad in air. Tissue dose is related to the dose in air by the ratio of energy absorption in the tissue to the energy absorption in air. Thus the ratio of the mass energy absorption coefficient of tissue to that of air multiplied by 0.869 is known as the *f*-factor, *f.*

$$f = 0.869 \frac{[(\mu_{en})_m]_{med}}{[(\mu_{en})_m]_{air}} \quad (1)$$

where $[(\mu_{en})_m]_{med}$ is the mass energy absorption coefficient of the medium for photons of the energy of interest and $[(\mu_{en})_m]_{air}$ describes the energy absorption in air. This relationship is illustrated in Figure 1.[4]

The quality factor for photons with energies between 100

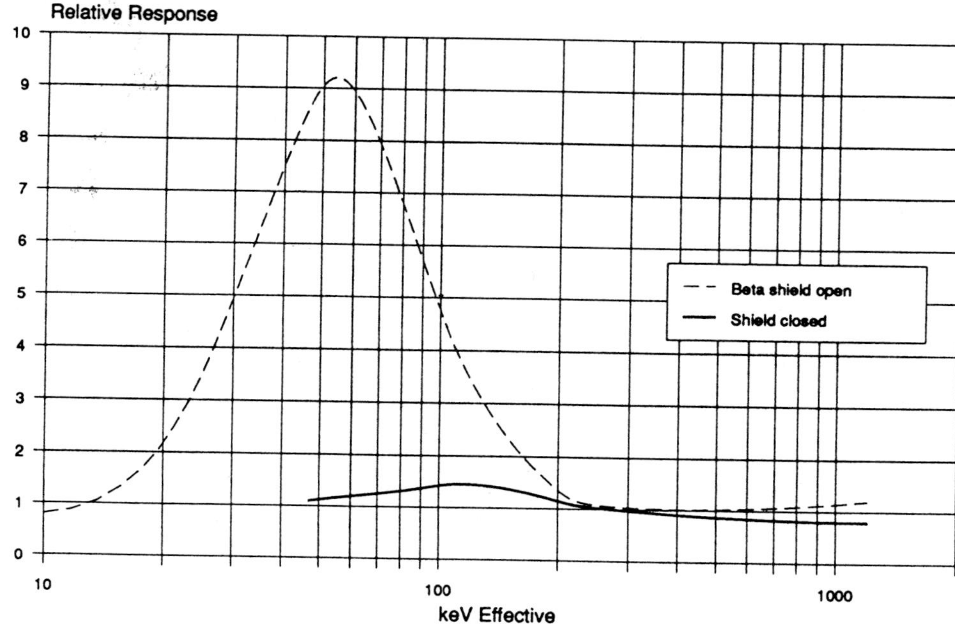

Figure 2. Typical response of an energy compensated G–M probe.

keV and 3 MeV is unity; therefore, the exposure (R), the absorbed dose (rad), and the dose equivalent (rem) are approximately equal for soft tissue.

Unfortunately the response of most survey meters used to measure exposure is not uniform relative to air at the lower end of the energy range of interest. Realizing this difficulty, instrument manufacturers produce survey instruments that are "energy compensated" to correct for over response at low energies. A typical response curve for such a Geiger-Müller (G–M) detector probe is shown in Figure 2. Knowing the detector's response and the energy of the radiation source, exposure may be used to estimate the dose equivalent. The reader is cautioned to verify these assumptions for the sources and conditions of their own measurements.

Most radiation survey meters used in nuclear medicine applications are calibrated with ^{137}Cs (E = 0.663 MeV). It can thus be assumed, as a reasonable approximation, that the values of exposure, absorbed dose, and dose equivalent are equal in the energy range of the calibration. This assumption can also be extended to the gamma emissions from most radionuclides currently used in nuclear medicine if the energy and the response of the detector to that energy are known.

Maximum Permissible Dose and Maximum Permissible Concentration

The standards adopted by the NRC, with its lead role in nuclear medicine safety and regulation, have been based on the recommendations of several national and international advisory bodies. The major advisory bodies are the National Council on Radiation Protection and Measurements (NCRP), the International Commission on Radiological Protection (ICRP), and the International Commission on Radiation Units and Measurements (ICRU). The current NCRP recommendations are displayed in Table 1. The current NRC occupational dose limits, adopted on January 1, 1994, are displayed in Table 2.

CONTROL OF EXTERNAL RADIATION EXPOSURE

In any work environment the control of external radiation exposure depends on all workers being aware of applicable regulations and means of controlling radiation exposure, that adequate procedures and equipment be available for measurement and control of personnel radiation exposures, and that work areas be designed to avoid unnecessary exposures. The degree of control required in any specific situation depends on the probability of exposure and the balancing of benefits and risks by the RSO. Control of exposure to sources of ionizing radiation includes the establishment of areas of restricted occupancy, limitations on the time an employee may spend in the radiation area, and shielding to minimize exposure to the source. Work areas must be designed with exposure factors in mind and may include areas designed to prevent either unauthorized access or limiting access when radiation sources are in use in the area.

Three methods of reducing the hazard from radiation sources are time, distance, and shielding. The simplest and cheapest method is to increase distance. The intensity of gamma- or x-ray exposure decreases roughly as the inverse of the distance squared. Although this inverse square law

Table 1. Summary of NCRP Recommendations[a]

A. Occupational exposures (annual)[b]		
1. Effective dose equivalent limit (stochastic effects)	50 mSv	(5 rem)
2. Dose equivalent limits for tissues and organs (nonstochastic effects)		
a. Lens of eye	150 mSv	(15 rem)
b. All others (eg, red bone marrow, breast, lung, gonads, skin, and extremities)	500 mSv	(50 rem)
B. Public exposures (annual)		
1. Effective dose equivalent limit, continuous or frequent exposure[b]	1 mSv	(0.1 rem)
2. Effective dose equivalent limit, infrequent exposure[b]	5 mSv	(0.5 rem)
3. Remedial action recommended when:		
a. Effective dose equivalent[c]	>5 mSv	(>0.5 rem)
b. Exposure to radon and its decay products	>0.007 Jhm^{-3}	(>2 WLM)
4. Dose equivalent limits for lens of eye, skin, and extremities[b]	50 mSv	(5 rem)
C. Embryo-fetus exposures[b]		
1. Total dose equivalent limit	5 mSv	(0.5 rem)
2. Dose equivalent limit in a month	0.5 mSv	(0.05 rem)

[a]Excluding medical exposures.

[b]Sum of external and internal exposures.

[c]Including background internal exposures.

holds rigorously only for the case of a point source and a point target, it is, in practice, a good approximation whenever the distance is much larger than the dimensions of the radiation source. Thus, moving from a position 1 m from a source to one 10 m away reduces the exposure by a factor of 100. Whenever possible, areas that contain radiation sources should be controlled. The degree of control required depends on the hazard and can range from conspicuously posted radiation area signs to complicated interlock systems that bar unauthorized access. In a typical nuclear medicine laboratory, control can be achieved by limiting access to dosing and storage areas and arranging patient waiting areas so that they are remote from sources of external radiation. On the other hand, protection from a multicurie therapy source requires extremely stringent restrictions to access. In handling radionuclides in the laboratory, the distance principle can be applied by requiring the use of forceps whenever possible.

Table 2. NRC Occupational Dose Limits

§ 20.1201 Occupational dose limits for adults.
§ 20.1201(a)
The licensee shall control the occupational dose to individual adults, except for planned special exposures under § 20.1206, to the following dose limits.
§ 20.1201(a)(1)
An annual limit, which is the more limiting of—
(i) The total effective dose equivalent and the committed dose equivalent to any individual organ or tissue other than the lens of the eye being equal to 50 rems (0.5 Sv).
§ 20.1201(a)(2)
The annual limits to the lens of the eye, to the skin, and to the extremities which are
(i) An eye dose equivalent of 15 rems (0.15 Sv), and
(ii) A shallow-dose equivalent of 50 rems (0.5 Sv) to the skin or to each of the extremities

Reducing the time of exposure is another effective way to decrease radiation exposures. In general, reduced exposure time can be accomplished by careful planning of all activities involving radiation sources. Whenever possible, planning should include not only detailed instructions for the operation, but also dry runs using nonradioactive materials until all aspects of the planned operation are familiar.

The use of shielding to reduce exposure has become a common practice. In general, shielding material has a high density and a large atomic number. Enclosing the source in a small container is the most efficient use of shielding. Examples of this approach include small lead containers for transport and storage of radionuclides and radiopharmaceuticals, "L" block shields for dose preparation, and syringe shields and vial shields to reduce exposure to patients and personnel during injection.[7] Other approaches include lead and leaded glass barriers to reduce exposure during radiopharmaceutical processing and the use of low-Z materials to shield high-energy beta-particle emitters. High-energy beta particles can be hazardous because of the production of bremsstrahlung radiation from interaction with high-Z materials. Shielding in these cases (eg, ^{32}P, ^{90}Sr) is best accomplished by absorbers with a low atomic number, such as lucite, to absorb beta particles with little bremsstrahlung production.

CONTROL OF INTERNAL RADIATION EXPOSURE

Radionuclides may be incidentally taken into the body by inhalation of aerosols or gases, by ingestion, through wounds or breaks in the skin, and, in some cases, directly through the skin. Internal contamination with radionuclides results in radiation exposures that may continue for long times after the contaminating event. The radionuclide may concentrate preferentially in specific organs or tissues, thus complicating evaluation of the hazard.

Once a radionuclide is deposited within the body, it may be difficult or impossible to remove. The radiation dose from internally deposited radionuclides contributes to the lifetime dose and so must be taken into consideration when determining whether an individual has exceeded the recommended dose limits. The total dose commitment is calculated from a summation of that dose resulting from internal as well as external exposure in the revision to 10 CFR Part 20 which became effective January 1, 1994. The methodology follows the recommendations of the ICRP for determining maximum permissible levels for internally deposited radionuclides. The development of these standards is explained in ICRP Publication Nos. 2 and 6 and current recommendations can be found in ICRP Publication No. 30.[8–10]

The ICRP Publication No. 2 calculates the amount of a radioactive isotope that can be present in the body throughout a working lifetime without exceeding the MPD to specific organs or tissues.[8] This amount is the maximum permissible body burden (MPBB). A related concept is the maximum permissible concentration (MPC) of radionuclide. These MPC values are the concentrations of a radionuclide in air or water that would result in acquisition of an MPBB over the course of a working lifetime.

The revised recommendations of ICRP Publication No. 30 are based on new information and changes in the Commission's methods for determining risk.[10] The concepts of MPC and MPBB have been replaced by that of annual limit on intake (ALI), a value equivalent to 0.05 Sv (5 rem) per year from all tissues irradiated. Complete details of methodology are available in ICRP Publication No. 26, and with limits for 187 radionuclides of 21 elements in part 1 of ICRP Publication No. 30.[10,11] Limits for the remaining radionuclides can be found in parts 2 and 3 of ICRP Publication No. 30. These limits have been adopted by many state and national regulatory agencies to form the basis for control of international and environmental radionuclide contamination.

Prevention of Internal Exposure

Because of the difficulty of reducing radiation exposure from internally deposited radionuclides, most effort should be concentrated on preventing their entry into the body. The development and enforcement of rules for safe handling of radionuclides can, in most cases, nearly eliminate the potential for hazard from either internal deposition or external contamination. Some common-sense rules for working safely with unsealed radionuclide sources include the following:

1. Always work in areas designed for handling radionuclides.
2. Never open sealed bottles or vials in open areas, especially if they contain such a volatile material as radioiodine. Use a well-designed hood or glove box.
3. Work areas should be covered with a plastic, glass, or stainless steel tray, preferably with absorbent paper covering the tray, to catch any spills and to prevent the spread of contamination.
4. Plan all procedures in advance to increase awareness of problem areas. A test run using nonradioactive materials prevents delays and pinpoints problems.
5. Do not eat or drink in areas where unsealed radionuclides are being used or stored.
6. Do not smoke in areas where radionuclides are being used or stored.
7. Clearly label all containers of radionuclides with isotope, date, and activity.
8. Work in a well-ventilated area, and use a hood or glove box designed for radiation control for all procedures that might release activity into the air.
9. Do not pipette by mouth.
10. Be aware of hazards and use good judgment.
11. Wear protective clothing and surgical gloves while working, and dispose of gloves before leaving the area.
12. Do not wear protective clothing outside the work area.
13. Keep all radionuclides in sealed containers when they are not in use.
14. Maintain high standards of cleanliness in the laboratory. Promptly clean up spills and dispose of wastes properly.
15. Survey the work area regularly for both contamination and exposure hazards. Conduct special surveys after operations that might result in contamination. Survey hands, clothing, shoes, etc.
16. Wash hands thoroughly before eating, drinking, or smoking.

Additional precautions to be considered by the individual responsible for radiation safety include air sampling where airborne contamination is possible, especially during radionuclide procedures; a routine program of personnel monitoring, including bioassay and whole body counting as appropriate; and routine education programs for all employees before they are allowed to use radionuclides. It is especially important for employee training programs to include detailed information about radionuclide handling techniques, radiation safety support, and specific steps to be taken in the event of spills or other emergencies.

MEASUREMENT OF RADIATION

Survey Instruments

Instruments designed to locate and measure radiation and radioactive material are discussed in Chapter 2. The type of monitoring required and the proper combination of detection instruments to use must be determined in order to perform surveys that map the distribution of radiation levels and contamination within the nuclear medicine facility. These surveys are essential in maintaining the safety of personnel, patients and the general public.

Basically, two types of surveys must be performed. *Exposure* or *radiation* surveys are performed to locate and quantify the radiation present in an area. The second type of survey is for *contamination* that results from loss of containment of radioactive material.

Various instruments are available for performing exposure surveys. Each of these instruments has its own distinctive advantages and disadvantages, so selecting the correct instrument for a particular application is important. An ideal instrument for radiation monitoring is small, light, rugged, stable over a wide range of environmental conditions, capable of measuring all types of radiation that might be encountered, capable of operating for long periods without depleting its batteries, and insensitive to intensity, pulse rate, and beam shape of the incident radiation. At present, no single instrument meets all of these requirements.

An ion chamber is the preferred instrument for exposure surveys because it can measure exposure directly. This is possible because the voltage at which an ion chamber operates is such that all primary ion pairs produced by the radiation in the sensitive volume are collected; however, there is no gas amplification because the voltage is not high enough to produce secondary ions. The current thus created is a direct measurement of exposure. Ion chambers are used in a wide variety of applications. When care is given to the size, shape, and composition of the chamber, the instrument can be calibrated for accurate measurements of absorbed dose; however, most are calibrated in roentgens per hour (R/h).

Measurement of exposure with an ion chamber is complicated by several factors. First, ion chambers under-respond to very high or very low energy radiation. Exposure due to low energy x-rays or gammas cannot be easily measured by an ion chamber. If the energy of the radiation is too low it will not penetrate the entrance window of the ion chamber. Conversely, the energy of the radiation cannot be so high that it will pass through the chamber without interacting. The most commonly used ion chambers are composed of plastic or aluminum walls that are approximately tissue equivalent. The sensitivity of these chambers drops for gamma energies less than 50 to 100 keV and greater than 3 MeV.[12] This is generally not a problem in nuclear medicine departments because most radionuclides used have energies within this range. However, attention must be paid to the response of an ion chamber when measuring the exposure from radionuclides such as ^{125}I with low-energy gammas or from beta emitters such as ^{90}Y. Most ion chambers have windows or caps that can be opened or removed to more accurately measure exposure from these sources.

A G–M detector can also be used to measure exposure. It may be necessary to apply correction factors to the GM exposure readings if the gamma energies of the radionuclides involved are significantly different from those of the calibration source. This may make use of a G–M calibrated for exposure impractical in nuclear medicine departments where a wide variety of radionuclides are used.

For contamination surveys it is necessary to amplify the small amount of ionization produced by potentially low levels of contamination into pulses that can be measured. Since ion chambers respond in a direct manner to radiation, they are not sensitive enough to be used for contamination surveys. Contamination surveys are conducted with either a G–M detector or a sodium iodide (NaI) scintillation detector which has been calibrated for contamination. A G–M detector is useful for locating contamination due to most gamma and/or beta emitters used in nuclear medicine such as ^{131}I and ^{99m}Tc. A G–M detector operates at a voltage that causes secondary ionization in the gas, which makes it sensitive to low levels of radiation. For low-energy gamma emitters such as ^{125}I, a thin NaI scintillation crystal is preferable because the crystal has higher density and mass than a gas and is more effective in stopping gammas. Since NaI crystals are sensitive and efficient detectors, problems may arise when they are used in high-background environments.

Surveys must be conducted to determine if removable contamination is present. This is done by wiping a piece of filter paper or a cotton swab across areas where contamination could potentially be found then measuring the amount of contamination removed. Special equipment, such as a gamma counter or a liquid scintillation counter, should be used to make this measurement. A properly calibrated thin end window G–M detector would also meet this requirement. The counter used depends on the types of radionuclides used and the detection sensitivities required in 10 CFR Part 35.[2] Contamination is first measured in units of counts per minute (cpm) per 100 square centimeters. These measurements must be converted to units of disintegrations per minute (dpm) per 100 square centimeters for recording purposes. The efficiency of the counting system, determined when the counter is calibrated, is used to make that conversion. For example, a calibrated source (standard) for a particular radionuclide with a known activity of 3.7×10^4 Bq (1 μCi or 2.22×10^6 dpm) is counted in a gamma counter. A count rate of 1.11×10^6 cpm is measured. The efficiency of that counter for that radionuclide is determined by dividing the measured cpm by the known dpm (corrected for decay). The efficiency of the counter in this example is 50%. The activity in dpm of samples containing this radionuclide can now be determined by dividing the measured cpm by 0.5.

Detectors must be properly calibrated to ensure meaningful results. Because of energy dependence and variations in response to different types of radiation, calibrations should always be done with standardized sources, under conditions that reflect those encountered in actual use. Separate calibrations may be necessary for each type of radiation that might be encountered. Routine calibration of instruments ensures that they are accurate and reliable over all instrument ranges.

Calibration can be performed by in-house staff or by vendors who are contracted to provide this service. Technical guidance and techniques for calibration of radiation survey

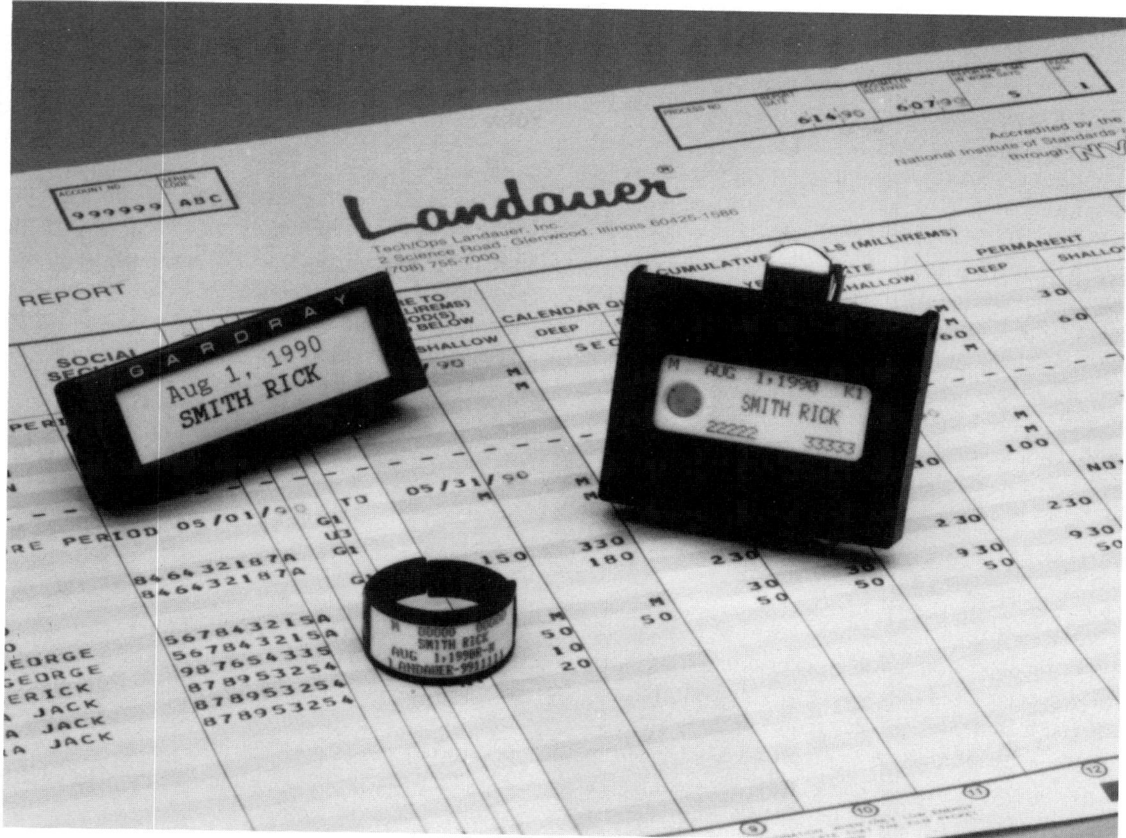

Figure 3. L to R: Whole body film monitor, TLD ring monitor, TLD whole body monitor.

instruments can be found in NCRP Report No. 112.[13] However, it is important to remember that detectors used to satisfy the survey requirements of 10 CFR Part 35 must be calibrated according to the regulations found in 10 CFR 35.51.[2] These requirements include annual calibration, use of a dedicated check source to verify proper operation on each day of use, and retention of calibration records for 3 years.

Personnel Dosimetry

To ensure that radiation exposures to personnel remain as low as possible and to fulfill legal and administrative requirements, radiation exposures to individuals must be monitored. Detectors used for this purpose include film badges, thermoluminescent dosimeters (TLDs), photoluminescent dosimeters, and various types of ionization chamber dosimeters (Fig. 3). In a complex working environment, there are few cases in which personnel monitoring devices accurately reflect total body exposure. Dosimeters can measure exposure only to the area of the body on which they are worn. Personnel monitoring devices do, however, reflect the exposure history of the worker. When dosimeter readings are considered in conjunction with area monitoring data, they can provide a basis for radiation control actions.

Film badges are the most widely used detectors for personnel monitoring of external exposure. They consist of a sealed packet of photographic film contained in a holder that includes a series of filters to aid in the separation of dose components from different radiation energies. The degree of darkening in various areas of the shielded film can be related to radiation exposure from x-ray and gamma radiation, beta particles, and slow neutrons. Special films are available for measuring exposure to fast neutrons.

The TLD uses a radiation-sensing element that when heated emits light in proportion to the radiation exposure it has received.[14] This instrument has an advantage over photographic film in that it is reusable. However, TLD dosimeters do not provide a permanent record because, once it has been read, no further readout of the dose can be made.

While film badges and TLDs provide accurate, sensitive measurements of personnel exposure, their results are not available to either the worker or radiation safety personnel until they can be developed or read. Ionization chamber devices, such as pocket electroscope dosimeters and integrating radiation meters (often equipped with audible alarms to signal a preset dose level), can be used to indicate radiation exposure while it is occurring. In general, these devices are used in addition to film badges or TLDs to provide rapid information about exposure levels or warnings of exposure hazards. They are, in general, more subject to damage and accidental loss of data than are film or TLD monitors and thus are unsuitable for long-term monitoring of personnel exposure levels.

Individuals must wear dosimeters if they are likely to receive more than 10% of the quarterly limits for occupational workers as specified in 10 CFR 20.1201(a). Individuals under the age of 18 and declared pregnant women who may receive more than 10% of of any of the applicable limits in 10 CFR 20.1207 or 20.1208, and individuals who enter high radiation areas must also be monitored. Records of individual exposure histories must be maintained until the NRC authorizes disposition. The regulations also require that all personnel dosimeters, except for pocket dosimeters and extremity dosimeters, must be evaluated by a dosimetry processor currently accredited by the National Voluntary Laboratory Accreditation Program (NAVLAP) of the National Institute of Standards and Technology (NIST).

BIOASSAY

It may be necessary to monitor the intake of radioactive material by workers to determine if exposure limits have been exceeded. Because of the potentially large commitment of monetary and technical resources required to establish a bioassay program, it is important to carefully determine the appropriate personnel to monitor, the frequency at which assays should be performed, and the monitoring method to use. These determinations must be based on ensuring regulatory compliance as well as consideration of the radionuclide and amounts being used, the effective half-lives, engineering controls available, results of surveys and air sampling, and the work practices of individuals with regard to contamination. Guidelines for monitoring workers can be found in ICRP Publication No. 35.[15] Information relating to methods of assessing internal contamination for occupational exposure are found in ICRP Publications Nos. 10 and 10A and NCRP Report No. 57.[16–18]

10 CFR 20.1204 delineates specific requirements for determination of internal exposure and the conditions under which measurements or calculations are required. Part 20.1502(b)(1) also requires monitoring the occupational uptake of radioactive material by assessing the committed effective dose equivalent to adults likely to receive, in 1 year, an intake in excess of 10% of the applicable annual limit on intake (ALI). 10 CFR 20.1502(b)(2) applies to minors and declared pregnant women likely to receive in 1 year a committed effective dose equivalent in excess of 0.05 rem (0.5 mSv). It is important to realize that 10 CFR Part 35.315 does specifically require the measurement of thyroid burdens of all individuals who helped prepare or administer 30 mCi or more of ^{131}I for therapy.[2]

Regulatory Guide 8.20 can be used to establish a bioassay program for individuals handling volatile or large quantities of bound, nonvolatile ^{125}I or ^{131}I.[19] Urine analyses may be required by the NRC as a license condition for use of large quantities of ^{3}H, ^{14}C, and ^{32}P. Criteria for establishing a bioassay program for ^{3}H can be found in Regulatory Guide 8.32.[20]

Several methods are suitable for the detection and evaluation of internal contamination. The method selected depends on the type of radiation emitted by the radionuclide in question and also the availability of detection equipment. In the case of gamma-, or x-ray emitters, direct measurements can be made since these radiations will penetrate the body and interact with an external detector. Bremsstrahlung x-rays produced in the body by very high-energy beta emissions may also be detected outside the body. If the radionuclide emits only alphas or weak energy betas, neither of which can penetrate the body, indirect methods, such as sampling of body fluids or tissues, are used. Another indirect method, environmental sampling, can be used to supplement other assay methods.[15]

Direct measurement of internally deposited gamma- or x-ray emitters can be made by whole body counters. Whole body counters, in general, do not define the distribution pattern of the nuclide, but they do provide rapid and accurate measurement of total body burden. Whole body counters are available in nearly every region of the United States and in many other countries. Since most of the counters are primarily research instruments, access for routine radiation monitoring measurements may be difficult to obtain. The cost of a whole body counting facility is prohibitive for most nuclear medicine facilities.

The least accurate method used for assessing internal uptake of radioactive materials is the calculation of body burden from such environmental measurements as air sampling, surface contamination levels, and measurements of skin contamination. All of these sources of data require assumptions that place the final estimate in doubt. Air sampling, especially in the breathing zone of workers throughout each procedure, probably yields the most accurate measurements in this indirect method.

TRAINING OF RADIATION WORKERS IN NUCLEAR MEDICINE

Nuclear Regulatory Commission regulations and policies and those of all Agreement States contain requirements for training and education of radiation workers in the safe use of radioactive materials. These requirements are specific to the individual worker's duties and are generally very specific in nature. The requirements cover formal education, on-the-job training, work experience, short courses and instructions, and annual refresher courses.

Training and Experience Requirements for Authorized Users in Nuclear Medicine

A physician may be qualified as an authorized user by one of three methods: an appropriate professional board certification, a specified combination of classroom and laboratory training and full time experience working under the supervision of a qualified authorized user who preceptors his work, or successful completion of a 6-month training program in nuclear medicine that has been approved by the Accreditation Council for Graduate Medical Education and which included classroom and laboratory training, work experience, and supervised clinical experience. There are lesser requirements for those physicians who may seek limited use of radioactive materials, eg, a physician who only desires to be authorized for treating hyperthyroidism with ^{131}I. These requirements are fully described in 10 CFR Part 35.[2]

In all cases, training and experience must have been obtained within 5 years of the date of the application or the individual must have had related continuing education and experience since the required training and experience was obtained.

RADIATION SAFETY PROCEDURES IN NUCLEAR MEDICINE

There are many procedures that must be followed by a nuclear medicine facility to ensure the safety of patients, workers, and the general public and to document regulatory compliance. The following is a general discussion of the most important of these procedures and the associated NRC regulatory requirements. (In order to be consistent with the current regulations, SI units will not be used in this section.) Since each NRC/agreement state license is in some ways unique, licensees *must* be familiar with the requirements in their own licenses.

Package Ordering, Receipt, and Opening Procedures

Regulations covering receipt and transfer of radioactive materials are found in 10 CFR Parts 20, 30, and 35.[2] These regulations state that procedures must be written and implemented for the purchase of radioactive materials, the receipt and opening of packages and inventory. Basically, the procedures require that packages containing specified quantities of radioactive materials must be monitored for external surface contamination and external radiation levels within 3 hours of receipt of the package if received during normal working hours or within 18 hours of receipt if received after normal working hours. The NRC and the carrier must be notified immediately if removable contamination exceeds 22,000 dpm per 100 cm^3 or if the external radiation level of the package is greater than 200 mrem/h at the surface or 10 mrem/h at 3 ft. A more-detailed description of an acceptable procedure for routine ordering and receipt of radioactive materials is found in Appendix K of Regulatory Guide 10.8. Safe opening procedures are detailed in Appendix L of that Guide.[1]

Surveys

The survey requirements for a nuclear medicine department are found in 10 CFR 35.70.[2] The acceptable procedure for implementation of these requirements is in Appendix N of Regulatory Guide 10.8.[1] The following surveys must be conducted:

1. Daily ambient exposure rate surveys of radiopharmaceutical elution, preparation, and administration areas, performed at the end of each day of use including after hours and weekend emergencies. These areas must also be surveyed for removable contamination once a week.
2. Weekly ambient exposure rate and removable contamination surveys of radiopharmaceutical storage and radiopharmaceutical waste storage areas.
3. Monthly ambient exposure rate and removable contamination surveys of laboratory areas where less than 200 μCi of radioactive material are used at one time.
4. Quarterly ambient exposure rate surveys of sealed source storage areas.

Ambient exposure rate surveys must be conducted with either an ionization chamber or an energy-compensated GM detector. The instrument used must be capable of measuring exposure rates as low as 0.1 mrem/h and must be calibrated for the range of gamma energies commonly used in nuclear medicine departments. Each survey instrument must be checked for proper operation with a dedicated check source at the beginning of each day of use as required by 10 CFR 35.51.[2]

Smears must be analyzed by an instrument capable of detecting 2000 dpm per 100 cm^2 (200 dpm per 100 cm^2 for radioiodines). As previously noted, smear analysis should be performed with a properly calibrated liquid scintillation or gamma counter or with a thin window GM detector.

Exposure rate and removable contamination trigger levels must be established by the licensee. The RSO must be notified when a trigger level has been exceeded.

Records of these surveys must be kept for 3 years and must include the date of the survey, a plan of the area surveyed, the trigger levels, exposure rates (in mrem per hour) or removable contamination (in dpm per 100 cm^2) found in several areas, detection instruments used, any corrective actions taken, and the initials of the surveyor.

Patient Dose Assays

The activity of every radiopharmaceutical dosage must be assayed in a dose calibrator prior to being administered to a patient. This assay is required by 10 CFR 35.53 and is necessary in order to verify that the correct patient is receiving the prescribed quantity of radioactivity. Records of these assays must be maintained for 3 years and must include the name of the radiopharmaceutical, patient's name, prescribed dose, measured activity, and date and time of assay.[2]

The regulations in 10 CFR 35.50 require that several quality control checks be performed on a routine basis.

1. Constancy—at the beginning of each day using a dedicated check source.
2. Accuracy—annually and after installation.
3. Linearity—quarterly and after installation.
4. Geometry (volume/count variation)—after installation.

The dose calibrator must be replaced or repaired if the constancy or accuracy error is greater than 10%. Dosages measuring more than 10 μCi (370 kBq) must be mathematically corrected if geometry or linearity errors exceed 10%. Records of geometry checks must be kept as long as the dose calibrator is in use. Records of all other dose calibrator checks must be kept for 3 years. Except for the daily constancy checks, all records must be signed by the RSO. Appendix C of Regulatory Guide 10.8 gives model procedures that satisfy the regulations in 10 CFR 35 for checking and testing dose calibrators.[1] The model procedures are somewhat more rigorous than the regulations.

Inventory and Leak Testing of Sealed Sources

Sealed sources, such as those used for calibration of gamma cameras, counters, and dose calibrators, may require periodic testing to determine if the integrity of the seal has been compromised. These sources can begin to leak because of rough handling during transport to the facility or during use. Also, routine inventories of sealed sources must be conducted and ambient dose rates must be measured in the source storage areas. The regulations for leak testing, inventory, and measurement of ambient dose rates are stated in 10 CFR 35.59 and include the following[2]:

1. All sealed sources must be leak tested every 6 months. Exceptions:
   a. Sealed sources with half-lives of less than 30 days.
   b. Sealed sources containing 100 μCi (3.7 mBq) or less of a beta or gamma emitter or 10 μCi (370 kBq) or less of an alpha emitter.
   c. Sources in the form of sealed gases.
   d. Stored sources that are not in use.
2. Sealed sources must be leak tested before the first use unless the supplier provides documentation of a leak test within 6 months before transferring the source to the licensee.
3. The leak test must be able to detect 0.005 μCi (0.185 kBq) of removable contamination. If the leak test shows 0.005 μCi or more of contamination the source must be taken out of use. The NRC must be notified within 5 days of discovery of the leak.
4. Physical inventories of each sealed source must be conducted quarterly.
5. Ambient dose rate measurements must be made quarterly at each sealed source storage site.
6. Records of leak tests and ambient dose rate measurements must be kept for 3 years. Inventory records must be kept for 5 years.

Appendix H of Regulatory Guide 10.8 can be used to develop a procedure for leak testing sealed sources.[1]

Gases and Aerosols

Xenon-133 is commonly used in nuclear medicine laboratories for pulmonary ventilation studies. The use of ^{127}Xe is not common, but it is increasing. The biologic properties of ^{133}Xe and ^{127}Xe are identical, but their physical characteristics require that they be handled differently. Xenon-133 has a half-life of 5.3 days and a gamma energy of 81 keV. These characteristics render shielding and disposal relatively easy. Xenon-127 has a 36.4-day half-life and gamma energies ranging from 58 to 375 keV. The long half-life and higher energies require heavier shielding and somewhat more careful handling than ^{133}Xe. Krypton-81m is in use in some nuclear medicine facilities; however, it poses no environmental hazard in the concentrations encountered clinically because of its half-life of 13 seconds.

Xenon-133 is supplied for medical use primarily in small, rubber-stoppered ampules containing 10 to 30 mCi (370 to 1110 MBq). Xenon-133 is also supplied in curie amounts in crushable ampules that require a mechanical dispensing system which may develop leaks. Transferring the gas into a syringe from the dispenser requires care and adequate ventilation to prevent the gas from escaping. According to 10 CFR 35.90, radioactive gases and volatile radiopharmaceuticals must be stored in the shipper's radiation shield and container. All multidose containers must be stored in a fume hood after the first use.[2] Single-use ampules should also be stored in a fume hood.

There are currently two types of xenon disposal methods. In one method, the xenon expired by the patient is exhausted to the outside atmosphere. This is sometimes accomplished by placing a hood over the patient and connecting it to a high-volume exhaust fan. The second disposal system employs a trap that contains activated charcoal as the collecting agent. Several commercial systems are available with up to 95% trapping efficiency.[21] The activated charcoal must be replaced periodically. Some commercial systems have a detector in the exhaust port of the trap to measure the concentration of xenon escaping from the charcoal filter. An alarm is meant to signal excessive exhaust concentrations, which indicates the need for replacing the charcoal cartridge. For hospitals in which a high volume of lung imaging is performed, some sort of trapping system may be required because of restrictions on exhausting to the outside.

The maximum permissible concentration of ^{133}Xe in air of a restricted area is 1×10^{-5} μCi/mL. While xenon gas is heavier than air, it will remain uniformly distributed once it is dispersed. Because of the low MPC of radioxenon, adequate ventilation with high room air turnover is desirable. Nishiyama has shown that differences in room air ventilation can effect a hundredfold reduction in xenon that is inhaled by technicians performing ventilation scans.[22] Commercial gas monitors are available to monitor a variety of radioactive gases, including ^{133}Xe, ^{14}C, and ^{3}H. Jacobstein has described a simple means of monitoring ^{133}Xe by measuring the activity taken up by 10-mL vacutainer tubes.[23] These can be punctured with a 20-gauge needle at the site to be monitored and measured in a well counter.

Table 3. Removable Contamination Limits Acceptable to the NRC*

TYPE OF SURFACE	TYPE OF RADIOACTIVE MATERIAL**					
	Alpha Emitters		*Beta- or x-Ray Emitters*		*Low-Risk Beta or x-Ray Emitters*	
	(μCi/cm²)	(dpm/100 cm²)	(μCi/cm²)	(dpm/100 cm²)	(μCi/cm²)	(dpm/100 cm²)
1. Unrestricted areas	10^{-7}	22	10^{-6}	220	10^{-5}	2,200
2. Restricted areas	10^{-6}	220	10^{-5}	2,200	10^{-4}	22,000
3. Personal clothing worn outside restricted areas	10^{-7}	22	10^{-6}	220	10^{-5}	2,200
4. Protective clothing worn only in restricted areas	10^{-6}	220	10^{-5}	2,200	10^{-4}	22,000
5. Skin	10^{-6}	220	10^{-6}	220	10^{-5}	2,200

*Averaging is acceptable over nonliving areas of up to 300 cm² or, for floors, walls, and ceiling, 100 cm². Averaging is also acceptable over 100 cm² for skin or, for the hands, over the whole area of the hand, nominally 300 cm².

**Beta- or x-ray emitter values are applicable for all beta- or x-ray emitters other than those considered low risk. Low-risk nuclides include C-14, H-3, S-35, Tc-99m, and others whose beta energies are less than 0.2 MeV maximum, whose gamma- or x-ray emission is less than 0.1 R/h at 1 meter per curie, and whose permissible concentration in air is greater than 10^6 μCi/ml.

From NRC.[24]

Decontamination Procedures

Surface contamination may originate as gases, liquids, or solids. It may react with surfaces to become relatively fixed or may remain removable. In all cases, cleaning up any spilled radioactive material as soon as possible is important.

Detection of contaminated areas can be accomplished quickly by means of a G–M or NaI detector and smears. Routine surveys combining these methods provide good indications of the extent of laboratory contamination. Standards should be established for permissible levels of contamination in various work areas. Areas in which permissible levels are exceeded should be decontaminated to acceptable levels. Table 3 lists contamination limits acceptable to the NRC. Other limits that can be justified may be found acceptable by the NRC.[24] Each nuclear medicine facility must be aware of the limits specified in their license conditions.

When contamination is found it should be clearly marked and promptly removed. It is important that contamination not be allowed to spread to new surfaces or personnel during the decontamination operation. Marking contaminated areas and posting warning signs helps to minimize the spread of contamination in most cases. When large areas are affected or high radiation levels are present, it may be necessary to restrict access to the area by means of barricades. Personnel involved in decontamination activities should wear protective clothing and appropriate personnel monitoring techniques should be applied. The degree of control and special precautions required depend on the extent and radiotoxicity of the contaminating event.

Methods of decontamination that reduce the potential for airborne radioactivity are preferred. Mild scrubbing with abrasive powders and scouring pads is acceptable. Vacuuming should be avoided unless the machine is equipped with absolute filters to prevent the exhaust from blowing radioactive dust into the air. Most contamination can be removed by gentle washing with soap and water. In the initial steps, scrubbing should be minimized and the primary effort directed toward removal of loose dirt and grease from the area. Commercial preparations of detergents and complexing agents are available for decontamination but these have little value over soap and water. Cleaners containing bleach should not be used to clean spills of radioiodine because bleach promotes volatility. Care should be exercised to prevent the washing solution from moving the contamination into inaccessible areas. After each washing survey the area to determine how much activity remains.

Spills, Personal Contamination, and Emergency Procedures

Spills involving small amounts of radioactive materials can occur in any nuclear medicine facility; however, this should be a rare occurrence in any efficient and well-designed department staffed by well-trained and competent personnel. Although the quantities involved are not expected to result in serious or lasting effects, these incidents must be taken seriously. Each facility should establish criteria for reporting spills to the RSO. This is important since additional assistance is sometimes required. It may also be necessary to report the incident to the NRC or other authorities.

These steps should be followed when cleaning a spill:

1. Place absorbent material over the spill to keep it from spreading.
2. Notify others in the area and limit access to the spill area.
3. Monitor personnel for contamination and, if necessary, decontaminate immediately.
4. Label the boundaries of the spill area.
5. Gather cleaning supplies; moistened paper towels and scouring powder or any commercially available detergent are recommended.
6. Do not ask untrained personnel to assist in the cleanup.
7. Wear protective clothing, such as lab coats and gloves,

while cleaning the spill area. Shoe covers may also be needed.

8. Begin the cleanup at the edges of the spill and work in toward the middle. Minimize the volume of water and other liquids used.
9. Dispose of all cleanup materials as radioactive waste.
10. Smear the area to ensure that removable contamination is within the regulatory limits for the facility.

It is important to remember that any serious injury or condition (heavy bleeding, heart attack, etc) that happens concurrent with a spill must be treated prior to initiation of decontamination efforts. Medical assistance should be obtained or first aid must be rendered immediately. For minor injuries such as puncture wounds, suspected inhalation or ingestion of radioactive materials, or skin contamination, decontamination should begin before seeking medical assistance. If the skin becomes contaminated, the affected area should be washed repeatedly in the nearest sink using soap and water. Unless quickly removed, external contamination of the skin can result in large radiation doses to the affected area. Beta-emitting radionuclides are especially hazardous in this respect. Do not abrade the skin while removing contamination because abrasions facilitate entry of the material into the body. A soft scrub brush may be used. Organic solvents should not be used on the skin. A G–M or NaI detector and smears can be used to determine when contamination can no longer be removed. Eye contamination can be removed by flushing the area with copious amounts of water. The eyelid and the skin under the eye can be smeared to determine when contamination is no longer removable. The RSO should be notified in all cases when personnel become contaminated. The staff health clinic should also be consulted.

Therapies

Nuclear medicine facilities frequently become involved with therapeutic uses of radiopharmaceuticals. Treatment of thyroid cancer with up to hundreds of millicuries of sodium iodide ^{131}I is a common procedure. The ^{131}I may be administered in liquid or capsule form. A relatively new type of therapy involves the labeling of monoclonal antibodies with ^{131}I or ^{90}Y for treatment of various types of cancer. Radionuclides unfamiliar to most nuclear medicine facilities, such as ^{186}Re and various alpha emitters, are also coming into use. These radionuclides present new and interesting radiation safety concerns that are not fully addressed by the current regulations and guides. The NRC is considering whether new regulations are needed for the use of radiolabeled monoclonal antibodies.[25]

The regulations covering the use of radiopharmaceuticals for therapy are found in 10 CFR 35.75, 10 CRF 35.300, and 10 CRF 20.1301 and 20.1302.[2] A model procedure for compliance with these regulations is found in Appendix P of Regulatory Guide 10.8.[1] Other valuable guidance is found in NCRP Report No. 37.[26] The regulations are summarized below.

1. A patient may not be released from his/her room until the measured dose rate from the patient is less than 5 mrem/h at 1 m *or* until the activity in the patient is less than 30 mCi. The following safety precautions must be taken while the patient is confined:
   a. The patient must be in a private room with private sanitary facilities.
   b. The door to the room must be posted with a "Radioactive Materials" sign. Instructions to visitors must be posted on the door or in the patient's chart.
   c. Dose rates in contiguous areas must be measured and recorded. These dose rates must be in compliance with the applicable limits. A record of this survey must be kept for 3 years.
   d. Items removed from the therapy room must be monitored or handled as radioactive waste.
2. The patient must be given guidance that will help reduce exposure to others when he/she is released from confinement.
3. The therapy room must be cleaned and surveyed before assigning it to another patient.
4. Thyroid counts must be performed on each individual who prepared or administered an ^{131}I therapy dose. The count must be obtained within 3 days of administration.
5. The RSO must be notified immediately if the patient dies or has a medical emergency.
6. Training must be provided to all personnel who care for the therapy patient. A record of this training must be kept for 3 years.

Fortunately emergency situations rarely occur during therapy procedures. However, if surgery is required on a patient containing high levels of radioactivity, the hazard to operating room personnel can be significantly reduced if the procedure can be delayed. Exposure to the hands can be high if they come into direct contact with highly radioactive organs or tissues. When surgery involves areas remote from the sites of deposition, the radiation hazard is much reduced and the presence of radioactivity is of much less concern.

The death of a patient who contains therapeutic amounts of radioactivity poses several problems from the standpoint of radiation safety. If an autopsy is to be performed, the pathologist and other personnel may receive appreciable radiation exposure. During embalming procedures, both personnel exposure hazards and danger of contamination exist. If the body is cremated, hazards include excessive release of radionuclides to the environment and inhalation of radioactive ashes by mortuary personnel. Because of the potential hazards involved, detailed procedures should be available to all persons who might be in contact with the patient. All procedures that might involve radiation risks to personnel or to members of the general public should be carried out under the supervision of the RSO.

QUALITY MANAGEMENT PROGRAM/ MISADMINISTRATIONS

The NRC recently modified existing regulations for therapeutic use of radioactive materials and some uses of radioiodine to require the establishment of a quality management program (QMP) to ensure that radiation and radioactive materials are used as intended by the prescribing physician. Effective January 1992, most nuclear medicine facilities were required to have an operational QMP in place. The regulations found in 10 CFR 35.32 require that a QMP be established if the following procedures are performed:[27]

1. Use of more than 30 μCi of sodium ^{125}I or sodium ^{131}I.
2. Any therapeutic use of a radiopharmaceutical other than sodium ^{125}I or sodium ^{131}I.
3. Certain teletherapy or brachytherapy procedures.

The QMP requires that written directives (prescriptions) must be prepared for the procedures covered by the program. The program must also ensure that the patient's identify is verified by more than one method prior to administration. A review of the program must be conducted at least annually to evaluate its effectiveness. Records of these reviews must be kept for 3 years. Figure 4 illustrates the written directive for radiophamaceutical administration used at the NIH.

An important change in the NRC regulations is the new definition of a misadministration and the addition of reportable events. Table 4 summarizes the types of incidents considered to be misadministrations or recordable events. Misadministrations must be reported to the NRC by telephone no later than the next calendar day after discovery of the incident. This must be followed by a written report within 15 days. Recordable events do not have to be reported to the NRC; however, they must be investigated within 30 days of discovery. Reports of recordable events must be kept for 3 years and misadministration records must be retained for 5 years.

PREGNANT PATIENTS AND WORKERS

Currently there are no regulations governing the limits for exposure to pregnant workers or the embryo/fetus. The *recommendations* found in NCRP Report No. 53 and NRC Regulatory Guide. 8.13 should be used by each nuclear medicine facility to develop a policy on pregnant or potentially pregnant workers.[28,29] It is recommended that the total dose to the fetus from the occupational exposure of the mother not exceed 0.5 rem during the entire gestation period. The exposure should be received at an even rate and should not be due to one or several large events. It is highly advisable that the pregnant worker notify the RSO of her condition so that her duties and past exposure history can be evaluated. In most cases, if the worker is involved with routine nuclear medicine procedures and the ALARA principle is being observed, she can continue her duties without major changes. If the pregnant worker is responsible for preparing radiopharmaceuticals or handles highly volatile material, she may wish to transfer to other duties. The worker should monitor herself and the work area frequently.

10 CFR 20 establishes a *limit* of 0.5 rem to the embryo/fetus during the gestation period.[3] However, this limit applies only if the mother has *declared* herself pregnant. This declaration must be made in writing.

Care should be taken to avoid administering radiopharmaceuticals to pregnant patients or to women who are breast-feeding. However, a nuclear medicine procedure should be performed if the physician considers it necessary for the well-being of the pregnant patient. NCRP Report No. 54 provides guidance on this issue.[30]

RADIOACTIVE WASTE

During the course of operation of a nuclear medicine laboratory, various types and quantities of radioactive wastes are produced. Examples of these wastes are used syringes and needles, dose vials, rubber gloves, unused radiopharmaceuticals, absorbent surface covers, and absorbent wipes from clean-up of spills. The radionuclides routinely used in nuclear medicine have short half-lives ranging from a few hours for ^{99m}Tc to a few days for others such as ^{131}I. The short half-lives of these materials' flexibility in disposal of nuclear medicine wastes and most nuclear medicine departments do not need to transfer radioactive wastes to commercial burial grounds.

The basic principles of disposal as given in IAEA Publication No. 38 are as follows:[31]

1. *Dilute and dispense* for low-level solid, liquid, and gaseous wastes.
2. *Delay and decay* for solid, liquid, and gaseous wastes that contain short-lived nuclides.
3. *Concentrate and contain* for intermediate and high-level solid, liquid, and gaseous wastes.

The design of waste disposal systems generally includes all of these methods, sometimes in combination. The procedures described in this section meet the requirements of the NRC and those of most agreement states.[1] In the text, references are keyed to the NRC regulations.

Several options for disposal of radioactive waste from nuclear medicine operations are available under current NRC regulations. It is important to recognize that patient excreta is not considered radioactive waste when disposed of through the sanitary sewer [10 CFR 20.2003(b)] Paragraph 20.2003 of 10 CFR also contains the authorization and limitations for the disposal by sewer of other radioactive wastes readily soluble or dispersible in water. Incineration of waste containing radioactivity is an option but requires specific NRC approval except for those wastes described in 10 CFR

Date ____________

WRITTEN DIRECTIVE FOR RADIOPHARMACEUTICAL ADMINISTRATION
NIH Quality Management Program for Radioisotopes

Patient's Full Name ______________________________

Hospital #______________________

Birth Date ______________________

MIS Request #:______________________

1. Dose Calibrator Printout Sheet Review ________
   Check Isotope; Dose; Initial Sheet

2. Radiopharmaceutical: ____________________________

   Dose: Prescribed:______________ Administered:________________

   Route of Administration: ______________

3. Methods of Identifying Patient:
   (Use at least two)

   Full Name: _____
   Birth Date: _____
   ID Bracelet: _____
   Signature: _____

______________________________ ________
Patient's Signature Date

4. Authorized User:

______________________________ ________
Authorized User's Signature **Date**

Figure 4. Example of a written directive for radiopharmaceutical administration.

20.2004. Waste described in that paragraph can be disposed of without regard to their radioactivity. The most widely employed technique for radioactive waste disposal in the nuclear medicine laboratory is decay-in-storage. In this method, short-lived radionuclides are stored until they decay to background. After a suitable period of decay, usually ten or more half-lives, the wastes are monitored with an appropriate radiation survey meter before being discarded as regular trash. The NRC also grants a general license to physicians for the use of certain in vitro test kits containing

Table 4. Types of Incidents Considered to be Misadministrations or Recordable Events in a Nuclear Medicine Department

PROCEDURE	RECORDABLE EVENT	MISADMINISTRATION
All diagnostic radiopharmaceuticals (including <30 μCi NaI, I-125 or I-131)		Wrong patient, radiopharm, route, or dosage *and* Dose >5 rem effective dose equivalent or 50 rem to organ
Sodium iodide radiopharmaceuticals (where >30 μCi NaI, I-125 or I-131)	Admin dosage differs by >10% of prescribed dosage *and* >15 μCi W/o written directive W/o daily dosage record	Wrong patient Wrong radiopharmaceutical Admin dosage differs by >20% of prescribed dosage *and* >30 μCi
Therapeutic radiopharmaceuticals	Admin dosage differs by >10% of prescribed dosage W/o written directive W/o daily dosage record	Wrong patient Wrong radiopharmaceutical Wrong route of administration Admin dosage differs by >20% of prescribed dosage

From NRC.[27]

very small quantities of radioactive materials. Under the provisions of 10 CFR 31.11(f), after use, these kits can be discarded in the regular trash. A nuclear medicine operation obtaining unit doses or other radiopharaceuticals from a nuclear pharmacy may return the used syringes and unused doses to the pharmacy for disposal.

The reader is reminded to carefully review the appropriate regulations before employing the techniques above. Following the general guidelines listed below is highly recommended.

1. Minimize radioactive waste as much as possible.
   a. Keep all extraneous, nonradioactive materials out of radioactive waste containers.
   b. Design work so as to confine contamination and minimize materials requiring disposal as radioactive waste.
2. Avoid mixing waste with short half-lives (2 days or less) with those containing longer-lived materials.
3. Prominently mark radioactive waste containers to avoid inadvertent removal as ordinary waste.
4. Allow only those personnel, in particular janitorial staff, who have had the proper instruction in recognizing radiation warning signs and labels, to service areas where the radioactive waste is stored.
5. Deface or remove all radiation warning signs and labels from materials being disposed of as ordinary trash.
6. Waste released to the sewer must be soluble or dispersible in water and must meet all other regulatory requirements.

REFERENCES

1. *Guide for the Preparation of Applications for Medical Use Programs.* NRC Regulatory Guide 10.8, Revision 2, Washington, DC: US Nuclear Regulatory Commission, 1987.
2. *Code of Federal Regulations.* Title 10-Energy (10 CFR). Office of the Federal Register, Washington, DC: US Government Printing Office, 1994.
3. *Standards for Protection Against Radiation.* 10 CFR Part 20, December 30, 1993.
4. Hendee, W.R. *Medical Radiation Physics.* 2nd ed. Chicago: Year Book Medical Publishers, 1979.
5. *Radiation Quantities and Units.* Report No. 33. Washington, DC: International Commission on Radiation Units and Measurements, 1980.
6. *Recommendations on Limits for Exposure to Ionizing Radiation.* Report No. 91. Washington, DC: International Commission on Radiation Units and Measurements, 1987.
7. Branson BM, Sodd VI, Nishiyama H, Williams CC. Use of syringe shields in clinical practice. *J Clin Nucl Med* 1976;1:56.
8. *Recommendation of the International Commission on Radiological Protection.* International Commission on Radiological Protection. Publication No. 2. London: Pergamon Press, 1959.
9. *Recommendations of the International Commission on Radiological Protection.* International Commission on Radiological Protection. Publication No. 6. London: Pergamon Press, 1962.
10. *Limits for Intakes of Radionuclides by Workers.* International Commission on Radiological Protection, Publication No. 30. London: Pergamon Press, 1979.
11. *Radiation Protection.* International Commission on Radiological Protection, Publication No. 26. London: Pergamon Press, 1977.
12. Knoll GF. *Radiation Detection and Measurement.* 2nd ed. New York: John Wiley & Sons, 1989.
13. *Calibration of Survey Instruments Used in Radiation Protection for the Assessment of Ionizing Radiation Fields and Radioactive Surface Contamination.* Report No. 112. Washington, DC: National Council on Radiation Protection and Measurements, 1991.
14. *Radiation Protection Instrumentation and Its Application.* Report No. 20. Washington, DC: International Commission on Radiation Units and Measurements, 1976.
15. *General Principles of Monitoring for Radiation Protection of Workers.* International Commission on Radiological Protection, Publication No. 35. London, Pergamon Press, 1982.
16. *Evaluation of Radiation Doses to Body Tissues from Internal Contamination Due to Occupational Exposure.* International Commission on Radiological Protection, Publication No. 10. London, Pergamon Press, 1968.
17. *The Assessment of Internal Contamination Resulting from Recurrent of Prolonged Uptakes.* International Commission on Radiological Protection, Publication No. 10A. London: Pergamon Press, 1971.
18. *Instrumentation and Monitoring Methods for Radiation Protection.* Report No. 57. Washington, DC: National Council on Radiation Protection and Measurements, 1978.

19. *Applications of Bioassay for ^{125}I and ^{131}I.* NRC Regulatory Guide 8.20. Washington, DC: US Nuclear Regulatory Commission, 1979.
20. *Criteria for Establishing a Tritium Bioassay Program.* Regulatory Guide 8.32. Washington, DC: US Nuclear Regulatory Commission, 1988.
21. McIlmoyle G, Holman BL, Davis M, Chandler HL. A portable radioxenon trap and patient ventilation system. *Radiology* 1978;127:544.
22. Nishiyama H, Lukes SJ. Exposure to xenon-133 in the nuclear medicine laboratory. *Radiology* 1982;143:243.
23. Jacobstein J. A simple method for the air monitoring of xenon-133. *J Nucl Med* 1979;20:159.
24. *Radiation Safety at Medical Institutions.* NRC Regulatory Guide 8.23. Washington, DC: US Nuclear Regulatory Commission, 1981.
25. Barber DE, Baum JW, Meinhold CB. *Radiation Safety Issues Related to Radiolabeled Antibodies.* NUREG/CR-4444, Office of Nuclear Regulatory Research, Washington, DC: US Nuclear Regulatory Commission, 1991.
26. *Precautions in the Management of Patients Who Have Received Therapeutic Amounts of Radionuclides.* Report No. 37. Washington, DC: National Council on Radiation Protection and Measurements, 1970.
27. *Quality Management Program and Misadministrations.* 10 CFR Parts 2 and 35, Federal Register, Vol. 56, No. 143, p. 34104-34122, July 25, 1991.
28. *Review of NCRP Radiation Dose Limit for Embryo and Fetus in Occupationally-Exposed Women.* Report No. 53. Washington, DC: National Council on Radiation Protection and Measurements, 1977.
29. *Instruction Concerning Prenatal Radiation Exposure.* NRC Regulatory Guide 8.13, Revision 2. Washington, DC: US Nuclear Regulatory Commission, 1987.
30. *Medical Radiation Exposure of Potentially Pregnant Women.* Report No. 54. Washington, DC: National Council on Radiation Protection and Measurements, 1977.
31. *Radiation Protection Procedures.* Safety Series No. 38, Vienna: International Atomic Energy Agency, 1973.

Section Two

Clinical Sciences

17 Neurological PET and SPECT

Michael J. Fulham, Giovanni Di Chiro

Positron emission tomography (PET) was developed in the mid-1970s with the promise of providing quantitative measurements and anatomical localization of biochemical processes in vivo.[1–3] PET began in a research environment, but the past decade has witnessed the application of PET to clinical management in a variety of neurological disorders.[4,5] In the same period, single photon emission computed tomography (SPECT) has been used to evaluate patients with stroke, epilepsy, dementia, traumatic brain injury, AIDS and, more recently, patients with movement disorders.[6–9] In the accompanying pages, the commonly used applications of PET and SPECT technology in neurological disorders are presented. For PET, the most widely used ligand is [^{18}F]-fluoro-2-deoxyglucose (FDG) and ^{99m}Tc-hexamethyl propylene amine oxime (HMPAO) for SPECT. Relevant applications of other tracers are listed but, unfortunately, a single chapter cannot adequately cover every current and potential application for the available PET and SPECT radiotracers.

GENERAL CONSIDERATIONS

For reliable interpretation of neurological functional imaging studies, there are a number of practical issues that should be considered. A sound understanding of normal and functional neuroanatomy, the limitations of the instrumentation used to acquire data, and the conditions under which the studies are performed are essential. PET, with its research background, the interest in quantification, and introduction of numerous radiotracers, has always had an emphasis on normal data collection even though differences in instrumentation used to acquire these data remain a significant factor for the comparison of data collected at different institutions. The need for a similar approach in SPECT has recently been discussed.[6,8] Although it is a significant undertaking, it is the authors' opinion that all centers committed to performing functional imaging, both for research and clinical applications, should acquire their own normative data.

The basics of PET and SPECT physics and instrumentation have already been outlined in Chapters 5 and 6, PET and Single Photon Imaging. It is important to remember that there continue to be major improvements in PET and SPECT instrumentation. SPECT was a major improvement over planar imaging; it produced better quality images because focal sources of activity were not superimposed on each other. Sensitivity was further improved by the routine use of multidetector gamma cameras, thus enabling improved resolution through the detection of a greater proportion of unscattered photons. Triple-head gamma cameras have resolution in the order of 8 to 10 mm full-width at half-maximum (FWHM) compared to 14 to 17 mm FWHM for single-head systems. HMPAO SPECT studies performed in the same patient on single, double, and triple-headed SPECT devices in Figure 1 illustrate the improvements in image quality. Ring-detector imaging devices have even better spatial resolution (7 to 8 mm FWHM), but these devices are not widely available. Meanwhile, similar advances have occurred with PET tomographs (Fig. 2) and the extended 15-cm field of view in current generation tomographs greatly simplify data acquisition without the need for multiple bed movements.[10] The next generation of PET scanners will approach the theoretical "finite" in-plane spatial resolution in PET of about 2 mm.[11]

Attention to the test environment is also critical for functional imaging modalities. Limitation of patient motion by attention to positioning and patient comfort with the utilization of some type of head restraint are important, but often overlooked factors, for the production of high quality images in both modalities. Physiological motion—myocardial contraction, diaphragmatic movement, intestinal peristalsis—is not a problem for neurological studies. However, head movement during data acquisition degrades image quality in PET and may produce image artifacts in SPECT. We routinely use a thermoplastic mask that is molded to the contours of the face and side of the head to limit head movement for all patients having cerebral SPECT and PET scans. Particular difficulties arise in patients who are demented or confused but, for most patients, a detailed explanation of the imaging procedure, a comfortable imaging bed, and knee support to prevent back discomfort are usually effective. Although there is considerable research in the detection, measurement, and correction of head motion during functional imaging, it should be emphasized that it is always better to limit motion during data collection than to try to correct for it during reconstruction.[12–14]

In neurology, SPECT has mainly assessed cerebral perfusion.[7–9] A list of commonly used SPECT and PET tracers are found in Table 1. More comprehensive lists for SPECT and PET ligands can be found in a number of recent textbooks.[15–19] SPECT tracers used to measure regional cerebral blood flow (rCBF) are assumed to accumulate in the brain

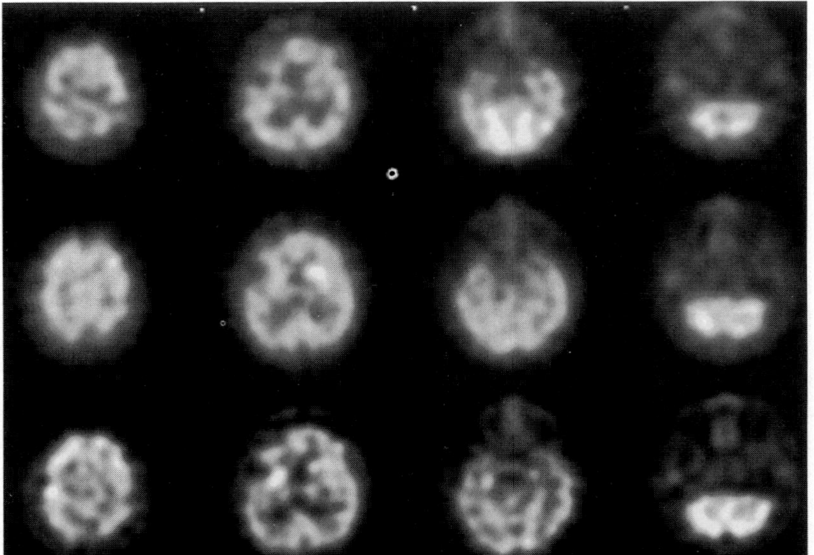

Figure 1. Representative HMPAO SPECT images of a 28-year-old woman with systemic lupus erythematosus studied on 3 different occasions with single-head (top row), dual-head (middle row), and triple-head (bottom) SPECT devices. Images show improved image quality with the multi-head devices, with better depiction of deep nuclei and better gray-to-white-matter contrast. (Note for this and all subsequent neurological studies, the patient's right side is on the reader's left.) (See Plate 8.)

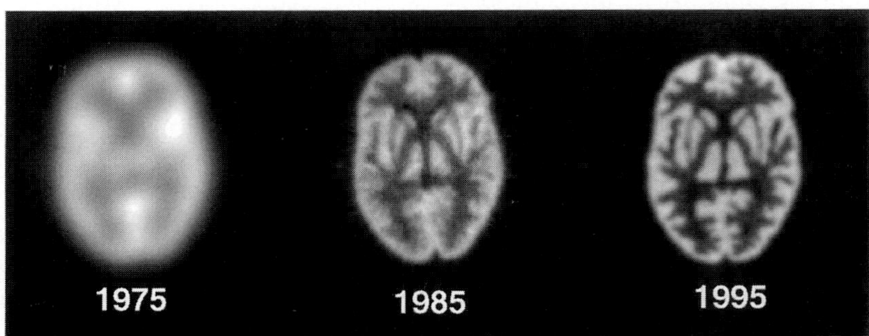

Figure 2. Hoffman brain phantom simulations, at level of the deep nuclei and insula, show the improvements in PET resolution over 2 decades. (See Plate 9.)

Table 1. Various SPECT and PET Radiotracers in Neurology

TECHNIQUE	RADIOTRACER NEURORECEPTOR LIGAND	RADIONUCLIDE HALF-LIFE	BIOLOGIC PARAMETER/RECEPTOR
SPECT	^{99m}Tc-hexamethyl propylene amine oxime (HMPAO)	^{99m}Tc = 6 hrs	regional cerebral blood flow
	^{201}Thallium	^{201}Tl = 73.1 hrs	K^+ analog-cellularity
	^{133}Xenon	^{133}Xe = 5.25 days	regional cerebral blood flow
	^{123}I-iodoamphetamine (IMP)	^{123}I ~ 13 hrs	regional cerebral blood flow
	^{123}I-iodo-α-methyl tyrosine (IMT)		amino acid transport
	^{123}I-iodoamphetamine (IMP)		regional cerebral blood flow
	^{123}I QNB		muscarinic cholinergic
	^{123}I-iodobenzamide (IBZM)		dopamine D2
	^{123}I-iomazenil		central benzodiazepine
	^{123}I-iododexetimide		muscarinic cholinergic
PET	[^{18}F]-fluorodeoxyglucose	^{18}F ~ 108 mins	glucose metabolism
	[^{18}F]-6-fluorodopa		presynaptic dopa uptake
	[^{11}C]-methionine	^{11}C = 20 mins	amino acid uptake
	[^{11}C]-raclopride		D2
	[^{11}C]-nomifensine		catecholamine reuptake sites
	[^{11}C]-flumazenil		central benzodiazepine
	[^{11}C]-PK 11195		peripheral benzodiazepine
	^{15}O-water	^{15}O ~ 2 mins	cerebral blood flow

in proportion to the rate of delivery of nutrients to a volume of brain tissue in units of mL/min/100 gm tissue. Measurement of rCBF is based on the microsphere model. This model assumes: (1) the injected tracer is freely diffusible from the blood pool into the brain, (2) there is complete extraction of the tracer by the brain, (3) once taken up by the brain, the tracer is "trapped," or that efflux from the brain to the blood pool is accounted for and, (4) following the initial tracer uptake, there is no subsequent redistribution.[18] In reality, however, many of these assumptions are violated to a degree by virtually all the available tracers. The application of FDG to the evaluation of cerebral glucose metabolism is based on the [^{14}C]deoxyglucose autoradiographic method developed by Sokoloff et al. in the albino rat.[12] The FDG PET method was validated in humans in the late 1970s.[19] FDG uptake is mainly localized in synaptic terminals,[20,21] rather than cell soma in mammalian nervous tissue. Thus, FDG PET images reflect synaptic activity, be it excitatory or inhibitory, because both require energy utilization, with the exception of high-grade cerebral tumors and epileptic seizure foci during the ictus, where somal glucose utilization predominates.

IMAGING PROTOCOLS

Although imaging protocols for PET and SPECT may vary from tracer to tracer, there are some common principles to both modalities.

FDG PET

Patients undergoing neurological FDG PET imaging are studied in a fasting state. Hyperglycemia results in decreased cerebral FDG uptake and "noisy" images because a tracer dose of FDG is administered. In patients with hyperglycemia a longer emission data collection may improve the image quality. Patients are advised not to eat for 6 hours prior to the study, but they may take their "usual" medication and drink water liberally. The exceptions to "usual" medication are the major tranquilizers because they depress glucose utilization. In small children, a 4-hour fast is acceptable. In children with epilepsy, a prolonged fast may promote seizure activity. Pregnancy tests are conducted prior to the study in all women of reproductive age. We routinely perform quantitative studies with blood sampling in all patients using a modification[22] of the Sokoloff three-compartment model[23] with standard gray matter rate constants ($k_1 = 0.1020$, $k_2 = 0.1300$, $k_3 = 0.0620$, $k_4 = 0.0068$) and a Lumped Constant value of 0.4180. We prefer the "arterialized venous" method[19] using hot water baths heated to 40°C because it is more convenient than placing a radial artery cannula and good quantitative data are obtained if the limb is allowed sufficient time to warm. Arterialization is better when the venous cannula is placed distally in the forearm and the dorsum of the hand is preferred. The venous cannula is positioned in the "reverse" direction; that is, with the tip pointing toward the fingertips. There are occasional patients who have very poor venous access and we then resort to arterial cannulation. Universal precautions are taken with every patient. For patients with refractory epilepsy and brain tumor patients with complex partial seizures, we perform video EEG monitoring throughout the study. Scalp surface EEG electrodes are positioned prior to the PET study and EEG monitoring is carried out for 1 hour before tracer injection and throughout the imaging to ensure that any seizures that may occur prior to or during the PET study are detected. Prior to the intravenous injection of tracer, the patient's eyes are patched and ears are plugged. The typical adult injected dose of FDG is 5.3 (140 μCi) MBq/kg for neurological studies performed with wide-aperture whole-body PET. An uptake period of 30 minutes is allowed before the patient is positioned on the imaging bed. Once the patient is on the bed, a thermoplastic mask is used to limit head movement. Care is taken to ensure the patient is comfortable, with attention to knee support and elbow padding for the arm from which blood is sampled. Attenuation can be corrected by a variety of methods but we prefer a postinjection methodology which, together with "off-camera" uptake, allows increased patient throughput without the errors introduced by a calculated method of attenuation correction or the lengthy study durations of preinjection transmission measurements.[24]

Young children pose a particular problem for any type of imaging. For computed tomography (CT) and magnetic resonance (MR) imaging, sedation is usually given 10 to 40 minutes prior to the study and can only improve image quality. But, for FDG PET, sedation prior to injection may affect uptake and violates the "steady state" assumptions of the FDG model.[23] Agents commonly used for sedating children, narcotics, short-acting barbiturates, and benzodiazepines, all depress cerebral glucose utilization; thus, our practice is to sedate young children at the end of the uptake period with a short-acting benzodiazepine. Respiration and oxygen saturation are monitored with a pulse oximeter and facilities to support respiration are always available.

SPECT

We also use a standardized approach for cerebral perfusion SPECT. Patients lie comfortably in a dimly lit room with eyes and ears patched for 15 minutes prior to and 15 minutes after tracer injection. Head restraint and a calculated method for attenuation correction are used for all studies. Blood sampling is not routinely performed. For patients with refractory epilepsy having an interictal HMPAO SPECT study, a routine identical to that for FDG PET is followed, including video EEG monitoring. One exception is that the patient is not required to fast. Attention is paid to patient positioning and comfort. Ictal SPECT images are only performed on inpatients who have been admitted for continuous EEG monitoring. In this situation, nursing staff reconstitute the tracer at the bedside and inject it soon after the onset of a clinical and EEG-verified seizure. The patient is later transported to

Table 2. The International League Against Epilepsy Classification of Seizures

- I Partial (focal) seizures
  - A. Simple partial seizures
  - B. Complex partial seizures (with impairment of consciousness)
  - C. Partial seizures evolving to secondary generalized seizures
- II Generalized seizures (convulsive or nonconvulsive)
  - A. Absence seizures
  - B. Myoclonic seizures
  - C. Clonic seizures
  - D. Tonic seizures
  - E. Tonic-clonic seizures
  - F. Atonic seizures
- III Unclassified seizures

the SPECT camera for data acquisition. We routinely align PET and SPECT images to one another and to anatomical imaging using software developed at our institution.[12]

EPILEPSY

In the United States, 1% of the population is affected by epilepsy. In at least 10% of these patients, seizures are poorly controlled with anticonvulsant medication. The majority of these patients with refractory epilepsy have partial or focal seizures at a significant personal and community cost. In the United States there are about 150,000 patients with refractory complex partial seizures.[25] The focal origin of these seizures make them amenable to surgical treatment by brain resection. Surgical excision of the epileptic focus provides the opportunity for cure, or at least a significant improvement in seizure frequency, for these patients. Seizure control also offers them the chance to lead normal and productive lives.

The majority of complex partial seizures arise from the temporal lobes but they can arise from other cortical areas, particularly frontal and occipital cortices. The International League Against Epilepsy classification of seizures is shown in Table 2. During a complex partial seizure, consciousness is impaired. The seizure may be preceded by an aura, or simple partial seizure, and can progress to become a secondarily generalized tonic-clonic seizure. Results from established Comprehensive Epilepsy Surgical Programs suggest that there is a greater than 70% seizure-free outcome after anterior temporal lobectomy with minimal morbidity.[26,27] The fundamental criterion for patients with refractory epilepsy who are potential surgical candidates is accurate localization of the seizure focus. The value of SPECT and PET for seizure focus localization of temporal lobe epilepsy is well established. These functional imaging tools have led to improved diagnosis and a reduction in invasive EEG monitoring (depth and subdural grid electrodes), with its attendant morbidity.

Interictal PET

Epileptic patients were among the first patients to be studied with PET.[28] The majority of PET studies in patients with refractory epilepsy have been done with FDG. Engel and co-workers at UCLA first demonstrated that in patients with temporal lobe epilepsy, in the interictal period, the seizure focus was characterized by reduced glucose metabolism (hypometabolism) and during a seizure there was increased glucose utilization (hypermetabolism), sometimes with propagation throughout the brain.[29–31] An example of a typical interictal study is shown in Figure 3. The patient is a 16-year-old boy with refractory complex partial seizures. His seizures began at 2 years of age and, in his teens, were refractory to medication. Surface and sphenoidal EEG recordings showed a seizure focus that was lateralized to the left temporal lobe. Left mesial temporal sclerosis was noted on MRI.

Interestingly, the zone of hypometabolism is usually much larger than the gliosis and neuronal loss found in the hippocampus histologically.[30] This finding has been consistently observed by other investigators, but remains unexplained.[32,33] It has been suggested that the interictal glucose hypometabolism is functional,[34] but the mechanism for diminished synaptic activity remains unanswered. Regional glucose hypometabolism outside the mesial and lateral temporal lobes is also found, and occurs in the ipsilateral thalamus and basal ganglia and, less commonly in frontal, parietal, and occipital lobes.[35]

In about 70% of surgical candidates with temporal lobe complex partial seizures, interictal FDG PET scans isolate regions of hypometabolism that correlate with the site of the epileptic focus determined by scalp and depth interictal and ictal EEG recordings.[34,36] At UCLA, this has resulted in a 30 to 50% reduction in the number of patients subjected to invasive depth electrode studies since the inclusion of PET in the preoperative evaluation.[37] Furthermore, in most studies that have compared structural imaging techniques, such as CT and MR imaging to PET,[30,33,38–42] PET is better able to localize the seizure focus. It should be noted, however, that the glucose hypometabolism observed interictally with FDG PET is nonspecific and, while it is found in mesial temporal sclerosis (the most common pathology underlying complex partial seizures which is not consistently recognized by anatomical imaging) it is also seen in low-grade gliomas and hamartomas where anatomical imaging is more sensitive.

The FDG PET method is useful in evaluating children with refractory complex partial seizures. It is useful in the classification and management of seizures that occur in the Lennox-Gastaut Syndrome (LGS), a childhood disorder characterized by recurrent atonic/myoclonic seizures, a distinctive spike-wave EEG pattern, and some degree of intellectual impairment.[43–46] Finally, it helps delineate the epileptic foci in intractable neonatal-onset seizures and infantile spasms that are amenable to surgery.[47–49]

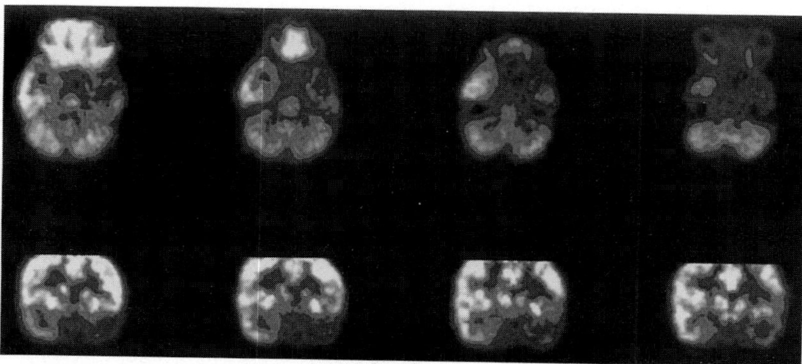

Figure 3. A 16-year-old boy with refractory complex partial seizures. Transaxial (top row) and coronal (bottom row) FDG PET images show marked left temporal lobe glucose hypometabolism involving mesial and lateral temporal neocortex consistent with an interictal epileptic focus. (See Plate 10.)

Ictal PET

Imaging a seizure during FDG PET is an infrequent occurrence. The nature of the FDG PET method and data acquisition means that a short-lived event, such as a seizure, may not be identified, even though it induces glucose hypermetabolism during the ictus, because of data averaging over the acquisition period. The possibility of a patient, particularly an inpatient who is undergoing evaluation while off or on reduced levels of anticonvulsant medication, having a seizure during the study underscores the importance of performing video EEG monitoring throughout the study. The longer the seizure and the earlier it occurs in the uptake period, the more likely a focus will be demonstrated. However, a note of caution: post-ictal glucose hypometabolism can be confused with ictal hypometabolism in patients who have periscan seizures. We have seen extensive hemispheric glucose hypometabolism 22 hours after a secondary generalized seizure in a child where the FDG PET scan overestimated the area of abnormality (see Fig. 4). The patient was a 32-month-old girl with refractory epilepsy from age 6 months. Multiple combinations of anticonvulsant medication had been tried, to no avail. The child was becoming mildly retarded. Seizures were preceded by anxiety, often a cry, then eye deviation to left, flexion of both upper limbs followed by extension, and elevation of the left arm and leg. The second FDG PET was done 3 months later because of the extensive abnormality found on the first study and the concern that some of the glucose hypometabolism may have been a post-ictal phenomenon. Before the second study, the child had been seizure-free for 1 week. We have altered our practice since this study and now do not perform PET studies within 24 hours of a secondary generalized or grand mal seizure.

There is limited experience with FDG PET in status epilepticus but we have found PET useful in delineating the epileptic focus, which may allow surgery to be performed in this potentially life-threatening illness. The ictal FDG PET of a 54-year-old man is shown in Figure 5 . He developed seizures 20 years after sustaining a right parietal subdural hematoma and brain abscess. After resolution of the abscess, the patient experienced occasional focal and generalized seizures. Three weeks before PET he was admitted with fever and confusion. Ten days after admission an EEG revealed complex partial status epilepticus. An ictal SPECT scan (not shown) revealed increased perfusion anterior to the patient's porencephalic cyst. Following the FDG PET, surgery was sucessfully performed to sever the association fibers in the right occipital cortex and parietal lobes.

Ictal SPECT

During a seizure, there is up to a 300% increase in regional cerebral blood flow (rCBF). This was first observed in humans with ^{133}Xe clearance techniques,[50] but this method is impractical for routine use. Ictal hyperperfusion using

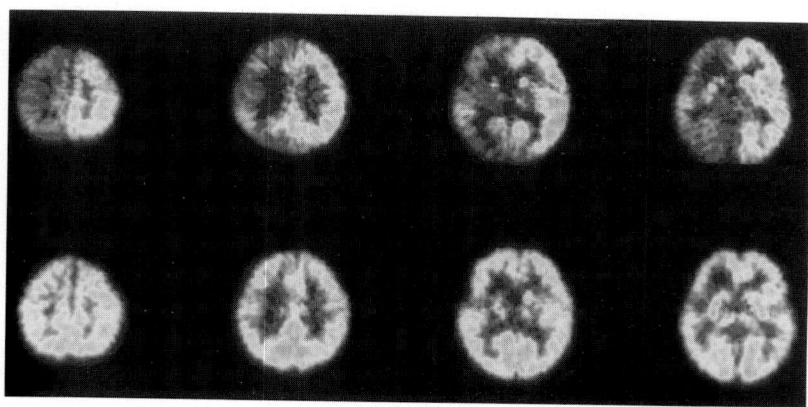

Figure 4. A 32-month-old child with refractory epilepsy. First FDG PET scan (top row) shows right hemispheric glucose hypometabolism suggesting an extensive interictal abnormality. Second study (bottom row) shows almost complete reversal of previous hemispheric hypometabolism except for reduced glucose utilization in right mid frontal lobe, indicating that most of the hypometabolism on first study was postictal. (See Plate 11.)

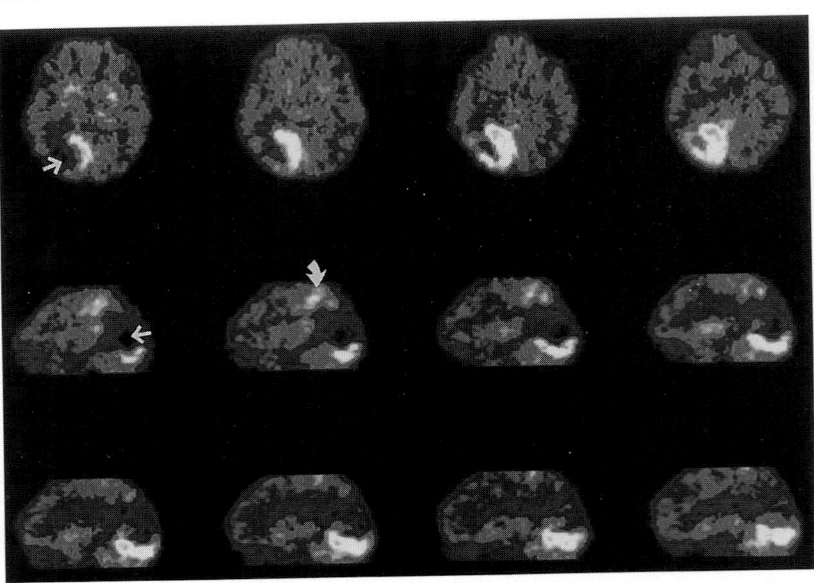

Figure 5. A 54-year-old man with complex partial status epilepticus. Transaxial (top row) and sagittal (middle and bottom rows) FDG PET images reveal glucose hypermetabolism in right mesial and infero-lateral occipital cortex. Glucose hypermetabolism is posterior and inferior to large ametabolic region (straight arrows) in right parieto-occipital lobe, the site of the previous trauma and brain abscess. Increased glucose metabolism (curved arrow) is also seen anterior to porencephalic cyst, but it is much less marked than in occipital lobe. Note: There is also a marked reduction in glucose metabolism throughout rest of the brain. (See Plate 12.)

SPECT and ^{123}I-iodoamphetamine in humans was first described in 1982.[51,52]

Since then, the use of ictal SPECT imaging in Comprehensive Epilepsy programs has become commonplace, notwithstanding the logistical difficulties of ictal tracer injections. The high first-pass extraction and prolonged retention of HMPAO, which allows for delayed imaging, has resulted in the widespread use of HMPAO as the preferred tracer for defining the epileptic focus. Training is required to rapidly reconstitute the tracer at the bedside to ensure that the ictus is captured; the timing of injection of the tracer is critical to the interpretation of the ictal studies. It is generally agreed that the tracer must be injected during the seizure or within 30 seconds of its completion. This method is very sensitive (83 to 95%) in detecting seizure foci.[53,54]

A visual side-to-side comparison is used to interpret images (i.e., left temporal vs. right temporal lobe). A typical example is shown in Figure 6, where the functional imaging studies are registered to the anatomical images. The scans are of a 31-year-old woman with complex partial seizures. Her seizures were preceded by nausea and an aura of impending events, whereupon witnesses reported the patient would stare blankly sometimes associated with facial grimacing and chewing movements that usually lasted 1 to 2 minutes. After the seizure the patient was confused and drowsy. The seizures were unresponsive to conventional anticonvulsant medication. Surface EEG showed a left temporal lobe seizure focus.

Generally, ictal SPECT interpretation is straightforward, as Figure 6 demonstrates. However, the distribution of hyperperfusion within the temporal lobe is variable. It may involve the entire temporal lobe or only the inferior or mesial structures. There can also be increased perfusion in the ipsilateral thalamus and basal ganglia when there is a motor accompaniment to the seizure, such as dystonic posturing of the arm.[55]

It should be emphasized that if the tracer injection is delayed, the changes detected with SPECT are more difficult to interpret. In the immediate post-ictal period, rCBF is reduced to a greater extent than is seen interictally and the onset, duration, and extent of this post-ictal depression varies from patient to patient. Policies for the incorporation of the ictal SPECT into the presurgical workup of patients with refractory epilepsy vary from institution to institution. However, an important principle is congruence of results. If all data, clinical, imaging, and ictal video EEG, point to one site and side then the matter is straightforward, but lack of congruence, in our experience, indicates the need for invasive monitoring.

Interictal SPECT

In the interictal period, rCBF and metabolism may be normal or reduced. Interictal SPECT has a sensitivity of 40 to 58% with a positive predictive value of 80 to 87% for partial seizures,[9] but it is the authors' impression that the detection of interictal hypoperfusion with HMPAO SPECT is improved with multidetector SPECT systems. As for FDG PET, the mechanism for reduced rCBF is unexplained and the region involved is more extensive than the pathological abnormalities found in resected specimens.

Other PET and SPECT Ligands

Unfortunately, a ligand that identifies the actual epileptic locus has yet to be developed and it remains the "holy grail" of neuroimaging in epilepsy. A number of ligands have been used to aid in seizure localization and, although some appear encouraging, none yet appear completely satisfactory.[56,57] The gamma-aminobutyric acid (GABA)/benzodiazepine-chloride ionophore complex is considered important in the genesis of epilepsy, and the selective reduction of GABA receptor density in human epileptic foci has been re-

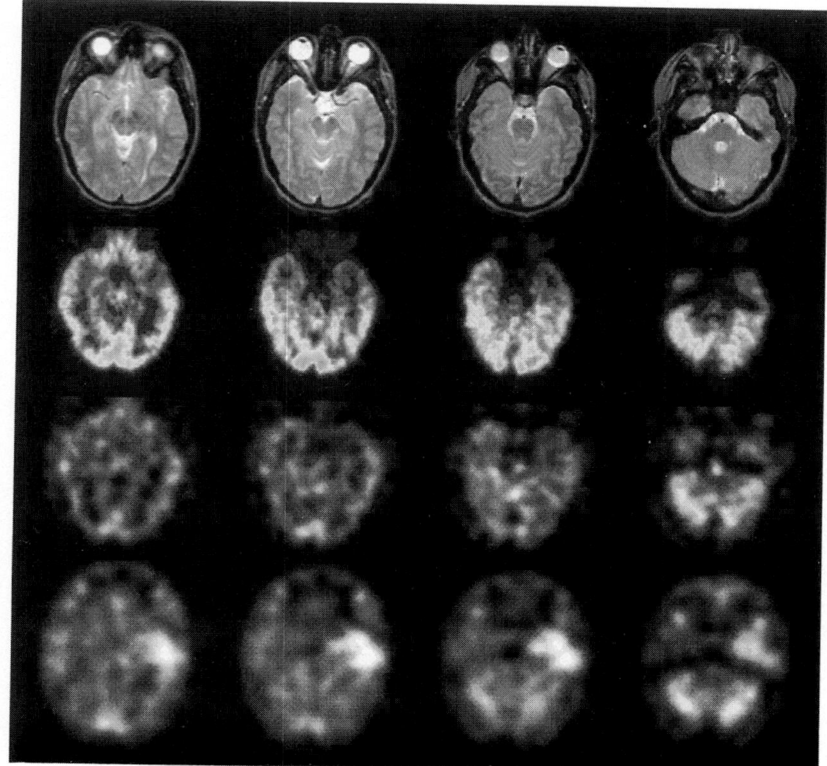

A

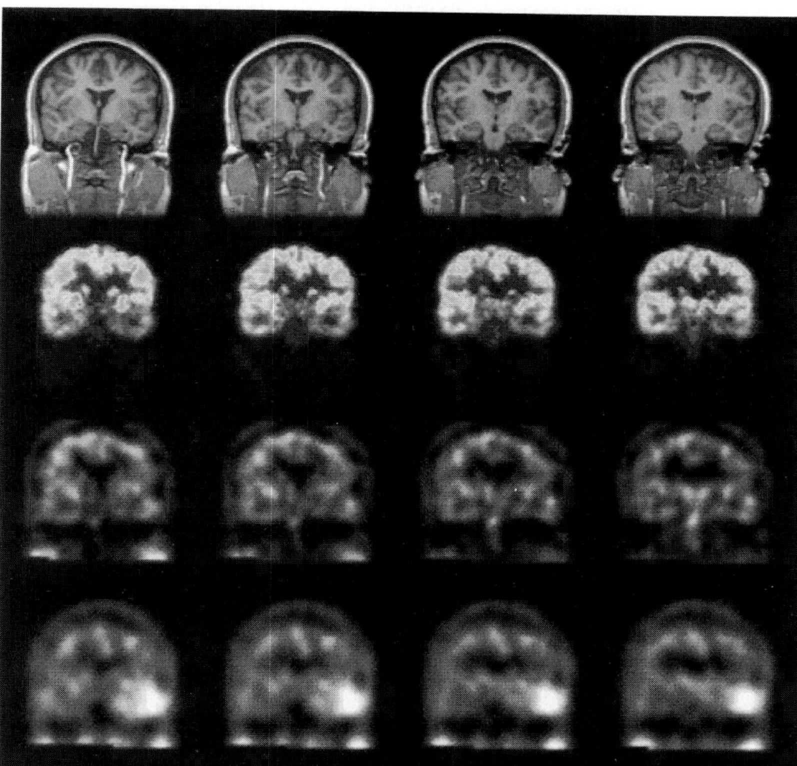

B

Figure 6. A 31-year-old woman with complex partial seizures. Multimodality registration of **(A)** transaxial and **(B)** coronal anatomical and functional images. Functional images are registered to MR dataset performed at 1.5 Tesla. **(A).** Transaxial T2-weighted MR images (top row) show slight left temporal lobe atrophy with prominence of left sylvian fissure; left hippocampal atrophy is not evident. FDG PET (second row) reveals glucose hypometabolism of left temporal lobe affecting mesial and lateral temporal neocortex. Interictal HMPAO SPECT (third row) shows mild left temporal lobe hypoperfusion. Ictal SPECT (fourth row) shows a marked increase in left temporal (mesial and lateral) perfusion maximal in inferior and mid temporal lobe. **(B).** Coronal images. T1-weighted MR images show subtle left to right temporal lobe asymmetry. On FDG PET hypometabolism affects inferomedial temporal lobe maximally. Asymmetric perfusion is difficult to appreciate on interictal SPECT but is clearly evident on ictal SPECT study, with markedly increased perfusion (lateral temporal neocortex > mesial). (See Plate 13.)

ported.[58,59] The peripheral benzodiazepine receptor ligands ^{11}C-flumazenil and ^{11}C-PK 11195 seem to bind to a smaller area than the area of glucose hypometabolism demonstrated in the same patients with FDG PET.[57] The iodinated derivative of flumazenil, ^{123}I-iomazenil, has been used with SPECT but preliminary data do not suggest that it is markedly better than interictal HMPAO SPECT for seizure localization.[60,61]

Opioid peptides that appear to have a role in post-ictal seizure inhibition rather than seizure initiation and propagation,[62,63] have been investigated with ^{11}C-carfentanil.[56] ^{11}C-carfentanil binds with high affinity to *mu*-opiate receptors and has much lower affinity for *delta*- and *kappa*-opiate receptors. In patients with partial epilepsy and a unilateral temporal lobe focus, Frost et al. showed that receptor binding is increased in the temporal cortex on the side of the seizure focus.[56] Recently, preliminary data showing reduced binding of ^{123}I-iododexetimide in the anterior hippocampus ipsilateral to the seizure focus of 4 patients with complex partial seizures, using SPECT, were reported.[64] However, these data require confirmation in a larger series of patients to determine ^{123}I-iododexetimide's real efficacy.

Extratemporal Lobe Epilepsy

The localization of partial seizures that originate outside the temporal lobe is a more difficult task, and further studies are needed to determine the role of functional neuroimaging in this situation. Interictal glucose hypometabolism, typically expected in temporal lobe epilepsy, is an uncommon finding in extratemporal lobe epilepsy unless a structural lesion is identified on anatomic imaging. There are limited data, but 3 patterns of glucose metabolism are reported with FDG PET: (1) normal glucose utilization; (2) focal areas of hypometabolism with clear margins from surrounding normal tissue, often associated with a structural lesion on anatomical imaging; (3) diffuse areas of reduced glucose utilization with a graded transition to surrounding cortex which may be unilateral or bilateral.[65] Ictal SPECT studies are similarly limited, but focal hyperperfusion may help guide the placement of grid or depth electrodes.[53,66,67] In the absence of a structural lesion, most centers would require depth or grid recordings in addition to focal hypometabolism on FDG PET or focal hyperperfusion on HMPAO SPECT prior to surgical resection. Functional and anatomic image superimposition and volumetric analyses with MR imaging may provide an additional aid to the evaluation of these cases.

BRAIN TUMORS

Major issues in the evaluation of patients with brain tumors include: (1) Grade of the tumor, is it a high- or low-grade glioma? Patient outcome and therapeutic options are determined largely by the histological grade. (2) How far does the tumor extend into surrounding neural tissue? (3) Is the tumor heterogeneous? Does it contain low- and high-grade cellular components that may affect pathologic classification, depending on the surgical tissue available to the pathologist? It is accepted that histologic grading based on small tissue samples provided by limited neurosurgical procedures is fraught with problems due to sampling error. (4) If a brain tumor patient deteriorates after surgery, radiation, and chemotherapy, is the deterioration due to recurrent tumor or is it because of the effects of treatment? (5) What is the best method to determine response or lack of response to new treatments?

In many institutions, surgical/radiation oncology planning and longitudinal follow-up of patients is based on anatomic (CT, MR) imaging before and after contrast agents. The presence of contrast enhancement in a mass lesion prior to and after treatment is usually accepted as indicating a high-grade tumor. Lack of contrast enhancement is generally regarded as indicating a low-grade lesion. Various pathologic classifications have been used for gliomas and, for practical purposes, the 3-tiered system of low-grade astrocytoma, anaplastic astrocytoma, and glioblastoma multiforme (GBM), initially proposed by Ringertz[68] has been adopted by several cooperative brain tumor groups.[69,70]

PET

In the research environment, PET using a variety of ligands has provided insights into many aspects of brain tumor biology, from glucose and oxygen metabolism, to blood flow, pH, status of the blood-brain barrier, amino acid uptake, presence/concentration of receptors, and pharmacokinetics of delivery of chemotherapeutic agents. However, to answer practical issues of patient management, the majority of work has been performed with FDG PET.[71–74] The application of the FDG PET method to brain tumors is based on the work of Warburg who demonstrated that "anaerobic glycolysis" increases with increasing grade or malignancy of tumors.[75,76]

FDG PET provides a noninvasive means of preoperative tumor grading on the basis of glucose utilization relative to normal white matter. High-grade tumors (anaplastic astrocytomas and GBMs) have markedly increased glucose utilization while low-grade tumors have reduced glucose metabolism. Figure 7 shows FDG PET in a 47-year-old woman with a low-grade astrocytoma. The patient had a CT scan performed because of unaccustomed headache 12 months earlier. CT revealed a hypodense area in the right frontal lobe. The headaches subsided with antimigrainous therapy and a PET scan was ordered to determine the grade of the presumed tumor. The lesion was later biopsied and proven to be a low-grade astrocytoma. Figure 8 shows the typical appearance of a hypermetabolic bifrontal "butterfly" malignant glioma. The patient was a 44-year-old man with a short history of severe unaccustomed headache and complex partial seizures. The images are scaled to the maximum pixel count in the image set, so that the surrounding brain appears

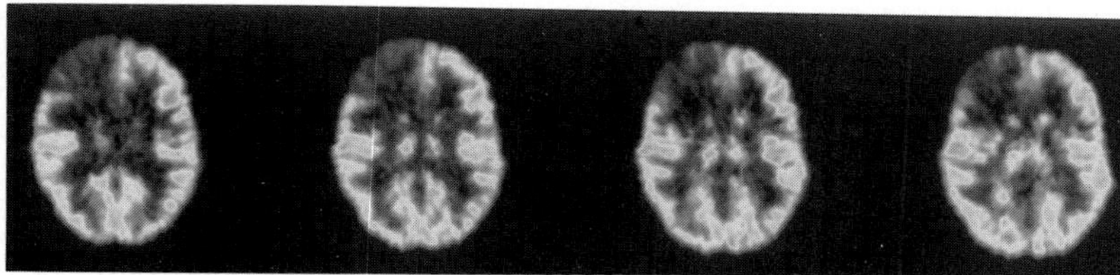

Figure 7. A 47-year-old woman with a low-grade glioma. Transaxial FDG PET scan shows an extensive area of glucose hypometabolism in right frontal lobe that affects white and gray matter. There are no foci of increased glucose metabolism to suggest a high-grade tumor. (See Plate 14.)

relatively hypometabolic, but it is only an artifact of the image scaling.

For the quantitative analysis of brain tumor metabolism our practice is to measure glucose metabolism in the most metabolically active region of the tumor and, then, to compare the tumoral glucose utilization to that of normal glia. The white matter of the centrum semi-ovale is used as the reference because it contains glia and the axons of afferent and efferent neurons. Because in neurons the bulk of glucose utilization is located in synaptic terminals[20] and, to a lesser extent, cell soma, white matter glucose utilization mainly reflects glial metabolism. FDG PET cannot distinguish between anaplastic astrocytomas and GBMs unless there is central ametabolism in the lesion indicating necrosis, which is a characteristic finding in GBMs. The highest glucose utilization we have seen in a tumor was in a GBM; however, the amount of glucose utilization in these tumors is extremely variable. If the tumor is growing so rapidly that it outgrows its blood supply there may be only a thin rim of active tumor surrounding a central region of necrosis. Glucose utilization in this rim is always greater than in white matter but may not be greater than normal contralateral cerebral cortex; PET underestimates true glucose utilization because of partial volume effects.

In the early postoperative period FDG PET can detect residual tumor bulk[77] that can be utilized for targeted radiosurgery or brachytherapy protocols. Patients with low-grade gliomas can remain asymptomatic for many years but, in a significant number of such patients, the tumor undergoes malignant degeneration which FDG PET is able to detect[78] earlier than structural imaging. Figure 9 shows malignant degeneration in a low-grade astroctyoma in a 51-year-old man who presented with a generalized tonic-clonic seizure 5 years earlier. At the time of the scan, seizures were controlled by anticonvulsant medication and he was asymptomatic. The tumor was located in the sensorimotor cortex and the focus of malignant degeneration was deep in the white matter. CT scan was unchanged. Despite the FDG PET findings, it was decided to observe the patient. Ten months later he developed right arm weakness and, on the second study, the focus of glucose hypermetabolism was much larger. Biopsy revealed a glioblastoma multiforme. In our opinion, FDG PET should be included in the routine follow-up imaging strategy for these patients.[74]

Clinical deterioration in a brain tumor patient months or years after treatment is generally due to tumor recurrence. Structural imaging usually reveals a mass lesion with surrounding edema and marked enhancement after injection of contrast media. Unfortunately, radiation and chemonecrosis have clinical and radiological pictures identical to that of

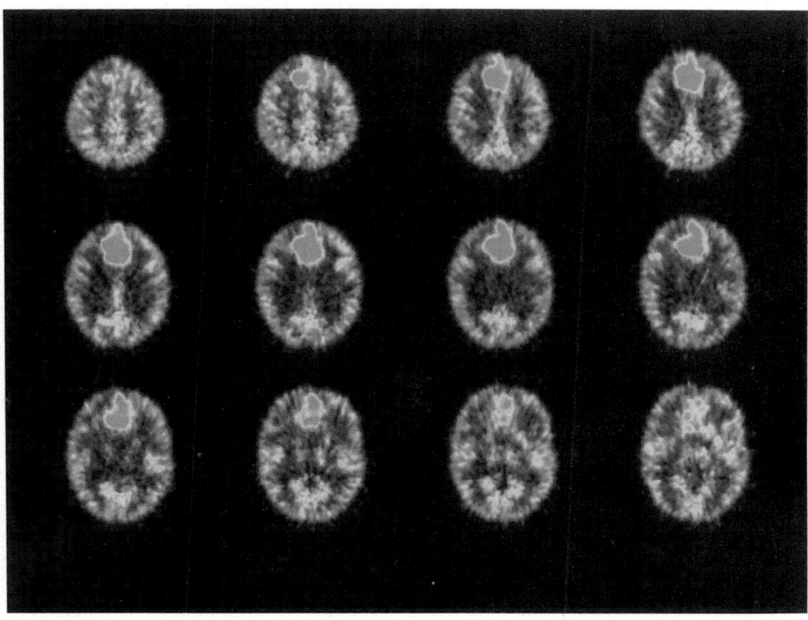

Figure 8. A 44-year-old man with a high-grade glioma. On transaxial FDG PET images, the tumor is markedly hypermetabolic and involves the corpus callosum and cortex and white matter of both mesial frontal lobes. (See Plate 15.)

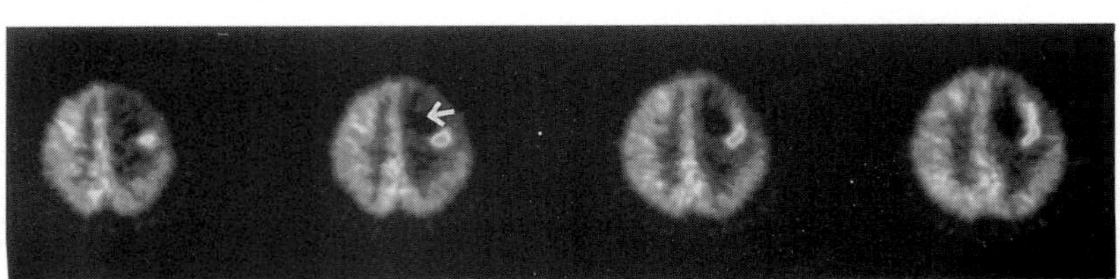

A

B

Figure 9. A 51-year-old man with malignant degeneration of a low-grade glioma. **(A).** Transaxial (top) and sagittal (bottom) FDG PET scans show a large area of hypometabolism in the left sensorimotor cortex with a deep focus (best seen on sagittal images) of markedly increased glucose metabolism consistent with malignant degeneration. **(B).** Transaxial FDG PET images 12 months later show the hypermetabolic lesion is more extensive and curves around a hypometabolic necrotic center (arrow) typical of a glioblastoma multiforme. (See Plate 16.)

recurrent tumor. However, FDG PET is able to separate recurrent hypermetabolic tumor from hypometabolic radiation or chemonecrosis. Figure 10 is a 48-year-old man with a parietal anaplastic astrocytoma that was diagnosed 5 years previously. He was treated with surgical resection, external beam radiotherapy (55 Gy), followed by a radiosurgery boost. He remained well until 4 months prior to PET, when he developed focal seizures, expressive aphasia, and right-sided weakness. CT showed a hypodense mass in the left parietal lobe with surrounding edema, contrast enhancement, and also calcification. FDG PET was ordered to determine if there was recurrent tumor. The extensive glucose hypometabolism seen on this scan was a combination of radiation necrosis and cerebral edema. The patient was taking 16 mg of dexamethasone, which has an additional negative effect on glucose metabolism. We recently reported the reduction of glucose metabolism secondary to corticosteroid therapy in a large group of brain-tumor patients. Patients who were cushingoid from corticosteroid therapy used in their management had markedly reduced glucose metabolism in the uninvolved hemisphere when compared to normal volunteers and other brain tumor patients who were not taking corticosteroids. Finally, FDG PET clearly documents tumor response or resistance to therapies; an example is illustrated in Figure 11.

Other Tumors

CEREBRAL METASTASES

MR imaging and thin-section CT are the imaging tools of choice for the detection of cerebral metastases because they have high resolution and sensitivity. In FDG PET neurological studies, the contrast between normal brain and a small hypermetabolic metastasis is poor because of normal brain glucose avidity. Lesions of 2 to 3 mm may be missed unless there is marked cerebral edema.

JUVENILE PILOCYTIC ASTROCYTOMAS

Juvenile pilocytic astrocytomas (JPAs) are regarded as low-grade brain tumors with a good prognosis. They occur in a younger age group than astrocytomas and are most

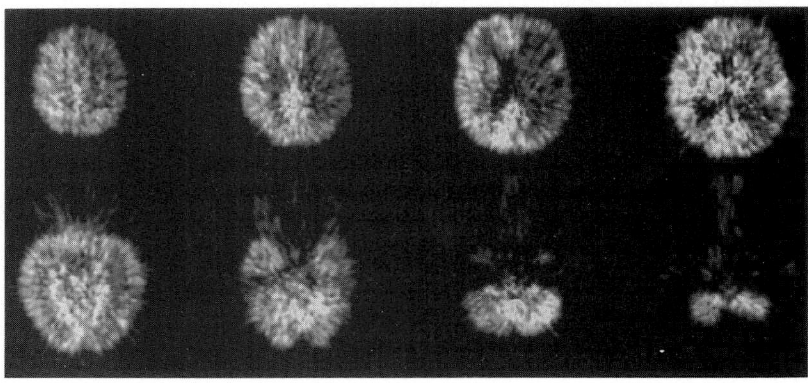

Figure 10. A 48-year-old man with an anaplastic astrocytoma of the left parietal lobe. Transaxial FDG PET scan shows extensive left fronto-parietal glucose hypometabolism without foci of glucose hypermetabolism to suggest recurrent tumor. In addition, there is a generalized reduction in cerebral glucose metabolism due to the effects of steroids. Left basal ganglia are hypometabolic and there is right crossed cerebellar diaschisis. (See Plate 17.)

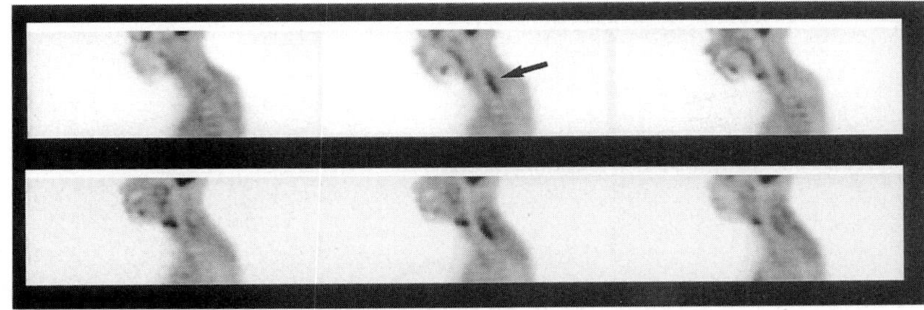

Figure 11. A 17-year-old woman with primitive neuroectodermal tumor of the cervical cord. Before chemotherapy and biopsy, sagittal FDG whole-body PET images (top row) show a hypermetabolic focus in mid cervical cord (black arrow). After chemotherapy (bottom row), there is little change in glucose utilization in the cervical cord lesion, consistent with poor response. (See Plate 18.)

commonly seen in midline cerebellum and hypothalamus, less frequently in the optic nerves and brainstem and, when found in the cerebral hemispheres, they usually occur in the temporal lobes.[79] However, we recently reported functional and structural imaging (CT and MR) results in 5 patients with JPAs where glucose metabolism in JPAs was significantly higher than in the low-grade astrocytomas and was similar to anaplastic astrocytomas.[80] All the tumors enhanced avidly after iodinated or paramagnetic contrast agents but there was little surrounding cerebral edema. In our experience, these data suggest that the prognosis for JPAs was not benign.[71,81] These results provoked a number of important questions: (1) Had we identified a subset of patients with JPAs whose tumors behave aggressively? (2) Conversely, did our data cast doubts on the value of FDG PET assessment of brain tumors and violate the general principles used in this evaluation (i.e., low-grade tumors are hypometabolic and high-grade tumors are hypermetabolic)? or (3) Did these data reveal an important exception to these principles and reflect a biological peculiarity in pilocytic tumors?

Our results indicated that all patients were stable and had no evidence of disease progression after a long follow-up period, despite the high tumoral glucose metabolism, and contrast enhancement on anatomic imaging indicating that these tumors were behaving in a benign fashion. However, it is apparent that JPAs are enigmatic tumors: (1) Although regarded as benign, they may undergo malignant degeneration and metastasize many years after the original diagnosis.[82–86] (2) High proliferative indices, using Ki-67 labeling, and chromosomal abnormalities that are usually seen in high-grade tumors have been reported for JPAs.[87–90] (3) JPAs would be incorrectly classified as aggressive tumors by a new glioma pathological grading system, based on morphological criteria, which correlates well with clinical outcome.[91] (4) JPA blood vessels have poorly developed tight junctions in their vascular endothelium, which explains the intense enhancement on structural imaging studies, but these are also usually found in malignant tumors.[92,93] Although the mechanism for the paradoxical increase in glucose utilization in these tumors is unexplained, we speculated that it was related to expression of the glucose transporter.[94–97] We believe that it is important to recognize that the combination of intense gadolinium enhancement on MR in a hypermetabolic tumor with little surrounding cerebral edema, in a younger patient, in the appropriate anatomical location does not always signify a high-grade tumor and pathological confirmation is needed for accurate prognosis.

SPINAL CORD TUMORS

The recent introduction of PET tomographs with wide apertures allows functional imaging of the spinal cord. Although there are few data on the role of FDG PET in the evaluation of spinal cord tumors, PET may allow the noninvasive grading of spinal tumors and also may be used to assess response to therapy and detect radiation necrosis. Figure 11 shows a spinal cord tumor in a 17-year-old woman before and after partially successful chemotherapy. The patient had a cervical intramedullary primitive neuroectodermal tumor. She initially presented 3 months prior to admission with sensory symptoms in the right arm and then the right leg. In the 2 weeks prior to admission, there was rapid deterioration with quadriparesis and sphincter disturbance. The second PET scan indicated a minimal response to an investigational chemotherapy regimen.

Other PET Ligands

Oxygen metabolism has been studied in gliomas. It has been shown that gliomas extract a lower fraction of oxygen than normal brain, suggesting that they are adequately oxygenated.[98] PET also demonstrated, surprisingly, that the pH of brain tumors was more alkaline than that of normal brain.[99] This was later confirmed with phosphorous MR spectroscopy.[100] The assessment of tumoral protein synthesis has been attempted with a number of amino acids. The largest experience has been obtained with ^{11}C-methionine. Its mechanism of uptake seems to be related mainly to a saturable process (capillary transport) rather than to increased amino acid requirements for protein synthesis. ^{11}C-methionine appears to be useful in defining the extent of tumors, but it cannot reliably separate low- from high-grade gliomas or recurrent tumor from radiation necrosis.[101,102] Other tracers (putrescine, tyrosine, pyruvate) have been proposed and tested, mostly in small series of patients; their use has not become widespread. Recently, attention has focused on imaging glioma peripheral benzodiazepine receptors (PBZ). Experimental evidence suggests that benzodiazepines may regulate glial cell proliferation via the PBZ.[103] PBZ ligands Ro5-4864 and PK 11195 have been labeled with ^{11}C. ^{11}C-

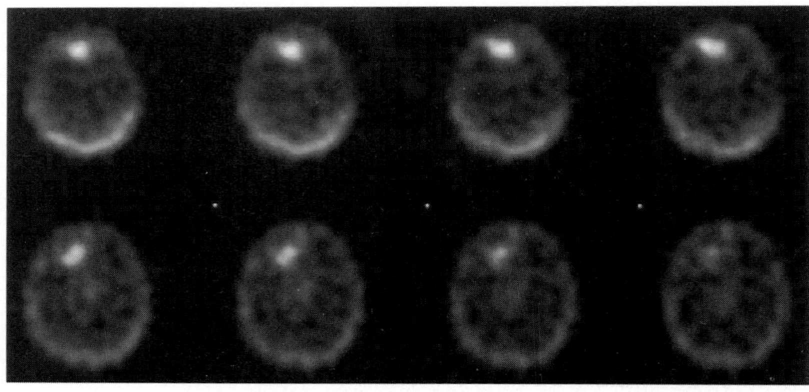
A

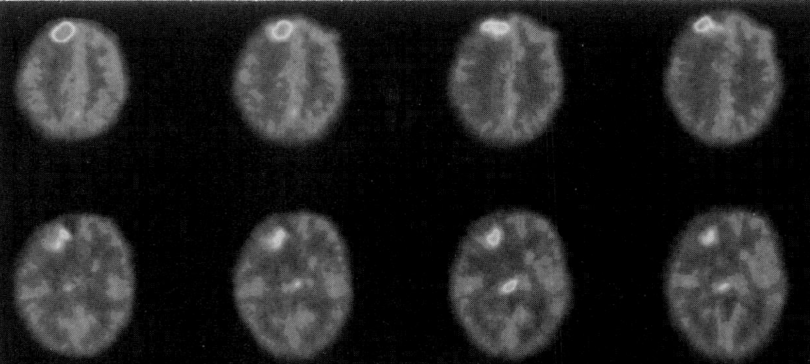
B

Figure 12. A 35-year-old woman with a right frontal anaplastic astrocytoma. **(A).** Thallium SPECT images show a large superficial focus of increased tracer uptake in the right frontal lobe. **(B).** Transaxial FDG PET images show the right frontal lesion is markedly hypermetabolic, consistent with recurrent tumor. In addition, another focus is seen in the right thalamus. The extension into the right thalamus was not detected with thallium SPECT. (See Plate 19.)

PK 11195 binds to human gliomas,[104] but specific binding to astrocytomas was not found with ^{11}CRo5-4864.[105]

SPECT

A number of SPECT radiotracers have been used in the evaluation of brain tumors.[106] Brain scintigraphy with ^{99m}Tc-pertechnetate was the single imaging technique for brain tumors prior to the advent of CT in the mid-1970s and perfusion agents such as IMP and HMPAO have been evaluated, but these ligands are generally not used for clinical management of patients with brain tumors.

Thallium-201 (^{201}Tl) and ^{123}I-IMT are used in a number of centers in patients with brain tumors. Thallium-201 is a K^+ analog with a high affinity for Na^+-K^+ ATPase and it has a slow cellular washout. The mechanism of ^{201}Tl uptake is uncertain, but it requires a disrupted blood-brain barrier to enter the central nervous system and uptake is also related to cotransport systems and facilitated diffusion, as well as Na^+-K^+ ATPase.[107–109] Kim et al.[110] concluded that ^{201}Tl was useful in separating high- from low-grade gliomas and Schwartz et al.[111] deduced that ^{201}Tl in combination with HMPAO SPECT could differentiate recurrent tumor from radiation necrosis. Thallium-201 SPECT and FDG PET images in a 35-year-old woman with an anaplastic astrocytoma are shown in Figure 12. The tumor was excised from the left frontal lobe after which she had postoperative radiotherapy (55 Gy). She re-presented 2 years later with headache. Anatomic imaging showed a right frontal mass, with mass effect, that enhanced avidly. Functional imaging was performed to differentiate recurrent tumor from radiation necrosis. The main problem with ^{201}Tl is illustrated in this patient; that is, poor resolution. ^{201}Tl SPECT missed the right thalamic extension that was clearly visible on PET and MR imaging. In addition, there is also evidence that ^{201}Tl is taken up in bacterial and fungal brain abscesses.[112,113] IMT appears to behave in a fashion similar to ^{11}C-methionine and, while there is avid IMT uptake into gliomas (even in tumors where there is no disruption of the BBB), preliminary evidence suggests that it cannot be used to grade gliomas.[106,114,115]

Cerebellar diaschisis

"Crossed" cerebellar diaschisis is an interesting physiologic phenomenon commonly seen with functional imaging modalities in patients with brain tumors and stroke. It refers to a reduction in blood flow and glucose metabolism in the cerebellar hemisphere contralateral, hence "crossed," to a supratentorial lesion. The term diaschisis was first introduced by Von Monakow in 1910 and his concept was that of a ". . . state of reduced or abolished function . . . after a brain injury and acting on a neural region remote from the lesion."[116,117] Diaschisis was first imaged in 1980 when Baron et al. used the term "cerebellar diaschisis" to denote the reduction in contralateral cerebellar hemisphere blood flow and oxygen utilization that they observed, using ^{15}O-PET, in patients with supratentorial infarction.[118] Their observation was confirmed by others and extended to cases of cerebral

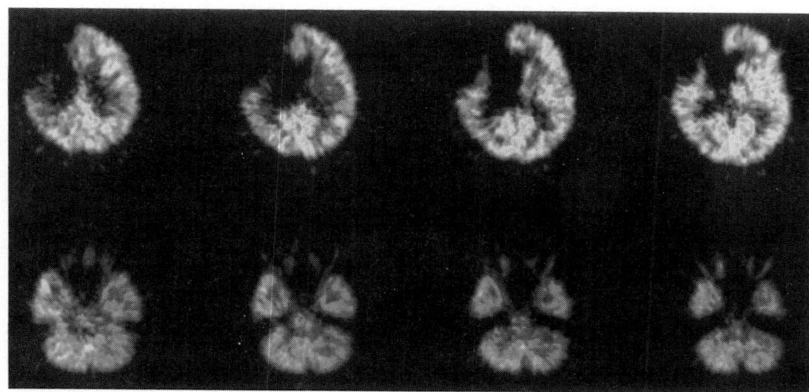

Figure 13. A 35-year-old man with unsuccessful right frontal lobectomy for refractory complex partial seizures. Transaxial FDG PET images show a large ametabolic right frontal lobe defect consistent with a frontal lobectomy. Left cerebellar hemisphere is relatively hypometabolic when compared to right. In addition, there is left temporal lobe glucose hypometabolism. (See Plate 20.)

glioma for both blood flow, using ^{15}O-PET, and for glucose utilization with FDG PET.[119–122] Crossed cerebellar diaschisis is also observed with ^{133}Xe and HMPAO SPECT.[123,124] The mechanism for this phenomenon appears to be interruption of the corticopontocerebellar (CPC) pathway. The CPC arises from all lobes of the cerebral hemispheres but with major inputs from prefrontal cortex, sensorimotor cortex, and occipital lobes.[118,127] The CPC has its first synapse in the pons and then second order neurons cross to the contralateral cerebellar hemisphere via the middle cerebellar peduncle to terminate in the cerebellar cortex. We recently demonstrated with FDG PET that there is ipsilateral pontine glucose hypometabolism in cerebellar diaschisis consistent with this hypothesis and, also, that there is relative preservation of glucose metabolism in the dentate nucleus of the hypometabolic cerebellar hemisphere.[122] A typical example is seen in Figure 13 in a 35-year-old man with refractory epilepsy who had an unsuccessful right frontal lobectomy in an attempt to control his seizures. Cerebellar diaschisis does not appear to have a clinical accompaniment and can be seen with any supratentorial injury, be it tumor, stroke, or trauma. Its time course is variable.[125] Reversibility has been noted in stroke but, with the fixed deficit induced by a tumor and probable permanent damage to the CPC, cerebellar diaschisis is persistent.

DEMENTIA

Accurate diagnosis is the most important issue in evaluating adults who present with progressive intellectual deterioration. Treatable causes of dementia, which comprise 20% of most series, should be excluded.[126,127] Thereafter, the most frequent causes of dementia in adults are Alzheimer's disease and multi-infarct dementia.[128]

Alzheimer's Dementia

Patients with presumed Alzheimer's disease have been studied extensively with PET in many centers, both with FDG and the steady-state ^{15}O technique.[129,130] Decreased glucose metabolism and reduced regional cerebral blood flow (rCBF) and regional cerebral oxygen utilization (rCMRO$_2$) were seen in frontal, parietal, and temporal lobes of demented patients.[129,130] Patients with multi-infarct dementia have focal and wedge-shaped reductions in glucose metabolism, rCBF, and rCMRO$_2$, which are related to arterial territories.[131,132] Later studies showed: (1) A direct relationship between the severity and type of clinical symptoms and the degree and location of glucose hypometabolism. (2) Asymmetric reductions in glucose metabolism are common, particular early in the course of the disease. (3) As the disease progresses and clinical symptoms worsen, there is a corresponding decline in glucose utilization.[133–142] (4) The association cortex of the postero-superior parietal lobes often have reduced glucose metabolism early in the course of the disease, although the patient's primary complaint may be memory disturbance. Focal reductions in hippocampal glucose utilization in such patients have been difficult to detect, probably because of the small size of the hippocampi and the relatively poor in-plane resolution of many of the PET tomographs. (5) With disease progression, glucose metabolism is reduced in the occipital association cortex, the temporal lobes, and frontal lobes with relative sparing of the deep nuclei, primary visual cortex, sensorimotor cortex, and cerebellar hemispheres.[143] Similar findings are seen with perfusion SPECT.[144–150] Close correspondence between FDG PET and HMPAO SPECT studies in a 70-year-old woman who presented initially with expressive aphasia are shown in Figure 14. She presented 5 years prior to the PET scan with nonfluent aphasia and, in the intervening years, there was progressive deterioration and dementia. We perform quantitative measurements of glucose metabolism in all patients with suspected dementia. In addition, absolute measurement of glucose utilization can document the serial decline over time and provides a tool to evaluate potential therapies for Alzheimer's disease.

There has been debate regarding accuracy of measurements of glucose metabolism in patients with presumed Alzheimer's disease in the presence of cerebral atrophy. Undoubtedly, in patients with severe cerebral atrophy partial volume effects would result in an exaggerated reduction in

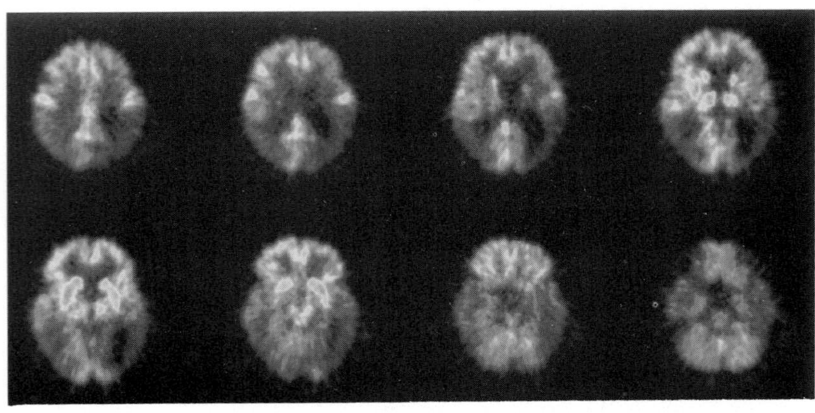
A

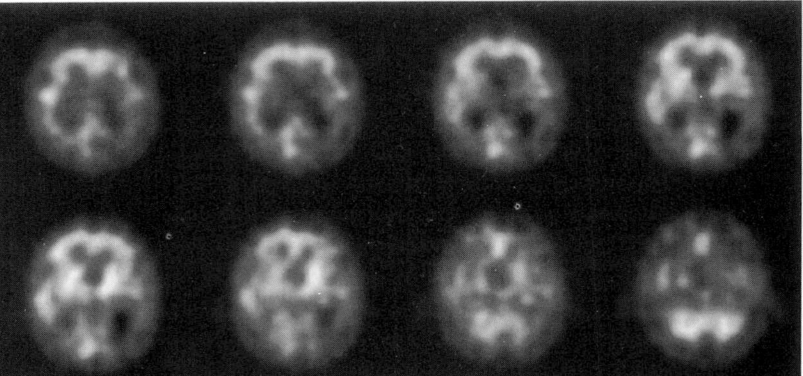
B

Figure 14. A 70-year-old woman with a 5-year history of progressive cognitive decline. **(A).** Transaxial FDG PET images show a marked bilateral reduction in parieto-temporal glucose metabolism. Occipital lobes, particularly association cortex, are also affected. Deep nuclei, inferior frontal lobes, sensorimotor cortices (top left images), and cerebellar hemispheres are relatively spared. **(B).** There is a close correspondence between reduced perfusion with HMPAO SPECT and FDG PET findings. (See Plate 21.)

glucose metabolism.[151] However, significant reductions in glucose metabolism are reported in mild cases of dementia where there is no structural evidence of cerebral atrophy, which suggests that reduced glucose metabolism is not a spurious finding.[135,141,142,152] An important question that has not yet been fully clarified is whether functional imaging can detect changes in cerebral glucose metabolism prior to the onset of clinical symptoms. A number of kindreds with autosomal dominant Familial Alzheimer's disease are currently being followed longitudinally with FDG PET.[153] The majority of patients are asymptomatic and are at risk of developing the disease. A preliminary report described a focal reduction in glucose metabolism in one of these asymptomatic patients.[154]

Non-Alzheimer-Type Dementias

FRONTAL LOBE DEMENTIAS

In recent years, there has been tremendous interest in subclassifying the dementia syndromes and, not surprisingly, it has accompanied recent developments in molecular biology. It is recognized that dementias are a heterogeneous group neuropathologically and, while Alzheimer's disease tends to affect temporoparietal and posterior cingulate regions, other less common dementias affect frontal, frontotemporal, and anterior cingulate regions.[155] In patients with frontal dementia, personality changes are early and progressive. Inappropriate and disinhibited behavior, lack of insight, and stereotyped speech are common. Preservation of spatial ability is a usual finding when compared to the spatial disorientation typically seen with nondominant parietal lobe involvement in Alzheimer's disease.[156] The organic dementias with prominent frontal lobe features include Pick's disease (or Pick's syndrome), frontal lobe dementia of non-Alzheimer type, motor neuron disease with dementia, progressive language disorder due to lobar atrophy, semantic dementia, and progressive aphasia.[155,157] The different patterns of involvement can be detected with SPECT and PET, but whether functional imaging can subclassify beyond a topographic pattern of involvement awaits further research.[156,158] Figure 15 illustrates a patient with frontal dementia who presented with a 1-year history of personality change characterized by disinhibition, impatience, irritability, and verbosity. He failed to respond to the usual medication for mania. MR imaging showed right mesial temporal lobe atrophy. Huntington's disease was considered because of caudate hypometabolism, despite the lack of chorea, but DNA testing was negative.

Few functional imaging findings have been reported in the transmissible spongiform encephalopathies characterized by Creutzfeldt-Jakob disease (CJD) and now referred to as human prion diseases.[159] CJD is a rapidly progressive dementia with myoclonus and is often accompanied by cerebellar ataxia, pyramidal, and extra-pyramidal involvement.

A 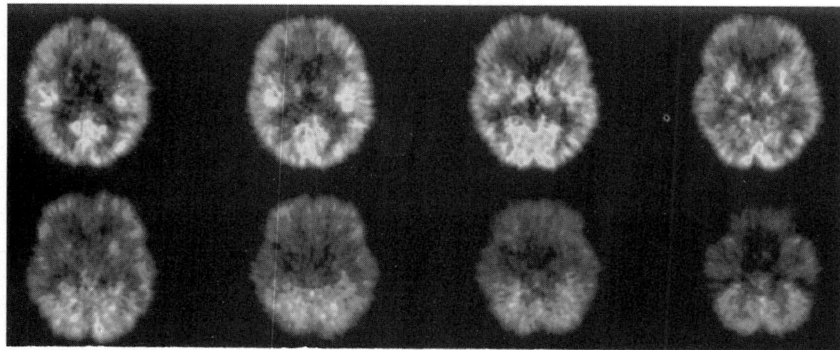

B 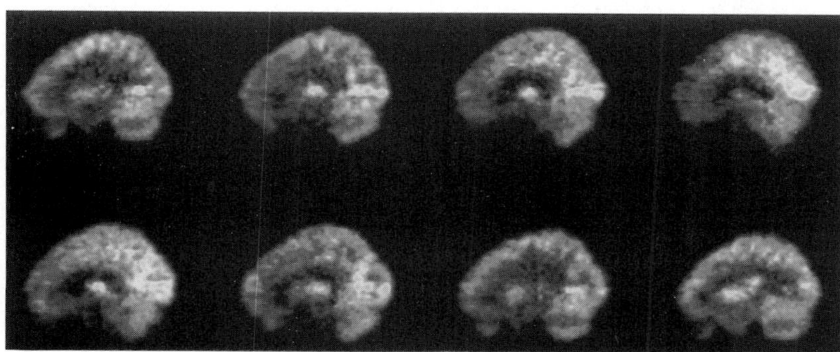

Figure 15. A 44-year-old man with frontal dementia. **(A).** Transaxial FDG PET images show marked glucose hypometabolism affecting both temporal and inferior frontal lobes with less severe involvement of superior frontal lobes. Basal ganglia are splayed laterally consistent with frontal lobe atrophy and caudate nuclei are markedly hypometabolic. There is relative sparing of primary visual cortex, precuneus, and posterior fossa structures. **(B).** Sagittal FDG PET emphasizes severe involvement of fronto-temporal lobes. (See Plate 22.)

Holtoff et al. reported a global, rather than focal, reduction in glucose metabolism with PET in a single patient.[160]

AIDS DEMENTIA

In AIDS-related dementia complex (ADC), FDG PET demonstrated a marked global, rather than focal, reduction in cerebral glucose metabolism that was reversed with AZT.[161] SPECT has also been reported to be sensitive for the detection of ADC[162–164] with multifocal areas of reduced cortical perfusion. As with FDG PET, perfusion SPECT may prove useful in evaluating the severity of dementia and the efficacy of newer therapies.

MOVEMENT DISORDERS

A number of the extrapyramidal movement disorders have been investigated with PET,[165] and the recent synthesis of ^{123}I-labeled compounds has allowed these disorders to be evaluated with SPECT.[166] In the main, movement disorders are diagnosed clinically and, with few exceptions, functional neuroimaging has provided insight into the pathophysiology and mechanisms of the disorders, rather than having improved diagnosis.

Parkinson's Disease

Idiopathic Parkinson's disease (PD) is characterized by tremor, bradykinesia, difficulty initiating and stopping movement, and rigidity.[167] It is due to degeneration of dopaminergic neurons in the pars compacta of the substantia nigra. Dopaminergic neurons represent <10% of striatal neurons; thus, it is not surprising that glucose metabolism, measured with FDG PET, is normal in the basal ganglia.[168,169] In 1984, Garnett et al. first reported PET findings using ^{18}F6-Fluorodopa (F-dopa) in patients with PD hemiparkinsonism,[170] and this heralded a decade of interest in this ligand and the dopaminergic system. F-dopa is taken up by dopaminergic neurons where it is decarboxylated to ^{18}F-dopamine, which is then stored and concentrated in terminal vesicles and, thus, reflects striatal dopamine storage capacity. In PD patients, F-dopa uptake is reduced in the putamen but normal in the caudate nuclei. The Hammersmith group have reported that the reduced striatal uptake of F-dopa correlates with degree of locomotor disability.[171,192] However, reduced putaminal F-dopa is not specific for PD and has been reported in neuroacanthocytosis, pallidopontonigral degeneration, and in Guamian patients with the motor neuron disease/parkinsonian-dementia complex.[173] Other PET ligands have been used to probe the biochemical defects in PD. ^{11}C-nomifensine binds to dopamine reuptake sites on nigro-striatal terminals in the striatum. Uptake in the striatum in PD is markedly reduced, suggesting that such patients are unable both to store dopamine and reaccumulate it after it is released. ^{11}C-Raclopride, a benzamide, binds to postsynaptic D2 receptors and increased binding to the striatum is reported in PD.[174] In Figure 16, F-dopa and ^{11}C-raclopride studies in a patient with PD show the differing distributions of these ligands. Preliminary SPECT studies using ^{123}I-iodo-

18F-6-Fluorodopa

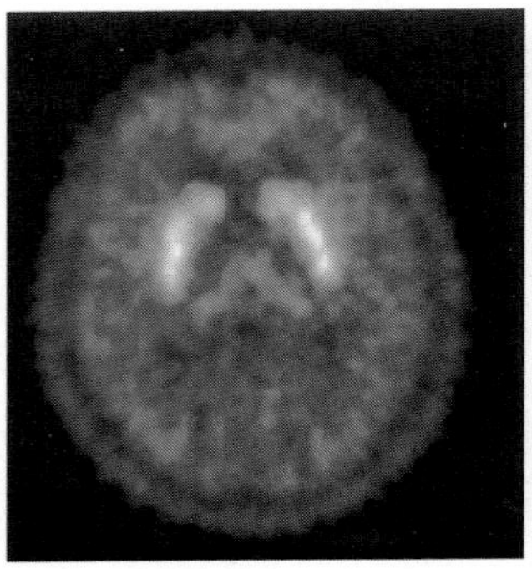

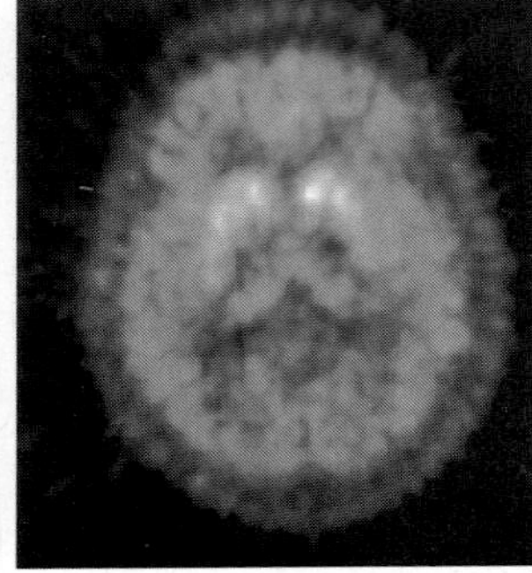

11C-Raclopride

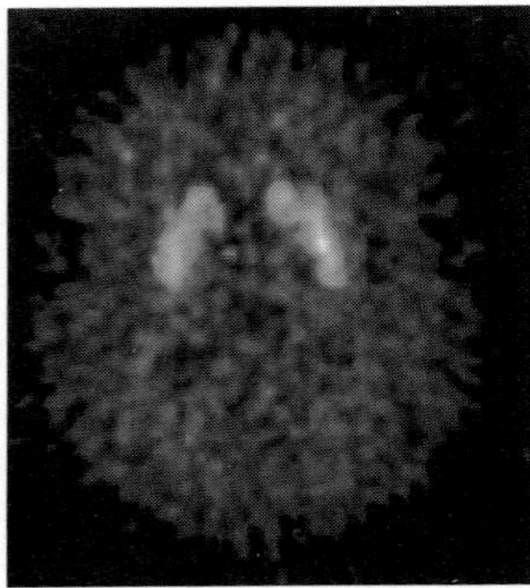

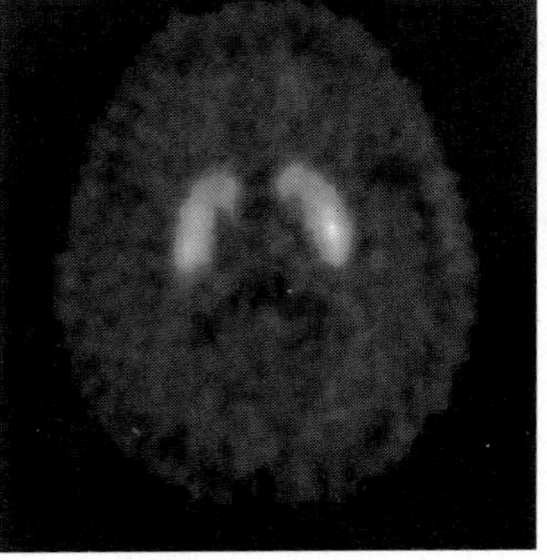

Figure 16. ^{18}F-6-fluorodopa (top) and ^{11}C-raclopride (bottom) PET scans in a normal volunteer (on left) and in a patient with Parkinson's disease (on right). Reduced putaminal F-dopa uptake and increased ^{11}C-raclopride uptake are seen in patient when compared to normal volunteer. (See Plate 23.)

benzamide (IBZM) have been reported,[175,176] and other studies are underway; at present, however, there is insufficient data to prescribe the role of IBZM in PD.

Multiple System Atrophy

Multiple system atrophy (MSA) is characterized by varying combinations of parkinsonism, cerebellar dysfunction, pyramidal signs, and autonomic failure.[177] It is sometimes difficult to distinguish patients with the striato-nigral type of MSA from those with PD because bradykinesia and rigidity are major features. However, unlike patients with PD, in patients with MSA there is generally a poor response to levodopa. MSA occurs, on average, a decade earlier than PD and it has a poorer prognosis. Early in the course of the disease, it can be difficult to distinguish MSA from patients with pure autonomic failure (PAF), who may have disabling autonomic failure but no neurological signs. However, MSA has characteristic functional imaging findings with FDG PET and [^{18}F]-6-F-dopa. Striatal uptake of F-dopa is more severely impaired in MSA than in Parkinson's disease and is normal in PAF,[172,178] and there is reduced glucose metabolism in the cerebellum, brainstem, frontal and motor cortices in patients with MSA when compared to PAF and PD.[172,177] In Figure 17, FDG PET scans of a 43-year-old woman with a 2-year history of rapidly progressive parkinsonism are shown. Her illness began with left hand tremor and bradykinesia that prevented her from playing the harp. She then developed severe postural hypotension, dysarthria, dysphagia, ataxia, and urinary incontinence. There was no response to antiparkinson medication.

Corticobasal Degeneration

Corticobasal degeneration (CBD) is characterized by focal frontal and parietal cortical atrophy together with atrophy of the basal ganglia and other subcortical nuclei.[179,180] The disease has an insidious onset dominated by asymmetric extrapyramidal and motor involvement, that includes upper limb apraxia, rigidity, myoclonus, dystonia, the alien limb sign, dysarthria, and a supranuclear disorder of eye movements. The condition is progressive and poorly responsive to antiparkinson medication and severe rigid immobility is the usual outcome 3 to 5 years after onset. Few neuroimaging reports are available and, although the clinical features are considered generally reliable, ultimate proof of the disorder remains neuropathologic. In suspected cases of CBD, Sawle et al. reported asymmetric ^{18}F-dopa uptake in the striatum with PET and Eidelberg et al. found decreased glucose utilization in the thalamus, inferior parietal lobule, and the hippocampus with FDG PET.[181,182] Figure 18 is an FDG PET scan of an 80-year-old man with clinical features of CBD. He had generalized rigidity and was virtually immobile at the time of the PET study. He required full nursing care. Five years earlier, he had developed stiffness in the right hand, followed by dystonic posturing, the alien hand sign, and gradual involvement of the left side. We have now studied a number of such cases of suspected CBD and have found such a striking uniformity in the FDG PET findings that we believe that this pattern is highly suggestive of CBD.

Progressive Supranuclear Palsy

Progressive supranuclear palsy (PSP) is a neurodegenerative condition characterized by vertical ophthalmoplegia, particularly in the downward direction, pseudobulbar palsy, severe nuchal rigidity, variable motor dysfunction due to pyramidal and extrapyramidal involvement, a tendency to retropulsion, and a mild dementia.[183,184] Neuronal loss and neurofibrillary tangles are found throughout the neuraxis but particularly in the tectum and midbrain tegmentum, the substantia nigra, the globus pallidus, Meynert's nucleus, and subthalamic nucleus. With FDG PET, a global reduction in cerebral glucose metabolism that is more marked in superior frontal cortex has been reported.[185–187] The dementia and frontal lobe hypometabolism in PSP is thought to be due to loss of afferent input to the frontal cortex from subcortical structures.[188,189] Figure 19 shows a 58-year-old woman with a 2-year history

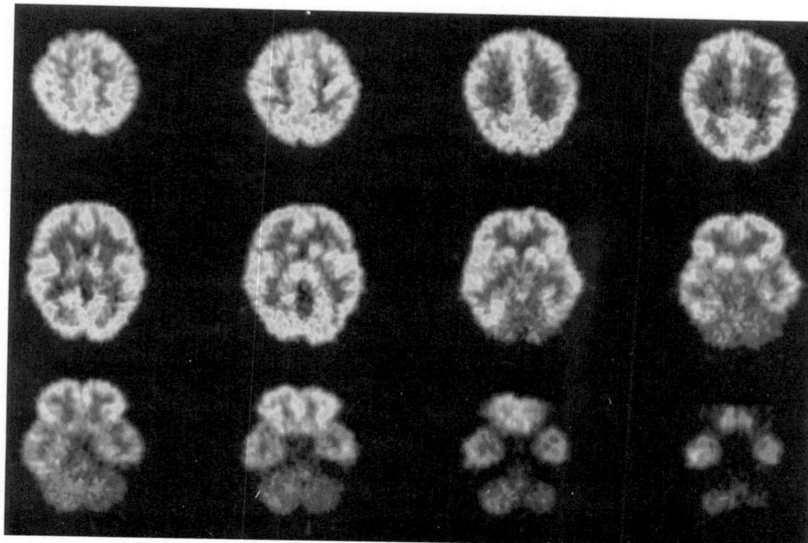

Figure 17. A 43-year-old woman with multiple system atrophy. Transaxial FDG PET images show marked glucose hypometabolism in the cerebellum (left > right), brainstem, both putamen (right > left), and a subtle but definite reduction in glucose metabolism in both superior frontal and parietal lobes. (See Plate 24.)

of vertigo, bradykinesia, a tendency to fall backward, and impaired memory. On examination she had marked axial rigidity with her head extended and there was a marked loss of upgaze.

Huntington's Disease

Huntington's disease (HD) is inherited in an autosomal dominant fashion with delayed penetrance. The neurological manifestations include choreiform involuntary movements, ocular motility disturbances, psychiatric symptoms that vary from altered personality to psychosis, and dementia.[190] The defective gene has been localized to chromosome 4. There is marked neuronal loss and gliosis in the caudate, putamen, globus pallidus, parts of the thalamus, and the frontal cortex. The first FDG PET report in HD appeared in 1982. The major findings were a marked reduction in glucose metabolism in the striatum (caudate more so than putamen) and in the late stage of the disease there can be hypometabolism in the frontal lobes.[191,192] Investigators at UCLA later reported that FDG PET could identify caudate glucose hypometabolism before the onset of structural changes in symptomatic patients and, also, in at-risk subjects before the onset of chorea.[193] The reduction in striatal glucose metabolism is also correlated with the degree of locomotor disability.[194]

Wilson's Disease

Hepatolenticular degeneration, or Wilson's disease, is an autosomal recessive disorder due to the abnormal deposition of copper in the liver and brain, particularly the lenticular (putamen and globus pallidus) nuclei. Neurological manifes-

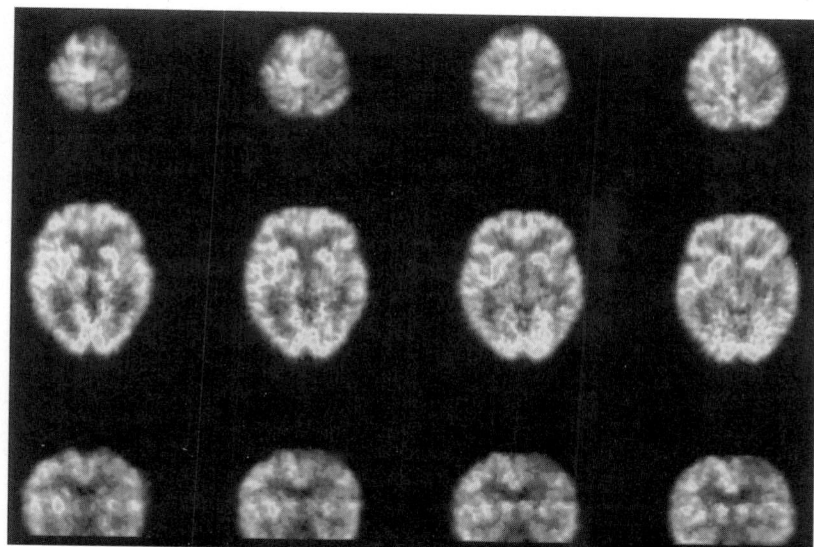

Figure 18. An 80-year-old man with suspected corticobasal degeneration. Transaxial (top and middle rows) FDG PET images reveal glucose hypometabolism involving the left Rolandic region together with hypometabolism of the ipsilateral putamen, particularly the posterolateral two thirds, and left thalamus. Coronal images (bottom) illustrate the marked glucose hypometabolism in the left superior frontoparietal lobes. (See Plate 25.)

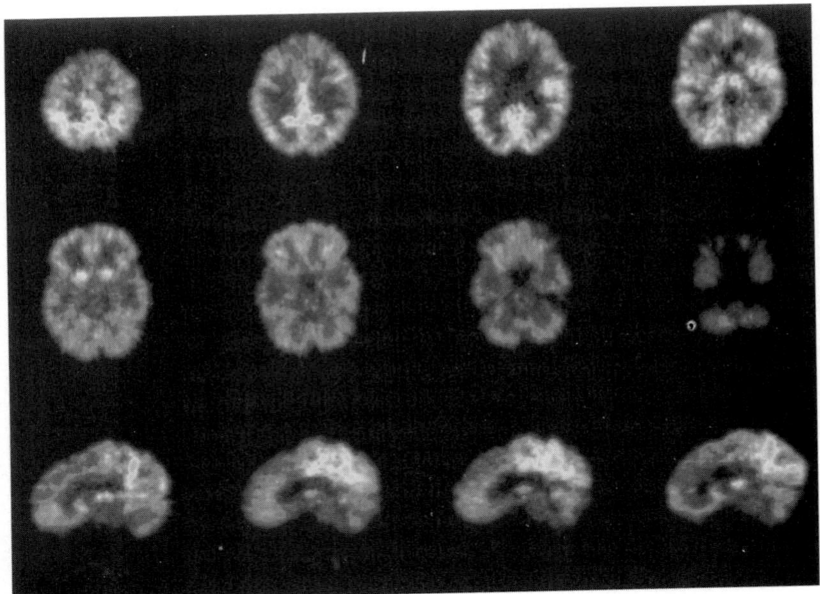

Figure 19. A 58-year-old woman with a clinical diagnosis of PSP. Transaxial (top and middle rows) and sagittal (bottom row) FDG PET images show reduced glucose metabolism in mid-frontal, superior frontal, and temporal cortices, putamina, and midbrain with relative sparing of parieto-occipital lobes and cerebellum. (See Plate 26.)

tations include rigidity, tremor, dysarthria, dystonia, gait disturbance, and corneal Kayser-Fleischer rings. Neuropathologically there is damage to the lenticular, caudate, red, and dentate nuclei, as well as the brainstem and frontal cortex. Hawkins et al. reported FDG PET findings in 4 patients with varying degrees of clinical involvement and noted diffuse symmetric reductions of glucose utilization in the frontal and parietal cortices and the caudate and lenticular nuclei, with sparing of the thalamus.[195] An example of an FDG PET scan in a young woman with Wilson's disease is shown in Figure 20.

CEREBROVASCULAR DISEASE

The physiology of cerebral ischemia and cerebral infarction has been studied extensively with PET, ^{133}Xe blood flow techniques, and SPECT methodology using a variety of tracers, and numerous reviews are available.[9,196–201] Cerebral hemodynamics including rCBF, $rCMRO_2$, regional oxygen extraction fraction (rOEF), and regional cerebral blood volume (rCBV) have been measured with ^{15}O-PET methodology.[202–204] The sequence of events that follows a drop in cerebral perfusion pressure has been extensively documented. After perfusion pressure drops, there is an "autoregulatory" compensatory vasodilatation to maintain a normal rCBF. When autoregulation fails, rCBF declines but $rCMRO_2$ is maintained by a progressive increase in rOEF. After rOEF is maximal, a further decrease in rCBF results in a disruption of normal function and metabolism. PET and SPECT depict "luxury" perfusion where there is increased rCBF, normal $rCMRO_2$, and decreased rOEF, together with "misery" perfusion where increased rOEF is accompanied by decreased rCBF.[205,206] In addition, SPECT is able to detect cortical supratentorial infarction earlier than anatomical imaging with CT, but it is much less sensitive in detecting posterior fossa and lacunar infarction.[207,208]

However, much of these data have not been translated into useful information for the clinical management of stroke patients.[209] The reasons for this are partly because much of the early work focused on attempts to explain the pathophysi-

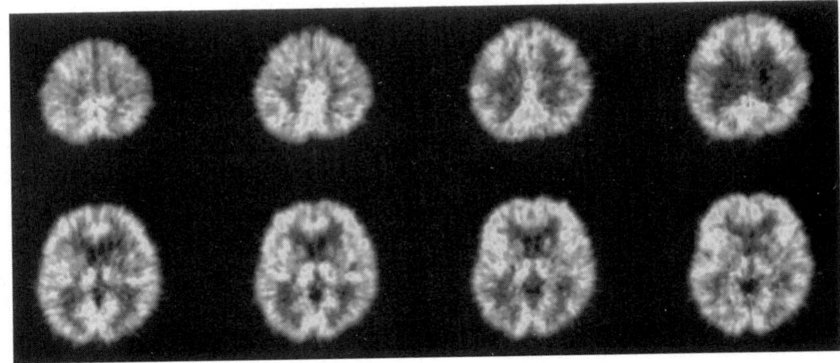

Figure 20. A 22-year-old woman with Wilson's disease and tremor and bradykinesia. Transaxial FDG PET scans show reduced cerebral cortical glucose metabolism together with a marked reduction in glucose utilization in the striatum. (See Plate 27.)

ology of transient ischemia attacks (TIA) and stroke in terms of hemodynamic variables. The aim was to identify patients at risk for stroke from poor perfusion. However, subsequent research has shown that hemodynamic factors play a small role in the genesis of stroke. For instance, in patients with carotid stenosis, TIAs and cerebral infarction are generally the result of embolism.[202,210] Caplan suggested 2 potential applications of SPECT and PET in patients with stroke: (1) If SPECT can identify the ischemic penumbra of cortical strokes reliably and an effective treatment for ischemic brain becomes available, then alteration in rCBF could be measured before and after intervention to assess efficacy of therapy. (2) The early identification of reduced rCBF, when the patient is asymptomatic, in patients with subarachnoid hemorrhage may alter patient outcome, if therapy could be delivered earlier.[209]

Further applications for SPECT and PET may reside at the receptor level of stroke. In vitro work has shown that ischemia provokes a massive release of glutamate from ischemic neurons.[211,212] This "glutaminergic storm" damages ischemic and surrounding cells through activation of glutamate receptors, in particular, the NMDA (N-methyl-D-aspartate) receptor.[213,214] The NMDA receptor can be blocked by a number of agents.[215] Research may allow the development of a PET or SPECT ligand to image ischemic tissue and, then, possibly determine the efficacy of pharmacological NMDA receptor blockade.

NEUROACTIVATION

Cerebral activation studies aimed at localizing specific neurologic functions through changes in cerebral blood flow have long been the domain of PET. Blood flow tracers, such as ^{15}O-water, have been used as indirect indicators of neuronal activity to investigate many aspects of neurological function, from simple motor behavior to complex cognitive function, Figure 21(A). In simple terms, the short half-life of ^{15}O is utilized to perform a series of imaging studies in one individual. Two states are usually studied: (a) a resting or control state and, (b) an activated state where a particular paradigm (or drug) is presented. The difference between "rest" and the "activated" state is hypothesized to be due to the paradigm (or drug), and any increased blood flow to particular parts of the brain is hypothesized to be the anatomical localization for that task. More recently, MR techniques (fMR imaging) have been used to similar effect.[216] With the wider availability of multidetector SPECT devices, there is a growing experience with SPECT in neuroactivation.[217–220] HMPAO is preferred because of its rapid uptake, high first-pass extraction, and prolonged retention in the brain. MR/functional imaging coregistration is now regarded as a necessity for the accurate localization of significant blood flow changes. An example of insula cortical activation to a strong rotational stimulus is shown for a single subject in Figure 21(B) where the HMPAO SPECT study is registered to the MR data. Neuroactivation with SPECT is in its infancy but, if it is validated for a number of different paradigms, it offers significant savings in cost and additional flexibility because the paradigm does not need to be carried out in the scanner as for PET and fMR.

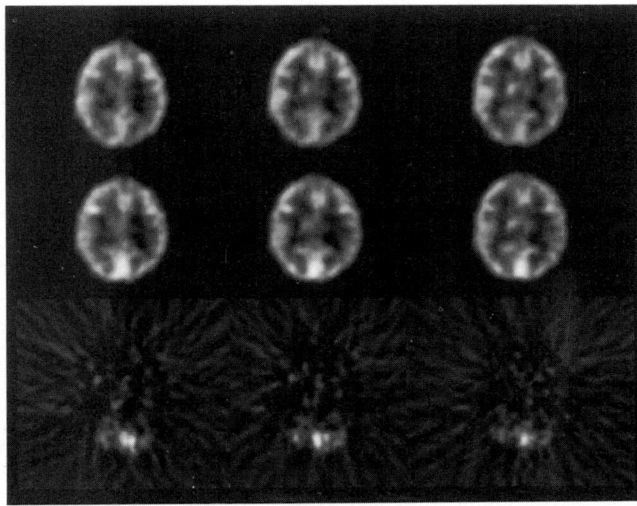
A

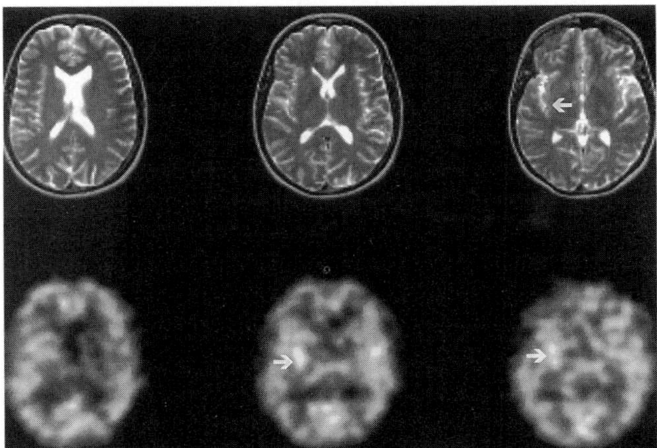
B

Figure 21. **(A).** ^{15}O-PET activation studies in a 24-year-old normal volunteer. Transaxial images demonstrate increased blood flow to primary visual cortex in response to a simple visual paradigm. Top row is control task with eyes staring at a fixed object, middle row is normal volunteer viewing a complex visual scene, and bottom row is subtraction images of activated minus control state. **(B).** HMPAO SPECT activation and MR studies in a 40-year-old normal volunteer. T2-weighted MR images (top) and registered HMPAO SPECT (bottom) studies are shown. Increased perfusion is seen in right insula (arrows on both MR and SPECT studies) after a strong rotational stimulus. (See Plate 28.)

Acknowledgments. We would like to thank Stefan Eberl, Senior Scientist, Department of Nuclear Medicine and Kim Silver, Senior PET Technologist, The PET Department, Royal Prince Alfred Hospital, Sydney, Australia, for help with the illustrations for this chapter.

REFERENCES

1. Phelps ME, Hoffman EJ, Mullani NA, Ter-Pogossian MM. Application of annihilation coincidence detection to transaxial reconstruction tomography. *J Nucl Med* 1975; 16:210–223.
2. Phelps ME, Mazziotta JC. Positron emission tomography: Human brain function and biochemistry. *Science* 1985; 228:799–809.
3. Ter-Pogossian MM, Phelps ME, Hoffman EJ, et al. A positron emission transaxial tomography for nuclear medicine imaging (PETT). *Radiology* 1975;114:39–93.
4. Kuhl DE, Wagner HN, Alavi A, Coleman RE, Gould L, et al. Positron emission tomography: Clinical status in the United States in 1987. *J Nucl Med* 1988;29:1136–1143.
5. Report of the Therapeutics and Technology Assessment Subcommittee of the American Academy of Neurology: Assessment: Positron Emission Tomography. *Neurology* 1991;41: 163–167.
6. Ell PJ. Editorial: Mapping cerebral blood flow. *J Nucl Med* 1992;33(10):1843–1845.
7. Holman BL, Devous Sr MD. Functional brain SPECT: The emergence of a powerful clinical method. *J Nucl Med* 1992;33:1888–1904.
8. Juni JE. Taking brain SPECT seriously: Reflections on recent clinical reports in The Journal of Nuclear Medicine. *J Nucl Med* 1994;35:1891–1895.
9. Masdeu JC, Brass LM, Holman BL, Kushner MJ. Brain single-photon emission computed tomography. *Neurology* 1994;44:1970–1977.
10. Weinhard K, Dahlbom M, Eriksson L, et al. The ECAT EXACT HR: Performance of a new high resolution positron scanner. *J Comput Assist Tomogr* 1994;18(1):110–118.
11. Phelps ME. Positron emission Tomography (PET), in Mazziotta JC, Gilman S (eds.): *Clinical Brain Imaging: Principles and Applications*. Philadelphia, FA Davis, 1992, pp 71–107.
12. Eberl S, Kanno I, Fulton RR, Ryan A, Hutton BF, Fulham MJ. An automated inter-study image registration technique for SPECT and PET studies. *J Nucl Med* (in press) 1995.
13. Fulton RR, Hutton BF, Braun M, Ardekani B, Larkin R. Use of 3D reconstruction to correct for patient motion in SPECT. *Phys Med Biol* 1994;39:563–574.
14. Green MV, Seidel J, Stein SD, et al. Head movement in normal subjects during simulated PET brain imaging with and without head movement. *J Nucl Med* 1994;35(9):1538–1546.
15. Phelps ME, Mazziotta JC, Schelbert HR (eds.): *Positron Emission Tomography and Autoradiography*. New York, Raven Press, 1986.
16. Murray IPC, Ell PJ (eds.): *Nuclear Medicine in Clinical Diagnosis and Treatment*. 1st ed. New York, Churchill Livingstone, 1994.
17. Early PJ, Sodee DB (eds.): *Principles and Practice of Nuclear Medicine*. 2nd ed. St Louis, Mosby-Year Book, Inc, 1995.
18. Kung HF, Ohmomo Y, Kung M-P. Current and future radiopharmaceuticals for brain imaging with single photon emission computed tomography. *Semin Nucl Med* 1990;20: 290–302.
19. Phelps ME, Huang SC, Hoffman EJ, Selin C, Sokoloff L, Kuhl DE. Tomographic measurement of local cerebral glucose metabolic rate in humans with [18F]2-fluoro-2-deoxy-d-glucose: Validation of method. *Ann Neurol* 1979;6: 371–388.
20. Kadekaro M, Ito M, Gross PM. Local cerebral glucose utilization is increased in acutely adrenalectomized rats. *Neuroendocrinology* 1988;47:329–334.
21. Schwartz WJ, Smith CB, Davidsen L, et al. Metabolic mapping of functional activity in the hypothalamo-neurohypophysial system of the rat. *Science* 1979;205:723–725.
22. Brooks RA. Alternate formula for glucose utilization using labelled deoxyglucose. *J Nucl Med* 1982;23:538–539.
23. Sokoloff L, Reivich M, Kennedy C, et al. The 14C-Deoxyglucose method for the measurement of local cerebral glucose utilization: Theory procedure and normal values in the conscious and anesthetized albino rat. *J Neurochem* 1977; 28:897–916.
24. Hooper PK, Meikle SR, Eberl S, Fulham MJ. Validation of post injection transmission measurements for attenuation correction in neurologic FDG PET studies. *J Nucl Med* 1995; (in press).
25. Mazziotta JC. Practical applications of positron emission tomography in epilepsy. *Am J Phys Imag* 1988;3:28–29.
26. Crandall PH, Rausch R, Engel J. Preoperative indicators for optimal surgical outcome for temporal lobe epilepsy, in Weiser HG, Elger CE (eds.): *Presurgical evaluation of epileptics*. Berlin, Springer, 1987, pp 325–344.
27. Weiser HG. Psychomotor seizures of hippocampal-amygdalar origin, in Pedley TA, Meldrum BS (eds.): *Recent advances in epilepsy*. Edinburgh, Churchill-Livingstone, 1986, pp 57–79.
28. Kuhl DE, Engel JJ, E PM, Selin C. Epileptic patterns of local cerebral metabolism and perfusion in humans determined by emission computed tomography of ^{18}FDG and $^{13}NH_3$. *Ann Neurol* 1980;8:348–60.
29. Engel JJ, Rausch R, Lieb JP, et al. Correlation of criteria used for localizing epileptic foci in patients considered for surgical therapy of epilepsy. *Ann Neurol* 1981;9:215–224.
30. Engel JJ, Brown WJ, Kuhl DE, Phelps ME, Mazziotta JC, et al. Pathological findings underlying focal temporal lobe hypometabolism in partial epilepsy. *Ann Neurol* 1982;12: 518–528.
31. Engel JJ, Kuhl DE, Phelps ME, Mazziotta JC. Interictal cerebral glucose metabolism in partial epilepsy and its relation to EEG changes. *Ann Neurol* 1982;12:510–517.
32. Theodore WH, Newmark ME, Sato S, Brooks R, Patronas N, et al. 18F-flourodeoxyglucose positron emission tomography in refractory complex partial seizures. *Ann Neurol* 1983;14:429–437.
33. Abou-Khalil BW, Siegel GJ, Sackellares JC, Gilman S, Hichwa R, et al. Positron emission tomography studies of cerebral glucose metabolism in chronic partial epilepsy. *Ann Neurol* 1987;22:480–486.
34. Engel JJ. The use of positron emission tomography scanning in epilepsy. *Ann Neurol* 1984;15(Suppl):S180–S191.
35. Henry TR, Mazziotta JC, Engel J. Interictal metabolic lobe anatomy of mesial temporal lobe epilepsy. *Arch Neurol* 1993;50:582–589.
36. Mazziotta JC, Engel JJ. The use and impact of positron emission tomography scanning in epilepsy. *Epilepsia* 1984; 25(Suppl 2):S86–104.
37. Engel JJ. The role of neuroimaging in the surgical treatment of epilepsy. *Acta Neurol Scand* 1988;117(Suppl 1):84–89.
38. Theodore WH, Dorwart R, Holmes M, Porter RJ, Di Chiro G. Neuroimaging in refractory partial seizures: comparison of PET, CT and MRI. *Neurology* 1986;36:750–759.
39. Sperling MR, Wilson G, Engel JJ, Babb TL, Phelps ME, et al. Magnetic resonance imaging in intractable partial epilepsy: Correlative studies. *Ann Neurol* 1986;20:57–62.
40. Kuzniecky R, de la Sayette V, Ethier R, et al. Magnetic resonance imaging in temporal lobe epilepsy: pathological correlations. *Ann Neurol* 1987;22:341–347.
41. Henry TR, Engel JJ, Sutherling WW, Risinger MR, Phelps ME. Correlation of structural and metabolic imaging with electrographic localization and histopathology in refractory complex partial epilepsy [abstract]. *Epilepsia* 1987;28:60.

42. Theodore WH, Katz D, Kufta C, Sato S, Patronas N, et al. Pathology of temporal lobe foci: correlation with CT, MRI, and PET. *Neurology* 1990;40:797–803.
43. Blume WT, David RB, Gomez MR. Generalized sharp and slow wave complexes: associated clinical features and long-term follow-up. *Brain* 1973;96:289–306.
44. Chevrie JJ, Aicardi J. Childhood epileptic encephalopathy with slow spike wave: a statistical study of 80 cases. *Epilepsia* 1972;13:250–271.
45. Chugani HT, Mazziotta JC, Engel JJ, Phelps ME. The Lennox-Gastaut syndrome: metabolic sub-types determined by 2-deoxy-2[18F]fluoro-D-glucose positron emission tomography. *Ann Neurol* 1987;21:4–13.
46. Theodore WH, Rose D, Patronas N, Sato S, Holmes M, et al. Cerebral glucose metabolism in the Lennox-Gastaut syndrome. *Ann Neurol* 1987;21:14–21.
47. Chugani HT, Shields WD, Shewmon DA, et al. Infantile spasms: I. PET identifies focal cortical dysgenesis in cryptogenic cases for surgical treatment. *Ann Neurol* 1990; 27:405–413.
48. Chugani HT, Shewmon A, Sankar R, Chen BC, Phelps ME. Infantile spasms: II. lenticular nuclei and brain stem activation on positron emission tomography. *Ann Neurol* 1992; 31:212–219.
49. Chugani HT, Shewmon DA, Peacock WJ, Shields WD, Mazziotta JC, et al. Surgical treatment of intractable neonatal-onset seizures: the role of positron emission tomography. *Neurology* 1988;38:1178–1188.
50. Hougaard K, Oikawa T, Sveinsdottir E, Skinhoj E, Ingvar DH, Lassen NA. Regional cerebral blood flow in focal cortical epilepsy. *Arch Neurol* 1979;33:527–535.
51. Uren RF, Magistretti PL, Royal HD, et al. Single photon emission computed tomography: preliminary results in patients with epilepsy and stroke. *Med J Aust* 1983;1:411–413.
52. Magistretti PL, Uren RF. Cerebral blood flow patterns in epilepsy, in Nistico G (ed.): *Epilepsy: an update on research and therapy.* New York, Alan R Liss, 1983, pp 241–247.
53. Duncan R, Patterson J, Roberts R, Hadley DM, Bone I: Ictal/postictal SPECT in the pre-surgical localization of complex partial seizures. *J Neurol Neurosurg Psychiat* 1993; 56:141–148.
54. Newton MR, Austin MC, Chan JG, McKay WJ, Rowe CC, Berkovic SF. Ictal SPECT using Tc-99m HMPAO: methods for rapid preparation and optimal deployment of tracer during spontaneous seizures. *J Nucl Med* 1993;34:666–670.
55. Newton MR, Berkovic SF, Austin MC, Reutens DC, McKay WJ, Bladin PF. Dystonia, clinical lateralization, and regional blood flow changes in temporal lobe seizures. *Neurology* 1992;42:371–377.
56. Frost JJ, Mayberg HS, Fisher RS, Douglass KH, Dannals RF, et al. Mu-opiate receptors measured by positron emission tomography are increased in temporal lobe epilepsy. *Ann Neurol* 1988;23:231–237.
57. Savic I, Persson A, Roland P, Pauli S, Sedvall G, et al. In-vivo demonstration of reduced benzodiazepine receptor binding in human epileptic foci. *Lancet* 1988;28616:863–6.
58. Lloyd KG, Munari C, Bossi L. Biochemical evidence for the alterations of GABA-mediated synaptic transmission in pathological brain tissue (stereo EEG or morphological definition) from epileptic patients, in Morselli PL, Lloyd KG, Loscher W, Meldrum B, Reynolds EM (eds.): *Neurotransmitters, seizures and epilepsy.* New York, Raven, 1981, pp 325–337.
59. Roberts E. Epilepsy and anti-epileptic drugs: a speculative synthesis, in Glaser G, Penry JK, Woodbury DM (eds.): *Anti-epileptic drugs: mechanism of action.* New York, Raven, 1980, pp 667–713.
60. Bartenstein P, Ludolph A, Schober O, Lottes G, et al. Benzodiazepine receptors and cerebral blood flow in partial epilepsy. *Eur J Nuc Med* 1990;18:111–118.
61. Ferstl FJ, Cordes M, Cordes I, Henkes H, et al. 123-I-iomazenil SPECT in patients with focal epilepsies—a comparative study with 99mTc-HMPAO SPECT, CT and MR, in Kito S (ed.): *Neuroreceptor mechanisms in brain.* New York, Plenum Press, 1991, pp 405–412.
62. Bajorek JG, Lee RJ, Lomas P. Neuropeptides: anticonvulsant and convulsant mechanisms in epileptic model systems and in humans, in Delgardo-Escueta AV, Ward AAJ, Woodbury DM, Porter RJ (eds.): *Advances in Neurology.* New York, Raven Press, 1986, pp 489–500.
63. Frenk H. Pro- and anticonvulsant actions of morphine and the endogenous opioids: involvement and interactions of multiple opiate and non-opiate systems. *Brain Res Rev* 1983;6: 197–210.
64. Muller-Gartner HW, Mayberg HS, Fisher RS, et al. Decreased hippocampal muscarinic cholinergic receptor binding measured by 123I-iododexetimide and single-photon emission computed tomography in epilepsy. *Ann Neurol* 1993; 34(2):235–238.
65. Henry TR, Sutherling WW, Engel JJ, Risinger MW, Levesque MF. The role of Positron Emission Tomography in presurgical evaluation of partial epilepsies of neocortical origin, in Luders H (ed.): *Epilepsy Surgery.* New York, Raven Press, 1991, pp 243–250.
66. Marks D, Katz A, Hoffer P, Spencer SS. Localization of extratemporal epileptic foci during ictal single photon emission computed tomography. *Ann Neurol* 1992;31:250–255.
67. Stefan H, Bauer J, Feistel H, et al. Regional cerebral blood flow during focal seizures of temporal and frontocentral onset. *Ann Neurol* 1990;27:162–166.
68. Ringertz N. Grading of gliomas. *Acta Pathol Microbiol* 1950;27:51–64.
69. Burger PC, Vogel FS, Green SB. Glioblastoma and anaplastic astrocytoma: pathologic criteria and prognostic considerations. *Cancer* 1985;56:1106–1111.
70. Nelson JS, Tsukada Y, Schoenfeld D, et al. Necrosis as a prognostic criterion in malignant supratentorial astrocytic tumors. *Cancer* 1983;52:550–554.
71. Di Chiro G. Positron emission tomography using [18F]Fluorodeoxyglucose in brain tumors. *Invest Radiol* 1987; 22:360–371.
72. Coleman RE, Hoffman JM, Hanson MW, Sostman HD, Schold SC. Clinical application of PET for the evaluation of brain tumors. *J Nucl Med* 1991;32:616–622.
73. Alavi JB, Alavi A, Chawluk J, et al. Positron emission tomography in patients with glioma: A predictor of prognosis. *Cancer* 1988;62:1074–1078.
74. Fulham MJ. PET with [18F]fluorodeoxyglucose (PET-FDG): An indispensable tool in the proper management of brain tumors, in Hubner KF, Collmann J, Buonocore E, Kabalka GW (eds.): *Clinical Positron Emission Tomography.* St. Louis, Mosby Year Book, 1992, pp 50–60.
75. Warburg O. *Metabolism of Tumors*. London, Arnold & Constable, 1930.
76. Warburg O. *On the origin of cancer cells. Science* 1956;123:309–314.
77. Glantz MJ, Hoffman JM, Coleman RE, et al. The role of F18 FDG PET imaging in predicting early recurrence of primary brain tumors. *Ann Neurol* 1991;29:347–355.
78. Francavilla TL, Miletich RS, Di Chiro G, Patronas NJ, Rizzoli HV, Wright DC. Positron emission tomography in the detection of malignant degeneration of low-grade gliomas. *Neurosurgery* 1989;24:1–5.
79. Russell DS, Rubinstein LJ. *Pathology of Tumours of the*

Nervous System. 5th ed. Baltimore, Williams & Wilkins, 1989, pp 83–350.
80. Fulham MJ, Melisi JW, Nishimiya J, Dwyer AJ, Di Chiro G. Neuroimaging of Juvenile Pilocytic Astrocytomas: An enigma. *Radiology* 1993;189:221–225.
81. Patronas NJ, Di Chiro G, Kufta C, et al. Prediction of survival in glioma patients by means of positron emission tomography. *J Neurosurg* 1985;62:816–822.
82. Bernell WR, Kepes JJ, Seitz EP. Late malignant recurrence of childhood cerebellar astrocytoma: A report of two cases. *J Neurosurg* 1972;37:470–474.
83. Kleinman GM, Schoene WC, Walshe TM, Richardson EP. Malignant transformation in benign cerebellar astrocytoma. *J Neurosurg* 1978;49:111–118.
84. Kocks W, Kalff R, Reinhardt V, et al. Spinal metastasis of pilocytic astrocytoma of the chiasma opticum. *Childs Nerv Syst* 1989;5:118–120.
85. Obana WG, Cogen PH, Davis RL, Edwards SB. Metastatic juvenile pilocytic astrocytoma: A case report. *J Neurosurg* 1991;75:972–975.
86. Mishima K, Nakamura M, Nakamura H, Nakamura O, Funata N, Shitara N. Leptomeningeal dissemination of cerebellar pilocytic astrocytoma. *J Neurosurg* 1992;77:788–791.
87. Murovic JA, Nagashima T, Hoshino T, Edwards MSB, Davis RL. Pediatric central nervous system tumors: A cell kinetic study with bromodeoxyuridine. *Neurosurgery* 1986;19: 900–904.
88. Tsanaclis AM, Robert F, Michaud J, Brem S. The cycling pool of cells within human brain tumors: In situ cytokinetics using the monoclonal antibody Ki-67. *Can J Neurol Sci* 1991;18:12–17.
89. Germano IM, Ito M, Cho KG, Hoshino T, Davis RL, Wilson CB. Correlation of histopathological features and proliferative potential of gliomas. *J Neurosurg* 1989;70:701–706.
90. Jenkins RB, Kimmel DW, Moertel CA, et al. A cytogenetic study of 53 gliomas. *Cancer Genet Cytogenet* 1989; 39:253–279.
91. Daumas-Duport C, Scheithauer B, O'Fallon J, Kelly P. Grading of astrocytomas: A simple and reproducible method. *Cancer* 1988;62:2152–2165.
92. Long DM. Capillary ultrastructure and the blood brain barrier in human malignant brain tumors. *J Neurosurg* 1970; 32:127–144.
93. Sato K, Rorke LB. Vascular bundles and wickerworks in childhood brain tumors. *Pediatr Neurosci* 1989;15:105–110.
94. Mueckler M, Caruso C, Baldwin S, et al. Sequence and structure of human glucose transporter. *Science* 1985;29:941–45.
95. Pessin JE, Bell GI. Mammalian facilitative glucose transporter family: Structure and molecular regulation. *Annu Rev Physiol* 1992;54:911–30.
96. Guerin C, Laterra J, Hruban RH, Brem H, Drewes LR, Goldstein GW. The glucose transporter and blood brain barrier of human brain tumors. *Ann Neurol* 1990;28:758–765.
97. Guerin C, Laterra J, Drewes LR, Brem H, Goldstein GW. Vascular expression of glucose transporter in experimental brain neoplasms. *Am J Path* 1992;140:417–425.
98. Rhodes CG, Wise RJ, Gibbs JM, Frackowiak RSJ, Hatazawa J, et al. In vivo disturbance of the oxidative metabolism of glucose in human cerebral gliomas. *Ann Neurol* 1983; 14:614–624.
99. Rottenberg DA, Ginos JZ, Kearfott KJ, Junck L, Dhawan V, et al. In vivo measurement of brain tumor pH using [11C]DMO and positron emission tomography. *Ann Neurol* 1985;17:70–79.
100. Radda G. The use of NMR spectroscopy for the understanding of disease. *Science* 1986;233:640–645.
101. Bergstrom M, Collins VP, Ehrin E, Ericson K, Eriksson L, et al. Discrepancies in brain tumor extent as shown by computed tomography and positron emission tomography using [68Ga]EDTA, [11C]glucose and [11C]Methionine. *J Comput Assist Tomogr* 1983;11:1062–1066.
102. Lilja A, Lundqvist H, Olsson Y, Spannare B, Gullberg P, et al. Positron emission tomography and computed tomography in differential diagnosis between recurrent or residual glioma and treatment-induced brain lesions. *Acta Radiol* 1989; 30:121–128.
103. Pawlikowski M, Kunert-Radek J, Radek A, Stepien H. Inhibition of cell proliferation of human gliomas by benzodiazepines in vitro. *Acta Neurol Scand* 1988;77:231–33.
104. Junck L, Olson JMM, Ciliax BJ, Koeppe RA, Watkins GL, et al. PET imaging of human gliomas with ligands for the peripheral benzodiazepine site. *Ann Neurol* 1989;26: 752–758.
105. Bergstrom M, Mosskin M, Ericson K, Ehrin E, Thorell J-O, et al. Peripheral benzodiazepine binding sites in human gliomas evaluated with positron emission tomography. *Acta Radiol* 1986;369:409–411.
106. Biersack HJ, Grunwald F, Kropp J. Single photon emission computed tomography imaging of brain tumors. *Semin Nucl Med* 1991;21:2–10.
107. Mountz JM, Raymond PA, McKeeven PE, et al. Specific localization of thallium-201 in human high grade astrocytoma by microautoradiography. *Cancer Res* 1989;49:4053–4056.
108. Sessler MJ, Geck P, Maul F-D, Hor G, Mung DL. New aspects of cellular thallium uptake: Tl+-Na+-2Cl-cotransport is the central mechanism of ion uptake. *Nucl Med* 1968;25:24–27.
109. Brismar T, Collins VP, Kesselberg M. Thallium-201 uptake relates to membrane potential and potassium permeability in human glioma cells. *Brain Res* 1989;500:30–36.
110. Kim T, Black KL, Marciano D, et al. Thallium-201 SPECT imaging of brain tumors: Methods and results. *J Nucl Med* 1990;31:965–969.
111. Schwartz RB, Carvalho PA, Alexander III E, Loeffler JS, Folkerth R, Holman LB. Radiation necrosis vs high-grade recurrent glioma: Differentiation by using dual-isotope SPECT with 201Tl and 99mTc-HMPAO. *AJNR* 1991;12: 1187–1192.
112. Tonami H, Matsuda H, Ooba H, et al. Thallium-201 accumulation in cerebral candidiasis. *Clin Nucl Med* 1990;15: 397–400.
113. Krishna L, Slizofski WJ, Katsetos CD, et al. Abnormal intracerebral thallium localization in a bacterial brain abscess. *J Nucl Med* 1992;33:2017–2019.
114. Langen K-F, Coenen HH, Roosen N, et al. Brain and brain tumor uptake of L-3[123I]iodo-alpha-methyl tyrosine: Competition with natural L-amino acids. *J Nucl Med* 1991;32:1225–1228.
115. Langen K-F, Coenen HH, Roosen N, et al. SPECT studies of brain tumors with L-3[123I]iodo-alpha-methyl tyrosine: Comparison with PET, 124IMT and first clinical results. *J Nucl Med* 1990;31:281–286.
116. von Monakow C. *Neue gesichtspunkte in der frage nach der lokalisation im grosshirm*. Wiesbaden, Bergman, J F, 1910.
117. West JR. The concept of diaschisis: A reply to Markowitsch and Pritzel. *Behav Biol* 1978;22:413–416.
118. Baron JC, Bousser MG, Comar D, Castaigne P. Crossed cerebellar diaschisis in human supratentorial infarction [abstract]. *Ann Neurol* 1980;8:128.
119. Martin WRW, Raichle ME. Cerebellar blood flow and metabolism in cerebral hemisphere infarction. *Ann Neurol* 1983;14:168–176.
120. Kushner M, Alavi A, Reivich M, Dann R, Burke A, Robinson G. Contralateral cerebellar hypometabolism following cere-

bral insult: A positron emission tomographic study. *Ann Neurol* 1984;15:425–434.

121. Patronas NJ, Di Chiro G, Smith BH, et al. Depressed cerebellar glucose metabolism in supratentorial tumors. *Brain Res* 1984;291:93–101.
122. Fulham MJ, Brooks RA, Hallett M, Di Chiro G. Cerebellar diaschisis revisited: Pontine hypometabolism and dentate sparing. *Neurology* 1992;42:2267–2273.
123. Meneghetti G, Vorstrup S, Mickey B, Lindewald H, Lassen NA. Crossed cerebellar diaschisis in ischemic stroke: A study of regional cerebral blood flow by 133Xe inhalation and single Photon Emission Computerized Tomography. *J Cereb Blood Flow Metab* 1984;4:235–240.
124. Perani D, Gerundini P, Lenzi GL. Cerebral hemispheric and contralateral cerebellar hypoperfusion during a transient ischemic attack. *J Cereb Blood Flow Metab* 1987;7:507–509.
125. Feeney DM, Baron JC. Diaschisis. *Stroke* 1986;17:817–830.
126. Marsden CD, Harrison MJG. Outcome of investigation of patients with presenile dementia. *Br Med J* 1972;2:249–252.
127. Smith JS, Kiloh LG. The investigation of dementia: results in 200 consecutive admissions. *Lancet* 1981;1:824–827.
128. Marsden CD. Assessment of dementia, in Frederiks JAM (ed.): *Handbook of Clinical Neurology*. New York, Elsevier, 1985, pp 221–232.
129. Alavi A, Ferris S, Wolf A, et al. Determination of cerebral metabolism in senile dementia using F-18-deoxyglucose and positron emission tomography. *J Nucl Med* 1980;21:21–5.
130. Frackowiak RSJ, Pozilli C, Legg NJ, Du Boulay GH, Marshall J, et al. Regional cerebral oxygen supply and utilization in dementia. *Brain* 1981;104:753–778.
131. Frackowiak RSJ, Lenzi GL, Jones T, Heather JD. Quantitative measurement of regional cerebral blood flow and oxygen metabolism in man using ^{15}O and positron emission tomography: Theory, procedure and normal values. *J Comput Assist Tomogr* 1980;4:727–736.
132. Kuhl DE, Metter EJ, Riege WH, Hawkins RA, Mazziotta JC, et al. Local cerebral glucose utilization in elderly patients with depression, multi-infarct dementia, and Alzheimer's disease. *J Cereb Blood Flow Metab* 1983;3(Suppl 1):S494–S495.
133. Friedland RP, Budinger TF, Ganz E, Yano Y, Mathis CA, et al. Regional cerebral metabolic alterations in dementia of the Alzheimer type: Positron emission tomography with [18F]Fluordeoxyglucose. *J Comput Assist Tomog* 1983;7:590–598.
134. Foster NL, Chase TN, Fedio P, Patronas NJ, Brooks RA, et al. Alzheimer's disease: Focal cortical changes shown by positron emission tomography. *Neurol* 1983;33:961–965.
135. de Leon MJ, Ferris SH, George AE, Reisberg B, Christman DR, et al. Computed tomography and positron emission transaxial tomography evaluations of normal ageing and Alzheimer's disease. *J Cereb Blood Flow Metab* 1983; 3:391–394.
136. Chase TN, Foster NL, Fedio P, Brooks RA, Mansi L, et al. Regional cortical dysfunction in Alzheimer's disease as determined by positron emission tomography. *Ann Neurol* 1984;15(suppl):S170–S174.
137. Cutler NR, Haxby JV, Duara R, Grady CL, Kay AD, et al. Clinical history, brain metabolism, and neuropsychological function in Alzheimer's disease. *Ann Neurol* 1985;18: 298–309.
138. Duara R, Grady C, Haxby J, Sundaram M, Cutler NR, et al. Positron Emission tomography in Alzheimer's disease. *Neurology* 1986;36:879–887.
139. Friedland RP, Budinger TF, Koss E, Ober BA. Alzheimer's disease: Anterior-posterior hemispheric alterations in cortical glucose utilization. *Neurosci Lett* 1985;53:235–240.
140. Haxby JV, Duara R, Grady CL, Cutler NR, Rapoport SI. Relations between neuropsychological and cerebral metabolic asymmetries in early Alzheimer's disease. *J Cereb Blood Flow Metab* 1985;5:193–200.
141. Haxby JV, Grady CL, Koss E, Horwitz B, Heston L, et al. Longitudinal study of cerebral metabolic asymmetries and associated neuropsychological patterns in early dementia of the Alzheimer type. *Arch Neurol* 1990;47:753–760.
142. McGeer EG, Peppard RP, McGeer PL, Tuokko H, Crockett D, et al. ^{18}Fluorodeoxyglucose positron emission tomography studies in presumed Alzheimer cases, including 13 serial scans. *Can J Neurol Sci* 1990;17:1–11.
143. Brun A, Gustafson L. Distribution of cerebral degeneration in Alzheimer's disease: a clinico-pathological study. *Arch Psychiatr Nervenkr* 1976;223:15–33.
144. Cohen MB, Graham LS, Lake R, et al. Diagnosis of Alzheimer's disease and multiple infarct dementia by tomographic imaging of iodine-123 IMP. *J Nucl Med* 1986;27:769–774.
145. Smith FW, Gemmell HG, Sharp PF. The use of Tc-99m-HM-PAO for the diagnosis of dementia. *Nucl Med Commun* 1987;8:525–533.
146. Jagust WJ, Budinger TF, Reed BR. The diagnosis of dementia with single photon emission computed tomography. *Arch Neurol* 1987;44:258–262.
147. Neary D, Snowden JS, Shields RA, et al. Single photon emission tomography using Tc-99m-HM-PAO in the investigation of dementia. *J Neurol Neurosurg Psychiat* 1987;50: 1101–1109.
148. Perani D, DiPiero V, Vallar G, et al. Technetium-99m HM-PAO SPECT study of regional cerebral perfusion in early Alzheimer's disease. *J Nucl Med* 1988;29:1507–1514.
149. Bonte FJ, Hom J, Tintner R, Weiner MF. Single photon tomography in Alzheimer's disease and dementia. *Semin Nucl Med* 1990;20:342–352.
150. Holman BL, Johnson KA, Garada B, Carvalho PA, Satlin A. The scintigraphic appearance of Alzheimer's disease: a prospective study using technetium-99m HMPAO SPECT. *J Nucl Med* 1992;33:181–185.
151. Herscovitch P, Auchus AP, Gado M, Chi D, Raichle ME. Correction of positron emission tomography data for cerebral atrophy. *J Cereb Blood Flow Metab* 1986;6:120–124.
152. McGeer PL, Kamo H, Harrop R, Li DKB, Tuokko H, et al. Positron emission tomography in patients with clinically diagnosed Alzheimer's disease. *Can Med Assoc J* 1986; 134:597–603.
153. Fulham MJ, Polinsky RJ, Nee L, Baser SM, Brooks RA, et al. Cerebral glucose metabolism in dominantly inherited Alzheimer's disease: A longitudinal PET study. *Neurology* 1990;40(Suppl 1):150.
154. Polinsky RJ, Noble H, Di Chiro G, Nee L, Feldman G, et al. Dominantly inherited Alzheimer's disease: cerebral glucose metabolism. *J Neurol Neurosurg Psych* 1987;50:752–757.
155. Gustafson L, Brun A, Passant U. Frontal lobe degeneration of non-Alzheimer type, in Rossor M (ed.): *Bailliere's Clinical Neurology*. vol. 1. London, Bailliere Tindall, 1992, pp 559–582.
156. Neary D, Snowden JS, Northen B, Gouldin P. Dementia of frontal lobe type. *J Neurol Neurosurg Psychiat* 1988; 51:353–361.
157. Brown J. Pick's disease, in Rossor M (ed.): *Bailliere's Clinical Neurology*. vol. 1. London, Bailliere Tindall, 1992, pp 535–557.
158. Heiss WD, Herholz K, Pawlik G, Hebold I, Klinkhammer P, et al. Positron emission tomography findings in dementia disorders: Contributions to differential diagnosis and objectivising of therapeutic effects. *Keio Med J* 1989; 38:111–135.
159. Palmer MS, Collinge J. Human prion disease, in Rossor M

(ed.): *Bailliere's Clinical Neurology.* vol. 1. London, Bailliere Tindall, 1992, pp 627–651.

160. Holthoff VA, Sandmann J, Pawlik G, Schroder R, et al. Positron emission tomography in Creutzfeldt-Jakob disease. *Arch Neurol* 1990;47:1035–1038.
161. Brunetti A, Berg G, Di Chiro G, et al. Reversal of brain metabolic abnormalities following treatment of AIDS Dementia Complex with 3′-azido-2′,3′-dideoxythymidine: A PET-FDG study. *J Nucl Med* 1989;30:581–590.
162. Ell PJ, Costa DC, Harrison M. Imaging cerebral damage in HIV infection. *Lancet* 1987;2:569–570.
163. Pohl P, Vogl G, Fill H, Rossler H, Zangerle R, Gerstenbrand F. Single photon emission computed tomography in AIDS dementia complex. *J Nucl Med* 1988;29:1382–1386.
164. Tran Dink YR, Mamo H, Cervoni C, Saimot AC. Disturbances in the cerebral perfusion of human immune deficiency virus-1 seropositive asymptomatic subjects: a quantitative tomography study of 18 cases. *J Nucl Med* 1990;31:1601–1607.
165. Brooks DJ, Frackowiak RSJ. PET and movement disorders. *J Neurol Neurosurg Psych* 1989;(Special Suppl):68–77.
166. Dannals RF, Ravert HT, Wilson AA. Radiochemistry of tracers for neurotransmitter receptor studies, in Frost JJ, Wagner HN, (eds.): *Quantitative Imaging: Neuroreceptors, neurotransmitters and enzymes.* New York, Raven, 1990, pp 19–35.
167. Duvoisin RC. Diseases of the extrapyramidal system, in Rosenberg RN (ed.): *The Clinical Neurosciences.* New York, Churchill Livingstone, 1983, p 441.
168. Kuhl DE, Metter EJ, Riege WH. Patterns of glucose utilization determined in Parkinson's disease by the [18F]Fluorodeoxyglucose method. *Ann Neurol* 1984;15:419–424.
169. Martin WRW, Beckman JH, Calne DB, Adam MJ, et al. Cerebral glucose metabolism in Parkinson's disease. *Can J Neurol Sci* 1984;11:169–173.
170. Garnett ES, Nahmias C, Firnau G. Central dopaminergic pathways in hemiparkinsonism examined by positron emission tomography. *Can J Neurol Sci* 1984;11:174–179.
171. Brooks DJ, Ibanez V, Sawle GV, et al. Differing patterns of striatal 18F-Dopa uptake in Parkinson's disease, Multiple System Atrophy, and Progressive Supranuclear Palsy. *Ann Neurol* 1990;28:547–555.
172. Brooks DJ, Salmon EP, Mathias CJ, Quinn N, et al. The relationship between locomotor disability, autonomic dysfunction, and the integrity of the striatal dopaminergic system in patients with multiple system atrophy, pure autonomic failure, and Parkinson's disease, studied with PET. *Brain* 1990;113:1539–1552.
173. Sawle GV. Nuclear medicine and the management of patients with Parkinson's movement disorders, in Murray IPC, Ell PJ, (eds.): *Nuclear Medicine in Clinical Diagnosis and Treatment.* vol. 1. New York, Churchill Livingstone, 1994, pp 589–598.
174. Leenders KL, Antonini A, Hess K. Brain dopamine D2 receptor density in Parkinsons's disease measured with PET using [11C]raclopride. *J Cereb Blood Flow Metab* 1991;11(Suppl 2):S818.
175. Tatsch K, Schwarz J, Oertal WH, Kirsch C-M. SPECT imaging of dopamine D2 receptors with 123-IBZM: initial experience in controls and patients with Parkinson's syndrome and Wilson's disease. *Nucl Med Commun* 1991;12: 699–707.
176. Brucke T, Podreka I, Angelberger P, et al. Dopamine D2 receptor imaging with SPECT: studies in different neuropsychiatric disorders. *J Cereb Blood Flow Metab* 1991; 11:220–228.
177. Fulham MJ, Dubinsky RM, Polinsky RJ, Brooks RA, Brown RT, et al. Computed tomography, magnetic resonance imaging and positron emission tomography with [^{18}F]Fluorodeoxyglucose in the assessment of Multiple System Atrophy and Pure Autonomic Failure. *Clin Auton Res* 1991;1:27–37.
178. Tedroff J, Aquilonius SM, Hartvig A, et al. Monoamine reuptake sites in the human brain evaluated in-vivo by means of ^{11}C-nomifensine and positron emission tomography: the effects of age and Parkinson's disease. *Acta Neurol Scand* 1988;77:192–201.
179. Riley RE, Lang AE, Lewis A, et al. Cortico-basal ganglionic degeneration. *Neurology* 1990;40:1203–1212.
180. Rebeiz JJ, Kolodny EH, Richardson EP. Corticodentatonigral degeneration with neuronal achromasia. *Arch Neurol* 1968;18:20–23.
181. Sawle GV, Brooks DJ, Marsden CD, Frackowiak RSJ. Corticobasal degeneration. A unique pattern of regional cortical oxygen hypometabolism and striatal fluorodopa uptake demonstrated by positron emission tomography. *Brain* 1991; 114:541–556.
182. Eidelberg D, Dhawan V, Moeller JR, et al. The metabolic landscape of corticobasal ganglionic degeneration: regional asymmetries studied with positron emission tomography. *J Neurol Neurosurg Psychiat* 1991;54:856–862.
183. Jackson JA, Jankovic J, Ford J. Progressive Supranuclear Palsy: Clinical features and response to treatment in 16 patients. *Ann Neurol* 1983;13:273–278.
184. Steele JC, Richardson JC, Olszewski J. Progressive supranuclear palsy. *Arch Neurol* 1964;10:333–359.
185. D'Antona R, Baron JC, Samson Y, et al. Subcortical dementia: frontal cortex hypometabolism detected by positron emission tomography in patients with progressive supranuclear palsy. *Brain* 1985;108:785–799.
186. Foster NL, Gilman SD, Berent S, Morin EM, Brown MB, et al. Cerebral hypometabolism in Progressive Supranuclear Palsy studied with positron emission tomography. *Ann Neurol* 1988;24:399–406.
187. Goffinet AM, De Volder AG, Gillain C, Rectem D, Michel C, et al. Positron tomography demonstrates frontal lobe hypometabolism in Progressive Supranuclear Palsy. *Ann Neurol* 1989;25:131–139.
188. Blin J, Baron JC, Dubois B, Pillon B, Cambon H, et al. Positron emission tomography study in Progressive Supranuclear Palsy: Brain hypometabolic pattern and clinicometabolic correlations. *Arch Neurol* 1990;47:747–752.
189. Albert ML, Feldman RG, Willis AL. The 'sub cortical dementia' of progressive supranuclear palsy. *J Neurol Neurosurg Psychiat* 1974;37:121–130.
190. Hayden MR. *Huntington's chorea.* Berlin, Springer-Verlag, 1981.
191. Hayden MR, Martin WRW, Stoessl AJ, Clark C, Hollenberg S, et al. Positron emission tomography in the early diagnosis of Huntington's disease. *Neurology* 1986;36:888–894.
192. Kuhl DE, Phelps ME, Markham CH, Metter EJ, Riege WH, Winter H. Cerebral metabolism and atrophy in Huntington's disease determined by FDG and computed tomographic scan. *Ann Neurol* 1982;12:425–434.
193. Mazziotta JC, Phelps ME, Pahl JJ, Huang SC, Baxter LR, et al. Reduced cerebral glucose metabolism in asymptomatic subjects at risk for Huntington's disease. *N Engl J Med* 1987;316:357–362.
194. Young AB, Penney JB, Starosta-Rubinstein S, et al. PET scan investigations of Huntington's disease: cerebral metabolic correlates of neurological features and functional decline. *Ann Neurol* 1986;20:293–303.
195. Hawkins RA, Mazziotta JC, Phelps ME. Wilson's disease studied with FDG and positron emission tomography. *Neurology* 1987;37:1701–1711.
196. Alavi A, Hirsch LJ. Studies of central nervous system disorders with single photon emission computed tomography and

positron emission tomography: evolution over the past two decades. *Semin Nucl Med* 1991;21:58–81.
197. Fayad PB, Brass LM. Single photon emission computed tomography in cerebrovascular disease. *Stroke* 1991;22: 950–954.
198. Frackowiak RSJ. PET scanning: Can it help resolve management issues in cerebral ischemic disease? *Stroke* 1986; 17:803–807.
199. Frackowiak RSJ, Wise RJS. Positron emission tomography in ischemic cerebrovascular disease. *Neurol Clin* 1983; 1:183–200.
200. Hellman RS, Tikofsky RS. An overview of the contributions of regional cerebral blood flow studies in cerebrovascular disease. Is there a role for single photon emission computed tomography? *Semin Nucl Med* 1990;20:303–324.
201. Powers WJ, Raichle ME. Positron emission tomography and its application to the study of cerebrovascular disease in man. *Stroke* 1985;16:361–376.
202. Powers WJ. Cerebral hemodynamics in ischemic cerebrovascular disease. *Ann Neurol* 1991;29:231–240.
203. Sette G, Baron JC, Mazoyer B, Levasseur M, Pappata S, et al. Local brain hemodynamics and oxygen metabolism in cerebrovascular disease. *Brain* 1989;112:931–951.
204. Wise RJS, Bernardi S, Frackowiak RSJ, Legg NJ, Jones T. Serial observations on the pathophysiology of acute stroke: transition from ischemia to infarction as reflected in the regional oxygen extraction. *Brain* 1983;106:197–222.
205. Lassen NA. The luxury-perfusion syndrome and its possible relation to metabolic acidosis located within the brain. *Lancet* 1966;2:1113–1115.
206. Baron JC, Bousser MG, Rey A, Guillard A, Comar D, et al. Reversal of focal 'misery perfusion syndrome' by extra-intraincranial arterial bypass in hemodynamic cerebral ischemia. *Stroke* 1981;12:454–459.
207. De Roo M, Mortelmans L, Devos P, et al. Clinical experience with Tc-99m HM-PAO high resolution SPECT of the brain in patients with cerebrovascular accidents. *Eur J Nucl Med* 1989;15:9–15.
208. Podreka I, Suess E, Goldenberg G, et al. Initial experience with technetium-99m HM-PAO brain SPECT. *J Nucl Med* 1987;28:1657–1666.
209. Caplan LR. Question-driven technology assessment: SPECT as an example. *Neurology* 1991;41:187–191.
210. EC-IC Bypass Study Group. Failure of extra-intracranial arterial bypass to reduce the risk of ischemic stroke. *N Engl J Med* 1985;313:1191–1200.
211. Greenmayre JT. The role of glutamate in neurotransmission and neurologic disease. *Arch Neurol* 1986;43:1058–1063.
212. Olney JW. Glutamate-induced neuronal necrosis in infant mouse hypothalamus: an electron microscopic study. *J Neuropathol Exp Neurol* 1971;30:75–90.
213. Rothman S. Synaptic release of excitatory amino acid transmitter mediates anoxic neuronal death. *J Neurosci* 1984; 4:1884–1891.
214. Wieloch T. Endogenous excitotoxins as possible mediators of ischemic and hypoglycemic brain damage. *Epilepsia* 1985;26:501.
215. Wieloch T. Hypoglycemia-induced neuronal damage prevented by an N-methyl-D-Aspartate antagonist. *Science* 1985;230:681–683.
216. Belliveau JW, Kennedy DN, McKinstry RC, et al. Functional mapping of the human visual cortex by magnetic resonance imaging. *Science* 1991;254:216–219.
217. Crosson B, Williamson DJG, Shukla SS, Honeyman JC, Nadeau SE. A technique to localize activation in the human brain with technetium-99m-HMPAO SPECT: A validation study using visual stimulation. *J Nucl Med* 1994;35:755–763.
218. Demonet J-F, Celsis P, Nespoulous J-L, Viallard G, Marc-Vergnes J-P, Rascol A. Cerebral blood flow correlates of word monitoring in sentences: influences of semantic incoherence. A SPECT study in normals. *Neuropsychologia* 1992;30:1–11.
219. Le Scao Y, Baulieu JL, Robier A, Pourcelot L, Beutter P. Increment of brain temporal perfusion during auditory stimulation. *Eur J Nucl Med* 1991;18:981–983.
220. Woods SW, Hegeman IM, Zubal IG, et al. Visual stimulation increases technetium-99m-HMPAO distribution in human visual cortex. *J Nucl Med* 1991;32:210–215.

18 Radionuclide Cisternography

John C. Harbert

The use of radiopharmaceuticals to image the cerebrospinal fluid (CSF) spaces was begun in 1953 by Bauer and Yuhl,[1] who were concerned about the hazards of conventional radiographic contrast agents in myelographic examinations. In 1955, Chou and French used external counting to follow the distribution and excretion of ^{131}I-human serum albumin (HSA) injected into the lumbar CSF spaces.[2] The next year, Crowe and colleagues demonstrated that ^{24}NaCl collected on cotton pledgets in the nose after cisterna magna injection in patients with CSF rhinorrhea.[3] Later, Rieselbach et al. used scintillation scanning to follow the ascent of intrathecally injected ^{198}Au colloid into the cerebral CSF spaces in patients with meningeal leukemia.[4]

Hydrocephalus was first studied scintigraphically by Bell, who injected radiopharmaceuticals directly into the ventricles.[5] Using a Geiger counter, he also used this method to demonstrate the patency of ventricular shunts. Mundinger in Germany performed similar studies using ^{131}I-labeled hippuran.[6] However, it was DiChiro in 1964, using external scanning of intrathecally injected ^{131}I-HSA, who developed the basic techniques of radionuclide cisternography and who demonstrated the marked changes in radionuclide patterns in obstructive hydrocephalus.[7]

CSF PHYSIOLOGY

The formation and flow of CSF has been termed the "third circulation." CSF is produced by the choroid plexus, the ventricular ependyma, and the arachnoid both by active secretion and passive diffusion. The largest amount, however, is secreted by the choroid plexus of the lateral, third, and fourth ventricles.[8] The CSF thus formed circulates within the ventricles and flows out of the fourth ventricular foramina into the subarachnoid spaces. Some of the CSF flows downward to bathe the spinal cord; the remainder ascends through the basal cisterns and incisura, then over the cerebral convexities, and is drained by bulk flow through the arachnoid villi into the superior longitudinal sinus (Fig. 1). The rate of production in adults is approximately 0.4 mL/min and is largely independent of CSF pressure, a critical factor in the development of hydrocephalus.[9] The rate of CSF reabsorption, on the other hand, is related directly to CSF pressure.[10] The chief clinical concerns related to the CSF circulation are anomalous structures, obstruction, and leakage. The radionuclide tests discussed here involve the identification and localization of these problems.

RADIOPHARMACEUTICALS

Early radionuclide tracer studies of the CSF were performed with ^{198}Au colloid and ^{131}I HSA; however, the beta-particle emissions of these radionuclides make them unsuitable CSF tracers. Occasional production problems resulted in contamination of ^{131}I-HSA with bacterial endotoxins that caused sporadic cases of aseptic meningitis.[11] Such mishaps led to the appreciation that radiopharmaceuticals injected into the CSF must be specifically prepared and tested for the presence of endotoxin. The intrathecal route is approximately 1000 times more sensitive to endotoxins than the intravenous route in producing a febrile response.[12] Endotoxin concentrations may be too low to be detected by USP rabbit testing, but they are readily detected by the more sensitive *Limulus* test. All radiopharmaceutical manufacturers observe this precaution.

Some acceptable radiopharmaceuticals are listed in Table 1. Radiolabeled chelates, especially DTPA, diffuse across the ependyma to some extent; however, this diffusion does not usually interfere with imaging. Currently, ^{111}In-DTPA is the most commonly used CSF tracer. The half-life of ^{99m}Tc is too short for the evaluation of adult hydrocephalus, in which 48-hour images may be needed. ^{97}Ru-DTPA delivers a somewhat lower radiation dose to the spinal cord than ^{111}In-DTPA because of a lower abundance of low-energy electron emissions, and possibly has better imaging qualities.[13] ^{99}Ru has a 2.9-day half-life and 88% 216-keV photon; however, it has not reached commercial production.

Techniques

Ordinarily, CSF radiopharmaceuticals are injected into the lumbar subarachnoid space. Cisterna magna and intraventricular injections are occasionally useful, however, depending upon the problem being investigated. The patient is prepared using standard lumbar puncture techniques. Children and agitated patients may require sedation. A 22-gauge needle should be used for the injection and the least possible manipulation (e.g., CSF manometry) is advised to avoid misinjection outside the subarachnoid space. Adding 2 to 3 mL of 10% dextrose solution to the injection and placing

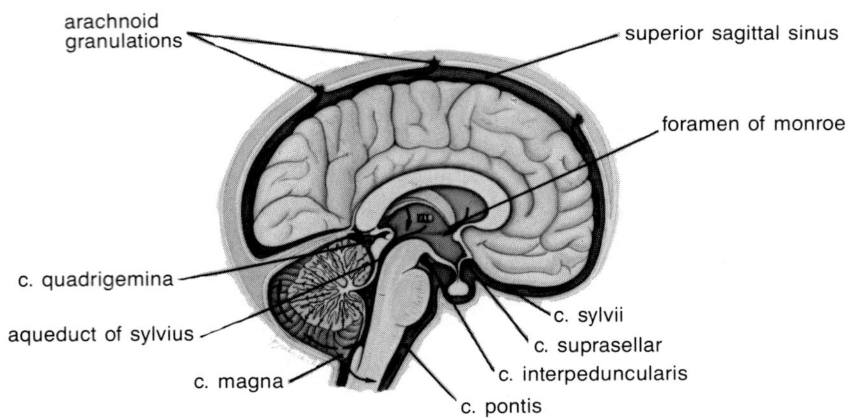

Figure 1. Cerebrospinal fluid circulation and the major intracranial cisterns.

the patient in the Trendelenburg position has been reported to reduce the number of misinjections.[14] The addition of this hyperbaric vehicle does not alter the subsequent cisternographic pattern, because the dextrose quickly diffuses out of the spinal CSF. In the injected radiopharmaceutical fails to reach the cisterns in satisfactory amounts, the spine should be scanned to rule out a subdural or epidural injection (Fig. 2).

High-quality images of the spinal and cerebral CSF spaces can be obtained with 30,000 to 50,000 counts. The usual imaging sequence is 1, 3, 6, 24, and 48 hours after injection. Early images are important because ventricular *reflux,* penetration of tracer into the ventricles and the hallmark of obstructive communicating hydrocephalus, usually is visualized early, if at all. The 48-hour images are useful in the diagnosis of porencephalic and subarachnoid cysts, and in ruling out the presence of a subarachnoid block in patients with a "delayed clearance" pattern, as in cerebral atrophy.

CLINICAL APPLICATIONS

Hydrocephalus

Hydrocephalus, a pathologic increase in the CSF volume, is associated with enlargement of the lateral ventricles. The following is a simple and useful classification:

1. Obstructive Hydrocephalus
   A. Noncommunicating: obstruction occurs between lateral ventricles and basal cisterns;
   B. Communicating: obstruction occurs in basal cisterns, cerebral convexities, or arachnoid villi;
2. Nonobstructive Hydrocephalus
   A. Generalized—due to cerebral atrophy;
   B. Localized—due to porencephaly.

Both Hakim et al. and Ommaya et al. have described the pathogenesis of obstructive hydrocephalus.[16,17] Only the briefest consideration is possible here. Some precipitating event (e.g., hemorrhage, infection, or tumor) blocks the CSF pathways. Cerebrospinal fluid formation continues undiminished, raising CSF pressure. As CSF volume increases and CSF pressure rises above venous pressure, the intracranial venous vascular volume decreases. Ultimately, interstitial water and cellular lipids are lost as the ventricles continue to expand. Alterations in the ventricular ependyma develop, so that the capillaries in the deep periventricular white matter, rather than the arachnoid villi, become the principal site of CSF absorption, causing an apparent reversal of normal CSF flow into the ventricles. If equilibrium is reestablished before brain hypoxia develops "compensated hydrocephalus" exists, sometimes without appreciable symptoms. Compensation is common in children with open fontanelles because the cranial vault can expand, relieving intracranial pressure and preserving brain substance. If ventricular expansion continues, however, progressive loss of brain substance occurs, and the characteristic features of overt hydrocephalus develop.

The cisternographic changes observed in hydrocephalus

Table 1. Properties of Some CSF Tracers

RADIOPHARMACEUTICAL	USUAL DOSE (μCi)	CSF T_{eff} (h)	SPINAL CORD RADIATION DOSE* (cGy)	WHOLE-BODY RADIATION DOSE (cGy)
^{99m}Tc-HSA	1000	5	2–5	0.03
^{99m}Tc-inulin or EDTA	1000	5	2–5	0.03
^{111}In-transferrin	500	21	7	0.26
^{111}In-DTPA or EDTA	500	10	2	0.04
^{169}Yb-DTPA	500	12	6–25	0.07

*Surface dose to spinal CSF at injection site in patients without spinal cord block.

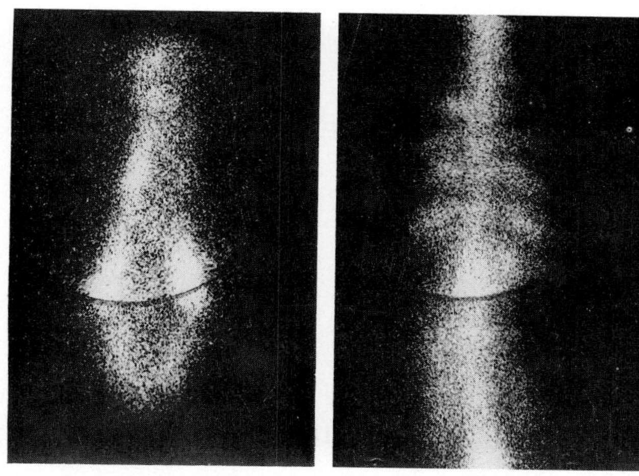

Figure 2. **(A)**. Lumbosacral region following subdural injection. **(B)**. Thoracolumbar region following epidural injection. Note the radiopharmaceutical outlining the thoracic nerve roots (from Larson SM, Schall GL, DiChiro G[15]).

are best understood by considering the normal pattern (Fig. 3). By 1 to 3 hours, the basal cisterns are visualized. Only the cisterna magna and quadrigeminal cistern are visualized distinctly. The pontine, interpeduncular, and suprasellar cisterns cannot be separately distinguished. By 3 to 6 hours, activity has entered the sylvian and interhemispheric fissures. By 24 hours, activity surrounds the hemispheres. Because of radiopharmaceutical diffusion into the cerebral cortex, images obtained after 24 hours increasingly reflect brain tissue rather than CSF space, and the residual tracer clears slowly.[18] At no time is activity seen within the ventricles.

The changes in the cisternographic pattern seen in hydrocephalus relate only to the presence or absence of ventricular reflux and to the relative rate of CSF clearance. In obstructive communicating hydrocephalus, ventricular reflux and delayed clearance occur (Fig. 4).[19,20] In noncommunicating hydrocephalus, the cisternographic pattern is normal or there may be delayed clearance, but no ventricular reflux occurs.

Normal Pressure Hydrocephalus Versus Cerebral Atrophy

After Hakim described the syndrome of *normal pressure hydrocephalus* (NPH), an enthusiastic effort was directed toward finding better methods for its diagnosis, because it is one of the few treatable dementias.[21,22] The cause and cisternographic finding of NPH do not differ essentially from those of obstructive communicating hydrocephalus with elevated pressure. Why the pressure is normal or only slightly elevated in NPH is not well understood. Nevertheless, as the obstructed ventricles expand and the ventricular wall area increases, lower pressures are required to maintain a given force acting against the walls.[16,23] Pascal's law, which states that force is the product of pressure and area, is a useful concept in obstructive hydrocephalus, even if it is an oversimplification of complex brain elastic dynamics. Thus, massively enlarged ventricles may be seen with only slightly elevated CSF pressures. Short of spontaneous remission, the only possibility for reversal of ventricular dilatation is by diversionary shunting which, by reducing CSF pressure, reduces the force acting against the ventricular walls, and allows the ventricles to return to normal volume. The symptoms associated with NPH are dementia, spastic gait, and urinary incontinence, progressing to coma in acute, untreated conditions. Computed tomography demonstrates ventricular dilatation, usually without cortical atrophy.

Bannister et al. first recognized the cisternographic pattern of ventricular reflux and delayed clearance.[24] Ependymal and/or choroid plexus reabsorption draws CSF into the ventricles where it clears, although more slowly than by the normal convexity route. Obstruction can occur anywhere within the subarachnoid space, a fact that accounts for the varying cisternographic patterns described in this condition. Obstruction at the level of either the basal cisterns or the incisura cerebelli (the notch in the tentorium through which the brain stem passes) is shown in Figure 4. This pattern is usually associated with clinical improvement following diversionary shunting, provided no brain damage coexists.[24–29] If the mechanical block is higher over the convexities, a "combination" pattern is seen (i.e., ventricular reflux and variable, but delayed, flow over the convexities) (Fig. 5). In this case, the prognosis following shunting is impossible to predict. In any event, the decision of whether or not to shunt adult patients almost always rests upon the clinical response to serial spinal taps and intracranial pressure monitoring.[30]

Cerebral atrophy or *hydrocephalus ex vacuo* results from a loss of brain substance by degenerative processes rather than by pressure expansion.[30] The symptoms associated with cerebral atrophy are often similar to those of NPH. Computed tomography (CT) scans demonstrate enlarged ventricles and dilated sulci and fissures; often, no other diagnostic procedure is needed. The most common cisternographic pattern associated with atrophy is normal or delayed tracer ascent without ventricular reflux. Transient ventricular reflux, when it occurs, does not persist at 24 hours.

CORRELATION WITH OTHER IMAGING MODALITIES

Computed tomography (CT) and magnetic resonance imaging (MRI) have largely replaced radionuclide cisternography as a screening test for hydrocephalus because of their precise definition of CSF spaces and surrounding structures. Too, MR can provide accurate information about CSF flow, using phase-contrast cine techniques.[31] In presenile dementia, the principle diagnostic problems to be excluded are cerebral atrophy, tumors, chronic subdural hematoma, deep white matter infarction (DWMI), and NPH. Computed tomography and MRI are sensitive in detecting all of these.

The MRI features that appear to correlate best with clinical improvement following shunting include: a) dilated ventri-

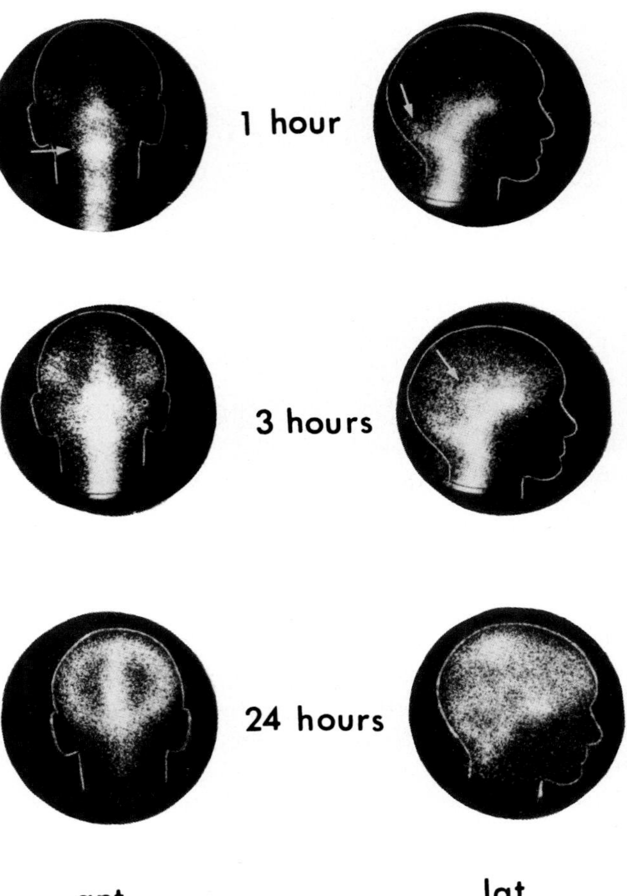

Figure 3. Normal radionuclide cisternogram showing anterior and right lateral views. At 1 hour, the cisterna magna (arrows) and basal cisterns are filled; by 3 hours, the large quadrigeminal cistern (arrow) is visible and, in the anterior view, the sylvian and interhemispheric fissures are well visualized. By 24 hours, activity is distributed completely over the hemispheres and has largely cleared from the basal cisterns.

cles out of proportion to any sulcal enlargement, b) upward bowing of the corpus callosum in sagittal sections, c) flattening of the cortical gyri against the inner table of the calvarium in parasagittal and coronal sections, d) prominent CSF *flow void* in the cerebral aqueduct and third ventricles, and e) absence of severe DWMI[32] (Fig. 6). The CSF flow void results from the pulsatile motion of CSF through the aqueduct. The magnitude of the flow void reflects ventricular size, size of the subarachnoid space, and cerebral blood flow; the MRI flow void is absent is atrophy and increased in obstructive hydrocephalus.[32]

Once the diagnosis of hydrocephalus without coexisting severe brain damage has been made, the question of patient management remains. There is broad consensus among neurosurgeons that, in the absence of significant CSF obstruction, the patient is not likely to benefit greatly from shunting. Radionuclide cisternography is very useful in estimating the CSF clearance capacity. The evaluation of CSF dynamics by CT and intrathecal metrizamide is complicated by continuing concern for the toxicity of metrizamide. The practicability of using gadolinium contrast agents intrathecally to add contrast to MR images has been demonstrated in animals,[33] but this is not yet the case for humans. For this reason, radionuclide cisternography remains a useful procedure in selecting patients for shunting. If atrophy or extensive brain damage is demonstrated by MRI, there is little indication for radionuclide cisternography. In significant ventricular dilation without atrophy, however, cisternography may be of value. Those patients with ventricular reflux and delayed clearance, especially with low subarachnoid blocks (Fig. 4) are probably candidates for shunting.

The value of SPECT in cisternography has yet to be determined. Rothenberg et al. reported its use in visualizing cisternal structures.[34] The anatomic detail may be superior to that of planar scans; however, its role in assessing CSF clearance has not been defined.

Pediatric Cisternography

The same technical principles that apply to adults pertain to infants and children, except that the dose of radiopharmaceutical is reduced. Good studies may be obtained using 0.4 to 0.6 MBq/kg (10 to 15 μCi/kg) ^{111}In-DTPA. In infants and young children, sedation may be needed. The normal cisternographic pattern is similar to that of adults, except that the tracer ascends more rapidly.[35] Activity reaches the basal cisterns by 15 to 30 min. and surrounds the convexities by 12 hours. Because early ventricular reflux is later ob-

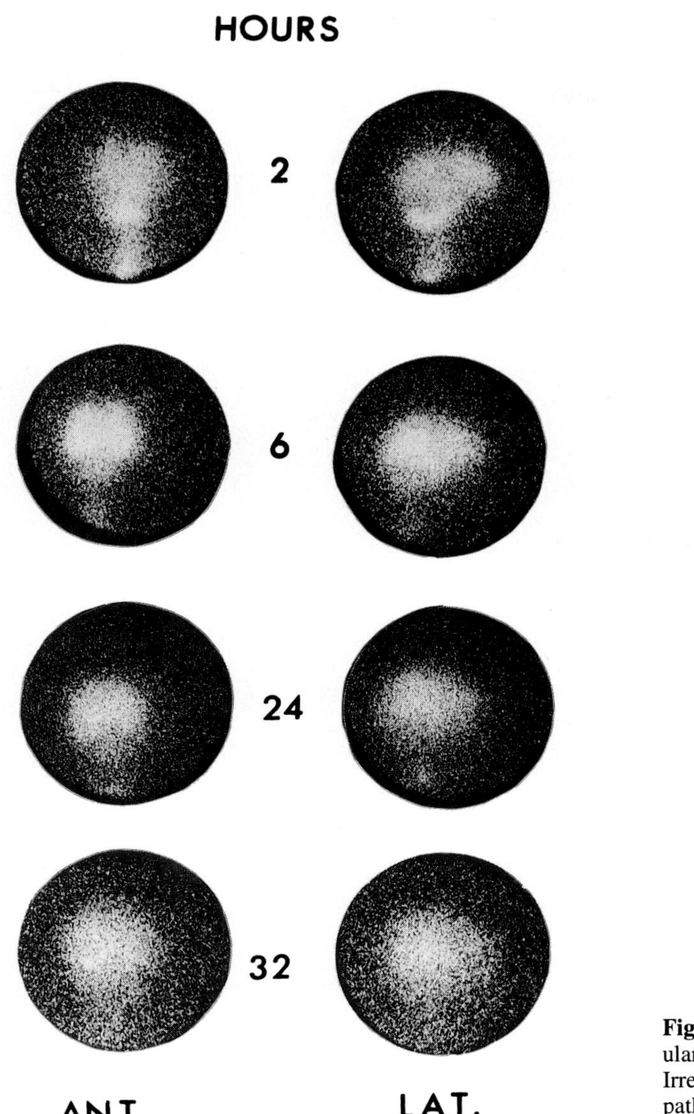

Figure 4. Communicating hydrocephalus with complete incisural block. Reflux into greatly enlarged ventricles is seen in all views. No activity ascends over the hemispheres. Note blurring of ventricular outline after 24 hours caused by diffusion of ^{111}In-DTPA into cerebral tissue.

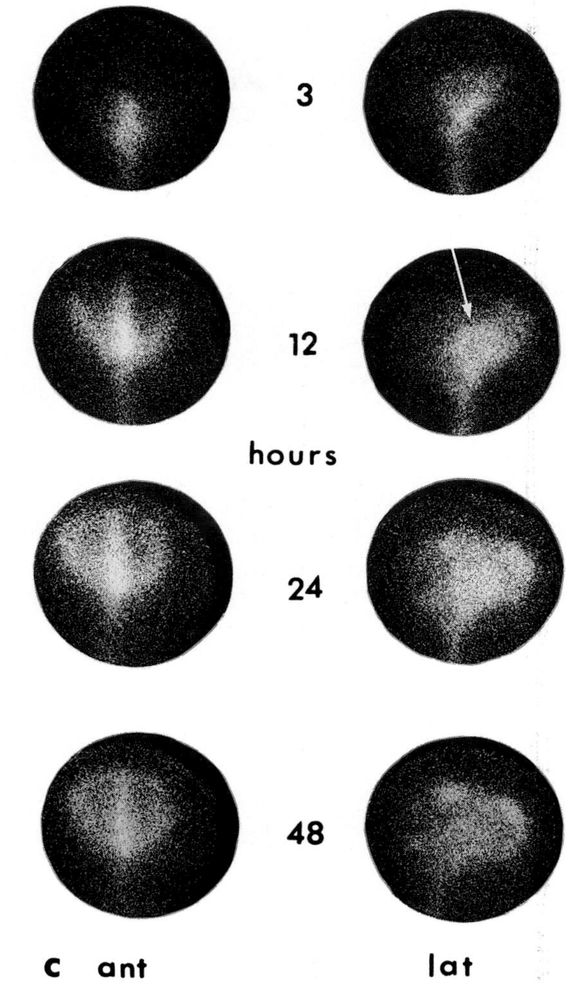

Figure 5. Communicating hydrocephalus demonstrating ventricular reflux (arrow) up to 12 hours, but not at 24 and 48 hours. Irregular hemispheric activity suggests partially occluded CSF pathways.

scured by activity in the quadrigeminal cistern and interhemispheric fissure, early scanning is essential.

In noncommunicating hydrocephalus, except for those cases caused by mass lesions, the usual sites of obstruction are the aqueduct and the outlets of the fourth ventricles. These infants require diversionary shunting. If a ventriculocisternal shunt is contemplated, the neurosurgeon must be assured that the CSF pathways over the convexities are patent. These patients ordinarily have increased intracranial pressure, and most neurosurgeons avoid lumbar puncture because of the danger of brain-stem herniation. The proper time to perform cisternography is after the pressure has been lowered by removal of ventricular fluid. This practice avoids the danger of brain-stem herniation and, by decreasing brain distention, affords a more reliable estimate of the functional patency of CSF pathways. If patients with noncommunicating hydrocephalus have normal cisternographic patterns under these conditions, they may respond satisfactorily to ventriculocisternal shunts or to ventriculocisternostomy.[36] However, the high incidence of complications associated with intracranial shunts restricts these procedures.[30] Patients with delayed clearance or a CSF pathway block after adjustment of CSF pressure must have extracranial (e.g., ventriculoatrial or ventriculoperitoneal) shunts.

In communicating hydrocephalus, the same cisternographic patterns seen in adults are found in children. In infants and younger children, CT scanning is satisfactory for evaluation because decision-making is supported by other factors, such as abnormal head size and growth pattern and

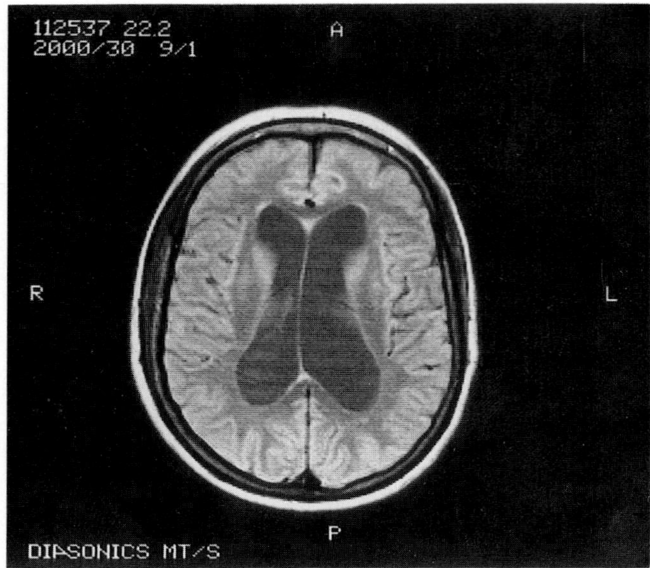

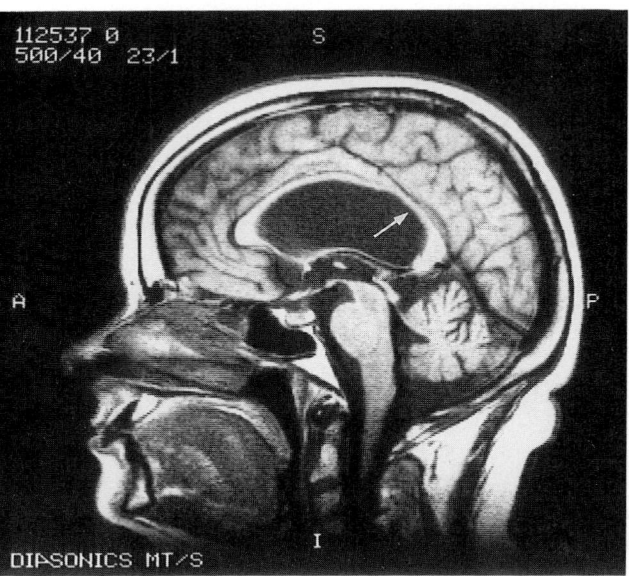

Figure 6. Normal pressure hydrocephalus: **(A)**. Axial section demonstrates dilatation of the lateral ventricles out of proportion to sulcal enlargement. The lack of a high-intensity border indicates that no interstitial edema is present and that the mean pressure is normal (spin echo [SE] 2000/30) (repetition time [Tr] msec/echo time [TE] msec); **(B)**. Midline sagittal section demonstrates upward bowing of the corpus callosum (arrow) and flattening of the cortical gyri against the inner table of the calvarium (SE 500/40). (Reproduced with permission of Bradley WG, et al.[32])

the tone of the anterior fontanelle, which are general signs of progression of the hydrocephalic condition.

Other Conditions

Several conditions give rise to focal abnormalities of the CSF spaces. Although the indications for cisternography in these cases are infrequent, the variations created in the cisternographic pattern are important to recognize:

1. Porencephalic cysts are the most frequently encountered focal CSF enlargements. They are caused by trauma (especially surgery), infection, or infarction, resulting in localized brain atrophy. They have pia-arachnoid linings and may or may not communicate with the ventricles. Those cysts that communicate with the subarachnoid spaces usually fill with the radionuclide tracer early and retain activity long after it has cleared from the rest of the CSF space (Fig. 7).
2. Leptomeningeal cysts are caused by traumatic dural rents. They are often associated with the basal cisterns and may require shunting if they create pressure on surrounding structures. In such cases, cisternography is useful in planning the most appropriate type of shunt procedure.[37] These cysts also tend to retain the injected radiopharmaceutical for prolonged periods, often in large, irregular collections.[20]
3. Posterior fossa abnormalities have several causes, including acquired and congenital cysts, osseous defects, and postoperative pseudocysts.[38,39] One of the most interesting, the Dandy-Walker cyst, is also associated with torcular elevation and with a marked decrease in the angle of the transverse sinuses on planar radionuclide brain scans (Fig. 8). For the most part, these posterior fossa abnormalities are better studied with CT and MRI.

SHUNT PATENCY STUDIES

Once the hydrocephalic patient has been shunted, regular examinations are required to assure shunt patency. Today, routine surveillance is usually undertaken through repeat CT scanning. However, these studies only demonstrate the increasing ventricular size associated with a malfunctioning shunt and not *why* the shunt is not functioning properly. Often too, a diagnosis of shunt patency and adequate CSF flow is made easily by examination of the patient and inspection of the subcutaneous CSF reservoir. If the patient is alert, is asymptomatic, and the reservoir readily rebounds after compression, the shunt cam be assumed to be functioning well. In cases of obvious neurological deterioration, with increased intracranial pressure and sluggish or unresponsive reservoirs, replacement is probably required and the final diagnosis of blocked shunt should be made in the operating room. Several conditions arise, however, in which the clinical diagnosis of shunt adequacy requires additional diagnostic information.

1. Signs of increased pressure or symptomatic progression with clinically functioning shunt. Dramatic or subtle progression of neurologic deficit may occur, even when the shunt reservoir appears to function normally. This condi-

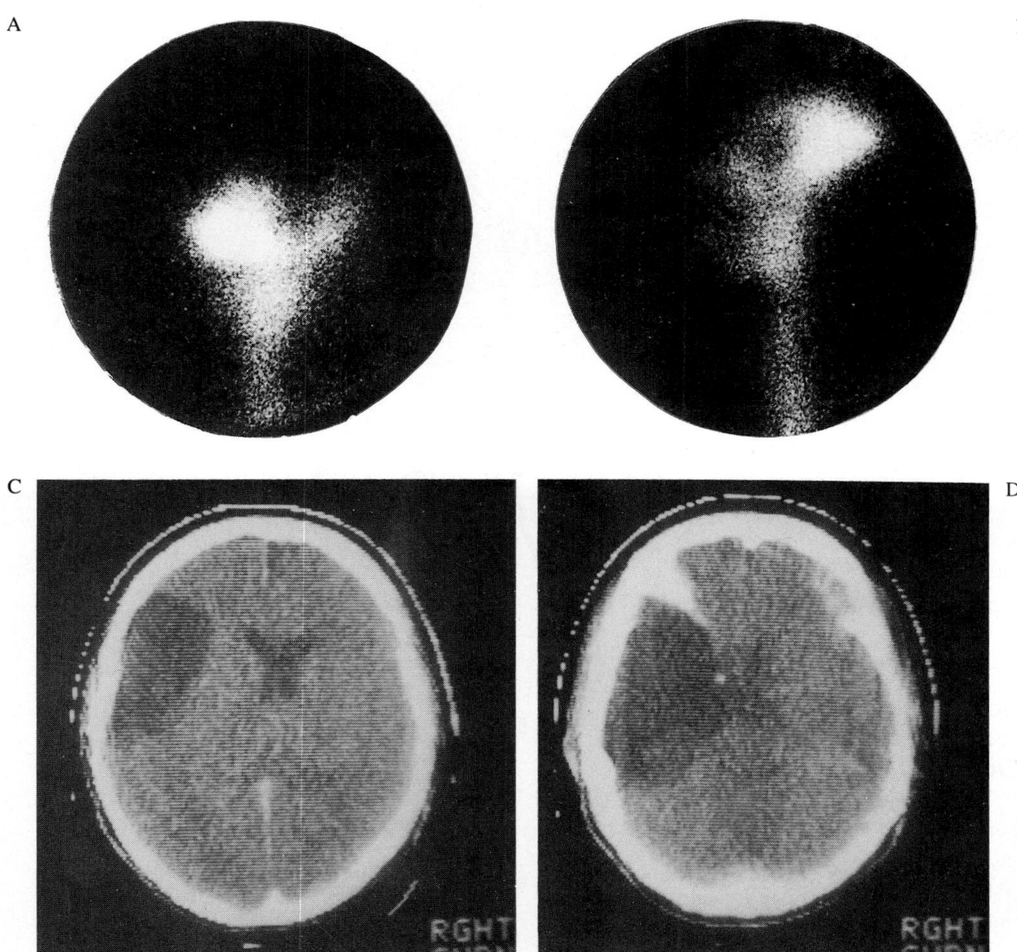

Figure 7. **(A)**. Anterior scintiphoto 3 hours after lumbar intrathecal injection of 20 MBq (500 μCi) ^{111}In-DTPA in a patient with right frontal porencephaly that developed after surgical excision of a meningioma; **(B)**. Right lateral; **(C, D)**. CT scans demonstrating communication with right ventricle.

tion is particularly likely to occur in the event of shunt or systemic infections, head trauma or acquired subdural hematomas, inappropriately high opening pressure in a *differential pressure valve,* and disconnection of the distal shunt catheter. All but the last two conditions dictate a course of action other than immediate shunt revision, and recognition of adequate shunt flow spares the patient both an unnecessary operation and delayed treatment of the precipitating cause.

2. Asymptomatic patient with clinically nonfunctioning shunt. CSF shunts usually require replacement at one time or another. The incidence of failed shunts increases with the length of follow-up. Young children frequently become shunt-dependent for life, but older children and adults with communicating hydrocephalus may eventually become shunt-independent. In the event of compensated hydrocephalus, the shunt is better left alone than replaced; however, one must be certain of shunt failure over a significant period of time before safely concluding that the patient has compensated hydrocephalus.
3. Ambiguous shunt function or unfamiliarity with shunt system. This category is perhaps the largest. Examples of ambiguity include shunted infants with failure to thrive, or adults with NPH who improve immediately

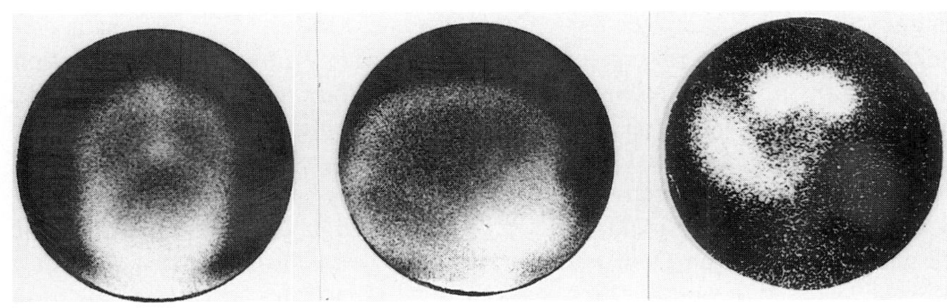

Figure 8. Posterior **(A)** and right lateral, **(B)** brain scans in 3-month-old patient with Dandy-Walker cyst, demonstrating elevation of the torcular and transverse sinus. **(C)**, Left lateral cisternogram 1 hour after lumbar intrathecal injection of ^{99m}Tc-HSA showing larger posterior fossa cyst.

after the surgical procedure and then become symptomatic again. Because so many different types of shunt systems are available, the clinician is unlikely to have evaluated all of them. Moreover, the function of Hakim and Holter valves is inherently difficult to judge by physical examination.

Techniques: Extracranial Shunts

The simplest method of measuring CSF shunt flow through extracranial shunts (i.e., ventriculoatrial, ventriculopleural, and ventriculoperitoneal shunts) involves the injection of a small amount of radionuclide (e.g., 3 MBq (100 μCi) of ^{99m}Tc-pertechnetate in 0.1 mL) directly into the subcutaneous shunt reservoir using a 25-gauge needle and sterile scalp preparation. A scintillation camera and computer are used to measure tracer clearance from the reservoir, and the clearance half-time is then determined.[40,41] Since the volume of each commercial reservoir is known, flow of CSF through the reservoir can be determined from the relationship:

$$F = \lambda V$$

where F = CSF shunt flow in mL/min, $\lambda = 0.693/T_{1/2}$, which is determined from the time-activity curve, and V = reservoir volume, which can be found from tables if the reservoir type is known.[40]

Figure 9 shows the usual placement of a ventriculoatrial shunt with the proximal arm extending through a burr hole into the lateral ventricle, and the distal arm running subcutaneously into the jugular vein. Figure 10 shows adequate clearance from a 16-mm Pudenz reservoir attached to a ventriculoperitoneal shunt. The scintiphoto is confirmatory evidence of an unobstructed distal catheter. The most common obstructive complications of ventriculoatrial shunts are (1) disconnection of the shunt tubing from the reservoir (either proximal or distal arms); (2) clotting of the distal shunt tubing; (3) retraction of the distal tubing from the venous channel; (4) blockage of the proximal arm with CSF debris or infection; and (5) impaction of the proximal tubing into brain tissue. If the injected radiopharmaceutical does not flow freely from the reservoir, have the patient execute a Valsalva maneuver or gently compress the reservoir several times to induce flow.

In Figure 10, the peritoneal end of a ventriculoperitoneal shunt is visualized for qualitative evidence of shunt function. Common complications of ventriculoperitoneal shunt catheters include mechanical failure by disconnection, knotting, kinking, and retraction from the abdomen with growth. The catheter tip may become occluded by fibrous encasement, infection, or pseudocyst formation. Intestinal obstruction, volvulus, intestinal perforation, ascites, and pleural effusions have also been reported.[42,43]

Some evidence suggests that valve systems, such as Holter valves, that are connected in series to a reservoir may slow tracer clearance from the reservoir.[44,45] The reasons for this prolonged clearance are not understood, but complex hydrodynamics set up in the reservoir may be the cause. The practical effect is an increase in the apparent reservoir volume. If CSF flow estimated from the above formula is unexpectedly low, use of the wrong value of V may be the cause of error. The only certain way of determining V is to measure clearance from the same shunt complex used in the patient under conditions of known flow rates. This has been done for combination valve-reservoir systems but not for multiple systems, where the reservoir and valve are connected in series.[40]

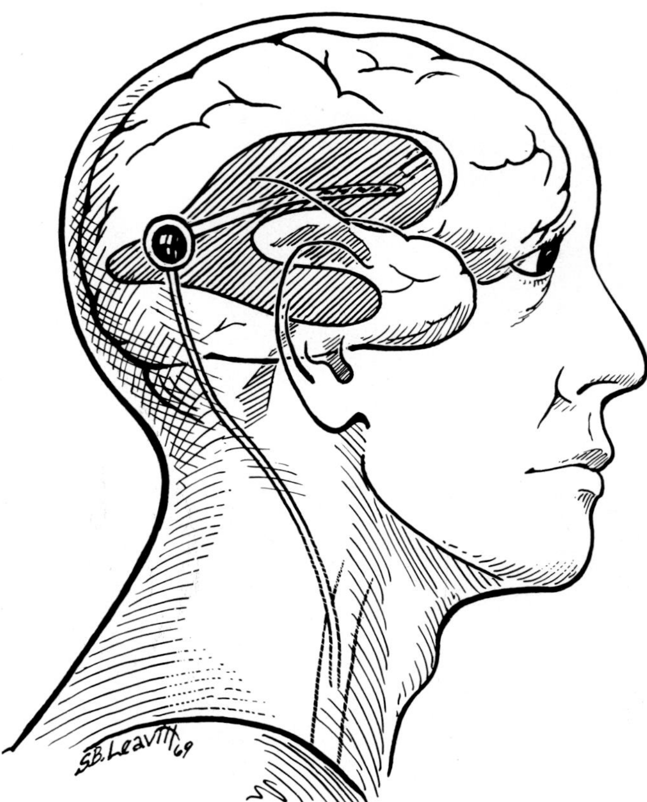

Figure 9. Ventriculoatrial shunt with proximal arm extending through a burr hole into the lateral ventricle and the distal arm running subcutaneously and into the atrium via the jugular vein.

Intracranial Shunts

Intracranial shunts, in which a catheter is inserted between the lateral ventricles and the cisterna magna or cervical spinal canal, and third *ventriculostomy,* in which a communication between the ventricular system and the CSF cisterns is created surgically, must be assessed by intraventricular injection of a *Limulus*-tested radiopharmaceutical, usually 4 MBq (100 μCi) ^{111}In-DTPA. Serial scintiphotos demonstrate flow of activity into the cisterna magna and, subsequently, over the convexities when the shunt is patent.

Similar studies are performed in assessing the patency of an Ommaya reservoir. This is a CSF access system with a

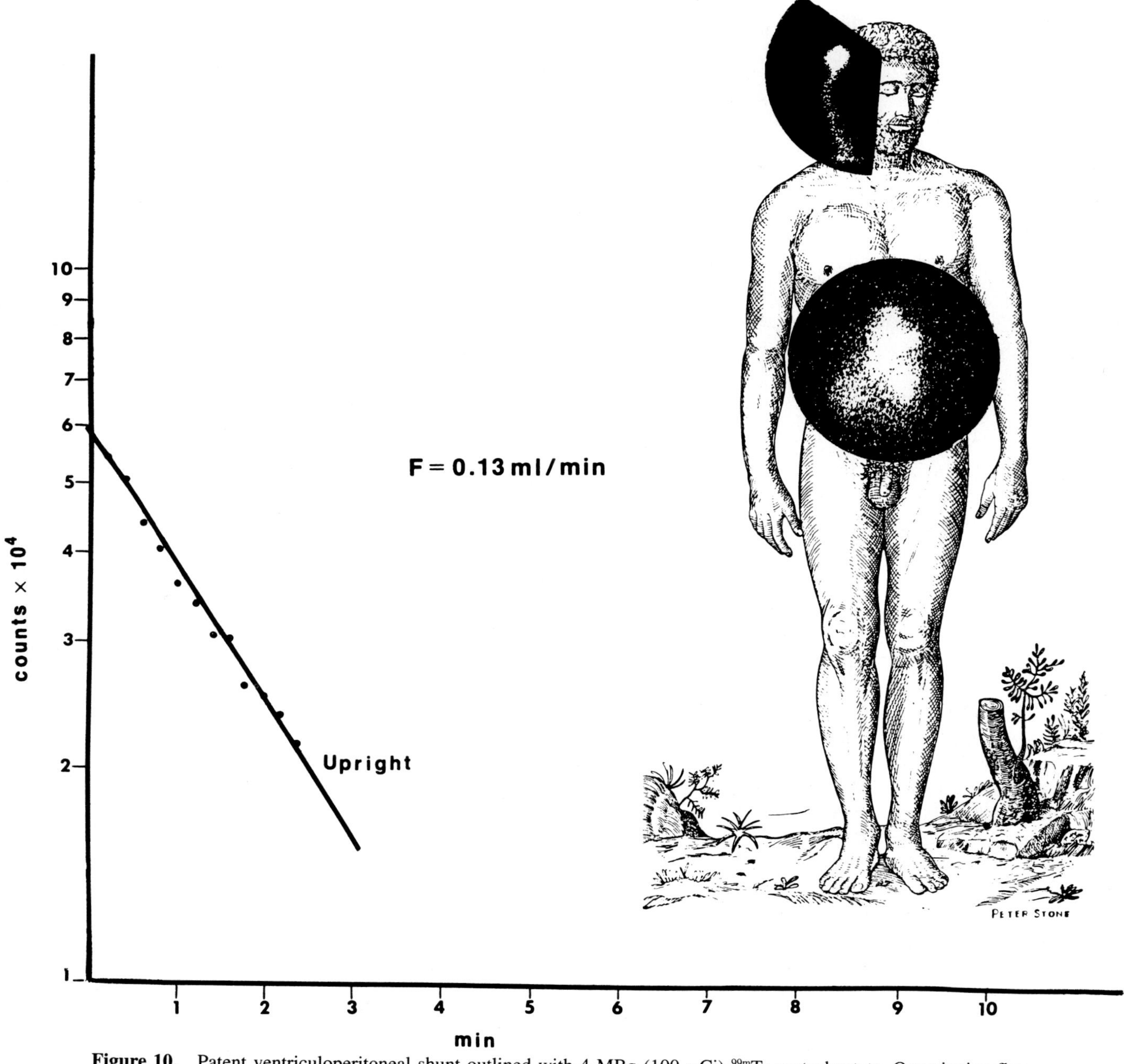

Figure 10. Patent ventriculoperitoneal shunt outlined with 4 MBq (100 μCi) ^{99m}Tc-pertechnetate. Quantitative flow study demonstrated a shunt flow of 0.13 mL.

reservoir implanted beneath the scalp and a single arm that is inserted through a burr hole and into the ventricle, used most often to deliver drugs intrathecally.[46] Such access ports can become blocked by CSF debris or by brain tissue, or become walled off by gliosis. Radionuclide ventriculography provides a convenient means of assessing patency of the CSF system from the reservoir to the cerebral and spinal subarachnoid spaces. Figure 11 demonstrates clear communication between an Ommaya reservoir and the basal cisterns following injection of 4 MBq (100 μCi) ^{111}In-DTPA.

Slow infusion devices for administering narcotic analgesia to patients with intractable pain can also be assessed by injection of radiopharmaceutical into the narcotic reservoir.[47] Apparent failure to control pain can be due to several causes, including pump system failure, progression of the disease, or to severe tachyphylaxis to the narcotic. Because of the

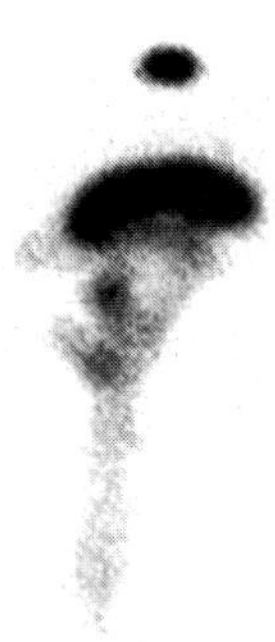

Figure 11. Patent Ommaya reservoir. 4 MBq (120 μCi) ^{111}In-DTPA injected into the reservoir, seen here at 15 min. filling the lateral ventricles, basal cisterns, and descending into the spinal subarachnoid space.

slow infusion rate and narrow tubing, higher doses of radiopharmaceutical (e.g., 40 to 80 MBq of ^{111}In-DTPA) must be administered, and overexposed film employed to image the transfer of the labeled reservoir contents into the spinal subarachnoid space.

CSF LEAKS

CSF Rhinorrhea and Otorrhea

CSF rhinorrhea and otorrhea pose difficult diagnostic problems. Occasionally, uncertainty that the rhinorrhea is of CSF origin exists and it is especially challenging to identify the exact site of leakage before surgery. Nuclear diagnostic techniques often are successful in proving the origin and many times can pinpoint the probable leak site.

Most cases of CSF rhinorrhea result from head trauma, although spontaneous CSF rhinorrhea also occurs. Several diagnostic procedures that have been developed to demonstrate the site of CSF leak include pneumoencephalography, various chemical and contrast dyes, radioactive tracers, and radionuclide scanning. Often, more than one procedure is required.

Crowe et al. introduced radionuclide tracers for detecting CSF leaks, using intrathecally injected ^{24}Na and counting pledgets placed in the nose.[3] Later, DiChiro introduced the use of ^{131}I-HSA for these studies.[48] Currently ^{111}In-DTPA is the most frequently used radiopharmaceutical.

If the patient is actively leaking, scintigraphy is used to localize the leak site.[49] ^{111}In-DTPA or ^{99m}Tc-HSA is injected in large doses (e.g., 75 to 100 MBq, 2 to 3 mCi) to achieve high counting rates and maximum resolution. The patient is injected in the lumbar space, then kept recumbent for 3 to 4 hours until images show activity well forward in the basal cisterns. The patient is then seated bent forward with head down to induce leaking. This maneuver draws the radioactivity into the leak tract where it can be imaged. Frequent images are taken with the head in the lateral position until the leak tract is demonstrated. Often this tract is visualized only transiently (Fig. 12).

The leak may take one of several pathways (Fig. 13). Perforations of the dura with communication through the petrous bone may give rise to otorrhea, although we have studied cases in which the CSF was diverted through the Eustachian tube to cause rhinorrhea (Fig. 14). Often, the actual leak "tract" is not visualized, but an abnormal accumulation is evident near the site of the leak, as shown in Figure 15 (which demonstrates a cribriform plate leak) or in Figure 16 (in which the leak sprang from a perforation of the petrous bone).

Magnaes and Solheim have reported the use of "overpressure" cisternography to localize CSF leaks.[51] In this technique, the lumbar infusion needle is connected to a pressure monitor and an infusion pump. Following injection of the radionuclide, artificial CSF is infused at a rate of 5 mL/min to maintain CSF pressure at up to 500 mm H_2O. This technique rapidly delivers the radiopharmaceutical to the leak site and increases the likelihood of demonstrating the leak tract.

Mamo et al. advocate frontal subarachnoid injections of radiopharmaceutical to increase the intracranial concentration of activity[52]; however, this more invasive technique is unlikely to become widespread.

Naidik and Moran reported the use of intrathecally injected metrizamide and CT to localize leak sites.[53] They recommended the "overpressure" technique with metrizamide when the usual Trendelenburg position fails to demonstrate the leak. Many patients suffer from nausea and headaches following intrathecal metrizamide and the sensitivity in localizing leaks varies from 20% to 87% in different centers.[54,55]

Whenever the diagnosis of CSF rhinorrhea is in doubt, the use of nasal pledgets is a useful procedure. These are placed in the anterior and posterior turbinates bilaterally following injection of the radiopharmaceutical and, subsequently, counted in a well counter. Because even "nondiffusible" tracers quickly reach the blood and then appear in mucous secretions,[51] corrections must be made. The cotton pledgets must be carefully weighed. The counts from the nasal pledgets are then compared with serum specimens drawn at the same time and expressed in terms of counts/fluid gram. This method will then account for normal nasal radioactivity as well as differences in pledget size and absorption. Nose-to-serum ratios under 1.5 should not be interpreted as evidence of CSF rhinorrhea.[57]

If all else fails to demonstrate the presence of a CSF leak, scan the abdomen. In some cases, the injected activity may leak into the posterior pharynx and appear in the gastrointestinal tract.[58] It may also be useful to perform SPECT scanning to better localize the site of the leak, because a tomographic slice through the plane of the leak may be more sensitive than planar imaging.[59]

CSF Fistulae

CSF rhinorrhea and otorrhea are the most common forms of CSF leak (Fig. 17), but CSF fistulae may communicate

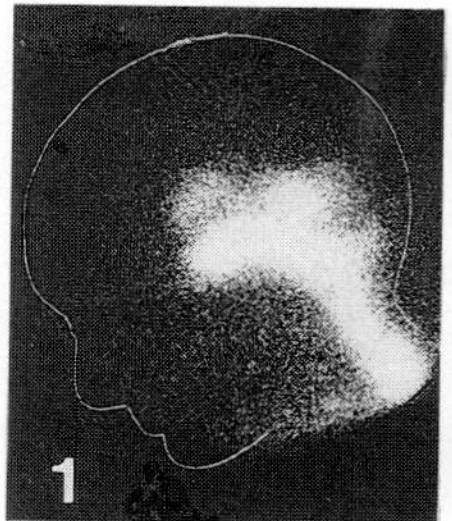

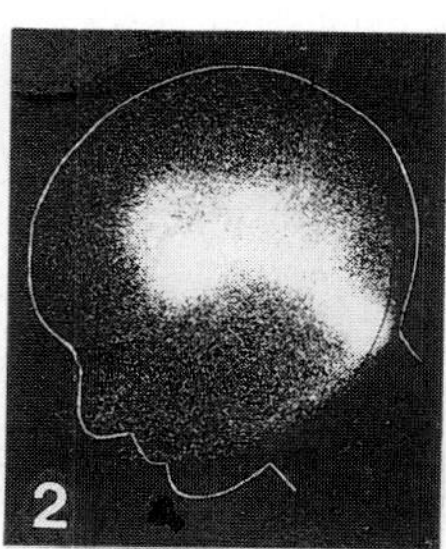

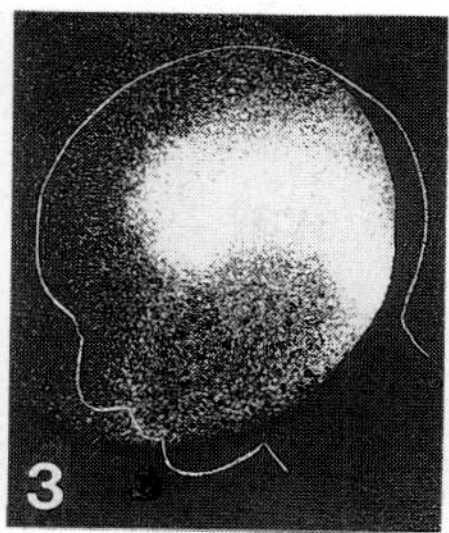

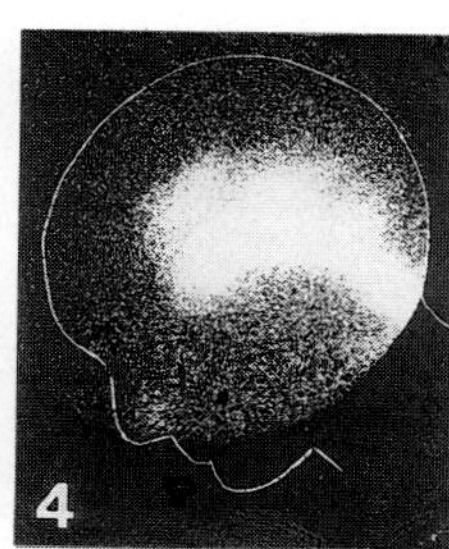

Figure 12. Sequential left lateral scintiphotos 3 hours after lumbar injection of 74 MBq (2 mCi) ^{99m}Tc-DTPA, showing ventricular reflux and abnormal accumulation of activity in the suprasellar cistern. In the third frame, a tract of activity is seen coming from the region of the ethmoid sinus and sella. (Courtesy of Dr. William Ashburn.)

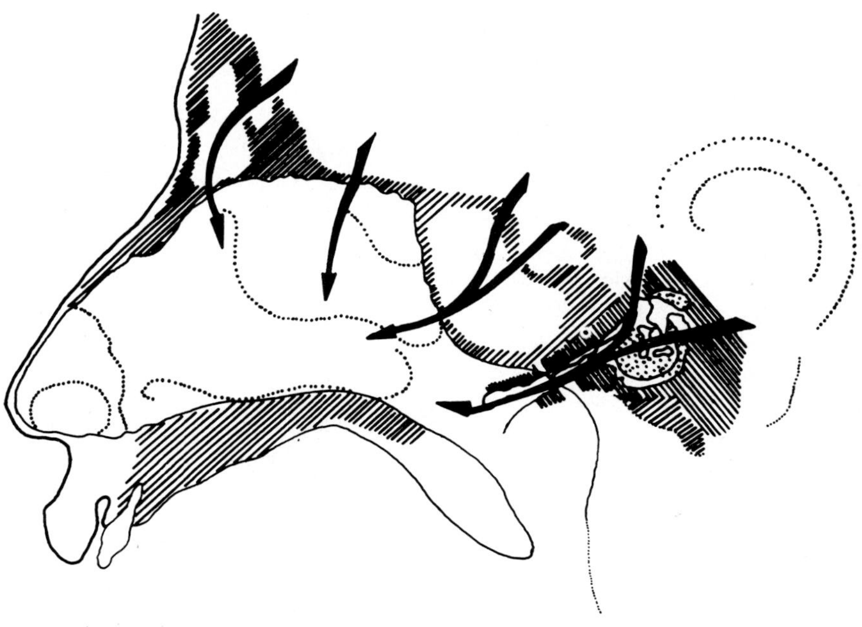

Figure 13. Schematic diagram indicating several possible routes of CSF rhinorrhea. (Courtesy of Dr. Giovanni DiChiro.)

with surgical wounds,[60] with the peritoneal and pleural cavities,[61–63] and with the epidural space.[64] Most often, CSF fistulae are caused by trauma and, because CSF pressure is dramatically lowered, are accompanied by headaches and slit-like ventricles. Most prolonged headaches that occur following lumbar puncture are caused by small CSF fistulae. Radionuclide studies can be performed using a lumbar intrathecal injection, or a cisterna magna or ventricular injection if access exists.[65] Figure 16 demonstrates a CSF fistula following trauma to the chest that resulted in leakage into the pleural cavity, causing persistent pleural effusion.

High tracer doses (e.g., 40 to 80 MBq ^{111}In-DTPA) and serial and delayed images are important because leaks may

Figure 14. The abnormal accumulation of activity in the left middle ear (arrow) in this posterior scintiphoto indicates a defect in the petrous bone from which CSF enters the nasal region via the eustachian tube.

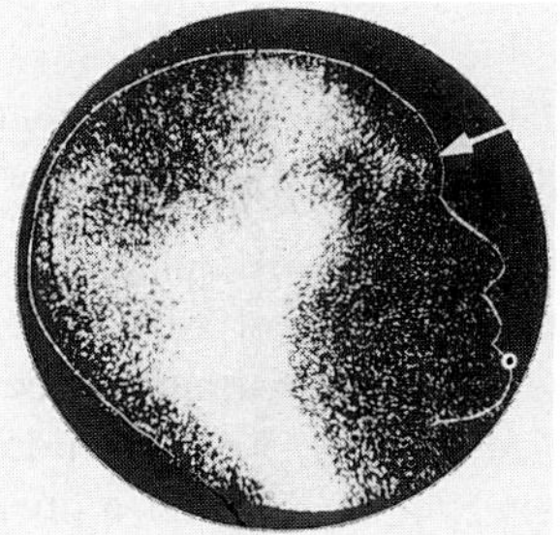

Figure 15. The abnormal accumulation of ^{99m}Tc-HSA far anteriorly (arrow) in this patient with CSF rhinorrhea suggests a cribriform plate leak.

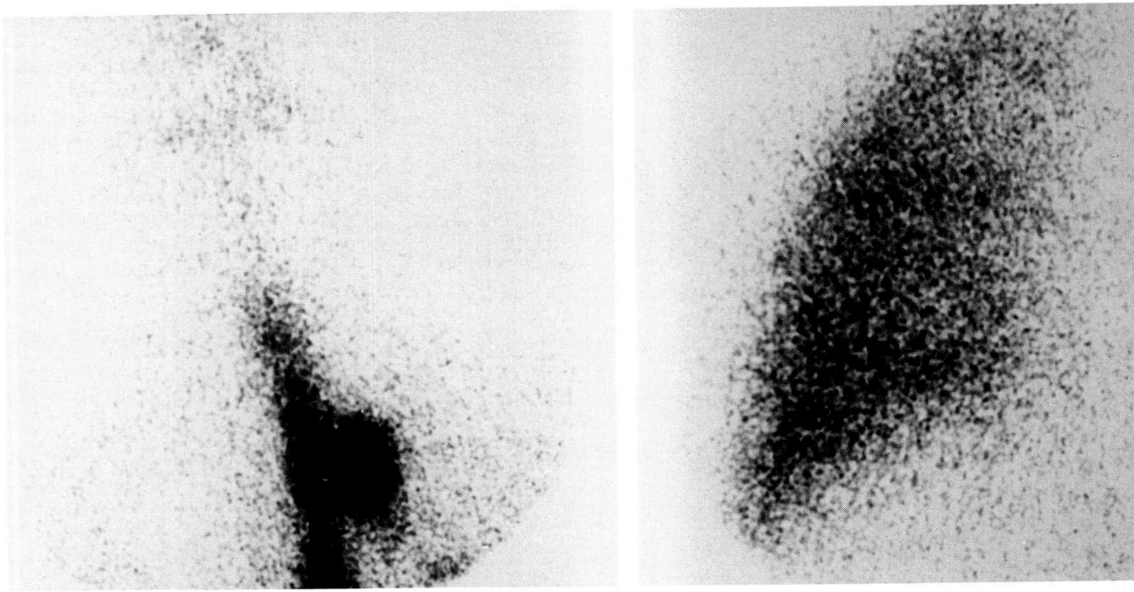

Figure 16. (**A**). Posterior scintiphoto with ^{111}In-DTPA in the upper thoracic intrathecal space demonstrates leakage of activity into a pleural CSF fistula on the right; (**B**). Anterior view of the lungs at 24 hours showing activity spread uniformly throughout the right pleural cavity. (Reprinted with permission of Dr. Arthur Krasnow, et al.[50])

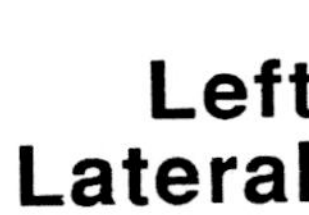

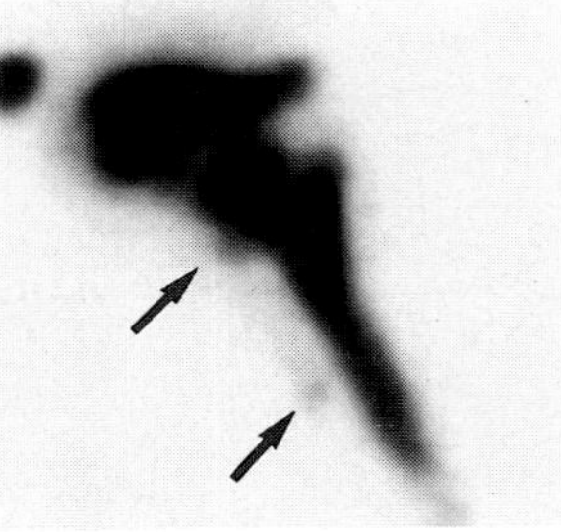

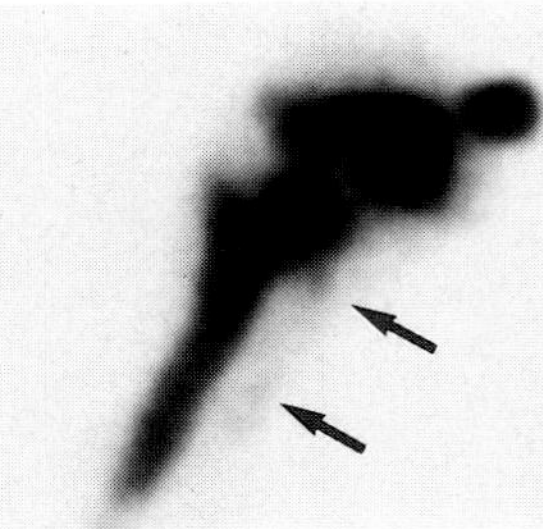

Figure 17. Summed, smoothed SPECT rotational images from a patient with CSF leak not visible on planar views. The thin tract of ^{99m}Tc-DTPA activity coming from the basal cisterns is well visualized. (Reproduced with permission from Reference 59.)

be intermittent and of small volume. When injecting into the lumbar space, early and frequent scintiphotos must be made to distinguish a misinjection into the epidural space (Fig. 2**B**) and a leak from the arachnoid into the epidural space.[66]

Radionuclide Ventriculography

We discussed earlier the usefulness of intraventricular injections of radionuclides in the evaluation of internal shunts. There are two other circumstances in which intraventricular injections may be helpful if transcranial access exists.

1. The communication of porencephalic cysts or an encysted temporal horn with the later ventricles may be demonstrated more easily by radionuclide techniques than by contrast ventriculography. Radionuclide techniques may be useful in determining whether a pressure cyst should be shunted, especially in patients with noncommunicating hydrocephalus who have been shunted and who continue to have symptoms. In these cases, it is useful to close off the ventricular shunt during the test, if possible, to encourage diffusion of the tracer into the cyst should a communication with the ventricle exist.
2. Documenting a communication between the lateral ventricles and a posterior fossa cyst may be useful in determining the shunting procedure to be undertaken. Contrast ventriculography is usually required in these cases, but the radionuclide ventriculogram may indicate the CSF communication and dynamics more effectively.[67]

REFERENCES

1. Bauer FK, Yuhl ET: Myelography by means of ^{131}I. The myeloscintigram. *Neurology* 1953;3:341.
2. Chou SN, French LA: Systemic absorption and urinary excretion of RISA from the subarachnoid space. *Neurology* 1955;5:555.
3. Crow HJ, Keogh C, Northfield DWC: The localization of cerebrospinal fluid fistulae. *Lancet* 1956;2:325.
4. Rieselbach RE, Di Chiro G, Freireich EJ, Rall DP: Subarach-

noid distribution of drugs after lumbar injection. *N Engl J Med* 1962;267:1273.

5. Bell RL: Isotope transfer test for diagnosis of ventriculosubarachnoidal block. *J Neurosurg* 1957;14:674.
6. Mundinger F, Anlauf M, Bouchard G: Die cardiale Impulsfrequenzmessung des Jod-131-hippuran, eine neue Methode zur passageprufung ventrikulo-atrialer shunts und die ventrikulare resorptionsprufung zur differentialdiagnose der hydrocephali. *Acta Neurochir* (*Wien*) 1963;11:272.
7. Di Chiro G, Reames PM, Matthews WB: RISA-ventriculography and RISA-cisternography. *Neurology* 1964;14:185.
8. Davson H: *Physiology of the Cerebrospinal Fluid.* Boston, Little, Brown, 1967.
9. Bering EA, Sato O: Hydrocephalus: Changes in formation and absorption of cerebrospinal fluid within the cerebral ventricles. *J Neurosurg* 1963;20:1050.
10. Cutler RWP, et al.: Formation and absorption of cerebrospinal fluid in man. *Brain* 1968;91:707.
11. Cooper JF, Harbert JC: Endotoxin as a cause of aseptic meningitis after radionuclide cisternography. *J Nucl Med* 1975;16:809.
12. Bennett IL, et al.: Pathogenesis of fever: Evidence for direct cerebral action of bacterial endotoxins. *Trans Assoc Am Physicians* 1957;70:64.
13. Oster ZH, Som P, Gil MG, et al.: Ruthenium-97 DTPA: A new radiopharmaceutical for cisternography. *J Nucl Med* 1981; 22:269.
14. Alazraki NP, Halpern SE, Ashburn WL, Coel M: Hyperbaric cisternography: Experience in humans. *J Nucl Med* 1973; 14:226.
15. Larson SM, Schall GL, DiChiro G: The unsuccessful injection in cisternography: Incidence, cause, and appearance, in Harbert, JC et al. (eds.): *Cisternography and Hydrocephalus.* Springfield, IL, Charles C Thomas, 1972, p 153.
16. Hakim S, Venegas JG, Benton JD: The physics of the cranial cavity, hydrocephalus and normal pressure hydrocephalus: Mechanical interpretation and mathematical mode. *Surg Neurol* 1976;5:187.
17. Ommaya AK, Metz H, Post KO: Observations on the mechanics of hydrocephalus, in Harbert, et al. (eds.): *Cisternography and Hydrocephalus.* Springfield, IL, Charles C Thomas, 1972, p 57.
18. Harbert JC, Reed V, McCullough DC: Comparison between ^{131}I-HSA and ^{169}Yb-DTPA for cisternography. *J Nucl Med* 1973;14:765.
19. James AE, et al.: Normal-pressure hydrocephalus: Role of cisternography in diagnosis. *JAMA,* 1970;213:1615.
20. Harbert JC: Radionuclide cisternography. *Semin Nucl Med* 1971;1:90.
21. Hakim S: *Some observation on CSF pressure. Hydrocephalic syndrome in adults with normal CSF pressure* (*recognition of a new syndrome*). Javeriana University School of Medicine, Bogata, Columbia. Thesis No. 957, 1964.
22. Hakim S, Adams RD: The special clinical problem of symptomatic hydrocephalus with normal cerebrospinal fluid pressure: Observations on cerebrospinal fluid hydrodynamics. *J Neurol Sci* 1965;2:307.
23. Breitz TVB: Effect of brain distension on cerebral circulation. *Lancet* 1969;1:863.
24. Bannister R, Gilford C, Kocen R: Isotope encephalography in the diagnosis of dementia due to communicating hydrocephalus. *Lancet* 1967;2:1014.
25. McCullough DC, Harbert JC, DiChiro G, Ommaya AK: Prognostic criteria for CSF shunting from isotope cisternography in communicating hydrocephalus. *Neurology* 1970;20:594.
26. Staab EV, Allen JH, Young AB, et al.: ^{131}I-HSA cisternograms and pneumoencephalograms in evaluation of hydrocephalus, in Harbert JC et al: *Cisternography and Hydrocephalus.* Springfield, IL, Charles C Thomas, 1972, p 235.
27. Flemming JFR, Sheppard RH, Turner VM: CSF scanning in the evaluation of hydrocephalus: A clinical review of 100 patients, in Harbert JC et al. (eds.) *Cisternography and Hydrocephalus.* Springield, IL, Charles C Thomas, 1972, p 261.
28. Heinz ER, Davis DO: Clinical, radiological, isotopic and pathologic correlation in normotensive hydrocephalus, in Harbert JC et al. (eds.): *Cisternography and Hydrocephalus.* Springfield, IL, Charles C Thomas, 1972, p 217.
29. Tator CH, Murray S: The value of CSF radioisotope studies in the diagnosis and management of hydrocephalus, in Harbert JC et al. (eds.): *Cisternography and Hydrocephalus.* Springfield, IL, Charles C Thomas, 1972, p 249.
30. Portnoy HD: Treatment of hydrocephalus, in McLauren RL (ed.): *Pediatric Neurosurgery.* New York, Grune and Stratton, 1982, p 211.
31. Enzmann DR, Pelc NJ: Normal flow patterns of intracranial and spinal cerebrospinal fluid defined with phase-contrast cine MR imaging. *Radiology* 1991;178:467.
32. Bradley WG, Whittemore AR, Kortman KE, et al: Marked cerebrospinal fluid void: indicator of successful shunt in patients with suspected normal-pressure hydrocephalus. *Radiology* 1991;178:459.
33. Di Chiro G, Knop RH, Girton ME, et al.: MR cisternography and myelography with Gd-DTPA in monkeys. *Radiology* 1985;157:373.
34. Rothenberg HP, Devenney J, Kuhl DE: Transverse-section scanning in cisternography. *J Nucl Med* 1976;17:924.
35. McCullough DC, Harbert JC: Pediatric radionuclide cisternography. *Semin Nucl Med* 1972;2:343.
36. Milhorat TH: *Hydrocephalus and the Cerebrospinal Fluid.* Baltimore, Williams & Wilkins, 1972, p 183.
37. McCullough DC, Manz HJ, Harbert JC: Large arachnoid cysts at the cranial base. *Neurosurgery* 1980;6:78.
38. James AE, Harbert JC, DeLand FH, et al.: Localized enlargement of the cerebrospinal fluid space demonstrated by cisternography. *Neuroradiology* 1971;2:184.
39. Harbert JC, James AE: Posterior fossa abnormalities demonstrated by cisternography. *J Nucl Med* 1972;13:73.
40. Harbert JC, Haddad D, McCullough DC: Quantitation of cerebrospinal fluid shunt flow. *Radiology* 1974;112:379.
41. Brendel AJ,Wynchank S, Castel J-P, et al.: Cerebrospinal patient position. *Radiology* 1983;149:815.
42. Agha FP, Amendola MA, Shirazi KK, et al.: Unusual abdominal complications of ventriculo-peritoneal shunts. *Radiology* 1983;146:323.
43. Norfray JF, Henry HM, Givens JD, et al.: Abdominal complications from peritoneal shunts. *Gastroenterology* 1979;77:337.
44. Chervu S, Chervu LR, Vallabhajosula B, et al.: Quantitative evaluation of cerebrospinal fluid shunt flow. *J Nucl Med* 1984;25:91.
45. Harbert JC, McCullough DC: Radionuclide tests of cerebrospinal fluid shunt patency. *J Nucl Med* 1984;25:112.
46. Ommaya AK: Subcutaneous reservoir and pump for sterile access to ventricular cerebrospinal fluid. *Lancet* 1963;2:983.
47. Hicks RJ, Kalff V, Brazenor G, et al.: The radionuclide assessment of a system for slow intrathecal infusion of drugs. *Clin Nucl Med* 1989;14:275.
48. DiChiro G, Reams PM, Matthews WB: RISA-ventriculography and RISA-cisternography. *Neurology* 1964;14:185.
49. Ashburn WL, et al.: Cerebrospinal fluid rhinorrhea studied with the gamma scintillation camera. *J Nucl Med* 1968;9:523.
50. Krasnow AZ, Collier BD, Isitman AT, et al.: The use of radionuclide cisternography in the diagnosis of pleural cerebrospinal fluid fistulae. *J Nucl Med* 1989;30:121.
51. Magnaes B, Solheim D: Controlled overpressure cisternogra-

phy to localize cerebrospinal fluid rhinorrhea. *J Nucl Med,* 1977;18:109.

52. Mamo L, Cophiznon T, Rey A, et al.: New radionuclide method for the diagnosis of post-traumatic cerebrospinal fistulas. A study of 308 cases. *J Neurosurg* 1982;57:92.
53. Naidich TP, Moran CJ: Precise anatomic localization of atraumatic sphenoethmoidal cerebrospinal fluid rhinorrhea by metrizamide CT cisternography. *J Neurosurg* 1980;53:222.
54. Chow JM, Goodman D, Mafee MF: Evaluation of CSF rhinorrhea by computerized tomography with metrizamide. *Otolaryngol Head Neck Surg* 1989;100:99.
55. Flynn BM, Butler SP, Quinn RJ, et al.: Radionuclide leaks: the test of choice. *Med J Aust* 1987;146:82.
56. DiChiro G, Stein SC, Harrington T: Spontaneous cerebrospinal fluid rhinorrhea in normal dogs. *J Neuropathol Exp Neurol* 1972;31:447.
57. McKusick KA, Malmud LA, Kordela PA, et al: Radionuclide cisternography: Normal values of nasal secretion of intrathecally injected In-111 DTPA. *J Nucl Med* 1973;14:933.
58. Zu'bi SM, Kirkwood R, Abbasy M, Bye R: Intestinal activity visualized on radionuclide cisternography in patients with cerebrospinal fluid leak. *J Nucl Med* 1991;32:151.
59. Lewis DH, Graham MM: Benefit of tomography in the scintigraphic localization of cerebrospinal fluid leak. *J Nucl Med* 1991;32:2149.
60. Maeda T, Ishida H, Matsuda H, et al.: The utility of radionuclide spinal fluid leaks. *Eur J Nucl Med* 1984;9:416.
61. Rosen PR, Chaudhuri TK: Radioisotope myelography in the detection of pleural-dural communication as a source of recurrent meningitis. *Clin Nucl Med* 1983;8:28.
62. Hoffstetter KR, Bjelland JC, Patton DD, et al.: Detection of bronchopleural-subarachnoid fistula by radionuclide myelography: case report. *J Nucl Med* 1977;18:981.
63. Krasnow AZ, Collier BD, Isitman AT, et al.: The use of radionuclide cisternography in the diagnosis of pleural cerebrospinal fluid fistulae. *J Nucl Med* 1989;30:120.
64. Kadrie H, Driedger AA, McInnis W: Persistent dural cerebrospinal fluid leak shown by retrograde radionuclide myelography: Case report. *J Nucl Med* 1976;17:797.
65. Silverman ED, Davis WB, Harbert JC, Levenson SM: Spinal cerebrospinal fluid leak demonstrated by retrograde myeloscintigraphy. *Clin Nucl Med* 1981;6:27.
66. Primeau M, Carrier L, Miletter PC, et al.: Spinal cerebrospinal fluid leak demonstrated by radioisotopic cisternography. *Clin Nucl Med* 1988;13:701.
67. Harbert JC, McCullough DC: Radionuclide studies in an unusual case of Dandy-Walker cyst. *Radiology* 1971;101:363.

19 The Eye

John C. Harbert

Choroidal melanoma is the most common primary intraocular tumor.[1] Despite significant advances in indirect ophthalmoscopy, ultrasound, computed tomography (CT), magnetic resonance imaging (MRI), and fluorescein angiography, choroidal melanomas may be difficult to distinguish from other malignant and nonmalignant eye lesions (Table 1).[3] Furthermore, approximately 10% of choroidal melanomas occur in eyes with opaque media, thus obviating the use of ophthalmoscopy.[4]

RADIONUCLIDES IN THE DIAGNOSIS OF CHOROIDAL MELANOMA

The ^{32}P Uptake Test

Numerous radionuclide tracers have been investigated as agents to help localize choroidal melanomas. Of the tracers listed in Table 2, only ^{32}P-orthophosphate has been used extensively. Phosphates are incorporated into dividing cells and play a role in the synthesis of deoxyribonucleic acid (DNA). As a tracer, ^{32}P-orthophosphate is incorporated into tissues and organs with rapidly dividing cells, which can distinguish them from more leisurely growing tissues.

The organ distribution of ^{32}P-orthophosphate cannot be imaged by conventional scintigraphy because it emits only beta particles (E_{max} = 1.7 MeV; average tissue penetration = 2.5 mm) and the bremsstrahlung radiations given off in the eye are not adequate for precise localization. Consequently, tumor detection must utilize probe counting with the detector in very close approximation to the lesion. This usually requires prior localization of the tumor by ultrasonography, MRI, transillumination, or by indirect ophthalmoscopy.[30] The outline of the tumor is then marked on the sclera with a marking pen or by diathermy. For posteriorly located tumors, the conjunctiva and Tenon's capsule must be dissected to gain access to the posterior sclera.[31]

In the ^{32}P uptake test 370 kBq/kg (10 μCi/kg) of ^{32}P-sodium orthophosphate is injected intravenously 24 to 72 hours before counting.[8,32] Counts are taken using a small, specially designed semiconductor probe positioned directly over the tumor, localized as described above, to measure the activity concentrated in the lesion.[8,33,34] Counts are taken for 60 to 100 sec. Background control counts are then measured on the opposite side of the globe. The tumor (T) and control area (C) counts are measured three times, and average counts are calculated. The ^{32}P uptake is expressed as a percent of the control counts:

$$\frac{T - C}{C} \times 100$$

Various criteria have been used to define a positive test. Most investigators consider a value of 100% or at least twice background as indicative of a melanoma.[6] Others have used 60% over background as indicating a positive test.[35]

There are obvious drawbacks to the ^{32}P uptake test, the most serious being the requirement that an opthalmic surgeon be present to locate the tumor margins, and the necessity of surgical incision for posterior tumors. The low counting rate and the need for precise positioning also increase the possibility of error. Numerous false-positive results have been reported, including both inflammatory lesions and other malignancies, especially metastases.[35,36] Today, such diagnostic tests as CT, ultrasound, fluorescein angiography, and indirect opthalmoscopy are mostly utilized to diagnose choroidal melanomas.[37]

Other Radiopharmaceuticals

1. Quinolines bind to melanin with a high degree of affinity, which has led to the use of ^{123}I-iodoquinoline to image choroidal melanomas.[9,16,25] However, this tracer binds to all melanin-containing structures in the eye and not just melanomas; hence sensitivity has not been high.
2. Thiouracil is covalently incorporated into melanin during melanin synthesis as a kind of "false precursor."[38] The attraction of radiolabeled thiouracils is that presumably they would bind only to synthesizing melanoma in a rapidly growing tumor, and not at all to the static melanin structures in the eye. Some success has been achieved, although high background of ^{123}I and ^{125}I-iodothiouracil in blood and surrounding tissues have limited the sensitivity of this tracer.[24,25]
3. Bomanji et al. have reported successful localization of choroidal melanomas using the ^{99m}Tc-labeled monoclonal antibody 225.28S, an antibody against cutaneous melanoma that also binds to elements in choroidal melanomas.[28] Using a combination of planar and SPECT scintigraphy, they reported a sensitivity of 93% with one false-positive and no false-negative results. Three ocular hemangiomas, two metastases, and one melanocytoma failed

Table 1. Lesions simulating ocular choroidal melanomas

Metastases	Hemangioma
Choroidal nevi	Melanocytoma
Disciform macular degeneration	Retinal detachment
Reactive retinal pigment epithelial hyperplasia	

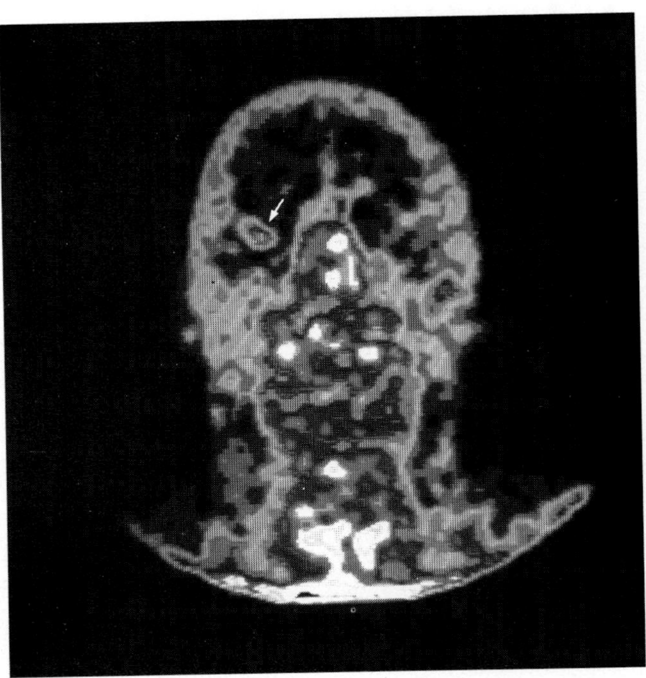

Figure 1. Anterior image of the head 7 hours following intravenous injection of 370 MBq (10 mCi) ^{99m}Tc labeled MoAb (Fab′)$_2$ against cutaneous melanoma. The image is positive for a right choroidal melanoma. (Reproduced from Reference 28 with permission.) (See Plate 29.)

to take up the labeled antibody. Tumor sizes ranged from $3 \times 5 \times 3$ mm to $18 \times 7 \times 11$ mm (Fig. 1). Further investigations are warranted with this promising technology.

Several techniques are being explored to improve immunodiagnosis of choroidal melanomas.[39] These include background substraction using ^{99m}Tc-human serum albumin, which identifies nonspecific blood background. A second means of decreasing blood background is to administer a second antibody that, after a period of localization, can be injected and clear the first antibody from the blood. The use of antibody fragments may also be useful, since the clear more rapidly than whole antibodies.

4. Iodoamphetamine has been used primarily to image regional cerebral perfusion, although it also distributes to sites of melanin production and has been used to detect malignant melanoma and its metastases.[40–42] Two reports have demonstrated uptake of ^{123}I-iodoamphetamine in

Table 2. Radiopharmaceuticals for Localization of Choroidal Melanoma

CATEGORY	RADIOPHARMACEUTICAL	REFERENCE*
Metabolite	^{32}P-orthophosphate	Thomas CI, et al.[5] (L); Shields JA, et al.[6] (C)
Metals	^{67}Ga-citrate	Packer S, et al.[7] (L); Packer S, et al.[8] (C); Langevelde et al.[9] (C)
	^{203}Pb-citrate	Packer S, et al.[7] (L)
	^{197}Hg-chlormerodrin	Greaves PP, Cappin JM[10] (C)
	^{111}In-chloride	Packer S, et al.[7] (L)
Antibiotics	^{131}I-tetracycline	Newell FW, et al.[11] (C)
	^{57}Co-bleomycin	Packer S, et al.[7] (L)
Quinolines	^{131}I-iodoquinoline	Beierwaltes WH, et al.[12] (C); Blanquet P, et al.[13] (C)
	^{125}I-iodoquinoline	Boyd CM, et al.[14] (C); Walsh IJ, Packer S[15] (C)
	^{123}I-iodoquinoline	Packer S, et al.[16] (C); Langevelde A, et al.[9] (C)
Dyes	^{125}I-diiodofluorescein	Newell FW, et al.[11] (C); Greaves DP, Cappin JM[10] (C)
	^{123}I-indocyanine green	Ansari A, et al.[17] (L)
Melanin precursors	^{3}H-tyrosine	Dencker L, et al.[18] (L); Kloss G, Leven M[19] (L)
	^{14}C-dopamine	Blois MS, Kallman RF[20] (L)
	^{3}H-dihydroxyindole	Pawelek JM, Lerner AB[21] (L)
"False" melanin precursors	^{35}S-thiouracil	Dencker L, et al.[18] (L); Fairchild RG, et al.[22] (L)
	^{3}H-methyltyrosine	Bockslaff H, et al.[23] (L)
	^{123}I-5-iodo-2-thiouracil	Packer S, et al.[24] (C); Langevelde A et al.[25]
	^{125}I-5-iodo-2-thiouracil	Packer S, et al.[24] (C)
Amine uptake process	^{123}I-iodoamphetamine	Ono S, et al.[26] (C); Dewey SH, Leonard JC[27] (C)
Antibody	^{99m}Tc-labeled 225.285 F(ab′)$_2$	Bomanji J et al.[28] (C)

(C) = clinical studies, (L) = laboratory studies (Modified from Packer S[29])

choroidal melanomas.[26,27] Because this perfusion agent is taken up in the brain, SPECT is necessary to separate ocular lesions, particularly those located nasally.

RADIONUCLIDE DACRYOCYSTOGRAPHY (DCG)

The use of radionuclides to study the lacrimal drainage apparatus was introduced by Rossomundo et al.[43] and has been modified by others.[44–47] This test, which is performed to evaluate obstructions of lacrimal drainage and excessive tearing (epiphora), is simple to perform and completely physiological, and provides a reasonably accurate image of the involved anatomy.

Techniques

The patient is seated in front of a scintillation camera fitted with a pinhole collimator and the smallest available (e.g., 1 mm) aperature. Radioactive markers are placed at the lateral margins of the eyes, so that both eyes just fill the field of view. It is convenient to immobilize the patient's head with a moldable vacuum pillow to prevent movement during the study. A droplet of sterile normal saline containing 4 to 8 MBq (100 to 200 μCi) of ^{99m}Tc-pertechnetate is placed onto the conjunctiva near the lateral canthus of both eyes. Timed, serial scintiphotos are then taken every 30 sec over the next 5 min.[48] Scintiphotos take only a few seconds to obtain 10 to 20×10^3 counts. If the eyes are studied separately, the asymptomatic eye should be studied first as a comparison and to get the patient accustomed to the procedure.

In a normal study, the lacrimal sac and nasolacrimal duct are visualized within 5 minutes after tracer instillation. An abnormal study is characterized by nonfilling of the sac or lack of complete filling of the nasolacrimal duct.

RADIATION DOSIMETRY

The radiation absorbed dose to the germinal epithelium of the lens from ^{99m}Tc-pertechnetate is approximately 0.04 μGy/kBq (0.14 mrad/μCi) in eyes with normal drainage, and about 1 μGy/kBq when complete blockage is present.[49] This exposure is substantially less than delivered during contrast dacryocystography.

Clinical Applications

The basic anatomy of the nasolacrimal drainage system is shown in Figure 2. Obstruction can occur at any point within the nasolacrimal duct system, and the nuclear study provides a simple noninvasive means of making the diagnosis (Fig. 3). Analysis of flow characteristics before and after surgery to unblock the drainage system is also helpful.[50] Partial or relative obstructions are often successfully treated with drugs such as pseudoephedrine. Radionuclide DCG provides objective evidence on the change in flow before and after therapy.[51]

Most non-nuclear tests used to evaluate obstruction, such as fluorescein dye tests and saline or glucose instillation tests, are neither sensitive nor physiological. They may miss low-grade mechanical or functional obstructions that result from mucus membrane folds within the lacrimal sac or ducts, ductal edema, or paralysis of the orbicularis oculi or facial muscles. In these types of partial or functional obstruction, certain interventional maneuvers in conjunction with radionuclide DCG may be useful: (1) compression of the lacrimal sac by digital massage may help overcome sluggish flow in the nasolacrimal duct; (2) augmentation of the tear film by 3 to 4 drops of saline may encourage flow of the radioactivity into the canaliculi; (3) ocular lavage, in which the remaining activity is washed out of the eye with saline and a sterile cellulose sponge to determine where radioactivity is stagnated may help distinguish obstruction from nonanatomical causes of reduced tear flow.[49]

Some investigators have attempted to quantify radionuclide DCG studies by timing the appearance of activity at various locations or plotting the disappearance time of activity from the eye.[46,52,53] In evaluating these techniques, Brown et al. found that only the appearance time in the lacrimal sac was a reliable indicator of obstruction.[48] Other measures are too dependent on blinking, gravity, and other nonpathologic conditions. Probably the most meaningful comparisons are made of activity clearances between the tearing and the normal eye.

COMPARISON WITH CONTRAST DACRYOCYSTOGRAPHY

Contrast DCG involves cannulation of the puncta and canaliculus and the injection of radiographic contrast material. This procedure provides exquisite detail of the lacrimal drainage anatomy. However, it usually requires the assistance of an ophthalmologist and injections may require pressure that is painful and may result in trauma to the puncta and canaliculi. In most cases, radionuclide DCG is the best initial study, because it is more physiological and is simpler to perform, it is a sensitive test for indicating serious nasolacrimal obstruction, it causes less discomfort, and delivers only a modest radiation dose to the lens. Furthermore, there are very few cases in which contrast DCG provides useful information when the radionuclide DCG is normal.[48,50]

Brown et al.[48] list the indications for contrast DCG as follows:

1. to define the pathologic anatomy of obstructive lesions of the nasolacrimal system,
2. to evaluate known lesions, such as sinus tracts or fistulae, arising from the nasolacrimal system,
3. to study patients with mass lesions (stone, tumor) of the nasolacrimal system,
4. to evaluate patients with epiphora in whom fluid passes

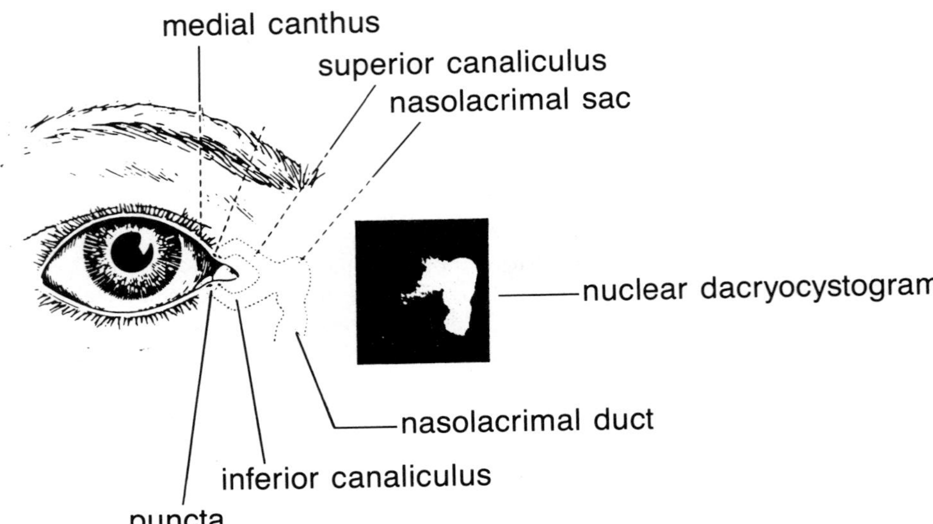

Figure 2. Normal lacrimal anatomy and nuclear dacryocystogram.

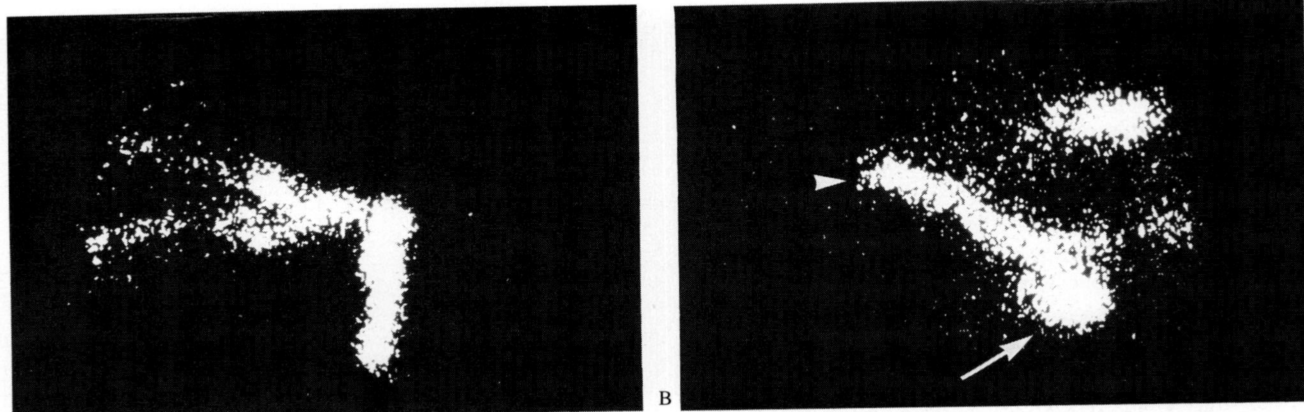

Figure 3. (**A**). Normal nuclear dacryocystogram of right eye well outling the superior and inferior canaliculi, nasolacrimal sac, and nasolacrimal duct, (**B**). Nuclear dacryocystogram of left eye demonstrating blockage at the nasolacrimal sac (arrowhead) and epiphora (arrow). (Reproduced by kind permission of George Burke, M.D.)

into the nose during irrigation, but in whom no flow can be demonstrated by radionuclide DCG.

REFERENCES

1. Hungerford JL: Current management of choroidal malignant melanoma. *Br J Hosp Med* 1985; 34:287.
2. Shields JA, Augsburger JJ, Brown GC, et al.: The differential diagnosis of posterior uveal melanoma. *Ophthalmology* 1980; 87:518.
3. Chang M, Zimmerman LE, McLean I: The persisting pseudomelanoma problem. *Arch Ophthalmol* 1984;102:726.
4. Shields JA, McDonald PR, Leonard BC, Canny CLB: The diagnosis of uveal malignant melanomas in eyes with opaque media. *Am J Ophthalmol* 1977;83:95.
5. Thomas CI, Bovington MS, MacIntyre WJ, et al: Experimental investigations on uptake of radioactive phosphorus in ocular tumors. *Arch Ophthalmol* 1959;61:464.
6. Shields JA, Hagler WS, Federman JL, et al.: The significance of the ^{32}P uptake test in the diagnosis of posterior uveal melanomas. *Trans Am Acad Ophthalmol Otolaryngol* 1975;79:297.
7. Packer S, Lambrecht RM, Christman DR, et al.: Metal isotopes used as radioactive indicators of ocular melanoma. *Am J Ophthalmol* 1977;83:80.
8. Packer S, Shilds JA, Christman DR, et al.: Radioactive phosphorus uptake test—an in vitro analysis of choroidal melanoma and ocular tissues. *Invest Ophthalmol Vis Sci* 1980;19:386.
9. Langevelde A van, Bakker CNM, Boer H, et al.: Potential radiopharmaceuticals for the detection of ocular melanoma. Part II. Iodoquinoline derivatives and ^{67}Ga-citrate. *Eur J Nucl Med* 1986;12:96.
10. Greaves DP, Cappin JM: The use of radioisotopes in the diagnosis of intraocular tumors. *Proc R Soc Med* 1968;61:1037.

11. Newell FW, Goren SB, Brizel HE, Harper PV: The use of iodine–125 as a diagnostic agent in ophthalmology. *Trans Am Acad Ophthalmol* 1963;67:177.
12. Beierwaltes WH, Varma VM, Lieberman LM, et al.: Scintillation scanning of malignant melanomas with radioiodinated quinoline derivatives. *J Lab Clin Med* 1968;72:485.
13. Blanquet P, Safi N. LeRebeller MJ: Ocular scintigraphy, in Croll MN et al. (eds): *Nuclear Ophthalmology.* New York, John Wiley & Sons, 1976.
14. Boyd CM, Beierwaltes WH, Lieberman LM, Bergstrom TJ: ^{125}I–labeled chloroquine analog in the diagnosis of ocular melanoma. *J Nucl Med* 1971;12:601.
15. Walsh TJ, Packer S: Radioisotope detection of ocular melanoma. *N Engl J Med* 1971;248:317.
16. Packer S, Redvanly C, Lambrecht RM, et al.: Quinoline analog labeled with iodine–123 in melanoma detection. *Arch Ophthalmol* 1975;93:504.
17. Ansari A, Lambrecht RM, Packer S, et al.: Note on the distribution of iodine-123-labeled indocyanine green in the eye. *Invest Ophthalmol Vis Sci* 1975;14:780.
18. Dencker L, Larsson B, Olander K, et al.: False precursors of melanin as selective melanoma seekers. *Br J Cancer* 1979; 39:449.
19. Kloss G, Leven M: Accumultion of radioiodinated tyrosine derivatives in the adrenal medulla and in melanomas. *Eur J Nucl Med* 1979;4:179.
20. Blois MS, Kallman RF: The incorporation of C^{14} from 3,4–2–C^{14} into the melanin of mouse melanomas. *Cancer Res* 1964;24:863.
21. Pawelek JM, Lerner AB: 5,6–dihydroxyindole is a melanin precursor showing potent cytotoxicity. *Nature* 1978;276: 627.
22. Fairchild RG, Packer S, Greenberg D, et al.: Thiouracil distribution in mice carrying transplantable melanoma. *Cancer Res* 1982;42:5126.
23. Bockslaff H, et al.: Studies on L–3–^{123}Ido-α-methyltyrosine: A new potential melanoma-seeking compound, in Schmidt W, Riccabona HAE eds.: *Nuklearmedizin.* Stuttgart, Schattaner, 1984, p 179.
24. Packer S, Fairchild RG, Coderre JA.: Radiopharmaceuticals and the Visual System *Nucl Med Biol* 1990;17:93.
25. Langevelde A van, Bakker CNM, Broxterman HJ, et al.: Potential radiopharmaceuticals for the detection of ocular melanoma. Part I. 5–iodo–2–thiouracil derivatives. *Eur J Nucl Med* 1983;8:45.
26. Ono S, Fukunaga M, Nobuaki O, et al.: Visulization of ocular melanoma with N-isopropyl-p-[123I]-iodoamphetamine. *J Nucl Med* 1988;29:1448.
27. Dewey SH, Leonard JC: Ocular melanoma: detection using iodine–123–iodoamphetamine and SPECT imaging. *J Nucl Med* 1990;31:375.
28. Bomanji J, Nimmon CC, Hungerford JL, et al.: Ocular radioimmunoscintigraphy: Sensitivity and practical considerations. *J Nucl Med* 1988;29:1038.
29. Packer S: The Eye, in Harbert J, Da Rocha AFG (eds): *Textbook of Nuclear Medicine,* Volume II: *Clinical Applications,* Philadelphia, Lea and Febiger, 1984, p 144.
30. Packer S, Lange R: Radioactive phosphorus for the detection of ocular melanomas. *Arch Ophthalmol* 1973;90:17.
31. Shields JA, Sarin LK, Federman JL, et al.: Surgical approach to the ^{32}P test for posterior uveal melanomas. *Ophthalmic Surg* 1974;5:13.
32. Dijk RA van: The ^{32}P test and other methods in the diagnosis of intraocular tumors. *Docum Ophthal* 1978;46:1.
33. Lommatzsch P, Ulrich C, Ulrich WD, et al.: Über eine neue Messonde zur Diagnostick intraocularer Tumoren. *Albrect Von Graefes Arch Kin Exp Ophthalmol* 1969;177:105.
34. Packer S, Goldberg H, Feldman M: The ultrasound guided ^{32}P test. *Ann Ophthalmol* 1978;10:1411.
35. Ruiz RS, Pernoud JM: Time and dose for optimum radioactive phosphorus uptake measurement in rabbit uveal melanoma. Am J Ophthalmol. 1976;82:218.
36. Goldberg B, Kara GB, Pervite LR: The use of radioactive phosphorus (^{32}P) in the diagnosis of ocular tumors. Am J Ophthalmol. 1980;90:817.
37. Char DH: *Clinical Ocular Oncology.* New York, Churchill Livingstone, 1989, 113.
38. Whittaker JR: Biosynthesis of thiouracil phenomelanin in embryonic pigment cells exposed to thioouracil. *J Biol Chem* 1976;246:6217.
39. Fairchild RG, Fand I, Laster BH: Monoclonal Antobodies, in *Encyclopedia of Medical Devices.* New York, Wiley, 1988. 1994.
40. Wada M Ichiya Y, Katsuragi M, et al.: Scintigraphic visualization of human malignant melanoma with N-isopropyl-p-(I-123)-iodoamphetamine. *Clin Nucl Med* 1985;10:415.
41. Liewendahl K, Kairento AL, Pyrhonen S, et al.: Localization of melanoma with radiolabelled monoclonal antibody fragments and iodoamphetamine. *Eur J Nucl Med* 1986;12:359.
42. Cohen MB, Saxton RE, Lake RR, et al.: Detection of malignant melanoma with iodine-123 iodoamphetamine. *J Nucl Med* 1988;29:1200.
43. Rossomondo RM, Carlton WH, Trueblood JH, Thomas RP: A new method of evaluating lacrimal drainage. *Arch Ophthalmol* 1972;88:523.
44. Denffer HV, Dressler J: Radionuklid-Dakryocystographie in der diagnostick von stenosen der tranenableitenden wege. *Albrech Von Graefes Arch Klin Exp Ophthalmol* 1974;191:321.
45. Hurwitz JJ, Welham RAN, Maisey MN: Intubation macrodacryocystography and quantitative scintillography. The complete lacrimal assessment. *Trans Am Acad Ophthalmol Otolaryngol* 1976;81:575.
46. Chavis RM, Welham RAN, Maisey MN: Quantitative lacrimal scintillography. *Arch Ophthalmol* 1978;96:2066.
47. Chaudhuri TK, Saparoff GR, Dolan KD, et al.: Comparative study of contrast dacryocystogram and nuclear dacryocystogram. *J Nucl Med* 1975;16:650.
48. Brown M, El Gammal TA, Luxenberg MN, Casimir E: The value, limitations and applications of nuclear dacryocystography. *Semin Nucl Med* 1981;11:250.
49. Robertson JS, Brown ML, Colvard DM: Radiation absorbed dose to the lens in dacryoscintigraphy with $^{99m}TcO_4^-$. *Radiology* 1979;133:747.
50. Nixon J, Birchall IWJ, Virjee J: The role of dacryocystography in the management of patients with epiphora. *Br J Radiol* 1990;63:337.
51. Kim CK, Palestro CJ, Solomon RW, Goldsmith SJ: Serial dacryoscintigraphy before and after treatment with pseudoephedrine. *Clin Nucl Med* 1987;10:734.
52. Hurwitz JJ, Maisey MN, Welham RAN: Quantitative lacrimal scintillography. I. Method and physiological application. *Br J Ophthalmol* 1975;59:308.
53. Hurwitz JJ, Maisey MN, Welham RAN: Quantative lacrimal scintillography. II. Lacrimal pathology. *Br J Ophthalmol* 1975; 59:313.

20 The Thyroid

John C. Harbert

The thyroid gland is situated in the anterior neck, immediately in front of the trachea, and below the thyroid cartilage. Its two lobes, united by an isthmus, form the shape of the Mycenean Greek shield; hence, its name is from the Greek *thyreos,* meaning shield. In adults, the gland weighs 20 to 25 g. Embryologically, the thyroid has a dual origin. One part derives from an evagination of pharyngeal entoderm in the vertex of the laryngeal pouch. The other derives from bilateral ectodermal buds from the last branchial clefts, which ultimately fuse in the midline. Cell remnants along the tract of the lingual evagination often connect with the thyroid to produce a "pyramidal lobe," the so-called pyramid of Lalouette. Occasionally, a lingual thyroid may persist, but it is almost never active in the presence of normal thyroid function. The same is true of thyroglossal duct remnants.

The thyroid cells derived from ectoderm form the *follicle cells,* which are responsible for the production of thyroid hormones. Those stemming from entoderm give rise to *parafollicular cells,* or clear cells, whose principal product is thyrocalcitonin.

The thyroid is under direct control of the pituitary through the secretion of thyrotropin, or *thyroid-stimulating hormone* (TSH). Secretion of TSH is stimulated in turn by thyrotropin-releasing hormone (TRH). This small tripeptide is formed by the hypothalamus and flows along the neurons to the median eminence (Fig. 1). Here, it enters the hypophyseal portal system, which serves as the arterial supply to the pituitary. These three organs, the thyroid, pituitary, and hypothalamus form a sensitive feedback system. The hypothalamus is extremely responsive to changes in serum thyroid hormone levels. With T_4 and T_3 deficiency, TRH secretion increases, stimulating release of TSH and, in turn, stimulating release of hormones from the thyroid. As T_4 and T_3 levels rise, TRH production decreases, TSH output falls, and thyroid hormone production and release fall. The integrity of this system is essential to the normal metabolic state.

Physiologically, the chief functions of the thyroid gland follicles are to synthesize, store, and secrete the iodinated hormones that are indispensable to cellular metabolism. For this role, the follicle cells must incorporate iodine into tyrosine. The metabolism of iodine was first explained in 1938, when Hertz et al garnered these facts largely through the use of radioactive isotopes of iodine.[1]

IODINE METABOLISM

It is difficult to formulate a compartmental model of iodine metabolism that, on the one hand, is simple and clinically useful and, on the other hand, permits a quantitative reconstruction of the metabolic cycle. The model in Figure 2, although a compromise, does show the interrelationships among extrathyroidal, intrathyroidal, and hormonal iodine. The fractions lost transplacentally and by mammary excretion are excluded because of their transitory nature.

Extrathyroidal Compartment

This small compartment (40 to 60 μg for a 70-kg man) has a high turnover rate. The absorption of dietary iodine and the deiodination of thyroid hormones are its principal input. Dietary iodine in the United States has increased greatly since 1960. With iodine supplementation programs and changes in food processing, dietary intake has increased from approximately 150 μg/day to 250 to 600 μg/day.[2] Ingested iodine is rapidly reduced to iodide in the upper intestine, and approximately 90% is absorbed in the first 60 min after ingestion. Once iodide reaches the blood, it is distributed as an extracellular ion in a pool similar to the chloride space. The plasma concentration of iodide fluctuates between 0.1 and 0.5 μg/dL, depending mostly on ingestion. Iodide leaves this compartment principally through thyroid uptake and urinary excretion. A small amount of plasma iodide is concentrated by the salivary glands and gastric mucosa; this quantity soon enters the digestive tract and is recycled rather than lost. Under normal plasma concentrations, the thyroid clearance of iodide is 5 to 40 mL per min, or between 7 and 58 liters of plasma per day. In chronic iodine deficiency, thyroid clearance can increase to 100 mL per min, and with iodine excess, it may fall as low as 2 to 5 mL per min.

Thyroid Compartment

Iodide trapped and organified by the thyroid gland is utilized in the synthesis of thyroid hormones. Iodine also is liberated by the intrathyroid deiodination of amino acids not utilized in hormone production. This compartment is large (10,000 μg) and has a slow turnover.[3] For didactic purposes, the steps in iodine utilization are represented schematically in Figure 3.

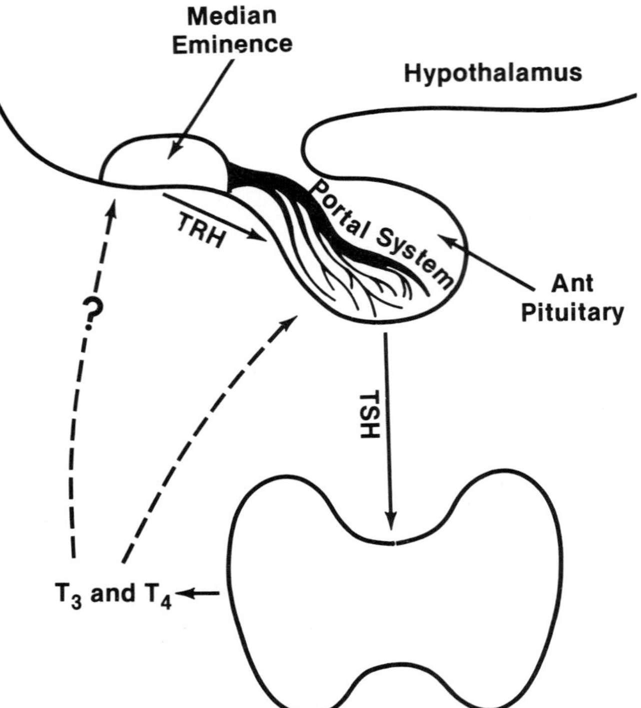

Figure 1. The hypothalamo-hypophyseal-thyroid axis. Thyrotropin-releasing hormone (TRH) is transported to the pituitary by way of the hypophyseal portal venous system, stimulating release of thyroid-stimulating hormone (TSH) into the circulation. TSH stimulates every step in the synthesis and release of T_3 and T_4. Through a sensitive negative-feedback relationship, circulating thyroid hormone suppresses release of TSH, and probably of TRH as well.

IODIDE TRAPPING

Iodide is trapped by means of a high-energy metabolic process known as the thyroid "pump," which permits intracellular concentrations 25 to 500 times the plasma concentration, depending upon the thyroid functional state. The trapping mechanism depends on oxidative phosphorylation and is inhibited by anoxia, cyanides, dinitrophenol, and hypothermia (Table 1). Iodide trapping can be blocked competitively by several monovalent anions, including the halides At and Br; peroxy anions, such as ReO_4^- and TcO_4^-; complex anions, such as perchlorate (ClO_4^-) and tetrafluoroborate (BF_4^-); and pseudohalides, such as thiocyanate (SCN^-). The effect of this blocking action is to return unbound thyroidal iodide to the plasma. This "washout" of thyroidal iodide serves as the basis for the *perchlorate washout test.* The fact that iodine can be displaced in this manner indicates that the trapping process is not unidirectional.

ORGANIFICATION

Once iodide has been incorporated into the cell, it is rapidly oxidized by enzymatic action. The oxidation process has not been well elucidated, but it is known that hydrogen peroxide is formed by a system of peroxidases and cytochrome oxidase, and hydrogen peroxide may be the oxidizing agent. Iodide is oxidized to neutral iodine (I) or to hypoiodide (IO^-), the only forms of iodine that can be utilized by the follicular cells. Soon after oxidation, iodine is incorporated by tyrosine, forming monoiodotyrosine (MIT) and diiodotyrosine (DIT), which are bound to thyroglobulin. The organification of iodine occurs within the follicle lumen. It is stimulated by TSH and blocked by thiourea. Thyroglobulin is a large glycoprotein (660 kD) composed of some 5000 amino acid elements, of which approximately 125 are tyrosine. Thyroglobulin is stored in the follicular lumen.

Table 1. Drugs That Interfere with Thyroid Hormone Synthesis and Metabolism

MECHANISM AFFECTED	DRUGS
Iodine trapping	Thiocyanate Perchlorate Nitroprusside
Organification	Propylthiouracil Tapazol Sulfonylureas Sulfonamides ρ-Aminosalicylic acid Phenylbutazone Aminoglutethimide
Hormone synthesis	Iodine
Hormone release	Iodine Lithium carbonate
Conversion of T_4 to T_3	Propylthiouracil Glucocorticoids Propranolol Iopanoic acid (Telepaque) Amiodarone

COUPLING

Following organification, coupling of MIT and DIT occurs by intramolecular rearrangement, or by intermolecular transfer, to form T_3 and T_4 (Fig. 4). Most evidence suggests that coupling occurs while tyrosine is bound to thyroglobulin and is catalyzed by thyroid peroxidase.[4] These thyronines remain bound to thyroglobulin in the follicular lumen until needed. As in the previous steps, the coupling process is stimulated by TSH.

STORAGE AND RELEASE

Microscopic sections through the thyroid reveal the gland's most prominent feature, the colloid-filled spherical sacs (acini). Colloid consists mostly of thyroglobulin. The normal thyroid gland contains at least a one-month supply of hormone. Hence, drugs preventing thyroid hormone synthesis do not become fully effective until intrathyroidal stores have been depleted. Ordinarily, thyroglobulin does not enter the bloodstream. Sensitive radioimmunoassay techniques, however, detect small amounts in normal individuals and

Table 2. Concentration and Thyroid-Binding Capacity of Serum Proteins

SERUM PROTEIN	CONCENTRATION mg/dL	BINDING CAPACITY μg/dL	BINDING OF T_4	BINDING of T_3
TBG	1.5	25	75%	85%
TBPA	15	300	15%	5%
Albumin	5000	Very great	10%	10%

larger amounts in patients with active thyroiditis and differentiated thyroid carcinoma.

Thyroid hormone release is stimulated by TSH, which acts upon the thyroid cell membrane. Adenyl cyclase is activated, resulting in a prompt rise in cyclic adenosine monophosphate (AMP), hydrolysis of thyroglobulin, and release of T_4 and T_3 (Fig. 3). This process may require only 20 to 30 minutes. Chlorpromazine inhibits the cell membrane activation, whereas lithium carbonate partially inhibits TSH stimulation of hormone release. Once released, T_3 and T_4 are bound to thyroid-binding proteins: thyroid-binding globulin (TBG), thyroid-binding prealbumin (TBPA), and albumin. Clearance half-times are approximately 1 day for T_3 and 7 days for T_4.

Average adult protein-binding capacities and concentrations are shown in Table 2. Binding of T_4 to TBG is strong, whereas binding of T_3 to this protein is somewhat weaker. Binding to TBPA is weak for both hormones. In addition, certain sex-linked disorders increase or decrease serum concentrations of TBG.[5]

Peripheral Metabolism

The exact mechanism whereby T_3 and T_4 increase global metabolic activity is not yet understood. Circulating thyroid hormones increase oxygen consumption (basal metabolic rate) and have a profound effect on growth and development. A lack of thyroid hormone at and after birth is particularly deleterious because the human brain at birth is not completely formed. Maternal thyroid hormone supports growth in utero. However, brain cell division continues 3 to 6 months after birth, and neonatal hypothyroidism results in cretinism. Early diagnosis of thyroid deficiency is therefore essential (see Neonatal Hypothyroidism below). The

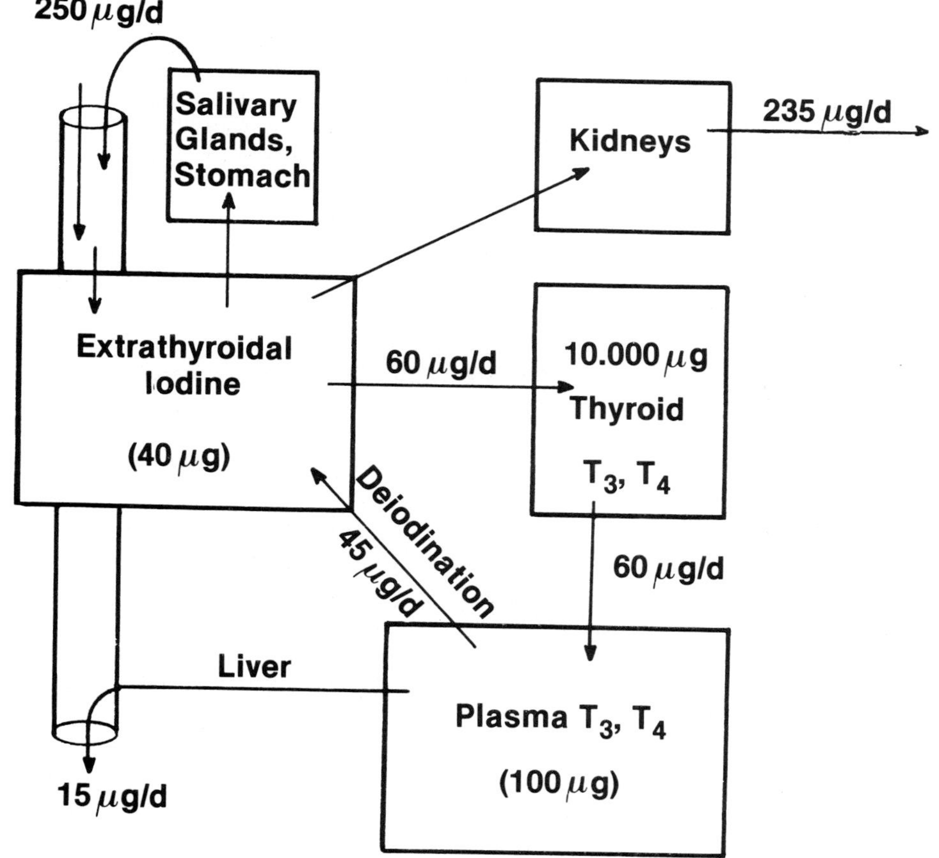

Figure 2. Schematic model of iodine metabolism.

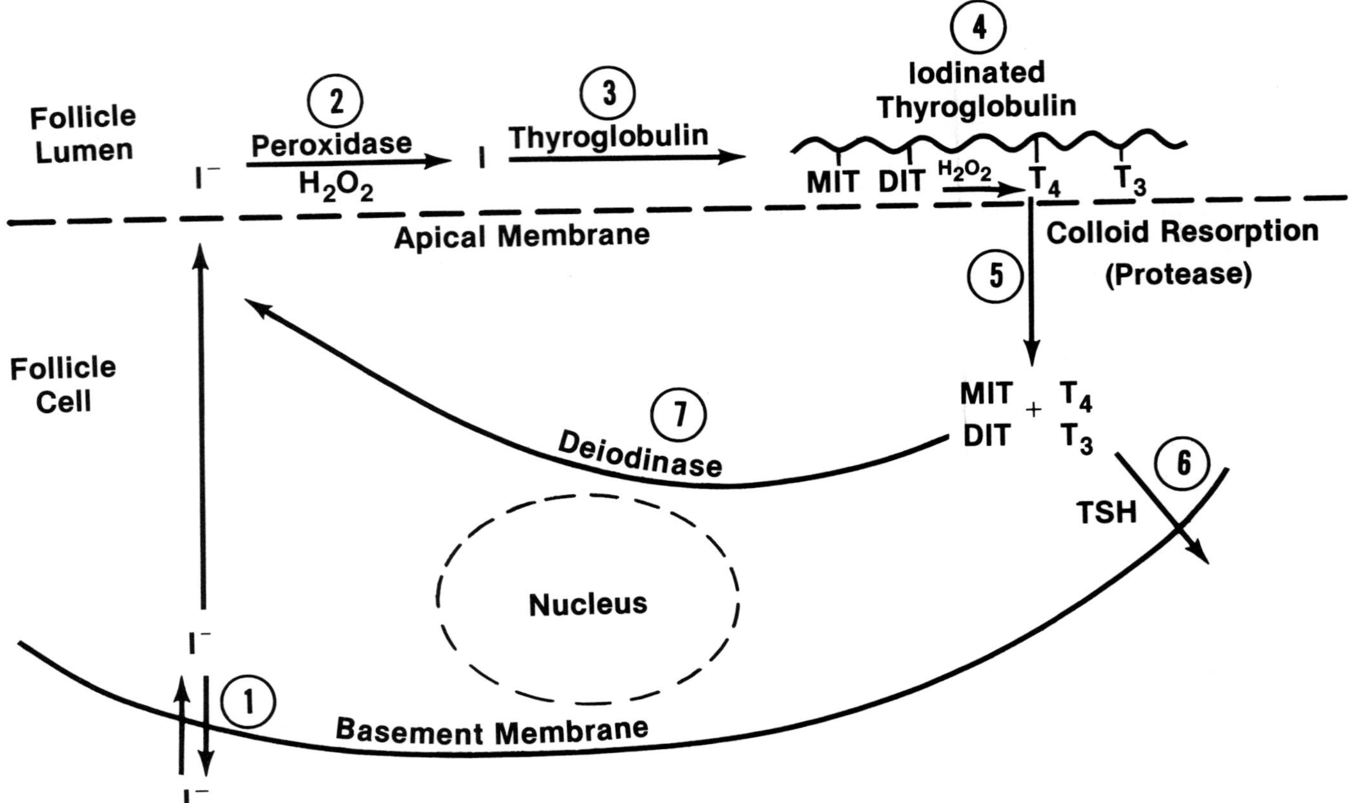

Figure 3. The follicle cell is polarized. Its base, which contains the nucleus, rests on the follicle basement membrane; the apex, composed of microvilli, projects into the follicle lumen. The steps in the intrathyroidal iodine cycle are numbered as follows: Iodine is trapped (1), oxidize to elemental I (2), organified to MIT and DIT (3), which are coupled to form T_3 and T_4, and bound to thyroglobulin (4). When resorption occurs (5), the iodine is either secreted as thyroid hormone (6) or deiodinated and recycled (7). I^- = iodide; DIT = diiodotyrosine; MIT = monoiodotyrosine; T_3 = triiodothyronine; and T_4 = thyroxine.

effects of exogenous thyroid hormone are not immediate. Peak clinical effect is not reached until 7 to 10 days after T_4 is administered, and the effects of T_3 are manifested within 2 to 3 days.

Effects on organ systems from alterations in thyroid hormone production are often profound. Hyperthyroidism increases cardiac output, decreases peripheral vascular resistance, and increases blood flow in most organs except the liver. Increased cutaneous blood flow, which is needed to dissipate excessive heat generation, leads to heat intolerance and warm, moist skin. Cortisol metabolism is accelerated, and serum levels of cortisol are normal or low. Conversely, hypothyroidism slows cortisol metabolism, resulting in hypercholesterolemia. Both glucose and protein metabolism are slowed in hypothyroidism.

The metabolism of T_3 and T_4 have important implications for therapy. T_3 is thought to be the tissue-active hormone, and T_4, merely a prohormone.[6] When radiolabeled T_4 is administered to athyreotic patients, substantial quantities of labeled T_3 are recovered.[7] The question might arise, why not treat patients who require thyroid hormone only with T_3? The answer is that often, after a single daily dose, serum levels of T_3 vary by an order of magnitude. Peak serum levels of T_3 after a single oral dose of 50 to 75 μg may reach 600 to 700 ng/dL. Such high peak levels are poorly tolerated, especially by older patients. Administration of T_4, on the other hand, results in more stable T_3 and T_4 levels, partly because of significantly greater TBG binding of T_4. Several drugs that affect metabolism by inhibiting conversion of T_4 and T_3 are listed in Table 1. Clinical conditions that inhibit conversion include chronic illness, starvation, and prolonged stress.

Both T_3 and *reverse* T_3 (rT_3) are derived primarily from peripheral deiodination of T_4. The serum concentration of rT_3 is only about 40 ng/dL in normal adults, and deiodination of T_4 at the 5′ position is favored over that at the 5 position (Fig. 4). Reverse T_3 is much less active metabolically; it is increased in patients with such conditions as hyperthyroidism, starvation, and severe illness. Its exact role in normal metabolism and disease states has yet to be defined.

IN VIVO FUNCTION STUDIES

Radiopharmaceuticals

Table 3 lists the most commonly used radiopharmaceuticals in thyroid studies along with recommended[8] adult and pediatric doses. The radiation absorbed doses from these radionuclides for various percent uptakes is given in the MIRD publications.[9]

IODINE-131

Using ^{131}I for thyroid diagnostic studies has several disadvantages. The long half-life and beta emissions increase the radiation dose to the thyroid. The high energy of the principal gamma photon (364-keV) is inefficiently collimated by most scintillation cameras. The long half-life also requires background corrections when repeat doses are administered for TSH stimulation and T_3 suppression tests. For these reasons, ^{123}I and ^{99m}Tc-pertechnetate are usually preferred.

IODINE-123

The principal advantages of ^{123}I are the low-energy gamma ray—159 keV (84%)—and the absence of beta emissions. The 13-hour half-life is ideal for most thyroid uptake and imaging studies. The emission of approximately 87% ^{123}Te X-rays, however, may present calibration problems, and contamination with other cyclotron-produced isotopes of iodine, notably ^{125}I, must be considered. Remember, that the longer ^{123}I is kept after delivery, the greater is the useless radiation to the patient from radioisotope contaminants, especially those associated with ^{123}I (p, 2n) production.

TECHNETIUM-99M

The physical characteristics of ^{99m}Tc make pertechnetate the radiopharmaceutical of choice for thyroid imaging in most cases. Generally, little background interference occurs with repeated studies, and both uptake and imaging can be completed within an hour.

Technetium-99m pertechnetate is trapped by the same mechanism as the iodide ion, and all conditions that interfere with iodide trapping also interfere with trapping of pertechnetate. The latter is not organified. Thus, while both agents are effective in separating degrees of thyroid function, they may yield different images in some conditions.[10] The most commonly encountered discrepancy is in chronic thyroiditis; in the recovery phase of this disease increased trapping occurs throughout the gland, with little or no organification. This combination of findings is practically diagnostic of thyroiditis in the absence of drugs that block hormone synthesis, such as propylthiouracil.

Intravenously administered ^{99m}Tc-pertechnetate is loosely bound to plasma proteins and moves rapidly out of the intravascular compartment. Compartmental analysis shows that 50 to 60% disappears with a $T_{1/2}$ of 1 to 2 min from plasma, 15% disappears with a $T_{1/2}$ of 5 to 7.5 min, and 20 to 30% disappears with a $T_{1/2}$ of 100 to 300 min.[11] Its distribution in the body is reflected by early concentration in salivary glands, gastric mucosa, choroid plexus, and thyroid gland. Pertechnetate also crosses the placenta. The pertechnetate ion is excreted primarily by the gastrointestinal tract and kidneys. Excretion occurs by filtration, with approximately 85% of the filtered ^{99m}Tc reabsorbed by the renal tubules. About 30% of the injected dose is excreted in urine during the first 24 hours. Fecal excretion is slower, with approximately 40% recovered by 4 days. Technetium activity appears in the left colon as early as 1 hour after injection, which suggests that a portion of this activity is transported and secreted from the bloodstream. Once secreted into the colon, it is not reabsorbed.

The biologic distribution of pertechnetate is altered by pretreatment of the patient with perchlorate (ClO_4^-),[12] a monovalent anion of approximately the same size as TcO_4^-. Perchlorate blocks the uptake of TcO_4^- in the thyroid gland, salivary glands, choroid plexus, and gastric mucosa by competitive inhibition.

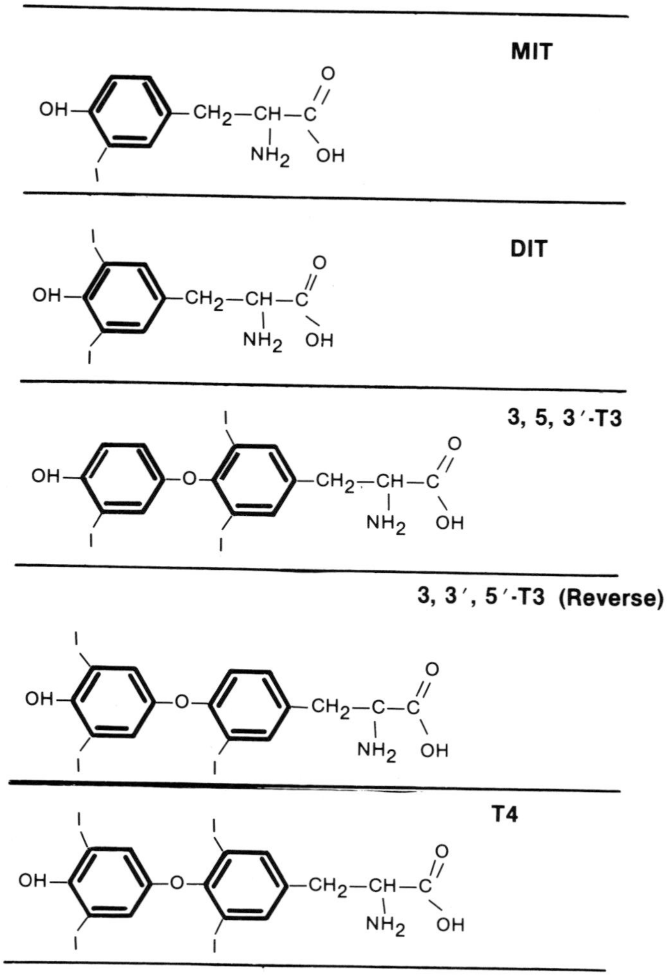

MIT

DIT

3, 5, 3′-T3

3, 3′, 5′-T3 (Reverse)

T4

Figure 4. Structures of the principal thyroid hormones.

Table 3. Recommended Administered Activity in Thyroid Function and Imaging Studies

AGE	^{131}I UPTAKE kBq (μCi)	^{131}I IMAGING kBq (μCi)	^{123}I UPTAKE kBq (μCi)	^{123}I IMAGING MBq (μCi)	^{99m}Tc MBq (mCi)
Adult	222 (6)	1110 (30)	740 (20)	7.4 (200)	185 (5.0)
15 yr	74 (2)	925 (25)	740 (20)	6.3 (170)	155 (4.2)
10 yr	74 (2)	666 (18)	370 (10)	4.4 (120)	111 (3.0)
5 yr	74 (2)	333 (9)	370 (10)	2.2 (60)	55 (1.5)
1 yr	74 (2)	148 (4)	370 (10)	1.0 (28)	30 (0.7)

OTHER RADIOPHARMACEUTICALS

Occasionally, ^{132}I is used in participants of survey studies, or in children, to whom it is important to administer a low absorbed dose. Iodine-125 has too long a half-life (60 days) and too weak photons (27.5 to 35.4 keV) for in vivo thyroid functions. It is most often used as an in vitro label.

Several investigators have used ^{67}Ga-citrate in an attempt to differentiate benign from malignant thyroid lesions. Although there is a higher incidence of positive scans in anaplastic carcinoma of the thyroid, the results in distinguishing differentiated thyroid carcinoma from benign processes are disappointing. Gallium-67 concentrates in a number of thyroid conditions, including subacute thyroiditis, Hashimoto's thyroiditis, anaplastic carcinoma and thyroid lymphoma.[13] Such findings are almost always found incidentally to gallium scintigraphy for other reasons.

Thallium-201 chloride localizes in normal thyroid tissue and in both primary and metastatic thyroid cancer.[14,15] Some data suggest that ^{201}Tl-chloride may be more sensitive than ^{131}I in localizing small thyroid metastases, eliminating the elaborate patient preparation required in using ^{131}I. More studies are required, however, to provide firm recommendations for its use. It is known, for example, that abnormal thyroid concentrations of ^{201}Tl are found in patients with thyroiditis.[15]

Some investigators have reported a high uptake of pentavalent ^{99m}Tc-dimercaptosuccinic acid (DMSA) by both primary and metastatic medullary carcinoma of the thyroid.[16,17] These authors have suggested that this tracer may be specific, because other thyroid malignancies fail to take it up.

Other reports document the use of ^{75}Se-selenomethionine, ^{131}Cs, ^{99m}Tc-bleomycin, and ^{99m}Tc-diphosphate for thyroid imaging.[18–21] None consistently distinguishes malignant from benign nodules.

Tests of Thyroid Function

The most commonly encountered tests of thyroid function are summarized in Table 4.

THYROID UPTAKE WITH RADIOIODINE

The thyroid uptake is the percentage of an administered radiopharmaceutical incorporated by the thyroid gland in a standard time period. If radioiodine is administered orally, the measured uptake increases progressively, reaching a plateau between 18 and 24 hours after intake (Fig. 5). If the dose is administered intravenously, the uptake is more rapid, and reliable measurements can be made 10 to 30 min after injection, although normal values must be established for each laboratory.

In the most common method of measuring thyroid uptake, Na^{123}I or Na^{131}I is administered orally in the doses shown in Table 3. The detector probe usually contains a 5-cm NaI (Tl) crystal and a small collimator angled sufficiently to visualize the entire gland easily from a thyroid-to-crystal distance of 35 cm. Even though the collimator is usually small, extrathyroidal neck activity is always detected. In practice, this error is negligible if the uptake is made 24 hours after administration of radioiodine. If earlier measurements are made, neck background may be appreciable and correction must be made. The usual method is to measure the thigh activity 10 cm above the patella, which reasonably approximates the neck structures in background activity. A known standard of radioiodine, placed in a plastic phantom that simulates the shape and diameter of the neck, is measured at the same time. The uptake is calculated as follows:

$$\% \text{ uptake} = \frac{\text{cpm in thyroid} - \text{cpm in thigh} \times 100}{\text{cpm standard} \times R}$$

where R is the ratio of dose administered to the dose in the standard.

A scintillation camera and pinhole collimator can also be used to measure uptake. This method yields values almost identical to standard probe measurements.[22]

It should be emphasized that ^{131}I uptake measurements will be subject to coincidence summing errors if ^{99m}Tc is injected on the same day for thyroid scintigraphy or other types of scintigraphy. Wasserman et al. found that when pre-dose measurements were subtracted, the 6-hour and 24-hour ^{131}I uptakes could be falsely decreased by up to 137 percentage points using a lower discriminator level of 250 keV, and by up to 35 percentage points with a discriminator level of 300 keV.[23] When pre-dose measurements from ^{99m}Tc were ignored, there was a general *increase* in ^{131}I uptake values at 6 hours. These errors can be eliminated by performing the ^{131}I uptake measurements through a 1-mm lead filter, which effectively excludes the 140-keV photons of ^{99m}Tc.

Table 4. Summary of Thyroid Function Studies

TESTS	USEFULNESS	DISADVANTAGES
A. IN VIVO STUDIES		
Radioiodine uptake Normal: Depends on dietary iodine. See text.	Easy to perform. In normal patients, uptake is proportional to hormone production and release.	Does not measure thyroid function directly because it often does not measure hormone production and release.
Plasma radioiodine Normal: Total ≦ 0.5%/L Organic fraction ≦ 0.2%/L	Dosimetry estimates and measuring iodine turnover.	Organic fraction depends on plasma protein concentration. Not reliable in renal diseases.
Urinary excretion of radioiodine Normal: Depends on dietary iodine	Indirect measure of thyroid function in incapacitated individuals. Estimates of radioiodine burden.	Depends on dietary iodine and renal function. Rarely used.
Absolute iodine uptake Normal: Less than 5 μg/h	Index of thyroid functional activity in endemic goiter.	Difficult to measure. Requires blood and urine determinations.
Perchlorate washout test Normal: No significant discharge	Useful in some forms of chronic thyroiditis and congenital goiter with iodide trapping defects.	
TSH stimulation test Normal: 50% increase over baseline uptake value	Differential diagnosis of primary and secondary hypothyroidism.	
T_3 suppression test Normal: 60% decrease from baseline uptake value	Differentiation of hyperthyroidism from euthyroidism.	Some euthyroid patients with endemic goiter do not suppress. May exaggerate toxic symptoms especially in elderly patients.
B. IN VITRO STUDIES		
T_3 by resin uptake Normal: 25–35 μg/dL	Easy to perform. Indirect measure of thyroid hormone binding proteins.	Results altered by several medications, pregnancy, and serum protein concentration.
T_4 by competitive binding Normal: 5–13 μg/dL (depends on the kit used)	Simple to perform, reliable, eliminates contamination from exogenous iodine. Especially useful in thyroid hyperfunction.	Affected by serum protein concentrations.
T_3 by competitive binding Normal: 150–450 ng/dL	T_3 thyrotoxicosis and euthyroidism in patients with diminished T_4.	Difficult to perform, high cost.
Free T_4 Normal: 2–3 ng/dL	Most exact method of measuring circulating hormone.	Difficult to perform. Not yet applicable to routine measurement.
Free thyroxine index Normal: 0.86–1.13	Compensates for changes in serum proteins in estimates of circulating thyroxine.	
T_3 and T_4 by radioimmunoassay Normal: Varies with laboratory Similar to CPB values	Precise measures of these hormones.	Results influenced by level of circulating proteins.
TSH by radioimmunoassay Normal: less than 10 μIU/mL	Differentiation of primary from secondary hypothyroidism. Borderline hyperthyroidism.	

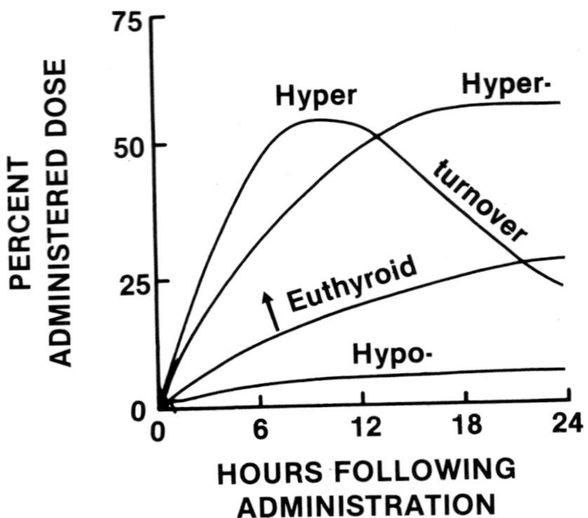

Figure 5. Characteristic curves of thyroid uptake of radioiodine after oral administration.

Table 6. Drugs That Interfere with Thyroid Uptake

TIME	MEDICATION	
About 1 week	Triiodothyronine Thiouracils Sulfonamides Cobaltous ion Thiocyanate Perchlorate Nitrates	Bromides Steroids ACTH Isoniazid Phenylbutazone Thiopental (Pentothal) Penicillin
2–3 weeks	Dinitrophenol Dinitrocresol	Iodides Some vitamin mixtures Some cough medications Seaweed
4–6 weeks	Thyroid extract Thyroxine	
About 2 months	Intravascular radiographic contrast media (e.g., Hypaque, Conray) Oral contrast media (e.g., Cholografin and Telepaque)	
>1 year	Oil-containing contrast media used in bronchography, myelography, arthography (e.g., Lipiodol and Pantopaque)	

The normal thyroid uptake values vary with the environment, so each laboratory must establish a normal range for its particular patient population. Higher levels of iodine in processed foods have substantially lowered the normal range in most developed countries. In Washington, D.C., the normal 24-hour ^{131}I thyroid uptake ranges from 6 to 30%. This wide variation produces some overlap between euthyroid and hyperthyroid ranges, and serves to emphasize that the uptake alone does not permit a definition of the functional thyroid state (Table 5). Low thyroid uptakes are especially meaningless because of the many sources of iodides that depress radioiodine uptake.

The 4-hour or 6-hour uptake is occasionally useful, especially in diagnosing thyroiditis in which trapping function is normal or increased and organification is impaired. This condition results in normal or elevated 4-hour uptake and low 24-hour uptake. Rarely, in Graves' disease with rapid turnover, the 4-hour uptake is elevated, and the 24-hour uptake normal (Fig. 5). Such high turnover is almost always associated with elevated serum thyroid hormones and obvious clinical hyperthyroidism.

Several foods and drugs interfere with the thyroid uptake test (Table 6). Ingestion of foods rich in iodine, such as seafood, may decrease uptake for up to 15 days. Iodinated medications, such as amebicides and antitussives, depress

Table 5. Thyroid Uptake in Relation to Thyroid Metabolic State

CLINICAL STATE	INCREASED	NORMAL	DECREASED
Hyperthyroid	Hyperthyroidism	Antithyroid drugs—propylthiouracil, Tapazol, thiocyanate	Expanded iodide pool Subacute thyroiditis, hyperthyroid phase Thyrotoxicosis factitia Antithyroid drugs Struma ovarii (rare)
Euthyroid	Rebound after thyroid hormone or antithyroid drug withdrawal Recovery from subacute thyroiditis Hashimoto's disease, early phase Compensated dyshormonogenesis	Euthyroidism	Decompensated dyshormonogenesis Hashimoto's disease
Hypothyroid	Decompensated dyshormonogenesis Hashimoto's disease	Hashimoto's disease After therapy for hyperthyroidism (^{131}I or surgery) Decompensated dyshormonogenesis Subacute thyroiditis, recovery phase	Hypothyroidism—primary, secondary

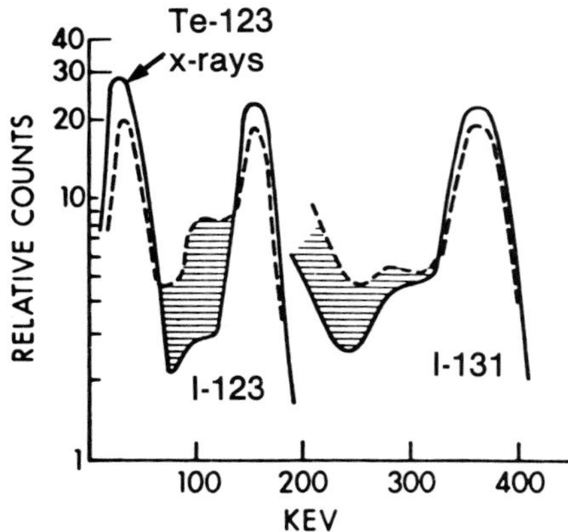

Figure 6. Relative spectra of ^{123}I and ^{131}I sources in air (solid lines) and in a plastic neck phantom (broken lines) obtained with a NaI(Tl) probe detector. The shaded area indicates the added Compton scatter. (Adapted from Chervu S., et al.[27])

uptake for up to 30 days. Iodinated contrast materials, including the nonionic compounds (because of dissociation), may decrease uptake from a few weeks, in cases of excretory urography and cholecystography, to several months and even years in cases of contrast myelography and bronchography.[24,25] Thyroid hormones such as T_3 and T_4 act to decrease TSH secretion, thus decreasing uptake. Such antithyroid drugs as propylthiouracil block thyroid hormone synthesis, but not trapping, therefore actually increasing uptake. Lithium carbonate inhibits thyroid hormone secretion from the gland, thereby elevating uptake moderately.[26] Other substances, such as steroids and phenylbutazone, may reduce uptake for a few days. Prolonged ingestion of such goitrogenic foods as turnips and cabbage liberate thiocyanates upon digestion. The latter compete with iodide trapping to decrease radioiodine uptake mildly.

Thyroid Uptake with Iodine-123. Some technical problems may be encountered when using ^{123}I to determine thyroid uptake. All are inherent in ^{131}I uptake determinations, but they are aggravated by the use of ^{123}I. The first problem relates to the separation of the Compton scatter from the photopeak. Figure 6 shows the photospectra of ^{123}I and ^{131}I sources in air and inside a plastic phantom, both obtained with a 5×5 cm NaI(Tl) probe. The Compton-scattered photons (shaded area) are considerably more abundant for ^{123}I with interposed scattering media than for ^{131}I. In addition, the Compton plateau is much closer to the ^{123}I photopeak. Consequently, any change in high voltage has a greater effect on ^{123}I recorded counts than on ^{131}I counts. Chervu et al. have suggested several modifications to the ^{131}I thyroid uptake protocol when using ^{123}I[27]:

1. Use a well-stabilized high-voltage supply,
2. Use the 250-keV range (higher gain setting in PHA) for counting ^{123}I, and avoid using the 1-MeV range when using a single-channel analyzer,
3. Perform high-voltage calibration each time the uptake probe is used,
4. If the ^{123}I capsule is placed inside the neck phantom during high-voltage calibration, use a 20-keV window,
5. If a 6-mm solid plastic rod is used for distance determination, remove it during measurements, or replace it with a hollow rod or thin bar (to reduce scatter),
6. Do not use integral mode for counting ^{123}I because of scatter from high-energy contaminants,
7. Count all capsules before administration to patients,
8. Do not use calculated counts (corrected for decay) when using ^{123}I, because of the variation of scatter component with high-voltage fluctuation,
9. Use a standard neck phantom,
10. Calculate the thyroid uptake by using the following formula:

$$\% \text{ uptake} = 100\ P_2S_1/S_2P_1$$

where:

P_1 = net dose counts before administration;
P_2 = patient neck counts, corrected for background counts obtained from the thigh;
S_1 = net standard-dose counts on the day of administration of capsule to the patient; and
S_2 = net standard-dose counts on the day of neck counting.

Wide fluctuations in line voltage are common in hospitals. The use of voltage stabilizer units with counting equipment and frequent HV calibrations, are therefore advisable.

Thyroid Uptake with Technetium-99m Pertechnetate. Thyroid uptake measurements obtained using ^{99m}Tc-pertechnetate to estimate thyroid functional status are usually satisfactory, except in thyroiditis and dyshormonogenesis. The maximum thyroid uptake occurs 10 to 20 min following injection.[28,29] The absolute uptake of pertechnetate by the thyroid is small, 0.3 to 3.0% of the administered dose. Neck background is relatively high and constantly changing, because of excretion into the salivary glands, stomach mucosa, and urine. Consequently, careful corrections must be made using computer subtraction of background if determination of absolute uptake is to be accurate. To avoid the errors inherent both in background subtraction and in administration of a variable amount of activity, neck-to-thigh ratios have been advocated.[29,30] The neck counts measured with a probe detector are compared with the activity measured 15 min after injection at the same distance from the thigh (35 cm), 10 cm above the patella. The normal ratio ranges from approximately 2.5 to 5.5, depending on technique and laboratory. A thyroid scan is obtained with the same 2 to 4 mCi (~75 to 150 MBq) of ^{99m}Tc-pertechnetate injected, and the entire procedure requires less than 45 min. This is an important consideration in cases of impending thyroid storm, when waiting 24 to 48 hours for radioimmunoassay results is out of the question.

Another index of thyroid function, proposed by Ashkar

and Smith, involves measuring the first transit of ^{99m}Tc-pertechnetate following injection from the carotid to the thyroid gland.[31] Changes in the carotid-to-thyroid transit time were found to reflect the relative metabolic function of the thyroid. This test has the advantage of simplicity, because it is easily combined with the pertechnetate thyroid scan. The test is probably no more nor less reliable than any of the thyroid uptake tests.

ABSOLUTE IODINE UPTAKE

The absolute iodine uptake measures the quantity of iodide extracted by the thyroid per unit time and, although it is used infrequently, it constitutes one of the most reliable indices of in vivo thyroid function.[32] Its utility has been particularly emphasized in the study of endemic goiter.[33] The test is seldom used because the method is laborious, requiring measures of plasma and urinary activity in addition to stable urinary iodide levels. Also, hormone assay methods have made the test unnecessary in most cases. The method developed by Alexander et al. and Wayne et al. allows calculation of absolute uptake through the determination of iodine clearance and plasma inorganic iodide concentration[32,34,35]:

$$\text{Absolute Uptake } (\mu\text{g/hr}) = C_{thy} \text{ (mL/min)} \times I^{-}_{plasma} \ (\mu\text{g/mL}) \times 0.6$$

where: C_{thy} = thyroid clearance of iodine, I^{-}_{plasma} = the plasma concentration of ^{127}I, and 0.6 = a correction factor to express the results in μg/hr.

The fasting patient is given 30 μCi (~1 MBq) of oral radioiodine. The thyroid uptake is measured at 60 and 150 min by an external probe. The patient empties his bladder at 60 min and the urine is discarded. The urine is collected at 150 min, and the % dose/mL is determined along with the total iodide content of the urine in μg/dL. At 105 min, a blood sample is drawn and the radioiodine is determined as % dose/mL. C_{thy} is determined from the following:

$$C_{thy} \text{ (mL/min)} = \frac{\text{150-min uptake} - \text{60-min uptake (\% dose)}}{\text{90 min} \times \text{total plasma level (\% dose/mL)}}$$

I^{-}_{plasma} is calculated indirectly because plasma inorganic iodide concentration is very low and difficult to measure:

$$I^{-}_{plasma} \ (\mu\text{g/dL}) = \frac{\text{Urine } ^{127}\text{I } (\mu\text{g/dL}) \times \text{plasma } ^{131}\text{I (\% dose/mL)}}{\text{Urine } ^{131}\text{I (\% dose/mL)}}$$

Thyroid clearance of radioiodine varies between 5 and 40 mL/min, depending upon the plasma concentration of iodide, which varies between 0.1 and 0.5 μg/dL. The absolute uptake of iodine, however, rarely exceeds 5 μg/hour and, in hyperthyroidism, rarely falls below 5 μg/hour.

PERCHLORATE WASHOUT TEST

Although it is not properly a test of thyroid function, the perchlorate washout test is useful in studies of congenital goiters and of Hashimoto's thyroiditis. The test is based on the fact that ClO_4^- is trapped by the thyroid and displaces iodide ions that have not been organified. In organification defects, such as peroxidase deficiency, iodide that has been trapped by the thyroid is discharged from the thyroid. Twenty microcuries (0.74 MBq) of ^{131}I are administered orally, and the uptake is measured 2 hours later. The patient is then given 1 g of $KClO_4$ orally, and the uptake is measured every 15 min for 90 min. Normally, no variation in the thyroid activity is found. If a significant organification defect exists, the thyroid activity falls at least 15% below the 2-hour value.[86]

FUNCTIONAL TESTS

Functional tests measure the organ's ability to respond to stimulation or suppression. They measure the integrity of the organ's inherent function and of the control mechanisms that regulate it.

TSH Stimulation Test. TSH stimulates all of the thyroid enzymatic processes from iodide trapping to hormone secretion, so that the effects of exogenous administration of this hormone can be evaluated at almost any level. This test was most commonly used to measure the change in thyroid uptake before and after TSH administration; occasionally the level of circulating T_3 was measured. The test is performed by first obtaining a baseline 24-hour radioiodine uptake. Immediately thereafter, the patient receives 10 units of bovine TSH intramuscularly for 3 days. On the fourth day, the radioiodine uptake test is repeated, with care taken to account for neck background if ^{131}I is used. Normally, thyroid uptake increases by greater than 50% above the baseline level.

In the past, this test was used to differentiate primary from secondary hypothyroidism. In secondary hypothyroidism inadequate TSH production occurs, but the thyroid can respond to exogenous TSH. In primary hypothyroidism (which is usually accompanied by high circulating levels of endogenous TSH), the defect is at the thyroid level and the gland is unable to respond. The same information about thyroid reserve is now obtained by measuring basal serum TSH concentrations. The TSH stimulation test also can be used to determine whether patients on thyroid replacement still require it. However, it is usually more convenient to discontinue hormone therapy and measure serum T_4 and TSH concentrations 4 to 6 weeks later.

T_3 Suppression Test. This test consists of measuring radioiodine uptake before and at the end of 7 days of administration of oral T_3. Normally, the uptake falls more than 60% below the baseline value. The principal value of the test was in distinguishing euthyroid from borderline hyperthyroidism. In the latter condition, the gland fails to suppress. This test has also been replaced largely by sensitive assays of TSH.[36]

TRH Stimulation Test. In this test, 500 μg of TRH is injected intravenously, and the serum TSH level is measured before and 30 and 120 min after injection. This test was used primarily to identify borderline hyperthyroidism and to distinguish among causes of hypothyroidism. However, its use has been disappointing[37] and it has been primarily replaced by sensitive assays of TSH. One exception is to assess whether TSH secretion is fully suppressed in patients on long-term T_4 treatment of differentiated thyroid carcinoma.[38]

IN VITRO FUNCTION STUDIES

The past several years have seen many changes in thyroid hormone assays. As these assays have become more sensitive, they have in many respects simplified the laboratory testing of thyroid disease. Most uncomplicated thyroid functional conditions can be described with sensitive assays of TSH and free T_4. In general, assays for free T_4 have replaced the combination of total T_4 and an index of binding. Assays for free T_3 are useful in the occasional case of hyperthyroidism with a normal T_4 when T_3 thyrotoxicosis is suspected.

Sensitive TSH Assays

The introduction of labeled antibody immunoassays, such as *immunoradiometric assay* (IRMA) has greatly increased the sensitivity of TSH assays. In IRMA an excess of labeled monoclonal antibody is incubated with the serum analyte. The labeled antibody-analyte complex is then removed from solution using an excess of a second, solid-phase antibody. The two antibodies recognize different epitopes on the analyte molecule. The concentration of analyte is thus directly proportional to the radioactivity in the analyte sandwich. The advantages are greater sensitivity and speed of assay. Earlier radioimmunoassays (RIA) had detection limits of 0.95 to 1.0 mU/L) and required about 4 days to complete. Current IRMAs have detection limits of 0.02 to 0.07 mU/L and can be completed in a day.[36] Such assays reliably separate euthyroid patients with previously undetectable TSH levels from patients with hyperthyroidism. TSH concentrations by such assays have replaced the TRH test in assessing the degree of thyrotrophe suppression in suspected hyperthyroidism. The normal range in serum is 0.5–5.0 μu/mL. A normal basal serum TSH value has the same significance as a normal serum TSH response to TRH, and excludes hyperthyroidism. A low or undetectable basal TSH level has the same significance as a reduced response to TRH, and indicates clinical hyperthyroidism.

Measurement of TSH is the most reliable method available for validating the adequacy of thyroid hormone replacement in hypothyroidism. Accurate measurements of TSH also allow the detection of more subtle forms of thyroid disease. The ability to assay the α-subunit of TSH has permitted identification of pituitary or TSH-induced hyperthyroidism, since TSH from pituitary adenomas contains more of the α-subunit.

Free T_3 and T_4

The original method of measuring free thyroid hormone was based on the fact that free, but not bound, hormone is dialyzable. It is important to know the free fraction, but this value eliminates interference with measurements of total hormone by the many conditions that alter serum concentrations of binding proteins. Because of the very small quantities of free T_3 and T_4, direct measurement is not possible without the use of radioactive tracers. Free T_3 and T_4 are now determined by kinetic assays, which use solid phase antibodies and radiolabeled T_3 and T_4. Dialysis assays are cumbersome and are no longer valid.

SCINTIGRAPHY

Indications

The following are the most frequent indications for thyroid scintigraphy:

1. Goiter
2. Palpable nodule in the neck
3. Clinical hypothyroidism or hyperthyroidism
4. Evaluation of the progress of thyroiditis
5. History of prior neck irradiation
6. Evaluation of substernal mass
7. Postoperative search for functioning metastases
8. Suspicion of occult malignancy
9. Evaluation of the effects of thyroid stimulating and suppressing medications
10. Search for thyroid tissue in neonatal and juvenile hypothyroidism.

In the past, thyroid scintigraphy was considered a routine part of the workup of most patients with thyroid disease. This practice has changed greatly with the growing skill of pathologists in interpreting needle biopsies, which can provide specific pathologic diagnoses; with the development of MRI which has much better anatomical resolution; and with the increasing realization that specific diagnoses cannot be made by thyroid scintigraphy in most instances. By far the most common uses of scintigraphy today relate to determining the functional status of thyroid nodules in euthyroid patients and, of course, in the search for functioning thyroid cancer metastases. This subject will be explored further under the discussion of thyroid nodules below.

Thyroid Imaging Agents

The most commonly used radiopharmaceuticals for thyroid imaging are listed in Table 7. Of these, ^{131}I is seldom used because of the high radiation absorbed dose and inferior image quality obtained with the 364-keV gamma emission.

Table 7. Thyroid Imaging Radiopharmaceuticals

AGENT	ADULT DOSE MBq (mCi)	THYROID ABSORBED DOSE (cGy)
$^{123}I^-$	11–15 (0.3–0.4)	2.25–3.0
$^{131}I^-$	2–4 (0.05–0.1)	3.4–6.8
$^{99m}TcO_4^-$	185–370 (5–10)	0.65–1.3
^{99m}Tc-MIBI	185–370 (5–10)	0.03–0.06
$^{201}Tl^-$	75–110 (2–3)	1.3–1.95

Thallium-201 and ^{99m}Tc-methoxyisobutyl isonitrile (MIBI) are used primarily to image suppressed thyroid tissue or when large doses of iodine have been recently administered.[39,40] Rather, $^{123}I^-$ and ^{99m}Tc-pertechnetate are almost universally used for routine thyroid imaging. Imaging is performed about 20 min after intravenous administration of ^{99m}Tc and 4 to 6 hours following oral administration of ^{123}I.

COMPARISON BETWEEN ^{123}I AND ^{99m}TC-PERTECHNETATE

Numerous comparative studies have attempted to determine the relative advantages of Na^{123}I and ^{99m}Tc for routine thyroid imaging. Some have claimed definite superiority of ^{123}I,[41–43] while others have found no significant difference.[44–47] Some images appear to have better contrast with ^{123}I because of higher thyroid:background ratio but, in other patients, the ^{99m}Tc images are preferred because of the higher count rate obtained with this radiopharmaceutical.

Of greater concern, however, have been occasional reports of discrepant uptake of the two radiopharmaceuticals in differentiated thyroid cancer. The most worrisome have been rare ^{99m}Tc images that revealed a "warm" or "hot" nodule because of intact trapping function, but radioiodine images revealed "cold" nodules because the organification function was not preserved by the cancer. The clear implication here is that the thyroid cancer would not have been followed up with biopsy because of the presumed benign nature of a functioning nodule. Thus, many[48–50] have recommended that all nodules that appear to trap pertechnetate should be additionally imaged with ^{123}I. Much more rarely, the opposite pattern has been reported.[51]

It is our conviction that these discrepancies are largely overblown. In a large, multi-institution study reported by Kusić et al.[47], comparing images in 316 patients with thyroid nodules, discrepancies were found in 5 to 8%, depending upon the reviewer. Most of these differences occurred in multinodular goiters and there were no discrepancies in the 12 lesions that contained differentiated thyroid carcinoma. In fact, in no case was a discrepancy in scintigraphic appearance judged to be of diagnostic significance. There was a slight preference among reviewers for ^{123}I scintigrams, but these authors concluded that there is no compelling reason to favor one agent over the other, or to routinely repeat imaging of ^{99m}Tc hot nodules with radioiodine.

Instrumentation

Nearly all thyroid scintigraphy is recorded with a scintillation camera fitted with a high-resolution pinhole collimator. With ^{123}I about 50,000 counts per image are collected, while with ^{99m}Tc-pertechnetate, approximately 150,000 counts per image are obtained. These count densities are comparable because the target-to-background ratio is higher with radioiodine. Normally, three views—anterior, left anterior oblique, and right anterior oblique—are obtained.

Tomographic Imaging of the Thyroid

Both PET[52] and SPECT[53] imaging of the thyroid have been reported. PET imaging of the thyroid uses ^{124}I, although the high radiation absorbed dose discourages most investigations with this isotope. Both ^{123}I and ^{99m}Tc-pertechnetate have been used with SPECT imaging. The increased contrast and resolution of tomographic imaging have been useful in:

1. Evaluation of small (<1 cm) nodules that are obscured by over- or underlying tissue in pinhole images. Such nodules are encountered with increasing frequency as ultrasonography, which can detect nodules of only a few millimeters in diameter, is used to evaluate the thyroid.
2. Detection of multinodularity in glands in which pinhole images demonstrate only a single cold nodule.
3. Demonstration of functional retrolaryngeal thyroid tissue in patients with dysphagia and airway obstruction. CT and MR imaging demonstrates the anatomical, but not the function of retropharyngeal and substernal tissue.[54,55]
4. Location of functioning thyroid metastases.

The SPECT methodology reported by Chen et al.[53] is typical of these techniques. They administered 15 MBq (400 μCi) of ^{123}I and imaged 5 hours later using a slant hole collimator, 180° rotation, 6° angle intervals and 40 sec per step. Reconstruction was performed through a combination of convolution technique and filtered backprojection using the Shepp and Logan filter. Figure 7 shows an example of SPECT imaging in a patient with retrolaryngeal extension.

Technique of Planar Thyroid Imaging

With scintillation cameras fitted with a pinhole collimator, approximately 50,000 counts are obtained for ^{123}I images and about 150,000 counts with ^{99m}Tc images. Three views are obtained routinely: anterior, left anterior oblique, and right anterior oblique.

NORMAL THYROID IMAGE

The thyroid gland has a homogeneous appearance, with sharply defined borders; the lateral margins are either straight or convex (Fig. 8). Left and right anterior oblique views are taken at angles of 30 to 45°. Figure 9 illustrates a small cold nodule on the posterior aspect of the left lower lobe, clearly visualized in the left anterior oblique view (at right) and only faintly so on the anterior image (left). Concave borders

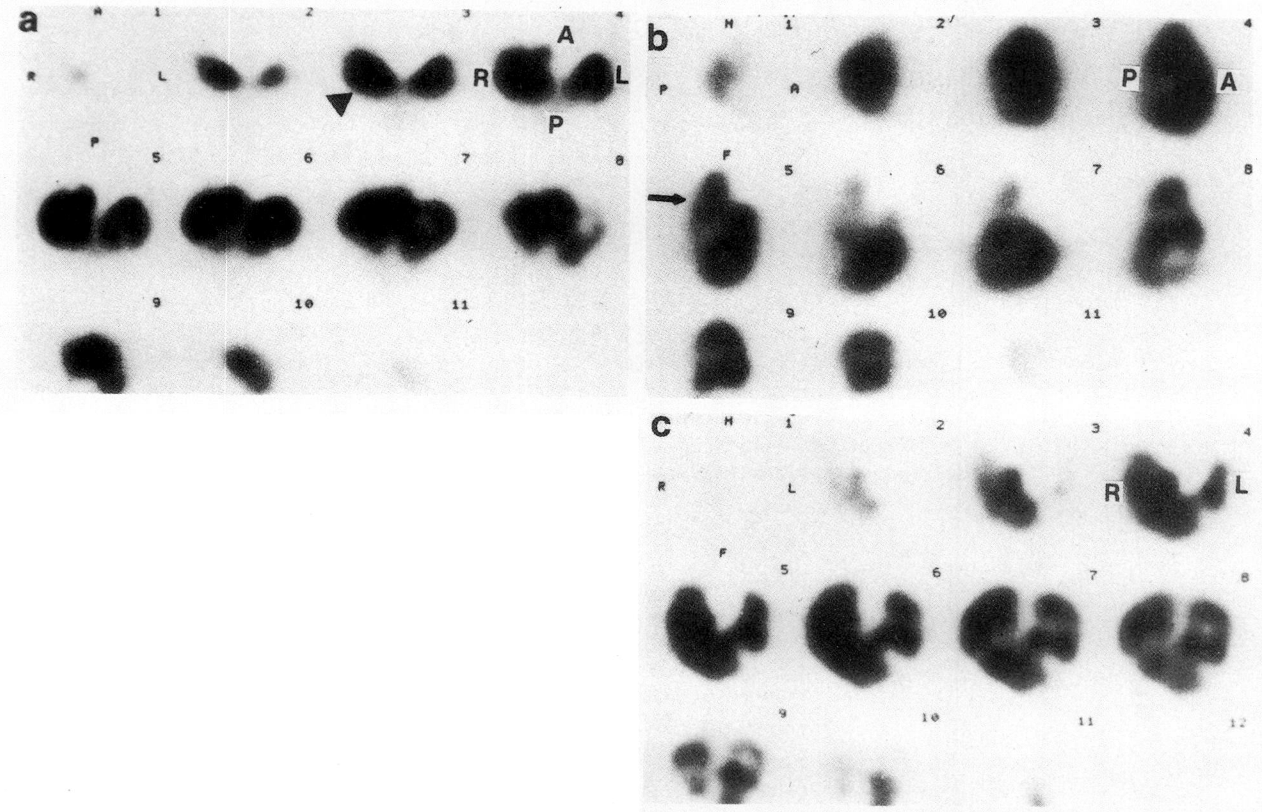

Figure 7. Transaxial (**a**), sagittal (**b**), and coronal (**c**) tomographic sections of SPECT imaging of the thyroid in a patient with toxic multinodular goiter with coexisting papillary carcinoma of the thyroid. Transaxial slices show retrolaryngeal extension of both lobes (slice numbers 2–5 and arrowhead) and tracheal space partially occupied and distorted by the goiter (slice numbers 6–9). Sagittal sections show posteriorly located thyroid tissue at the level of the isthmus (slice numbers 5–6, and arrow). A. anterior; P, posterior; R, right; L, left. Reproduced from Reference 53 by permission.

should arouse suspicion of an extrinsic mass. A pyramidal lobe (Fig. 10) is visualized in thyroid scans in approximately 17% of normal glands and in as many as 43% of patients with toxic goiters.[56]

Several methods of estimating gland size using scintigraphic parameters have been proposed to help estimate therapeutic doses of radioiodine. Surgical and autopsy correlations with these methods have been disappointing, however. In one large series in autopsy-measured glands, du Cret and colleagues[57] found that the best formula to predict thyroid lobar mass (in grams) was: $4.9D + (0.07L \times 2W) - 2.3$ (in cms) with depth, D, to be determined by ultrasound. Without knowing lobar depth they found the best formula for mass (g) to be $0.1L \times 2W$ (in cm).

The best judgment of gland size is probably that made by palpation, with use of the scintigram or ultrasound reserved for orientation in unusually shaped glands or substernal extension. The thyroid must be palpated carefully before scintigraphy, because the combination of scintigraphy and physical examination best clarifies the relationship between

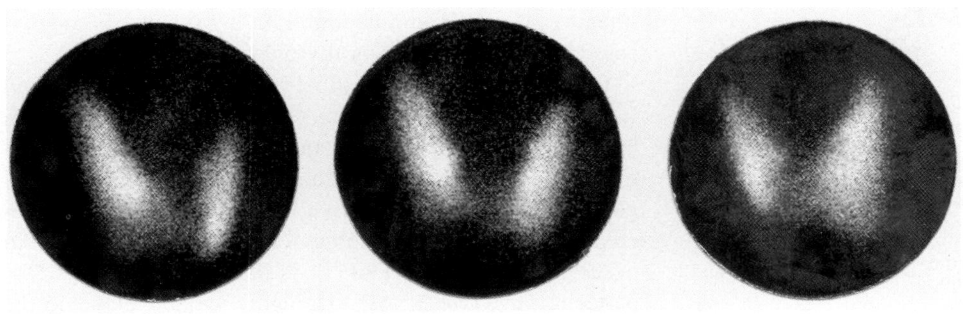

Figure 8. Normal RAO, anterior, and LAO thyroid images obtained using ^{99m}Tc-pertechnetate and pinhole collimator.

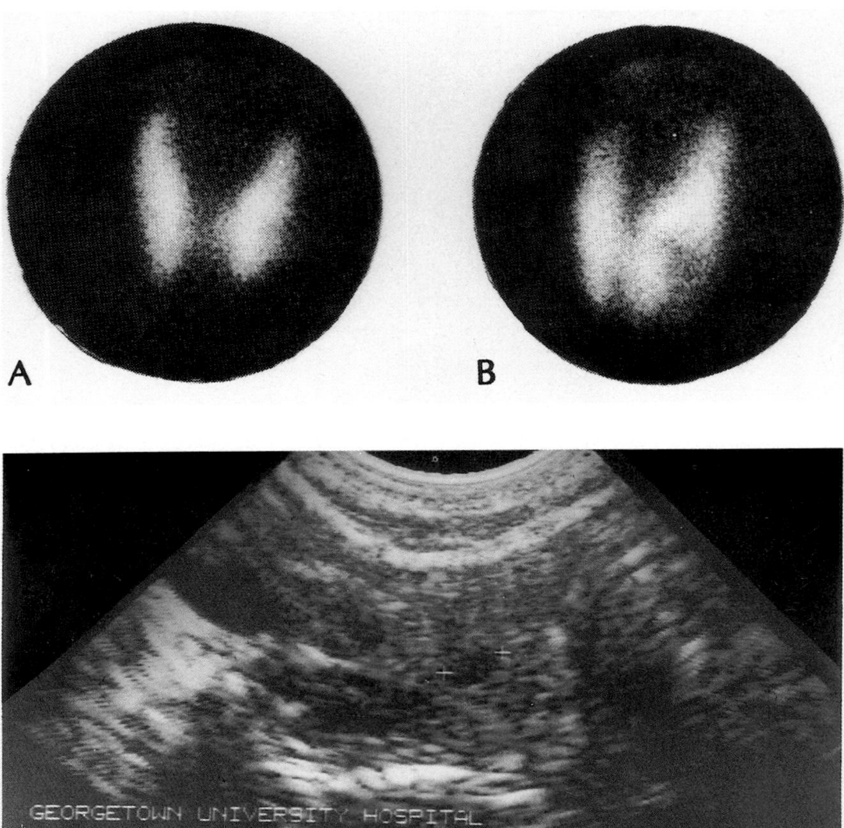

Figure 9. (**A**). Anterior ^{99m}Tc-pertechnetate thyroid image with poorly defined irregularity in left lobe; (**B**). left anterior oblique better demonstrates a solitary cold nodule, which proved to be a thyroid adenoma; **(C)**. ultrasound demonstrates other nodules, some as small as 2 mm.

the thyroid parenchyma and masses or structures within and surrounding the gland. The gland should be palpated with the patient in the upright, rather than recumbent, position because separating the lower margin of the gland from the clavicle is difficult when the patient is recumbent.

Unusual variants include congenital absence of one lobe (hemiagenesis), sublingual thyroid (Fig. 11), or substernal extension of the gland. Lateral thyroid rests may occur, but they almost always fail to function in the presence of normal thyroid activity. If they do demonstrate iodine uptake, they must be considered metastases from well-differentiated thyroid carcinoma.

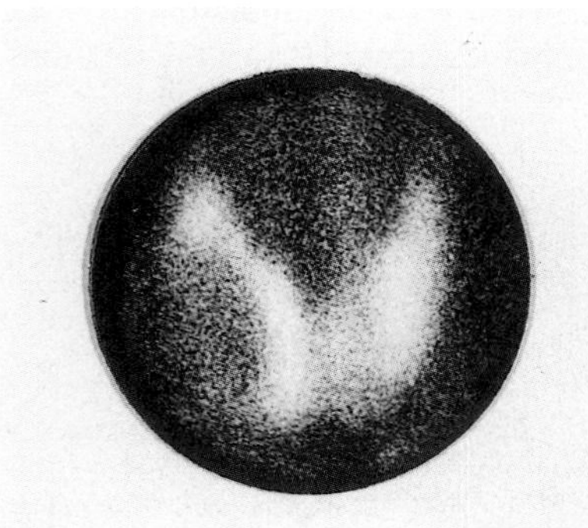

Figure 10. Colloid cyst involving right lobe; note small pyramidal lobe extending superiorly from left lobe.

Hemiagenesis was found in 4 of 7000 scintiscans by Hamburger and Hamburger[58]; however, the true incidence in asymptomatic populations is not known. The characteristic scintigraphic appearance is shown in Figure 12; it has been called the "hockey-stick" sign.[59] Methods of demonstrating absence versus suppression of a lobe include ultrasonography, ^{201}Tl scintigraphy,[39] ^{99m}Tc-MIBI scintigraphy,[40] and reimaging after TSH stimulation. Both thyrotoxicosis and thyroid cancer can develop in thyroid hemiagenesis.[60,61]

Rarely, detached mediastinal remnants, ovarian thyroid rests, struma cordis, or struma ovarii occur.[62–64] All of these abnormal rests may function and give rise to thyrotoxicosis or malignancy. In the presence of a functioning thyroid gland, all functioning extrathyroidal tissue should be considered metastases. In searching for ectopic foci of thyroid tissue, use of either ^{131}I or ^{123}I is important because ^{99m}Tc-pertechnetate concentrates to a highly variable extent in the

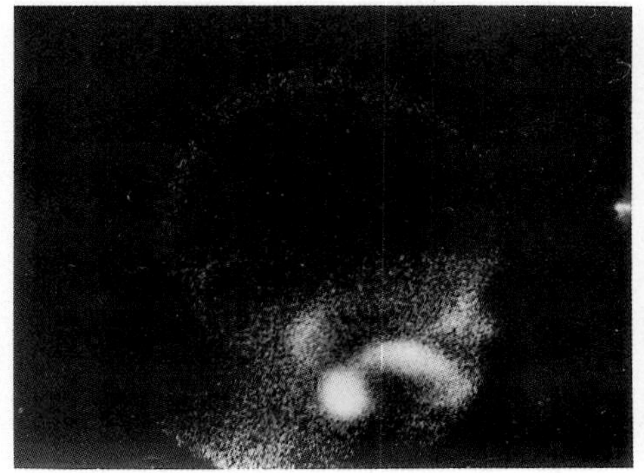
A

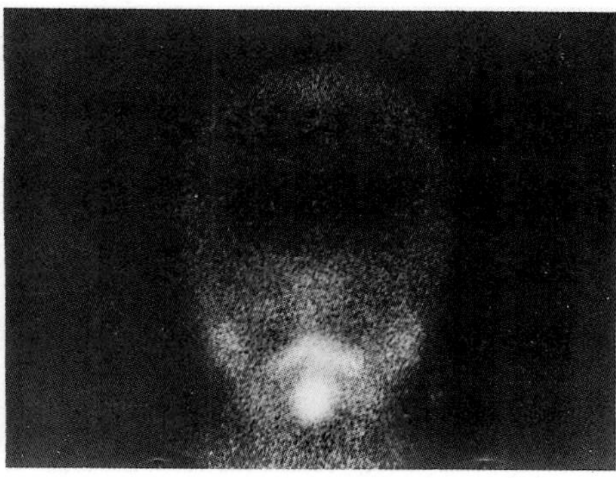
B

Figure 11. Sublingual thyroid in a 5-year-old child imaged with ^{99m}Tc-pertechnetate. **(A)**. Anterior view. **(B)**. Right lateral view. Activity in the mouth and faint parotid activity are normal.

vicinity of ectopic thyroid tissue (the salivary gland and esophagus in the neck; esophagus and blood pool of the mediastinum; colon and bladder in the pelvis).

NONVISUALIZING THYROID

When the thyroid uptake is low, scintigraphy may fail to visualize the gland, or it may visualize the gland only faintly. The following are causes of a nonvisualizing thyroid:

1. Increased iodine pool,
2. Acute thyroiditis; often, local signs and symptoms occur,
3. Chronic thyroiditis; in some cases, low iodine uptake is associated with an elevated trapping index, and the gland is better visualized with ^{99m}Tc-pertechnetate,
4. Suppressing or antithyroid medication,
5. Surgical or radioiodine ablation,
6. Congenital absence of one or both lobes (rare).

NODULES

The clinical finding of a palpable nodule is the most frequent indication for thyroid scintigraphy. Determining whether the nodule is functioning and whether the nodule is solitary or multiple is important. These considerations largely determine the subsequent therapy.

The term *nodule* is nonspecific and embraces a variety of pathologic processes, including adenomas, carcinomas, cysts, or merely ill-defined lumps resulting from a process of cyclical hyperplasia and involution. Nodules are usually classified according to their scintigraphic appearance: "cold," "warm," or "hot." Occasionally, cold nodules may be identified as warm nodules because overlying or underlying functional tissue has masked their true nature. Therefore, they are often better identified by oblique views (Fig. 9). In general, warm nodules are best regarded as if they were cold nodules. Nonfunctioning nodules may represent simple cysts, degenerative changes (including hemorrhage, edema, and fibrosis), thyroiditis, benign adenoma, or carcinoma.

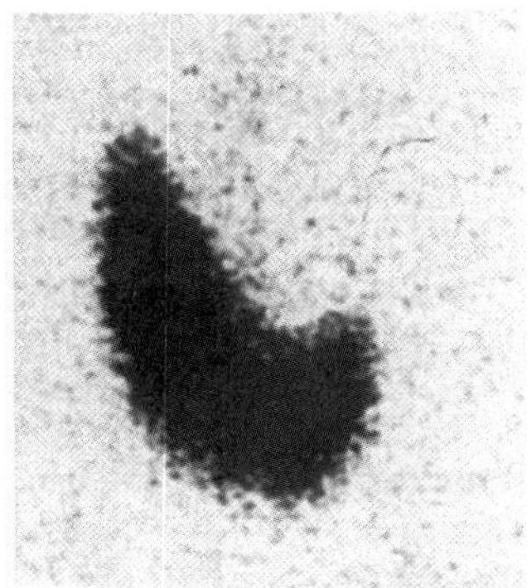

Figure 12. Hemiagenesis of the left thyroid lobe.

Thyroid nodules are common. In as many as 50% of autopsies, the gland contains nodules that had not been suspected clinically and in three fourths of these cases multiple nodules are found.[65] The incidence of nodules increases with age, and they are more common in women than in men. Atkins reviewed several studies reporting the incidence of malignancy in thyroid nodules.[66] In over 2000 solitary nodules, thyroid cancer was found in 2% of hot nodules, 4% of warm nodules, and 20% of cold nodules.

COLD NODULES

Thyroid scintigraphy is not particularly useful in distinguishing benign from malignant cold nodules. Furthermore, palpable nodules less than 1 cm in diameter may be missed. The presenting characteristics often weigh heavily in the decision to operate.

Most thyroid nodules are found in patients over 40 years of age. Most cases of well-differentiated thyroid cancer, however, occur in patients under 40. Solitary cold nodules in young patients, therefore, have a high likelihood of containing cancer.

While nodular thyroid disease is four times more prevalent in females, the approximate female-to-male ratio for thyroid cancer is only two to one. Thus, solitary cold nodules are more likely to be malignant in males than in females. A history of radiation exposure to the neck, voice changes suggesting vocal cord paresis, Horner's syndrome suggesting cervical nerve involvement, dysphagia suggesting esophageal compression, and superior vena cava syndrome all increase the likelihood of malignancy.

Rapid growth of a nodule, especially when accompanied

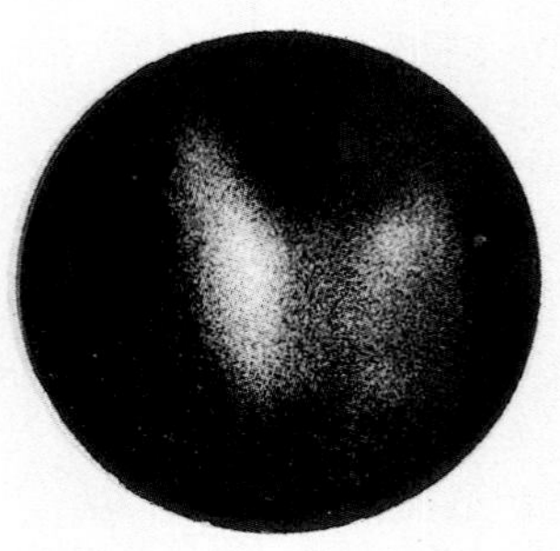

Figure 13. Thyroid carcinoma involving the left lobe.

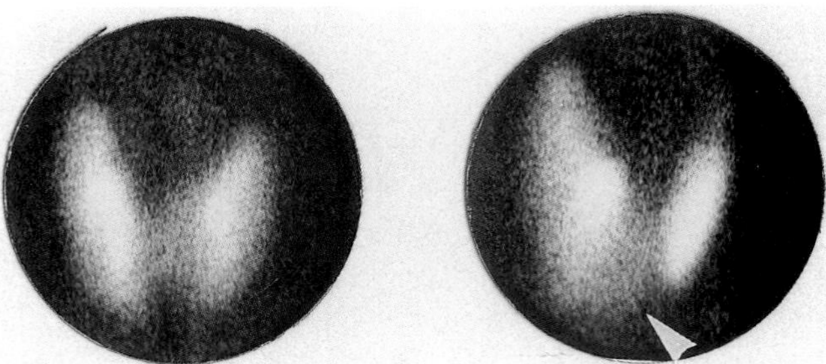

Figure 15. Warm nodule of the right lower thyroid lobe seen only in the right anterior oblique view (arrow).

by local tenderness, is usually caused by hemorrhage into a benign lesion. Hemorrhage can occur in malignant lesions, however, especially in nodules greater than 2.5 cm in diameter. Fixation of the thyroid to surrounding neck structures and the presence of enlarged cervical or laryngeal lymph nodes is an ominous sign of metastatic spread.

The probability of malignancy increases in nodules that fail to decrease (or that actually increase in size) after several months of thyroid suppression, and in multinodular glands in males under 40 who do not live in a goitrous area and who have not had a history of thyroiditis.

Figures 9, 10, 13, and 14 show several cold nodules imaged with ^{99m}Tc pertechnetate. Figure 15 shows a warm nodule in the right lower pole.

Cold nodules that have a low incidence of malignancy are included in the following:

1. Nodules that involve an entire lobe are most likely to be caused by subacute thyroiditis;
2. Large, soft nodules with smooth borders are most often benign cysts (Fig. 10);
3. Nodules associated with hyperthyroidism are most often benign cysts.[67,68]

The Use of Ultrasound and Fine-needle Biopsy. The use of high-resolution real-time ultrasound has greatly increased the ability to define thyroid morphology and to detect nodules too small to be imaged by radionuclide imaging. The range of ultrasonographic patterns in benign adenomatous and malignant nodules is too great to make this distinction.[69] The principle uses of ultrasound are (1) scanning to distinguish between cystic and solid solitary lesions that are nonfunctioning; (2) to detect multinodular disease when only one nodule is suspected clinically; (3) to characterize palpable thyroid nodules that are not visualized by radionuclide scanning; (4) guiding needle biopsy of nodules too small to palpate; and (5) screening patients with prior history of childhood neck irradiation. Ultrasound cannot, however, distinguish between benign and malignant nodules.

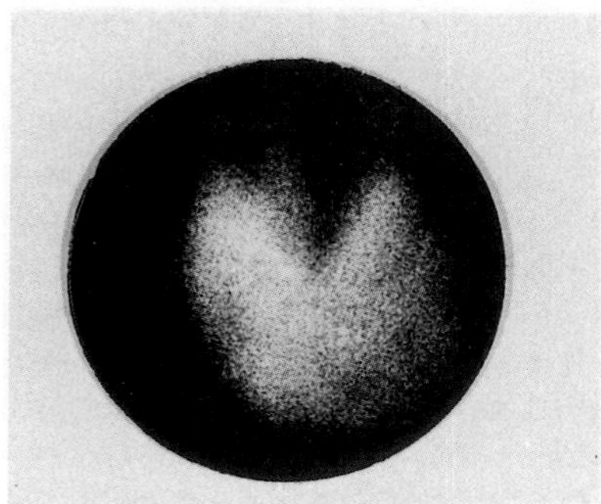

Figure 14. Multinodular goiter.

Fine-needle aspiration is of great value in the histological diagnosis of thyroid nodules. This technique is simple and almost free of complications. Seeding of the biopsy tract is not an important consideration.[70] An interested pathologist with extensive experience in thyroid cytology is essential to proper interpretation of needle aspirations. Crile (who generally favors a Vim-Silverman needle) believes that needle biopsy can eliminate 90% of thyroid nodule surgery.[71] However, in many large series, both false-positive and false-negative rates have been high. The latter is more serious and ranges from 2 to 37%.[72–74] When unsatisfactory smears and cores of normal thyroid tissue (occurring when the needle misses the lesion) are eliminated and categorization is made merely on the basis of malignant versus nonmalignant nodules, the false-negative rate appears to be about 5%. Because approximately 20% of solitary cold nodules are malignant, only about 1% of malignant lesions would thus be missed. If these nodules are carefully followed, the risk of delayed surgery appears to be small.

Hamburger et al.[75] point out that biopsies are not required for all nodules. For example, they do not biopsy autonomously functioning thyroid nodules, functional hyperplastic nodules, or purely cystic nodules that disappear after aspiration, because of the low probability of cancer occurring in these categories. On the other hand, they generally recommend surgery for young patients with a histological diagnosis of follicular adenoma, because approximately 10% of these nodules are found at surgery to harbor papillary, follicular, or Hürthle cell carcinoma.

Other Tests. Measurement of serum titers of antimicrosomal and antithyroglobulin antibodies sometimes helps to identify patients with a nodule caused by thyroiditis, but the presence of circulating antibodies is so frequent that it limits the value of this test. Measurement of serum calcitonin is useful. When serum calcitonin is elevated, the presence of medullary carcinoma or premalignant parafollicular hyperplasia must be suspected. Soft-tissue roentgenograms of the neck may be useful. Psammomatous calcifications within the nodule increase the likelihood of papillary carcinoma. Serum calcium measurements are essential in ruling out a parathyroid adenoma.

Several investigators have attempted to differentiate benign from malignant thyroid nodules by their uptake and retention of ^{201}Tl-chloride.[76–79] In general, these studies have shown that the majority of benign nodules either do not take up ^{201}Tl, or that there is rapid washout so that early, but not late (3-hour), images show activity within the nodules. Conversely, differentiated thyroid cancers tend to take up the tracer and exhibit prolonged washout, so that delayed images have a higher lesion-to-nonlesion ratio. The problem, of course, is that while sensitivity is generally high, specificity is not.

Figure 16 illustrates a practical approach to the management of solitary cold and hypofunctioning nodules.

HOT NODULES

Hyperfunctioning nodules may be multiple or solitary. Charkes et al. found that more than 50% of these nodules suppress with T_3.[80] In Plummer's disease, the hot nodules are autonomous (i.e., they do not suppress with T_3, but they do suppress surrounding normal tissue, which can be demonstrated by TSH stimulation) (Fig. 17).

About half of all autonomous functioning nodules occur in association with hyperthyroidism. In these patients, distinguishing Plummer's disease from Graves' disease is important because patients with the former generally require much more ^{131}I for adequate treatment and the incidence of ultimate hypothyroidism is considerably lower. In Graves' disease, the gland is usually larger and more uniform in size (Fig. 18). In Plummer's disease, the nodularity is usually prominent and often single, although multiple hot nodules are common. Even when several nodules are present, the scan demonstrates some suppressed tissue that responds to TSH stimulation, even though the increase may not be reflected by the uptake.[81]

The use of both ^{201}Th and ^{99m}Tc-MIBI have been suggested as an alternative to TSH stimulation in demonstrating suppressed thyroid tissue[39,40]; however, at this time the reliability of these agents has not been established.

MULTINODULAR GOITER

Multinodular goiters are common. Vander et al. found that approximately 3% of the population of Framingham, Massachusetts, a nongoitrous region, had multinodular goiters (in all, 4% had thyroid nodules).[82] The most common cause of multinodular goiter is dietary iodine deficiency, which is also known as *endemic goiter* or *colloid nodular goiter*.[83] Hypothyroidism is rare in these patients and, when it develops, the underlying process is presumed to be Hashimoto's disease. On the other hand, a large proportion of patients with multinodular goiter later develop hyperthyroidism.

The thyroid varies in size from a barely enlarged gland to one with great disfiguring masses, as found in endemic goitrous regions. The nodules also vary in size, from a few millimeters to several centimeters. The scintigraphic appearance is equally varied; it is characteristically variegated, with normally homogeneous appearance deformed by the presence of nodules (Fig. 19). The differential diagnosis includes Hashimoto's thyroiditis, multiple adenomas, and carcinoma.

The question of thyroid cancer in multinodular goiter has long been debated. If surgical specimens of multinodular goiter are examined, histological evidence of thyroid cancer is found in 4 to 17%.[84,85] Most studies that have followed large series of cases for several years, however, have found a low emergence of thyroid cancer.[82]

DeGroot and Stanbury advance a persuasive argument that there is minimal risk of thyroid carcinoma in multinodular goiter.[86] From U.S. Public Health Service Survey data, only 25 new thyroid tumors appear per year per 10^6 population. If the incidence of clinical nodularity is 4% or 40,000 per 10^6 population, an emergence of approximately 1600 new tumors per year would be expected. Thus, there appears to be a great discrepancy between the incidence of thyroid carcinoma in surgical specimens and the appearance of clinically significant thyroid carcinoma. Two reasons for this variance seem likely. One reason is selection; patients who are selected for surgery have a high clinical suspicion of malignancy. The second factor is that the histological diagnosis of thyroid carcinoma may not correlate well with clinical invasiveness. In summary, then, the suspicion of thyroid carcinoma in patients with multinodular goiter is much lower than in patients with solitary cold nodules.

With regard to the utility of thyroid scintigraphy in clinically apparent nontoxic multinodular goiter, most studies have found that scintigraphy seldom affects management of the disease.[87] An exception is in the identification of function in a substernal goiter. Ultrasound is more useful in characterizing gland consistency and changes in size with time.

THYROIDITIS

Thyroid inflammatory disease may be acute (viral or bacterial), subacute (of unknown cause), or chronic (the most common form). Often known as lymphocytic or Hashimoto's disease, chronic thyroiditis is thought to be an autoimmune disease. Histologically, Hashimoto's thyroiditis is characterized by diffuse lymphocytic infiltration, fibrosis, atrophy of

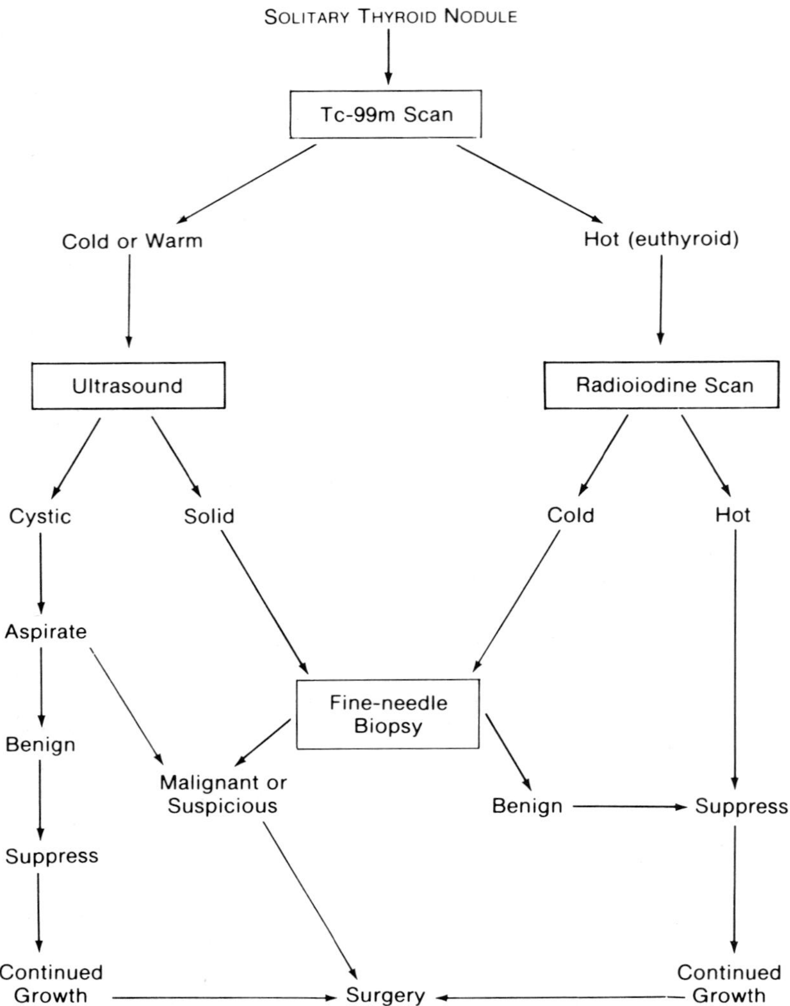

Figure 16. Disposition of solitary cold (or warm) nodules; the term "solitary nodule" includes a single dominant nodule within a multinodular goiter.

follicular cells, and an eosinophilic change in some of the follicular cells.[88]

The scintigraphic pattern is highly variable.[89] The most common pattern is that of an enlarged gland with diffusely increased uptake, a pattern very like that of Graves' disease. In other cases, the gland may be completely nonvisualized, may have only a faint outline of an enlarged gland or, more commonly, may show patchy irregularity consisting of cold areas interspersed with areas of hyperplasia (Fig. 20).

In acute and subacute thyroiditis, the uptake is usually low, although circulating levels of thyroid hormone may be elevated. Elevation of serum thyroglobulin during the initial stages is caused by inflammatory destruction of the gland

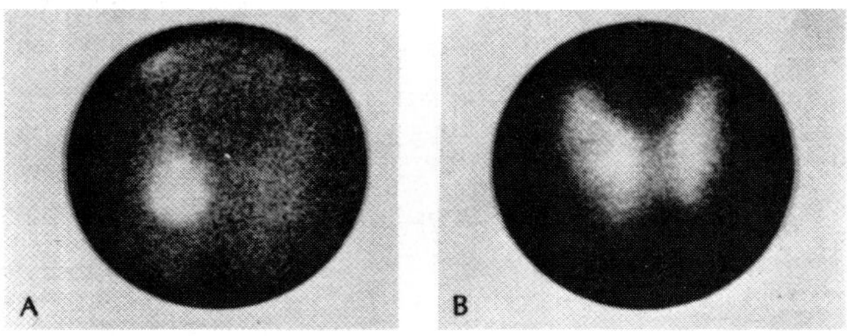

Figure 17. Nontoxic autonomous functioning nodules imaged with ^{99m}Tc-pertechnetate: (**A**), before TSH stimulation; (**B**), after TSH stimulation.

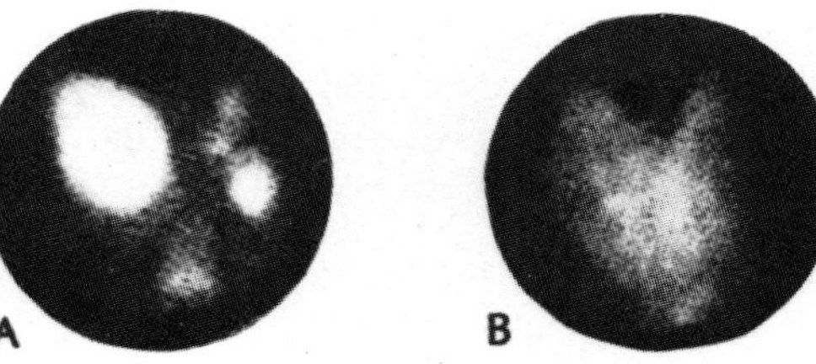

Figure 18. (**A**). Toxic nodular goiter (multiple). (**B**). Graves' disease with nodularity.

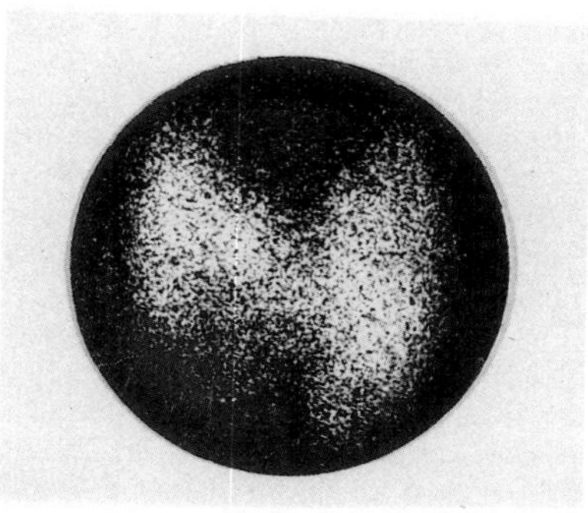

Figure 19. Large multinodular goiter imaged with ^{123}I.

with leakage of colloid—along with MIT, DIT, T_3, and T_4—into the serum. During the recovery phase, serum concentrations of these elements return to normal. During the acute phase, the patient may present with typical symptoms of thyrotoxicosis and with reduced thyroid uptake. The elevated serum thyroglobulin may help distinguish subacute thyroiditis from *thyrotoxicosis factitia*.

In Hashimoto's disease, the 24-hour uptake is usually lower, and radioiodine imaging may be unsatisfactory. Trapping may be increased, as evidenced by elevated 2-hour radioiodine or 20-min ^{99m}Tc-pertechnetate uptake. Levels of circulating hormone may be normal or low. These patients are seldom clinically hypothyroid, however, because they have a disproportionate production of T_3 in relation to T_4.

CONGENITAL HYPOTHYROIDISM

Most developed countries and most states in the United States have newborn screening programs for congenital hypothyroidism. Congenital *primary* hypothyroidism is associated with an elevated TSH level and reduced T_4. However, these findings fail to distinguish between transient hypothyroidism, ectopic or hypoplastic thyroid, athyrosis, dyshormonogenesis, and transient hyperthyrotopinemia.[90] A classification of congenital hypothyroidism suggested by Dussault[91] is shown in Table 8.

Table 8. Classification of Congenital Hypothyroidism

Permanent	Transient
Dysgenetic	Iatrogenic
Athyreotic	Exposure to iodine
Hypoplastic	Antithyroid drugs to the mother
Ectopic	Autoimmune
Eutopic	Blocking antibodies
Dyshormonogenesis	Iodine deficiency
Autoimmune	

Dyshormonogenesis and most cases of *transient* hypothyroidism are associated with goiter. Thyroid scintigraphy (with ^{123}I at 4–6 hours) is a highly useful means of identifying athyreosis, hypoplastic, and ectopic thyroid dysgenesis (Fig. 11). When these conditions are identified, lifelong thyroid replacement can be started immediately. Dyshormonogenesis and most cases of transient hypothyroidism are associated with congenital goiter. Therefore, scintigraphy should be reserved for those hypothyroid neonates without goiter. Pertechnetate should not be used for these studies because ectopia in areas of high blood background may be missed. Eutopic glands with depressed uptake are almost always visualized with ^{123}I scintigraphy.

An incorrect diagnosis of athyreosis has been reported in a neonate *without goiter* born of a mother with thyroxine-treated hypothyroidism and high circulating levels of *thyrotropin-binding inhibitory immunoglobulins* (TBII).[92] Routine measurements of autoimmune and blocking antibodies in the mothers of presumed athyreotic neonates will guard against this misdiagnosis.

HYPERTHYROIDISM AND THYROID CANCER

These conditions are discussed in detail in chapters 39 and 40.

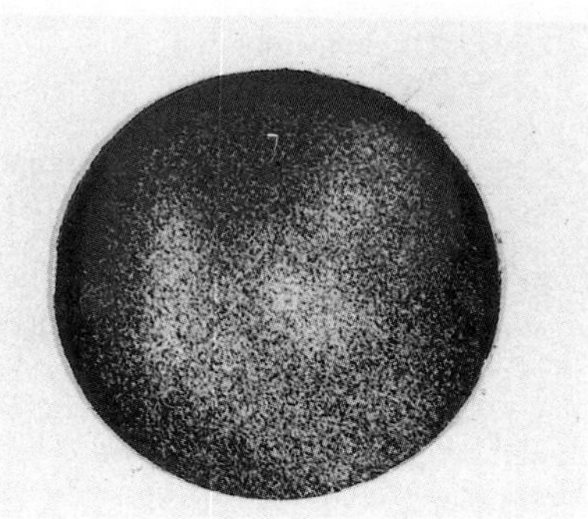

Figure 20. Hashimoto's thyroiditis (^{99m}Tc-pertechnetate).

REFERENCES

1. Hertz S, Roberts A, Evan RD: Radioactive iodine as an indicator in thyroid physiology. *Proc Soc Biol Med* 1938;38:510.
2. Robbins J, Rall JE, Gorden P: The thyroid and iodine metabolism, in Bondy PK, Rosenberg LE (ed): *Metabolic Control and Diseases*. Philadelphia, WB Saunders, 1980, pp 1325–1425.
3. Wideman JC, Powsner ER, Plato PS: Long-term clearance of iodine from the thyroid. *Int J Appl Radiat Isot* 1980;21:375.
4. Taurog A: Thyroid hormone synthesis and release. in Werner SG and Ingbar SH (eds): *The Thyroid*. New York, Harper & Row, 1978.
5. Kitchin FD, Weinstein IB: Genetic factors in thyroid disease. in Werner SC, Ingbar SH (eds): *The Thyroid*, 4th ed. New York, Harper & Row, 1978.

6. Oppenheimer JH, Schwartz HL, Surks ML: Propylthiouracil inhibits the conversion of L-thyroxine to L-triiodothyronine: An explanation of the antithyroxine effect of propylthiouracil and evidence supporting the concept that triiodothyronine is the active thyroid hormone. *J Clin Invest* 1972;51:2492.
7. Braverman LE, Ingbar SH, Sterling K: Conversion of thyroxine (T4) to triiodothyronine (T3) in athyreotic human subjects. *J Clin Invest* 1970;49:855.
8. Task Force on Short-lived Radionuclides for Medical Applications: Evaluation of diseases of the thyroid gland with the in vivo use of radionuclides. *J Nucl Med* 1978;19:107.
9. Loevinger R, Budinger TF, Watson EE: *MIRD Primer for Absorbed Dose Calculations.* Society of Nuclear Medicine, New York, 1988.
10. Shambaugh GE, et al: Disparate thyroid imaging. Combined studies with sodium pertechnetate Tc-99m and radioactive iodine. *JAMA,* 1974;228:866.
11. Lathrop KA, Harper PV: Biological behavior of ^{99m}Tc and ^{99m}Tc-pertechnetate ion. *Progr Nucl Med* 1972;1:145.
12. Welch MF, Adatepe M, Potchen EJ: An analysis of technetium kinetics. The effect of perchlorate and iodide pretreatment. *Int J Appl Radiat Isot* 1969;20:437.
13. Stadalnick RC: Thyroid localization of Ga-67 citrate. *Semin Nucl Med* 1985;15:224.
14. Hisada K et al.: Clinical evaluation of tumor imaging with 201Tl-chloride. *Radiology* 1978;129:497.
15. Tonami N, Hisada K: ^{201}Tl scintigraphy in postoperative detection of thyroid cancer: A comparative study with ^{131}I. *Radiology* 1980;136:461.
16. Ohta H, Yamamoto K, Endo K, et al.: A new imaging agent for medullary carcinoma of the thyroid. *J Nucl Med* 1984;25:323.
17. Clarke SEM, Lazarus CR, Wraight P, et al.: Pentavalent (99mTc) DMSA, (131I)MIBG, and (99mTc) MDP—An evaluation of three imaging techniques in patients with medullary carcinoma of the thyroid. *J Nucl Med* 1988;29:33.
18. Rosenberg IN: Newer methods for evaluating thyroid nodules. *N Engl J Med* 1972;287:1197.
19. Koutras DA, Pandos PG, Sfontaouris J, et al.: Thyroid scanning with gallium-67 and cesium-131. *J Nucl Med* 1976;17:268.
20. Mori T, Hamamoto K, Onoyama Y, et al.: Tumor imaging after administration of ^{99m}Tc-labeled bleomycin. *J Nucl Med* 1975;16:414.
21. Wellman HN, Siddiqui AR, Burt RW, et al.: Simultaneous I-123 and "early" Tc-99m EHDP scintiimaging in the differential diagnosis of solid vs. cystic thyroid nodules. *J Nucl Med* 1978;19:741.
22. Prince JR, et al.: An evaluation of the 24-hour RAIU test performed with an Anger camera and a pinhole collimator. *Clin Nucl Med* 1979;4:471.
23. Wasserman HJ, Muller C, Klopper JF: The elimination of errors caused by prior technetium-99m scintigraphy on iodine-131 thyroid uptake measurements. *S Afr Med J* 1987;72:496.
24. Grayson RR: Factors influencing I-131 thyroidal uptake. *Am J Med* 1960;28:397.
25. Laurie AJ, Lyon SG, Lasser EC: Contrast material iodides: potential effects on radioactive iodine thyroid uptake. *J Nucl Med* 1992;33:237.
26. Sedvall G, Jonsson B, Petterson U: Evidence of an altered thyroid function in man during treatment with lithium carbonate. *Acta Psychiatr Scand* 1969;297(suppl):59.
27. Chervu S, Chervu LR, Goodwin PN, Blaufox MD: Thyroid uptake measurements with I-123: Problems and pitfalls. *J Nucl Med* 1982;23:667.
28. Maisey MN, et al.: Validation of a rapid computerized method of measuring Tc-99m pertechnetate uptake for routine assessment of thyroid structure and function. *J Clin Endocrinol Metab* 1973;36:317.
29. Schneider PB: Simple, rapid thyroid function testing with ^{99m}Tc-pertechnetate thyroid uptake ratio and neck/thigh ratio. *Am J Roentgenol* 1979;132:249.
30. Selby JB, Buse MG, Gooneratne NS, et al.: The anger camera and the pertechnetate ion in the routine evaluation of thyroid uptake imaging. *Clin Nucl Med* 1979;4:233.
31. Ashkar FS, Smith EM: The dynamic thyroid study. *JAMA* 1971;217:441.
32. Alexander WD, et al.: Quantitative studies of iodine metabolism in thyroid diseases. Q J Med 1962;31:281.
33. Beckers C, et al.: Endemic goiter in Pedregoso (Chile). 2: Dynamic studies on iodine metabolism. *Acta Endocrinol (Kbh)* 1967;54:591.
34. Alexander WD, et al.: Development of thyroidal suppression by triiodothyronine (T3) during 6 month treatment of thyrotoxicosis with antithyroid drugs. *J Clin Endocrinol Metab* 1967;27:1682.
35. Wayne ES, Koutras DA, Alexander WD: *Clinical Aspects of Iodine Metabolism.* Philadelphia, F.A. Davis, 1964.
36. Toft AD: Thyrotropin: Assay, secretory physiology, and testing of regulation. in Braverman LE, Utiger RD (eds): *Werner and Ingbar's The Thyroid,* 6th ed. Philadelphia, J.B. Lippincott, 1991, p 287.
37. Snyder PJ, Jacobs LS, Rabello MM, et al.: Diagnostic value of thyrotropin-releasing hormone in pituitary and hypothalamic diseases: assessment of thyrotrophin and prolactin secretion in 100 patients. *Ann Intern Med* 1974;81:751.
38. Lamberg B-A, Helenius T, Leiwendahl K: Assessment of thyroxine suppression in thyroid carcinoma patients with sensitive immunoradiometric assay. *Clin Endocrinol (Oxf)* 1986;25:259.
39. Corstens F, Huysmans D, Kloppenberg P: Thallium-201 scintigraphy of the suppressed thyroid: an alternative for iodine-123 scanning after TSH. *J Nucl Med* 1988;29:1360.
40. Ramanathan P, Patel RB, Subrahmanyaml N, et al.: Visualization of suppressed thyroid tissue by technetium-99m-tertiary butyl isonitrile: an alternative to post-TSH stimulation scanning. *J Nucl Med* 1990;31:1163.
41. Atkins HL, Klopper JF, Lambrecht RM, Wolf AP: A comparison of technetium-99m and iodine-123 for thyroid imaging. *Am J Roentgenol* 1973;117:195.
42. Prince JR, Zubi SM, Haag BL: Thyroid imaging with iodine-125 and technetium-99m. *Eur J Nucl Med* 1979;4:37.
43. Shapiro B, Britton K, Fountos A, et al.: A multiobserver comparison of $99mTcO_4$ and 123I thyroid imaging. *Eur J Nucl Med* 1981;6:135.
44. Arnold JE, Pinsky S: Comparison of 99mTc and 123I for thyroid imaging. *J Nucl Med* 1976;17:261.
45. Dige-Petersen H, Kroon S, Vadstrup S, et al.: A comparison of 99mTc and 123I scintigraphy in nodular thyroid disorders. *Eur J Nucl Med* 1978;3:1.
46. Ryo UY, Vaidya PV, Schneider AB, et al.: Thyroid imaging agents: a comparison of I-123 and Tc-99m pertechnetate. *Radiology* 1983;148:819.
47. Kusic Z, Becker DV, Saenger EL, et al.: Comparison of Technetium-99m and Iodine-123 imaging of thyroid nodules: Correlation with pathologic findings. *J Nucl Med* 1990;31:393.
48. Steinberg M, Cavalieri RR, Choy SH: Uptake of technetium-99m pertechnetate in a primary thyroid carcinoma: need for caution in evaluating nodules. *J Clin Endocrinol* 1970;31:81.
49. Shambaugh GE, Quinn JL, Oyasu R, Freinkel N: Disparate thyroid imaging. Combined studies with sodium pertechnetate Tc-99m and radioactive iodine. *JAMA* 1974;228:866.
50. O'Connor MK, Cullen MJ, Malone JF: A kinetic study of 131I iodide and 99mTc pertechnetate in thyroid carcinomas

to explain a scan discrepancy: case report. *J Nucl Med* 1977;18:796.

51. Tennvall J, Cederquist E, Moller T, et al: Preoperative scintigraphy with correlation to cytology and histopathology in carcinoma of the thyroid. *Acta Radiol Oncol* 1983;22:183.
52. Frey P, Townsend D, Flattet A, et al.: Tomographic imaging of the human thyroid using 124I. *J Clin Endocrinol Metab* 1986;63:918.
53. Chen JJS, LaFrance ND, Rippin R, et al.: Iodin-123 SPECT of the thyroid in multinodular goiter. *J Nucl Med* 1988;29:110.
54. Blum M, Reede DL, Seltzer TF, et al.: Computerized axial tomography in the diagnosis and management of thyroid and parathyroid disorders. *Am J Med Sci* 1984;187:34.
55. Sandler MP, Patton JA, Sacks GA, et al.: Evaluation of intrathoracic goiter with I-123 scintigraphy and nuclear magnetic resonance imaging. *J Nucl Med* 1984;25:874.
56. Levy HA, Sziklas JJ, Rosenberg RJ, Spencer RP: Incidence of a pyramidal lobe on thyroid scans. *Clin Nucl Med* 1982;7:560.
57. duCret RP, Choi RE, Roe SJ, et al.: Improved prediction of thyroid lobar mass from parameters obtained by routine thyroid scintigraphy. *Clin Nucl Med* 1987;12:436.
58. Hamburger JI, Hamburger SW: Thyroidal hemiagensis. *Arch Surg* 1970;100:319.
59. Melnick JC, Stemkowski PE: Thyroid hemiagenesis (hockey stick sign): a review of the world literature and a report of four cases. *J Clin Endocrinol Metab* 1981;52:247.
60. Schechner C, Kraiem Z, Zuckerman E, Dickstein KG: Toxic Graves' disease with thyroid hemiagenesis: diagnosis using thyroid-stimulating immunoglobulin measurements. *Thyroid* 1992;2:133.
61. Khatri VP, Espinosa MH, Harada WA: Papillary adenocarcinoma in thyroid hemiagenesis. *Head Neck* 1992;14:312.
62. Enge LA: Functional and growth characteristics of struma ovarii. *Am J Obstet Gynecol* 1940;40:738.
63. Pelmutter M, Mufson M: Inhibition of a cervical thyroid gland by a functioning struma ovarii. *J Clin Endocrinol* 1951;11:621.
64. Rieser GD, Ober KP, Cowan RJ, Cordell AR: Radioiodide imaging of struma cordis. *Pediatrics* 1987;80:745.
65. Mortensen JD, Woolner LB, Bennet WA: Gross and microscopic findings in clinically normal thyroid glands. *J Clin Endocrinol Metab* 1955;15:1270.
66. Atkins HL: The thyroid, in Freeman LM, Johnson PM (eds): *Clinical Scintillation Imaging*. 2nd ed. New York, Grune and Stratton, 1975.
67. Molnar GD, et al.: On the hyperfunctioning solitary thyroid nodule. *Mayo Clin Proc* 1965;40:665.
68. Dische S: The radioiosotope scan applied to the detection of carcinoma in thyroid swellings. *Cancer* 1964;17:473.
69. Simeone JF, Daniels GH, Mueller PR, et al.: High resolution real-time sonography of the thyroid. *Radiology* 1982;145:431.
70. Frable WJ: *Thin-needle Aspiration Biopsy.* Philadelphia, W.B. Saunders, 1983, p 152.
71. Crile G, Hawk WA: Aspiration biopsy of thyroid nodules. *Surg Gynecol Obstet* 1973;136:241.
72. Tennvall J, Cederquist E, Moller R, et al.: Preoperative scintigraphy with correlation to cytology and histopathology in carcinoma of the thyroid. *Acta Radiol Oncol* 1983;22:183.
73. Russ JE, Scanlon EF, Christ MA: Aspiration cytology of head and neck masses. *Am J Surg* 1978;136:342.
74. Friedman M, Shimaoka K, Getaz P: Needle aspiration of 310 thyroid lesions. *Acta Cytol* 1979;23:194.
75. Hamburger JI, Kaplan MM, Husain M: Diagnosis of thyroid nodules by needle biopsy, in Braverman LE, Utiger RD (eds): *Werner and Ingbar's The Thyroid,* 6th ed. Philadelphia, J.B. Lippincott, 1991, p 544.
76. Tonami N, Bunko H, Michigishi T, et al.: Clinical application of Tl scintigraphy in patients with cold thyroid nodules. *Clin Nucl Med* 1978;3:217.
77. Ochi H, Sawa H, Fukuda T, et al.: Thallium-201-chloride thyroid scintigraphy to evaluate benign and/or malignant nodules. *Cancer* 1982;50:236.
78. Hardoff R, Baron E, Sheinfeld M: Early and late lesion-to-non-lesion ratio of thallium-201-chloride uptake in the evaluation of "cold" thyroid nodules. *J Nucl Med* 1991; 32:1873.
79. el-Desouki M: Tl-201 thyroid imaging in differentiating benign from malignant thyroid nodules. *Clin Nucl Med* 1991;16:425.
80. Charkes ND, Cantor RE, Goluboff B: A three day, double isotope, 1-triiodothyronine suppression test of thyroid anatomy. *J Nucl Med* 1967;8:627.
81. Charkes ND: Scintigraphic evaluation of nodular goiter. *Semin Nucl Med* 1971;1:316.
82. Vander JB, Gaston EA, Dawber TR: The significance of nontoxic thyroid nodules. Final report of a 15-year study of the incidence of thyroid malignancy. *Ann Intern Med* 1968;69:537.
83. Taylor S: Sporadic nontoxic goiter, in Werner SC, Ingbar SH (eds): *The Thyroid,* 4th ed. New York, Harper & Row, 1978.
84. Tellem M, Stahl T, Meranze DR: Carcinoma of the thyroid gland: An explanation for its varying incidence in surgically removed nodular thyroids. *Cancer* 1961;14:67.
85. Veith FJ, et al.: The nodular thyroid gland and cancer: A practical approach to the problem. *N Engl J Med* 1964;270:431.
86. DeGroot LJ, Stanbury JB: *The Thyroid and Its Diseases,* 4th ed. New York, John Wiley & Sons, 1975.
87. Tindall H, Griffiths AP, Penn ND: Is the current use of thyroid scintigraphy rational? *Postgrad Med J* 1987;63(744):869.
88. Volp R: Autoimmune thyroiditis, in Braverman LE, Utiger RD (eds): *Werner and Ingbar's The Thyroid,* 6th ed. Philadelphia, J.B. Lippincott, 1991.
89. Ramtoola S, Maissey MN, Clarke SE, Fogelman I: The thyroid scan in Hashimoto's thyroiditis: the great mimic. *Nucl Med Commun* 1988;9:639.
90. Schoen EJ, dos Remedios LV, Backstrom M: Heterogeneity of congenital primary hypothyroidism: the importance of thyroid scintigraphy. *J Perinat Med* 1987;15:137.
91. Dussault JH: Congenital hypothyroidism, in Braverman LE, Utiger RD (eds): *Werner and Ingbar's The Thyroid.* Philadelphia, J.B. Lippincott, 1991.
92. Connors MH, Styne DM: Transient neonatal 'athyreosis' resulting from thyrotropin-binding inhibitory immunoglobulins. *Pediatrics* 1986;78:287.

21 Parathyroid Scintigraphy

Clara C. Chen

The parathyroid glands play a key role in the maintenance of calcium homeostasis through the production of parathyroid hormone (PTH), a 34-amino acid polypeptide with an active N-terminal end.[1] Abnormal parathyroid function is reflected in under- or over-production and secretion of this hormone. Hypoparathyroidism occurs infrequently except in its iatrogenic forms, but hyperparathyroidism is a common disorder, particularly among the elderly.

Hyperparathyroidism occurs both as a primary disorder and secondarily in association with other disease states, including chronic renal insufficiency, malabsorption, and Vitamin D deficiency. In most of these patients, surgical intervention with removal of the abnormal parathyroid tissue offers the only real cure. Preoperative parathyroid imaging plays an important role in ensuring surgical success and decreasing morbidity.

PRIMARY HYPERPARATHYROIDISM

Primary hyperparathyroidism has an approximate incidence of 28 cases per 100,000 persons per year.[2] The disease is most commonly seen in females and in the elderly, and is a component of the Multiple Endocrine Neoplasias (MEN) Types I and IIa. Approximately 82% of cases are due to the presence of a solitary hyperfunctioning parathyroid adenoma, 15% to multiple gland hyperplasia (sporadic, familial MEN-related, familial non-MEN-related), and 3% to parathyroid carcinoma.[1] Almost all cases of MEN-1 (Wermer's syndrome) and approximately 50% of cases of MEN-IIa (Sipple's syndrome) are associated with diffuse parathyroid hyperplasia and hyperparathyroidism.[3]

The diagnosis of primary hyperparathyroidism is based upon findings of persistently elevated serum calcium and PTH levels. Symptomatic patients often present with a variety of non-specific complaints, such as weakness and fatigue, whereas more serious complications include the development of significant hypercalcemia, renal calculi, and bone disease secondary to calcium resorption. Surgery is the treatment of choice in these patients. In recent years, however, hyperparathyroidism has been diagnosed with increasing frequency in asymptomatic patients, in whom hypercalcemia is incidentally discovered on routine lab tests.[2] It is thought that many of these individuals can be safely managed with periodic follow-up.[4–6] Indications for surgery in this group include the development of significant hypercalcemia, renal, or bone disease, even if the patient remains "asymptomatic." Surgery must also be considered in patients who request it, those who are unlikely to receive adequate follow-up, those with coexisting conditions that could complicate medical management, and younger patients (<50 years old), as the consequences of long-term untreated hyperparathyroidism are unknown.[6]

Parathyroid Surgery

In patients undergoing an initial operation for primary hyperparathyroidism, experienced surgeons generally achieve a 95% or greater surgical success rate without any preoperative localization studies.[7,8] Consequently, there is much controversy as to the need for and cost-effectiveness of preoperative localization in most of these patients. One proposed justification involves performing scintigraphy-directed unilateral surgery,[9–11] as opposed to the conventional surgical strategy of identifying and biopsying all 4 glands[12] to ensure that multiple-gland disease is not overlooked. This approach has been shown in a limited number of studies to decrease mean operative time by approximately 25 minutes without significantly effecting surgical success,[9,10] but is controversial and not widely adopted.

In contrast, the usefulness of preoperative localization studies in reoperative surgery is well recognized. Approximately 30% of patients presenting for reoperative surgery will eventually undergo 2 or more additional operations before a cure is achieved.[13,14] Reoperative surgery is successful in 62%[15] to 90%[13] of cases without extensive preoperative imaging. Not only are problems secondary to scarring encountered, but ectopic glands account for 24 to 39% of missed lesions in this patient population, while they account for only 4 to 8% of glands in those undergoing initial surgery.[8,16] Multiglandular disease occurs in approximately 37%[14] of cases compared to 15% in the general population with primary hyperparathyroidism.[1] Reoperative surgery is also associated with a ten-fold increase in morbidity compared to initial operations,[17] primarily recurrent laryngeal nerve injury and permanent hypoparathyroidism. Preoperative localization can be useful in decreasing these complications by directing the surgeon's attention to a specific area, reducing the amount of surgical exploration required, and decreasing operative time.

Parathyroid Anatomy

The problems encountered with parathyroid localization are closely related to the anatomy and embryology of these glands. Usually, the two superior and two inferior glands are located near the upper and lower poles of the thyroid gland. The number of glands range from 1 to 12; approximately 2 to 6.5% of the population have more than four glands.[1] On average, each parathyroid gland measures 5 × 3 × 1 mm and weighs approximately 35 to 40 mg.[18] It is this small size and flat shape that account for the nonvisualization of normal parathyroid glands on most imaging studies.

The superior parathyroid glands are derived embryologically from the fourth branchial cleft pouch, as is the thyroid gland. The inferior parathyroid glands are derived from the third branchial cleft pouch, as is the thymus gland. During development, these structures migrate caudally, with the embryonic parathyroid and thyroid glands normally coming to rest in the anterior neck, and the thymus continuing into the chest. Thus, ectopic parathyroid glands are found anywhere along this migration route, from the angle of the jaw (undescended) to the level of the pericardium. Autopsy series of patients without parathyroid disease have confirmed this variability in location. In a study of 156 patients with 624 individual glands, Wang[18] found 77% of superior glands located posteriorly at the crico-thyroidal junction, 22% behind the upper poles of the thyroid, and 1% located in a retropharyngeal or retroesophageal position. An even greater variability was noted in the positions of the inferior glands, 42% of which were found near the lower poles of the thyroid, 39% in the lower neck at the thoracic inlet, 15% lateral to the lower poles of the thyroid, and 4% in the mediastinum associated with the thymus gland or elsewhere.

Another factor that contributes to the problem of parathyroid localization is that these glands are often mobile. In particular, heavy, enlarged glands may migrate from their original positions as they hypertrophy, often descending posteriorly (superior glands) or anteriorly (inferior glands) into the mediastinum.[19] Tracing the blood supply of these ectopic glands at the time of surgery allows identification as to their embryological origin.

Radionuclide Imaging

The ideal radiopharmaceutical for parathyroid imaging should not only have favorable imaging characteristics and dosimetry, but also high sensitivity and specificity for parathyroid tissue. Unfortunately, a parathyroid-specific agent has yet to be found. The first radiopharmaceutical used for parathyroid localization in humans was ^{75}Se-selenomethionine, sometimes combined with thyroid suppression using exogenous thyroid hormone. This met with limited success and delivered a relatively high radiation burden.[20,21] Other agents used in the past have included ^{131}Cs-chloride,[22,23] ^{67}Ga-citrate,[24] and ^{99m}Tc-pertechnetate ($^{99m}TcO_4$).[25–27] However, it was not until 1981, when Ferlin et al.[23] described the use of a ^{99m}Tc-pertechnetate/^{201}Tl-chloride (Tc/Tl) subtraction method, that radionuclide localization of parathyroid abnormalities became widely accepted. Most recently, ^{99m}Tc-sestamibi has shown promise as an alternative to ^{201}Tl.[28,29]

SUBTRACTION SCANNING

Because of their location and the lack of a parathyroid-specific imaging agent, subtraction scanning is an important technique in the scintigraphic localization of parathyroid abnormalities. In brief, subtraction allows one to differentiate activity in a parathyroid abnormality from that in adjacent or superimposed thyroid tissue. Normal parathyroid glands are generally too small to be detected by these techniques, while lesions distant from the thyroid can be appreciated without subtraction.[30,31] Additionally, subtraction scanning of the neck is supplemented by ^{201}Tl or ^{99m}Tc-sestamibi imaging of the chest in these studies, for detection of mediastinal abnormalities (Fig. 1). If parathyroid autotransplants are present, these, too, can also be imaged.[32–34]

TC/TL SUBTRACTION SCANNING

To date, most reports of parathyroid scintigraphy have focused on the Tc/Tl subtraction scanning method. With this method, $^{99m}TcO_4$, an iodide analog, is concentrated by the thyroid gland, whereas ^{201}Tl, a potassium ion analog, is taken up by thyroid and parathyroid tissue.[35] When the $^{99m}TcO_4$ image (thyroid gland) is "subtracted" from the ^{201}Tl (thyroid + parathyroid) image, areas of excess ^{201}Tl accumulation that would be consistent with parathyroid tissue are revealed (Fig. 2). Similarly, ^{123}I/^{99m}Tc-sestamibi subtraction can be performed using sestamibi in place of ^{201}Tl and ^{123}I in place of $^{99m}TcO_4$ for thyroid imaging and subtraction (Fig. 3).

Over the years, numerous variations of the Tc/Tl subtraction scanning procedure have been developed. Differences in techniques include injection of ^{201}Tl versus ^{99m}Tc first,[36] sequential versus simultaneous image acquisition,[37] use of ^{123}I vs. $^{99m}TcO_4$ for thyroid imaging,[30] color vs. gray-scale analysis,[38] and use of different motion correction techniques.[39–41] At NIH, the Tc/Tl method used is a dual-isotope simultaneous acquisition procedure that minimizes motion artifacts.[42] The patient is positioned under the scintillation camera using a pinhole collimator with neck extended, as for a thyroid scan. Approximately 15 minutes following injection of 2 mCi (74 MBq) $^{99m}TcO_4$, an image that includes the submandibular glands and lower neck is obtained. A marker view of the thyroid cartilage and sternal notch is sometimes obtained to define regional landmarks. Next, a 28-minute (4 min./frame) dynamic acquisition is begun, during which counts are simultaneously collected in both the ^{99m}Tc (140 keV +/− 10%) and ^{201}Tl (70 keV +/− 10%) windows. 3 mCi (111 MBq) ^{201}Tl is injected 5 minutes into this acquisition program. The first pair of simultaneous images thus provides a ^{99m}Tc image of the thyroid and ^{99m}Tc downscatter information. Processing involves correction for ^{99m}Tc

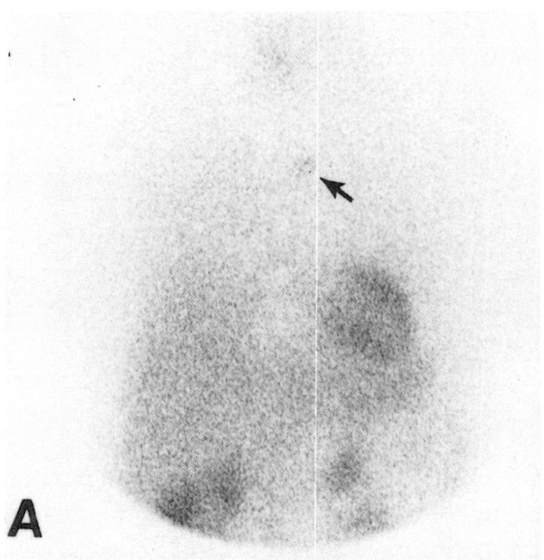

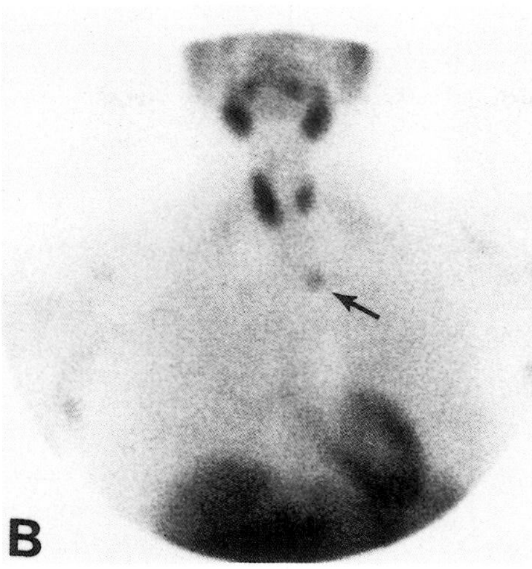

Figure 1. Thallium **(A)** and sestamibi **(B)** images of the chest revealing mediastinal parathyroid lesions (arrows) in 2 patients presenting for reoperative parathyroid surgery.

down-scatter into the ^{201}Tl window, normalization, motion correction, and subtraction. Additionally, a ^{201}Tl image of the chest is obtained at the end of the study. The ^{201}Tl injection is performed via a temporary, indwelling peripheral line to prevent patient motion caused by a needlestick. This line is inserted in the foot whenever possible, to avoid injection artifacts due to ^{201}Tl in the vasculature of the upper chest and neck (Fig. 4). A 10-cc saline flush is also used after injection.

Because the success of subtraction scanning requires thyroid uptake of $^{99m}TcO_4$, each patient's history with respect to thyroid disease, prior surgery, or thyroid suppression (e.g., by exogenous thyroid hormone or other medications, recent IV contrast, etc.) should be obtained prior to all studies. In patients who have undergone total thyroid ablation for thyroid cancer, the $^{99m}Tc0_4$ portion of the study can be eliminated. However, in other situations where the full extent of thyroid resection or suppression is unknown, $^{99m}Tc0_4$ scanning should usually be performed. In many cases, patients have only undergone subtotal thyroidectomies or are only partially suppressed, and thus will continue to demonstrate residual thyroid activity.

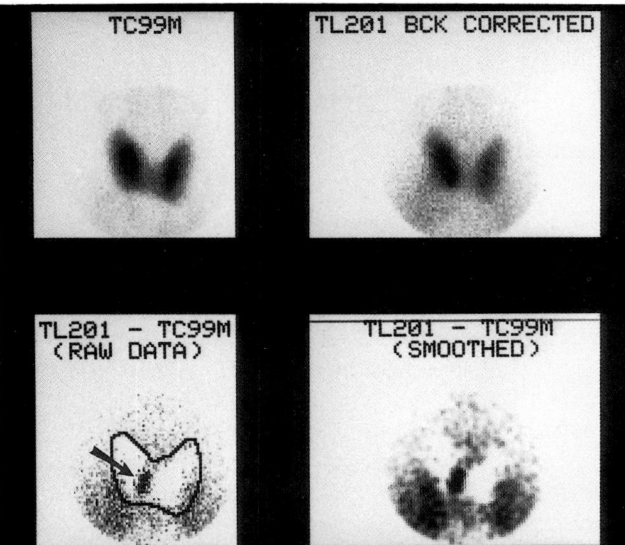

Figure 2. Tc/Tl subtraction study in a reoperative patient with recurrent hypercalcemia. After background correction and normalization of counts within the thyroid region of interest, the Tc image (upper left) is subtracted from Tl image (upper right), revealing excess Tl activity at the level of the right lower lobe of the thyroid (arrow).

Reported sensitivities for Tc/Tl scanning range widely, from 25 to 100% as tabulated by Hauty et al.[43] and Sandrock et al.[44] Many factors account for this variability, including differences in imaging protocols, patient populations, scoring systems, skill of the surgeons, and histological criteria used. Patient population variables include factors such as primary vs. secondary hyperparathyroidism, initial vs. reoperative surgery, and whether or not patients with concomitant thyroid pathology are included. The classification of lesions as true-positive, false-positive, etc., is also performed in different ways; some choosing to accept localization to predetermined zones in the neck as adequate,[45] while most require more exact localization.

In calculating the sensitivity of a parathyroid localization procedure, direct communication with the surgeon is recommended to determine the exact position of a lesion found at surgery, as reliance on the operative note alone may lead to inaccuracies. For instance, an adenoma found in the lower neck may represent a superior gland that has migrated inferiorly. If this lesion is identified in the operative note as a superior gland, one might falsely conclude that a localization study which demonstrated an abnormality in an inferior position was inaccurate, unless the actual position of the

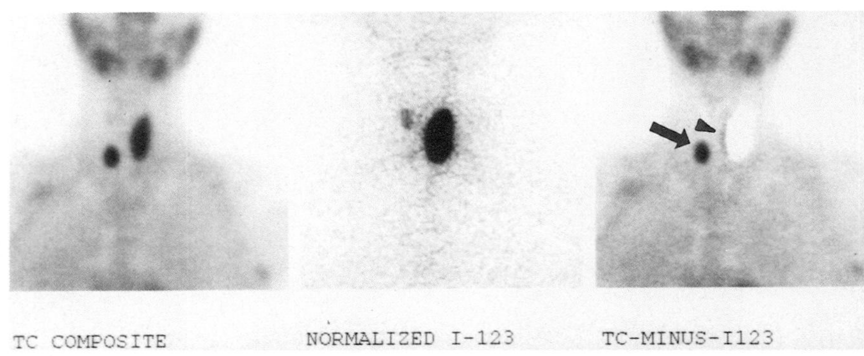

Figure 3. $^{123}I/^{99m}Tc$-sestamibi subtraction study in a patient with 2 prior neck explorations; most of the right lobe of the thyroid has been removed. After motion correction and normalization of counts within the thyroid region of interest, the ^{123}I image (middle) is subtracted from the ^{99m}Tc-sestamibi image (left), revealing excess sestamibi uptake at the level of the missing right lower lobe of the thyroid (arrow). A motion artifact is seen along the medial edge of the left lobe of the thyroid on the subtraction image (arrowhead) despite attempted motion correction.

lesion was also described.[46,47] An example is provided in Figure 5.

As for specificities, these are difficult to calculate for parathyroid imaging studies because the number of "true negative" foci is unknown. First, over 6% of the population has either less than or more than the norm of 4 parathyroid glands.[1] Second, in reoperative patients, the number of glands that have previously been removed is often unknown. Last, despite the high surgical success rate of >95% at first operations, the reciprocal "failure" rate indicates that approximately 5% of lesions are missed, and that not all areas deemed "negative" by the gold standard of surgical exploration are truly free of abnormalities. This is an even greater problem with reoperative surgery, in which the success rate is often lower.

One of the major factors in determining the success or failure of most non-invasive imaging modalities is the size of the lesion in question—large masses are more easily detected than small ones. With Tc/Tl, lesions >1 g are generally detected with a >90% sensitivity, while those <0.5 g are detected <50% of the time.[9,38,48,49] However, localization of lesions as small as 60 mg has been reported,[38,50] whereas adenomas as large as 5 g have been missed.[39,51]

In almost all reported series of Tc/Tl imaging, detection rates for adenomas are higher than those for hyperplasias, as reviewed by Hauty et al.[43] and Sandrock et al.[44] Size alone is often enough to explain these differences, however, as solitary adenomas are usually larger than the individual glands seen in multiple gland hyperplasia.[38,52,53] (The pathologic distinction between adenoma and hyperplasia is difficult, both appearing hypercellular with variable numbers of chief, transitional, and oxyphil cells.[1] At NIH, solitary lesions are classified as adenomas, whereas lesions in multiglandular disease are classified as "hyperplasias.") Measurements of mean % uptake of ^{201}Tl injected dose (ID)/gram of tissue have shown no significant differences between adenomas and hyperplasias.[49] Recently, scintigraphic detectability using Tc/Tl has been linked to the presence of mitochondria-rich oxyphil cells, but no significant differences between adenomas and hyperplasias were found.[54] Neverthe-

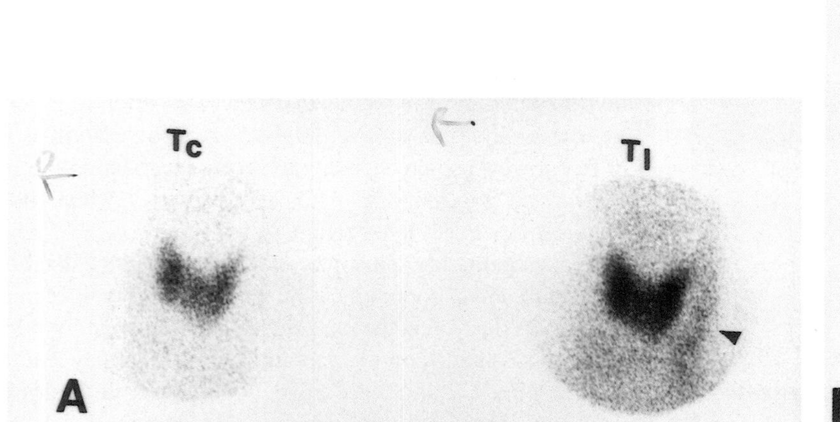

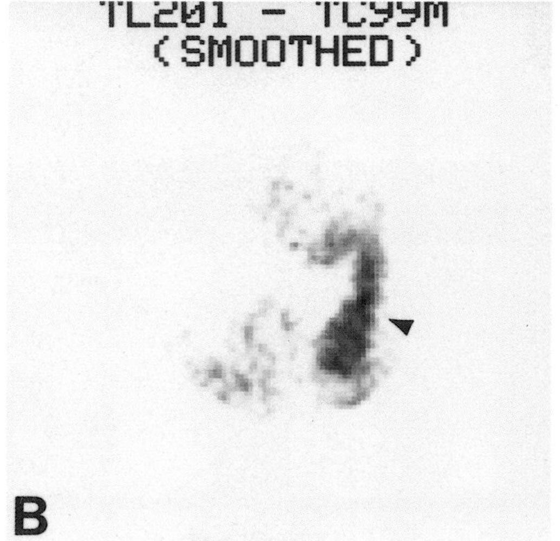

Figure 4. Tc/Tl subtraction study demonstrating a Tl injection artifact (arrowheads). Subtraction image **(B)** also shows excess Tl uptake at the level of the left upper pole of the thyroid (arrow), where a 2.5 × 2 × 1.5 cm parathyroid adenoma was found at surgery.

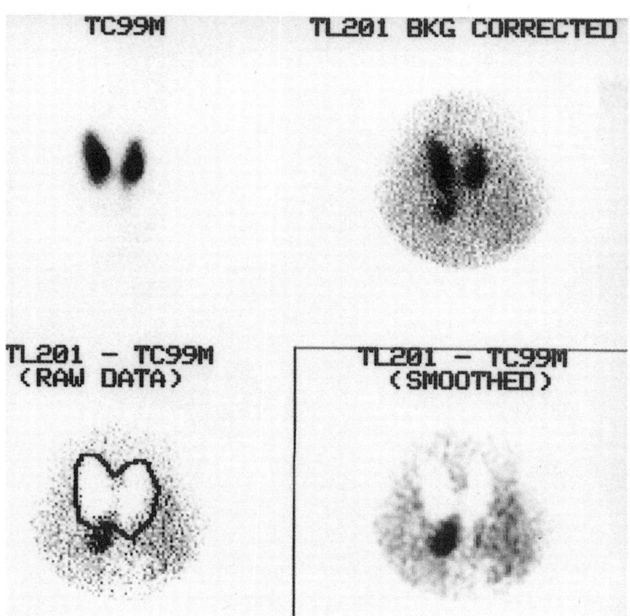

Figure 5. Tc/Tl subtraction study in a reoperative patient. Obvious excess Tl uptake is seen below the right lobe of the thyroid. At surgery, a 4 × 3.5 × 3 cm right superior parathyroid gland adenoma was found in the right tracheoesophageal groove.

less, pathophysiological differences between the 2 types of lesions that may account for differences in Tc/Tl detection rates cannot be ruled out.

^{99m}TC-SESTAMIBI IMAGING

Since its introduction as a myocardial perfusion agent, ^{99m}Tc-sestamibi has been successfully used in place of ^{201}Tl for parathyroid imaging.[28,29,55–57] This agent can be used in conjunction with ^{123}I Na for thyroid subtraction[29,55–58] or as a single agent in the "double-phase technique",[59,60] and has several advantages over ^{201}Tl. These include superior imaging characteristics, improved dosimetry, and a better target-to-background (parathyroid:thyroid) ratio at different time points.

For ^{123}I/sestamibi subtraction scanning, reported sensitivities range from 88 to 100% for parathyroid adenomas[29,55,56] and from 53 to 67% in patients with diffuse parathyroid hyperplasia.[29,55] These studies have been performed primarily in patients prior to initial surgery and in conjunction with ^{123}I thyroid scanning for subtraction. With the double-phase technique, parathyroid abnormalities are generally characterized by early uptake and persistent late (2–3 hour) retention of sestamibi compared to thyroid tissue, which usually exhibits a more rapid wash-out of the radiotracer (Figs. 6, 7). In some cases, however, parathyroid lesions also demonstrate rapid washout, and may only be seen on the early images (unpublished observation). Taillefer et al.[59] studied 21 patients with parathyroid adenomas who had not had prior neck surgery and reported a sensitivity of 90%. In 71% of these cases, the adenoma was evident on the early images, with delayed imaging contributing to adenoma detection in an additional 19%. Imaging was successful in two patients with hyperplasia, and there were two false-positive results, one of which was caused by a thyroid adenoma.

The imaging protocol used for ^{123}I/sestamibi subtraction scanning at NIH is as follows: as with Tc/Tl, information as to any known thyroid disease, etc., is obtained before each study. ^{123}I scanning is performed in most cases despite histories of thyroid surgery or suppression, as residual uptake is often present in these settings. For imaging, the patient is positioned under a scintillation camera with the neck extended approximately 4 hours after p.o. ingestion of 300 uCi ^{123}I Na. Using a LEAP collimator and 1.5 magnification, a 5-minute ^{123}I image (159 keV, 15% window) of the neck that includes the salivary glands and upper chest is obtained. This is immediately followed by a 5-min. image taken in the ^{99m}Tc window (140 keV, 15% window) for down-scatter information. Without moving the patient, ^{99m}Tc-sestamibi is injected (20 mCi) and a 20-minute (1 min./frame) dynamic acquisition is begun in the ^{99m}Tc window. Additional 5-min. anterior oblique neck and anterior chest images are obtained at the end of the dynamic study. Approximately 2 hours later, 5-min. neck and chest images are repeated. Processing involves optional correction for ^{123}I down-scatter into the ^{99m}Tc window (usually insignificant), motion correction, normalization, and subtraction. As with Tc/Tl scanning, radionuclide injections are performed via temporary, indwelling peripheral lines to prevent patient motion caused by needlesticks during a study.

Studies are interpreted as positive if there are areas of excess sestamibi uptake seen compared to ^{123}I (Fig. 3), and/or if areas of increased or separate sestamibi uptake relative to thyroid tissue are seen on either the early or delayed Sestamibi images, or both (Figs. 6 and 7). In selected patients, the ^{123}I part of the study may be omitted and a single-agent sestamibi study performed. This is done primarily in patients without prior neck surgery or history of thyroid disease who presumably have normal thyroid morphology, and in patients with a history of total thyroid ablation for thyroid cancer. In other patients, and particularly in reoperative patients whose thyroid anatomy is likely to be distorted, knowledge of thyroid morphology is very important, and an ^{123}I study is obtained.

Given its advantages over ^{201}Tl and the ease of the single agent method, use of ^{99m}Tc-sestamibi is likely to increase in the future. Initial reports seem to indicate that sestamibi scanning is at least as good as Tc/Tl imaging. Whether thyroid imaging for subtraction purposes is necessary or the single-agent method proves adequate remains to be determined.

PITFALLS IN SUBTRACTION SCANNING

One major problem with parathyroid scintigraphy is the occurrence of false-positive and false-negative studies. There are many documented causes of such results in Tc/

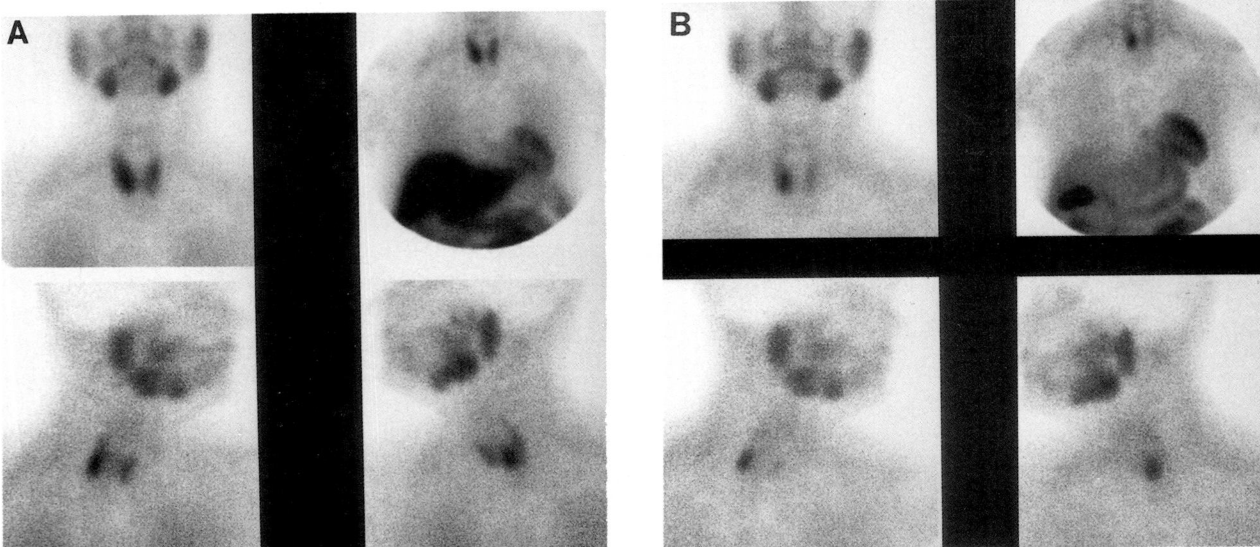

Figure 6. Early **(A)** and 2-hour delayed **(B)** ^{99m}Tc-sestamibi images in a patient with recurrent hyperparathyroidism. Anterior neck (upper left), chest (upper right), RAO (bottom left), and LAO (bottom right) views provided. Delayed images show retention of activity in the region of the lower pole of the right thyroid lobe in the same area as seen on this patient's Tc/Tl study (see Fig. 2).

Tl subtraction imaging. With sestamibi, the number of such causes has been limited to date, but can be expected to increase as experience with that agent increases. With both agents, thyroid abnormalities (which are present in approximately 40% of patients with hyperparathyroidism[61]) are the major source of false positive findings. Thyroid adenomas and other abnormalities which appear as "cold" nodules on the ^{99m}Tc or ^{123}I images often continue to take up ^{201}Tl and sestamibi, resulting in false-positive scans (Fig. 8).[31,39,55,59,62] Other causes of false-positive Tc/Tl scans include Hashimoto's thyroiditis,[63] inflamed cervical lymph nodes,[31] cervical metastases,[31,64] sarcoidosis,[65] and brown tumors of bone.[66]

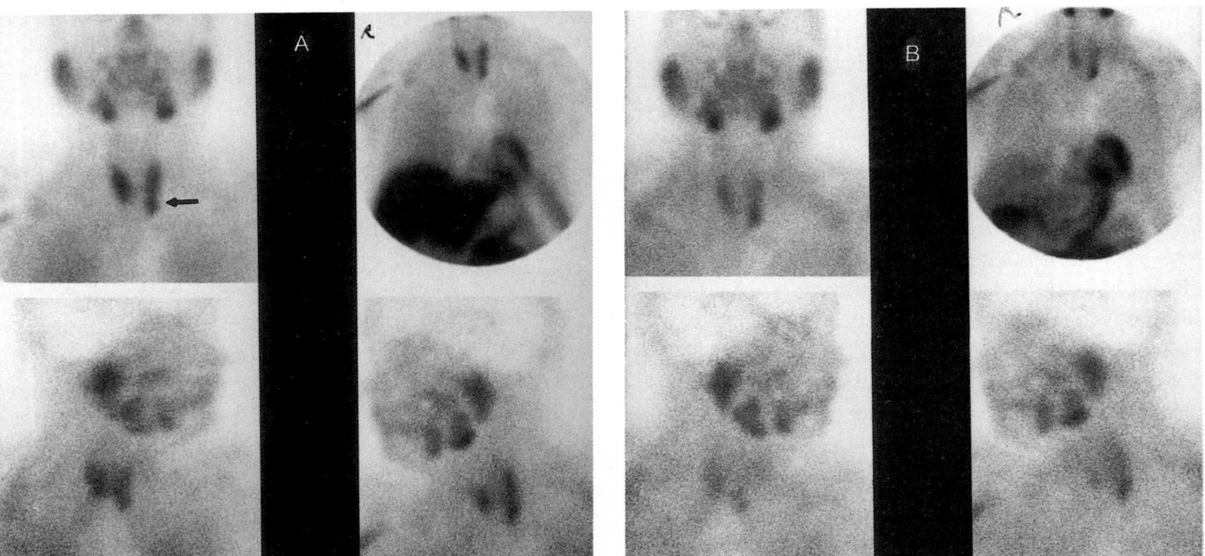

Figure 7. Early **(A)** and 2 hour delayed **(B)** ^{99m}Tc-sestamibi images in a patient with hyperparathyroidism and no previous neck surgery. Anterior neck (upper left), chest (upper right), RAO (bottom left), and LAO (bottom right) views provided. Abnormal uptake extending inferiorly from the left lobe of the thyroid on the early images (arrow) is consistent with a parathyroid lesion at this level, as confirmed on the delayed images.

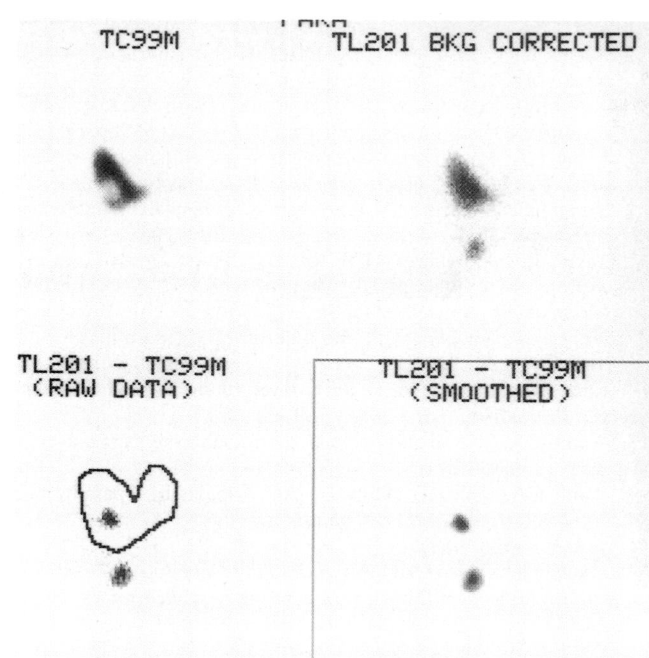

Figure 8. Tc/Tl subtraction study in a patient whose left thyroid lobe has been previously resected. Tc image (upper left) shows a cold defect in the right thyroid lobe. Tl image (upper right) shows uptake in thyroid tissue, "filling in" of the cold defect, and an additional focus in the right superior mediastinum. Subtraction confirms 2 areas of Tl excess—one in the right lobe of the thyroid gland which was a thyroid adenoma, and another in a mediastinal parathyroid adenoma.

These entities also take up ^{201}Tl while failing to concentrate ^{99m}Tc pertechnetate. Technical factors, such as patient movement, normalization artifacts, and image distortion by pinhole collimation, may also lead to false-positive results.[31,39,41] Injection artifacts caused by ^{201}Tl retention in blood vessels (Fig. 4) should also be recognized.

As for false-negatives, these may occur when lesions are small or located deep within the neck or chest, thereby subject to increased amounts of attenuation by overlying tissues. (This is less of a problem with ^{99m}Tc-sestamibi than with ^{201}Tl, since the 140 keV gamma emission of ^{99m}Tc is less effected by attenuation.) Failure to image the upper cervical region or the mediastinum will obviously lead to missed lesions in those areas, and myocardial uptake of ^{201}Tl or sestamibi can also theoretically mask a low-lying ectopic parathyroid lesion. Other documented causes of false-negative studies with Tc/Tl include ^{99m}Tc accumulation by parathyroid adenomas[67] and rapid washout of ^{201}Tl from parathyroid tissue.[68] Lack of retention of sestamibi on the delayed views can also lead to missed lesions on double-phase sestamibi scanning.

Another major limitation of subtraction scanning is that planar images provide no information about the depth of a gland. Lesions that lie within or adjacent to the thyroid gland may, in reality, be situated deep in the neck. Oblique views and/or tomography (SPECT) can help.[69,70] In this respect, ultrasound and other radiographic imaging modalities can provide more accurate information.

Table 1. Tc/Tl Imaging in Secondary Hyperparathyroidism

REFERENCE (#)	# GLANDS	# TP	SENS (%)
Okerlund et al., 1984[38]	23	19	83
Goggin et al., 1987[71]	66	18	27
Carmalt et al., 1988[72]	85	22	26
Moolenaar et al., 1988[52]	43	19	44
Borsato et al., 1989[31]	120	67	56
Rademaker et al., 1990[73]	37	20	54
Cumulative	374	165	44%

Secondary and Tertiary Hyperparathyroidism

In secondary hyperparathyroidism, parathyroid hyperplasia results as a compensatory response to the hypocalcemic effects of the primary disease process. Unfortunately, treatment of the underlying disease is not always accompanied by a return of the hyperfunctioning parathyroid tissue to normal. In addition, hyperplastic parathyroid glands in secondary hyperparathyroidism may become "autonomous," resulting in an inappropriately high secretion of PTH, hypercalcemia, and tertiary hyperparathyroidism.

To date, reports of ^{123}I/sestamibi imaging have focused heavily on patients with primary hyperparathyroidism. However, Tc/Tl scintigraphy has been used in a small number of patients with secondary and tertiary hyperparathyroidism, primarily those with chronic renal failure. In general, sensitivities fall between those seen in primary hyperparathyroidism for adenomas and hyperplasias, ranging from 26 to 83% (Table 1). One factor that may account for this is the observation that ^{201}Tl uptake varies inversely with serum potassium levels,[31] which are often higher than normal in patients requiring dialysis. Another factor is that hyperplastic glands in secondary and tertiary hyperparathyroidism are, on average, larger than those seen in patients with primary multiple-gland disease.[38,52,53]

Other Imaging Modalities

In addition to radionuclide scintigraphy, a number of other imaging modalities are currently available for parathyroid localization. These include ultrasound, computed tomography (CT), magnetic resonance imaging (MRI), angiography, and venous sampling. Numerous studies have been performed to determine the relative sensitivities of these techniques, and several reviews of this literature have recently been published.[53,74]

High-resolution ultrasound is non-invasive, readily available, and relatively inexpensive. In patients with primary hyperparathyroidism, comparative studies[72,75–81] have reported sensitivities of 34 to 92% and 36 to 56% for lesions in previously unexplored and reoperative patients, respectively.

This compares to 48 to 92% and 27 to 73% for Tc/Tl subtraction imaging in those populations. Drawbacks to ultrasound include the inability to locate deep-seated neck lesions or those in the chest, the high false-positive rate, and non-specificity.

Although the modality of choice is debated, most agree that either ultrasound or radionuclide scintigraphy should be used as first-line studies in parathyroid localization. Many recommend using both techniques, and have shown that this increases detection rates. Gooding et al.[76] found that overall sensitivities for adenomas in primary hyperparathyroidism were 78% and 74% for ultrasound and Tc/Tl scanning, respectively, compared to 91% when both were used. The disadvantages of such an approach are the combined high false-positive rates and costs involved.

In comparative studies, computed tomography is reported to have sensitivities of 41 to 86% and 47 to 57% in primary hyperparathyroidism for previously unexplored and reoperative patients, respectively.[72,77,79–81] MRI data in such studies is limited, but at least one found MRI to have a sensitivity of 80%, both in previously unexplored and reoperative patients.[79] Both modalities provide detailed anatomic information, but also involve added costs and administration of i.v. contrast media. More invasive studies include angiography and selective venous sampling of PTH levels.[53,82] These procedures are associated with a small, but real, risk of significant morbidity, and are usually reserved for difficult cases. Lastly, radiographic contrast ablation,[53,83] or percutaneous intratumoral injection of ethanol[84] can obviate the need for surgery in selected patients.

REFERENCES

1. Roth SI: The parathyroid gland in Silverberg SG (ed.): *Principles and Practice of Surgical Pathology*, John Wiley & Sons, 1983, p. 1443.
2. Heath H, Hodgeson SF, Kennedy MA: Primary hyperparathyroidism. Incidence, morbidity, and potential economic impact in a community. *N Engl J Med* 1980;302:189.
3. Wells SA Jr: Multiple endocrine neoplasia type II. *Recent Results Cancer Res* 1990;118:70.
4. Scholz DA, Purnell DC: Asymptomatic primary hyperparathyroidism. *Mayo Clin Proc* 1981;56:473.
5. Bilezikian JP: The medical management of primary hyperparathyroidism. *Ann Intern Med* 1982;96:198.
6. NIH Consensus Panel: Diagnosis and management of asymptomatic primary hyperparathyroidism, *NIH Consensus Statement* 1990;8:1.
7. Bruining HA, van Houten H, Juttmann JR, et al.: Results of operative treatment of 615 patients with primary hyperparathyroidism. *World J Surg* 1981;5:85.
8. Gaz RD, Doubler PB, Wang CA: The management of 50 unusual hyperfunctioning parathyroid glands. *Surgery* 1987; 102:949.
9. Maltby C, Russell CFJ, Laird JD, Ferguson WR: Thallium-technetium isotope subtraction scanning in primary hyperparathyroidism. *J R Coll Surg Edinb* 1989;34:40.
10. Russell CFJ, Laird JD, Ferguson WR: Scan-directed unilateral cervical exploration for parathyroid adenoma: A legitimate approach? *World J Surg* 1990;14:406.
11. Davis RK, Hoffmann J, Dart D, Datz FL: Unilateral parathyroidectomy: The role of thallium-technetium subtraction scans. *Otolaryngol Head Neck Surg* 1990;102:635.
12. Norton JA: Reoperative parathyroid surgery: Indications, intraoperative decision-making and results. *Prog Surg* 1986;18:133.
13. Wang CA: Parathyroid reexploration—a clinical and pathologic study of 112 cases. *Ann Surg* 1977;186:140.
14. Brennan MF, Norton JA: Reoperation for persistent and recurrent hyperparathyroidism. *Ann Surg* 1985;201:40.
15. Satava RM Jr, Beahrs OH, Scholz DA: Success rate of cervical exploration for hyperparathyroidism. *Arch Surg* 1975;110:625.
16. Brennan MF, Marx SJ, Doppman J, Costa J, et al.: Results of reoperation for persistent and recurrent hyperparathyroidism. *Ann Surg* 1981;194:671.
17. Katz AD, Formichella D: Fifty-three reoperations for hyperparathyroidism. *Am J Surg* 1989,158:385.
18. Wang CA: The anatomic basis of parathyroid surgery. *Ann Surg* 1976;183:271.
19. Wang CA, Gaz RD, Moncure AC: Mediastinal parathyroid exploration: A clinical and pathologic study of 47 cases. *World J Surg* 1986;10:687.
20. Potchen EJ, Sodee DB: Selective isotopic labeling of the human parathyroid; a preliminary case report. *J Clin Endocr* 1964; 24:1125.
21. Waldorf JC, van Heerden JA, Gorman CA, et al.: Se75 selenomethionine scanning for parathyroid localization should be abandoned. *Mayo Clin Proc* 1984;59:534.
22. Ferlin G, Borsato N, Perelli R: Positive 131-cesium scanning in parathyroid adenoma. *Eur J Nucl Med* 1977;2:153.
23. Ferlin G, Conte N, Borsato N, et al.: Parathyroid scintigraphy with 131Cs and Tl201. *J Nucl Med Allied Sci* 1981;25:119.
24. Cann CE, Prussin SG: Possible parathyroid imaging using Ga67 and other aluminum analogs. *J Nucl Med* 1980;21:471.
25. Arkles LB: Experience in parathyroid scanning. *Am J Roentgenol Radium Ther Nucl Med* 1975;125:634.
26. Alagumalai K, Avramides A, Carter AC, et al.: Uptake of Technetium pertechnetate in a parathyroid adenoma presenting as an Iodine 131 "cold" nodule. *Ann Intern Med* 1979;90:204.
27. Naunheim KS, Kaplan EL, Kirchner PT: Preoperative Technetium-99m imaging of a substernal parathyroid adenoma. *J Nucl Med* 1982;23:511.
28. Coakley AJ, Kettle AG, Wells CP: Tc99m sestamibi—a new agent for parathyroid imaging. *Nucl Med Commun* 1989; 10:791.
29. O'Doherty MJ, Kettle AG, Wells P, Collins RE, Coakley AJ: Parathyroid imaging with technetium-99m-sestamibi: preoperative localization and tissue uptake studies. *J Nucl Med* 1992;33:313.
30. MacFarlane SD, Hanelin LG, Taft DA, Ryan JA Jr, Fredlund PN: Localization of abnormal parathyroid glands using thallium-201. *Am J Surg* 1984;148:7.
31. Borsato N, Zanco P, Camerani M, Saitta B, Ferlin G: Scintigraphy of the parathyroid glands with 201Tl: experience with 250 operated patients. *Nuklearmedizin* 1989;28:26.
32. McCall AR, Calandra D, Lawrence AM, Henkin R, Paloyan E: Parathyroid autotransplantation in forty-four patients with primary hyperparathyroidism; The role of thallium scanning. *Surg* 1986;4:614.
33. Fronistas O, Stavraka-Kakavaki A, Giougi A, Papatheophanis J: Evaluation of parathyroid tissue transplants by Tl-201 scintigraphy. *Clin Nucl Med* 1992;17:954.
34. Chen CC, Premkumar A, Hill SC, et al.: Tc-99m Sestamibi Imaging of a Hyperfunctioning Parathyroid Autograft with Doppler Ultrasound and MRI Correlation. *Clin Nucl Med* 1995;20:222.
35. Oster ZH, Strauss HW, Harrison K, et al.: Thallium 201 distri-

bution in the thyroid: Relationship to thyroidal trapping function. *Radiology* 1978;126:733.
36. Brownless SM, Gimlette TMD: Comparison of techniques for thallium-201-technetium-99m parathyroid imaging. *Br J Radiol* 1989;62:532.
37. Arndt JW, Heslinga JM, Bolk JH, et al.: Thallium-201-technetium-99m parathyroid subtraction scintigraphy: Dual channel acquisition or sequential imaging? *Diagn Imag Clin Med* 1986;55:236.
38. Okerlund MD, Sheldon K, Corpuz S, et al.: A new method with high sensitivity and specificity for localization of abnormal parathyroid glands. *Ann Surg* 1984;200:381.
39. Basarab RM, Manni A, Harrison TS: Dual isotope subtraction parathyroid scintigraphy in the preoperative evaluation of suspected hyperparathyroidism. *Clin Nucl Med* 1985;10:300.
40. Conte FA, Orzel JA, Weiland SL, Borchert RD: Prevention of motion artifacts on dual isotope subtraction parathyroid scintigraphy. *J Nucl Med* 1987;28:1335.
41. Foster GS, Bekerman C, Blend MJ, et al: Preoperative imaging in primary hyperparathyroidism. *Arch Otolaryngol Head Neck Surg* 1989;115:1197.
42. Sandrock D, Dunham RG, Neumann RD: Simultaneous dual energy acquisition for Tl201/Tc99m parathyroid subtraction scintigraphy: Physical and physiologic considerations. *Nucl Med Commun* 1990;11:503.
43. Hauty M, Swartz K, McClung M, Lowe DK: Technetium-Thallium scintiscanning for localization of parathyroid adenomas and hyperplasia. *Am J Surg* 1987;153:479.
44. Sandrock D, Merino MJ, Norton JA, Neumann RD: Parathyroid imaging by Tc/Tl scintigraphy. *Eur J Nucl Med* 1990; 16:607.
45. Krubsack AJ, Wilson SD, Lawson TL, et al.: Prospective comparison of radionuclide, computed tomographic, and sonographic localization of parathyroid tumors. *World J Surg* 1986;10:579.
46. Skibber JM, Reynolds JC, Spiegel AM, et al.: Computerized technetium/thallium scans and parathyroid reoperation. *Surgery* 1985;98:1077.
47. Chan TYK, Serpell JW, Chan O, Gaunt JI, et al.: Misinterpretation of the upper parathyroid adenoma on thallium-201/technetium-99m subtraction scintigraphy. *Br J Radiol* 1991;64:1.
48. Percival RC, Blake GM, Urwin GH, et al.: Assessment of thallium-pertechnetate subtraction scintigraphy in hyperparathyroidism. *Br J Radiol* 1985;58:131.
49. Gimlette TMD, Brownless SM, Taylor WH, et al.: Limits to parathyroid imaging with thallium-201 confirmed by tissue uptake and phantom studies. *J Nucl Med* 1986;27:1262.
50. Gupta SM, Belsky JL, Spencer RP, Frias J, et al.: Parathyroid adenomas and hyperplasia. Dual radionuclide scintigraphy and bone densitometry studies. *Clin Nucl Med* 1985;10:243.
51. Manni A, Basarab RM, Plourde PV, Koivunen D, et al.: Thallium-technetium parathyroid scan. A useful noninvasive technique for localization of abnormal parathyroid tissue. *Arch Intern Med* 1986;146:1077.
52. Moolenaar W, Heslinga JM, Arndt JW, et al.: Tl201-Tc99m subtraction scintigraphy in secondary hyperparathyroidism of chronic renal failure. *Nephrol Dial Transplant* 1988;2:166.
53. Eisenberg H, Pallotta J, Sacks B, Brickman, AS: Parathyroid localization, three-dimensional modeling, and percutaneous ablation techniques. *Endocrinol Metab Clin N Amer* 1989; 18:659.
54. Sandrock D, Merino MJ, Norton JA, Neumann RD: Ultrastructural histology correlates with results of thallium-201/technetium-99m parathyroid subtraction scintigraphy. *J Nucl Med* 1993;34:24.
55. Wei JP, Burke GJ, Mansberger AR Jr: Prospective evaluation of the efficacy of technetium 99m sestamibi and iodine 123 radionuclide imaging of abnormal parathyroid glands. *Surgery* 1992;112:1111.
56. Casas AT, Burke GJ, Sathyanarayana, Mansberger AR, Jr, Wei JP: Prospective comparison of Technetium-99m-Sestamibi/Iodine-123 radionuclide scan versus high-resolution ultrasonography for the preoperative localization of abnormal glands in patients with previously unoperated primary hyperparathyroidism. *Am J Surg* 1993;166:369.
57. Weber CJ, Vansant J, Alazraki N, Christy J, et al.: Value of technetium 99m sestamibi iodine 123 imaging in reoperative parathyroid surgery. *Surgery* 1993;114:1011.
58. Halvorson DJ, Burke GJ, Mansberger AR Jr, Wei JP: Use of technetium Tc 99m sestamibi and iodine 123 radionuclide scan for preoperative localization of abnormal parathyroid glands in primary hyperparathyroidism. *South Med J* 1994;87:336.
59. Taillefer R, Boucher Y, Potvin C, Lambert R: Detection and localization of parathyroid adenomas in patients with hyperparathyroidism using a single radionuclide imaging procedure with technetium-99m-sestamibi (double-phase study). *J Nucl Med* 1992;33:1801.
60. Irvin GL III, Prudhomme DL, Deriso GT, Sfakianakis G, Chandarlapaty SK: A new approach to parathyroidectomy. *Ann Surg* 1994;219:574.
61. Laing VO, Frame B, Block MA: Associated primary hyperparathyroidism and thyroid lesions. *Arch Surg* 1969;98:709.
62. Blue PW, Crawford G, Dydek GJ: Parathyroid subtraction imaging—pitfalls in diagnosis. *Clin Nucl Med* 1989;14:47.
63. Shimaoka K, Parthasarathy KL, Friedman M, Rao U: Disparity of radioiodine and radiothallium concentrations in chronic thyroiditis. *J Med* 1980;11:401.
64. Maslack MM, Brosbe RJ: Dual isotope parathyroid imaging. *Clin Nucl Med* 1986;11:622.
65. Young AE, Gaunt JI, Croft DN, et al.: Location of parathyroid adenomas by thallium 201 and technetium 99m subtraction scanning. *Br Med J* 1983;286:1384.
66. Yang CJC, Seabold JE, Gurll NJ: Brown tumor of bone: A potential source of false-positive thallium 201 localization. *J Nucl Med* 1989;30:1264.
67. Chen CC, Irony I, Jaffe GS, Norton JA: Tc-99m uptake in a parathyroid adenoma. Potential pitfall in Tc-99m/Tl-201 subtraction imaging. *Clin Nucl Med* 1992;17:539.
68. Greenberg SB, Park CH, Intenzo C: Dynamic or early imaging in dual-tracer parathyroid scintigraphy. *Clin Nucl Med* 1986; 11:627.
69. Jenkins BJ, Newell MS, Goode AW, Boucher BJ, et al.: Impact of conventional and three-dimensional thallium-technetium scans on surgery for primary hyperparathyroidism. *J Royal Soc Med* 1990;83:427.
70. Neumann DR: Simultaneous dual-isotope SPECT imaging for the detection and characterization of parathyroid pathology. *J Nucl Med* 1992;33:131.
71. Goggin MJ, Black DA, Wells CP, et al.: Thallium 201 and technetium 99m subtraction scanning of the parathyroid glands in patients with hyperparathyroidism due to renal osteodystrophy. *Contr Nephrol* 1987;56:196.
72. Carmalt HL, Gillett DJ, Chu J, Evans RA, Kos S: Prospective comparison of radionuclide, ultrasound, and computed tomography in the preoperative localization of parathyroid glands. *World J Surg* 1988;12:830.
73. Rademaker P, Meijer S, Piers DA: Parathyroid localization by Tl201-Tc99m subtraction scintigraphy: Results in secondary hyperparathyroidism. *Acta Endocrinol* 1990;123:402.
74. Miller DL: Preoperative localization and interventional treatment of parathyroid tumors: when and how? *World J Surg* 1991;15:706.
75. Winzelberg GG, Hydovitz JD, O'Hara KR, et al.: Parathyroid adenomas evaluated by Tl-201/Tc-99m pertechnetate, subtrac-

tion scintigraphy and high-resolution ultrasonography. *Radiology* 1985;155:231.
76. Gooding GAW, Okerlund MD, Stark DD, Clark OH: Parathyroid imaging: Comparison of double-tracer (Tl-201, Tc-99m) scintigraphy and high-resolution US. *Radiology* 1986;161:57.
77. Miller DL, Doppman JL, Shawker TH, et al.: Localization of parathyroid adenomas in patients who have undergone surgery. Part I: Noninvasive imaging methods. *Radiology* 1987; 162:133.
78. Attie JN, Khan A, Rumancik WM, Moskowitz GW, et al.: Preoperative localization of parathyroid adenomas. *Am J Surg* 1988;156:323.
79. Erdman WA, Breslau NA, Weinreb JC, et al.: Noninvasive localization of parathyroid adenomas: A comparison of X-ray computerized tomography, ultrasound, scintigraphy, and MRI. *Magn Reson Imaging* 1989;7:187.
80. Roses DF, Sudarsky LA, Sanger et al.: The use of preoperative localization of adenomas of the parathyroid glands by thallium-technetium subtraction scintigraphy, high resolution ultrasonography and computed tomography. *Surg Gynecol Obstet* 1989;168:99.
81. Kohri K, Ishikawa Y, Kodama M, Katayama Y, et al.: Comparison of imaging methods for localization of parathyroid tumors. *Am J Surg* 1992;164:140.
82. Miller DL, Doppman JL, Krudy AG, et al.: Localization of parathyroid adenomas in patients who have undergone surgery. Part II. Invasive procedures. *Radiology* 1987;162:138.
83. Geelhoed GW, Krudy AG, Doppman JL: Long-term follow-up of patients with hyperparathyroidism treated by transcatheter staining with contrast agent. *Surgery* 1983;94:849.
84. Takeda S, Michigishi T, Takazakura E: Successful ultrasonically guided percutaneous ethanol injection for secondary hyperparathyroidism. *Nephron* 1992;62:100.

22 The Salivary Glands

Bruce J. Baum, Philip C. Fox, Ronald D. Neumann

Salivary glands can be divided into two classes based on their size and fluid output, so-called major and minor glands. There are three bilateral pairs of major salivary glands, the parotid, submandibular, and sublingual glands. The parotid glands are located anteriorly and inferiorly to the external ear. Parotid saliva enters the mouth through Stensen's duct, the orifice of which is located in the buccal mucosa roughly opposite the maxillary first molar. The submandibular glands are located beneath the floor of the mouth and their saliva exits via Wharton's duct adjacent to the lingual frenum, just posterior to the mandibular incisors. The sublingual glands are the smallest of the major glands. They are located on the anterolateral margin of the submandibular glands and often share the latter's main excretory duct. There are literally hundreds of minor salivary glands scattered throughout the oral cavity. They are named for their anatomic locations (e.g., labial, buccal, and palatal glands).

Each salivary gland consists of two regions, the acinar region or secretory endpiece, and the ductal region. The parotid, sublingual, and minor glands each contain a single acinar cell type; serous, mucous, and mucous, respectively. The submandibular gland contains a mixture of serous and mucous acini. Acinar cells are the site of all fluid transport in salivary glands (i.e., the acinus is water permeable and the ducts are water impermeable). Acinar cells also secrete 85 to 90% of the exocrine proteins found in saliva. The initial acinar cell secretion is termed the primary saliva and is isotonic to plasma (i.e., ~140mEq NaCl/L). The ductal region of the major glands includes multiple cell types. The minor glands have extremely short duct segments, lying just beneath the oral mucosa. Duct cells, in addition to conducting the saliva into the mouth, secrete some exocrine proteins (10 to 15%) but, most importantly, reabsorb NaCl. The final saliva that enters the mouth is markedly hypotonic (~25mEq NaCl/L).

Each gland type makes a distinctive secretion, primarily because of the differing macromolecular composition. These gland salivas mix in the mouth to form what is commonly called whole saliva. Whole saliva is not the simple additive sum of individual gland secretions. For example, some exocrine proteins are degraded upon entering the mouth, others bind to the teeth or the oral mucosa to provide protective, semipermeable barriers. Further, whole saliva also contains many nonsalivary gland products, such as desquamated mucosal epithelial cells, food debris, oral bacterial components, sputum, and blood elements. Under basal or resting conditions, the parotid gland contributes ~30% to the forming saliva, the submandibular and sublingual glands ~40%, and the aggregate minor glands ~30%. This basal secretion is considered essential for protecting the oropharyngeal and esophageal tissues. The resting saliva keeps teeth mineralized, lubricates and repairs the mucosa, modulates microbial populations, and buffers local acid production. Under stimulated conditions, such as during a meal, output may increase by 10 to 20-fold and saliva functions mainly in food bolus formation and translocation, thus facilitating swallowing. The parotid gland contributes ~45% of the stimulated secretion, the submandibular/sublingual glands ~45%, and the minor glands ~10%.

All saliva is secreted in response to neural activation; there is no spontaneous secretion.[1] At rest, low level neurotransmitter release regulates acinar cell secretion, while high levels of neurotransmitters are released during stimulation. Both sympathetic and parasympathetic nerves innervate salivary glands. Norepinephrine and acetylcholine, respectively, are the principal neurotransmitters involved. These neurotransmitters form the first message or signal for an acinar cell to secrete (Fig. 1). There are two major intracellular signaling mechanisms in these cells: cyclic AMP (3′, 5′-cyclic adenosine monophosphate, primarily related to protein secretion); and IP_3 (inositol 1,4,5-trisphosphate, primarily related to fluid secretion).[2] The latter pathway is most relevant to salivary gland ^{99m}Tc-pertechnetate handling and, accordingly, will be reviewed in some detail.

The ability of acinar cells to secrete fluid depends on their ability to transport anions in a directional fashion.[3] Anion movement (the principal anions being Cl^- and HCO_3^-) and, thus, fluid secretion require mobilization of intracellular Ca^{2+} and the subsequent entry of extracellular Ca^{2+}. IP_3 induces the release of free Ca^{2+} from an intracellular storage pool (part of the endoplasmic reticulum).[2] This step results in three key ion transport events: the opening of two Ca^{2+}-activated ion channels (one for Cl^- in the apical membrane, the other for K^+ in the basolateral membrane) and the activation of the basolateral membrane Ca^{2+} entry pathway.[2,3] Loss of K^+ from the cell provides the K^+ source to be utilized to help drive Cl^- into the cell against its electrochemical gradient. Cl^- entry takes place via a loop-diuretic sensitive, $Na^+/K^+/2Cl^-$ cotransporter, energized by the Na^+/K^+ ATPase.[3] For each Cl^- entering the cell, another Cl^- exits into the

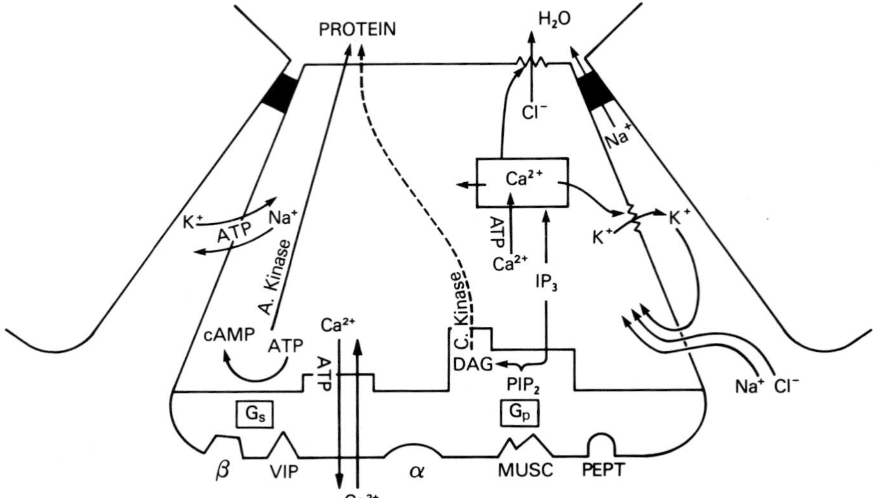

Figure 1. Schematic depiction of secretory events in acinar cells. β = β-adrenoreceptor, VIP = vasoactive intestinal polypeptide receptor; α = α-adrenoreceptor, MUSC = muscarinic-cholinergic receptor, PEPT = substance *P* receptor; G_s and G_p are signal transducing *G* proteins; PIP_2 = phosphatidylinositol 4,5-bisphosphate. Right side of figure depicts events involved in fluid secretion. See text for details.

acinar lumen via the apical Ca^{2+}-activated channel. Na^+ is believed to enter the lumen across the intercellular tight junctions, electrically neutralizing the released Cl^- and, thus, providing the osmotic gradient driving water movement.

^{99m}Tc-pertechnetate is a pseudo-halide that is used extensively to study salivary gland function (see below). Experiments with rat parotid acinar cells suggest that this radionuclide enters acinar cells via the $Na^+/K^+/2Cl^-$ cotransporter, substituting for Cl^- and, likely, exits the cell via the Ca^{2+}-activated Cl^- channel.[4,5] Although studies with a laboratory model tissue are unlikely to yield an exact picture of human cell function, such results are consistent with the notion that ^{99m}Tc-pertechnetate is handled by the acinar cell anion transport pathways involved in fluid secretion. Thus, normal ^{99m}Tc-pertechnetate uptake and release would appear to indicate the presence of functional salivary gland parenchyma capable of fluid secretion. Indeed, scintigraphic studies with healthy, nonmedicated control subjects and with xerostomic (dry mouth) patients, demonstrate strong correlations between ^{99m}Tc-pertechnetate uptake and major salivary gland flow rates.[6]

As discussed below, the primary diagnostic value of scintigraphy is in the evaluation of patients with xerostomic complaints or frank salivary hypofunction. The most common cause of dry mouth complaints is the iatrogenic use of pharmaceuticals with anticholinergic effects[7]: antidepressants, antihypertensives, antispasmodics and antihistamines. Salivary hypofunction frequently results from therapeutic head and neck irradiation.[7] The most common disease resulting in decreased salivary secretion is Sjögren's syndrome, an autoimmune exocrinopathy affecting predominantly postmenopausal women.[7] Scintigraphy is particularly valuable for the latter two conditions, both of which show quite heterogenous presentations. The demonstration of potentially functional glandular tissue by ^{99m}Tc-pertechnetate uptake in such patients indicates the possibility of therapeutic intervention with the use of systemically administered sialogogues, such as the partial muscarinic agonist pilocarpine.[6,8]

The evaluation of salivary function in patients complaining of dry mouth (xerostomia) is a major indication for ^{99m}Tc-pertechnetate scintiscanning. Other conditions that can be evaluated with pertechnetate imaging include acute, chronic, or recurrent salivary gland swellings, focal masses, and salivary obstructions.[9–13]

^{99m}Tc-pertechnetate scintigraphy is a particularly valuable tool for evaluating the dynamics of the salivary secretory process. The uptake phase represents the transport of tracer from the vasculature into the salivary tissues. This aspect of secretion can be distinguished easily from the subsequent secretory phase, in which tracer is transported from the salivary glands into the oral cavity.[6] Salivary gland performance should be examined first in an unstimulated state, to evaluate basal secretory function. Patients should be instructed to refrain from eating, drinking, or performing any oral hygiene for at least 90 minutes prior to scintigraphy to assure a resting secretory state. After the unstimulated study, a stimulus (usually gustatory or masticatory) is applied intraorally. Increased activity demonstates clearance of tracer in response to a physiological stimulus and, thus, the integrity of the secretory system. The main ducts of the parotid glands can be seen clearly (Fig. 2).

Modern computer-interfaced gamma cameras are capable of both functional salivary analysis and morphological imaging of the gland with resolution approaching 4 to 5mm. The recommended techniques that follow are those used in our NIH Nuclear Medicine Clinic.

To study gland function, an intravenous dose (260 to 370 MBq) of ^{99m}Tc-pertechnetate is usually sufficient. The scintillation camera-computer system is set for dynamic acquisition with 120 seconds per image for about 1 hour. A low energy LEAP or high-sensitivity collimator can be used for flow analysis but, if morphological detail is required, a high-resolution collimator is better. The patient is positioned

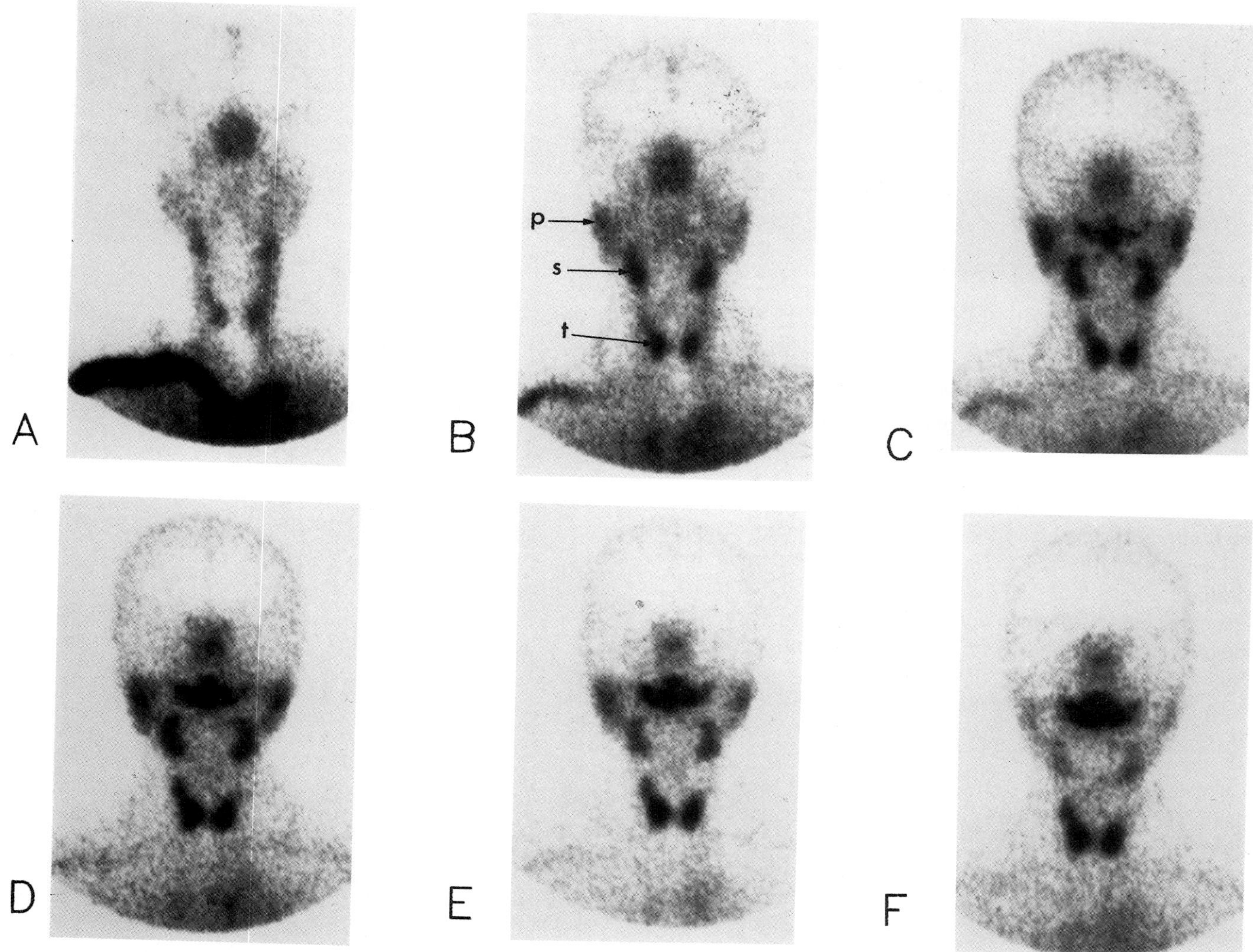

Figure 2. Selected frames from a representative normal salivary scintiscan demonstrating the major secretory events. **(A).** 0–2 min, vascular phase with tracer present in major vessels. **(B).** 2–4 min, initial salivary gland uptake (p = parotid, s = submandibular/sublingual, t = thyroid). **(C).** 12–14 min, secretion noted in oral cavity and major excretory ducts visualized (oral bridging). **(D).** 24–26 min, maximal tracer density in the glands. Note the relative density versus the thyroid. **(E).** 38–40 min, 2% citric acid rinse is given at this time. **(F).** 40–42 min, tracer is cleared rapidly from the glands and the oral activity is increased following stimulation.

comfortably with the collimator over the anterior face and neck. The ^{99m}Tc-pertechnetate is given as a bolus in an arm vein. After 40 minutes of acquisition, the patient receives 0.5mL 2% sodium citrate solution by carefully squirting this fluid into the patient's mouth, without any movement of the patient's head position relative to the camera. The patient is allowed to swallow the solution after 30 seconds.

To include morphological images, high-resolution anterior, lateral, and Water's radiographic projections are obtained. Each lateral must be controlled for time of acquisition to the desired total counts. At least 400K counts are recorded for the anterior and Water's views, as well as for the first lateral view. The opposite lateral view is obtained for the same time as the first lateral. Anterior and posterior oblique projection images sometimes provide better definition of suspicious findings. A second set of images is obtained after the salivary glands are emptied by oral citrate stimulation.

Only the parotid glands and the submandibular/sublingual gland complex are visualized with ^{99m}Tc-pertechnetate.[14] The minor glands are not seen, although radioactivity can be detected in minor gland saliva collected following stimulation (unpublished observations). Failure to visualize these glands is likely the result of relatively low tracer uptake, as well as an inability to resolve very small structures. Also, the activity in the oral cavity adherent to mucosa can obscure activity contributed by the minor glands that line the oral mucosa.

Recent work has characterized the range of times for uptake and clearance of pertechnetate from the major salivary glands in a group of 33 nonmedicated, healthy volun-

SCINTISCAN RATING SCALE

	Points		Points
UPTAKE PAROTID		CONCENTRATION TRACER PAROTID VS. THYROID	
0-06 MINUTES	2	› 50 PERCENT	1
07-40 MINUTES	1	‹ 50 PERCENT	0
› 40 MINUTES	0		
UPTAKE SUBMANDIBULAR		CONCENTRATION TRACER SUBMANDIBULAR VS. THYROID	
0-06 MINUTES	2		
07-40 MINUTES	1	› 50 PERCENT	1
› 40 MINUTES	0	‹ 50 PERCENT	0
FIRST APPEARANCE IN ORAL CAVITY		RESPONSE TO STIMULATION	
		YES	1
		NO	0
0-32 MINUTES	2		
33-40 MINUTES	1		
Post-stimulation	0	MAXIMUM SCORE	9

Figure 3. A clinically applicable grading scale for salivary scintiscans based on results from a series of healthy controls.

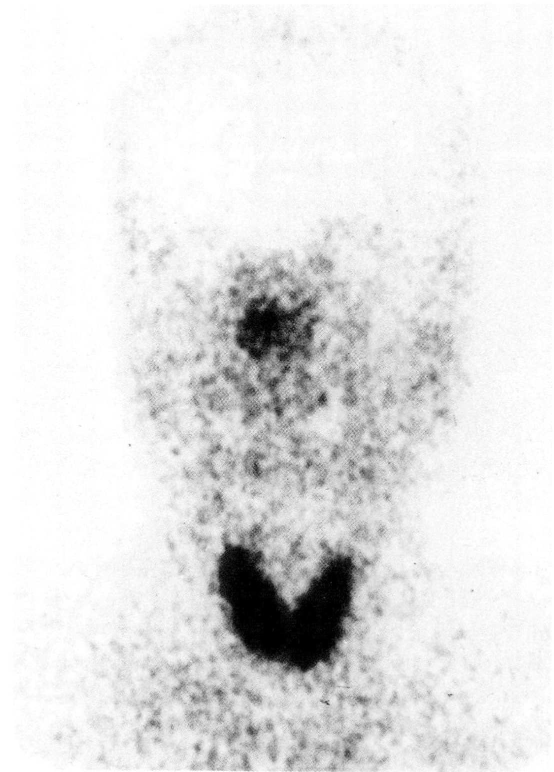

Figure 5. A salivary scintiscan of a patient with endstage Sjögren's syndrome. There is complete absence of tracer uptake or secretion into the oral cavity seen in this frame, taken immediately following citric acid stimulation.

teers with normal salivary function.[6] Normal uptake is rapid and symmetrical (Fig. 2). Tracer is seen in the parotid and submandibular/sublingual glands, on average, in 3 minutes. The outer limit of normal, defined as 2 standard deviations above the group mean, was 6 minutes. Without exogenous stimulation, ^{99m}Tc-pertechnetate appeared in the oral cavity in 13 minutes, with a wide normal range. It was considered abnormal (mean + 2SD) if oral tracer was not seen within 32 minutes. In 94% of the subjects, the density of tracer in the major glands was >50% of the density in the thyroid gland. The response of the salivary glands to stimulation was also examined. In normally functioning glands, a gustatory stimulus (2% citric acid orally) induced a prompt increase in oral tracer density and/or decreased concentration in the major glands (Fig. 2). These results were used to develop a clinically applicable rating scale (Fig. 3) for ^{99m}Tc-pertechnetate scintiscans. Scores derived from the rating scale were found to correlate well with salivary function in a mixed patient group with clinically determined normal and diminished salivary gland function.[6] ^{99m}Tc-pertechnetate scintigraphy was a reliable indicator of salivary gland performance. This scale was designed to be used clinically and to require no specialized equipment.

More quantitative information can be derived from ^{99m}Tc-pertechnetate scans using region-of-interest (ROI) techniques.[15] Individual major gland activity can be visualized and the time to maximum tracer uptake, start of secretion, and response to stimulation calculated with accuracy. An obvious drawback is the time required and the hardware and software necessary for these analyses. Because the borders of the salivary glands are scintigraphically indistinct and there is significant background tracer, the assignment of regions-of-interest boundaries is somewhat subjective. This introduces uncontrolled variability into the procedure. Region-of-interest analyses of salivary function have been used in experimental investigations, but have little clinical utility.

^{99m}Tc-pertechnetate scintiscans are useful to evaluate salivary gland masses, both for diagnostic and for presurgical planning purposes.[16] The size and location of the glands can be seen. More importantly, the secretory function of a gland

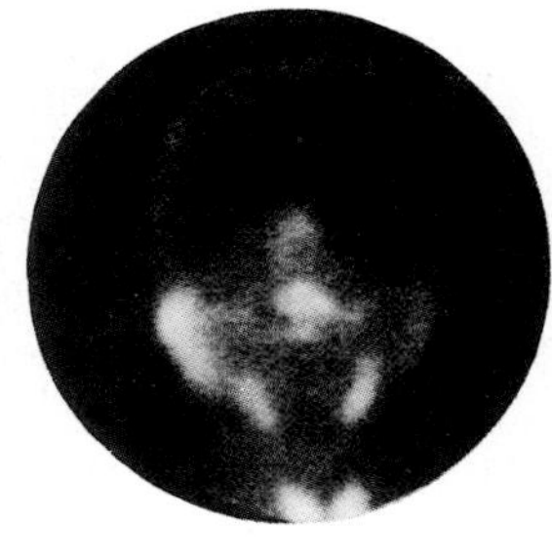
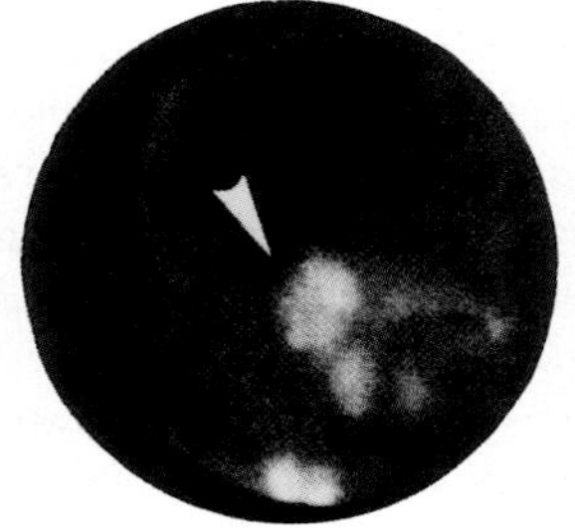
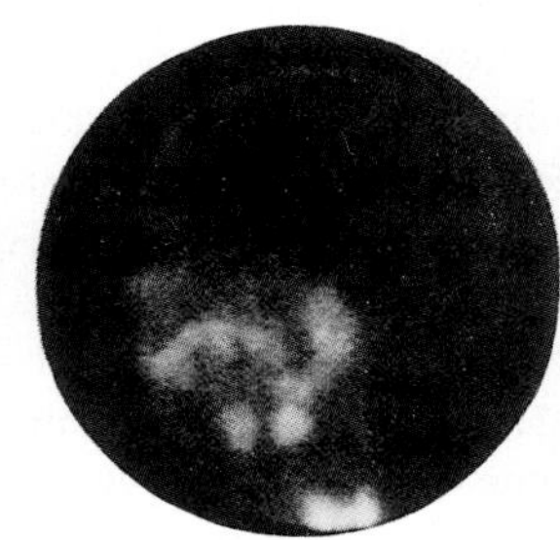

Figure 4. Warthin's tumor demonstrates increased activity in the right parotid gland (arrow). Images are from left to right: anterior, right lateral, and left lateral.

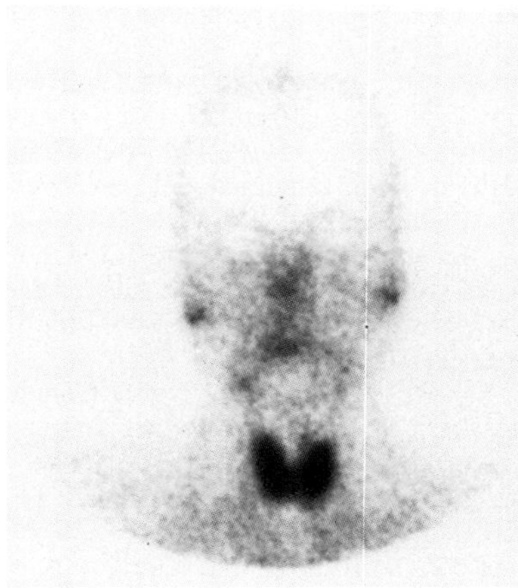
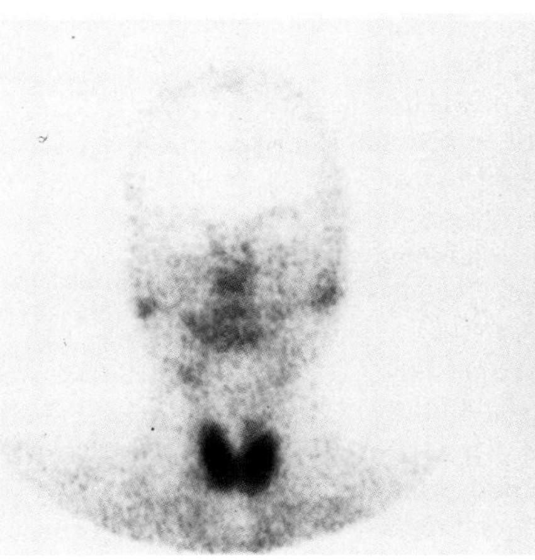

Figure 6. A salivary scintiscan of a patient with severe Sjögren's syndrome, but with some remaining salivary function. The left frame is immediately prior to stimulation (38–40 min). There is reduced uptake of tracer (parotid uptake > submandibular/sublingual). In the right frame, after stimulation, there is evidence of some response with decreased tracer density in the glands and an increase of tracer in the oral cavity.

mass can be determined. It should be remembered that 70 to 80% of salivary gland tumors are benign. The most common salivary tumor, the pleomorphic adenoma ("mixed tumor"), generally appears as a "cold" focal lesion with a smooth outline. Nonfunctioning masses with irregular borders are more frequently associated with malignant lesions. In general, functioning (or "hot") masses are benign. An example of this is the papillary cystadenoma lymphomatosum (Warthin's tumor), which demonstrates focally increased tracer activity (Fig. 4).

Scintiscans are often used to evaluate inflammatory disease. Acute sialadenitis usually causes increased tracer activity in the involved gland. If the inflammation continues, as in chronic sialadenitis, sarcoidosis, and connective tissue diseases, activity is decreased as gland function declines. Acute obstruction by a sialolith will often initially show good uptake and increased density of tracer with no secretion after stimulation. With time, as the gland undergoes pressure atrophy, activity decreases and the gland eventually has no uptake.

^{99m}Tc-pertechnetate scintiscanning has been utilized frequently to evaluate salivary gland involvement in Sjögren's syndrome.[17] There is no consistent pattern that can be described for this disorder, as the extent of salivary dysfunction in Sjögren's varies greatly, ranging from normal to no function. The scintigraphic appearance reflects the severity of salivary hypofunction and is not specific for diagnostic purposes. In early involvement, one sees normal tracer uptake with a delay in secretion. With increasing gland dysfunction, uptake decreases and secretion is prolonged. In end-stage disease (Fig. 5), there is no tracer uptake as salivary epithelium has been lost and replaced with a mononuclear cell infiltrate. As noted earlier, ^{99m}Tc-pertechnetate scintiscanning has been useful in identifying patients with remaining functional salivary tissues (Fig. 6) who are candidates for treatment with sialogogues.[6,8]

Other diagnostic techniques used to evaluate salivary gland pathology include collection of whole or gland salivas (sialometry), sialochemical analyses, contrast sialography (conventional or CT), MRI, ultrasound, and aspiration or incisional biopsy. Each of these has strengths and drawbacks.

Saliva collection provides objective measurement of gland output. However, it requires specialized training and equipment and provides no information on the glandular site of any dysfunction found.[18] There are also the considerations of handling a potentially infectious body fluid. Analysis of the composition of the secretions can help pinpoint a glandular region of dysfunction, but alterations detected usually lack diagnostic specificity. Salivary analysis is not routinely available in clinical pathology laboratories.

Sialography clearly visualizes the ductal anatomy of the major salivary glands. It is useful to localize regions of obstruction (such as sialoliths or strictures), displacement of glandular tissue by tumors, and loss of normal parenchymal architecture (Fig. 7). Limitations to contrast sialography are

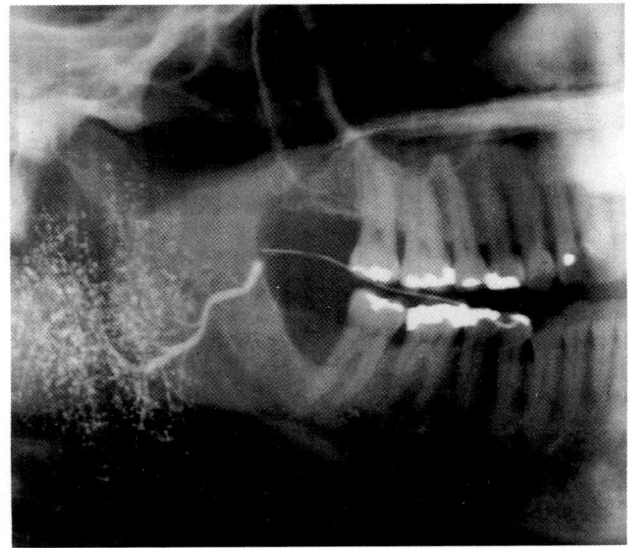

Figure 7. A sialogram of a patient with Sjögren's syndrome. The main duct structure is intact but there is loss of acinar structure and punctate sialectasis.

the technical difficulties of cannulating the ducts (particularly Wharton's duct), the invasiveness of the procedure, the radiation exposure, and a lack of diagnostic specificity. Also, sialography is contraindicated in the presence of infection or acute inflammation. An additional consideration is that, in nonfunctioning glands, the contrast material may persist in the tissues indefinitely and has been implicated in granuloma formation. Contrast sialography provides little definitive information concerning gland function.

Both MRI and ultrasound are useful in distinguishing between solid and cystic masses, but there is little additional diagnostic specificity. Incisional biopsy provides diagnostic certainty, but is invasive and carries a risk of complications from the close proximity of major nerves. Aspiration biopsy is often nondiagnostic and may create draining fistulae or seed tumor cells. Although the salivary glands are superficial in location and are amenable to evaluation with numerous diagnostic techniques, the assessment of salivary gland dysfunction still presents many difficulties.

REFERENCES

1. Garrett JR: Adventures with autonomic nerves. Perspectives in salivary gland innervations. *Proc R Microscop Soc* 1982;17:242.
2. Baum BJ: Principles of saliva secretion. *Ann NY Acad Sci* 1993;694:17.
3. Turner RJ: Ion transport related to fluid secretion in salivary glands, in Vergona K (ed.): *The Biology of Salivary Glands.* Caldwell, NJ, Telford Press, 1993, p 105.
4. Helman J, Turner RJ, Fox PC, Baum BJ: ^{99m}Tc-pertechnetate uptake in parotid acinar cells by the $Na^+/K^+/Cl^-$ co-transport system. *J Clin Invest* 1987;79:1310.
5. Fox PC, Bodner L, Bowers MR, Baum BJ: Uptake and secretion of technetium pertechnetate by the rat parotid gland. *Comp Biochem Physiol* 1986;83A:579.
6. Kohn WG, Ship JA, Atkinson JC, Patton LL, Fox PC: Salivary gland ^{99m}Tc-scintigraphy: a grading scale and correlation with major salivary gland flow rates. *J Oral Pathol Med* 1992;21:70.
7. Atkinson JC, Fox PC: Salivary gland dysfunction. *Clin Geriatr Med* 1992;8:499.
8. Fox PC, Atkinson JC, Macynski AA, Wolff A, Kung DS, Jackson W, Delapenha RA, Shiroky J, Baum BJ: Pilocarpine treatment of salivary hypofunction and dry mouth (xerostomia). *Arch Intern Med* 1991;151:1149.
9. Grove AS, DiChiro G: Salivary gland scanning with technetium-99m pertechnetate. *Am J Roentgenol* 1968;102:109.
10. Abramson AL, Levy LM, Goodman M, Attie JN: Salivary gland scintiscanning with technetium-99m pertechnetate. *Laryngoscope* 1969;79:1105.
11. Fletcher MM, Workman JB: Salivary gland scintigrams in inflammatory disease. *Am Surg* 1969;35:765.
12. Schall GL, DiChiro G: Clinical usefulness of salivary gland scanning. *Semin Nucl Med* 1972;2:270.
13. Ohrt HJ, Shafer RB: An atlas of salivary gland disorders. *Clin Nucl Med* 1982;7:370.
14. van der Akker HP, Busemann-Skole E, van der Schoot JB: Origin and localization of the oral activity in sequential salivary scintigraphy with ^{99m}Tc-pertechnetate. *J Nucl Med* 1976; 17:959.
15. Schall GL, Larson SM, Anderson LG, Griffith JM: Quantification of parotid uptake of pertechnetate using a gamma scintillation camera and a "region of interest" system. *Am J Roentgenol* 1972;115:689.
16. Schall GL: The role of radionuclide scanning in the evaluation of neoplasms of the salivary glands: a review. *J Surg Oncol* 1971;3:699.
17. Daniels TE, Powell MR, Sylvester RA, Talal N: An evaluation of salivary scintigraphy in Sjögren's syndrome. *Arthritis Rheum* 1979;2:809.
18. Fox PC, van der Ven PF, Sonies BC, Weiffenbach JM, Baum BJ: Xerostomia: evaluation of a symptom with increasing significance. *J Am Dent Assoc* 1985;110:519.

23 The Heart

Section 1: Myocardial Perfusion Imaging

Frans J. Th. Wackers

Since the mid-1970s thallium-201 (^{201}Tl) has been widely used to image the heart and assess regional myocardial perfusion at rest and during exercise.[1–4] Because ^{201}Tl has less than optimum physical characteristics, substantial research has been directed toward developing ^{99m}Tc-labeled myocardial perfusion agents, better suited for imaging with conventional scintillation cameras. In recent years, the U.S. Food and Drug Administration (FDA) approved 2 new ^{99m}Tc-labeled myocardial perfusion imaging agents, ^{99m}Tc-sestamibi, which has rapidly gained wide acceptance,[5,6] and ^{99m}Tc-teboroxime, which is less widely used.[7,8] Although the ^{99m}Tc-labeled agents are better suited for imaging, they are not ideal. Because of the short residence time of ^{99m}Tc-teboroxime in the heart, adequate imaging is technically difficult. Furthermore, the occasionally intense, subdiaphragmatic activity of ^{99m}Tc-sestamibi poses a problem in interpreting images. Accordingly, a new generation of ^{99m}Tc-labeled agents with the potential of further improved imaging characteristics, such as tetrofosmine[9] and furifosmine[10] are currently under clinical evaluation.

IMAGING

Planar Imaging

Using conventional planar imaging, the relative distribution of a radiopharmaceutical is projected on images acquired from 3 different angles.[11] The configuration of the heart on such images depends on the amount of myocardial mass perpendicular to the camera face, regional myocardial uptake of radiopharmaceutical, and the effect of tissue attenuation (Fig. 1). The familiar horseshoe appearance of the heart on ^{201}Tl and ^{99m}Tc-sestamibi images is the result of (a) attenuation of radiation from the distant myocardial wall by the left ventricular blood pool, (b) the relatively low concentration of radiopharmaceutical in the blood pool and, (c) the relatively greater mass of walls perpendicular to the plane of view. The "left ventricular cavity" (center of the horseshoe) that appears to be visualized on planar images, is an illusion caused by fewer photons emanating from the facing left ventricular wall.

Single Photon Emission Tomography (SPECT Imaging)

In SPECT imaging, the scintillation camera rotates around the heart in a 180° arc.[12,13] While traveling through this orbit, multiple planar projections (usually 32) are obtained. After applying a filter to the raw projection images, back projection is performed to produce the images. Subsequently, further filtering and three-dimensional computer reconstruction is performed. Tomographic slices are reconstructed perpendicular to the anatomical axis of the heart itself: short axis slices, vertical long axis slices, and horizontal long axis slices.

As with planar imaging, SPECT images are affected by the relative distribution of radiopharmaceutical in the heart, as well as by the effect of radiation attenuation. The major advantage of SPECT imaging is that surrounding organs are separated in space from the heart, which allows more precise analysis of the regional distribution of radiopharmaceutical within the heart.

IMAGING TECHNIQUES

Planar Imaging

To acquire optimum planar myocardial perfusion images, careful attention to detail is required. The most frequent causes of suboptimum image quality are: (1) insufficient count density within the heart; (2) inconsistent patient positioning and repositioning; (3) the use of too large a zoom factor and, (4) inadequate display of images.[10]

COUNT DENSITY

At least 600,000 counts in the field of view should be collected for planar images (Fig. 2). When substantial extracardiac activity is present (e.g., increased lung uptake or subdiaphragmatic uptake), greater count density in the entire image is needed. Using the standard dose of 2.5 mCi (92 MBq) of ^{201}Tl, the acquisition time of planar images should be approximately 8 to 10 minutes per view. Using ^{99m}Tc-sestamibi, the dose ranges from 10 to 25 mCi (370 to 925 MBq). Each planar view should then be acquired for 5 minutes, accumulating 1.5 to 2 million counts per image.

PATIENT POSITIONING

Planar imaging is routinely performed in 3 projections (Fig. 3).[11] The left anterior oblique (LAO) projection or view is acquired with the patient lying supine. The camera face should be positioned so that the cardiac septum appears to

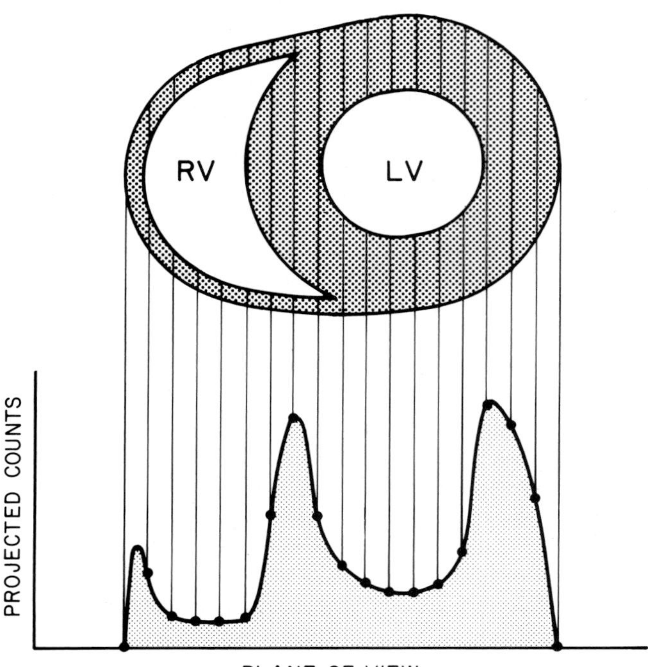

Figure 1. Schematic representation of the generation of a planar image. The projection of radioactivity on the planar view is demonstrated for the left anterior oblique projection (see text). (From Wackers FJTh: Thallium-201 myocardial imaging, in Wackers FJTh (ed): *Thallium-201 and Technetium-99m Pyrophosphate Myocardial Imaging in the Coronary Care Unit*. The Hague, Martinus Nijhoff, 1980, pp 70–104.)

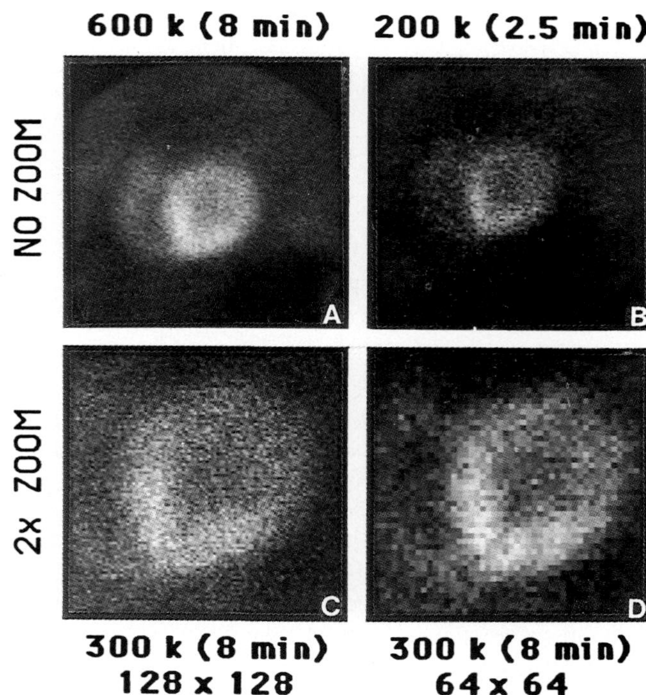

Figure 2. Effect of varying count density and zoom factor on image quality. LAO image of the same patient acquired in 4 different ways. **(A)** Optimal image: 600,000 counts were acquired over 8 min using a 128 × 128 matrix. Maximum count per pixel in the heart is 191. The heart occupies approximately 1/3 of the field of view. **(B)** Suboptimum image: because of the shorter acquisition time, only 200,000 counts are obtained in the field of view. The maximum count per pixel in the heart is only 65. **(C)** Acquisition with a 2X zoom factor: 128 × 128 matrix. Although the image was acquired over the same time as image **(A),** a lower count density is obtained in the field of view. The maximum count per pixel in the heart was only 52. This image is of suboptimum quality. **(D)** Acquisition with a 2X zoom factor: 64 × 64 matrix. Although the count per pixel is higher (159), the resulting coarse and "boxy" image is of unsatisfactory quality (from reference 11).

be vertical, with good separation between right and left ventricular cavities. The anterior view is obtained with the patient lying supine with the camera angled 45° to the right of the LAO projection. For the left lateral view, the patient is turned on the right side with the camera head in the same position as for the anterior view.[14] The detector head should be angulated so that it is as close as possible to the patient's chest wall. On all projections, the heart should lie in the center of the field of view. For delayed or rest imaging, the patient should be repositioned as close as possible to the exercise images.

ZOOM FACTOR

When a large-field-of-view camera is used, the zoom factor should not exceed 1.2 times (Fig. 2). On optimum planar images, the heart is approximately 1/3 to 1/4 the diameter of the field of view.

PLANAR IMAGE DISPLAY

The method of display of planar myocardial perfusion images is important for consistent interpretation. The images are preferably displayed white on black using a linear gray scale. The images should be normalized to the "hottest" pixel within the heart, so that the gray scale is utilized fully to represent relative count density in the heart. This is particularly important for images acquired with ^{99m}Tc agents, in which there may be substantial subdiaphragmatic activity, exceeding the count density within the heart (Fig. 4). Finally, exercise/rest or delayed images should be displayed side by side for comparison.

SPECT Imaging

Careful attention to technical details is even more important for SPECT than for planar imaging. The patient is positioned supine on the imaging table. The camera head rotates in a 180° arc around the patient, acquiring 32 stop images. For thallium imaging, each stop is usually 40 seconds. For imaging with sestamibi, each stop is either 20 seconds (high dose) or 30 seconds (low dose). Adequate count density is especially important for good quality SPECT imaging.

Patient positioning is also important in SPECT imaging. The most common cause of suboptimum SPECT images is *patient motion*. The patient should be lying comfortably on

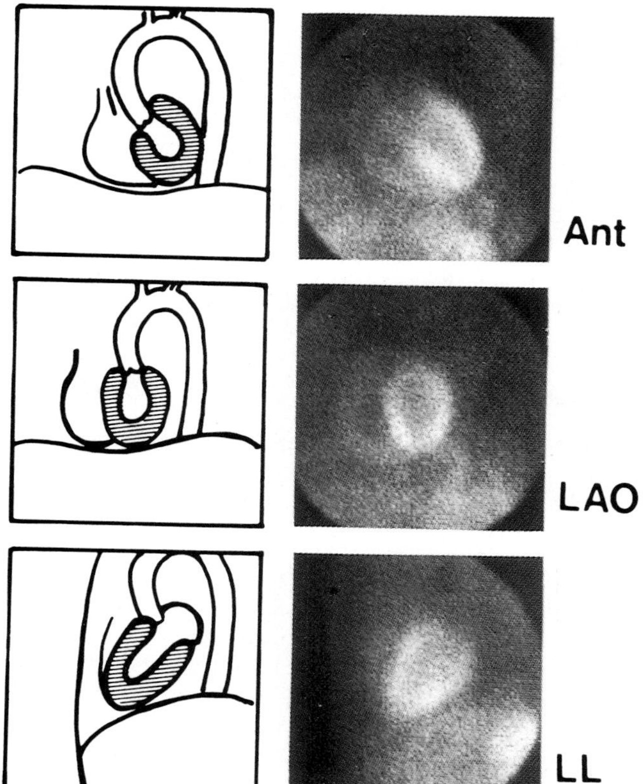

Figure 3. ^{201}Tl images in three planar projections of a normal subject. On the left schematic representations of cardiac anatomy. The left ventricle is well visualized, the right ventricle is only faintly visible. Accumulation of ^{201}Tl in the left ventricle is almost homogeneous. The central area of decreased activity is the left ventricular cavity. Ant, anterior; LAO, left anterior oblique; LL, left lateral (from reference 11).

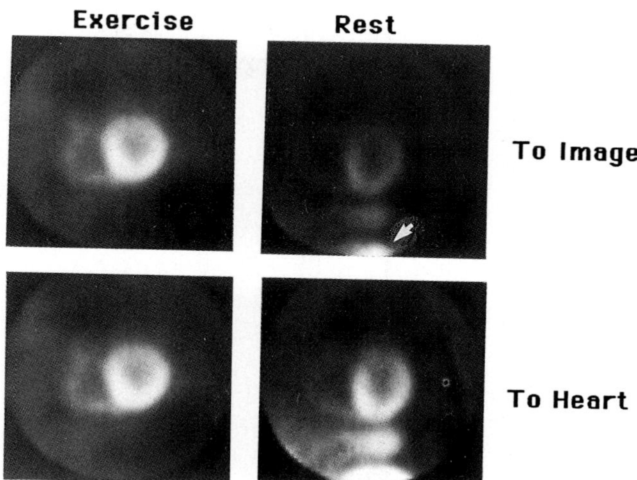

Figure 4. Normalization of exercise/rest ^{99m}Tc-sestamibi images. Intense subdiaphragmatic activity (arrow) may prevent adequate display of the heart image. Radionuclide images are usually normalized to the "hottest" area in the field of view. On the exercise sestamibi images, the heart is the "hottest" organ. However, on the rest image, the gastrointestinal tract is the "hottest" area (arrow). Consequently, when the rest image is normalized to subdiaphragmatic activity, the heart is only faintly visualized (top). Using ^{99m}Tc-labeled myocardial perfusion imaging agents, images should be normalized to the heart, as shown in the bottom panel (from reference 11).

the table with the arms over the head. Velcro straps may be helpful in immobilizing the patient. The phenomenon of "upward creep" has been observed after strenuous exercise. This can be minimized by *delaying* exercise SPECT imaging until 10 minutes after terminating exercise. The first 10 minutes may be utilized to acquire a *planar* anterior image to assess lung uptake.

TECHNICAL CONSIDERATIONS IN MYOCARDIAL PERFUSION IMAGING

Scintillation Camera

For planar imaging, a camera with a 10-inch diameter detector and a 1/4-inch thick crystal is preferred. Low-energy photons of ^{201}Tl do not adequately penetrate thicker crystals, which reduces count density. For tomographic imaging, cameras with a large field of view are used. These cameras usually have 3/8-inch thick crystals and, therefore, are less suited to ^{201}Tl imaging than to ^{99m}Tc imaging. Recently, multidetector camera systems have been introduced with advanced electronics and significantly improved sensitivity, resolution, and overall image quality. Although multihead systems permit shorter imaging times, it is more appropriate to take advantage of the higher counting statistics than shortening image acquisition time.

Collimation

For planar ^{201}Tl and sestamibi imaging, an all-purpose, parallel-hole collimator is used. Using ^{201}Tl for SPECT imaging, the all-purpose, parallel-hole collimator assures adequate count density. With ^{99m}Tc-labeled imaging agents, the count rate is sufficiently high to use a high-resolution, parallel-hole collimator for SPECT imaging.

Energy Window

For ^{201}Tl imaging, a dual window with a 25% window over the 80-keV x-ray peak and a 20% window over the 167-keV gamma peak is used. For ^{99m}Tc-labeled imaging agents, a single 20% window is placed over the 140-keV peak.

Computer Acquisition

Images should be acquired on computer disk or magnetic tape for data processing. For planar myocardial perfusion imaging, the acquisition is usually performed in 128 × 128 matrix; for tomographic imaging, a 64 × 64 matrix is most commonly used.

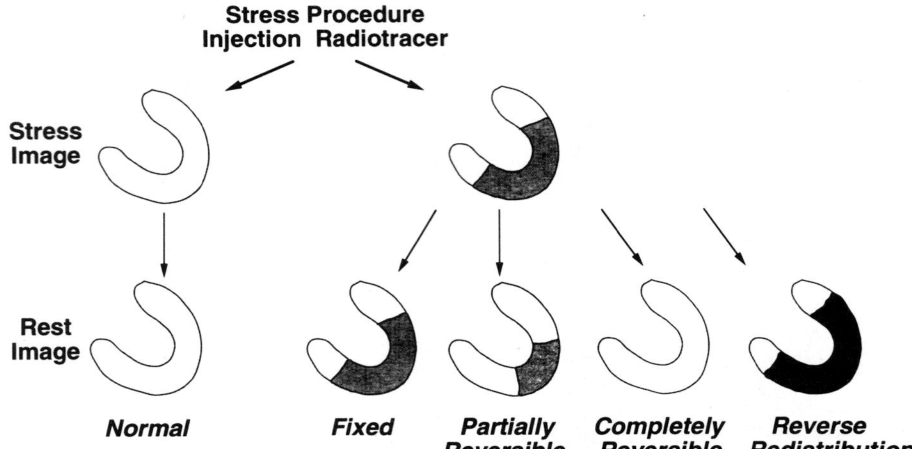

Figure 5. Schematic representation of myocardial perfusion defects (shaded areas) (from reference 25).

Imaging Protocol

For ^{201}Tl stress imaging, a single dose of ^{201}Tl (2.5 to 4.0 mCi) is injected at peak exercise. The patient should be encouraged to continue exercising for another 1 to 2 minutes. Stress imaging is started within 5 minutes after the injection. Delayed or redistribution imaging is usually performed 3 to 4 hours later. Other imaging protocols are discussed in the next section. For complete assessment of the presence of viable myocardium, a second injection of ^{201}Tl may be administered at rest in selected patients.

For myocardial perfusion imaging with ^{99m}Tc-sestamibi, 2 injections are given, 1 during exercise and a second at rest. Again, it is important that the patient continues to exercise for another 1 to 2 minutes after injection. Rest/exercise ^{99m}Tc-sestamibi imaging may be performed on 1 or 2 days. When a 1-day protocol is used, the first injection (usually at rest) is 10 mCi (370 MBq) of ^{99m}Tc-sestamibi, whereas the second injection during exercise is 25 mCi (925 MBq) of ^{99m}Tc-sestamibi. If the patient is imaged on 2 different days, 30 mCi (1.1 GBq) of sestamibi is administered on each day. In contrast to the ^{201}Tl imaging protocol, ^{99m}Tc-sestamibi exercise imaging is started 15 to 30 minutes after termination of exercise. After a resting injection of sestamibi a 60- to 90-minute delay is necessary before imaging can be started. These delays are necessary to allow for clearance of sestamibi from the liver.

Image Interpretation

Planar and SPECT images are interpreted qualitatively by visual analysis, often aided by computer quantification.

Images are usually characterized as follows (Fig. 5): (1) *normal*, homogeneous uptake of radiopharmaceutical throughout the myocardium. Quantitatively, the regional distribution of the radiopharmaceutical is within the range of the normal. (2) *defect*, a localized myocardial area with relatively decreased tracer uptake. Defects may vary in intensity from slightly reduced activity to almost total absence of activity. Quantitatively, defects are characterized as areas with less uptake than the lower limit of normal radiotracer distribution. The severity and intensity of the defect can be quantified relative to the lower limit of normal. (3) *reversible defect*, a defect that is present on the initial stress image and no longer present, or present to a lesser degree, on the resting or delayed image. This pattern indicates myocardial ischemia. The change of defects with time is termed "redistribution" using ^{201}Tl, and "reversibility" using sestamibi. (4) *fixed defects*, a defect is present and unchanged on both exercise and rest or delayed images. This pattern generally indicates infarction or scar tissue. However, some patients with fixed ^{201}Tl defects on the 3 to 4 hour delayed images may show improved uptake after resting reinjection of ^{201}Tl. (5) *reverse redistribution*, the initial stress images are either normal or show a defect, whereas the delayed or rest images show a more severe defect. This pattern is typically seen in patients who have a history of myocardial infarction and/or reperfusion of the infarct artery either by thrombolytic therapy or percutaneous transluminal coronary angioplasty. (6) *transient left ventricular dilation*, occasionally the left ventricle is noted to be larger following exercise than on the rest or delayed image. This pattern indicates severe exercise-induced left ventricular dysfunction. (7) *increased lung uptake* is a pattern typically observed using ^{201}Tl and, occasionally, using ^{99m}Tc-sestamibi. Normally no, or very little, uptake of radiopharmaceutical is noted in the lungs and its presence on exercise images is markedly abnormal. Increased lung uptake can be quantified as lung/heart ratio (normal <0.5). This abnormal pattern indicates exercise-induced left ventricular dysfunction.

Image Quantification

Visual interpretation of myocardial perfusion images has considerable inter- and intraobserver variability, even among experienced readers. Quantification of images is a means to reduce this variability. Quantification should consist of (1) graphic display of relative count distribution and, (2) a normal reference database.

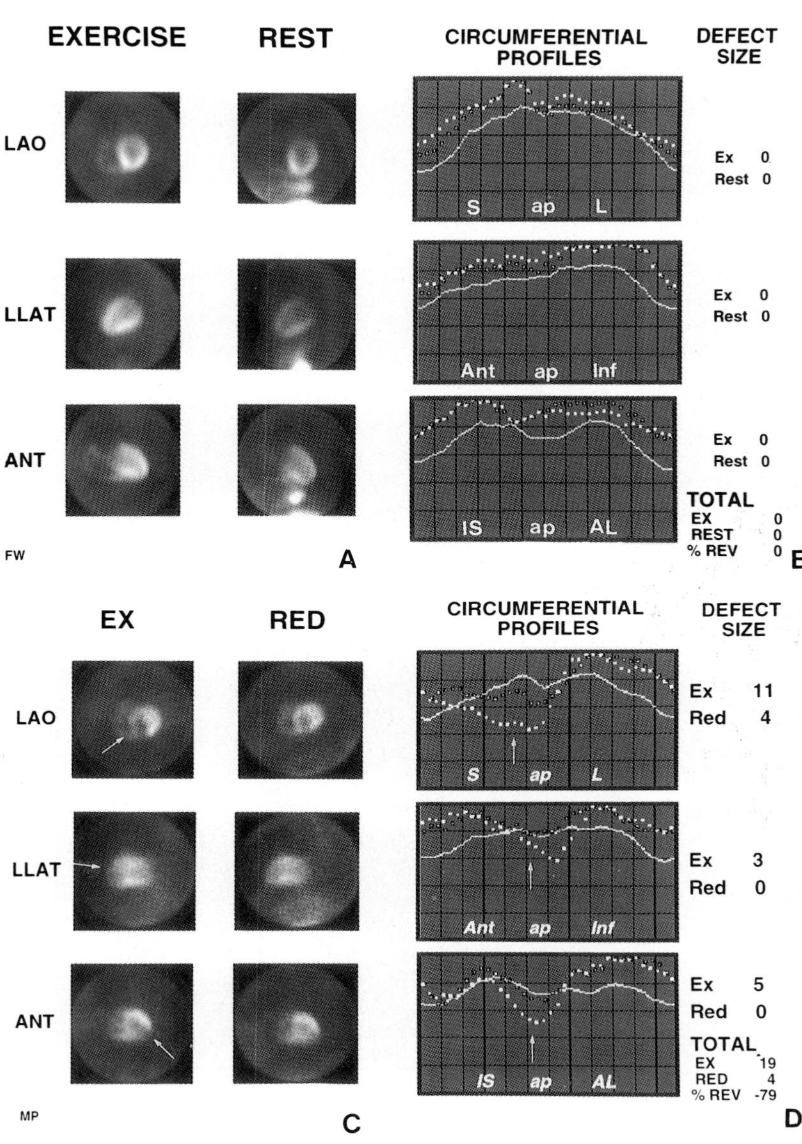

Figure 6. (A), (B). Normal planar quantitative myocardial perfusion imaging with ^{99m}Tc-sestamibi. **(A).** The images on the left are normal: no myocardial perfusion defects on exercise or rest images. **(B).** The relative distribution of counts is quantified as circumferential profiles on the right. The large white dots represent the exercise image; the small white dots represent the resting image. On all 3 views, all data points are above the lower limit of normal (white line). **(C), (D).** Planar quantitative myocardial perfusion imaging with ^{201}Tl in the patient with a reversible anteroseptal myocardial perfusion defect. **(C).** The image on the left shows a myocardial perfusion defect in the inferoseptal and anteroapical and apical area (arrows) with substantial improvement on the redistribution images. **(D).** Circumferential profiles at the right show the graphic display of an almost completely reversible defect. Abbreviations: Ant, anterior wall; AL, anterolateral wall; ap, apex; IS, inferoseptal wall; Inf, inferior wall; S, septal wall; L, lateral wall.

QUANTIFICATION OF PLANAR IMAGES

For quantification of planar images, background correction is necessary to account for differences in background activity on exercise and delayed or rest images. Background correction is performed by creating an interpolative background image that is subtracted from the original raw images. Subsequently, the relative distribution of myocardial uptake of radiopharmaceutical can be displayed as *circumferential count profiles*.[15] These profiles are displayed simultaneously with a lower-limit-of-normal radiotracer distribution, derived from normal subjects with low likelihood of coronary artery disease (Fig. 6). Usually, mean minus 2 standard deviations is used as a lower-limit-of-normal distribution on planar images. Defect size and defect reversibility can be quantified in a reproducible manner.

QUANTIFICATION OF SPECT IMAGING

SPECT imaging creates a set of multiple images (Fig. 7).[12,13] Typically, an exercise and rest SPECT study is displayed as 25 to 40 paired slices. For quantification of SPECT images, usually short axis slices are used. The relative count distribution on the short axis images can be displayed as concentric color coded rings around the apex, creating a "*polar map*" or "*bull's eye*" display (Fig. 7). The relative distribution of count activity can, thus, be related to a normal database. Areas that are lower than normal can be coded as "blackout" regions. These defects can also be quantified in terms of extent and severity. As with planar imaging, the relative count distribution of the short axis slices can be displayed as *circumferential count profiles* and superimposed on a lower limit of normal. The advantage of dis-

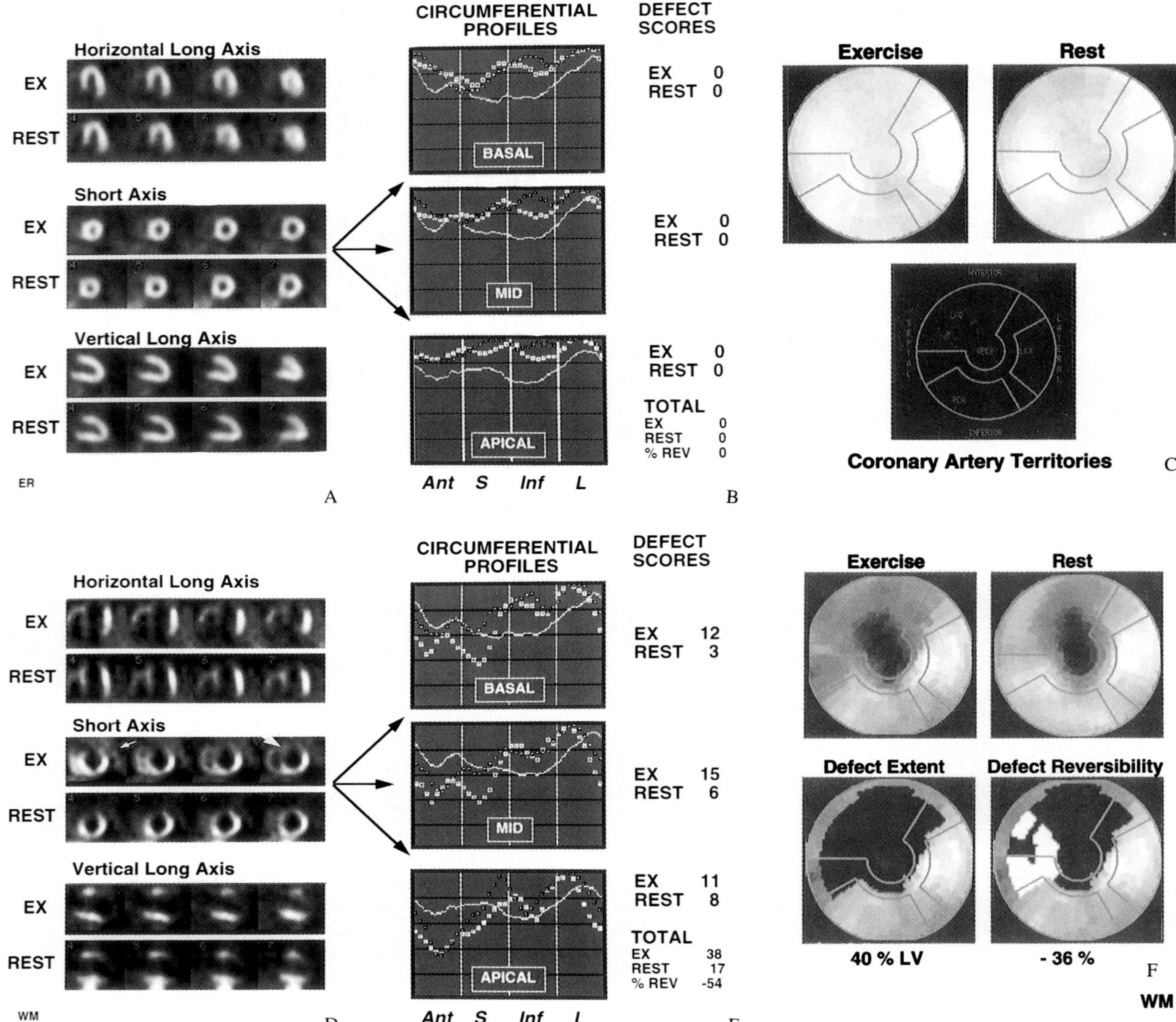

Figure 7. (A), (B). Quantitative SPECT myocardial perfusion imaging with ^{99m}Tc-sestamibi in a normal subject. **(A).** The images (left) are normal. **(B).** All short axis slices are quantified using circumferential profile analysis. Quantification of 3 representative apical, midventricular, and basal slices is shown (right). The exercise profile (large white dots) and rest profile (small dots) are displayed normalized to the area with maximum activity and compared to lower-limit-of-normal distribution (white curve). In this example of a normal subject, all data points are above the lower limit of normal. Defect scores are tabulated at the far right (from reference 11). **(C).** Bull's eye or polar map display of normal SPECT images in **(A), (B).** The coronary artery territories are shown. **(D).** High-risk quantitative SPECT myocardial perfusion imaging with ^{99m}Tc-sestamibi. The images (left) show post-exercise dilation on short axis slices and increased lung uptake (small arrow). There is a partially reversible (basal and midventricular) anteroseptal myocardial perfusion defect (arrow). **(E).** This is confirmed by quantitative circumferential profile analysis. The defect is large (total integral: 38) with 54% defect reversibility. **(F).** Polar map display of exercise and rest images. The defect is in shades of blue and red. Defect extent (40% LV) is indicated in black; defect reversibility (36%) in white (from reference 11). (See Plate 30.)

playing circumferential profiles is that the graphic display can be related directly to the images. In contrast, the "bull's eye" or "polar map" display is a *summarizing image* that is more difficult to relate to the original images. Moreover, artifacts are more difficult to recognize on *polar map* display.

NORMAL VARIATIONS ON PLANAR AND SPECT IMAGING

Interpretation of planar and SPECT imaging cannot be performed without an understanding of the normal patterns and variations of perfusion images.[11,16]

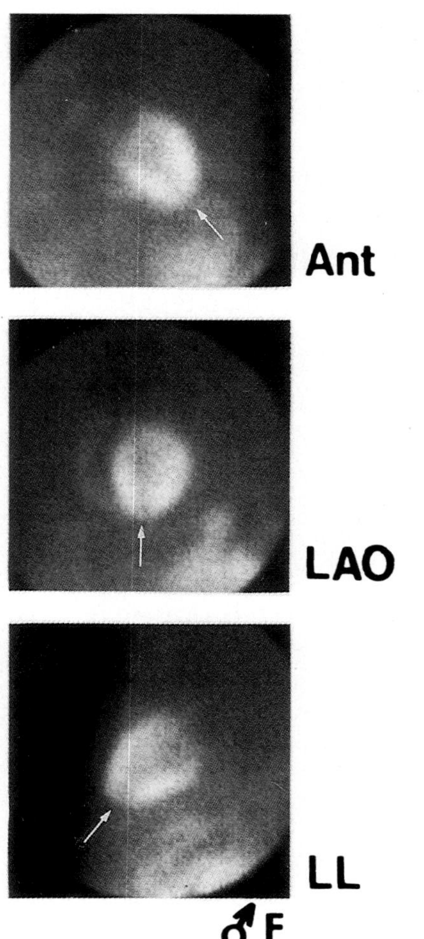

Figure 8. Apical thinning. Planar ^{201}Tl image of a subject with normal apical thinning (*arrows*), best appreciated in the LAO and LL projections, although it is also present in the anterior projection. Note that this cleft-like defect is aligned with the long axis of the heart (from reference 11).

A well-known normal variation on planar myocardial perfusion images is that of *apical thinning* (Fig. 8). This is a narrow slit-like area of diminished activity at the apex. An apical normal variant can be identified as being relatively small and being aligned along the long axis of the left ventricle. True apical myocardial perfusion defects (caused by coronary artery disease) typically extend from the apex in either the anterior wall or inferior wall. Apical variants can be seen on both ^{201}Tl and ^{99m}Tc-sestamibi planar images.

On LAO planar images, the heart appears as a horseshoe or a doughnut-like structure. The open end of the horseshoe is the base of the heart with aortic and mitral valve planes.

On the anterior and left lateral planar images, slightly less accumulation of radiopharmaceutical in the inferior wall and the inferoseptal wall is a normal variant. On planar sestamibi imaging, a typical variant may occur on the left lateral images. Due to scatter from subdiaphragmatic radioactivity into the inferior wall, the anterior wall may appear to have significantly less activity, mimicking a defect.

On SPECT imaging, normal variations of tracer uptake occur as well (Fig. 9). Uptake of radiopharmaceutical in the septal area is *frequently* less than in the lateral wall. Furthermore, the inferior wall may have apparently less uptake than the septum, anterior, and lateral walls due to the diaphragmatic attenuation. Finally, the most basal portion of the septum on the short axis slices may have a definite septal defect that represents the membranous septum. For the same reason, the septum is shorter than the lateral wall on horizontal long slices.

ARTIFACTS COMMON TO PLANAR AND SPECT IMAGING

Diaphragmatic Attenuation

Artifacts due to attenuation of radiation emanating from the heart may occur on both planar and SPECT images.[16] A notorious artifact on planar imaging is attenuation of activity in the inferior wall on *supine* steep (70°) LAO images.[14] When a patient is imaged in the supine position, such artifactual defects occur in approximately 20% of patients (Fig. 10). These artifacts can be avoided by turning the patient into a *right-side-down decubitus* position. Not surprisingly, inferior wall attenuation defects can also be seen on SPECT imaging, which is usually performed in the supine position. Slightly decreased uptake in the inferior wall on the short axis slices and on the vertical long axis slices should be considered normal variants. Recently, SPECT imaging in a different position (either prone or upright) has been proposed as a means of avoiding, or at least minimizing, inferior wall attenuation artifacts.

Breast Artifacts

Attenuation of radiation by overlying (breast) tissue occurs frequently in obese patients and in patients with large breasts.[11,16] On planar imaging, such attenuation can cause artifactual defects in the upper septum and/or upper lateral wall on the LAO view, and apparent anterior and anterolateral perfusion defects on the left lateral and anterior views (Fig. 11). On SPECT images, artifactual defects can be observed in the anterior area. One would expect that breast attenuation artifacts occur in all women with large breasts. Unfortunately, breast attenuation cannot be predicted from the patient's weight or bra size. The degree of radiation attenuation is extremely variable among patients. Furthermore, one would expect that such breast attenuation artifacts are fixed (i.e., the same on both the exercise and rest study). This is not the case. The breast may shift in position relative to the heart and cause different artifacts when repeat imaging is performed. To recognize breast artifacts, one can use radioactive line sources to outline the contour of the breast. This is particularly helpful in planar imaging. Alternatively, one can flatten the breast against the chest using a wide strap. In SPECT imaging, the best means of recognizing breast attenuation is to inspect

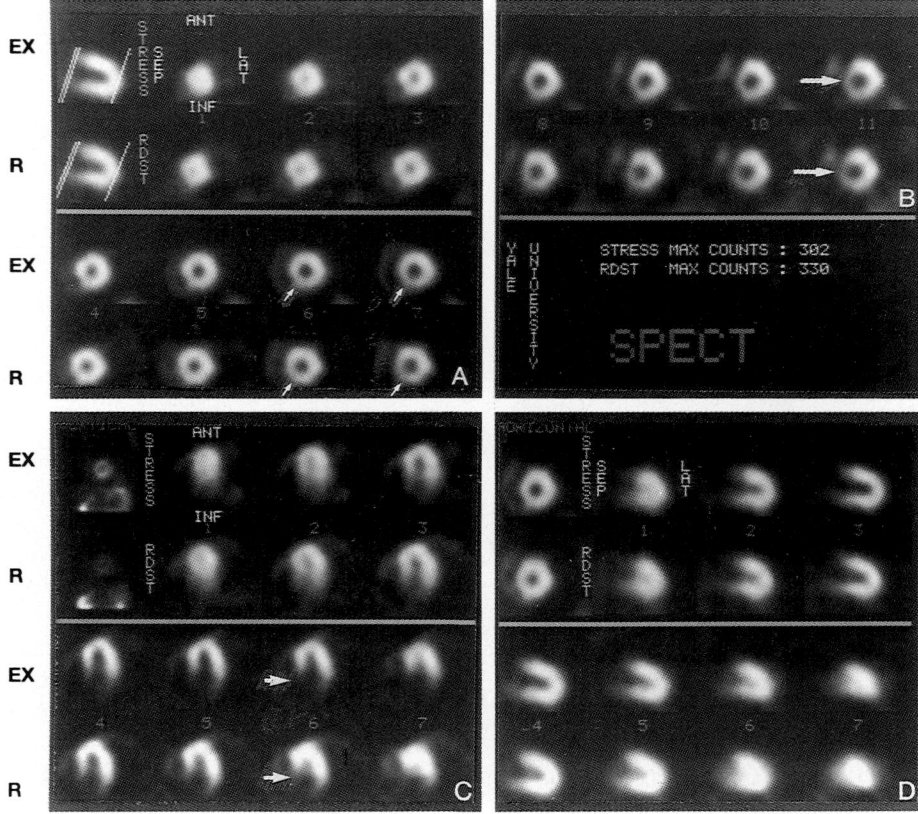

Figure 9. SPECT ^{99m}Tc-sestamibi myocardial images after exercise and at rest in a normal subject, showing normal variations of radiopharmaceutical distribution. On the midventricular short axis slices **(A)** the inferior septal areas (small arrows) have slightly less activity than the lateral wall. This is a normal variation. The hottest area is in the lateral wall. On the basal slices **(B)** an apparent septal defect is present (large arrow). This is the membranous portion of the septum. This "septal defect" and normal variation is also seen in the horizontal long axis slices **(C)** where the septum is shorter (arrow) than the lateral wall. Vertical long axis slices. are shown in **(D)** (from reference 16).

the cine display of the rotating planar projection images, where breast attenuation appears as a shadow moving over the heart.

Artifacts Specific for SPECT Imaging

Artifacts are particularly troublesome with SPECT imaging.[15] They are frequently difficult to recognize after tomographic reconstruction has been performed. Careful analysis of the rotating planar projection images is an essential step in quality control *before interpretation*. From the cine display, the overall quality of the image can be judged. The rotating images should be checked for the following: (1) Is there motion? This can consist of either *patient motion* (e.g., a sudden change in position on the imaging table), or it can

Figure 10. Vertical long axis ^{201}Tl SPECT images of the same patient. Images acquired with the patient lying on his back (supine) are shown in the top panel. An inferior wall myocardial perfusion defect is present (arrow). The patient was turned on the right side (lateral) and SPECT imaging was repeated. This time, the vertical long axis images are normal. The erroneous inferior wall artifact on supine imaging is caused by attenuation by the left hemidiaphragm. Turning the patient on the right side diminishes diaphragmatic attenuation (from reference 16).

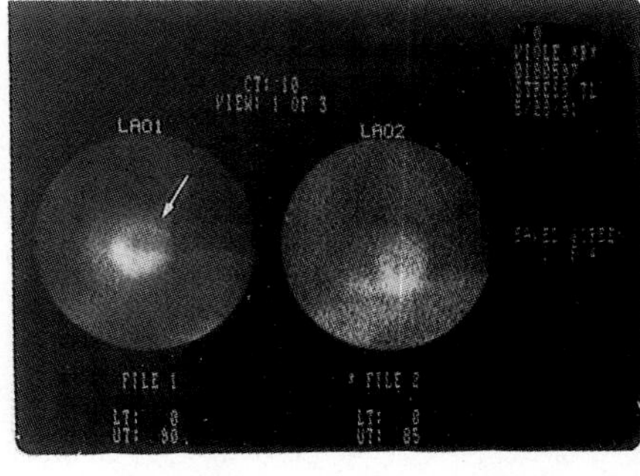

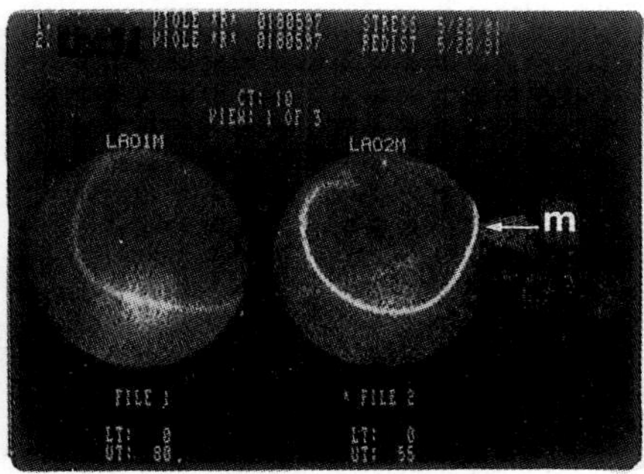

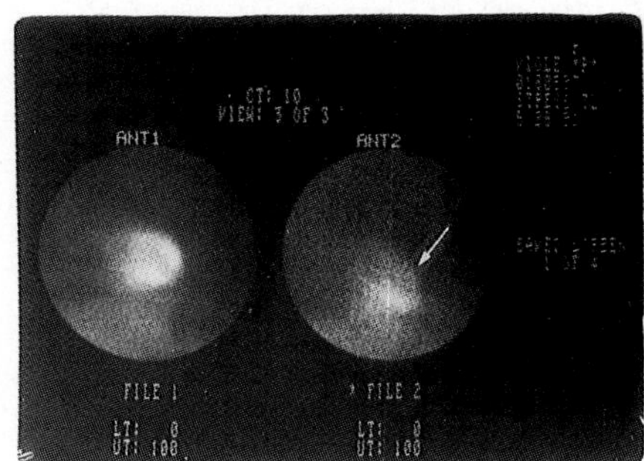

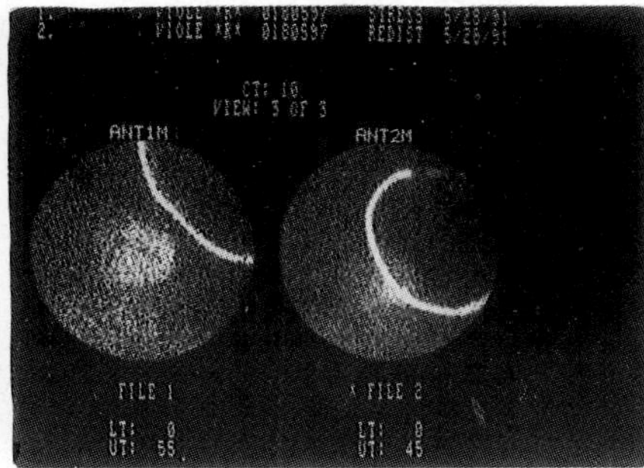

Figure 11. Planar ^{201}Tl LAO and anterior images in a woman with large breasts (LAO1, ANT1, exercise images; LAO2, ANT2, delayed images). The breasts are marked with radioactive line markers (m) in the images on the right. On the LAO exercise images (top), a definite attenuation artifact is present (arrow). At delayed imaging, the breast contour is lower and is visualized as a linear area (arrow) with increased activity due to "small-angle scatter." The exercise anterior view (bottom) is normal, because the breast did not cover the heart. However, at delayed imaging, the contour of the breast is across the heart, causing an attenuation artifact (arrow). This is an example of how breast attenuation artifacts can vary in the same view due to different breast positions. Note that on the delayed LAO image, unequal attenuation mimics an image with increased lung uptake of ^{201}Tl (from reference 16).

be a slow shift in the *position of the heart* (i.e., from a vertical to a more horizontal position, "upward creep"). Motion and upward creep can cause serious artifacts on the reconstructed images. (2) It is important to assess whether the heart is in the center of the camera orbit. When the heart is in the center of acquisition orbit, the heart "pivots" in the center of the image. When the heart is eccentric in the orbit, the heart "runs" across the field of view, from one side to the other, causing small defects located on the short axis slices at the 11 o'clock and 6 o'clock positions (Fig. 12). They are most frequently seen in the short axis *apical* slices. Another recently described artifact on reconstructed SPECT slices may be noted in patients with intense subdiaphragmatic radiotracer uptake. Back projection may cause an apparent myocardial defect adjacent to intense extracardiac activity (Fig. 13).

Artifacts are plentiful in both planar and SPECT images. Artifacts are somewhate easier to recognize in planar imaging than on reconstructed SPECT slices.

COMPARISON OF ^{201}THALLIUM AND ^{99m}TECHNETIUM AGENTS

The problems and artifacts described above are, to a great extent, related to the low-energy background scatter and relatively low count density typical of ^{201}Tl. The newly developed ^{99m}Tc-labeled myocardial perfusion imaging agents,

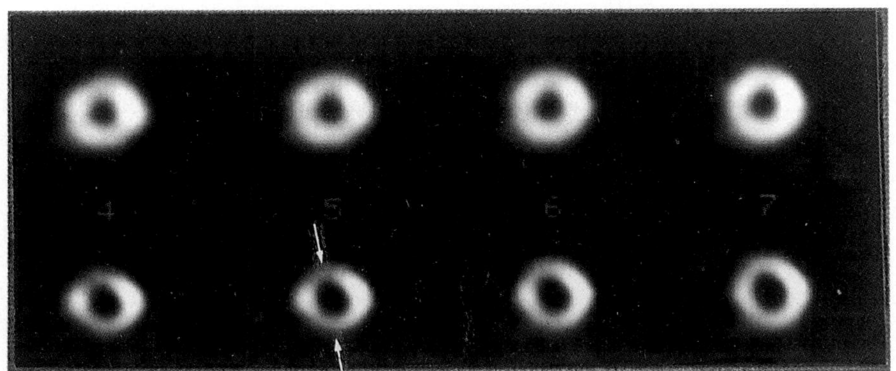

Figure 12. Effect of gamma camera orbit. Short axis SPECT slices using a circular orbit (i.e., the heart is in the center of rotation of the camera head) are shown (top). The images are normal. Short axis SPECT slices using a body contour orbit are shown in bottom panel. Varying spatial resolution causes a typical artifact of 180° diametrical defects (arrow) (from reference 16).

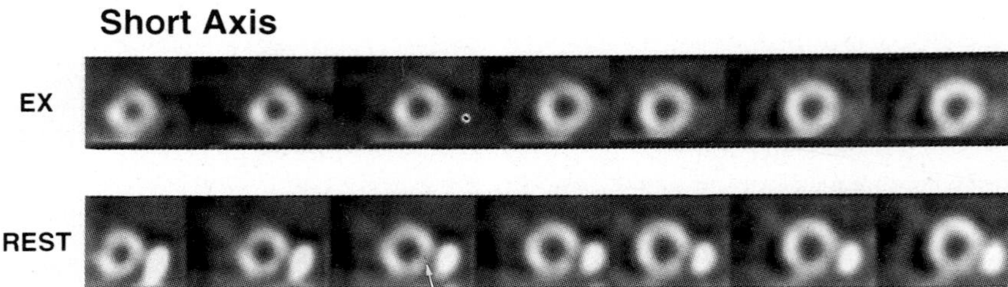

Figure 13. SPECT reconstruction artifact due to intense hepatic and intestinal activity. Exercise/rest short-axis ^{99m}Tc-sestamibi SPECT images in patient with intense bowel activity at rest. The exercise (EX) images are normal. The septum on the EX image is relatively "hot" due to hypertrophy in this patient with hypertension. The resting images show intense uptake adjacent to the inferior lateral wall. Filtered back projection using a standard Butterworth filter causes an artifactual defect in the inferior lateral wall (arrow). In patients with intense activity adjacent to the heart, the filter should be adjusted (from reference 11).

such as ^{99m}Tc-sestamibi, overcome some of these problems.[5] The relatively high dose (25 to 30 mCi) and favorable energy (140 keV) of ^{99m}Tc result in images with better count statistics, improved image resolution, and less low energy background scatter than with ^{201}Tl images. Because of significantly improved image quality, interpretation of sestamibi images is generally easier, and can be performed with greater confidence than that of ^{201}Tl images. Unfortunately, some tissue attenuation also occurs with ^{99m}Tc-labeled agents. The tissue attenuation factor of ^{99m}Tc is only 1/7 less than that of ^{201}Tl.

The most important cause for improved image quality using ^{99m}Tc-sestamibi is the relative high count density. As a result, sestamibi images can be described as being crisper and less grainy than ^{201}Tl images. In particular, for SPECT imaging the development of sestamibi signifies a major improvement in image quality. On the other hand, ^{99m}Tc-sestamibi images also have drawbacks. Resting dipyridamole sestamibi images have substantial diaphragmatic activity which, at times, may interfere with image interpretation.[16] This is particularly true for planar imaging, where superimposition of extracardiac radioactivity cannot be avoided. However, SPECT images, intense subdiaphragmatic activity adjacent to the heart may give problems with interpretation of the inferior wall.

STRESS MODALITIES WITH MYOCARDIAL PERFUSION IMAGING

Myocardial perfusion imaging is most often performed in conjunction with physical stress, using either treadmill or bicycle exercise. Stress testing is usually performed employing a graded protocol, in which the workload is increased every 3 minutes until the patient reaches an exercise endpoint, such as severe fatigue, severe angina, ventricular arrhythmias, or decreased blood pressure. The majority of patients referred to a nuclear imaging laboratory are able to perform physical exercise. However, in approximately 25% of patients, because of neurological, orthopedic, or peripheral vascular problems, physical exercise may not be an option. In these patients, *pharmacological vasodilation* with dipyridamole can be used as an alternative stress method.[17–19] The mechanism of action in brief is as follows: dipyridamole blocks the reabsorption of endogenous adenosine, causing increased serum levels of adenosine and vasodilation of the coronary resistance vasculature (Fig. 14). If a hemodynami-

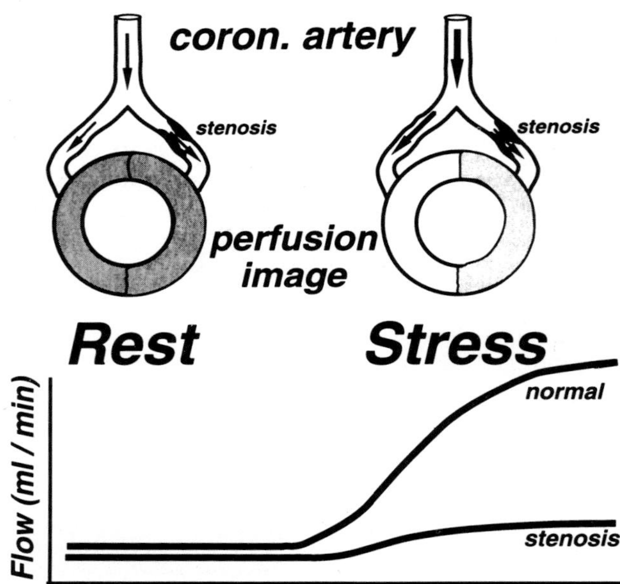

Figure 14. Schematic representation of the principle of rest/stress myocardial perfusion imaging. (top) Two branches of a coronary artery are schematically shown, the left branch is normal, the right branch has a significant stenosis. Myocardial perfusion images of the territories supplied by the two branches. (bottom) Schematic representation of coronary blood flow in the branches at rest and during stress. At rest, myocardial blood flow is similar in both coronary artery branches. When a myocardial perfusion imaging agent is injected at rest, myocardial uptake is homogenous (normal image). During stress, coronary blood flow increases 2.0 to 2.5 times in the normal branch, but not to the same extent in the stenosed branch, resulting in heterogenous distribution of blood flow. This heterogeneity of blood flow can be visualized with ^{201}Tl or ^{99m}Tc-sestamibi as an area with relatively decreased radiotracer uptake (myocardial perfusion defect). (From Wackers FJTh: Exercise myocardial perfusion imaging, *J Nucl Med* 1994;35: 726.)

cally significant stenosis is present, the distal coronary resistance vessels have already dilated and no further dilation can occur by dipyridamole. In contrast, the distal blood flow of normal coronary arteries increases by dipyridamole 3 to 4 times. This creates a *heterogeneity* of regional myocardial blood flow that is detected with myocardial perfusion imaging. Recently adenosine has been used for the same purpose. Adenosine has the advantage of a very short half-life of approximately 30 seconds. In contrast, the effect of dipyridamole may last for 20 to 30 minutes. Pharmacological vasodilation is not true myocardial stress testing because metabolic demand is not increased.

An alternative stress modality recently introduced is that of dobutamine infusion.[20,21] Dobutamine is a B1 agonist and a true myocardial stressor. Dobutamine increases heart rate and blood pressure, and increases metabolic demand. As with physical exercise, there is a secondary increase in blood flow that can be visualized with myocardial perfusion imaging. In most laboratories, dobutamine stress is reserved for patients who have contraindications to dipyridamole, such as patients with severe chronic obstructive lung disease and bronchospasm.

Pharmacological stress testing is as efficient as exercise imaging for detecting coronary artery disease. However, a disadvantage is that important functional information derived from physical exercise is not obtained.

CLINICAL APPLICATIONS OF MYOCARDIAL PERFUSION IMAGING

Chronic Coronary Artery Disease

During the late 1970s and early 1980s, myocardial perfusion imaging in conjunction with stress testing was used mainly to evaluate patients suspected of having coronary artery disease. Numerous studies have documented the clinical accuracy of myocardial perfusion imaging, both with ^{201}Tl[11] and the newer ^{99m}Tc-labeled myocardial perfusion imaging agents, such as ^{99m}Tc-sestamibi,[5,6,22] ^{99m}Tc-tetrofosmine,[9] and ^{99m}Tc-furifosmine.[10] The sensitivity and specificity of planar ^{201}Tl imaging using visual analysis alone was reported to be approximately 80 and 90%. Using computer quantification of planar images, the overall detection of coronary artery disease improved to over 90%, without loss of specificity.[15,23,24] The sensitivity of SPECT imaging for the detection of coronary artery disease has been reported to be better than 90%, with either ^{201}Tl or ^{99m}Tc-sestamibi.[25] On the other hand, the specificity of SPECT imaging was observed to be relatively low, ranging from 60 to 70%. The apparent decrease in specificity of SPECT imaging can be explained by referral bias (i.e., only patients with abnormal myocardial perfusion imaging are referred for cardiac catheterization). Thus, the occasional patient with angiographically normal coronary arteries is usually referred because of abnormal myocardial perfusion stress imaging. With both ^{201}Tl and ^{99m}Tc-sestamibi imaging the *normalcy rate*, that is the rate of normal studies in subjects with $<$5% likelihood of coronary artery disease, is 90% or better.

A major advantage of SPECT over planar imaging is the ability to separate coronary territories in space without overlap. When both planar and SPECT techniques are applied to the same patient, SPECT has been shown to have a slight, but definite, superiority over planar imaging.[26] However, SPECT is far more demanding than planar imaging, both in acquisition and interpretation. One must be constantly aware of the possibility of artifacts.

Prognosis of patients with coronary artery disease

There is extensive evidence in the literature that the more severe the myocardial perfusion abnormality, the more severe angiographic coronary artery disease is present. Moreover, the more abnormal myocardial perfusion images are, the poorer the prognosis and the greater the incidence of the future coronary events (i.e., nonfatal myocardial infarction and/or death).[27,28]

Abundant reports have been published with regard to the prognostic value of planar imaging. In recent years, also, similar prognostic information has been reported for SPECT imaging.[29] Because the extent of a perfusion abnormality is directly related to a patient's prognosis, quantification of myocardial perfusion images is important.[13,30] High-risk myocardial perfusion images, associated with poor prognosis can be characterized by (1) multiple reversible defects; (2) large defects; (3) increased lung uptake of ^{201}Tl, or transient left ventricular dilatation after exercise.[24] Iskandrian et al.[29] demonstrated that SPECT ^{201}Tl imaging, moreover, has independent and incremental prognostic value over the other diagnostic modalities, including cardiac catheterization.

On the other hand, normal ^{201}Tl or sestamibi planar or SPECT images, even if angiographic coronary artery disease is present, indicate extremely good and favorable prognosis.[31,32]

SELECTION OF PATIENTS FOR MYOCARDIAL PERFUSION IMAGING

For the detection of coronary artery disease, myocardial perfusion imaging should not be used in patients with *very high* or *very low likelihood* of disease. In these conditions, the results of perfusion imaging are not likely to make a significant contribution to overall patient evaluation. In contrast, it is in the group of patients with an intermediate (30 to 60%) likelihood of coronary disease that myocardial perfusion imaging can make a substantial difference in patient management. Furthermore, myocardial perfusion imaging is useful in patients with a recent coronary event, such as recent myocardial infarction,[33] or in patients who had a recent change in clinical symptoms. Myocardial perfusion imaging is also valuable in patients who are to undergo noncardiac surgery.[34] On the other hand, myocardial perfusion imaging is not very useful in *stable patients* with known chronic coronary artery disease. In such patients, the coro-

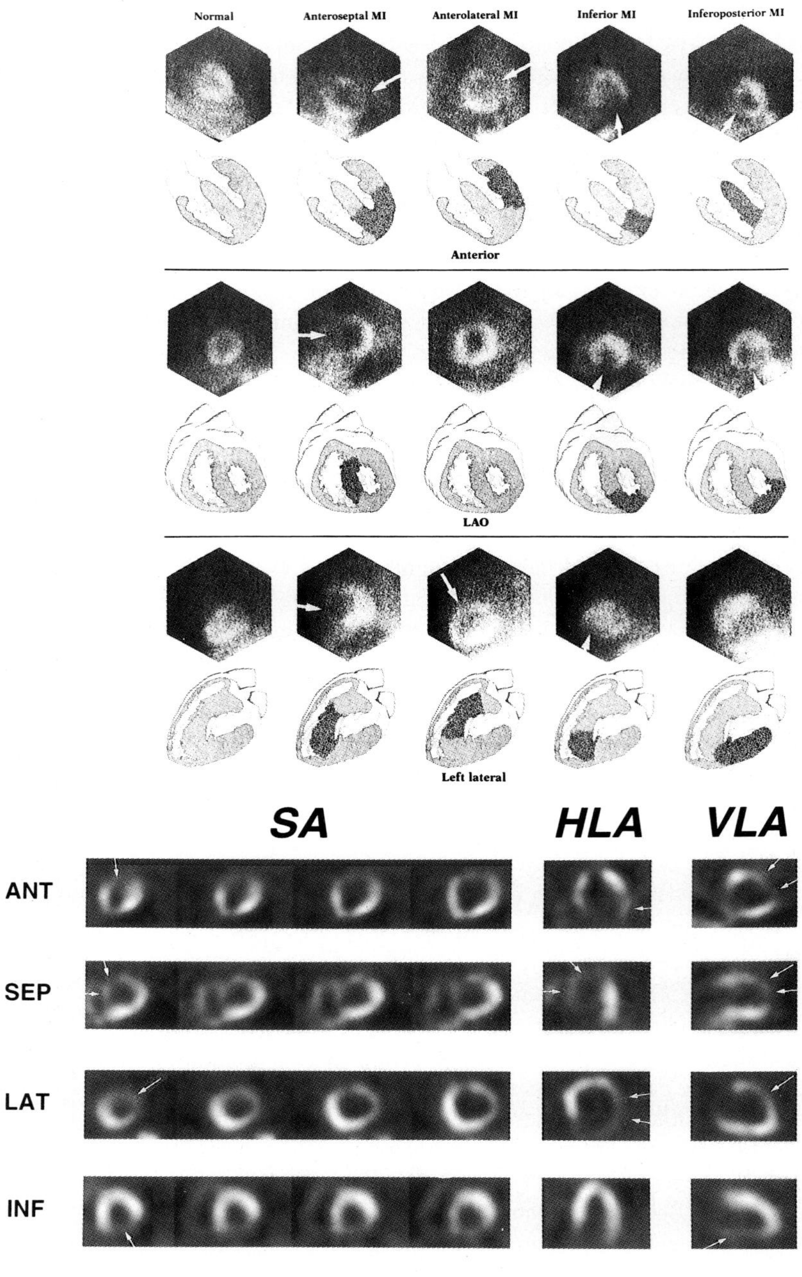

Figure 15. (A). Planar ^{201}Tl images of acute myocardial infarction. Typical planar ^{201}Tl images of acute myocardial infarction in three projections: anterior (top panel), left anterior oblique (LAO) (middle panel), and left lateral (lower panel). The first column shows normal planar ^{201}Tl images. The second to fourth columns show abnormal planar ^{201}Tl images with defects (arrows) caused by acute myocardial infarction. Shown are examples of acute anteroseptal, anterolateral, inferior, and inferoposterior myocardial infarctions. Schematic representations of the infarcted area are shown on the diagrams below each ^{201}Tl image. (Modified from Wackers FJTh, Busemann Sokole E, Samson G, van der Schoot JB, Lie KI, Liem KL, Wellens HJJ: Value and limitations of thallium-201 scintigraphy in the acute phase of myocardial infarction. *N Engl J Med* 1976;295:1. **(B).** SPECT ^{99m}Tc-sestamibi images of acute myocardial infarction. Typical ^{99m}Tc-sestamibi SPECT images of acute myocardial infarction, in short axis (SA) horizontal long axis (HLA) and vertical (VLA) slices. From top to bottom: anterior (ANT), anteroseptal (SEP), lateral (LAT) and inferior (INF) infarctions. Defects are indicated by arrows (from reference 11).

nary event rate is low and the predictive value of myocardial perfusion imaging is limited.[35]

Myocardial Perfusion Imaging After Coronary Angioplasty

A substantial number of patients (20 to 40%) have restenosis after successful angioplasty. Myocardial perfusion imaging is an effective method of detecting restenosis, even in the absence of symptoms. Some investigators have suggested that imaging early after the performance of angioplasty is not useful because images may still be abnormal.[36] Others, however, have shown that even early after coronary angioplasty, myocardial perfusion imaging is highly predictive of coronary restenosis.[37] In our experience, most patients with successful angioplasty have normal stress myocardial perfusion images in the first 2 to 5 days after the procedure.

Myocardial Perfusion Imaging in Acute Ischemic Syndromes

UNSTABLE ANGINA

In patients with unstable angina, without prior myocardial infarction, resting myocardial perfusion imaging can document objectively the presence of resting hypoperfusion and ischemia.[38] In these patients, ^{201}Tl or ^{99m}Tc-sestamibi may be injected at rest either *during* pain or *shortly after* pain. Using ^{201}Tl, imaging should be performed immediately after injection and again approximately 4 hours later. The early image may demonstrate resting hypoperfusion, whereas the 4-hour delayed image visualizes the total extent of viable myocardium. Using sestamibi, 2 injections may be necessary: 1 during or immediately after chest pain, and a second one when the patient is pain-free. Bilodeau et al.[39] have demonstrated that myocardial perfusion imaging with sestamibi in this clinical setting is highly sensitive and specific for the presence of significant coronary artery disease on subsequent coronary angiography. Myocardial perfusion imaging in patients with unstable angina is clinically useful because it provides a means to *objectively visualize* the presence of ischemia. In many patients, this may not be obvious from clinical observation alone. The electrocardiogram is rather insensitive under these circumstances.

ACUTE MYOCARDIAL INFARCTION

Radionuclide myocardial perfusion imaging is a sensitive and reliable method for visualizing acute myocardial infarction (Fig. 15).[40] During the early hours (within 6 hours) of onset of chest pain, almost all patients will have perfusion abnormalities, irrespective of the presence of either Q-wave or non-Q-wave infarcts. Consequently, myocardial perfusion imaging has potential value as a means of triaging patients with chest pain in the emergency department.[41] Recent data in limited numbers of patients suggest that it is feasible to distinguish between patients who have true ongoing myocardial ischemia and those who have not.[42] Furthermore, the presence or absence of myocardial perfusion defects at the time of presentation in the emergency department was predictive of subsequent cardiac events.

Myocardial perfusion imaging in patients with acute myocardial infarct reliably documents the location and extent of myocardial infarction. Quantification of defect size also has prognostic significance.[43,44] ^{99m}Tc-sestamibi has been used to document the area at risk and the amount of salvage by thrombolytic therapy of patients with acute myocardial infarction.[45] For this purpose, ^{99m}Tc-sestamibi is administered *prior* to initiation of thrombolytic therapy and *again after* completion of therapy (Fig. 16). The initial area at risk is quite variable in patients who meet criteria for thrombolytic therapy. The area at risk is not related to the site of occlusion in the infarction artery, but is determined by the presence or absence of collateral circulation.[46] A significant change in defect size before and after thrombolytic therapy predicts noninvasively reperfusion of the infarct artery. Radionuclide myocardial perfusion imaging with sestamibi has provided important insight into the pathophysiology of acute myocardial infarction.

Assessment of myocardial viability

Accurate assessment of myocardial viability has become increasingly important in management of patients with severe coronary artery disease. This is particularly relevant in patients with multiple infarcts and global left ventricular dysfunction and ongoing ischemia. Frequently, it is important to assess objectively whether these patients may benefit from revascularization, either by coronary bypass surgery or coronary angioplasty. A number of investigators have shown that fixed ^{201}Tl defects after exercise do not reliably indicate the presence of scar.[47–49] However, ^{201}Tl uptake after a repeat injection at rest, provides an accurate image of the distribution of viable myocardium. At the present time, ^{201}Tl imaging is considered the single photon imaging "gold standard" for assessing myocardial viability. The accuracy of ^{99m}Tc-sestamibi to identify viable myocardium is presently under investigation. Preliminary data suggest that, in most patients populations, resting images with ^{201}Tl and ^{99m}Tc-sestamibi are comparable, although quantitatively, differences occur in individual patients.

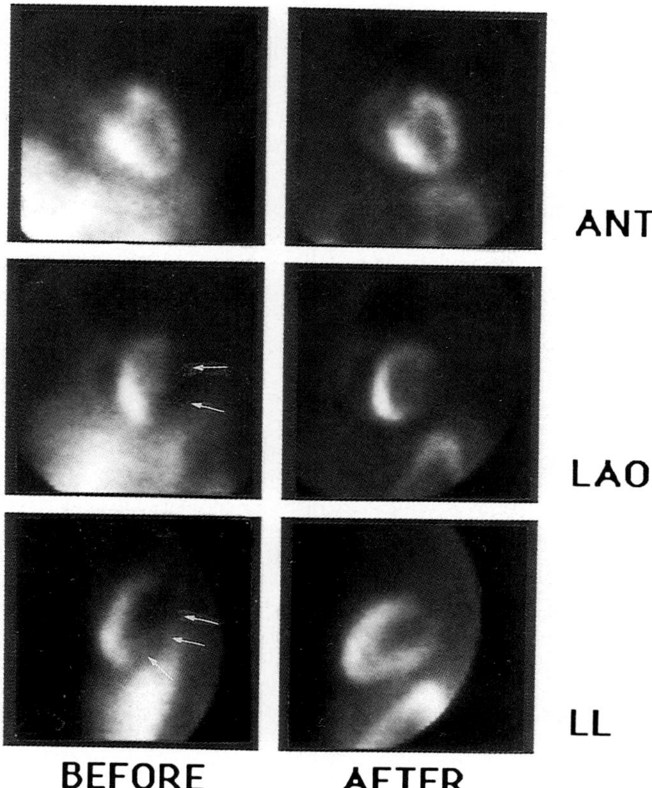

Figure 16. Planar myocardial perfusion imaging with ^{99m}Tc-sestamibi before and after thrombolytic therapy in a patient with a large posterior and lateral infarct. The images obtained with injection prior to thrombolytic therapy show a large inferoposterior myocardial perfusion defect (arrow), quantified as 49. After thrombolytic therapy, there is evidence of successful reperfusion of the infarct artery. The inferoposterior wall is now visualized, although the posterolateral wall still shows a defect. The defect after thrombolytic therapy was 28, indicating 42% of myocardial salvage (from reference 45).

CONCLUSION

Radionuclide myocardial perfusion imaging provides a unique means to noninvasively visualize relative regional myocardial blood flow. In conjunction with stress testing, radionuclide myocardial perfusion imaging provides unique physiological information regarding the functional significance of anatomic coronary artery disease. This information is quantitative and reproducible. Importantly, radionuclide myocardial perfusion imaging provides information that has independent, incremental prognostic value over other diagnostic modalities.

REFERENCES

1. Bailey J, Griffith L, Rouleau J, et al. Thallium-201 myocardial perfusion imaging at rest and during exercise. Comparative sensitivity to electrocardiography in coronary artery disease. *Circulation* 1977;55:79.
2. Verani M, Marcus M, Razzak M, et al. Sensitivity and specificity of thallium-201 perfusion scintigrams under exercise in diagnosis of coronary artery disease. *J Nucl Med* 1978;19:773.
3. Pohost G, Zir L, Moore R, et al. Differentiation of transiently ischemic from infarcted myocardium by serial imaging after a single dose of thallium-201. *Circulation* 1977;55:294.
4. Ritchie J, Zaret B, Strauss H, et al. Myocardial imaging with thallium-201: a multicenter study in patients with angina pectoris or acute myocardial infarction. *Am J Cardiol* 1978; 42:345.
5. Wackers F, Berman DS, Maddahi J, et al. Technetium-99m hexakis 2-methoxyisobutyl isonitrile: human biodistribution, dosimetry, safety, and preliminary comparison to thallium-201 for myocardial perfusion imaging. *J Nucl Med* 1989;30:301.
6. Kiat H, Maddahi J, Roy L, et al. Comparison of technetium 99m methoxy isobutyl isonitrile and thallium-201 for evaluation of coronary artery disease by planar and tomographic methods. *Am Heart J* 1989;117:1.
7. Seldin D, Johnson L, Blood D, et al. Myocardial perfusion imaging with technetium-99m SQ30217: comparison with thallium-201 and coronary anatomy. *J Nucl Med* 1989;30:312.
8. Hendel R, McSherry B, Karimeddini M, et al. Diagnostic value of a new myocardial perfusion agent, teboroxime (SQ30,217), utilizing a rapid planar imaging protocol. *J Am Coll Cardiol* 1990;16:855.
9. Jain D, Wackers F, Mattera J, et al. Biokinetics of ^{99m}Tc-tetrofosmin, a new myocardial perfusion imaging agent: implications for a one day imaging protocol. *J Nucl Med* 1993;34:1254.
10. Hendel RC, McSherry B, Karimeddini M, et al. Diagnostic value of a new myocardial perfusion agent, teboroxime (SQ30,217), utilizing a rapid planar imaging protocol: Preliminary results. *J Am Coll Cardiol* 1990;16:855.
11. Wackers FJTh. Myocardial perfusion imaging, in Sandler MP, Coleman RE, Wackers FJTh, et al. (eds): *Diagnostic Nuclear Medicine* 3rd ed. Baltimore, Williams & Wilkins, 1995, in press.
12. Ritchie J, Williams D, Harp G, et al. Transaxial tomography with thallium-201 for detecting remote myocardial infarction. Comparison with planar imaging. *Am J Cardiol* 1982;50:1236.
13. Wackers F. Single photon emission computed tomography, in Zaret BL, Kaufman L, Berson AS, Dunn RA (eds): *Frontiers in Cardiovascular Imaging*. New York, Raven Press, 1993, p 85.
14. Johnstone D, Wackers F, Berger H, et al. Effect of patient positioning on left lateral thallium-201 images. *J Nucl Med* 1979;20:183.
15. Wackers F, Fetterman R, Mattera J, et al. Quantitative planar thallium-201 stress scintigraphy: a critical evaluation of the method. *Semin Nucl Med* 1985;15:46.
16. Wackers FJTh. Artifacts in planar and SPECT myocardial perfusion imaging. *Am J Cardiac Imaging* 1992;6:42–58.
17. Leppo J. Dipyridamole-thallium imaging: the lazy man's stress test. *J Nucl Med* 1989;30:281.
18. Wackers F. Pharmacologic stress with dipyridamole: how lazy can one be? Editorial. *J Nucl Med* 1990;31:6.
19. Wackers F. Adenosine-thallium imaging: faster and better? Editorial. *J Am Coll Cardiol* 1990;16:1384.
20. Wackers F. Which pharmacological stress is optimal? A technique dependent choice. *Circulation* 1993;87:646.
21. Pennell D, Underwood R, Swanton R, et al. Dobutamine thallium myocardial perfusion tomography. *J Am Coll Cardiol* 1991;18:1471.
22. Iskandrian A, Heo J, Kong B, et al. Use of technetium-99m isonitrile (RP-30A) in assessing left ventricular perfusion and function at rest and during exercise in coronary artery disease and comparison with coronary arteriography and exercise thallium-201 SPECT imaging. *Am J Cardiol* 1989;64:270.
23. Watson D, Campbell N, Read E, et al. Spatial and temporal quantitation of plane thallium myocardial images. *J Nucl Med* 1981;22:577.
24. Garcia E, Maddahi J, Berman D, et al. Space/time quantitation of thallium-201 myocardial scintigraphy. *J Nucl Med* 1981; 22:309.
25. Wackers F, Soufer R, Zaret B. Nuclear cardiology, in Braunwald E (ed): *Heart Disease, A Textbook of Cardiovascular Medicine*. 5th ed. Vol. 1. Philadelphia, W.B. Saunders, 1995, in press.
26. Fintel D, Links J, Brinker J, et al. Improved diagnostic performance of exercise thallium-201 single photon emission computed tomography over planar imaging in the diagnosis of coronary artery disease: a receiver operating characteristic analysis. *J Am Coll Cardiol* 1989;13:600.
27. Brown K. Prognostic value of thallium-201 myocardial perfusion imaging. A diagnostic tool comes of age. *Circulation* 1991;83:363.
28. Ladenheim M, Pollock B, Rozanski A, et al. Extent and severity of myocardial hypoperfusion as predictors of prognosis in patients with suspected coronary artery disease. *J Am Coll Cardiol* 1986;7:464.
29. Iskandrian A, Chae S, Heo J, et al. Independent and incremental prognostic value of exercise single-photon emission computed tomographic (SPECT) thallium imaging in coronary artery disease. *J Am Coll Cardiol* 1993;22:665.
30. Chae S, Heo J, Iskandrian A, et al. Identification of extensive coronary artery disease in women by exercise single-photon emission computed tomographic (SPECT) thallium imaging. *J Am Coll Cardiol* 1993;21:1305.
31. Wackers F, Russo D, Russo D, et al. Prognostic significance of normal quantitative planar thallium-201 stress scintigraphy in patients with chest pain. *J Am Coll Cardiol* 1985;6:27.
32. Pamelia F, Gibson R, Watson D, et al. Prognosis with chest pain and normal thallium-201 exercise scintigrams. *Am J Cardiol* 1985;55:920.
33. Gibson R, Watson D, Craddock G, et al. Prediction of cardiac events after uncomplicated myocardial infarction: a prospective study comparing predischarge exercise thallium-201 scintigraphy and coronary angiography. *Circulation* 1983;68:321.
34. Hendel R, Layden J, Leppo J, et al. Prognostic value of dipyridamole thallium scintigraphy for evaluation of ischemic heart disease. *J Am Coll Cardiol* 1990;15:109.
35. Moss A, Goldstein R, Hall W, et al. Detection and significance

of myocardial ischemia in stable patients after recovery from an acute coronary event. *J Am Med Assoc* 1993;269:2379.
36. Manyari D, Knudtson M, Kloiber R, et al. Sequential thallium-201 myocardial perfusion studies after successful percutaneous transluminal coronary artery angioplasty: delayed resolution of exercise-induced scintigraphic abnormalities. *Circulation* 1988;77:86.
37. Hardoff R, Shefer A, Gips S, et al. Predicting late restenosis after coronary angioplasty by very early (12 to 24 hr) thallium-201 scintigraphy: implications with regard to mechanisms of late coronary restenosis. *J Am Coll Cardiol* 1990;15:486.
38. Wackers F, Lie K, Liem K, et al. Thallium-201 scintigraphy in unstable angina pectoris. *Circulation* 1978;57:738.
39. Bilodeau L, Theroux P, Gregoire J, et al. Technetium-99m sestamibi tomography in patients with spontaneous chest pain: Correlations with clinical, electrocardiographic and angiographic findings. *J Am Coll Cardiol* 1991;18:1684.
40. Wackers F, Busemann Sokole E, et al. Value and limitations of thallium-201 scintigraphy in the acute phase of a myocardial infarction. *N Engl J Med* 1976;295:1.
41. Varetto T, Cantalupi D, Altiero, et al. Emergency room technetium-99m-sestamibi imaging to rule out acute myocardial ischemic events in patients with nondiagnostic electrocardiograms. *J Am Coll Cardiol* 1993;22:1804.
42. Hilton TC, Thompson RC, Williams HJ, et al. Technetium-99m-sestamibi myocardial perfusion imaging in the emergency room evaluation of chest pain. *J Am Coll Cardiol* 1994; 23:1016.
43. Silverman K, Becker L, Bulkley B, et al. Value of early thallium-201 scintigraphy for predicting mortality in patients with acute myocardial infarction. *Circulation* 1980;61:996.
44. Cerqueira M, Maynard C, Ritchie J, et al. Long term survival in 618 patients from the western Washington streptokinase in myocardial infarction trials. *J Am Coll Cardiol* 1992; 20:1452.
45. Wackers F, Gibbons R, Verani M, et al. Serial quantitative planar technetium-99m isonitrile imaging in acute myocardial infarction: efficacy for noninvasive assessment of thrombolytic therapy. *J Am Coll Cardiol* 1989;14:861.
46. Christian T, Schwartz R, Gibbons R. Determinants of infarct size in reperfusion therapy for acute myocardial infarction. *Circulation* 1992;86:81.
47. Dilsizian V, Rocco T, Freedman N, et al. Enhanced detection of ischemic but viable myocardium by the reinjection of thallium after stress redistribution imaging. *N Engl J Med* 1990;323:141.
48. Kayden D, Sigal S, Soufer R, et al. Thallium-201 for assessment of myocardial viability: quantitative comparison of 24 hour redistribution imaging with imaging after reinjection at rest. *J Am Coll Cardiol* 1991;18:1480.
49. Kiat H, Berman D, Maddahi J, et al. Late reversibility of tomographic myocardial thallium-201 defects: an accurate marker of myocardial viability. *J Am Coll Cardiol* 1988;12:1456.

23 *Section 2:* Nuclear Imaging Techniques for Assessing Myocardial Ischemia and Viability

Vasken Dilsizian

In patients with ischemic heart disease, the distinction between ischemic, but viable, from nonviable myocardium is an issue of increasing clinical relevance in guiding interventional therapy (angioplasty, coronary artery bypass surgery). Approximately half a million of these interventional procedures are performed in the United States annually. However, until recently, determining whether impaired myocardial contractile function at rest might be reversed could be made only retrospectively, after patients had undergone myocardial revascularization.[1–6] Because enhanced global left ventricular function after revascularization is associated with improved survival,[7–11] prospective identification of viable myocardium in patients with coronary artery disease and left ventricular dysfunction has important clinical and prognostic implications.

ASSESSMENT

Radionuclide imaging techniques are the most widely used diagnostic studies for assessing myocardial viability (Table 1). More conventional approaches for identifying scarred and necrotic myocardium include the presence of occluded coronary artery, regional contractile dysfunction, and electrocardiographic Q-wave. However, it is now well established that dysfunctional myocardium subtended by an occluded epicardial coronary artery does not necessarily indicate scarred tissue, because coronary collateral circulation is capable of sustaining myocardial function at rest[12–14] and even during exercise.[14–16] Conversely, dysfunctional myocardium perfused by a patent coronary artery after thrombolytic or interventional therapy is insufficient evidence that the myocardium is viable.[17] Electrocardiographic Q-wave criteria are also imprecise for identifying scarred myocardium. Although dysfunctional myocardium is more likely to improve after revascularization in patients with nonQ-wave rather than Q-wave infarctions,[18] the accuracy of such electrocardiographic criteria in reliably predicting recovery of function after revascularization is limited.[3,19–21]

Since the late 1970s, both animal and clinical studies have demonstrated that regional myocardial contractile dysfunction at rest does not necessarily represent an irreversible process.[22–26] Under certain conditions, when viable myocytes are subjected to ischemia, prolonged alterations in myocyte function leading to regional left ventricular dysfunction can occur, and this dysfunction may be completely reversible.[27–30] At present, 2 pathophysiologic states have been described in which impaired regional contractile function at rest may be partly or completely reversible, and that may cause diagnostic difficulties in terms of myocardial viability. The first, *hibernating myocardium*,[27] has been described in patients with left ventricular dysfunction secondary to chronic hypoperfusion. The second condition, *stunned myocardium*,[29] has

Table 1. Myocardial Perfusion Tracers

SINGLE PHOTON (SPECT)	POSITRON-EMITTING (PET)
^{201}Thallium	^{15}Oxygen-water
Isonitriles	^{13}N-ammonia
^{99m}Technetium-sestamibi	^{82}Rubidium
BATO Compounds	^{38}Potassium
^{99m}Technetium-teboroxime	^{62}Copper-PTSM
Diphosphines	
^{99m}Technetium-tetrofosmin	
^{99m}Technetium-phosfurimine (Q12)	

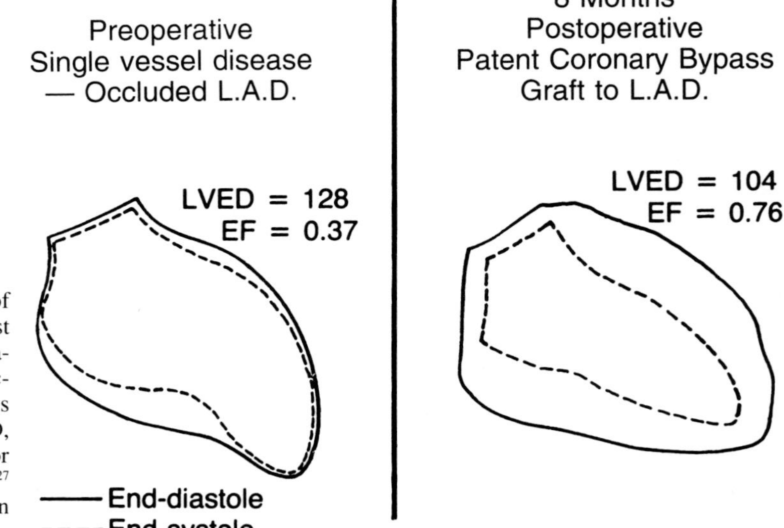

Figure 1. End-diastolic and end-systolic silhouettes of the left ventricle from the right anterior oblique contrast ventriculography are shown. Preoperatively, the anteroapical region is akinetic associated with an ejection fraction of 37%. Postoperatively, the anteroapical region is normal and the ejection fraction increased to 76%. LVED, left ventricular end-diastolic volume; LAD, left anterior descending coronary artery. (From Rahimtoola SH,[27] modified and reprinted with permission of the American Heart Association.)

been observed in patients with prolonged, but reversible, postischemic left ventricular dysfunction following a brief period of transient coronary occlusion. This chapter will focus on the application of nuclear imaging techniques to address myocardial ischemia and viability in patients with coronary artery disease.

Hibernating Myocardium

For many years, left ventricular dysfunction at rest was considered to be an irreversible process. Recovery of regional and global left ventricular function at rest following revascularization in some patients with chronic left ventricular dysfunction (Fig. 1) suggested that many myocardial regions that are asynergic before revascularization may represent viable myocardium.[1–6,27,28,30] Reversible left ventricular dysfunction at rest arising from prolonged chronic myocardial hypoperfusion, in which myocytes remain viable but contraction is chronically depressed, has been termed hibernating myocardium (Fig. 2).[27] Upon restoration of myocardial blood flow, the function of hibernating myocardium may improve immediately.[28] Because there are no adequate animal models of hibernation, the precise pathophysiology responsible for the depressed contractile function has not been established. However, it has been suggested that hibernation is a protective response of the myocytes to decrease oxygen demand in the setting of decreased oxygen availability, thereby establishing perfusion-contraction coupling.[31] At this time, there are no serial studies in patients in whom hibernating myocardium has been shown to be a truly chronic condition. It is conceivable that some cases of hibernation may represent stunning, while others may represent hibernation with intermittent stunning.[32]

In our experience at the National Institutes of Health, nearly one third of patients with preoperative left ventricular dysfunction exhibited a significant increase in global left ventricular ejection fraction after coronary artery bypass surgery (Fig. 3). The severity of the left ventricular dysfunction at rest did not predict the results of revascularization. In a different group of patients,[5] the increase in global left ventricular ejection fraction at rest was shown to be related

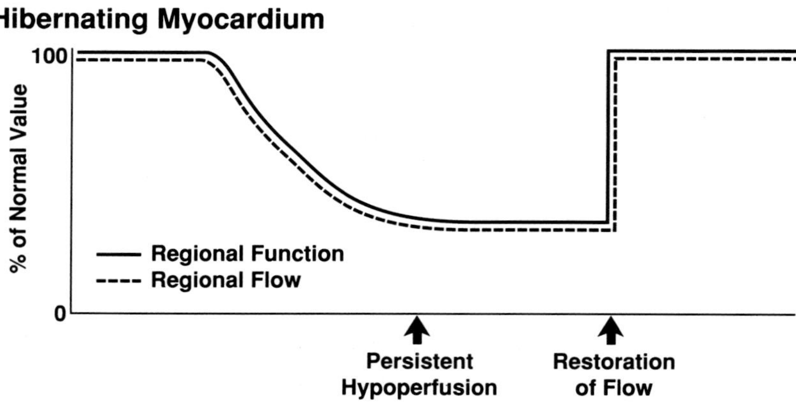

Figure 2. A schematic diagram of hibernating myocardium.

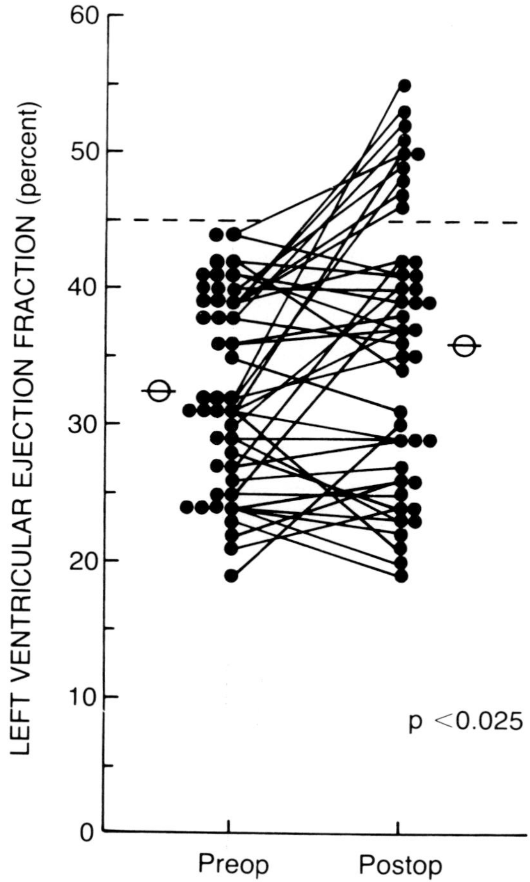

Figure 3. The prevalence of improvement in left ventricular ejection fraction at rest in 43 patients with preoperative (Preop) left ventricular dysfunction. Left ventricular ejection fraction was assessed 6 months after (Postop) coronary artery bypass surgery. The dashed line at 45% indicates the lower limit of normal resting ejection fraction for the National Institutes of Health. Substantial increases in ejection fraction were observed in 15 patients (35%), and the Postop ejection fraction was normal in 10 patients (23%). (Reprinted[33] with permission of Seminars in Nuclear Cardiology.)

to the extent of ischemic regions manifesting an improvement in systolic function after coronary artery bypass surgery (Fig. 4). Hence, distinction between hibernating myocardium and myocardial fibrosis among patients with chronic coronary artery disease and left ventricular dysfunction, prospectively, can be difficult clinically.

Stunned Myocardium

The phenomenon of prolonged, but reversible, left ventricular dysfunction after a period of transient, severe myocardial ischemia is known as myocardial stunning (Fig. 5).[29] Regional dysfunction associated with stunning represents the combined effects of transient ischemic injury and reperfusion injury. Myocardial stunning can occur secondary to reduced oxygen supply or increased demand in the presence of severe coronary artery stenosis. Recovery of regional dysfunction in patients after thrombolytic therapy for acute myocardial infarction indicates that many asynergic myocardial regions in such patients represent viable but stunned myocardium.[29,34–36] Although the actual pathophysiological basis for myocardial stunning is not well understood, several mechanisms have been proposed to explain this phenomenon. These include abnormal myocardial energy production and utilization[37,38]; detrimental effects of cytotoxic oxygen-derived free radicals during reperfusion[39,40]; altered calcium flux, sensitivity, and overload at the myofilament level[41–43]; microvascular accumulation of neutrophils in previously ischemic tissue[44]; extracellular collagen matrix abnormalities[45]; and impairment of sympathetic nerve activity as a result of ischemic damage.[46]

In the current era of thrombolytic therapy, accurate assessment of myocardial salvage after reperfusion may provide important clinical and prognostic information in patients with acute myocardial infarction.[47–49] In many instances, this assessment cannot wait the several days or weeks necessary for recovery of wall motion. For example, among hemodynamically unstable patients in the early post-thrombolytic period, the accurate distinction between postischemic left ventricular dysfunction due to viable but stunned myocardium from that of extensive scar greatly affects decisions regarding revascularization. Urgent revascularization will benefit patients with postischemic stunned myocardium, but not those with scarred myocardium. Myocardial stunning may also occur in those patients who have experienced unstable angina[50,51] or developed exercise-induced ischemia.[52,53] Thus, the presence of regional dysfunction at rest does not necessarily indicate irreversible disease in patients with these ischemic syndromes.

Considering the uncoupling of blood flow and function, measures of blood flow and vascular patency are insufficient to assess viability. Recently, nuclear imaging techniques that evaluate myocardial viability on the basis of myocardial cell membrane integrity and metabolic activity have gained substantial clinical success. These methods provide greater precision in this assessment than can be achieved by analyzing electrocardiographic Q-waves, regional contraction, or coronary anatomy.

^{201}THALLIUM SCINTIGRAPHY

For the last 2 decades, ^{201}Tl myocardial imaging has been a clinically important method with which to assess perfusion and sarcolemmal membrane integrity and, hence, to address myocardial viability. Myocardial uptake early after intravenous injection of thallium is proportional to regional blood flow, with a first-pass extraction fraction in the range of 85%.[54] Experimental studies with thallium have suggested that the cellular extraction of thallium across the sarcolemmal membrane is unaffected by hypoxia unless irreversible injury is present.[55,56] Similarly, pathophysiological conditions of chronic hypoperfusion (hibernating myocardium) and postischemic dysfunction (stunned myocardium) do not ad-

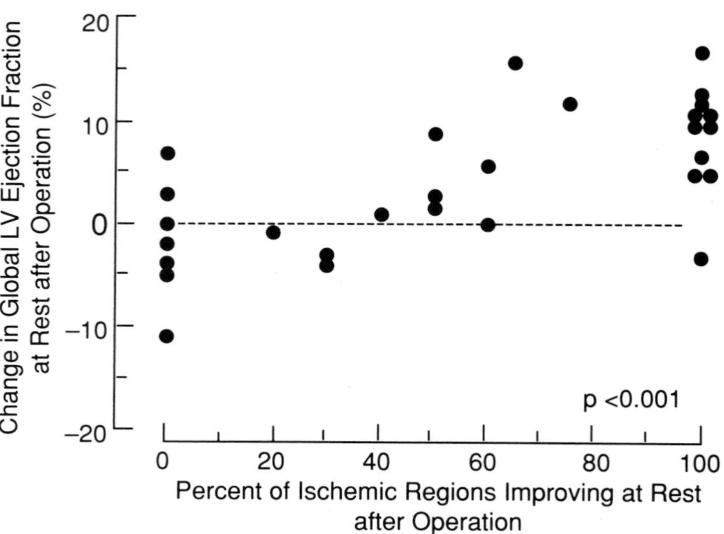

Figure 4. Change in left ventricular (LV) ejection fraction after coronary artery bypass surgery as a function of the percent of ischemic LV regions manifesting improved regional function after operation. The ischemic regions were defined as those in which the ejection fraction decreased during exercise before surgery more than 2 standard deviations below the mean change observed in that region in normal volunteers during exercise. (Reprinted[5] with permission of The American Journal of Cardiology.)

versely alter extraction of thallium.[57–59] Thus, like potassium, intracellular uptake of thallium across the sarcolemmal membrane is maintained for as long as sufficient blood flow is present to deliver thallium to the myocardial cell.

The period that follows early myocardial uptake of thallium is termed the delayed or redistribution phase. Regional thallium activity on delayed or redistribution images, acquired either 2 to 4 hours or 8 to 72 hours after stress, has been used to demonstrate the distribution of viable myocardial cells and the extent of myocardial fibrosis. During the redistribution phase, there is a continuous exchange of thallium from the myocardial to the extracardiac compartments, driven by the concentration gradient of the tracer and presence or absence of myocyte viability. The extent of defect resolution on the initial images over time reflects the degree of thallium redistribution on the delayed images and, hence, viability. When only scarred myocardium is present, the degree of the initial thallium defect persists over time and no redistribution is detected on delayed images. When both ischemic but viable and scarred myocardium are present, the degree of thallium redistribution is incomplete, giving the appearance of partial reversibility on delayed images. Hence, thallium scintigraphy has the rather unique potential for distinguishing viable from scarred myocardium with greater precision than can be achieved by the assessment of regional anatomy or function alone. Advantages and disadvantages of stress-redistribution, late (8- to 72-hour) redistribution, thallium reinjection, and rest-redistribution methods for assessing myocardial viability (Table 2) are reviewed.

Stress-Redistribution Imaging

In 1977, Pohost and coworkers reported that thallium defects on immediate postexercise images may normalize or redistribute if images were repeated several hours after the initial stress study.[60] This was followed by several animal studies showing that redistribution on a delayed image represented reduced thallium concentration in the normal segments, along with increased thallium concentration in ischemic segments.[60–66] The presence of thallium redistribution was subsequently confirmed in patients with ischemic heart disease undergoing exercise or pharmacological stress testing, as well as after the injection of thallium at rest. Hence, the acquisition of redistribution images 3 to 4 hours after stress

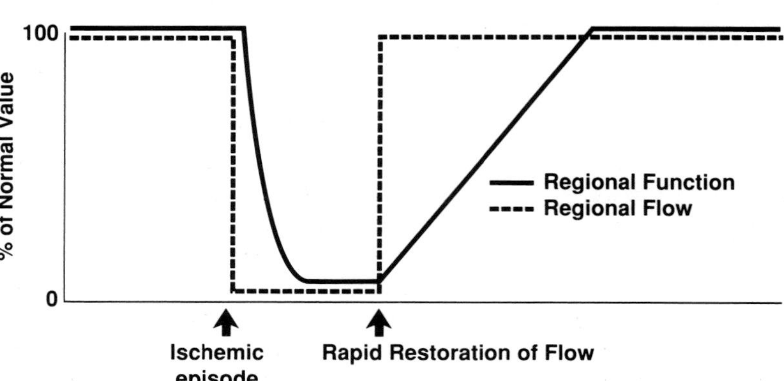

Figure 5. A schematic diagram of stunned myocardium.

Table 2. ^{201}Tl Protocols for Assessing Myocardial Viability

Early (3–4 hour) redistribution after stress
Late (8–72 hour) redistribution after stress
Rest-redistribution
Reinjection after stress 3–4-hour redistribution
Late redistribution after stress 3–4-hour reinjection

became the standard for thallium scintigraphic studies. However, further experience indicated that there are limitations of stress 3- to 4-hour redistribution imaging in differentiating viable from scarred myocardium.

Thallium defects on stress images that redistribute on 3- to 4-hour delayed images are accurate indicators of ischemic but viable myocardium. However, the converse, abnormal thallium uptake during stress and lack of redistribution on delayed images, does not necessarily indicate myocardial scar. Severely ischemic but viable myocardium as well as admixture of scar and viable myocardium may also appear irreversible on stress-redistribution studies (Fig. 6). A large number of myocardial regions with irreversible thallium defects on stress-redistribution imaging will exhibit normal thallium uptake after revascularization.[67–72] Using thallium quantification, Gibson and coworkers demonstrated that 45% of segments with irreversible defects had improved thallium uptake after coronary artery bypass surgery (Fig. 7).[68] Segments that were likely to improve had thallium activity that was >50% of the activity in normal regions. Similar results were obtained after successful percutaneous coronary angioplasty.[69,72] Thus, standard stress 3- to 4-hour redistribution thallium scintigraphy may fail to differentiate viable from scarred myocardium in many patients with coronary artery disease.

Late Redistribution Imaging

Among patients demonstrating apparent irreversible thallium defects on conventional stress-redistribution studies,

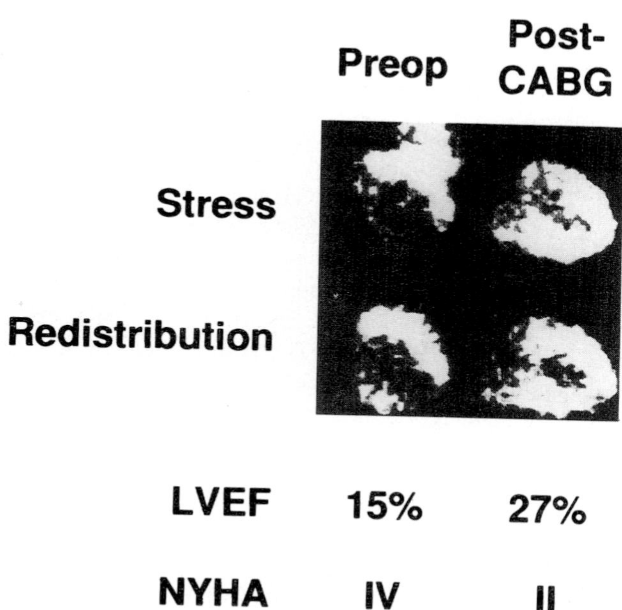

Figure 6. Evidence for viable myocardium in a region with irreversible thallium defect. Pre- and postoperative anterior planar thallium images demonstrate partially reversible inferior and fixed apical thallium defects preoperatively that normalize after coronary artery bypass surgery. The left ventricular ejection fraction increased from 15% before to 27% after surgery. (From Akins et al.,[67] modified and reprinted with permission of The American Journal of Cardiology.)

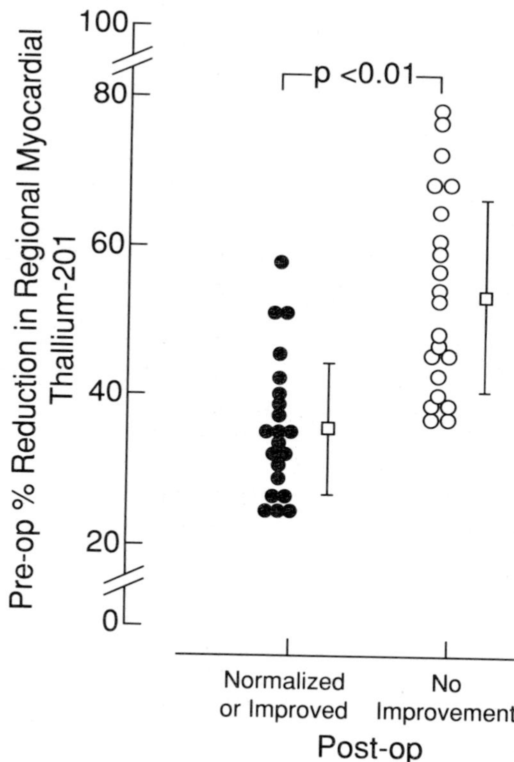

Figure 7. Percentage of reduction in regional thallium uptake for irreversible defects that normalized or improved after revascularization (solid circles) as compared with irreversible defects that did not improve after revascularization (open circles). Note that the irreversible defects that normalized or improved after surgery had a significantly smaller reduction in regional myocardial thallium activity preoperatively (Preop). (From Gibson et al.,[68] reprinted with permission of the Journal of the American College of Cardiology.)

the identification of viable myocardium may be improved by acquiring a third set of late (8- to 24-hour) images, which permits a longer period of thallium redistribution (Fig. 8). In a series of patients with coronary artery disease, when late images were obtained 18 to 24 hours after exercise, 21% of the segments with irreversible thallium defects on the 3- to 4-hour delayed images showed redistribution on the late images.[73] Myocardial segments with such late thallium redistribution were usually perfused by significantly narrowed coronary arteries. These initial observations, using planar imaging techniques, were confirmed by a number of subsequent studies using SPECT imaging.[70–74] To determine the frequency of late redistribution in a nonselected patient population, Yang et al.[74] performed late redistribution using SPECT in 118 consecutive patients with irreversible thallium defects on standard stress-redistribution studies. In this prospective study, late redistribution was observed in 53% of the patients and in 22% of the segments with 4-hour irreversible defects (Fig. 9). However, a potential limitation of late imaging are the suboptimal count statistics at 24 hours, even when 50% longer imaging time is employed.

A possible explanation for late redistribution may be that, in certain ischemic myocardial regions supplied by critically stenosed coronary arteries, both the initial uptake of thallium and the rate of delivery of thallium during the 3- to 4-hour redistribution period is significantly reduced. Hence, ischemic but viable myocardium may mimic the appearance of scarred myocardium. However, if a greater time is allowed for redistribution, a greater number of viable myocardial regions may be discriminated from fibrotic or scarred myocardium.

Late thallium redistribution, when present, is an accurate marker of ischemic and viable myocardium. Kiat and coworkers reported that 95% of segments that exhibited late redistribution at 18 to 24 hours improved after revascularization.[71] However, as with early redistribution imaging, the absence of late redistribution remains an inaccurate marker for scarred myocardium; 37% of segments that remained irreversible on both 3- to 4-hour and 24-hour studies also improved after revascularization.[71] These data suggest that although late thallium imaging improves the identification of viable myocardium when compared to 3- to 4-hour redistribution imaging, it continues to underestimate segmental improvement after revascularization.

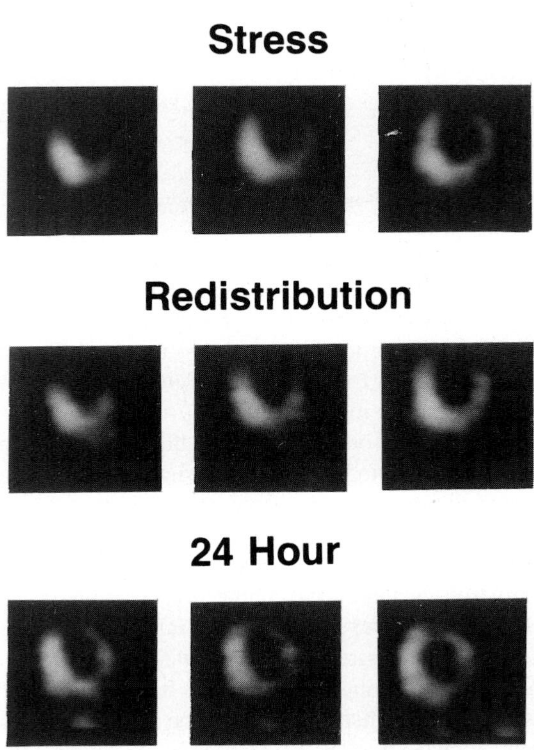

Figure 8. Short-axis thallium tomograms during stress, redistribution, and 24-hour imaging from a patient with coronary artery disease. There are extensive anterior and lateral thallium abnormalities during stress, which persist on redistribution images but improve at 24 hours. (Modified and reprinted[99] with permission of the American Heart Association.)

THALLIUM REINJECTION IMAGING

Recently, we introduced the concept that reinjection of thallium at rest after stress-redistribution imaging improves the assessment of myocardial viability.[75,76] Among 100 patients with coronary artery disease studied using SPECT thallium scintigraphy, 33% of abnormal myocardial regions identified by stress imaging appeared to be irreversible on 3- to 4-hour redistribution imaging. However, after a second dose of 1 mCi (37 MBq) of ^{201}Tl was reinjected at rest, 49% of the apparently irreversible defects on conventional stress-redistribution images demonstrated improved or normal thallium uptake.[75] Furthermore, in the subgroup of patients who

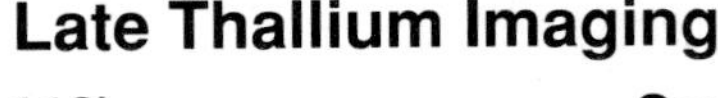

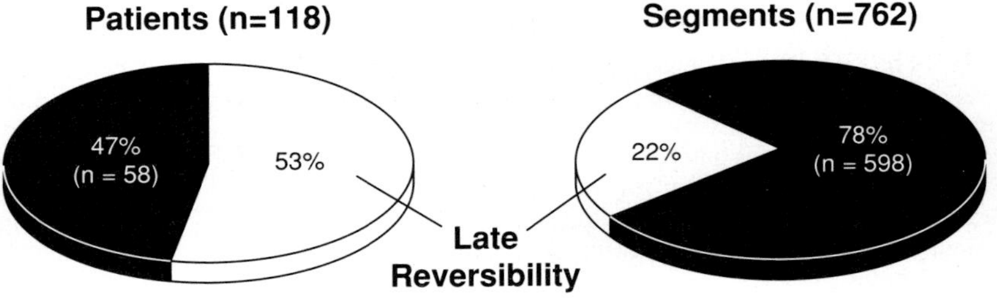

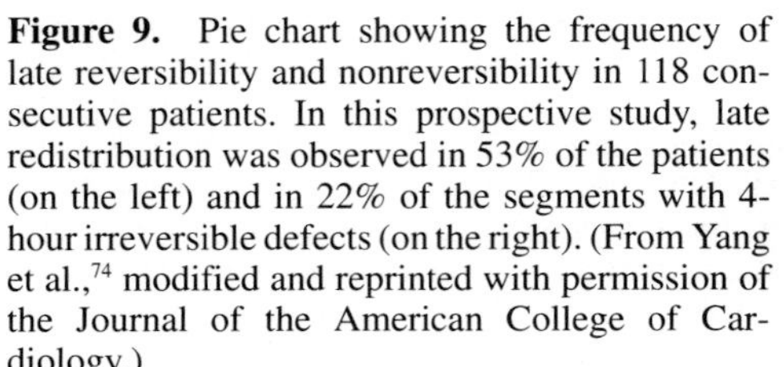

Figure 9. Pie chart showing the frequency of late reversibility and nonreversibility in 118 consecutive patients. In this prospective study, late redistribution was observed in 53% of the patients (on the left) and in 22% of the segments with 4-hour irreversible defects (on the right). (From Yang et al.,[74] modified and reprinted with permission of the Journal of the American College of Cardiology.)

underwent coronary angioplasty, 87% of myocardial regions identified as viable by reinjection studies had normal thallium uptake and improved regional wall motion after coronary angioplasty. In contrast, all regions with irreversible defects on reinjection imaging before coronary angioplasty had abnormal thallium uptake and abnormal regional wall motion after coronary angioplasty. These findings were subsequently confirmed by a number of other medical centers,[76–84] as well as a recent multicenter trial, undertaken in Italy, involving 402 consecutive patients with ischemic heart disease recruited from 12 hospitals.[85] In the Italian multicenter study, thallium reinjection identified ischemic but viable myocardium in approximately 31% of irreversible defects and 48% of patients with only irreversible defects on stress-redistribution studies. Examples of the thallium reinjection effect are shown in Figures 10 and 11. Similar results were obtained when thallium reinjection was performed immediately after pharmacological stress-redistribution studies.[81,86,87]

The experience with thallium reinjection before and after revascularization now totals 161 patients in the literature, performed in 5 different medical centers.[75,77,81–84] The available data suggest that enhanced thallium uptake after reinjection in otherwise irreversible defects predicts improvement in regional contraction at rest after revascularization in 80 to 91% of regions. In contrast, among regions that remained irreversible after reinjection, regional function improved after revascularization in only 0 to 18% of myocardial regions.

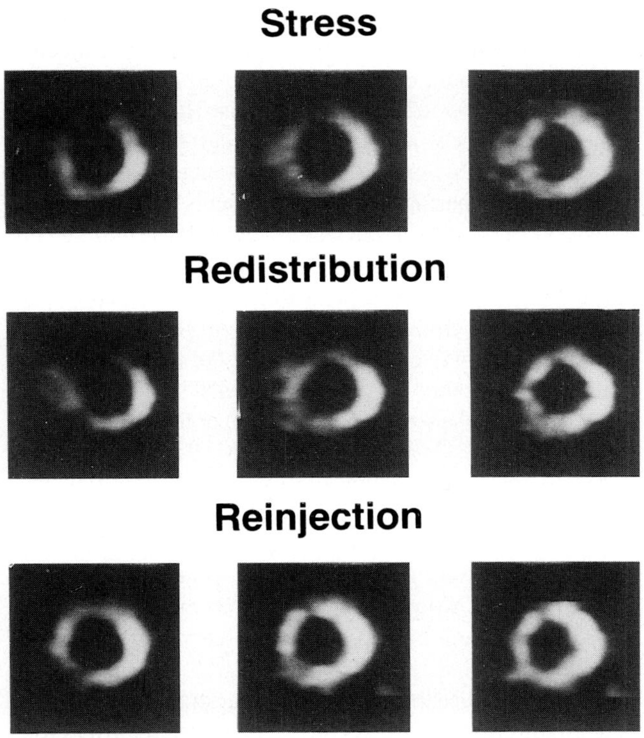

The following is a possible explanation for the success of thallium reinjection clinically. The *initial* myocardial uptake of thallium depends on regional perfusion and the *delayed* redistribution of thallium depends on the presence of viable myocytes, the concentration of the tracer in the blood,[88] and the rate of decline of thallium levels in the blood.[89–92] Therefore, the heterogeneity of regional myocardial blood flow and flow reserve observed on the initial thallium images (stress-induced defects) may be independent of the subsequent extent of thallium redistribution.[64,93] Thallium redistribution in a given defect depends on the continuing delivery of thallium over the subsequent 3 to 4 hours, as reflected by serum thallium levels,[94] as well as the capacity of the myocytes to retain the tracer.[95] Retention of thallium by myocytes requires intact sarcolemmal cell membrane and preserved transmembrane potential gradient. In regions with impaired myocardial blood flow, modest levels of metabolic activity, approximately one fifth of basal myocardial oxygen consumption is required to sustain sarcolemmal cell membrane integrity.[96] If the blood thallium level remains the same (or increases) during the period between stress and 3- to 4-hour redistribution imaging, then an apparent defect in a region with viable myocytes that can retain the thallium should improve. On the other hand, if the serum thallium concentration decreases during the imaging interval, the delivery of thallium may be insufficient, and the thallium defect may remain irreversible even though the underlying myocardium is viable.[97] This suggests that some ischemic but viable regions may never redistribute, even with late imaging, unless serum levels of thallium are increased. This hypothesis is supported by a study where thallium reinjection was performed immediately after 24-hour redistribution images were obtained.[98] Improved thallium uptake after reinjection occurred in 39% of defects that appeared irreversible both on the 4-hour and 24-hour redistribution images. This percentage is quite similar to the 37% of irreversible defects at 24 hours that improve after revascularization, as previously reported.[71]

Stress

Redistribution

Reinjection

Figure 10. Short-axis thallium tomograms during stress, redistribution, and reinjection imaging in a patient with coronary artery disease. There are extensive thallium abnormalities in the anterior and septal regions during stress that persist on redistribution images but improve markedly on reinjection images. (Reprinted[75] with permission of the New England Journal of Medicine.)

Is Late Redistribution Imaging Necessary After Reinjection? If thallium reinjection after stress 3- to 4-hour redistribution improves detection of hibernating and viable myocardium, it is possible that delaying the period between reinjection and repeat imaging from 10 minutes to 24 hours allows for further redistribution of the reinjected thallium dose. In a study of 50 patients with chronic coronary artery disease who underwent 4 sets of images (stress, 3- to 4-hour redistribution, reinjection, and 24-hour redistribution images), only 11% of myocardial regions (involving 6% of patients) that remained irreversible after both 3- to 4-hour redistribution and reinjection showed evidence of late redistribution.[99] It was concluded that all clinically relevant information pertaining to viability was obtained by stress-redistri-

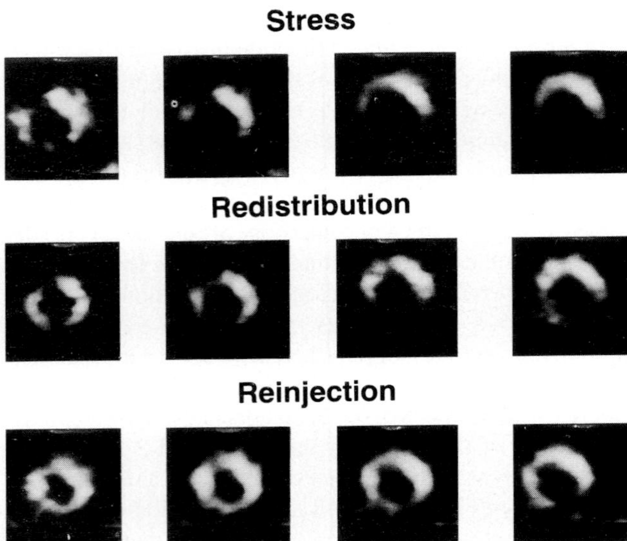

Figure 11. Short-axis tomograms during stress, redistribution, and reinjection imaging in a patient with coronary artery disease. Thallium stress-redistribution images reveal partially reversible septum and fixed inferior defects that improve after reinjection of thallium at rest. (Reprinted[33] with permission of Seminars in Nuclear Cardiology.)

bution-reinjection protocol (Figs. 12 and 13). Therefore, late imaging after the reinjected dose is not necessary. These observations have been confirmed by 2 subsequent studies.[100,101]

Stress-Reinjection Protocol: Should 3- to 4-Hour Redistribution Imaging be Eliminated? In view of the clinical success of thallium reinjection, many laboratories have adopted the practice of performing reinjection imaging instead of 3- to 4-hour redistribution imaging. This approach

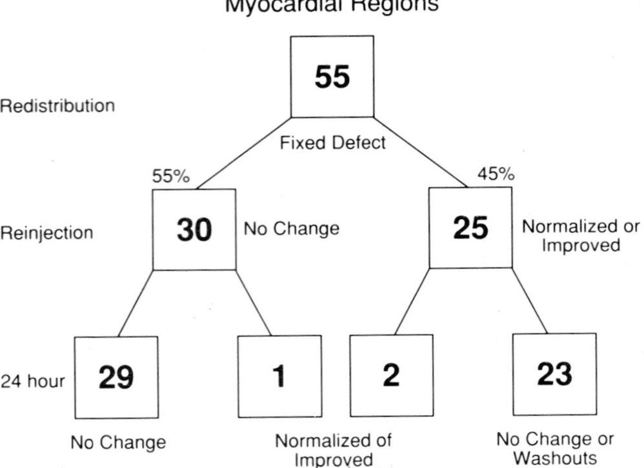

Figure 12. Flow diagram displaying the fate of "irreversible" thallium defects on the 3–4 hour standard redistribution studies after reinjection and at 24 hours. (Reprinted[99] with permission of the American Heart Association.)

assumes that a stress-reinjection protocol (without the 3- to 4-hour redistribution image) provides the same information regarding both exercise-induced ischemia and myocardial viability as a stress-redistribution followed by reinjection protocol. However, further analysis of the 50 patients with chronic coronary artery disease who underwent 4 sets of images (stress, 3- to 4-hour redistribution, reinjection, and 24-hour redistribution images) revealed that there are drawbacks in not performing redistribution images.[102]

Reliance on reinjection images alone (eliminating 3- to 4-hour redistribution image) may incorrectly assign up to 25% of reversible thallium defects on stress-redistribution images to be "irreversible" after reinjection.[75,102] Reversible stress-redistribution defects, that appear to wash out after reinjection, result from a disproportionately smaller increment in regional thallium activity after reinjection in some ischemic regions compared to the uptake in normal regions, a phenomenon we have termed "differential uptake."[75,102] Unlike conventional redistribution imaging, in which washout reflects an actual net loss of thallium activity between stress and redistribution imaging, it is the low differential uptake of thallium after reinjection that is responsible for the appearance of washout. At 24 hours after reinjection, redistribution of the reinjected thallium dose occurs simulating the reversible defect observed on stress 3- to 4-hour redistribution images (Fig. 14).

Despite the logistic concerns of performing reinjection imaging after 3- to 4-hour redistribution, elimination of the 3- to 4-hour redistribution images and reliance on reinjection images alone would overestimate scarred myocardium in a substantial number of ischemic regions. However, a stress-reinjection protocol appears to be a reasonable alternative to stress-redistribution-reinjection imaging, as long as 24-hour imaging is performed in those patients with irreversible defects on stress-reinjection studies. Thus, these data suggest that high predictive accuracy for ischemic and viable myocardium can be achieved with thallium scintigraphy with either stress-redistribution-reinjection or stress-reinjection-late redistribution imaging. The third set of images for either of the above protocols is necessary only if an irreversible defect exists on the stress-redistribution or the stress-reinjection images.

Does Early (Post-Stress) Thallium Reinjection Protocol Provide the Same Information as Reinjection After Delayed (3- to 4-hour) Redistribution Images? To avoid acquiring 3 sets of images, an alternative method would be to reinject thallium immediately after the stress images and acquire a modified redistribution image 3 to 4 hours later, representing redistribution of both the stress and the reinjected thallium doses. Applying such an early thallium reinjection protocol, Kiat and coworkers reported that 24% of irreversible thallium defects on 4-hour modified redistribution images became reversible on late redistribution studies.[103] Van Eck-Smit and coworkers reported that after early reinjection, there was good agreement between 1-hour and

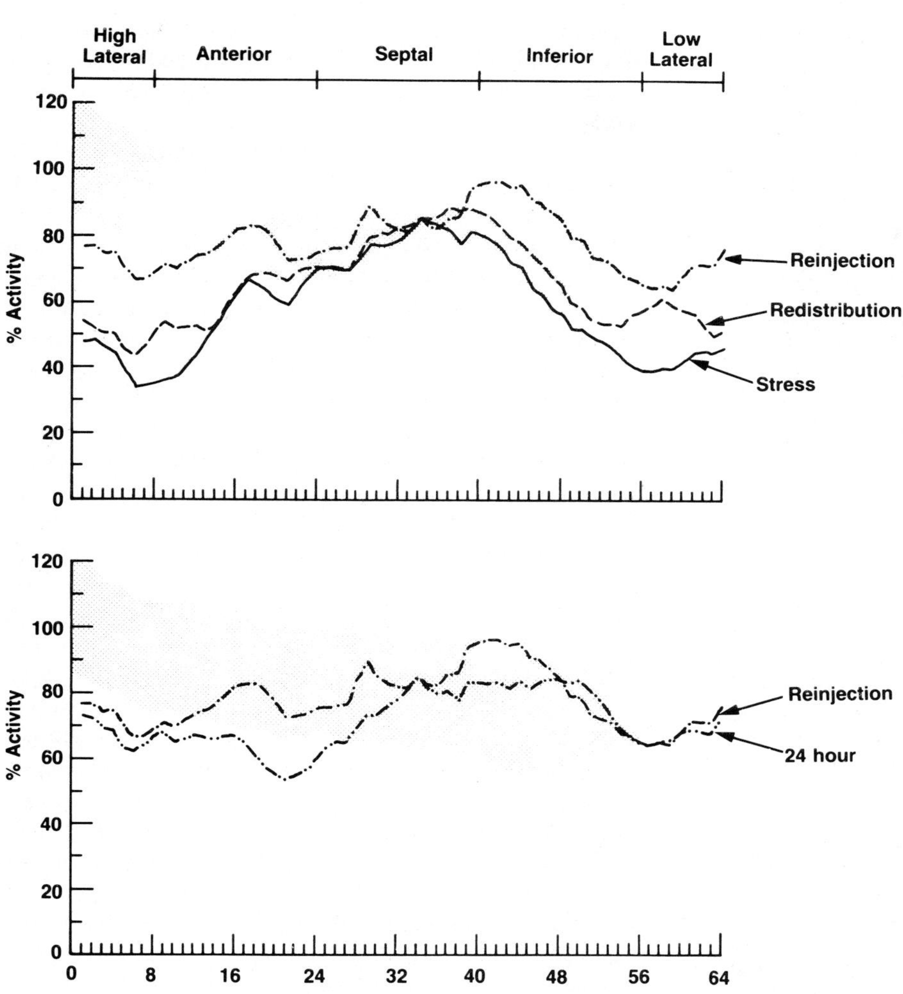

Figure 13. Quantitative regional thallium activity. The myocardial sectors in the anterior and inferior regions remain irreversible on the redistribution study but improve after reinjection and do not change at 24 hours. In addition, the anterolateral and inferolateral regions demonstrate partial reversibility on the redistribution study, improve further after reinjection, but show no further improvement after 24 hours. (Reprinted[99] with permission of the American Heart Association.)

3-hour modified redistribution images.[104] However, in this latter study, an independent validation of the accuracy of the early reinjection technique was not provided. In a subsequent publication, Klingensmith and Sutherland compared early and standard 3-hour reinjection protocols among 2 groups of patients with similar clinical parameters.[105] Their study confirmed previous observations that the frequency of reversible defects was significantly less with early reinjection compared to the standard 3-hour reinjection protocol. More recently, in addition to acquiring stress and 3- to 4-hour modified redistribution images, a second 1 mCi (37 MBq) dose of ^{201}thallium was reinjected after the modified redistribution images and a third set of 3- to 4-hour reinjection images were acquired in patients with chronic coronary artery disease.[106] When modified redistribution images after early reinjection were compared with 3- to 4-hour reinjection images, early thallium reinjection overestimated myocardial fibrosis in about 25% of irreversible defects. These preliminary data suggest that 3 to 4 hours delay after exercise is necessary to accurately determine myocardial ischemia and viability.

The Utility of Thallium Reinjection in Patients with Reverse Redistribution. The clinical significance of reverse redistribution in patients with chronic coronary artery disease is uncertain. On conventional stress-redistribution imaging, reverse redistribution indicates either the worsening of a defect apparent on stress images or the appearance of a new defect on the redistribution images. However, it remains unclear whether regions demonstrating the phenomenon of reverse redistribution represent areas of myocardial necrosis or ischemic but viable myocardium.

Because thallium reinjection is a useful technique for detecting myocardial viability, the effect of thallium reinjection was evaluated among patients with chronic coronary artery disease, all of whom demonstrated reverse redistribution on standard stress-redistribution studies.[107] The results of this investigation showed enhanced thallium uptake in the majority (82%) of regions with reverse redistribution (Fig. 15). Regions with reverse redistribution and improved thallium uptake after reinjection were supplied by severely stenosed coronary arteries with prominent collateral circulation, and associated with absence of electrocardiographic

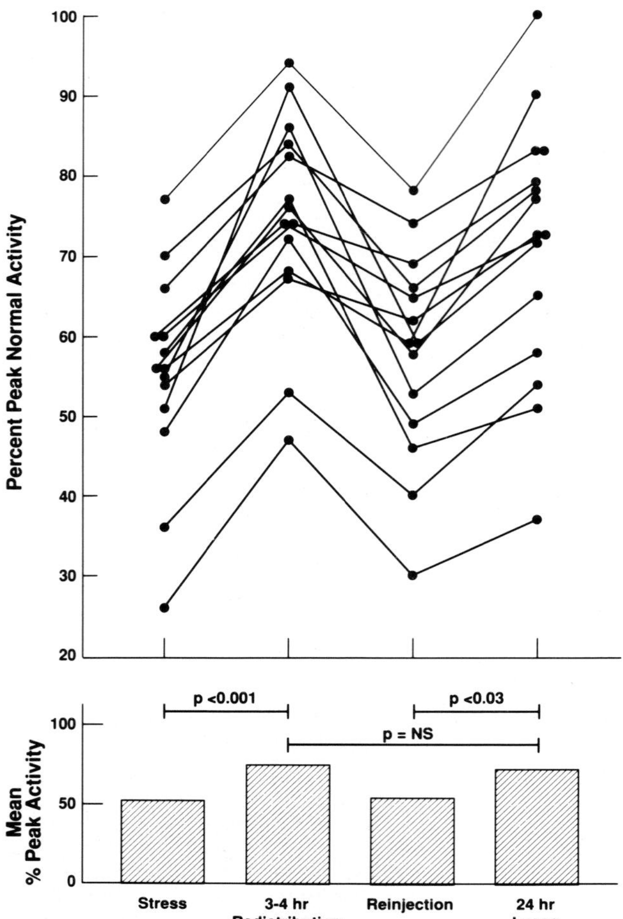

Figure 14. Relative regional thallium activity (presented as a percent of normal activity) in 14 regions demonstrating the phenomenon of apparent thallium washout due to low differential uptake. *Top panel*: Individual data points are displayed for stress, 3–4 hour redistribution, reinjection, and 24-hour images. *Bottom panel*: Mean thallium activity in relation to each of the 4 corresponding images. If the 3–4 hour redistribution images were eliminated and the reinjection images were acquired alone, these regions would be incorrectly assigned to be irreversible. On the 24-hour images, redistribution is again apparent, indicating reversibility of the defect, and the relative thallium activity is similar to that observed on the 3–4 hour redistribution studies. (Reprinted[102] with permission of the American Heart Association.)

and functional indices of myocardial necrosis. Furthermore, normal ^{18}F-fluorodeoxyglucose (FDG) uptake or FDG/blood flow mismatch were observed by positron emission tomography (PET) in such regions. In contrast, regions with reverse redistribution in which thallium activity failed to increase after reinjection were associated with pathological Q-waves, severely impaired wall motion, and severely reduced FDG uptake and blood flow (FDG/blood flow match) by PET. These observations indicate that reverse redistribution in chronic coronary artery disease usually reflects viable myocardium, critically dependent upon collateral circulation.[107]

Magnitude of Change in Thallium Activity After Reinjection Distinguishes Viable from Nonviable Myocardium. From the comparative FDG PET and thallium SPECT studies, evidence of metabolic activity and, hence, viability, have been observed in regions in which thallium defects remain irreversible despite reinjection by using analysis of *relative* regional thallium activity. This is particularly the case in regions with only mild-to-moderate reduction in thallium activity. Among 150 patients with chronic ischemic coronary artery disease who underwent stress-redistribution-reinjection thallium protocol, the increase in regional thallium activity from redistribution to reinjection was computed, normalized to the increase observed in a normal region, and termed "differential uptake."[108] The study demonstrated that a substantial increase in thallium activity may occur after reinjection in thallium defects that appear irreversible, and that the magnitude of increase in thallium activity in regions that appeared to remain irreversible despite reinjection was significantly greater in mild-to-moderate defects than in severe irreversible defects (Fig. 16). All regions with mild-to-moderate defects demonstrated ≥50% differential uptake after reinjection. The substantial uptake of thallium after reinjection in mild-to-moderate irreversible defects, even though relative thallium activity may not appear to increase (and the defect appears to remain irreversible), suggests that these regions represent viable myocardium. This was confirmed by the PET data; in regions with mild-to-moderate reduction in thallium activity, FDG uptake was preserved in 91% of the regions and the results of differential uptake and FDG were concordant in 81% of the regions.[108] When relative thallium activity was assessed in comparison to normal regions, increased thallium activity after reinjection occurred in a similar percentage of mild-to-moderate and severe irreversible defects (Fig. 17).

These initial observations were supported by a recent comparative clinicopathological study by Zimmermann et al.[109] Among 37 patients with significant left anterior descending coronary artery disease undergoing coronary artery bypass surgery, the magnitude of thallium activity within irreversible preoperative stress-redistribution and reinjection thallium images was correlated with the extent of interstitial fibrosis, determined from intraoperative transmural left ventricular biopsies of the anterior wall (Fig. 18). Although there was a good overall inverse correlation between percent thallium uptake on 4-hour redistribution and percent interstitial fibrosis, the inverse relation was significantly better after thallium reinjection. Similar results were obtained in our laboratory.[110] These data indicate that residual thallium activity after reinjection is proportional to the mass of preserved viable myocardium and confirm the value of thallium reinjection for assessing viability.

Prognostic Value of Thallium Reinjection. There are only preliminary data to indicate the prognostic contribution of thallium reinjection.[111,112] After excluding patients with early coronary artery revascularization (within 30 days of

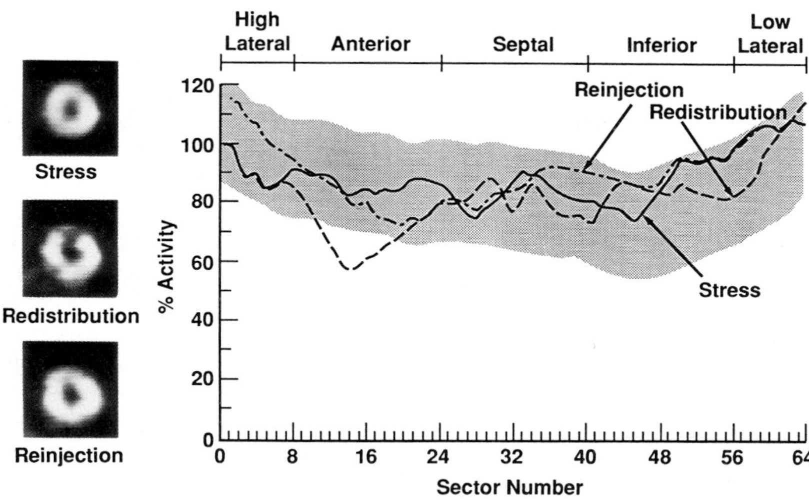

Figure 15. An example of reverse redistribution in the anterior region with enhanced thallium uptake after thallium reinjection. Representative short-axis tomograms obtained during stress, redistribution, and reinjection are shown on the left. On the right, plots of quantitative regional thallium activity during stress, redistribution, and reinjection are compared to the normal range (mean ± 2 SD for normal subjects), represented as the shaded area. (From Marin-Neto et al.,[107] reprinted with permission of the American Heart Association.)

scintigraphic evaluation), Miller et al. examined the late prognostic value of thallium reinjection in 50 consecutive patients with coronary artery disease followed for a mean of 9 months.[111] When the subgroup of patients with cardiac events (death, myocardial infarction, or late coronary revascularization; n = 22) were compared with those without events (n = 38), there were marked differences between the groups in: (1) number of segments with irreversible defects, (2) lung uptake and, (3) transient left ventricular cavity dilatation. Although conventional stress-redistribution studies predicted 13 of the 22 patients (60%) with cardiac events, thallium reinjection predicted additional events in 7 of 9 patients (78%) not identified by stress-redistribution studies alone. Similar findings were reported by Pieri et al.[112] When Cox multivariate analysis was applied to the data, the best predictor of hard cardiac events (death or myocardial infarction) was the number of irreversible defects after thallium reinjection. Hence, these preliminary data suggest that in addition to its well-established value as a viability marker, thallium reinjection may help assess risk in patients with chronic coronary artery disease.

Rest-Redistribution Imaging

Thallium imaging using the stress-redistribution-reinjection protocol provides important diagnostic and prognostic information regarding both inducible ischemia and myocardial viability. However, in a subset of patients with known multivessel disease and left ventricular dysfunction, the clinical question to be addressed is one of the presence and

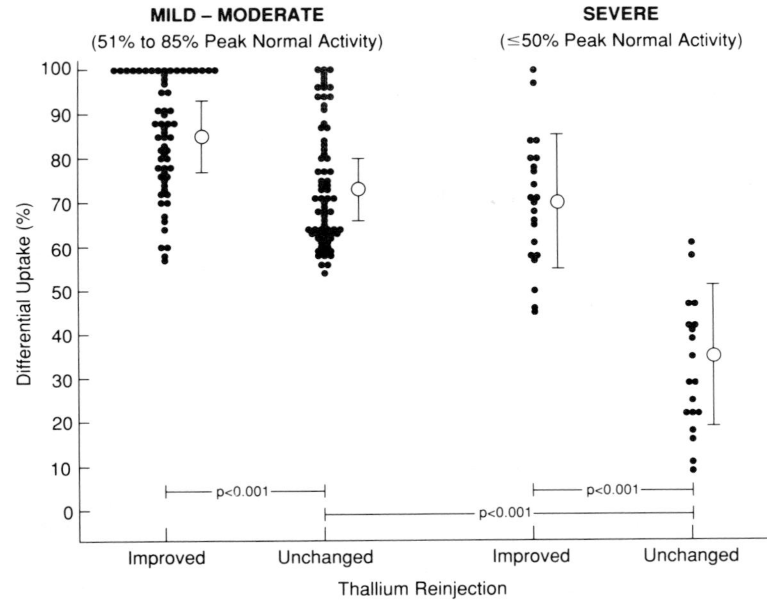

Figure 16. Plots show differential regional uptake of thallium after reinjection based on analysis of changes in the *magnitude* of regional thallium activity in regions with irreversible thallium defects on redistribution imaging. *Left panel*: regions with mild-moderate reduction in thallium activity on redistribution images (ranging from 51 to 85% of peak normal activity). *Right panel*: regions with severe reduction in thallium activity (≤50% of peak activity). Within each panel, regions are further subdivided on the basis of improved or unchanged *relative* thallium activity after reinjection. Mild-moderate defects in which relative thallium activity was unchanged after reinjection had significantly greater increase in absolute thallium activity than similar regions that represented severe irreversible defects. (Reprinted[108] with permission of the American Heart Association.)

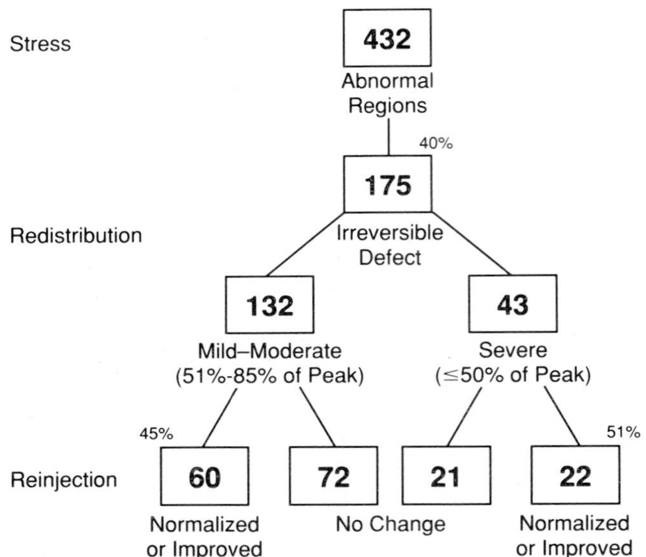

Figure 17. Flow diagram displaying the prevalence of irreversible thallium defects on conventional redistribution imaging and subsequent improvement after reinjection in mild-moderate and severe irreversible defects. (Reprinted[108] with permission of the American Heart Association.)

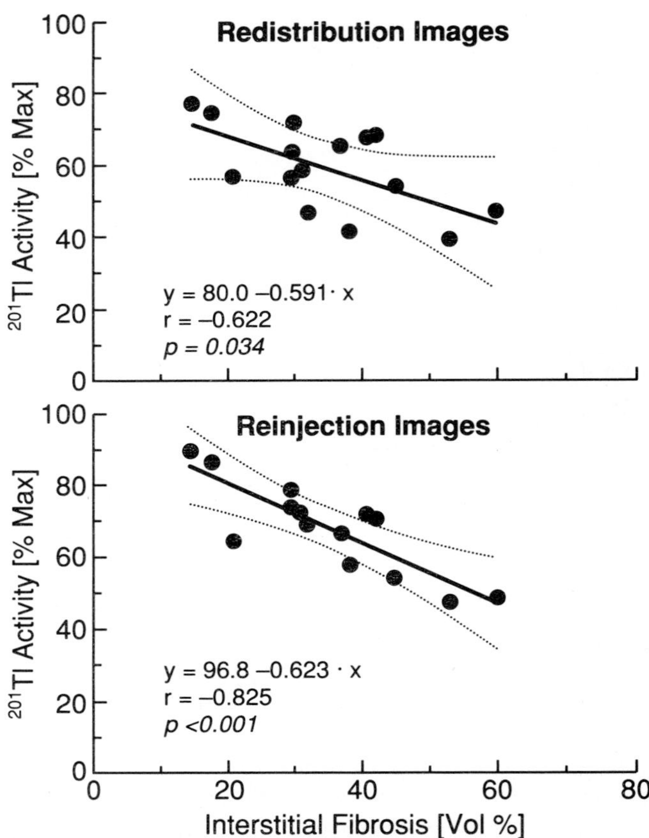

Figure 18. Graphs showing the relation between regional thallium activity on redistribution (top panel) and reinjection (bottom panel) images and regional volume fraction of interstitial fibrosis in patients with chronic stable coronary artery disease undergoing coronary artery bypass surgery. Two transmural biopsy specimens were taken during surgery and volume fraction of interstitial fibrosis was assessed by use of light microscopic morphometry. Dotted lines indicate 95% confidence limits for the regression line. % Max indicates percentage of maximum normal activity. When compared to redistribution images, regression analysis reveals a significantly improved correlation ($p < 0.01$) between thallium reinjection and regional volume fraction of interstitial fibrosis. (From Zimmerman et al.,[109] modified and reprinted with permission of the American Heart Association.)

extent of viable myocardium within dysfunctional regions, and not inducible ischemia. In such patients, it is reasonable to perform only rest-redistribution thallium imaging.

In 1978, Wackers et al. reported resting thallium defects during angina-free periods in patients with unstable angina and without myocardial infarction.[113] One year later, Gewirtz et al. demonstrated that thallium defects may also occur on resting images in patients with severe coronary artery disease in the absence of an acute ischemic process or previous myocardial infarction.[114] They also recognized that many of these defects redistribute over the next 2 to 4 hours. Since this initial report, 3 other studies evaluated the efficacy of rest-redistribution imaging in predicting the outcome of myocardial regions after revascularization.[115–117] These studies demonstrated that the majority (77 to 86%) of regions with reversible rest-redistribution thallium defects preoperatively have normal thallium uptake and/or improved left ventricular function postoperatively. However, 22 to 38% of regions with irreversible rest-redistribution defects preoperatively also showed improved left ventricular contraction after revascularization.

It should be emphasized, however, that none of the 3 studies used quantitative thallium scintigraphic methods to assess the severity of the irreversible thallium defects. Thallium defects in each of these studies were classified as being reversible, partially reversible, or irreversible. More recently, improved results were obtained using quantitative analysis in which the severity of reduction in thallium activity was considered within irreversible rest-redistribution thallium defects.[83,118] When myocardial viability was defined as thallium activity greater than 50% of activity in normal regions, 57% of severely asynergic regions that were viable by thallium demonstrated improved wall motion after surgery, compared to only 23% of severely asynergic regions that were considered to be nonviable by thallium.[118] Furthermore, the number of asynergic but viable myocardial segments correlated well with postoperative improvement in global left ventricular function.

In another study, quantitative regional thallium levels obtained from patients undergoing both stress-redistribution-reinjection and rest-redistribution SPECT imaging were compared with metabolic activity determined by PET.[83] Among 41 patients studied, when the outcome of 91 irreversible regions on stress-redistribution images were assessed after reinjection and compared with rest-redistribution images, there was concordance of data regarding myocardial

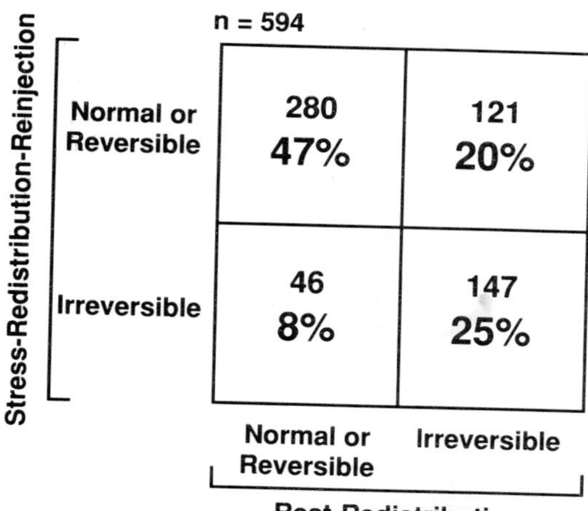

Figure 19. Chart showing concordance and discordance between stress-redistribution-reinjection and rest-redistribution thallium images in 20 patients who underwent positron emission tomographic studies. Five myocardial regions of interest were drawn on the transaxial tomograms from the 5 sets of thallium images, and thallium activities were then computed within each region. Thallium defects were classified as normal/reversible or irreversible. (Reprinted[83] with permission of the American Heart Association.)

viability (normal/reversible or irreversible) in 72 of the 91 (79%) irreversible defects (Fig. 19). However, when the irreversible defects were further analyzed according to the severity of the thallium defect, the concordance between stress-redistribution-reinjection and rest-redistribution imaging regarding myocardial viability increased to 94%.[83]

HIBERNATING MYOCARDIUM: THALLIUM PROTOCOLS

In most cases, identifying inducible myocardial ischemia is much more important clinically in terms of patient management and risk assessment than knowing myocardial viability. The influence of exercise stress in differentiating an asynergic region with mixed scarred and viable myocardium from a region with underperfused but viable (hibernating) myocardium is outlined in Figure 20. It has been established that an asynergic segmental contraction itself could influence the appearance of myocardial perfusion images.[119–123] A region with minimal or absent systolic wall thickening (hibernating but viable region) may appear to have reduced and irreversible thallium activity on a rest-redistribution study as a result of partial volume and recovery coefficient effects, in the presence of thinned or nonthickening myocardium. Hence, an asynergic segment with an irreversible rest-redistribution thallium pattern may represent either mixed scarred and viable myocardium (nonischemic), or a region with predominantly underperfused but viable myocardium (hibernating). These 2 hypocontractile segments may be differentiated by demonstrating exercise-induced ischemia (reversible thallium defect) in the case of hibernating myocardium and absence of ischemia (irreversible thallium defect) in the case of mixed fibrotic and viable myocardium. Accurate distinction between these 2 hypocontractile segments has important clinical implications because impaired regional function can be reversed in the case of hibernating myocardium, but not in regions with mixed viable and scarred myocardium.

Therefore, if the clinical question is one of myocardial viability within dysfunctional regions, a simplified rest-redistribution thallium protocol along with an assessment of the severity of reduction in thallium activity may suffice. On the other hand, if the clinical question is one of inducible ischemia and viability, stress-redistribution-reinjection or stress-reinjection-late redistribution imaging provides a more comprehensive assessment of the extent and severity of coronary artery disease by demonstrating regional myocardial ischemia without losing information on myocardial viability.

STUNNED MYOCARDIUM: THALLIUM PROTOCOLS

Several animal studies have shown that myocardial thallium extraction and washout kinetics are unaffected in stunned myocardium.[57,58,124] Studies in animals have also shown a good correlation between pathological infarct size and thallium defects.[125] Using intravenous thallium injections during occlusion and intracoronary injections after reperfusion, Maddahi and colleagues found that in persistently occluded coronary artery vascular territories, the absence of thallium uptake correlated with myocardial necrosis as assessed by histochemical staining.[126] In contrast, when the coronary artery occlusion was limited to 30 minutes, the reperfused myocardium had normal thallium uptake. Hence, these studies in animals suggest that thallium uptake in the early postinfarction period may be useful in estimating myocardial infarct size and the extent of myocardial salvage.

In patients with acute infarction, studied 2.5 hours and 5 hours from onset of symptoms to reperfusion, intracoronary thallium images immediately after reperfusion showed normal or improved thallium uptake in the 2.5-hour group along with recovery of regional function. In contrast, in the 5-hour group, irreversible thallium abnormalities associated with persistent wall motion abnormalities were observed, which persisted up to 10 days thereafter.[126] These findings were confirmed by other investigators among patients studied before and after intracoronary streptokinase infusion.[127] Thus, a severe thallium defect that remains irreversible after thrombolytic therapy is predictive of necrotic myocardium, with no potential for recovery in regional wall motion 10 days to 3 months after infarction. Despite the good correlation between thallium uptake after reperfusion and recovery of regional wall motion, subsequent studies have suggested that early postreperfusion thallium uptake appears to overestimate myocardial viability.

The discrepancy among published studies probably relates to the timing of thallium injection after reperfusion. If thallium is injected immediately after reperfusion,[126,127] the initial uptake of thallium may reflect hyperemic flow and thereby

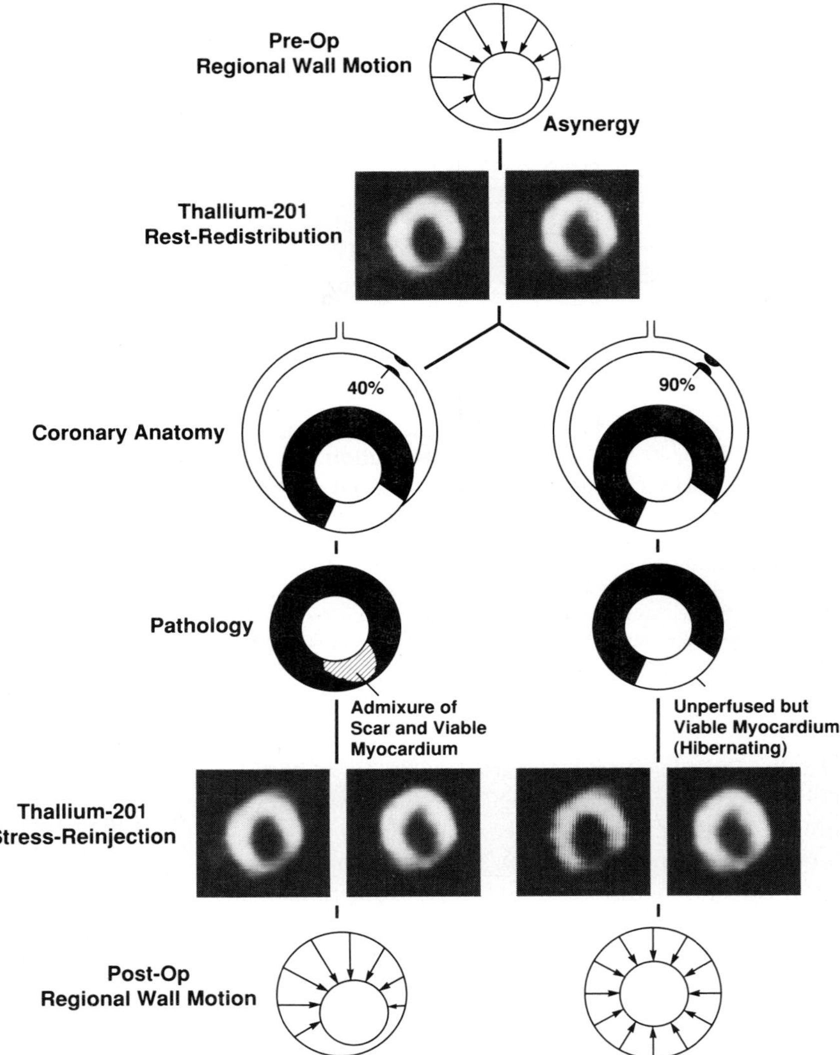

Figure 20. A schematic diagram of how exercise stress may produce greater regional myocardial blood flow heterogeneity when compared to rest-redistribution imaging and thereby differentiate an asynergic region with mixed scarred and viable myocardium from a region with underperfused but viable (hibernating) myocardium. A preoperative asynergic myocardial region that exhibits reduced thallium uptake at rest and remains irreversible on the redistribution study may represent a region with patent (40% stenosis) coronary artery after thrombolytic therapy (on the left) or a region with critically narrowed (90% stenosis) coronary artery without myocardial infarction (on the right). In a patient with 40% coronary artery stenosis and prior myocardial infarction, the dysfunctional myocardium (assessed several months after the acute infarction) represents mixed scarred and viable myocardium that will *not* recover after revascularization. In contrast, in the patient with 90% coronary artery stenosis without prior myocardial infarction, the dysfunctional myocardium perfused by this artery represents underperfused but viable myocardium that will recover completely after revascularization. These 2 situations can be differentiated by performing a stress-redistribution-reinjection study but not by a rest-redistribution study. (Reprinted[83] with permission of the American Heart Association.)

overestimate the extent of myocardial salvage.[128] In a canine model of thallium injection during rapid reperfusion, uptake of thallium immediately after reperfusion was very high, overestimating the amount of viable myocardium when compared to histochemical evidence of necrosis.[129] Even in regions with frankly necrotic myocardium, thallium may accumulate in the interstitium, driven primarily by hyperemic flow.[126,130] Therefore, initial thallium uptake following reperfusion cannot distinguish viable from necrotic myocardium.[129–132] However, necrotic myocardium cannot retain thallium and, despite its initial uptake, early rapid thallium washout occurs in necrotic tissue.[129,132] Consequently, accelerated kinetics of thallium washout might indicate nonviability after reperfusion therapy.[129,133]

These studies indicate that by allowing enough time for thallium to wash out from necrotic myocardium and to "wash in" in regions with viable myocardium, delayed redistribution images may play a more important role than early postreperfusion imaging for assessing myocardial viability. Several experimental studies support and emphasize the importance of acquiring redistribution images following the initial, early reperfusion thallium images. In a canine model, in which thallium was administered intravenously after 1 or 3 hours of coronary artery occlusion, Granato and coworkers demonstrated that the extent of thallium redistribution in the reperfused vascular territory correlated with the degree of myocardial salvage as assessed by regional blood flow and histochemical staining.[129] Similarly, in patients treated with thrombolytic therapy, the acquisition of a thallium redistribution image has been shown to accurately differentiate viable from scarred myocardium.[33,134–136] Among patients with successful reperfusion, the final thallium infarct size on redistribution images was smaller when compared to those with unsuccessful thrombolysis and totally occluded coronary arteries. Furthermore, in patients who did not receive thrombolytic therapy for their acute myocardial infarction, a good

Table 3. Advantages of ^{99m}Tc over ^{201}Tl

Higher photon energy (140 KeV)	→	Less attenuation and scatter
Shorter half-life (6 hours)	→	Permits higher imaging dose –Improved resolution –ECG Gated acquisition –First pass function

correlation was observed between tomographic thallium infarct size, enzymatic estimates of infarct size, and left ventricular ejection fraction.[137,138]

However, there are obvious limitations in performing rest (prethrombolysis) and redistribution (post-thrombolysis) thallium images in patients with acute myocardial infarction. The 30-minute delay for acquiring prethrombolysis thallium images may be detrimental for a patient with evolving acute myocardial infarction. On the other hand, if thallium is imaged immediately after thrombolytic therapy, then the extent of myocardial salvage could be overestimated, due to hyperemia. Thus, late (24 hours) redistribution imaging after thrombolysis is recommended.[139] Others have proposed delaying the assessment of myocardial salvage in the peri-infarct period and, instead, obtain a predischarge submaximal exercise thallium study to determine both the extent of myocardial salvage and residual myocardial ischemia in the infarct-related vascular territory.[128,130]

^{99m}Tc-LABELED PERFUSION TRACERS

Advantages of ^{99m}Tc over ^{201}Tl

Despite the excellent physiological characteristics of thallium for imaging myocardial perfusion and viability, its low-energy gamma spectrum is suboptimal for scintillation camera imaging. In 1981, Deutsch and coworkers described a series of ^{99m}Tc-labeled myocardial perfusion tracers.[140] ^{99m}Tc-sestamibi, ^{99m}Tc-teboroxime, ^{99m}Tc-tetrofosmin, and ^{99m}Tc-phosfuramine (Q12) overcome 2 major limitations of ^{201}thallium; long physical half-life (73 hours) and low photon energy (69 to 80 keV mercury x-rays). The short 6-hour half-life of ^{99m}Tc permits the administration of doses 10 times higher than ^{201}Tl, thereby improving the resolution of the images (higher photon flux and count statistics) without increasing radiation burden to the patient. Photon attenuation as a function of tissue depth is also less for ^{99m}Tc, resulting in improved spatial resolution and less prominent soft-tissue artifacts (Table 3).

Similar to thallium, these tracers are taken up by the myocardium in proportion to regional blood flow, and recent studies have indicated that the accuracy of these technetium-labeled perfusion tracers for detecting coronary artery disease is analogous (but not superior) to that of thallium.[141–143] However, the application of these tracers for the assessment of myocardial viability remains an area of uncertainty.

^{99m}Tc-Sestamibi for Identifying Myocardial Viability

^{99m}Tc-sestamibi is a lipophilic perfusion tracer extracted by the myocardium differently from thallium. Unlike thallium, which (like potassium) requires predominantly active transport systems,[144,145] the uptake of sestamibi is passive across mitochondrial membranes but, at equilibrium, sestamibi is retained within the mitochondria due to a large negative transmembrane potential.[146] Transcapillary transport and myocardial retention of both sestamibi and thallium are affected by the perfusion rate, capillary permeability, and by the binding characteristics within the myocardium.[147,148] Despite the differences in kinetics between sestamibi and thallium, the initial regional myocardial uptake of the 2 tracers is similar and both agents have similar accuracy for detecting coronary artery disease.[149–152]

Although published reports to date have demonstrated a good correlation between rest sestamibi uptake and degree of coronary artery stenosis,[153] the correlation between sestamibi uptake and viability as assessed by wall motion is less impressive.[154] Among regions with only moderate (50 to 67% of peak activity) reduction in sestamibi activity, 80% had improved sestamibi activity after coronary artery bypass surgery. However, 39% of regions with severe (<50% of peak) reduction in sestamibi activity also showed improved regional perfusion postoperatively.[154]

SESTAMIBI IMAGING IN STUNNED MYOCARDIUM

In stunned but viable myocardium, in which coronary flow has been restored by reperfusion, sestamibi uptake should be an accurate marker of cellular viability; this has been confirmed in several studies.[58,155–161] In experimental models of stunned myocardium, the retention of sestamibi has been comparable to that of thallium.[58,156] In contrast, in regions of necrotic myocardium, the retention of sestamibi is negligible and parallels indices of viability, such as FDG uptake and histochemical staining.[156] Furthermore, after acute reperfusion in animal models, a close correlation between sestamibi autoradiographic images and pathologic infarct size has been demonstrated,[157,158] independent of regional blood flow.

In patients studied within the first week of thrombolytic therapy for acute myocardial infarction, sestamibi defect size correlates well with regional wall motion at the time of discharge,[159] with late ejection fraction measurements,[159] and with peak release of creatine kinase.[160] These confirma-

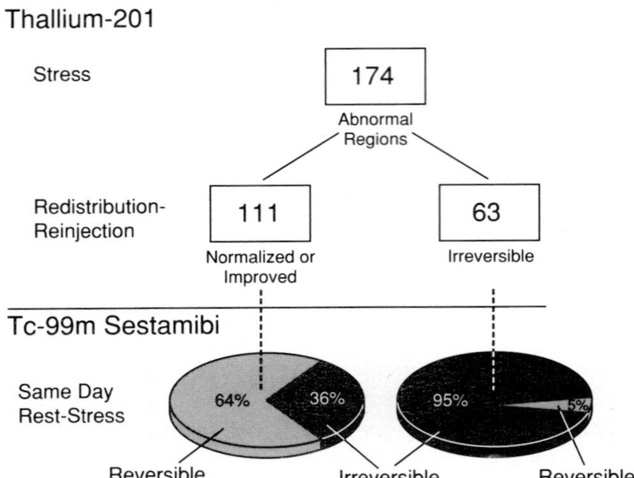

Figure 21. Flow diagram displaying the prevalence of reversible and irreversible thallium perfusion defects by stress-redistribution-reinjection and same-day rest-stress sestamibi studies in 54 patients with chronic coronary artery disease with a mean left ventricular ejection fraction of 34 ± 14%. (Reprinted[169] with permission of the American Heart Association.)

tory clinical studies suggest that sestamibi may be useful as a viability marker of stunned myocardium after reperfusion therapy for acute myocardial infarction.

SESTAMIBI IMAGING IN HIBERNATING MYOCARDIUM

Unlike stunned myocardium, the role of sestamibi imaging for identifying hibernating myocardium in patients with chronic coronary artery disease and left ventricular dysfunction is limited. There are a growing number of studies to suggest that sestamibi overestimates irreversible defects and myocardial scarring in patients with chronic coronary artery disease.[154,162–173]

Using conventional planar imaging and qualitative analysis in patients with chronic coronary artery disease, Cuocolo and coworkers reported that 29% of reversible myocardial regions by thallium reinjection appeared irreversible when a 2-day stress-rest sestamibi protocol was performed.[162] In our laboratory,[169] 36% of myocardial regions that were classified as ischemic but viable by the thallium stress-redistribution-reinjection protocol were misclassified as irreversible defects on the sestamibi rest-stress protocol (Fig. 21). Viability of these regions was confirmed by PET imaging.[169] These initial observations were confirmed by subsequent studies.[163–168,170–173]

If the mechanism of the thallium reinjection effect is merely that the reinjected thallium dose provides a better assessment of resting myocardial perfusion than redistribution images, thallium reinjection results should be equivalent to results obtained when sestamibi is injected at rest. It is likely that the period of thallium redistribution after exercise may be the key factor, with the images after reinjection incorporating resting blood flow along with the metabolic information inherent in the redistribution data. Thus, thallium reinjection images are not merely measures of resting blood flow.[83] Thallium and sestamibi uptake, like that of all other tracers, reflects both regional blood flow and myocardial extraction; these vary depending upon the retention mechanism involved for each individual tracer. However, despite the recognized metabolic or transmembrane trapping of these tracers, the relationship between myocardial tracer uptake and blood flow is not significantly altered except during (1) acute myocardial ischemia, (2) conditions of extremely low pH or, (3) hyperemic flow.

Previous studies have shown that thallium reinjection more accurately reflects myocardial viability (as confirmed by FDG:blood flow mismatch by PET) than images obtained in the same patients immediately after a separate resting injection of thallium one week later.[83] These observations imply that perfusion agents that measure coronary blood flow alone may not assess myocardial viability as well as an agent that redistributes, such as thallium. Thus, sestamibi may underestimate viable myocardium in regions with chronic reduction in blood flow.

Severity of Regional Sestamibi Activity. One approach that may surmount, in part, the limitations of sestamibi in assessing viable myocardium is to quantify the severity of regional sestamibi activity. Such quantitative methods have been useful in thallium imaging for identifying viable myocardium within apparently irreversible thallium defects.[83,108,174] In one study, among regions that were considered viable by thallium imaging and PET, but possibly nonviable on the basis of an irreversible defect on rest-stress sestamibi images, 78% had sestamibi activity that was >50% of the activity in normal territories.[169] If such mild-to-moderate sestamibi defects are considered to represent viable (nonischemic) myocardial tissue on the basis of sestamibi activity alone, and only severe reduction in activity (≤50% of normal) is considered evidence of nonviability, then the overall concordance between thallium and sestamibi studies was increased to 93% (Fig. 22). Despite the application of quantitative techniques, other studies have demonstrated that rest sestamibi imaging underestimates myocardial viability when compared to PET.[166,171] In patients with chronic coronary artery disease undergoing both rest sestamibi SPECT and FDG PET studies, Altehoefer et al.[166,173] found discordance between the magnitude of reduction in sestamibi activity and FDG uptake (Fig. 23). Using quantitative analysis of rest sestamibi, ^{13}N-ammonia and FDG PET images, and the same threshold values for viability, Sawada et al.[171] found that the sestamibi defect size at rest was larger than that of ammonia PET. Furthermore, 47% of segments with severe sestamibi defects (<50% of peak activity) had preserved metabolic activity as assessed by FDG PET.[171]

It is important to keep in mind, however, that the mere presence of viable myocardium (quantitative analysis of the severity of sestamibi defect) does not necessarily indicate ischemic myocardium (stress-induced reversible defects).

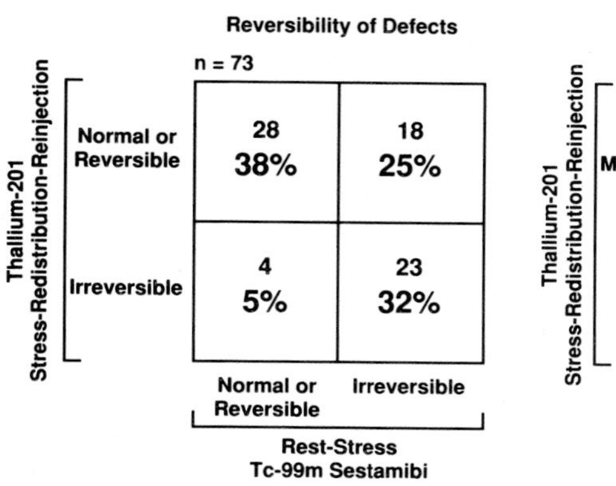

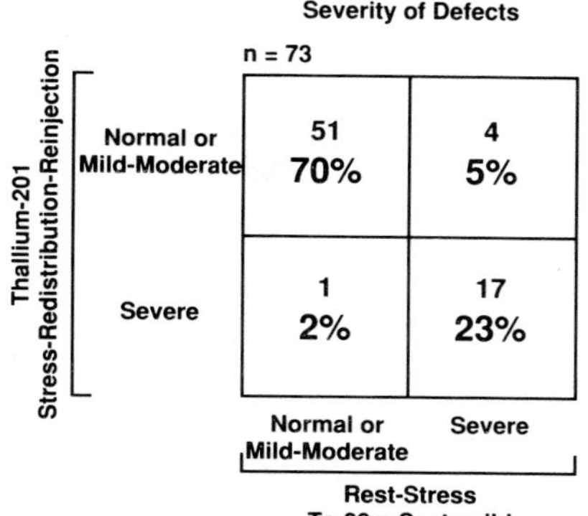

Figure 22. Diagram showing concordance and discordance between thallium stress-redistribution-reinjection and sestamibi rest-stress images in 25 patients who also underwent PET studies. Data on reversibility of defects (normal/reversible or irreversible) are shown on the left, and severity of defects (normal/mild-to-moderate or severe) is shown on the right. Eighteen of 22 discordant regions between thallium and sestamibi studies are reversible by thallium redistribution-reinjection studies. Myocardial viability was confirmed in 17 of 18 regions by PET. (Reprinted[169] with permission of the American Heart Association.)

It is more likely for an ischemic region to improve after revascularization than nonischemic but viable myocardium (mild-to-moderate reduction in tracer activity). In the study by Marzullo et al., 32% of segments exhibiting sestamibi activity of >55% of peak normal (viable at rest) showed no improvement in regional contraction after revascularization.[164] Conversely, 25% of segments with normal wall motion had severely reduced (≤55% of peak) sestamibi activity at rest (nonviable). Therefore, the distinction between ischemic myocardium (stress-induced reversible defect) and viable myocardium (severity of defect at rest) has important clinical implications (Table 4).

Sestamibi Redistribution. Sestamibi does redistribute after a resting injection in some patients with left ventricular dysfunction.[175–178] Following injection of sestamibi at peak exercise, minimal but clinically relevant redistribution occurs in ischemic myocardium of patients with coronary artery disease.[177] In an animal model of sustained low-flow ischemia,[178] sestamibi redistribution was observed over 2.5 hours in a manner comparable to thallium (Fig. 24). In clinical studies of patients undergoing an additional redistribution sestamibi study 4 hours after injecting the tracer at rest, sestamibi redistribution occurred in 38% of regions with perfusion defects on the initial rest image that were identified as viable by thallium and PET studies (Fig. 25). Such redistribution was observed in 22% of patients, and increased the overall concordance between thallium and sestamibi imaging regarding defect reversibility to 82%.[169] The clinical relevance of rest sestamibi redistribution has been confirmed by others.[179]

Pre- and Postrevascularization Studies. Only a few studies have evaluated sestamibi uptake before and after revascularization. In 1992, Lucignani et al. studied patients with sestamibi SPECT before and after coronary artery bypass surgery.[165] Of the 54 asynergic regions before surgery, 42 had normal or reduced perfusion at rest and developed stress-induced ischemia, and 11 had markedly reduced or absent perfusion at rest. After revascularization, recovery of wall motion was observed in 79% of regions with stress-induced ischemia. However, 72% of regions with markedly reduced or absent perfusion at rest also showed improved wall motion after surgery. In another study, using planar imaging and quantitative analysis, Marzullo and coworkers reported 79% positive predictive and 76% negative predictive values for recovery of regional left ventricular dysfunction after revas-

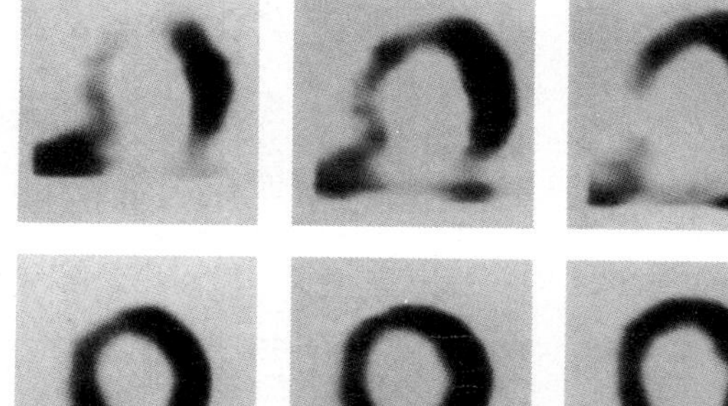

Figure 23. Discordance between PET and rest sestamibi SPECT imaging is demonstrated in this patient with three-vessel coronary artery disease. Three consecutive short-axis tomograms are displayed for ^{99m}technetium-sestamibi (top), with corresponding FDG PET tomograms (bottom). Rest sestamibi images reveal extensive perfusion abnormalities involving the anteroapical, septal, and inferior regions with preserved viability in the posterolateral region and mixed viable and scarred myocardium in the septal region. FDG uptake in the corresponding regions demonstrate preserved metabolic activity and viability in all 3 coronary artery vascular territories. The patient had totally occluded but collateralized left anterior descending and right coronary arteries and severe stenosis of the left circumflex artery. (From Altehoefer et al.,[173] modified and reprinted with permission of The Journal of Nuclear Medicine.)

Table 4. Definitions of Myocardial Viability with Single–Photon Tracers

SCINTIGRAPHIC INTERPRETATION		CLINICAL INTERPRETATION
Reversibility of defects –Stress-induced myocardial ischemia	→	Ischemic but viable myocardium
Severity of defects		
–Mild-moderate (51–85% of normal activity)	→	Nonischemic, viable myocardium
–Severe (≤50% of normal activity)	→	Nonischemic, scarred myocardium

cularization.[164] Recently, among 18 patients with coronary artery disease undergoing revascularization, more favorable positive (80%) and negative (96%) predictive accuracy was attained by Udelson et al. when the severity of sestamibi defect was quantified at rest.[180] A patient with discordant thallium stress-redistribution-reinjection and 2-day rest-stress sestamibi imaging studied before and after revascularization is shown in Figure 26.

In summary, sestamibi appears to underestimate myocardial ischemia and viability in patients with chronic coronary artery disease and left ventricular dysfunction compared to thallium scintigraphy and FDG PET. Whether or not

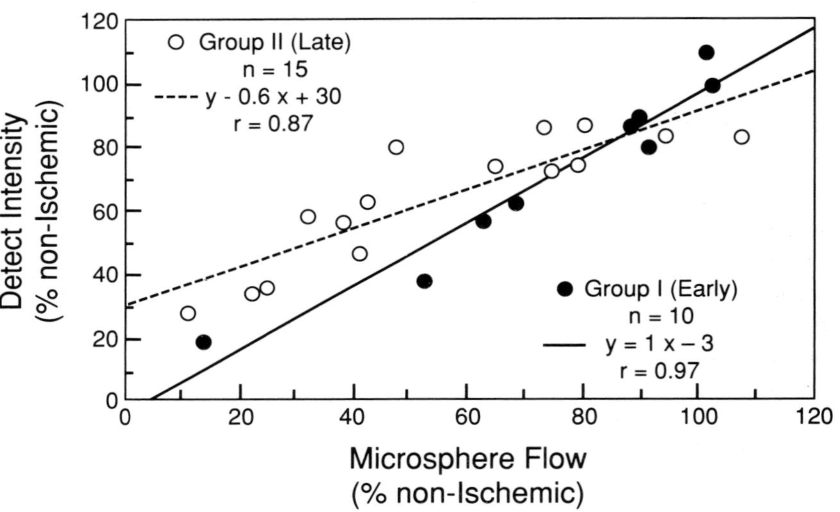

Figure 24. Scatterplot of transmural defect intensity (% nonischemic) from gamma camera images of ex vivo myocardial slices. Ten slices from 5 group I dogs and 15 slices from 8 group II dogs were analyzed. The relative defect intensity correlates well with the relative transmural microsphere flow deficit in identical regions early after sestamibi injection (group I). In group II, there was also good correlation between relative defect intensity and the flow deficit in the corresponding region. However, the defect was less pronounced than the flow deficit at the time of injection, suggesting that redistribution of sestamibi was detectable by quantitative analysis of high-resolution ex vivo images. (From Sinusas et al.,[178] reprinted with permission of the American Heart Association.)

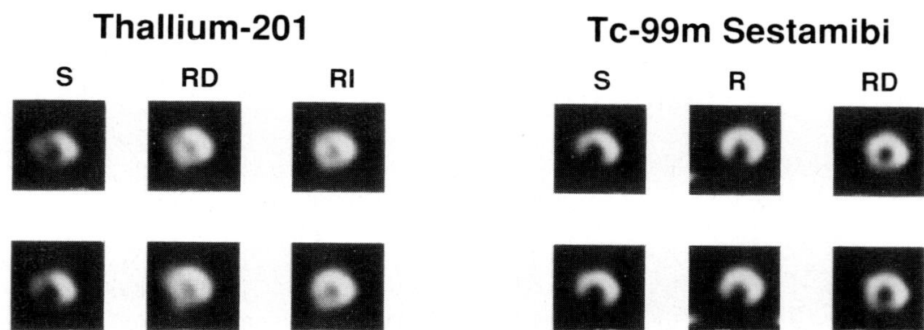

Figure 25. An example of a patient with reversible thallium defects and irreversible defects on rest-stress sestamibi imaging. The same level of exercise was achieved with both studies. Two consecutive short-axis tomograms are displayed for thallium stress (S), redistribution (RD), and reinjection (RI) with corresponding sestamibi tomograms of stress, rest (R), and redistribution. Thallium SPECT images reveal extensive inferior and septal perfusion defects during stress that are reversible on redistribution and reinjection images. Same day rest-stress sestamibi images, performed 3 days after the thallium study, show extensive inferior and septal perfusion defects, with partial reversibility in the upper septum but irreversibility in the lower septum and inferior regions. Sestamibi redistribution images acquired 4 hours following injection of the tracer at rest show partial reversibility in the lower septum and inferior regions. (Reprinted[169] with permission of the American Heart Association.)

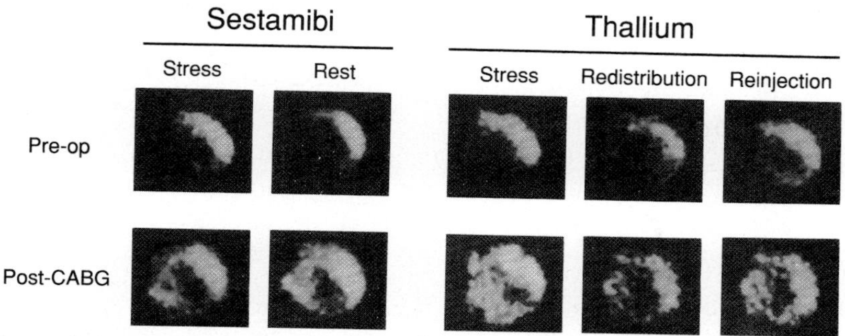

Figure 26. Evidence of viable myocardium in a region with irreversible sestamibi defect. Preoperative anterior planar thallium images on the right demonstrate severe irreversible inferior thallium defect on stress-redistribution images that becomes reversible after reinjection and improves after coronary artery bypass surgery. Two-day rest-stress sestamibi images (on the left), performed 5 days after the thallium study, show severe irreversible inferior defect preoperatively that improves after coronary artery bypass surgery. The left ventricular ejection fraction increased from 40% before to 55% after surgery. (From Maurea et al.,[170] modified and reprinted with permission of The Journal of Nuclear Medicine.)

measuring redistribution of sestamibi after rest injections will enhance assessment of viable myocardium is a subject of ongoing investigation. Perhaps a more likely improvement could be achieved through combined sestamibi perfusion and functional imaging or ECG gated myocardial perfusion studies.

^{99m}Tc-Teboroxime and Viability

^{99m}Tc-teboroxime is a neutral lipophilic compound that is avidly extracted by the myocardium and its extraction remains linear even at high-flow conditions.[181,182] In studies with cultured myocardial cells, the accumulation of teboroxime is approximately 4 times greater than that of thallium or sestamibi,[183,184] and permits accurate assessment of coronary blood flow even during pharmacological hyperemia.[185–188] Unlike sestamibi, teboroxime washes out rapidly from the myocardium at a rate proportional to regional blood flow. Both uptake and washout of teboroxime depend predominantly upon regional myocardial blood flow and are not confounded by tissue metabolism or other binding characteristics within the myocardium.[189–194] However, despite its rapid washout, some reports suggest that teboroxime may underestimate myocardial ischemia and viability compared with thallium scintigraphy.[185,195–198] Its role in assessing myocardial viability awaits further study.

^{99m}Tc-Tetrofosmin

^{99m}Tc-tetrofosmin is a lipophilic phosphine dioxo cation that is distributed within the myocardium in proportion to regional myocardial blood flow.[199,200] However, unlike thallium, tetrofosmin does not redistribute significantly over time, thereby requiring injections of the tracer at both peak exercise and at rest.[201] Tracer uptake in the heart and blood clearance kinetics of tetrofosmin are similar to those of sestamibi. However, the clearance of tetrofosmin from lungs and liver is faster than that of sestamibi, which improves early image resolution. The more rapid excretion of tetrofosmin compared to sestamibi may also reduce the radiation absorbed dose.[202] Multicenter phase III clinical trials comparing the efficacy of tetrofosmin with thallium show an overall concordance for defining normal or abnormal regions of about 80%.[143] However, when patients were catergorized as showing normal, ischemia, infarction, or mixed (infarction and viable) myocardium, the concordance between tetrofosmin and thallium was only 59.4%.

^{99m}Tc-Phosfurimine (Q12)

^{99m}Tc-phosfurimine (Q12) is a mixed-ligand cationic complex used as a myocardial imaging agent. After injection of Q12, it is avidly taken up by the myocardium and rapidly cleared from the blood. Q12 is cleared primarily by the hepatobiliary system and approximately 30% by the kidneys. Q12 myocardial distribution is proportional to regional myocardial blood flow, as measured by the radioactive microsphere technique for flows up to 2 ml/gm/min.[203] However, with pharmacological stress (myocardial blood flow above 2 ml/gm/min), Q12 activity does not increase proportionately. Unlike thallium, Q12 does not redistribute significantly from the time of injection.[203] Imaging with both thallium and Q12 was performed in a pilot study including patients with coronary artery disease and control subjects.[204] Identification of angiographically documented coronary disease in individual coronary arteries was 80 and 82% for thallium and 73 and 87% for Q12. Agreement between thallium stress-redistribution-reinjection protocol and rest-stress Q12 studies for detecting myocardial ischemia and viability (defect reversibility) was poor. However, there was good overall concordance between thallium and Q12 in normal and irreversible regions. Multicenter clinical trials are currently underway comparing Q12 with thallium in the same patients.

INFARCT-AVID MYOCARDIAL SCINTIGRAPHY

In contrast to tracers that concentrate in perfusable myocardium, infarct-avid tracers, such as ^{99m}Tc-pyrophosphate and ^{111}In- or ^{99m}Tc-labeled antimyosin, are sequestered by necrotic

Table 5. Infarct-Avid Myocardial Scintigraphy

^{99m}Technetium-pyrophosphate
^{111}Indium-labeled antimyosin antibody
^{99m}Technetium-labeled antimyosin antibody

myocardium and are used to evaluate the presence and extent of necrotic myocardium after acute myocardial infarction or in patients with cardiomyopathy (Table 5).

The diagnosis of acute myocardial infarction is based on clinical presentation, electrocardiography, and serum levels and isoenzymes of creatine kinase and lactic dehydrogenase. The MB isoenzyme of creatine kinase provides the most sensitive and specific marker for acute myocardial infarction if the diagnosis is made within the first 24 hours after the onset of initial symptoms. The creatine kinase-MB isoenzyme constitutes approximately 20% of cytosolic creatine kinase in adult human myocardium, with the remaining 80% representing creatine kinase-MM isoenzyme. Lactic dehydrogenase levels begin to increase approximately 10 hours after the onset of clinical symptoms of acute myocardial infarction and peak at 24 to 48 hours. As with creatine kinase, lactic dehydrogenase isoenzymes are assayed as markers of acute myocardial infarction. A ratio of lactic dehydrogenase-1 to lactic dehydrogenase-2 greater or equal to 1 indicates acute myocardial infarction.

^{99m}Tc-Pyrophosphate

Imaging myocardial infarctions with ^{99m}Tc-pyrophosphate is based on the fact that calcium accumulates in necrotic myocardial cells and pyrophosphate is avidly taken up by crystalline or amorphous calcium phosphate.[205,206] In patients presenting late, 24 to 72 hours after the onset of chest pain, myocardial uptake of pyrophosphate may be useful in identifying acute myocardial necrosis, particularly if the elapsed time is beyond the time course for cardiac enzymes to be diagnostic.[207–210]

Cardiac imaging after the injection of ^{99m}Tc-pyrophosphate is delayed for at least 3 hours to allow clearance of the tracer from blood. Normal pyrophosphate images exhibit no activity in the region of the heart, with clear outline of bony structures. On the other hand, abnormal pyrophosphate scans may show localized tracer uptake in a specific vascular territory or myocardial region, as shown in Figure 27, or diffuse uptake throughout the myocardium. SPECT imaging may facilitate detection of small, nontransmural myocardial infarction, especially when combined with a gated blood pool overlay.[211]

The sensitivity of pyrophosphate imaging is greater in Q-wave compared to nonQ-wave myocardial infarctions.[212,213] The myocardial necrosis should be at least 3 grams to detect pyrophosphate uptake by planar imaging.[210,214] On the other hand, myocardial necrosis as small as 1 gram can be detected when imaged by SPECT.[211] Sensitivities and specificities of pyrophosphate imaging in myocardial necrosis vary greatly in the literature depending on the technology, diagnostic criteria, and the prevalence of myocardial infarction in the patient population studied. For example, if both focal and diffuse patterns of pyrophosphate uptake are considered diagnostic for recent myocardial infarction, the overall sensitivity of pyrophosphate imaging may be as high as 93%, but at the expense of lower specificity.[212,215] On the other hand, exclusion of the diffuse pattern improves specificity but lowers sensitivity to approximately 66%.[213,216] Although focal pyrophosphate activity usually corresponds to myocardial necrosis, several other conditions simulate myocardial necrosis, including (1) old myocardial infarctions with or without left ventricular aneurysms,[217] (2) acute pericarditis and myocarditis, (3) valvular calcification,[218] (4) calcified fibrosis around prosthetic valves,[219] (6) cardiac contusion,[220] (7) high-voltage electrical injury[221] or electrical cardioversion, and (8) metastatic cardiac tumor.[222]

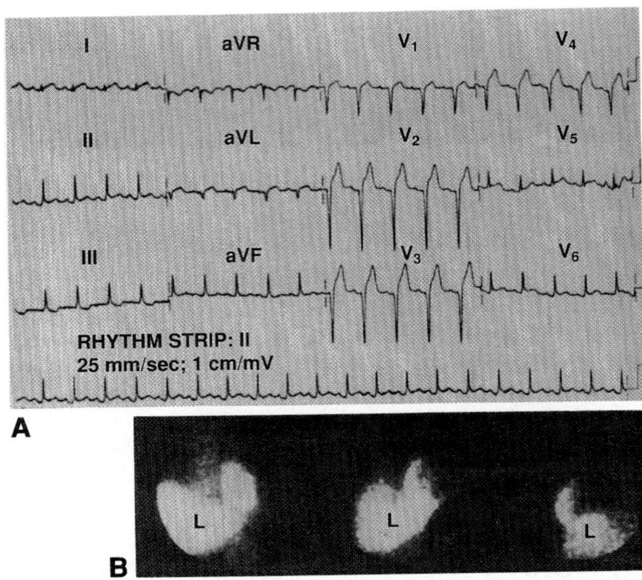

Figure 27. An example of a patient with acute anterior Q-wave myocardial infarction (panel A) and corresponding ^{111}indium-labeled antimyosin uptake in the anterior, septal, and apical regions of the left ventricle (panel B). Planar images in the anterior, best septal left anterior oblique, and left lateral projections are shown. L, liver. (From Johnson et al.,[227] reprinted with permission of the Journal of the American College of Cardiology.)

^{111}In- and ^{99m}Tc-Labeled Antimyosin Antibodies

Antimyosin monoclonal antibodies and their Fab fragments may be more specific markers of myocardial necrosis than pyrophosphate imaging.[223–225] Following acute myocardial infarction, myocardial cell membrane disruption exposes cardiac myosin to the extracellular space. Myosin heavy chains are abundant in the myocytes, relatively insoluble, and remain within the necrotic myocyte. Radiolabeled antimyosin antibody will bind to the exposed myosin molecules

Table 6. Commonly Used PET Radionuclides

RADIONUCLIDE	HALF-LIFE (min)
Generator-produced	
^{82}Rubidium	1.3
^{62}Copper	9.7
Cyclotron-produced	
^{15}Oxygen	2.1
^{13}Nitrogen	10.0
^{11}Carbon	20.3
^{18}Fluorine	110.0

in sufficient concentrations for imaging. Even with a totally occluded coronary artery, antimyosin antibody can identify necrotic myocardium by way of diffusion.[226]

In a multicenter study of 50 patients with transmural Q-wave infarction, ^{111}In-DTPA-antimyosin Fab identified myocardial necrosis in 46 (92%) patients; 2 had diffuse uptake and 44 had focal antimyosin uptake.[227] Focal myocardial uptake of antimyosin corresponded to electrocardiographic infarct localization (Fig. 27). Preliminary studies also suggest a role for antimyosin in detecting ongoing cell necrosis in patients with myocarditis,[228,229] dilated cardiomyopathy,[230] hypertrophic cardiomyopathy,[231] and cardiac transplant rejection.[229]

POSITRON EMISSION TOMOGRAPHY

Viable myocardium is identified by PET tracers on the basis of preserved or enhanced metabolic substrate utilization in hypoperfused and dysfunctional myocardial regions. Compared to SPECT imaging, PET provides high spatial resolution and high count density cardiac images, as well as quantitative assessment of regional myocardial tissue function under various physiological conditions.

PET Perfusion

Myocardial blood flow tracers include ^{15}O-water, ^{13}N-ammonia, and ^{82}Rb (Table 6). Although ^{38}K and ^{62}Cu-PTSM have also been used for assessment of myocardial perfusion, they are considered investigational. Noninvasive quantitation of regional blood flow in milliliters per minute per gram of tissue can be obtained with these PET tracers. As a result of their short physical half-lives, repeat blood flow measurements in response to physiological or pharmacological interventions can be assessed at relatively short time intervals.

^{15}O-WATER

^{15}O-water is a freely diffusable tracer, the kinetics of accumulation and clearance of which are less complicated than tracers that are partially extractable. Quantitative assessment of regional ^{15}O-water perfusion correlates closely with perfusion as assessed by microspheres.[232] Because ^{15}O-water is in both the vascular space and myocardium, visualization of myocardial activity requires correction for activity in the vascular compartment. This is accomplished by acquiring a separate scan after inhalation of ^{15}O-carbon monoxide, which labels red blood cells and delineates the vascular space. Subtraction of ^{15}O-carbon monoxide images from the ^{15}O-water images results in visualization of the myocardium.[232,233] To eliminate a second scan with ^{15}O-carbon monoxide, the early phase of ^{15}O-water distribution, which reflects first pass of the tracer through the cardiac blood pool, may be analyzed separately.[234] Myocardial uptake of ^{15}O-water parallels regional blood flow even at hyperemic ranges.[235–237]

^{13}N-AMMONIA

^{13}N-ammonia is the most commonly used extractable perfusion tracer with PET.[238,239] At physiological pH, ammonia is in its cationic form with a physical half-life of 10 minutes. Myocardial distribution of ammonia is inversely and nonlinearly related to blood flow and its uptake is thought to involve carrier-mediated transport.[240,241] The kinetics of accumulation and clearance from myocardium depends on the conversion of ammonia to glutamine via the glutamine synthetase pathway. Hence, absolute quantification requires two- and three-compartment kinetic models that incorporate both extraction and retention rate constants.[242,243] Quantification of ammonia is further complicated by the rapid degradation of ammonia, which occurs within 5 minutes after administration, producing metabolic intermediates, such as urea and glutamine, that are also extracted by the heart.[244–247] Experimental studies suggest that myocardial uptake of ammonia reflects absolute blood flows of up to 2 to 2.5 ml/gm/min and plateaus at flows in the hyperemic range.[240,241] Qualitative estimates of myocardial perfusion have been used in a number of clinical studies to assess myocardial viability. Ischemic regions are defined in terms of % peak activity ammonia values 2 standard deviations below the regional mean activity in healthy, human subjects. Such qualitative estimates result in high sensitivities and specificities for detecting coronary artery disease.[238,248–250]

Gewirtz et al.[251] reported that quantitative assessment of absolute regional myocardial blood flow with ammonia permits differentiation of viable from scarred myocardium in

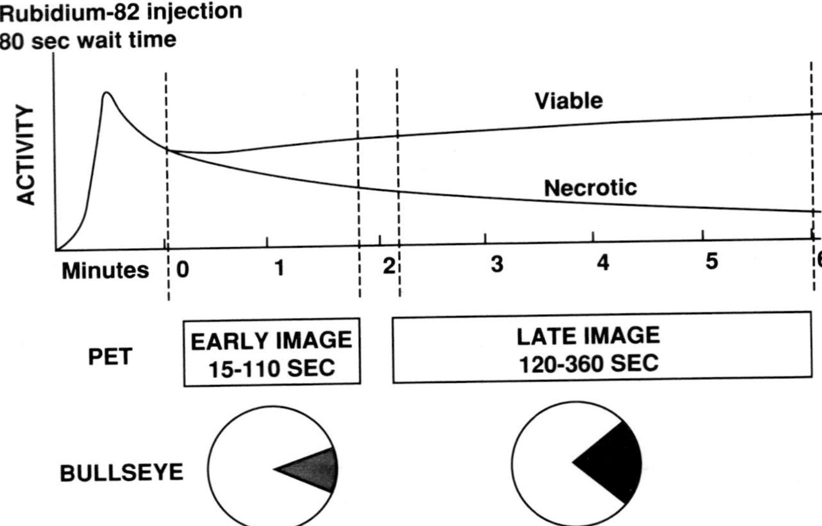

Figure 28. Schematic protocol utilizing the kinetic changes of rubidium-82 after intravenous injection to assess myocardial viability. (From Gould et al.,[263] modified and reprinted with permission of The Journal of Nuclear Medicine.)

asynergic myocardial regions. All dyskinetic regions demonstrated ammonia blood flow values less than 0.25 ml/gm/min, and all but one region determined to be metabolically active and viable by PET had blood flow values of more than 0.25 ml/gm/min. In contrast, regional blood flow values were greater than 0.39 ml/gm/min (average flow of 0.78 ml/gm/min) in 43 of 45 regions with normal or hypokinetic contraction. However, among patients with chronic coronary artery disease studied before and after revascularization, the positive and negative predictive values of ammonia perfusion studies for improvement in regional asynergy were reported to be only 48 and 87%, respectively.[252]

^{82}RUBIDIUM

^{82}Rb is a generator-produced, short-lived (1.3 minute half-life) cation, whose uptake depends on myocardial perfusion.[253] As with potassium and thallium, intracellular uptake of rubidium across the sarcolemmal membrane reflects active cation transport. Experimental studies have suggested that myocardial uptake of rubidium reflects absolute blood flows of up to 2 to 3 ml/gm/min. However, net uptake of rubidium plateaus at hyperemic flows with pharmacological stress.[254,255] There are several studies that suggest that myocardial ischemia or ischemia followed with reperfusion reduces the extraction fraction of rubidium, presumably due to diminished cation transport across the sarcolemmal membrane.[254–257] Nonetheless, qualitative assessment of relative rubidium perfusion defects have correlated well with those obtained from microspheres.[258] Clinically, rubidium PET has both high sensitivity and specificity for detecting coronary artery disease.[248,259–261] As a result, clinical assessment of myocardial perfusion with rubidium PET has received U.S. Food and Drug Administration (FDA) approval.

With regard to viability assessment in patients with chronic coronary artery disease, uptake of rubidium is severely reduced in regions with scarred myocardium and preserved in viable myocardium, demonstrating regional heterogeneity. In the setting of acute myocardial infarction and reperfusion, initial ^{82}Rb uptake like ^{201}Tl reflects restored blood flow. However, necrotic myocardium cannot retain rubidium and, despite its initial uptake, the tracer rapidly washes out resulting in an image defect. Hence, rubidium is taken up by both viable and necrotic myocardium, but is not retained by necrotic myocardium.[262]

Based on these observations, Gould et al.[263] have suggested that the kinetics of rubidium washout may be used as an index of myocardial viability (Fig. 28). Applying such analyses of washout kinetics in patients with acute myocardial infarction, they demonstrated that ^{82}Rb provides information regarding myocardial viability comparable to that of FDG PET.[263] This suggests that early after myocardial infarction, myocardial viability may be evaluated either by the behavior of potassium analogues (such as ^{201}Tl and ^{82}Rb), as indices of cell membrane integrity, or by measures of metabolic activity with FDG or ^{11}C-acetate.

PET Metabolism

PET has emerged as a useful technology for demonstrating myocardial viability in patients with left ventricular dysfunction,[21,264–268] as PET can demonstrate preserved metabolic activity in regions with reduced perfusion (Table 7). At rest and in the fasting state, the respiratory quotient (the rate of oxygen uptake divided by carbon dioxide release) of myocardium is approximately 0.7 in man,[269] indicating that

Table 7. PET Assessment of Myocardial Viability

^{18}F-deoxyglucose metabolism-perfusion mismatch
^{82}Rb uptake and washout
Regional oxidative metabolism assessed by ^{11}C-acetate
^{15}O-water perfusable tissue index

the primary substrates of myocardial energy production in the normal myocardium are fatty acids.[270] Upon feeding, circulating levels of insulin increase, stimulating glucose metabolism and diminishing free fatty acid metabolism.[271] Breakdown of fatty acids occurs in the mitochondria via beta-oxidation.

During hypoxia or myocardial ischemia, beta-oxidation of fatty acids in the mitochondria is reduced. Myocytes compensate for the loss of oxidative potential by shifting toward glucose utilization to generate high-energy phosphates.[271–273] Although the amount of energy produced by glycolysis may be adequate to maintain myocyte viability and preserve the electrochemical gradient across the cell membrane, it may not be sufficient to sustain mechanical work. However, it is important to recognize that glycolysis can be maintained for as long as end-products of the glycolytic pathway (lactate and hydrogen ion) are removed and do not accumulate intracellularly.[271,273] Therefore, in order to maintain myocyte viability, adequate blood flow is necessary both to deliver the tracer to the myocyte and to remove the metabolites of the glycolytic pathway. If regional blood flow is severely reduced or absent, then byproducts of glycolysis accumulate, causing inhibition of the glycolytic enzymes, depletion of high-energy phosphates, cell membrane disruption, and cell death.

^{11}C-PALMITATE

Because fatty acids are the primary source of myocardial energy production, early studies focused on the characterization of myocardial kinetics of ^{11}C-palmitate. Uptake of fatty acids across the sarcolemmal membrane is thought to occur along a concentration gradient, possibly through a facilitated transport. After extraction by normal myocardium, ^{11}C-palmitate is cleared biexponentially.[274,275] The first, rapid-clearance phase represents oxidative metabolism of ^{11}C-palmitate through beta-oxidation and the tricarboxylic acid cycle. The second, slower-clearance phase of the tracer represents the turnover of ^{11}C-palmitate in the endogenous pool of phospholipids and triglycerides.[272,275] During hypoxia or myocardial ischemia, both myocardial extraction and clearance of ^{11}C-palmitate are reduced.[276] In a canine model, Schwaiger et al. demonstrated that reperfusion after experimental coronary artery occlusions of 3 hours duration resulted in altered kinetics and delayed clearance of ^{11}C-palmitate from myocardium, suggesting reduced fatty acid utilization.[277] However, under ischemic conditions, myocardial kinetics of ^{11}C-palmitate are not specific for oxidative metabolism but, rather, reflect the overall metabolic function of the myocardium. In a reperfused working swine heart model, Liedtke et al. demonstrated that fatty acid oxidation actually increases during early reflow.[278] Despite conflicting data in experimental animals, impaired fatty acid oxidation has been shown in patients with acute myocardial ischemia.[279] However, the kinetics of myocardial extraction and clearance of ^{11}C-palmitate can be markedly altered by arterial substrate concentration, myocardial ischemia and reperfusion, and hormonal environment.[280–282] As a result, the application of ^{11}C-palmitate oxidation has been limited in the clinical evaluation of patients with chronic coronary disease or acute myocardial ischemia.

Currently, several radioiodine-labeled fatty acid analogs have been used to assess myocardial fatty acid metabolism by SPECT technology. The 2 most widely accessible tracers are iodophenylpentadecanoic acid (IPPA) and beta-methyliodopentadecanoic acid (BMIPP). Studies are now in progress to investigate myocardial tissue kinetics and substrate utilization by the human heart.

^{18}F-FLUORODEOXYGLUCOSE

^{18}F-2-fluoro-2-deoxyglucose (FDG) is a glucose analog that competes with glucose for hexokinase and tracks transmembranous exchange and phosphorylation of glucose.[283] After it is phosphorylated, FDG-6-phosphate does not enter glycolysis, fructose-pentose shunt, or glycogen synthesis.[284] Thus, myocardial uptake of FDG reflects the overall rate of transmembrane exchange and phosphorylation of glucose, but is unable to track the glycolytic and glycogen synthesis pathways. Because the dephosphorylation rate of glucose is slow, FDG becomes essentially trapped in the myocardium, reflecting regional glucose utilization. Glucose utilization, in turn, is influenced by several factors such as coronary perfusion, cardiac work, competitive substrates, insulin, and neurohormonal effects.[272,285,286] Quantification of glucose utilization rates requires a constant that relates the kinetic behavior of FDG to naturally occurring glucose for transmembrane exchange and phosphorylation by hexokinase. Because this constant may vary under different pathophysiological conditions, kinetic modeling that attempts to quantify glucose utilization rates should be treated with appropriate caution.

^{11}C-ACETATE IMAGING

^{11}C-acetate is taken up by myocardium in proportion to blood flow, and its washout rate is directly related to oxidative tricarboxylic acid cycle flux.[287–289] Given the close link between the tricarboxylic acid cycle and oxidative phosphorylation, it has been suggested that the myocardial turnover and clearance of ^{11}C-acetate in the form of ^{11}Carbon dioxide reflects overall oxidative metabolism. Hence, ^{11}C-acetate may provide insight into the mitochondrial function of ischemic but viable myocardium.

Laboratory investigations have demonstrated that preservation of myocardial oxidative metabolism using ^{14}C-acetate predicts restoration of mechanical function after acute ischemia.[287] In 2 separate studies involving small numbers of patients with recent myocardial infarction[290] and chronic stable angina,[291] preservation of myocardial oxidative metabolism was also shown to predict functional recovery after revascularization. When clearance rates of ^{11}C-acetate were within 2 standard deviations of the normal mean, the positive predictive accuracy for recovery of function after revascularization was 84% in patients with recent myocardial infarction and 79% in patients with chronic stable angina. Conversely, when clearance rates of ^{11}C-acetate were more than 2 standard deviations below the normal mean, the negative predictive values were 70% in patients with recent myocardial infarction and 83% in patients with chronic stable angina.[290,291] In another study of patients with reperfused anterior myocardial infarction studied between 2 weeks and 3 months after the acute event, regional oxidative metabolism assessed by ^{11}C-acetate was reduced in proportion to residual myocardial blood flow.[289] Furthermore, regional oxidative metabolism did not differ among similarly hypoperfused segments with and without perfusion-metabolism mismatch. The authors concluded that because regional oxidative metabolism is intimately coupled to myocardial blood flow, it is unlikely that such studies will provide additional independent information in terms of myocardial viability beyond that of residual blood flow and glucose metabolism.[289]

Relation of Metabolic Activity to Perfusion. The dependence of glucose utilization on blood flow suggests that myocardial perfusion tracers that accurately measure blood flow may also reflect myocardial viability. This is likely to be the case at either extreme of the perfusion range, so that regions with severely reduced or absent blood flow would represent scarred myocardium and regions with only mildly reduced blood flow would represent viable myocardium. In regions of intermediate blood flow reduction, perfusion information alone may be insufficient to differentiate hibernating myocardium from mixed scarred (endocardium) and viable (epicardium) myocardium. In such regions, additional data, such as metabolic indices, would improve the diagnostic accuracy of perfusion tracers.

Recent studies have explored the ability of ^{15}O-water to assess myocardial viability through modification of the blood flow information (Fig. 29). Rather than reliance on the net transmural blood flow, Iida et al. have proposed measuring the volume of perfusable and nonperfusable tissue within a myocardial region.[292,293] When this perfusable tissue index method of ^{15}O-water was tested in patients with acute and chronic ischemic heart disease, the determination of myocardial viability was comparable to that obtained using FDG.[293]

Because the integrity of sarcolemmal membranes depends on preserved intracellular metabolic activity, tracers that reflect cell membrane cation flux as well as perfusion should parallel viability information provided by markers of metabolic activity. ^{201}Tl, ^{82}Rb, and ^{38}K are such tracers. Recent data suggest that thallium uptake is related to the regional metabolic activity assessed by FDG PET.[108,174,294] Furthermore, the magnitude of thallium activity within perfusion defects correlates inversely with the extent of interstitial fibrosis determined by histomorphological studies.[109,110]

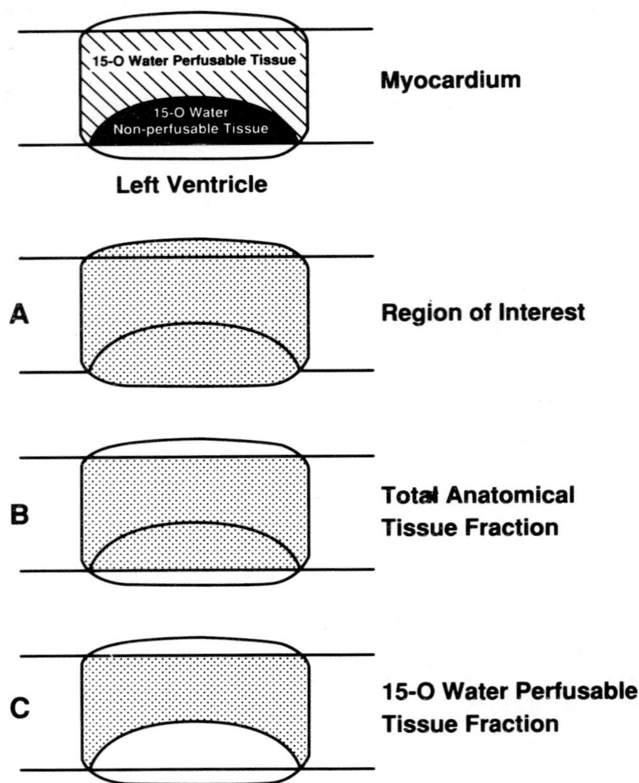

Figure 29. Schematic of a myocardial region of interest containing a mixture of ^{15}O-water perfusable and nonperfusable tissue. *Panel A:* Volume of the region of interest. *Panel B:* Anatomic tissue fraction for the region of interest produced by subtraction of the blood pool (^{15}O-carbon monoxide) from the transmission images after normalization of the latter to tissue density (1.04 gm/ml). Total anatomic tissue fraction represents the total extravascular tissue and contains both perfusable and nonperfusable tissue components. *Panel C:* ^{15}O-water perfusable tissue fraction for the region of interest that is calculated from the ^{15}O-water data set and identifies the mass of tissue within the region of interest that is capable of rapid transsarcolemmal exchange of water. Note that the nonperfusable or necrotic region is excluded from this parameter. The ^{15}O-water perfusable tissue index is calculated by dividing ^{15}O-water perfusable tissue fraction (panel C) by the total anatomic tissue fraction (panel B) and represents the fraction of the total anatomic tissue that is perfusable by water. (From Yamamoto et al.,[293] modified and reprinted with permission of the American Heart Association.)

Chronic Coronary Artery Disease and Hibernating Myocardium. Although the metabolic shift from fatty acids to glucose has been well characterized in experimental models of ischemia,[295,296] these metabolic alterations may not apply to patients with chronic coronary artery disease and hibernating myocardium. It is conceivable that when regional contractile function in hibernating myocardium is downregulated to conserve energy expenditure and adapt to regional reduction of blood flow, a new state of perfusion-contraction coupling is achieved to ensure myocyte survival. In patients with

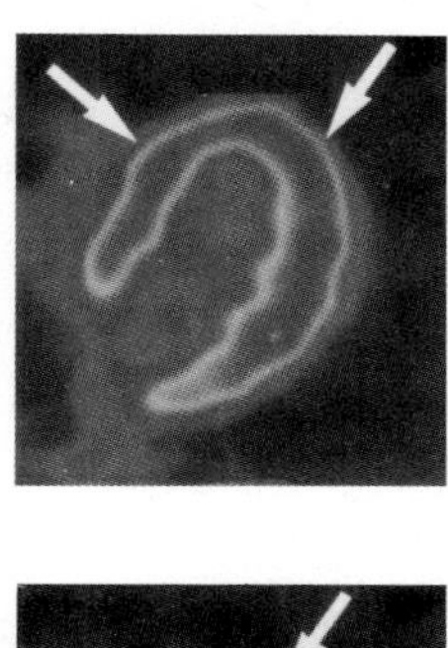

Figure 30. Cross-sectional PET images are shown for ^{13}N-ammonia and ^{18}FDG. Top panel shows discordance between ^{18}FDG uptake and ^{13}N-ammonia uptake (FDG-blood flow mismatch) in the apical and septal regions (arrows). Lower panel shows concordant ^{13}N-ammonia and ^{18}FDG uptake (FDG-blood flow match) in the apical region. (From Maddahi et al.,[267] modified and reprinted with permission of The Journal of Nuclear Medicine.)

coronary artery disease, Marshall et al.[265] proposed that ischemic and scarred myocardium could be differentiated by evaluating regional FDG uptake in hypoperfused myocardial regions (assessed by ^{13}N-ammonia). Among regions with reduced myocardial perfusion at rest, a concordant reduction in FDG uptake (termed FDG-blood flow "match") was considered to represent scarred myocardium, and discordant increase in FDG uptake (termed FDG-blood flow "mismatch") was considered to represent ischemic but viable myocardium. Examples of FDG-blood flow mismatch and match are shown in Figure 30. To determine whether preserved or enhanced FDG uptake in dysfunctional regions identifies potentially reversible and viable myocardium, Tillisch et al.[21] and Tamaki et al.[268] evaluated metabolism and blood flow before and after revascularization, with glucose loading and after overnight fasting, respectively. In these 2 studies, preoperative identification of enhanced FDG uptake relative to blood flow was associated with functional improvement in 78 to 85% of regions after revascularization. Conversely, contractile function did not improve in 78 to 92% of regions demonstrating reduced FDG uptake and concomitant reduction in blood flow.[21,268] In Tillisch's study, 22 (63%) of the 35 dysfunctional regions that demonstrated improved contractile function after revascularization demonstrated normal blood flow preoperatively.[297] Because dysfunctional regions with normal blood flow at rest are more likely to represent stunned, rather than hibernating, myocardium, it underscores the importance for consistent definition of "mismatch" regions in different publications (Table 8). Tillisch et al. also demonstrated a correlation between the extent of myocardial mismatch regions and improvement of global left ventricular ejection fraction 12 to 18 weeks after revascularization.[21] In patients demonstrating 2 or more regions with FDG-blood flow mismatch, left ventricular ejection fraction improved from a mean of 30% before to 45% after surgery. Significantly increased global left ventricular ejection fraction was also observed in 2 subsequent studies.[298,299]

Studies with FDG PET before and after revascularization have a positive predictive accuracy of functional recovery after surgery in regions with FDG-blood flow mismatch patterns of approximately 80% and negative predictive accuracy in regions with match patterns of about 83%.[21,268,291,289–303] More recently, vom Dahl et al. reported an association between the severity of wall motion abnormality at rest and recovery of function after revascularization in regions with PET mismatch.[303] Among 37 patients with coronary artery disease and left ventricular dysfunction (mean ejection frac-

Table 8. Variable Definitions and Interpretations for ^{18}F-Deoxyglucose (FDG) PET Viability

BLOOD FLOW	FDG UPTAKE	INTERPRETATION
Normal	Normal	Normal
	Increased	Mismatch—stunned myocardium
	Decreased	Admixture of scarred/viable myocardium
Abnormal	Normal Increased	Mismatch—hibernating myocardium
	Decreased	
	–moderate	Match—admixture of scarred/viable myocardium
	–severe	Match—scarred/nonviable myocardium

tion of 34%), the positive predictive accuracy for PET mismatch was only 48% in regions with mild hypokinesis at rest and 67% in regions with severe wall motion abnormalities at rest. Despite the less impressive positive predictive accuracy, the negative predictive accuracy of PET match pattern was 86%, which is consistent with prior publications.[303] It is noteworthy, too, that the predictive accuracies reported with PET are quite similar to those achieved with thallium reinjection: positive predictive values of 80 to 87% and negative predictive values of 82 to 100%.[75,77,81–84]

Although there are several studies that characterize metabolic alterations in patients with chronic coronary artery disease and hibernating myocardium preoperatively, only a few studies have reevaluated substrate utilization after revascularization.[300,302] To examine the effects of angioplasty on regional coronary blood flow, metabolism, and contractile function, Nienaber and coworkers studied 12 patients with PET and echocardiography before and within 72 hours after revascularization.[300] In a subset of patients, PET and echocardiography were repeated approximately 2 months after coronary angioplasty. Despite restoration of blood flow, both regional contractile function and absolute glucose utilization rates remained abnormal within 72 hours after revascularization and normalized only at late (mean 2 months) follow-up. In a similar study, Marwick and colleagues reported that most mismatch regions that demonstrate improved perfusion and function postoperatively also show reduced FDG activity, reflecting metabolic shift back to fatty acids.[302] However, despite improved regional blood flow, some myocardial regions continue to utilize FDG as late as 5 months after the surgery. Such persistent FDG utilization after revascularization was more prevalent among severely hypoperfused regions preoperatively. An example of a patient with persistent FDG utilization in a region with improved blood flow after revascularization is shown in Figure 31.

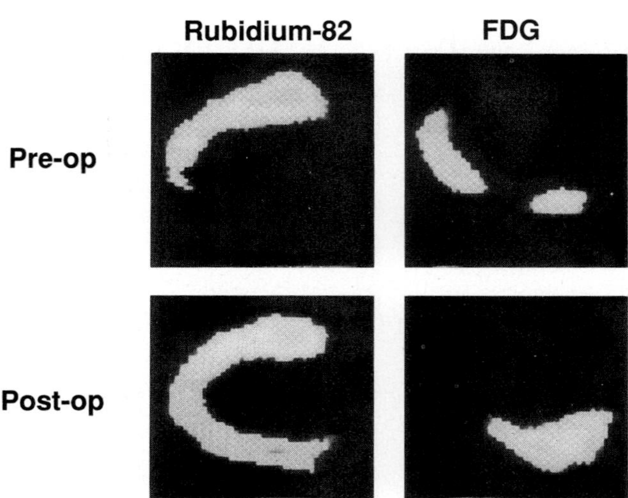

Figure 31. Evidence for persistent FDG utilization in the inferior region, despite improved blood flow after revascularization. Preoperative sagittal PET images show severely reduced perfusion defects in the inferoapical and inferior regions associated with enhanced FDG uptake (mismatch) in both regions. Despite improved perfusion and contraction in the inferoapical and inferior regions after surgery, FDG activity is reduced in the inferoapical region, but not in the inferior region. (From Marwick et al.,[302] modified and reprinted with permission of the American Heart Association.)

It has been hypothesized that chronically depressed wall motion abnormalities may be the consequence of repeated episodes of ischemia, rather than chronic hypoperfusion. To explore this possibility, Vanoverschelde and coworkers studied 26 patients with chronic occlusion of a major coronary artery, but without prior myocardial infarction, by measuring absolute regional myocardial blood flow with ammonia at rest and after intravenous dipyridamole using PET.[304] The kinetics of ^{11}C-acetate and FDG were also assessed at rest. In a subgroup of 11 patients, global and regional left ventricular function was evaluated by contrast ventriculography before and after revascularization. Transmural myocardial biopsies were obtained from the collateral dependent regions during coronary artery bypass surgery and were analyzed by optical and electron microscopy. When data were analyzed according to resting regional wall motion, in patients demonstrating normal wall motion (Group I); regional myocardial blood flow, FDG uptake, and oxidative metabolism were similar among collateral dependent and remote regions. In contrast, in patients with regional wall motion abnormality (Group II); collateral dependent segments had lower myocardial blood flow, higher FDG uptake, and smaller slope of ^{11}C-acetate clearance (k) when compared to remote regions. Following intravenous dipyridamole infusion, there was a significant inverse correlation between wall motion abnormality and collateral flow reserve. Despite the demonstration of marked ultrastructural alteration on morphological analysis, regional wall motion abnormalities improved significantly in the subgroup of patients who underwent revascularization. Based on these preliminary data, the authors propose that chronically depressed wall motion abnormalities in collateral dependent regions may be the consequence of repeated episodes of ischemia, rather than chronic hypoperfusion.

Metabolic Imaging Compared with Thallium Studies. Because, in theory, delayed thallium images reflect cation flux and sarcolemmal membrane integrity, thallium perfusion imaging and metabolic imaging with FDG should yield comparable results in differentiating viable from nonviable myocardium. In a canine model of 2 hours coronary occlusion and reflow, thallium was injected before reperfusion and FDG was administered 3 hours after reflow.[305] Both thallium redistribution and preserved FDG uptake accurately identified viable myocardium after reperfusion. Conversely, lack of redistribution and reduced FDG uptake identified irreversibly injured, necrotic myocardium. However, early studies employing conventional stress 3- to 4-hour redistribution thallium imaging in patients with coronary artery disease showed the superiority of metabolic PET imaging

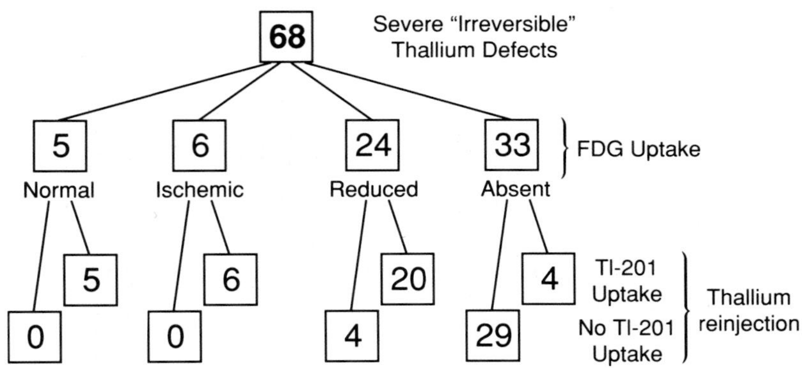

Figure 32. FDG uptake in 68 regions with severe "irreversible" thallium defects on redistribution imaging. FDG uptake, when present, usually represented a reduction in FDG activity in proportion to reduced blood flow, rather than an ischemic pattern of increased FDG uptake relative to blood flow. All but 4 regions with FDG uptake also had enhanced thallium uptake after reinjection. (From Bonow et al.,[174] reprinted with permission of the American Heart Association.)

with FDG compared to that of thallium.[306–309] When thallium defects were visually classified as being reversible, partially reversible or irreversible, 38 to 58% of regions with apparently "irreversible" thallium defects were identified as viable by PET. These findings are consistent with previous investigations demonstrating that up to 50% of regions with visually assigned "irreversible" thallium defects on preoperative stress 3- to 4-hour redistribution images have normal thallium uptake and improved regional contraction postoperatively.[3,68,71]

However, conventional stress-redistribution thallium imaging without late (24-hour) redistribution or reinjection studies will seriously overestimate the frequency and extent of myocardial fibrosis.[68,75,77,81–84] In addition, the severity of thallium activity within irreversible thallium defects assessed quantitatively may reflect myocardial viability.[68,108–110,174,294] When late redistribution thallium images were compared with PET among patients with coronary artery disease and left ventricular dysfunction, PET identified more viable regions than late redistribution thallium imaging.[310] However, when the severity of thallium activity within fixed 24-hour thallium defects was assessed, there was an inverse correlation between the severity of 24-hour thallium defect score and presence of myocardial viability by PET.[310] Among regions with profoundly reduced 24-hour thallium scores, the probability of PET demonstrating viability was less than 15%.

PET Compared with Thallium Reinjection and Rest-Redistribution Imaging. The similar predictive accuracies of PET imaging and thallium reinjection for assessing myocardial viability have prompted comparative studies of the 2 imaging techniques in the same patients.[83,174,311] In 1991, studies from our laboratory showed that FDG uptake was present in 94% of regions demonstrating either complete or partial reversibility on standard stress 3- to 4-hour redistribution thallium studies, confirming that such regions represent viable myocardium.[174] Among regions considered "irreversible" on redistribution images, the magnitude of reduction in thallium activity correlated with the likelihood of metabolic

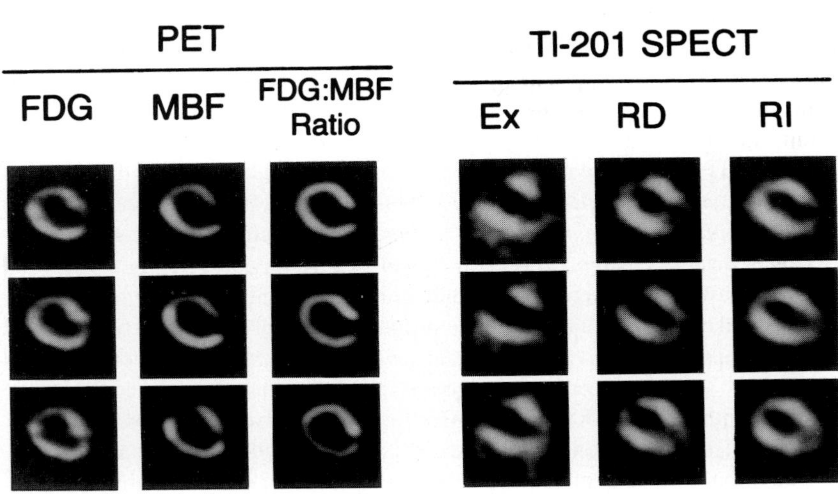

Figure 33. Concordance of PET and thallium reinjection data. Tomographic FDG, myocardial blood flow (MBF), and FDG to blood flow ratio (FDG:MBF), generated from the quantitative ^{15}O-water data with partial volume and spillover correction are shown on the left panel. The corresponding thallium data for exercise (Ex), 3–4-hour redistribution (RD), and reinjection (RI) are shown on the right panel. Standard exercise-redistribution thallium studies demonstrate an apparently irreversible anteroapical defect. Myocardial blood flow is reduced in this region and in the septum according to PET. However, FDG images demonstrate uptake and, hence, viability in all regions, most notably the anteroapical region. Functional images of FDG-to-blood-flow ratio demonstrate enhanced FDG uptake relative to blood flow (mismatch) involving the apex and septum. Thallium reinjection images mirror the FDG images, with evidence of enhanced thallium uptake and, hence, viability in the anteroapical region. (From Bonow et al.,[174] reprinted with permission of the American Heart Association.)

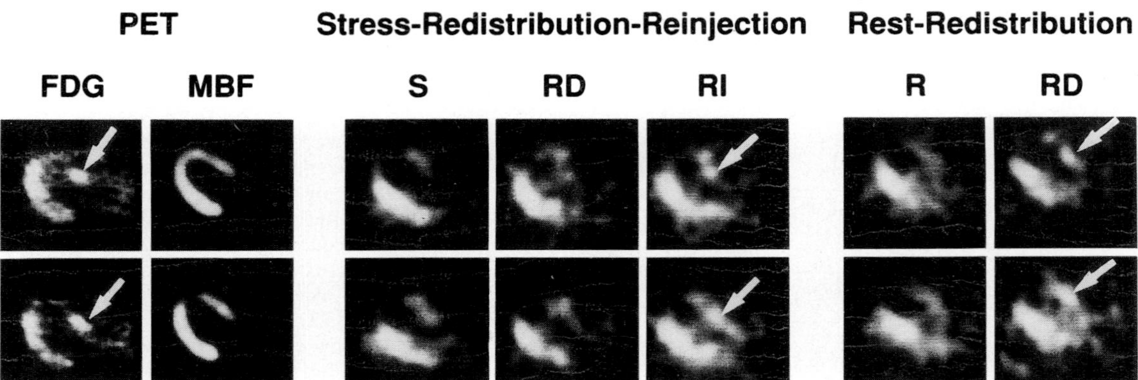

Figure 34. Concordance between PET, stress-redistribution-reinjection, and rest-redistribution imaging is demonstrated in this patient example. Two consecutive transaxial tomograms are displayed for FDG and myocardial blood flow (MBF) by PET, with corresponding thallium tomograms of stress (S), redistribution (RD), reinjection (RI), and rest(R)-redistribution. On the PET study, myocardial blood flow is reduced in the anteroapical, anteroseptal, and posteroseptal regions. FDG uptake in the corresponding regions demonstrate a *mismatch* in the posteroseptal region (arrowhead) and a *match* between FDG uptake and blood flow in the anteroapical and anteroseptal regions. Corresponding SPECT thallium images reveal extensive perfusion abnormalities involving the apical and septal regions during stress, which persist on redistribution images. However, thallium reinjection images show improved thallium uptake in the posteroseptal region (arrowhead), and the apical region remains fixed. On rest-redistribution images, the apical region has severely reduced thallium activity that remains fixed, while the posteroseptal region that was abnormal on the initial rest study shows significant improvement on 3–4-hour redistribution study, suggesting viable myocardium. (Reprinted[83] with permission of the American Heart Association.)

activity as assessed by FDG uptake. Preserved FDG activity was shown in 91% of mildly reduced (60 to 84% of peak activity) and 84% of moderately reduced (50 to 59% of peak activity) irreversible thallium regions. Hence, these data suggest that the level of thallium activity itself in mild-to-moderate defects might be a clinically reliable marker of myocardial viability. Among regions with severe irreversible thallium defects (≤50% of peak activity), the results of thallium reinjection were comparable to those of PET (Fig. 32). Both techniques provided evidence of viable myocardium in 51% of regions, and with a concordance between the 2 techniques of 88% for viable or nonviable myocardium.[174] An example of this concordance is demonstrated in Figure 33.

These initial observations were subsequently confirmed by other investigators.[311,312] In Tamaki's study, the concordance of viable or nonviable myocardium for thallium reinjection and PET was 85%.[311] Of 48 regions that appeared irreversible on standard stress 3-hour redistribution studies, thallium reinjection identified viable myocardium in 20 (42%), all of which were confirmed to be viable by PET. In contrast, of the 28 regions that remained irreversible after reinjection, only 7 (25%) were identified to be viable by PET. However, the severity of the irreversible thallium defects was not quantified in this study. It is possible that the level of thallium activity or the magnitude of differential uptake within these defects might have provided additional evidence of viability.

Data comparing rest-redistribution thallium imaging with PET are limited.[83,308] Recently, we reported 94% concordance between stress-redistribution-reinjection and rest-redistribution imaging regarding myocardial viability as defined by PET in 41 patients with chronic coronary artery disease.[83] Considering the concordance between the 2 approaches, either thallium protocol might yield clinically satisfactory information as long as the severity of thallium defect is quantified within rest-redistribution images (Fig. 34). However, if there are no contraindications to stress testing, stress-redistribution-reinjection imaging provides a more comprehensive assessment of the extent and severity of coronary artery disease by demonstrating regional myocardial ischemia, without jeopardizing information on myocardial viability. The relation between PET criteria of viability, stress-redistribution-reinjection and rest-redistribution thallium studies is shown in Tables 9 and 10.

PET Characterization of Stunned Myocardium

Glucose metabolism during reperfusion has also been evaluated by PET using FDG. The initial impetus for using FDG as a viability marker came from experimental studies during acute myocardial ischemia. In canine models and in isolated arterially perfused, heart preparations, a metabolic switch from fatty acid to glucose utilization was observed.[272,273] Although the kinetics of glycolysis during early myocardial reperfusion are not completely understood, attenuated or decreased glucose utilization as well as reduced oxidation of pyruvate and lactate have been reported.[313–315] Such abnormal utilization of glucose and/or its intermediates could be the result of competitive inhibition caused by the preferred oxidation of fatty acids.[315] In a canine model of transient ischemia and reperfusion, Schwaiger et al. demonstrated that

Table 9. Relation of Stress-Redistribution-Reinjection Thallium Results to Patterns of PET Viability

STRESS-REDISTRIBUTION-REINJECTION THALLIUM SPECT*	PET							
	Normal		*FDG*: blood flow mismatch*		*Moderately reduced FDG*		*Severely reduced FDG*	
	No.	*%*	*No.*	*%*	*No.*	*%*	*No.*	*%*
Regional analysis								
n*	209		188		138		59	
Normal	98	47	38	20	26	19	1	2
Reversible	65	31	115	61	48	35	7	12
Irreversible								
Mild-to-moderate	42	20	28	15	46	33	1	2
Severe	4	2	7	4	18	13	50	85
Patient analysis								
N*	20		20		20		10	
Viable	19	95	18	90	17	85	2	20
Nonviable	1	5	2	10	3	15	8	80

*SPECT, single photon emission computed tomography; FDG, [^{18}F]-fluorodeoxyglucose; n, number of myocardial regions; N, number of patients in whom the corresponding positron emission tomography (PET) category was observed. (Reprinted[83] with permission of the American Heart Association.)

although FDG activity was depressed early after reperfusion, FDG utilization was elevated at 24 hours after reperfusion.[277]

In patients with acute anterior myocardial infarction, metabolic imaging with FDG was able to differentiate viable from nonviable myocardium in regions with decreased blood flow and impaired contraction.[316] When PET was performed within 72 hours after the onset of their acute symptoms, all regions determined to have matched reduction in perfusion and metabolism manifested either no change or a deterioration in regional function when reevaluated 6.0 ± 4.6 weeks later by two-dimensional echocardiography. However, despite the excellent negative predictive accuracy, the positive predictive accuracy of metabolic imaging with FDG PET was less impressive. Among regions exhibiting perfusion-metabolism mismatch, only 50% demonstrated spontaneous improvement of function, suggesting that in the early postinfarction period, metabolic imaging with FDG identifies necrotic myocardium accurately, but substantially overestimates the presence and extent of viable myocardium. This lack of specificity of FDG utilization by PET among patients with recent myocardial infarction has been confirmed by other investigators.[290,317] These clinical data are supported by the findings of Sebree et al.,[318] in rabbits undergoing coronary artery occlusion and reperfusion. Twenty-four hours after reperfusion, myocardial concentrations of ^{14}C-deoxyglucose and ^{201}Tl in macroautoradiograms were correlated quantitatively with evidence of myocardial necrosis by light microscopy. Discordance between accumulation of ^{14}C-deoxyglucose and thallium was observed in reperfused myocardium; many myocardial regions with severely reduced thallium activity and histological evidence of necrosis had deposition of ^{14}C-deoxyglucose. The mechanism responsible for FDG uptake in recently infarcted necrotic myocardium is not well understood and awaits further study.

PROGNOSTIC VALUE OF PET

Recent retrospective analyses of data have indicated that patients with FDG-blood flow mismatch regions have greater cardiac morbidity and mortality when compared to patients exhibiting only FDG-blood flow matched regions.[319–320] Among medically treated patients with moderate-to-severely depressed left ventricular dysfunction (ejection fraction <35%) who were followed for a mean of approximately one year, the group with a mismatched PET pattern had a higher incidence of myocardial infarction or revascularization than those with only a matched PET pattern (92% versus 50%). Moreover, when the subgroup of patients with mismatch were further analyzed according to treatment received, the mortality rates were significantly higher in the group receiving medical therapy (33 to 41%) compared with those undergoing revascularization (4 to 12%).

PET AND SPECT: COMPARISON OF 2 TECHNOLOGIES

Compared to SPECT, PET provides (1) enhanced image resolution and contrast, (2) routine correction for scatter and body attenuation and, (3) quantification of regional blood flow and metabolism. In addition, PET permits the noninvasive assessment of regional metabolic activity independent of blood flow. Given the technical superiority of PET over SPECT, PET would appear to be the preferred technique to assess both perfusion and metabolism in patients with coronary artery disease. However, with the exception of FDG, most PET tracers have very short half-lives, and require an on-site cyclotron facility.

By serving as a reference standard, PET has played an important role in recent modifications and improvements of

Table 10. Relation of Rest-Redistribution Thallium Results to Patterns of PET Viability

REST-REDISTRIBUTION THALLIUM SPECT*	PET: Normal No.	%	FDG*: blood flow mismatch No.	%	Moderately reduced FDG No.	%	Severely reduced FDG No.	%
Regional analysis								
n*	209		188		138		59	
Normal	108	52	56	30	19	14	0	0
Reversible	48	23	50	26	26	19	8	14
Irreversible								
Mild-to-moderate	49	23	73	39	57	41	2	3
Severe	4	2	9	5	36	26	49	83
Patient analysis								
N*	20		20		20		10	
Viable	18	90	16	80	12	60	2	20
Nonviable	2	10	4	20	8	40	8	80

*SPECT, single photon emission computed tomography; FDG, [^{18}F]-fluorodeoxyglucose; n, number of myocardial regions; N, number of patients in whom the corresponding positron emission tomography (PET) category was observed. (Reprinted[83] with permission of the American Heart Association.)

SPECT technology and protocols. However, there are other considerations, unrelated to technology and cost-effectiveness, that might favor the use of stress thallium scintigraphy. Stress-redistribution-reinjection thallium imaging provides a comprehensive evaluation of the presence and extent of exercise-induced myocardial ischemia and identifies patients who are at high risk for future cardiac events. In most cases, the presence of inducible myocardial ischemia in a patient with coronary artery disease and impaired left ventricular function is a much more significant clinical variable, in terms of patient management and risk assessment, than the knowledge of myocardial viability. Because reversible ischemia on thallium scintigraphy is evidence for the presence of viable myocardium, PET would not be required in the majority of such patients. Furthermore, the rigid standards of dietary and metabolic environment that are necessary to maximize the diagnostic accuracy obtained by PET do not apply to thallium imaging. For example, in patients with diabetes mellitus, the application of PET imaging with FDG requires insulin administration to normalize plasma glucose levels. Finally, regional heterogeneity of FDG uptake has been reported in normal volunteers, which may complicate image interpretation in some patients with coronary artery disease.[321,322]

REFERENCES

1. Rees G, Bristow JD, Kremkau EL, Green GS, Herr RH, Griswold HE, Starr A. Influence of aortocoronary bypass surgery on left ventricular performance. *N Engl J Med* 1971;284:1116–1125.
2. Chatterjee K, Swan HJC, Parmley WW, Sustaita H, Marcus HS, Matloff J. Influence of direct myocardial revascularization on left ventricular asynergy and function in patients with coronary heart disease. *Circulation* 1973;47:276–86.
3. Rozanski A, Berman DS, Gray R, Levy R, Raymond M, Maddahi J, Pantelo N, Waxman AD, Swan HJC, Matloff J: Use of thallium-201 redistribution scintigraphy in the preoperative differentiation of reversible and nonreversible myocardial asynergy. *Circulation* 1981;64:936–944.
4. Brundage BH, Massie BM, Botvinick EH. Improved regional ventricular function after successful surgical revascularization. *J Am Coll Cardiol* 1984;3:902–8.
5. Dilsizian V, Bonow RO, Cannon RO, Tracy CM, Vitale DF, McIntosh CL, Clark RE, Bacharach SL, Green MV. The effect of coronary artery bypass grafting on left ventricular systolic function at rest: evidence for preoperative subclinical myocardial ischemia. *Am J Cardiol* 1988;61:1248–1254.
6. Brill DA, Deckelbaum LI, Remetz MS, Soufer R, Elefteriades JA, Zaret BL. Recovery of severe ischemic ventricular dysfunction after coronary bypass grafting. *Am J Cardiol* 1988;61:650–651.
7. Nesto RW, Cohn LH, Collins JJ Jr, Wynne J, Holman L, Cohn PF. Inotropic contractile reserve: a useful predictor of increased 5-year survival and improved postoperative left ventricular function in patients with coronary artery disease and reduced rejection fraction. *Am J Cardiol* 1982;50:39–44.
8. Alderman EL, Fisher LD, Litwin P, Kaiser GC, Myers WO, Maynard C, Levine F, Schloss M. Results of coronary artery surgery in patients with poor left ventricular function (CASS). *Circulation* 1983;68:785–95.
9. Pigott JD, Kouchoukos NT, Oberman A, Cutter GR. Late results of surgical and medical therapy for patients with coronary artery disease and depressed left ventricular function. *J Am Coll Cardiol* 1985;5:1036–45.
10. Mock MB, Ringqvist I, Fisher LD, Davis KB, Chaitman BR, Kouchoukos NT, Kaiser GC, Alderman E, Ryan TJ, Russell RO, Mullin S, Fray D, Killip T. Survival of medically treated patients in the coronary artery surgery study (CASS) registry. *Circulation* 1982;66:562–68.
11. Sheehan FH, Doerr R, Schmidt WG, et al. Early recovery of left ventricular function after thrombolytic therapy for acute myocardial infarction: an important determinant of survival. *J Am Coll Cardiol* 1988;40:633–644.
12. Knoebel SB, Henry PL, Phillips JF, Pauletto FJ. Coronary collateral circulation and myocardial blood flow reserve. *Circulation* 1972;46:84–94.
13. Levin DC. Pathways and functional significance of coronary collateral circulation. *Circulation* 1974;50:831–7.

14. Schwarz F, Flameng W, Ensslen R, Sesto M, Thormann J. Effects of coronary collaterals on left ventricular function at rest and during stress. *Am Heart J* 1978;95:570–7.
15. Goldberg HL, Goldstein J, Borer JS, Moses JW, Collins MB. Functional importance of coronary collateral vessels. *Am J Cardiol* 1984;53:694–9.
16. Dilsizian V, Cannon RO, Tracy CM, McIntosh CL, Clark RE, Bonow RO. Enhanced regional left ventricular function after distant coronary bypass via improved collateral blood flow. *J Am Coll Cardiol* 1989;14:312–318.
17. DeWood MA, Spores J, Notske R, Mouser LT, Burroughs R, Golden MS, Lang HT. Prevalence of total coronary occlusion during the early hours of transmural myocardial infarction. *N Engl J Med* 1980;303:897–902.
18. Banka VS, Bodenheimer MM, Helfant RH. Determinants of reversible asynergy. The native coronary circulation. *Circulation* 1975;52:810–816.
19. Popio KA, Gorlin R, Bechtel D, Levine JA. Postextrasystolic potentiation as a predictor of potential myocardial viability: preoperative analysis compared with studies after coronary bypass surgery. *Am J Cardiol* 1977;39:944–53.
20. Rozanski A, Berman D, Gray R, Diamond G, Raymond M, Prause J, Maddahi J, Swan HJC, Matloff J. Preoperative prediction of reversible myocardial asynergy by postexercise radionuclide ventriculography. *N Engl J Med* 1982; 307:212–216.
21. Tillisch JH, Brunken R, Marshall R, Schwaiger M, Mandelkorn M, Phelps M, Schelbert H. Reversibility of cardiac wall-motion abnormalities predicted by positron tomography. *N Engl J Med* 1986;314:884–888.
22. Heyndrickx GR, Baig H, Nelkins P, Leusen K, Fishbein MC, Vatner SF. Depression of regional blood flow and wall thickening after brief coronary occlusions. *Am J Physiol* 1978;234:H653–H659.
23. Matsuzaki M, Gallagher KP, Kemper WS, White F, Ross J Jr. Sustained regional dysfunction, produced by prolonged coronary stenosis: Gradual recovery after reperfusion. *Circulation* 1983;68:170–182.
24. Rahimtoola SH. Coronary bypass surgery for chronic angina—1981: A perspective. *Circulation* 1982;65:225–241.
25. Ross J Jr. Mechanisms of regional ischemia and antianginal drug action during exercise. *Prog Cardiovasc Dis* 1989;31:455–466.
26. Perrone-Filardi P, Bacharach SL, Dilsizian V, Maurea S, Marin-Neto JA, Arrighi JA, Frank JA, Bonow RO. Metabolic evidence of viable myocardium in regions with reduced wall thickness and absent wall thickening in patients with chronic ischemic left ventricular dysfunction. *J Am Coll Cardiol* 1992;20:161–168.
27. Rahimtoola SH. A perspective on the three large multicenter randomized clinical trials of coronary bypass surgery for chronic stable angina. *Circulation* 1985;72(suppl V):V-123–V-135.
28. Topol EJ, Weiss JL, Guzman PA, et al. Immediate improvement of dysfunctional myocardial segments after coronary revascularization: detection by intraoperative transesophageal echocardiography. *J Am Coll Cardiol* 1984;4:1123–1134.
29. Braunwald E, Kloner RA. The stunned myocardium: prolonged, postischemic ventricular dysfunction. *Circulation* 1982;66:1146–9.
30. Braunwald E, Rutherford JD. Reversible ischemic left ventricular dysfunction: evidence for the "hibernating myocardium". *J Am Coll Cardiol* 1986;8:1467–1470.
31. Ross J Jr. Myocardial perfusion-contraction matching: Implications for coronary heart disease and hibernation. *Circulation* 1991;83:1076–1082.
32. Bolli R. Myocardial "stunning" in man. *Circulation* 1992;86:1671–1691.
33. Bonow RO, Dilsizian V. Thallium-201 for assessment of myocardial viability. *Semin in Nucl Med* 1991;11:230–241.
34. Reduto LA, Freund GC, Gaeta JM, Smalling RW, Lewis B, Gould KL. Coronary artery reperfusion in acute myocardial infarction: beneficial effects of intracoronary streptokinase on left ventricular salvage and performance. *Am Heart J* 1981;102:1168–1177.
35. Anderson JL, Marshall HW, Bray BE, Lutz JR, Frederick PR, Yanowitz FG, Datz FL, Klausner SC, Hagan AD. A randomized trial of intracoronary streptokinase in the treatment of acute myocardial infarction. *N Engl J Med* 1983;308:1312–8.
36. Stack RS, Phillips HR III, Grierson DS, Behar VS, Kong Y, Peter RH, Swain JL, Greenfield JC. Functional improvement of jeopardized myocardium following intracoronary streptokinase infusion in acute myocardial infarction. *J Clin Invest* 1983;72:84–95.
37. Greenfield RA, Swain JL. Disruption of myofibrillar energy use: dual mechanisms that may contribute to post-ischemic dysfunction in stunned myocardium. *Circ Res* 1987;60:283–289.
38. Swain JL, Sabina RL, McHale PA, Greenfield JC, Holmes EW. Prolonged myocardial nucleotide depletion after brief ischemia in the open-chest dog. *Am J Physiol* 1982;242:H818–H826.
39. McCord JM. Oxygen-derived free radicals in postischemic tissue injury. *N Engl J Med* 1985;312:159–163.
40. Przyldenk K, Kloner RA. Superoxide dismutase plus catalase improve contractile function in the canine model of "stunned myocardium." *Circ Res* 1986;58:148–56.
41. Krause SM, Jacobus WE, Becker LC. Alterations in sarcoplasmic reticulum calcium transport in the post-ischemic "stunned" myocardium. *Circ Res* 1989;65:526–530.
42. Kusuoka H, Porterfield JK, Weisman HF, Weisfeldt ML, Marban E. Pathophysiology and pathogenesis of stunned myocardium. Depressed Ca+2 activation of contraction as a consequence of reperfusion-induced cellular calcium overload in ferret heart. *J Clin Invest* 1987;79:950–61.
43. Przyldenk K, Kloner RA. Effects of verapamil on post-ischemic "stunned" myocardium: Importance of timing of treatment. *J Am Coll Cardiol* 1988;11:614–623.
44. Engler R, Covell JW. Granulocytes cause reperfusion ventricular dysfunction after 15-minute ischemia in the dog. *Circ Res* 1987;61:20–28.
45. Zhao M, Zhang H, Robinson TF, Factor SM, Sonnenblick EH, Eng C. Profound structural alterations of the extracellular collagen matrix in postischemic dysfunction ("stunned") but viable myocardium. *J Am Coll Cardiol* 1987;10: 1322–34.
46. Ciuffo AA, Ouyang P, Becker LC, Levin L, Weisfeldt ML. Reduction of sympathetic inotropic response after ischemia in dogs: contributor to stunned myocardium. *J Clin Invest* 1985;75:1504–1509.
47. Ritchie JL, Davis KB, Williams DL, Caldwell J, Kennedy JW. Global and regional left ventricular function and tomographic radionuclide perfusion: the Western Washington intracoronary streptokinase in myocardial infarction trial. *Circulation* 1984;70:867–875.
48. Gruppo Italiano per lo Studio della Streptochinasi Nell'Infarto Miocardico (GISSI). Effectiveness of intravenous thrombolytic treatment in acute myocardial infarction. *Lancet* 1986;1:397–401.
49. Simoons ML, Serruys PW, van den Brand M, Res J, Verheugt FWA, Krauss XH, Remme WJ, Bar F, deZwaan C, van der Laarse A, Vermeer F, Lubsen J. Early thrombolysis in acute

myocardial infarction: limitation of infarct size and improved survival. *J Am Coll Cardiol* 1986;7:717–728.
50. Nixon JV, Brown CN, Smitherman TC. Identification of transient and persistent segmental wall motion abnormalities in patients with unstable angina by two-dimensional echocardiography. *Circulation* 1982;65:1497–1503.
51. Renkin J, Wijns W, Ladha Z, Col J. Reversal of segmental hypokinesis by coronary angioplasty in patients with unstable angina, persistent T wave inversion, and left anterior descending coronary artery stenosis: additional evidence for myocardial stunning in humans. *Circulation* 1990;82:913–921.
52. Camici P, Araujo LI, Spinks T, Lammertsma AA, Kaski JC, Shea MJ, Selwyn AP, Jones T, Maseri A. Increased uptake of ^{18}F-fluorodeoxyglucose in postischemic myocardium of patients with exercise-induced angina. *Circulation* 1986;74:81–88.
53. Katsiyiannis PT, Arrighi JA, Quyyumi AA, Bonow RO, Bacharach SL, Stuhlmuller JE, Dilsizian V. Do persistent regional wall motion abnormalities after exercise represent stunned myocardium? (abstr) *J Am Coll Cardiol* 1994;23:79A.
54. Weich HF, Strauss HW, Pitt B. The extraction of thallium-201 by the myocardium. *Circulation* 1977;56:188–191.
55. Leppo JA, Macneil PB, Moring AF, Apstein CS. Separate effects of ischemia, hypoxia, and contractility on thallium-201 kinetics in rabbit myocardium. *J Nucl Med* 1986;27:66–74.
56. Leppo JA. Myocardial uptake of thallium and rubidium during alterations in perfusion and oxygenation in isolated rabbit hearts. *J Nucl Med* 1987;28:878–885.
57. Moore CA, Cannon J, Watson DD, Kaul S, Beller GA. Thallium-201 kinetics in stunned myocardium characterized by severe postischemic systolic dysfunction. *Circulation* 1990;81:1622–1632.
58. Sinusas AJ, Watson DD, Cannon JM, Beller GA. Effect of ischemia and postischemic dysfunction on myocardial uptake of technetium-99m-labeled methoxyisobutyl isonitrile and thallium-201. *J Am Coll Cardiol* 1989;14:1785–1793.
59. Granato JE, Watson DD, Flanagan TL, Beller GA. Myocardial thallium-201 kinetics and regional flow alterations with 3 hours of coronary occlusion and either rapid reperfusion through a totally patent vessel or slow reperfusion through a critical stenosis. *J Am Coll Cardiol* 1987;9:109–118.
60. Pohost GM, Zir LM, Moore RH, McKusick KA, Guiney TE, Beller GA. Differentiation of transiently ischemic from infarcted myocardium by serial imaging after a single dose of thallium-201. *Circulation* 1977;55:294–302.
61. Schwartz JS, Ponto R, Carlyle P, Forstrom L, Cohn JN. Early redistribution of thallium-201 after temporary ischemia. *Circulation* 1978;57:332–5.
62. Beller GA, Watson DD, Ackell P, Pohost GM. Time course of thallium-201 redistribution after transient myocardial ischemia. *Circulation* 1980;61:791–7.
63. Pohost GM, Okada RD, O'Keefe DD, Gewirtz H, Beller G, Strauss HW, Leppo J, Daggett WM. Thallium redistribution in dogs with severe coronary artery stenosis of fixed caliber. *Circ Res* 1981;48:439–446.
64. Okada RD, Leppo JA, Boucher CA, Pohost GM. Myocardial kinetics of thallium-201 after dipyridamole infusion in normal canine myocardium and in myocardium distal to a stenosis. *J Clin Invest* 1982;69:199–209.
65. Okada RD, Leppo JA, Strauss HW, Boucher CA, Pohost GM. Mechanism and time course of the disappearance of thallium-201 defects at rest in dogs. *Am J Cardiol* 1982;49:699–706.
66. Mays AE Jr, Cobb FR. Relationship between regional myocardial blood flow and thallium-201 distribution in the presence of coronary artery stenosis and dipyridamole induced vasodilation. *J Clin Invest* 1984;73:1359–1366.
67. Akins CW, Pohost GM, Desanctis RW, Block PC. Selection of angina-free patients with severe left ventricular dysfunction for myocardial revascularization. *Am J Cardiol* 1980;46:695–700.
68. Gibson RS, Watson DD, Taylor GJ, Crosby IK, Wellons HL, Holt ND, Beller GA. Prospective assessment of regional myocardial perfusion before and after coronary revascularization surgery by quantitative thallium-201 scintigraphy. *J Am Coll Cardiol* 1983;1:804–815.
69. Liu P, Kiess MC, Okada RD, Block PC, Strauss HW, Pohost GM, Boucher CA. The persistent defect on exercise thallium imaging and its fate after myocardial revascularization: Does it represent scar or ischemia? *Am Heart J* 1985;110:996–1001.
70. Cloninger KG, DePuey EG, Garcia EV, Roubin GS, Robbins WL, Nody A, DePasquale EE, Berger HJ. Incomplete redistribution in delayed thallium-201 single photon emission computed tomographic images: An overestimation of myocardial scarring. *J Am Coll Cardiol* 1988;12:955–963.
71. Kiat H, Berman DS, Maddahi J, Yang LD, Van Train K, Rozanski A, Friedman J. Late reversibility of tomographic myocardial thallium-201 defects: An accurate marker of myocardial viability. *J Am Coll Cardiol* 1988;12:1456–63.
72. Manyari DE, Knudtson M, Kloiber R, Roth D. Sequential thallium-201 myocardial perfusion studies after successful percutaneous transluminal coronary artery angioplasty: delayed resolution of exercise-induced scintigraphic abnormalities. *Circulation* 1988;77:86–95.
73. Gutman J, Berman DS, Freeman M, Rozanski A, Maddahi J, Waxman A, Swan HJC. Time to completed redistribution of thallium-201 in exercise myocardial scintigraphy: Relationship to the degree of coronary artery stenosis. *Am Heart J* 1983;106:989–995.
74. Yang LD, Berman DS, Kiat H, Resser KJ, Friedman JD, Rozanski A, Maddahi J. The frequency of late reversibility in SPECT thallium-201 stress-redistribution studies. *J Am Coll Cardiol* 1989;15:334–340.
75. Dilsizian V, Rocco TP, Freedman NM, Leon MB, Bonow RO. Enhanced detection of ischemic but viable myocardium by the reinjection of thallium after stress-redistribution imaging. *N Engl J Med* 1990;323:141–146.
76. Rocco TP, Dilsizian V, McKusick KA, Fischman AJ, Boucher CA, Strauss HW. Comparison of thallium redistribution with rest "reinjection" imaging for the detection of viable myocardium. *Am J Cardiol* 1990;66:158–163.
77. Ohtani H, Tamaki N, Yonekura Y, Mohiuddin IH, Hirata K, Ban T, Konishi J. Value of thallium-201 reinjection after delayed SPECT imaging for predicting reversible ischemia after coronary artery bypass grafting. *Am J Cardiol* 1990;66:394–399.
78. Kuijper AF, Vliegen HW, van der Wall EE, Oosterhuis WP, Zwinderman AH, van Eck-Smit BL, Niemeyer MG, Pauwels EK. The clinical impact of thallium-201 reinjection scintigraphy for detection of myocardial viability. *Eur J Nucl Med* 1992;19:783–789.
79. Bartenstein P, Schober O, Hasfeld M, Schafers M, Matheja P, Breithardt G. Thallium-201 single photon emission tomography of myocardium: Additional information in reinjection studies is dependent on collateral circulation. *Eur J Nucl Med* 1992;19:790–795.
80. Maublant JC, Lipiecki J, Citron B, Karsenty B, Mestas D, Boire JY, Veyre A, Ponsonnaille J. Reinjection as an alternative to rest imaging for detection of exercise-induced ischemia with thallium-201 emission tomography. *Am Heart J* 1993;125:330–335.
81. Nienaber CA, de la Roche J, Carnarius H, Montz R. Impact of ^{201}thallium reinjection imaging to identify myocardial viability after vasodilation-redistribution SPECT (abstr). *J Am Coll Cardiol* 1993;21:283A.

82. Bartenstein P, Hasfeld M, Schober O, Matheja P, Schafers M, Budde T, Hammel D, Scheld H, Breithardt G. Tl-201 reinjection predicts improvement of left ventricular function following revascularization. *Nucl Med* 1993;32:87–90.
83. Dilsizian V, Perrone-Filardi P, Arrighi JA, Bacharach SL, Quyyumi AA, Freedman NMT, Bonow RO. Concordance and discordance between stress-redistribution-reinjection and rest-redistribution thallium imaging for assessing viable myocardium: Comparison with metabolic activity by PET. *Circulation* 1993;88:941–952.
84. Melin JA, Marwick T, Baudhuin T, DeKock M, D'Hondt A, Vanoverschelde JL. Assessment of myocardial viability with thallium-201 imaging and dobutamine echocardiography: a comparative patient analysis (abstr). *Circulation* 1993;88:I-535.
85. Inglese E, Brambilla M, Dondi M, Pieri P, Bisi G, Sara R, Cannizzaro G, Cappagli M, Giordano A, Moscatelli G, Arrigo F, Tarolo G. Assessment of myocardial viability after thallium-201 reinjection or rest-redistribution imaging: a multicenter study. *J Nucl Med* 1995;36(4):555–563.
86. Lekakis J, Vassilopoulos N, Germanidis J, Theodorakos A, Nanas J, Kostamis P, Moulopoulos S. Detection of viable tissue in healed infarcted myocardium by dipyridamole thallium-201 reinjection and regional wall motion studies. *Am J Cardiol* 1993;71:401–404.
87. Kennedy NSJ, Cook B, Choy AM, Bridges AB, Hanson JK, McNeill GP, Pringle TH. A comparison of the redistribution and reinjection techniques in dipyridamole thallium tomography. *Nuc Med Commun* 1993;14:479–484.
88. Budinger TF, Pohost GM. Indication for thallium reinjection by 3 hour plasma levels (abstr). *Circulation* 1993;88:I-534.
89. Gewirtz H, Sullivan MJ, Shearer DR, Ohley W, Most AS. Analysis of proposed mechanisms of thallium redistribution: comparison of a computer model of myocardial thallium kinetics with quantitative analysis of clinical scans, in *Computers in Cardiology.* IEEE, 1981, pp 75–80.
90. Grunwald AM, Watson DD, Holzgrefe HH Jr, Irving JF, Beller GA. Myocardial thallium-201 kinetics in normal and ischemic myocardium. *Circulation* 1981;64:610–618.
91. Okada RD, Jacobs ML, Daggett WM, et al. Thallium-201 kinetics in nonischemic canine myocardium. *Circulation* 1982;65:70–77.
92. Nelson CW, Wilson RA, Angello DA, Palac RT. Effect of thallium-201 blood levels on reversible thallium defects. *J Nucl Med* 1989;30:1172–1175.
93. Leppo JA, Okada RD, Strauss HW, Pohost GH. Effect of hyperaemia on thallium-201 redistribution in normal canine myocardium. *Cardiovasc Res* 1985;19:679–685.
94. Budinger TF, Pohost GM. Thallium "redistribution"—an explanation (abstr). *J Nucl Med* 1986;27:996.
95. Goldhaber SZ, Newell JB, Alpert NM, Andrews E, Pohost GM, Ingwall JS. Effects of ischemic-like insult on myocardial thallium-201 accumulation. *Circulation* 1983;67:778–786.
96. Mckeever NP, Gregg DE, Caney PC. Oxygen uptake of nonworking left ventricle. *Circ Res* 1958;6:612–623.
97. Budinger TF, Knittel BL. Cardiac thallium redistribution and model (abstr). *J Nucl Med* 1987;28:588.
98. Kayden DS, Sigal S, Soufer R, Mattera J, Zaret BL, Wackers FJ. Thallium-201 for assessment of myocardial viability: Quantitative comparison of 24-hour redistribution imaging with imaging after reinjection at rest. *J Am Coll Cardiol* 1991;18:1480–1486.
99. Dilsizian V, Smeltzer WR, Freedman NMT, Dextras R, Bonow RO. Thallium reinjection after stress-redistribution imaging: Does 24 hour delayed imaging following reinjection enhance detection of viable myocardium? *Circulation* 1991;83:1247–1255.
100. Dae MW, Botvinick EH, Starksen NF, Zhu YY, Lapidus A. Do 4-hour reinjection thallium images and 24-hour thallium images provide equivalent information? (abstr) *J Am Coll Cardiol* 1991;17:29.
101. McCallister BD, Clemments IP, Hauser MF, Gibbons RJ. The limited value of 24-hour images following 4-hour reinjection thallium imaging (abstr). *Circulation* 1991;84:II-533.
102. Dilsizian V, Bonow RO. Differential uptake and apparent thallium-201 "washout" after thallium reinjection: Options regarding early redistribution imaging before reinjection or late redistribution imaging after reinjection. *Circulation* 1992;85:1032–1038.
103. Kiat H, Friedman JD, Wang FP, Van Train KF, Maddahi J, Takemoto K, Berman DS. Frequency of late reversibility in stress-redistribution thallium-201 SPECT using an early reinjection protocol. *Am Heart J* 1991;122:613–619.
104. van Eck-Smit BLF, van der Wall EE, Kuijper AFM, Zwinderman AH, Pauwels EKJ. Immediate thallium-201 reinjection following stress imaging: A time-saving approach for detection of myocardial viability. *J Nucl Med* 1993;34:737–743.
105. Klingensmith WC III, Sutherland JD. Detection of jeopardized myocardium with Tl-201 myocardial perfusion imaging: comparison of early and late reinjection protocols. *Clin Nucl Med* 1993;18:487–490.
106. Dilsizian V, Bonow RO, Quyyumi AA, Smeltzer WR, Bacharach SL. Is early thallium reinjection after post-exercise imaging a satisfactory method to detect defect reversibility? *Circulation* 1993;88(4):I-199.
107. Marin-Neto JA, Dilsizian V, Arrighi JA, Freedman NMT, Perrone-Filardi P, Bacharach SL, Bonow RO. Thallium reinjection demonstrates viable myocardium in regions with reverse redistribution. *Circulation* 1993;88:1736–1745.
108. Dilsizian V, Freedman NMT, Bacharach SL, Perrone-Filardi P, Bonow RO. Regional thallium uptake in irreversible defects: Magnitude of change in thallium activity after reinjection distinguishes viable from nonviable myocardium. *Circulation* 1992;85:627–634.
109. Zimmermann R, Mall G, Rauch B, Zimmer G, Gabel M, Zehelein J, Bubeck B, Tillmanns H, Hagl S, Kubler W. Residual Tl-201 activity in irreversible defects as a marker of myocardial viability: clinicopathological study. *Circulation* 1995;91:1016–1021.
110. Dilsizian V, Quigg RJ, Shirani J, Lee J, Alavi K, Pick R, Bacharach SL. Histomorphologic validation of thallium reinjection and fluorodeoxyglucose PET for assessment of myocardial viability (abstr). *Circulation* 1994;90:I-314.
111. Miller DD, Kemp DL, Armbruster RW, Younis LT, Liu J, Byers S, Bonow RO. Prognostic synergy of thallium-201 stress/redistribution and reinjection protocols in revascularization candidates (abstr). *J Nucl Cardiol* 1995;2:S70.
112. Pieri PL, Tisselli A, Moscatelli G, Spinelli A, Riva P. Prognostic value of Tl-201 reinjection in patients with chronic myocardial infarction. *J Nucl Cardiol* 1995;2:S89.
113. Wackers FJ, Lie KI, Liem KL, Sokole EB, Samson G, van der Schoot JB, Durrer D. Thallium-201 scintigraphy in unstable angina pectoris. *Circulation* 1978;57:738–742.
114. Gewirtz H, Beller GA, Strauss HW, Dinsmore RE, Zir LM, McKusick KA, Pohost GM. Transient defects of resting thallium scans in patients with coronary artery disease. *Circulation* 1979;59:707–713.
115. Berger BC, Watson DD, Burwell LR, Crosby IK, Wellons HA, Teates CD, Beller GA. Redistribution of thallium at rest in patients with stable and unstable angina and the effect of coronary artery bypass surgery. *Circulation* 1979;60:1114–1125.
116. Iskandrian AS, Hakki A, Kane SA, Goel IP, Mundth ED, Hakki A, Segal BL, Amenta A. Rest and redistribution thal-

lium-201 myocardial scintigraphy to predict improvement in left ventricular function after coronary artery bypass grafting. *Am J Cardiol* 1983;51:1312–1316.

117. Mori T, Minamiji K, Kurogane H, Ogawa K, Yoshida Y. Rest-injected thallium-201 imaging for assessing viability of severe asynergic regions. *J Nucl Med* 1991;32:1718–24.
118. Ragosta M, Beller GA, Watson DD, Kaul S, Gimple LW. Quantitative planar rest-redistribution ^{201}Tl imaging in detection of myocardial viability and prediction of improvement in left ventricular function after coronary artery bypass surgery in patients with severely depressed left ventricular function. *Circulation* 1993;87:1630–1641.
119. Hoffman EJ, Huang SC, Phelps ME. Quantitation in positron emission tomography: 1. Effect of object size. *J Comput Assist Tomog* 1979;3:299–308.
120. Gewirtz H, Grotte GJ, Strauss HW, et al. The influence of left ventricular volume and wall motion on myocardial images. *Circulation* 1979;59:1172–1179.
121. Parodi AV, Schelbert HR, Schwaiger M, Hansen H, Selin C, Hoffman EJ. Cardiac emission computed tomography: estimation of regional tracer concentrations due to wall motion abnormality. *J Comput Assist Tomogr* 1984;8:1083–1092.
122. Sinusas AJ, Shi QX, Vitols PJ, et al. Impact of regional ventricular function, geometry and dobutamine stress on quantitative 99mTc-sestamibi defect size. *Circulation* 1993; 88:2224–2234.
123. Eisner RL, Schmarkey S, Martin SE, Carey D, Worthy MA, Chu TH, Horowitz SF, Patterson RE. Defects on SPECT "perfusion" images can occur due to abnormal segmental contraction. *J Nucl Med* 1994;35:638–643.
124. Krivokapich J, Watanabe CR, Shine KI. Effects of anoxia and ischemia on thallium exchange in rapid myocardium. *Am J Physiol* 1985;249:H620–H628.
125. Prigent F, Maddahi J, Garcia EV, Saitoh Y, Van Train K, Berman D. Quantification of myocardial infarct size by thallium-201 single photon emission computerized tomography: experimental validation in the dog. *Circulation* 1986; 74:852–861.
126. Maddahi J, Ganz W, Ninomiya K, Hashida J, Fishbein MC, Mondkar A, Buchbinder N, Shah PK, Swan HJC, Berman DS. Myocardial salvage by intracoronary thrombolysis in evolving myocardial infarction: evaluation using intracoronary injection of thallium-201. *Am Heart J* 1981; 102:664–674.
127. Markis JE, Malagold M, Parker JA, Silverman KJ, Barry WH, Als AV, Paulin S, Grossman W, Braunwald E. Myocardial salvage after intracoronary thrombolysis with streptokinase in acute myocardial infarction. *N Engl J Med* 1981;305:777–782.
128. Beller GA. Role of myocardial perfusion imaging in evaluating thrombolytic therapy for acute myocardial infarction. *J Am Coll Cardiol* 1987;9:661–668.
129. Granato JE, Watson DD, Flanagan TL, Gascho JA, Beller GA. Myocardial thallium-201 kinetics during coronary occlusion and reperfusion: influence of method of reflow and timing of thallium-201 administration. *Circulation* 1986; 73:150–160.
130. Melin JA, Becker LC, Bukley BH. Differences in thallium-201 uptake in reperfused and nonreperfused myocardial infarction. *Circ Res* 1983;53:414–419.
131. Forman R, Kirk ES. Thallium-201 accumulation during reperfusion of ischemic myocardium: dependence on regional blood flow rather than viability. *Am J Cardiol* 1983; 54:659–663.
132. Okada RD, Pohost GM. The use of preintervention and postintervention thallium imaging for assessing the early and late effects of experimental coronary arterial reperfusion in dogs. *Circulation* 1984;69:1153–1160.
133. Okada RD. Kinetics of thallium-201 in reperfused canine myocardium after coronary artery occlusion. *J Am Coll Cardiol* 1984;3:1245–1251.
134. Schuler G, Schwarz F, Hofmann M, Mehmel H, Manthey J, Maurer W, Rauch B, Herrmann HJ, Kubler W. Thrombolysis in acute myocardial infarction using intracoronary streptokinase: assessment by thallium-201 scintigraphy. *Circulation* 1982;66:658–664.
135. Simoons ML, Wijns W, Balakumaran K, Serruys PW, van den Brand M, Fioretti P, Reiber JHC, Lie P, Hugenholtz PG. The effect of intracoronary thrombolysis with streptokinase on myocardial thallium distribution and left ventricular function assessed by blood-pool scintigraphy. *Eur Heart J* 1982;3:433–440.
136. DeCoster PM, Melin JA, Detry JMR, Brasseur LA, Beckers C, Col J. Coronary artery reperfusion in acute myocardial infarction: Assessment by pre- and post-intervention thallium-201 myocardial perfusion imaging. *Am J Cardiol* 1985;55:889–895.
137. Tamaki S, Nakajima H, Murakami T, Yui Y, Kambara H, Kadota K, Yoshida A, Kawai C, Tamaki N, Mukai T, Ishi Y, Torizuka K. Estimation of infarct size by myocardial emission computed tomography with thallium-201 and its relation to creatine kinase-MB release after myocardial infarction in man. *Circulation* 1984;66:994–1001.
138. Mahmarian JJ, Pratt EM, Borges-Neto S, Cushion WR, Roberts R, Verani MS. Quantification of infarct size by thallium-201 single-photon emission computed tomography during acute myocardial infarction in humans: Comparison with enzymatic estimates. *Circulation* 1988;78:831–839.
139. Schwartz F, Schuler G, Katus H, Mehmel HC, von Olshausen K, Hofmann M, Hermann H-J, Kubler W. Intracoronary thrombolysis in acute myocardial infarction: correlation among serum enzyme, scintigraphic and hemodynamic findings. *Am J Cardiol* 1982;50:32–38.
140. Deutsch E, Bushong W, Glavan KA, et al. Heart imaging with cationic complexes of technetium. *Science* 1981;214:85–86.
141. Leppo JA, DePuey EG, Johnson LL. A review of cardiac imaging with sestamibi and teboroxime. *J Nucl Med* 1991;32:2012–2022.
142. Maddahi J, Kiat H, Berman DS. Myocardial perfusion imaging with technetium-99m-labeled agents. *Am J Cardiol* 1991;67:27D–34D.
143. Zaret BL, Rigo P, Wackers FJT, et al. Myocardial perfusion imaging with Tc-99m tetrofosmin: comparison to Tl-201 imaging and coronary angiography in a phase III multicenter trial. *Circulation* 1995;91:313–319.
144. Mullins LJ, Moore RD. The movement of thallium ions in muscle. *J Gen Physiol* 1960;43:759–773.
145. Gehring PJ, Hammond PB. The interrelationship between thallium and potassium in animals. *J Pharmacol Exp Ther* 1967;155:187–201.
146. Piwnica-Worms D, Kronauge JF, Chiu ML. Uptake and retention of hexakis (2-methoxyisobutyl isonitrile) technetium (I) in cultured chick myocardial cells. Mitochondrial and plasma membrane potential dependence. *Circulation* 1990;82: 1826–1838.
147. Leppo JA, Meerdink DJ. Comparison of the myocardial uptake of a technetium-labeled isonitrile analogue and thallium. *Circ Res* 1989;65:632–639.
148. Meerdink DJ, Leppo JA. Comparison of hypoxia and ouabain effects on the myocardial uptake kinetics of technetium-99m hexakis 2-methoxy-isobutyl isonitrile and thallium-201. *J Nucl Med* 1989;30:1500–1506.
149. Wackers FJ, Berman DS, Maddahi J, Watson DD, Beller GA,

Strauss HW, Boucher CA, Picard M, Holman BL, Fridrich R, Inglese E, Delaloye B, Bischof-Delaloye A, Camin L, McKusick K. Technetium-99m hexakis 2-methoxyisobutyl isonitrile: human biodistribution, dosimetry, safety, and preliminary comparison to thallium-201 for myocardial perfusion imaging. *J Nucl Med* 1989;30:301–311.
150. Kiat H, Maddahi J, Roy LT, Van Train K, Friedman J, Resser K, Berman DS. Comparison of technetium-99m methoxy isobutyl isonitrile and thallium 201 for evaluation of coronary artery disease by planar and tomographic methods. *Am Heart J* 1989;117:1–11.
151. Kahn JK, McGhie I, Akers MS, Sills MN, Faber TL, Kulkarni PV, Willerson JT, Corbett JR. Quantitative rotational tomography with Tl-201 and Tc-99m 2-methoxy-isobutyl-isonitrile: a direct comparison in normal individuals and patients with coronary artery disease. *Circulation* 1989;79:1282–1293.
152. Iskandrian AS, Heo J, Kong B, Lyons E, Marsch S. Use of technetium-99m isonitrile (RP-30A) in assessing left ventricular perfusion and function at rest and during exercise in coronary artery disease, and comparison with coronary arteriography and exercise thallium-201 SPECT imaging. *Am J Cardiol* 1989;64:270–275.
153. Dilsizian V, Rocco TP, Strauss HW, Boucher CA. Technetium-99m isonitrile myocardial uptake at rest: I. Relation to severity of coronary artery stenosis. *J Am Coll Cardiol* 1989;14:1673–1677.
154. Rocco TP, Dilsizian V, Strauss HW, Boucher CA. Technetium-99m isonitrile myocardial uptake at rest: II. Relation to clinical markers of potential viability. *J Am Coll Cardiol* 1989;14:1678–1684.
155. Beanlands RSB, Dawood F, Wen WH, Mclaughlin PR, Butany J, D'Amati G, Liu PP. Are the kinetics of technetium-99m methoxyisobutyl isonitrile affected by cell metabolism and viability? *Circulation* 1990;82:1802–1814.
156. Li QS, Matsumura K, Dannals R, Becker LC. Radionuclide markers of viability in reperfused myocardium: comparison between ^{18}F-2-deoxyglucose, ^{201}Tl, and ^{99m}Tc-sestamibi (abstr). *Circulation* 1990;82:III-542.
157. Verani MS, Jeroudi MO, Mahmarian JJ, Boyce TM, Borges-Neto S, Patel B, Bolli R. Quantification of myocardial infarction during coronary occlusion and myocardial salvage after reperfusion using cardiac imaging with technetium-99m hexakis 2-methoxybutyl isonitrile. *J Am Coll Cardiol* 1988;12:1573–1581.
158. Sinusas AJ, Trautman KA, Bergin JD, Watson DD, Ruiz M, Smith WH, Beller GA. Quantification of "area at risk" during coronary occlusion and degree of myocardial salvage after reperfusion with technetium-99m-methoxyisobutyl-isonitrile. *Circulation* 1990;82:1424–1437.
159. Gibbons RJ, Verani MS, Behrenbeck T, Pellikka PA, O'Connor MK, Mahmarian JJ, Chesebro JH, Wackers FJ. Feasibility of tomographic technetium-99m-hexakis-2-methoxy-2-methylpropyl-isonitrile imaging for the assessment of myocardial area at risk and the effect of acute treatment in myocardial infarction. *Circulation* 1989;80:1277–1286.
160. Behrenbeck T, Pellikka PA, Huber KC, Bresnahan JF, Gersh BJ, Gibbons RJ. Primary angioplasty in myocardial infarction: assessment of improved myocardial perfusion with technetium-99m isonitrile. *J Am Coll Cardiol* 1991; 17:365–372.
161. Beller GA, Glover DK, Edwards NC, Ruiz M, Simanis JP, Watson DD. ^{99m}Tc-sestamibi uptake and retention during myocardial ischemia and reperfusion. *Circulation* 1993; 87:2033–2042.
162. Cuocolo A, Pace L, Ricciardelli B, Chiariello M, Trimarco B, Salvatore M. Identification of viable myocardium in patients with chronic coronary artery disease: comparison of thallium-201 scintigraphy with reinjection and technetium-99m methoxyisobutyl isonitrile. *J Nucl Med* 1992;33: 505–511.
163. Bonow RO, Dilsizian V. Thallium-201 and technetium-99m-sestamibi for assessing viable myocardium. *J Nucl Med* 1992;33:815–818.
164. Marzullo P, Sambuceti G, Parodi O. The role of sestamibi scintigraphy in the radioisotopic assessment of myocardial viability. *J Nucl Med* 1992;33:1925–1930.
165. Lucignani G, Paolini G, Landoni C, et al. Presurgical identification of hibernating myocardium by combined used of technetium-99m-hexakis-2-methoxyisobutylisonitrile single photon emission tomography and fluorine-18-fluoro-2-deoxy-D-glucose positron emission tomography in patients with coronary artery disease. *Eur J Nucl Med* 1992;19: 874–881.
166. Altehoefer C, Kaiser HJ, Dorr R, Feinendegen C, Beilin I, Uebis R, Buell U. Fluorine-18 deoxyglucose PET for assessment of viable myocardium in perfusion defects in 99mTc-MIBI SPET: a comparative study in patients with coronary artery disease. *Eur J Nucl Med* 1992;19:334–342.
167. Ferreira J, Gil VM, Ventosa A, Calqueiro J, Seabra-Gomes R. Reversibility in myocardial perfusion scintigraphy after myocardial infarction: comparison of SPECT 99mTc-sestamibi rest-stress single day protocol and thallium-201 reinjection. *Rev Port Cardiol* 1993;12:1013–1021.
168. Marzullo P, Parodi O, Reisenhofer B, Sambuceti G, Picano E, Distante A, Gimelli A, L'Abbate A. Value of rest thallium-201/technetium-99m sestamibi scans and dobutamine echocardiography for detecting myocardial viability. *Am J Cardiol* 1993;71:166–172.
169. Dilsizian V, Arrighi JA, Diodati JG, Quyyumi AA, Bacharach SL, Alavi K, Marin-Neto JA, Katsiyiannis PT, Bonow RO. Myocardial viability in patients with chronic coronary artery disease: comparison of ^{99m}Tc-sestamibi with thallium reinjection and ^{18}F-fluorodeoxyglucose. *Circulation* 1994;89: 578–587.
170. Maurea S, Cuocolo A, Pace L, et al. Left ventricular dysfunction in coronary artery disease: comparison between rest-redistribution thallium-201 and resting technetium-99m methoxyisobutyl isonitrile cardiac imaging. *J Nucl Cardiol* 1994;1:65–71.
171. Sawada SG, Allman KC, Muzik O, Beanlands RS, Wolfe ER, Gross M, Fig L, Schwaiger M. Positron emission tomography detects evidence of viability in rest technetium-99m sestamibi defects. *J Am Coll Cardiol* 1994;23:92–98.
172. Maurea S, Cuocolo A, Nicolai E, Salvatore M. Improved detection of viable myocardium with thallium-201 reinjection in chronic coronary artery disease: comparison with technetium-99m-MIBI imaging. *J Nucl Med* 1994;35:621–624.
173. Altehoefer C, vom Dahl J, Biedermann M, Uebis R, Beilin I, Sheehan F, Hanrath P, Buell U. Significance of defect severity is technetium-99m-MIBI SPECT at rest to assess myocardial viability: comparison with fluorine-18-FDG PET. *J Nucl Med* 1994;35:569–574.
174. Bonow RO, Dilsizian V, Cuocolo A, Bacharach SL. Identification of viable myocardium in patients with coronary artery disease and left ventricular dysfunction: Comparison of thallium scintigraphy with reinjection and PET imaging with ^{18}F-fluorodeoxyglucose. *Circulation* 1991;83:26–37.
175. Canby RC, Silber S, Pohost GM. Relations of the myocardial imaging agents ^{99m}Tc-MIBI and ^{201}Tl to myocardial blood flow in a canine model of myocardial ischemic insult. *Circulation* 1990;81:289–296.
176. Li QS, Solot G, Frank TL, Wagner HN, Becker LC. Myocardial redistribution of technetium-99m-methoxyisobutyl isonitrile (sestamibi). *J Nucl Med* 1990;31:1069–1076.

177. Taillefer R, Primeau M, Costi P, Lambert R, Leveille J, Latour Y. Technetium-99m-sestamibi myocardial perfusion imaging in detection of coronary artery disease: Comparison between initial (1-hour) and delayed (3-hour) postexercise images. *J Nucl Med* 1991;32:1961–1965.
178. Sinusas AJ, Bergin JD, Edwards NC, Watson DD, Rutz M, Makuch RW, Smith WH, Beller GA. Redistribution of 99mTc-sestamibi and 201Tl in the presence of a severe coronary artery stenosis. *Circulation* 1994;89:2332–2341.
179. Maurea S, Cuocolo A, Soricelli L, Castelli M, Imbriaco F, Squame E, Nicolai C, Morisco C, Salvatore M. Resting technetium-99m MIBI redistribution in patients with chronic coronary artery disease (abstr). *J Nucl Med* 1994;35:114P.
180. Udelson JE, Coleman PS, Metherall JA, Pandian NG, Gomez AR, Griffith JL, Shea NL, Oates E, Konstam MA. Predicting recovery of severe regional ventricular dysfunction: comparison of resting scintigraphy with ^{201}Tl and ^{99m}Tc-sestamibi. *Circulation* 1994;89:2552–2561.
181. Weinstein H, Reinhardt CP, Leppo JA. Teboroxime, sestamibi and thallium-201 as markers of myocardial hypoperfusion: comparison by quantitative dual-isotope autoradiography in rabbits. *J Nucl Med* 1993;34:1510–1517.
182. DiRocco RJ, Rumsey WL, Kuczynski BL, et al. Measurement of myocardial blood flow using a coinjection technique for technetium-99m teboroxime, technetium-99m sestamibi and thallium-201. *J Nucl Med* 1992;33:1152–1159.
183. Maublant JC, Moins N, Gachon P. Uptake and release of two new Tc-99m labeled myocardial blood flow imaging agents in cultured cardiac cells. *Eur J Nucl Med* 1989;15: 180–182.
184. Kronauge JF, Chiu ML, Cone JS, et al. Comparison of neutral and cationic myocardial perfusion agents: characteristics of accumulation in cultured cells. *Nucl Med Biol* 1992; 19:141–148.
185. Seldin DW, Johnson L, Blood DK, et al. Myocardial perfusion imaging with technetium-99m SQ30217: comparison with thallium-201 and coronary anatomy. *J Nucl Med* 1989;30:312–319.
186. Iskandrian AS, Heo J, Nguyen T, Mercuro J. Myocardial imaging with Tc-99m teboroxime: technique and initial results. *Am Heart J* 1991;121:889–894.
187. Iskandrian AS, Heo J, Nguyen T. Tomographic myocardial perfusion imaging with technetium-99m teboroxime during adenosine-induced coronary hyperemia: correlation with thallium-201 imaging. *J Am Coll Cardiol* 1992;19:307–312.
188. Henzlova MJ, Machac J. Clinical utility of technetium-99m teboroxime myocardial washout imaging. *J Nucl Med* 1994;35:575–579.
189. Stewart RE, Schwaiger M, Hutchins GD, Chiao PC, Gallagher KP, Nguyen N, Petry NA, Rogers WL. Myocardial clearance kinetics of technetium-99m SQ30217: A marker of regional myocardial blood flow. *J Nucl Med* 1990;31:1183–1190.
190. Gray WA, Gewirtz H. Comparison of ^{99m}Tc-teboroxime with thallium for myocardial imaging in the presence of a coronary artery stenosis. *Circulation* 1991;84:1796–1807.
191. Weinstein H, Dahlberg ST, McSherry BA, Hendel RC, Leppo JA. Rapid redistribution of teboroxime. *Am J Cardiol* 1993;71:848–852.
192. Beanlands R, Muzik O, Nguyen N, Petrey N, Schwaiger M. The relationship between myocardial retention of technetium-99m teboroxime and myocardial blood flow. *J Am Coll Cardiol* 1992;20:712–719.
193. Maublant JC, Moins N, Gachon P, Renoux M, Zhang Z, Veyre A. Uptake of technetium-99m teboroxime in cultured myocardial cells: comparison with thallium-201 and technetium-99m sestamibi. *J Nucl Med* 1993;34:225–229.
194. Smith AM, Gullberg GT, Christian PE, Data FL. Kinetic modeling of teboroxime using dynamic SPECT imaging of a canine model. *J Nucl Med* 1994;35:484–495.
195. Fleming RM, Kirkeeide RL, Taegtmeyer H, Adyanthaya A, Cassidy DB, Goldstein RA. Comparison of technetium-99m teboroxime tomography with automated quantitative coronary arteriography and thallium-201 tomographic imaging. *J Am Coll Cardiol* 1991;17:1297–1302.
196. Hendel RC, Dahlberg ST, Weinstein H, Leppo JA. Comparison of teboroxime and thallium for the reversibility of exercise-induced myocardial perfusion defects. *Am Heart J* 1993;126:856–862.
197. Johnson LL, Seldin DW. Clinical experience with technetium-99m teboroxime, a neutral, lipophilic myocardial perfusion imaging agent. *Am J Cardiol* 1990;66:63E–67E.
198. Bisi G, Sciagra R, Santoro GM, Zerauschek F, Fazzini PF. Evaluation of 99mTc-teboroxime scintigraphy for the differentiation of reversible from fixed defects: comparison with 201Tl redistribution and reinjection imaging. *Nucl Med Commun* 1993;14:520–528.
199. Kelly JD, Forester AM, Higley B, et al. Technetium-99m tetrofosmin as a new radiopharmaceutical for myocardial perfusion imaging. *J Nucl Med* 1993;34:222–227.
200. Sinusas AJ, Shi QX, Saltzberg MT, et al. Technetium-99m tetrofosmin to assess myocardial blood flow: experimental validation in an intact canine model of ischemia. *J Nucl Med* 1994;35:664–671.
201. Jain D, Wackers FJ, Mattera J, et al. Biokinetics of 99m Tc-tetrofosmin, a new myocardial perfusion imaging agent: implications for a one day imaging protocol. *J Nucl Med* 1993;34:1254–1259.
202. Higley B, Smith FW, Smith T, Gemmell HG, Das Gupta P, Gvozdanovic DV, Graham D, Hinge D, Davidson J, Lahiri A. Technetium-99m-1,2-bis[bis(2-ethoxyethyl)phosphino] ethane: human biodistribution, dosimetry and safety of a new myocardial perfusion imaging agent. *J Nucl Med* 1993; 34:30–38.
203. Gerson MC, Millard RW, Roszell NJ, McGoron AJ, et al. Kinetic properties of 99mTc-Q12 in canine myocardium. *Circulation* 1994;89:1291–1300.
204. Gerson MC, Lukes J, Deutsch E, BiniakieWicz D, Rohe RC, Washburn LC, Fortman C, Walsh RA. Comparison of technetium-99m Q12 and thallium-201 for detection of angiographically documented coronary artery disease in humans. *J Nucl Cardiol* 1994;1:499–508.
205. D'Agostino AN. An electron microscopic study of cardiac necrosis produced by 9a-fluorocortisol and sodium phosphate. *Am J Pathol* 1964;45:633–644.
206. Shen AC, Jennings RB. Myocardial calcium and magnesium in acute ischemic injury. *Am J Pathol* 1972;67:417–440.
207. Bonte FJ, Parkey RW, Graham KD, Moore J, Stokely EM. A new method for radionuclide imaging of myocardial infarcts. *Radiology* 1974;110:473–474.
208. Buja JL, Tofe AJ, Kulkarni PV, Mukherjee A, Parkey RW, Francis MD, Bonte FJ, Willerson JT. Sites and mechanisms of localization of technetium-99m phosphorous radiopharmaceuticals in acute myocardial infarcts and other tissues. *J Clin Invest* 1977;60:724–740.
209. Chien KR, Reeves JP, Buja LM, Bonte F, Parkey RW, Willerson JT. Phospholipid alterations in ischemic myocardium: Temporal and topographical correlations with Tc-99m PPi accumulation and an in vitro sarcolemmal Ca+2 permeability defect. *Circ Res* 1981;48:711–719.
210. Willerson JT, Parkey RW, Bonte FJ, Lewis SE, Corbett J, Buja LM. Pathophysiologic considerations and clinicopathological correlates of technetium-99m stannous pyrophosphate myocardial scintigraphy. *Semin Nucl Med* 1980;10:54–69.
211. Corbett JR, Lewis M, Willerson JT, et al. Tc-99m pyrophos-

phate imaging in patients with acute myocardial infarction: comparison of planar imaging with single-photon tomography with and without blood pool overlay. *Circulation* 1984; 69:1120–1128.

212. Ahmed M, Dubiel JP, Logan KW, Verdon TA, Martin RH. Limited clinical diagnostic specificity of technetium-99m stannous pyrophosphate myocardial imaging in acute myocardial infarction. *Am J Cardiol* 1977;39:50–54.
213. Massie BM, Botvinick EH, Werner JA, Chatterjee K, Parmley WW. Myocardial scintigraphy with technetium-99m stannous pyrophosphate: An insensitive test for nontransmural myocardial infarction. *Am J Cardiol* 1979;43:186–192.
214. Willerson JT, Parkey Rw, Stokely EM, Bonte FJ, Lewis S, Harris RA, Blomqvist G, Poliner LR, Buja LM. Infarct sizing with technetium-99m stannous pyrophosphate scintigraphy in dogs and man: Relationship between scintigraphic and precordial mapping estimates of infarct size in patients. *Cardiovasc Res* 1977;11:291–298.
215. Wynne J, Holman BL. Acute myocardial infarc scintigraphy with infarct-avid radiotracers. *Med Clin North Am* 1980; 64:119–144.
216. Lyons KP, Olson HG, Aronow WS. Pyrophosphate myocardial imaging. *Semin Nucl Med* 1980;10:168–177.
217. Ahmed M, Dubiel JP, Verdon TA Jr, Martin RH. Technetium 99m stannous pyrophosphate myocardial imaging in patients with and without left ventricular aneurysm. *Circulation* 1976;53:833–838.
218. Jengo JA, Mena I, Joe SH, Criley JM. The significance of calcific valvular heart disease in Tc-99m pyrophosphate myocardial infarction scanning: Radiographic, scintigraphic, and pathological correlation. *J Nucl Med* 1977;18:776–781.
219. Seo I, Donoghue G. Tc-99m-pyrophosphate accumulation on prosthetic valves. *Clin Nucl Med* 1980;5:367–369.
220. Go RT, Doty DB, Chiu CL, Christie H. A new method of diagnosing myocardial contusion in man by radionuclide imaging. *Radiology* 1975;116:107–110.
221. Datz FL, Lewis SE, Parkey RW, Bonte FJ, Buja LM, Willerson JT. Radionuclide evaluation of cardiac trauma. *Semin Nucl Med* 1980;10:187–192.
222. Hartford W, Weinberg MN, Buja LM, Parkey RW, Bonte FJ, Willerson JT. Positive Tc-99m stannous pyrophosphate myocardial image in a patient with carcinoma of the lung. *Radiology* 1977;122:747–748.
223. Khaw BA, Beller GA, Haber E, Smith TW. Localization of cardiac myosin-specific antibody in myocardial infarction. *J Clin Invest* 1976;58:439–446.
224. Beller GA, Khaw BA, Haber E, Smith TW. Localization of radiolabeled cardiac myosin-specific antibody in myocardial infarcts: Comparison with technetium-99m stannous pyrophosphate. *Circulation* 1977;55:74–78.
225. Khaw BA, Fallon JT, Strauss HW, Haber E. Myocardial infarct imaging of antibodies to canine cardiac myosin with indium-111-diethylene-triamine pentaacetic acid. *Science* 1980;209:295–297.
226. Khaw BA, Yasuda T, Gold HK, Leibach RC, Johns JA, Kanke M, Barlai-Kovach M, Strauss HW, Haber E. Acute myocardial infarct imaging with indium-111-labeled monoclonal antimyosin Fab. *J Nucl Med* 1987;28:1671–1678.
227. Johnson LL, Seldin DW, Becker LC, LaFrance ND, Liberman HA, James C, Mattis J, Dean R, Brown J, Reiter A, Arneson V, Cannon PJ, Berger HJ: Antimyosin imaging in acute transmural myocardial infarctions: Results of a multicenter clinical trial. *J Am Coll Cardiol* 1989;13:27–35.
228. Yasuda T, Palacios IF, Dec GW, Fallon JT, Gold HK, Leinbach RC, Strauss HW, Khaw BA, Haber E. Indium-111 monoclonal antimyosin antibody imaging in the diagnosis of acute myocarditis. *Circulation* 1987;76:306–311.
229. Carrio I, Berna L, Ballester M, Estorch M, Obrador D, Cladellas M, Abudal L, Ginjaume M. Indium-111 antimyosin scintigraphy to assess myocardial damage in patients with suspected myocarditis and cardiac rejection. *J Nucl Med* 1988;29:1893–1900.
230. Obrador D, Ballester M, Carrio I, Berna L, Pons-Llado G. High prevalence of myocardial monoclonal antimyosin antibody uptake in patients with chronic idiopathic dilated cardiomyopathy. *J Am Coll Cardiol* 1989;13:1289–1293.
231. Dec GW, Palacios I, Yasuda T, Fallon JT, Khaw BA, Strauss HW, Haber E. Antimyosin antibody cardiac imaging: Its role in the diagnosis of myocarditis. *J Am Coll Cardiol* 1990;16:97–104.
232. Bergmann SR, Fox KAA, Rand AL, McElvany KD, Welch MJ, Markham J, Sobel BE. Quantification of regional myocardial blood flow in vivo with O-15 water. *Circulation* 1984;70:724–733.
233. Walsh MN, Bergmann SR, Steele RL, Kenzora JL, Ter-Pogossian MM, Sobel BE, Geltman EM. Delineation of impaired regional myocardial perfusion by positron emission tomography with O-15 water. *Circulation* 1988;78:612–620.
234. Bacharach SL, Cuocolo A, Bonow RO, et al. Arterial blood concentration curves by cardiac PET without arterial sampling or image reconstruction, in: *Computers in Cardiology* 1988, Washington, DC, IEEE Computer Society Press, 1989, p 219.
235. Bergmann SR, Herrero P, Markham J, Weinheimer CJ, Walsh MN. Noninvasive quantitation of myocardial blood flow in human subjects with oxygen-15-labeled water and positron emission tomography. *J Am Coll Cardiol* 1989;14:639–652.
236. Iida H, Kanno I, Takahashi A, Miura S, Murakami M, Takahashi K, Ono Y, Shishido F, Inugami A, Tomura N, Higano S, Fujita H, Sasaki H, Nakamichi H, Mizusawa S, Kondo Y, Uemura K. Measurement of absolute myocardial blood flow with O-15 water and dynamic positron emission tomography. *Circulation* 1988;78:104–115.
237. Araujo LI, Lammertsma AA, Rhodes CG, McFalls EO, Iida H, Rechavia E, Galassi A, DeSilva R, Jones T, Maseri A. Noninvasive quantification of regional myocardial blood flow in coronary artery disease with oxygen-15-labeled carbon dioxide inhalation and positron emission tomography. *Circulation* 1991;83:875–885.
238. Schelbert HR, Wisenberg G, Phelps ME, Gould KL, Henze E, Hoffman EJ, Gomes A, Kuhl DE. Noninvasive assessment of coronary stenoses by myocardial imaging during pharmacologic coronary vasodilation. VI. Detection of coronary artery disease by human beings with intravenous N-13 ammonia and positron computed tomography. *Am J Cardiol* 1982;49:1197–1206.
239. Tamaki N, Senda M, Yonekura Y, Saji H, Kodama S, Konishi Y, Ban T, Kambara H, Kawai C, Torizuka K. Dynamic positron computed tomography of the heart with a high sensitivity positron camera and nitrogen-13 ammonia. *J Nucl Med* 1985;26:567–575.
240. Schelbert HR, Phelps ME, Huang S-C, MacDonald NS, Hansen H, Selin C, Kuhl DE. N-13 ammonia as an indicator of myocardial blood flow. *Circulation* 1981;63:1259–1272.
241. Shah A, Schelbert HR, Schwaiger M, Henze E, Hansen H, Selin C, Huang S-C. Measurement of regional myocardial blood flow with N-13 ammonia and positron emission tomography in intact dogs. *J Am Coll Cardiol* 1985;5:92–100.
242. Krivokapich J, Smith GT, Huang S-C, Hoffman EJ, Ratib O, Phelps ME, Schelbert HR. N-13 ammonia myocardial imaging at rest and with exercise in normal volunteers. *Circulation* 1989;80:1328–1337.
243. Hutchins GD, Schwaiger M, Rosenspire KC, Krivokapich J, Schelbert HR, Kuhl DE. Noninvasive quantification of re-

gional blood flow in the human heart using N-13 ammonia and dynamic positron emission tomographic imaging. *J Am Coll Cardiol* 1990;15:1032–1042.
244. Rosenspire KC, Schwaiger M, Mangner TJ, Hutchins GD, Sutorik A, Kuhl DE. Metabolic fate of [N-13] ammonia in human and canine blood. *J Nucl Med* 1990;31:163–167.
245. Bergmann SR, Hack S, Tewson T, Welch MJ, Sobel BE. The dependence of accumulation of N-13 ammonia by myocardium on metabolic factors and its implications for quantitative assessment of perfusion. *Circulation* 1980;61:34–43.
246. Krivokapich J, Huang S-C, Phelps ME, MacDonald NS, Shine KI. Dependence of N-13 ammonia myocardial extraction and clearance on flow and metabolism. *Am J Physiol: Heart Circ Physiol* 1982;242:H536–H542.
247. Rauch B, Helus F, Grunze M, Braunwell E, Mall G, Hasselbach W, Kubler W. Kinetics of N-13 ammonia uptake in myocardial single cells indicating potential limitations in its applicability as a marker of myocardial blood flow. *Circulation* 1985;71:387–393.
248. Gould KL, Goldstein RA, Mullani NA, Kirkeeide RL, Wong W-H, Tewson TJ, Berridge MS, Bolomey LA, Hartz RK, Smalling RW, Fuentes F, Nishikawa A. Noninvasive assessment of coronary stenoses by myocardial perfusion imaging during pharmacologic vasodilation. VIII. Clinical feasibility of positron cardiac imaging without a cyclotron using generator-produced rubidium-82. *J Am Coll Cardiol* 1986;7:775–789.
249. Yonekura Y, Tamaki N, Senda M, Nohara R, Kambara H, Konishi Y, Koide H, Kureshi SA, Saji H, Ban T, Kawai C, Torizuka K. Detection of coronary artery disease with N-13 ammonia and high-resolution positron emission computed tomography. *Am Heart J* 1987;13:645–654.
250. Tamaki N, Yonekura Y, Senda M, Yamashita K, Koide H, Saji H, Hashimoto T, Fudo T, Kambara H, Kawai C, Konishi J. Value and limitation of stress thallium-201 single photon emission computed tomography: Comparison with nitrogen-13 ammonia positron tomography. *J Nucl Med* 1988; 29:1181–1188.
251. Gewirtz H, Fischman AJ, Abraham S, Gilson M, Strauss HW, Alpert NM. Positron emission tomographic measurements of absolute regional myocardial blood flow permits identification of nonviable myocardium in patients with chronic myocardial infarction. *J Am Coll Cardiol* 1994;23:851–859.
252. Tamaki N, Kawamoto M, Tadamura E, Magata Y, Yonekura Y, Nohara R, Sasayama S, Nishimura K, Ban T, Konishi J. Prediction of reversible ischemia after revascularization: perfusion and metabolic studies with positron emission tomography. *Circulation* 1995;91:1697–1705.
253. Love WD, Burch GE. Influence of the rate of coronary plasma flow on the extraction of rubidium-86 from coronary blood. *Circ Res* 1959;7:24–30.
254. Selwyn AP, Allan RM, L'Abbate A, Horlock P, Camici P, Clark J, O'Brien HA, Grant PM. Relation between regiona myocardial uptake of rubidium-82 and perfusion: Absolute reduction of cation uptake in ischemia. *Am J Cardiol* 1982;50:112–121.
255. Goldstein RA, Mullani NA, Marani SK, Fisher DJ, Gould KL, O'Brien HA Jr. Myocardial perfusion with rubidium-82. II, Effects of metabolic and pharmacologic interventions. *J Nucl Med* 1983;24:907–915.
256. Fukuyama T, Nakamura M, Nakagaki O, Matsuguchi H, Mitsutake A, Kikuchi Y. Reduced reflow and diminished uptake of rubidium-86 after temporary coronary occlusion. *Am J Physiol: Heart Circ Physiol* 1978;234:H724–H729.
257. Wilson RA, Shea M, De Landsheere C, Deanfield J, Lammertsma AA, Jones T, Selwyn AP. Rubidium-82 myocardial uptake and extraction after transient ischemia: PET characteristics. *J Comput Assist Tomogr* 1987;11:60–66.
258. Jeremy RW, Links JM, Becker LC. Progressive failure of coronary flow during reperfusion of myocardial infarction: documentation of the no reflow phenomenon with positron emission tomography. *J Am Coll Cardiol* 1990;16:695–704.
259. Demer LL, Gould LK, Goldstein RA, Kirkeeide RL, Mullani NA, Smalling RW, Nishikawa A, Merhige ME. Assessment of coronary artery disease severity by positron emission tomography. Comparison with quantitative arteriography in 193 patients. *Circulation* 1989;79:825–835.
260. Go RT, Marwick TH, MacIntyre WJ, Saha GB, Neumann DR, Underwood DA, Simpfendorfer CC. A prospective comparison of rubidium-82 PET and thallium-201 SPECT myocardial perfusion imaging utilizing a single dipyridamole stress in the diagnosis of coronary artery disease. *J Nucl Med* 1990;31:1899–1905.
261. Stewart RE, Schwaiger M, Molina E, Popma J, Gacioch GM, Kalus M, Squicciarini S, al-Aouar ZR, Schork A, Kuhl DE. Comparison of rubidium-82 positron emission tomography and thallium-201 SPECT imaging for detection of coronary artery disease. *Am J Cardiol* 1991;67:1303–1310.
262. Goldstein RA. Kinetics of rubidium-82 after coronary occlusion and reperfusion: assessment of patency and viability in open-chested dogs. *J Clin Invest* 1985;75:1131–1137.
263. Gould KL, Yoshida K, Hess MJ, Haynie M, Mullani N, Smalling RW. Myocardial metabolism of fluorodeoxyglucose compared to cell membrane integrity for the potassium analogue rubidium-82 for assessing infarct size in man by PET. *J Nucl Med* 1991;32:1–9.
264. Schelbert HR, Phelps ME, Hoffman E, Huand SC, Kuhl DE. Regional myocardial blood flow, metabolism, and function assessed noninvasively with positron emission tomography. *Am J Cardiol* 1980;46:1269–1277.
265. Marshall RC, Tillisch JH, Phelps ME, Huang SC, Carson R, Henze E, Schelbert HR. Identification and differentiation of resting myocardial ischemia and infarction in man with positron emission tomography, F-18 labeled fluorodeoxyglucose and N-13 ammonia. *Circulation* 1983;67:766–778.
266. Schelbert HR, Buxton D. Insights into coronary artery disease gained from metabolic imaging. *Circulation* 1988;78: 496–505.
267. Maddahi J, Schelbert H, Brunken R, DiCarli M. Role of thallium-201 and PET imaging in evaluation of myocardial viability and management of patients with coronary artery disease and left ventricular dysfunction. *J Nucl Med* 1994;35:707–715.
268. Tamaki N, Yonekura Y, Yamashita K, Saji H, Magata Y, Senda M, Konishi Y, Hirata K, Ban T, Konishi J. Positron emission tomography using fluorine-18 deoxyglucose in evaluation of coronary artery bypass grafting. *Am J Cardiol* 1989;64:860–865.
269. Ferrannini E. The theoretical bases of indirect calorimetry: a review. *Metabolism* 1981;63:1273–1279.
270. Neely JR, Rovetto MJ, Oram JF. Myocardial utilization of carbohydrate and lipids. *Prog Cardiovasc Dis* 1972; 15:289–329.
271. Camici P, Ferrannini E, Opie LH. Myocardial metabolism in ischemic heart disease: basic principles and application to imaging by positron emission tomography. *Prog Cardiovas Dis* 1989;32:217–238.
272. Liedtke AJ. Alterations of carbohydrate and lipid metabolism in the acutely ischemic heart. *Prog Cardiovasc Dis* 1981; 23:321–336.
273. Opie LH. Effects of regional ischemia on metabolism of glucose and fatty acids: relative rates of aerobic and anaerobic energy production during myocardial infarction and comparison with effects of anoxia. *Circ Res* 1976;38:I-52–74.
274. Schon HR, Schelbert HR, Najafi A, et al. C-11 labeled pal-

mitic acid for the noninvasive evaluation of regional myocardial fatty acid metabolism with positron computed tomography, I: kinetics of C-11 palmitic acid in normal myocardium. *Am Heart J* 1982;103:532–547.

275. Rosamond TL, Abendschein DR, Sobel BE, Bergmann SR, Fox KAA. Metabolic fate of radiolabeled palmitate in ischemic canine myocardium: implications for positron emission tomography. *J Nucl Med* 1987;28:1322–1329.
276. Lerch RA, Bergmann SR, Ambos HD, Welch JM, Ter-Pogossian MM, Sobel BE. Effect of flow-independent reduction of metabolism on regional myocardial clearance of C-11 palmitate. *Circulation* 1982;65:731–738.
277. Schwaiger M, Schelbert HR, Ellison D, Hansen H, Yeatman L, Vinten-Johansen J, Selin C, Barrio J, Phelps ME. Sustained regional abnormalities in cardiac metabolism after transient ischemia in the chronic dog model. *J Am Coll Cardiol* 1985;6:336–347.
278. Liedtke AJ, DeMaison L, Eggleston AM, Cohen LM, Nellis SH. Changes in substrate metabolism and effects of excess fatty acids in reperfused myocardium. *Circ Res* 1988; 62:535–542.
279. Schelbert HR, Henze E, Schon HR, et al. C-11 palmitic acid for the noninvasive evaluation of regional myocardial fatty acid metabolism with positron computed tomography, IV: in vivo demonstration of impaired fatty acid oxidation in acute myocardial ischemia. *Am Heart J* 1983;106:736–750.
280. Schelbert HR, Henze E, Schon HR, et al. Carbon-11 palmitate for the noninvasive evaluation of regional myocardial fatty acid metabolism with positron computed tomography, III: in vivo demonstration of the effects of substrate availability on myocardial metabolism. *Am Heart J* 1983;105:492–504.
281. Fox KAA, Abendschein D, Ambos HD, Sobel BE, Bergmann SR. Efflux of metabolized and nonmetabolized fatty acid from canine myocardium. Implications for quantifying myocardial metabolism tomographically. *Circ Res* 1985;57:232–243.
282. Myears DW, Sobel BE, Bergmann SR. Substrate use in ischemic and reperfused canine myocardium: quantitative considerations. *Am J Physiol: Heart Circ Physiol* 1987;253: H107–H114.
283. Sokoloff L, Reivich M, Kennedy C, et al. The [14C]-deoxyglucose method for the measurement of local cerebral glucose utilization: Theory, procedure and normal values in the conscious and anesthetized albino rat. *J Neurochem* 1977; 28:897–916.
284. Phelps ME, Schelbert HR, Mazziotta JC. Positron computer tomography for studies of myocardial and cerebral function. *Ann Intern Med* 1983;98:339–359.
285. Neely JR, Rovetto MJ, Oram JF. Myocardial utilization of carbohydrate and lipids. *Prog Cardiovasc Dis* 1972; 15:289–329.
286. Neely JR, Morgan HE. Relationship between carbohydrate and lipid metabolism and the energy balance of heart muscle. *Annu Rev Physiol* 1974;36:413–459.
287. Taegtmeyer H, Robers AFC, Raine AEG. Energy metabolism in reperfused heart muscle: Metabolic correlates of return of function. *J Am Coll Cardiol* 1985;6:864–870.
288. Armbrecht JJ, Buxton DB, Schelbert HR. Validation of [1-^{11}C] acetate as a tracer for noninvasive assessment of oxidative metabolism with positron emission tomography in normal, ischemic, postischemic, and hyperemic canine myocardium. *Circulation* 1990;81:1594–1605.
289. Vanoverschelde JJ, Melin JA, Bol A, Vanbutsele R, Cogneau M, Labar D, Robert A, Michel C, Wijns W. Regional oxidative metabolism in patients after recovery from reperfused anterior myocardial infarction: Relation to regional blood flow and glucose uptake. *Circulation* 1992;85:9–21.
290. Gropler RJ, Siegel BA, Sampathkumaran K, Perez JE, Sobel BE, Bergmann SR, Geltman EM. Dependence of recovery of contractile function on maintenance of oxidative metabolism after myocardial infarction. *J Am Coll Cardiol* 1992; 19:989–997.
291. Gropler RJ, Geltman EM, Sampathkumaran K, Perez JE, Moerlein SM, Sobel BE, Bergmann SR, Siegel BA. Functional recovery after coronary revascularization for chronic coronary artery disease is dependent on maintenance of oxidative metabolism. *J Am Coll Cardiol* 1992;20:569–577.
292. Iida H, Rhodes CG, de Silva R, Yamamoto Y, Araujo LI, Maseri A, Jones T. Myocardial tissue fraction: Correction of partial volume effects and measure of tissue viability. *J Nucl Med* 1991;32:2169–2175.
293. Yamamoto Y, de Silva R, Rhodes CG, Araujo LI, Iida H, Rechavia E, Nihouannopoulos P, Hackett D, Galassi AR, Taylor CJV, Lammertsma AA, Jones T, Maseri A. A new strategy for the assessment of viable myocardium and regional myocardial blood flow using 15O-water and dynamic positron emission tomography. *Circulation* 1992;86:167–178.
294. Perrone-Filardi P, Bacharach SL, Dilsizian V, Maurea S, Frank JA, Bonow RO. Regional left ventricular wall thickening: Relation to regional uptake of 18-Fluorodeoxyglucose and thallium-201 in patients with chronic coronary artery disease and left ventricular dysfunction. *Circulation* 1992;86: 1125–1137.
295. Krivokapich J, Huang SC, Phelps ME, Barrio JR, Watanabe CR, Selin CE, Shine KI. Estimation of rabbit myocardial metabolic rate for glucose using fluorodeoxyglucose. *Am J Physiol* 1982;243:H884–H895.
296. Ratib O, Phelps ME, Huang SS, Henze E, Selin CE, Schelbert HR. Positron tomography with deoxyglucose for estimating local myocardial glucose metabolism. *J Nucl Med* 1982;23:577–586.
297. Schelbert HR. Metabolic imaging to assess myocardial viability. *J Nucl Med* 1994;35(suppl):8S–14S.
298. Luciganani G, Paolini G, Landoni C, Zuccari M, Paganelli G, Galli L, DiCredico G, Vanoli G, Rossetti C, Mariani MA, Gilardi MC, Colombo F, Grossi A, Fazio F. Presurgical identification of hibernating myocardium by combined use of technetium-99m hexakis 2-methoxyisobutylisonitrile single photon emission tomography and fluorine-18-fluoro-2-deoxy-D-glucose positron emission tomography in patients with coronary artery disease. *Eur J Nucl Med* 1992;19:874–881.
299. Carrel T, Jenni R, Haubold-Reuter S, Von Schulthess G, Pasic M, Turina M. Improvement of severely reduced left ventricular function after surgical revascularization in patients with preoperative myocardial infarction. *Eur J Cardiothorac Surg* 1992;6:479–484.
300. Nienaber CA, Brunken RC, Sherman CT, Yeatman LA, Gambhir SS, Krivokapich J, Demer LL, Ratib O, Child JS, Phelps ME, Schelbert HR. Metabolic and functional recovery of ischemic human myocardium after coronary angioplasty. *J Am Coll Cardiol* 1991;18:966–978.
301. Tamaki N, Ohtani H, Yamashita K, Magata Y, Yonekura Y, Nohara R, Kambara H, Kawai C, Hirata K, Ban T, Konishi J. Metabolic activity in the areas of new fill-in after thallium-201 reinjection: comparison with positron emission tomography using fluoro-18-deoxyglucose. *J Nucl Med* 1991; 32:673–678.
302. Marwick TH, MacIntyre WJ, LaFont A, Nemec JJ, Salcedo EE. Metabolic responses of hibernating and infarcted myocardium the revascularization: a follow-up study of regional perfusion, function, and metabolism. *Circulation* 1992; 85:1347–1353.
303. vom Dahl J, Eitzman DT, Al-Aouar ZR, Kanter HL, Hicks RJ, Deeb GM, Kirsh MM, Schwaiger M. Relation of regional function, perfusion, and metabolism in patients with advanced

coronary artery disease undergoing surgical revascularization. *Circulation* 1994;90:2356–2366.

304. Vanoverschelde JJ, Wijns W, Depre C, Essamri B, Heyndrickx GR, Borgers M, Bol A, Melin JA. Mechanisms of chronic regional postischemic dysfunction in humans: new insights from the study of noninfarcted collateral-dependent myocardium. *Circulation* 1993;87:1513–1523.
305. Melin JA, Wijns W, Keyeux A, Gurne O, Cogneau M, Michel C, Bol A, Robert A, Charlier A, Pouleur H. Assessment of thallium-201 redistribution versus glucose uptake as predictors of viability after coronary occlusion and reperfusion. *Circulation* 1988;77:927–934.
306. Brunken R, Schwaiger M, Grover-McKay M, Phelps ME, Tillisch J, Schelbert HR. Positron emission tomography detects tissue metabolic activity in myocardial segments with persistent thallium perfusion defects. *J Am Coll Cardiol* 1987;10:557–567.
307. Tamaki N, Yonekura Y, Yamashita K, Senda M, Saji H, Hashimoto T, Fudo T, Kambara H, Kawai C, Ban T, Konishi J. Relation of left ventricular perfusion and wall motion with metabolic activity in persistent defects on thallium-201 tomography in healed myocardial infarction. *Am J Cardiol* 1988;62:202–208.
308. Brunken RC, Kottou S, Nienaber CA, Schwaiger M, Ratib OM, Phelps ME, Schelbert HR. PET detection of viable tissue in myocardial segments with persistent defects at Tl-201 SPECT. *Radiology* 1989;65:65–73.
309. Tamaki N, Yonekura Y, Yamashita K, Mukai T, Magata Y, Hashimoto T, Fudo T, Kambara H, Kawai C, Hirata K, Ban T, Konishi J. SPECT thallium-201 tomography and positron tomography using N-13 ammonia and F-18 fluorodeoxyglucose in coronary artery disease. *Am J Cardiac Imaging* 1989;3:3–9.
310. Brunken RC, Mody FV, Hawkins RA, Nienaber C, Phelps ME, Schelbert HR. Positron emission tomography detects metabolic viability in myocardium with persistent 24-hour single-photon emission computed tomography TL-201 defects. *Circulation* 1992;86:1357–1369.
311. Tamaki N, Ohtani H, Yamashita K, Magata Y, Yonekura Y, Nohara R, Kambara H, Kawai C, Hirata K, Ban T, Konishi J. Metabolic activity in the areas of new fill-in after thallium-201 reinjection: Comparison with positron emission tomography using fluorine-18-deoxyglucose. *J Nucl Med* 1991;32:673–678.
312. Ogiu N, Nakai K, Hiramori K. Thallium-201 reinjection images can identify the viable and necrotic myocardium similarly to metabolic imaging with glucose loading F-18 fluorodeoxyglucose (FDG)-PET. *Ann Nucl Med* 1994;8:171–176.
313. Myears DW, Sobel BE, Bergmann SR. Substrate use in ischemic and reperfused canine myocardium: Quantitative considerations. *Am J Physiol* 1987;253:H107–H114.
314. Renstrom B, Nellis SH, Liedtke AJ. Metabolic oxidation of glucose during early myocardial reperfusion. *Circ Res* 1989;65:1094–1101.
315. Renstrom B, Nellis SH, Liedtke AJ. Metabolic oxidation of pyruvate and lactate during early myocardial reperfusion. *Circ Res* 1990;66:282–288.
316. Schwaiger M, Brunken R, Grover-McKay M, Krivokapich J, Child J, Tillisch JH, Phelps ME, Schelbert HR. Regional myocardial metabolism in patients with acute myocardial infarction assessed by positron emission tomography. *J Am Coll Cardiol* 1986;8:800–808.
317. Pierard LA, De Landsheere CM, Berthe C, Rigo P, Kulbertus HE. Identification of viable myocardium by echocardiography during dobutamine infusion in patients with myocardial infarction after thrombolytic therapy: comparison with positron emission tomography. *J Am Coll Cardiol* 1990; 15:1021–1031.
318. Sebree L, Bianco JA, Subramanian R, Wilson MA, Swanson D, Hegge J, Tschudy J, Pyzalski R. Discordance between accumulation of C-14 deoxyglucose and Tl-201 in reperfused myocardium. *J Mol Cell Cardiol* 1991;23:603–616.
319. Eitzman D, Al-Aouar Z, Kanter HL, vomDahl J, Kirsh M, Deeb GM, Schwaiger M. Clinical outcome of patients with advanced coronary artery disease after viability studies with positron emission tomography. *J Am Coll Cardiol* 1992;20:559–565.
320. DiCarli M, Davidson M, Little R, Khanna S, Mody FV, Brunken RC, Czernin J, Rokhsar S, Stevenson LW, Laks H, Hawkins R, Schelbert HR, Phelps ME, Maddahi J. Value of metabolic imaging with positron emission tomography for evaluating prognosis in patients with coronary artery disease and left ventricular dysfunction. *Am J Cardiol* 1994; 73:527–533.
321. Gropler RJ, Siegel BA, Lee KJ, Moerlein SM, Perry DJ, Bergmann SR, Geltman EM. Nonuniformity in myocardial accumulation of fluorine-18-fluorodeoxyglucose in normal fasted humans. *J Nucl Med* 1990;31:1749–1756.
322. Berry JJ, Baker JA, Pieper KS, Hanson MW, Hoffman JM, Coleman RE. The effect of metabolic milieu on cardiac PET imaging using fluorine-18-deoxyglucose and nitrogen-13-ammonia in normal volunteers. *J Nucl Med* 1991; 32:1518–1525.

23 *Section 3:* Radionuclide Angiography in Coronary and Noncoronary Heart Disease: Technical Background and Clinical Applications

James A. Arrighi, Vasken Dilsizian

Radionuclide angiography is an important clinical tool for defining the functional impact of coronary artery disease, valvular heart disease, or systemic illness on cardiac ventricular function. Because left ventricular function is a powerful predictor of prognosis, this technique has also been used to evaluate the functional outcome of cardiac interventions such as thrombolysis, coronary artery angioplasty, or bypass surgery. Assessment of systolic and diastolic ventricular function by radionuclide angiography is accurate and reproducible. Such tests can be performed serially to assess changes in ventricular performance over time, thereby providing a means to objectively follow the effects of a disease or therapy on heart function in individual patients. This discussion will consider first the technical aspects of radionuclide angiography, and then the clinical applications of this technique.

TECHNICAL ASPECTS OF DATA ACQUISITION

Radionuclide angiography may utilize either *first-pass* or *equilibrium* techniques. Although both methods produce similar results with regard to quantification of ventricular function, each technique has advantages and limitations that will be discussed below. For both methods, the clinical goal is to assess ventricular function with the injection of a radiopharmaceutical intravenously. Data are collected with a scintillation camera coupled to a computer that controls data collection, processing, and analysis. Studies are then analyzed both qualitatively by the observation of closed-loop cinematic display, and quantitatively by the calculation of various parameters of ventricular function.

Data may be acquired in either *frame mode* or *list mode* (Fig. 1). In frame-mode acquisition, the cardiac cycle is divided into a prespecified number of time intervals, based on an operator-defined number of frames per cycle or time interval per frame. Usually, the beginning of each cycle corresponds to the R-wave on the electrocardiogram (ECG). Counts are collected into each frame over a number of cardiac cycles. In list-mode acquisition, data are collected with time data (relative to the ECG). The advantage of list mode is that data can be reformatted retrospectively, after the study has been completed. This will permit filtration of arrhythmias or modification of the temporal resolution before formatting data. List-mode acquisition requires a large amount of computer memory and more processing time compared to frame-mode acquisition. For practical purposes, frame-mode acquisition is adequate for most clinical studies. List-mode acquisition may be preferred in some cases, particularly research protocols in which there is a potential need for multiple analyses of the original data.

First-Pass Radionuclide Angiography

RADIOPHARMACEUTICALS

In first-pass studies, the bolus of radioactivity passes initially through the right chambers of the heart, and through the lungs to the left chambers of the heart. Images must be acquired rapidly (less than 10 seconds for ventricular function data) as the radiopharmaceutical passes through the heart chambers of interest. Separation of the right- and left-sided chambers is achieved as a result of the temporal separation of the bolus. Radiopharmaceuticals used for this purpose must produce adequate counts in a short period of time at an acceptably low radiation dose to the patient. ^{99m}Technetium-labeled compounds are ideally suited for this purpose (Table 1).

In clinical practice, first-pass studies are often used to evaluate right ventricular function after injection of ^{99m}Tc-labeled red blood cells (RBCs); left ventricular function is subsequently measured with an equilibrium study. If this technique of using labeled RBC is used, only single first-pass measurements of right and/or left ventricular function are possible, with further measurements obtained from the equilibrium phase. However, assessment of both right and left ventricular function can be obtained by first-pass techniques if compounds with short intravascular residence times, such as ^{99m}Tc-labeled sulfur colloid or diethylenetri-

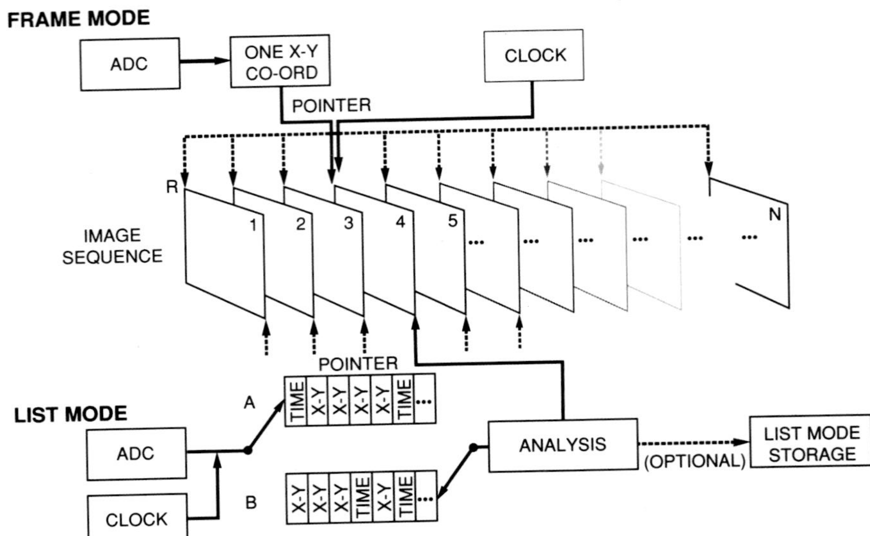

Figure 1. Comparison of frame-mode and list-mode data acquisition (modified from Bacharach et al,[52] reprinted with the permission of *Seminars in Nuclear Medicine*).

aminepentaacetic acid (DTPA) are used, thereby permitting multiple observations using multiple injection of a radiopharmaceutical within a short time interval.

Recently, ^{99m}Tc-labeled myocardial perfusion agents, such as sestamibi and tetrafosmin, have also been used to assess left ventricular function at rest and during exercise, using first-pass radionuclide angiography. These tracers allow for evaluation of myocardial function and perfusion using a single injection. Exercise radionuclide angiography can be obtained by this technique using a portable gamma camera, with correction for motion using a fixed radioactive point source on the patient's chest.

Image Acquisition. A single or multiple crystal scintillation camera may be used for image acquisition, although multiple-crystal cameras are preferred because of their ability to efficiently collect the high count rates over a brief period of time in first-pass studies. Newer digital single-crystal cameras also may be used, having intermediate count rate capabilities. The 30° right anterior oblique projection is usually used to optimize separation of the atria and great vessels from the ventricles, and to view the ventricles parallel to their long axes. Although the right anterior oblique view maximizes overlap of the right and left ventricles, the timing of tracer appearance reliably identifies each chamber sequentially. Other views can be obtained, depending on the area of interest. If multiple views are desired with the first-pass technique, rapidly cleared radiopharmaceuticals must be employed (^{99m}Tc-sulfur colloid or DTPA).

Images are acquired in the seated or supine position following the rapid injection of 10 to 20 mCi (370 to 740 MBq) of radiopharmaceutical through an intravenous catheter (usually 20-gauge or larger) placed in the median antecubital vein. Image quality is related to the injection technique; this should be rapid and even in order to achieve an uninterrupted bolus.[1] ECG gating is not required to perform first-pass studies, but sometimes is utilized to achieve more precise summation of cardiac cycles and, thus, improve the statistical accuracy of the ejection fraction calculation.

Radionuclide data can be recorded in the frame mode or list mode (Table 2). The optimal framing interval depends on the heart rate. At rest, in the absence of significant tachycardia, a minimum framing rate of 25 frames/sec (40 msec/frame) is recommended to permit accurate determination of end-systole and end-diastole. With exercise, higher framing rates are necessary to achieve adequate temporal resolution, with a resultant decrease in counting statistics. Counting statistics also are influenced by ejection fraction. For opti-

Table 1. Radiopharmaceuticals for Blood Pool Imaging

FIRST PASS	EQUILIBRIUM
^{99m}Tc Sulfur Colloid	^{99m}Tc Albumin
^{99m}Tc Diethylenetriaminepentaacetic acid (DTPA)	^{99m}Tc Red Blood Cells
^{99m}Tc Sestamibi	

Table 2. Image Acquisition in Frame and List Mode

	FRAME MODE	LIST MODE
Size of computer memory required	Small	Large
Computer processing time	Short	Long
Ability to correct for arrhythmias	Minimal, predefined windows	Possible, during formatting
Temporal resolution	Fixed	Variable
Data reformatting	None	Possible

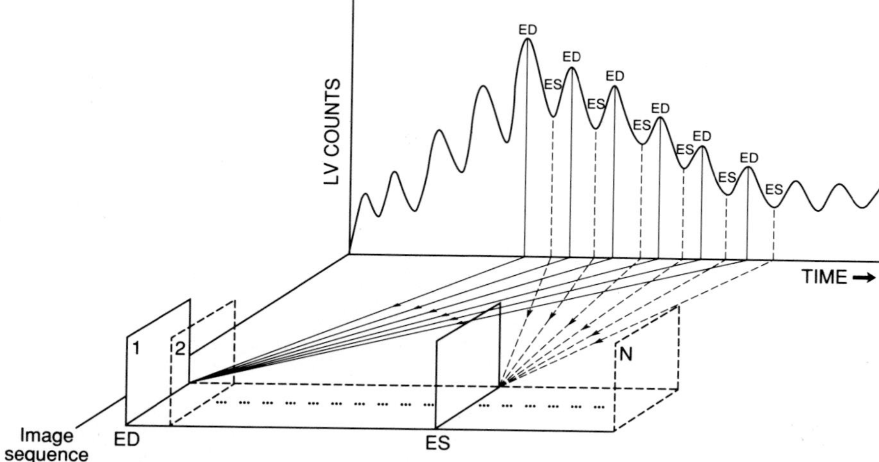

Figure 2. First-pass image acquisition and analysis (modified from Bacharach et al,[52] reprinted with the permission of *Seminars in Nuclear Medicine*).

mum statistical reliability, peak count density should be at least 3000 counts per 40 msec frame for the right ventricular phase and 1000 counts per frame for the left ventricular phase. In patients with left ventricular dysfunction (low ejection fractions), higher count densities are required to reduce statistical error.[2]

Image Analysis. Initial time-activity curves are generated for the entire cardiac region to identify the right and left ventricular phases. Data are separated into the right heart phase (from bolus injection to lung visualization) and left heart phase (from left atrium to aortic visualization). Regions of interest are drawn around the left ventricle (usually at end-diastole) and right ventricle (at end-diastole or using the stroke-volume image). Background subtraction often is employed to correct for activity within the lungs and left atrium (for left ventricle) and within the right atrium (for right ventricle). Time-activity curves can be generated for each ventricle, and cycles around and including the peak time-activity curve are used to calculate ejection fraction (Fig. 2). In general, 2 to 3 cardiac cycles are summed for the right ventricular phase, and 5 to 7 cycles are summed for the left ventricular phase. Cardiac cycles are summed in order to compute ejection fraction.

The primary advantages of the first-pass technique are the rapidity of imaging, which may be important in very sick patients, and the temporal separation of left and right ventricles. The latter is more important with the quantitative assessment of right ventricular ejection fraction. Although sequential assessment of cardiac function is possible with multiple injections of radiopharmaceuticals, with short intravascular residence times, the radiation burden increases with each injection. An alternative approach utilizes multiple acquisitions after injection of an equilibrium tracer. Also, complete assessment of regional wall motion from multiple views is more practical with equilibrium studies (Table 3).

Equilibrium Radionuclide Angiography

RADIOPHARMACEUTICALS

The ideal radiopharmaceutical for equilibrium radionuclide angiography should have a constant concentration in the blood over the interval of measurement. The two most commonly used agents are ^{99m}Tc-labeled RBCs and ^{99m}Tc-labeled albumin. ^{99m}Tc-labeled RBCs are preferred in most situations, because of greater intravascular retention and target-to-background ratio that results in better image contrast compared to albumin. However, ^{99m}Tc-labeled albumin may be preferable in patients in whom it is difficult to achieve adequate labeling of RBCs (Table 4). Poor RBC labeling is indicated by high background activity and accumulation of ^{99m}Tc-pertechnetate in the stomach, kidneys and bladder.

Labeling RBCs with ^{99m}Tc-pertechnetate requires administration of a reducing agent, stannous pyrophosphate, 15 to 30 minutes prior to pertechnetate injection. The usual dose of stannous pyrophosphate is 10 to 20 μg/kg; alternatively, 1 to 1.25 mg per 3 to 10 ml of blood is used for in vitro methods.[3] ^{99m}Tc-pertechnetate is administered either directly into a peripheral vein ("in vivo labeling") or after a brief incubation with approximately 5 mL of blood in a shielded syringe containing anticoagulant ("modified in vivo labeling"). Red blood cell labeling efficiencies of 85 to 95% can

Table 3. Advantages and Disadvantages of First-Pass Radionuclide Angiography

ADVANTAGES	DISADVANTAGES
Rapidity of imaging	Limited views of ventricle
Temporal separation of ventricles	High radiation dose with multiple injections
Can be performed in conjunction with ^{99m}Tc perfusion study	Technically demanding

Table 4. RBC Labeling With ^{99m}Tc: Factors That May Decrease Labeling Efficiency

Drugs:	Digoxin Doxorubicin Hydralazine, methyldopa Antibiotics Quinidine Anti-inflammatory
RBC antibodies:	Leukemia, lymphoma Immune disorders
Anemia (Hematocrit <30%)	
Hemolysis (sickle cell disease, immune disorders)	
Injection of Sn-pyrophosphate and ^{99m}Tc-pertechnetate in the same IV line	
Excess or insufficient Sn	

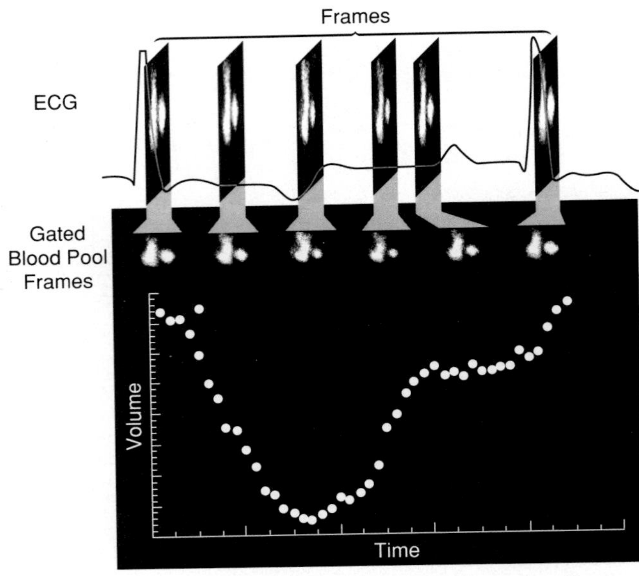

Figure 3. An example of electrocardiographic gating. Data are collected from each defined electrocardiographic interval and summed over multiple cardiac cycles to obtain a representative image for each interval.

be expected with these methods.[3,4] In vitro labeling methods have not gained wide acceptance because they involve multiple steps with only marginal improvement in labeling efficiency over the technically easier in vivo methods. It is important to note that, for studies in which background counts may interfere with proper study interpretation, such as GI bleeding studies, the improved labeling efficiency of in vitro labeling is desirable.

A number of drugs and diseases may cause poor RBC labeling (Table 4).[5,6] Drugs that interfere with labeling include digoxin, doxorubicin, hydralazine, methyldopa, antibiotics, anti-inflammatory agents, and quinidine.[5,6] Diseases that result in the development of RBC antibodies may interfere with labeling, such as lymphoma, leukemia, and immune system disorders. Labeling efficiency also is reduced in anemia (with hematocrit <30%), sickle cell disease, and hemolytic conditions. Injection of ^{99m}Tc-pertechnetate through an intravenous line containing heparin or dextrose may also decrease labeling efficiency.[7,8] If injection through intravenous lines is necessary, it is preferable to inject the stannous pyrophosphate and ^{99m}Tc-pertechnetate in different lines; this minimizes local reduction and trapping of ^{99m}Tc at the injection site. For the modified in vivo and in vitro methods, acid-citrate-dextrose is the preferred anticoagulant, because heparin may complex with ^{99m}Tc-pertechnetate, reducing labeling efficiency.

Image Acquisition. Rest images are acquired using a gamma camera linked to a computer synchronized to the patient's ECG (Fig. 3). For most studies, a parallel-hole, all-purpose collimator produces good resolution with acceptable imaging times (Table 5). For exercise studies, in which it is preferable to shorten the time of image acquisition, a high sensitivity collimator is preferred (Table 6). In most cases, a 64 × 64 pixel matrix is used to achieve adequate spatial resolution. Acquisition of images in a "zoom mode" may decrease the memory requirements while maintaining resolution by utilizing a smaller matrix (32 × 32) in one quarter of the camera's field of view.

The triggering signal for the computer usually is the R-wave of the patient's ECG, which generally is easily identifiable because of its high amplitude. However, ECG gating may be adversely affected by a low-voltage or poor quality tracing, or by such physiologic situations as peaked T-waves or a functioning pacemaker. If gating is inadequate, image interpretation will be inaccurate and may lead to erroneous (usually low) measurements of ventricular function. Therefore, it is essential to assess the adequacy of ECG gating prior to data acquisition, and to record a brief rhythm strip for the patient's file.

Images are acquired in 3 or 4 standard views: anterior, 45-degree left anterior oblique, and left lateral and/or 30-degree left posterior oblique (Fig. 4). The left anterior oblique view gives the best separation of the left and right ventricles and is used for quantification of left ventricular function. Exact camera position is modified to achieve opti-

Table 5. Imaging Protocol for Rest Equilibrium Radionuclide Angiography

Parallel-hole, LEAP collimator
Adequate ECG signal
3 or 4 standard views: –45° LAO, anterior, left lateral, (30° LPO) –Caudal tilt or slant hole collimator (5–10°)
Minimum framing rate 16 frames/cycle (about 50 msec/frame) –Increase temporal resolution for assessment of diastolic function, regional ejection fraction, or with tachycardia
250,000 cts per frame or count density of 300 cts per pixel (5–10 min acquisition time per view).

Table 6. Imaging Protocol for Exercise Equilibrium Radionuclide Angiography

LAO view
Supine or semierect
Graded bicycle ergometry, increasing workload every 2 minutes by 25 watts
Imaging during final 2–3 minutes of exercise
–Importance of continuation of exercise during imaging
High sensitivity collimator
150,000 cts per frame typically

mum ventricular separation using the persistence oscilloscope. To minimize overlap of atria and ventricles, a caudal tilt (5 to 10 degrees) is utilized. The left lateral and left posterior oblique views are obtained with the patient in the right lateral decubitus position; depending on the orientation of the heart, one or the other of these two views may better assess inferior wall motion.

Exercise radionuclide angiography is carried out in the left anterior oblique view, with the patient in the supine or semierect position (Table 6). Graded exercise is performed with a bicycle ergometer, usually increasing workload every 2 minutes in 25-watt increments. Imaging should ideally be performed during the final 2 to 3 minutes of exercise to

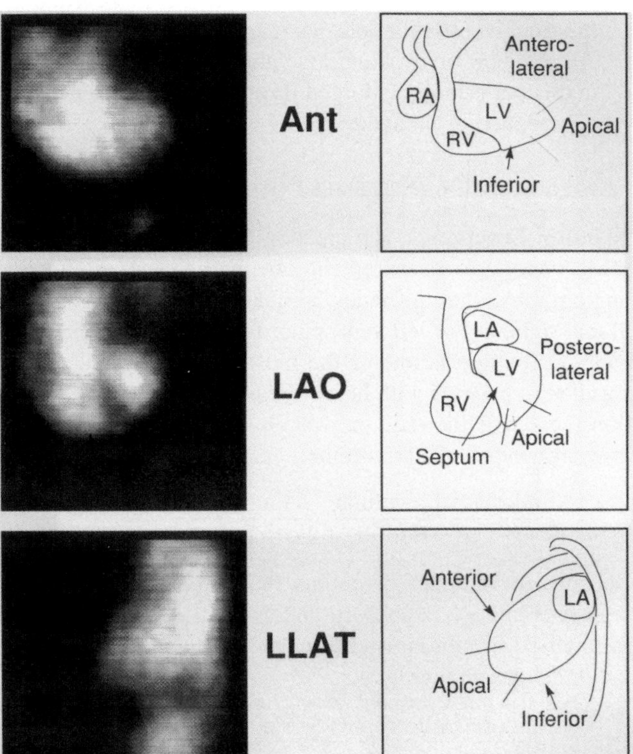

Figure 4. Three standard projections obtained with equilibrium radionuclide angiography: left anterior oblique (LAO), anterior (Ant), and left lateral (LLat). Corresponding left ventricular walls visualized are depicted in Figure 6.

reflect maximum stress. If the patient fatigues before imaging is completed, it is preferable to continue a lower level of exercise until the study is completed, because the time required for left ventricular function to return to normal may be variable.

The minimum framing rate for resting equilibrium radionuclide angiography is 16 frames/cycle (approximately 50 msec/frame). If quantitative assessment of regional ejection fraction or diastolic filling is desired, it is preferable to increase the temporal resolution (e.g., 32 frames/cycle or 25 msec/frame). In the presence of tachycardia, such as during exercise, the higher framing rate should be utilized.

For adequate counting statistics, images usually are acquired for a preset count of at least 250,000 per frame (count density of about 300 cts/pixel), corresponding to a 5 to 10-minute acquisition time. For exercise studies, adequate counts can be obtained in most cases with a 2-minute acquisition using a high–sensitivity collimator.

As noted above, arrhythmias can affect the accuracy of radionuclide angiography. The most commonly encountered arrhythmia is multiple premature supraventricular or ventricular contractions. In general, the study will not be adversely affected if these beats account for $<10\%$ of the total. If premature beats occur frequently, arrhythmia filtering is required. In frame mode acquisition, this is accomplished by rejecting of beats outside of a predetermined R-R interval; the more beats rejected, the longer the acquisition time required. Alternatively, studies obtained in list mode can be analyzed after acquisition to determine the R-R interval distribution by histogram. Aberrant beats can easily be excluded from analysis after examining the histograms (Fig. 5).

Atrial fibrillation has varying affects on radionuclide angiography, depending on the magnitude of heart rate variability. When left ventricular ejection fraction is recorded continuously using a nonimaging probe, considerable beat-to-beat variability is observed, even in patients with marked left ventricular dysfunction.[9] The ejection fraction obtained from equilibrium radionuclide angiography can be considered to represent the mean ejection fraction over the period of acquisition; as such, it may underestimate left ventricular performance in patients with atrial fibrillation.[9]

Analysis of First-Pass and Equilibrium Studies

QUALITATIVE ASSESSMENT

Both first-pass and equilibrium studies can be viewed qualitatively, although equilibrium studies are superior in quality for visual analysis. Images are displayed as an endless cinematic loop of the cardiac cycle. Images should be viewed in a systematic fashion:

1. **Quality of the images.** Poor-quality images (high background) may result from improper RBC labeling or radiopharmaceutical injection. Image "flickering" may result from arrhythmias.
2. **Extracardiac uptake.** Normally, there is some activity in

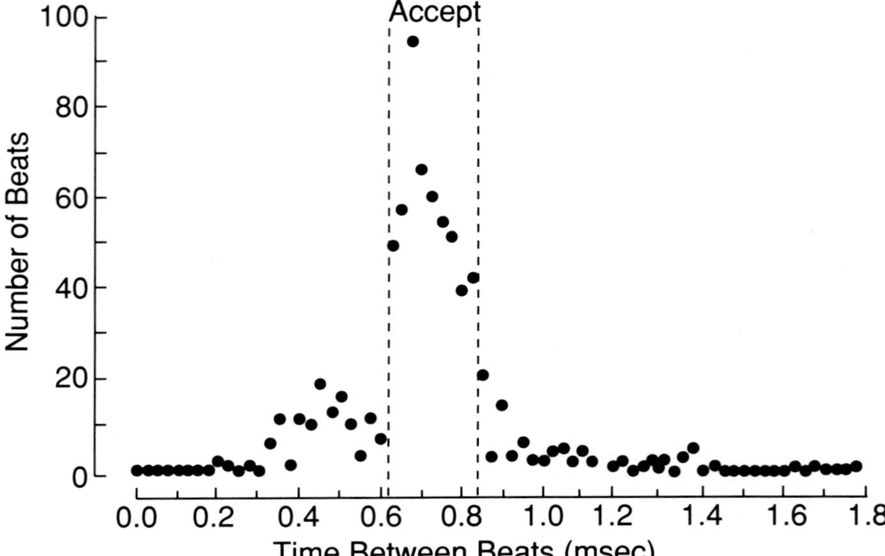

Figure 5. List mode: aberrant beats can easily be excluded from analysis after examining the R-R interval distribution by histogram.

the liver, spleen, and stomach. If these structures partially overlap the heart, particularly in the left anterior oblique view, background activity may be elevated which, in turn, affects ejection fraction.

3. **Size of great vessels and heart chambers.** The images are examined for atrial or ventricular enlargement, as well as dilatation of the pulmonary artery or aorta. The right atrium is best visualized in the anterior view where it lies superior and lateral to the right ventricle. The left atrium is seen best on the lateral view posterior, superior to the left ventricle.
4. **Abnormal photopenia around the heart.** Ventricular hypertrophy, pericardial effusion, or a prominent pericardial fat pad may cause an increased photopenic zone around the heart. With hypertrophy, the interventricular septum appears thickened, whereas the septum appears normal with effusion or enlarged fat pad. Left ventricular hypertrophy should be expected when the photopenic zone around the left ventricle is >4 pixels wide (using a 64 × 64 matrix, 25-cm field of view camera unzoomed) and thickens during systole. This finding is specific, but not sensitive, for left ventricular hypertrophy; echocardiography is the most accurate noninvasive means to evaluate left ventricular hypertrophy and pericardial effusion.
5. **Regional wall motion.** Right ventricular wall motion is assessed best by first-pass studies in the anterior projection. In equilibrium studies, overlap of the right ventricle with other cardiac structures limits the utility of visual analysis; the inferoapical segment can usually be assessed on the anterior or left anterior oblique view. Sometimes the only clue to right ventricular hypokinesis on an equilibrium study is delayed contraction of the inferoapical segment relative to the left ventricle. Left ventricular wall motion is assessed on all views, and graded into normal (regional shortening of a radius of at least 25%), *hypokinetic* (regional shortening 10 to 25%), *akinetic* (absent shortening), or *dyskinetic* (systolic expansion). Specific attention is given to the regional nature of wall motion abnormalities, because such regional left ventricular dysfunction suggests coronary artery disease. *Paradoxical* septal motion can be caused by conduction system disease (in particular, left bundle branch block), myocardial infarction, ventricular pacing, and prior cardiac surgery. An akinetic or dyskinetic segment of the left ventricle that is persistently enlarged throughout the cardiac cycle is evidence of an aneurysm.

QUANTITATIVE ASSESSMENT OF SYSTOLIC FUNCTION

Ejection Fraction. The ejection fraction is clinically the most important measurement obtained from radionuclide angiography, and provides a quantitative assessment of global right and/or left ventricular function. Left ventricular ejection fraction is one of the most powerful predictors of survival in patients with heart disease.[10–24] The ejection fraction represents the ratio between left ventricular *stroke volume* and end-diastolic volume:

$$\frac{\text{End-diastolic volume} - \text{End-systolic volume}}{\text{End-diastolic volume}}$$

Because the number of counts recovered in a ventricular region of interest is proportional to ventricular volume, the following formula is used to calculate ejection fraction by radionuclide angiography:

$$\frac{\text{End-diastolic counts} - \text{End-systolic counts}}{\text{End-diastolic counts} - \text{Background counts}}$$

Because this count-based technique yields volumetric measurements, it more accurately reflects ejection fraction, compared to techniques based on geometric measurements (such

End-diastole

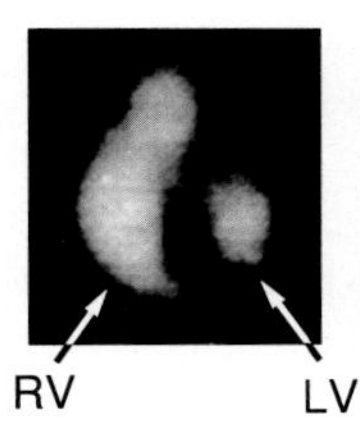

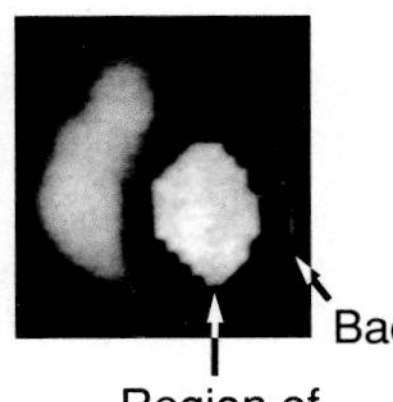

Time-Activity Curve

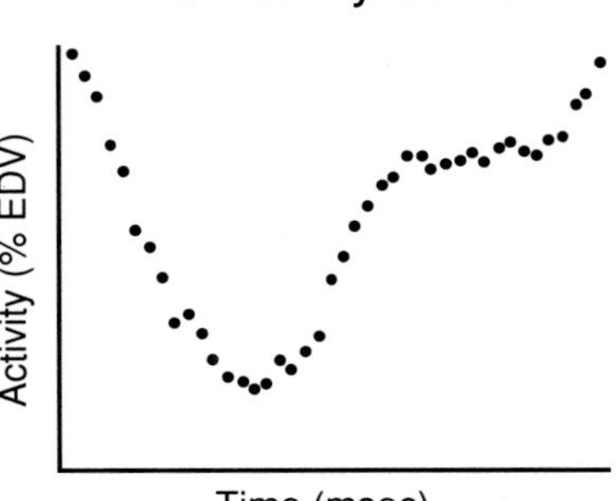

Figure 6. Example of drawing a region of interest around the left ventricle (LV) and background in the left anterior oblique view. The corresponding left ventricular time-activity curve (on the right) reflects volume within the ventricle (modified from Bacharach et al,[52] reprinted with the permission of *Seminars in Nuclear Medicine*).

as echocardiography or contrast ventriculography), which require mathematical assumptions to calculate volumes.

To calculate ejection fraction, a region of interest is drawn around the left ventricle in the left anterior oblique image (Fig. 6). This region can be drawn manually or by using automatic edge detection programs that employ threshold or second derivative of phase analysis techniques.[25] Regions can be drawn on all frames, at end-diastole and end-systole, or at end-diastole alone. Although a single region of interest produces smoother time-activity curves, the calculated ejection fraction is about 5% lower than that obtained from the multiple region-of-interest technique. Background subtraction is performed using a region of interest one or more pixels lateral to the posterolateral left ventricular blood pool. After background subtraction is applied to all pixels within the region of interest, a time-activity curve is generated, which closely parallels the angiographic time-volume curve. Ejection fraction and rates of ejection and filling are obtained from these curves (Fig. 6). The lower limit of normal ejection fraction may vary from laboratory to laboratory, depending on the methods used for data acquisition and analysis. In most laboratories, the normal resting left ventricular ejection fraction is ≥45 to 50%, and the right ventricular ejection fraction is >40 to 45%. If the background region is placed manually, care must be taken not to place the region in an area of increased activity, such as the spleen, because this results in a spuriously increased ejection fraction. Although background activity accounts for about 50% of activity within the ventricular region of interest, it rarely should exceed 60 to 65%.

Regional left ventricular function can be assessed quantitatively by calculating regional left ventricular ejection frations. Usually, this is achieved by dividing the left ventricle into a number of sectors emanating from the center of the ventricle. Regional ejection fraction is calculated based on changes in counts in each sector during the cardiac cycle (Fig. 7). Quantification of regional left ventricular function may increase the specificity of radionuclide angiography in detecting coronary disease.[26–28]

Ventricular Volume. Absolute left ventricular volumes can be calculated by either geometric[29] or count-based[30] methods. Geometric methods rely on assumptions of the ventricular area-length relationship. The gamma camera is calibrated to determine ventricular size in 2 views, and volume of the chamber is then calculated using the Simpson rule, as used in contrast ventriculography. For geometric methods, a first-pass right anterior oblique study is preferred to project the greatest area of the left ventricle over the gamma camera. The application of geometric methods is limited by the often inaccurate definition of myocardial edges. Equilibrium gated blood-pool scintigraphy is not well suited for geometric volume determinations, because the left anterior oblique projection, although separating the ventricles, does not allow accurate definition of the long axis of the left ventricle.

Count-based methods are potentially more accurate for determining absolute left ventricular volume, but require measurement of blood activity and a correction for attenuation. Left ventricular volume is calculated from the actual count rate from the left ventricle (cps) divided by the product of the blood activity (mCi/mL blood) and the expected count recovery per millicurie (cps/mCi). The standard method requires blood sampling and, although more precise than geometric methods (standard error 10 to 35 mL), may have significant inaccuracy because it is difficult to estimate attenuation and background activity. Attenuation may be measured directly by swallowing a low-activity radioactive capsule and measuring esophageal or gastric recovery, because these structures are in close proximity to the heart. Because this method usually is not practical, it is more common to assess attenuation based on estimates of left ventricular depth.[31] The critical step in this method, estimation of left ventricular depth, is performed by imaging the ventricle in 2 views with a superimposed point source (or lead marker) on the chest wall. A trigonometric calculation then is performed to estimate ventricular depth, which is combined with an estimation of the linear attenuation coefficient for the chest wall. Attenuation-corrected ventricular activity then can be calculated according to the following formula:

$$A_0 = \frac{Ad}{e^{-\mu l}}$$

where A_0 = ventricular activity (corrected for attenuation), Ad = activity measured by the camera, μ = linear attenua-

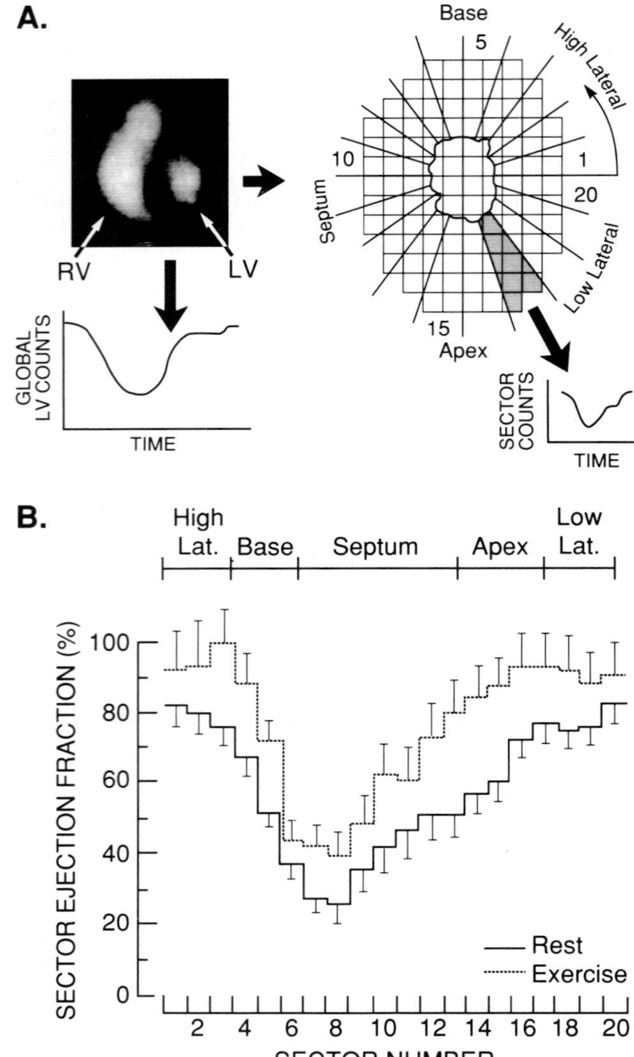

Figure 7. Calculation of regional left ventricular ejection fraction using sector analysis. In panel **(A)**, the radionuclide end-diastolic image is shown (upper left), from which the global time-activity curve was generated (lower left). The left ventricular region of interest was then subdivided into 20 annular sectors (upper right), from which sector time-activity curves were generated (lower right) to compute the sector ejection fraction. In this normal subject **(B)**, ejection fraction increases during exercise in all sectors (modified from Vitale et al,[27] reprinted with the permission of the *American Journal of Cardiology*).

tion coefficient, and p = distance from source (ventricle) to camera.

Other methods of assessing absolute left ventricular volume have been proposed that do not require blood sampling or attenuation correction.[32,33] The technique of Massardo and colleagues is based on *reference volume* theory, in which the ratio of total counts to peak pixel counts is a function of ventricular volume. This method is reproducible and correlates well with angiographic volumes, and does not require blood sampling or attenuation correction.[33] These techniques may result in more widespread use of the noninvasive measurement of preload and contractility, and may become important in the assessing progression of disease and/or response to therapy, especially in patients with heart failure.

Stroke-Volume Ratio: The stroke-volume ratio has been proposed as a method of quantifying the severity of valvular regurgitation. It is defined as the ratio of left-to-right ventricular stroke volume (which should be 1.0 in normals), and can be estimated by measuring the relative stroke counts (end-diastole minus end-systole) with separate region of interests for each ventricle.[34] In the presence of unilateral valvular regurgitation, the ventricular stroke volume on the affected side is increased in proportion to the severity of regurgitation. The ability of radionuclide angiography to detect regurgitation is limited by underestimation of right ventricular stroke counts (due to right atrial and ventricular overlap), resulting in calculated left-to-right ventricular stroke-volume ratios of 1.1 to 1.4 in normals.[35] This technique also is limited in patients with severe left ventricular dysfunction or bilateral regurgitant lesions.[36] Despite the limitations of stroke-volume ratio to accurately detect valvular regurgitation, it may be useful in the serial assessment of patients with known valvular disease.

FUNCTIONAL IMAGES

Stroke-Volume and Paradox Images. Functional images are used to evaluate regional ventricular function by condensing data from several images into a composite image that reflects a particular parameter. The stroke-volume image is a graphical representation of the difference between background-corrected end-diastolic and end-systolic counts on a pixel-by-pixel basis, which reflects the volume of blood ejected from the ventricle during systole. In this way, regional wall motion abnormalities appear as areas of reduced activity. The paradox image, which represents the difference between end-systolic and end-diastolic counts (the converse of the stroke-volume image), reflects regions in which blood volume increases during systole, such as left ventricular aneurysms or the left atrium in mitral regurgitation.

Phase Analysis. Phase analysis applies Fourier techniques to the images on a pixel-by-pixel basis. From each pixel within the blood pool image, an individual time-activity curve is generated. This curve is then fitted to a symmetrical cosine curve (the first harmonic Fourier transform), defined by an amplitude (magnitude of maximum deflection) and a phase angle (angular location of the maximal deflection). This curve makes one complete cycle for each cardiac cycle and, by definition, starts at an angular location of 0° and ends at 360°. The amplitude image, therefore, is similar to the stroke-volume image because each curve's amplitude is proportional to each pixel's "stroke volume," but is computed from the entire cardiac cycle rather than just from end-diastolic and end-systolic images. Each pixel is assigned an amplitude and displayed on a grey- or color-scale image.

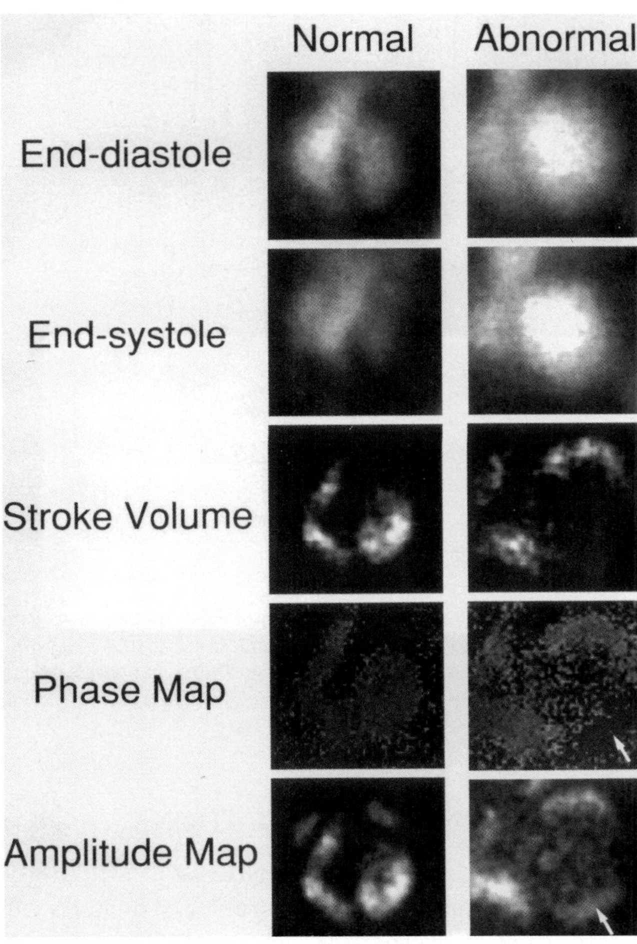

Figure 8. Examples of end-diastole, end-systole, stroke volume, phase map, and amplitude map from a normal subject on the left, and from a patient with coronary artery disease on the right. In the normal subject (left column), the left ventricular contraction from end-diastole to end-systole is preserved, and the stroke volume image is normal. The phase image shows a uniform contraction pattern and in the amplitude image both the atria and ventricles are visualized. In the patient with coronary artery disease (right column), the end-diastolic and end-systolic images demonstrate dilated left ventricle with severely reduced contraction except for the base of the ventricle, as shown in the stroke volume image. The phase image shows nonuniform contraction pattern, worse in the apex (shown by the arrows), and the amplitude image shows contraction in the same region, suggestive of apical dyskinesis.

Because the amplitude image represents maximum amplitude on a pixel-by-pixel basis at any time in the cardiac cycle, both the atria and ventricles are visualized in a normal image (Fig. 8).

Similarly, the phase image is a graphic representation of the phase angle for each pixel. The phase angle depends on the timing of contraction and, therefore, the usefulness of this image is in analyzing the synchrony of ventricular contraction. For example, the pixel in the region of earliest ventricular contraction would have the earliest phase angle, and a pixel in an area which contracts later would have a later phase angle. These phase angles (0° to 360°) are displayed with proportionate intensities in a single image. In general, the sequence of activation of the left ventricle is fairly uniform. Nonuniformity of the phase image identifies abnormal sequences of ventricular activation, as may occur in conduction disturbances, myocardial ischemia, or left ventricular aneurysm (Fig. 8).

ASSESSING DIASTOLIC FUNCTION

Physiology. The physiology of diastole involves a complex interaction of physical properties of the left ventricle, venous inflow and transvalvular pressure gradients, afterload, and interventricular interaction. In addition to these "passive" determinants of left ventricular filling, recent studies have determined that myocardial relaxation is an active, energy-dependent process that may be altered in a variety of diseases, including hypertension,[37,38] hypertrophic cardiomyopathy,[39,40] infiltrative/restrictive cardiomyopathies,[41] acromegaly,[42] and ischemic heart disease.[43,44] Changes in diastolic function may be clinically significant, as diastolic dysfunction may antedate systolic dysfunction or, by itself may be responsible for symptoms of congestive heart failure in the absence of systolic dysfunction.[45]

The phases of diastole[46] are illustrated in a plot of left ventricular volume versus time in Figure 9. Immediately after the completion of systole, left ventricular volume is at its minimum, and the first phase, *isovolumic relaxation*, begins. This phase is brief, and is a period of ventricular relaxation without increase in volume, resulting in a rapid decline of pressure. When the ventricular pressure falls below the atrial pressure, the atrioventricular valves open and the second phase, *rapid ventricular filling*, commences. During this phase, the majority of ventricular filling takes place, and the rate of decline in left ventricular pressure may be greater than corresponding increase in filling. In this manner, negative ventricular pressure ("suction") may contribute importantly to ventricular filling.[47] As atrial and ventricular pressures begin to equalize, filling ceases, and there is a period of "diastasis" reflected by the flat segment of the volume curve. Finally, atrial systole occurs, resulting in additional ventricular filling and the conclusion of diastole. In normal subjects, only 10 to 20% of ventricular filling occurs in this phase.

Parameters of Diastolic Function. Quantitative parameters of left ventricular filling are derived from the time-activity curve (Fig. 10), which closely approximates left ventricular volume changes described above. High temporal resolution methods are preferred to avoid underestimation of filling.[48] Peak filling rate (PFR) is the most widely used parameter of diastolic function, and represents the maximum value of the first derivative of the time-activity curve. It is expressed in units of end-diastolic volumes (or sometimes stroke-volumes) per second. The time to peak filling rate (TPFR) is the time of PFR relative to end-systole, expressed in milliseconds. The filling fraction method separates dias-

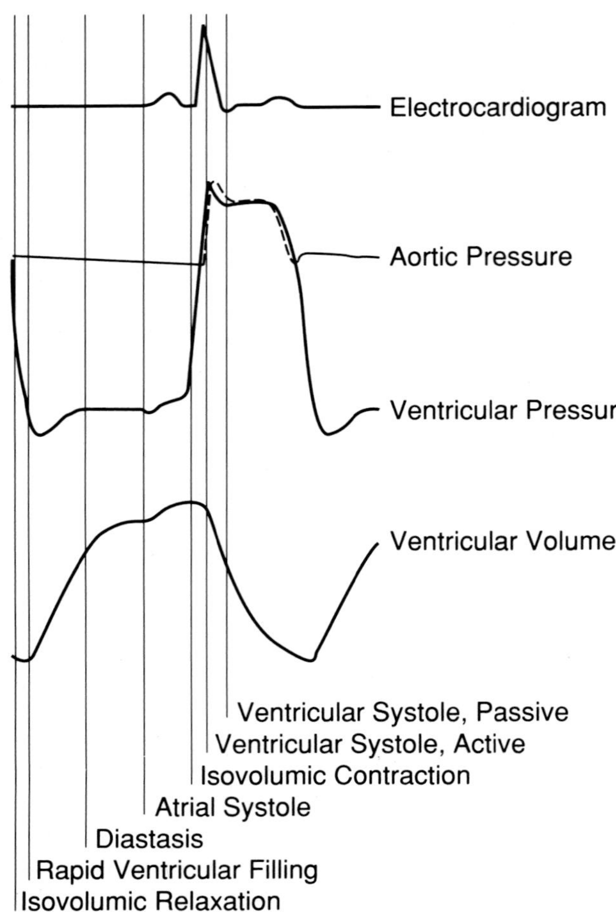

Figure 9. Schematic representation of the temporal relationship of left ventricular pressure and volume to surface electrocardiogram for a single cardiac cycle.

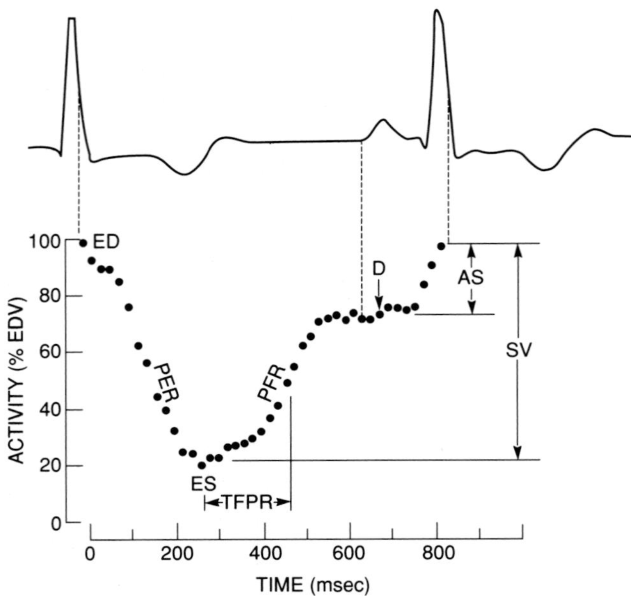

Figure 10. Left ventricular time-activity curve and diastolic filling parameters. ED, end-diastole; ES, end-systole; EDV, end-diastolic volume; PER, peak ejection rate; PFR, peak filling rate; TPFR, time to PFR; SV, stroke volume; D, diastasis; AS, atrial systole.

tole into several time intervals and determines the percentage of stroke volume at one third, one half, and two thirds of diastole. The atrial contribution to filling can be assessed by quantification of the time spent and/or increase in ventricular volume (counts) that is due to atrial systole.

Although PFR is viewed as an index of early left ventricular filling, it is widely appreciated that PFR depends upon relaxation (loading conditions, energy-dependent processes),[48,49] ejection fraction and heart rate.[50] As a result, this value is influenced by factors other than left ventricular filling. In particular, the extreme sensitivity of PFR measurements to relatively small changes in heart rate during exercise tachycardia limits the usefulness of this technique in exercise studies.[51] To minimize the effects of heart rate variability, careful attention must be focused on excluding extrasystolic and postextrasystolic beats, often through list-mode acquisition[52] or by rejecting beats outside of a narrowly defined R-R interval during frame-mode acquisition. Temporal smoothing of time-activity curves may result in significant underestimation of PFR, and the magnitude of the error varies among patients.[53]

CLINICAL APPLICATIONS

Coronary Artery Disease

Radionuclide angiography is frequently used to assess left ventricular function in patients with coronary artery disease. The degree of left ventricular systolic dysfunction, which reflects the extent of infarcted or severely ischemic myocardium, is a powerful prognostic indicator in these patients. Exercise radionuclide angiography has also been used to detect coronary disease, although it has been replaced in most centers with exercise perfusion scintigraphy which has better specificity.

DETECTION OF CORONARY ARTERY DISEASE

Stress-induced left ventricular dysfunction is the principal indicator of coronary artery disease by radionuclide angiography, and is more sensitive than standard exercise electrocardiography for detecting coronary artery disease (CAD). This is based on the observation that regional wall motion abnormalities appear before angina or electrocardiographic abnormalities.[54,55]

Exercise Stress Testing. Exercise studies are performed in the modified left anterior oblique position, using a high sensitivity collimator and graded supine or semierect bicycle ergometry.[56] The sensitivity and specificity of radionuclide angiography for detecting coronary artery disease was initially reported to be excellent (95 and 100%, respectively) in a selected group of patients with a high likelihood of coronary artery disease.[56] Compared with normal subjects, in which exercise ejection fraction increased by at least 5%, patients with coronary artery disease demonstrated a fall or no change in ejection fraction from rest to exercise. However, it was subsequently appreciated that a blunted response in ejection fraction to exercise was not specific for coronary artery disease. In an unselected population, sensitivity remained high (90%) but specificity fell to 58%.[57] This lack of specificity can be explained by many cardiac and noncardiac factors that affect the response of left ventricular contraction during exercise. Abnormal response of the ventricle to exercise may be observed in valvular heart disease, cardiomyopathies, and hypertension.[58] Furthermore, even in healthy subjects, the increase in ejection fraction to exercise may be blunted, particularly in the elderly[59] and in women.[60]

In addition to low specificity, the sensitivity of exercise radionuclide angiography may be lower than initially indicated in patients with limited coronary artery disease. Because only one view is obtained during exercise, limited vascular territories are represented: the septum (left anterior descending artery), posterolateral wall (left circumflex artery), and apex (varies depending on individual coronary anatomy). Exercise-induced ischemia must be of sufficient magnitude to affect regional contraction in these visualized vascular territories, which is critically dependent on achieving an adequate level of stress (rate-pressure product ≥25,000) or clinical ischemia (ECG changes or chest pain).[61] In particular, the right coronary artery is underrepresented in the left anterior oblique view, unless this vessel is very dominant and supplies the posterolateral wall. As such, although the sensitivity for detecting left anterior descending or 3-vessel coronary disease is good (80 to 96%), it is considerably lower for disease of the left circumflex or right coronary arteries.[28,56,62,63] The assessment of the right ventricular response to exercise provides evidence of right coronary artery disease, but an abnormal response may be nonspecific.[64]

Thus, although exercise radionuclide angiography is sensitive for detecting left anterior descending or 3-vessel coronary artery disease, its use is limited for lesser degrees of coronary artery disease. Additionally, the finding of abnormal left ventricular ejection fraction response to exercise is nonspecific. However, exercise radionuclide angiography remains useful in assessing the functional impact of coronary artery disease on left ventricular function.

Pharmacological Stress Testing. Dipyridamole radionuclide angiography is an alternative to exercise in certain patients who are intolerant to physical activity. Intravenous administration of dipyridamole indirectly results in coronary vasodilation by inhibiting phosphodiesterase and increasing levels of adenosine monophosphate (AMP), a potent vasodilator. Alternatively, adenosine can be infused directly in doses of up to 140 μg/kg/min with effects similar to dipyridamole. The main advantage of adenosine is its shorter half-life (<10 sec), but adverse effects are more common than with dipyridamole. These agents are most commonly used in conjunction with myocardial perfusion imaging. In patients with coronary artery disease, they induce regional heterogeneity of myocardial blood flow that can be imaged using ^{201}Tl, ^{99m}Tc-sestamibi, or other perfusion tracers. These agents also may induce regional wall motion abnormalities that can be detected by radionuclide angiography.[65] As in exercise studies, failure to increase ejection fraction and/or the appearance of new wall motion abnormalities are indicators of coronary artery disease. Although this technique appears to be quite specific for coronary artery disease, its sensitivity is only 60 to 70%,[65] which is lower than dipyridamole perfusion scintigraphy. Furthermore, the dose of dipyridamole required is larger than that used for perfusion studies (0.84 mg/kg versus 0.57 mg/kg). Additional studies are needed in order to define the role of dipyridamole or adenosine radionuclide angiography for coronary artery disease detection.

Dobutamine also can be used as a pharmacological stressor during radionuclide angiography, although it is more commonly combined with echocardiographic or perfusion imaging. Dobutamine is a beta-agonist that has positive inotropic and chronotropic effects. During radionuclide angiography, dobutamine generally increases global left ventricular ejection fraction, even in patients with coronary artery disease.[66,67] Variable effects have been noted with regard to regional function in such patients. From the more extensive experience with dobutamine echocardiography, it appears that high-dose dobutamine causes regional wall motion abnormalities to develop in most patients with coronary artery disease[68] and may be useful as a diagnostic test. The unaffected regions with increased contractility, and therefore global ejection fraction, may remain the same or increase even in the presence of a new wall-motion abnormality. Although it is unlikely that dobutamine radionuclide angiography will become a widely used diagnostic test for coronary artery disease, it may have a role in the assessment of "contractile reserve" in patients with certain cardiomyopathies.[69]

Risk Stratification in Chronic Coronary Artery Disease. The prognosis in patients with chronic coronary artery disease is determined by the interaction of many factors, most importantly the extent of coronary artery stenoses, the degree of left ventricular dysfunction at rest, and the presence of inducible myocardial ischemia. Although 1-year mortality increases with the extent of coronary artery disease,[70] prognosis is worse for patients with impaired resting left ventricular function for any given degree of coronary artery disease.[14] For medically treated patients in the Coronary Artery Surgery Study (CASS) registry, 4-year mortality was 8% overall in patients with resting ejection fractions ≥50%, 17% with ejection fractions 35 to 49%, and 42% with ejection fractions <35%.[14] The negative prognostic influence of left ventricular dysfunction was more evident in patients with multivessel disease than with single-vessel disease. Similarly, in patients with chronic stable angina, mortality is higher in patients with severe left ventricular dysfunction at rest.[71] Thus, rest radionuclide angiography provides powerful prognostic information in patients with coronary artery disease.

Exercise radionuclide angiography also provides prognostic information in chronic coronary artery disease patients.[19,21–24] When subgrouped according to coronary anatomy, high-risk patients were those with (1) three-vessel disease and normal left ventricular function,[19] and (2) one- or two-vessel disease and impaired left ventricular function.[21,22] Data from the National Heart, Lung, and Blood Institute in patients with 3-vessel coronary artery disease and normal resting left ventricular function indicate that those patients with inducible ischemia identified by a decrease in left ventricular ejection fraction during exercise, positive ST-segment response on ECG, or poor exercise capacity have a 4-year mortality of 29%, compared to 0% in all other patients without evidence of inducible ischemia.[19] Furthermore, in another study of medically treated patients with coronary artery disease, exercise ejection fraction was the most powerful predictor of subsequent cardiac events, stronger than extent of coronary artery disease, exercise duration of ECG changes, and resting left ventricular function.[18] Patients with exercise ejection fractions <35% were at highest risk of death or nonfatal myocardial infarction (52% at 4-year follow-up compared to 13% for ejection fraction ≥50%). Similarly, Lee and coworkers reported a linear relationship between exercise ejection fraction and cardiovascular events (death or nonfatal myocardial infarction). The risk of death increased as ejection fraction decreased, with the highest risk occurring at the lowest ejection fractions.[23] More recently, the prognostic significance of exercise radionuclide angiography has been confirmed in a population-based cohort of 536 patients with known or suspected coronary artery disease. In this study, over a 4-year follow-up period, exercise ejection fraction, exercise heart rate, and age were independent predictors of cardiac events.[72] Exercise left ventricular ejection fraction greater than 58% and peak heart rate greater than 122 were associated with 98% infarct-free survival, suggesting that exercise radionuclide angiography may have considerable prognostic value in community practice.

Exercise radionuclide angiography also may be useful in predicting restenosis after coronary angioplasty. Studies indicate that if exercise radionuclide angiography is normal within the first month after angioplasty, significant late restenosis is rare (0 to 7%). In contrast, if exercise radionuclide angiography is abnormal, the restenosis rate is 42 to 43%.[73,74]

Risk Stratification in Myocardial Infarction. Following myocardial infarction, the major prognostic determinants are left ventricular size and function, presence of inducible ischemia, and occurrence of arrhythmias. The assessment of ventricular function after myocardial infarction is one of the most prognostically important applications of radionuclide angiography. Larger infarcts usually result in more extensive regional or global left ventricular dysfunction.[75] Depending on the size and location of the infarct, ventricular function may be severely depressed, preserved globally but with regional dysfunction, or entirely normal.[76,77] As with patients with chronic coronary artery disease, the severity of left ventricular dysfunction correlates negatively with survival. In the Multicenter Post-Infarction Research Group study, 1-year mortality was 2 to 4% in patients with left ventricular ejection fraction (EF) ≥40%, 12% in patients with ejection fraction 20 to 39%, and 47% in patients with ejection fraction <20%.[78] Exercise ejection fraction has also been associated with an adverse outcome after myocardial infarction.[79]

It is important to realize that ventricular function may change during the first few days or weeks postinfarction. Within the first 2 weeks, left ventricular function improves in most patients, but may not change or may deteriorate in others.[80] In the current era of acute revascularization or pharmacological thrombolysis, reperfusion of the infarct zone may result in a more rapid improvement of ventricular function. Following successful thrombolysis, left ventricular function usually begins to improve within 3 to 5 days.[81] Global ventricular function may actually decline initially, as hyperkinetic regions in the noninfarct zone return to normal function before recovery of function in the infarct zone is complete.[82] Therefore, single measurements of ventricular function should be viewed with caution, particularly when obtained within the first week after infarction. Recent studies have indicated that use of angiotensin-converting enzyme (ACE) inhibitors early after infarction improves survival in patients with left ventricular systolic dysfunction early after myocardial infarction.[83] Thus, despite its limitations, the early assessment of left ventricular function postinfarction has therapeutic, as well as prognostic, implications.

Right ventricular dysfunction may be observed in patients with right ventricular infarction, and is associated with hemodynamic compromise if right ventricular ejection fraction is less than 35%.[84] Although usually associated with inferior infarction, it may occur with extensive anterior infarction.[85] In most patients, right ventricular function improves within several weeks, although it is unclear whether recanalization of the infarct-related artery is required for this improvement to occur.[86,87]

Diastolic Function in Coronary Artery Disease. A number of studies have shown abnormalities of left ventricular relaxation in patients with coronary disease, even in the absence of prior myocardial infarction or unstable angina.[88,89] These abnormalities in filling improved after medical[90] and mechanical[91] coronary artery disease treatment (Fig. 11). The reversibility of the diastolic filling abnormalities suggests that they are a manifestation of myocardial ischemia that is alleviated by medical therapy. Abnormalities in regional diastolic filling (regional asynchrony) also have been reported in coronary artery disease patients, and may contribute to global diastolic dysfunction.[88] Such asynchronous filling in patients with single-vessel coronary artery disease is reversible following successful angioplasty.[92] Blunting of the

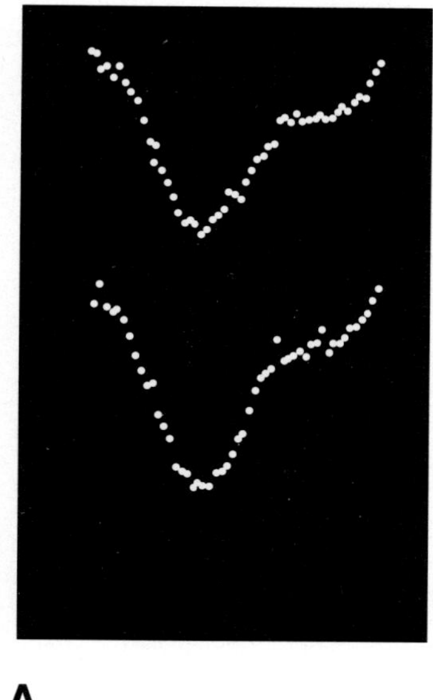

A

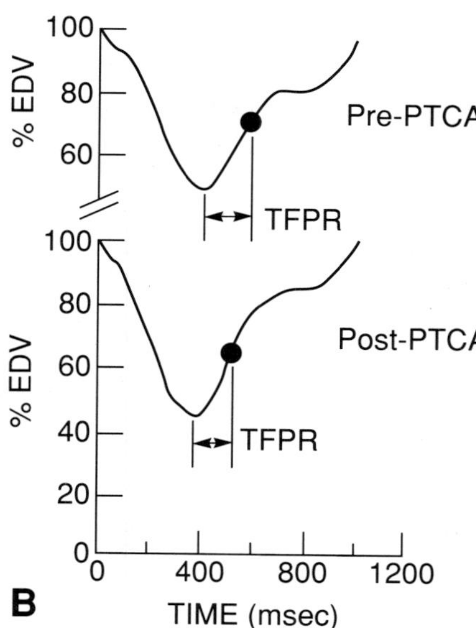

B

Figure 11. **(A).** Left ventricular time-activity curves at rest from a patient with coronary artery disease before and after percutaneous transluminal coronary angioplasty (PTCA). **(B).** Schematic representations of the two curves. Before and after PTCA, heart rate (57 vs 58 beats/min), ejection fraction (53% vs 55%), peak ejection rate (2.3 vs 2.2 EDV/sec), and ejection time (400 vs 380 msec) are similar. However, after PTCA, peak filling rate is greater (1.1 vs 2.3 EDV/sec) and time to peak filling rate (TPFR) is lower (186 vs 166 msec). EDV, end-diastolic volume. (From Bonow et al,[91] reprinted with the permission of the *American Heart Association.*)

expected increment of left ventricular filling during exercise was observed in patients with coronary artery disease compared to controls.[93] However, as noted previously, the assessment of PFR during exercise is technically difficult and is influenced significantly by variability in exercise heart rate and ejection fraction.

Effects of Aging on Left Ventricular Function. Numerous studies have documented age-related deterioration in left ventricular diastolic function,[94–97] even in the absence of coronary artery disease (Table 7). These changes must be taken into account when interpreting studies in the elderly. With increasing age, the rate and extent of rapid diastolic filling declines, and the atrial contribution to filling increases (Fig. 12). The age-related changes in left ventricular relaxation may place some elderly individuals at risk for developing symptoms of pulmonary congestion despite normal systolic function, particularly if additional deterioration in diastolic function occurs as a result of cardiac disease or hypertrophy. These effects on diastolic filling may be due to alterations in myocardial stiffness from changes in interstitial collagen composition and/or alterations in active myocardial relaxation from changes in calcium metabolism. Preliminary data indicate that these age-related changes in diastolic filling may be, in part, reversible with verapamil; although the mechanism of verapamil's effect is unclear, it may involve alterations in intracellular calcium metabolism and/or ventricular loading.[97] Exercise training also may improve diastolic filling through unknown mechanisms.[98]

The effect of aging on systolic left ventricular performance is variable. At rest, systolic function usually is preserved, but the response of left ventricular ejection fraction to exercise may be blunted.[59] Exercise training results in greater ability to increase left ventricular ejection fraction during exercise in elderly subjects.[99]

Table 7. Effects of Age on Indexes of Left Ventricular Function in Normal Subjects

	YOUNG (20–33 yrs)	MIDDLE (37–53 yrs)	ELDERLY (61–71 yrs)
LVEF (%)	53 ± 4	52 ± 7	56 ± 10
PER (EDV/sec)	2.9 ± .3	2.6 ± .3	2.6 ± .6
PFR			
(EDV/sec)	4.1 ± .6	3.0 ± .8	2.5 ± 1.0
(SV/sec)	7.8 ± 1.2	5.8 ± 1.2	4.3 ± 1.0

LVEF, left ventricular ejection fraction; PER, peak ejection rate; PFR, peak filling rate; EDV, end-diastolic volume; SV, stroke volume.

Valvular Heart Disease

Valvular pathology alters the hemodynamics of blood flow through the heart, which may result in heart failure manifested as pulmonary congestion and/or low cardiac output. Heart failure observed in valvular disease may be due to hemodynamic abnormalities alone or in combination with myocardial failure as a result of chronic ventricular overload. Applications of radionuclide angiography in valvular heart disease[100] are related to the evaluation of ventricular function and its change over time, which are major determinants of surgical and long-term mortality (Table 8). As such, monitoring of ventricular function is important in assessing the functional significance of valvular pathology in both symp-

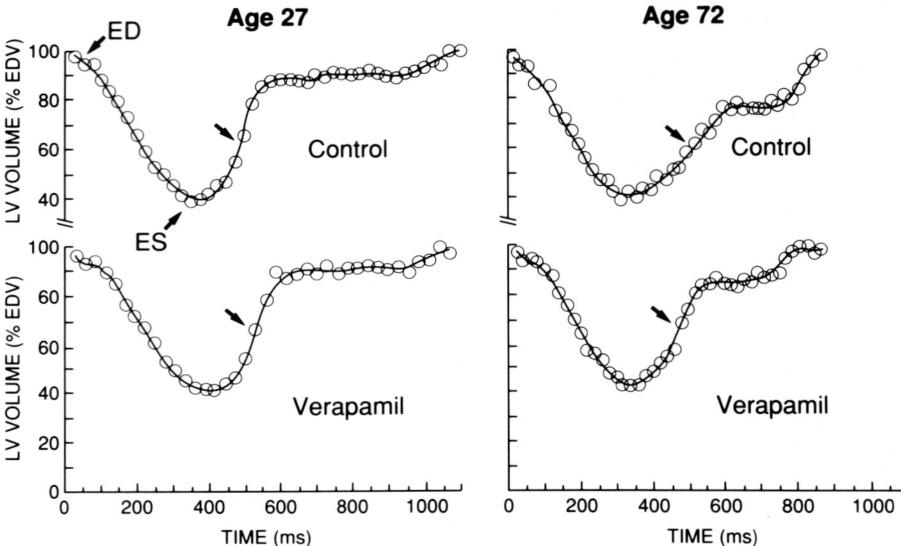

Figure 12. Left ventricular (LV) time-activity curves from normal subjects of different ages. Aging is associated with a reduction in the rate and extent of diastolic filling (indicated by arrows), and an increase in the atrial contribution to filling. The effect of verapamil on left ventricular diastolic filling is shown in 2 representative subjects. In the younger patient, LV filling is normal before verapamil (top left) and is unaffected by verapamil (bottom left). In the older patient, LV filling is reduced before verapamil (top right) and improves with verapamil (bottom right). %EDV indicates percent of end-diastolic volume; ED, end-diastole; and ES, end-systole (reprinted from reference 97).

tomatic and asymptomatic patients with valvular heart disease.

MECHANISMS

There are 2 major mechanisms of myocardial failure in patients with valvular disease: *volume overload* and *pressure overload*. Volume overload may be acute or chronic, and is usually the result of regurgitant valves or ventricular septal defects. When volume overload occurs acutely, as may happen as a complication of myocardial infarction or bacterial endocarditis, the hemodynamic consequences are profound and mortality is high. Because the heart and pulmonary vasculature cannot accommodate the sudden volume load, large increases in left heart and pulmonary pressures results in sudden pulmonary congestion. However, ventricular function, per se, usually is preserved and, therefore, blood pool imaging plays a limited role in these circumstances.

Volume Overload. In chronic volume overload, the ventricle dilates to accommodate the increased volume. Initially, as chamber size increases, the ventricle operates at the upper limit of the Starling curve, and left ventricular ejection fraction is maintained.[101] In the next phase, a degree of left ventricular hypertrophy occurs[102] that results in a modest increase in wall thickness, reduced wall stress, and maintenance of normal ejection fraction with increasing stroke volume.[103] If volume overload persists for a prolonged period, a final phase of progressive myocardial failure will occur when the heart can no longer compensate. Correction of the valvular abnormality may result in improved ventricular function if timed appropriately.[104–106] However, at some point, the myocardial failure will become irreversible. Although the pathophysiological basis of reversibility of ventricular dysfunction is incompletely understood, factors that may be involved include the duration of volume overload,[103] alterations in ventricular shape,[107] myofibrillar slippage,[108] and myocardial cellular degeneration and/or fibrosis.[109]

Pressure Overload. In pressure overload, as occurs in aortic stenosis or systemic hypertension, ventricular pressure must rise to meet the demands of a sustained increase in afterload. Initially, increased contractility through pressure-dependent mechanisms occurs and greatly increases wall stress, a major determinant of myocardial oxygen consumption. The increased wall stress may result in myocardial ischemia in some patients even in the absence of coronary artery disease.[110] Left ventricular ejection fraction may decline as wall stress increases.[111] If the pressure overload is sustained, wall thickness increases to restore normal wall stress and systolic function,[112] and concentric hypertrophy develops. Some patients may progress to a final, late stage of myocardial failure and dilatation through poorly understood mechanisms.

The scintigraphic findings of volume and pressure overload states are summarized in Table 9. In chronic volume overload, the left ventricular cavity is often enlarged, ejection fraction is normal or increased until late in the disease, stroke volume is increased, and concentric left ventricular hypertrophy is absent. In contrast, with pressure overload, left ventricular size, ejection fraction, and stroke volume are preserved in most patients; concentric hypertrophy is commonly observed. The scintigraphic findings of concentric hypertrophy have been described above.

AORTIC REGURGITATION

Chronic aortic regurgitation creates a state of volume overload that may remain asymptomatic for many years. When symptoms develop, valve replacement may be indicated to improve functional status, preserve left ventricular function, and enhance survival (Fig. 13). The assessment

Table 8. Approaches to Evaluation of the Gated Blood Pool Scan in Patients with Noncoronary Heart Disease*

CHAMBER	FINDING *Size*	FINDING *Contraction*	POSSIBLE ETIOLOGIES
Left:			
Atrium	Dilated	Decreased	Mitral regurgitation Mitral stenosis Constrictive pericarditis Restrictive cardiomyopathy
Ventricle	Normal	Increased	Hypertrophic cardiomyopathy Systemic hypertension Aortic stenosis Anemia Renal failure
	Dilated	Normal	Chronic aortic insufficiency Chronic mitral regurgitation Systemic hypertension Renal failure
	Dilated	Decreased	Dilated cardiomyopathy Coronary artery disease Prolonged aortic insufficiency Prolonged mitral insufficiency Prolonged aortic stenosis Prolonged systemic hypertension
Right:			
Atrium	Dilated	Decreased	Tricuspid regurgitation Tricuspid stenosis Constrictive pericarditis Restrictive cardiomyopathy Atrial septal defect Atrial fibrillation
Ventricle	Dilated	Normal	Left-sided failure Tricuspid regurgitation
	Dilated	Decreased	Pulmonary stenosis Pulmonary hypertension Dilated cardiomyopathy

*Reprinted from reference 100.

of left ventricular function in aortic regurgitation serves 2 purposes: in symptomatic patients, to evaluate surgical and postoperative risk and, in asymptomatic patients, to identify the subgroup in whom left ventricular dysfunction may develop prior to the onset of symptoms.

Left Ventricular Function at Rest. In symptomatic patients, preoperative parameters of left ventricular systolic function, including ejection fraction and end-systolic volume, are major determinants of postoperative heart failure and survival.[113–118] Patients with reduced preoperative systolic function have reduced postoperative survival compared to survival in those with normal preoperative left ventricular function. Left ventricular dilatation is not as predictive as left ventricular function; studies indicate that preoperative end-systolic volume is more predictive of postoperative heart failure than end-diastolic volume.[115,116,119]

In addition to left ventricular systolic performance, the duration of left ventricular dysfunction and the preoperative functional capacity are determinants of postoperative recovery of function. Patients with left ventricular dysfunction of limited duration (< about 1 year) show a greater improvement in ejection fraction and ventricular dilatation after surgery than patients with more prolonged dysfunction.[120,121] In addition, left ventricular function in patients who have lim-

Table 9. Characteristic Findings on Gated Blood Pool Imaging in Patients with Noncoronary Heart Disease

VALVULAR LESION	FINDINGS
Aortic regurgitation	Dilated LV cavity with hypertrophy Normal or decreased LVEF
Aortic stenosis	Normal LV cavity and EF LV hypertrophy Dilated LA
Mitral regurgitation	Dilated LV cavity and normal or decreased LVEF Normal LV wall thickness Dilated LA
Mitral stenosis	Normal left and right cavity size and EF Severely dilated LA
Tricuspid regurgitation	Dilated RV cavity and decreased RVEF Dilated RA
Hypertensive	LV concentric hypertrophy Normal or supranormal LVEF
Cardiomyopathy	
Dilated (congestive)	Dilatation of all four chambers Decreased LVEF and RVEF Decreased LV wall thickness
Ischemic	Normal or dilated LV cavity and decreased LVEF Decreased LV wall thickness Normal or dilated LA
Hypertrophic	Normal or small LV cavity Normal or supranormal LVEF Severe LV hypertrophy Normal or dilated LA
Restrictive	Normal LV cavity and normal or decreased LVEF Normal or increased RV cavity and normal or decreased RVEF Normal or increased LV wall thickness Dilated LA
Septal defect:	
Atrial	Dilated RV cavity and decreased RVEF Dilated RA with normal or dilated LA
Ventricular	Normal or increased LV cavity and normal or increased LVEF Dilated RV and normal or decreased RVEF Dilated LA

LV, left ventricle; RV, right ventricle; LA, left atrium; RA, right atrium; EF, ejection fraction (Reprinted from reference 100.)

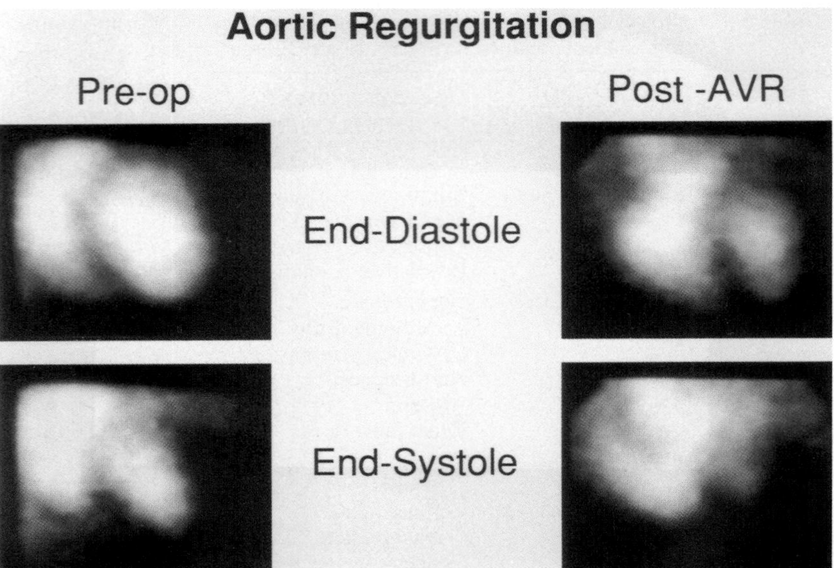

Figure 13. Chronic aortic regurgitation: an example of left ventricular volume overload. Preoperative (left) end-diastolic and end-systolic rest blood pool images show dilated left ventricle with reduced contraction. Postoperative images (right) show normal left ventricular cavity and contraction.

ited functional capacity preoperatively is less likely to improve after valve replacement.[116,118,121]

These data suggest that: (1) measurement of systolic function provides an estimate of operative and postoperative risk in patients with symptomatic aortic regurgitation and, (2) early surgery in asymptomatic or mildly symptomatic patients preserves left ventricular function and is associated with improved survival. Once left ventricular dysfunction develops, two thirds of asymptomatic patients will then develop symptoms requiring surgery within 2 to 3 years.[122]

It must be emphasized that asymptomatic patients with normal left ventricular function have an excellent prognosis with conservative medical management.[123] Such patients develop symptoms and/or left ventricular dysfunction at a rate of about 4% per year. In one study, no mortality was observed during 4 years of follow-up.[124] These patients can be followed clinically for symptom development, and by echocardiography and/or radionuclide angiography for the development of left ventricular dilatation and systolic dysfunction. Once left ventricular dysfunction is identified, it is prudent to recommend surgery; significant delay increases the risk of operative mortality or irreversible left ventricular dysfunction.[104,115,116,121–123]

Left Ventricular Function During Exercise. Many patients with aortic regurgitation, both symptomatic and asymptomatic, have an abnormal ejection fraction response to exercise.[121,124] This abnormal response is related to the severity of regurgitant volume and ventricular dilatation,[125] and may improve after surgery.[126] Although abnormalities of exercise ejection fraction may precede resting left ventricular dysfunction, exercise ejection fraction does not appear to add to the prognostic information derived from the resting variables.[121] In addition, abnormal exercise ejection fraction is not specific for myocardial contractile dysfunction, as it is greatly influenced by alterations in loading conditions as a result of exercise and regurgitant volume.[125,127]

Changes In Ventricular Function after Surgery. Shortly after aortic valve replacement, left ventricular function may decrease.[128] However, within 6 to 12 months after surgery, left ventricular function at rest and during exercise improve, but often do not normalize.[126,129] In severe aortic regurgitation, improvement in left ventricular function at 6 to 8 months after surgery predicts further improvement in left ventricular ejection fraction and end-diastolic volume at 3 to 7 years after surgery. In contrast, patients without some improvement in left ventricular function at 6 months are unlikely to improve later.[130]

MITRAL REGURGITATION

As with aortic regurgitation, mitral regurgitation results in left ventricular volume overload. Volume overload may be tolerated for many years if it develops gradually, and may result in progressive left ventricular dilatation and heart failure. As the degree of regurgitation worsens, stroke volume and end-diastolic volume increase. The left atrium is usually markedly dilated, and patients have a propensity to develop atrial fibrillation, both of which may complicate the measurement of left ventricular function (Fig. 14). Although determining the optimum time of surgery in patients with mitral regurgitation has been difficult, the preoperative evaluation of left ventricular performance provides useful prognostic information. This evaluation may include measurements of left ventricular size, ejection fraction, and right ventricular function.

Left Ventricular Size. Data from echocardiographic and angiographic studies suggest that symptomatic patients with severe left ventricular dilatation preoperatively are at high

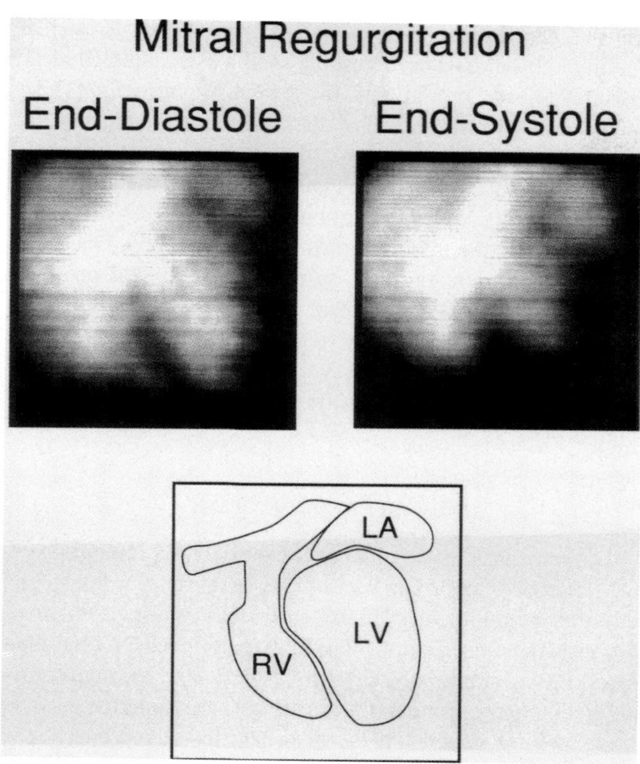

Figure 14. Chronic mitral regurgitation: an example of left ventricular volume overload. End-diastolic and end-systolic blood pool images obtained at rest in the left anterior oblique view demonstrate dilated left atrium and left ventricle.

risk for left ventricular failure postoperatively.[131] Although guidelines based on echocardiographic end-diastolic and end-systolic dimensions have been proposed, the prognostic significance of left ventricular dilatation and its applicability to asymptomatic patients is unclear. Since radionuclide measurements of left ventricular dimensions are imprecise, echocardiography better estimates ventricular volume.

Left Ventricular Function. The ejection fraction may overestimate systolic function in patients with mitral regurgitation because a certain percentage of stroke volume is ejected into the left atrium, which is a low-impedance structure and constitutes a form of "endogenous" afterload reduction.[132] Left ventricular ejection fraction may be maintained within the normal range, even with depressed systolic function. Thus, low-normal ejection fractions should be considered abnormal in patients with significant mitral regurgitation. Despite this inaccuracy, depressed left ventricular ejection fraction preoperatively is associated with reduced survival of medically treated patients[133] and patients after mitral valve replacement.[134]

Right Ventricular Function. Because chronic mitral regurgitation results in elevation of pulmonary arterial pressure, right ventricular dysfunction may develop as a complication. In medically treated patients, a right ventricular EF $\leq$ 30% is a specific indicator of reduced survival, and correlates with functional status.[133] In patients who undergo mitral valve replacement, preservation of right ventricular function is associated with excellent survival.[133] Thus, a high-risk subgroup of patients can be identified on the basis of reduced left and/or right ventricular ejection fraction.

Changes in Ventricular Function after Surgery. Correction of mitral regurgitation by valve replacement or repair acutely removes the low-impedance circuit, and left ventricular ejection fraction declines in almost all patients immediately after surgery.[134,135] Therefore, patients with depressed ejection fraction preoperatively may not tolerate the further reduction in ejection fraction postoperatively. There is a general consensus that mitral valve surgery should be performed before left ventricular function deteriorates significantly. In symptomatic patients, surgery should be performed while left ventricular function is normal; in asymptomatic patients, surgery is usually recommended when left ventricular function falls below normal or when a decline in function is observed on serial evaluations. However, definitive data regarding the significance of pre- and postoperative left ventricular dysfunction are lacking. Left ventricular dysfunction may persist after mitral valve replacement, particularly in patients with low-normal or abnormal preoperative left ventricular ejection fraction.[128] Mitral valve repair, which preserves the native architecture of the valve and its attachments to the myocardium, may lessen the decline in left ventricular function postoperatively.

AORTIC STENOSIS

Aortic stenosis places considerable pressure overload on the left ventricle due to mechanical obstruction to blood flow through the aortic valve. The ventricle hypertrophies to maintain normal wall stress, and left ventricular ejection fraction usually remains within normal range until late in the disease. Symptoms include angina, syncope, and heart failure, even in the absence of systolic dysfunction. Elevated left ventricular filling pressures are common, and contribute to the congestive symptoms.

Typical findings on radionuclide angiography include normal left ventricular systolic function, left ventricular hypertrophy, and widening of the aortic root (post-stenotic dilatation). Parameters of diastolic function are often abnormal; early in the course of the disease, atrial contribution to filling may be increased. With time, peak filling rate becomes abnormal.[136,137] In some patients, systolic dysfunction develops late in the disease and is typically global, without significant regional abnormalities. Echocardiography often is the preferred method for evaluating aortic stenosis because severity can be estimated noninvasively by this technique.

Unlike aortic regurgitation, the evaluation of left ventricular function is not useful in predicting postoperative risk of death in aortic stenosis. Patients with preoperative left ventricular systolic dysfunction, even with severe congestive symptoms, usually have improved function after surgery.[138,139] Asymptomatic patients can be managed conservatively until symptoms develop.[140]

Significant aortic stenosis generally is considered a contraindication to exercise testing, and exercise radionuclide angiography usually is not recommended. However, in a study by Milanes and coworkers, in which rest and exercise radionuclide angiography was performed safely in patients with aortic stenosis who also underwent contrast angiography, an increase of left ventricular ejection fraction of >5% during exercise implied an aortic valve area of >0.8 cm^2 and absence of significant coronary artery disease.[141] Thus, exercise studies with careful monitoring may be considered in selected patients in whom stenosis severity is in question.

MITRAL STENOSIS

Unlike the valvular lesions discussed above, mitral stenosis results in neither volume nor pressure overload of the left ventricle. Isolated mitral stenosis places a pressure burden on the left atrium, which may lead to pulmonary hypertension, pulmonary congestion and, eventually, right ventricular dysfunction. As in mitral regurgitation, left atrial dilatation and atrial fibrillation often develop, and may make accurate assessment of left ventricular function difficult. Thus, the radionuclide angiographic appearance of preserved left ventricular function, dilated left atrium, and right ventricular systolic dysfunction characterize mitral stenosis.

Left Ventricular Function. Because the left ventricle is not subjected to abnormal demands with mitral stenosis, ejection fraction is usually preserved and left ventricular size is normal. However, a few patients do develop systolic dysfunction,[142] which may be due to prior rheumatic myocarditis or chronic ventricular underfilling. In such patients, the degree of left ventricular dysfunction is usually mild in comparison to the elevation of pulmonary pressures from the stenosis itself and, therefore, may be of little clinical significance.

Right Ventricular Function. The right ventricle may become dilated and hypocontractile from secondary pulmonary hypertension. In patients with preserved right ventricular ejection fraction at rest, right ventricular response to exercise may be abnormal.[143] Preliminary data indicate that the right ventricular ejection fraction response to exercise may normalize after successful percutaneous balloon mitral valvuloplasty.[144] The prognostic utility of measuring right ventricular function preoperatively is unknown. Currently, the timing of surgery is based on symptoms and severity of stenosis.

Cardiomyopathies and Myocarditis

The cardiomyopathies are a group of disorders characterized by primary myocardial involvement of a disease process that often results in functional impairment. Although this term is used sometimes to connote systolic dysfunction of the left ventricle as a result of a known disorder (e.g., ischemic or hypertensive cardiomyopathy), the etiology is often unknown. Myocarditis refers to an inflammatory disorder affecting the heart. The cardiomyopathies are classified according to the predominant functional impairment: (1) Dilated (congestive) cardiomyopathy, characterized by left ventricular dilation, systolic dysfunction, and congestive heart failure; (2) restrictive, characterized by impairment of diastolic filling; (3) hypertrophic, characterized by inappropriate and prominent left ventricular hypertrophy. Diagnosis of these disorders is made primarily on clinical grounds, often with hemodynamic and/or imaging data. Because these disorders affect cardiac function, radionuclide angiography is useful in determining the severity of impairment in systolic and diastolic function and the response to therapy in afflicted patients.

DILATED CARDIOMYOPATHY

Dilated cardiomyopathy is characterized by impaired systolic function and dilatation of one or both ventricles. The etiology is unknown in many cases, but a large number of diseases have been implicated in its pathogenesis, including alcohol, various toxins, nutritional deficiencies, neuromuscular disorders, connective tissue disease, pregnancy, and infections. In general, these disorders result in generalized myocardial dysfunction, and focal abnormalities are less commonly observed compared with ischemic cardiomyopathy.[145] The observation of striking regional wall motion abnormalities should raise the suspicion of ischemic heart disease. However, it is important to note that regional dysfunction of a lesser degree can be observed in idiopathic cardiomyopathy.[146] Both ventricles are usually involved, whereas the right ventricle tends to be spared in coronary artery disease.[147] Survival is influenced negatively by the degree of left ventricular dysfunction, although not to the same extent as in coronary artery disease.[148,149] Interestingly, resting left ventricular ejection fraction does not correlate with response to exercise in these patients.[150]

Radionuclide angiography may be useful in assessing response to therapy in patients with dilated cardiomyopathy. Several groups have documented improved left ventricular ejection fraction with therapy for congestive heart failure (afterload reduction and/or inotropic drugs).[151–155] However, the favorable response in systolic function to therapy may not predict a favorable clinical or hemodynamic response.[155,156] Although the utility of measuring changes in left ventricular volumes with therapy is unclear, recent data from the SOLVD (Studies of Left Ventricular Dysfunction) investigation suggest that such measurements may be clinically important. In this trial, patients with significant left ventricular dysfunction (left ventricular ejection fraction ≤35%) who were treated with the ACE inhibitor enalapril had decreases in end-diastolic and end-systolic left ventricular volumes, whereas patients given placebo had no such changes.[157] The favorable changes in the treatment group were accompanied by decreased left ventricular wall stress and a trend toward a reduction in cardiac events.

who are monitored serially by radionuclide angiography may have significant spontaneous changes in left and right ventricular ejection fractions over a relatively short period of time. In a study of patients with significant left ventricular dysfunction (left ventricular ejection fraction mean 27%), one third of patients had an absolute change in left ventricular ejection fraction of greater than 5% over a 12-week period, during which therapy and clinical status were not changed.[158] A similar proportion of patients had significant changes in right ventricular ejection fraction. The mean ejection fractions did not change over the follow-up interval. Thus, serial changes in such patients must be interpreted with caution.

In patients with idiopathic dilated cardiomyopathy, left ventricular function may spontaneously improve in 20 to 50% of patients. While ejection fraction often normalizes in such patients, left ventricular peak filling rate and end-diastolic and end-systolic volumes usually remain abnormal for a prolonged period of time.[159]

Some patients with dilated cardiomyopathy ultimately will require cardiac transplantation. Implantable left ventricular assist devices sometimes are used as a life-saving "bridge" as the patient awaits transplantation. In such patients, radionuclide angiography may be useful in monitoring the effects of these devices. Dramatic improvements in left ventricular ejection fraction (from 17 to 47%) and right ventricular ejection fraction (from 21 to 32%) have been observed in a study of 10 patients using the Novacor device.[160] After transplantation, radionuclide angiography may be performed for a variety of indications. The right atrium usually is enlarged, due to the presence of a portion of the patient's own right atrium and that of the orthotopic transplanted heart. Although the left ventricular ejection fraction invariably improves after transplantation, rest left ventricular ejection fraction, as well as end-diastolic volume and stroke volume indexes, are significantly lower than in normal control subjects.[161]

Exercise radionuclide angiography generally is not useful in the evaluation of patients with dilated cardiomyopathy. Cardiovascular response to exercise in these patients is highly variable and depends on loading conditions. Thus, changes in left ventricular function to exercise may not be specific for myocardial disease progression.

Anthracycline Cardiotoxicity. The most commonly used anthracycline, doxorubicin, is a potent anticancer chemotherapeutic agent. However, its use often is limited by myocardial toxicity. Doxorubicin myocardial toxicity can be divided into early and late forms. Acute toxicity may include arrhythmias, myocarditis, and left ventricular dysfunction. Serious acute toxicity is rare, but may cause sudden death.

The major limitation to doxorubicin use is its dose-dependent late cardiotoxicity that results in dilated cardiomyopathy. In patients without cardiac disease, this rarely occurs if the cumulative dose is less than 500 mg/m^2, but is progressive with larger cumulative doses.[162] Cardiotoxicity may be observed at lower doses (<450 mg/m^2) if other therapeutic modalities, such as radiation or cyclophosphamide, are used with conjunction with doxorubicin.[163] Patients in whom left ventricular function progressively deteriorates during therapy are at high risk for developing congestive heart failure.[164] If doxorubicin therapy is stopped, however, ventricular function usually stabilizes.[164–166]

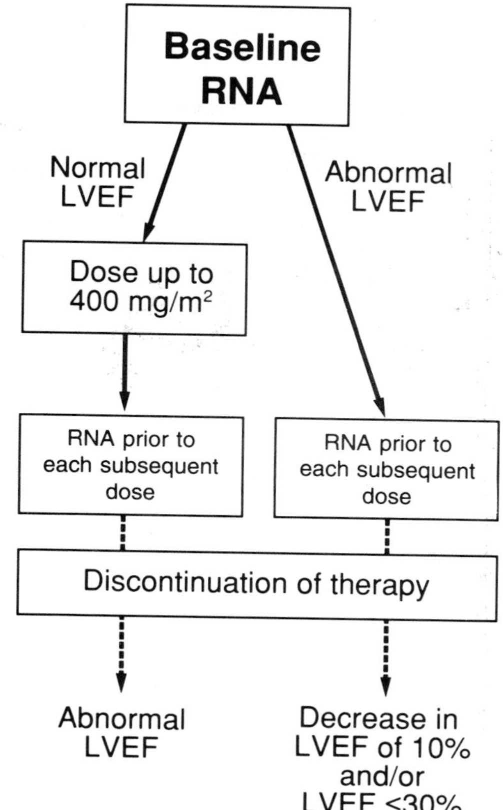

Figure 15. Guidelines for monitoring patients for doxorubicin cardiotoxicity.

Because the cardiotoxicity of doxorubicin is highly variable, a set of guidelines have been developed to monitor patients.[167] Baseline radionuclide angiography should be performed prior to initiation of therapy. In patients with normal left ventricular function, ejection fraction should be measured after a cumulative dose of 400 to 450 mg/m^2, and sequentially (prior to each dose) thereafter. The risk/benefit ratio for continued therapy should be reassessed when cardiotoxicity develops, indicated by a decline in ejection fraction below normal. In patients with an abnormal baseline ejection fraction, left ventricular function should be assessed prior to each dose, and discontinuation of therapy should be considered when there is an absolute decrease of 10% in left ventricular ejection fraction, or left ventricular ejection fraction falls below 30% (Fig. 15).

Following these guidelines, patients can be monitored for evidence of progressive cardiotoxicity. Therapy can be

Hypertrophic Cardiomyopathy

End-Diastole End-Systole

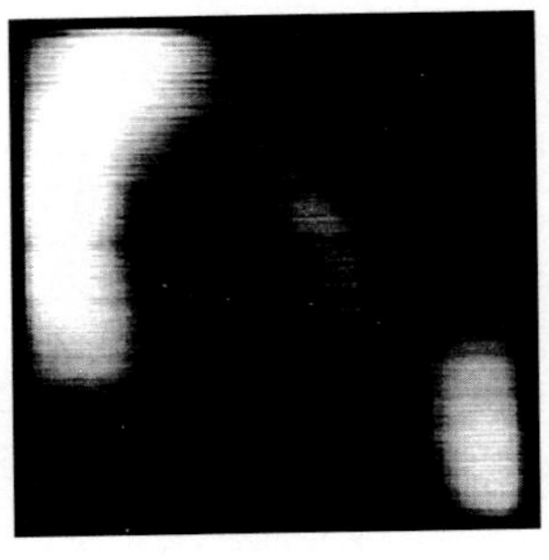

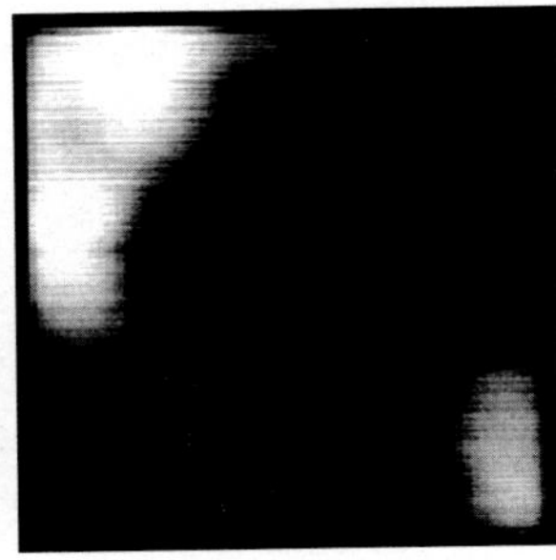

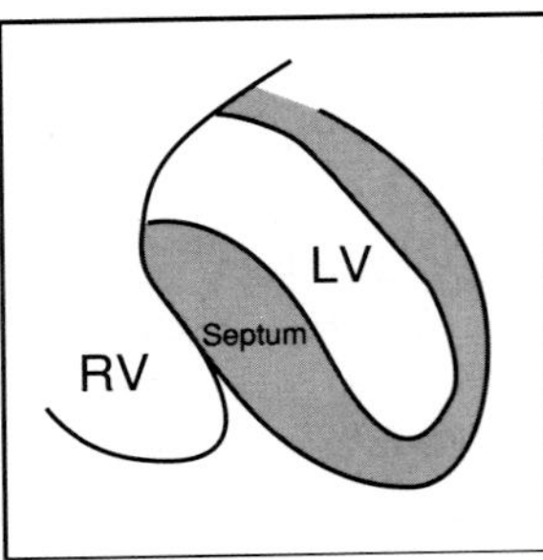

Figure 16. Hypertrophic cardiomyopathy: an example of disproportionate severe hypertrophic process. End-diastolic and end-systolic blood pool images obtained at rest in the left anterior oblique view demonstrate supranormal left ventricular systolic function, disproportionate septal thickening, and systolic ventricular cavity obliteration.

continued in cumulative doses over 500 mg/m^2 if cardiotoxicity is not observed. Patients with baseline cardiac dysfunction or mild cardiotoxicity can continue to receive doxorubicin safely as long as cardiac function is monitored closely.

HYPERTROPHIC CARDIOMYOPATHY

Hypertrophic cardiomyopathy is characterized by thickened myocardium without a definable cause, usually in an asymmetrical pattern with predominant septal involvement. These gross changes are accompanied by cellular abnormalities that include sarcomere hypertrophy, fiber disarray, and abnormalities of calcium metabolism. Pathophysiological hallmarks of the disorder are hyperdynamic left ventricular function,[160] impaired ventricular relaxation,[169–172] and dynamic subaortic obstruction.[173–175] It occurs at all ages and may be familial. Recent advances have been made in our understanding of the genetic and molecular abnormalities in hypertrophic cardiomyopathy.[176–180] Clinical manifestations include angina, dyspnea, and syncope. In most patients, radionuclide angiographic findings suggestive of hypertrophic cardiomyopathy include normal or supranormal left ventricular systolic function, disproportionate septal thickening, and systolic ventricular cavity obliteration (Fig. 16). A small subset of patients develop left ventricular systolic dysfunction late in the course of disease; in such patients, ejection fraction falls below normal, and the ventricular cavity dilates; in effect transforming into a dilated cardiomyopathy.[181] The identification of such transformation is important because therapy in these patients is markedly different from that of hypertrophic cardiomyopathy with normal or supranormal systolic function.

Diastolic filling abnormalities are a characteristic feature of hypertrophic cardiomyopathy.[182–184] The observed diastolic dysfunction is most likely caused by the complex interaction of reduced distensibility (or compliance) related to the passive properties of a hypertrophied ventricle, abnormal cellular architecture, and impaired in active (energy-requiring) ventricular relaxation. In some patients, increased atrial contribution to filling is the only manifestation of diastolic dysfunction. The clinical significance of diastolic dysfunction in hypertrophic cardiomyopathy is suggested by its correlation to diminished exercise tolerance[185] and poor prognosis.[186] Improvement in left ventricular filling and symptoms has been observed after therapy with calcium blockers such as verapamil.[183–186] Thus, radionuclide angiography is useful both to assess the severity of diastolic dysfunction and the response to therapy (Fig. 17).

RESTRICTIVE CARDIOMYOPATHY

Restrictive cardiomyopathies are the least common cardiomyopathy seen in the Western hemisphere, and are characterized by impaired ventricular filling with relative preservation of systolic function. The causes are numerous, and include amyloidosis, sarcoidosis, hemachromatosis, carcinoid disease, and radiation therapy. There are no distinctive findings on radionuclide angiography; left ventricular size and systolic function are often normal, and the ventricular wall may be thickened. Diastolic function is usually abnormal, and assessment of the time-activity curve may help to differentiate restrictive cardiomyopathy from constrictive pericarditis, a disorder with similar clinical presentation.[187] In the former condition, the initial filling is usually abnormally slow whereas, in the latter disorder, the initial component of filling is rapid.

MYOCARDITIS

Myocarditis is a disorder characterized by inflammation of the myocardium, and may be caused principally by viral, bacterial, or protozoal infections, depending on geography. In North America, viruses are responsible for most cases, and Chagas' disease predominates in South America. The clinical manifestations are widely varied; the disease may be asymptomatic, as it is in most patients, or it may present with progressive congestive heart failure, arrhythmias, or chest pain. Myocarditis is the initial event in many patients with idiopathic dilated cardiomyopathy. Radionuclide angiography is helpful in defining the extent of systolic dysfunction in such patients. Because most patients with viral myocarditis recover over several weeks, serial testing is used to

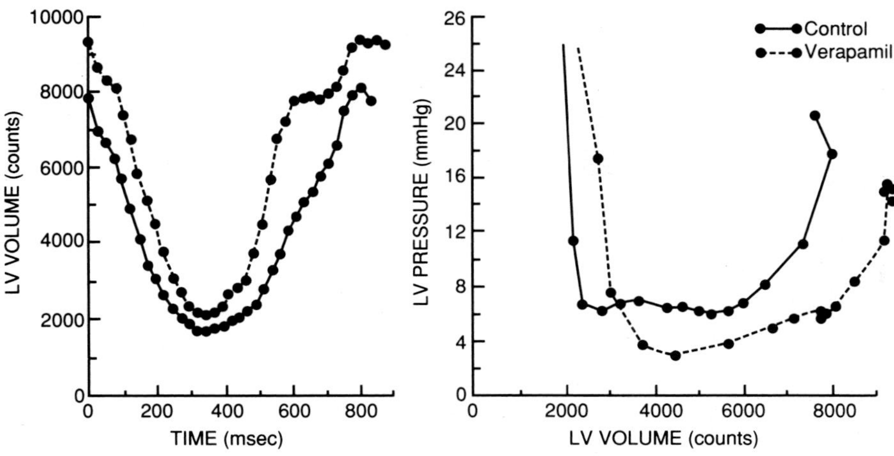

Figure 17. Time-activity curves before and after verapamil (left). Verapamil caused increases in left ventricular (LV) systolic and diastolic counts, stroke counts, and peak filling rate, and a decrease in ejection fraction. These changes were associated with a downward and rightward shift in the diastolic pressure-volume relation (right). (From Bonow et al,[184] reprinted with the permission of the *American Heart Association.*)

document recovery of ventricular function. In patients with Chagas' disease, regional left or right ventricular wall motion abnormalities may result from focal myocardial involvement.[188]

SYSTEMIC HYPERTENSION

Hypertension is a common disorder characterized by elevated systemic vascular resistance to varying degrees. Many patients with hypertension, even if only mild, demonstrate left ventricular hypertrophy by electrocardiographic or echocardiographic criteria. Investigations by Sasayama[189] and Pfeffer and Pfeffer[190] have demonstrated that an acute increase in afterload results in transiently impaired systolic performance that "normalizes" with the development of left ventricular hypertrophy, and that once left ventricular hypertrophy develops, contractile performance is maintained, despite progressive increases in systemic vascular resistance. These studies suggest that left ventricular hypertrophy represents a compensatory response to chronic pressure overload, as in aortic stenosis. However, recent evidence indicates that ventricular hypertrophy may be intrinsically related to the pathogenesis of hypertension, and may develop simultaneously with the associated vascular changes.[191,192]

Left ventricular systolic function is usually normal in patients with systemic hypertension.[37,193–197] However, the increase in ejection fraction to exercise may be blunted, even in the absence of coronary disease.[198] End-diastolic volume may be increased at rest, and may not increase normally during exercise; this may be the mechanism for the abnormal ejection fraction response with exercise in these patients. Left ventricular hypertrophy is suggested on radionuclide angiography by a photopenic zone around the left ventricular blood pool, as described earlier. In some patients, systolic dysfunction may develop late in the course of disease.

Diastolic filling abnormalities are common in patients with essential hypertension,[197,199–201] especially among hypertensive patients with left ventricular hypertrophy,[38,199] although they can be found even in the absence of hypertrophy.[199] Regression of hypertrophy with antihypertensive therapy has been associated with improved left ventricular filling.[201] On the basis of these findings, some have argued that filling rate abnormalities are important early indices (i.e., predating clinically detectable systolic dysfunction) of the hemodynamic impact of left ventricular pressure loading. Further, the use of the filling parameters as a means of choosing and/or evaluating antihypertensive therapy is an area needing more study. Note, however, that patients with hypertension are also at risk for coronary disease, and careful attention must be given to exclude patients with coronary artery disease in investigations of diastolic function in hypertension.

CONGESTIVE HEART FAILURE WITH NORMAL SYSTOLIC FUNCTION

Recent studies have indicated that up to 40% of patients with congestive heart failure have normal systolic function, and most of these patients have abnormalities of diastolic function.[45,202] Systemic hypertension was the underlying etiology in over half of these patients (see above). Treatment with calcium blockers may improve symptoms and exercise capacity, as well as left ventricular filling, in hypertensive patients with left ventricular hypertrophy who present with heart failure and normal systolic function.[203] Thus, although definitive studies are lacking, distinguishing systolic from diastolic dysfunction appears to be important, as the management of symptoms arising from each may be quite different.[196] The radionuclide parameters of diastolic function in patients with significant systolic dysfunction must be interpreted with caution because of the interdependence of systolic and diastolic function.

Evaluation of Right Ventricular Function

The right ventricle, in comparison to the left, is a thin-walled structure that generates much lower pressures. Under normal circumstances, the vascular resistance of the pulmonary circulation is very low. However, with elevated pulmonary vascular resistance, right ventricular function becomes important in maintaining transpulmonary flow and, therefore, cardiac output. This adaptation must take place gradually; if pulmonary pressures increase suddenly and severely, the right ventricle fails rapidly, resulting in hemodynamic collapse.

The evaluation of right ventricular function is complicated by its unusual pyramidal shape, which makes geometric methods impractical. Radionuclide angiography can be used to accurately assess right ventricular function by count-based methods that do not rely on geometric assumptions. First-pass or equilibrium studies are often used to assess right ventricular function.

First-pass radionuclide angiography is better suited for the evaluation of right ventricular function because the left and right ventricles can be temporally separated and, in the right anterior oblique position the overlap between right atrial and ventricular chambers is minimized.[204]

Count-based methods, using attenuation corrections, have also been developed using equilibrium studies.[205,206] It is important to emphasize that attenuation correction is necessary for greatest accuracy, particularly when right ventricular volume measurements are made.[205] Several modifications to the usual acquisition and analysis may improve accuracy further. A slant-hole collimator better separates right atrium from right ventricle in the left anterior oblique position.[207] A dual region-of-interest method may further minimize the effects of atrial-ventricular overlap.[208] In a study by Maddahi and colleagues, the single-region-of-interest method significantly underestimated right ventricular ejection fraction, whereas the dual method correlated well with first-pass measurements.[209]

CORONARY ARTERY DISEASE

Chronic Coronary Artery Disease. In normal subjects, right ventricular ejection fraction increases with exercise.[210,211] Some investigators have reported an abnormal response of the right ventricle to exercise in patients with proximal right coronary artery disease.[210,211] However, this abnormal response also has been observed in patients with left ventricular dysfunction, even in the absence of right coronary stenosis.[212] This illustrates that the right ventricle is very sensitive to loading conditions, and an abnormal ejection fraction at rest or during exercise must be interpreted with caution.

Right Ventricular Infarction. Hemodynamically significant right ventricular infarction usually occurs as a complication of inferior left ventricular infarction, although it can occur in isolation or associated with anterior infarction. Its occurrence is associated with a poor prognosis, and is diagnosed on the basis of hemodynamic and electrocardiographic criteria. Hemodynamically significant right ventricular infarction is associated with right ventricular regional wall motion abnormalities and/or a right ventricular ejection fraction of less than 40%.[208,213] Although most patients with acute right ventricular infarction recover function with time,[84,214] dysfunction may persist in some patients, particularly those with large infarcts.[215] Thus, radionuclide angiography may be useful in both the identification and follow-up of hemodynamically significant right ventricular infarction.

RIGHT VENTRICULAR DYSFUNCTION AND LEFT HEART FAILURE

Impaired right *and* left ventricular function suggests cardiomyopathy. In contrast, coronary artery disease usually is associated with preserved right ventricular function and impaired left ventricular function. Right ventricular systolic dysfunction does have important prognostic and therapeutic implications in patients with congestive heart failure. In patients with chronic left ventricular dysfunction, an abnormal right ventricular ejection fraction is associated with reduced survival and functional class compared to those with preserved right ventricular function.[216] Furthermore, the reduced functional capacity in patients with heart failure may be related to impaired right ventricular function caused by chronically elevated pulmonary resistance.[150] In addition, both right and left ventricular function may improve with afterload reduction in heart failure patients,[217,218] which may translate into improved functional status.

CHRONIC OBSTRUCTIVE PULMONARY DISEASE

The assessment of right ventricular function in patients with chronic obstructive pulmonary disease (COPD) is useful in evaluating suspected cor pulmonale, prognosis, and response to therapies. Although right ventricular ejection fraction varies in COPD patients, cor pulmonale is invariably associated with right ventricular systolic dysfunction.[219] Furthermore, nearly half of patients with right ventricular dysfunction subsequently develop cor pulmonale. The presence of right ventricular failure is also associated with reduced survival.[220] With exercise, patients with moderate to severe COPD tend to have abnormal right ventricular ejection fraction responses to exercise, whereas left ventricular response remains normal in the absence of concomitant coronary or left ventricular disease.[221] Radionuclide angiography is used to demonstrate improvement in rest and exercise right ventricular function with a variety of therapies, including digoxin,[222] aminophylline,[223] oxygen,[224] and vasodilators.[225]

VALVULAR HEART DISEASE

Mitral Regurgitation. As left atrial and pulmonary vascular pressures rise in chronic mitral regurgitation, right ventricular afterload increases, which may result in right ventricular failure. A study by Hochreiter and colleagues demonstrated an inverse relationship between right ventricular ejection fraction and pulmonary artery systolic and pulmonary capillary wedge pressures.[133] Furthermore, impaired right ventricular ejection fraction was associated with adverse prognosis. Medically treated patients with right ventricular ejection fraction of less than 30% were at higher risk of death. In this study, resting left ventricular ejection fraction also was associated with increased mortality, although it did not add to the prognostic information available from right ventricular ejection fraction alone. Importantly, surgically treated patients with right ventricular and/or left ventricular dysfunction had a favorable prognosis. Thus, this study suggests that assessment of both right and left ventricular function may provide useful prognostic information, and possibly aid in determining the optimum time of surgery in patients with chronic mitral regurgitation.

Mitral Stenosis. As in patients with lung disease or mitral regurgitation, right ventricular dysfunction may develop as a result of secondary pulmonary hypertension. While right ventricular function at rest usually is preserved in mitral stenosis, the response to exercise is often abnormal.[143] The prognostic significance of right ventricular dysfunction in this disorder is unknown.

Tricuspid Regurgitation. Although echocardiography may be more useful in detecting tricuspid regurgitation, first-pass techniques may demonstrate severe tricuspid regurgitation.[226] Severe tricuspid regurgitation in ungated first-pass studies is characterized by inability to deliver an intact bolus to the left ventricle. In gated first-pass studies, reflux of the radiotracer in great veins of the right atrium may be visualized.

CONGENITAL HEART DISEASE

Atrial Septal Defect. Atrial septal defect may cause right ventricular volume overload due to the left-to-right shunting, which results in right ventricular dilatation and systolic dysfunction. Depressed right ventricular function is associated with increased symptoms and, once it develops, may not normalize even after correction of the atrial septal defect.[227] Thus, assessment of right ventricular function may identify patients at risk for persistent right ventricular failure postoperatively.

Right Ventricular Dysplasia. Right ventricular dysplasia is a form of cardiomyopathy affecting the right ventricle and is an important cause of arrhythmias in young patients. Radionuclide angiography findings suggestive of right ventricular dysplasia include right ventricular wall motion abnormalities, exercise right ventricular ejection fraction less than 50%, and right ventricular dilatation out of proportion to the left ventricle.[228]

Other Congenital Disorders. Right ventricular dysfunction is caused by several congenital heart diseases, including tetralogy of Fallot, double-outlet right ventricle, Epstein's anomaly of the tricuspid valve, pulmonic stenosis, and transposition of the great vessels. In general, echocardiography is the diagnostic modality of choice in infants with these disorders. However, radionuclide angiography may be useful later in life, after surgical correction, if reassessment of ventricular function is clinically indicated.

Ambulatory Monitoring of Ventricular Function

Continuous monitoring of left ventricular function may provide important information in assessing the functional significance of coronary disease. It is likely that most episodes of myocardial ischemia in patients with coronary artery disease are "silent," not associated with symptoms. Changes in left ventricular function may be more sensitive indicators of ischemia than symptoms or electrocardiographic abnormalities.[229]

The technique of ambulatory monitoring is based on equilibrium radionuclide angiography, and was first described by Wilson and colleagues.[230] A nonimaging gamma detector is placed over the patient's left ventricle, using a standard gamma camera to aid in identification of the ventricle on the left anterior oblique projection, after labeling of red blood cells. The probe is suspended in a vest-like apparatus, and the entire apparatus is referred to as a "VEST." Background activity is measured with a small detector over the right lung field. Simultaneous electrocardiographic monitoring is also performed, and the data are stored on cassette tape for 4 to 6-hour periods. Measurements of left ventricular ejection fraction by the VEST correlate well with standard measurements by radionuclide angiography.[231,232] Measurement of peak filling rate, an index of diastolic function, also can be measured accurately using the VEST.[233,234]

Patients with coronary artery disease often have abnormal left ventricular ejection fraction responses to mild-to-moderate activities. Tamaki and colleagues observed that approximately two thirds of episodes of transient left ventricular dysfunction were asymptomatic, and most were not accompanied by electrocardiographic abnormalities.[232] These data suggest that ambulatory monitoring of left ventricular function may be more sensitive than ambulatory electrocardiographic monitoring for the detection of myocardial ischemia. Kayden and coworkers showed that transient ambulatory left ventricular dysfunction in patients after myocardial infarction, who were treated with thrombolytics, predicts subsequent cardiac events.[235] Thus, ambulatory monitoring of left ventricular function provides a useful research tool to evaluate the effects of ischemia on ventricular function under various conditions.

Because the VEST allows continuous assessment of left ventricular function in the ambulatory patient, it may have unique research and clinical applications. The VEST has been used in the assessment of therapeutic interventions in patients with heart disease. In a study of patients with coronary artery disease, Mohuiddin and colleagues used the VEST to demonstrate improvement in cardiac function during therapy with nitroglycerin or nifedipine.[236] No such improvement was observed in controls without coronary artery disease. In another recent study in coronary artery disease patients, Burg and colleagues used the VEST during a mental stress test, and showed that patients with certain psychological profiles were more likely to have mental stress-induced myocardial ischemia, as indicated by a decrease in left ventricular ejection fraction during mental stress.[237] Future applications of the VEST outside of the laboratory setting may include its use as a monitor of myocardial ischemia during routine daily activities, which is more sensitive than current approaches using Holter (ECG) monitoring alone.[238]

Tomographic Radionuclide Angiography

Efforts to expand the utility of gated blood pool imaging from simple measures of global left ventricular function have led to several methods of regional wall motion quantification using planar techniques. These methods include (1) a centerline method based on end-diastolic and end-systolic contours[239]; (2) phase analysis based on the onset, timing, and extent of contraction at rest[240]; and (3) sector analysis based on dividing the blood pool activity into a number of sectors in the left anterior oblique projection.[26,27,241] However, despite these quantitative techniques, accurate assessment of regional function remains suboptimal. This is due to the inherent limitation of applying two-dimensional images to assess the function of a three-dimensional organ, such as the heart.[242] Other disadvantages of planar imaging include: (1) poor resolution and inadequate separation of the myocardial segments; (2) the tissue underlying and overlying each pixel are blurred together, thereby preventing the exact location of a regional wall motion abnormality; (3) geometry prohibits positioning the camera perpendicular to the heart's long axis; (4) only one planar view of the heart can be imaged during exercise; and (5) superimposition of overlying structures.

The application of single photon emission computed tomography (SPECT) in myocardial perfusion studies has enhanced the localization of individual diseased coronary arteries when compared with planar scintigraphy.[243–245] Similar to perfusion imaging, SPECT radionuclide angiography may prove to be superior to currently applied planar imaging techniques. The potential advantages of SPECT imaging over planar imaging are as follows: (1) SPECT allows for three-dimensional reconstruction of the entire heart with the ability to reproject the data to obtain all possible planar views with a single acquisition; (2) improved segmental resolution; (3) permits independent assessment of regional contraction, slice by slice, from apex to the base of the left ventricle; and (4) improved separation of overlapping structures. For example, a true left ventricular long axis view can be reconstructed from SPECT without overlying right ventricular activity. In addition, an apical four-chamber view of the heart can be displayed to evaluate simultaneous contraction of the atria and the ventricles. Currently, there are only few reports in the literature that utilize SPECT radionuclide angiography for the evaluation of regional and global left ventricular function and determination of ventricular volumes at rest.[242,246–251] By constructing a beating heart phantom, Bartlett and coworkers recently confirmed that SPECT may be superior to planar radionuclide angiography for visual assessment of regional wall motion abnormalities.[252] Furthermore, when SPECT gated blood pool studies were performed among patients with coronary artery disease undergoing positron emission tomography (PET), there was a good correlation between quantitative measures of regional contraction by SPECT and regional blood flow by PET.[252]

CONCLUSION

Radionuclide angiography provides important mechanistic insight into the right and left ventricular diastolic and systolic function in patients with coronary and noncoronary heart disease. The technology is safe, noninvasive, quantitative, highly reproducible, widely accessible, and relatively inexpensive when compared to other emerging technologies. With the changing emphasis of medical health care, advances in new technology as well as currently available technologies will be viewed from the perspective of (1) cost-effectiveness, (2) independent information and, (3) patient outcomes. Radionuclide angiography provides important diagnostic, prognostic, and therapeutic information in patients with coronary artery disease. In addition, it provides quantitative and highly reproducible assessment of left ventricular function among patients with noncoronary heart disease. For example, sequential assessment of left ventricular function among patients with left-sided valvular regurgitation has played an important role in determining whether a patient should undergo valve replacement surgery or be maintained on medical therapy. Radionuclide assessment of left ventricular relaxation and diastolic filling indices has provided insight into the pathophysiology of hypertrophic cardiomyopathy and hypertensive heart disease. Monitoring cardiac function among patients receiving potent anticancer chemotherapeutic agents has prevented potential dose-dependent cardiotoxicity. Thus, radionuclide evaluation of cardiac function has been assured a clinically significant role for the evaluation and management of patients with heart disease well into the next century. In the future, with increasing emphasis on image fusion and correlation of anatomy, physiology, and metabolism, ambulatory ventricular function monitors and tomographic gated cardiac blood pool imaging may play an important role in providing tomographic functional correlates to myocardial perfusion and metabolism.

REFERENCES

1. Dymond DS, Elliott A, Stone D, et al. Factors that affect the reproducibility of measurements of left ventricular function from first-pass radionuclide ventriculograms. *Circulation* 1982;65:311.
2. Green MV, Bacharach SL, Borer JS, Bonow RO. A theoretical comparison of first-pass and gated equilibrium methods in the measurement of systolic left ventricular function. *J Nucl Med* 1991;32:1801–1807.

3. Kato M. In vivo labeling of red blood cells withTc-99m with stannous pyrophosphate. *J Nucl Med* 1979;20:1071.
4. Callahan RJ, Froelich JW, McKusick KA, et al. A modified method for the in vivo labeling of red blood cells with Tc-99m: Concise communication. *J Nucl Med* 1982;23:315.
5. Hladik WB, Ponto JA, Stathis VJ. Drug-radiopharmaceutical interactions, in Thrall JH and Swanson DP (eds): *Diagnostic Interventions in Nuclear Medicine*. Chicago: Year Book Medical Publishers, 1985, pp 226–246.
6. Zanelli GD. Effect of certain drugs used in the treatment of cardiovascular disease on the "in vitro" labeling of red blood cells with Tc-99m. *Nucl Med Commun* 1982;3:155.
7. Hladik WB, Nigg KK, Rhodes BA. Drug induced changes in the biologic distribution of pharmaceuticals. *Semin Nucl Med* 1982;12:184.
8. Hegge FN, Hamilton GW, Larson SM, et al. Cardiac chamber imaging: A comparison of red blood cells labeled with Tc-99m in vitro and in vivo. *J Nucl Med* 1978;19:129.
9. Schneider J, Berger HJ, Sands MJ, Lachman AB, Zaret BL. Beat-to-beat left ventricular performance in atrial fibrillation: Radionuclide assessment with the computerized nuclear probe. *Am J Cardiol* 1983;51:1189–95.
10. Burggraf GW, Parker JO. Prognosis in coronary artery disease: Angiographic, hemodynamic, and clinical factors. *Circulation* 1975;51:146.
11. Proudfit WL, Bruschke AVG, Sones FM. Natural history of obstructive coronary artery disease: ten-year study of 601 nonsurgical cases. *Prog Cardiovasc Dis* 1978;21:53.
12. Harris PJ, Harrell FE, Lee KL, Behar VS, Rosati RA. Survival in medically treated coronary artery disease. *Circulation* 1979;60:1259.
13. Hammermeister KE, DeRouen TA, Dodge HT. Comparison of survival of medically and surgically treated coronary disease patients in Seattle Heart Watch: a non-randomized study. *Circulation* 1982;65:53.
14. Mock MB, Ringqvist I, Fisher LD, et al. Survival of medically treated patients in the Coronary Artery Surgery Study (CASS) registry. *Circulation* 1982;66:562.
15. European Coronary Surgery Study Group: Long-term results of prospective randomized study of coronary artery bypass surgery in stable angina pectoris. *Lancet* 1982;2:1173.
16. Jones RH, Floyd RD, Austin EH, Sabiston DC. The role of radionuclide angiocardiography in the preoperative prediction of pain relief and prolonged survival following coronary artery bypass grafting. *Ann Surg* 1983;197:743.
17. Gohlke H, Samek L, Betz P, et al. Exercise testing provides additional prognostic information in angiographically defined subgroups of patients with coronary artery disease. *Circulation* 1983;68:979.
18. Pryor DB, Harrell FE, Lee KL, et al. Prognostic indicators from radionuclide angiography in medically treated patients with coronary artery disease. *Am J Cardiol* 1984;53:18.
19. Bonow RO, Kent KM, Rosing DR, et al. Exercise-induced ischemia in mildly symptomatic patients with coronary artery disease and preserved left ventricular function: identification of subgroups at risk of death during medical therapy. *N Engl J Med* 1984;311:1339.
20. Weiner DA, Ryan TJ, McCabe CH, et al. Value of exercise testing in determining the risk classification and the response to coronary artery bypass grafting in three-vessel coronary artery disease: a report from the Coronary Artery Surgery Study (CASS) registry. *Am J Cardiol* 1987;60:262.
21. Mazzotta G, Bonow RO, Pace L, Brittian E, Epstein SE. Relation between exertional ischemia and prognosis in mildly symptomatic patients with single or double vessel coronary artery disease and left ventricular dysfunction at rest. *J Am Coll Cardiol* 1989;13:567–573.
22. Miller TD, Taliercio CP, Zinsmeister AR, Gibbons RJ. Risk stratification of single or double vessel coronary artery disease and impaired left ventricular function using exercise radionuclide angiography. *Am J Cardiol* 1990;65:1317–1321.
23. Lee KL, Pryor DB, Pieper KS, Harrell FE, Califf RM, Mark DB, Hlatky MA, Coleman RE, Cobb FR, Jones RH. Prognostic value of radionuclide angiography in medically treated patients with coronary artery disease: a comparison with clinical and catheterization variables. *Circulation* 1990;82: 1705–1717.
24. Miller TD, Christian TF, Taliercio CP, Zinsmeister AR, Gibbons RJ. Severe exercise-induced ischemia does not identify high risk patients with normal left ventricular function and one- or two-vessel coronary artery disease. *J Am Coll Cardiol* 1994;23:219–224.
25. Berman DS, Maddahi J, Garcia EV, et al. Assessment of left and right ventricular function with multiple gated equilibrium cardiac blood pool scintigraphy. *Clin Nucl Cardiol* 1981;224.
26. Steckley RA, Kronenberg MW, Born ML, et al. Radionuclide ventriculography: Evaluation of automated and visual methods for regional wall motion analysis. *Radiology* 1982; 142:179.
27. Vitale DF, Green MV, Bacharach SL, Bonow RO, Watson RM, Findley SL, Jones AE. Assessment of regional left ventricular function by sector analysis: a method for objective evaluation of radionuclide blood pool studies. *Am J Cardiol* 1983;52:1112–1119.
28. Dilsizian V, Perrone-Filardi P, Cannon RO, Freedman NMT, Bacharach SL, Bonow RO. Comparison of exercise radionuclide angiography with thallium SPECT imaging for detection of significant narrowing of the left circumflex coronary artery. *Am J Cardiol* 1991;68:320–328.
29. Strauss HW, Zaret BL, Hurley PJ, et al. A scintigraphic method for measuring left ventricular ejection fraction in man without cardiac catheterization. *Am J Cardiol* 1971;28:575.
30. Massie BM, Kramer BL, Gertz EW, Henderson SG. Radionuclide measurements of left ventricular volume: comparison of geometric and count based methods. *Circulation* 1982; 65:725.
31. Links JM, Becker LC, Shindledecker JG, et al. Measurement of absolute left ventricular volume from gated blood pool studies. *Circulation* 1982;65:82–90.
32. Nichols K, Adatepe MH, Isaacs GH, et al. A new scintigraphic method for determining left ventricular volumes. *Circulation* 1984;70:672.
33. Massardo T, Gal RA, Grenier RP, et al. Left ventricular volume calculation using a count-based ratio method applied to multigated radionuclide angiography. *J Nucl Med* 1990; 31:450.
34. Rigo P, Alderson PO, Robertson RM, et al. Measurement of aortic and mitral regurgitation by gated blood pool scans. *Circulation* 1979;60:306.
35. Urquhart J, Patterson RE, Packer M, et al. Quantification of valve regurgitation by radionuclide angiography before and after valve replacement surgery. *Am J Cardiol* 1981;47:287.
36. Lam W, Pavel D, Byrom E, et al. Radionuclide regurgitant index: value and limitation. *Am J Cardiol* 1981;47:292.
37. Fouad FM, Tarazi RC, Gallagher JH, et al. Abnormal left ventricular relaxation in hypertensive patients. *Clin Sci* 1980; 59:411S.
38. Fouad FM, Slominshi JM, Tarazi RC. Left ventricular diastolic function in hypertension: relation to left ventricular mass and systolic function. *J Am Coll Cardiol* 1984;3:1500.
39. Stewart S, Mason DT, Braunwald E. Impaired rate of left ventricular filling in idiopathic hypertrophic subaortic stenosis and valvular aortic stenosis. *Circulation* 1968;37:8.
40. Sanderson JE, Traill TA, St John Sutton MG, et al. Left

ventricular relaxation and filling in hypertrophic cardiomyopathy. *Br Heart J* 1978;40:596.
41. Tyberg TI, Goodyer AVN, Hurst JW, et al. Left ventricular filling in differentiating restrictive amyloid cardiomyopathy and constrictive pericarditis. *Am J Cardiol* 1981;47:791.
42. Fazio S, Cittadini A, Cuocolo A, et al. Impaired cardiac performance is a distinct feature of uncomplicated acromegaly. *J Clin Endocrinol Metab* 1994;79:441–446.
43. Bristow JD, Van Zee BE, Judkins MP. Systolic and diastolic abnormalities of the left ventricle in coronary artery disease. *Circulation* 1970;42:219.
44. Barry WH, Broomer JE, Alderman EL, Harrison DC. Changes in diastolic stiffness and tone of the left ventricle during angina pectoris. *Circulation* 1974;49:255.
45. Soufer R, Wohlgelernter D, Vita NA, et al. Intact systolic left ventricular function in clinical congestive heart failure. *Am J Cardiol* 1985;55:1032.
46. Wiggers CJ, Katz LN. The contour of the ventricular volume curve under different conditions. *Am J Physiol* 1922;58:439.
47. Hori M, Yellin EL, Sonnenblick EH. Left ventricular diastolic suction as a mechanism of ventricular filling. *Circulation* 1982;42:124.
48. Bacharach SL, Green MV, Borer JS. Left ventricular peak ejection rate, peak filling rate, and ejection fraction: frame rate requirements at rest and during exercise. *J Nucl Med* 1979;20:189.
49. Brutsaert DL, Housmans PR, Goethals MA. Dual control of relaxation: its role in the ventricular function in the mammalian heart. *Circ Res* 1980;47:637.
50. Bianco JA, Filiberti AW, Baker SP, et al. Ejection fraction and heart rate correlate with diastolic peak filling rate at rest and during exercise. *Chest* 1985;88:107.
51. Bacharach SL, Green MV, Bonow RO, Larson SM. Maximal filling rate during exercise: RR interval normalization, in: *Computers in Cardiology.* Long Beach CA, IEEE Computer Society, 1984, pp 207–210.
52. Bacharach SL, Green MV, Borer JS. Instrumentation and data processing in cardiovascular nuclear medicine: evaluation of ventricular function. *Semin Nucl Med* 1979;9:257–274.
53. Bonow RO, Bacharach SL, Crawford-Green C, Green MV. Influence of temporal smoothing on quantitation of left ventricular function by gated blood pool scintigraphy. *Am J Cardiol* 1989;64:921.
54. Scheuer J, Brachfeld N. Coronary insufficiency: relations between hemodynamic, electrical, and biochemical parameters. *Circ Res* 1966;18:178.
55. Upton MT, Rerych SK, Newman GE, Port S, Cobb FR, Jones RH. Detecting abnormalities in left ventricular function during exercise before angina and ST-segment depression. *Circulation* 1980;62:341–349.
56. Borer JS, Kent KM, Bacharach SL, et al. Sensitivity, specificity, and predictive accuracy of radionuclide cineangiography during exercise in patients with coronary artery disease. *Circulation* 1979;60:572.
57. Jones RH, McEwan P, Newman GE, et al. Accuracy of diagnosis of coronary artery disease by radionuclide measurement of left ventricular function during rest and exercise. *Circulation* 1981;64:586.
58. Rozanski A, Diamond GA, Berman D, et al. Declining specificity of exercise radionuclide ventriculography. *N Engl J Med* 1983;309:518.
59. Port S, Cobb FR, Coleman RE, et al. Effect of age on the response of the left ventricular ejection fractions to exercise. *N Engl J Med* 1980;303:1133.
60. Greenberg PS, Berge RD, Johnson KD, et al. The value and limitations of radionuclide angiocardiography with stress in women. *Clin Cardiol* 1983;6:312.
61. Brady TJ, Thrall JH, Lo K, et al. The importance of adequate exercise in the detection of coronary heart disease by radionuclide ventriculography. *J Nucl Med* 1980;2:1115.
62. Elkayam U, Weinstein M, Berman D, et al. Stress thallium-201 myocardial scintigraphy and exercise technetium ventriculography in the detection and location of chronic coronary artery disease: Comparison of sensitivity and specificity of these noninvasive tests alone and in combination. *Am Heart J* 1981;101:657.
63. Stone D, Dymond D, Elliot AT, et al. Exercise first-pass radionuclide ventriculography in detection of coronary artery disease. *Br Heart J* 1980;44:208.
64. Maddahi J, Berman DS, Matsuoka DT, et al. Right ventricular ejection fraction during exercise in normal subjects and in coronary artery disease patients: assessment by multiple-gated equilibrium scintigraphy. *Circulation* 1980;62:133.
65. Cates CU, Kronenberg MW, Collins HW, Sandler MP. Dipyridamole radionuclide ventriculography: A test with high specificity for severe coronary artery disease. *J Am Coll Cardiol* 1989;13:841–51.
66. Movahed A, Reeves WC, Rose GC, Wheeler WS, Jolly SR. Dobutamine and improvement of regional and global left ventricular function in coronary artery disease. *Am J Cardiol* 1990;65:375–377.
67. Freeman ML, Palac R, Mason J, et al. A comparison of dobutamine infusion and supine bicycle exercise for radionuclide cardiac stress testing. *Clin Nucl Med* 1984;9:251–255.
68. Mazeika PK, Nadazdin A, Oakley CM. Dobutamine stress echocardiography for detection and assessment of coronary artery disease. *J Am Coll Cardiol* 1992;19:1203–1211.
69. Hurwitz RA, Siddiqui A, Caldwell RL, Weetman RM, Girod DA. Assessment of ventricular function in infants and children: Response to dobutamine infusion. *Clin Nucl Med* 1990;15:556–559.
70. Humphries JO. Expected course of patients with coronary artery disease, in Rahimtoola SH (ed): *Coronary Bypass Surgery, Cardiovascular Clinics*, Vol. 8. Philadelphia, FA Davis Co., 1977, p 41.
71. Borer JS, Wallis J, Hochreiter C, Moses JW. Prognostic value of left ventricular dysfunction at rest and during exercise in patients with coronary artery disease. *Adv Cardiol* 1986; 34:179.
72. Iqbal A, Gibbson RJ, Zinsmeister AR, Mock AB, Ballard DJ. Prognostic value of exercise radionuclide angiography in a population-based cohort of patients with known or suspected coronary artery disease. *Am J Cardiol* 1994;74:119–124.
73. DePuey EG, Leatherman LL, Leachman RD, et al. Restenosis after transluminal coronary angioplasty detected with exercise gated radionuclide ventriculography. *J Am Coll Cardiol* 1984;4:1103.
74. O'Keefe JH, Lapeyre AC, Holmes DR, Gibbons RJ. Early radionuclide angiography identifies low risk patients for late restenosis after transluminal coronary angioplasty. *Am J Cardiol* 1988;61:51.
75. Morrison J, Coromilas J, Munsey D, et al. Correlation of radionuclide estimates of myocardial infarction size and release of creatine kinase MB in man. *Circulation* 1980;62: 277.
76. Rigo P, Murray M, Strauss HW, et al. Left ventricular function in acute myocardial infarction evaluated by gated scintiphotography. *Circulation* 1974;50:678.
77. Sanford CF, Corbett J, Nicod P, et al. Value of radionuclide ventriculography in the immediate characterization of patients with acute myocardial infarction. *Am J Cardiol* 1982;49:637.
78. Multicenter Postinfection Research Group: Risk stratification and survival after myocardial infarction. *N Engl J Med* 1983;309:331.

79. Morris KG, Palmeri ST, Califf RM, et al. Value of radionuclide angiography for predicting specific cardiac events after acute myocardial infarction. *Am J Cardiol* 1985;55:318.
80. Schelbert HR, Henning H, Ashburn WL, et al. Serial measurements of left ventricular ejection fraction by radionuclide angiography early and late after myocardial infarction. *Am J Cardiol* 1976;38:407.
81. Sheehan FH, Doerr R, Schmidt WG, et al. Early recovery of left ventricular function after thrombolytic therapy for acute myocardial infarction: An important determinant of survival. *J Am Coll Cardiol* 1988;12:289.
82. Schmidt WG, Sheehan FH, von Essen R, et al. Evolution of left ventricular function after intracoronary thrombolysis for acute myocardial infarction. *Am J Cardiol* 1989;63:497.
83. Pfeffer MA, Braunwald E, Moye LA, et al. Effect of captopril on mortality and morbidity in patients with left ventricular dysfunction after myocardial infarction. Results of the Survival and Ventricular Enlargement Trial. *N Engl J Med* 1992;327:669.
84. Dell'Italia LJ, Starling MR, Crawford MH, et al. Right ventricular infarction: Identification by hemodynamic measurements before and after volume loading and correlation with noninvasive techniques. *J Am Coll Cardiol* 1984;4:931.
85. Cabin HS, Clubb KS, Wackers FJ, et al. Right ventricular myocardial infarction with anterior wall left ventricular infarction: An autopsy study. *Am Heart J* 1987;113:16.
86. Schuler G, Hoffmann M, Schwarz F, et al. Effect of successful thrombolytic therapy on right ventricular function in acute inferior wall myocardial infarction. *Am J Cardiol* 1984; 54:951.
87. Verani MS, Tortoledo FE, Batty JW, et al. Effect of coronary artery recanalization on right ventricular function in patients with acute myocardial infarction. *J Am Coll Cardiol* 1985; 5:1029.
88. Yamagishi T, Ozaki M, Kumada T, et al. Asynchronous left ventricular diastolic filling in patients with isolated disease of the left anterior descending coronary artery: assessment with radionuclide ventriculography. *Circulation* 1984;69:933.
89. Polak JF, Kemper AJ, Bianco JA, Parisi AF, Tow DE. Resting early peak diastolic filling rates: a sensitive index of myocardial dysfunction in patients with coronary artery disease. *J Nucl Med* 1982;23:471.
90. Bonow RO, Leon MB, Rosing DR, et al. Effects of verapamil and propranolol on left ventricular systolic function and diastolic filling in patients with coronary artery disease: radionuclide angiographic studies at rest and during exercise. *Circulation* 1981;65:1337.
91. Bonow RO, Kent KM, Rosing DR, et al. Improved left ventricular diastolic filling in patients with coronary artery disease after percutaneous transluminal coronary angioplasty. *Circulation* 1982;66:1159.
92. Bonow RO, Vitale DF, Bacharach SL, et al. Asynchronous left ventricular regional function and impaired global diastolic filling in patients with coronary artery disease: reversal after coronary angioplasty. *Circulation* 1985;71:297.
93. Reduto LA, Wichemyer WJ, Young JB, et al. Left ventricular diastolic performance in patients with coronary artery disease: assessment with first pass radionuclide angiography. *Circulation* 1981;63:1228.
94. Gerstenblith G, Fredericksen J, Yin FCP, et al. Echocardiographic assessment of a normal aging population. *Circulation* 1977;56:273.
95. Miller TR, Grossman SJ, Schechtman KB, et al. Left ventricular diastolic filling and its association with age. *Am J Cardiol* 1986;58:531.
96. Bonow RO, Vitale DF, Bacharach SL, Maron BJ, Green MV. Effects of aging on asynchronous left ventricular regional function and global ventricular filling in normal human subjects. *J Am Coll Cardiol* 1988;11:50.
97. Arrighi JA, Dilsizian V, Perrone-Filardi P, Diodati JG, Bacharach SL, Bonow RO. Improvement of the age-related impairment in left ventricular diastolic filling with verapamil in the normal human heart. *Circulation* 1994;90:213–219.
98. Levy WC, Cerquira MD, Abrass IB, Schwartz RS, Stratton JR. Endurance exercise training augments diastolic filling at rest and during exercise in healthy young and older men. *Circulation* 1993;88:116–126.
99. Ehsani AA, Ogawa T, Miller TR, Spina RJ, Jilka SM. Exercise training improves left ventricular systolic function in older men. *Circulation* 1991;83:96–103.
100. Dilsizian V, Rocco TP, Bonow RO, Fischman AJ, Boucher CA, Strauss HW. Cardiac blood pool imaging II: Applications in noncoronary heart disease. *J Nucl Med* 1990;31:10–22.
101. Ross J. Afterload mismatch and peload reserve: a conceptual framework for the analysis of ventricular function. *Prog Cardiovas Dis* 1976;18:255.
102. McCullagh WH, Covell JW, Ross J. Left ventricular dilatation and diastolic compliance changes during chronic volume overloading. *Circulation* 1972;45:943.
103. Ross J, McCullagh WH. Nature of enhanced performance of the dilated left ventricle in the during chronic volume overloading. *Circ Res* 1972;30:549.
104. Kennedy JW, Doces J, Steward DK. Left ventricular function before and following aortic valve replacement. *Circulation* 1977;31:944.
105. O'Toole JD, Geiser EA, Reddy S, et al. Effect of preoperative ejection fraction on survival and hemodynamic improvement following aortic valve replacement. *Circulation* 1978;58: 1175.
106. Clark DG, McAnulty JH, Rahimtoola SH. Valve replacement in aortic insufficiency with left ventricular dysfunction. *Circulation* 1980;61:411.
107. Fischi SJ, Gorlin R, Herman MV. Cardiac shape and function in aortic valve disease: physiologic and clinical implications. *Am J Cardiol* 1977;39:170.
108. Ross J, Sonnenblick EH, Taylor RP, Covell JW. Diastolic geometry and sarcomere lengths in the chronically dilated canine left ventricle. *Circ Res* 1971;28:49.
109. Maron BJ, Ferrans VJ, Roberts WC. Myocardial ultrastructure in patients with chronic aortic valve disease. *Am J Cardiol* 1975;35:725.
110. Pichard AD, Gorlin R, Smith H, et al. Coronary flow studies in patients with left ventricular hypertrophy of the hypertensive type. Evidence for impaired coronary vascular reserve. *Am J Cardiol* 1981;47:547.
111. Strauer BE. Myocardial oxygen consumption and chronic heart disease: role of wall stress, hypertrophy and coronary reserve. *Am J Cardiol* 1979;44:730.
112. Grossman W, Jones D, McLauren LP. Wall stress and patterns of hypertrophy in the human left ventricle. *J Clin Invest* 1975;56:56.
113. Cohn PF, Gorlin R, Cohn LH, Collins JJ. Left ventricular ejection fraction as a prognostic guide in surgical treatment of coronary and valvular heart disease. *Am J Cardiol* 1974;34:136.
114. Copeland JG, Griepp RB, Stinson EB, Shumway NE. Long-term follow-up after isolated aortic valve replacement. *J Thorac Cardiovasc Surg* 1977;74:875.
115. Forman R, Firth BG, Barnard MS. Prognostic significance of preoperative left ventricular ejection fraction and valve lesion in patients with aortic valve replacement. *Am J Cardiol* 1980;45:1120.
116. Greves J, Rahimtoola SH, McAnulty JH, et al. Preoperative criteria predictive of late survival following valve replacement for severe aortic regurgitation. *Am Heart J* 1981;101:300.

117. Henry WL, Bonow RO, Borer JS, et al. Observations on the optimum time for operative intervention for aortic regurgitation. I. Evaluation of the results of aortic valve replacement in symptomatic patients. *Circulation* 1980;61:471.
118. Cunha CLP, Giuliani ER, Fuster V, et al. Preoperative M-mode echocardiography as a predictor of surgical results in chronic aortic insufficiency. *J Thorac Cardiovasc Surg* 1980; 79:256.
119. Boucher CA, Bingham JB, Osbakken MD, et al. Early changes in left ventricular size and function after correction of left ventricular volume overload. *Am J Cardiol* 1981; 47:991.
120. Bonow RO, Rosing DR, Maron BJ, et al. Reversal of left ventricular dysfunction after aortic valve replacement for chronic aortic regurgitation: Influence of duration of preoperative left ventricular dysfunction. *Circulation* 1984;70:570.
121. Bonow RO, Picone AL, McIntosh CL, et al. Survival and functional results after valve replacement for aortic regurgitation from 1976 to 1983: impact of preoperative left ventricular function. *Circulation* 1985;72:1244.
122. Bonow RO, Rosing DR, Kent KM, Epstein SE. Timing of operation for chronic aortic regurgitation. *Am J Cardiol* 1982;50:325.
123. Bonow RO, Rosing DR, McIntosh CL, et al. The natural history of asymptomatic patients with aortic regurgitation and normal left ventricular function. *Circulation* 1983;68:509.
124. Borer JS, Bacharach SL, Green MV, et al. Exercise-induced left ventricular dysfunction in symptomatic and asymptomatic patients with aortic regurgitation: assessment with radionuclide cineangiography. *Am J Cardiol* 1978;42:351.
125. Steingart RM, Yee C, Weinstein L, et al. Radionuclide ventriculographic study of adaptations to exercise in aortic regurgitation. *Am J Cardiol* 1983;51:483.
126. Borer JS, Rosing DR, Kent KM, et al. Left ventricular function at rest and during exercise after aortic valve replacement in patients with aortic regurgitation. *Am J Cardiol* 1979; 44:1297.
127. Kawinishi DT, McKay CR, Chandraratna AN, et al. Cardiovascular responses to dynamic exercise in patients with chronic symptomatic mild-to-moderate and severe aortic regurgitation. *Circulation* 1986;73:62.
128. Boucher CA, Bingham JB, Osbakken MD, et al. Early changes in left ventricular size and function after correction of left ventricular volume overload. *Am J Cardiol* 1981;47:991.
129. Iskandrian AS, Hakki AH, Kane SA, et al. Left ventricular pressure-volume relationship in aortic regurgitation. *Am Heart J* 1985;110:1026.
130. Bonow RO, Dodd JT, Maron BJ, et al. Long-term serial changes in left ventricular function and reversal of ventricular dilatation after valve replacement for chronic aortic regurgitation. *Circulation* 1988;78:1108.
131. Zile MR, GaaschWH, Carroll JD, et al. Chronic mitral regurgitation: Predictive value of preoperative echocardiographic indexes of left ventricular function and wall stress. *J Am Coll Cardiol* 1984;3:235–42.
132. Berko B, Gaasch WH, Tanigawa N, et al. Disparity between ejection and end-systolic indexes of left ventricular contractility in mitral regurgitation. Circulation 1987;75:1310–19.
133. Hochreiter C, Niles N, Devereux RB, et al. Mitral regurgitation: relationship of noninvasive descriptors of right and left ventricular performance to clinical and hemodynamic findings and to prognosis in medically and surgically treated patients. *Circulation* 1986;73:900.
134. Phillips HR, Levine FH, Cartes JE, et al. Mitral valve replacement for isolated mitral regurgitation: analysis of clinical course and late postoperative left ventricular ejection fraction. *Am J Cardiol* 1981;48:647.
135. Schuler G, Peterson KL, Johnson A, et al. Temporal response of left ventricular performance to mitral valve surgery. *Circulation* 1979;59:1218–31.
136. Lavine SJ, Follansbee WP, Schreiner DP, Amidi M. Left ventricular diastolic filling in valvular aortic stenosis. *Am J Cardiol* 1986;57:1349–53.
137. Clyne CC, Arrighi JA, Maron BJ, Dilsizian V, Bonow RO, Cannon RO. Systemic and left ventricular responses to exercise stress in asymptomatic patients with valvular aortic stenosis. *Am J Cardiol* 1991;68:1469–1476.
138. Smith N, McAnulty JH, Rahimtoola SH. Severe aortic stenosis with impaired left ventricular function and clinical heart failure: Results of valve replacement. *Circulation* 1978; 58:255–64.
139. Redicker DE, Boucher CA, Block PC, et al. Degree of reversibility of left ventricular systolic dysfunction after aortic valve replacement for isolated aortic stenosis. *Am J Cardiol* 1987;60:112–18.
140. Kelly TA, Rothbart RM, Cooper CM, et al. Comparison of outcome of asymptomatic to symptomatic patients older than 20 years of age with valvular aortic stenosis. *Am J Cardiol* 1988;61:123.
141. Milanes JC, Paldi J, Romero M, Goodwin D, Hultgren HN. Detection of coronary artery disease in aortic stenosis by exercise gated nuclear angiography. *Am J Cardiol* 1984; 54:787–791.
142. Heller SJ, Carleton RA. Abnormal left ventricular contraction in patients with mitral stenosis. *Circulation* 1970;42: 1099–1110.
143. Morise AP, Goodwin C. Exercise radionuclide angiography in patients with mitral stenosis: Value of right ventricular response. *Am Heart J* 1986;112:509–13.
144. Dilsizian V, Rocco TP, Palacios IF, Strauss HW, Boucher CA. Enhanced right ventricular exercise performance following percutaneous balloon valvotomy in patients with severe mitral stenosis. *J Nucl Med* 1988;29:945A (abstract).
145. Greenberg JM, Murphy JH, Okada RD, et al. Value and limitations of radionuclide angiography in determining the cause of reduced left ventricular ejection fraction: comparison of idiopathic dilated cardiomyopathy and coronary artery disease. *Am J Cardiol* 1985;55:541.
146. Greenberg JM, Murphy JH, Okada RD, et al. Value and limitations of radionuclide angiography in determining the cause of reduced left ventricular ejection fraction: Comparison of idiopathic dilated cardiomyopathy and coronary artery disease. *Am J Cardiol* 1985;55:541.
147. Bulkley BH, Hutchins GM, Bailey IK, et al. Thallium-201 imaging and gated blood pool scans in patients with ischemic and idiopathic congestive cardiomyopathy. *Circulation* 1977; 55:753.
148. Franciosa JA, Wilen M, Ziesche S, et al. Survival in men with severe chronic left ventricular failure due to either coronary heart disease or idiopathic dilated cardiomyopathy. *Am J Cardiol* 1983;51:831.
149. Hofmann T, Meinertz T, Kasper W, Geibel A, Zehender M, Hohnloser S: Mode of death in idiopathic dilated cardiomyopathy: A multivariate analysis of prognostic determinants. *Am Heart J* 1988;116:1455–1463.
150. Franciosa JA, Park M, Levine TB. Lack of correlation between exercise capacity and indexes of resting left ventricular performance in heart failure. *Am J Cardiol* 1981; 47:33.
151. Colucci WS, Wynne J, Holman BL, et al. Long-term therapy of heart failure with prazosin: a randomized double blind trial. *Am J Cardiol* 1980;45:337.
152. LeJemtel TH, Keung E, Ribner HS, et al. Sustained beneficial effects of oral amrinone on cardiac and renal function in

patients with severe congestive heart failure. *Am J Cardiol* 1980;45:123.

153. Dzau VJ, Colucci WS, Williams GH, et al. Sustained effectiveness of converting-enzyme inhibition in patients with severe congestive heart failure. *N Engl J Med* 1980;302:1373.
154. Arnold SB, Byrd RC, Meister W, et al. Long-term digitalis therapy improves left ventricular function in heart failure. *N Engl J Med* 1980;303:1443.
155. Goldberg MJ, Franklin BA, Rubenfire M, et al. Hydralazine therapy in severe chronic heart failure: inability of radionuclide left ventricular ejection fraction measurement to predict the hemodynamic response. *J Am Coll Cardiol* 1983; 2:887.
156. Firth BG, Dehmer GJ, Markham RV, et al. Assessment of vasodilator therapy in patients with severe congestive heart failure: limitations of measurements of left ventricular ejection fraction and volumes. *Am J Cardiol* 1982;50:954.
157. Pouleur H, Rosseau MF, van Eyll C, et al. Effects of long-term enalapril therapy on left ventricular diastolic properties in patients with depressed ejection fraction: SOLVD Investigators. *Circulation* 1993;88:481–491.
158. Narahara KA. Spontaneous variability of ventricular function in patients with chronic heart failure: The Western enoximone study group and the REFLECT investigators. *Am J Med* 1993;95:513–518.
159. Semigran MJ, Thaik CM, Fifer MA, Boucher CA, Palacios IF, Dec GW. Exercise capacity and systolic and diastolic ventricular function after recovery from acute dilated cardiomyopathy. *J Am Coll Cardiol* 1994;24:462–470.
160. Charron M, Follansbee W, Ziady GM, Kormos RL. Assessment of biventricular cardiac function in patients with a Novocor left ventricular assist device. *J Heart Lung Transplant* 1994;13:263–267.
161. Verani MS, Nishimura S, Mahmarian JJ, Hays JT, Young JB. Cardiac function after orthotopic heart transplantation: Response to postural changes, exercise, and beta-adrenergic blockade. *J Heart Lung Transplant* 1994;13:181–193.
162. Greene HL, Reich SD, Dalen JE. How to minimize doxorubicin toxicity. *J Cardiovasc Med* 1982;7:306.
163. Merrill J, Greco FA, Zimbler H, et al. Adriamycin and radiation: synergystic cardiotoxicity. *Ann Intern Med* 1975;85:122.
164. Alexander J, Dainiak N, Berger HJ, et al. Serial assessment of doxorubicin cardiotoxicity with quantitative radionuclide angiocardiography. *N Engl J Med* 1979;300:278.
165. Gottdiener JS, Mathisen DJ, Borer JS, et al. Doxorubicin cardiotoxicity: assessment of late left ventricular dysfunction by radionuclide cineangiography. *Ann Intern Med* 1981; 94:430.
166. Palmeri ST, Bonow RO, Myers CE, et al. Prospective evaluation of doxorubicin cardiotoxicity by rest and exercise radionuclide angiography. *Am J Cardiol* 1986;58:607.
167. Schwartz RG, McKenzie WB, Alexander J, et al. Congestive heart failure and left ventricular dysfunction complicating doxorubicin therapy. *Am J Med* 1987;82:1109–18.
168. Pouleur H, Rousseau MF, Van Eyll C, et al. Force-velocity-length relations in hypertrophic cardiomyopathy: evidence of normal or depressed myocardial contractility. *Am J Cardiol* 1983;52:813.
169. Gaasch WH, Levine HJ, Quinones MA, Alexander JK. Left ventricular compliance: mechanisms and clinical implications. *Am J Cardiol* 1976;38:645–53.
170. Sanderson JE, Gibson DG, Brown DJ, Goodwin JF. Left ventricular filling in hypertrophic cardiomyopathy: an angiographic study. *Br Heart J* 1977;39:661–70.
171. Alvares RF, Shaver JA, Gamble WH, Goodwin JF. Isovolumic relaxation period in hypertrophic cardiomyopathy. *J Am Coll Cardiol* 1984;3:71–81.
172. Betocchi S, Bonow RO, Bacharach SL, Rosing DR, Maron BJ, Green MV. Isovolumic relaxation period in hypertrophic cardiomyopathy: assessment by radionuclide angiography. *J Am Coll Cardiol* 1986;7:74–81.
173. Goodwin JF, Hollman A, Cleland WP, Teare D. Obstructive cardiomyopathy simulating aortic stenosis. *Br Heart J* 1960; 22:403–14.
174. Wigle ED, Heimbecker RO, Gunton RW. Idiopathic ventricular septal hypertrophy causing muscular subaortic stenosis. *Circulation* 1962;26:325–40.
175. Braunwald E, Lambrew CT, Rockoff SD, Ross J Jr, Morrow AG. Idiopathic hypertrophic subaortic stenosis: I. A description of the disease based upon an analysis of 64 patients. *Circulation* 1964;30(Suppl 4):IV-3–IV-19.
176. Jarcho JA, McKenna W, Pare JAP, Solomon SD, Levi T, Donis-Keller H, Seidman JG, Seidman CE. Mapping a gene for familial hypertrophic cardiomyopathy to chromosome 14ql. *N Engl J Med* 1990;321:1372–1378.
177. Solomon SC, Jarcho JA, McKenna W, Geisterfer-Lowrance A, Germain R, Salerni R, Seidman JH, Seidman CE. Familial hypertrophic cardiomyopathy is a genetically heterogenous disease. *J Clin Invest* 1990;86:993–999.
178. Hejtmancik JF, Brink PA, Towbin J, Hill R, Brink L, Tapscott T, Trakhtenbroit A, Roberts R. Localization of gene for familial hypertrophic cardiomyopathy to chromosome 14a1 in a diverse US population. *Circulation* 1991;83:1592–1597.
179. Epstein ND, Cohn GM, Cyran F, Fananapazir L. Differences in clinical expression of hypertrophic cardiomyopathy associated with two distinct mutations in the β-myosin heavy chain gene: a 908*Leu*→*Val* mutation and a 403*Arg*→*Gln* mutation. *Circulation* 1992;86:345–352.
180. Thierfelder L, MacRae C, Watkins H, Tomfohrde J, Williams M, McKenna W, Bohm K, Noeske G, Schlepper M, Bowcock A, Vosberg H-P, Seidman JG, Seidman C. A familial hypertrophic cardiomyopathy locus maps to chromosome 15q2. *Proc Natl Acad Sci, USA* 1993;90:6270–6274.
181. Ciro E, Maron BJ, Bonow RO, et al. Relation between marked changes in outflow tract gradient and disease progression in patients with hypertrophic cardiomyopathy. *Am J Cardiol* 1984;53:1103.
182. Sanderson JE, Gibson DG, Brown DJ, Goodwin JF. Left ventricular filling in hypertrophic cardiomyopathy: an angiographic study. *Br Heart J* 1977;39:661.
183. Bonow RO, Rosing DR, Bacharach SL, et al. Effect of verapamil on left ventricular systolic function and diastolic filling in patients with hypertrophic cardiomyopathy. *Circulation* 1981;64:787.
184. Bonow RO, Ostrow HG, Rosing DR, Cannon RO, Lipson LC, Maron BJ, Kent KM, Bacharach SL, Green MV. Effects of verapamil on left ventricular systolic and diastolic function in patients with hypertrophic cardiomyopathy: pressure-volume analysis with a nonimaging scintillation probe. *Circulation* 1983;68:1062–1073.
185. Bonow RO, Dilsizian V, Rosing DR, et al. Verapmil-induced improvement in left ventricular diastolic filling and increased exercise tolerance in patients with hypertrophic cardiomyopathy: short- and long-term effects. *Circulation* 1985;72:853.
186. Hanrath P, Schluter M, Sonntag F, Diemert J, Bleifeld W. Influence of verapamil therapy on left ventricular performance at rest and during exercise in hypertrophic cardiomyopathy. *Am J Cardiol* 1983;52:544.
187. Aroney CN, Ruddy TD, Dighero H, et al. Differentiation of restrictive cardiomyopathy from pericardial constriction: Assessment of diastolic function by radionuclide angiography. *J Am Coll Cardiol* 1989;13:1007.
188. Marin-Neto JA, Marzullo P, Sousa AC, et al. Radionuclide angiographic evidence for early predominant right ventricular

involvement in patients with Chagas' disease. *Can J Cardiol* 1988;4:231.

189. Sasayama S, Ross J, Franklin D, et al. Adaptation of the left ventricle to chronic pressure overload. *Circulation Res* 1976;38:172.
190. Pfeffer MA, Pfeffer JM, Frolich ED. Pumping ability of the hypertrophying left ventricle of the spontaneously hypertensive rat. *Circulation Res* 1976;38:423.
191. Gottdiener JS, Brown J, Zoltick J, Fletcher RD. Left ventricular pressure in men with normal blood pressure: Relation to exaggerated blood pressure response to exercise. *Ann Intern Med* 1990;112:161–6.
192. Devereux RB. Does increased blood pressure cause left ventricular hypertrophy or vice versa? *Ann Intern Med* 1990; 112:157–9.
193. Karliner JS, Williams D, Gorwit J, et al. Left ventricular performance in patients with left ventricular hypertrophy caused by systemic arterial hypertension. *Br Heart J* 1976;39:1239.
194. Savage DD, Drayer JIM, Henry WL, et al. Echocardiographic assessment of cardiac anatomy and function in hypertensive subjects. *Circulation* 1979;49:623.
195. Guazzi M, Fiorentine C, Olivari MT, Polese A. Cardiac load and function in hypertensive subjects. *Am J Cardiol* 1979; 44:1007.
196. Topol EJ, Traill TA, Fortuin NJ. Hypertensive hypertrophic cardiomyopathy of the elderly. *N Engl J Med* 1985;312:277.
197. Miller DD, Ruddy TD, Zusman RM, et al. Left ventricular ejection fraction response during exercise in asymptomatic systemic hypertension. *Am J Cardiol* 1987;59:409.
198. Wasserman AG, Katz RJ, Varghese PJ, et al. Exercise radionuclide ventriculographic response in hypertensive patients with chest pain. *N Engl J Med* 1984;311:1276.
199. Cuocolo A, Sax FL, Brush JE, Maron BJ, Bacharach SL, Bonow RO. Left ventricular hypertrophy and impaired diastolic filling in essential hypertension: diastolic mechanisms for systolic dysfunction during exercise. *Circulation* 1990; 81:978.
200. Inouye I, Massie B, Loge D, et al. Abnormal left ventricular filling: an early finding in mild to moderate systemic hypertension. *Am J Cardiol* 1985;53:120.
201. Smith VE, White WB, Meeran MK, Karimeddini MK. Improved left ventricular filling accompanies reduced left ventricular mass during therapy of essential hypertension. *J Am Coll Cardiol* 1986;8:1449.
202. Dougherty AH, Naccarelli GV, Gray EL, Hicks CH, Goldstein RA. Congestive heart failure with normal systolic function. *Am J Cardiol* 1984;54:778.
203. Setaro JF, Zaret BL, Schulman DS, Black HR, Soufer R. Usefulness of verapamil for congestive heart failure associated with abnormal left ventricular diastolic filling and normal left ventricular systolic performance. *Am J Cardiol* 1990; 66:981.
204. Nusynowitz ML, Benedetto AR, Walsh RA, Starling MR. First-pass anger camera radiocardiography: biventricular ejection fraction, flow, and volume measurements. *J Nucl Med* 1987;28:950–959.
205. Dell'Italia LJ, Starling MR, Walsh RA, et al. Validation of attenuation-corrected equilibrium radionuclide angiographic determinations for right ventricular volume: Comparison with cast-validated biplane cineventriculography. *Circulation* 1985;72:317.
206. Parrish MD, Graham TP, Born ML, et al. Radionuclide ventriculography for assessment of absolute right and left ventricular volumes in children. *Circulation* 1982;66:811.
207. Dehmer GJ, Firth BG, Hillis LD, et al. Nongeometric determination of right ventricular volumes from equilibrium blood pool scans. *Am J Cardiol* 1982;49:78.
208. Tobinick E, Schelbert HR, Henning M, et al. Right ventricular ejection fraction in patients with acute anterior and inferior myocardial infarction assessed by radionuclide angiography. *Circulation* 1978;57:1078.
209. Maddahi J, Berman DS, Matsuoka DT, et al. A new technique for assessing right ventricular ejection fraction using rapid multiple-gated equilibrium cardiac blood pool scintigraphy. *Circulation* 1979;60:581.
210. Berger HJ, Johnstone DE, Sands JM, et al. Response of right ventricular ejection fraction to upright bicycle exercise in coronary artery disease. *Circulation* 1979;60:1292.
211. Maddahi J, Berman DS, Matsuoka DT, et al. Right ventricular ejection fraction during exercise in normal subjects and in coronary artery disease patients: Assessment by multiple-gated equilibrium scintigraphy. *Circulation* 1980;62:133.
212. Johnson LL, McCarthy DM, Sciarra RR, et al. Right ventricular ejection fraction during exercise in patients with coronary artery disease. *Circulation* 1979;60:1284.
213. Starling MR, Dell'Italia LJ, Chaudhuri TK, et al. First transit and equilibrium radionuclide angiography in patients with inferior transmural myocardial infarction: Criteria for the diagnosis of associated hemodynamically significant right ventricular infarction. *J Am Coll Cardiol* 1984;4:923.
214. Steele P, Kirch D, Ellis J, et al. Prompt return to normal of depressed right ventricular ejection fraction in acute inferior infarction. *Br Heart J* 1977;39:1319.
215. Marmor A, Geltman EM, Biello DR, et al. Functional response of the right ventricle to myocardial infarction: Dependence on the site of left ventricular infarction. *Circulation* 1981;64:1005.
216. Polak JF, Holman BL, Wynne J, et al. Right ventricular ejection fraction: An indicator of increased mortality in patients with congestive heart failure associated with coronary artery disease. *J Am Coll Cardiol* 1983;2:217.
217. Konstam MA, Cohen SR, Salem DN, et al. Comparison of left and right ventricular end-systolic pressure-volume relations in congestive heart failure. *J Am Coll Cardiol* 1985;5:1326.
218. Baker BJ, Wilen MM, Boyd CM, et al. Relation of right ventricular ejection fraction to exercise capacity in chronic left ventricular failure. *Am J Cardiol* 1984;54:596.
219. Berger HJ, Matthay RA, Loke J, et al. Assessment of cardiac performance with quantitative radionuclide angiography: right ventricular ejection fraction with reference to findings in chronic obstructive pulmonary disease. *Am J Cardiol* 1978;41:897.
220. Renzetti AD, McClement JH, Litt BD: The Veterans Administration Cooperative Study of Pulmonary Function. Mortality in relation to respiratory function in chronic obstructive pulmonary disease. *Am J Med* 1966;41:115.
221. Matthay RA, Berger HJ, Davies RA, et al. Right and left ventricular exercise performance in chronic obstructive pulmonary disease: Radionuclide assessment. *Ann Intern Med* 1980;93:234.
222. Mathur PN, Powles ACP, Pugsley SO, et al. Effect of digoxin on right ventricular function in severe chronic airflow obstruction. *Ann Intern Med* 1981;95:283.
223. Matthay RA, Berger HJ, Loke J, et al. Effects of aminophylline upon right and left ventricular performance in chronic obstructive pulmonary disease: Noninvasive assessment by radionuclide angiocardiography. *Am J Med* 1978;65:903.
224. Olvey SK, Reduto LA, Stevens PM, et al. First pass radionuclide assessment of right and left ventricular ejection fraction in chronic pulmonary disease: Effect of oxygen upon exercise response. *Chest* 1980;78:4.
225. Brent BN, Berger HJ, Mathay RA, et al. Contrasting acute effects of vasodilators (nitroglycerin, nitroprusside, and hydralazine) on right ventricular performance in patients with

chronic obstructive pulmonary disease and pulmonary hypertension: A combined radionuclide-hemodynamic study. *Am J Cardiol* 1983;51:1682.

226. Winzelberg GG, Boucher CA, Pohost GM, et al. Right ventricular function in aortic and mitral valve disease. *Chest* 1981;79:520.
227. Konstam MA, Idoine J, Wynne J, et al. Right ventricular function in adults with pulmonary hypertension with and without atrial septal defect. *Am J Cardiol* 1983;51:1144.
228. Manyari DE, Duff HJ, Kostuk WJ, et al. Usefulness of noninvasive studies for diagnosis of right ventricular dysplasia. *Am J Cardiol* 1986;57:1147.
229. Hung GJ, Goris ML, Nash E, et al. Comparative value of maximal treadmill testing, exercise thallium myocardial perfusion scintigraphy and exercise radionuclide ventriculography for distinguishing high and low risk patients soon after myocardial infarction. *Am J Cardiol* 1984;53:1221.
230. Wilson RA, Sullivan PJ, Moore RH, et al. An ambulatory ventricular function monitor: Validation and preliminary clinical results. *Am J Cardiol* 1983;52:601.
231. Tamaki N, Yasuda T, Moore RH, et al. Continuous monitoring of left ventricular function by an ambulatory radionuclide detector in patients with coronary artery disease. *J Am Coll Cardiol* 1988;12:669.
232. Yang L, Bairey CN, Rozanski A, et al. Validation of the ambulatory ventricular function (VEST) for measuring exercise left ventricular ejection fraction. *J Nucl Med* 1988; 29:741.
233. Pace L, Cuocolo A, Nappi A, Nicolai E, Trimarco B, Salvatore M. Accuracy and repeatability of left ventricular systolic and diastolic function measurements using ambulatory radionuclide monitor. *Eur J Nucl Med* 1992;19:800–806.
234. Pace L, Cuocolo A, Stefano ML, et al. Left ventricular systolic and diastolic function measurements using an ambulatory radionuclide monitor: Effects of different time averaging on accuracy. *J Nucl Med* 1993;34:1602–1606.
235. Kayden DS, Wackers FJ, Zaret BL: Silent left ventricular dysfunction during routine activity following thrombolytic therapy for acute myocardial infarction. *J Am Coll Cardiol* 1990;15:1500.
236. Mohuiddin IH, Kambara H, Ohkusa T, et al. Clinical evaluation of cardiac function by ambulatory ventricular scintigraphic monitoring (VEST): Validation and study of the effects of nitroglycerin and nifedipine in patients with and without coronary artery disease. *Am Heart J* 1992;123: 386–394.
237. Burg MM, Jain D, Soufer S, Kerns RD, Zaret BL: Role of behavioral and psychological factors in mental stress-induced silent left ventricular dysfunction in coronary artery disease. *J Am Coll Cardiol* 1993;22:440–448.
238. Vassiliadis IV, Machac J, Sharma A, Horowtiz SF, Goldsmith SJ: Detection of silent left ventricular dysfunction during daily activities in coronary artery disease patients by the nuclear VEST. *J Nucl Biol Med* 1993;37:198–206.
239. Zaret BL, Wackers FJ. Radionuclide methods for evaluating the results of thrombolytic therapy. *Circulation* 1987; 76(suppl II):8–16.
240. Starling MR, Walsh RA, Lasher JC, et al. Quantification of left ventricular regional dyssynergy by radionuclide angiography. *J Nucl Med* 1987;28:1725–1735.
241. Wackers FJ, Terrin ML, Kayden DS, et al. Quantitative radionuclide assessment of regional ventricular function after thrombolytic therapy for acute myocardial infarction: Results of phase 1 thrombolysis in myocardial infarction (TIMI) trial. *J Am Coll Cardiol* 1989;13:998–1005.
242. Corbett JR, Jansen DE, Lewis SE, et al. Tomographic blood pool radionuclide ventriculography: Analysis of wall motion and left ventricular volumes in patients with coronary artery disease. *J Am Coll Cardiol* 1985;6:349–358.
243. Nohara R, Kambara H, Suzuki Y, Tamaki S, Kadota K, Kawai C, Tamaki N, Torizuka K. Stress scintigraphy using single-photon emission computed tomography in the evaluation of coronary artery disease. *Am J Cardiol* 1984;53:1250–1254.
244. Tamaki N, Yonekura Y, Mukai T, Fujita T, Nohara R, Kadota K, Kambara H, Kawai C, Torizuka K, Ishii Y. Segmental analysis of stress thallium myocardial emission tomography for localization of coronary artery disease. *Eur J Nucl Med* 1984;9:99–105.
245. Fintel DJ, Links JM, Brinker JA, Frank TL, Parker M, Becker LC. Improved diagnostic performance of exercise thallium-201 single photon emission computed tomography over planar imaging in the diagnosis of coronary artery disease: A receiver operating characteristic analysis. *J Am Coll Cardiol* 1989;13(3):600–612.
246. Stadius ML, Williams DL, Harp G, Cerqueira M, Caldwell JH, Stratton JR, Ritchie JL. Left ventricular volume determination using single photon emission computed tomography. *Am J Cardiol* 1985;55:1185–1191.
247. Gill JB, Moore RH, Tamaki N, et al. Multigated blood-pool tomography: New methods for the assessment of left ventricular function. *J Nucl Med* 1986;27:1916–1924.
248. Faber TL, Stokely EM, Templeton GH, et al. Quantification of three dimensional left ventricular segmental wall motion and volumes from gated tomographic radionuclide angiograms. *J Nucl Med* 1989;30:638–649.
249. Honda N, Machida K, Takishima T, et al. Cinematic three-dimensional surface display of cardiac blood pool tomography. *Clin Nucl Med* 1991;16:87–91.
250. Cerqueira MD, Harp GD, Ritchie JL. Quantitative gated blood pool tomographic assessment of regional ejection fraction: Definition of normal limits. *J Am Coll Cardiol* 1992; 20:934–941.
251. Metcalfe MJ, Norton MY, Jennings K, Walton S. Improved detection of abnormal left ventricular wall motion using tomographic radionuclide ventriculography compared with planar radionuclide and single plane contrast ventriculography. *Br J Radiol* 1993;66:986–993.
252. Bartlett ML, Bacharach SL, Barker C, Unger E, Carson J, Kitsiou N, Smeltzer W, Elliot E, Pettiford M, Katsiyiannis PT, Dilsizian V. SPECT gated blood pool—potentials and problems. Computers in Cardiology, IEEE Computer Society Press, 1994;197–200.

24 Vascular Diseases

John C. Harbert

Reduced blood flow to the extremities may be either acute or chronic. The major causes of acute arterial occlusion are *embolism, thrombosis*, and *vascular injury*. Radionuclide diagnostic procedures rarely figure in the diagnosis of acute occlusions, because other procedures, especially contrast arteriography and doppler ultrasound, provide more specific information about the causes and precise locations that are needed to make surgical and angioplastic decisions. Large vessel anomalies and occlusions are often recognized as patterns of absent blood flow coincidentally in the course of some other diagnostic procedure, whence they provide the grist for endless clinical case reports (Fig. 1).

ARTERIAL OCCLUSIVE DISEASES

Chronic and progressive arterial occlusive disease is much more common than acute occlusions and the most prevalent of these by far is *arteriosclerosis obliterans*, found most often in atheromatous disease and diabetes mellitus. Less common forms of chronic symptomatic occlusive disease are *thromboangiitis obliterans* (*Buerger's disease*), vasospastic disorders (Raynaud's disease, acrocyanosis), arteriovenous fistulas, aneurysms, and extrinsic compressions. There are two types of blood-flow techniques that have provided clinically useful information in these conditions: measures of the local distribution and clearance of diffusible tracers and arterial injections of nondiffusible particles.

RADIOPHARMACEUTICALS

Table 1 lists several radiopharmaceuticals that have been used to assess arterial perfusion. These are usually classified as particulate and nonparticulate tracers. Particulate tracers, being larger in diameter than capillaries, are trapped within the first capillary bed they reach and, if adequately mixed, are distributed in proportion to regional perfusion.[1]

Nonparticulate tracers can be used to assess relative distribution of blood flow, e.g., ^{201}Tl-chloride or ^{99m}Tc-isonitriles (sestamibi), that are extracted by organ tissues during first passage through the circulation and clear with a long half-life; intravascular blood pool tracers (^{99m}Tc-HSA, ^{113m}In-transferrin; ^{99m}Tc-RBCs or ^{99m}Tc-pertechnetate immediately postinjection) or freely diffusible tracers that measure blood flow per weight of tissue, as with ^{133}Xe.

Clinical Applications

The applications for such studies include:

1. the regional distribution of capillary perfusion under various stresses to determine the physiological significance of arteriographically demonstrable small vessel disease;
2. to determine vascular graft patency;
3. to predict the healing potential of ischemic ulcers;
4. to quantify the magnitude of arteriovenous shunts;
5. to determine the skin perfusion in selecting the level of limb amputation.

EVALUATION OF MUSCLE BLOOD FLOW IN PERIPHERAL VASCULAR DISEASE

Almost invariably, surgical decisions in occlusive arterial disease in the legs are made on the basis of angiographic findings. Significant narrowing or blockage of vessels in the context of claudication, diminished pulses, or poorly healing ulcers supposes a causative relationship that dictates surgical relief of obstruction. However, the correlation between structure and function is by no means perfect and the contribution of collateral circulation to capillary perfusion is not well evaluated by angiography. Numerous physiological studies have been developed in an attempt to find sensitive tests that are less invasive than contrast angiography and more appropriate for following the course of disease.

Historical Methods. The earliest studies of extremity muscle perfusion were undertaken by Kety, who measured the local clearance of ^{24}NaCl following intramuscular injection.[32] Using the clearance of small ionic tracers, blood flow is calculated by plotting on semilog paper the activity versus time data from a simple probe and analyzer. During the initial monoexponential phase, the clearance half-time is determined and flow, F (mL/min/100g) is calculated from the Schmidt-Kety equation:

$$F = \frac{0.693\lambda}{T_{1/2}} \times 100$$

where λ is the partition coefficient for the tissue being studied.

Such ionic tracers as ^{24}Na and ^{99m}Tc-pertechnetate are seldom used for these studies, because they are severely *diffusion limited*, which means that during hyperemia, their disappearance is limited by their rate of diffusion into sur-

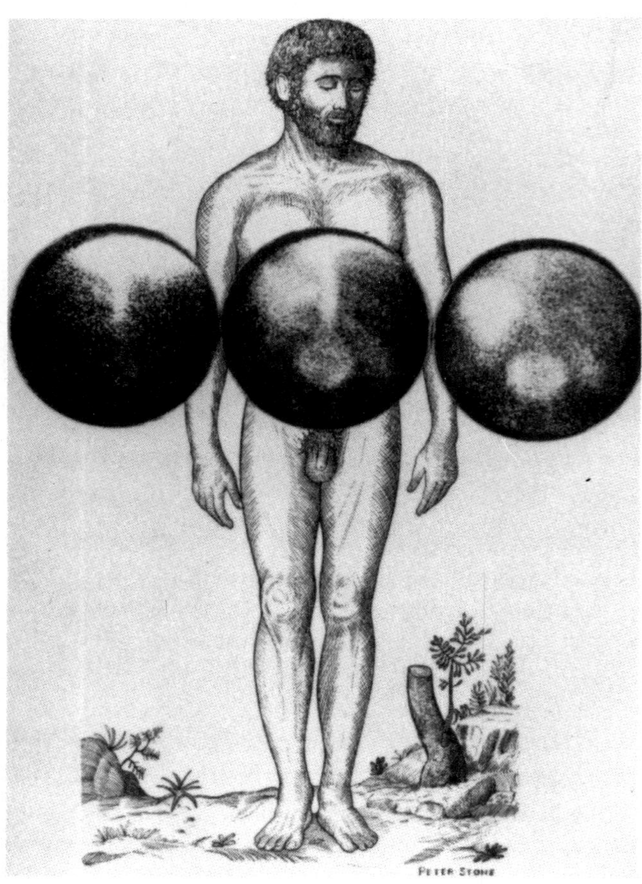

Figure 1. Anterior 3-s scintiphotos beginning 12 s following intravenous injection of 740 MBq (20 mCi) ^{99m}Tc-DTPA in a patient with a hepatic mass lesion. The dynamic flow study demonstrates the incidental finding of a large aortic aneurysm.

rounding capillaries. Only at very low blood flow rates are these tracers *flow limited*, (i.e., their clearance depends upon regional blood flow).[17] Consequently, when blood flow is determined by local clearance, such freely diffusible tracers as ^{133}Xe in saline are used.[14,15]

Xenon Clearance Studies. In this technique, approximately 0.1 mL of sterile saline containing 3.5 MBq (~100 μCi) of ^{133}Xe is injected intramuscularly. The injection is made through a 27-gauge needle inserted 1 to 2 cm deep into the muscle being investigated, taking care to avoid subcutaneous fat which results in slow, nonreproducible clearance curves. The needle is left in place for approximately 30 seconds after the injection to prevent escape of the tracer. A collimated detector or scintillation camera is positioned above the injection site, and constant geometry is maintained during the measurement.

The declining activity at the injection site is plotted as a function of time on semilog paper. Blood flow is determined by the Schmidt-Kety equation above, using a value of $\lambda = 0.7$. The needle injection creates a small amount of local trauma, which may increase the initial portion of the slope. Therefore, the "second slope" beginning 2 to 3 minutes after injection is used. Usually, both resting and exercise flows are determined because the resting blood flow alone is insensitive.[33] Exercising is accomplished with a treadmill for 5 to 6 minutes, or until claudication develops. In healthy persons, resting and maximally exercised (hyperemic) muscle blood flows are about 2 and 50 mL/min/100 g, respectively,[33] while maximum blood flow to the lower extremity muscles in patients with peripheral vascular disease is less than 20 mL/min/100 g and is reached later after injection than in normal subjects. In the lower extremity, the anterior tibialis muscle is preferred over the gastrocnemius because it contains less fat.[33] However, when these studies are performed with the patient walking, the gastrocnemius should be injected.[16]

What is the sensitivity of this test? Lassen found significantly decreased blood flow in about 95% of patients with arterial occlusion between the heart and the site of measurement.[17] False-negative results are encountered in subjects with good collateral circulation and in patients with occlusions close to the site of measurement. The fact that there is approximately 25% variability in reproducibility is largely offset by the large differences in blood flow between normal subjects and patients with symptomatic peripheral vascular disease.

The problems with xenon clearance techniques are that

Table 1. Radiotracers Used to Evaluate Arterial Disease

RADIOPHARMACEUTICALS	INDICATION
Particulate	
macroaggregates—^{131}I[2]	Determine relative distribution of perfusion
^{99m}Tc[3]	
microspheres—^{99m}Tc[4,5]	
^{113m}In[3]	
Nonparticulate	
Serum albumin—^{131}I[6]	
^{99m}Tc	
Transferrin—^{131m}In	Blood pool imaging
^{99m}Tc-pertechnetate (immediately postinjection)[7]	
DTPA—^{99m}Tc	
^{113m}In	
^{81m}Kr[8]	
^{43}K[9]	Relative distribution of perfusion in muscle
^{201}Tl-chloride[3,4,10–12]	
^{99m}Tc-isonitrile[13]	
^{133}Xe (in solution)[14–16]	
4-iodo-antipyrine—^{131}I[17]	Blood flow per weight of tissue
Platelets—^{111}In[18–20]	
^{99m}Tc[21]	Bind to atheromas
Low-Density Lipoprotein—^{123}I[22,23]	
^{125}I[24]	
^{131}I[25]	
^{99m}Tc[26–28]	
^{111}In[29,30]	
Immunoglobulin G—^{111}In[31]	

multiple injections must be made if more than one vascular territory is to be investigated and no images are obtained. Too, the exact location of the injection site is difficult to determine. Today, these studies are seldom performed.

Arterial Perfusion Using Labeled Microspheres. The distribution of radiolabeled particles following intraarterial injection has been studied in many organs.[34,35] The basic assumptions upon which the particle distribution method is based are (1) that the particles do not alter blood flow, (2) that the particles are trapped and removed from circulation by the first capillary bed they encounter and thus there is no recirculation, (3) that the particles have the same distribution pattern as red blood cells and, (4) that the particles are adequately mixed in the blood. Only the fourth assumption has been challenged. To achieve "complete" mixing, a Reynold value (turbulence coefficient) of a least 2000 must be obtained.[36] This value might not be achieved if injections are made below the descending aorta; however, in studies that utilized multiple sites and directions for injecting microspheres into peripheral arteries, the same patterns of distribution were found as in studies using intracardiac injections.

Siegel et al. injected ^{99}Tc-labeled microspheres into the descending aorta or the femoral artery in a large number of patients that were undergoing contrast angiography at the same time.[5,13] They injected microspheres both at rest and after the reactive hyperemia that occurs following release of vascular occlusion that induced temporary ischemia of the lower limbs. This is a method of increasing regional blood flow that simulates exercise and increases the sensitivity of the test. Using this technique, the authors identified several distinguishable patterns that characterized large vessel occlusive disease, small vessel disease, ischemic ulcers, and other conditions. Nevertheless, this technique has not enjoyed widespread adoption because of the requirement of arterial injections.

Perfusion Studies with Diffusible Tracers. The use of intravenously administered diffusible tracers such as ^{43}K or ^{201}Tl to image the distribution of perfusion among the muscles of the leg was proposed by Miyamoto et al.[9] Thallium-201 has been extensively studied in the heart. The immediate postinjection pattern of uptake has been shown to portray the fractional distribution of cardiac output and is directly related to relative regional perfusion.[10] The extraction of ^{201}Tl and its persistent localization within muscle ($T_{\text{eff}} \approx 2$ d) permits assessment of relative perfusion. Just as in cardiac testing, measures at rest and after stress intervention greatly increase the sensitivity of the test for detecting reduced arterial perfusion.[12,37–39]

In the studies of Segall et al.[12] whole-body scans were obtained immediately after exercise stress and 4 hours later. The latter "redistribution" patterns are equivalent to the resting distribution, so that rest and exercise patterns can be recorded using a single injection. ^{201}Thallium activity in the gluteal, thigh, and calf regions was measured and expressed in terms of total body activity. In normal subjects total leg activity represented about 25% of total activity (Fig. 2). Resting and exercise images in normal subjects are qualitatively similar, although muscle activity is much higher after exercise. In patients with peripheral vascular disease, rest and exercise distribution patterns are dissimilar and the fractional activity at rest is usually higher than with exercise. The value of expressing regional uptake as a fraction of whole-body activity is that bilaterally diminished activity can be detected when age- and sex-adjusted normal values have been determined.[12] Merely comparing extremity counts with the contralateral side may not detect bilateral disease.[40] To date, these studies have been used only to detect the presence or probable absence of lower extremity ischemic disease. However, they may prove useful to help select candidates and evaluate the effect of revascularization procedures. Such studies require both resting and exercise measurements, because resting studies alone reveal few differences before and after revascularization.[41]

SPECT Imaging. Oshima and colleagues have evaluated muscle distribution of ^{201}Tl using SPECT images of the lower legs in patients with occlusive vascular disease.[11] They found significantly decreased uptake of ^{201}Tl in muscles supplied by narrowed arteries. Figure 3 shows several tomographic slices through the legs of a patient with arteriosclerosis obliterans. Quantitative uptake of thallium in these images is determined by normalizing against total body thallium activity summed in separate whole-body planar views.

At this time, preliminary studies of lower extremity perfusion using the isonitrile, ^{99m}Tc-MIBI, have been reported.[42,43] Qualitative images may be somewhat superior to ^{201}Tl images because of the 140-keV energy of ^{99m}Tc. Rest and stress images are quite similar to ^{201}Tl images, although far greater count rates are obtained (Fig. 4).

QUANTITATIVE MEASUREMENTS OF SKIN PERFUSION

Measurements of skin perfusion with radiopharmaceuticals have been used (1) to select the level of amputation in ischemic limb disease,[44] (2) to assess the vascularization of pedicle flaps in reconstructive surgery[45] and, (3) to select appropriate treatment for chronic skin ulcers.[46]

Determination of Amputation Level

It is generally believed that the *appearance* of healthy skin at a proposed amputation level is no guarantee of adequate blood flow for wound healing, because the perfusion required to heal a surgical wound is greater than that required merely to maintain viability of intact skin.[47] Such objective criteria as skin temperature, level of distal pulse, or angiographic patterns are not reliable in estimating skin perfu-

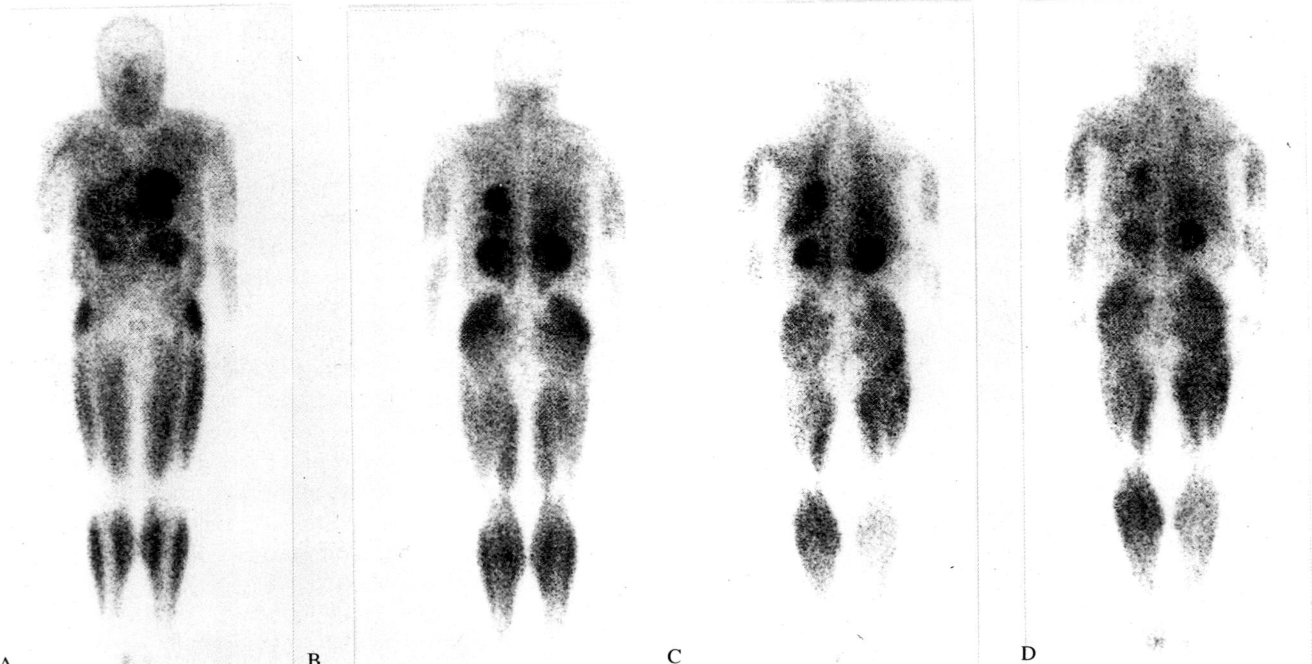

Figure 2. **(A)** and **(B)**. Early postexercise anterior **(A)** and posterior **(B)** whole-body ^{201}Tl images of a man with no vascular disease. The gluteal muscles are not well seen on the anterior view and activity in the thigh and calf muscles is significantly attenuated by the long bones. In contrast, muscle groups are clearly defined in the posterior view. **(C)** and **(D)**. Early **(C)** and 4-hour **(D)** postexercise posterior whole-body ^{201}Tl images in a patient with bilateral intermittent claudication of the buttocks and calves. Decreased activity in the right calf and left thigh is apparent in the early exercise scan. Quantitative analysis also reveals decreased activity in the left gluteal region on the early scan. The 4-hr redistribution image shows some increase in activity in the left thigh and right calf. However, quantitative analysis indicates higher than normal redistribution to both thighs and both calves, indicating extensive occlusive arterial disease. (Reproduced by permission from Reference 12.)

sion.[48] A variety of radiopharmaceuticals and techniques have been used. In the earliest studies, Lassen and others used skin perfusion pressures as measured by xenon or iodo-antipyrine to predict the healing ability of amputation stumps.[17] Lassen preferred ^{131}I or ^{125}I iodo-antipyrine to ^{133}Xe because of xenon's significant diffusion into subcutaneous fatty tissue, in which it is highly soluble. Iodo-antipyrine was injected intradermally, and pressure applied over the injected radioactivity with a blood pressure cuff (Fig. 5A). The skin perfusion pressure is the pressure at which perfusion stops (i.e., at which the clearance of radioactivity ceases). In normal individuals, this pressure approximates diastolic pressure. Lassen found that stumps healed well when skin perfusion pressures exceeded 40 mmHg.

Most of these studies have used measurements of the skin clearance of ^{133}Xe in saline following intradermal injection.[49,50] The washout of ^{133}Xe when injected intradermally in a saline solution is biexponential. The initial fast component is probably caused by the temporary hyperemia of trauma.[17] The second, slower component is free of the effects of trauma, but underestimates dermal blood flow, probably because of accumulation of xenon in subcutaneous fat. However, errors in estimating skin blood flow using the exponential derived from the first 10 minutes appear to be small.

In the clearance method proposed by Daly and Henry, 0.05 mL of ^{133}Xe in saline (0.5 to 1.0 MBq) is injected intradermally in the anterior skin of the legs, just as a tuberculin test would be administered.[47] Washout of activity is measured for 10 minutes, at four frames per minute, using a scintillation camera and computer to generate time-activity curves. A least-squares fit for a monoexponential function is determined, and the slope constant, λ ($0.693/T_{1/2}$) is determined from the first 6 minutes after injection. This value is then entered into the Schmidt-Kety equation given above to derive blood flow in mL/100 g/min.

The three sites of injection usually selected are the typical amputation levels 10 cm above the knee, 10 cm below the tibial tuberosity, and at the dorsal junction of the foot and ankle. The skin perfusion rates, expressed in mL/min/100 g, for 5 normal male volunteers studied by Daly and Henry were 8.9 above the knee (range: 6.1 to 14.5), 10.8 below the knee (range 8.6 to 14.5), and 14.3 at the ankle (range: 10.4 to 18.8).[47] These results were reproducible when injection volumes and ambient temperature were held constant, and they agree with data from normal subjects in probe-ratemeter studies.

An advantage of this technique is that it permits examination of several sites simultaneously, without interference from previous injections. Malone et al. found that when skin

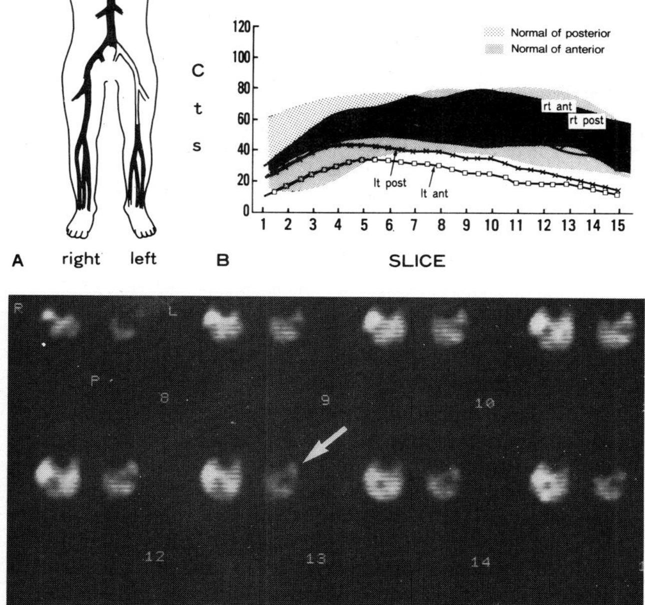

Figure 3. A 70-year-old patient with intermittent claudication of the left calf. Contrast arteriography **(A)** showed occlusion of the left iliac artery and normal right femoral and leg arteries. Stress profile curves **(B)** show abnormal ^{201}Th activity in both anterior and posterior tibial muscle groups on the left compared with normal limits (mean $\pm$ 2 S.D.). Stress SPECT **(C)** shows markedly decreased uptake in the left muscle groups (arrow). (Reproduced by permission from Reference 11.)

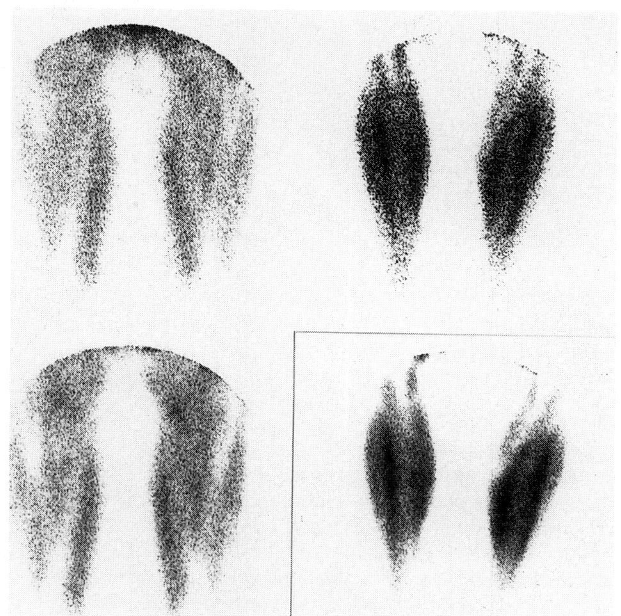

Figure 4. Posterior ^{201}Tl rest (upper) and stress (lower) images of the thighs (left) and calves (right) in a patient without evidence of arteriovascular disease. The stress images appear more intense, but the distribution of activity is the same as in the resting images.

flow rates exceeded 2.2 mL/min/100 g tissue, 95% of 137 lower extremity amputations healed primarily.[51] Roon et al. confirmed these findings in below-knee amputations.[52]

Assessment of Skin Graft Viability

There are two basic types of skin grafts: free and distant grafts. Free skin grafts are completely detached from donor sites and applied to recipient sites. These grafts seldom require radionuclide studies. Distant grafts are formed by incising a flap of skin, which is attached by a pedicle to the intact base through which arterial and venous supplies pass, until the grafted flap becomes revascularized from the recipient vessels. The pedicle graft is then sutured to the recipient site and the donor site closed primarily or covered with a free skin graft. Generally two or three weeks are required to establish adequate revascularization to maintain pedicle viability. Because the revascularization period is variable, tests have been devised to assess viability before detaching the pedicle vessels.

The most commonly used test of pedicle viability is the fluorescein test in which 15 mg/kg of body weight of fluorescein in 10% solution is injected intravenously over about 5 minutes. Twenty minutes later, the skin flap is examined under ultraviolet light which reveals a gold-greenish glow over the perfused region of the flap. Usually this test is safe and, in uncomplicated cases, gives a good visual impression of viability. In doubtful cases, however, a radionuclide clearance test can provide more precise quantitative measurements of blood flow. These tests have been reviewed recently by Wahner.[53] We will only describe two tests.

1. ^{133}Xe clearance. In this method, a dose of about 1 MBq (40 μCi) of ^{133}Xe dissolved in sterile saline is injected intradermally using a tuberculine syringe and 26–gauge needle. Preparation of ^{133}Xe in saline has been described by Herold.[54] The time-activity curve of ^{133}Xe disappearance is then measured using a probe and strip-chart recorder or gamma camera and computer. The raw data for the first 30 minutes are plotted on semilogarithmic paper and the slopes calculated. The blood flow can then be calculated as follows:

$$F = \frac{100\ \lambda\ \log C_1 - \log C_2}{t_2 - t_1}$$

where F is the blood flow in mL/100 g/min, λ is the partition coefficient between skin and blood for xenon = 0.7 mL/g, C_1 is the natural log of counts at the beginning of the study t_1, and log C_2 is the natural log of counts at the end of the study, t_2. Normal intact skin blood flow is quite variable, ranging from about 5 mL/100 g/min to about 20 mL/110 g/min.[55] Poor skin flap survival has been found with blood flow below about 0.5 mL/100 g/min.[56]

2. ^{99m}Tc-pertechnetate clearance. Wahner and others have developed another clearance technique using ^{99m}Tc-pertechnetate, which is much more readily available in the average nuclear medicine laboratory.[57,58] In this method, a similar preparation of the flap and recording devices as described above for ^{133}Xe are used. Approximately 1.25 MBq (50 μCi)

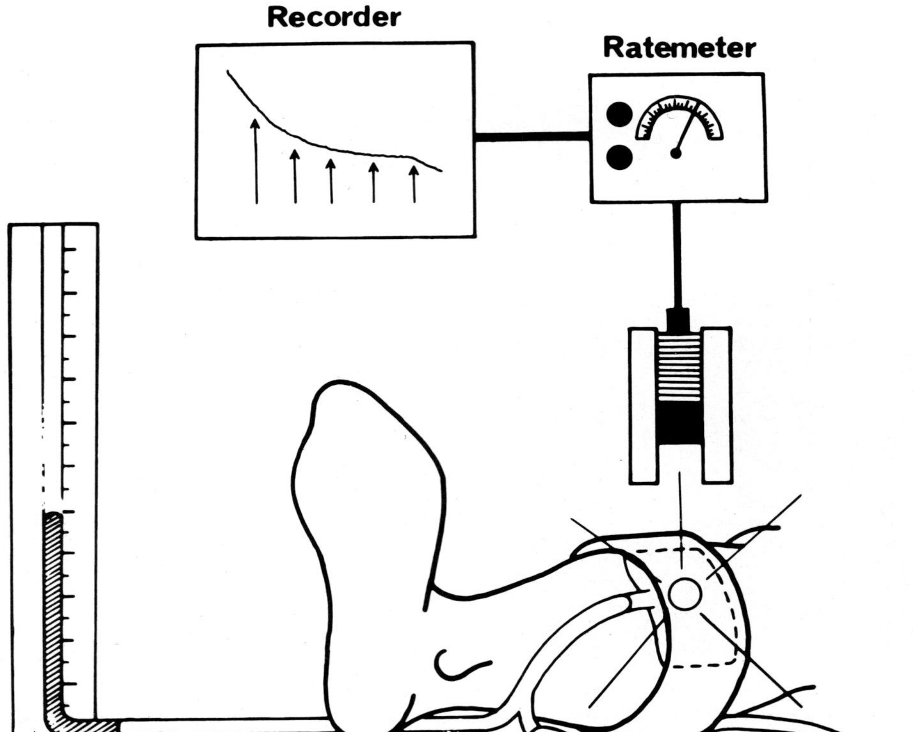

Figure 5A. Method of measuring skin perfusion pressure by recording the disappearance of intradermally injected diffusible tracer. As can be seen in the "recorder," the disappearance slope, y/x decreases and approaches zero as the increasing pressure (arrows) approximates the "skin perfusion pressure." With release of the pressure (last vertical arrow) y/x increases as perfusion resumes. (From reference 17.)

of ^{99m}Tc-pertechnetate are injected intradermally to form a wheal. Any fluid that seeps from the injection site is carefully removed with a gauze sponge. Counts are recorded for 5 to 10 minutes. The pedicle is then clamped with a sterile Young pedicle clamp to cut off the pedicle blood supply. Counts are recorded for another 5 to 10 minutes and the clamp removed. This reestablishes blood flow and counts are recorded for another 5 to 10 minutes.

The points from each of the three recording periods are then fitted by a straight line as shown in Fig. 5B. The $T_{1/2}$ of each slope is then determined graphically. The half-times before and after clamping are averaged to determine a mean "unclamped" half-time (value A in Fig. 5B). The blood flow F derived from the new host site is determined from:

$$F = \frac{\text{half-time (min) unclamped}}{\text{half-time (min) clamped}} \times 100$$

The blood flow contributed by the donor site ("Block" in Fig. 5B) is calculated as:

$$F_{\text{block}} = 100 - F$$

Blood flow from the donor site is, of course, blocked by clamping the pedicle. Presumably, one would like to have host blood flow rates of about 20% before severing the pedicle from the flap.

Ischemic Ulcers

Siegel et al. first described the use of ^{201}Tl to determine the healing potential of ischemic ulcers.[59] They found that tissue hyperemia surrounding the ulcer correlated generally with healing through conservative treatment.

Subsequently, Ohta used ^{201}Tl after reactive hyperemia and redistribution to predict the healing of ischemic ulcers of the feet.[60] In these studies, reactive hyperemia of the skin was produced by applying a pressure cuff above the ankle and raised above systolic pressure for 3 minutes. Upon release of the cuff, 75 MBq (2 mCi) ^{201}Thallium was injected into an arm vein. Plantar views of the feet were recorded for the first 15 minutes and redistribution views were obtained 3 hours later. Four different patterns of uptake (Fig. 6) were observed and found to correlate with healing:

1. Type I pattern consisted of localized increased thallium accumulation (a hot spot) in the postocclusive initial distribution, and relatively *decreased* uptake in the redistribution image. Ulcers of Type I healed with conservative treatment.
2. Type II pattern consisted of relatively increased uptake in the ulcer region initially, with sustained *increased* uptake during redistribution. Type II ulcers also healed with conservative treatment.
3. Type III pattern consisted of *decreased* initial activity followed by *increased* activity during redistribution. These ulcers healed, but required surgical treatment to avoid protracted hospitalization.
4. Type IV pattern consisted of *decreased* uptake in both initial and redistribution images. Type IV ulcer did not heal without surgical treatment.

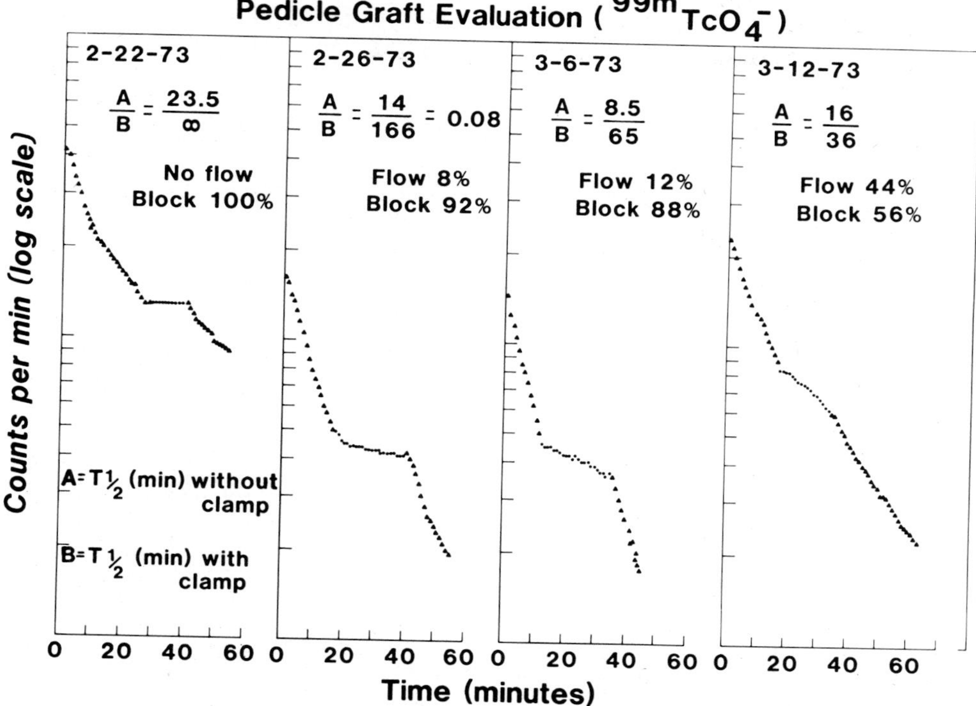

Figure 5B. Flow rates determined by the disappearance of ^{99m}Tc-pertechnetate from pedicle injection sites at various times following grafting. See text for description. (Reproduced by kind permission of Dr. Heinz Wahner.)

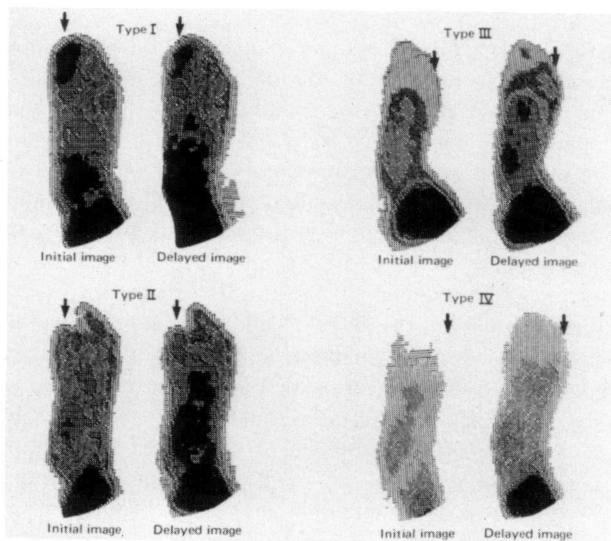

Figure 6. Plantar views of the feet 15 min (initial) and 3 hrs (delayed) following intravenous injection of 74 MBq (2 mCi) ^{201}Tl. The images are computer-generated isocount depictions. See text for a description of ulcer types. (Reproduced by permission from Reference 60.)

In another study, Siegel and colleagues found that ^{201}Tl studies were more sensitive than Doppler ultrasound in predicting ulcer healing.[61] Using a minimum postocclusive hyperemia of 1.5:1, thallium perfusion imaging correctly predicted healing in 20 of 23 ulcers. Doppler alone predicted only 15 of 23 of the eventually healed ulcers. Doppler ultrasound correctly predicted nonhealing of 3 of 6 cases, while thallium perfusion correctly predicted nonhealing of 5 of 5 ulcers. The overall accuracy of thallium imaging was 86 versus 62% for Doppler ultrasound.[62]

Preliminary studies suggest that ^{201}Tl perfusion imaging may be useful in predicting the outcome of lumbar sympathectomy as a procedure to increase peripheral circulation.[13] In a small group of patients in whom extremity perfusion increased after anesthetic block of sympathetic ganglia, subsequent lumbar sympathectomy was generally successful in helping to heal ulcers. In a few patients in whom the block *decreased* perfusion, lumbar sympathectomy was not successful.

OTHER APPLICATIONS

Frostbite. ^{99m}Technetium-pertechnetate scintigraphy has been used to differentiate viable from nonviable tissues injured by frostbite.[64] Images of the involved extremities with 555 MBq (15 mCi) reveal a persistent perfusion defect in nonviable tissues of the fingers and toes.

Electrical Burns. Hunt et al. have described the use of ^{99m}Tc-pyrophosphate to determine the extent of muscle damage resulting from electrical burns.[65] They found several characteristic scintigraphic patterns:

1. areas with no uptake, indicating absence of blood flow and obvious necrosis,
2. a "donut" pattern consisting of a central cold area surrounded by increased tracer uptake,
3. focal hot spots, and
4. homogeneous tracer uptake both adjacent and proximal to areas of focally increased uptake.

The fourth pattern presumably represents hyperemia. The authors defined the level of amputation by the area of diffuse homogeneous tracer uptake proximal to areas of intense uptake.

Atheromatous Lesions. Recently, a number of radiopharmaceuticals have been developed in an effort to label atherosclerotic plaques. These include low-density lipoproteins (LDL) labeled with ^{123}I,[22,23] ^{125}I,[24] ^{131}I,[25] ^{99m}Tc,[26–28] and ^{111}In[29–30]; polyclonal immunoglobulin G and Fc fragments labeled with ^{111}In.[31] When atherosclerotic plaques become eroded with disruption of endothelium, they can be imaged with labeled platelets.[18,19]

The mechanism of labeled LDL entry into atherosclerotic plaques appears to be as a metabolic substrate, since cholesterol deposits contain LDL. While carotid plaques can be imaged as early as 30 minutes,[66] delayed images are more practical because high residual blood background interferes with visualization in earlier images.

The uptake of radiolabeled IgG and Fc fragments is based on the fact that foam cells, another component of atherosclerotic plaques, contain abundant Fc receptors.[18] Preliminary animal studies suggest sufficiently high accumulation of ^{111}In-labeled IgG to permit external imaging.

Therapeutic Embolization Monitoring. Ivalon is the trade name for polyvinyl alcohol in the form of inert, nonresorbable, spongelike particles (250 to 1000 μm diameter) that are used in transcatheter embolizations to occlude arteriovenous malformations and vascular tumors.[67–69] One of the most serious complications of therapeutic embolization with Ivalon is inadvertent passage of the particles into the lungs, causing (sometimes fatal) pulmonary embolization. Because Ivalon particles are radiolucent, they cannot be monitored by fluoroscopy, unless specially impregnated. Fortunately, Ivalon is efficiently labeled with ^{99m}Tc-sulfur colloid and can be monitored by a portable scintillation camera.[68,69]

In this technique, Ivalon particles (Fig. 7) are labeled with ^{99m}Tc-sulfur colloid and injected in small doses (100 to 300 MBq) after initial catheter placement and, subsequently, at various intervals during the therapeutic embolization. The distribution of activity is monitored over the lungs and over the site of the vascular malformation (Fig. 8). If excessive lung activity accumulates at some point in the procedure, the catheter tip can be readjusted and therapeutic embolization continued. The radiation absorbed dose has been determined by Johnson.[70]

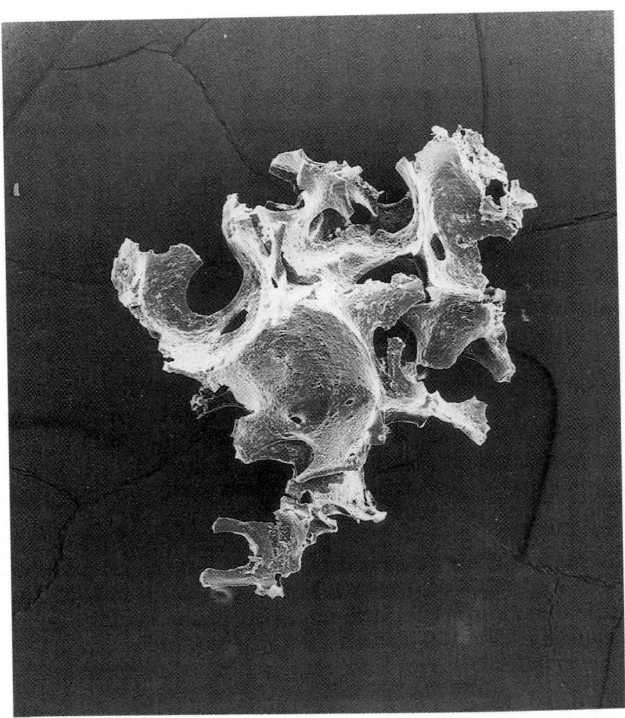

Figure 7. Scanning electron micrograph of an Ivalon particle. (Reproduced by permission from Reference 68.)

PATENCY OF MAJOR ARTERIES AND GRAFTS

Radionuclide scintiangiograms are obtained following a bolus intravenous injection of 750 to 925 MBq (20 to 25 mCi) of in vivo-labeled ^{99m}Tc-red blood cells (or other suitable nonparticulate tracer) (Fig. 9). Serial images are obtained at 2- to 3-second intervals. Creating a closed loop cine of the dynamic phase of the study often aids in the interpretation of the radionuclide angiogram. Immediately following the dynamic phase of the study, a single 500,000-count blood-pool image is obtained. If bleeding is expected, a second static image is taken 10 to 15 minutes later. Using this technique, Moss et al. found that in normal subjects' arteries are visualized to the level of the popliteal artery in the leg and to the ulnar and radial arteries in the arm.[71,72] Unimpeded flow is interpreted as absence of significant intraluminal disease. Total occlusions are readily apparent. Greater than 30% stenosis is detectable in larger vessels. Aneurysms are characterized by widening of the lumen, representing the aneurysmal sac, or as a narrowed tortuous lumen surrounded by an area of relatively decreased activity, which represents clot within the aneurysm. In cases of trauma, extraluminal accumulations may represent acute hemorrhage or false aneurysms.[73,74] These findings usually are apparent on the dy-

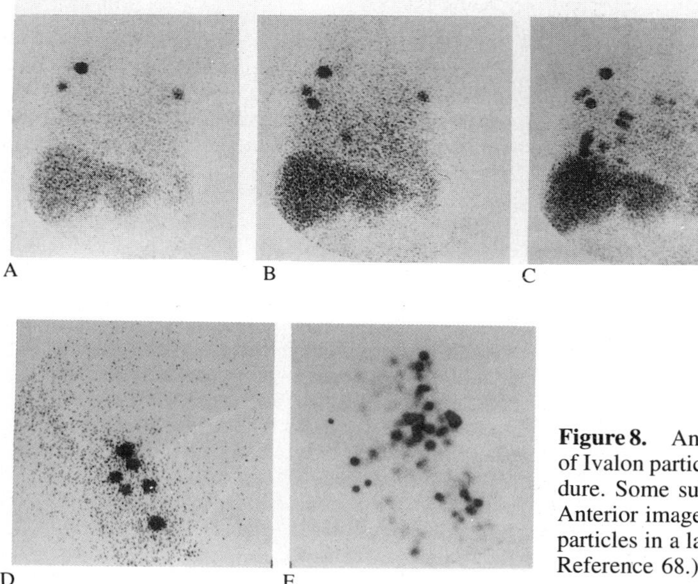

Figure 8. Anterior views of the lungs **(A,B,C)** showing progressive accumulation of Ivalon particles labeled with ^{99m}Tc-sulfur colloid during the embolization procedure. Some sulfur colloid dissociated from the Ivalon can be seen in the liver. Anterior images of the left thigh **(D,E)** show progressive accumulation of Ivalon particles in a large arteriovenous malformation. (Reproduced by permission from Reference 68.)

namic studies, but sometimes may be demonstrated only on delayed static images (Fig. 10).

In a group of 70 patients studied by Rudavsky et al., who were suspected of having traumatic arterial injury, radionuclide angiography demonstrated 22 lesions with a 90% true-positive rate, as confirmed by contrast angiography[75]; 47 studies yielded true-negative results. Thus, radionuclide angiography can be an accurate screening procedure for traumatic arterial injury and can aid in the selection of patients requiring contrast angiography. An example of arteriovenous fistula is shown in Figure 11.

Radionuclide angiography is useful in the postoperative evaluation of surgical bypass graft patency. In the postoperative period, when the limb is swollen and obscured by dress-

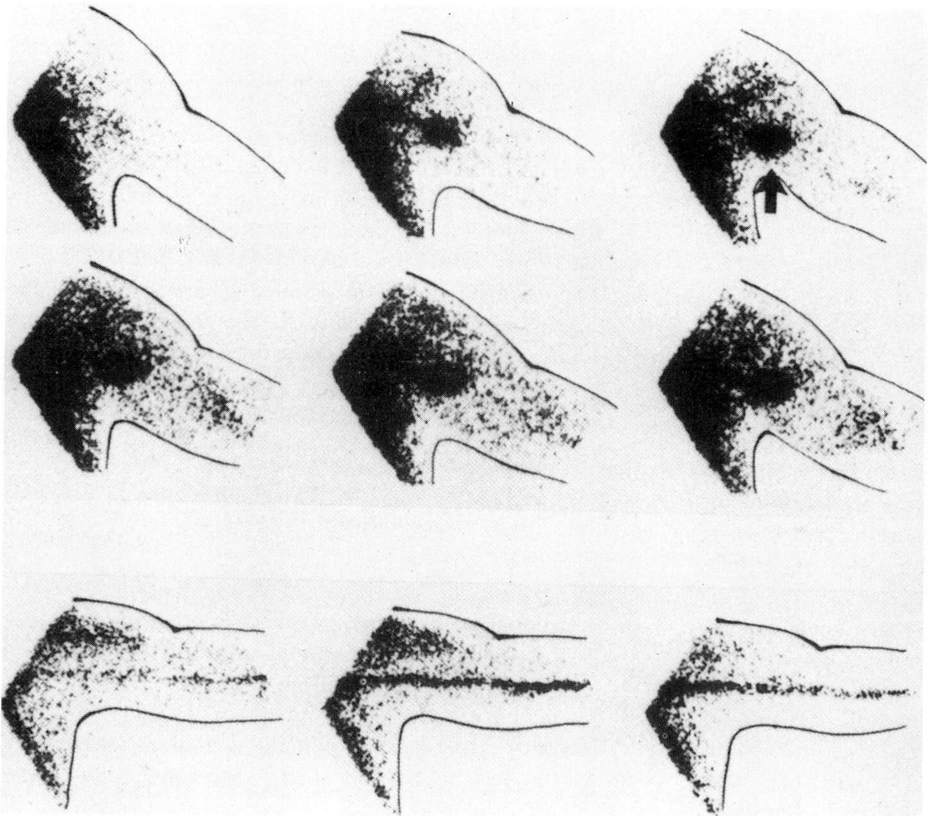

Figure 9. Left axillary artery aneurysm. *Top*, 6 serial 3-s anterior images over the left axilla following injection of 750 MBq (20 mCi) ^{99m}Tc-RBCs into the right antecubital vein. The aneurysm (arrow) severely inhibits distal flow into the arm. *Bottom*, normal axillary and brachial artery restored after aneurysmectomy. (Reproduced by kind permission of Dr. Michael Siegel.)

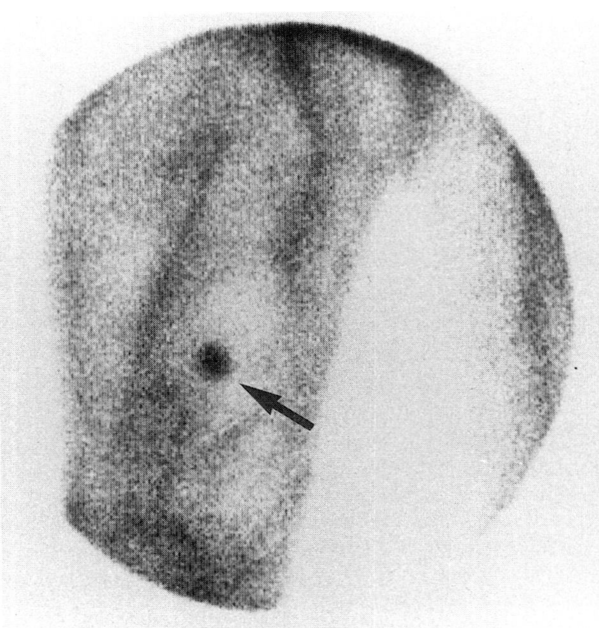

A

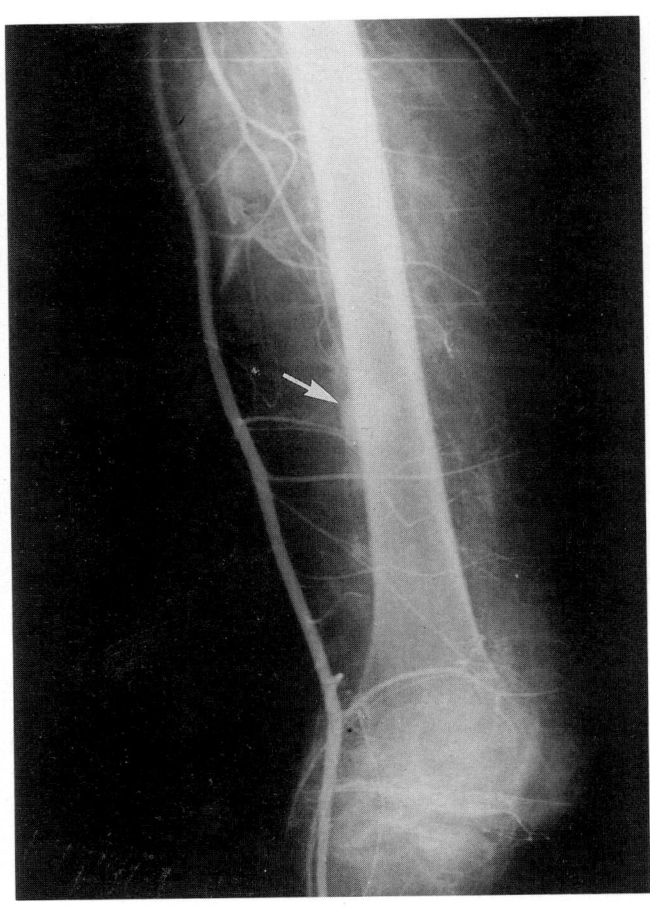

B

Figure 10. A 29-year-old male paraplegic was studied for acute bleeding in the right thigh: **A.** The static blood flow image following intravenous injection of 750 MBq (20 mCi) ^{99m}Tc-RBCs demonstrates a focus of increased activity with a photopenic halo, suggesting an active bleeding site. **B.** Angiography showed a 2-cm region of increased opacification fed by a branch of the superficial femoral artery. No extravasation of contrast was seen. The radiological diagnosis was false aneurysm, possibly mycotic. (Reproduced by permission from Reference 75.)

ings, assessment by palpation of pulses is difficult. Intraarterial catheterization is better avoided in patients with preexisting arterial disease and in patients receiving anticoagulation therapy. Radionuclide studies can be repeated frequently and are better tolerated than contrast angiography.[71,72] Patent grafts as far distal as the tibial vessels in the legs can be visualized.[78]

ARTERIOVENOUS SHUNT QUANTIFICATION

Intraarterially injected particles are trapped in the distal microcirculation in proportion to regional blood flow, as discussed earlier. Blood flow through arteriovenous (A-V) communications larger than capillaries carries a fraction of the injected particles past this capillary bed to the lungs, where they are removed from circulation. The number of particles that bypass the peripheral capillary bed depends on the fraction of blood flowing through the communication and on the size of the particles relative to the communicating vessels. If the particles used are large enough to be trapped by the normal microcirculation, but small enough to pass through abnormal A-V communications, the estimated peripheral perfusion represents nutritive flow, and the presence of A-V communications can be quantified. The following procedure is used to estimate the fraction of A-V shunting.

1. A known quantity of labeled washed particles (25 to 40 μm diameter) is injected intraarterially, and the activity over a selected region of the lungs is measured. Ideally 100,000 to 300,000 particles should be injected, labeled with 75 to 150 MBq (2 to 4 mCi) of ^{99m}Tc.
2. Approximately the same quantity of labeled, washed particles is injected *intravenously.* This injection represents 100% shunting. A second count over the same lung region is made. Then, by the use of the following formula, the percentage of blood shunted through the A-V communication is determined:

$$\%\ \text{shunting} = \frac{C_a A_a}{C_v A_v} \times 100$$

where:

C_a = counting rate after arterial injection,
C_v = counting rate after venous injection,
A_a = activity of the arterial injection,
A_v = activity of the venous injection.

The reason that *washed* particles are specified is that if there is significant activity in the suspending fluid, back-

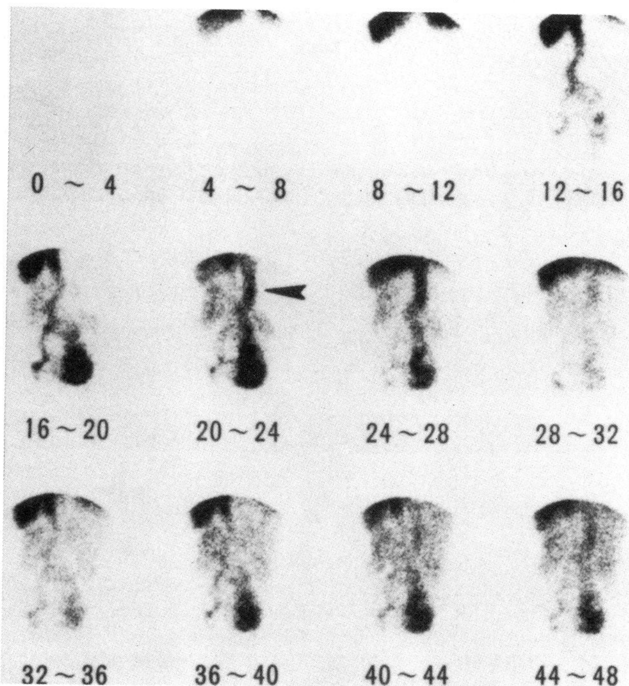

Figure 11. Arteriovenous fistula. Serial posterior abdominal scintiphotos taken at 4-s intervals following injection of 750 MBq (20 mCi) ^{99m}Tc-RBCs show abnormal blood pool in the right pelvis and rapid filling of a dilated inferior vena cava (arrow). The bottom row shows the malformation refilling with recirculation of tracer. (Reproduced by permission from Reference 77.)

ground corrections are required.[63] For these studies, sieved albumin microspheres of 15 to 25 μm are preferred, because they have a narrower size range than macroaggregated albumin (MAA). However, because these are no longer commercially available, most laboratories use ^{99m}Tc-MAA. It is advisable to measure the unbound activity in the suspending fluid and resuspend the MAA particles if it contains more than 10% of total activity.

This technique has been useful in confirming and quantifying the degree of shunting in arteriovenous malformations and fistulae, as well as some hypernephromas. It has also been used to document shunting in pulmonary osteoarthropathy.[79] On the other hand, it has confirmed that no A-V shunting can be demonstrated in patients with Paget's disease.[80]

EVALUATION OF VENOUS DISEASE

Deep Venous Thrombosis

Deep venous thrombosis (DVT) and pulmonary embolism remain a major cause of morbidity and mortality throughout the world. A review of autopsy series in the United States shows that from 8 to 52% of patients autopsied can be demonstrated to have evidence of pulmonary embolism.[81] Of these, between 2 and 14% were thought to have contributed to the patient's death. The wide variation in these estimates relates in part to autopsy techniques. The more detailed the dissection of the pulmonary vascular tree, the more pulmonary emboli will be found. As predisposing factors, a history of (DVT) as well as the postoperative state appear to be most influential.[82]

NONRADIONUCLIDE TESTS OF DVT

The clinical diagnosis of DVT remains highly uncertain. Half of all patients with objective evidence of DVT are asymptomatic, while as many as 70% of patients with symptoms of DVT have no demonstrable evidence of thrombosis.[83] Therefore, objective tests for the diagnosis of DVT are essential. Of these, only 3 are in widespread use: contrast venography, impedance plethysmography (IPG), and Doppler ultrasonography.

Contrast Venography. For many years, contrast venography has been considered the "gold standard" for the diagnosis of DVT. In this procedure, approximately 100 mL of water-soluble iodinated contrast agent are injected into a vein on the dorsum of the foot to obtain anterior and lateral views of the leg veins.[84] Venous thrombi are seen as discrete filling defects within vessels, as abrupt cutoff of the vessels, or as nonfilling of the deep veins with diversion of contrast through the superficial veins.[85]

The principle advantages of contrast venography are that the entire lower extremity is visualized with a high degree of detail, and false-negative examinations are rare. False-positive test results occur in less than 5% of cases, in which there is inadequate mixing of contrast medium with blood or there are technical flaws in the injection technique.[85]

The principal disadvantages of contrast venography are that it is an invasive procedure resulting in patient discomfort, and contrast media-induced thrombophlebitis develops in from 7 to 24% of patients, depending upon the type and concentration of the agent used.[86] Consequently, the test is not appropriate for repeated studies. In some patients, contrast venography cannot be performed because of swelling of the feet, and a small number cannot be studied because of sensitivity to the contrast agent. Moreover, patients with a prior history of deep venous thrombosis may have residual venous occlusion, so that acute thrombosis may be impossible to distinguish from old disease.

Impedance Plethysmography (IPG). This is a noninvasive test that measures venous outflow from the lower extremity. When a thigh cuff is inflated, the venous blood volume increases along with increased electrical resistance (impedance) through the thigh, which is easily and reproducibly detected. When the cuff is then released and venous outflow is restricted by thrombosis, the normal decrease in impedance fails to occur.

IPG detects only thrombi that obstruct venous outflow from the thigh. Therefore, calf thrombi are not detected. Hull combined IPG with the ^{125}I-fibrinogen uptake test to increase the sensitivity for thrombus detection[87]; however, this test takes at least 24 hours and ^{125}I-fibrinogen is no long marketed in the United States and some other countries. Like contrast venography, IPG does not distinguish acute from residual occlusions from prior episodes of deep venous thrombosis. False-negative tests can be obtained in cases with well-established collateral vessels and in cases in which thrombosis does not completely occlude the outflow vessels.[88]

Ultrasound. Recent advances in ultrasound techniques have greatly enhanced the ability of this noninvasive imaging modality to detect DVT. Conventional B-mode scanning is used to outline the vessels, while pulsed Doppler detects movement of blood within the vessel (*duplex imaging*). The addition of color Doppler detects the direction of imaging, and assigns a color value to the direction, so that arteries and veins can be easily discriminated. Color Doppler is also more sensitive for detecting patency of veins in the calf than is older duplex imaging, particularly when combined with compression and valsalva techniques.[89] Many investigators now consider color Doppler with compression techniques the procedure of choice for detecting DVT in the legs.

Nevertheless, assessment of all of the calf veins is tedious and difficult under the best of circumstances; fewer than 60% of calf vessels can be visualized.[90] Obesity and edema also impair delineation of structure by ultrasound. And, there is again the problem of distinguishing recent from prior causes of obstruction. In a study by Cronan and Leen, who followed 60 patients for 6 to 21 months after onset of acute DVT, nearly one half of patients had evidence of residual venous obstruction.[91]

Thus, most commonly employed techniques for diagnosing DVT suffer drawbacks: they rely upon indirect evidence for the presence of thrombosis, they do not distinguish between acute and residual DVT, and the procedures must be repeated if both legs or multiple sites are to be sampled.

RADIONUCLIDE TECHNIQUES

Early radionuclide studies attempted to duplicate contrast venography without the necessity of pedal injections and the use of irritating contrast media. The most commonly used tracer has been ^{99m}Tc-labeled RBCs to image the intravascular blood.[92–95] A reliable use of this type of study is in the diagnosis of superior vena cava thrombosis (Fig. 12). However, the use of labeled RBC venography in detecting DVT in the legs has been relatively disappointing, both for lack of sensitivity and specificity (Fig. 13). In a study by Leclerc et al., the sensitivity for proximal DVT in the lower extremity was 68% and specificity was 88%.[95] Some studies have found radionuclide venography to compare favorably with contrast venography[92,93]; however, most studies to date have used small numbers of patients and widely varying techniques to derive their conclusions.[96]

In recent years, the principal thrust in the nuclear medicine diagnosis of deep venous thrombosis has been the search

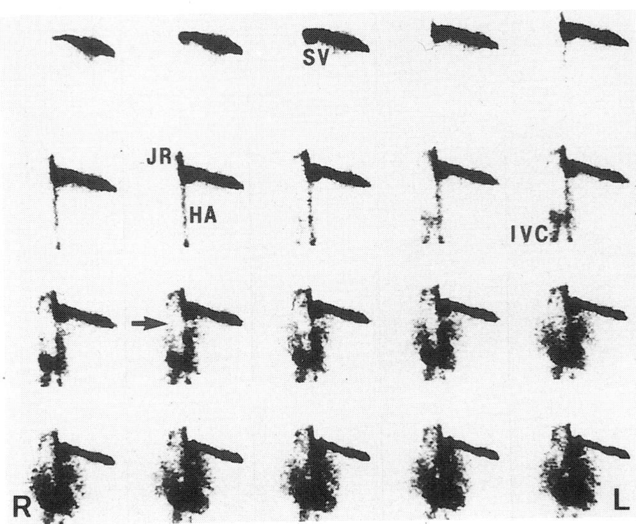

Figure 12. Radionuclide angiogram in a 43-year-old female with swollen neck veins suspected of having superior vena cava obstruction. Following the intravenous injection of 370 MBq (10 mCi) ^{99m}Tc-DTPA into the left antecubital vein, serial 2-s images were taken over the thorax and lower neck. The study demonstrates stasis within the left axillary and subclavian veins (SV), retrograde flow into the left jugular (JR) and hemiazygous (HA) veins, absence of the superior vena cava (arrow), filling of the inferior vena cava (IVC), and subsequent return to the heart and lungs. An identical study (not shown) performed from the right antecubital vein, revealed normal blood flow through the heart and lungs, thus excluding an obstruction of the superior vena cava. (Reproduced with permission from Reference 97.)

for radiolabeled agents that would specifically combine with newly formed or forming thrombi. Such an agent would not only provide a means of surveying the entire venous system, but would also be able to distinguish between acute and residual DVT. Table 2 lists several radiopharmaceuticals that have been investigated for this purpose.

Radionuclide Venography with Radiolabeled Particles

Radionuclide venography using radiolabeled particles has been described by several investigators.[91,95,113,114] In this technique, 5 to 7 MBq (1.5 to 2.0 mCi) ^{99m}Tc-MAA are injected into the dorsal pedal veins bilaterally. Subsequently, serial scintiphotos are taken over the legs and pelvis in search of focal retention of particles (Fig. 14). Presumably, electrostatic forces between the thrombus and the MAA particles account for adherence of the particles.[114] Some investigators use tourniquets and multiple injections for these studies.[115] Although ^{99m}Tc-microspheres may be somewhat superior to MAA, they are no longer commercially available.

The chief advantage of this method over contrast venography is that, technically, it is easier to perform in patients who have obese or edematous extremities. A much smaller volume of radionuclide is injected, and it may be introduced through a 23- or even 25-gauge needle rather than the 19-gauge needle used for contrast venography. A baseline lung

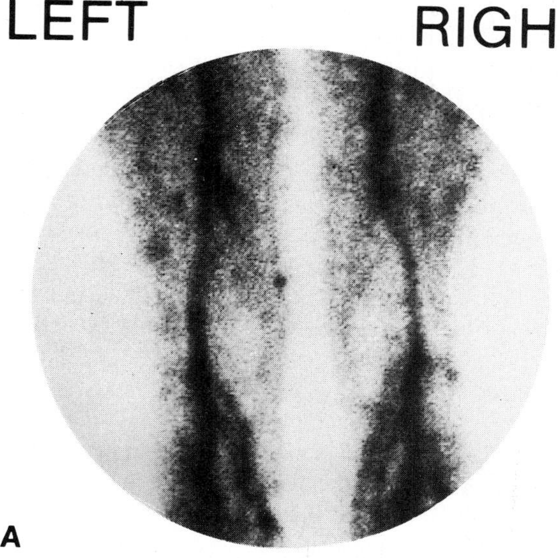

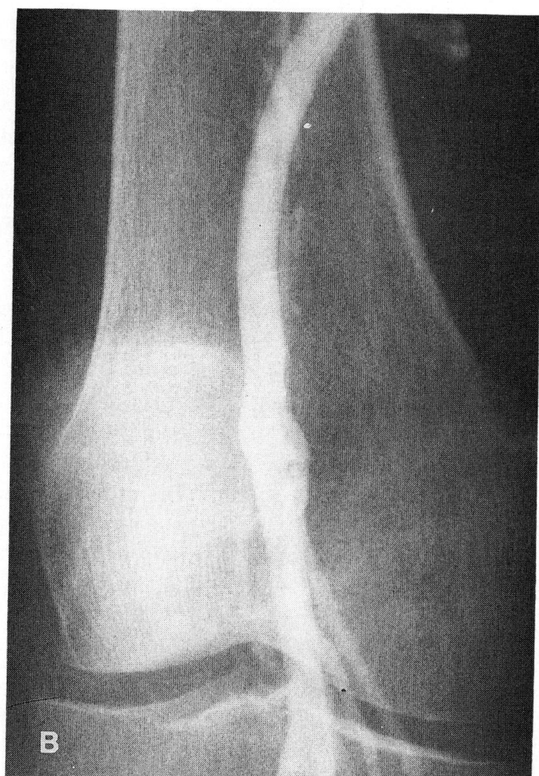

Figure 13. **(A)**. Posterior scintigram of the vessels of the midleg (knees) following the intravenous injection of 750 MBq (20 mCi) ^{99m}Tc-RBCs; there is decreased activity in the right popliteal vein compared to the left. **(B)**. Contrast venography of the right leg was normal and showed no intraluminal filling defect in the popliteal vein. (Reproduced with permission from Reference 95.)

Table 2. Thrombus-Seeking Radiopharmaceuticals

RADIOPHARMACEUTICAL	MECHANISM OF LOCALIZATION
MAA—^{131}I,[95] ^{99m}Tc[81,82]	Physical (electrostatic?) attachment
Albumin microspheres—^{99m}Tc[91]	
Platelets—^{111}In[20], ^{99m}Tc[21]	Incorporation into forming thrombi
Fibrinogen—^{131}I,[97] ^{123}I,[20] ^{125}I,[97] ^{99m}Tc[98]	
Plasmin—^{99m}Tc[99]	
Streptokinase—^{131}I, ^{99m}Tc[100,101]	Fibrinolytic (?)
Urokinase—^{111}In, ^{131}I, ^{99m}Tc[102]	
Antifibrin—^{111}In,[103] ^{99m}Tc[103]	Fibrin epitope and platelet membrane attachment
Antiplatelet MoAbs—^{111}I,[104,105] ^{123}I,[104] ^{99m}Tc[106,107]	
Anti-Activated platelet MoAbs—^{123}I,[108] ^{99m}Tc[109]	Binds to epitope of activated platelets
Anti-t-PA—^{111}In[110]	Binds to formed and lysing thrombi(?)
Fibronectin—^{131}I[111]	Binds to atheroma elements (?)
Fragment E_1—^{123}I[112]	Binds to fibrin polymers

scan is also obtained with no additional radiation exposure. Most studies comparing radionuclide venography with contrast venography have demonstrated a sensitivity of about 90% and false-positive and false-negative rates averaging about 5% each. A significant problem with radionuclide venography is that it is difficult to achieve uniform distribution of the MAA throughout the veins of the calf, which accounts for many false-negative examinations and one reason this test is now seldom performed. One possible application is its use in pregnancy in detecting obstruction of the deep pelvic veins.[116] These veins are not well visualized by other imaging modalities, including ultrasound.

Fibrinogen Uptake Test

Fibrinogen is transformed by thrombin cleavage into fibrin, which mechanically blocks the flow of blood through damaged blood vessels. The incorporation of radiolabeled fibrinogen provides the basis for the fibrinogen uptake test, a relatively sensitive means for detecting DVT. The principle radiopharmaceutical used for this test has been ^{125}I-fibrinogen, although it is no longer produced commercially in the U.S.A. In this test, 3 to 5 MBq (100 to 200 μCi) of ^{125}I-fibrinogen are injected intravenously after oral thyroid blocking dose of 100 mg NaI. The legs are marked at sequential 2-inch segments from the inguinal ligament along the medial thigh and posteriorly from the popliteal fossa down the dorsal aspect of the calf to the ankle, and these points are counted at intervals. Counts are taken using a hand-held probe. After 10 minutes of elevating the legs to reduce background from circulating fibrinogen, counts are taken over each segment and over the precordial blood pool, which is used as the denominator for count ratios in the leg. Routinely, two 5-second counts are obtained 4 hours after injection and are repeated daily for 5 to 6 days. The results are plotted on graph paper and expressed as a percentage of precordial activity.

A normal pattern consists of gradually diminishing activ-

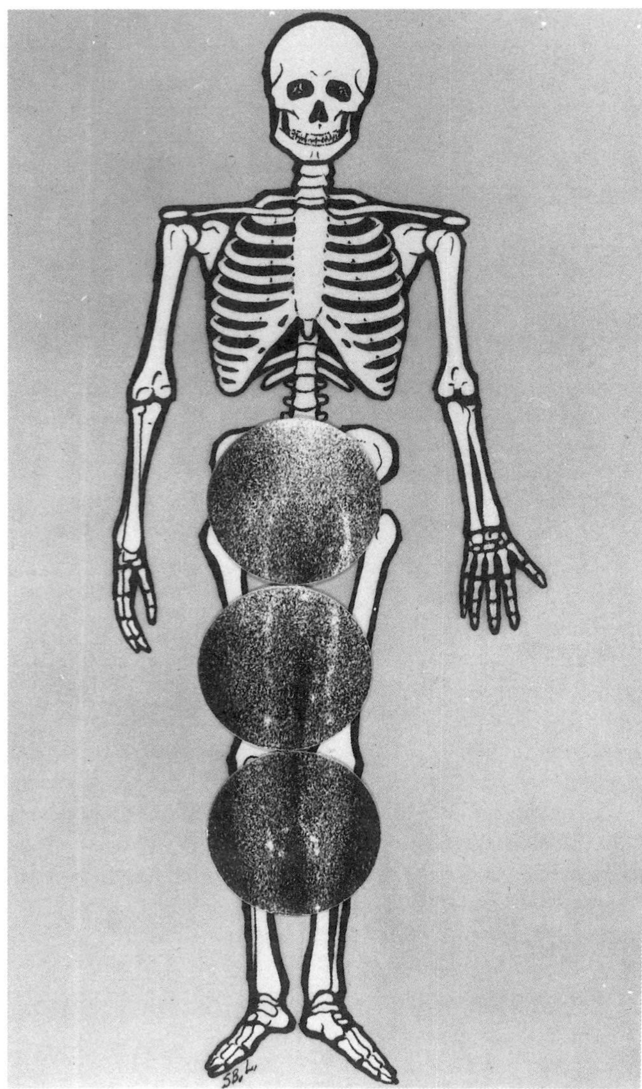

Figure 14. Deep venous thrombosis: Multiple thrombi are well outlined 20 min following injection of ^{99m}Tc-MAA into both dorsalis pedis veins.

ity from the inguinal ligament down to the ankle, except for a slight increase frequently observed in the popliteal fossa. A positive test is determined by any of three criteria: (1) a difference of 20% between adjacent sites on the same leg, (2) a difference of 20% between the same sites on opposite legs or, (3) a consistent increase greater than 15% over any site as compared with the same site on previous observations. Any abnormality should be confirmed by testing for persistence at 24 hours.

In several studies summarized by Kakkar, the agreement between ^{125}I-fibrinogen tests and contrast venography was 92%.[97] False-positive results were found in 7% of patients; false-negative results were found in 4%. The chief limitations of the test are the long period of time (at least 24 hours) to complete the test, and the fact that pelvic vein thrombosis cannot be detected both because of high bladder activity and because of the low, 27-keV energy of ^{125}I. A serious production problem with fibrinogen is that it must be obtained from hepatitis-free and HIV-free donors.

Labeled Platelets

With the development of ^{111}In-labeling of platelets by Thakur et al., imaging of platelet depositions within venous thrombi became possible.[117] Platelet labeling techniques are discussed in Chapter 32 and will not be addressed here, except to observe that platelet viability and spleen dosimetry considerations limit the labeling dose of ^{111}In to about 20 MBq (0.5 mCi) in platelet imaging studies. Both early (2 to 4 hours) and delayed (24 to 96 hours) imaging have been reported.[118–123]

In the study by Farlow et al.,[123] 65 patients with clinically suspected DVT (mean symptom duration = 8 days) were studied within 2 hours of injection of 150 MBq (0.4 mCi) ^{111}In-labeled autologous platelets. In comparison with contrast venography performed at the same time, the sensitivity was 40%, and specificity was 95%. These results contrast sharply with those of Seabold et al.,[121] who studied 31 nonheparinized patients with suspected DVT, presenting 1 to 6 days after onset of symptoms and imaged 4 and 24 hours after injection. They found sensitivities of 69% at 4 hours vs 100% at 24 hours and specificities of 92% vs 89%, respectively. From these and other studies, a number of generalizations can be made:

1. Delayed labeled platelet images are more sensitive than early images, primarily because reduced blood background permits visualization of smaller, less active "hot spots." The principle question from a clinical point of view remains, "Can one justify withholding anticoagulants for 24 hours when DVT is suspected?"
2. Early images appear to be somewhat more specific, because fewer sources of false-positive images interfere with interpretation. Causes of false-positive images include[124]:
   - hematomas
   - hemangiomas[125]
   - varicose veins (increased blood background)
   - inflammation
3. Heparin therapy interferes with platelet localization.
4. ^{111}In-labeled platelets appear to be an accurate means of detecting the *development* of DVT in asymptomatic high-risk patients postoperatively.[126,127] In a study by Siegel et al., who studied 473 patients who had undergone extensive orthopedic surgery, no patient who had negative imaging, nor any patient who had verified positive scintigraphy and received appropriate heparin therapy, subsequently developed symptoms or signs of pulmonary embolism.[126]

Monoclonal Antibodies

Two major types of antithrombus antibodies have been developed to detect both venous and arterial thrombi—

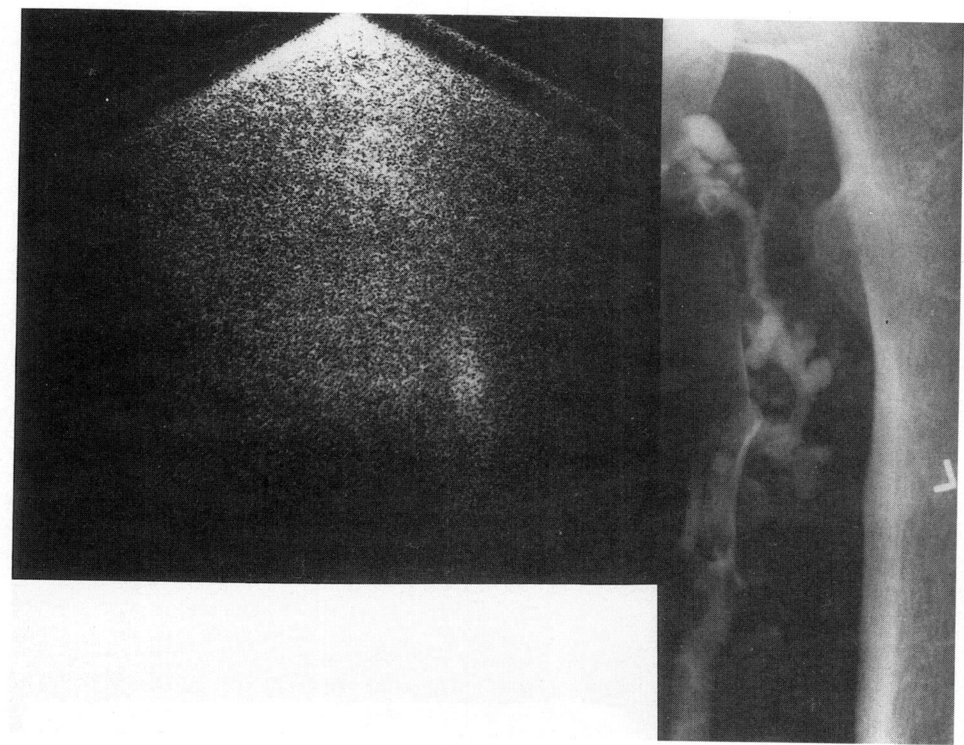

Figure 15. Anterior scintiphoto of the pelvis showing ^{111}In-F(ab′)2 GC4 thrombus accumulation in the patient's left upper groin. Venography reveals a large thrombus in the femoral vein. (Reproduced by courtesy of Dr. Scott F. Rosebrough.)

antiplatelet antibodies and antifibrin antibodies. The first report on successful thrombus radioimmunoimaging was published by Oster and colleagues in 1985 using the 7E3 antibody that binds to a glycoprotein complex on the platelet membrane.[128] Subsequently, several antiplatelet antibodies and fragments have been developed labeled with ^{111}In, ^{123}I, and ^{99m}Tc.[109,129–131] Some of the most promising studies have been reported with antibody fragments labeled with ^{99m}Tc.[130] These antibodies have shown high immunoreactivity to platelets and clots, but no binding to other blood elements. Blood half-disappearance times have been short and thrombus:blood ratios up to 15 have been demonstrated. More recent studies have examined the use of antibodies only to *activated* platelets.[109] It is hoped that such tracers will constitute highly specific tests for both arterial and venous thrombi, and possibly even be used to monitor thrombus dissolution with thrombolytic therapy.

Antibodies have also been labeled that bind specifically to activated platelets,[108,109] or to the protein, thrombospondin, secreted in alpha granules by activated platelets and thought to be a kind of extracellular "glue."[132] Koblick et al. have written a good review of various immunoscintigraphic agents used in the detection of DVT.[133] MoAbs are most useful during the acute phase of thrombogenesis when active platelet aggregation and stimulation are occurring. In experimental studies, clots older than 24 to 48 hours are seldom imaged.[134]

Antifibrin Antibodies

Antifibrin monoclonal antibodies were first reported by Hui et al., and denominated the 59D8 antibody.[135] Subsequently, the T2G1s antibody was developed by Kudryk, probably to the same epitope.[136] Since then, several whole antibodies and various monomeric and dimeric fragment preparations (Fab, Fab′, and F(ab′)2) labeled with ^{111}In and ^{99m}Tc have been reported.[136–141] For the most part, these antibodies bind to an epitope on the fibrin molecule exposed only after the action of thrombin on fibrinogen (i.e., the fibrin monomer that results after thrombin cleavage of fibrinogen). Thus, they do not label circulating fibrinogen. Furthermore, the T2G1s antibody, with which most clinical work has been done, does not bind to fibrin that has undergone fibrinolysis, because the specific epitope is cleaved by plasmin. Thus, this antibody is specific for freshly formed thrombi.

In general, Fab fragments without the Fc portion are preferred, because they clear from the blood more rapidly, their lower molecular weight may permit greater penetration into thrombus, and they are less likely to cause immune reactions. Knight has also shown that Fab fragments labeled with ^{99m}Tc clear faster than those labeled with ^{111}In.[142]

In clinical trials using ^{99m}Tc-labeled T2G1s antifibrin Fab′, a multicenter study of patients with signs and symptoms of DVT found an overall sensitivity of 80% and a specificity of 82% when compared with contrast venography.[142,143] However, when only the results for thrombi in the thighs were considered, the sensitivity was 94%, which is very high indeed. Depending upon the antibody selected, both forming and old thrombi can be targeted.[141]

One approach to imaging older thrombi has been developed by Rosebrough and colleagues.[140] They developed an antibody, GC4, that reacts with an epitope on the D fragment of fibrin, which becomes exposed after plasmin digestion later in the history of thrombus aging. In animal comparisons with the T2G1s antibody, the relative uptake of GC4 rises with increasing age of thrombus. Fig. 15 shows uptake of ^{111}In-F(ab')2 GC4 in the left groin of a patient with angiographically proven DVT.

Recently, antibodies to tissue plasminogen activator (t-PA) have been labeled for imaging thrombi.[110] This antibody has a relatively rapid blood clearance half-time and background can be dramatically reduced by subsequent administration of the t-PA antigen in subtherapeutic doses.[144] Another apparent advantage of anti-t-PA is that its uptake in thrombi may be independent of circulating anticoagulants, which interfere with labeling of most antiplatelet and antifibrin antibodies.

Radiolabeled E_1 Fragment

Knight and colleagues have described thrombus imaging with radiolabeled E_1 fragment.[112] This is a protein derived from the digestion of cross-linked fibrin and is believed to contain a pair of binding sites important for the formation of lateral polymers of fibrin. Clot-to-blood ratios reported for fragment E_1 are similar to those reported for antifibrin antibodies. In animal models, blood clearance of fragment E_1 is somewhat faster than that of antifibrin antibodies or antibody fragments and clots may be imaged somewhat sooner. The major disadvantages of fragment E_1 appear to be that isolation and preparation of the product is difficult and binding to clots is transient.

REFERENCES

1. Wagner HN, Rhodes BA, Sisaki Y, Ryan JP. Studies of the circulation with radioactive microspheres. *Invest Radiol* 1969;4:374.
2. Rhodes BA, Rutherford RB, Lopez-Majano U, et al. Arteriovenous shunt measurements in extremities. *J Nucl Med* 1972;13:357.
3. Webber MM. Labeled albumin macroaggregates for detection of clots. *Semin Nucl Med* 1977;7:253.
4. Rhodes BA, Greyson ND, Siegel ME, et al. The distribution of radioactive microspheres after intra-arterial injection in the legs of patients with peripheral vascular disease. *Am J Roentgenol* 1973;118:820.
5. Siegel ME, Giorgiana FA, Rhodes BA, et al. Effect of reactive hyperemia on the distribution of radioactive microspheres in patients with peripheral vascular disease. *Am J Roentgenol* 1974;118:814.
6. Cuypers Y, Merchie G. Etude de la circulation sanguine peripherique a l'aide de serum albumine humaine marlfuee a ^{131}I. La circulation an neereau du mollet. *Cardiology* 1962;41:166.
7. Muroff LR, Freedman GS. Radionuclide angiography, *Semin Nucl Med* 1976;6:217.
8. Kaplan E, Mayron LW. Evaluation of perfusion with the ^{81}Rb-^{81m}Kr generator. *Semin Nucl Med* 1976;6:163.
9. Miyamoto AT, Mishkin FA, Maxwell T. Noninvasive study of extremity perfusion by potassium-43 scanning. *J Nucl Med* 1974;15:518.
10. Strauss HW, Harrison K, Pitt B. Thallium-201: noninvasive determination from the regional distribution of cardiac output. *J Nucl Med* 1977;18:1167.
11. Oshima M, Akanabe H, Sadayuki S, et al. Quantification of leg muscle perfusion using thallium-201 single photon emission computed tomography. *J Nucl Med* 1989;30:458.
12. Segall GM, Lennon SE, Stevick CD. Exercise whole-body thallium scintigraphy in the diagnosis and evaluation of occlusive arterial disease in the legs. *J Nucl Med* 1990;31:1443.
13. Siegel ME, Wagner HN. Radioactive tracers in peripheral vascular disease. *Semin Nucl Med* 1976;6:253.
14. Lassen NA, Lindbjerg IF, Dahn I. Validity of the ^{133}Xe method for measurement of muscle blood flow evaluated by simultaneous venous occlusion plethysmography: Observations in the calf of normal man and patients with occlusive vascular disease. *Circ Res* 1965;16:287.
15. Tonnesen KH. The blood flow through calf muscle during rhythmic contraction and in rest and in patients with occlusive arterial disease measured by Xe-133. *Scand J Clin Lab Invest* 1965;17:433.
16. Alpert JS, Larsen OA, Lassen NA. Exercise and intermittent claudication. Blood flow in the calf muscle during walking studied by xenon-133 clearance method. *Circulation* 1969;39:353.
17. Lassen NA, Holstein P. Use of radioisotopes in assessment of distal blood flow and distal blood pressure in arterial insufficiency. *Surg Clin North Amer* 1974;54:39.
18. Ritchie JL, Stratton JR, Thiele B, et al. Indium-111 platelets imaging for detection of platelet deposition in abdominal aneurysms and prosthetic grafts. *Am J Cardiol* 1981;47:884.
19. Davis HH, et al. Scintigraphic detection of carotid, atherosclerosis with indium-111 labeled autologous platelets. *Circulation* 1980;61:982.
20. DeNardo SJ, DeNardo GL. Iodine-123-fibrinogen scintigraphy. *Semin Nucl Med* 1977;7:245.
21. Hardeman MR. Thrombocytes labelled with 99mTc-HMPAO in vitro studies and preliminary clinical experience. *Prog Clin Biol Res* 1990;355:49.
22. Kaliman J, Sinzinger H, Bergmann H, Kolbe C. Value of ^{123}I-low-density lipoprotein (LDL) in the diagnosis of human atherosclerotic lesions. *Circulation* 1987;72:789.
23. Sinzinger H, Angelberger P, Pesl H, Flores J. Further insight into lipid lesion imaging by means of ^{123}I-labeled autologous low-density lipoproteins (LDL). VIII, in Crepaldi G, Gotto AM, Baggio G, (eds.): *Atherosclerosis VIII*. Amsterdam, New York, Oxford, Excerpta Medica, 1989, p 645.
24. Lees RS, Lees AM, Strauss HW. External imaging of human atherosclerosis. *J Nucl Med* 1985;24:154.
25. Lupattelli G, Palumbo R, Deleide G, Ventura S. Radiolabelled LDL in the in vivo detection of human atherosclerotic plaques, in Crepaldi E, Gotto AM, Manzato E, Baggio G (eds.): *Atherosclerosis VIII*. Amsterdam, New York, Oxford, Excerpta Medica, 1989.
26. Lees RS, Garabedian HD, Lees AM. Technetium-99m-low density lipoproteins: preparation and biodistribution. *J Nucl Med* 1985;26:1056.
27. Lees AM, Lees RS, Schön FJ. Imaging human atherosclerosis with ^{99m}Tc-labeled low-density lipoprotein in human subjects. *Arteriosclerosis* 1988;8:461.
28. Vallabhajosula S, Paidi M, Badimon JJ, Ginsberg H. Radiotracers for low-density lipoprotein biodistribution studies in vivo: technetium-99m-low-density lipoprotein versus radioiodinated low-density lipoprotein preparations. *J Nucl Med* 1988;29:1237.
29. Rosen JM, Butler SP, Heinken GE, et al. Indium-111-labeled LDL: a potential agent for imaging atherosclerotic disease and lipoprotein biodistribution. *J Nucl Med* 1990;31:343.
30. Virgolini I, Angelberger P, Li SR, et al. Indium-111-labeled

low-density lipoprotein binds with higher affinity to the human liver as compared to iodine-123-low-density-labeled lipoprotein. *J Nucl Med* 1991;32:2132.

31. Fischman AJ, Rubin RH, Khaw BA, et al. Radionuclide imaging of experimental atherosclerosis with nonspecific, polyclonal immunoglobulin G. *J Nucl Med* 1989;30:1095.
32. Kety SS. Measurement of regional circulation by the local clearance of radioactive sodium. *Am Heart J* 1949;38:321.
33. Lassen NA, Henriksen O. Tracer studies of peripheral circulation, in: Lambrecht RM, Rescigno A (eds.). *Tracer Kinetics and Physiologic Modeling*. Berlin, Springer-Verlag, 1983, p 235.
34. Wagner HN Jr. Regional pulmonary blood flow in man by radioisotope scanning. *JAMA* 1964;187:601.
35. Bassingthwaighte JB, Holloway GA. Estimation of blood flow with radioactive tracers. *Semin Nucl Med* 1976;6:141.
36. Krovetz L, Benson R. Mixing of dy in the canine aorta. *J Appl Physiol* 1950;20:922.
37. Siegel ME, Stewart CA. Tl-201 peripheral perfusion scans: Feasibility of single dose, single-day, rest and stress study. *Am J Roentgenol* 1981;136:1179.
38. Glass EC, DeNardo GL. Abnormal peripheral distribution of thallium-201 due to arteriosclerosis. *Am J Roentgenol* 1978;131:718.
39. Hamanaka D, Odori T, Maeda H, et al. A quantitative assessment of scintigraphy of the legs using ^{201}Tl. *Eur J Nucl Med* 1984;9:12.
40. Seder JS, Botvinick EH, Rahimtoola SH, et al. Detecting and localizing peripheral arterial disease: Assessment of ^{201}Tl scintigraphy. *AJR* 1981;137:373.
41. Earnshaw JJ, Hardy JG, Hopkinson BR, Makin GS. Noninvasive investigation of lower limb revascularisation using resting thallium peripheral perfusion imaging. *Eur J Nucl Med* 1986;12:443.
42. Christian WJ, Schieper CA, Siegel ME. Assessment of peripheral vascular perfusion of the lower extremities with hexa-MIBI (RP-30): a new noninvasive approach (Abst). *Radiology* 1988;169(suppl):336.
43. Sayman HB, Urgancioglu I. Muscle perfusion with technetium-MIBI in lower extremity peripheral arterial diseases. *J Nucl Med* 1991;32:1700.
44. Moore WS. Determination of amputation level. *Arch Surg* 1973;107:798.
45. Tauxe WN, Simons JN, Lipscomb PR, et al. Determination of vascular status of pedicle skin flaps by use of radioactive pertechnetate (^{99m}Tc). *Surg Gynecol Obstet* 1970;130:87.
46. Siegel ME, Williams GM, Giorgiana FA, et al. A useful, objective criterion for determining the healing potential of an ischemic ulcer. *J Nucl Med* 1975;16:993.
47. Daly MJ, Henry RE. Quantitative measurement of skin perfusion with Xenon-133. *J Nucl Med* 1980;21:156.
48. Romano RL, Burgess EM. Level selection in lower extremity amputations. *Clin Orthop Related Res* 1971;74:177.
49. Bohr H. Measurement of the blood flow in the skin with radioactive xenon. *Scan J Clin Lab Invest* (Suppl) 1967;93:60.
50. Sejrsen P. Measurement of cutaneous blood flow by freely diffusible radioactive isotopes. *Dan Med Bull* 1971; 18(Suppl 3):9.
51. Malone JM, Leal JM, Moore WS, et al. The "gold standard" for amputation level selection: Xenon-133 clearance. *J Surg Res* 1981;30:449.
52. Roon AJ, Moore WS, Goldstone H. Below-knee amputation: a modern approach. *Am J Surg* 1977;134:153.
53. Wahner HW. Assessment of the viability of skin grafts. *Semin Nucl Med* 1988;18:255.
54. Herold TJ, Dewanjee MK, Wahner HW. Preparation of xenon-133 solution for intravenous administration. *J Nucl Med Tech* 1985;13:72.
55. Tsuchida Y. Rate of skin blood flow in various regions of the body. *Plast Reconstr Surg* 1979;64:505.
56. Snelling CFT, Poomee A, Sutherland JB, et al. Timing of distant flap pedicle division using Xenon-133 clearance. *Ann Plast Surg* 1980;5:201.
57. Wahner HW, Robertson JS. Skin graft viability test, in Wahner H (ed.): *Nuclear Medicine: Quantitative Procedures*. Boston, Little, Brown, 1983, p 407.
58. Tauxe WN, Simons JN, Lipscomb PR, et al. Determination of vascular status of pedicle skin flaps by use of radioactive pertechnetate (^{99m}Tc). *Surg Gynecol Obstet* 1970;130:87.
59. Siegel ME, Stewart CA, Wagner W, et al. A new objective criteria for determining, noninvasively, the healing potential of an ischemic ulcer. *J Nucl Med* 1981;22:187.
60. Ohta T. Non-invasive technique using 201Tl for predicting ischaemic ulcer of the healing of the foot. *Br J Surg* 1985;72:892.
61. Siegel ME, Stewart CA, Kwong P, Sakimura I. ^{201}Thallium perfusion study of ischemic ulcers of the leg: Prognostic ability compared with Doppler ultrasound. *Radiology* 1982; 143:233.
62. Siegel ME, Stewart CA, Wagner FW Jr, Sakimura I. An index to measure the healing potential of ischemic ulcers using thallium-201. *Prosthet Orthot Int* 1983;7:67.
63. Siegel ME, Stewart CA. The role of nuclear medicine in evaluating peripheral vascular disease, in Freeman LM, Weissmann HS (eds.): *Nuclear Medicine Annual 1984*. New York: Raven Press, 1984, p 227.
64. Salimi Z, Vas W, Tang-Barton P et al. Assessment of tissue viability in frostbite by ^{99m}Tc-pertechnetate scintigraphy. *Am J Roentgenol* 1983;142:415.
65. Hunt J, et al. The use of technetium-99m stannous pyrophosphate scintigraphy to identify muscle damage in acute electric burns. *J Trauma* 1979;19:409.
66. Sinzinger H, Bergmann H, Kaliman J, Angelberger P. Imaging of human atherosclerotic lesions using ^{123}I-low-density lipoprotein. *Eur J Nucl Med* 1986;12:291.
67. Tadavarthy SM, Moller JH, Amplatz K. Polyvinyl alcohol (Ivalon): a new embolic material. *AJR* 1975;125:609.
68. duCret RP, Adkins MC, Hunter DW, et al. Therapeutic embolization: enhanced radiolabeled monitoring. *Radiology* 1990;177:571.
69. Sirr SA, Johnson TK, Stuart DD, et al. An improved radiolabeling technique of Ivalon and its use for dynamic monitoring of complications during therapeutic transcatheter embolization. *J Nucl Med* 1989;30:1399.
70. Johnson TK. MABDOS: a generalized program for internal radionuclide dosimetry. *Comput Meth Programs Biomed* 1988;27:159.
71. Moss CM, Rudavsky AZ, Veith FJ. Value of scintiangiography in arterial disease. *Arch Surg* 1976;111:1235.
72. Moss CM, et al. Isotope angiography: Techniques, validation, and value in assessment of arterial reconstruction. *Ann Surg* 1976;184:116.
73. Royal H, et al. Scintigraphic identification of bleeding duodenal varices. *Am J Gastroenterol* 1980;74:173.
74. Powers TA, Harolds JA, Kadir S, Grover RB. Pseudoaneurysm of the profunda femoris artery diagnosed on angiographic phase of bone scan. *Clin Nucl Med* 1979;4:422.
75. Wallace JC. First Impressions. *J Nucl Med* 1990;31:429.
76. Rudavsky AZ, Moss CM, Veith FJ. Arterial visualization by isotope angiography, in Dietrich EB (ed.): *Non-Invasive Cardiovascular Diagnosis*. Baltimore, University Park Press, 1978.
77. Miyamae T, Fujioka M, Tsubogo Y, et al. Detection of a large

arteriovenous fistula between the internal iliac vessels by radionuclide angiography. *J Nucl Med* 1979;20:36.

78. Rudavsky AZ. Radionuclide angiography in the evaluation of arterial and venous grafts. *Semin Nucl Med* 1988; 18:261.
79. Rutherford RB, Rhodes BA, Wagner HN. The distribution of extremity blood flow before and after vagectomy in a patient with hypertrophic pulmonary osteoarthropathy. *Dis Chest* 1969;56:19.
80. Rhodes BA, Greyson NP, Hamilton CR, et al. Absence of anatomic arteriovenous shunts in Paget's disease of bone. *N Engl J Med* 1972;287:686.
81. Goldhaber SZ. Strategies for diagnosis, in Goldhaber SZ (ed.): *Pulmonary embolism and deep venous thrombosis*. Philadelphia, PA, Saunders, 1985, p 79.
82. Goldhaber SZ, Hennekens CH, Evans DA, et al. Factors associated with correct antemortem diagnosis of major pulmonary embolism. *Am J Med* 1982;73:822.
83. Hirsch J, Hull RD, Raskob GE. Clinical features and diagnosis of venous thrombosis. *J Am Coll Cardiol* 1986;8:114B.
84. McLachlan MSF, Thomson JG, Taylor DW, et al. Observer variation in the interpretation of lower limb venograms. *AJR* 1979;132:227.
85. Rabinov K, Paulin S. Roentgen diagnosis of venous thrombosis in the leg. *Arch Surg* 1972;104:134.
86. Bettmann MA, Robbins A, Braun SD, et al. Contrast venography of the leg: Diagnostic efficacy, tolerance, and complication ratio with ionic and non-ionic contrast media. *Radiology* 1987;165:113.
87. Hull R, Hirsh J, Sackett DL, et al. Combined use of leg scanning and impedance plethysmography in suspected venous thrombosis: An alternative to venography. *N Engl J Med* 1977;296:1497.
88. Hull RD, Carter CJ, Jay RM, et al. The diagnosis of acute, recurrent deep vein thrombosis: A diagnostic challenge. *Circulation* 1983;67:901.
89. Cronan JJ, Dorfman GS. Advances in ultrasound imaging of venous thrombosis. *Semin Nucl Med* 1991;21:297.
90. Rose SC, Zwiebel WJ, Nelson BD, et al. Symptomatic lower extremity deep venous thrombosis: Accuracy, limitations, and role of color Duplex flow imaging in diagnosis. *Radiology* 1990;175:639.
91. Webber MM, Resnick LH, Victory WK, et al. Thrombosis scanning: its reliability and usefulness, *J Nucl Med* 1972;13:476.
92. Beswick W, Chmiel R, Booth R, et al. Detection of deep venous thrombosis by scanning of ^{99m}technetium-labelled-red-cell venous pool. *Br Med J* 1979;1:82.
93. Lisbona R, Stern J, Derbekyan D. Tc-99m red blood cell venography in deep vein thrombosis of the leg: a correlation with contrast venography. *Radiology* 1982;143:771.
94. Singer I, Royal HD, Uren RF, et al. Radionuclide plethysmography and Tc-99m red blood cell venography in venous thrombosis: comparison with contrast venography. *Radiology* 1984;150:213.
95. Rosenthall L, et al. Measurement of lower extremity arteriovenous shunting with ^{131}I macroaggregates of albumin. *J Can Assoc Radiol* 1970;21:153.
96. Henkin RE, Rao JST, Quinn JL, et al. Isotope venography in lower extremity vascular disease. *J Nucl Med* 1973;14:407.
97. Kakkar V. 125-Iodine-fibrinogen uptake test. *Semin Nucl Med* 1977;7:229.
98. Wong DW, Mishkin FS. Technetium-99m-human fibrinogen. *J Nucl Med* 1975;16:343.
99. Deacon JM, En PJ, Anderson P, Khan O. Technetium 99m-plasmin: a new test for the detection of deep vein thrombosis. *Br J Radiol* 1980;53:673.
100. Siegel ME, et al. Scanning of thromboembolism with I-131 streptokinase. *Radiology* 1972;103:695.
101. Dugan MA, et al. Localization of deep venous thrombosis using radioactive streptokinase. *J Nucl Med* 1973;14:233.
102. Millar WT, Smith JF. Localization of deep-venous thrombosis using technetium-99m-labelled urokinase. *Lancet* 1974;2:695.
103. Schaible TF, Alavi A. Antifibrin scintigraphy in the diagnostic evaluation of acute deep venous thrombosis. *Semin Nucl Med* 1991;21:313.
104. Oster ZH, Srivastava SC, Som P, et al. Thrombus radioimmunoscintigraphy: an approach using monoclonal antiplatelet antibody. *Proc Natl Acad Sci USA* 1985;82:3456.
105. Peters AM, Lavender LP, Needham SG, et al. Imaging thrombus with radiolabeled monoclonal antibody to platelets. *Br Med J* 1986;293:1525.
106. Som P, Oster ZH, Zamora PO, et al. Radioimmunoimaging of experimental thrombi in dogs using technetium-99m-labeled monoclonal antibody fragments reactive with human platelets. *J Nucl Med* 1986;27:1315.
107. Oster ZH, Som P. Editorial: Of monoclonal antibodies and thrombus-specific imaging. *J Nucl Med* 1990;31:1055.
108. McEver RP, Martin MN. A monoclonal antibody to a membrane glycoprotein binds only to activated platelets. *J Biol Chem* 1984;259:9799.
109. Palabrica TM, Furie BC, Konstam MA, et al. Thrombus imaging in a primate model with antibodies specific for an external membrane protein of activated platelets. *Proc Natl Acad Sci USA* 1989;86:1036.
110. Tromholt N, Hesse B, Folkenborg O, et al. Immunoscintigraphic detection of deep venous thrombophlebitis in the lower extremities with indium-111 labeled monoclonal antibody against tissue plasminogen activator. *Eur J Nucl Med* 1991;18:321.
111. Uehara A, Isaka Y, Hashikawa K, et al. Iodine-131-labeled fibronectin: potential agent for imaging atherosclerotic lesion and thrombus. *J Nucl Med* 1988;29:1264.
112. Knight LC, Maurer AH, Robbins PS, et al. Fragment E_1 labeled with I-123 in the detection of venous thrombosis. *Radiology* 1985;156:509.
113. Duffy GJ, et al. New radioisotope test for detection of deep venous thrombosis in the legs. *Br Med J* 1973;1:712.
114. Webber MM, et al. Demonstration of thrombophlebitis and endothelial damage by scintiscanning. *Radiology* 1971; 100:93.
115. Henkin RE. Radionuclide detection of thromboembolic diseases, in Kwaan HC, Bowle EJW (eds.): *Thrombosis*. Philadelphia, W.B. Saunders, 1982.
116. Dhekne RD, Barron BJ, Koch ER. Radionuclide venography in pregnancy. *J Nucl Med* 1987;28:1290.
117. Thakur ML, et al. Indium-111 labeled platelets: Preparation, function studies and in vivo evaluation. *J Nucl Med* 1976;17:561.
118. Grimely RP, Rafiqi E, Hawker RJ, Drolc Z. Imaging of indium-111 labeled platelets—a new method for the diagnosis of deep venous thrombosis. *Br J Surg* 1981;68:714.
119. Fenech A, Hussey JK, Smith FW, et al. Diagnosis of deep vein thrombosis using autologous indium-111-labeled platelets. *Br Med J* 1981;282:1020.
120. Ezekowitz MD, Pope CF, Sostman HD, et al. Indium-111 platelet scintigraphy for the diagnosis of acute venous thrombosis. *Circulation* 1986;73:667.
121. Seabold JE, Conrad GR, Ponto JA, et al. Deep venous thrombophlebitis: detection with 4-hour versus 24-hour platelet scintigraphy. *Radiology* 1987;165:355.
122. Davis HH, Siegel BA, Sherman LA, et al. Scintigraphy with indium-111-labeled platelets in venous thromboembolism. *Radiology* 1980;136:203.

123. Farlow DC, Ezekowitz MD, Rao SR, et al. Early image acquisition after administration of Indium-111 platelets in clinically suspected deep venous thrombosis. *Am J Cardiol* 1989; 64:363.
124. Sinzinger H, Virgolini I. Nuclear medicine and atherosclerosis. *Eur J Nucl Med* 1990;17:160.
125. Shulkin BL, Argenta LC, Cho KJ, Castle VP. Kasabach-Merritt syndrome: treatment with epsilon aminocaproic acid and assessment by indium 111 platelet scintigraphy. *J Pediatr* 1990;1217:746.
126. Siegel RS, Rae JL, Ryan NL, et al. The use of Indium-111 labeled platelet scanning for the detection of asymptomatic deep venous thrombosis in a high risk population. *Orthopedics* 1989;12:1439.
127. Clarke-Pearson KL, Coleman RE, Siegel RS, et al. Indium-111 platelet imaging for the detection of deep venous thrombosis and pulmonary embolism in patients without symptoms after surgery. *Surgery* 1985;98:98.
128. Oster ZH, Srivastava SC, Som P, et al. Thrombus radioimmunoscintigraphy: an approach using monoclonal antiplatelet antibody. *Proc Natl Acad Sci USA* 1985;82:3465.
129. Peters AM, Lavender LP, Needham SG, et al. Imaging thrombus with radiolabeled monoclonal antibody to platelets. *Br Med J* 1986;293:1525.
130. Som P, Oster ZH, Zamora PO, et al. Radioimmunoimaging of experimental thrombi in dogs using technetium-99m-labeled monoclonal antibody fragments reactive with human platelets. *J Nucl Med* 1986;27:1315.
131. Oster ZH, Som P, Zamora PO. Mesenteric vascular occlusion: a new diagnostic method using a radiolabeled monoclonal antibody reactive with platelets. *Radiology* 1989;171:653.
132. Legrand C, Dubernard V, Kieffer N, et al. Use of a monoclonal antibody to measure the surface expression of thrombospondin following platelet activation. *Eur J Biochem* 1988; 171:393.
133. Koblik PD, DeNardo GL, Berger HJ. Current status of immunoscintigraphy in the detection of thrombosis and thromboembolism. *Semin Nucl Med* 1989;19:221.
134. Knight LC, Primeau JL, Siegel BA, et al. Comparison of In-111 labeled platelets and iodinated fibrinogen for the detection of deep vein thrombosis. *J Nucl Med* 1978;19:391.
135. Hui KY, Haber E, Matusueda GR. Monoclonal antibodies to a synthetic fibrin-like peptide bind to human fibrin, but not fibrinogen. *Science* 1983;222:1129.
136. Kudryk BJ, Rohoza A, Ahadi M, et al. Specificity of a monoclonal antibody for the NH_2 terminal region of fibrin. *Mol Immunol* 1984;21:89.
137. Jung M, Kletter K, Dudczak R, et al. Deep vein thrombosis: scintigraphic diagnosis with In-111 labeled monoclonal antifibrin antibodies. *Radiology* 1989;173:469.
138. Rosebrough SF, Grossman ZD, McAfee JG, et al. Aged venous thrombi: radioimmunoimaging with fibrin-specific monoclonal antibody. *Radiology* 1987;162:575.
139. Knight LC, Maurer AH, Ammar IA, et al. Evaluation of indium-111-labeled anti-fibrin antibody for imaging vascular thrombi. *J Nucl Med* 1988;29:494.
140. Rosebrough SF, Grossman ZD, McAfee JG, et al. Thrombus imaging with indium-111 and iodine-131-labeled fibrin-specific monoclonal antibody and its $F(ab')_2$ and F(ab) fragments. *J Nucl Med* 1989;29:1212.
141. Rosebrough SF, McAfee JG, Grossman ZD, et al. Thrombus imaging: a comparison of radiolabeled GC4 and T2GIs fibrin-specific monoclonal antibodies. *J Nucl Med* 1990;31: 1048.
142. Schaible T, DeWoody K, Dann R, et al. Technetium-99m antifibrin scintigraphy accurately diagnoses acute recurrent deep venous thrombosis. *J Nucl Med* 1991;32:967.
143. Schaible T, DeWoody K, Dann R, et al. Accurate diagnosis of acute deep venous thrombosis with technetium-99m antifibrin scintigraphy: Results of phase III trial. *J Nucl Med* 1991;32:1020.
144. Tromholt N, Selmer J. Biological background subtraction improves immunoscintigraphy by subsequent injection of antigen. *J Nucl Med* 1991;32:2318.

25 The Respiratory System

H. Dirk Sostman, Ronald D. Neumann

The clinical use of radionuclides to study regional lung function and pulmonary diseases has become commonplace. The impetus for these studies stems from the work of Knipping and his colleagues, who first used ^{133}Xe to examine regional ventilation more than 40 years ago.[1] Later, Dyson et al. and West and Dollery used ^{15}O as $C^{15}O_2$ to study pulmonary blood flow.[2,3] Since that time, much work has been done using various radionuclides to study both regional ventilation and blood flow.[4–8] In the past few decades, there has been a great increase in understanding of regional pulmonary blood flow and ventilation,[9,10] of lung anatomy and morphology,[11–13] of the mechanical factors that influence lung function[14–16] and, more recently, of the biochemical and other nonrespiratory functions of the lung.[17–19] The relationships between structure and function are remarkable, and a clear understanding of them throws much light on the disturbances seen in pulmonary diseases.

ANATOMY

A knowledge of the lobular, segmental, and lobar structures of the lungs, with their airways, dual blood supply, and lymphatic drainage, provides a useful framework on which to base our short discussion of lung pathophysiology.

Airways and Alveoli

The bronchial tree is formed by the fourth month of intrauterine life. Although rudimentary alveoli appear during fetal development, most of the increase in their number occurs within the first few years of birth, and it continues until about 8 years of age. Alveoli continue enlarging in size until growth of the thorax is complete.[20] The bronchial tree divides irregularly; before the peripheral alveoli are reached, there are up to 16 divisions to the terminal bronchioles, plus 3 or more divisions of the respiratory bronchioles and their alveolar ducts and sacs. Alveoli line the respiratory bronchioles in increasing numbers as the distal bronchial tree is approached. Cartilaginous support ends where the bronchioles begin; the whole bronchial tree, however, is enveloped in smooth muscle, even as far as the entrance to alveolar ducts. In addition, a meshwork of connective tissue, collagen, and elastic fibers spreads around and along the entire bronchial tree and is continuous with the meshwork that surrounds the alveoli.

The intimate relationships between alveoli and airways within the lung parenchyma play an important part in maintaining the stability and patency of both airways and alveoli during respiration.[15]

The conducting airways contain approximately 70 to 80 ml of air and are lined by ciliated epithelium interspersed with a very few goblet cells and, toward the terminal bronchioles, the nonciliated Clara cells. Beneath the mucosa are bronchial glands. A thin layer of mucus moves continuously from the terminal bronchioles toward the larynx because of mucociliary transport.

Alveoli number approximately 250 to 300 million in the adult.[11] The alveolus is the functional end unit that composes the air-blood barrier formed by an alveolar type I cell, the basement membrane, and a capillary endothelial cell. Alveolar type II cells are cuboidal cells that synthesize and secrete pulmonary surfactant, which is spread in a thin film over the entire alveolar surface. Alveolar macrophages are also found within the alveoli.

Intercommunications called the pores of Kohn exist between alveoli. The canals of Lambert, which connect alveoli and neighboring respiratory bronchioles, also provide passages for gas transfer. Both types of communication allow for collateral air drift, which permits air to enter a part of the lung whose bronchus (segmental or smaller) is obstructed, thereby preventing atelectasis.[16,21]

Blood Vessels and Lymphatics

During childhood, the number of small pulmonary arteries increases as the number of alveoli increases. Branches of the pulmonary arteries follow the bronchial tree and divide 22 to 24 times before the terminal arterioles are reached. These latter vessels are about 35 μm in diameter and give rise to a dense capillary network in the walls of each alveolus. Supernumerary pulmonary arteries, which outnumber the pulmonary vessels accompanying the airways, are usually closed but can provide extensive collateral channels between neighboring vessels.[22,23] Alveolar capillaries are 7 to 10 μ in diameter and have tight endothelial junctions. Approximately one thousand capillaries line the surface of each alveolus, so that blood flows around the alveolus nearly like a sheet.

The pulmonary veins drain blood from the alveolar capillaries, the capillaries of the respiratory bronchioles and alveoli, and also from the pleura. These veins run along the edges of lobules toward the hilum before draining into the left atrium.

The bronchial arteries arise from the aorta and travel along the airways, branching with them and nourishing the tissues.[24] Anastomoses between the pulmonary capillaries and bronchial capillaries are found along the respiratory bronchioles.

PHYSIOLOGY

Ventilation

The exchange of air during tidal breathing is accompanied by remarkably small pressure changes within the chest. At functional residual capacity, that is, at the end of a normal expiration when lung elastic recoil balances chest wall recoil, the intrapleural pressure is about 5 cm H_2O less than atmospheric pressure. By convention, atmospheric pressure is called 0, so that intrapleural pressure is -5 cm H_2O. As the intercostal muscles and diaphragm contract, the chest expands and intrapleural pressure falls by approximately 3 cm H_2O. Part of this fall in pressure overcomes the elastic recoil forces in the lung, and part the resistance to airflow drawing air into the lungs. Expiration is a passive process: the pressure necessary to expel the air comes from elastic recoil forces.

Intrapleural pressure is not evenly distributed from the top to the bottom of the lung. It is more negative at the top—approximately -10 cm H_2O compared with -2.5 cm H_2O at the bases—and falls in proportion to the increase in weight of the lungs within the chest. This means that the transpulmonary pressure (the force between alveoli and pleura) is greater at the apex of the lung than at the base and, therefore, that alveoli at the apex of the lung are more expanded than those at the base. In the upright position, alveoli lie on different parts of the lung's compliance or pressure-volume curve, depending on their position in the lung. Those at the top are near the plateau of the curve and expand only slightly for a small change in pressure, while those toward the base of the lung are on a steeper portion of the curve and expand more for the same pressure change (Fig. 1). At total lung capacity, all alveoli have expanded to the same size, but the increase in volume is greater at the base compared to the apex.[25]

At residual volume, the intrapleural pressure at the base of the lung is positive in relation to the atmosphere, and many of the airways are closed. When inhalation starts from residual volume, air preferentially enters the upper parts of the lung where the airways are still open. The basal regions receive air later, as these airways open.

Although the weight of the lung (and hence gravity, acceleration, and posture) is an important determinant of the distribution of pleural pressure, other less defined factors are involved (e.g., the shape and uneven support of the lung within the chest, the presence of ribs and intercostal spaces along the chest wall, which cause subtle changes of pleural pressure, and the mechanical stresses and strains, which are more pronounced over the upper parts of the lung than the lower.[26]

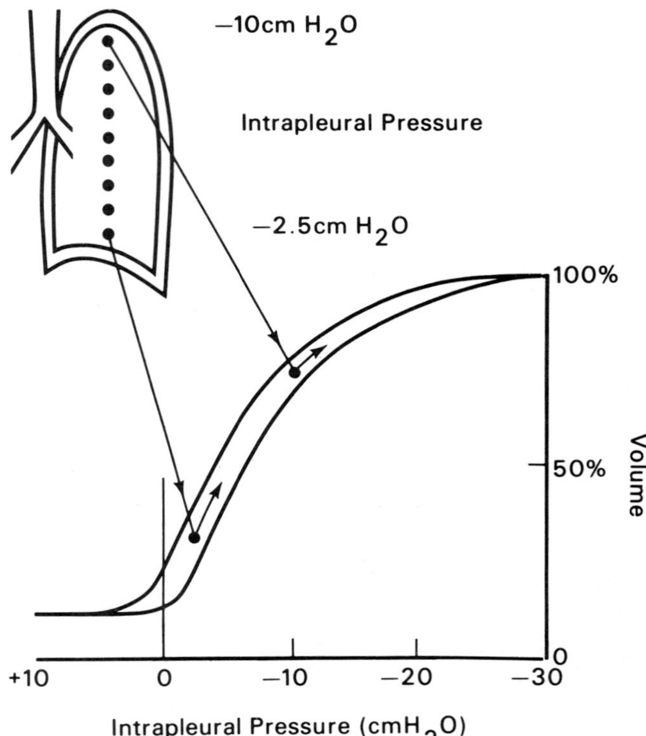

Figure 1. Distribution of regional ventilation differences within the lung. The intrapleural pressure is less negative at the lung base than at the apex because of lung weight, and because the alveoli at the base are smaller than those at the top. For the same change in intrapleural pressure, a greater change in volume occurs in the basal than in the apical alveoli (from West JB[25]).

The distribution of ventilation also depends on airway resistance, that is, the relationship between driving pressure and airflow rate. Most of the resistance to airflow is located in the larger bronchi. Resistance in the smaller bronchi (those less than 2 mm in diameter) accounts for only 10 to 20% of resistance in the airways.[27] Airflow in the larger bronchi is turbulent, and the resistance to flow is related to the square of the velocity and also to gas density and viscosity. In the smaller bronchioles, airflow is thought to be laminar, and the resistance here is independent of gas density but proportional to the length of the airway and inversely proportional to the fourth power of the radius.

Airway resistance increases at low lung volumes as the airways are compressed, and decreases at high volumes as they expand. In addition, increasing rates of breathing increase resistance by increasing turbulent flow, and this increase is more marked at the bases, so that the overall distribution of ventilation is more even.[28] For an expanded discussion of ventilation, refer to Hlastala's review.[29]

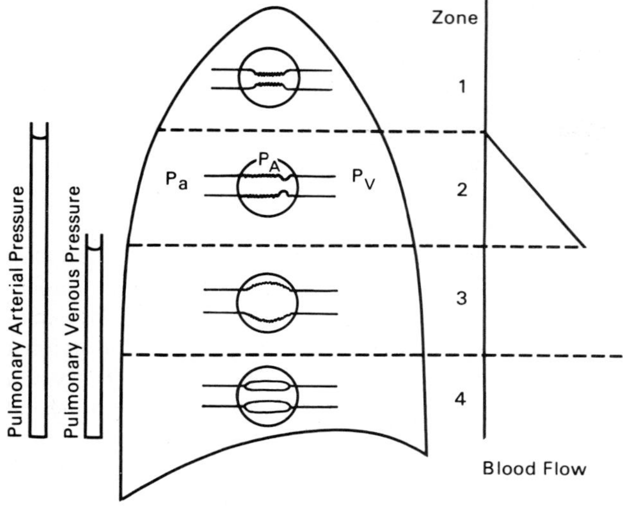

Figure 2. Cause of regional differences in blood flow within the lung. The diagram within each lung zone represents the effects of alveolar pressure (P_A), pulmonary arterial pressure (P_a), and pulmonary venous pressure (P_V) on pulmonary capillaries. In zone 4, the thickened walls of the vessel symbolize the edema found in extra-alveolar vessels. (Modified from West JP[6] and Hughes JMB et al.[34])

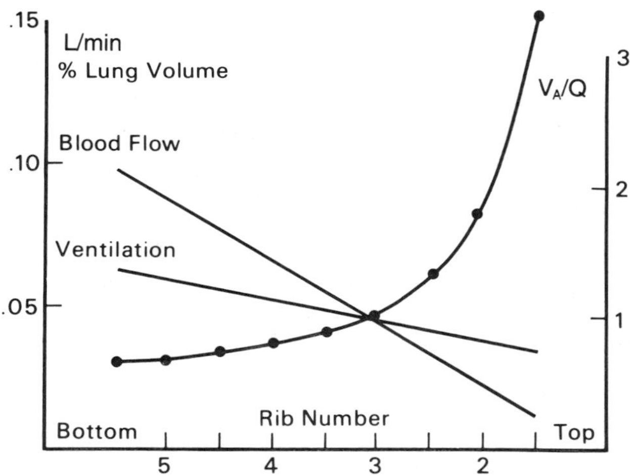

Figure 3. Distribution of ventilation and blood flow within the upright lung. The ventilation-perfusion ratio decreases down the lung (from West JP[25]).

Blood Flow

The normal pulmonary vasculature offers little resistance to blood flow. The entire cardiac output is propelled through the lungs by a mean driving pressure of only 10 to 15 mmHg. Pulmonary vascular resistance falls during exercise, when cardiac output may increase severalfold with only a small increase in pulmonary arterial pressure.

The regional distribution of blood flow is markedly uneven in the upright position, with a threefold to fivefold increase in blood flow per unit volume between the upper and lower zones. This effect is due primarily to gravity.[9,30–32] More blood flows to the dependent portions of the lungs in whatever position the subject lies. In any region of the lung, blood flow is determined by the balance between alveolar pressure, pulmonary arterial pressure, pulmonary venous pressure, and interstitial pressure.[33]

In the upper parts of the upright lung, alveolar pressure exceeds pulmonary arterial pressure, and the capillaries are collapsed (Fig. 2). Blood passes through only at the peaks of the pulsatile pressure wave (West's zone 1).[34] Further down, pulmonary arterial pressure exceeds alveolar pressure, and flow then depends on the difference between these 2 pressures (zone 2). When pulmonary venous pressure exceeds alveolar pressure, flow depends on the difference between pulmonary arterial and venous pressures. In this region of the lung (zone 3), blood flow continues to increase as the difference between these 2 pressures and alveolar pressure increases. The capillaries are more dilated and offer less resistance to blood flow. In the lowermost reaches of the lung, extra-alveolar vascular resistance increases, so that blood flow diminishes (zone 4).

At functional residual capacity, blood flow per unit lung volume is greatest at approximately the level of the fourth rib anteriorly, but at residual volume, the gradient is almost even from top to bottom of the lung.[8,9,28,32,35]

During exertion, the distribution of blood flow rapidly becomes more even and the vertical gradient is lost.[25] Local hypoxia causes constriction of the local pulmonary arterioles and a diversion of blood flow away from the hypoxic region, so that the ratio of ventilation to blood flow tends to return to normal.[36–38] With increasing age, both ventilation and blood flow tend to decrease at the bases of the lungs.[39] In the normal upright lungs, the gradient of ventilation increases 1.5- to 2-fold from the upper third to the lower third (Fig. 3). Blood flow per unit volume increases from threefold to fivefold at functional residual capacity, so that ventilation-perfusion ratios fall from 2 to 3 in the apices to about 0.6 at the base. In fact, at functional residual capacity, the ratio increases slightly again at the base, because blood flow begins to diminish here while ventilation is still increasing slowly.

The concentration or partial pressures of oxygen and carbon dioxide in the alveoli and pulmonary capillary blood depend not on the absolute quantities of ventilation and blood flow, but on the ratio at which ventilation and blood flow are mixed. As the ventilation-perfusion ratio falls, hypoxemia ensues. The oxygen content of the blood that leaves a region with a low ventilation-perfusion ratio cannot be compensated for by a region with a high ventilation-perfusion ratio because of the shape of the oxygen-hemoglobin dissociation curve (Fig. 4). The carbon dioxide level can be corrected, however, because the carbon dioxide-blood dissociation curve is more nearly linear over its working range.

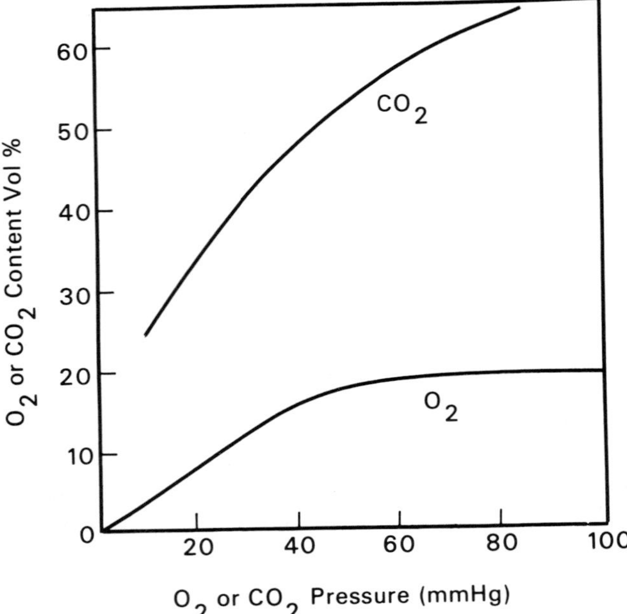

Figure 4. Typical O_2 and CO_2 dissociation curves plotted with the same scales. Note that over the normal working range of pCO_2, 40 to 45 mmHg, the CO_2 curve is steeper and more linear than the O_2 curve over its normal working range, pO_2 40 to 100 mmHg (from West JB[39]).

PATHOPHYSIOLOGY

Abnormal patterns of blood flow are seen in conditions affecting the pulmonary vasculature, such as pulmonary embolism (from thrombus, tumor, amniotic fluid, parasites, air, or fat), vasculitis, arteriovenous fistulae, or the changes that take place with pulmonary hypertension. In addition, compression or invasion of the pulmonary vessels, particularly in the hilum, by tumors, or granulomata can alter the distribution of blood flow. In emphysema, extensive loss of alveolar capillary bed occurs—most markedly in bullous disease—which contributes to the alterations of blood flow seen in these conditions. Similarly, in diseases associated with diffuse interstitial fibrosis, loss of capillary bed and severe reductions of local blood flow occur.

Regional hypoxia, causing reflex pulmonary arteriolar constriction, plays an important part in the changes in blood flow seen in chronic bronchitis, emphysema, bronchial asthma, and cystic fibrosis, as well as in localized bronchial obstruction. In bronchiectasis, there is virtually no pulmonary arterial blood flow to the affected segments, but extensive bronchial collateral vessels are found, instead.

In pneumonic consolidation and atelectasis, blood flow is reduced and acts as a right-to-left shunt, because no ventilation takes place in these areas. In pulmonary infarction, pulmonary blood flow to the infarcted lung segments is virtually absent.

Increasing left atrial pressure is associated with a redistribution of blood flow toward the upper lung zones. The redistribution is proportional to the elevation of left atrial pressure, but is greater for any given pressure in mitral stenosis than in other causes of raised left atrial pressure, such as left ventricular failure.[39]

Cardiomegaly, pleural effusion, emphysematous bullae, and pneumothorax are all conditions in which the lung is compressed or displaced. As would be expected, these conditions are associated with diminished blood flow.

Abnormal regional ventilation is seen most commonly in such chronic obstructive pulmonary diseases as chronic bronchitis, emphysema, and bronchial asthma. Bronchiectasis and cystic fibrosis also cause abnormalities of regional ventilation. Similarly, airway obstructions by tumors, foreign bodies, or mucous plugs cause localized abnormalities of ventilation, the extent of which depends on the completeness of the obstruction (Fig. 5). When alveolar consolidation occurs, as in pneumonia, infarction, or severe pulmonary edema, no ventilation of the affected region exists. In the presence of diffuse interstitial lung diseases, such as fibrosing alveolitis or pulmonary edema, lung compliance is decreased and alveolar ventilation increased, so that the clearance of tracer gases is more rapid. Patients who hyperventilate also have a more rapid clearance than normal, but this aspect can be difficult to appreciate from routine studies of regional ventilation.

TECHNIQUES

Perfusion Lung Scintigraphy

Intravenous injections of radioactive particles have been used extensively to study regional pulmonary blood flow. The principle underlying their use is simple and depends on the observation that blood flow can be determined when a tracer is completely removed from the bloodstream in a single passage through an organ.[40] In these circumstances, if the tracer is evenly mixed with blood its distribution within the lungs is proportional to blood flow.

Following intravenous injection, macroaggregates of albumin (MAA) are well mixed with blood in their passage through the heart.[41] These particles are too large to pass through the pulmonary capillaries and become impacted in the terminal arterioles and other precapillary vessels. Their distribution is, thus, proportional to pulmonary arterial blood flow.[42–44] Early experimental work using ceramic particles in dogs showed that the idea was feasible.[45] The technique was successfully transferred to human beings with the development of radiolabeled macroaggregates.[46,47] However, the images obtained by this technique show only the relative distribution of pulmonary arterial blood flow. Absolute blood flow to any region can be determined only if cardiac output is measured at the same time.

Regional pulmonary perfusion has been conveniently studied following the intravenous injection of labeled macroaggregates and, previously, microspheres of human serum albumin.[48,49] The usual adult dose of ^{99m}Tc-labeled particles

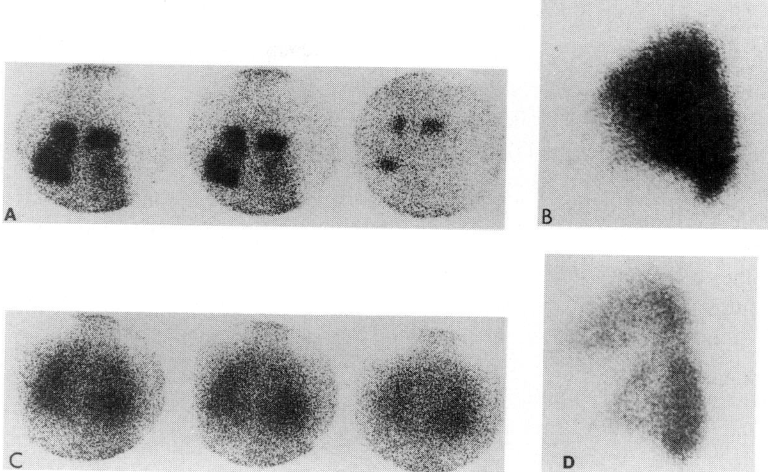

Figure 5. Transient perfusion defect secondary to rapidly changing ventilatory pattern. These studies were done shortly after this young diabetic suffered a cardiac arrest and probably aspiration during renal hemodialysis. **(A).** Initial ventilation study images (30–120 sec) show multiple zones of air trapping. **(B).** Initial left lateral perfusion image is normal. This study was "indeterminate" because the amount of air trapping made it impossible to determine the significance of perfusion defects apparent in other views. It was not possible to obtain an immediate pulmonary angiogram, but because anticoagulation was contraindicated, a repeat V-Q study was requested 14 hr after the initial series. **(C).** Comparable views from the second ventilation study show less trapping than seen initially. Note the scatter introduced by ^{99m}Tc activity remaining from the initial perfusion scan. The scatter makes the lung borders "fuzzy" and complicates interpretation. **(D).** Left lateral view from second perfusion study. Both segments of the lingula are no longer perfused. Because of these new lingular perfusion defects, this second study was interpreted as "high probability of PE." However, the obvious transient ventilation changes caused concern, and selective angiography of the left lung was strongly recommended. Pulmonary arteriography was negative for emboli.

is 1 to 4 mCi (~37 to 148 MBq). MAA has become the radiopharmaceutical of choice because of fewer reported reactions to this product. After impaction, most MAA particles are believed to break up and eventually pass through the lungs to be removed from circulation by reticuloendothelial cells of the liver and spleen.[50–52] Some studies have shown little liver activity, but increased intestinal and bladder activity.[53,54] In the presence of cardiac disease or obstructive airway disease, clearance from the lungs is often slower, presumably due to decreased pulmonary blood flow.

^{99m}Tc-MAA particles typically should be injected with the subject supine. Some physicians prefer that half the injection be given in the supine position and half in the prone position, to ensure the most even distribution of blood flow. When the injection is given in the upright position, the effect of gravity on pulmonary blood flow is often quite apparent. In whatever position the patient is injected, he or she should be asked to take 2 or 3 deep breaths during the injection to promote even distribution of particles. Immediately prior to injection, the particles should be shaken gently in a shielded syringe and then given slowly. Ideally, the patient should rest quietly for several minutes before the injection to stabilize physiological conditions. No blood should actually be permitted to enter the syringe; any blood clotting within the radiopharmaceutical may clump the particles, forming large aggregates that produce "hot" spots in perfusion images.

Perfusion images can be made immediately after injection. They are most conveniently and rapidly obtained with a large-field-of-view scintillation camera. Anterior, posterior, and both lateral projections must be obtained whenever possible. Posterior oblique views are necessary to enhance the accuracy with which defects can be localized in the posterior and basal segments.[55] Perfusion images are collected for a fixed time, based upon the time required to collect at least 500,000 counts for the posterior view. Between 25 and 30% of the counts detected in a typical lateral view actually come from the opposite lung as "shine through." The posterior oblique views are often even more useful than lateral views. They are favored because the opposite lung contributes little or no photons to the image; thus, small peripheral perfusion defects are better visualized. Some clinics also use anterior oblique views for the same purpose.

^{81m}Kr in saline solution has also been used for perfusion studies, given by continuous i.v. infusion. Because of its short physical half-life (13 sec), the counting rate at equilibrium in any lung region is proportional to blood flow. Images of regional lung perfusion can then be made in each projection.[50]

When the radiolabeled particles are injected in the supine position, activity is evenly distributed in the anterior and posterior projections. The outlines of the lungs are smooth, and the posterior and lateral costophrenic angles are only slightly rounded. Less activity is seen in the upper lung zones. If the particles are injected in the upright position, the effect of gravity on the distribution of blood flow is usually readily apparent, with virtually no apparent flow to the apical parts of the lung and apparent increased flow to the lower lung zones. The heart produces a clearly defined defect in the anterior and left lateral views. A smaller defect due to the heart is seen in most posterior views and occasionally, faintly, on the right lateral view as well. Usually, the lower and upper borders of each lung are at the same level on the posterior view. On the lateral views, more activity can be seen along the posterior aspect of each lung. In general, the outline of the lungs as seen on the perfusion images corresponds closely to the outlines seen on the chest radiograph (Fig. 6).

In obese subjects, the lungs can look smaller and the costophrenic angles are usually blunted. Additional minor variations in the pattern of blood flow are detected in about 20 to 25% of apparently healthy subjects.[56] These variations are more frequent in the right upper lobe. When an azygos lobe is present, it may show diminished perfusion.[57] Other minor irregularities in the pattern of perfusion need to be recognized, such as central defects on the lateral views ascribed to the hilar vessels and a curious artifact sometimes seen on posterior oblique views ascribed to the overlying scapula and its surrounding musculature.[54] Minor defects in perfusion images in elderly subjects are probably related to unrecognized obstructive airway disease.[58–60]

Perfusion scintigraphy has a reputation for great safety and has been performed on many severely ill patients without apparent harm. A few patients with severe pulmonary hypertension have died, however, perhaps as a direct result of the injection of these particles.[61,62] It has been postulated that their already compromised pulmonary vascular bed becomes critically obstructed, causing acute right heart failure. Other mechanisms, such as a pulmonary chemoreflex that is associated with bradycardia, hypotension, and apnea, may be involved.

In normal lungs, fewer than 1 in 1000 pulmonary arterioles are obstructed by the injected MAA, so a large safety margin exists.[63] No changes in pulmonary hemodynamics or diffusing capacity have been demonstrated following injection of the usual quantities of particulate radiopharmaceuticals.[64–67] The safe amount apparently lies between 200,000 and 700,000 particles for adults and proportionately less for children.[68,69] The particle numbers suggested for children of various ages is specified in the package insert for the MAA radiopharmaceuticals.

The presence of severe pulmonary hypertension in a patient should be regarded as a contraindication to MAA perfusion imaging. More caution should also be exercised in patients with right-to-left shunts (Fig. 7). Patients with prior hypersensitivity reactions to products containing human serum albumin should not normally be given MAA. Even nonsensitized individuals can occasionally react to MAA, and the nuclear medicine physician must be prepared to treat such reactions as necessary.

A

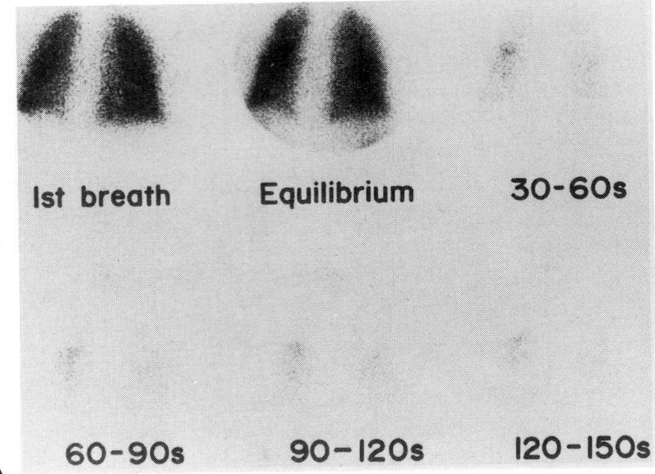

B

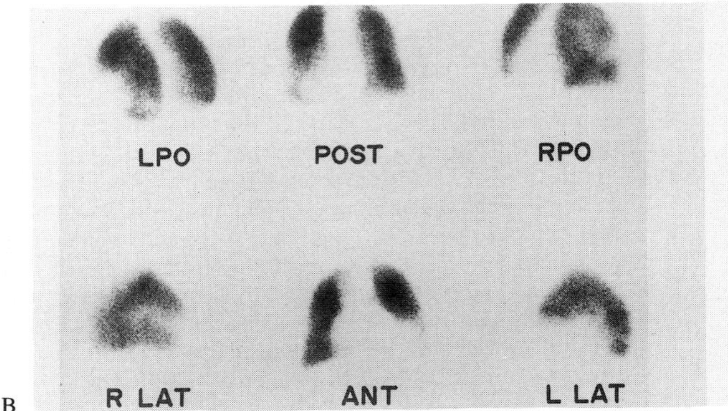

C D

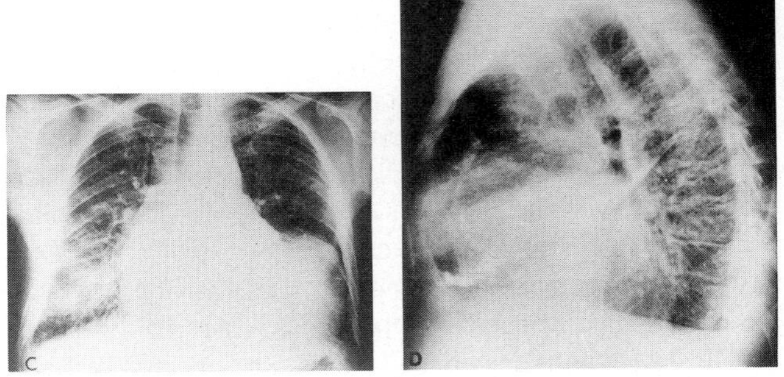

Figure 6. Perfusion defects caused by a cardiac abnormality. **(A).** ^{133}Xe ventilation study shows slight retention in the left lung. **(B).** Perfusion images demonstrate a large defect in the left lung and a smaller defect in the right lung. **(C)** and **(D).** AP and lateral radiographs demonstrate massive cardiomegaly with a deformed cardiac silhouette caused by a calcified left ventricular aneurysm and pulmonary edema in the right lung. This case illustrates the importance of interpreting V-Q studies with a high-quality radiograph. The V-Q studies show a significant mismatch that could be incorrectly diagnosed as PE without the chest film.

With the use of commercially prepared MAA radiopharmaceuticals, most artifacts related to the preparation of the particle aggregates have become uncommon. If too many small particles are present (i.e., those less than 10 μm in diameter), the RE cells of the liver and spleen are visualized,

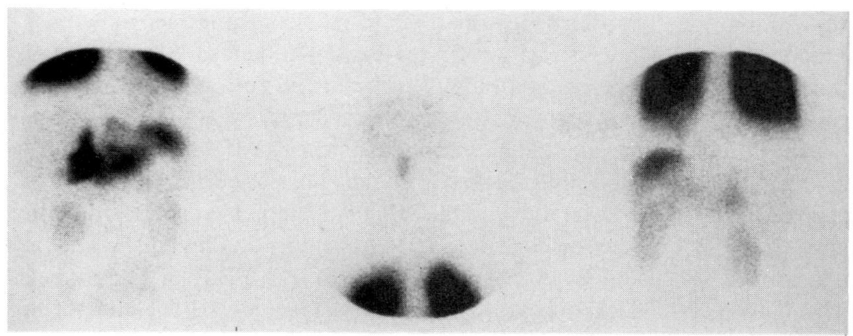

Figure 7. Anterior images of the upper abdomen (left), head and upper thorax (center), and a posterior upper abdomen image (right) show the typical findings present when a right-to-left shunt is present in a patient given an intravenous injection of ^{99m}Tc-MAA.

making the lung bases difficult to define. If a few large particles are given or if small clots form in the syringe at the time of injection, several large "hot" spots are seen on subsequent images. If too few particles are given, their distribution appears inhomogeneous in the resultant perfusion image.[68] Usually, artifacts in the perfusion images caused by attenuating objects overlying the lungs, such as pacemakers, some breast prostheses, Harrington rods used for spinal support in kyphoscoliosis, etc., are easily recognized by their particular shapes.

Ventilation Lung Studies

Regional ventilation can be best assessed with the use of radioactive inert gases. ^{133}Xenon is the most widely used, although its suboptimal gamma-ray energy and modest solubility in blood and fat are disadvantages. ^{127}Xenon, if available, has the same solubility disadvantage but it has more desirable energy peaks for imaging with conventional gamma cameras. Better quality images are obtained with a smaller radiation dose to the patient. Radioxenon's long half-life requires methods for trapping or safely venting this gas.[70–75] In addition, appropriate radioxenon collimators are required. With some available medium-energy collimators, system resolution for ^{127}Xe is lower than the resolution of ^{133}Xe using low-energy collimators.[75]

Interest developed in ventilation studies with ^{81m}Kr; this gas has a 13-second half-life and is obtained from a ^{81}Rb generator. Ventilation studies can be made in projections similar to perfusion studies and, thus, can be directly compared with them.[50,76–79] At present, widespread use of this gas is limited by the fact that the ^{81}Rb generator has a half-life of only 4.5 hours.

The short half-life of ^{81m}Kr has some subtle physiological implications, however. Theoretical studies based on a single-compartment model of well-mixed gas indicate that during tidal breathing of ^{81m}Kr, equilibrium is reached when the counting rate is almost directly proportional to ventilation. Studies in dogs, however, have shown that the situation is more complex than this. Tidal volume, the frequency of ventilation, and length of inspiration all influence the counting rate observed over the lungs and suggest that either the ^{81m}Kr is not distributed to the entire resident gas volume or that its distribution changes with lung volume. In both cases, the use of this gas for quantitative studies of regional ventilation would be limited.[79]

Regional ventilation is generally studied using a large-field gamma scintillation camera, so that both lungs are visualized simultaneously. If numerical analysis is required, the data are best stored in digital format for subsequent computer analysis.

RADIOGASES

The simplest ventilation technique is the single-breath method, in which a radioactive gas is inhaled to total lung capacity. An image of the gas distribution is taken during breath-holding, followed by serial washout images during which the patient breathes room air.[80] A more satisfactory technique provides for an equilibrium study between the washin and the washout phases.[17,29,81] During an equilibrium phase, the patient rebreathes radioxenon in a spirometer system for several minutes while carbon dioxide is chemically absorbed and oxygen added. If equilibrium is reached, the counting rate over the lungs is proportional to lung volume, and the changing activity during washout is related to regional ventilation or to air exchange.

Inhalation of boluses of radioxenon during particular phases of respiration can be used to study the distribution of air under special circumstances and also to measure closing volume.[32,38,82,83]

In clinical practice, a single-breath image, an equilibrium image of 3 to 5 minutes, followed by a washout period of up to 10 minutes, with serial 60-second images taken at intervals during this time, provide sufficient information for the majority of studies. Serial images obtained over the first 5 minutes of washout are more sensitive in detecting regions of impaired ventilation than shorter washout times. Serial images are also more sensitive than single-breath images.[84]

At the end of the washin, there should be an even distribution of activity, which corresponds to lung volume. Clearance during washout is rapid, and the lung outlines are usually no longer visible 2 to 3 minutes after washout begins. It is sometimes possible to see that clearance is faster from the lower lung zones. Clearance from a single-breath study is more rapid because the alveoli are not completely filled in a single breath.

Normal ventilation studies with radiogases show lung outlines corresponding to the patient's chest radiograph. The trachea is sometimes faintly visible on the anterior views. In the upright position, the gradient of ventilation is barely visible between the upper and lower zones.

A number of devices are available from commercial sources for administering radioxenon and for performing rebreathing and washout studies. They range from disposable devices and simple manually operated machines to complex computer-controlled systems. Exhaust systems for radioxenon must be vented properly or the radioxenon trapped efficiently and disposed of safely.[85,86]

Ventilation studies should be performed in the upright position, where ventilation is most efficient. The posterior projection encompasses the largest volume of lung and is the preferred view for radioxenon studies. Turning the patient for images in each posterior oblique view during the later minutes of washout scan provide valuable information that enables regions of radioxenon retention to be localized more accurately within each lung.[87] Patients are sometimes too ill to be studied while seated, however, and in this situation posterior views from beneath the scanning table are preferred to anterior views.[88]

Most children above the ages of 5 or 6 can cooperate adequately for ventilation studies. In younger children or in stuporous or uncooperative patients, the radioxenon can actually be given intravenously and the clearance from perfused alveoli studied or, more commonly, a close-fitting anesthetic mask can be tried.[89] In all of these methods, efficient room exhaust systems must be used, as the radioxenon will be freely exhaled by such patients in spite of one's best efforts.

Two approaches to measuring regional ventilation have been described in the literature. In the quasi-static methods, the distribution of a single breath of radioxenon is compared to its distribution at equilibrium to give an index of ventilation per unit lung volume. If the distribution of blood flow is also measured, an index of blood flow per unit lung volume can be obtained.[5,19]

Methods based on the washin and washout of the tracer gas may use the time to 50 or 90% of the equilibrium counting rate during the washin.[7,81] The time to 50% of the equilibrium value during the washout is the most commonly used "dynamic index" of ventilation.[90] More elaborate calculations may be made to determine regional clearance. Of greatest practical importance, however, is the observation that serial images of radioxenon washin and washout provide excellent qualitative evidence of both normal and abnormal ventilation.

RADIOAEROSOLS

Aerosol inhalation studies have also been used as an indicator of regional lung ventilation.[91,92] A number of radiopharmaceuticals have been used, including ^{198}Au colloid, ^{197}Hg-chlormerodrin, ^{99m}Tc-albumin, ^{99m}Tc-pertechnetate, ^{113m}In-chloride, and ^{99m}Tc-labeled minimicrospheres.[92–95] More recently, ^{99m}Tc-DTPA and Technegas® have emerged as the aerosol radiopharmaceuticals of choice.

An aerosol can be administered by a positive-pressure ventilator fitted with ultrasonic or gas-jet nebulization. The aerosol is breathed through a mouthpiece or face mask. Bacterial filters in the exhaust system prevent contamination of the surrounding area. Satisfactory studies can be obtained using 20 to 30 mCi (~0.7 to 1.1 GBq) of ^{99m}Tc-labeled DTPA in a volume of 3 to 4 ml. Only about 10% of this activity actually reaches the lungs.

Removing the larger aerosol particles by using a settling bag in line with the nebulizer did much to improve the quality of earlier aerosol inhalation scans.[96–98] Newer systems generate particles of smaller median diameter and eliminate the need for a settling bag. Semiquantitative scoring of regional ventilation has shown close correspondence between ^{81m}Kr ventilation and ^{113m}In aerosol inhalation images in both normal subjects and patients with a variety of lung diseases.[98] The multi-view aerosol inhalation procedure takes only 5 to 10 minutes.

The biologic half-life of ^{99m}Tc-DTPA aerosol (median mass diameter ~0.6 μm) is about 0.75 hours in healthy subjects.[99] In smokers, however, clearance is greatly increased because of increased alveolar membrane permeability.[100] Clearance may be so rapid, in fact, as to make six-view ventilation studies nearly impossible. In such cases, the most promising views must be predetermined by the perfusion study. Rapid clearance is not a problem when colloidal aerosols are used because they are cleared by ciliary action, which is much slower.

A normal aerosol study looks much like a perfusion study but, often, the trachea and major airways are visible, together with portions of the esophagus and stomach (Fig. 8). Hyperventilation produces considerable central deposition of aerosol, which usually then clears in delayed images. Asymptomatic cigarette smokers can also show more irregular central deposition.

Quantitative information on clearance rates from central and peripheral areas of the lungs can be gained from serial images obtained at intervals after inhalation of the aerosol.[101] Such studies have been performed in healthy nonsmoking subjects, in smokers, in patients with airway obstruction, in children with cystic fibrosis, and in a few patients with the immobile cilia syndrome.[102–105]

Such small molecules as ^{99m}Tc-pertechnetate and ^{99m}Tc-DTPA appear to clear the alveoli by passive diffusion through the alveolar epithelium. Their rate of clearance is proportional to their molecular size. On the other hand, large particles, such as ^{99m}Tc-albumin, are thought to be cleared by pinocytosis or phagocytosis. The ability to use particles <1.0 μm, which deposit beyond the ciliated airways, provides a useful means of studying alterations in alveolar epithelium.

Aerosol deposition depends on a number of factors, including the size, shape, density, and electrostatic charge on

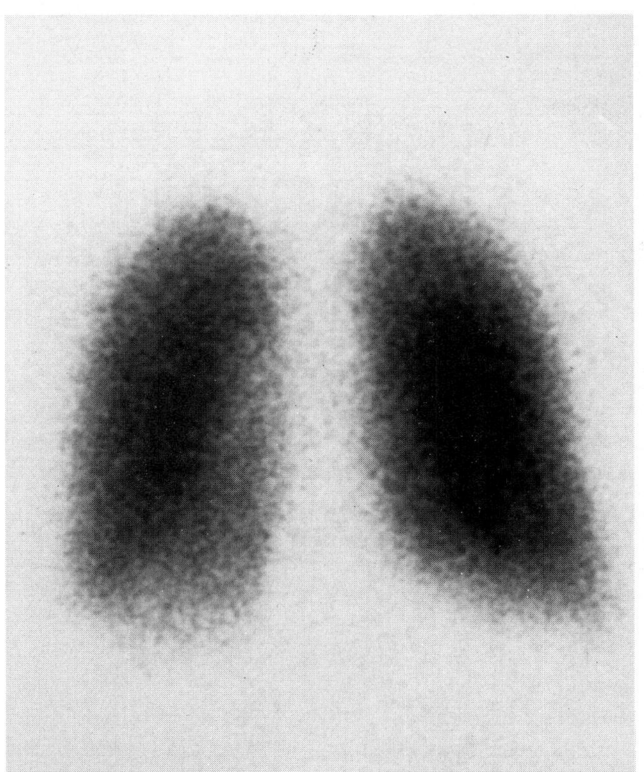
A

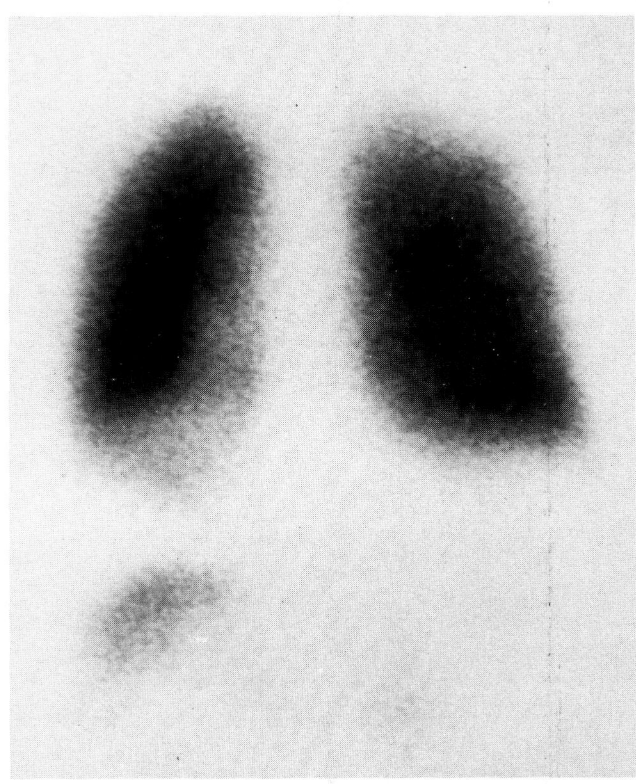
B

Figure 8. **(A).** Posterior view from a ^{99m}Tc-MAA perfusion study shows a normal pattern of lung perfusion. **(B).** Posterior view from the corresponding ^{99m}Tc-DTPA aerosol ventilation study shows good correspondence, although there is a small amount of swallowed ^{99m}Tc-DTPA in the stomach.

the particle, as well as lung geometry and the pattern of ventilation. Deposition of aerosol particles occurs by impaction, sedimentation, or diffusion. Deposition by impaction depends on velocity, change of direction, density, and the square of the diameter of the particle. It is the principal mode of deposition for particles larger than 10 μm. Smaller particles (between 1 and 5 μm) tend to be deposited by sedimentation, which is also related to the density and square of the particle diameter. For particles less than 1 μm, diffusion is the chief method of deposition. Diffusion is inversely proportional to the diameter of the particle. Particles 0.5 μm in diameter are deposited more than those of other sizes.[106]

Because airflow rates are slow in the distal airways, sedimentation and diffusion play important roles in particle deposition there. In general, particles larger than 10 to 15 μm are removed by the nose or deposited in the larger airways. Smaller particles (less than 2 to 4 μm) reach the alveoli, and even smaller ones may be exhaled. Deposition takes place during both inspiration and expiration. A greater proportion of inhaled particles are deposited with deep slow breathing and when the forced expiratory volume at 1 second, FEV_1, is low in relation to more normal patterns of breathing.

Radioaerosols were first proposed and demonstrated by Pircher et al.[91] and Taplin and Poe[92] as early as 1965, but required several technical advances before the radioaerosol methods gained widespread clinical application. The early aerosols were produced from colloidal solutions like human serum albumin, which was radiolabeled. In the 1970s, Isitman et al.[107] suggested solutions of ^{99m}Tc-MDP and ^{111}In-DTPA because these could be aerosolized to produce smaller droplets. Finally in the 1980s, reliable commercial radioaerosol generators and delivery systems became available; and this technique gained wider acceptance for application in ventilation studies. Although radiolabeled aerosol particles are delivered to the peripheral lungs with inspiratory air flow, because they deposit in the lungs by sedimentation and gravitational inpaction, they do not behave as a gas in the strictest sense. Nonetheless, ventilation images generated by radioaerosol methods have for the most part been practically applicable in many diseases.

Alderson et al.[108] compared ^{133}Xe ventilation studies with postperfusion ^{99m}Tc-DTPA aerosol studies, and found overall good agreement. Rammanna et al.[109] re-examined these studies on a zone-by-zone basis and also found little discrepant data. Hull et al.,[110] agreed that there was little difference between results when ^{133}Xe ventilation studies were compared to radioaerosols.

The majority of reported radioaerosol ventilation studies have used ^{99m}Tc-DTPA as the radiopharmaceutical. This includes studies measuring alveolar capillary membrane permeability. But Isitman et al.[111] have produced good results

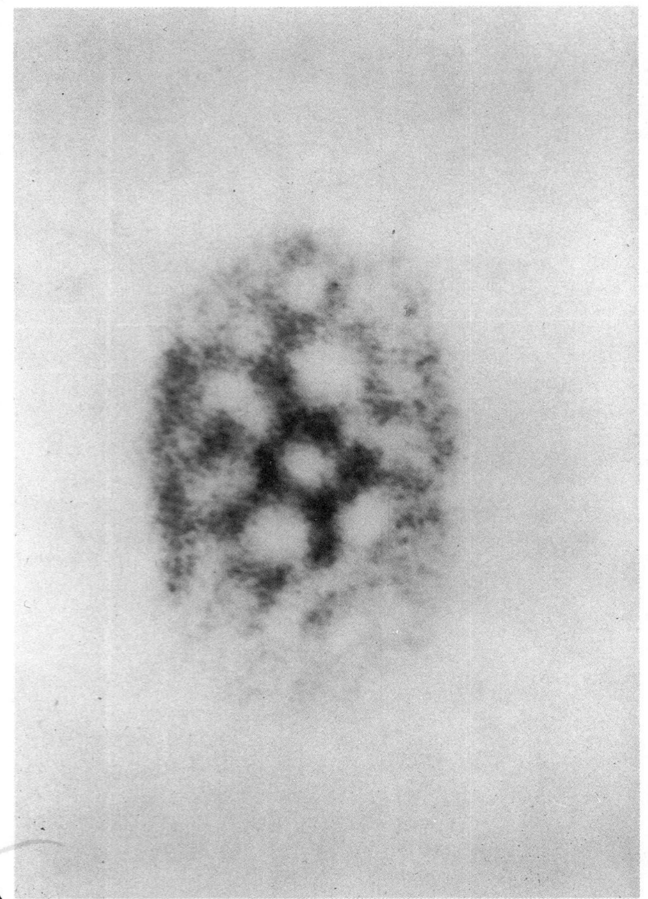

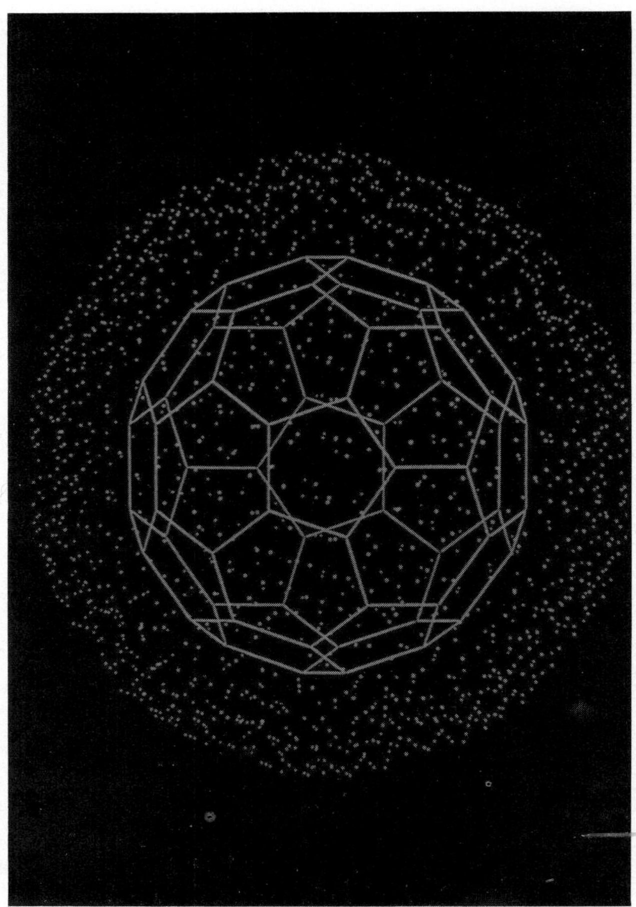

A B

Figure 9. **(A).** This electron photomicrograph of a Technegas® carbon particle shows the fullerene-like structure that is presumed to carry the ^{99m}Tc. (Courtesy W Burch and J McAfee.) **(B).** Artist's rendering of a sixty-carbon cluster initially termed a "buckministerfullerene (Nature 1985;318:162–163.)" The Technegas® particles were later shown to be agglomerated graphite particles 60–160 nm in size (EJNM 1993;20:576–579).

using ^{99m}Tc-pyrophosphate, as well. ^{99m}Tc-pyrophosphate aerosol produces a longer lung retention time that facilitates SPECT lung studies. Radioaerosol ventilation studies have also been reported using a number of liquid radiopharmaceuticals[112] and, more recently, dry particles.

^{99m}Tc-Technegas® was first developed in 1984 in Australia and has been used in tens of thousands of patient studies worldwide, except in the United States. Technegas ventilation images are considered superior to those obtained with ^{133}Xe gas or ^{99m}Tc-liquid aerosols. The dispersal of radioactivity throughout the lungs is faster and more homogeneous using Technegas®. Hence, the ventilation study is quicker and more convenient; an especially important aspect for acutely ill, dyspneic patients. Unfortunately, this radiopharmaceutical has not yet been approved by the FDA for use in the U.S. Technegas® is reported to be particularly good for ventilation imaging of the lungs before ^{99m}Tc-MAA perfusion imaging when V-Q studies are used to detect perfusion defects produced by pulmonary emboli.

Technegas® is a dry aerosol of ^{99m}Tc-labeled minute carbon particles (Fig. 9). It is generated in a proprietary system (Technegas Generator®, Tetly Technologies, Sydney, Australia) during the electrostatic heating of a graphite crucible containing a saline solution of ^{99m}Tc-pertechnetate. The details of this process are described in several articles.[113,114] The unusually consistent small particles pass quickly into the alveoli with only small amounts remaining in the central airways.[115] This characteristic permits generally good ventilation images even in patients with COPD.[116]

Technegas® ventilation studies are usually performed by having the patient already positioned before a gamma camera, maximally expire, then inspire to tidal volume, followed by a short breath hold. This is repeated a few times until the desired counts/second/unit lung volume is reached in the image. Alternatively, the patient can be asked to breathe at tidal volume for approximately 30 to 40 seconds until an adequate count rate is obtained. Both methods are reportedly quicker and easier to perform than studies using liquid aerosols, and patients seem to tolerate the Technegas® procedure with little difficulty (Fig. 10).

Retention of the carbon particles in the lungs means that ventilation images can be obtained in any projection for

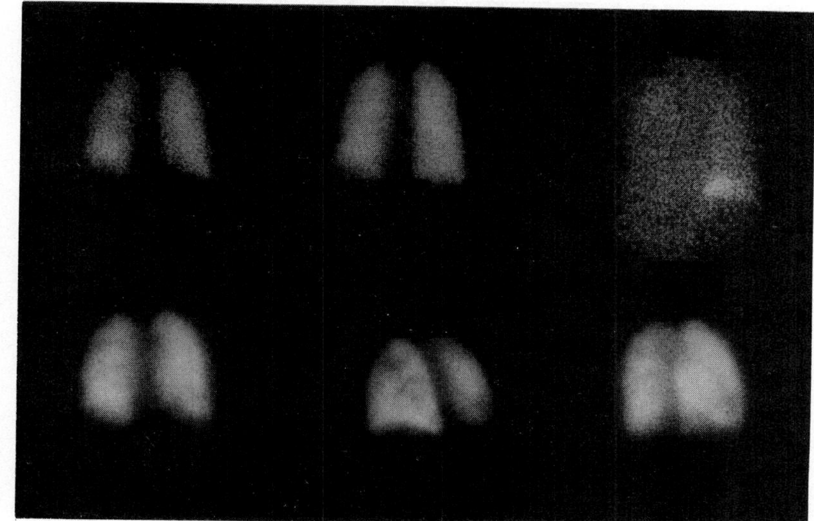

A

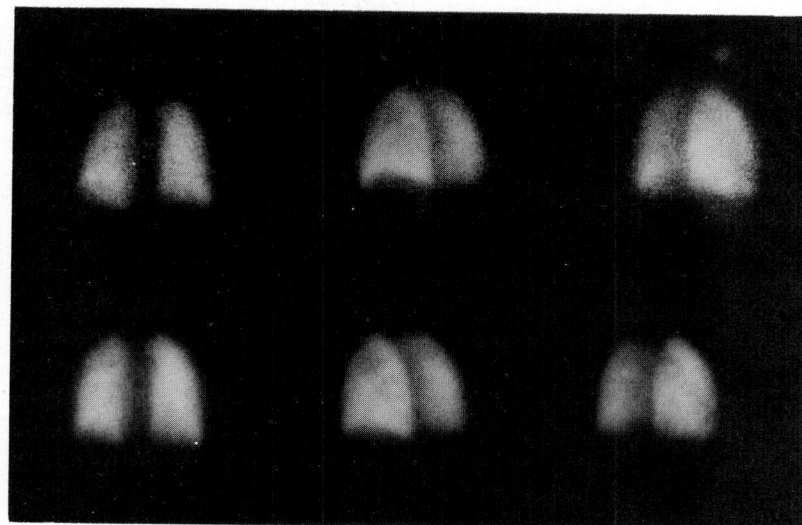

B

Figure 10. (A). The upper panel shows the ^{133}Xe washin (left) equilibrium (center), and washout (right) images from a 47-year-old patient with a small-cell lung carcinoma and congestive heart failure. The lower panel shows selected ^{99m}Tc-MAA perfusion images: (L—R) posterior and the 2 posterior obliques. Attempting to correlate the perfusion defects with ventilation abnormalities is made more difficult because only the posterior view was available with ^{133}Xe. **(B).** The same patient was re-studied with a Technegas® ventilation procedure. The upper panel shows the technegas images (L—R) posterior and the 2 posterior obliques. The lower panel shows the corresponding ^{99m}Tc-MAA images. Correlation of the abnormalities in ventilation and perfusion images is made easier by aligning the corresponding projections. (Courtesy of J. McAfee)

many minutes after inhalation. Most investigators have administered Technegas® first to obtain a ventilation study, and then followed with the perfusion study using 5-mCi of ^{99m}Tc-MAA.[117] Successful postperfusion-study Technegas® ventilation imaging has also been reported[118] (Fig. 11).

CLINICAL APPLICATIONS

Pulmonary Embolism

Pulmonary embolism (PE) is not, in itself, a disease. Rather, it is a potentially fatal complication of deep vein thrombosis (DVT). Accordingly, these 2 processes must be considered together. Although effective therapy is available for venous thromboembolism, the therapy itself can produce significant morbidity. Thus, an accurate diagnosis is mandatory. The clinical presentation and laboratory findings in pulmonary embolism are nonspecific, so that additional evaluation with imaging studies is essential. The most accurate imaging test, pulmonary arteriography is invasive and the noninvasive imaging tests, the V-Q study in particular, are still not perfectly accurate.

PRETEST PROBABILITY OF PULMONARY EMBOLI

Subclinical pulmonary emboli may be extremely common if the autopsy data represent the true picture, since pathologic studies have shown PE to be present in up to 70% of autopsies when they are searched for zealously.[119] However, the occurrence of clinically significant pulmonary embolism probably depends upon several factors. These include the degree of vascular occlusion produced by the emboli, the pulmonary vascular reserve, the age of the embolized thrombus, and the presence of associated medical or surgical conditions affecting cardiac function, pulmonary vascular smooth muscle function and fibrinolytic activity. There is uncertainty about patient selection and about the accuracy of diagnostic

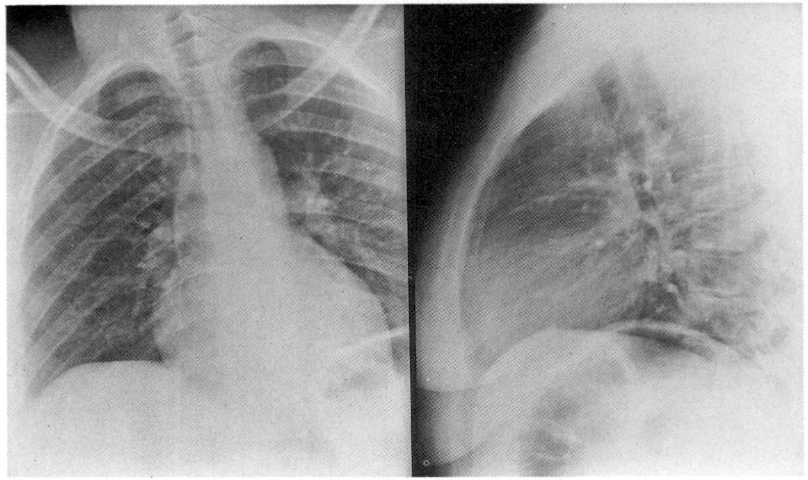

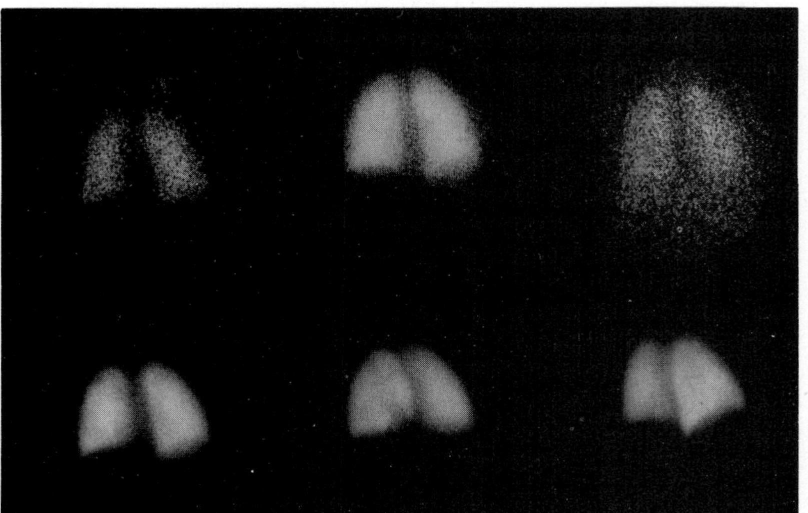

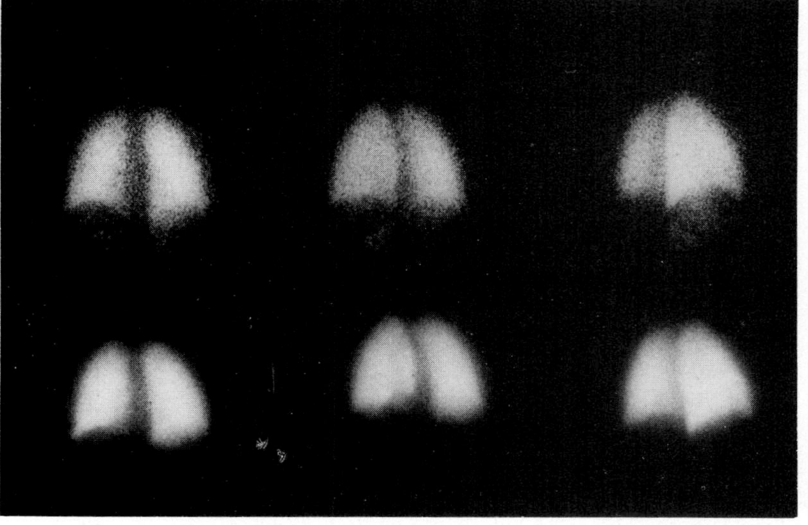

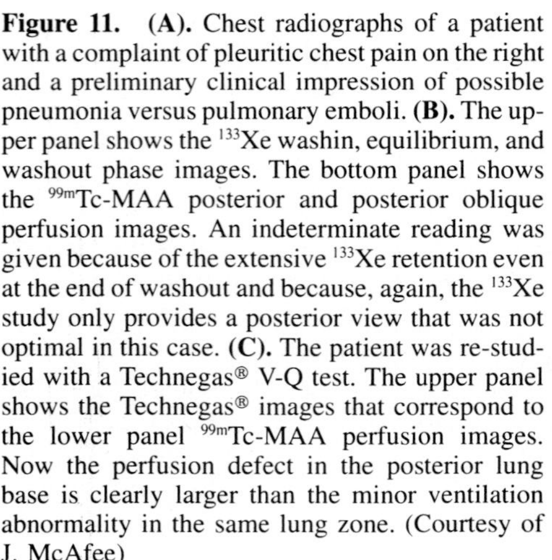

Figure 11. **(A).** Chest radiographs of a patient with a complaint of pleuritic chest pain on the right and a preliminary clinical impression of possible pneumonia versus pulmonary emboli. **(B).** The upper panel shows the ^{133}Xe washin, equilibrium, and washout phase images. The bottom panel shows the ^{99m}Tc-MAA posterior and posterior oblique perfusion images. An indeterminate reading was given because of the extensive ^{133}Xe retention even at the end of washout and because, again, the ^{133}Xe study only provides a posterior view that was not optimal in this case. **(C).** The patient was re-studied with a Technegas® V-Q test. The upper panel shows the Technegas® images that correspond to the lower panel ^{99m}Tc-MAA perfusion images. Now the perfusion defect in the posterior lung base is clearly larger than the minor ventilation abnormality in the same lung zone. (Courtesy of J. McAfee)

tests as applied in clinical studies that define the frequency of pulmonary emboli. Therefore, interpretation of their results is not straightforward. The prevalence of PE in large series of patients who were suspected clinically of having PE and referred for V-Q imaging has ranged from 25 to 50%. A reasonable point estimate would be about 33%, which was the frequency observed in the Prospective Investigation of Pulmonary Embolism Diagnosis (PIOPED) study.[120] However, it should be recalled that most of the prevalence data in the literature emanates from academic, tertiary-care hospitals, and associated clinics. It is possible that the prevalence of pulmonary embolism in other types of inpatient and outpatient settings is quite different.

One would like to know the actual pretest probability in an individual patient. If this, and the operating characteristics of the diagnostic test (e.g., the likelihood ratios for positive and negative results) are known, a reasonable estimate of the probability of the disease in an individual patient can be derived. The starting point for the assessment of pretest probability is the relative risk of venous thrombosis in certain groups to which individual patients may belong.

The clinical presentations seen in patients with PE are variable and relatively nonspecific.[121,122] Although numerous signs and symptoms have been touted as diagnostic, none have been found truly discriminatory after objective assessment. The "classic" triad of dyspnea, pleurisy, and hemoptysis was present in only 22% of patients with confirmed pulmonary emboli in the Urokinase Pulmonary Embolism Trial. However, some characteristic clinical features do occur in many patients. In patients with confirmed pulmonary emboli without preexisting cardiac or pulmonary disease, either dyspnea or tachypnea occurred in 96%. When the clinical diagnosis of deep venous thrombosis was also present, 99% of patients with a positive diagnosis of pulmonary embolism were included. Unfortunately, dyspnea and tachypnea may be seen in a wide variety of both serious and trivial clinical disorders and, thus, these findings are not specific for PE.

Reliable exclusion or confirmation of acute PE by the ECG or by any blood chemistry is not currently possible. The pCO_2 and pO_2 lack sensitivity and specificity, although they can serve to assess the severity of the acute event. The pO_2 cannot be used to exclude an embolus, as up to 15% of patients with PE may have pO_2 tensions greater than 80 torr when breathing ambient air. The use of blood markers for coagulation has been studied extensively and may have an adjunctive role in clinical evaluation, but low specificity vitiates their usefulness.

The clinical examination also has been shown to be inaccurate for deep vein thrombosis (DVT). The signs and symptoms used to make a clinical diagnosis of DVT (calf pain and tenderness, unilateral lower limb swelling, positive Homan sign) occur with equal frequency in patients with and without confirmed thrombi. In about 50% of cases with clinically suspected DVT, no thrombus will be demonstrated on further testing. Autopsy series demonstrate the poor sensitivity of clinical examination. In only 11 to 25% of patients with autopsy-proven deep vein thrombi is the diagnosis suspected prior to death. However, if the clinical picture suggests DVT, there is a greater chance that a thrombus will be present than in patients having a normal clinical examination. Recent analysis suggests that a limited number of clinical findings can predict the occurrence of DVT with relative accuracy,[123] but this remains to be confirmed by independent evaluations.

Table 1. Positive predictive values in the PIOPED study for PE of the Pretest Clinical Assessment (which was given as 80–100%, 20–79%, and 0–19%) and the V-Q categories of high, intermediate, and low-through-normal.*

V-Q SCINTIGRAPHY		CLINICAL ASSESSMENT	
Category	*PPV*	*Category*	*PPV*
High	87%	80–100%	74%
Intermediate	29%	20–79%	31%
Low-Normal	11%	0–19%	9%

*Data from reference 120.

In the PIOPED study, the pretest estimate of the likelihood of PE by experienced clinicians was almost as accurate as the V-Q categorization of patients (Table 1). Unfortunately, these clinical estimates were not made according to set criteria and thus it is impossible for them to be tested or improved upon by other studies.

Chest Radiograph. The chest radiograph is not an accurate means of diagnosing PE,[124] although it may on occasion be suggestive. Most patients with PE, and many patients who undergo a negative workup for PE, have abnormal chest radiographs. The radiographic changes are nonspecific. Common findings include consolidation, various manifestations of atelectasis, pleural effusion (usually small), and diaphragmatic elevation. Less common findings include nodules, focal oligemia, proximal pulmonary artery enlargement, and acute congestive heart failure. Some of the previously described "diagnostic" signs (particularly focal oligemia or changes in proximal pulmonary artery size) can be extremely subtle and difficult to interpret unless good comparison films are available (Fig. 12). Resolution of the parenchymal abnormalities usually occurs within 1 to 4 weeks; residual abnormalities may include pleural reaction and linear scars. Cavitation may occur in bland infarcts, but is uncommon in the absence of secondary infection.

However, the chest radiograph is an essential component in the imaging evaluation of a patient clinically suspected of having PE for 2 reasons: it is needed to establish or exclude some of the clinical simulators of PE, such as pneumonia, rib fracture, or pneumothorax, and it is essential for adequate evaluation of the lung scintigram, which is interpreted by comparing the chest radiographic and V-Q images in the same areas of the lung. One should obtain a high-quality PA and lateral examination at the same time as the lung

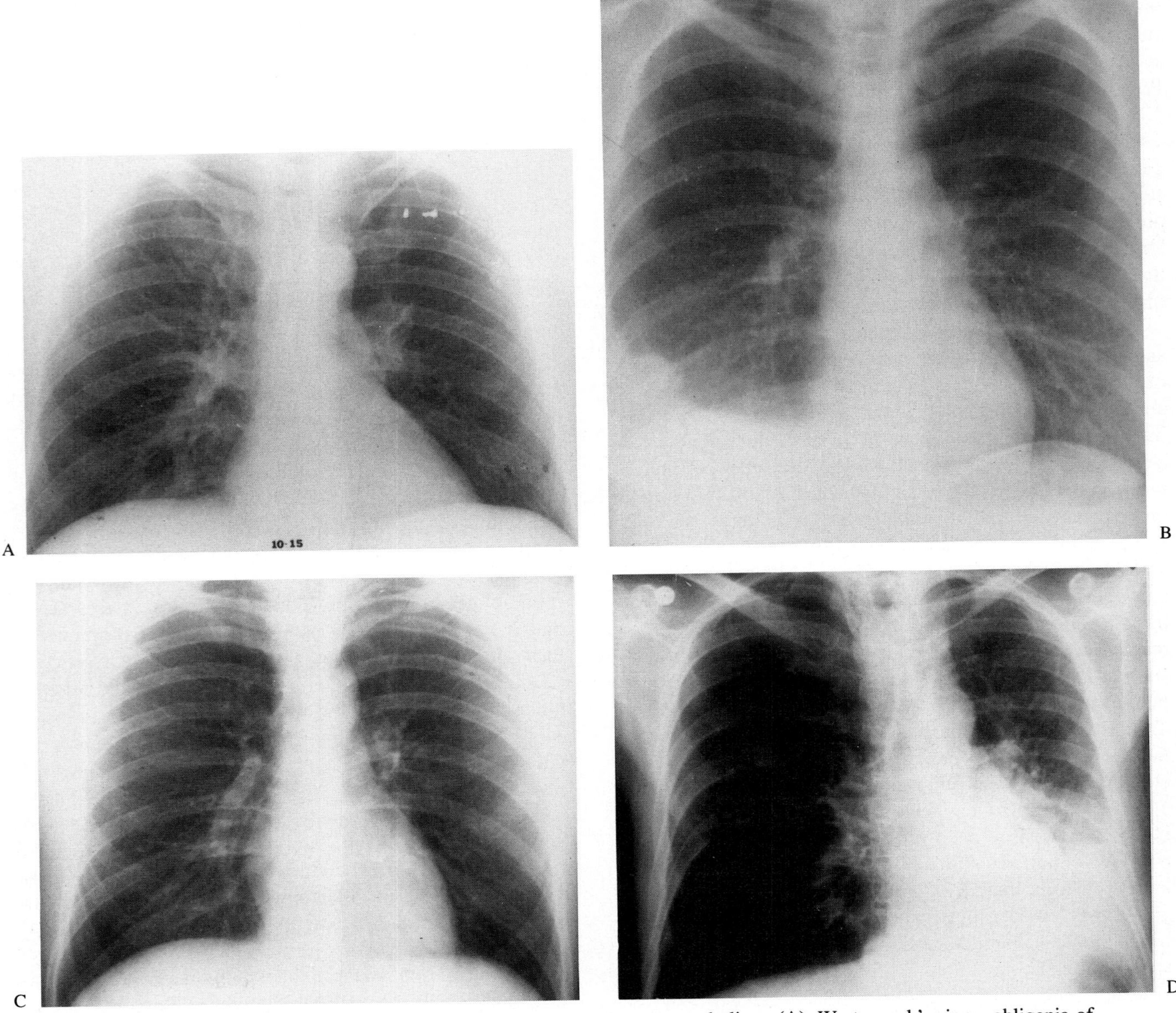

Figure 12. Some radiographic findings associated with pulmonary embolism: **(A).** Westermark's sign—obligenia of the lung (L) after a large pulmonary embolus. **(B).** Hampton's hump—infiltrate in the right lung base at the costophrenic angle. **(C).** "Sausage" sign—an enlarged right lower lobe pulmonary artery after an embolus to the right lower lobe. **(D).** Atelectasis—seen here in the region of a recent embolus.

scan. Portable AP films are a poor substitute, and films more than a few hours old should not be used when interpretating lung scintigraphy. If a portable film must be used, the patient's position should be accurately recorded so that account may be made for layering of pleural fluid.

Ventilation-Perfusion Scintigraphy. Normal lung scintigraphy demonstrates homogeneous patterns of evenly matched ventilation (V) and perfusion (Q). Pathophysiological states commonly are associated with scintigraphically detectable perturbations of ventilation and/or perfusion. These perturbations generally result in regional heterogeneity of pulmonary perfusion and ventilation, rather than overall changes.

Vascular occlusive processes include PE, extrinsic vascular compression (Fig. 13), and pulmonary vasculitis. These processes usually leave alveoli structurally intact and, thus, ventilation usually is preserved in regions of vascular occlusion. Accordingly, V-Q mismatch is the hallmark of this type of pathophysiology. Airspace occlusion may be associated with pneumonia, pulmonary infarction, and other airspace disorders. The degree of ventilation and perfusion loss can vary independently, but both usually are reduced concomitantly. Therefore, a V-Q match typically is present,

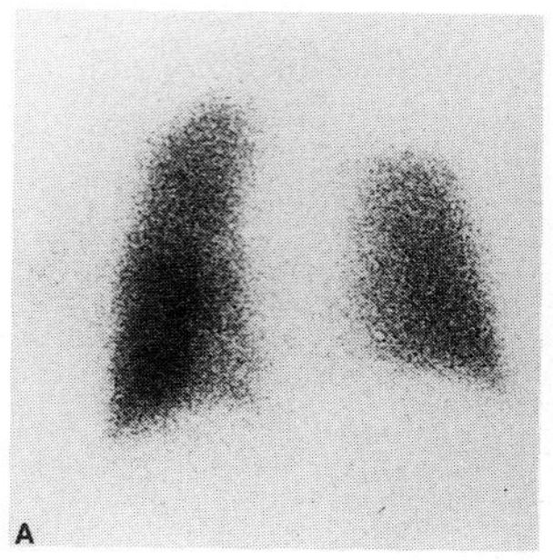

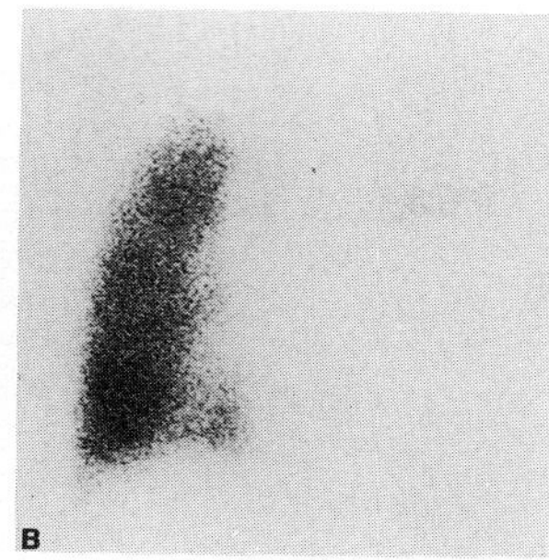

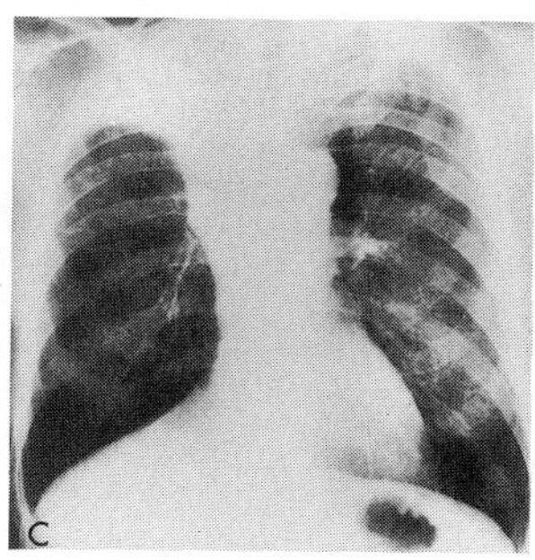

Figure 13. Nonembolic V-Q mismatch. **(A).** Posterior view ^{133}Xe equilibrium image. **(B).** Posterior view ^{99m}Tc-MAA perfusion image. **(C).** Radiograph showing right upper lobe collapse and consolidation and a right hilar mass. There is compensatory hyperinflation of the right lower and middle lobes. Strong cartilage rings maintain bronchial patency, even when this lung carcinoma has caused enough compression of the main pulmonary artery to stop pulmonary artery blood flow to the entire right lung.

usually associated with a radiographic opacity. Obstructive physiology is seen in such disorders as emphysema, bronchitis, bronchiectasis, and asthma, which predominately affect the conducting and exchanging air spaces. Alveolar hypoxia results, and the corresponding pulmonary arteries constrict, thereby redistributing blood to better ventilated alveoli and preserving the matching of ventilation and blood flow. Thus, matched V-Q abnormalities are seen in this type of physiology as well, but corresponding radiographic opacities are less common. In restrictive lung disease, chronic inflammation and fibrosis may eventually obliterate alveoli and capillaries. However, the airways remain functional and, therefore, regional ventilation usually may be increased relative to perfusion. The configuration and pattern of perfusion abnormalities is usually different from the vascular occlusive state.

Of course, combinations of these pathophysiological states can be present.

V-Q Criteria—Older Data. A truly normal perfusion study has long been accepted as excluding PE for practical purposes (that is, the morbidity and mortality of missed PE has been thought to be less than that from pulmonary arteriography or anticoagulant therapy). Theoretical reasons for PE with a "normal" perfusion study are central, nonobstructing PE which causes a subtle decrease in whole lung perfusion, or minimal defects that are not appreciated. However, perfusion images should be interpreted very conservatively, and a "normal" diagnosis reserved for unequivocally normal perfusion studies because (1) it has been demonstrated experimentally that perfusion scintigraphy is not perfectly sensitive and (2) great weight is placed upon normal scan interpretations in clinical management. In dogs, the sensitivity of perfusion imaging is about 80% for emboli that completely occlude pulmonary vessels, but only about 30% for partially occluding emboli.[125] The high sensitivity of perfusion scintigraphy for PE in the patient, as opposed to an individual site in the patient, results from the occurrence of multiple emboli in most patients. Usually, a normal perfusion pattern stops the workup for PE and diverts attention to other diagnostic possibilities.

Although it is sensitive, perfusion scintigraphy is not specific for pulmonary embolism. Nearly all pulmonary diseases, including neoplasms, infections, and chronic obstructive pulmonary disease (COPD), can produce decreased pulmonary blood flow to affected regions.[126] To overcome this problem, Wagner[127] and DeNardo[128] suggested combined ventilation-perfusion lung imaging. McNeil et al.[129] highlighted the findings of numerous investigators by pointing out that abnormalities in perfusion images that are matched by abnormal ventilation usually are not due to pulmonary embolism, but that mismatched abnormalities, coexisting with a normal chest radiograph, have a high correlation with angiographically demonstrated pulmonary embolism. Alderson and coworkers[130] later showed that the overall diagnostic accuracy for scintigraphic detection of pulmonary emboli was significantly improved when ^{133}Xe ventilation studies were added to the perfusion image and chest radiograph (Fig.14).

Neumann and colleagues[130] introduced the concept of "segmental equivalents"—that 2 subsegmental perfusion defects may be added to produce the same diagnostic significance as a single segmental defect. A subsequent retrospective study by Kotlyarov and Reba supported the usefulness of this approach.[132]

Extensive work by Biello and collaborators[133,134] further categorized perfusion defects matched by ventilatory or radiographic abnormalities and provided grounds for reducing the number of "indeterminate" diagnoses. Further evaluation of this work[135] indicated that this diagnostic scheme provides improved interobserver consistency and a 30% reduction in "indeterminate" readings compared with the results from an older scheme. The diagnostic criteria of Biello and coworkers are summarized in Table 2.

Experience has clearly shown that a scintigraphic study demonstrating multiple large, wedge-shaped, pleural-based perfusion defects (Fig. 17) with normal ventilation and a clear chest radiograph in the corresponding areas has a high correspondence with PE. The major cause of error in this situation is prior, unresolved PE (see "Conditions That Mimic Pulmonary Embolism"). Normally, a pattern of this type results in a diagnosis of PE, followed by appropriate therapy.

Intermediate patterns on V-Q studies are less diagnostic (Fig. 15), and must be interpreted with care. As discussed below, the degree of pretest clinical probability of PE must

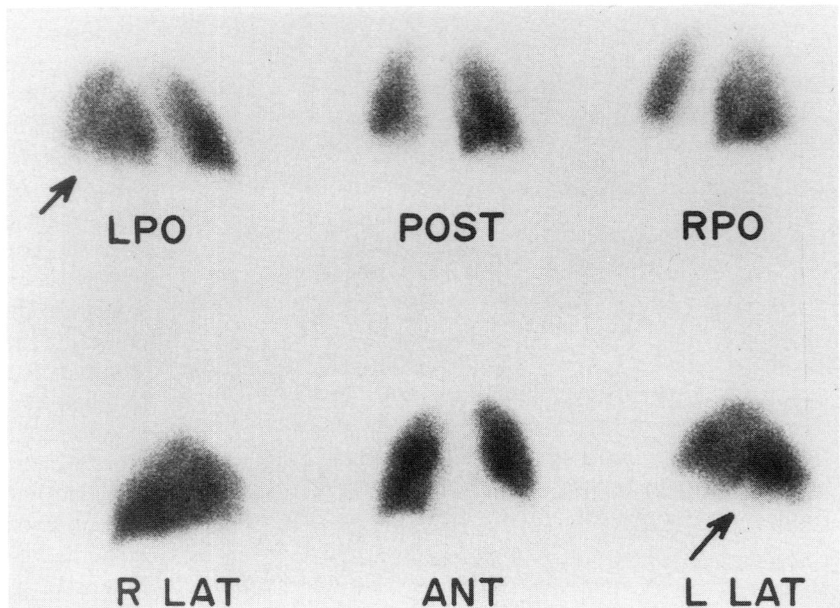

Figure 14. "Low probability of pulmonary emboli." This 6-view perfusion study contains a subsegmental defect (arrow). The corresponding ventilation study is normal. Note that the depicted arrangement of perfusion images follows a clockwise rotation of the patient and permits easy visual comparison of adjacent lung segments. We routinely position our patients in this order for multiformat viewing to facilitate interpretation.

be taken into account in deciding upon management of patients in this group. Often another study, such as pulmonary angiography, is required.

Table 2 shows two sets of commonly used diagnostic criteria. The "Biello" criteria (named for the late Daniel Biello, who was instrumental in formulating them) are simpler and probably more useful in clinical practice, as the PIOPED criteria were developed for research purposes. Ta-

Table 2. Older Diagnostic Criteria for Scintigraphic Detection of Pulmonary Embolism

CATEGORY	ESTIMATED PROBABILITY OF PE	SCINTIGRAPHIC FINDINGS	
		Biello (134)	*Pioped (120)*
Normal	<2%	Normal perfusion	Normal perfusion
Low	<15%	1. Small V-Q mismatches 2. Q defect substantially smaller than CXR opacity 3. V-Q match <50% of one lung field	1. Small Q defects regardless of number, V, or CXR findings 2. Q defect substantially smaller than CXR defect (V irrelevant) 3. V-Q match in <50% one lung or <75% of one lung zone; CXR normal or nearly normal 4. Single moderate Q with normal CXR (V irrelevant) 5. Nonsegmental Q defects
Intermediate	15–85%	1. Diffuse V-Q match 2. Matched Q and CXR 3. Single V-Q mismatch (one segment or smaller) with CXR normal in area	Abnormality that is not defined by either "high" or "low"
High	>85%	1. Q substantially larger than CXR opacity, which shows some area of mismatch 2. Two or more large or moderate V-Q mismatches, CXR normal in corresponding area	1. Two or more large Q; V and CXR normal 2. Two or more large Q where Q substantially larger than either matching V or CXR 3. Two or more moderate Q and one large Q; V and CXR normal 4. Four or more moderate Q; V and CXR normal

CXR, chest X-ray; V, ventilation; Q, perfusion.

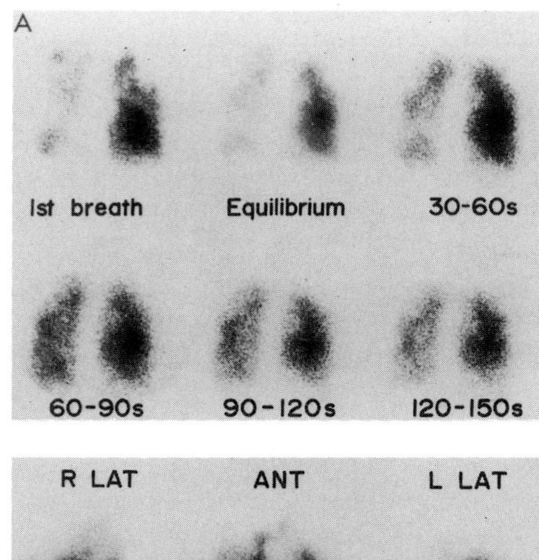

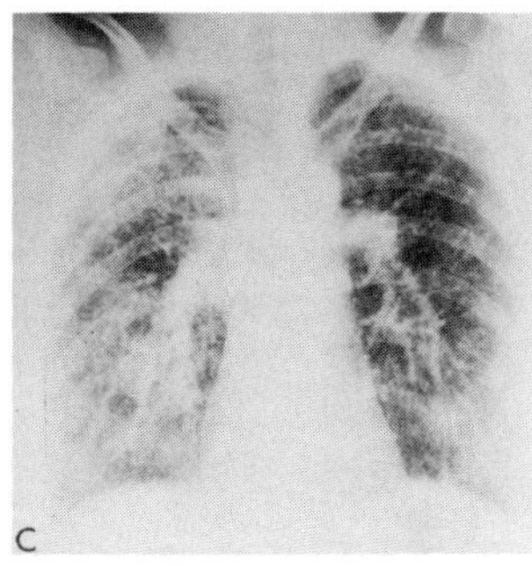

Figure 15. "Indeterminate study." The extensive radiographic and ventilation abnormalities prevent an accurate interpretation of this perfusion study. The angiogram was negative for pulmonary emboli. **(A).** ^{133}Xe ventilation study with washout to 3 min. The 5-min image was unchanged. **(B).** Selected ^{99m}Tc-MAA perfusion images. **(C).** Chest radiograph shows diffuse reticulonodular infiltrates and elevation of both hila. This pattern is consistent with diffuse parenchymal disease.

ble 3 shows the revised PIOPED criteria, with modifications based upon retrospective review of the large database of proven cases provided by the PIOPED study.[136,137]

Certain definitions are important to understanding and proper use of these criteria. In all these criteria, "small" is defined as a lesion involving less than 25% of the area of an average-sized pulmonary arterial segment; "moderate" is equivalent to 25 to 75% of the area of a segment; and "large" means more than 75% of a segment. Figure 16 shows examples of different sizes of perfusion defects. A chest X-ray (CXR) defect indicates a radiographic opacity in the region related to the Q or V lesion. When CXR is called "normal" this also alludes to the CXR appearance in the same region as the V or Q defect. Finally, a lung zone is one third of a lung divided craniocaudally (i.e., upper, middle, and lower zones).

V-Q Criteria—Newer Data. Interestingly, there are data to indicate that some experienced individuals can achieve more accurate results using their own experience than the reference criteria cited here.[136–140] Nevertheless, diagnostic reference criteria can be extremely useful, particularly for observers who do not have extensive and ongoing experience in interpreting V-Q studies. Use of reference criteria has been shown to reduce the number of indeterminate readings. In addition, if all the physicians in a group practice use the same reference criteria, standardization of the V-Q interpretations is likely to improve. In the PIOPED study, pairs of independent readers achieved high levels of prospective agreement (90 to 95%) for high probability and normal-near normal diagnoses, but lesser agreement (70 to 75%) for intermediate and low probability. The implications of these findings for clinical interpretations are obvious. It is worth noting that the good agreement between readers was only achieved after several practice sessions in which the description of findings and assignment of diagnostic categories were standardized.

The above discussion suggests that further refinement of diagnostic criteria is possible and there have been several attempts to do this recently. The PIOPED Nuclear Medicine Working Group revised the PIOPED criteria as described above and in Tables 2 and 3. A recent trial at Duke University[139] tested the revised PIOPED criteria (Table 3) and found that they were more accurate than the original PIOPED criteria, but that the "gestalt" impression of experienced readers remains the most accurate diagnostic impression (Table 4). The V-Q studies of 104 consecutive patients who underwent clinically motivated pulmonary angiography were reviewed by 2 experienced readers who had participated in the PIOPED study. The images were described using the PIOPED scan description method. The scans were categorized according to the original PIOPED and the revised PIOPED criteria and a "gestalt" percent probability estimate was also made. In addition, the official clinical reading (original PIOPED criteria, by one of a larger group of nuclear medicine physicians) was recorded. The "gestalt" impression was the most accurate for assessing the likelihood of PE from the V-Q study (Mann-Whitney ROC curve area = 0.836). The revised PIOPED criteria (area = 0.753) were more accurate than the original PIOPED criteria used either by the 2 study investigators (area = 0.650) or by the clinical nuclear medicine physicians (area = 0.584). Recent papers by Stein et al.[140,141] helped in making the criteria for "high probability" easier to apply and more sensitive. A subset of their data is shown in Tables 5 and 6. Their contribution has been to indicate (1) that the segmental equivalent concept[137] does not really add to diagnostic accuracy and that the total number of large or moderate defects is the important finding and (2) that patients who have had cardiopulmonary disease previously need to have more mismatched perfusion defects to achieve the same positive predictive value as those patients who have no history of cardiopulmonary disease. A study by Worsley et al.[142] inves-

Table 3. Revised PIOPED V-Q Scan Criteria

High Probability (≥80%)

- ≥2 Large mismatched segmental perfusion defects or the arithmetic equivalent in moderate or large + moderate defects*

Intermediate Probability (20–79%)

- 1 moderate to 2 large mismatched segmental perfusion defects or the arithmetic equivalent in moderate or large + moderate defects*
- Single matched ventilation-perfusion defect with clear chest radiography†
- Perfusion defects with matching chest radiographic abnormality in the lower lung zones
- Difficult to categorize as low or high, or not described as low or high

Low Probability (≤19%)

- Nonsegmental perfusion defects (e.g., cardiomegaly, enlarged aorta, enlarged hila, elevated diaphragm)
- Any perfusion defect with a substantially larger chest radiographic abnormality
- Perfusion defects with matching chest radiographic abnormality in the upper or middle lung zones
- Perfusion defects matched by ventilation abnormality† provided that there are (1) clear chest radiograph and (2) some areas of normal perfusion in the lungs
- Any number of small perfusion defects with a normal chest radiograph

Normal

- No perfusion defects—perfusion outlines exactly the shape of the lungs seen on the chest radiograph (note that hilar and aortic impressions may be seen, and the chest radiograph and/or ventilation study may be abnormal)

*Two large mismatched perfusion defects are borderline for "high probability." Individual readers may correctly interpret individual scans with this pattern as "high probability." In general, it is recommended that more than this degree of mismatch be present for the "high probability" category.

†Very extensive matched defects can be categorized as "low probability." Single V-Q matches are borderline for "low probability" and should be considered "intermediate" in most cases by most readers, although individual readers may correctly interpret individual scans with this pattern as "low probability."

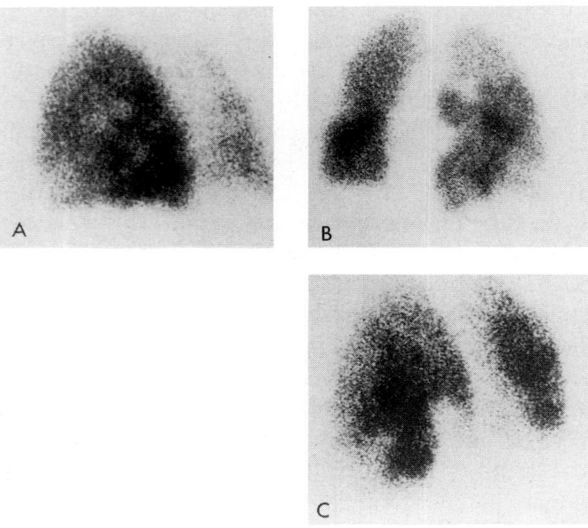

Figure 16. Perfusion defect patterns **(A).** This LPO view demonstrates nonsegmental "Swiss cheese" perfusion defects. These defects are small, rounded, and randomly distributed throughout the lung and are not always associated with "air trapping" on the ventilation study. **(B).** This RPO view demonstrates a geometric, pleural-based subsegmental perfusion defect. Note that this defect is smaller in volume than a full segment but clearly "segmental" in shape and position. The posterior contour of the lung image is definitely interrupted by this defect. Real lesions in the apical and posterior basal segments always interrupt the lung contour in this manner. "Artifacts" produced by enlarged mediastinal structures (e.g., hila or aorta), leave the posterior surface intact on the oblique views. **(C).** This LPO view demonstrates a full segmental perfusion defect in the posterior basal segment of the left lower lobe.

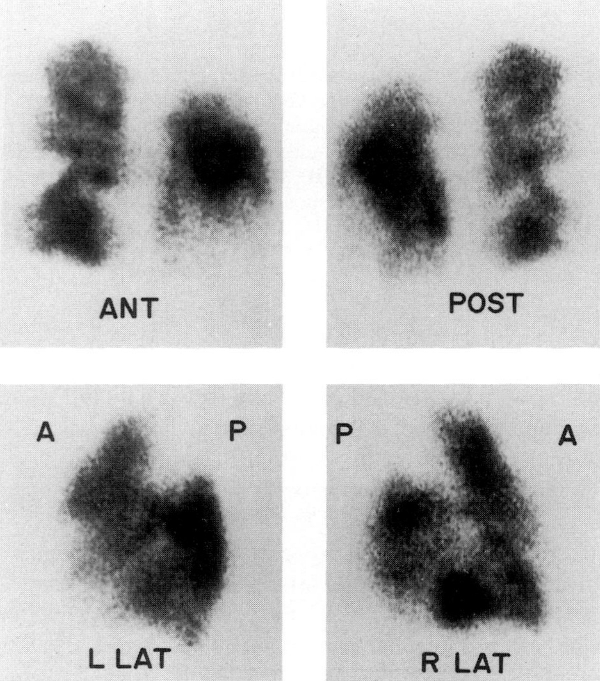

Figure 17. "High probability of pulmonary emboli." Selected views from the perfusion study show multiple segmental defects. Note that the right middle lobe defect is not as apparent in the right lateral image because of "shine through" from normal lung medial to the unperfused segment. The ventilation study was completely normal.

Table 4. Accuracy (area under the ROC curve) in 104 patients at Duke University for the original PIOPED criteria (as used in the official hospital report and as used by 2 experienced observers) and for the revised PIOPED criteria (2 experienced observers) are compared with the "gestalt" probability estimates of 2 experienced observers. The differences are statistically significant.*

CATEGORY	AREA UNDER ROC CURVE
Hospital report	0.584
Original PIOPED	0.650
Revised PIOPED	0.753
Gestalt	0.836

*Data from reference 139.

Table 5. Number of mismatched moderate or large-size perfusion defects compared with the sensitivity, specificity, and positive predictive value (PPV) for PE in patients with no history of prior cardiopulmonary disease.*

NUMBER OF DEFECTS	SENSITIVITY	SPECIFICITY	PPV (95% C.I.)
≥1	71%	88%	80% (74–86)
≥2	54%	95%	89% (83–95)
≥3	46%	97%	85% (85–97)
≥4	39%	97%	87% (81–97)
≥5	32%	98%	92% (84–100)

*Data from reference 141.

tigated whether the location of matched perfusion-radiographic abnormalities could be used to reduce the number of intermediate-probability characterizations. Their data suggest that perfusion-radiographic matches in the upper and middle lung zones have a low likelihood (11 to 12%) of being associated with PE in the same zone, but those in the lower zones have a higher likelihood (33%); the data are

Table 6. Number of mismatched moderate or large-size perfusion defects compared with sensitivity, specificity, and positive predictive value for PE in patients with a history of prior cardiopulmonary disease.*

NUMBER OF DEFECTS	SENSITIVITY	SPECIFICITY	PPV (95% C.I.)
≥1	63%	86%	68% (62–74)
≥2	51%	93%	77% (69–85)
≥3	44%	95%	80% (72–88)
≥4	40%	96%	84% (76–92)
≥5	37%	98%	89% (83–95)

*Data from reference 141.

Table 7. Positive predictive value for PE *in Individual Perfusion Defects* when perfusion defects matched by ventilation defects and radiographic abnormalities and are located in the upper, middle, or lower lung zones.*

ZONE	PERCENT OF DEFECTS DUE TO PE	(95% C.I.)
Upper	11%	3–26%
Middle	12%	4–23%
Lower	33%	27–41%

*Data from reference 142.

shown in Table 7. Although the differences in frequency of PE between different zones are statistically significant, due to the small number of cases the confidence intervals are quite large and we do not yet feel comfortable incorporating this very promising work into clinical diagnosis.

Table 8 lists the criteria we currently use to interpret V-Q studies in patients suspected of having PE. Among many issues that still need to be resolved, we mention only two. First, the significance of a single matched V-Q defect with clear chest radiograph is still not clear. The data from the PIOPED study suggest that this should be intermediate probability; however, this finding is without a medical rationale and a small prospective study at Duke did not necessarily confirm the PIOPED data (Table 9). However, in both instances, the confidence intervals are very wide. Second, it is not clear whether or not to recommend use of the "stripe sign"[143] in routine V-Q interpretation. The data shown in Table 10 seem to support its use, but the stripe sign is more accurate when used by experienced observers[143] and exercise appropriate caution.

Conditions That Mimic Pulmonary Embolism. Numerous disease processes can result in V-Q mismatch but, fortunately, most of them are quite uncommon. The pathology of these lesions involves the pulmonary vessels, whether in the lumen, the vessel wall, or the perivascular tissues, to produce vascular occlusion.

The most common cause of V-Q mismatch not due to acute PE is unresolved prior PE (Fig. 18). One study[144] showed that as many as 35% of patients with acute pulmonary embolism have incomplete scintigraphic resolution. Data from the PIOPED study also imply that prior PE is one of the most common causes of false-positive "high-probability" scans (the positive predictive value of a "high-probability" study was 91% in patients with no history of prior PE and only 74% in those with that history, $p < 0.05$). Other processes occurring in the pulmonary arterial lumen (embolism of material other than thrombus, in situ thrombosis or pulmonary artery tumor), processes involving the arterial wall (vasculitis, connective tissue disorder, tuberculosis, or irradiation), vascular anomalies (pulmonary artery agenesis, peripheral coarctations, arteriovenous malformations, or surgical pulmonic-systemic shunts) and extrinsic compres-

Table 8. Current Duke/PIOPED V-Q Criteria[1]

High Probability (>80%)

No prior cardiopulmonary disease: ≥2 mismatched moderate or large perfusion defects

Prior cardiopulmonary disease or uncertain: ≥4 mismatched moderate or large perfusion defects

Intermediate Probability (20–80%)

Difficult to categorize, or not described as low or high

Single perfusion defect matched by ventilation abnormality[2]

Low Probability (<20%)

Nonsegmental perfusion defects (e.g., cardiomegaly, enlarged hila, elevated diaphragm)

Perfusion defect with a substantially larger chest radiographic abnormality

Perfusion defects matched by ventilation abnormality of equal or larger size, provided that there are (1) clear chest radiograph and (2) some areas of normal perfusion in the lungs

Any number of small perfusion defects with a normal chest radiograph

Normal

No perfusion defects—perfusion outlines exactly the shape of the lungs seen on the chest radiograph (normal hilar and aortic impressions may be seen, and the chest radiograph and/or ventilation study may be abnormal)

[1]Presence of "stripe sign" can be used to eliminate a perfusion defect from consideration (essentially relegating it from the "segmental" to the "nonsegmental" category)

[2]Single perfusion defect matched by ventilation abnormality requires more investigation and is likely appropriate for low probability—may depend on coexisting factors

Table 9. Positive predictive value for PE *in Individual Perfusion Defects* when single perfusion defects are matched by ventilation defects in zones that are radiographically normal.*

STUDY	NO. OF PATIENTS	PERCENT OF DEFECTS DUE TO PE (95% C.I.)
PIOPED	23	26% (8–44%)
Duke	8	0% (0–37%)

*Data from references 137 and 139.

Table 10. Positive predictive value for PE *in Individual Perfusion Defects* when perfusion defects exhibit the stripe sign.*

STUDY	NO. OF DEFECTS	PERCENT OF DEFECTS DUE TO PE (95% C.I.)
Yale	17	6% (0–20%)
PIOPED	85	7% (3–15%)

*Data from reference 143 and reference 1 therein.

Table 11. Positive predictive value of combined scintigraphic and clinical assessment in the PIOPED study is shown together with number of patients in category.*

SCAN CATEGORY	CLINICAL PROBABILITY		
	80–100%	20–79%	0–19%
High	95% (29)	85% (80)	83% (9)
Intermediate	71% (41)	29% (236)	14% (68)
Low	43% (15)	16% (191)	4% (90)
N-NN	0% (5)	7% (62)	2% (61)

*Data from reference 120.

sion of pulmonary arteries or veins (mediastinal or hilar carcinomas or fibrosis) can result in segmental or lobar perfusion deficits. In some of the above pathologic entities, the perfusion deficits may be matched by ventilatory or radiographic abnormalities, but V-Q mismatch mimicking acute PE can be seen in all of them.

In spite of the extensive list of possibilities, we have found that most PE mimics are due to: (1) unresolved PE, (2) intravenous drug abuse or, (3) hilar or mediastinal involvement (usually by bronchogenic carcinoma). Clues to the correct diagnosis often can be found on the chest radiograph and the history is of paramount importance because unresolved PE appears to be the most common cause of false-positive studies.

If a PE mimic is possible, it is essential to alert the referring physician to this fact. Additionally, many authorities advise a "baseline" V-Q study on all patients with PE about 3 months after the acute episode to avoid confusion in future interpretations.

Interpretive Pitfalls. Some readers have considered perfusion defects as large or segmental only if perfusion was completely absent. This will lead to error in the application of modern diagnostic criteria, in which only the area of the perfusion deficit is considered. The rationale for this is that a partially occluding embolus often produces diminished, rather than absent, perfusion in the involved segments.

We caution against interpreting as "real" a lesion that is visible on only a single view of the perfusion series, because this results in overcalling perfusion defects. The most common mistakes of this type are interpreting defects caused by prominent aortic arch or pulmonary hila as due to PE. With eight-view lung scintigraphy, virtually any real lesion can be identified on 2 of the 8 views.

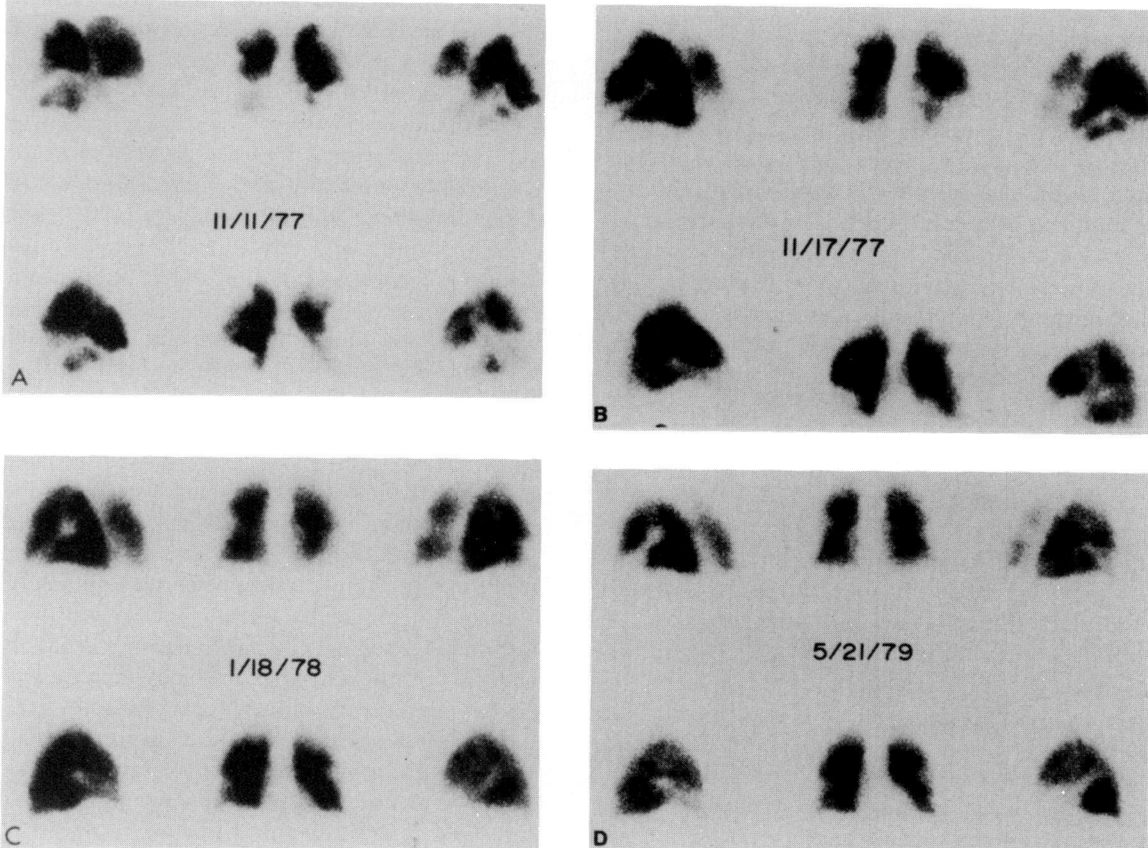

Figure 18. Resolution patterns. This series of perfusion studies in a 39-year-old male illustrates the temporal pattern of resolution after pulmonary emboli. Most resolution has occurred within 1 wk of the initial study; only minor changes are apparent between **(B)** and **(C)**. Study **(C)** (1/18/78) demonstrates this patient's new baseline perfusion status. On 5/21/79, study **(D),** he presented with new pleuritic chest pain. The radiograph was normal and the ventilation study on 5/21/79 showed slight slow washout in the right upper lung zone, but was normal in the area of the lingula and right middle-lobe sites of the apparent segmental perfusion defects. Without study **(C)** for comparison, study **(D)** would be considered "high probability" for PE. Residual perfusion defects like those shown here can occur in 10–20% of embolism patients and provide a constant source of confusion or overdiagnosis of PE when "baseline" perfusion has not been redetermined after an episode of pulmonary emboli.

The chest radiograph may become a serious pitfall in the interpretation of V-Q studies. A poor quality radiograph may not show parenchymal opacities or pleural effusions that correspond to perfusion defects. Whenever possible, a standard chest radiograph should be obtained.

Finally, it is difficult to diagnose recurrent PE utilizing V-Q studies alone. If a central embolus is present, it has the potential to fragment during its resolution (which may take days to weeks), potentially causing a variety of different perfusion patterns. Furthermore, differential clot lysis and varying pulmonary arterial pressures may cause changing perfusion patterns.[65] Only when the V-Q pattern has been stable for at least 3 months can acute changes support the diagnosis of recurrent PE.

The decision to perform pulmonary angiography depends on the degree of diagnostic certainty needed. Patients in whom the clinical and scintigraphic probabilities are concordant seldom require angiographic confirmation (Table 11). The categories that most often need angiographic confirmation are intermediate-probability scintigraphy and a low-probability V-Q study with high clinical suspicion. Newer diagnostic algorithms add venous imaging to the decision tree, which increases the complexity of the decision process, but allows conclusive, noninvasive diagnosis in a larger number of patients.

Chronic Bronchitis and Emphysema

Chronic bronchitis and emphysema are now common conditions caused, for the most part, by cigarette smoking. Both are more prevalent in older smokers. The prevalence of these diseases and of others, such as asthma and bronchiectasis, makes an assessment of the patient's ventilation an important test and an integral part of the interpretation of clinical perfusion studies. The chest radiograph may be normal in each of these conditions, and clinical evidence of airway obstruction cannot prove which defects in pulmonary blood flow are due to obstructive airway disease.

In chronic bronchitis, the pathologic lesions are found in the airways, with an increase in mucous glands, thickening of the mucosa, excessive secretion of mucus, and irregular narrowing of the airways.[146] Goblet cells spread to the periphery of the lung, and ciliated epithelium and Clara cells are reduced.[147] Viral and other infections of the respiratory passages may result in the production of more mucus, secondary infection, inflammatory infiltration of bronchial walls, and sometimes bronchospasm. The disease mainly affects the airways, causing an increase in airway obstruction and, hence, airway resistance, which leads to abnormalities of regional ventilation.[148] The earliest changes take place in the smaller airways and, because these contribute so little to airway resistance, the routine pulmonary function tests may be normal in young cigarette smokers.

The washout of radioxenon can be used to demonstrate abnormalities of regional ventilation and, although it is not an ideal screening test for small airway disease, it is one of the most sensitive.[149] Images made after the inhalation of labeled aerosols also have similar sensitivity, although the mechanism underlying the clearance of the aerosol particles is quite different from the delayed clearance seen with the radioxenon studies.

In emphysema, dilatation and destruction of the alveoli occur with loss of alveolar surface area and pulmonary capillary bed. Elastic recoil forces are diminished, and the support of the small airways by neighboring alveoli is weakened, causing narrowing and irregularity of these structures. Airflow rates and gas exchange are thus reduced by the increase in airway resistance, the loss of driving force of expiration, and the reduced alveolar surface area and capillary bed.

Occasionally, patients seem to have chronic bronchitis alone (i.e., without emphysema), and others may have emphysema with little chronic bronchitis. Most patients, however, have evidence of both disease processes, as would be expected because smoking is their common etiologic factor.[150]

Widely differing patterns of regional ventilation are seen, ranging from predominantly upper lobe disease in centrilobular emphysema and predominantly lower lobe disease in panlobular emphysema, to diffuse involvement. All grades of severity, as measured by retention of radioxenon, may be found.[151,152] In emphysema associated with α_1 antitrypsin deficiency, the disease process is most severe in the lower lobes.[153] Symptomless heterozygotic patients usually show abnormalities of ventilation, particularly as they age.[154] In general, both lungs are affected to a similar, though rarely identical, degree. Predominantly unilateral disease may be attributable to the Swyer-James syndrome, a constellation of signs and symptoms including hyperlucent lung and angiographic loss of small vessels, which is thought to result from chronic bronchial infections during childhood.

Usually, the defects in ventilation are patchy and nonsegmental. Studies with radiogases show that such defects often cross lobar boundaries, but discrete subsegmental, segmental, or lobar defects can also be seen. Emphysematous bullae and other severely affected lung regions usually fail to fill evenly during a single-breath study, or during a prolonged "washin," in which case they can be recognized as defects in the "equilibrium" image.

In these 2 diseases, the basic problem is in the airways but, in emphysema, the alveoli are also destroyed. Blood vessels are lost in emphysema and narrowed in both diseases when hypoxia ensues. Structural changes take place in the pulmonary arteries and arterioles when pulmonary hypertension develops.

In early or mild airway obstruction, little disturbance of the blood flow can be appreciated. As the disease progresses, alterations in blood flow become more apparent. Perfusion changes are, however, usually less than the defects in ventilation.[155] Several studies have shown that the defects are patchy and nonsegmental in most patients, whereas in a small percentage the defects are seen in anatomically recognizable subdivisions of the lung. These latter cases are accompanied by the most severe derangements of regional ventilation. The matching of ventilation and blood flow is less common in chronic bronchitis, in which it depends primarily on hypoxic vasoconstriction, while in emphysema the loss of capillary bed tends to compensate for abnormalities in ventilation. Usually, the failure to match these 2 aspects of lung function can be appreciated from studies of regional lung function and, in some instances, the predominant regions of physiological shunting can be identified.

In the lung apices, the effect of posture on the distribution of blood flow may give the appearance of reduced blood flow. Even when airway obstruction occurs in these regions, the local ventilation-perfusion ratios are high. High ventilation-perfusion ratios are rarely seen in other parts of the lung in patients with chronic bronchitis or emphysema. If they are seen, the possibility of concomitant pulmonary embolism, or even carcinoma of the bronchus, should be considered.

The overall clearance of radioxenon from the lungs of patients with chronic bronchitis and emphysema has been shown to be significantly correlated with forced expiratory volume (FEV_1) at 1 second ($r = 0.7$), with maximum midflow rates ($r = 0.7$), with FEV_1/forced vital capacity ratio ($r = 0.5$), and with arterial $PaCO_2$ ($r = -0.67$).[155]

Asthma

The obstruction to airflow that occurs during attacks of asthma is due to edema of the bronchial mucosa, spasm of the bronchial smooth muscles, and mucus plugging of airways. Abnormalities of regional ventilation and perfusion are apparent at the onset of an attack. Often, the defects in ventilation are local and more severe than the accompanying defect in perfusion, in keeping with the hypoxemia that is seen during episodes of asthma.[156–160]

The defects in perfusion are characteristically subsegmental, segmental, or lobar and are indistinguishable from those associated with pulmonary embolism. Ventilation studies are, therefore, essential for correct interpretation. As the attack of asthma subsides, defects in both ventilation and perfusion improve. The time course of this improvement in blood flow may mimic that of pulmonary embolism (see Fig. 5).

Some asthmatic patients show normal regional ventilation and perfusion between attacks, but others, even when asymptomatic, continue to show defects of both. As would be expected, the induction of an asthma attack by inhalation of an instigator is accompanied by readily visible abnormalities of ventilation and perfusion,[161] whereas the administration of such bronchodilator drugs as aminophylline improves both ventilation and perfusion. Usually, the degree of improvement parallels that seen clinically and by pulmonary function tests.[162,163]

Cystic Fibrosis

Although this disease usually occurs in childhood, an increasing number of patients with this condition are diagnosed in their late teens and early adulthood. Inappropriate secretions are produced by most of the exocrine glands of the body. In the lungs, the bronchial mucus is more viscid, which leads to early widespread airway obstruction with recurrent episodes of infection and inflammation, local scarring, and destruction of bronchi and lung parenchyma.

Studies from infancy through the second decade show a pattern of steadily increasing abnormalities of ventilation and perfusion.[164–167] Usually, the upper lobes are affected most severely. The defects in ventilation and perfusion are patchy, irregular, and not necessarily symmetrical. The overall clearance of radioxenon from the lungs of such patients is an excellent guide to the severity of the condition and correlates reasonably well with FEV at 1 second and peak flow.[166]

Deterioration in the perfusion images may occur 6 months to 2 years before clinical deterioration, and the extent of the defects in blood flow have been correlated more closely with survival than either clinical scores or radiographic scores.[167]

Bronchiectasis may be cylindrical, varicose, or saccular. The affected lung regions have progressively fewer demonstrable branches of the airways, from approximately 12 branches in cylindric bronchiectasis to as few as 4 branches in saccular bronchiectasis. The bronchi are dilated, tortuous, and surrounded by chronic inflammatory tissue and fibrosis. The bronchial arteries are enlarged. Such regions of the lung scarcely ventilate and have virtually no pulmonary arterial blood flow.[168] They appear in an equilibrium image as a region without activity, which corresponds to the involved segment. During washout, some retention of radioxenon is seen, reflecting the marked delay in clearance of what little radioxenon reaches the affected area. Some radioxenon may, in fact, arrive through the bronchial circulation.

Studies in which macroaggregates have been injected into catheterized bronchial arteries have shown little overlap between blood flow to the bronchiectatic regions of lung, which are supplied from the bronchial arteries, and blood flow to the normal lung, which is perfused from the pulmonary arteries.

Bronchial Obstruction

Bronchial obstruction may be caused (1) by processes within the bronchial lumen, such as a foreign body or mucus plug, (2) by processes arising in the wall of the bronchus, such as a tumor or, (3) by conditions compressing the bronchus from without. The disturbances in ventilation and perfusion depend on the extent of the obstruction to airflow, unless the process also involves the pulmonary vessels accompanying the bronchus.

In the same manner in which gas exchange is diminished because of airway obstruction, local hypoxia causes pulmonary arteriolar constriction and, thus, a reduction in blood flow. The defects in ventilation and perfusion scans correspond to the anatomic distribution of the involved lung segment or lobe. Complete lobar obstruction is followed by atelectasis, with absent ventilation and greatly diminished blood flow. In segmental obstruction, there may be no loss of volume because collateral ventilation can take place from neighboring segments, through the pores of Kohn. Such segments are readily recognized on a ventilation study, because their clearance of radioxenon is much delayed. When the obstruction is due to a foreign body, removal of the object is followed by return of perfusion over several days.[169]

Carcinoma of the Bronchus

Carcinoma of the bronchus may also alter both ventilation and perfusion. Because these tumors derive their blood supply from the bronchial arteries, they may appear as defects on perfusion scans. Usually, small tumors (less than 2.0 or 3.0 cm in diameter) are not detected unless they involve vessels at the pulmonary hilum. Larger tumors produce perfusion defects corresponding to the size of the tumor, in the involved segment or lobe, or even to the entire lung.[170–172] The larger the perfusion defect is in relation to the size of the tumor, the greater is the involvement of the hilar vessels by the tumor.[173–175] Such involvement may be attributable to metastatic spread to the lymph nodes, direct invasion of the mediastinum or, less commonly, invasion and thrombosis of the pulmonary veins. More rarely still, it may be due to invasion and thrombosis of the pulmonary arteries.[176,177]

Ventilation defects depend on the degree of bronchial obstruction and are confined to the affected segment or lobe, or the whole lung when the tumor is in a mainstem bronchus. The defect in ventilation is often less than that of perfusion, because extrabronchial spread of tumor is usually much greater than intrabronchial protrusion (Fig. 13).

Other defects in both ventilation and perfusion are seen in other parts of pulmonary cancer patient's lungs; in general, such abnormalities are related to the concomitant existence of chronic bronchitis and emphysema. Abnormalities of radioxenon clearance are seen in the contralateral lung in approximately three quarters of such patients, and abnormalities of blood flow are seen in approximately half.[173,179] In 10 to 15% of these patients, unexpectedly large defects in blood flow may be found in the nontumor-bearing lung. These problematic defects may be so large that a more conservative surgical approach is taken, or the decision to operate may even be abandoned.[180,181]

Ventilation-perfusion studies can play an important role in demonstrating the functional integrity of each lung prior to thoracotomy. Perfusion scans can be used to predict postoperative pulmonary function with considerable accuracy. Regional ventilation studies prior to thoracotomy are of less value in this regard.

In patients about to undergo pneumonectomy, postoperative forced expiratory volume in one second (FEV_1) can be estimated by multiplying the preoperative FEV_1 by the proportion of counts in the contralateral lung. In patients with compromised lung function, surgery is undertaken if the calculated postoperative FEV_1 is 800 mL or greater.[183,184] Although lung function after lobectomy can be predicted in a similar fashion, calculations based on the theoretic contribution of segments involved in the proposed resection—regardless of their functional status—are reported to be just as good.[184]

The relative distribution of pulmonary blood flow also has been suggested as a means of predicting resectability. The greater the reduction in blood flow, the more extensively are the hilar structures involved with tumor, and the less chance there is of complete surgical removal of the tumor.[184,185] A number of other studies, however, showed that tumors have been successfully resected when the blood flow to the tumor-bearing lung was much diminished; consequently, decreased perfusion to the involved lung should not be considered an absolute contraindication to resection.[183,184,187] Mediastinoscopy, however, more accurately determines resectability in patients who, by clinical, radiologic, bronchoscopic, or V-Q criteria, are apparently resectable.[188]

Occasionally, V-Q studies can localize the site of an otherwise occult carcinoma of the bronchus (i.e., a tumor that has been found by positive cytology but whose exact location cannot be determined by radiologic or bronchoscopic techniques). The primary site may be indicated by localized disturbance of perfusion or ventilation or by abnormal deposition of an aerosol. Unfortunately, the frequent coexistence of chronic bronchitis and emphysema in lung cancer patients, with their associated abnormalities of ventilation and perfusion, usually makes it impossible to determine which defect corresponds to a tumor.[173,189] Thus, ventilation-perfusion studies are of no real value in the early detection of lung cancer.[179]

Following radiation therapy for cancer of the bronchus, some return of perfusion may be seen in up to 80% of patients. The remainder show either no change or progressive reduction in perfusion. Ventilation tends to return earlier and more frequently.[190–193] The restoration of blood flow has been of no demonstrable prognostic significance.[194,195] Perfusion also decreases in radiation pneumonitis, which may result in severe damage to the pulmonary vasculature.[196] Although the lung may lose volume, little permanent damage is done to the airways and, thus, the clearance of radioxenon is not usually impaired. Experiments with dogs have shown that fast-neutron irradiation produces greater changes in blood flow, in the distribution of a single breath, and in aerosol disposition than ^{60}Co-photon irradiation does. These changes, which are of a restrictive nature, are 4 to 5 times more prominent with fast neutrons than with photons.[197] Perfusion lung scintigraphy is more sensitive than chest x-rays in detecting radiation changes.[198] Perfusion defects may be observed soon after radiation treatments and may appear to be maximum after 2 months, whereas the earliest evident fibrotic response apparent on X-ray to teletherapy is typically 2 to 4 months.

Pneumonia

Areas of pneumonia have both absent ventilation and diminished perfusion. Perfusion studies typically show defects that correspond closely in size to the radiologic infiltrate. Hyperperfusion has rarely been seen early in the course of pneumonia; the usual finding is reduced perfusion. The disparity between absent ventilation and some retained perfusion accounts for the shunting of blood and low PaO_2 found in patients with this pneumonia.

The pneumonic segment or lobe can be seen on a radioxenon ventilation study as a defect in the single breath or equilibrium image. Unless associated chronic bronchitis or emphysema is present, clearance from the lungs is rapid. Occasionally, some retention of radioxenon can be seen in or immediately adjacent to the pneumonic area, possibly from peripheral blood releasing xenon into this poorly ventilated space.

The findings in pneumonia are somewhat similar to those found in zones of pulmonary infarction. Although blood flow and ventilation should be completely absent in the zone of the infarct, it may not be possible to distinguish these solely on the basis of the ventilation-perfusion study. The finding of additional defects in perfusion associated with normal ventilation should strongly suggest the diagnosis of pulmonary embolism with infarction.

Pulmonary Tuberculosis

In pulmonary tuberculosis, defects in blood flow are present almost invariably and are often larger than the radiographic extent of the disease. Although a surgical procedure is now rarely used in the management of this disease, the extent of the defects in blood flow have been used to aid in decisions over the extent of such resections.[199,200] Usually, ventilation is markedly impaired in the involved segments, with poor filling during washin and delayed clearance during washout, as would be expected in a region of the lung affected by secondary bronchiectasis.

Pneumoconiosis

In general, the defects in blood flow seen in nonsmoking workers with pneumoconioses correspond to the abnormalities seen on the chest radiograph and usually are extensive only in progressive massive fibrosis.[201] The findings are often complicated by the presence of chronic bronchitis and emphysema, which are common in coal workers and others exposed to these occupational lung diseases. The abnormalities of ventilation and perfusion are more often due to the associated chronic bronchitis and emphysema than to the pneumoconiosis itself.

Impaired ventilation accompanying parenchymal changes has been demonstrated in the lower lung zones of asbestos workers.[202] Blood flow is diminished in those regions of the lung where diffuse fibrotic changes are seen radiographically. The extent of these defects correlates with the years of exposure to asbestos fiber. In cigarette-smoking asbestos workers with radiographic evidence of pulmonary fibrosis, perfusion scintigraphy may distinguish between the effects of asbestos exposure and those of cigarette smoking or other causes of pulmonary dysfunction.[203]

Acute Smoke Inhalation

Inhalation of smoke and other noxious products of combustion may cause an acute chemical laryngotracheobronchitis. The severity of the injury is presumably related to concentration and duration of contact with the offending agents. Early recognition of impending laryngeal obstruction is of great importance and is best accomplished by inspection of the larynx. Usually, patients with early severe laryngeal edema require tracheostomy.[204]

Clearance of radioxenon from the lungs following its intravenous injection has been shown to be sensitive in detecting injury to the bronchial mucosa after smoke inhalation. Studies within 48 hours of thermal injury have shown that those patients with delayed clearance of radioxenon are twice as likely to die as those with normal studies. Two thirds of these patients have infiltrates or atelectasis on their radiographs.[205] The airflow rate is decreased, pulmonary resistance is increased, and the single-breath nitrogen test is more abnormal in those patients with abnormal radioxenon studies.[206]

Pulmonary Manifestations of Drug Addiction

Ventilation-perfusion studies have been used to examine intravenous drug users. Perfusion studies are most sensitive in showing abnormalities in such patients, even when standard pulmonary function tests, including the diffusing capacity, are normal. The number of perfusion defects is inversely related to the diffusing capacity; however, defects in ventilation bear no relationship to perfusion defects, in keeping with the vascular damage caused by the injected substances.[207,208]

Kyphoscoliosis

In kyphoscoliosis blood flow and ventilation are both disturbed. Usually, the vertical gradient of blood flow is less apparent than in healthy people, and regions of impaired ventilation may be seen. These areas tend to be more prominent in the lung zone adjacent to the greatest convexity of the scoliosis.[209] Some evidence suggests that fixing the spine by operative procedures may improve the regional efficiency of ventilation, although the overall pulmonary function tests may show little change.[210]

Pleural Effusions and Pleural Thickening

Pleural effusions are associated with diminished perfusion and ventilation in proportion to effusion size. Underlying parenchymal or embolic disease may cause the functional defects to be more widespread. If the pleural fluid is freely mobile, the pattern changes, depending on the position in which the injection is given and the position in which the patient is imaged. Unilateral pleural thickening can affect the performance of both lungs. Ventilation and blood flow are shifted away from the affected lung base; also, blood flow is shifted away from the opposite lung base. Alveolar expansion is diminished in both lungs compared to healthy lungs.[211]

Pneumothorax

A chest radiograph is the best way to confirm the presence of a pneumothorax. But, characteristic ventilation and perfusion patterns have been described in patients with relatively small pneumothoraces. Single-breath images and perfusion images at total lung capacity show the lungs to be of almost equal size, with the lung on the side of the pneumothorax being slightly smaller. Images of both ventilation and perfusion made during tidal breathing, however, show the lung on the side of the pneumothorax to have a faster washout time and to be considerably smaller than the other lung.[212]

Bronchopleural Fistula

^{133}Xe can be used to identify the presence of bronchopleural fistulae.[213,214] In one case, the ^{133}Xe was instilled through a fiberoptic bronchoscope into different segments of the lung, and its efflux was monitored in the chest tube. A rapid increase in counting rate occurred in the chest tube when a bolus of ^{133}Xe was instilled into the appropriate segmental bronchus.[213] In addition, Skorodin et al. have documented closure of a bronchopleural fistula using ^{133}Xe ventilation studies,[214] although closure was also evident on clinical and radiologic grounds.

Congenital Heart Disease

Redistribution of blood flow between the lungs is often present in patients with congenital heart disease and can be easily recognized by perfusion lung scintigraphy. Right-to-left shunts of more than 10 to 15% are readily apparent because of activity trapped in the kidneys, brain and, to a lesser extent, the spleen. Occasionally, myocardial activity is also seen.[215] Measurement of the degree of shunting, using whole-body imaging, may be of some value in detecting faulty anastomoses postoperatively for congenital heart disease. This method correlates reasonably well with the Fick method.[216,217] Chest radiographs are considerably less sensitive and require a 2.5-fold difference between the lungs before the discrepancy can be appreciated.[218–220]

Shunt patency has been studied after Blalock-Taussig anastomoses, Potts anastomoses, Waterston-Cooley anastomoses, and the Glen shunt procedure using labeled macroaggregates. Interpretation of the results requires accurate knowledge of the presence and severity of any associated pulmonic stenosis or peripheral pulmonary artery stenosis, of the extent of any bronchial collaterals, and of the nature of the operative procedure.[221]

Usually, vascular anomalies are readily recognized by their associated perfusion defect. Pulmonary arteriovenous malformations produce localized perfusion defects when they are more than 2 to 3 cm in diameter. Smaller ones are not detected. An anomalous origin of the pulmonary artery may be accompanied by a profound reduction in blood flow with normal ventilation. This finding should lead to pulmonary angiography to demonstrate the faulty anatomy. Similarly, the stenosis that may occur in the anastomotic channel following repair of anomalous venous return can be recognized by reduced blood flow to that lung, while ventilation is preserved.

Pediatric Applications

Perfusion studies in children present no special problems, except that the number of particles injected must be reduced, in keeping with the smaller number of blood vessels within the lung. Studies of regional ventilation may be performed during tidal breathing. Radioxenon may be administered by nasal prongs or face mask, provided there is adequate room exhaust.[89]

Studies have been performed in children with agenesis of the lung, congenital lobar emphysema,[222] pulmonary papillomatosis,[223] bronchiectasis, inhaled foreign bodies, Macleod's syndrome, bronchomalacia, and a variety of cystic lesions, as well as the Wilson-Mikity syndrome and hyaline membrane disease.[224–226] Studies of perfusion alone have been reported in children with lobar pneumonia, bronchopneumonia, asthma, chronic bronchitis, and pleural effusion.[227–229]

As would be expected, such studies provide information about the severity and localization of the functional deficit, and also show the functional status of the rest of the lungs. Such information can be of considerable benefit, particularly when surgery is being considered.

Bronchopulmonary Sequestration

Bronchopulmonary sequestration is a congenital malformation that may present as a chest mass in childhood or later in life. This developmental abnormality derives its blood supply from the systemic circulation and can be recognized by radionuclide angiography. The mass seen on the chest radiograph, which is usually in one or the other lower lobe (the left more often than the right), appears as a perfusion defect and also on the radionuclide angiogram during the pulmonary phase. Perfusion is seen early in the systemic phase of the angiogram, however.[230,231] If surgery is to be performed, aortography is usually required to define the origin and course of the systemic arterial supply to the sequestrated portion of the lung. This radionuclide technique does not differentiate between bronchopulmonary sequestration and such conditions as intrathoracic kidney, hepatic herniation through the diaphragm, and the anomalous pulmonary venous drainge that occurs in scimitar syndrome.

Special Applications

Radionuclides have been used in several other ways to study the lung. For instance, pulmonary extravascular lung water has been measured by comparing the mean transit times of a vascular or nondiffusible indicator with those of water and other diffusable tracers.[232–234] Extensions of this method have been used to study pulmonary capillary permeability.[235] Regional extravascular lung water has been studied using cyclotron-produced tracers: $H_2{}^{15}O$ as the diffusible indicator and $C^{15}O$–labeled red cells as the nondiffusible indicator.[236,237]

$C^{15}O$ has been used to study regional clearance of carbon monoxide in normal subjects, in patients with mitral stenosis and chronic obstructive lung disease,[238] and in patients with intrapulmonary hemorrhage from Goodpasture's syndrome.[239] Radiolabeled red cells have also been shown to accumulate in the lungs of such patients.[240]

QUANTITATIVE ASPECTS OF VENTILATION-PERFUSION STUDIES

Several systems and analytic methods have been described for quantifying V-Q studies.[241,243] Ventilation can be evaluated in a quasistatic fashion, as the distribution of a single breath of radioxenon at tidal lung capacity compared with the distribution after equilibrium. This equilibrium image represents lung volume. Such images are usually normalized by expressing the regional counting rate as a proportion of the total counting rate. The figures derived by this method give an indication of relative ventilation per unit lung volume. The ventilation indices, initially described by Ball et al.,[4] allow for more accurate comparisons in the same individual, or between individuals, by taking into account both the concentration of radioxenon in the spirometer and the volume of air in the lungs.

Perfusion per unit lung volume can be described in the same way, by recording the distribution of intravenously injected radioxenon while the patient holds his breath at total lung capacity, and then comparing this to the distribution of lung volume obtained after a rebreathing period. In patients with obstructive airway disease, equilibrium may not be reached, so that ventilation and perfusion per unit volume are overestimated. Regional V-Q ratios are obtained by dividing the regional figures for ventilation per unit volume by those for perfusion per unit volume. The figures obtained are rather different from the proper physiological V-Q ratios because the real values for alveolar ventilation or pulmonary blood flow are not taken into account. The distribution of radioactive particles labeled with ^{99m}Tc is often substituted for intravenous radioxenon for the perfusion studies, and the differences in energy and volume of tissue counted are ignored. ^{127}Xe is more comparable to ^{99m}Tc in these respects than is ^{133}Xe. Studies of regional ventilation and blood flow during normal tidal breathing have been shown to provide similar information to the breath-holding techniques and to require less patient cooperation.

More dynamic assessments of regional ventilation can be made from the changing activity during either a washin or a washout study. In their simplest forms, these can be the time to 50 or 90% of the equilibrium counting rate or, as is most commonly used, the time to 50% of the equilibrium counting rate during a washout procedure. Regional rate constants may be determined from the first 50 or 60% of the washout curves from either inhaled or intravenously injected radioxenon,[244–248] but such an analysis tends to ignore the later parts of the curve and, hence, underestimates the more poorly ventilated regions. The regional mean rate constants using whole washout curves have been determined using the Stewart-Hamilton equation. A background subtraction technique is necessary in those circumstances.[245,247] Also, Kety's model has been applied successfully with a multidetector system.[246]

The mean transit time for ^{133}Xe in the lungs can be measured accurately from the slope of the washout or desaturation curve, by calculating the initial washout rate. Studies in both normal patients and a few patients with pulmonary disease have shown excellent agreement with measurements of the mean transit time for helium. Measurement of the mean washout time in these same patients showed it to be significantly longer than the mean transit time for helium, implying that the use of the mean washout time would underestimate ventilation per unit volume.[249]

Differences are found between the quasistatic and the dynamic measurements in patients with obstructive airway disease, because the quasistatic methods show how much air enters a region in relation to its volume, while the latter indicate how much air is actually exchanged. In healthy lungs, the two techniques give comparable results.

Although washout procedures provide the most useful clinical information, they do have the disadvantage of the radioxenon being dissolved in the tissues of the chest wall and blood.[250] Thus, measurement from this part of the study is inaccurate unless a correction can be made for the tissue and blood contributions. The magnitude of this effect has been studied in comparisons with ^{13}N. These comparisons suggest that one quarter of the delay in radioxenon clearance is accounted for by chest wall activity and three quarters by radioxenon dissolved in the blood.

The results of these quantitative studies, which can provide figures for relative blood flow, ventilation, lung volume, regional ventilation and blood flow indices, regional V-Q ratios, and regional V-Q products, may be expressed either numerically or as functional or parametric images. Parametric images have the advantage of showing a large amount of information on function relationships in a readily assimilated form. Contour images, three-dimensional images, color images, gray-scale images, and cinematic images have all been used. A critical evaluation of their use in patient care has yet to be undertaken.

Acknowledgment. The authors wish to thank Roger H. Secker-Walker for allowing us to use substantial portions of his previous chapter as the framework for this version.

REFERENCES

1. Knipping HW, et al. Eine neue methode zur prufung der Herz- und lungerfunktion: die regionale funktionsanalyse in der lungen-und Herz-Klinik mit Hilfe desradioactiven Edengases Xenon 133 (isotopen-Thorakographie). *Dtsch Med Wochenschr* 1955;80:1146.
2. Dyson NA, et al. Studies of regional lung function using radioactive oxygen. *Br Med J* 1960;1:231.
3. West JB, DolleryCT. Distribution of blood flow and ventilation-perfusion ratio in the lung, measured with radioactive CO_2. *J Appl Physiol* 1960;15:405.
4. Ball WC Jr, et al. Regional pulmonary function studied with xenon-133. *J Clin Invest* 1962;41:519.
5. Dollery CT, Gillam PMS. The distribution of blood and gas within the lungs measured by scanning after administration of ^{133}Xe. *Thorax* 1963;18:316.
6. West JB. Distribution of gas and blood in the normal lungs. *Br Med Bull* 1963;19:53.
7. Bryan AC, et al. Factors affecting regional distribution of ventilation and perfusion in the lung. *J Appl Physiol* 1964;19:395.
8. West JB, Dollery CT, Naimark A. Distribution of blood flow in isolated lung: relation to vascular and alveolar pressures. *J Appl Physiol* 1964;19:713.
9. West JB. Pulmonary function studies with radioactive gases. *Ann Rev Med* 1967;18:459.
10. Integrated physiology and pastbiophysiology, in Crystal RG, West JB (eds.): *The Lung—Scientific Foundations*, Vol. 1, Section 5, New York, Raven Press, 1991, pp 807–1207.
11. Weibel ER. *Morphometry of the Human Lung*. New York, Academic Press, 1963.
12. Horsfield K, Cumming G. Functional consequences of airway morphology. *J Appl Physiol* 1968;24:384.
13. Horsfield K, Cumming G. Morphology of the bronchial tree in man. *J Appl Physiol* 1968;24:373.
14. Peters RM. Coordination of ventilation and perfusion. *Ann Thorac Surg* 1968;6:570.
15. Mead J, Takishima T, Leith D. Stress distribution in lungs: A model of pulmonary elasticity. *J Appl Physiol* 1970;28:596.
16. Macklem PT. Airway obstruction and collateral ventilation. *Physiol Rev* 1971;51:368.
17. Heinemann HO, Fishman AP. Nonrespiratory functions of mammalian lung. *Physiol Rev* 1969;49:1.

18. Said SI. Endocrine role of the lung in disease. *Am J Med* 1974;57:453.
19. General cell biologic processes in the lung, in Crystal RG, West JB (eds.): *The Lung—Scientific Foundations*. Vol. 1, Section 2. New York, Raven Press, 1991, pp 3–153.
20. Davies G, Reid L. Growth of the alveoli and pulmonary arteries in childhood. *Thorax* 1970;25:669.
21. Henderson R, Horsfield K, Cumming G. Intersegmental collateral ventilation in the human lung. *Respir Physiol* 1968;6:128.
22. Elliott FM, Reid L. Some new facts about the pulmonary artery and its branching pattern. *Clin Radiol* 1965;16:193.
23. Hislop A, Reid L. Intra-pulmonary arterial development during fetal life-breathing pattern and structure. *J Anat* 1972;113:35.
24. Daly IdeB, Hebb C. *Pulmonary and bronchial vascular systems; their reactions under controlled conditions*. London, Edward Arnold, 1966.
25. West JB. *Respiratory Physiology*, 5th Ed. Baltimore, Williams & Wilkins, 1995, pp 61, 99.
26. West JB. Distribution of mechanical stress in the lung, a possible factor of localization of pulmonary disease. *Lancet* 1969;1:839.
27. Macklem PT, Mead J. Resistance of central and peripheral airways measured by a retrograde catheter. *J Appl Physiol* 1967;22:395.
28. Jones JG, Clarke SW. The effect of expiratory flow rate on regional lung emptying. *Clin Sci* 1969;37:343.
29. Hlastala MP. Ventilation, in Crystal RG, West JB (eds.): *The Lung—Scientific Foundations*, Chap. 5.3.1. New York, Raven Press, 1991, pp 1209–1214.
30. Anthonisen NR, Milic-Emili J. Distribution of pulmonary perfusion in erect man. *J Appl Physiol* 1966;21:760.
31. Kaneko K, et al. Regional distribution of ventilation and perfusion as a function of body position. *J Appl Physiol* 1966;21:767.
32. Maloney JE, et al. Transmission of pulsatile pulmonary artery pressure on distribution of blood flow in isolated lung. *Respir Physiol* 1968;4:154.
33. West JB, Wagner PD. Ventilation-perfusion relationships, in Crystal RG, West PB (eds.): *The Lung—Scientific Foundations*. Chap. 5.34. New York, Raven Press, 1991 pp 1289–1305.
34. Hughes JMB, et al. Effect of lung volume on the distribution of pulmonary blood flow in man. *Respir Physiol* 1968;4:58.
35. Glazier JB, et al. Measurements of capillary dimensions and blood volume in rapidly froxen lungs. *J Appl Physiol* 1968;26:65.
36. Glazier JB, Murray JE. Sites of pulmonary vasomotor reactivity in the dog during alveolar hypoxia and serotonin and histamine infusion. *J Clin Invest* 1971;50:2550.
37. Arborelius M. Influence of unilateral hypoventilation on distribution of pulmonary blood flow in man. *J Appl Physiol* 1969;26:101.
38. Arborelius M Jr, Lilja B. Effect of sitting, hypoxia, and breath-holding on the distribution of pulmonary blood flow in man. *Scand J Clin Lab Invest* 1969;24:261.
39. West JB. *Respiratory Physiology—The Essentials, 5th Ed.* Baltimore, Williams & Wilkins, 1995, p 79.
40. Saperstein LA, Moses LE. Cerebral and cephalic blood flow in man; basic considerations of the indicator fractionation technique in dynamic clinical studies with isotopes, in *Proceedings of Symposium held at Oak Ridge Institute of Nuclear Studies*, October 21–25, 1963.
41. Tow DE, et al. Validity of measuring regional pulmonary arterial blood flow with macroaggregates of human serum albumin. *Am J Roentgenol Radium Ther Nucl Med* 1966;96:664.
42. Chernick V, et al. Estimation of differential pulmonary blood flow by bronchospirometry and radioisotope scanning during rest and exercise. *Am Rev Respir Dis* 1965;92:958.
43. Rogers RM, et al. Measurement of the vital capacity and perfusion of each lung by fluoroscopy and macroaggregated albumin lung scanning. An alternative to bronchospirometry for evaluating individual lung function. *Ann Intern Med* 1967;67:947.
44. Garnett ES, et al. Quantitated scintillation scanning for the measurement of lung perfusion. *Thorax* 1969;24:372.
45. Haynie TP, et al. Visualization of pulmonary artery occlusion by photoscanning. *JAMA* 1963;185:306.
46. Taplin GV, et al. Lung photoscans with macroaggregates of human serum radioalbumin. Experimental basis and initial clinical trials. *US 82 AEC UCLA School Med Lab Nucl Med* 1964;April:1.
47. Wagner HN Jr, et al. Diagnosis of massive pulmonary embolism scanning. *N Engl J Med* 1964;271:377.
48. Harper PV, et al. Technetium-99m as a scanning agent. *Radiology* 1965;85:101.
49. Wagner HN Jr, Hosain F, Rhodes BA. Recently developed radiopharmaceuticals; ytterbium-169 DTPA and technetium-99m microspheres. *Radiol Clin North Am* 1969;7:233.
50. Fazio F, Jones T. Assessment of regional ventilation by continuous inhalation of radioactive krypton-81m. *Br Med J* 1975;3:673.
51. Taplin GV, MacDonald NS. Radiochemistry of macroaggregated albumin and newer lung scanning agents. *Semin Nucl Med* 1971;1:132.
52. Goodwin DA. Lung retention of labeled ferric hydroxide macroaggregates used in lung scanning. *J Nucl Med* 1971;12:580.
53. Galt JM, Tothill P. The fate and dosimetry of two lung scanning agents: ^{131}IMAA and ^{99m}Tc ferrous hydroxide. *Br J Radiol* 1973;46:272.
54. Malone LA, Malone JF, Ennis JT. Kinetics of technetium 99m labelled macroaggregated in humans. *Br J Radiol* 1983;56:109.
55. Nielsen PE, Kirchner PT, Gerger FH. Oblique views in lung perfusion scanning: Clinical utility and limitations. *J Nucl Med* 1977;18:967.
56. Tetalman MR, et al. Perfusion lung scans in normal volunteers. *Radiology* 1973;106:593.
57. Polga JP, Drum DE. Abnormal perfusion and ventilation scintigrams in patients with azygos fissures. *J Nucl Med* 1972;13:633.
58. Secker-Walker RH. The value of lung scanning in the diagnosis of pulmonary embolism in the elderly. *Geriatrics* 1969;24:81.
59. Friedman SA, et al. Perfusion defects in the aging lung. *Am Heart J* 1968;79:160.
60. Kronenberg RS, et al. The effect of aging on lung perfusion. *Ann Intern Med* 1972;76:413.
61. Vincent WR, Goldberg SJ, Desilets D. Fatality immediately following rapid infusion of macroaggregates of ^{99m}Tc-albumin (MAA) for lung scan. *Radiology* 1968;91:1181.
62. Child JS, et al. Fatal lung scan in a case of pulmonary hypertension due to obliterative pulmonary vascular disease. *Chest* 1975;67:308.
63. Harding LK, et al. The proportion of lung vessels blocked by albumin microspheres. *J Nucl Med* 1973;14:579.
64. Gold WM, McCormack KR. Pulmonary function response to radioisotope scanning of the lungs. *JAMA* 1966;197:146.
65. Rootwelt K, Vale JR. Pulmonary gas exchange after intravenous injection of 99mTc-sulphur-colloid albumin macroag-

gregates for lung perfusion scintigraphy. *Scand J Clin Lab Invest* 1972;30:17.

66. Allen DR, et al. Critical evaluation of acute cardiopulmonary toxicity of microspheres. *J Nucl Med* 1978;19:1202.
67. Davis MA, Taube RA. Pulmonary perfusion imaging: Acute toxicity and safety factor as a function of particle size. *J Nucl Med* 1978;19:1209.
68. Heck LL, Duley JW Jr. Statistical considerations in lung imaging with ^{99m}Tc-albumin particles. *Radiology* 1974; 113:675.
69. Dworkin HJ, et al. Effect of particle number on lung perfusion images: concise communication. *J Nucl Med* 1977;18:260.
70. Ackery DM, Goddard BA. Proceedings: Advantage of ^{127}Xe over ^{133}Xe for measurements of regional ventilation. *Bull Physiopathol Respir* 1975;11:123.
71. Atkins HL, et al. A clinical comparison of Xe-127 and Xe-133 for ventilation studies. *J Nucl Med* 1977;18:653.
72. Coates G, Nahmias C. Xenon-127, a comparison with xenon-133 for ventilation studies. *J Nucl Med* 1977;18:221.
73. Atkins HL, et al. Estimates of radiation absorbed doses from radioxenons in lung imaging. *J Nucl Med* 1980;21:459.
74. Chu RYL, et al. The heatlh physics of xenon-127. *Radiology* 1980;134:493.
75. Chu RYL, et al. Collimator and xenon-127 for ventilation studies. *Radiology* 1980;137:819.
76. Weber PM, dos Remedios LV. Kr-81m versus Xe-133 for ventilation imaging in suspected pulmonary embolism. *J Nucl Med* 1977;18:625.
77. Fazio F, Lavender PJ, Steiner RE. ^{81m}Kr ventilation and ^{99m}Tc perfusion scans in chest disease: Comparison with standard radiographs. *An J Roentgenol* 1978;130:421.
78. Lavender JP (ed.). *Clinical and experimental applications of Krypton 81m.* Br J Radiol Spec Rep No. 15, 1978.
79. Modell HI, Graham MM. Limitations of Kr-81m for quantitation of ventilation scans. *J Nucl Med* 1982;23:301.
80. Taplin GV, Chopra SK, Elam D. Imaging experimental pulmonary ischemic lesions after inhalation of a diffusible radioaerosol: concise communication. *J Nucl Med* 1977; 18:250.
81. Anthonisen NR, et al. Regional lung function in patients with chronic bronchitis. *Clin Sci* 1968;35:495.
82. Dollfuss RE, Milic-Emili J, Bates DV. Regional ventilation of the lung studied with boluses of ^{133}xenon. *Respir Physiol* 1967;2:234.
83. Milic-Emili J. Radioactive xenon in the evaluation of regional lung function. *Semin Nucl Med* 1971;1:246.
84. Alderson PO, et al. Comparison of ^{133}Xe single-breath and washout imaging in the scintigraphic diagnosis of pulmonary embolism. *Radiology* 1980;137:481.
85. Corrigan KE, Mantel J, Corrigan HH. Trapping system for radioactive gas. *Radiology* 1970;96:571.
86. Luizzi A, Keaney K, Freedman G. Use of activated charcoal for the collection and containment of Xe-133 exhaled during pulmonary studies. *J Nucl Med* 1972;13:673.
87. Alderson PO, Line BR. Scintigraphic evaluation of regional pulmonary ventilation. *Semin Nucl Med* 1980;10:218.
88. Suprenant EL, Wilson A, Bennett LR. Clinical application of regional pulmonary function studies. *Radiology* 1971; 99:623.
89. Treves S, et al. Radionuclide evaluation of regional lung function in children. *J Nucl Med* 1974;15:582.
90. Dollery CT, Hugh-Jones P, Matthews CME. Use of radioactive xenon for studies of regional lung function: a comparison with oxygen-15. *Br Med J* 1962;5311:1006.
91. Pircher FJ, et al. Distribution of pulmonary ventilation determined by radioisotope scanning—a preliminary report. *Am J Roentgenol Radium Ther Nucl Med* 1965;94:807.
92. Taplin GV, Poe ND, Greenberg A. Lung scanning following radioaerosol inhalation. *J Nucl Med* 1966;7:77.
93. Cook DJ, Lander H. Inhalation lung scanning using carrier-free ^{113m}In. *J Nucl Med* 1971;12:765.
94. Santolicandro A, et al. Uneven deposition of inhaled minimicrospheres related to lung disorders. *Bull Physiopathol Respir* 1976;12:203.
95. Taplin GV, et al. Radioaerosol inhalation scanning, in Gilson AJ, Smoak W (eds.): *Pulmonary Investigation and Radionuclides*. Springfield IL, Charles C. Thomas, 1970.
96. Taplin GV, Chopra SK. Lung perfusion inhalation scintigraphy in obstructive airways disease and pulmonary embolism. *Radiol Clin North Am* 1978;16:491.
97. Hayes M, et al. Improved radioaerosol administration system for routine inhalation lung imaging. *Radiology* 1979;131:256.
98. Fazio F, et al. Clinical ventilation imaging with In-113m aerosol: A comparison with Kr-81m. *J Nucl Med* 1982;23:306.
99. Selby JB, Kaiser ML, Hunter GO. Inhalation lung imaging with ^{99m}Tc DTPA aerosol. *Clin Nucl Med* 1983;8:60. NO
100. Jones JG, Lawler P, Crawley JCW. Increased alveolar epithelial permeability in cigarette smokers. *Lancet* 1980;1:66.
101. Sanchis J, et al. Quantitation of regional aerosol clearance in the normal human lung. *J Appl Physiol* 1972;33:757.
102. Lourenco RV, Klimek MF, Borowski CJ. Deposition and clearance of 2 m particles in the tracheobronchial tree of normal subjects, smokers and non-smokers. *J Clin Invest* 1971;50:1411.
103. Ramanna L, et al. Radioaerosol lung imaging in chronic obstructive pulmonary lung disease. Comparison with pulmonary function tests and roentgenography. *Chest* 1975; 68:634.
104. Sanchis J, et al. Pulmonary mucociliary clearance in cystic fibrosis. *N Engl J Med* 1973;288:651.
105. Eliasson R, et al. The immotile-cilia syndrome. A congenital ciliary abnormality as an etiologic factor in chronic airway infections and male sterility. *N Engl J Med* 1977;297:1.
106. Morrow PF. Evaluation of inhalation hazards based upon the respirable dust concept and the philosophy and application of selective sampling. *Am Ind Hyg Assoc J* 1964;25:213.
107. Isitman AT, Manoli R, Schmidt GH, et al. An assessment of alveolar deposition and pulmonary clearance of radiopharmaceuticals after nebulization. *Ann J Roentgenol* 1974; 120:776–781.
108. Alderson PO, Kotlyarov EV, Loken MK, et al. A comparison of Xe-133 ventilation and Tc-99m aerosol inhalation imaging as aids to perfusion scanning in the scintigraphic detection of pulmonary embolism. *J Nucl Med* 1981;22:42–43.
109. Ramanna L, Alderson PO, Waxman AD, et al. Regional comparison of Tc-99m DTPA aerosol and radioactive gas ventilation (xenon and krypton) studies in patients with suspected pulmonary embolism. *J Nucl Med* 1986;27:1391–1396.
110. Hull RD, Hirsh J, Carter CJ, et al. Diagnostic value of ventilation-perfusion lung scanning in patients with suspected pulmonary embolism. *Chest* 1985;88:819–828.
111. Isitman AT, Collier BD, Palmer DW, et al. Comparison of Tc-99m PYP and Tc-99m DTPA aerosols for SPECT ventilation lung imaging. *J Nucl Med* 1988;29:1761–1767.
112. Krasnow AZ, Isitman AT, Collier BD, et al. Diagnostic applications of radioaerosols in nuclear medicine, in Freeman LM (ed.): *Nuclear Medicine Annual.* New York, Raven Press, 1993, pp 123–193.
113. Burch WM, Sullivan PJ, McLaren CJ. Technegas—a new ventilation agent for lung scanning. *Nucl Med Commun* 1986;7:865–871.
114. Monaghan P, Provan I, Murray C, et al. An improved radionu-

clide technique for the detection of altered pulmonary permeability. *J Nucl Med* 1991;32:1945–1949.
115. Strong JC, Agnew JE. The particle size distribution of technegas and its influence on regional lung deposition. *Nucl Med Commun* 1989;10:425–430.
116. Crawford AB, Davison A, Anis TC, et al. Intrapulmonary distribution of Tc-99m labeled ultrafine carbon aerosol (technegas) in severe airflow obstruction. *Eur Respir J* 1990; 3:686–692.
117. Sullivan PJ, Burke WM, Burch WM, et al. A clinical comparison of technegas and xenon-133 in 50 patients with suspected pulmonary embolus. *Chest* 1988;94:300–304.
118. James JM, Hermen KJ, Lloyd JJ, et al. Evaluation of Tc-99m technegas ventilation scintigraphy in the diagnosis of pulmonary embolism. *Br J Radiol* 1991;64:711–719.
119. Morrell MT, Dunnill MS. The post mortem incidence of pulmonary embolism in a hospital population. *Br J Surg* 1968;55:347–352.
120. The PIOPED Investigators. Value of the ventilation/perfusion scan in acute pulmonary embolism. *JAMA* 1990;263: 2753–2759.
121. Humphries JO, Bell WR, White RI. Criteria for the recognition of pulmonary emboli. *JAMA* 1976;235(18):2011–2012.
122. Bell WR, Simon TL, DeMets DS. The clinical features of submassive and massive pulmonary emboli. *Am J Med* 1977;62:355–359.
123. Landefeld CS, McGuire E, Cohen AM. Clinical findings associated with acute proximal deep venous thrombosis: a basis for quantifying clinical judgment. *Am J Med* 1990;88:382–388.
124. Greenspan RH, Ravin CE, Polansky SM, McLoud TC. Accuracy of the chest radiograph in diagnosis of pulmonary embolism. *Invest Radiol* 1982;17:539–543.
125. Alderson PO, Doppman JL, Diamond SS, Mendenhall KG, Barron EL, Girton M. Ventilation-perfusion lung imaging and selective pulmonary angiography in dogs with experimental pulmonary embolism. *J Nucl Med* 1978;19:164–171.
126. Secker-Walker RH, Siegel BA. The use of nuclear medicine in the diagnosis of lung disease. *Radiol Clin North Am* 1973;11:215–241.
127. Wagner HN Jr, Lopez-Majano V, Langan JK, et al. Radioactive xenon in the differential diagnosis of pulmonary embolism. *Radiology* 1968;91:1168–1174.
128. DeNardo GL, Goodwin DA, Ravasini R, et al. The ventilatory lung scan in the diagnosis of pulmonary embolism. *N Engl J Med* 1970;282:1334–1336.
129. McNeil BJ, Holman L, Adelstein J. The scintigraphic definition of pulmonary embolism. *JAMA* 1974;227:753–756.
130. Alderson PO, Rejanavech N, Secker-Walker RH, et al. The role of 133-xenon ventilation studies in the scintigraphic detection of pulmonary embolism. *Radiology* 1976;120:633–640.
131. Neumann RD, Sostman HD, Gottschalk A. Current status of ventilation-perfusion imaging. *Semin Nucl Med* 1980;10: 198–217.
132. Kotlyarov EV, Reba RC. The concept of using abnormal V/Q segment equivalents to refine the diagnosis of pulmonary embolism (abstr). *Invest Radiol* 1981;16:383.
133. Alderson PO, Biello DR, Sachariah KG, et al. Scintigraphic detection of pulmonary embolism in patients with obstructive pulmonary disease. *Radiology* 1981;138:661–666.
134. Biello DR, Mattar AG, McKnight RC, et al. Ventilation-perfusion studies in suspected pulmonary embolism. *AJR* 1979;133:1033–1037.
135. Carter WD, Brady TM, Keyes JW, et al. Relative accuracy of two diagnostic schemes for detection of pulmonary embolism by ventilation-perfusion scintigraphy. *Radiology* 1982; 145:447–451.
136. Gottschalk A, Juni JE, Sostman HD, et al. Ventilation-perfusion scintigraphy in the PIOPED study. Data collection and tabulation. *J Nucl Med* 1993;34:1109–1118.
137. Gottschalk A, Sostman HD, Juni JE, et al. Ventilation-perfusion scintigraphy in the PIOPED study. Evaluation of the scintigraphic criteria and interpretations. *J Nucl Med* 1993;34:1119–1126.
138. Sullivan DC, Coleman RE, Mills SR, Ravin CE, Hedlund LW. Lung scan interpretation: Effect of different observers and different criteria. *Radiology* 1983;149:803–807.
139. Sostman HD, Coleman RE, DeLong DM, Newman GE, Paine SS. Evaluation of revised criteria for ventilation-perfusion scintigraphy in patients with suspected pulmonary embolism. *Radiology* 1994;193:103–107.
140. Stein PD, Gottschalk A, Henry JW, Shivkumar K. Stratification of patients according to prior cardiopulmonary disease and probability assessment based on the number of mismatched segmental equivalent perfusion defects. *Chest* 1993;104:1461–1467.
141. Stein PD, Henry JW, Gottschalk A. Mismatched vascular defects. *Chest* 1993;104:1468–1472.
142. Worsley DF, Kim CK, Alavia A, Palevsky HI. Detailed analysis of patients with matched ventilation-perfusion defects and chest radiographic opacities. *J Nucl Med* 1993;34:1851–1853.
143. Sostman HD, Gottschalk A. Prospective validation of the stripe sign in ventilation-perfusion scintigraphy. *Radiology* 1992;184:455–459.
144. Paraskos VA, Adelstein SJ, Smith RE, Richman RD, et al. Late prognosis of acute pulmonary embolism. *N Engl J Med* 1973;289:55–58.
145. Alderson PO, Dzebolo NN, Biello DR, Seldin DW, et al. Serial lung scintigraphy: utility in diagnosis of pulmonary embolism. *Radiology* 1983;149:797–802.
146. Reid LM. Pathology of chronic bronchitis. *Lancet* 1954; 1:275.
147. Ebert RV, Terracio MI. The bronchiolar epithelium in cigarette smokers. Observations with the scanning electronic microscope. *Am Rev Respir Dis* 1975;111:4.
148. Hogg JC, Macklem PT, Thurlbeck WM. Site and nature of airway obstruction in chronic obstructive lung disease. *N Engl J Med* 1968;278:1355.
149. McKusick KA, et al. Measurement of regional lung function in the early detection of chronic obstructive pulmonary disease. *Scand J Respir Dis* 1974;85(Suppl):51.
150. Burrows B, et al. The emphysematous and bronchial types of chronic airway obstruction—a clinicopathological study of patients in London and Chicago. *Lancet* 1966;1:830.
151. Bentivoglio LG, et al. Studies of regional ventilation and perfusion in pulmonary emphysema using xenon-133. *Am Rev Respir Dis* 1963;88:315.
152. Pain MC, et al. Regional and overall inequality of ventilation and blood flow in patients with chronic airflow obstruction. *Thorax* 1967;22:453.
153. Welch MH, et al. The lung scan in alpha-1-antitrypsin deficiency. *J Nucl Med* 1969;10:687.
154. Fallat RJ, et al. ^{133}Xe-ventilatory studies in a1,-antitrypsin deficiency. *J Nucl Med* 1973;14:5.
155. Alderson PO, Secker-Walker RH, Forrest JV. Detection of obstructive pulmonary disease. Relative sensitivity of ventilation-perfusion studies and chest radiography. *Radiology* 1974;112:643.
156. Novey HS, et al. Early ventilation-perfusion changes in asthma. *J Allergy* 1970;46:221.
157. Bentivoglio LG, et al. Regional pulmonary function studied

with xenon-133 in patients with bronchial asthma. *J Clin Invest* 1963;42:1193.

158. Mishkin FS, Wagner HN. Regional abnormalities in pulmonary arterial blood flow during acute asthmatic attacks. *Radiology* 1967;88:142.
159. Heckscher T, et al. Regional lung function in patients with bronchial asthma. *J Clin Invest* 1968;47:1063.
160. Wilson AF, et al. The significance of regional pulmonary function changes in bronchial asthma. *Am J Med* 1970;48:416.
161. Riley DJ, et al. Regional bronchoconstriction in asthma. 133-xenon washout scans following parenteral methacholine. *Chest* 1976;70:715.
162. Fazio F, et al. Aerosol versus gaseous tracers for imaging regional ventilation: A comparison of Tc-99m-minimicrospheres nebulization and continuous inhalation of Kr-81m. *Bull Physiopathol Respir* 1976;12:205.
163. Fazio F, et al. Imaging of pulmonary ventilation in asthma assessed with continuous inhalation of Kr-81m. *Bull Physiopathol Respir* 1976;12:202.
164. Gyepes MT, Bennett LR, Hassakis PC. Regional pulmonary blood flow in cystic fibrosis. *Am J Roentgenol Radium Ther Nucl Med* 1969;106:567.
165. Samánek M, et al. Distribution of pulmonary blood flow in children with cystic fibrosis. *Acta Paediatr Scand* 1971;60:149.
166. Alderson PO, et al. Quantitative assessment of regional ventilation and perfusion in children with cystic fibrosis. *Radiology* 1974;111:151.
167. Piepsz A, et al. Critical evaluation of lung scintigraphy in cystic fibrosis: Study of 113 patients. *J Nucl Med* 1980;21:909.
168. Dollery CT, Hugh-Jones P. Distribution of gas and blood in the lungs in disease. *Br Med Bull* 1963;19:59.
169. Moncada R, et al. Reversible unilateral pulmonary hypoperfusion secondary to acute check-valve obstruction of a main bronchus. *Radiology* 1973;106:361.
170. Hatch HB Jr, Maxfield WS, Ochsner JL. Radioisotope lung scanning in bronchogenic carcinoma. *J Thorac Cardiovasc Surg* 1965;50:634.
171. Wagner HN Jr, et al. Radioisotope scanning of lungs in early diagnosis of bronchogenic carcinoma. *Lancet* 1965;1:344.
172. Maxfield WS, Hatch HG, Ochsner JL. Perfusion lung scanning in evaluation of patients with bronchogenic carcinoma. *Surg Clin North Am* 1966;46:1389.
173. Secker-Walker RH, et al. Lung scanning in carcinoma of the bronchus. *Thorax* 1971;26:23.
174. Arborelius M Jr, et al. ^{133}Xe-radiospirometry and extension of lung cancer. *Scand J Respir Dis* 1971;52:145.
175. Rosler H, Schnaars P, Kinser J. ^{133}Xenon lung scintigraphy: results in 86 patients with bronchial carcinoma. *Helv Med Acta* 1972;56:307.
176. Vassallo CL, et al. Lung scanning in hilar bronchogenic carcinoma. *Am Rev Respir Dis* 1968;97:851.
177. Macumber HM, Calvin JM. Perfusion lung scan patterns in 100 patients with bronchogenic carcinoma. *J Thorac Cardiovasc Surg* 1976;72:299.
178. Sarlin RF, et al. Focal increased lung perfusion and intrapulmonary venoarterial shunting in broncho-alveolar cell carcinoma. *Am J Med* 1980;68:618.
179. Katz RD, et al. Ventilation-perfusion lung scanning in patients detected by a screeing program for early lung carcinoma. *Radiology* 1981;141:171.
180. Garnett ES, et al. Lung perfusion patterns in carcinoma of bronchus. *Br Med J* 1968;2:209.
181. Fraser HS, et al. Lung scanning in the preoperative assessment of carcinoma of the bronchus. *Am Rev Respir Dis* 1970;101:349.
182. Kristersson S. Prediction of lung function after lung surgery. A ^{133}Xe-radiospirometric study of regional lung function in bronchial cancer. *Scand J Thorac Cardiovasc Surg* 1974;18(Suppl):5.
183. Boysen PG, et al. Prospective evaluation for pneumonectomy using the ^{99m}technetium quantitative perfusion lung scan. *Chest* 1977;72:422.
184. Wernley JA, et al. Clinical value of quantitative ventilation-perfusion lung scans in the surgical management of bronchogenic carcinoma. *J Thorac Cardiovasc Surg* 1980;80:535.
185. Maynard CD, et al. Pulmonary scanning in bronchogenic carcinoma. *Radiology* 1969;92:903.
186. Secker-Walker RH, Provan JL. Scintillation scanning of lungs in preoperative assessment of carcinoma of bronchus. *Br Med J* 1969;3:327.
187. Lefrac SS. Preoperative evaluation for pulmonary resection. The role of radionuclide lung screening (editorial). *Chest* 1977;72:419.
188. Sealy WC. Mediastinoscopy: Does it have a place in the management of carcinoma of the lung? *Ann Thorac Surg* 1974;18:433.
189. Lindell L, Lindell SE, Svanberg L. Regional lung function in roentgenologically occult lung cancer. *Scand J Respir Dis* 1972;53:109.
190. Germon PA, Brady LW. Physiologic changes before and after radiation treatment for carcinoma of the lung. *JAMA* 1968;206:809.
191. Johnson PM, Sagerman RH, Jacos HW. Changes in pulmonary arterial perfusion due to intrathoracic neoplasia and irradiation of the lung. *Am J Roentgenol Radium Ther Nucl Med* 1968;102:637.
192. Secker-Walker RH, Goodwin J. Quantitative aspects of lung scanning. *Proc R Soc Med* 1971;64:344.
193. Fazio F, et al. Improvement in regional ventilation and perfusion after radiotherapy for unresectable carcinoma of the bronchus. *Am J Roentgenol* 1979;133:191.
194. Tauxe WN, Carr DT, Thorsen HC. Perfusion lung scans in patients with inoperable primary lung cancer. *Mayo Clin Proc* 1970;45:337.
195. McCormack KR, Cantril ST, Kamenetsky S. Serial pulmonary perfusion scanning in radiation therapy for bronchogenic carcinoma. *J Nucl Med* 1971;12:800.
196. Goldman SM, et al. Effects of thoracic irradiation on pulmonary arterial perfusion in man. *Radiology* 1968;93:289.
197. Alderson PO, et al. Pulmonary ventilation perfusion and radioaerosol deposition in dogs following hemithorax irradiation with Co-60 or fast neutrons. *J Nucl Med* 1977;18:625.
198. Todorov J, et al. Comparative radiological and scintigraphic examination of radiation pneumonitis with postoperative ^{60}Co-telegamma therapy of patients with breast cancer. *Radiobiol Radiother (Berlin)* 1981;22:69.
199. Lopez-Majano V, et al. Radioisotope scanning of the lungs in pulmonary tuberculosis. *JAMA* 1965;194:1053.
200. Isawa T. Studies on the distribution of the pulmonary arterial blood flow with special reference to pulmonary function. II. Pulmonary tuberculosis. *Sci Rep Res Inst Tohoku Univ (Med)* 1966;13:123.
201. Seaton A, Lapp NL, Chang CHJ. Lung perfusion scanning in coal workers pneumoconiosis. *Am Rev Respir Dis* 1971;103:338.
202. Seaton D. Regional lung function in asbestos workers. *Thorax* 1977;32:40.
203. Secker-Walker RH, Ho JE. Regional lung function in asbestos workers: Observations and speculations. *Respiration* 1982;43:8.
204. Wanner A, Cutchavaree A. Early recognition of upper airway

obstruction following smoke inhalation. *Am Rev Respir Dis* 1973;108:1421.
205. Moylan JA, et al. Early diagnosis of inhalation injury using ^{133}xenon lung scan. *Ann Surg* 1972;176:477.
206. Petroff PA, et al. Pulmonary function studies after smoke inhalation. *Am J Surg* 1976;132:346.
207. Soin JS, et al. Increased sensitivity of regional measurements in early detection of narcotic lung disease. *Chest* 1975;67:325.
208. Thomashow D, et al. Lung disease in reformed drug addicts: Diagnostic and physiologic correlations. *Johns Hopkins Med J* 1977;141:1.
209. Secker-Walker RH, Ho JE. Observations on regional ventilation and perfusion in kyphoscoliosis. *J Nucl Med* 1977;18:606.
210. Shannon DC, Riseborough EJ, Kazemi H. Ventilation-perfusion relationships following correction of kyphoscoliosis. *JAMA* 1971;217:579.
211. Davidson FF, Glazier JB. Unilateral pleuritis and regional lung function. *Ann Intern Med* 1972;77:37.
212. Dhekne RD, Burdine JA. The diagnosis of pneumothorax by ventilation-perfusion imaging. *Radiology* 1978;129:119.
213. Lillington GA, et al. Bronchoscopic location of bronchopleural fistula with xenon-133. *J Nucl Med* 1982;23:322.
214. Skorodin MS, et al. Xenon-133 evidence of bronchopleural fistula healing during treatment of mixed aspergillus and tuberculous emphysema. *J Nucl Med* 1982;23:688.
215. Weissman HS, et al. Myocardial visualization on a perfusion lung scan. *J Nucl Med* 1980;21:745.
216. Gates GF, Orme HW, Dore EK. Surgery of congenital disease assessed by radionuclide scintigraphy. *J Thorac Cardiovasc Surg* 1975;69:767.
217. Gates GE, Orme HW, Dore EK. The hyperperfused lung. Detection in congenital heart disease. *JAMA* 1975;233:782.
218. Haroutunian LM, Neill CA, Wagner HN Jr. Radioisotope scanning of the lung in cyanotic congenital heart disease. *Am J Cardiol* 1969;23:387.
219. Gluck MC, Moser KM. Pulmonary artery agenesis—Diagnosis with ventilation and perfusion scintiphotography. *Circulation* 1970;41:859.
220. Arborelius M Jr, et al. Xe-133 radiospirometry for evaluation of congenital malformations of pulmonary arteries. *Pediatrics* 1971;47:529.
221. Hurley PJ, Wesselhoeft JH, James AE Jr. Use of nuclear imaging in the evaluation of pediatric cardiac disease. *Semin Nucl Med* 1972;2:353.
222. Mauney FM, Sabiston DC. The role of pulmonary scanning in the diagnosis of congenital lobar emphysema. *Am Surg* 1970;36:20.
223. Espinola D, Rupani H, Camargo EE, Wagner HN. Ventilation-perfusion imaging in pulmonary papillomatosis. *J Nucl Med* 1981;22:975.
224. Ronchetti R, et al. Clinical application of regional lung function studies in infants and small children using ^{13}N. *Arch Dis Child* 1975;50:595.
225. McKenzie SA, Godfrey S, Singh MP. A new method for investigating regional lung function in children with localized lung disease. *J Pediatr Surg* 1977;12:177.
226. Koch G. Proceedings: Regional lung function in the newborn infant assessed by means of 133Xe. *Bull Physiopathol Respir* 1975;11:132.
227. Pendarvis BC, Swischuk LE. Lung scanning in the assessment of respiratory disease in children. *Am J Roentgenol Radium Ther Nucl Med* 1969;107:313.
228. Robinson AE, Goodrich JK, Spock A. Inhalation and perfusion radionuclide studies of pediatric chest diseases. *Radiology* 1969;93:1123.
229. Schmidt BJ, et al. Scintillography in children's lung diseases; some clinical observations. *Clin Pediatr* 1976;15:845.
230. Gooneratne N, Conway JJ. Radionuclide angiographic diagnosis of bronchopulmonary sequestration. *J Nucl Med* 1976;17:1035.
231. Kawakami K, et al. Radionuclide study in pulmonary sequestration. *J Nucl Med* 1978;19:287.
232. Chinard FP, Enns T, Nolan MF. Pulmonary extravascular water volumes from transit time and slope data. *J Appl Physiol* 1962;17:179.
233. Goresky CA. A linear method for determining liver sinusoidal and extravascular volumes. *Am J Physiol* 1963;204:626.
234. Even P, et al. Proceedings: On-line measurement of extravascular lung water in man with gamma emitting tracers. *Bull Physiopathol Respir* 1975;11:135.
235. Harris TR, Rowlett RD, Brigham KL. The identification of pulmonary capillary permeability from multiple-indicator data. Effects of increased capillary pressure and alloxan treatment in the dog. *Microvasc Res* 1976;12:177.
236. Fazio F, et al. Proceedings: Measurement of total and regional lung water in vivo. *Bull Physiopathol Respir* 1975;11:136.
237. MacArthur CGC, et al. Regional distribution of extravascular lung water in man. *Bull Physiopathol Respir* 1976;12:193.
238. Pande JN, et al. Distribution of diffusing capacity using $C^{15}O$. *Bull Physiopathol Respir* 1976;12:196.
239. Ewan PW, et al. Intraregional inhomogeneity of ventilation and perfusion. *Bull Physiopathol Respir* 1976;12:195.
240. Morita R, et al. Lung scintigraphy with ^{51}Cr erythrocytes in Goodpasture's syndrome; case report. *J Nucl Med* 1976;17:702.
241. Kingaby GP, et al. Automation of data collection and analysis in lung scanning with radioactive gases. *Med Biol Engl* 1968;6:403.
242. Wilson JE III, Bynum LJ, Ramanathan M. Dynamic measurement of regional ventilation and perfusion of the lung with Xe-133. *J Nucl Med* 1977;18:660.
243. Jones RH, et al. Radionuclide quantitation of lung function in patients with pulmonary disorders. *Surgery* 1971;70:891.
244. DeRoo MJK, et al. Computerized dynamic scintigraphy of the lungs. *Respiration* 1969;26:408.
245. MacIntyre WJ, et al. Spatial recording of disappearance constants of xenon-133 washout from the lung. *J Lab Clin Med* 1970;76:701.
246. Alpert NM, et al. Initial assessment of a simple functional image of ventilation. *J Nucl Med* 1976;17:88.
247. Secker-Walker RH, et al. The measurement of regional ventilation in man: A new method of quantitation. *J Nucl Med* 1973;14:725.
248. Peset R, et al. The measurement of regional alveolar ventilation in liters per minute and dead space ventilation using xenon-133 during spontaneous breathing (the xenon-133 dead space). *Scand J Respir Dis* 1974;85(Suppl):38.
249. Henriksen O, Lonborg-Jensen H, Rasmussen FV. Evaluation of a method for determination of mean transit time of xenon-133 in the lungs. *J Nucl Med* 1980;21:333.
250. Matthews CME, Dollery CT. Interpretation of ^{133}Xe lung washin and washout curves using an analogue computer. *Clin Sci* 1965;28:573.

26 The Gastrointestinal Tract

Harvey A. Ziessman

Gastrointestinal transit studies highlight the ability of nuclear medicine to noninvasively study physiology and the mechanisms of disease. This chapter will discuss the use of radionuclide techniques to study esophageal transit, gastroesophageal reflux, and gastric emptying.

ESOPHAGEAL TRANSIT

Radionuclide esophageal transit scintigraphy has theoretical advantages over other methods of evaluating esophageal motility. It is noninvasive, relatively simple to perform, and quantitative. However, the exact clinical role of this technique has yet to be clearly defined. This section will review radionuclide techniques used for evaluating esophageal transit, quantitative methods, and the role of these studies in evaluating various esophageal motility disorders.

Anatomy and Physiology of the Esophagus

The esophagus transports liquids and solids from the mouth to the stomach, clears regurgitated substances, and prevents tracheobronchial aspiration and acid reflux. Located in the posterior mediastinum, the esophagus can be divided into three anatomic regions. The upper esophageal sphincter (UES) consists of striated muscle that tonically contracts and relaxes, allowing swallowed food to pass from the mouth to the proximal esophagus. The esophageal body has striated muscle proximally and smooth muscle distally. Swallowing initiates a coordinated persistaltic contraction that propagates down the esophagus. The lower esophageal sphincter (LES) is a high-pressure smooth muscle region that prevents gastric reflux, but relaxes during swallowing to allow food passage into the stomach. The separate physiological functions of these three regions are coordinated by myogenic, neural, and hormonal mechanisms.

Disorders of Esophageal Motility

Discomfort during swallowing (dysphagia) is the most common complaint of patients with abnormal esophageal motility. Esophageal motor disorders can be classified as primary (e.g., achalasia, esophageal spasm, nutcracker esophagus) or secondary (e.g., scleroderma or diabetic enteropathy) or, alternatively, by the type of dysfunction (e.g., amotility, achalasia and scleroderma; hypomotility, presbyesophagus; and hypermotility, diffuse spasm and the nutcracker esophagus).

Non-Radioisotopic Evaluation of Esophageal Function

The evaluation of esophageal motor disorders often requires the use of multiple diagnostic modalities. Each method has certain advantages and disadvantages, and information that it can and cannot furnish. Barium radiography is useful for excluding structural lesions of the esophagus and detecting mucosal changes. However, cinefluorography provides only qualitative, not quantitative, information about function. Endoscopy is also commonly used to detect structural and mucosal changes, but is of no value in diagnosing disorders of motility. Esophageal manometry provides useful information on amplitude, duration, and velocity of peristaltic contractions and on sphincter pressure and the ability of the UES and LES to relax. It serves as the standard for making the definitive diagnosis of esophageal motility disorders and specific manometric criteria exist for each entity (Table 1). Since manometry requires passing a catheter through the nose or mouth, patients are often not thrilled with the technique. Provocative pharmacological testing is also sometimes used (e.g., edrophonium to repro-

Table 1. Definitions of Esophageal Motor Disorders

Achalasia
Absence of esophageal peristalsis
Transient or incomplete LES relaxation
Elevated resting intraesophageal pressure
A positive bethanechol chloride test result
Diffuse esophageal spasm
Repetitive nonperistaltic contractions of increased amplitude in the distal 2/3 of the esophagus accompanying more than 30% of wet swallows, but with retention of some peristaltic function
Normal LES relaxation
Normal resting intraesophageal pressure
The presence of chest pain and/or dysphagia with or without a positive bethanechol chloride test
Hypertensive LES
LES pressure >35 mmHg above intragastric pressure
Normal LES relaxation
Normal peristalsis
Normal intraesophageal resting pressure
High-amplitude peristaltic contractions ("nutcracker" esophagus)
Mean contraction amplitude >140 mmHg at 5 cm above the LES; peak contraction amplitude >165 mmHg
Normal peristalsis
Normal LES relaxation

duce noncardiac chest pain or bethanecol to help aid in diagnosis of achalasia).

Radionuclide Esophageal Transit Studies

In 1972, Kazem et al.[1] described the use of radionuclides to evaluate esophageal transit. Many variations on that technique have been described since (e.g., the radionuclide used, bolus content, patient positioning, method of acquisition, and analysis, Table 2).

Although the specifics may differ, a general protocol for esophageal transit studies could be described as follows: A radioactive marker is placed on the cricoid cartilage. In the supine position, practice swallows are performed, then ^{99m}Tc–sulfur colloid (SC), 150 to 300 μCi in 10 to 15 mL water is swallowed as a bolus. Dynamic images are acquired (0.1 to 0.8 frames/sec) on a computer. Dry swallows follow at defined intervals (e.g., 30 sec). The individual images and cinematic display is reviewed. Regions of interest can be drawn on the computer and time-activity curves generated. Quantification may be performed (transit time or percent clearance) and functional images (e.g., condensed dynamic images) constructed and reviewed.

RADIONUCLIDES

^{99m}Tc-sulfur colloid (^{99m}Tc-SC) in water is the most commonly used radiopharmaceutical for esophageal transit studies due to its property of nonabsorbability, although adherence of ^{99m}Tc-SC to areas of esophagitis has been described.[2] An interesting alternative is ^{81m}Krypton in solution, eluted from a ^{81}Rb/^{81m}Kr generator.[3] It has the advantage of a high counting rate and minimal radiation absorbed dose because of its 13 second half-life. However, it is expensive and not widely available.

RADIATION DOSIMETRY

The radiation absorbed dose to patients from radionuclide esophageal transit studies is low (Table 3 A,B), particularly when compared to that received from fluoroscopy and cine-esophagography.

BOLUS COMPOSITION

A swallowed liquid bolus, usually water, is most commonly used to evaluate esophageal transit. However, semisolid boluses of jam, gelatin, hamburger, chelex resin in oatmeal, cold cereal with milk, and others, have been used.[6–9] Recent reports suggest that semisolid boluses may be more sensitive than liquids for detecting abnormal esophageal transit.[6]

An interesting study investigating non-liquid boluses by Fisher et al.[10] found that gelatin capsules and chicken liver cubes transitted best with the patient upright, by first ingesting a prelubricating sip of water, and by swallowing water

Table 2. Different Methodologies for Performing Esophageal Transit Studies

AUTHOR	BOLUS	DOSE	POSITION	ACQUISITION METHOD	DRY SWALLOWS	METHOD OF QUANTITATION
Kazem[1]	Tc-O_4^-	0.5–1.0 mCi in 10–20 mL tea	erect	0.4 s per frame × 1.0 to 1.5 min		time/activity curves
Tolin[11]	Tc-SC	150 μCi in 15 mL H_2O	supine	1 s per frame × 15, then 15 s per frame × 10	q 15 s × 10 min	% emptying
Russell[16]	Tc-SC	250 μCi in 10 mL H_2O	supine	0.4 s per frame × 50 s	1 @ 30 s	transit time
Blackwell[18]	Tc-SC	500 μCi in 10 mL H_2O	supine	list mode 0.3–5.0 s/ frame	q 30 s × 2 min	transit time
Klein and Wald[19]	Tc-SC	300 μCi in 15 mL H_2O	supine	0.2 s per frame × 30 s, then 1 s per frame × 15 s for 2–4th swallow	at 30 s, then q 15 s × 10 min	transit time centroid of mass late swallow indices, condensed images
Taillefer[17]	Tc-SC	0.5–1.0 mCi in 15–20 mL H_2O	supine	0.5 s × 60 per frame	at 30 s, then q 15 s × 2 min	time-activity curves
Tatsch[6]	Tc-Sc	250 μCi in 10 mL H_2O	supine	0.8 s per frame × 240	none	transit time condensed images
Drane[39]	Tc-SC	100–300 μCi	supine	0.5 s per frame × 50 s	every 30 s	transit time percent emptying

Table 3A. Radiation Absorbed Dose with ^{99m}Tc-SC Gastroesophageal Scintigraphy for Various Ages of Children

ORGAN*	cGy/37 MBq					
	Newborn	*1 yr*	*5 yr*	*10 yr*	*15 yr*	*Adult*
STO	0.383	0.093	0.050	0.031	0.022	0.018
SI	0.372	0.164	0.090	0.058	0.036	0.032
ULI	0.596	0.267	0.164	0.090	0.054	0.052
LLI	0.927	0.380	0.194	0.120	0.072	0.033
Ovaries	0.099	0.042	0.033	0.072	0.002	0.010
Testes	0.018	0.007	0.003	0.011	0.001	0.000
Thyroid	0.002	0.0006	0.0002	0.0001	0.000	0.000
Whole body	0.020	0.011	0.006	0.004	0.003	0.002

*Abbreviations: Stomach (STO), small intestine (SI), upper large intestine (ULI), lower large intestine (LLI); modified from Castranovo FP: Gastroesophageal scintiscanning in a pediatric population: Dosimetry. *J Nucl Med* 1986; 27:1212–1214.[43]

Table 3B. Dosimetry for Esophageal and Gastric Scintigraphy in Adults*

	10^{-5} Gy/STUDY MEAL						
	STO	*SI*	*ULI*	*LLI*	*Ovaries*	*Testes*	*Total Body*
Liquid							
300 μCi ^{99m}Tc-SC	28	83	160	97	29	2	5
1 mCi ^{99m}Tc-DTPA	93	280	520	320	98	5	20
250 μCi ^{111}In-DTPA	110	490	1100	2000	420	27	60
500 μCi ^{113}In-DTPA	170	280	270	68	20	1	10
Solid							
500 μCi ^{99m}Tc (or Tc-SC) ovalbumin	120	120	230	140	42	2	9
250 μCi ^{111}In-chicken liver	240	480	1100	1900	400	28	58
500 μCi ^{99m}Tc-chicken liver	120	120	230	140	42	2	9

*Modified from Siegel JA, et al.: Radiation dose estimates for oral agents used in upper gastrointestinal diseases. *J Nucl Med* 1983; 24:835–837.[5]

with and after the bolus. Even so, the gelatin capsules, often used for medication, may be retained unknowingly within the esophagus.

POSITION

The supine position is usually advocated because it eliminates the effect of gravity on esophageal emptying[11] (Fig. 1 **A,B**). However, the upright position may help distinguish achalasia (where the LES does not relax) from systemic sclerosis (with a hypotensive LES), since a liquid bolus may not empty from the esophagus in achalasia in the supine position. Lamki et al.[12] found that quantitative grading is best performed with the patient upright because some emptying will occur in that position. Both anterior and posterior imaging have been used for transit studies.

Factors in Bolus Transit. Consistency, position, and volume all influence normal esophageal transit. Transit is faster for (1) liquids than for more viscous material, (2) with the patient upright compared to supine positioning and, (3) for smaller volumes (10 mL) compared to larger volumes (20 ml). Multiple swallows are often required for even healthy people to completely empty the esophagus. A high incidence of "aberrant" swallows (up to 25%) has been noted in normal people.[13–15] These extra swallows, occurring between two prescribed swallows, can result in inhibition of the initial swallow (deglutitive inhibition), thereby delaying the transit of the bolus. Careful patient instruction and observation are necessary to prevent misinterpretation of this common occurrence. Because of the poor reproducibility of single swallows, multiple swallows (4 to 6) have been suggested in order to obtain sufficient data to establish an accurate diagnosis.[3,6] Valid quantitative analysis requires that the patient swallow the tracer bolus in a single swallow; pharyngeal time-activity curves can help establish that this has occurred.[16]

Analysis and Quantification

Although analog film or cine image interpretation is often adequate to diagnose severe abnormalities[17] (Fig. 1 **C,D**), some form of quantitative analysis is commonly used to diagnose less severe abnormalities and is particularly helpful in the follow-up of patients after therapy (Fig. 2 **A,B**).

An estimate of esophageal emptying can be quantified by calculating (1) the residual activity in the esophagus; and/

Figure 1 A. Upright esophageal transit study: a normal volunteer ingested 25 MBq ^{99m}Tc-SC in 10 mL water while standing in front of the gamma camera. Scintigraphy was performed at 2-s intervals. The liquid radionuclide bolus is sipped into the mouth through a straw and held there (arrow) for at least 2 s. Then the patient is asked to swallow the entire bolus. Global esophageal clearance is rapid, completed within 8 s after ingestion. Only the fundus of the stomach is seen in the field of view due to the patient's height. (With permission, Taillefer R, Beauchamp G, Duranceau A: Radionuclide esophageal transit studies, in Van Nostrand D, Baum S (eds.): *Atlas of Nuclear Medicine*. Philadelphia, J.B. Lippincott Company, 1988.[17])

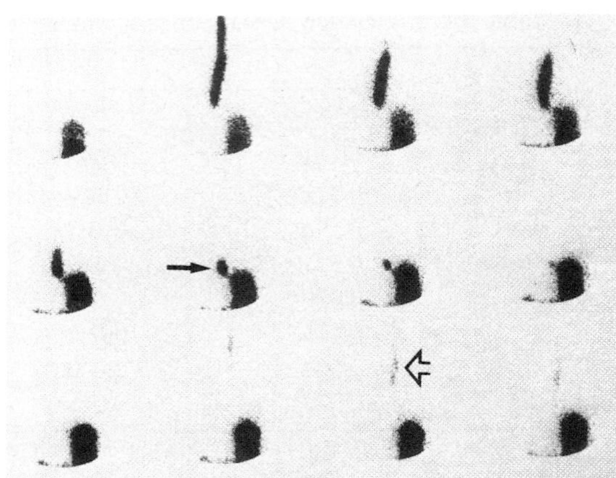

Figure 1 B. Supine esophageal transit study: images are obtained at 2-s per frame. The bolus travels rapidly through the upper esophagus; at midesophagus, the bolus moves less rapidly. There is also a normal slight delay in the distal esophageal lumen (closed arrow). The transit time is 13 s (normal, <15 s). Gastric activity seen on the first frame represents residual activity originating from a previous study performed in the upright position. At 18 s, there is a second swallow (open arrow), which is less than 10% of the initial activity. (With permission, Taillefer, Beauchamp G, Duranceau A, Lafontaine E: Nuclear medicine and esophageal surgery. *Clin Nucl Med* 1986;11:445–459.)

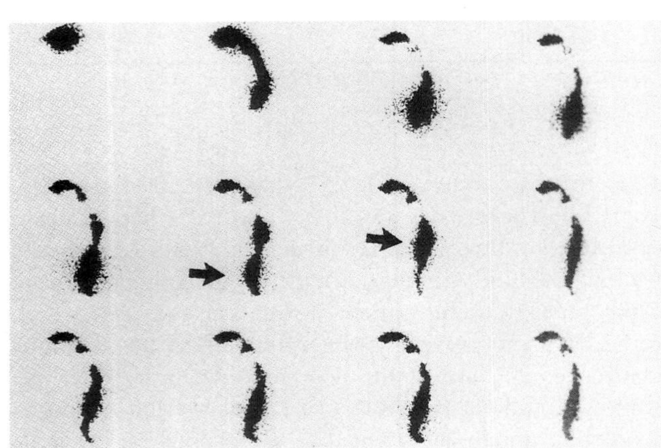

Figure 1 C. Diffuse esophageal spasm: radionuclide transit scintigraphy shows a global and segmental incoordinate passage through the esophageal lumen, accompanied by fragmentation and retrograde movement of the bolus (arrows). (With permission, Taillefer R, Jadliwalla M, Pellerin E, et al.: Radionuclide esophageal transit study in detection of esophageal motor dysfunction: comparison with motility studies (manometry). *J Nucl Med* 1990;31:1921–1926.[2])

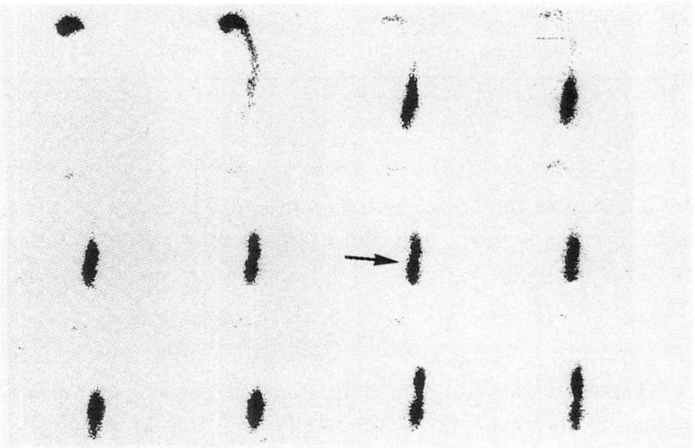

Figure 1 D. Achalasia: two-s analog images. There is significant radiotracer stasis (arrow) at the level of the distal esophageal lumen. More than 80% of the activity remained in the esophagus at the end of the study. (With permission, Taillefer R, Jadliwalla M, Pellerin E, et al.: Radionuclide esophageal transit study in detection of esophageal motor dysfunction: comparison with motility studies (manometry). *J Nucl Med* 1990;31:1921–1926.[2])

or (2) the transit time through the esophagus. In 1979, Tolin et al.[11] first quantified esophageal emptying using the formula: $[(E_{max} - E_t)/E_{max} \times 100\%]$, where E_{max} represents the maximum counting rate in the esophagus (counts per 15-sec interval), and E_t represents the counting rate after dry swallow number t. That study found decreased emptying in achalasia, diffuse spasm, and scleroderma. (Fig. 3 **A,B**).

Russell et al.[14] defined esophageal transit time as the time from initial entry of the bolus into the esophagus until total clearance from the esophagus. Patients with achalasia, diffuse spasm, scleroderma, aperistalsis associated with diabe-

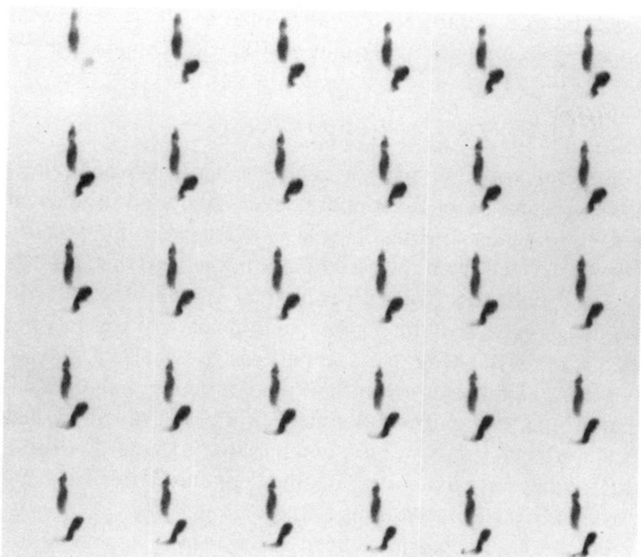

Figure 2 A. Quantitative analysis: this study in a patient with achalasia serves as a baseline for follow-up investigations to evaluate the effectiveness of therapy. One-minute images are acquired for 30 min. There is significant radionuclide stasis at the level of the distal esophageal lumen. Some early emptying into the stomach is noted; however, there is minimal further esophageal clearance for the remainder of the 30-minute study.

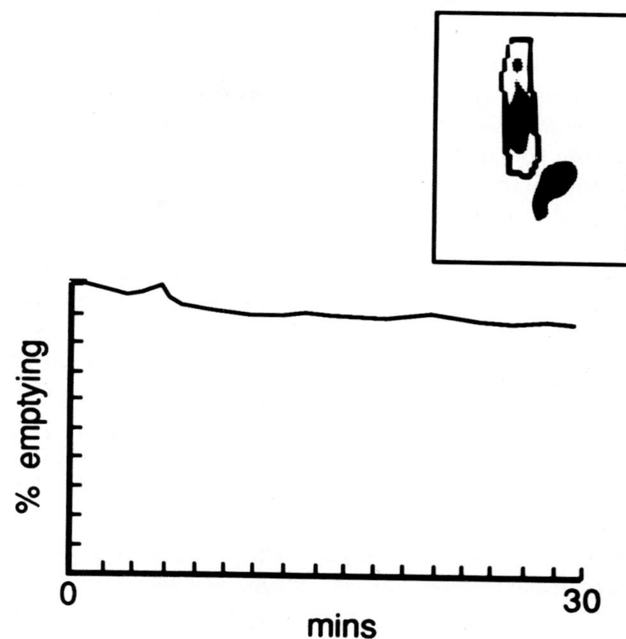

Figure 2 B. The time-activity curve from a region of interest for the entire esophagus confirms minimal emptying during the 30-minute transit study. The percent esophageal emptying was calculated to be only 10%.

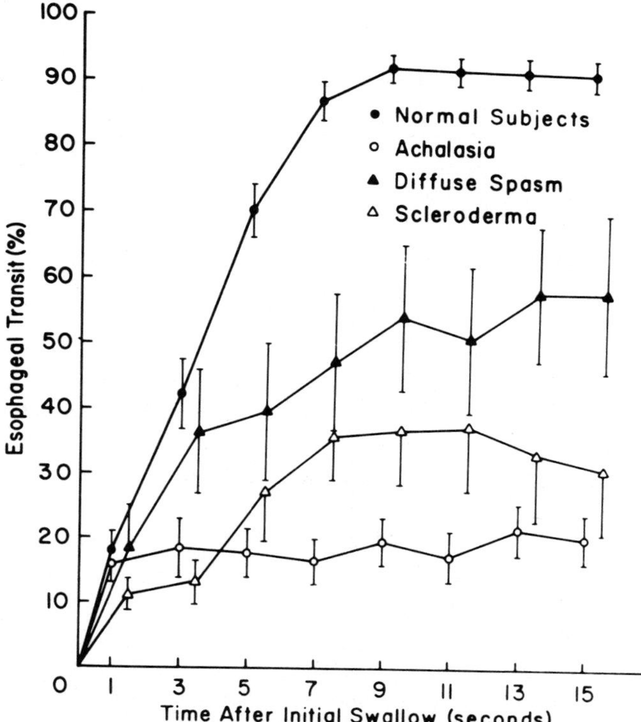

Figure 3 A. Mean esophageal transit time-activity curves after single swallow in 15 normal subjects, 8 patients with achalasia, 10 patients with diffuse esophageal spasm, and 5 patients with scleroderma. Error bars represent ± SEM.

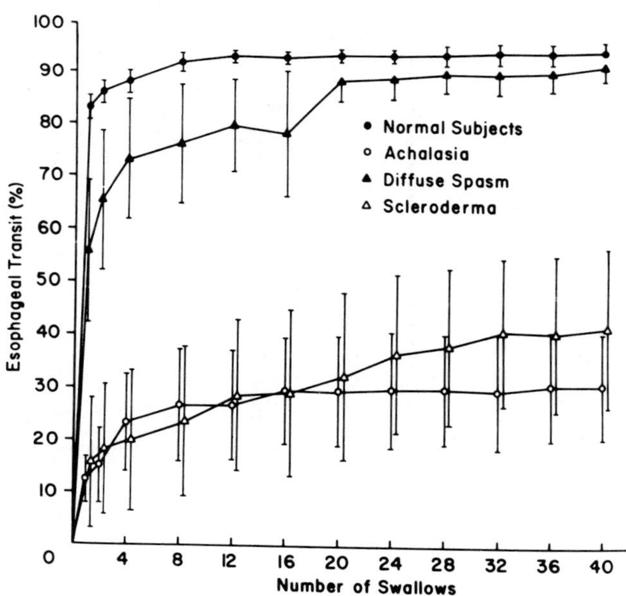

Figure 3 B. Mean esophageal transit time-activity curves after multiple swallows in the same patients. Each swallow represents a 15-s time interval. As a group, patients with achalasia and scleroderma were clearly seaprated from healthy persons and those with esophageal spasm. (With permission, Tolin RD, Malmud LS, Reilley J, Fisher RS: Esophageal scintigraphy to quantitate esophageal transit (quantitation of esophageal transit). *Gastroenterology* 1979;76:1402–1408.[11])

tes, and nonspecific motor disorders had transit times longer than 15 seconds (normal mean 7 ± 3 seconds SD). Patients with achalasia often had transit times greater than 50 seconds, limiting this method's ability to estimate the severity of disease. Blackwell et al.[18] used a similar method, but a different endpoint. Since the time-activity curve frequently did not return to zero, the time required for all but 10% of peak activity to be cleared from the lower third of the esophagus was used.

The esophageal residual that remains after an initial swallow will often clear if followed by a second dry swallow, and the results of the study must be interpreted with knowledge of the swallowing schedule.[19,20] Klein and Wald[19] developed a method of quantitative analysis for both the initial swallow of a bolus and subsequent dry swallows. After curve processing and measuring a transit time and residual fraction (Fig. 4), the vertical component of the center of mass of the spatial distribution of radioactivity for each 0.2-second image frame is determined and the mean location of the bolus tracked.[21,22] De Vincentis et al.,[23] calculated the transit time as the point of maximum slope of the esophagus and stomach. These various quantitative methods have been compared and analyzed.[19] Normal mean liquid esophageal transit times vary somewhat depending on the technique used, but are usually in the range of 6 to 10 seconds with an accepted upper normal range of 10 to 15 seconds.[8,16,20,23,24]

PATTERN ANALYSIS AND FUNCTIONAL IMAGING

Several kinds of pattern analyses based on computer-generated curves or functional images have been used as an aid to diagnosis. Russell et al.[16] evaluated time-activity curves derived from the proximal, middle, and distal thirds of the esophagus. Normal people had a peak of activity in sequence in each of the regions, but this pattern was lacking in disease states (Fig. 5). The patterns of achalasia, scleroderma, and diabetes were described as being "adynamic," and esophageal spasm and nonspecific motor disorders had "incoordination." However, another study found that these differences were not always distinct, nor could specific diagnoses be based on the transit study alone.[25]

Functional images have been found useful by several investigators.[3,21,22,26] As an alternative or aid to viewing the many images acquired in a single transit study, the dynamic data can be condensed into a single image (condensed dynamic images or CDIs) with one spatial dimension (vertical) and one temporal dimension (horizontal) (Fig. 6). The technique is based on the fact that one is interested only in

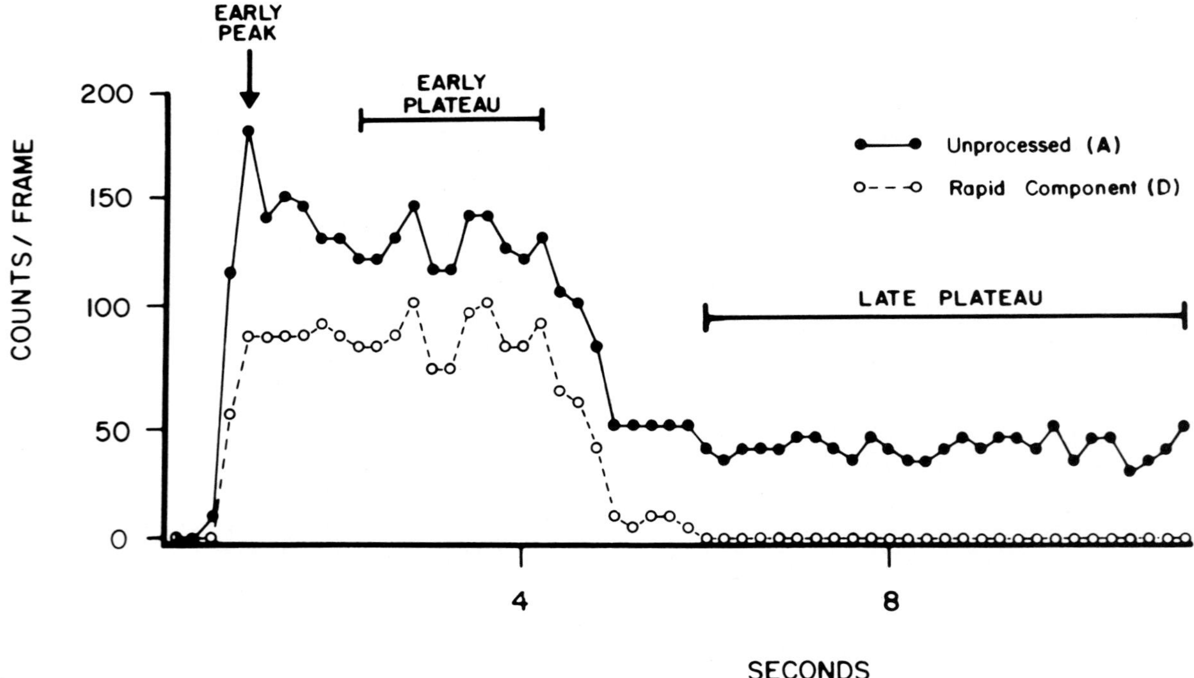

Figure 4. Measurement of a Residual Fraction (RF) for the first swallow in a patient with a motility disorder associated with reflux. A whole esophagus time-activity curve (0.2 s/point) is used. The unprocessed curve shows an initial peak due to an artifact caused by a proximal region of decreased attenuation that occurs with anterior imaging. The curve is then processed (19), resulting in a constant plateau of activity that shows the continued presence of the entire bolus in the esophagus. The RF is calculated (defined as the ratio of late to early plateau mean counting rates expressed as a percentage). A second swallow curve (not shown) revealed no reduction in counting rate. In this case the RF = 28.9%, which is abnormal. (With permission, Klein HA, Wald A: Normal variation in radionuclide esophageal transit studies. *Eur J Nucl Med* 1987;15:115–120.[20])

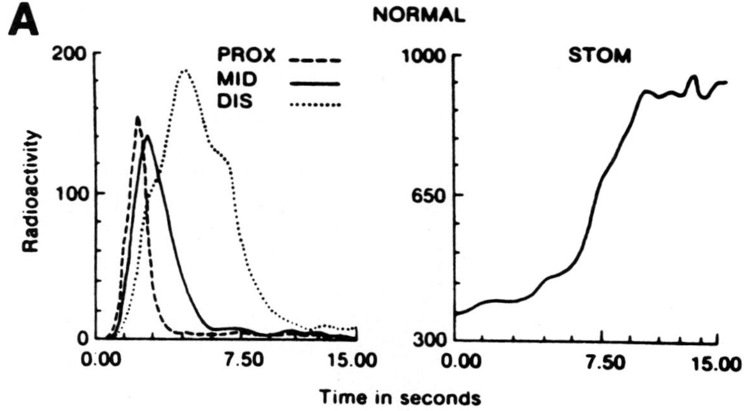

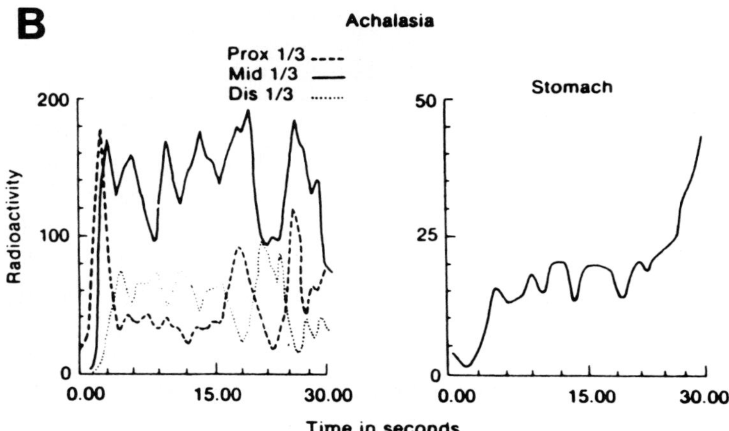

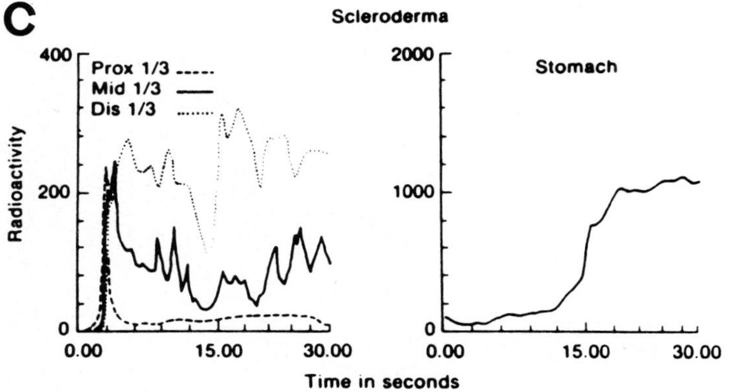

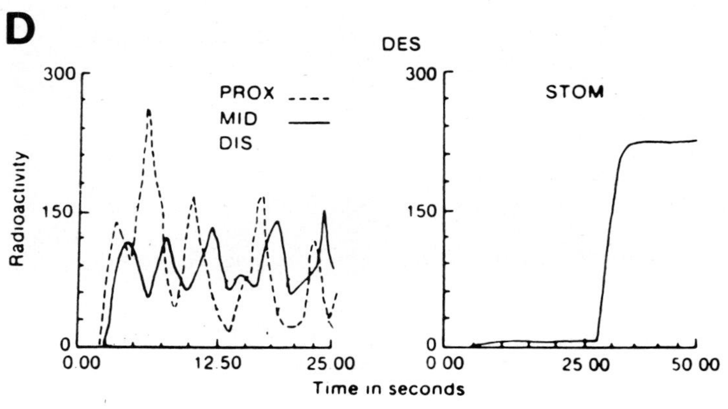

Figure 5 A,B,C,D. Pattern Analysis. **(A).** Normal volunteer; three regions of interest (proximal, mid, and distal esophagus) were selected with resulting transit time-activity curves. Note sequential peaks in the 3 regions indicating smooth passage of the bolus in an aboral direction with early complete entry into the stomach; **(B).** Achalasia; there is no progression of the bolus beyond the midsegment at 30 s. This is an "adynamic pattern." Note the relative lack of radioactivity entering the stomach. **(C).** Scleroderma; note the loss of proper bolus progression at 30 s and entry of substantial portion of the bolus into stomach. **(D).** Diffuse esophageal spasm; note multiple peaks of activity representing disorganized bolus transit. Some of the bolus, however, reached the stomach within the 30-s time period. (With permission, Russell COH, Hill LD, Holmes ER, et al.: Radionuclide transit: a sensitive screening test for esophageal dysfunction. *Gastroenterology* 1981;80:887–892.[16])

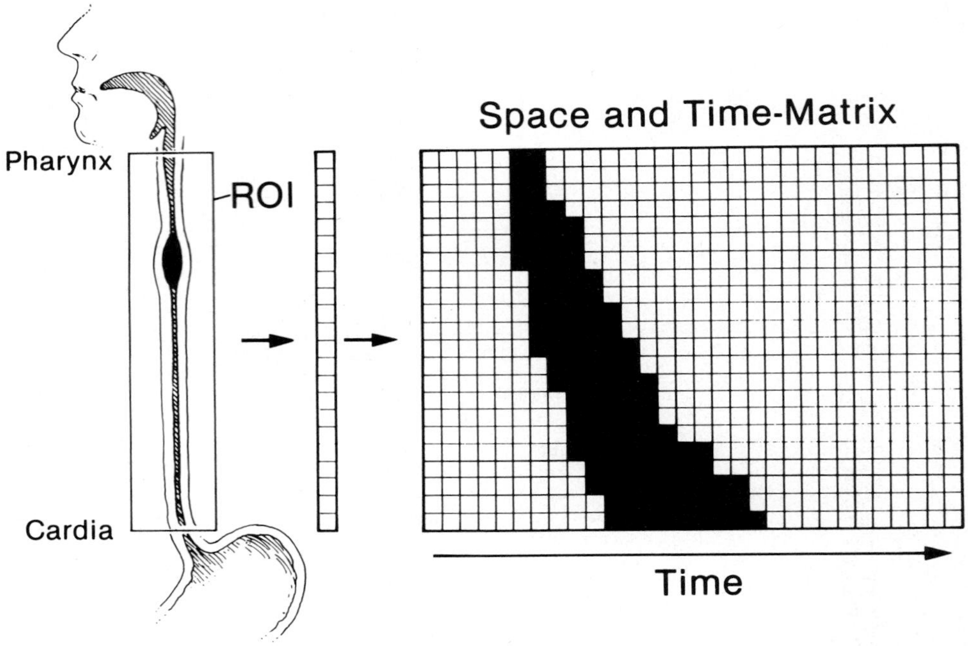

Figure 6. Schematic diagram illustrating the generation and display of condensed dynamic images (CDIs). In each consecutive frame of the study ($n = 240$), the information in an esophageal region of interest is compressed into a single column, displaying the distribution of the tracer from the pharynx to the proximal stomach within a 0.8-s interval. The columns are arranged consecutively, thus generating a space-and-time matrix whose vertical and horizontal dimensions represent spatial and temporal activity changes, respectively.

craniocaudal transit, not lateral motion. Klein and Wald[19,21] have used this technique extensively and have described characteristic disease patterns for the initial swallow as well as subsequent dry swallows (Fig. 7 **A–C**).

FINDINGS IN ESOPHAGEAL MOTILITY DISORDERS

Achalasia is characterized by the absence of peristalsis in the distal two thirds of the esophagus, increased LES pressure, and incomplete relaxation with swallowing. The result is dilatation and retention of food. Patients complain of dysphagia with both liquids and solids, weight loss, nocturnal regurgitation, cough, and occasional aspiration. The etiology is unknown. A barium swallow shows esophageal dilatation with smooth tapering at the gastroesophageal junction. Tumors can be excluded by endoscopy. The diagnosis of achalasia is confirmed by manometry, which shows aperistalis and incomplete LES relaxation. Elevated LES pressure is common. Radionuclide esophageal transit studies are very sensitive (93 to 100%) for making the diagnosis noninvasively.[11,16,27–29]

Diffuse esophageal spasm is characterized by intermittent chest pain and/or dysphagia without a demonstrable organic lesion. The symptoms are produced by abnormal nonperistaltic contractions of the esophageal body, which can be demonstrated by manometry or radiological studies. Specific manometric criteria are required to make this diagnosis[30]: nonperistaltic contractions occurring in greater than 30% of wet swallows with some normal peristaltic waves. Repetitive contractions and increased amplitude and duration of contractions may be present. Radionuclide transit studies have a moderate sensitivity (67 to 77%) for detecting this condition.[18,28]

The "*nutcracker esophagus*" is a somewhat controversial diagnosis.[31–33] These patients typically have noncardiac chest pain and normal radiographic studies. High-amplitude peristaltic contractions, sometimes of prolonged duration, are

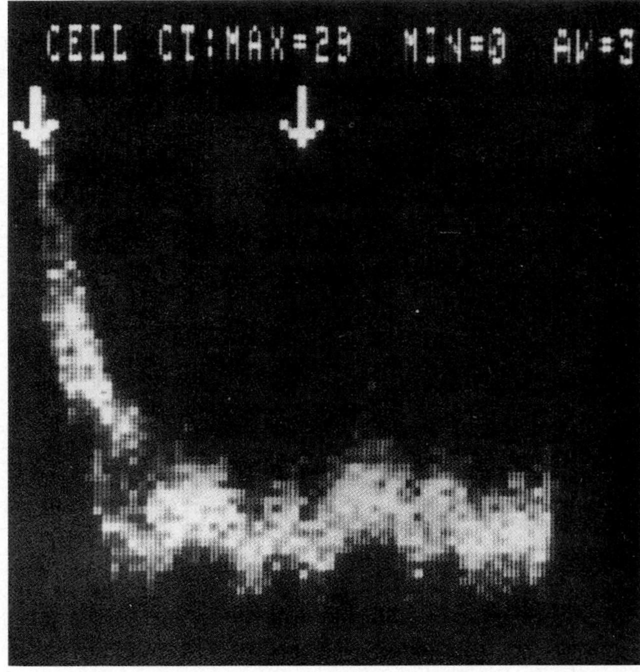

Figure 7 A. Condensed dynamic image (CDI) of a normal swallow sequence. There is smooth uninterrupted transit of the bolus down the esophagus. Vertical arrows indicate the timing of swallows.

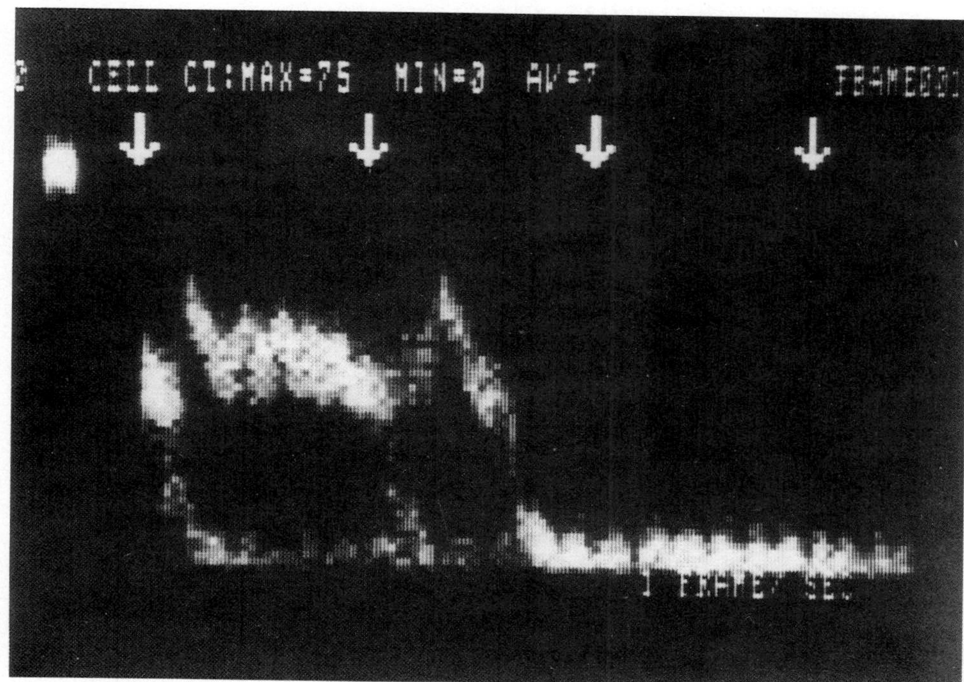

Figure 7 B. CDI from a patient with diffuse esophageal spasm. After the initial swallow, part of the bolus remains in the mid-esophagus, the remainder being transported to the stomach. A subsequent dry swallow propels the rest of the bolus into the stomach. Vertical arrows indicate the timing of swallows.

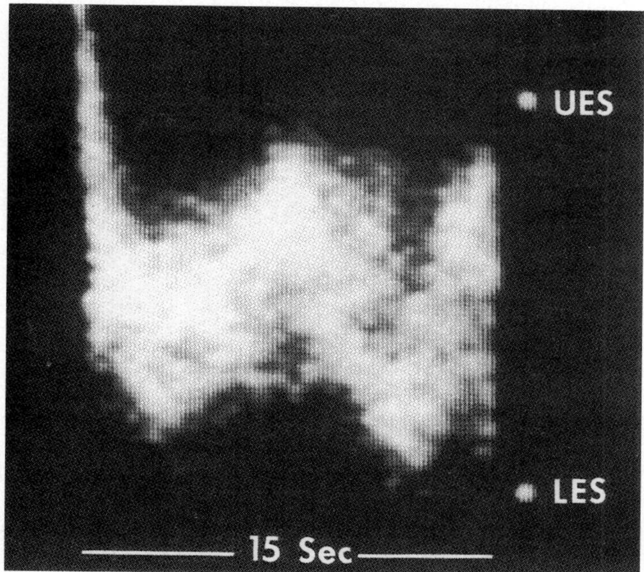

Figure 7 C. CDI of the initial swallow in a patient with achalasia and retention of the bolus in esophagus and oscillatory motion. (With permission, Klein HA, Wald A: Esophageal transit scintigraphy, in: *Nuclear Medicine Annual 1988.* New York, Raven Press, 1988.[19])

found at manometry.[34] The sensitivity for radionuclide transit studies has ranged from 0 to 94%.[35–38]

Nonspecific motor disorder is a diagnosis used in patients who have abnormal manometry but do not fit into other well-defined categories. The sensitivity of radionuclide transit studies for detecting this entity has been variable (42 and 100%).[25,38]

Scleroderma, a systemic disease involving the smooth muscle of the esophagus, often shows aperistalsis, a dilated esophagus, and retention of barium and gastroesophageal relux on barium radiographs. Manometry may demonstrate decreased or absent LES pressure and decreased amplitude of peristaltic contractions, or aperistalsis confined to the smooth muscle portion of the esophagus. Radionuclide transit studies have found delayed emptying.[39] *Systemic lupus erythematosus* and *polymyositis* may also be associated with smooth muscle disease of the esophagus and abnormal esophageal transit studies.[40] Striated muscle abnormalities of *muscular dystrophy, myasthenia gravis, dermatomyositis/polymyositis*, and *myotonia dystrophica* can cause loss of propulsive force in the pharyngeal muscles and impairment of the coordinated transfer of food from pharynx to esophagus, manifested by difficulty in initiating the act of swallowing. Radionuclide transit studies may detect abnormalities in these patients.[41]

Diabetes and *alcoholism* are often associated with abnormalities of esophageal motor function. In diabetics, this is associated with a gastroenteropathy.[42,43] Esophageal motility disorders have also been described with *gastroesophageal reflux* and *esophagitis*.

Clinical Role of Esophageal Transit Studies

The role of radionuclide esophageal transit studies has not yet been fully defined. Although this noninvasive study can detect achalasia with high sensitivity, a lower or more variable detection rate is reported in other conditions, limiting its use as a screening test. The most clearcut indication is for monitoring the disease process over time and for evaluating response to therapy, whether pharmacological, medical, or surgical. For example, improvement has been documented in achalasia following pneumatic dilatation, myotomy with fundoplication, and the use of isosorbide dinitrate[27,29,44] (Fig. 8). Studies have also shown improvement in patients with systemic sclerosis using metoclopramide.[37]

A number of studies have described patients with esophageal symptoms and normal esophageal manometry, but abnormal radionuclide esophageal transit studies.[8,16,18,24,25,38] Because the positive rates for esophageal transit scintigraphy were considerably greater than the false-positive rates derived from asymptomatic controls, it has been argued that esophageal transit studies can detect disease missed by manometry,[16] although others feel that the findings merely denote a lack of specificity for the test.[38]

GASTROESOPHAGEAL REFLUX DISEASE

Symptomatic reflux of gastric contents into the esophagus is one of the most common gastrointestinal disorders. *Gastroesophageal reflux disease* (GERD) refers to a symptomatic clinical condition and/or the histological changes that result from episodes of gastroesophageal reflux (GER), while *reflux esophagitis* refers to the mucosal changes of inflammation, hyperplasia, and erosions that often occur secondary to GER. Only 30 to 40% of patients with heartburn have mucosal injury.

Pathophysiology

GERD is not usually caused by a single abnormality. Although acid alone may produce esophagitis, pepsin in small amounts often contributes substantially. Esophageal clearance is a critical factor because this determines the duration of exposure of the esophagus to a reflux event. With normal esophageal motor activity, the reflux volume clears within seconds; however, acid takes several minutes to clear, because it must be neutralized by swallowed saliva. Other contributing factors include the efficacy of the antireflux mechanism, the volume of gastric contents, the potency of refluxed material, the resistance of the mucosa to injury, and its reparative ability (Table 4).

Although lower esophageal sphincter (LES) pressure is reduced in groups of patients with GER, there is considerable overlap between normal people and patients with GER. GER does not occur when basal LES pressure is above a minimal value ($\geq$10 mm Hg); however, many patients with GER have normal resting LES pressure. Reflux occurs either as a result of transient LES relaxation not associated with swallowing, stress reflux due to transient increases in intra-abdominal pressure, or free reflux across an atonic sphincter[45] (Fig. 9). Although the relationship between a sliding hiatus hernia and esophagitis is controversial, the consensus is that most patients with moderate to severe esophagitis have a

A

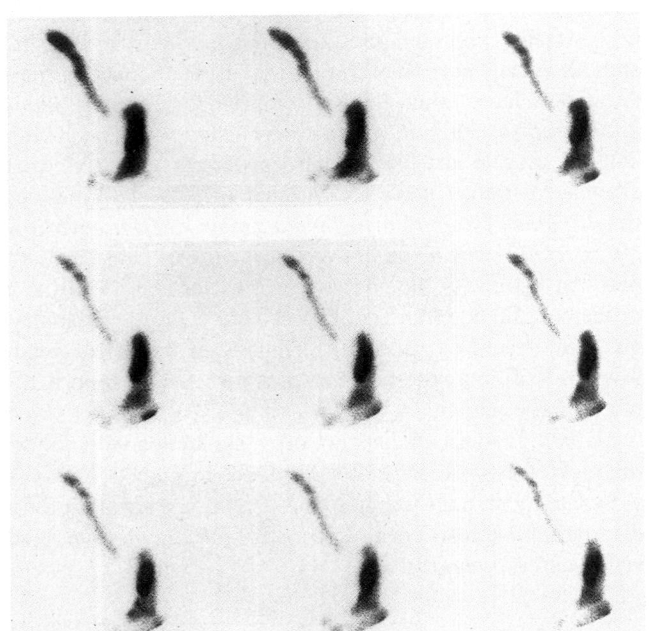

B

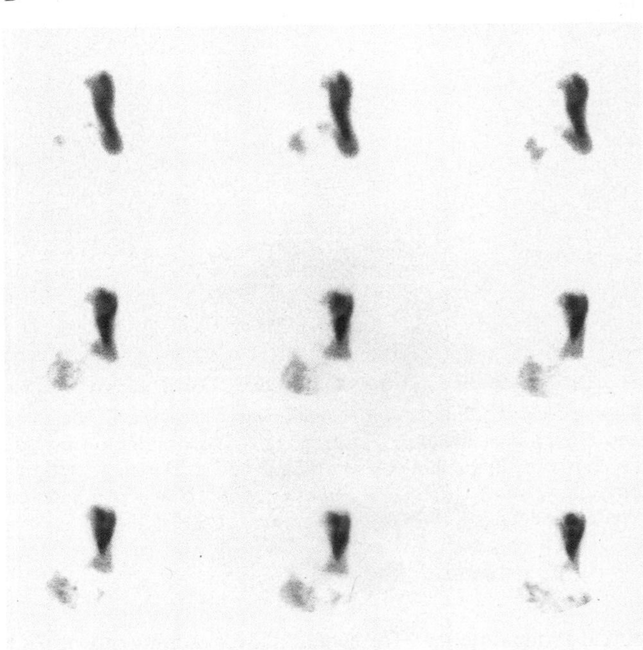

Figure 8 A,B. Serial images of esophageal transit in a patient with achalasia pre- and postesophageal dilitation; **(A).** The pretherapy study shows significantly delayed esophageal clearance during the 30-minute study; **(B).** The posttherapy repeat study shows essentially normal esophageal clearance. No esophageal retention is seen.

Table 4. Pathophysiological Factors Associated with GERD

1. Reduced LES pressure or inappropriate relaxation
2. Defective esophageal clearance mechanisms (peristalsis, saliva)
3. Increased gastric secretion (acid, pepsin)
4. Delayed gastric emptying
5. Impaired esophageal epithelial resistance
6. Hiatal hernia

sliding hiatus hernia; however, the majority of individuals with a hiatus hernia do not have GERD.

Clinical Presentation and Complications

Heartburn is the most common clinical complaint. Other symptoms include chest pain, regurgitation, and sour breath. Regurgitation and aspiration may cause respiratory symptoms of asthma and recurrent pneumonia. Other serious complications of GERD include stricture, bleeding, and perforation. Dysphagia is usually a symptom of stricture. A peculiar reparative process occurs in some patients, whereby squamous epithelium of the esophagus is replaced by metaplastic columnar-type epithelium, *Barrett's esophagus*. This entity is important because it is associated with a 10% incidence of adenocarcinoma. The symptoms of GER in infants and children differ considerably from those in adults. In addition to excessive regurgitation, the predominant symptoms are respiratory distress, iron deficiency anemia, and failure to thrive.

Diagnostic Tests for GER

A variety of tests have been used to diagnose GERD. *Barium esophagography* can detect severe grades of reflux, mucosal damage, strictures, and tumors; however, it has a low overall sensitivity for detecting GERD. This is not surprising because the morphological changes of esophagitis are difficult to detect even at endoscopy without the benefit of biopsy. It also has a high false-positive rate if hiatus hernia is used as a diagnostic criteria. *Endoscopy* is commonly used, provides a direct view of the esophageal mucosa, and allows biopsy. The *Bernstein acid infusion test* attempts to reproduce the patient's symptoms and confirm their esophageal origin by infusing 0.1 N hydrochloric acid into the distal esophagus. *Esophageal manometry* can produce a quantitative assessment of esophageal body motor function in response to swallowing and acid infusion. A subset of patients with reflux disease have abnormal peristalsis, which is reported to be as high as 50% in patients with moderate to severe esophagitis. Manometry can also assess LES pressure, but this can not discriminate between patients with reflux disease and normal controls.

The *Tuttle acid reflux test* requires that a pH electrode be positioned in the distal esophagus 5 cm above the LES. An abrupt drop of esophageal pH to less than 4.0 is associated with GER (Fig. 9). Proper placement is a critical factor in correct interpretation of this test. This study is performed during basal conditions and after acid loading. To detect recurrent events requires clearance of the previous acid reflux event. Although false-negatives and false-positives occur, it is generally considered the "gold standard" for diagnosis of GER. A test increasingly used is *extended* (12 to 24

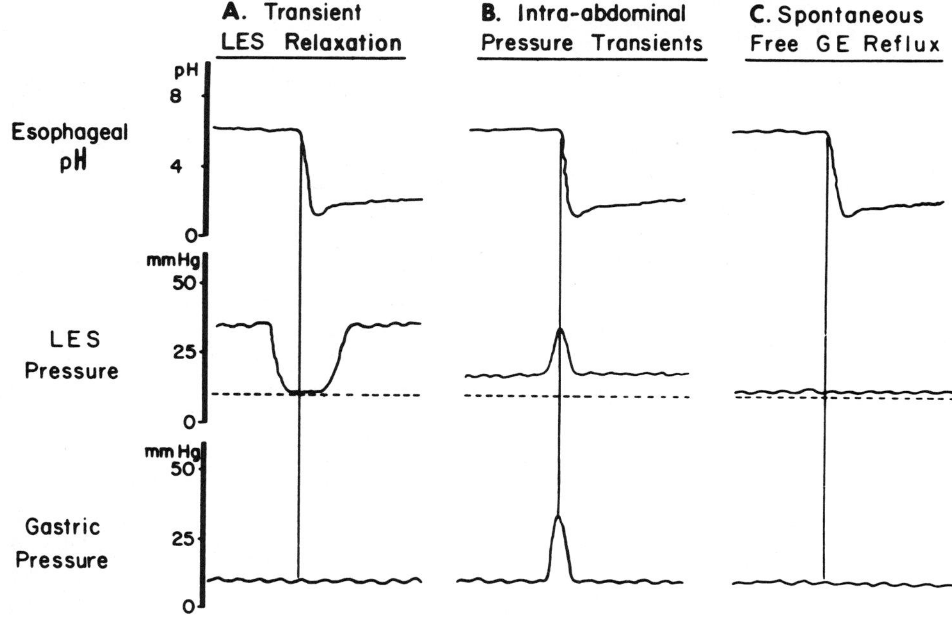

Figure 9. Schematic representation of 3 different mechanisms for gastroesophageal (GE) reflux. GE reflux events (shown as vertical lines) may accompany a transient lower esophageal sphincter (LES) relaxation **(A)**, develop as stress reflux during a transient increase in intra-abdominal pressure that overcomes LES resistance **(B)**, or occur as spontaneous reflux across an atonic sphincter **(C).** (With permission, Dodds WJ, Dent J, Hogan WJ, et al.: Mechanisms of gastroesophageal reflux in patients with reflux esophagitis. *N Engl J Med* 1982;307:1547–1552.)

Table 5. Sensitivity of GER Scintigraphy in Adults

REFERENCE	SENSITIVITY (%)			
	Scintigraphy	*Acid Reflux*	*Radiography*	*Endoscopy*
Fisher[50]	27/30 (90%)	30/30 (100%)	15/30 (50%)	14/30 (47%)
Kaul[51]	59/69 (86%)	48/69 (70%)	19/69 (28%)	69/69 (100%)
Velasco[52]	40/54 (74%)	38/49 (78%)	20/53 (38%)	–
Styles[53]	12/17 (71%)	–	–	17/17 (100%)
Fung[54]	7/48 (15%)	–	–	48/48 (100%)
Hoffman[57]	4/29 (14%)	4/29 (14%)	18/29 (62%)	20/29 (69%)
Jenkins[41]	9/15 (60%)	–	–	15/15 (100%)

hour) *pH monitoring*. It is typically performed in a symptomatic patient without evidence of esophagitis by esophagography or endoscopy. Continuous pH monitoring is now possible while the patient continues his normal daily activities.

Of these diagnostic procedures, barium studies and the acid reflux tests provide direct evidence of GER, and manometry, esophagoscopy, and biopsy only suggest reflux indirectly. Esophageal pH monitoring is simple in principle, but fraught with technical problems.

Radionuclide Investigation of GER

Radionuclide GER scintigraphy has a number of potential advantages over the other diagnostic procedures discussed. It is more physiological, easily performed, well tolerated by the patient, and quantitative. The radiation exposure is considerably lower than that associated with other radiographic procedures commonly used to evaluate the esophagus (Table 3 A,B). Despite these advantages, radionuclide studies do not play a major role in the evaluation of most adult GER patients. One reason for this seems to be a perception by the gastroenterology community that radionuclide scintigraphy has a poor sensitivity for detecting GERD.[46] Although its sensitivity has been reported to be as high as 90%, other studies have found it to be considerably poorer, 14 to 78% (Table 5). Some recent reviews of GER either do not even mention it as a diagnostic option[47], describe radionuclide methods as "obsolete and replaced by pH monitoring"[48], reserve its role for a subgroup of select patients (e.g., those with alkaline reflux or atrophic gastritis), or use it solely for investigational purposes.[45] An important reason seems to be the existence of many competing modalities performed by the gastroenterologist. In contrast, pediatricians seem to believe that scintigraphy is very useful for evaluating GER in children.[1,45,49] It is interesting to note that the accuracy in adults and children appears to be quite similar (Tables 5, 6).

ADULT RADIONUCLIDE GER STUDIES

Much of the original adult investigation and validation of adult GER scintigraphy was performed at Temple University.[50] Several reviews have updated their results.[61–64] Initially, they studied 30 patients with symptoms of GER and a positive acid-reflux test. Scintigraphy was found to have a sensitivity of 90% for detecting GER, better than the other methods used, for example, hiatal hernia seen on radiography (60%), fluoroscopic reflux (50%), LES pressure ≤ 15 mmHg (77%), acid perfusion test (63%), histological esophagitis (47%) and endoscopic esophagitis (40%). They have now studied over 1000 patients and report an overall sensitivity of 88 to 91%.[64]

Their scintigraphic method is as follows; after an overnight fast, the patient drinks a solution containing 150 mL of orange juice, 150 mL of 0.1 N HCl, and 300 μCi ^{99m}Tc-SC. In the upright position, a 30-second image is obtained to ensure that the solution transits the esophagus. If not, the patient is given 30 mL of water to clear any residual esophageal activity. The patient is then placed supine under a scintillation camera interfaced with a computer. A valsalva is performed and an image acquired. An abdominal binder is then placed below the rib cage and attached to a sphygmomanometer to increase the pressure in 20 mmHg increments from 0 to 100 mmHg. Timed 30-second images are obtained at each pressure gradient. Total study time is less than 5 minutes.

GER is calculated at each pressure step using the formula: $R = (E_t - E_b) \times 100/G_o$ where R = %GEF index, E_t = esophageal counts at time t, E_b = esophageal background counts, and G_o = gastric counts at the beginning of the study. Activity above the gastroesophageal junction is interpreted as reflux. In the Temple University experience, the mean reflux index for symptomatic patients was 11.7 ± 1.8% compared to 2.7 ± 0.3% for the 20 normal controls ($p < .001$). The upper limit of normal used was 4%, although two of the controls had GER greater than 4%.

Others have used similar methods. Kaul et al.[51] studied 69 adults with GER symptoms and endoscopic esophagitis. The sensitivity for scintigraphy was 86%, significantly higher than 70% for intraesophageal pH measurements, and 28% for contrast esophagography. The severity of esophagitis correlated with positive GER scintigraphy. Spontaneous reflux was greatly increased by the presence of acid. Two of 22 normal controls had a positive study. A follow-up study by these investigators compared esophageal biopsy

Table 6. Sensitivity and Specificity of GER Scintigraphy in Children

AUTHOR	#PTS	SENS	SPEC	ACQUISITION PARAMETERS	GOLD STANDARD
Rudd[56]	25	80%	–	30-s images 25 to 100 mm Hg abdominal binder	acid reflux test Ba radiography pH probe
Heyman[57]	39	88%	–	1 min frames × 60	Ba radiography
Blumhagen[58]	65	75%	71%	30-s frames × 30–60 min; manual pressure intermittently	acid reflux test Ba radiography
Arasu[59]		57%	100%	1-min images for unstated time	acid reflux (Tuttle)
Seibert[60]	49	79%	93%	30-s frames × 1 hr	24-hr pH probe

with GER scintigraphy in 101 patients with symptoms strongly suggestive of GERD.[65] Scintigraphy was positive in 86%, endoscopy in 58%, and histological esophagitis was present in 58%. They concluded that scintigraphy is of particular value in patients in whom endoscopy and histology cannot confirm the presence of suspected GERD.

In contrast, Hoffman et al.,[55] using a similar method, were able to identify GER in only 4 of 29 patients who showed other evidence of reflux by either fluoroscopically monitored barium swallow, esophagogastroscopy, or esophageal biopsy. Interestingly, the pH reflux study had a similar low sensitivity. They concluded that both tests were too insensitive to be of value in the diagnosis of GERD. Fung et al.[54] studying 51 subjects who presented with heartburn and endoscopic evidence of reflux esophagitis, had similarly disappointing results. The scintigraphic sensitivity for reflux was only 17% with moderate and 11% with severe esophagitis.

Styles et al.[53] studied 32 patients with symptoms of GER and 15 healthy volunteers. The sensitivity of reflux scintigraphy as determined by esophageal histology was 70% and its specificity, 87%. They concluded that GER scintigraphy was unsuitable as a single screening test. Other studies have been equally unenthusiastic about the sensitivity (70 to 78%) of GER scintigraphy.[46,53,66,67]

Velasco et al.[52] described a modification of the previously described method that did not require the use of an abdominal binder and allowed recognition of both reflux episodes and clearance rates. They studied 54 patients with symptoms of GER, 26 were classified as moderate and 28 as severe reflux, and compared the results of scintigraphy with radiographic studies, manometry, and pH probe studies. Continuous acquisition, 5-second frames for 7 minutes, then 10-second valsalva maneuvers every 30 seconds for 2 minutes, were acquired on a computer. Scintigraphy was positive in 74% (62% with moderate reflux and 85% with severe reflux). The results were found to be more sensitive than radiography and approximately equal to pH testing. They felt that their sensitivity was similar to Fisher et al.[50] because the patients in that study all had pH-proven reflux, comparable to their "severe" group.

In an interesting study, Shay et al.[68] performed simultaneous pH monitoring and continuous scintigraphy (5-frame) for 40 minutes in 9 patients with histologically proven severe reflex esophagitis. Scintigraphy detected 61% of all events as opposed to 16% for pH monitoring. The two techniques detected the same events in only 23% of 218 reflex events. GER scintigraphy detected more reflux events during the first 20 minutes, and pH monitoring detected more events during the second 20 minutes. The reflux episodes detected by scintigraphy, but not pH monitoring, usually occurred while the intraesophageal pH was <4 (Fig. 10). This highlights the fact that these techniques measure different components of refluxate (i.e., volume vs. acid concentration) and are influenced by different physiological events, such as ingestion of a meal, gastric emptying, and esophageal acid clearance.

In summary, when scintigraphy has been compared to short-term pH probe monitoring, considered the "gold standard," it has been shown to be quite sensitive,[50–52] certainly more sensitive than the only other technique that directly measures reflux, radiography with fluoroscopy. The poor results in some studies[54,55] distort the overall results (Table 5). The reasons for this are unclear although, in one of these studies, pH monitoring curiously had a similar low sensitivity.[55] Esophagitis has been used as the "gold standard" in some of the latter studies; however, esophagitis is only found in 40% of patients with symptoms of GER. The presence of esophagitis may be more a function of other factors (e.g., the potency of refluxate, delayed clearance, esophageal dysmotility, etc). Because up to 50% of patients with esophagitis exhibit some impairment of esophageal peristalsis,[69] the additional information available from a radionuclide esophageal transit study may be clinically valuable as an adjunct to the GER study.

PEDIATRIC GER STUDIES

Radionuclide GER studies play a much more important clinical role in pediatrics. This is probably due to pediatrician's preference for non-invasive procedures and the difficulties involved in performing invasive and technically demanding studies in children.

Pediatric GER is most common in infants 6 to 9 months

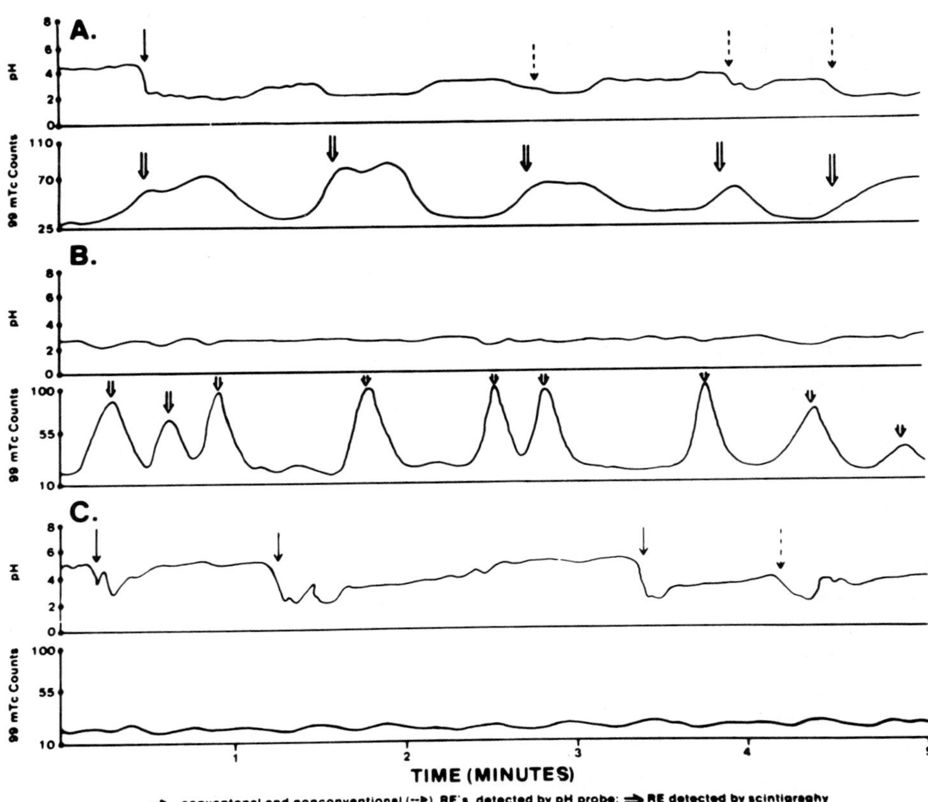

Figure 10. Comparison of reflux events detected by an intra-esophageal pH probe and scintigraphic monitoring in 3 patients **(A,B,C).** The tracing from patient **(A)** obtained during the initial 20 mins shows 4 reflux events simultaneously detected by the pH probe and scintigraphy. One reflux event is detected only by scintigraphy (second from left). Only one of four reflux events detected by the pH probe met the pH probe conventional criteria for gastroesophageal reflux (solid arrow). On the tracing from patient **(B)**, also obtained during the first 20 mins, 9 reflux events met the scintigraphic criteria at a time when the esophageal pH was <4 due to a previous reflux event (not shown). On the tracing from patient **(C)** obtained during the second 20-min interval, 4 reflux events were detected by the pH probe at a time when no scintigraphic reflux event was observed. (With permission, Shay SS, Eggli D, Johnson LF: Spontaneous esophageal pH monitoring and scintigraphy during the postprandial period in patients with severe reflux esophagitis. *Dig Dis Sci* 1991;36:558–564.[68])

of age. It usually becomes apparent by the age of 2 months but, in the majority, is self-limited, resolving spontaneously by the end of infancy. Approximately a third have persistent symptoms until 4 years of age. A smaller percentage develop significant sequelae, for example, strictures (5%) and even death (5%) due to inanition or recurrent pneumonia.[70] Older children have a much lower incidence of reflux and more closely resemble the adult population. Since small amounts of GER occur as a normal physiological event, the clinician must pinpoint those with significant reflux that require intensive therapy.

GER has been implicated as a cause of recurrent respiratory infections, asthma, failure to thrive, esophagitis, esophageal stricture, chronic blood loss, and the sudden infant death syndrome. Symptoms and signs of GER in children include chronic nocturnal cough, poor weight gain, vomiting, aspiration or choking, asthmatic episodes, stridor, and apnea. As in adults, a variety of diagnostic methods have been used, with the 24-hour pH probe being the "gold standard."

Methodology. The radionuclide method involves feeding the infant a meal that approximates its normal feeding, usually formula or milk, although juice has been used, with 4 to 40 MBq ^{99m}Tc-SC as the radiomarker. A concentration of 200 kBq/mL has been recommended for optimum imaging.[57] After the infant burps, the patient is placed supine, with the scintillation camera positioned either anteriorly[57,71] or posteriorly[60,72] and the chest and upper abdomen in the field of view. Abdominal compression is not usually used because it is considered "nonphysiological"; it is poorly tolerated in infants, and there is evidence that it does not increase the detection rate for reflux.[58,73] Data is acquired on computer and the study lasts 60 to 120 minutes.[71,74] An acquisition time of 60 minutes compared to 30 minutes has been shown to increase the detection rate for GER by 25%.[75] The framing rate used has varied from 20 to 60 seconds/frame to 5 to 10 seconds/frame. Shorter time intervals seem to increase the sensitivity of the test and allow a better estimate of the frequency of reflux and esophageal clearance following each episode.

All images should be reviewed frame by frame with contrast enhancement and/or by cinematic display (Fig. 11 **A,B**). Quantitation may also be helpful. Reflux events are graded as low or high level, by duration (e.g., less or greater than 10 seconds), and by their temporal relationship to meal ingestion. Longer reflux events increase the risk of esophagitis; events with smaller gastric volumes may have more clinical significance because reflux is occurring without the increased pressure effect of a full meal volume and lack of an acid buffering effect. Evidence of pulmonary aspiration is sought in the dynamic study, although infrequently found. For maximum sensitivity, static high count images are obtained at 1 and 2 to 4 hours, and sometimes the next morning (Table 7).

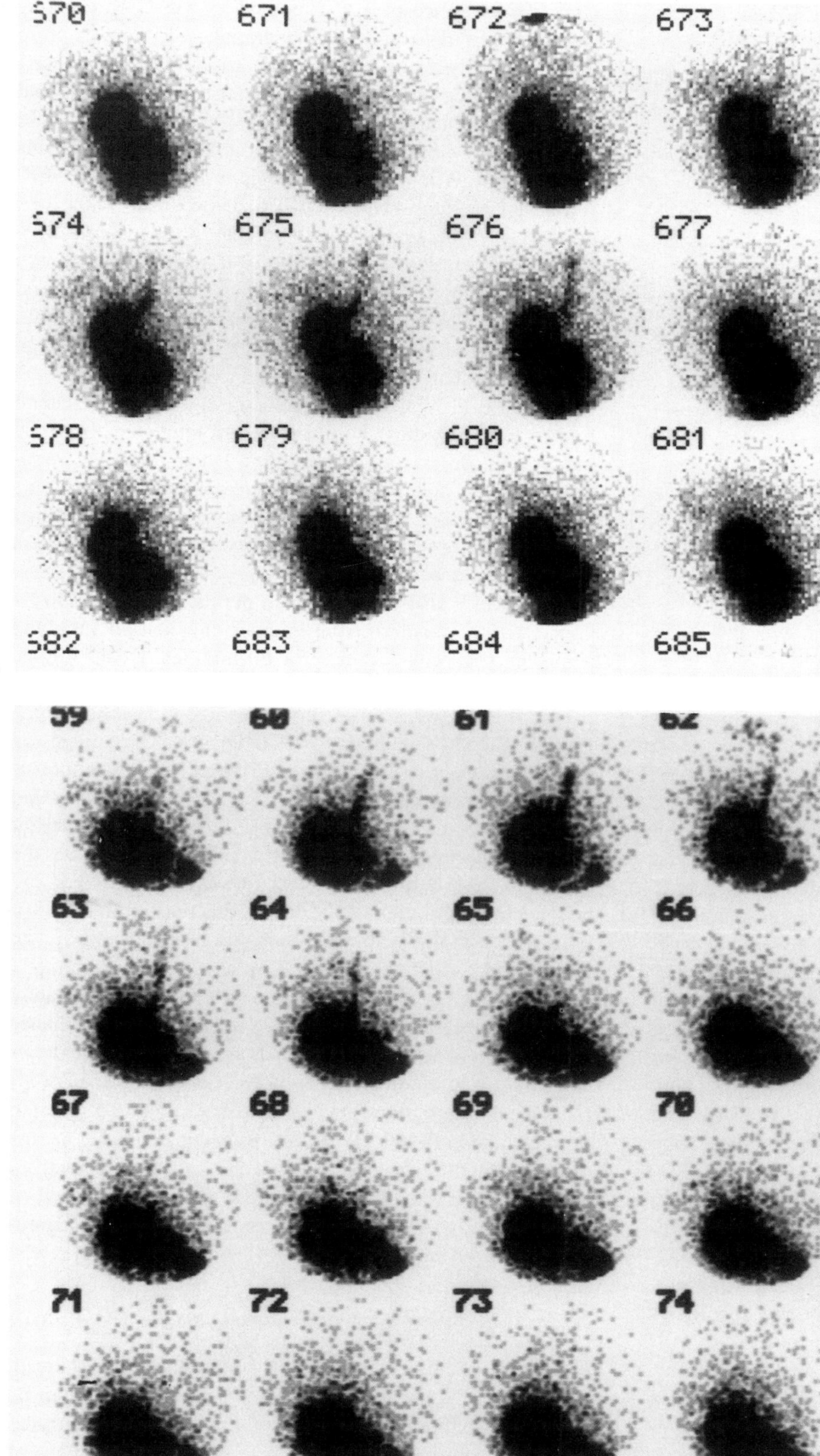

Figure 11 A,B. Gastroesophageal Reflux; five-second frames for 1 hour. Review of the individual frames demonstrates episodes of high level reflux of >10 s duration in 2 different patients **(A** and **B).**

Table 7. Detection of Aspiration in Children

	SENSITIVITY	DELAYED IMAGE TIME
Heyman[57]	2/29 (6.9%)	2 hrs
Arasu[59]	0/30 (0%)	4 and 24 hrs
Blumhagen[58]	0/10 (0%)	2 hrs
Boonyaprapa[76]	5/20 (25%)	5 min, 4 hours, and overnite AM images
Jona[77]	18/125 (14%)	8–24 hrs
Piepsz[75]	0/35 (0%)	4 hours
MacFayden[78]	3/9 (33%)	6 hours
Berger[79]	3/18 (17%)	12–24 hours
McVeagh[80]	23/120 (19%)	2 hrs and AM

An esophageal transit study can be performed either before[74] or after[71] the reflux study. In addition to diagnosing an associated motility disorder, the "salivagram" can detect pulmonary aspiration often when the GER study is negative[81] (Fig. 12 **A,B**). ^{99m}Tc-SC (250 μCi) in 10 to 15 mL sterile water is given in bolus form via a feeding tube placed in the posterior pharynx. Once the transit study is performed, the remainder of the meal can be fed for volume. Esophageal transit, reflux, and gastric emptying can all be quantitated.

Clinical Studies

Rudd et al.[56] studied 25 infants and children with recurrent symptoms of GER. Using a method similar to that used in adults with an abdominal binder, reflux was demonstrated in 20 patients (80%) who had a positive acid reflux test.

Heyman et al.[57] reported a new scintigraphic technique for detecting GER in 48 children. After ingestion of a normal milk feeding with ^{99m}Tc-SC, images were obtained on computer at a rate of 1 frame/minute for 60 minutes. Computer processing and calculation of GER and gastric emptying were performed. Radiographic studies were available for comparison in 39 patients. There was agreement in 20, both showing reflux in 7 (18%) and no reflux in 13 (33%). The radionuclide study was positive in 59%, barium radiography was positive in 26%.

Blumhagen et al.[58] used the acid reflux test as the standard for evaluating 65 infants and children with GER scintigraphy. After ingesting labeled apple juice, the study was acquired continuously (30 seconds/frame) for 30 to 60 minutes. The overall sensitivity for GER was 75% and specificity was 71%.

Arasu et al.[59] prospectively evaluated GER scintigraphy. After distending the stomach with saline (^{99m}Tc-SC) via a nasogastric tube, serial one-minute gamma camera images were obtained with the patient in the upright and supine positions, with and without manual abdominal pressure. Demonstration of esophageal activity was considered indicative of GER. Compared with the acid reflux test, the sensitivity of scintigraphy was 55%, radiography 52%, and endoscopy 70%. In retrospect, the method for GER scintigraphy was probably inadequate. Saline empties very rapidly from the stomach compared to formula or milk, and the long acquisition times and lack of computer enhancement would all tend to reduce sensitivity.

Jona et al.[77] performed GER scintigraphy on 125 infants and children with symptoms and signs suggestive of GER. A normal feeding volume of 5% dextrose in water was inserted into the stomach with a feeding tube. Serial one-minute images were obtained for 30 minutes. If reflux was not demonstrated, the patient was placed in the left lateral position for 10 minutes. GER was demonstrated in 96 (77%), 18 had pulmonary aspiration, and 38 (41%) had reflux on barium examination; none aspirated.

Seibert et al.[60] compared GER scintigraphy (30-second frames × 60 minutes) with 24-hour continuous pH probe monitoring. All patients with positive 1-hour pH probe monitoring also had positive scintigraphy. Four additional patients that were positive only with the 24-hour pH probe test had negative scintigraphy. The sensitivity for scintigraphy was 79% and the specificity 93%.

Tolia et al.[82] also used extended pH monitoring (16 to 24 hour) as the standard. Scintigraphic acquisition involved acquiring 60-second frames for 60 minutes. Of 69 infants younger than 1 year of age; 482 showed reflux by extended pH monitoring, whereas 46 showed reflux with scintigraphy. However, the two methods correlated poorly. They suggested that the two techniques were measuring different pathophysiological phenomena, that the tests are complementary and should not be used interchangeably. It is likely that infant formula temporarily buffers gastric contents and reduces the ability of the pH probe to detect reflux, whereas GER can be detected scintigraphically during this period. In contrast, GER scintigraphy is likely to become less sensitive as the labeled meal empties from the stomach.

In summary, it is generally agreed that GER scintigraphy is a valuable and clinically useful technique for pediatric patients. Rapid acquisition methods are more sensitive; however, the exact cutoff between normal and abnormal in infants is uncertain. Increased significance should be given to frequent and high-level GER, reflux as the stomach contents diminish, and associated delayed clearance or a motility disorder. A radionuclide transit study performed as part of the same study can both evaluate motility and detect aspiration with high sensitivity.

ANALYSIS OF GER STUDIES

All images of the dynamic GER study should be reviewed. Cine display is often helpful. Time-activity curves can be generated from regions of interest drawn for the oropharynx, esophagus, and stomach. GER is seen as distinct spikes of activity into the esophagus (Fig. 10). The time-activity curves should be evaluated in conjunction with the images because patient movement may result in gastric activity appearing in the esophageal region. Some do not consider

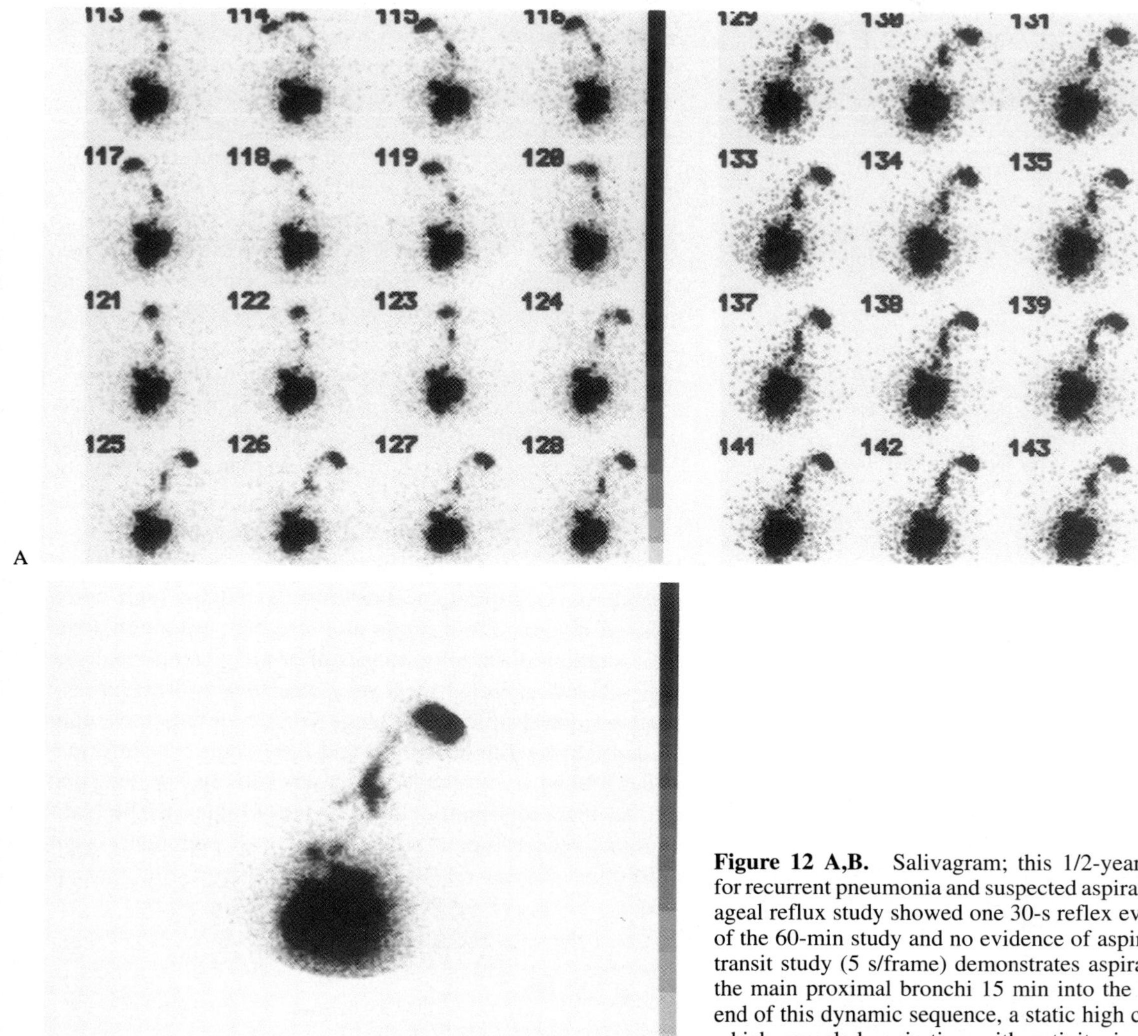

Figure 12 A,B. Salivagram; this 1/2-year-old patient was studied for recurrent pneumonia and suspected aspiration. A prior gastroesophageal reflux study showed one 30-s reflex event during the first 5 min of the 60-min study and no evidence of aspiration. **(A).** This dynamic transit study (5 s/frame) demonstrates aspiration with tracer entering the main proximal bronchi 15 min into the transit study; **(B).** At the end of this dynamic sequence, a static high count image was acquired which revealed aspiration with activity in the right and left upper bronchi and left lower lobe. (Courtesy of Kenneth Levin, MD).

episodes of GER in the first 5 minutes to be abnormal unless prolonged,[74,75] while others believe that all episodes are abnormal.[71]

A variety of quantitative indices used in adult populations may also be useful for pediatric studies (Table 8). Devos et al.[83] modified the method of Fisher et al.,[50] expressing the mean value of the esophageal time-activity curve as a percentage of the initial gastric activity. A significant difference was found between normal people (0.66 ± 0.12%) and those with peptic esophagitis (3.66 ± 0.81%). Heyman et al.[57] derived a reflux index by integrating the esophageal time-activity curve over 60 minutes and dividing this by the initial gastric activity. In patients judged to have significant reflux by 24-hour pH probe monitoring, an initial assessment showed the index to be 2.3 ± 1.1 compared to 0.9 ± 0.3 in those without reflux. Piepsz et al.[84] determined the percent activity in a specific episode relative to the gastric activity at that time, multiplied by the duration of the episode in multiples of 20 seconds. The resultant values were summed for the 60-minute study. Peaks greater than 5% generally corresponded to reflux. The index was not predictive of esophagitis. Blumhagen et al.[58] graded the severity of reflux by the number of episodes.

The gastric emptying portion of the study can be quantified by drawing a region of interest around the stomach and generating a time-activity curve; then, after correction for physical decay, emptying can be expressed as the time required to reach one half emptying or, as is more commonly done, the percent of initial activity remaining at 1 and 2 hours can be calculated. Normal asymptomatic children have not been studied. However, Heyman[74] states that, in his experience, the normal residual of milk feedings appears to be 50 to 75% of the initial value after 1 hour. Others use normal values of 40 to 50% emptying at 1 hour and 60 to

Table 8. Techniques for Quantifying Reflux

STUDY	TECHNIQUE	INDEX*
Fisher	30-s images with increasing abdominal pressure	C_e–C_b%/G
Devos[83]	30-min study	Mean of esoph TAC%/G
Blumhagen[58]	30-s images 30–60 min study	Number of episodes (1–2 in 0–5 min)
Piepz[75]	20-s images 60-min study	$\frac{\Sigma\, C_e\% \times d}{G}$
Heyman[74]	3-s images 60-min study	Number of episodes delayed clearance $\int C_e/G$

*Abbreviations: C_e, esophageal activity; C_b, background; G, gastric activity. Modified, with permission, from Heyman S: Pediatric nuclear gastroenterology: evaluation of gastroeosophageal reflux and gastrointestinal bleeding, in Freeman LM, Weissman HS (eds.): New York, Raven Press, 1985.[74]

75% at 2 hours.[71] Emptying in preterm infants is more rapid. Infant formula empties with a half-time of 52 ± 9 minutes, compared to human milk (25 ± 12 minutes). Human milk empties more rapidly in older infants, with a half-time of 48 ± 15 minutes, compared to 78 ± 16 for formula feedings.[85,86]

Gelfand et al.[87] recently pointed out that it is not uncommon for the 1-hour gastric emptying to appear delayed, but at 2 hours emptying has significantly improved. They recommend the latter time interval as a better indicator for separating normal from abnormal.

Relationship Between Gastric Emptying and GER

An increased incidence of a delayed gastric emptying has been reported in patients with GER; however, the data is conflicting. In adults, McCallum et al.[88] described delayed solid gastric emptying in 41% of 100 patients with a positive Bernstein test and endoscopic or histological evidence of esophagitis. The mean percent emptying was 52% ± 8% compared to 65 ± 21% for 26 healthy controls ($p < 0.05$). Maddern et al.[89] studied 72 patients with symptomatic GER and a positive acid reflux test or endoscopy; 44% had delayed solid and 37% had delayed liquid emptying. A significant difference was found between normal controls and patients with GER ($p < 0.01$). In contrast, Shay et al.[90] studied 33 patients with symptoms of GER, a positive Bernstein test, and 24-hour pH testing. They found no significant difference in the gastric emptying rate between those patients with and without endoscopic esophagitis compared to 15 normal controls. Another study by Johnson et al.[91] found delayed solid gastric emptying in only 2 of 17 patients with a history of severe reflux and Barrett's esophagus. Therefore, the role of delayed gastric emptying in the pathophysiology of adult GER is uncertain and controversial.

There is similar conflicting data on the relationship between GER and gastric emptying in pediatric patients with GER. Hillemeier et al.[92] found gastric emptying (cow milk formula meal) to be significantly less in 13 infants with severe reflux and recurrent pulmonary disease or failure to thrive (mean 20%), compared to 10 infants with mild disease (mean 44%) ($p < 0.05$). They postulated that abnormal gastric function may be a factor in the pathogenesis of gastroesophageal reflux of infancy. However, Rosen et al.[93] found no significant difference in gastric emptying between 126 infants and children with and without GER. DiLorenzeo et al.,[94] in a study of 477 infants and children, found no difference in gastric emptying in children under 3 years of age, regardless of the presence or absence of GER. However, in children over 6 years, gastric emptying was delayed in those with reflux. Tolia et al.[68] found no significant correlation between GER diagnosed by extended pH monitoring and gastric emptying in 69 infants less than 12 months old.

Pulmonary Aspiration

Delayed images are routinely obtained to search for evidence of pulmonary aspiration. Best results require high count delayed images 2 to 4 hours after feeding. Although some have suggested morning images after an evening meal, the radiolabeled aspirated meal may clear due to its relatively short residence time in the lung. Several authors have concluded that overnight images add little additional information.[80,95] Most studies have shown a relatively low detection rate for the 2 to 4-hour delayed images (Table 7). The "salivagram" seems to be a better indicator of pulmonary aspiration.[81]

GASTRIC EMPTYING

Background

Radionuclide gastric emptying studies allow the noninvasive evaluation of the transit of a physiological meal through the

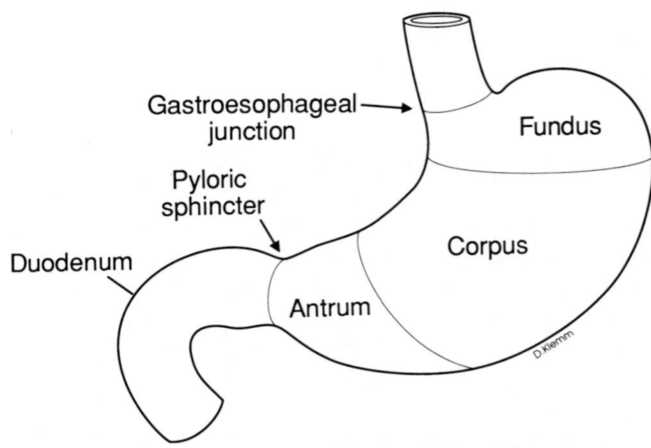

Figure 13. Gastric anatomy and function. The proximal stomach (fundus) accomodates and stores food; the distal stomach (antrum) acts as a preparatory chamber where mixing and grinding of food occurs.

stomach. In the past, a variety of non-isotopic techniques have been used for measuring gastric emptying. Gastric intubation methods with serial aspiration and marker-dilution techniques with duodenal recovery are cumbersome, disliked by patients, and the tubing itself can alter emptying. Radiographic methods can define anatomy and diagnose mechanical obstruction, but are insensitive to motor disturbances of the stomach and cannot provide quantitative information on gastric emptying. Radionuclide studies are, by their nature, quantitative and are the most sensitive method for detecting gastric stasis. The first radionuclide gastric emptying study was performed in 1966 by Griffith et al. who used an external scintillation detector to detect ^{57}Cr markers instilled in the stomach.[96]

Anatomy and Physiology of the Stomach

From the viewpoint of gastric physiology, the stomach is composed of two functionally distinct regions (Fig. 13). The proximal stomach (fundus) can accept large volumes of fluid with only minimally increased pressure. This property of receptive relaxation and accomodation occurs by the way of the vagus nerve and is impaired after vagotomy. Regular slow tonic muscular contractions in the proximal stomach produce a pressure gradient between the stomach and duodenum, moving the stomach contents toward the more distal stomach (Fig. 14). The emptying of liquids is largely due to this fundal mechanism, which is volume dependent; that is, the larger the volume the more rapid the emptying (exponential emptying) (Fig. 15). Nutrients, salts, and acidity all tend to slow liquid emptying.

While the proximal stomach acts mainly as a reservoir, the antrum plays an active role in grinding and regulating the emptying of solid food. Muscular contractions of the antrum sweep down in a ring-like pattern after ingestion of solid food, squeezing the food toward the pylorus. Large food particles are not allowed to pass, but are retropelled toward the gastric antrum and become progressively ground up and mixed, until finally this chyme mixture (particle size <1 to 2 mm) is able to pass through the pylorus. After an initial delay before emptying (lag phase), solids typically empty linearly (Fig. 16) and the rate of emptying depends to a large extent on the meal content (Table 9). Inhibitory receptors for fat, acid, amino acids, and osmolality located in the duodenum and jejunum all act to slow gastric emptying of solids.

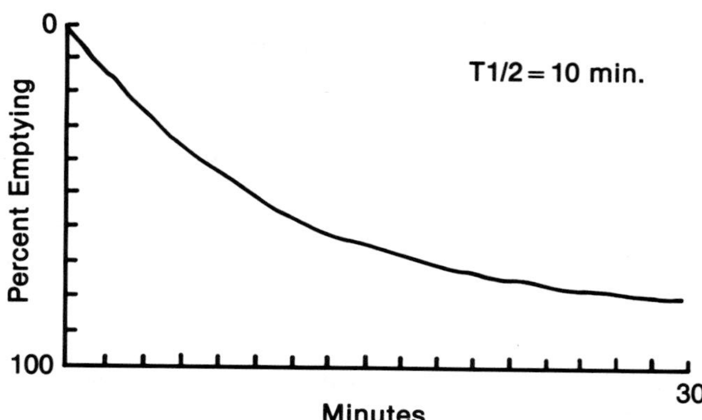

Figure 15. Normal liquid-only time-activity curve; the ingested water with ^{99m}Tc as a marker empties rapidly and monoexponentially.

In the fasting state, "phase-III interdigestive contractions" empty nondigestible debris from the stomach.[97] These contractions are forceful lumen-obliterating peristaltic waves that sweep down the gastric contents through the open pylorus. Motilin, a peptide hormone secreted by the mocosa of the upper small bowel, is responsible for producing this interdigestive motility pattern.[98]

Although isolated antral motility disorders that result in gastric stasis of solids, but not liquids, are well recognized, there is no known clinical entity that produces isolated liquid retention. In severe cases of gastroparesis, both liquid and solid emptying may be delayed. After partial gastric resection or Billroth anastomoses with or without vagotomy, emptying of liquids and solids may both be more rapid than normal ("dumping syndrome"), although a subgroup of patients have slow solid emptying due to an atonic antrum.[99,100]

Gastric function is controlled by both neural and hormonal

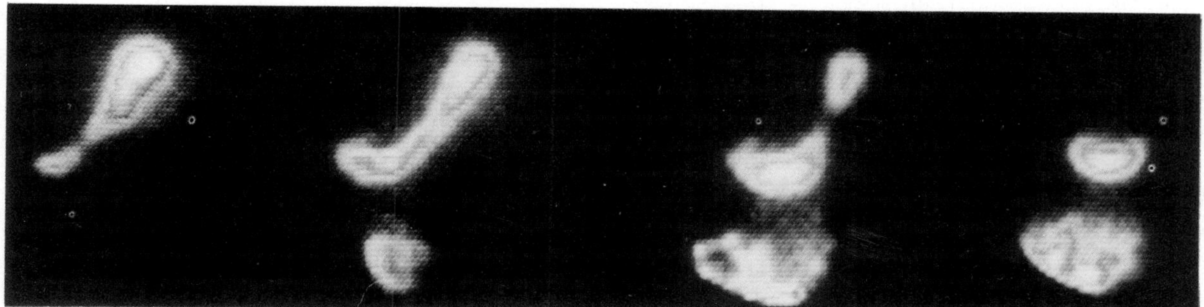

Figure 14. Normal movement of stomach contents during a solid radionuclide gastric emptying study. Four selected images, the first immediately after ingestion, and then one every 15 min (15, 30, 45 min). The labeled meal can be seen to pass from the proximal fundus to the more distal antrum.

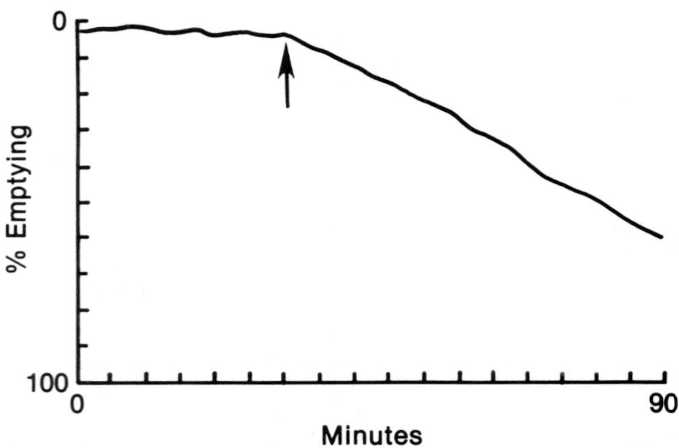

Figure 16. Solid emptying time-activity curve. The ^{99m}Tc-labeled egg sandwich must be broken down into small particles that can pass through the pylorus. The time required is represented on the emptying curve as a lag phase (arrow), followed by a linear pattern of emptying.

Table 9. Gastric Emptying

A. Rate of gastric emptying depends on meal composition
  Fastest to slowest:
    Water
    Clear liquids with nutrients (orange juice)
    Full liquids with nutrients (Ensure)
    Semisolids (eggs, oatmeal)
    Solids (meat)
B. Meal composition effect on gastric emptying
  Emptying half-time increases with increasing:
    Volume
    Weight
    Caloric density
    Particle size
    Fat content
    Fatty acid chain length
    Amino acid concentration
    Osmolality
    Acidity
C. Other factors affecting the rate of gastric emptying
  Time of day
  Metabolic state
  Position, e.g. standing, sitting, supine
  Gender
  Stress
  Medications, drugs
  Alcohol, cigarettes
  Hormones
    Secretin
    Gastric inhibitory peptide
    Motilin
    Vasoactive intestinal peptide
    Neurotensin
    Glucagon
    Serotonin
    Somatostatin
    Cholecystokinin

mechanisms. Vagal and sympathetic inervation of the stomach have long been appreciated. The proximal one third of the stomach is electrically silent. However, the distal two thirds undergoes repeated electrical discharges from a pacemaker located in the greater curvature of the midcorpus, which generates the rhythmic gastric slow waves and occasional intense phasic contractions after ingestion of food. Many hormones are known to affect gastric function (Table 9). The interaction between neural and hormonal factors is complex and incompletely understood.

Gastric Stasis Syndromes

Patients with delayed gastric emptying often have *symptoms* of early satiety, bloating, nausea and, occasionally, vomiting. Symptomatic gastroparesis may occur in the acute or chronic clinical setting due to several causes (Table 10). For example, delayed emptying may occur acutely with viral gastroenteritis, postoperatively, or due to metabolic derangements, such as hyperglycemia and hypokalemia. *Mechanical* obstruction (e.g., due to tumor or peptic ulcer disease) must be excluded with endoscopy or a contrast barium study. Chronic *functional* gastric paresis has been associated with a large number of diseases. Some are of metabolic origin (diabetes, hypothyroidism, uremia), others neurological (Fabry's disease), systemic (lupus, scleroderma), or primarily gastric (pernicious anemia, gastric ulcer). Many are of undetermined etiology. Chronic forms of gastric stasis may initially be asymptomatic, but usually become clinically manifest with time. Rapid emptying may also produce severe symptoms (e.g., the palpitations, diaphoresis, weakness, and diarrhea of the "dumping syndrome" seen after gastric resection).

Diabetic gastroparesis is a well-recognized clinical entity that has been traditionally thought to reflect vagal damage, occurring as part of a generalized autonomic neuropathy. However, no morphological abnormality in the gastric wall or abdominal vagus has been identified. Gastroparesis is more frequent in patients with long-standing insulin-dependent diabetes and other evidence of autonomic nerve dysfunction, but there is a relatively poor correlation between the severity of autonomic nerve dysfunction and gastric emptying. Because delayed emptying may be impaired by hyperglycemia alone,[101] optimum diabetic control is needed prior to performing a radionuclide gastric emptying study to differentiate acute hyperglycemic dysfunction from chronic gastric stasis. Although the onset of diabetic gastroparesis may be insiduous and asymptomatic, it can progress to a complicated course of persistent vomiting and weight loss. Surprisingly, there is not a good correlation between the degree of gastric stasis and symptoms.

Gastroparesis can make diabetic control more difficult because timing of the insulin dose with food intake and absorption is critical for the care of brittle insulin-dependent diabetics. Reports on the incidence of gastroparesis in diabetics have varied and seem to depend on the population studied (e.g., whether most are symptomatic, asymptomatic, or have

Table 10. Causes of *Delayed* Gastric Emptying

Mechanical
- Tumors
- Obstructing duodenal or pyloric channel ulcer
- Hypertrophic pyloric stenosis
- Radiotherapy

Functional
- *Acute* states or diseases
  - Trauma
  - Postoperative ileus
  - Gastroenteritis
  - Hyperalimentation
  - Metabolic disorders (hyperglycemia, acidosis, hypokalemia, hypercalcemia hepatic coma, myxedemia)
  - Physiological effects (labryinth stimulation, gastric distention, increasing intragastric pressure, stress, physical and mental)
  - Drug effects (anticholinergics, antidepressants, nicotine (cigarettes), narcotics (opiates), levodopa, progesterone, birth control pills, beta adrenergic agonists)
  - Hormones (gastrin, secretin, glucagon, cholecystokinin, somatostatin, estrogen, progesterone)
- *Chronic* Diseases
  - Diabetes mellitus (diabetic gastroparesis)
  - Hypothyroidism
  - Fabry's Disease
  - Progressive systemic sclerosis
  - Myotonic dystrophy, familial dysautonomia
  - Systemic lupus, dermatomyositis
  - Amyloidosis
  - Pernicious anemia
  - Anorexia nervosa
  - Bulbar poliomyelitis
  - Gastric ulcer
  - Post-vagotomy for obstruction with or without pyloroplasty
  - Tumor-associated gastroparesis
  - Idiopathic

Causes of *Increased* Gastric Emptying
- Postoperative
  - Pyloroplasty
  - Hemigastrectomy (Billroth I or II)
- Diseases
  - Duodenal ulcer
  - Gastrinoma (Zollinger-Ellison syndrome)
  - Hyperthyroidism
- Hormones
  - thyroxine
  - motilin
  - entergastrone
- Drugs
  - Metoclopramide
  - Domperidone
  - Cisapride
  - Erythromycin

evidence of autonomic, cardiac, or peripheral neuropathy, etc.).[102–105] In a group of 20 insulin-dependent diabetics referred to us for symptoms suggestive of gastroparesis who were having difficulty in achieving good blood glucose control, solid gastric emptying was delayed in 10, normal in 8, and rapid in 2 (Fig. 17).[106] This highlights the need to perform a gastric emptying study to determine gastric function, because similar symptoms may have a variety of causes in diabetics and therapy will be difficult for each. Most studies have shown liquid emptying to be less sensitive than solid emptying for making the diagnosis of gastroparesis.

Medication and Drug Effects on Gastric Emptying

A number of drugs and common medications may also cause delayed emptying. A primary gastroparesis could be incorrectly diagnosed if it is not appreciated that the patient is taking medication that could adversely affect emptying. Data on the effect of drugs on gastric emptying is important; however, it is somewhat limited. Table 11 lists the effects of several commonly used medications. The effect of cigarettes, alcohol, and coffee on gastric emptying seems particularly pertinent but, here also, data is limited and sometimes conflicting. One study has found that cigarettes can stimulate duodenogastric reflux and inhibit antral motility.[107] Caffeine, a theophylline, has unknown effects. Drinks with a high concentration of alcohol can delay emptying of a standard meal,[108] but the amount found in wine does not.[109] Morphine and other narcotic analgesics, including pentazocine, delay emptying. Cocaine and cannabis have not been well studied.

Pharmacological Therapy of Gastroparesis

A number of pharmacological agents have been used to treat gastroparesis. The gastrokinetic properties of these drugs are mediated by different mechanisms. *Metoclopramide* has both central and peripheral antidopaminergic properties and releases acetylcholine from the myenteric plexus.[111] It also has central antiemetic properties. Neurological adverse effects (e.g., drowsiness, anxiety, and lassitude) are seen in up to 20% of patients. *Domperidone* is a peripheral dopamine antagonist that penetrates the blood-brain barrier poorly; therefore, neurological side effects are rare.[112] Both occasionally cause adverse effects due to hyperprolactinemia (e.g., breast tenderness, galactorhea, and menstrual irregularity). *Cisapride* releases acetylcholine from the myenteric plexus and is devoid of antidopaminergic properties and side effects.[113] Both metoclopramide and cisapride are also dependent on serotonergic mechanisms. *Erythromycin* acts as an agonist of the gastrointestinal peptide motilin.

The motor mechanisms by which these drugs improve gastric emptying is poorly understood. They all increase the amplitude of antral contractions. Metoclopramide, domperidone, and cisapride improve the coordination between antral, pyloric, and duodenal contractions. All are more effective than placebo in improving symptoms and have been studied most extensively for treatment of diabetic gastroenteropathy.[114–121] With metoclopramide and domperidone, symptomatic improvement may occur in the absence of documented alleviation of gastric stasis, due to the drug's central antiemetic properties. The gastrokinetic efficacy of these drugs often diminishes during prolonged administration.

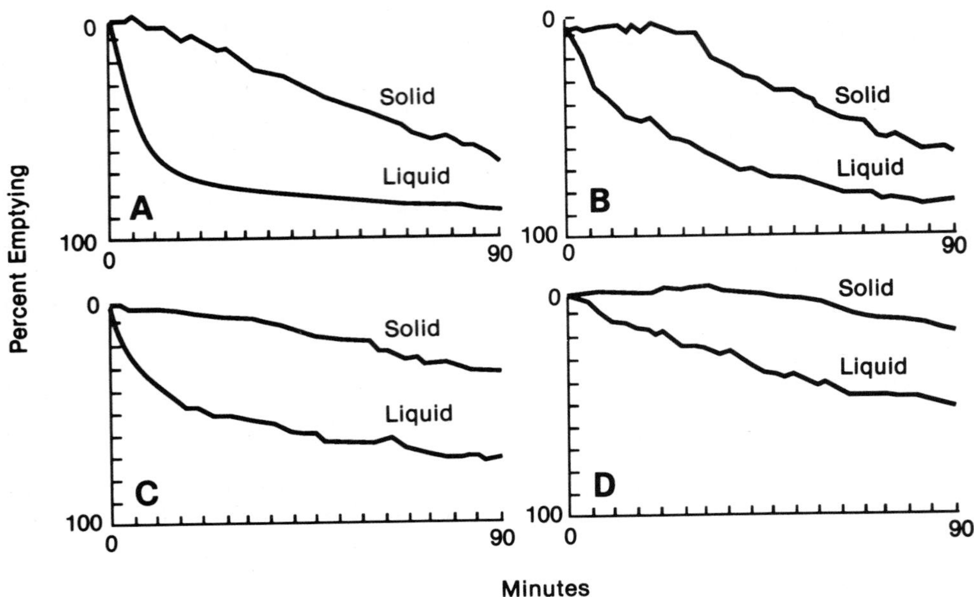

Figure 17. Dual-phase solid-liquid gastric emptying study in a normal control and 3 diabetics: **(A).** Normal; a short solid lag phase (5 min) is followed by linear emptying (66% at 90 min). The liquid phase has rapid early emptying phase (T1/2 = 3 min) followed by a much slower, normal second exponential clearance rate (T1/2 = 59 min). **(B).** Diabetic with a longer, but normal solid lag phase (23 min) and normal emptying (57% emptying at 90 min). Liquid emptying is also normal and has a single exponential clearance rate (T1/2 = 41 min). **(C).** Diabetic with delayed solid emptying at 90 min (21%). Liquid emptying is borderline abnormal (T1/2 = 93 min). Note the biphasic pattern of liquid emptying. **(D).** Diabetic with very delayed solid (17% at 90 min) and liquid gastric emptying (T1/2 = 139 min). The rates of solid and liquid emptying are quite similar during the latter portions of the studies. (Reprinted with permission, Ziessman HA, Fahey FH, Collen MJ: Biphasic solid and liquid gastric emptying in normal controls and diabetics using continuous acquisition in the LAO view. *Dig Dis Sci* 1992;37:744–750.)

Table 11. Commonly Used Medicines that Affect Gastric Emptying*

DRUG	THERAPEUTIC USE	GASTRIC EMPTYING	MODE OF ACTION
		CARDIOVASCULAR	
Potassium	Electrolyte replacement	Delay	Unknown
Dopamine	Vasopressor	Slow	Via dopamine receptors
Levodopa	Parkinson's	Delay	Via dopamine receptors
Nifedipine	Antihypertensive, antianginal	Delay or no effect	Ca++ blocker
		RESPIRATORY	
Isoproterenol	Asthma	Delay	Beta-adrenergic
Theophylline	Asthma	Not known	Smooth muscle relaxant
		GASTROINTESTINAL	
Sucralfate	Peptic ulcer	Delay or no effect	Mucosal coating and antacid
Aluminum OH	Peptic ulcer	Delay	Antacid
Propantheline	Peptic ulcer	Delay	Anticholinergic
Cimetidine	Peptic ulcer	No effect	H_2-blocker
Bulk laxatives	Constipation	Accelerates	Gastric distention
Opiates	Diarrhea	Delay	Increased smooth muscle tone
		PSYCHIATRIC	
Chlordiazepoxide	Anxiety	No effect	
Tricyclics	Antidepressant	Delay	Anticholinergic, norepinephrine-enhancing
Phenothiazines	Psychosis	Delay	Anticholinergic
Diazepam	Anxiety	Accelerates	Spasmolytic
		NONSTEROIDAL ANTI-INFLAMMATORY	
Indomethacin	Anti-inflammatory	No effect	Prostaglandin inhibitor
		MISCELLANEOUS	
Estrogens	Hormonal therapy	Delay	?gastric sex hormone receptors
Acetaminophen	Analgesic, antipyretic	Unknown	Prostaglandin synthetase inhibitor

*With permission, modified from Chaudhuri TK and Fink S: Update: Pharmaceuticals and gastric emptying. *Am J Gastroenterol* 1990; 85:223–230.[110]

Table 12. Various Solid-liquid Meals and their Normal Emptying Half-Times*

WEIGHT/VOLUME OF MEAL	MEAL SOLID/LIQUID	RADIONUCLIDE SOLID/LIQUID	MEAN t1/2 (MIN) SOLID/LIQUID	REF.
15 g/100 mL	oat and resin/milk	Tc-O4	44/	132
150 g/150 mL	chicken liver and beef/ water	Tc-SC	106/	145
300 g/150 mL	chicken liver and beef/ orange juice	Tc-SC/ ^{111}Ind-DTPA	77/38	136
105 g/200 mL	chicken liver (A) and noodles (B)/water	^{111}Ind (A) ^{123}Ind (B)	72/ 47/	159
110 g/240 mL	egg salad/milk	Tc-SC	80/17	170
255 g/200 mL	chicken liver and beef stew/water	Tc-SC/ ^{113m}Ind	110/	148
265 g/200 mL	chicken liver 0.25 (A) and 10-mm pieces (B) plus beef/water	Tc-SC (A) ^{113m}Ind (B)	69/ 114/	159
450 g/450 mL	chicken liver and beef/ orange juice	Tc-SC/ ^{111}Ind-DTPA	100/58	126
1692 g/150 mL	chicken liver and beef/ orange juice	Tc-SC/ ^{111}Ind-DTPA	277/178	136
150 g/300 mL	scrambled egg sandwich/water	Tc-SC/ ^{111}Ind-DTPA	88/23	5
150 gm/250 mL	egg white sandwich/ water	Tc-SC/ ^{111}Ind-DTPA	80/88	106

*With permission, modified from Maurer AH, Heyman S, Vitti RA, Winzelberg GG: Gastrointestinal nuclear medicine, in Siegel BA, Kirchner PT (eds.): New York, Nuclear Medicine: Self Study Program I, Society of Nuclear Medicine, 1988

Radionuclide Gastric Emptying Studies

RADIOPHARMACEUTICALS AND MEALS

A wide variety of radiolabeled meals have been used for investigative as well as clinical purposes. Solid meals have included meat, potatoes, porridge, pancakes, corn flakes, chicken liver, eggs, and chemical resins in oatmeal, to name a few (Table 12). However, to accurately quantify solid emptying, a radioactive marker must be tightly bound to the meal. Elution of the radiolabel in vivo results in a partially solid, partially liquid labeling mixture, which produces an erroneously shortened solid emptying time.

A physiologically exquisite method for labeling chicken liver in vivo was described by Meyer et al.[123] ^{99m}Tc-sulfur colloid (^{99m}Tc-SC) is injected into the wing vein of a chicken; the chicken is then killed, and the liver removed and cooked. The intracellular ^{99m}Tc-SC label is tightly bound to the cytoplasm of the Kupffer cells and does not dissociate after ingestion by the patient. The labeled chicken liver is often mixed with beef or chicken stew for palatability and volume. In spite of the logic and proven utility of this technique, it has not been adopted for routine clinical testing, for obvious reasons.

Alternative acceptable in vitro methods of labeling liver have been developed and are more commonly used (Table 13). Cooking injected or surface-labeled liver cubes or liver paté traps the radionuclide within the meat. The labeling efficiency and in vivo stability are good (Table 14).[124–126] Labeling of fried whole eggs or egg whites, often served as a sandwich, has been found to be convenient, easy to prepare, and palatable. The labeled eggs have a high labeling efficiency and good stability.[127,128] Of various foods tested, in vivo labeled chicken liver is the most stable in gastric juice,

Table 13. Preparation of Different Solid Gastric Emptying Meals

1. In vivo chicken liver.[123] ^{99m}Tc-SC is injected into the wing vein of a live chicken. Fifteen to 30 min later, the chicken is slaughtered, the liver removed and placed in water bath for 5 min. It is then wrapped in aluminum foil and baked in a preheated broiler for 20 min at 350 degrees. It is cut into 0.5-cm cubes and added to an 8-ounce can of chicken stew.
2. Surface-labeled in vitro chicken liver. Raw liver is cut into 1 cm-cubes. ^{99m}Tc-SC is squirted onto the surface of the cubes, then they are wrapped in foil and cooked as in 1.[124,125]
3. Injected in vitro chicken liver. Same as 2 except that ^{99m}Tc-SC is injected into each cube of liver before cooking.[124,125]
4. Canned liver paté is mixed homogenously with ^{99m}Tc-SC, incubated for 10 min, then fried for 10–15 min.[126]
5. Sulfur colloid egg. ^{99m}Tc-SC is injected into a beaten raw egg. The egg is cooked until firm in consistency.[127]
6. Egg white sulfur colloid egg; similar to 5 except only the whites are used.[128]
7. MAA egg. Tc-MAA is mixed with a beaten raw egg and cooked as in 5.[129]
8. HSA egg. ^{99m}Tc-labeled human serum albumin is mixed with a beaten raw egg and cooked as above.[129]
9. Ovalbumin egg. ^{99m}Tc-ovalbumin is prepared by labeling purified ovalbumin with ^{99m}Tc in an electrolytic method similar to a kit for ^{99m}Tc-HSA.[127,130]

Table 14. Stability of Radiolabeled Solid Foods

MEAL	PERCENT BOUND AFTER 3 hr IN GASTRIC JUICE*
Chelex resin	98%
In vivo-labeled chicken liver	
baked	98
fried	97
In vitro surface-labeled liver cubes	
baked	91
In vitro injected cubes of liver	
baked	78
fried	84
Tc-SC egg	81
Tc-OA egg	78
Tc-HSA	65

*Values from Knight et al.,[131] Christian et al.,[126] Wirth et al.,[132] and Brown et al.[133]

followed by cubes of liver injected with the radiolabel, and then eggs mixed with ^{99m}Tc-SC before cooking (Table 14). Surface-labeled fried liver paté is also acceptable.

A ^{99m}Tc-labeled polystyrene resin mixed with oatmeal has been used as a semisolid meal; however, it is not physiological and offers few advantages.[132] Radioiodinated fiber has been shown to have a stable label for tracing the fiber component of a solid meal; however, fiber is processed differently from digestible solid foods and is not simple to prepare.[134] In an attempt to measure the gastric emptying of fat, olive oil has recently been labeled with ^{99m}Tc (V)thiocyantate and ingested with soup.[135] It has a high labeling efficiency and is reasonably stable in vivo.

Liquid phase markers must equilibrate rapidly, be nonabsorbable, and not bind to the solid phase in a combined solid-liquid meal. ^{99m}Tc-SC meets these criteria and is most commonly used to measure liquid-only emptying. In dual isotope solid-liquid studies, ^{111}In-DTPA is often used because of its higher photopeaks (171 and 247 keV) when used in conjunction with ^{99m}Tc-labeled solids.[136,137] Concern has been raised as to whether it might bind or absorb to the solid component in the stomach. However, in vitro studies show that less than 2% of the ^{111}In becomes associated with the solid phase.[136]

TECHNICAL FACTORS IN GASTRIC EMPTYING STUDIES

To date, there is no generally accepted standard with regard to the composition of the meal, the method of data acquisition, or the quantitative parameters used to characterize gastric emptying. Therefore, no generally applicable "normal" values are valid. Normal values have to be determined either in one's own laboratory using a standard meal and technique, or one must closely follow a method described in the literature and use their values. Generally, the larger the meal, the slower the emptying and, therefore, the longer the study. A number of factors need to be considered before deciding on a particular protocol (Table 15).

Patient Positioning. Supine, sitting, semi-upright, and standing imaging positions have all been advocated and are used in different laboratories. Upright imaging may be more physiological to some; however, others might find reclining after a meal preferable and just as physiological. Personal preference and the instrumentation available will usually determine the method. For example, many two-headed cameras require supine imaging. Imaging position and activity influence emptying, e.g., the stomach empties faster when the patient is upright compared to recumbent[140,141] and walking enhances emptying.[142] Soft tissue attenuation effects may also vary depending on patient positioning.[143] Therefore, whichever imaging protocol is chosen should be used exclusively to maximize reproducibility.

Decay, Downscatter, Septal Penetration, and Attenuation. Because solid gastric emptying study protocols require 1.5 to 3 hours of imaging, correction for radioactive decay is necessary for short-lived radiopharmaceuticals such as ^{99m}Tc. Ideally, studies should be carried out until half-emptying has occurred, although this is not always practical in patients with very delayed emptying.

Dual tracer studies for combined solid-liquid phase studies may require scatter correction (e.g., from the ^{111}In photopeak down into the ^{99m}Tc window). If radionuclide energies are close, significant scatter into both windows may occur. Malmud et al.[137] found that 23% of the ^{99m}Tc counts were the result of downscatter from the ^{111}In window and 8% of the ^{111}In counts were due to the ^{99m}Tc. However, the amount of scatter depends on multiple factors, including the radiopharmaceuticals used, window width, and the relative amounts of activity. Since these parameters likely differ for each laboratory, the scatter fraction should be determined based on patient or phantom studies and each study corrected accordingly. Scatter correction should be performed before decay corrections when the two decay rates are dissimilar. A simple alternative method for minimizing the problem of scatter is to use larger amounts of activity for the lower energy radionuclide (e.g., 37 MBq ^{99m}Tc and 7 MBq ^{111}In). Using these doses, we have found that the amount of downscatter is negligible with only 1% of the ^{99m}Tc counts scattered up into the ^{111}In window and 3% of the ^{111}In counts downscattered into the ^{99m}Tc window[106] and, therefore, do not perform routine scatter correction. Others[125] have also found <5% downscatter if the ratio of ^{99m}Tc to ^{111}In radioactivity is high.

High-energy radionuclides (e.g., ^{113m}In (392 keV), may also require correction for *septal penetration* of the collimator.[144] ^{113m}In is a generator-produced radiopharmaceutical (^{113}Sn/^{113m}In) used as a liquid marker (^{113m}In-DTPA) in regions of the world where shorter-lived radiotracers are not readily available. The tin parent has a 115-day half-life; therefore, the generator requires replacing only 2 to 3 times per year.

For accurate quantification of solid gastric emptying studies, *attenuation correction* is frequently required. If the scintillation camera is positioned anteriorly, an artificial increase in counts will often result as the stomach contents move

Table 15. Gastric Emptying Protocols*

	GEORGETOWN UNIVERSITY	TEMPLE UNIVERSITY	UNIVERSITY OF UTAH
References:	Ziessman et al.[106]	Urbaine et al.[138]	Christian et al.[139]
Preparation	Overnite fast	Overnite fast	8-hr fast
Marker	Ant ^{99m}Tc point source on right lower chest		1.5–3 mCi (50–100 MBq) ^{99m}Tc taped to right ant. rib margin away from stomach and post. marker similarly placed for image repositioning
Meal	^{99m}Tc-SC egg-white sandwich 200 mL water	^{99m}Tc-SC whole egg sandwich 300 cc water	^{99m}Tc-SC in vitro labeled fried liver paté mixed with beef stew, orange juice
Dose	^{99m}Tc-SC 37 MBq ^{111}In 7 MBq	^{99m}Tc-SC 18.5 MBq ^{111}In-DTPA 5 MBq	^{99m}Tc-SC 22 MBq ^{111}In-DTPA 3.7 MBq
Camera	Single-head LFOV	Dual-head camera	Single-head LVOF
Window	15% 140 keV 15% 247 keV 10% 172 keV	10% 140 keV 20% 247 keV	20% 140 keV 20% 247 keV
Patient position	semi-upright (60 degrees) on gurney	Seated	Upright
Projections	Left ant oblique	Ant and post simultaneously	Ant and post sequentially
Framing rate	90 sec/frame for 90 min	60 sec/frame × 2 hr	40 s/frame q 15 min × 1 hr, then q 30 min until 50% emptying
Bkgd correct	no	yes	no
Decay correct	yes	yes	yes
Scatter correct	no	yes	yes
Attenuation correction	LAO view	Geometric mean	Geometric mean
Computer processing	ROI around summed gastric image	ROI around summed gastric image	ROI around each image and counts obtained
Data presentation	Time-activity curve of percent emptying vs. time	Time-activity curve of GM cts	Percent of counts remaining at each time interval
Quantitation	Solid: Percent emptying at 90 min Liquid: half-emptying time	Curve fit to a modified power exponential with estimation of lag phase and rate of emptying	Half-emptying time for solids and liquids

*Note: These three protocols are abstracted from the referenced papers, but modified to fit into this protocol comparison. The exact method may not reflect that institution's usual or present protocol.

from the fundus, which is located relatively posteriorly, to the more anteriorly positioned antrum due to depth-related varying soft-tissue attenuation (Fig. 18). Emptying may be underestimated. Likewise, posterior imaging overestimates emptying. Solid emptying half-times may be in error by 10 to 34% with anterior imaging alone, and considerably larger errors can occur in individual patients.[136,143,145] The amount of error depends on meal size, patient size, patient position, stomach orientation, and other factors that cannot be reliably predicted. Liquid emptying does not require attenuation correction because the liquid moves so rapidly to the distal stomach.[144,146]

The generally accepted "gold standard" for attenuation correction is the *geometric mean* method. Opposed anterior and posterior images are acquired, either simultaneously with a dual-headed camera or, more commonly, sequentially with a single-headed camera. The geometric mean (square root of the product of the anterior and posterior counts) is determined for each imaging set. Phantom studies indicate that the calculated geometric mean method gives count rates that vary less than 2 to 4% for depths of 2.5 to 27.0 cm[136,145] (Fig. 19).

Because most laboratories use a single-headed scintillation camera for gastric emptying studies, geometric mean correction is performed by acquiring sequential anterior and posterior images, typically every 15 to 30 minutes for the duration of the study (1.5 to 2.5 hours). This technique has drawbacks. Frequent repositioning can be demanding on both patient and technologist. Gastric regions of interest must be drawn on the computer for each image; careful repositioning of the patient or realignment of images is important. Most important, infrequent intermittent imaging

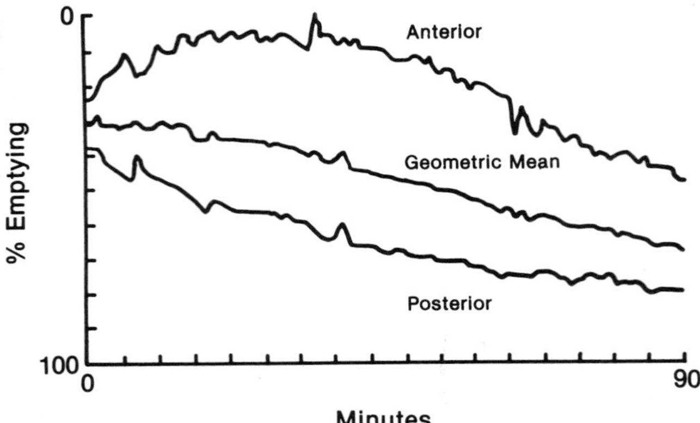

Figure 18. Anterior and posterior acquisition with geometric mean correction. This solid gastric emptying study shows the effect of varying soft-tissue attenuation due to movement of the stomach contents from the reltively posterior gastric fundus to the more anteriorly positioned antrum. The upper curve is the result of imaging anteriorly only and the lower curve from posterior imaging. The middle curve is the geometric mean (square root of the product of the ant and post views) correction at each data point. Note the flat lag phase before linear emptying begins.

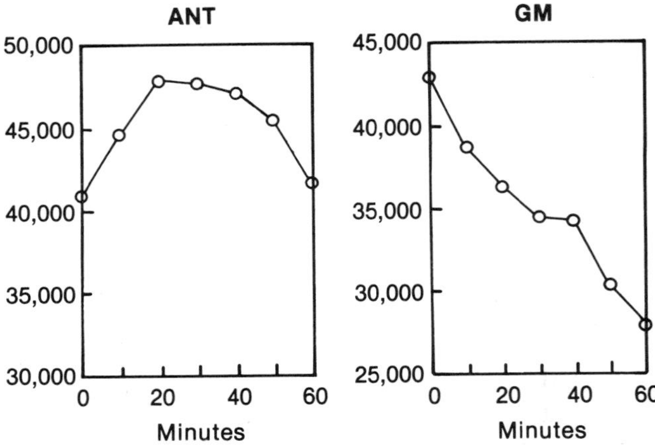

Figure 20. Geometric mean correction using limited data points: Left, data acquired in the anterior view every 15 min for 1 hour. The curve initially rises as a result of movement of the labeled stomach contents toward the scintillation camera. Right, geometric mean correction shows no lag phase and linear emptying. Although it seems that attenuation correction has eliminated the lag phase, this is merely the result of infrequent and inadequate data points during the early phase of the study. Curve fitting to calculate a rate of emptying with this limited data is also subject to error.

results in few data points from which to estimate an emptying rate (Fig. 20). Of course, continuous imaging is not possible with a single-headed camera using this method.

Alternative methods of attenuation correction using a single-headed camera have been sought. Collins et al.[147] have described a method of attenuation correction that requires a *lateral image* to estimate depth and then attenuation is mathematically corrected at each data point. This method has not been generally used or validated by others. Another approach using a single-headed gamma camera is the *peak-to-scatter* (P/S) ratio method. The rationale for this method is that with increasing thickness of overlying soft tissue, there is increasing scattered radiation; therefore, the ratio between the photopeak counts and a lower energy scatter window should be negatively correlated with the thickness of the overlying attenuating material. This ratio is used to estimate and mathematically correct for depth. Initial studies showed results similar to the geometric mean.[148] However, the P/S ratio can be affected by scatter from sources outside the field of view of the stomach (e.g., small bowel activity or a radioactive marker). We have not found this method sufficiently accurate when compared with the geometric mean technique.[146]

Another approach to the problem of attenuation that requires only a single-headed camera and no mathematical

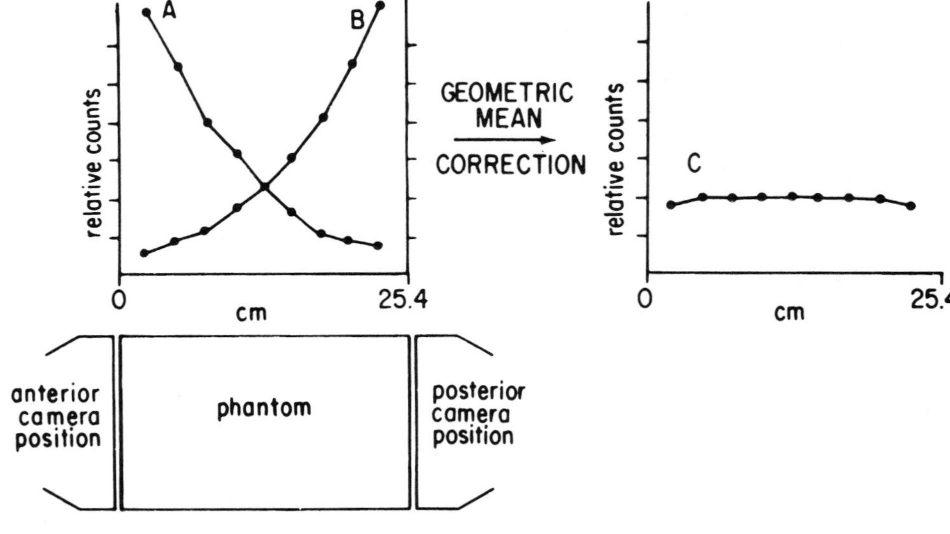

Figure 19. Phantom study illustrates varying sensitivity at depth for a ^{99m}Tc point source in tissue-equivalent polystyrene. Counts were obtained with the source at increasing distance, for both anterior **(A)** and posterior imaging **(B)**, and the geometric mean correction **(C).** Calculation of the geometric mean results in uniform sensitivity independent of depth. (With permission, Christian PE, Moore JG, Sorensons JA, et al.: Effects of meal size and correction technique on gastric emptying time: Studies with two tracers and opposed detectors. *J Nucl Med* 1980;21: 883–885.)

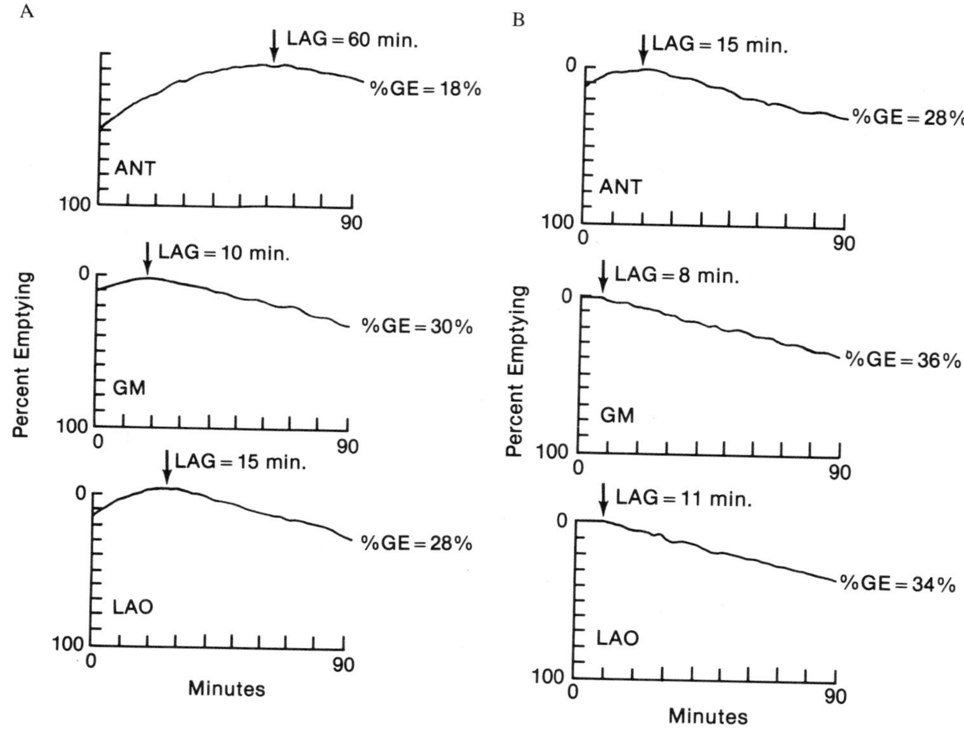

Figure 21 A,B. Comparison of anterior, LAO, and geometric mean (GM) time-activity curves in two patients: **(A).** In the anterior view (top), the lag phase is very prolonged (58 min) and the rate of emptying slow, resulting in poor overall emptying. The GM curve (middle) corrects the effect of varying attenuation substantially, although incompletely. The lag phase is much shorter (10 min), the slope of emptying steeper, and the overall emptying much improved. The LAO view (bottom) also substantially corrects for attenuation, but not quite as well as the GM. **(B).** This patient has a more typical lag phase of about 15 min in the anterior view. Both the geometric mean and LAO methods correct for attenuation similarly, with a short flat lag phase and better emptying.

correction is to acquire the study in the left anterior oblique (LAO) projection.[146] In this view, the radiolabeled meal in the stomach moves essentially parallel to the face of the scintillation camera, thus minimizing the effect of attenuation. In a preliminary study, Fahey et al.[146] found that gastric emptying using the LAO method highly correlated with and was not significantly different than the geometric mean method. These results have been confirmed by others.[106,149,150] However, one study has noted that the lag phase in the LAO view may be overestimated when compared to that of the geometric mean method,[149] suggesting incomplete attenuation correction (Fig. 21 **A,B**). Physiologically, the lag phase is the time required for the gastric contents to move from the proximal to distal stomach and for the food to be ground up into small enough particles to pass through the pylorus. Unfortunately, there is no generally agreed upon method for calculating the lag phase.[151] For routine clinical use and investigation where exact measurement of the lag phase is not critical, the LAO method is a simple and accurate way to compensate for attenuation. For investigative studies requiring precise quantification, the geometric mean method may be preferable.

Continuous Versus Intermittent Imaging. Continuous imaging allows more complete characterization of the phases of gastric emptying and provides many more data points from which to accurately quantify the rate of emptying. For routine clinical studies, this detailed information may not be vital but, for physiological and pharmacological studies, intermittent imaging is often not adequate. For example, the lag phase (mean 10 minutes, range 5 to 25 minutes) cannot be accurately determined with intermittent imaging every 15 to 30 minutes. From a technical standpoint, a study acquired continuously is usually easier to perform. Once the patient is positioned comfortably, minimal technologist interaction is required. The main disadvantage is that the patient must remain in the same position for the duration of the study. With proper positioning for comfort (e.g., pillow under the knees) and occasional reminders and encouragement, this is usually easily accomplished.[106] A single summed image can be used for drawing a region of interest. Computer correction for patient motion may occasionally be necessary; therefore, a radioactive marker is routinely placed in the field of view away from the stomach during acquisition.[152]

Variability. Reproducibility data for gastric emptying studies is somewhat limited; however, it has generally been found to be good with a mean difference of about 5 to 15% on repeated testing, although larger variations have been reported.[153,154] Normal diurnal variation can affect emptying; therefore, studies should always be performed at the same time of day,[155] preferably in the morning after an overnite fast. A difference in the rate of normal emptying between men and women has been reported.[156]

ANALYSIS OF GASTRIC EMPTYING DATA

Unfortunately, but not surprisingly, analysis and quantification of gastric emptying data has been done differently at various institutions. No consensus has been reached, although various attempts have been made.[157]

Computer processing varies, depending on the method

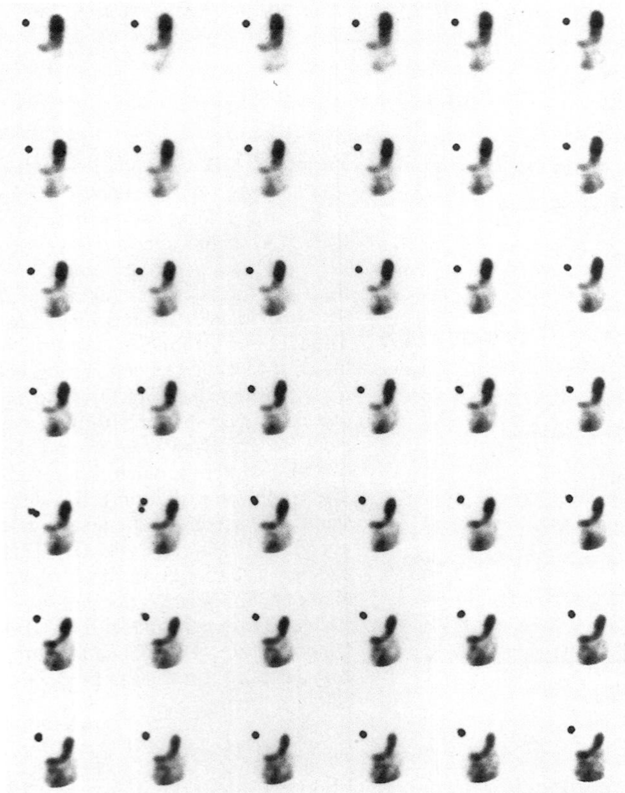

Figure 22. Sequential serial images (90 sec) during continuous dynamic imaging of a solid gastric emptying study. These images could also be viewed as a cinematic display. Note the slight patient movement as indicated by the radioactive marker on the patient's chest seen on the first two images of the 5th line.

of acquisition. With continuous acquisition, review of the images helps to get a feel for the pattern of emptying and detect any potential quantitative problems (e.g., patient motion or overlapping bowel and stomach, Fig. 22). A region of interest (ROI) can then be drawn around a summed gastric image (Fig. 23). In addition, a ROI can be drawn for the radionuclide body marker to detect movement and also used to reorient the images if movement has occurred. If intermittent acquisition is used, ROIs can be drawn for all images, or for a summed image if the images have been realigned. This procedure must be done for both the anterior and posterior images if opposing images are acquired for geometric mean correction.

Liquid emptying is the most straightforward. Emptying of a single radiotracer in water or saline usually begins immediately after ingestion although, occasionally, a short pause is seen, probably due to reflex relaxation. Emptying is rapid and monoexponential (Fig. 15). The time of half-emptying (time required for peak counts to decrease by half) is easily calculated. Normal liquid emptying time is in the range of 10 to 20 minutes, although it is slowed by the presence of nutrients.

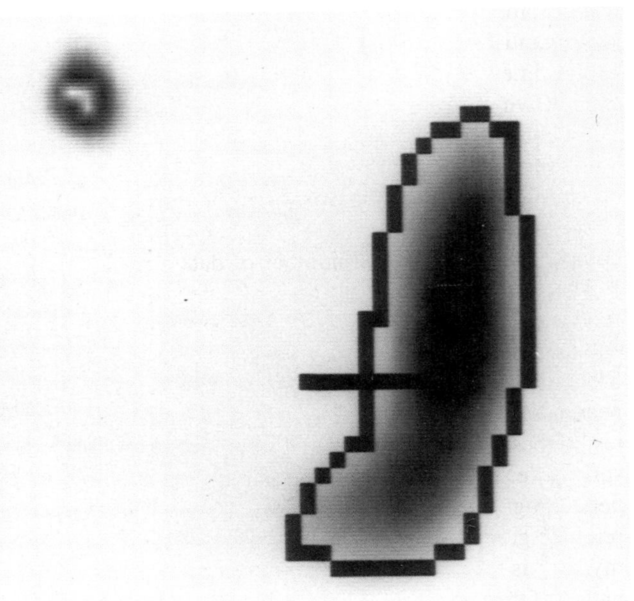

Figure 23. Gastric region of interest (ROI) drawn on computer. A ROI could also be drawn for the radioactive marker to check for patient motion.

Solid emptying is more complex. A time delay (mean 10 to 15 minutes) before solid emptying begins has often been reported (Fig. 16).[114,147,158,159] However, there has been considerable controversy regarding the reason for this so-called lag phase. Physiologically, it has been described as the time required for the stomach to break down solid food into particles small enough to pass through the pylorus (grinding and sieving of the distal stomach).[158] However, some investigators have failed to detect a lag phase during radionuclide gastric emptying studies[143,160–162] and one group concluded that the lag phase seen on radionuclide gastric emptying studies is usually due to a lack of adequate attenuation correction.[160] On the other hand, several recent studies have clearly demonstrated the consistent presence of a solid lag phase, even when adequate attenuation correction was performed.[106,151,163] The difference in the study results seems to be due to the sampling interval used. Frequent imaging is required to regularly detect a normal lag phase of 5 to 25 minutes. It is easy to see how it may be missed entirely with intermittent imaging performed every 15 to 30 minutes.

The lag phase has been measured differently by various investigators. The following are 3 definitions proposed[151]: (1) subjective visual inspection of the time-activity curve to identify the starting time of emptying (inflection point), (2) time at which a defined percent decrease from maximum activity is measured (e.g., $<2\%$) and, (3) time of visual appearance of duodenal activity determined on enhanced computer images. Using these 3 definitions, the mean lag phase was found to be 8.3 (range 4 to 14), 10.3 (range 6 to 15), and 7.4 min (range 4 to 16), respectively.[151] Another study has shown that the time of maximum filling of the distal stomach corresponds to the duration of the lag phase.[138] One quantitative approach fits a modified power exponential to the time-activity curve and defines the lag phase as the time at which the second derivative of the filling function is equal to zero, and represents the time at which the gastric emptying process switches from a variable to a constant emptying rate.[163] This latter method has been mainly used in studies acquired every 15 to 30 minutes in an attempt to compensate for a limited number of data points.

The length of the lag phase is affected by differences in food particle size, caloric content of the meal, and the type and amount of solid food ingested.[136,159,164,165] An abnormally prolonged lag phase as a cause for delayed emptying has been associated with certain disease processes (e.g., diabetes,[114] obesity[166]; loss of the lag phase has been reported with surgery (e.g., vagotomy and antrectomy[100]; certain gastrokinetic drugs seem to work by shortening a prolonged lag phase (e.g. metoclopramide and domperidone[114,117]); erythromycin[120] is reported to abolish normal solid-liquid discrimination of the stomach, even in healthy people. Further studies are needed using frequent image acquisition to confirm these individual reports.

After the lag phase, solid food empties in a linear manner (Figs. 16, 17). The time of half-emptying has often been used to characterize this rate; however, since the terminology suggests exponential rather than linear emptying, others have recommended calculating the percent emptying (or percent gastric residual) at specific time intervals (e.g., at the end of the study). The rate of emptying (e.g., percent per minute) may be a more correct way to reflect the linear character of this emptying.[167] More complex methods of calculating emptying have been used. Siegel et al. has used a modified power exponential to characterize the biphasic character of the gastric emptying curve, providing an estimate of both the lag phase and the rate of emptying.[163]

Dual tracer studies are evaluated similarly. Since emptying of liquids is slowed in the presence of food,[168] the emptying of liquids is considerably slower in dual-phase meals than with clear liquids only. Numerous reports have described the liquid-phase component of a dual tracer study as having a single exponential emptying rate that empties faster than the solid meal.[137] However, when continuous imaging is performed, we have found that liquid emptying may often be biexponential, with an early rapid component (mean 5.3 min) and a second slower component (mean 48 $\pm$ 7 min).[106] The second slower exponential liquid emptying rate correlates with the rate of solid emptying, confirming a previous report by Siegel et al.[169] which found that the major difference between solid and liquid phase emptying times was that solids have a lag phase before emptying begins. Physiologically, this similar rate of emptying may be due to the fact that the liquid and solid phases become a mixture and, essentially, empty together. Therefore, they have suggested that perhaps only the liquid component need be labeled. The advantage of this approach would be that the study would take less time and result in less radiation dose to the patient. Further study of this intriguing but controversial suggestion is needed.

GASTRIC EMPTYING PROTOCOLS

Three different protocols that have been used at institutions with considerable experience in performing gastric emptying studies are summarized for comparison (Table 15). All three of these protocols is applicable to single or dual tracer imaging. Combined solid and liquid gastric emptying studies are probably unnecessary for routine clinical work, although they may sometimes be important for investigative studies. Dual radionuclide imaging with ^{99m}Tc and ^{111}In requires a medium energy collimator. *Liquid-only* studies are indicated for patients who cannot ingest solids. Liquid studies must be acquired rapidly (1-minute frames $\times$ 30 minutes) because normal water and saline empty very fast ($t_{1/2}$ of 10 to 20 minutes).

Evaluation of Therapy and Pharmacological Interventions

The various gastrokinetic drugs previously discussed have proven effective for therapy of diabetic gastroenteropathy[114–121] as well as for a variety of other causes of gastroparesis, including tumor-associated gastroparesis,[131,170] amyloidosis,[171] scleroderma, anorexia nervosia, postviral and postoperative pseudo-obstruction,[111,133] Fabry's disease,[172] and idiopathic gastric stasis and gastric ulcer.[173]

However, some of these therapeutic drugs may relieve patients of their symptoms without producing a concomitant improvement in gastric emptying, and vice versa. For example, metoclopramide has a central-nervous-system antinausea effect that, by itself, may result in clinical improvement. Only by repeating a gastric emptying study after initiation of therapy can one determine if the desired gastrokinetic effect has been achieved (Fig. 24).

Pharmacological intervention can predict the potential effectiveness of a particular therapy. For example, if poor emptying is observed, metoclopramide could be given intravenously during the study (10 mg).[174] A change to a steeper emptying slope confirms a positive response to the drug (Fig. 25). A single oral dose might not be predictive because a response requires that the drug first be emptied from the stomach, before it can be absorbed to produce the desired gastrokinetic effect. To see a definite pharmacological effect may require multiple doses over a period of days. Parenteral administration can sometimes initiate the process sooner. Alternatively, the effectiveness of a particular therapy can be evaluated with a repeat gastric emptying study after a short course of a trial drug (Fig. 26). If the effectiveness of oral therapy is to be investigated, the patient should ingest his usual dose 15 to 30 minutes prior to the study. Gastric emptying studies have been used to evaluate the effectiveness of various interventional therapies for morbid obesity (e.g., gastroplasty[139,175,176] and the Garren-Edwards Balloon[177]).

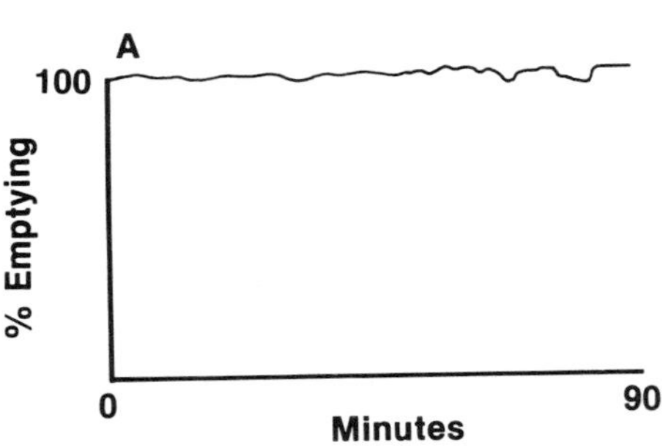

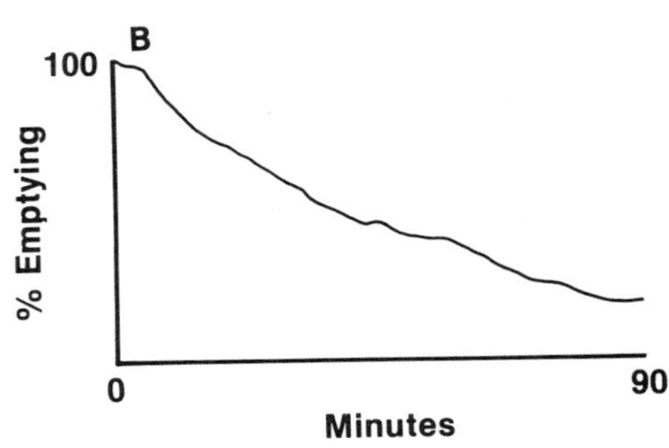

Figure 24. Time-activity curves before and after surgery in a fifty-five-year-old male with pyloric stenosis secondary to peptic ulcer disease: **(A).** The baseline study shows no gastric emptying during the 90 min study. **(B).** A repeat study after surgery (partial gastrectomy) shows rapid gastric emptying after a short lag phase.

Post Operative Gastric Emptying

Some patients who have had truncal vagotomy with subtotal gastrectomy (both Billroth I and II) performed for gastric outlet obstruction, as a complication of peptic ulcer disease, may have rapid early emptying of liquids and solids. Gastric sieving of food is impaired and a significant portion of solid food enters the bowel as large particles of food.[158] However, other patients who had this same surgery have chronic gastric atony and stasis postoperatively,[178] probably due to damaged gastric smooth muscles from a chronically distended and dilated preoperative state. Patients with rapid emptying due to the Zollinger-Ellison or the dumping syndrome can be similarly evaluated to find an effective therapy (Fig. 27).

Dosimetry

Radiation absorbed dose calculations for various radiopharmaceuticals and meals are listed in Table 3 B. Generally, the overall radiation dose is low. The large intestine receives the highest dose. Any factor that delays gastric emptying and intestinal transit increases the estimated dose. The ^{111}In-label results in considerably more radiation absorbed dose than ^{99m}Tc.

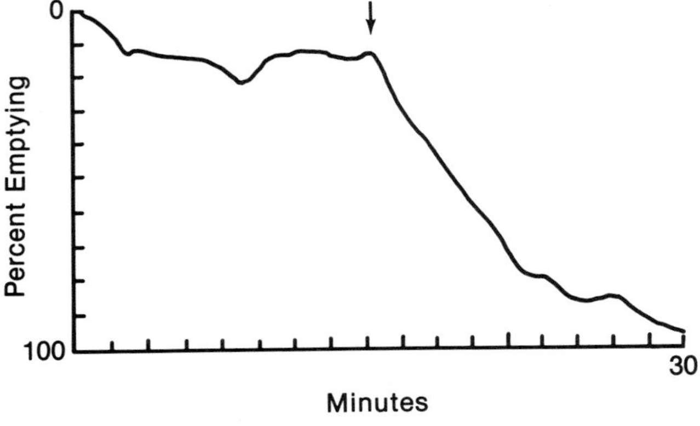

Figure 25. Metoclopramide intervention: this diabetic had very delayed liquid-only emptying that was noted by the physician viewing the persistence scope during the study. After intravenous injection of 10 mg metoclopramide (arrow), prompt and rapid emptying ensues as illustrated by the change to a steep slope and resulting nearly complete emptying by 30 min.

BREATH TESTS IN GASTROINTESTINAL DISEASES

Of the five gases produced in the gastrointestinal tract (hydrogen (H_2), carbon dioxide (CO_2), methane, nitrogen, and oxygen), CO_2 and H_2 are the only ones used extensively to measure metabolic breakdown products by breath analysis.

Hydrogen Breath Tests

Because human cells are incapable of producing H_2, the appearance of H_2 in the breath in concentrations greater than the 0.5 ppm found naturally in air must represent a fermentation product of some intestinal bacteria. The exhaled H_2 is measured relatively straightforwardly by gas chromatography using thermoconductivity detectors. Generally, abnormal H_2 concentrations in the breath indicate either carbohydrate malabsorption (with consequent fermentation in the colon) or excessive bacterial colonization within the small intestine.[179] Thus, this test is often used to measure bacterial overgrowth, even though it lacks sensitivity because about 25% of bacteria in the small intestine do not produce H_2.

The most common use of hydrogen breath tests is in suspected lactase deficiency. Lactose metabolism is mediated by lactase, present in small bowel mucosa. In lactase deficiency, the lactose (especially in milk) passes undigested to the colon where it is fermented by colonic bacteria producing H_2, and causes such symptoms as cramps, bloating, and diarrhea. The appearance of abnormal concentrations of H_2 in the breath following a lactose challenge meal is a highly sensitive indication of lactase deficiency and distinguishes that condition from milk allergy.[180]

Carbon Dioxide Breath Tests

In labeled carbon breath tests a substrate labeled either with radioactive ^{14}C, or with stable carbon ^{13}C that is metabolized to CO_2, is administered orally to the subject and the quantity of labeled CO_2 exhaled is measured as a function of time. Carbon-11 can be used; however, the short 20-minute half-life imposes special technical problems of measurement and, of course, requires direct access to a cyclotron and rapid synthesis of substrate compounds.

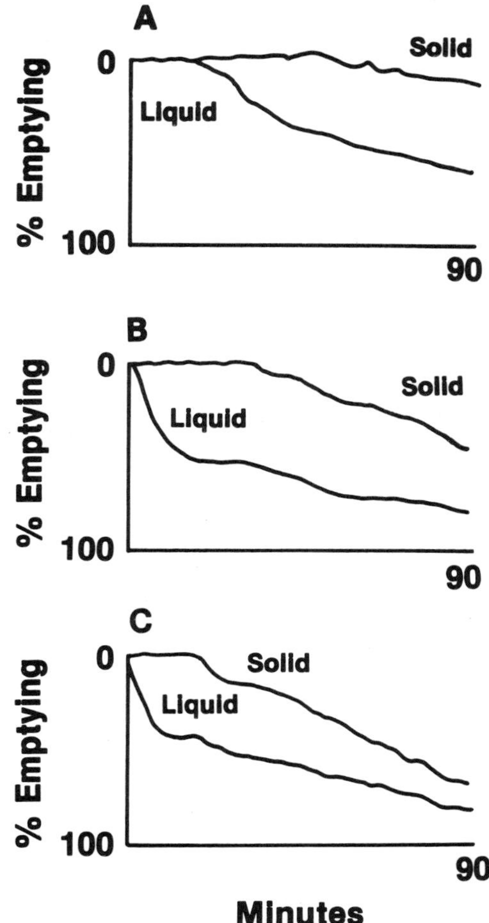

Figure 26. Therapeutic trials in a patient with diabetic gastroparesis. The upper time-activity curve **(A)** is the baseline study prior to therapy showing very delayed solid gastric emptying. The middle curve **(B)** shows improved emptying after 2 weeks of oral metoclopramide. The bottom study **(C)** shows even better gastric emptying after one week of oral cisapride therapy.

METHODS

Carbon-14. Most labeled carbon breath tests have used ^{14}C, which, with its low-energy (150 keV) beta ray and 5700-year half-life allows relatively uncomplicated substrate preparation and low radiation absorbed doses. These studies require small radionuclide dosages of 80 to 800 kBq (2 to 20 μCi) that deliver absorbed radiation doses of 0.2 to 10 mSv.[181–183] In early studies, the exhaled $^{14}CO_2$ was collected in large Douglas bags and then percolated through a solution of $Ba(OH)_2$ and precipitated onto plates as $Ba^{14}CO_2$. These plates could then be counted in gas-flow proportional counters or thin end-window G-M counters.[184,185] Later, LeRoy et al. developed at 4π G-M counter that could record continuous activity as it was exhaled.[186] Tolbert et al. developed an elegant, although complex, ionization chamber that measures $^{14}CO_2$ continuously as well as cumulative expired CO_2 that provides peak activity, specific activity, and computer-programmed readouts of time-activity curves.[187]

The most commonly used technique for measuring exhaled $^{14}CO_2$ is that introduced by Abt and von Schuching, in which the gas is collected in a liquid scintillation vial containing a measured amount of organic base (e.g. Hyamine) and some pH indicator such as phenolphthalein.[188] The subject exhales into the collecting vial until the indicator just changes color as the solution goes from base to acid. Multiple samples are obtained at various times to construct a timed excretion curve. The duration of collection depends on the normality of the hyamine. The pH indicator quantifies the total CO_2 collected so that specific activity can be determined. A water trap is often added to remove water and prevent later quenching when the sample is counted. Liquid scintillation cocktail is then added to the vial and the total activity determined in a liquid scintillation counter. Figure 28 shows a diagram of the steps involved in measuring the metabolism of ^{14}C-urea by *Helicobacter* (formerly *Campylobacter*) *pylori*.

To normalize for body size, the results may be expressed in terms of body weight. The percent dose excreted is determined by calculating: DPM × 100 × body weight (kg)/ DPM administered × mmol CO_2 collected. An example of a calculation is given below:

- DPM of standard = 176,000;
- Proportion of dose administered in standard = 1/125;
- Weight of patient = 82 kg;
- Concentration of hyamine = 0.25 mmol;
- Volume of collecting solution = 2 mL;
- DPM of sample at time t = 6400.

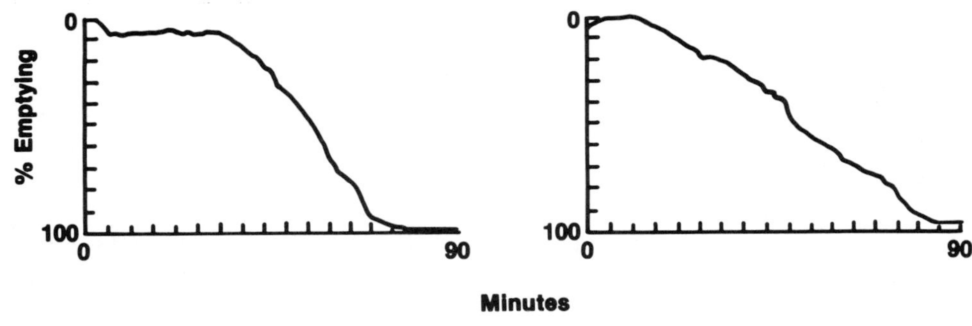

Figure 27. Dumping syndrome in a patient with a Billroth II gastrojejunostomy: Left, the baseline postoperative study shows a long lag phase followed by very rapid complete emptying. Right, on oral therapy with Donnatal, the lag phase has shortened and emptying is more gradual; the patient's symptoms improved as well.

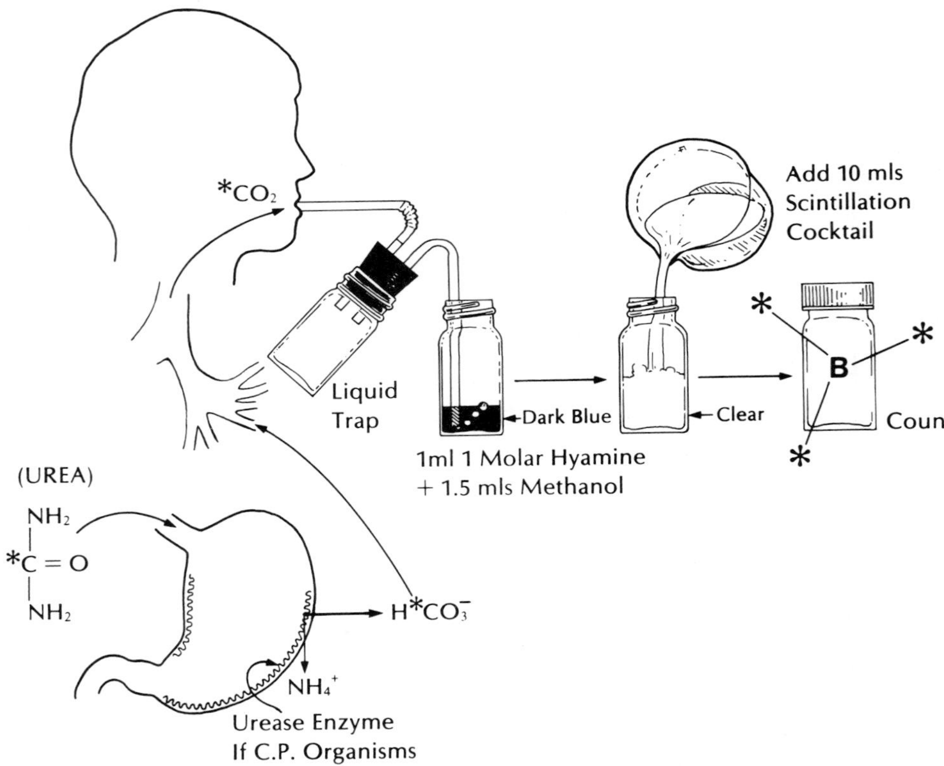

Figure 28. If urease-producing organisms are present in the gastric mucosa, ^{14}C urea is hydrolyzed, forming $^{14}CO_2$ which is expired in the breath. Patients exhale through a water trap, into a 20-mL vial containing methanol, hyamine, and a pH indicator until the blue (alkaline) solution becomes colorless upon CO_2 saturation. Scintillation cocktail is added to the sample and counted in a liquid scintillation counter. (Reproduced with permission of Marshall, et al[202]).

Then,

$$\% \text{ dose excreted} = \frac{6400 \times 100 \times 82}{(176{,}000 \times 125) \times (2 \times .25)} = 4.77$$

Carbon-13. Stable ^{13}C has a natural abundance of about 1.1%, so that labeled substrates must utilize enriched ^{13}C. Because ^{13}C is not radioactive, $^{13}CO_2$ must be measured by other means than radiation detection. It is possible to measure $^{13}CO_2$ using mass spectrometry[189] or by infrared spectroscopy.[190,191] Because $^{13}CO_2$ occurs naturally in the breath, the "background" concentration must be determined for each individual.[189] Because C-13 does not involve any radiation hazard, its use may be more acceptable for children, pregnant women, and mass screening. The techniques involved in measuring ^{13}C are somewhat more complex than is entailed in the use of ^{14}C, the tests may be less sensitive, and they are often more expensive.

CLINICAL APPLICATIONS

Several potential clinical applications exist for breath tests. However, it must be kept in mind that all uses must be regulated by institutional review committees, because no radiolabeled substrates have been approved by the US Food and Drug Administration (FDA) for routine diagnostic use.

Intestinal Absorption. In labeled carbon tests of malabsorption states, a labeled substrate is administered orally and the quantity of labeled CO_2 liberated is measured over several hours. It is then compared with the time-activity curves from normal controls. Malabsorption of fats has been extensively studied using ^{14}C trioctanoin,[192] ^{14}C glyceryl-tripalmitate[193,194] and ^{14}C triolein.[195,196] Figure 29 shows the time-activity curves of expired $^{14}CO_2$ after ingestion of ^{14}C tripalmitin by healthy subjects and patients with fat malabsorption. These tests have largely been developed to replace the 72-hour fecal fat test.

Deficiency States. Fish et al. demonstrated that the metabolism of ^{14}C propionic acid is decreased in vitamin B_{12} deficiency because B_{12} is utilized in the metabolism of methylmalonyl CoA to succinyl CoA.[197] Folic acid deficiency can be distinguished from B_{12} deficiency because propionic acid is metabolized normally in that condition. On the other hand, the metabolism of ^{14}C histidine is decreased in folic acid deficiency and normal in B_{12} deficiency. Lactase deficiency has also been studied using ^{14}C-l-lactose as the substrate.[198] However, as discussed above, this test has largely been replaced by the hydrogen breath test.

Bacterial Overgrowth. The excessive deconjugation and absorption of bile salts have been studied with a number of abnormalities of the enterohepatic circulation, including "blind-loop" syndrome, ileal resection, bypass operations, and excessive bacterial colonization using glycine-^{14}C-cholate or glycine-^{13}C-cholate. Currently the most sensitive test for bacterial colonization is the ^{14}C xylose breath test.[199] Xylose is absorbed in the small bowel and not hydrolyzed to CO_2. In small bowel bacterial colonization, $^{14}CO_2$ of fer-

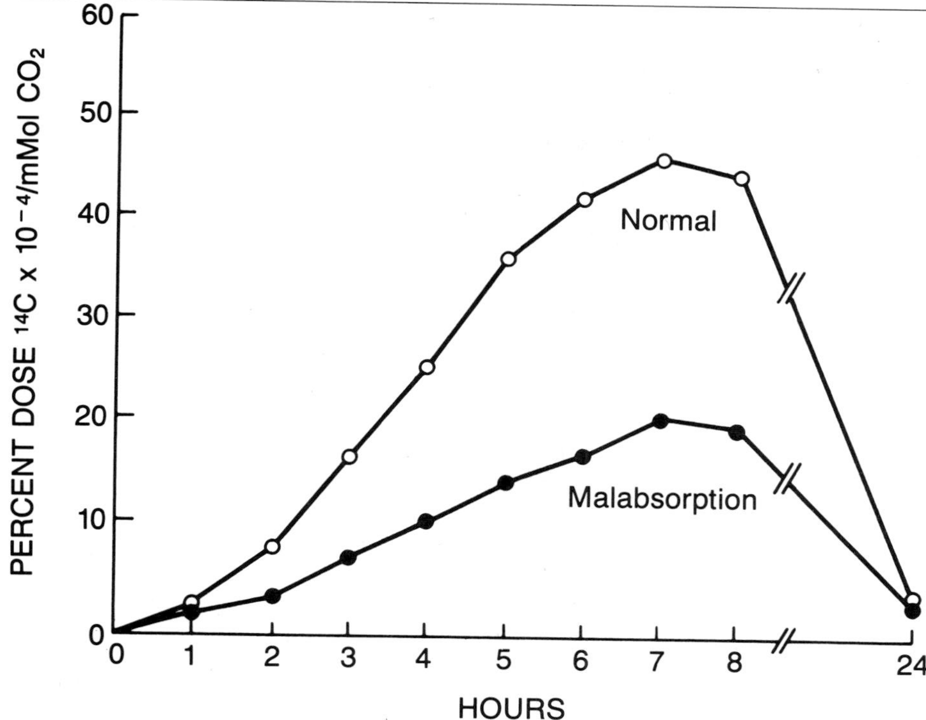

Figure 29. Time course of specific activity of expired $^{14}CO_2$ after oral ^{14}C tripalmitin by normal subjects and patients with fat malabsorption (Courtesy of Dr. Walton Shreeve).

mentation is produced and detected in the breath. In fact, the ^{14}C xylose test may be more sensitive for detecting small bowel bacteria than cultures of small bowel aspirates.

Recently, a relation between peptic ulcer disease and the presence of *Helicobacter pylori* has been demonstrated.[200] These organisms contain plentiful quantities of urease, an enzyme not present in mammalian cells and absent from the normal human gastric mucosa.[201] Identification of these bacteria by nonradiometric techniques generally requires intestinal biopsy, hardly a convenient screening test. Oral administration of ^{14}C urea, which is metabolized by the bacteria, provides the substrate for a convenient breath analysis[202–204] (Figs. 28 and 30).

Other carbon dioxide breath tests that have been shown to have clinical or research utility include:

- labeled aminopyrine to assess microsomal liver function in cirrhosis and hepatitis,[205–208]
- labeled galactose to study galactose tolerance in cirrhotic patients,[209–211]
- labeled glucose to study altered glucose metabolism in diabetics and obesity,[212–214]
- labeled glycine to study hyperglycinemia,[215]
- labeled hydroxytryptopan in depression,[216]
- labeled asparagine in neoplasia,[217]
- labeled phenylalanine in phenylketonuria.[218]

GASTROINTESTINAL BLEEDING

Effective therapy of acute gastrointestinal bleeding depends on accurate localization of the site of bleeding. The history and clinical findings can usually distinguish upper from lower gastrointestinal bleeding. Upper tract bleeding can often be confirmed with gastric intubation and localized with flexible fiberoptic endoscopy; however, lower gastrointestinal bleeding is more problematic. During active hemorrhage, endoscopy and barium studies are of limited value in the small bowel and colon. Angiography can only be successful in detecting the site of bleeding if contrast injection coincides with active bleeding; however, hemorrhage is typically intermittent. The clinical determination of whether the patient is actively bleeding is difficult because the signs of active bleeding are often present only after the hemorrhage has ceased. Because repeated angiographic studies are not practical, it is often the angiographers who request radionuclide gastrointestinal bleeding studies prior to performing angiography. This is to insure that the patient is, indeed, actively bleeding and to localize the approximate site of bleeding so that the length of the angiographic study and the amount of contrast used can be minimized.

Radionuclide Studies

Chromium-51 labeled red blood cells (RBCs) was the first radiopharmaceutical used to detect and quantify gastrointestinal bleeding.[219] Although this non-imaging method allowed quantification of blood loss by measuring stool samples, and localization of bleeding by withdrawing samples from various regions of the gastrointestinal tract, it was not found to be clinically practical or very accurate and, therefore, was not widely used. In 1977, Alavi et al.[220] first described the scintigraphic imaging of active gastrointestinal bleeding with ^{99m}Tc-sulfur colloid (^{99m}Tc-SC) and, in 1979, Winzelberg et al.[221] described the use of ^{99m}Tc-labeled red blood cells (^{99m}Tc-RBC), leading to our present day approach for localizing the site of active bleeding noninvasively.

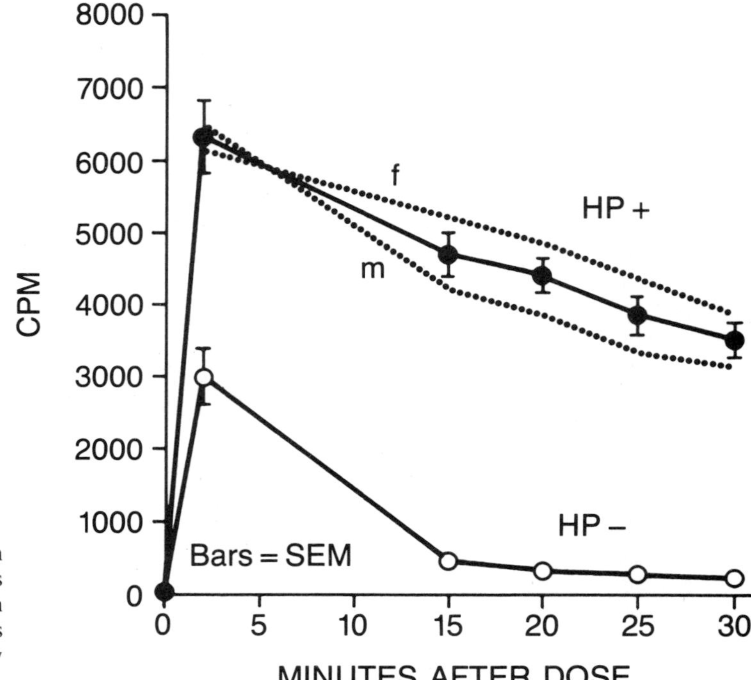

Figure 30. Time-activity curve displaying the $^{14}CO_2$ excretion after oral administration of 185 kBq (5μCi) ^{14}C urea in subjects with and without positive cultures for *H. pylori*. Females with *H. pylori* give slightly higher cpm due to lower endogenous $^{14}CO_2$ production. (Reproduced with permission of Dr. Barry Marshall.)

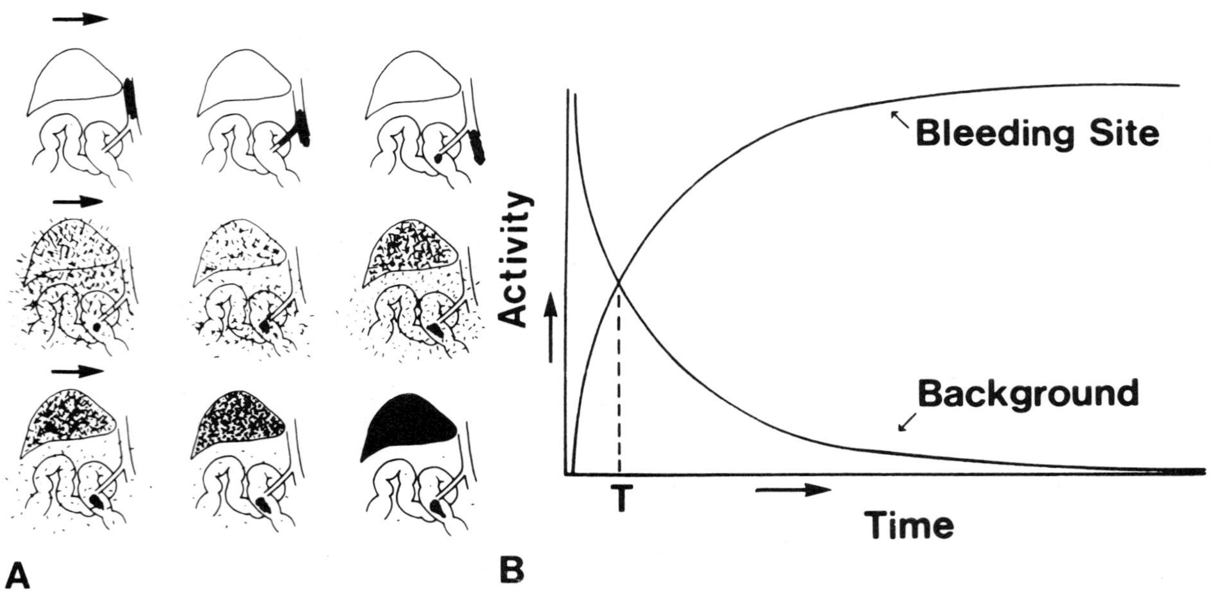

Figure 31. Theoretical basis for ^{99m}Tc-SC gastrointestinal bleeding study. **(A).** The intravenously injected ^{99m}Tc-SC is cleared by the reticuloendothelial system with a clearance half-life of 2.5–3.5 min, so that by 15 min after injection most activity is cleared from the vascular system. With active bleeding, a fraction of injected radioactivity will extravasate at the site of bleeding. Because of the rapid background clearance, a high contrast between the bleeding site and surrounding background results. **(B).** Time activity-curves demonstrate the exponential clearance of background after injection and exponential increase in activity at the bleeding site. Detectability begins when the two curves cross (point T). (With permission, Alavi A, Ring EJ: Localization of gastrointestinal bleeding: superiority of 99mTc sulfur colloid compared with angiography. *AJR* 1981;137:741–748.[222])

Table 16. Technique for ^{99m}Tc-SC Gastrointestinal Bleeding Scintigraphy

1. The patient is placed supine before injection under a large-field-of-view gamma camera with a high-resolution, low-energy parallel-hole collimator interfaced with a computer.
2. The field-of-view should include the entire abdomen and pelvis.
3. ^{99m}Tc-SC, 10 mCi (370 MBq), is injected as a bolus and 1 s flow images obtained for 1 min.
4. 500,000 to 750,000 count anterior images of the abdomen are acquired every 1–2 min for 20 min with the intensity setting set so that bone marrow is visualized.
5. Oblique, lateral, and posterior views are obtained as needed to confirm the site of bleeding.
6. If no bleeding site is detected, 10^6-count image of the upper abdomen is obtained with obliques to evaluate the hepatic and splenic flexures. If negative, repeat views of the lower abdomen are taken 15 min later to check for activity that may have been obscured in the hepatic and splenic flexures.
7. If the patient has a bowel movement during the study, this should be scanned to detect a low rectal source of bleeding.
8. If the scan is negative and recurrent active bleeding suspected, a repeat dose of ^{99m}Tc-SC is given and the same protocol repeated.

The use of ^{99m}Tc-SC for detecting acute gastrointestinal hemorrhage was based on the following theoretical considerations: after intravenous injection, this radiopharmaceutical is rapidly extracted by the reticuloendothelial cells of the liver, spleen, and bone marrow with a clearance half-time of 2.5 to 3.5 minutes; by 12 to 15 minutes after injection most of the activity is cleared from the vascular system. During active gastrointestinal bleeding, a fraction of the radiotracer will extravasate at the site of bleeding into the gastrointestinal lumen with each recirculation of blood. The continued extravasation and simultaneous background clearance results in a high target-to-background ratio, allowing visualization of the active bleeding site (Fig. 31).

Details of the "Alavi" method[222] are described in Table 16. In experimental animal studies, bleeding rates as low as 0.05 to 0.1 mL/min have been detected in dogs.[220]

Although not part of the originally described protocol, an initial flow study is sometimes helpful. Rapid bleeding may be detected on the 1 second/frame blood flow images. This may be particularly helpful in confirming the site of bleeding in easily obscured areas (e.g., the hepatic and splenic flexures). In addition, vascular blushes of tumors, angiodysplasia, and arteriovenous malformations may be visualized in the absence of active bleeding. Active hemorrhage is most commonly detected in the first 5 to 10 minutes of imaging on the static high-count images. The site of bleeding is identified as a focal area of radiotracer accumulation which increases in intensity and moves through the intestinal tract during the course of the study (Fig. 32). Because blood acts as an intestinal irritant, movement is often rapid and *bidirectional*. A fixed region of radiotracer accumulation that does not move is not likely to represent intraluminal hemorrhage. An ectopic spleen is a common cause for this finding. Renal transplants may accumulate radiocolloid. Asymmetric marrow activity can also be misleading. For example, marrow replacement by tumor, infarction, or fibrosis may make the adjacent marrow appear as focal uptake and suggest a bleeding site. The critical diagnostic point is that this uptake does not move. If the initial study is negative, but recurrent active bleeding is suspected clinically, a repeat study using a second dose of ^{99m}Tc-SC is recommended.[223]

Due to the large amount of uptake in the liver and spleen, this method is recommended primarily for evaluating lower gastrointestinal bleeding. Detection of bleeding in the splenic flexure and transverse colon can sometimes be difficult, although flow images, frequent repeated static images, and the rapid movement of intraluminal contents may detect the bleeding site.

CLINICAL RESULTS

Alavi et al.[222] initially studied 43 patients using ^{99m}Tc-SC and compared the results with contrast angiography. Of 23 patients with a positive ^{99m}Tc-SC study in the first 5 to 10 minutes, the etiology of the bleeding was determined in 19 using various correlative modalities. Extravasation of contrast was detected angiographically at sites corresponding to those detected by scintigraphy in 11 patients. Both studies were negative in 20 patients.

Winn et al.,[224] using a similar technique, visualized images in 63 patients with 82 studies. Thirteen studies were positive for lower gastrointestinal bleeding; angiography was positive in only three. Of 69 negative studies in 50 patients, 13 had angiography; 10 were negative, two positive, and one equivocal. The authors found this method to be a good screening test and particularly helpful in directing the angiographer to the site of active bleeding.

Other investigators have also found the ^{99m}Tc-SC method useful.[225–227] In one report,[227] 4 of 5 patients had positive studies, 2 with intermittently bleeding hypervascular lesions were positive only on the flow images, and 2 others had both positive flow and static phases.

^{99m}Tc-RBCs. The use of ^{99m}Tc-labeled red cells to diagnose gastrointestinal bleeding has the theoretical advantage over ^{99m}Tc-SC that extravasation at the site of bleeding can be detected over a much longer period of time, dependent only on the physical half-life of ^{99m}Tc and the stability of the radiolabel. This could be an important advantage because gastrointestinal bleeding is typically intermittent and often not active at the time of radiotracer injection.

RBC labeling. A high labeling efficiency is important for proper interpretation of the ^{99m}Tc-RBC bleeding study. Free unbound ^{99m}Tc-pertechnetate is taken up by the salivary glands and gastric mucosa and then secreted into the gastrointestinal tract, potentially complicating interpretation of the study. Various labeling techniques have been used. All de-

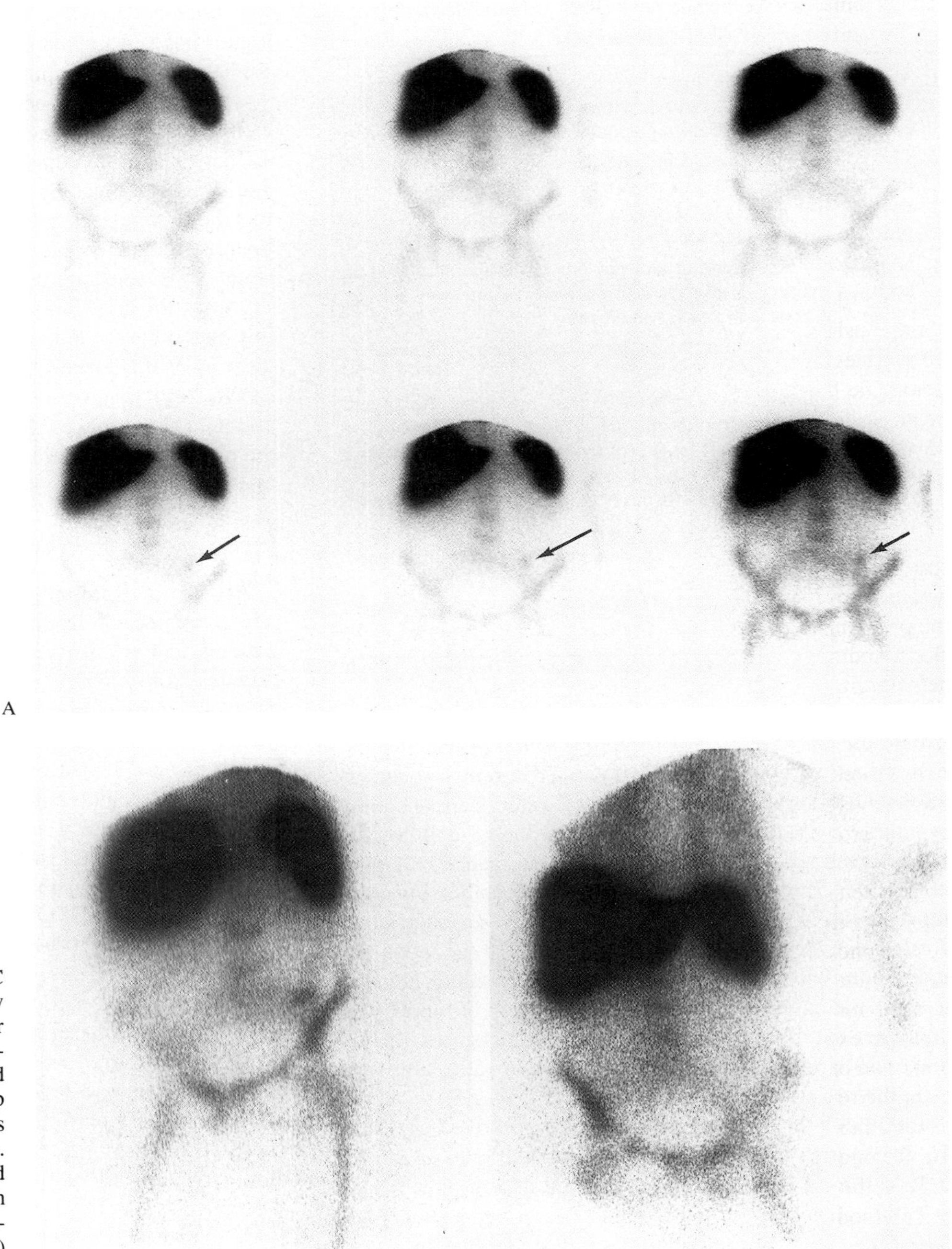

Figure 32. Positive ^{99m}Tc-SC study: **(A).** Images every 3 min show increasing activity in the left lower quadrant between 12–15 min (bottom 3 images). **(B).** LAO (left) and RAO (right) images at 30 min help confirm that the site of bleeding is in the region of the sigmoid colon. Some retrograde movement of blood can be seen on the LAO view. (With permission, Patrick Peller, MD, Walter Reed Hospital, Washington, DC.)

pend on the ability of the stannous ion to reduce ^{99m}Tc intracellularly, thereby binding to hemoglobin.[228] Extracellular stannous ion in the serum can cause unwanted reduction of ^{99m}Tc-pertechnetate prior to its entry into RBCs. Only the oxidized form of ^{99m}Tc can be transported into the erythrocyte.

The in vivo labeling method[229] was originally used because of its clinical simplicity. Nonradioactive (cold) tin as stannous chloride (in a stannous pyrophosphate complex) is injected intravenously, followed 10 to 20 minutes later by injection of the ^{99m}Tc-pertechnetate. However, the labeling efficiency (fraction of totally administered pertechnetate incorporated into the red cells) is variable, ranging from 60 to 90%.[230] For cardiac wall motion studies this may be adequate, but not for gastrointestinal bleeding studies. Alternatively, in vitro red blood cell labeling uniformly achieves >98% labeling, minimizing the likelihood of false-positive studies from free ^{99m}Tc-pertechnetate, and greatly improves the target-to-background ratio. However, until recently, in vitro labeling methods required multiple manipulations of red cells in a sterile laboratory environment, blood centrifugation, and cell washing before reinjection. It was time consuming, had potential for contamination, and was not commercially available.

A modified in vivo labeling method has been popularized.[231] Similar to the in vivo method, patients first receive an intravenous injection of cold stannous ion. Then several milliliters of blood are drawn into a heparinized syringe containing ^{99m}Tc-pertechnetate, which remains attached to the patient via a butterfly and stopcock assembly; the syringe is never disconnected. Incubation takes place within the syringe using gentle inversion to ensure good mixing. After 10 minutes, the tagged red cells are reinjected into the patient. The labeling efficiency of this method is reported to be 90%[231] after 10 minutes, although others have found that 45 minutes of incubation is required to achieve this high labeling efficiency.[232] Although this method was clearly superior to the in vivo method, free pertechnetate can still be a problem. A further modification of this method[233] requires spinning down and disposing of the untagged ^{99m}Tc-pertechnetate before reinjection. This modified method minimizes the problem of poor tagging often caused by blood transfusions, iodinated contrast, circulating antibodies, or a low hematocrit.[230] Drugs that reduce RBC labeling efficiency include heparin, methyldopa, hydralazine, doxorubicin (Adriamycin), quinidine, digoxin, prazosin, and propranolol.

A kit technique for in vitro red blood cell labeling has been developed[234] and a commercial version has recently been approved by the FDA and is now available (Fig. 33). This method uses whole blood, does not require centrifugation (potentially damaging to red cells) or transferring red cells into sterile containers. The in vivo and modified in vivo method depend on biological clearance of undesirable extracellular reduced stannous ion and the laboratory in vitro method removes it by centrifugation, but the kit method prevents extracellular reduction of stannous ion by the addition of an oxidizing agent (sodium hypochlorite) that cannot enter the red cell. A labeling efficiency of greater than 98% results. Table 17 summarizes and compares the various labeling techniques. The radiation dose to the patient using the ^{99m}Tc-sulfur colloid technique and the ^{99m}Tc-labeled red blood cell method is quite low compared to that with contrast angiography.

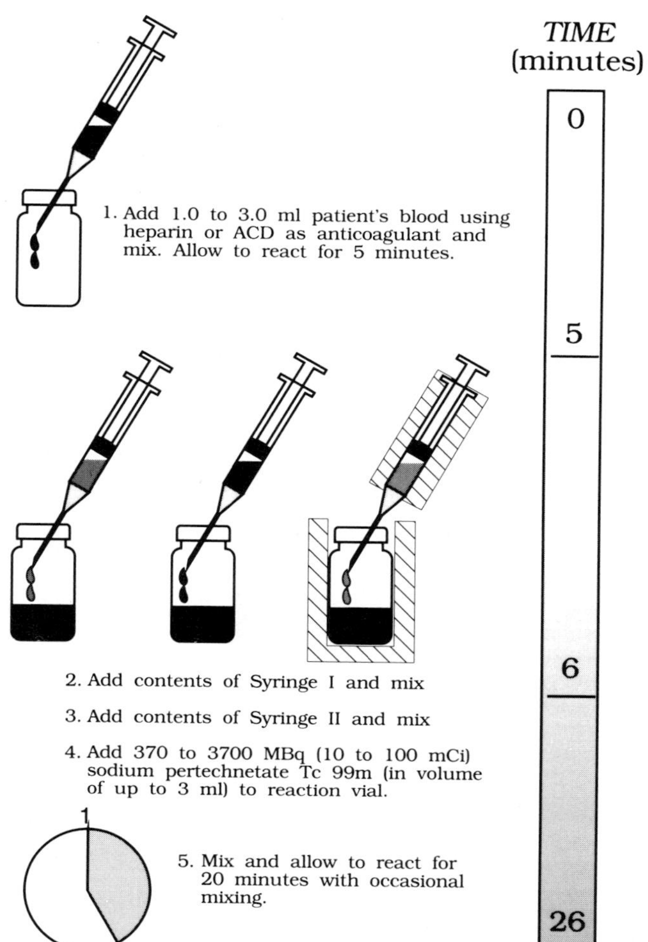

Figure 33. Simple kit technique preparation of in vitro ^{99m}Tc-labeled red blood cells (UltraTag RBC, Mallinkrodt Medical, Inc., St. Louis, MO). Each kit consists of 3 nonradioactive components: 1. A 10 mL vial containing stannous chloride, syringe I containing sodium hypochlorite, and syringe II containing citric acid, sodium citrate and dextrose. The percent labeling efficiency is greater than 98%.

^{99m}Tc-RBC Imaging Technique

A detailed imaging protocol is outlined in Table 18. The field of view should include the entire abdomen and pelvis so that the stomach, as well as the rectosigmoid colon, can be seen. The intensity is set so that the aorta, inferior vena cava, and iliac vessels are well visualized.

The radionuclide angiogram may detect vascular bleeding sources that are not actively bleeding at the moment (e.g., angiodysplasia or tumors) (Fig. 34); may define vascular structures, such as the uterus, kidneys, ectatic vessels (Fig. 35); may occasionally be helpful for detecting bleeding sites difficult to see on later dynamic imaging (e.g., those adjacent to the bladder).[235] High-count oblique or lateral images are sometimes helpful in differentiating rectosigmoid bleeding from bladder and genital activity (Figs. 36 and 37). If the initial study is negative, delayed acquisitions are obtained at intervals (e.g., 2, 4, and 24 hours) if there is clinical suspicion of recurrent bleeding. Dynamic computer acquisition is also suggested at these times.

IMAGE INTERPRETATION

Active bleeding can often be diagnosed from intermittent static images during the first 60 minutes of acquisition. To make this diagnosis, the extravascular activity (1) must be judged to be intraluminal, (2) must be increasing over time and, (3) must be moving through the gastrointestinal tract (Figs. 36 to 42). Activity that does not move should not be

Table 17. Methods for ^{99m}Tc-Red Blood Cell Labeling

In vivo method
1. Inject stannous pyrophosphate,
2. wait 10–20 minutes,
3. inject ^{99m}Tc-sodium pertechnetate.

Modified in vivo method
1. Inject stannous pyrophosphate,
2. wait 10–20 minutes,
3. withdraw 5–8 mL whole blood into shielded syringe containing ^{99m}Tc-sodium pertechnetate,
4. gently mix syringe contents for 10 min at room temperature.

In vitro (Brookhaven) method
1. Add 4 ml heparinized whole blood to reagent vial containing: 2.0 mg Sn+2, 3.67 mg Na citrate, 5.5 mg dextrose, 0.11 mg NaCl,
2. incubate at room temperature for 5 min,
3. add 2.0 mL 4.4% EDTA,
4. centrifuge tube for 5 min at 1300 G,
5. withdraw 1.25 mL of packed red cells, transfer to sterile vial containing 1–3 mL ^{99m}Tc-sodium pertechnetate,
6. incubate at room temperature for 10 min.

In vitro commercial kit method 2
1. Add 1.0 to 3.0 mL of whole blood (heparin or ACD as anticoagulant) to reagent vial (50–100 μg stannous chloride, 3.67 sodium citrate) and mix; allow to react for 5 min,
2. add contents of syringe 1 (0.6 mg sodium hypochlorite) and mix by gently inverting 4–5 times,
3. add contents of syringe 2 (citric acid 8.7 mg, sodium citrate 32.5 mg, dextrose) and mix,
4. add 370 to 3700 MBq (10–100 mCi) sodium pertechnetate ^{99m}Tc to reaction vial,
5. mix and allow to react for 20 min with occasional mixing.

diagnosed as an active bleeding site, and is often due to a fixed vascular structure, as described above. "Pitfalls" in diagnosis are listed in Table 19. For example, poor labeling can result in bladder activity; lateral images may be needed

Table 18. Technique for ^{99m}Tc-RBC Scintigraphy

1. Camera: large field-of-view scintillation camera with parallel hole high-resolution collimator and computer.
2. Computer settings: 1 s frames × 60, then 1 min frames for 60–90 min. Each subsequent delayed imaging period (e.g., at 2 and 4 hrs and up to 24 hrs) is acquired continuously on computer at 1 min/frame for 20–30 min.
3. Patient is positioned supine and imaged anteriorly. The field-of-view should include the entire abdomen and pelvis.
4. The ^{99m}Tc-RBCs are injected as a bolus.
5. Analog images are acquired as 2-s flow images and 10^6-count images every 5 min.
6. After the initial acquisition, selected oblique and lateral images are obtained as required.
7. Additional images to include the areas of the salivary and thyroid glands, heart, and stomach to evaluate the adequacy of labeling and the presence of free pertechnetate.

to differentiate rectosigmoid bleeding from radioactivity in the bladder, uterus, or penis (Fig. 36). Free pertechnetate can be a particularly troublesome problem due to gastric uptake simulating a gastric bleed or bleeding more distally, particularly on delayed images (Fig. 37).

Frequent imaging is critical for determining the site of bleeding. Review of computer-acquired images on cinematic display can aid in detecting the bleeding source and anatomically defining the bowel involved, confirm suspected retrograde movement of blood, and help differentiate ureteral clearance from gastrointestinal bleeding.

Small bowel bleeding can be particularly troublesome to localize. The cecum is often the site of pooling of a more proximal small bowel bleed. Glucagon has been advocated as a method to aid in the diagnosis of small bowel bleeds.[236] After injection, bowel peristalsis is inhibited, resulting in pooling of the radiotracer in the small bowel at the site of the active bleed. Note should be made of any evidence of bleeding from the stomach and duodenum. Although an upper gastrointestinal bleed should be detected clinically by aspiration from a nasogastric tube placed in the stomach prior to scintigraphy, this is not always the case. Images of the thyroid, salivary glands, and heart at the end of the 60 to 90-minute acquisition can help evaluate the red cell labeling efficiency and the presence or absence of free pertechnetate (Fig. 38). Recommendations in the past have suggested nasogastric suction, perchlorate, or cimetidine administration to minimize the problem of free pertechnetate.[237–239] With the use of the new in vitro kit technique, this is rarely a problem.

Intraluminal radioactivity first detected on delayed images can be a diagnostic dilemma. Blood first seen in the sigmoid colon or rectum on a single delayed image at 18 to 24 hours could have originated from anywhere in the gastrointestinal tract, or be due to the transit of free pertechnetate. The study can sometimes turn out to be an expensive alternative to a stool guiaiac, and this has caused some clinical skepticism on the utility of this technique. Extreme caution is urged in overinterpreting the site of bleeding based on delayed images only, unless active bleeding is observed. A recent report suggests that, when the first evidence of bleeding is seen on delayed images, it may be helpful to reinject the patient at that time and reimage.[240] Some of these patients will demonstrate active bleeding with reinjection. The origin of activity seen only on delayed images is more likely to be from the stomach or small bowel than from the colon.[241]

Efficacy of Scintigraphy

In 1979, Winzelberg et al.[221] first described the use of in vivo labeled RBCs in 10 patients for the diagnosis of acute gastrointestinal bleeding. Although able to localize angiographically confirmed bleeding sites in the duodenum, small bowel, and colon, gastric activity occurred in 50% of patients. In a subsequent larger series[242] these investigators used the modified in vivo method of red cell labeling, which

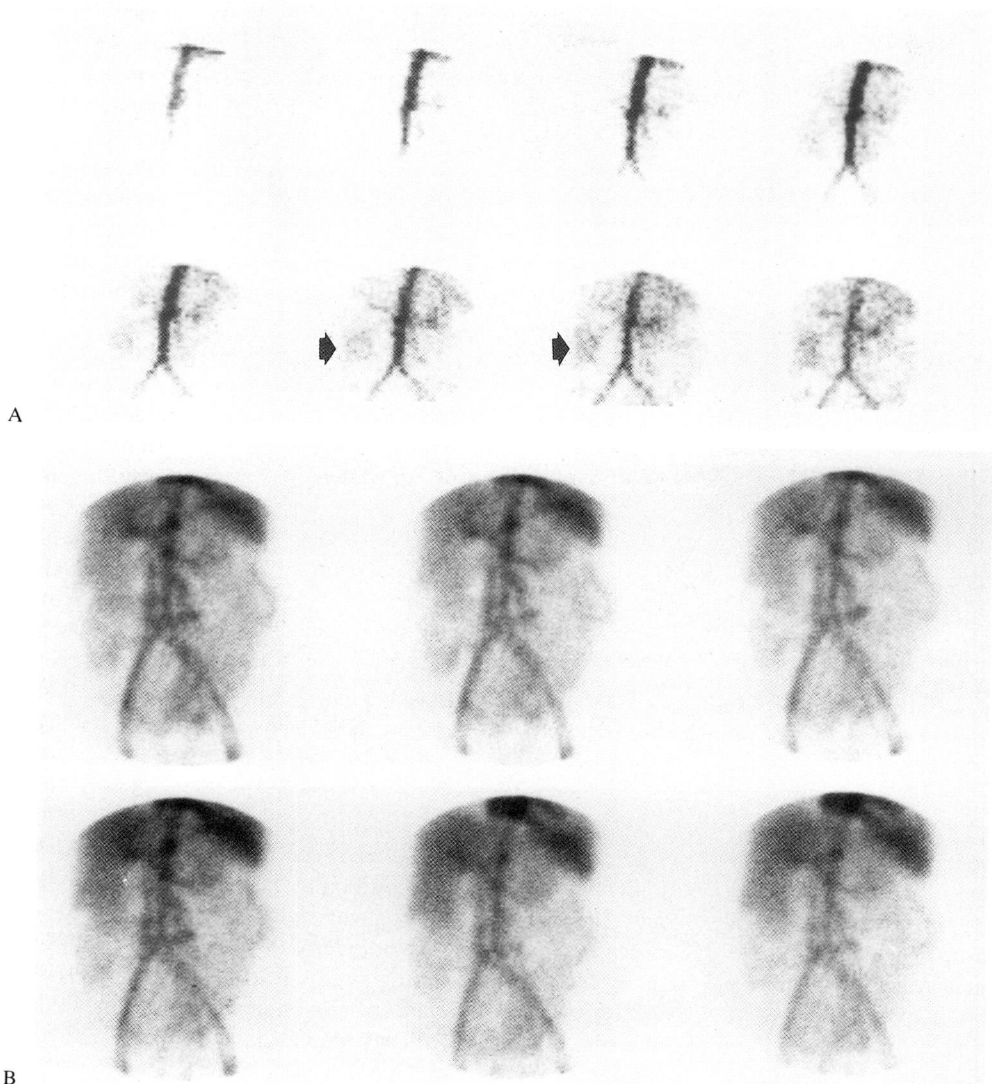

Figure 34. Utility of the radionuclide angiogram phase of the ^{99m}Tc-RBC study. This 72-year-old female has had several brief episodes of gastrointestinal bleeding, the most recent one being 3 hours prior to this study. **(A).** The flow study shows hyperperfusion in the region of the right lower quadrant (arrow heads). **(B).** The 90-min dynamic study shows no definite bleeding site, although some mildly increased blood pool is seen in the same region. Exploratory laparotomy due to recurrent bleeding revealed an inflamed diverticulum in the right colon as the source.

significantly reduced this problem.[231] Of 32 patients with documented active gastrointestinal bleeding, 29 had positive studies (91% sensitivity). Of 18 patients without confirmed bleeding, 17 had negative studies (95% specificity). Twelve of 29 patients had positive studies at 6 to 24 hours. The authors recommend that if initial scintigraphy is negative, emergency angiography should not be performed because the likelihood of a diagnostic study is low. Later elective angiography might be indicated in those with suspected angiodysplasia or small-bowel tumors. A positive scan was found especially helpful to the angiographer for determining which vessel to study. In a updated report of 80 patients at the same institution,[243] bleeding was detected in 65% of patients with bright red blood per rectum, 71% of patients with melena, and in none with occult bleeding and chronic anemia. No further hemorrhage occurred in 26 of 27 patients who had negative studies.[243] In their review of 100 accumulated patients,[244] these investigators noted that in 83% of patients tagged red blood cell studies had correctly located the site of bleeding when compared to angiography, endoscopy, or surgery. Over 80% of studies were positive after the first hour, although misinterpretation occurred regarding the exact bleeding site when frequent images were not obtained. In 2 of 12 patients with a gastric or duodenal origin of bleeding, scintigraphy incorrectly identified the cecum as the source, and in 3 of 9 patients with small bowel pathology bleeding was incorrectly localized to the colon. Five patients with occult bleeding and chronic anemia had negative studies. In 33 patients with a colonic source, the abnormality on scintigraphy was proximal to the proven lesion in 2 and distal in 3. All 5 studies localizing bleeding to the rectosigmoid colon were correct.

Other investigators have reported similar results. Smith and Arterburn[239] also used in vivo ^{99m}Tc-RBCs for diagnosing

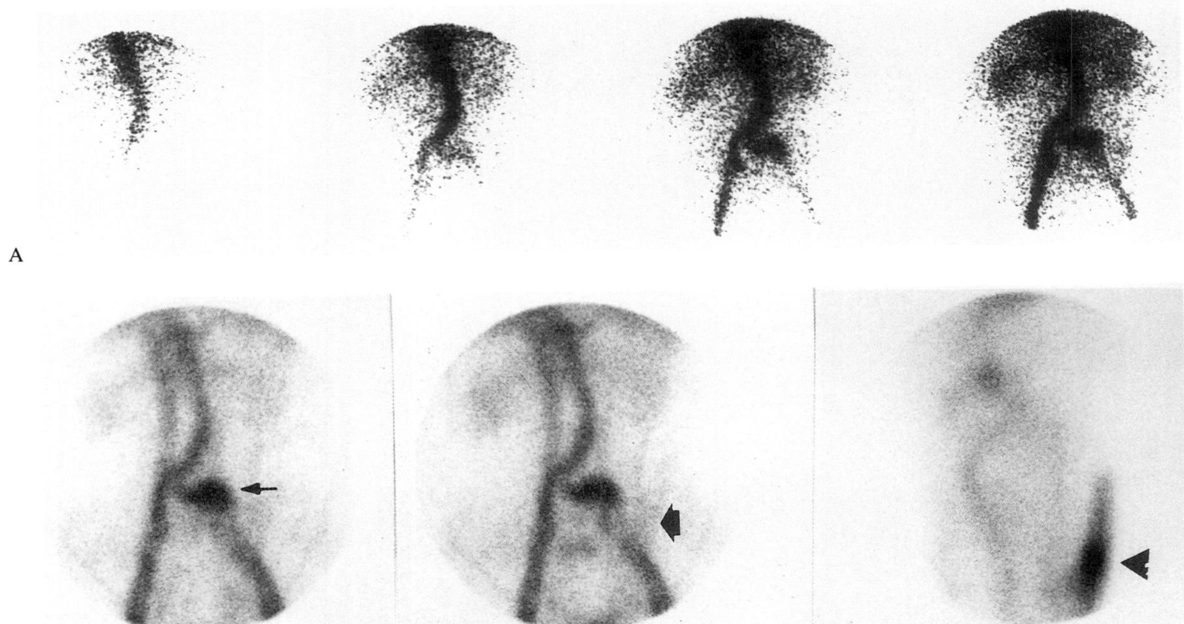

Figure 35. Aneurysmal dilatation of the left iliac artery as a potential cause of a false-positive ^{99m}Tc-RBC study. **(A).** The radionuclide angiogram is helpful in delineating the anatomical vascular abnormality. **(B).** Images obtained at 15 min (left) and 3 hr (middle) show no change in the focal iliac activity (arrow). Low-intensity activity consistent with bleeding is seen in the rectosigmoid area at 3 hours (arrowhead). A left lateral view (right) shows blood between the gluteal folds (triangle).

suspected active bleeding. They were able to distinguish upper gastrointestinal bleeding from colonic bleeding and left colon from right colon bleeding in most cases. One volunteer whose blood was labeled in vivo had a sample withdrawn by venipuncture and drank increasing volumes of the labeled blood. They were able to image activity in the epigastric area after ingestion of only 5 ml.

Markisz et al.[245] studied 39 patients with lower gastrointestinal bleeding using in vitro labeled RBCs; 17 (44%) of 39 were positive. Of those with positive studies, angiography was performed in 11; 4 were positive. Nine (82%) of 11 patients whose bleeding sites were localized by independent means had positive scintigraphy within the first 90 minutes of this study, although 8 (47%) of 17 patients with positive

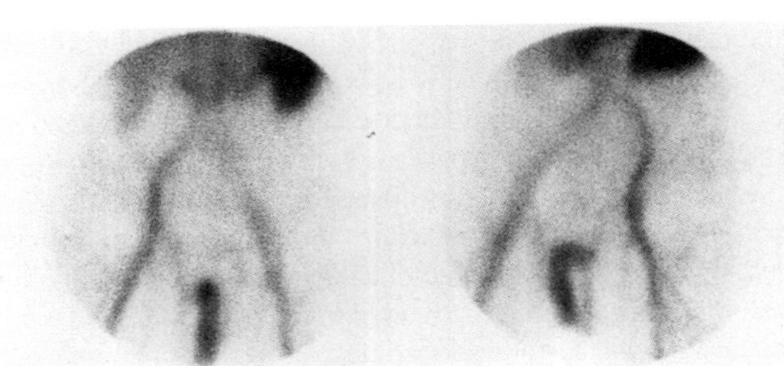

Figure 36. Normal penile activity, anterior (left) and LAO (right) views. Oblique or lateral views can differentiate rectal bleeding from bladder and penile activity.

studies were first positive between 6 and 24 hours. All 8 patients with negative scintigraphy had negative angiography. In a subset of 11 patients whose bleeding site was confirmed by surgery, angiography, or colonoscopy, scintigraphy located the bleeding site in 10 (91%). There were 6 deaths in patients with positive and none in those with negative studies. Similar efficacy studies have been reported by Bunker et al.[246] and by Gupta et al.[247]

Experimental studies using labeled RBCs[248] have detected and localized bleeding rates as low as 0.04 ml/min by 60 minutes after initiation of a simulated hemorrhage in dogs with a catheter inserted into the sigmoid lumen. Bleeding rates from 0.2 to 4.6 mL/min were all detected by 10 minutes. Only 2 to 3 ml of extravasated blood was necessary for scintigraphic detection. This was clinically validated in 62 patients by calculating mean bleeding rates.[249] The patient's transfusion volume requirements were divided by the duration of active bleeding. The minimum mean bleeding rate detectable by scintigraphy was calculated to be 0.1 mL/min.

^{99m}Tc-RBCs VS. ^{99m}Tc-SC

Considerable controversy has resulted over which radiopharmaceutical, ^{99m}Tc-SC or ^{99m}Tc-RBC is best for detection of acute gastrointestinal bleeding.[250-252] A comparison of the two methods and the theoretical advantages and disadvantages are listed in Table 20. Although the controversy has not completely abated, a general consensus has evolved in

A

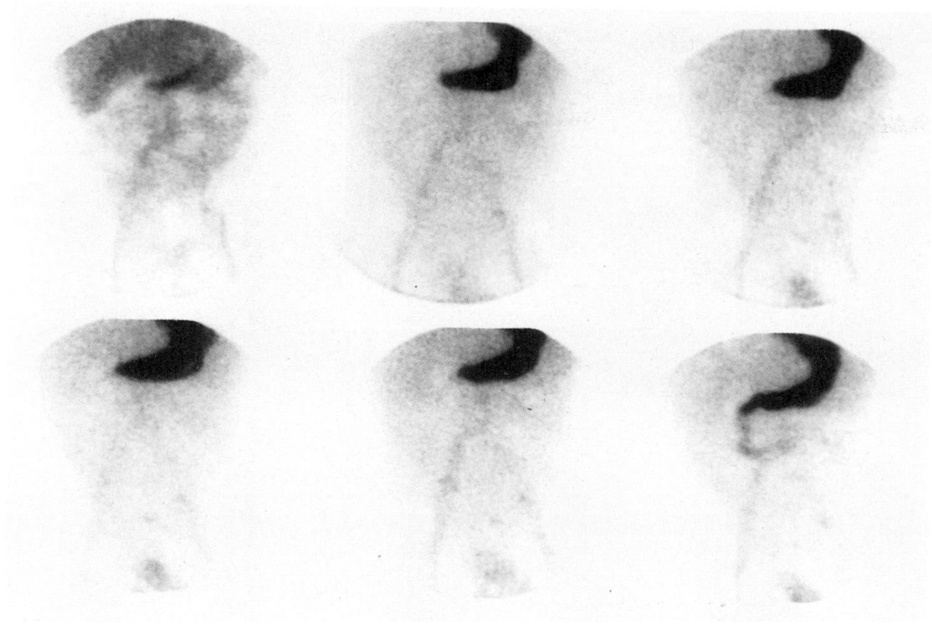

B

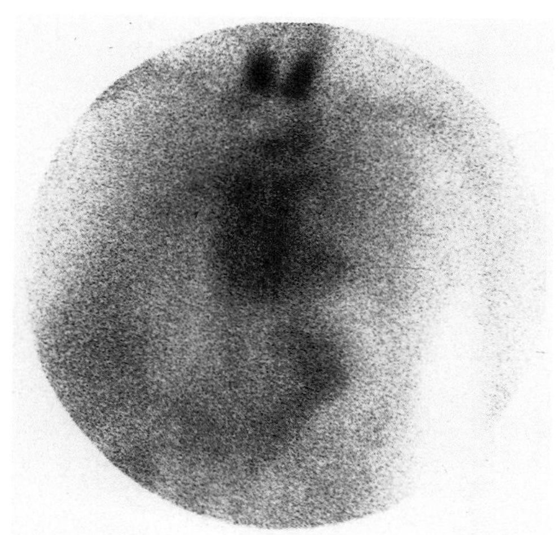

Figure 37. Hemorrhagic gastritis vs free ^{99m}Tc-pertechnetate. Although hemorrhagic gastritis may occasionally be diagnosed with a labeled red cell study, evidence for free pertechnetate should be sought. **(A).** Prominent gastric uptake increases over 60 min and moves distally. However, the target-to-background ratio is poor (e.g., the iliac and femoral vessels are poorly visualized). **(B).** Prominent uptake within the thyroid confirms the presence of free pertechnetate.

favor of ^{99m}Tc-RBC from several comparison studies described below.[253–255]

Tanasescu et al.[253] compared the results of ^{99m}Tc-SC and ^{99m}Tc in vitro-labeled RBC in 26 patients. The results were correlated with clinical, arteriographic, endoscopic, and surgical results. The ^{99m}Tc-RBC study correctly located the site of bleeding in 9 of 10 patients but no ^{99m}Tc-SC study was positive. Siddiqui et al.[254] also compared these two radiotracers in 27 bleeding patients. Only 2 ^{99m}Tc-SC studies were positive. Both of these studies were also positive with ^{99m}Tc-RBC; an additional 15 patients were positive with RBC studies. Seventy percent of the positive studies occurred after the first hour. Contrast angiography was performed following 6 positive RBC studies; no active bleeding site was visualized, although one case of angiodysplasia and another of severe gastritis were diagnosed. Colonoscopy detected bleeding sites in 3 patients correctly identified only on the ^{99m}Tc-RBC studies. Surgery confirmed the bleeding site in 1 of 2 patients that were positive on the ^{99m}Tc-RBC study.

Bunker et al.[255] reported similar comparative findings in 100 patients referred with clinical evidence of gastrointestinal bleeding. A 20-minute ^{99m}Tc-SC study was performed first, followed by an in vitro labeled ^{99m}Tc-RBC study. The reported sensitivity was 93% and specificity 95% for the ^{99m}Tc-RBC studies. The sensitivity of the ^{99m}Tc-SC studies was only 13%.

Although there appears to be convincing evidence that ^{99m}Tc-RBCs are superior to ^{99m}Tc-SC for detecting the site of active bleeding, several factors should be kept in mind. First, the "gold standard" is a poor one. Angiography is best but, because it is considerably less sensitive than scintigraphy, it cannot corroborate many positive cases. Definite endoscopic visualization or surgical confirmation of a bleed-

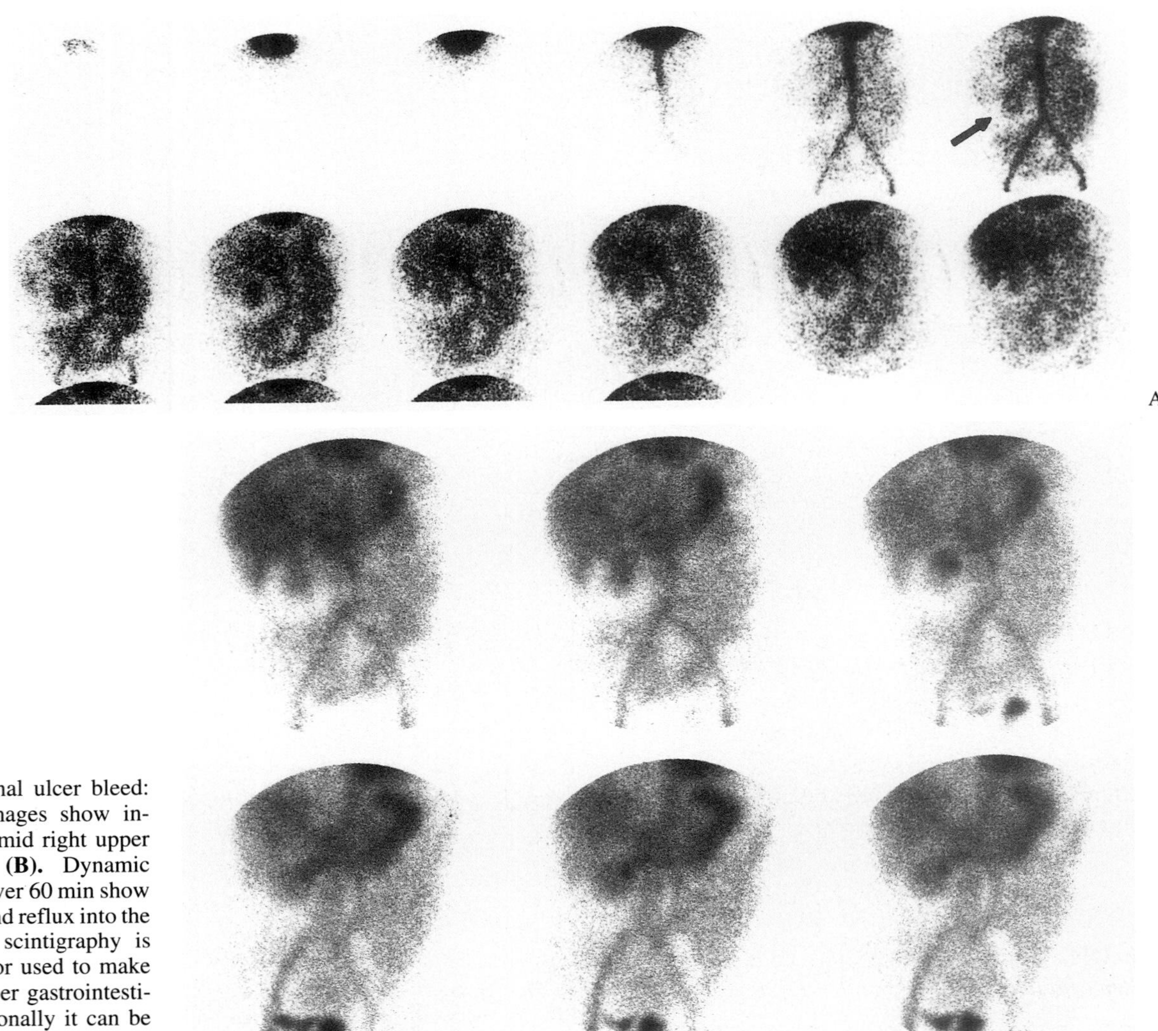

Figure 38. Duodenal ulcer bleed: **(A).** Blood flow images show increased flow to the mid right upper abdomen (arrow). **(B).** Dynamic ^{99m}Tc-RBC images over 60 min show increasing activity and reflux into the stomach. Although scintigraphy is not usually needed or used to make the diagnosis of upper gastrointestinal bleeding, occasionally it can be useful when the diagnosis is not suspected.

ing site is also adequate confirmation. However, clinical criteria, barium studies, or other methods for defining lesions but not actually proving active bleeding are inadequate. In fact, most reported studies do not have optimal confirmation for most patients, leaving room for argument. It has been argued that the comparative studies were biased against ^{99m}Tc-SC because the protocols allowed for no repeat injections of this radiotracer. On the other hand, ^{99m}Tc-RBC studies have been criticized for the problem of false-positive studies. These may occur because of (1) misinterpretation of "pitfalls" (Table 19), (2) free ^{99m}Tc-pertechnetate or, (3) over-interpretation of delayed images. In summary, ^{99m}Tc-RBC scintigraphy seems to be more sensitive than ^{99m}Tc-SC. However, its specificity is poorer because of a greater number of false-positives.

OTHER RADIOPHARMACEUTICALS FOR IMAGING GASTROINTESTINAL BLEEDING

Although only the methods of Alavi et al.[220] and Winzelberg et al.[221] have become widely used, other radiopharmaceuticals have been described for imaging gastrointestinal bleeding. ^{99m}Tc-HSA[237] has been used to detect bleeding from the esophagus, stomach, duodenum, and colon. However, the marked liver accumulation and substantial amount of free pertechnetate gives this method no theoretical advantage.[256] Large series have not been reported.

Heat-treated ^{99m}Tc-RBCs have been used[257] but limited data is available. Because of enhanced splenic clearance, a high target-to-nontarget ratio can be achieved, so that small bleeding sites may theoretically be imaged. ^{111}Indium-oxine labeled RBCS have been proposed to image intermittent

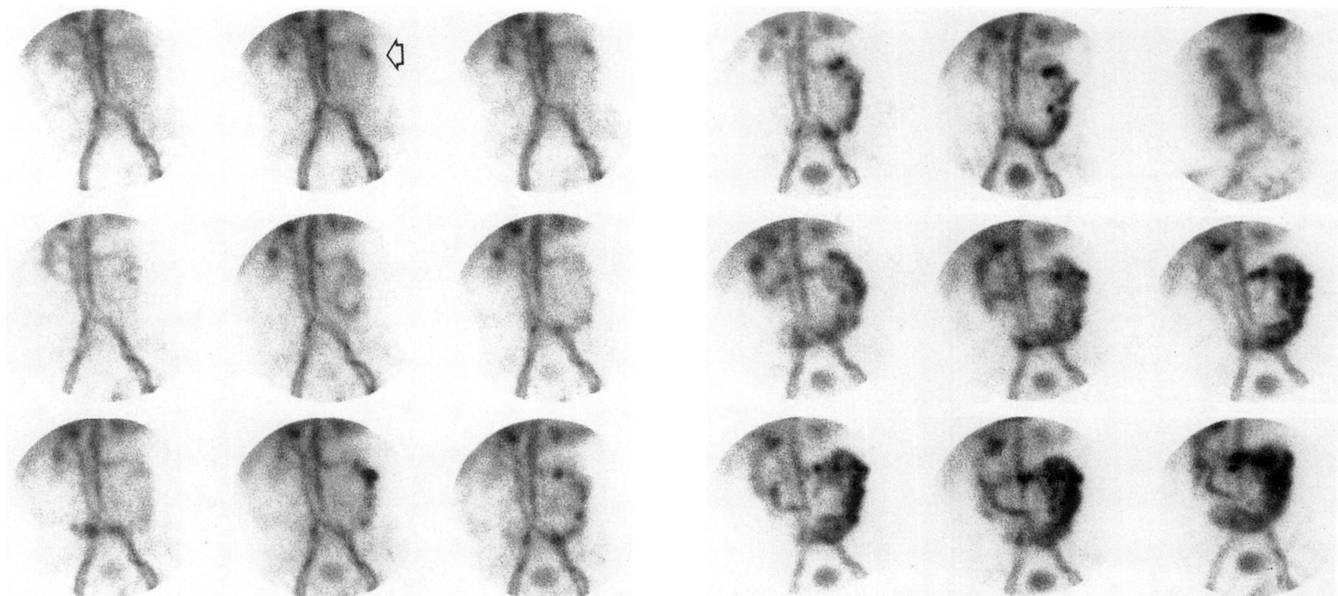

Figure 39. Active small bowel bleeding is noted in the region of the ligament of Treitz (open arrowhead). The activity increases and moves through the small bowel over 90 min.

gastrointestinal bleeding because of its long physical half-life (2.7 days).[258] ^{111}In-labeled platelets have also been used in an attempt to diagnose chronic bleeding sources.[259]

ECTOPIC GASTRIC MUCOSA

Ectopic gastric mucosa can be found in *Meckel's diverticulum*, *duplication of the gastrointestinal tract*, and *Barrett's esophagus*. A *retained gastric antrum* containing gastric mucosa may inadvertently be left behind after performing a partial gastrectomy for peptic ulcer disease. In all of these clinical situations, acid and pepsin secretion from the gastric mucosa can produce ulceration of adjacent tissue and result in serious complications. ^{99m}Tc-pertechnetate scintigraphy has been successfully used to help make these diagnoses.

Normal mucosa of the gastric fundus contains *parietal*

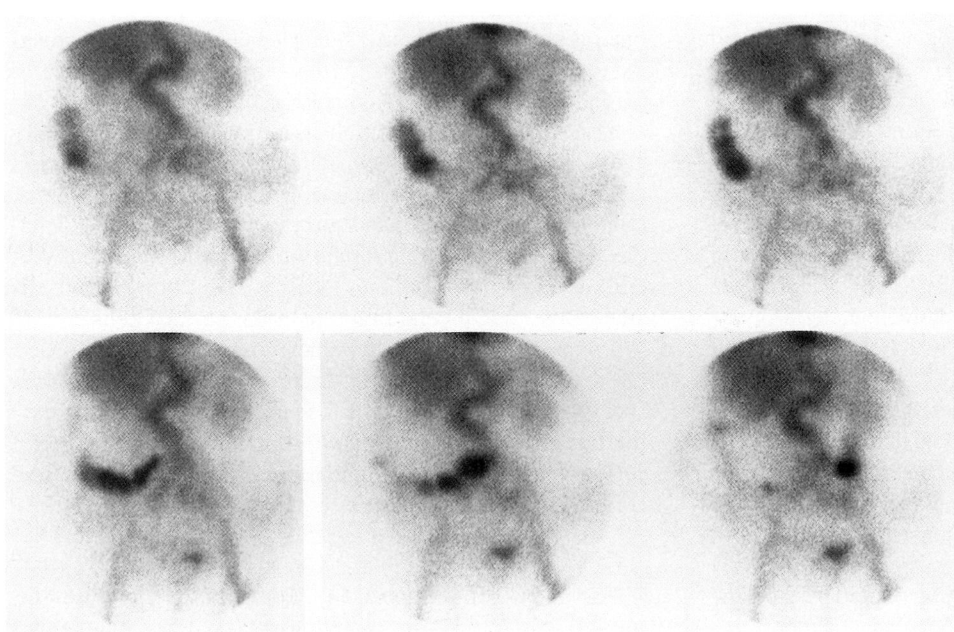

Figure 40. Hepatic flexure bleed: this elderly male has evidence of active bleeding in the region of the hepatic flexure. The blood can be seen to move along the low-lying transverse colon and into the left colon by the end of 60 min. A tortuous aorta is noted. The source of bleed in this elderly man was cancer of the colon.

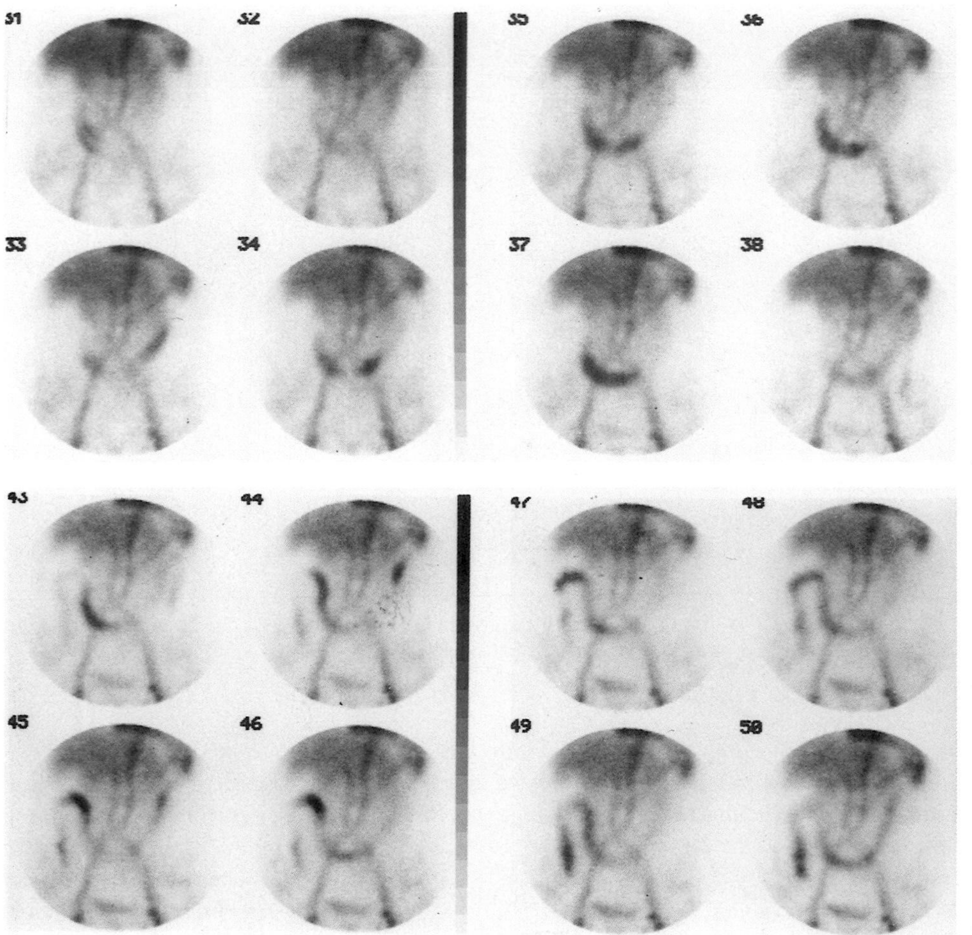

Figure 41. Sequential 1-min dynamic images show a site of active bleeding from the beginning of the study. Attention to the course of blood flow allows anatomical definition of the bleeding site to be in the proximal transverse colon. The activity moves both distally to the splenic flexure and proximally to the cecum over 10 mins.

cells, which secrete hydrochloric acid and intrinsic factor, and *chief cells* which secrete pepsinogen. The antrum and pylorus contain *G cells*, which secrete the hormone gastrin. Columnar *mucin-secreting epithelial cells* may be found throughout the stomach. Gastric secretions in both normal and ectopic gastric mucosa are stimulated by neural and hormonal mechanisms in response to the ingestion of food, serving to increase the volume and acidity of gastric secretions over the basal fasting state. The presence or absence of symptoms, the clinical presentation (e.g., bleeding vs. obstruction), and the ability of ^{99m}Tc-pertechnetate to image ectopic gastric mucosa all depend on which gastric mucosal cell types are present.

As early as 1967, it was found that the stomach could be imaged with ^{99m}Tc-pertechnetate.[260] Since that time, there has been considerable controversy as to the mechanism of gastric mucosal uptake and secretion. It was initially assumed that the parietal cells were responsible. The pertechnetate ion, in the same periodic table group as chloride, might be expected to compete with chloride in the formation of acid by the parietal cell. There is some experimental evidence to support this hypothesis. Gastric acid output parallels ^{99m}Tc-pertechnetate output, both are stimulated by pentagastrin and histamine, and one autoradiographic study in man localized ^{99m}Tc-pertechnetate to the parietal cells.[261–264] However, the predominance of evidence lies with the mucin-secreting cells. These cells excrete an alkaline juice that protects the mucosa from the highly acidic gastric fluid. Pertechnetate uptake has been found in gastric tissue with no parietal cells (e.g., pernicious anemia, retained gastric antrum, and some cases of Barrett's esophagus).[265–267] A number of animal studies confirm this, and several autoradiographic studies localize ^{99m}Tc-pertechnetate uptake to the mucin cells rather than the parietal cells.[265,268,269] Williams has proposed a hypothesis explaining this conflicting data.[270] He suggests that the predominant mechanism is specific mucin cell uptake and secretion, which is suppressible by perchlorate in a manner similar to iodide, while parietal cell uptake is a minor factor, nonspecific, secondary and, like chloride uptake, not suppressed by perchlorate.

Meckel's Diverticulum

Meckel's diverticulum is the most common congenital anomaly of the gastrointestinal tract, occurring in 1.0 to

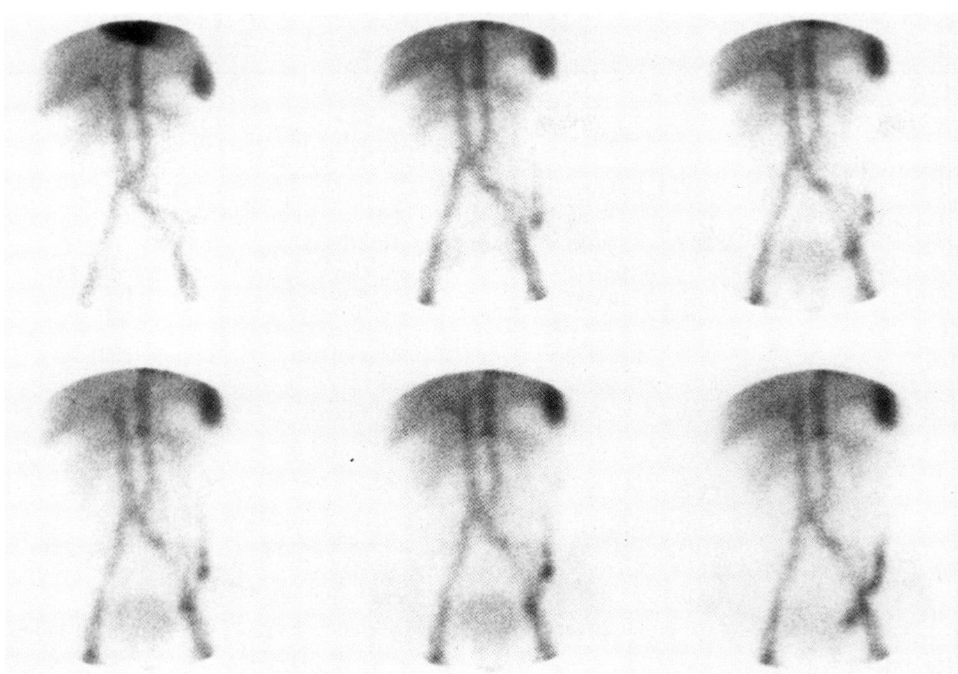

Figure 42. Left colon bleed: dynamic images over 60 min show increasingly activity in the region of the sigmoid colon that moves distally.

3.0% of the population. It results from embryonic failure of closure of the omphalo-mesenteric duct, which connects the yolk sac to the primitive foregut via the umbilical cord. This true diverticulum arises on the antimesenteric side of the small bowel, usually 80 to 90 cm proximal to the ileocecal valve, is usually only 2 to 3 cm in size, but may be considerably larger.[271,272] Gastric mucosa is present in 10 to 30% of all cases, in approximately 60% of symptomatic patients, and in about 98% of those with bleeding.[273]

CLINICAL MANIFESTATIONS

Gastric mucosa is responsible for most symptoms of Meckel's diverticulum. Gastric secretions may cause peptic ulceration of the diverticulum itself or adjacent ileum, resulting in pain, bleeding, or perforation. Sixty percent of all patients presenting with complications of Meckel's diverticulum are under the age of 2 and bleeding accounts for the majority of cases.[273]

Other manifestations of a Meckel's diverticulum, seen most commonly in adults, include intussusception, obstruction, infection, and abnormal fixation of the diverticulum. Bleeding from a Meckel's diverticulum after age 40 is unusual.

DIAGNOSIS

The preoperative diagnosis of Meckel's diverticulum was quite difficult prior to scintigraphy. It is often not identified on small bowel follow-through films because the diverticulum may have a narrow or stenotic ostium; they are often not well filled and empty rapidly.[274] Small bowel enteroclysis is felt to be a better method for detection because the higher pressure of the barium column more reliably fills the diverticulum. It is reported to have a sensitivity as high as 87%.[275] Angiography is useful only if there is brisk active bleeding and is rarely used.[276]

SCINTIGRAPHY

^{99m}Technetium-pertechnetate scanning, when first introduced in 1970 by Jewett et al., represented a major advance in the diagnosis of Meckel's diverticulum.[277] Attention to patient preparation is important. Fasting 3 to 4 hours prior to the study to decrease the size of the stomach or continuous nasogastric aspiration is recommended. A full stomach or urinary bladder may obscure an adjacent Meckel's diverticulum. Therefore, voiding prior, possibly during, and also at the end of the study is important. Sodium or potassium perchlorate is not recommended because it may block gastric mucosa uptake as it does with thyroid uptake. However, perchlorate may be administered after the study to clear the radiotracer from the thyroid, reducing radiation exposure to the gland. Barium studies should not be performed for several days prior to scintigraphy because attenuation by the contrast material may prevent lesion detection. Procedures (endoscopy) or drugs (laxatives) that irritate the intestinal mucosa may result in nonspecific ^{99m}Tc-pertechnetate uptake and should be avoided. Certain drugs, for example, ethosuximide (Zarontin), may also cause unpredictable uptake. A typical imaging protocol is described in Table 21.

Table 19. Pitfalls in Interpretation of Gastrointestinal Bleeding Scintigraphy

- Common
  - Physiological
    - Gastrointestinal
      - Stomach, small intestine, bowel (due to free pertechnetate)
    - Genitourinary
      - Pelvic kidney
      - Ectopic kidney
      - Renal pelvic activity
      - Ureter
      - Bladder
      - Uterine blush
      - Male genitalia
- Uncommon
  - Accessory spleen
  - Hepatic hemangioma
  - Varices, esophageal and gastric
- Rare
  - Vascular
    - Abdominal aortic aneurysm
    - Gastroduodenal artery aneurysm
    - Abdominal varices
    - Caput medusae and dilated mesenteric veins
    - Gallbladder varices
    - Pseudoaneurysm
    - Hemobilia from false hepatic artery aneurysm
    - Arterial grafts
    - Cutaneous hemangioma
    - Ovarian vein
    - Duodenal telangiectasia
    - Angiodysplasia
  - Miscellaneous
    - Leiomyoma
    - Leiomyosarcoma
    - Metastatic implants
    - Metastatic choriocarcinoma
    - Hamartoma
    - Adenoma
    - Angiomylipomas of tuberous sclerosis
    - Gallbladder (heme products)
    - Gluteal hematoma
    - Nonhemorrhagic gastritis
    - Factitious gastrointestinal bleeding
    - Sarcoidosis

Pharmacological Augmentation. Various pharmacological maneuvers have been evaluated to improve detectability (e.g., pentagastrin, glucagon, and cimetidine). Although some authors recommend routine premedication with one or a combination of these drugs, we reserve their use for situations where an initial false-negative study is suspected. No large series have evaluated their effectiveness.

Treves et al.[278] found that pretreatment with *pentagastrin* experimentally increased the rapidity, duration, and intensity of ^{99m}Tc-pertechnetate uptake by 65% and reported one case where this drug converted an initially false-negative scan to positive. The mechanism is uncertain, but may be the result of increased acid production, leading to increased activity of the mucous-producing cells and increased tracer uptake.

Table 20. Comparison of ^{99m}Tc-SC and ^{99m}Tc-RBC Scintigraphy for Gastrointestinal Bleeding*

	^{99m}Tc-SC	^{99m}Tc-RBCs
Dose	370 MBq (10 mCi) (may be repeated)	925 MBq (25 mCi)
Dosimetry		
whole body	0.2 cGy	0.3 cGy
target organ	3.6 cGy (liver)	1.2 cGy (heart)
Minimal bleeding detectable	0.1 mL/min	0.05–0.4 mL/min
Labeling	Commercial kit	Commercial kit
Imaging duration	30 min Repeat study if needed	60–90 min, then 20–30 min acquisition 2 and 4 hrs later and up to 24 hrs, as needed
Advantages	Short imaging time High target-to-background ratio	Repeat imaging up to 24 hrs
Disadvantages	Difficulty detecting hepatic and splenic flexure bleeding Only detects bleeding over short time	False-positive studies due to excretion of free $^{99m}TcO_4$

*With permission, modified from Winzelberg GG, Froelich JW, McKusick KA, et al.: Scintigraphic detection of gastrointestinal bleeding: A review of current methods. *Am J Gastroenterol* 1983; 78:324–327.[256]

Table 21. Meckel's Scan Protocol

Patient preparation:
- 4–6 hour fasting reduce size of stomach prior to study,
- No pretreatment with perchlorate, but it may be given after completion of study
- No barium studies should be performed within 3–4 days of scintigraphy
- Void prior to study

Premedication:

None (or)	
Pentagastrin	6 μg/kg subcutaneously 5–15 min before study
Cimetidine	20 mg/kg orally for 2 days prior to study
Glucagon	50 μg/kg intravenously 10 min before study

Radiopharmaceutical:

^{99m}Tc-pertechnetate	Children	1–3 KBq/kg
	Adults	200–500 MBq IV

Procedure:
- LFOV scintillation camera with low energy all-purpose or high-resolution collimator interfaced with computer
- Place patient supine under camera with xiphoid to symphysis pubis in field of view
- Flow: 60 1-s frames
- Static: 500,000 counts for first image, others for same time every 5–10 min for 1 hr
- Erect, right laterals, posteriors or obliques may be helpful at 30–60 min
- Postvoid image

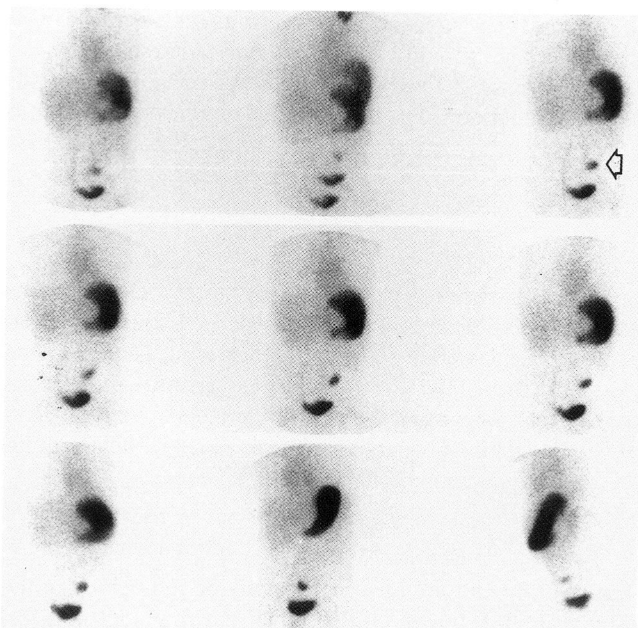

Figure 43. Meckel's diverticulum: sequential images over 60 min in this 6-year-old child shows focal uptake in the left lower quadrant (open arrowhead) increasing over time simultaneously with gastric uptake. The last image is a left lateral view. The diagnosis was confirmed pathologically.

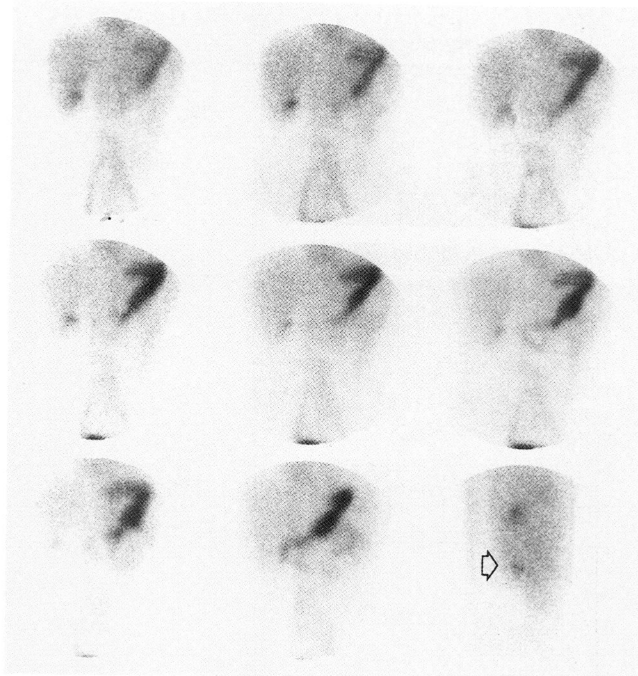

Figure 44. This figure illustrates the potential for misinterpretation. Renal pelvis activity on the right could be misinterpreted as consistent with a Meckel's diverticulum. A right lateral view (last image) confirms that the activity is posterior and of renal origin (open arrowhead).

However, pentagastrin also increases intestinal motility, leading to rapid movement into the small bowel. The antiperistaltic effect of *glucagon* has been used to prevent washout of pertechnetate from the stomach and from the Meckel's diverticulum. One study reported optimum visualization of Meckel's diverticulum with a combination of pentagastrin and glucagon.[279] The use of *cimetidine*, a histamine H_2 receptor antagonist, has also been reported to improve detection of ectopic gastric mucosa.[279,280] The more intense and prolonged uptake of ^{99m}Tc-pertechnetate by gastric mucosa is thought to be due to inhibition of its release from the gastric mucosa. Although no controlled studies have been performed, some investigators recommend its routine use because it has no significant risks or adverse effects.[281]

Image Interpretation. On scintigraphy, a Meckel's diverticulum appears as a focal area of increased intraperitoneal activity, usually in the right lower quadrant, although it may be seen anywhere within the abdomen (Fig. 43). Increased activity is usually first seen 5 to 10 minutes after injection simultaneously with gastric uptake, and persists or increases in activity over time. Lateral or oblique views are sometimes helpful in confirming the anterior position of a Meckel's diverticulum. Lateral and posterior images can help confirm renal or ureteral origin of activity (Fig. 44). Upright views can help distinguish fixed activity (e.g., duodenum) from ectopic gastric mucosa, which moves inferiorly in response to the altered position; it also serves to empty renal pelvis activity. The intensity of activity within the lesion may sometimes fluctuate due to intestinal secretions, hemorrhage, or increased intestinal motility which carries the radiotracer away. Postvoiding images are suggested to help empty collecting system activity and better identify uptake adjacent to the bladder.

Diagnostic Accuracy. False-negative studies may result from poor technique, washout of the secreted ^{99m}Tc-pertechnetate, or to the lack of sufficient gastric mucosa. Experimentally, an area smaller than 2 square centimeters cannot be detected scintigraphically.[282] A Meckel's diverticulum with impaired blood supply due to intussusception, volvulus, or infarction may also result in a false-negative study.[283]

False-positive studies have been reported from a variety of causes (Table 22). Normal structures can be confused with ectopic gastric mucosa if careful technique is not followed. False-positives often result from inflammatory or obstructive lesions. Lesions with increased blood pool (e.g., arteriovenous malformation and tumors) may be seen on flow and blood pool images, but do not take up ^{99m}Tc-pertechnetate; therefore, they are seen early and then fade.

The reported accuracy of Meckel's scanning has varied considerably and seems to depend, at least in part, on the referral population studied (e.g., children or adults), the presenting symptom (rectal bleeding or abdominal pain), and

Table 22. Causes for False-Positive Meckel's Scans and Their Mechanisms

Urinary tract
Ectopic kidney
Extrarenal pelvis
Hydronephrosis
Vesicoureteral reflux
Horseshoe kidney
Bladder diverticulum
Hyperemia and inflammatory
Peptic ulcer
Crohn's Disease
Ulcerative colitis
Abscess
Appendicitis
Colitis
Vascular
Arteriovenous malformation
Hemangioma
Aneurysm of intrabdominal vessel
Angiodysplasia
Neoplasm
Carcinoma of sigmoid colon
Carcinoid
Lymphoma
Jejunal neurinoma
Leiomyosarcoma
Small bowel obstruction
Intussusception, volvulus
Other areas of ectopic gastric mucosa
Gastrogenic cyst
Enteric duplication
Duplication cysts
Barrett's esophagus
Retained gastric antrum
Pancreas
Duodenum
Colon

on the technology used. Sfakianakis et al. summarized the results in 954 patients, mostly pediatric, using modern imaging methods, who had scintigraphy for suspected Meckel's diverticulum and found an overall sensitivity of 85% and specificity of 95%.[284,285] He emphasizes that experience in differentiating "nonspecific" accumulation of pertechnetate from true ectopic gastric mucosa has made this high specificity possible. Earlier studies, often using rectilinear scanner equipment, noted sensitivities and specificities in the range of 78%.[286] Meckel's scans in adults appear to have a poorer accuracy than in children. One retrospective study of Meckel's scintigraphy in an adult population reported a sensitivity of only 63%.[287] There were ten false-positives, although seven had surgically treatable disease. The lower sensitivity may be related to the fact that adults often do not have gastric mucosa in their diverticula.

Gastrointestinal Duplications

Duplications are cystic or tubular lesions of congenital origin, composed of gastrointestinal muscular walls with mucosal linings. Fifty percent occur in the small bowel, most in the ileum, and 20% in the mediastinum. Although most are symptomatic by the age of 2 years, some remain asymptomatic into adulthood. The presenting symptoms are similar to a Meckel's diverticulum because 30 to 50% have gastric mucosa.

DIAGNOSIS

The diagnosis is usually made at surgery. Occasionally, a preoperative diagnosis may be made by barium radiography or ultrasonography. Scintigraphy has occasionally been reported to be helpful.[288–291] Mediastinal gastrointestinal cysts have been diagnosed with ^{99m}Tc-pertechnetate scintigraphy.[292,293] Duplications often appear as large areas of increased activity, sometimes multilobulated.

Retained Gastric Antrum

The gastrum antrum may occasionally be left behind in the afferent loop following a Billroth II gastrojejunostomy for peptic ulcer disease. The antrum continues to produce gastrin, which is no longer inhibited by acid in the stomach because it is diverted through the gastrojejunostomy. The resulting high acid production often leads to marginal ulcers. Other etiologies for recurrent ulcers in postpartial gastrectomy patients include an incomplete vagotomy and the Zollinger-Ellison syndrome. In this last syndrome, a pancreatic gastrinoma secretes gastrin. The diagnosis is usually based on the response of serum gastrin to intravenous calcium or secretion infusions. In the Zollinger-Ellison syndrome, serum gastrin levels increase following these infusions; serum gastrin levels will decrease with a retained gastric antrum.

Endoscopy or barium radiography can often demonstrate the retained gastrum antrum. However, ^{99m}Tc-pertechnetate scintigraphy can be confirmatory. The protocol used is similar to that for Meckel's diverticulum. Uptake in the gastric remnant occurs simultaneously with gastric uptake and is seen as a collar of radioactivity in the area of the duodenal stump of the afferent loop. The retained antrum usually lies to the right of the gastric remnant. Several cases diagnosed with ^{99m}Tc-pertechnetate have been reported[294,295] as well as a series of Billroth II patients where 16 of 22 patients with a retained antrum demonstrated ^{99m}Tc-pertechnetate uptake.[296]

Barrett's Esophagus

Barrett's esophagus is a condition in which the distal esophagus becomes lined by columnar epithelium, rather than the usual esophageal squamous epithelium. It is generally thought to be secondary to chronic gastroesophageal reflux and is associated with ulcers, high strictures, and esophageal adenocarcinoma in 8.5% of cases.[297]

The diagnosis is usually made today by endoscopy and mucosal biopsy. ^{99m}Tc-pertechnetate scintigraphy first detected Barrett's esophagus in 1973.[267] The study is usually performed with the patient erect to decrease gastroesophageal reflux. Left anterior oblique views may be helpful. It has been recommended that a chest/abdominal radiograph be performed after a barium swallow to localize the gastroesophageal junction or, alternatively, to compare it with a prior upper gastrointestinal series.[267,298] The normal esophagus ends at the esophagogastric junction. Positive scintigraphy shows dense intrathoracic uptake contiguous with the stomach, but conforming to the shape and posterior location of the esophagus. Scintigraphy should be interpreted in conjunction with the upper gastrointestinal series to differentiate Barrett's esophagus from a simple hiatal hernia. False-negatives have been reported and the scan does not replace endoscopic biopsy. At best, it is a complementary or confirmatory procedure.

INTESTINAL TRANSIT STUDIES

Introduction

The study of small and large intestine transit times by radionuclide scintigraphy is relatively new and techniques are still being developed. However, there is considerable interest and active investigation into the physiology, pathophysiology, and clinical utility of intestinal transit times. This section will try to summarize that work, emphasizing the various methodologies used and their clinical relevance.

Unique technical problems exist in the study of intestinal transit. To accurately measure the movement of intestinal contents, the radiolabeled meal must be able to withstand the acid environment of the stomach and the alkaline environment of the small bowel. In contrast to gastric emptying, where the breakdown of food in the stomach into small enough particles to pass through the pylorus is part of the physiological process being studied, the absorption of ingested meal nutrients in the small bowel hinders intestinal transit scintigraphy.

One of the difficulties in studying intestinal transit is determining the starting point (e.g., there is no clearcut time zero). In contrast to gastric emptying where, after ingestion of a radiolabeled meal (5 to 10 minutes) all the food resides within the stomach and measurement of gastric transit depends only on the rate of clearance, intestinal transit is more complex. The input into the intestines is not a single bolus, but rather a protracted infusion from the stomach. This must be taken into account in quantifying small and large bowel transit.

Small Intestinal Transit

The importance of small bowel transit and its relationship to absorption and digestion of food are not well understood. The study of normal intestinal physiology and pathophysiology has been hampered by the lack of good quantitative methods for investigating this important gastrointestinal process. Intestinal transit time alone does not necessarily define the underlying process. For example, small bowel transit time may be accelerated and contact time reduced due to an increase in the propulsive motor activity, an increase in secretion, a reduction in epithelial absorption, or a combination of these factors.

NONSCINTIGRAPHIC METHODS

The transit of barium through the small intestine during a routine small bowel follow-through study does not give quantitative transit information. Mixing barium with food and plotting its progress through the bowel on a monitor using image intensification can provide a more accurate index of the rate of food emptying into the colon. However, the radiation exposure required is relatively high and the results cannot be extrapolated to other meals because of its nonphysiological nature.

Nonimaging radionuclide intestinal absorption studies have been used as an indicator of intestinal transit. For example, breath analysis tests measure the $^{14}CO_2$ produced when a carbohydrate (^{14}C–lactose) is fermented by colonic bacteria.[299,300] It is a measurement of the transit time of the leading edge of the meal from the mouth to cecum and does not provide an index of the transit of the bulk of the meal. The study has other limitations (e.g., lactose itself may alter transit, the resulting transit time is to some extent determined by the rate of gastric emptying, and the test requires an appropriate population of fermentative bacteria in the colon which may be absent in up to 25% of the population). As a result, the data is not always reproducible. Measuring *plasma sulfapyridine* after ingestion of salicylazosulfapyridine has been proposed as a method for measuring intestinal transit, but requires repeated blood sampling.[301]

RADIONUCLIDE SCINTIGRAPHY

In spite of the problems discussed, radionuclide scintigraphy has the potential to noninvasively quantify small bowel transit. Various radiopharmaceuticals, meals, and methods have been investigated.

RADIOPHARMACEUTICALS, MEALS, AND SMALL BOWEL PHYSIOLOGY

Table 23 lists the various radiopharmaceuticals and carrier meals that have been utilized for studies of small intestinal transit. Nonabsorbable radiotracers such as ^{99m}Tc-sulfur colloid (^{99m}Tc-SC) or ^{99m}Tc-DTPA in isotonic water or mixed with a semisolid meal have been used to measure the transit of water-soluble nutrients within the small bowel lumen.[302–304] The study of the movement of the semi-solid phase of the intestinal contents is more complex. Radiolabeled digestible food (e.g., ^{99m}Tc-labeled chicken liver or egg) used for gastric emptying studies cannot measure the intestinal transit of solids because the food carrier is hydrolyzed and absorbed. Accurate measurement requires stable nondigestible markers. An ideal solid particle for bowel transit studies has been

Table 23. Radiopharmaceuticals and Meals: Small Intestinal Transit

RADIOPHARMACEUTICAL	CARRIER MEAL	REFERENCE
^{99m}Tc-SC	Mashed potatoes	Read et al. 1982[306]
^{99m}Tc-SC	Steak, bread, butter	Jian et al. 1984[304]
^{51}Cr	Egg, milk	
^{99m}Tc-DTPA	Isosomotic liquid	Caride et al. 1984[302]
^{99m}Tc-DTPA	Triscuits®, cheese	Malagelada et al. 1984[307]
^{131}I-fiber		
^{111}In-resin pellets	Scrambled egg, bread,	Camilleri et al. 1989[308]
^{131}I-labeled fiber	Milk	
^{99m}Tc-cellulose	Cheese, butter	Madsen et al. 1989[309]
^{111}In-plastic particles	Yogurt, bread	
^{111}In-plastic particles	Cheese, butter	Madsen et al. 1991[310]
^{99m}Tc-DTPA	Yogurt, bread	

described as one that can be labeled with high efficiency, is unaltered by changes in intraluminal pH, and has a size that mimics that of triturated solid food.[305]

Fiber is the only normal dietary constituent that is unaffected by gastric antral mechanical grinding, and progresses along the small intestine in solid form without hydrolytic digestion.[311,312] Therefore, ^{131}I-fibrin is an attractive radiopharmaceutical for measuring small and large intestinal transit.[313] It has a high labeling efficiency and is quite stable in acid and alkaline environments.[308,312,313] However, it has drawbacks, including a laborious synthesis, and entails a relatively high radiation absorbed dose from the beta emission.

A study comparing ^{99m}Tc-DTPA and ^{131}I-fibrin transit through the gastrointestinal tract has demonstrated that, although ^{131}I-fibrin acts like a solid in the stomach (emptying from the stomach slower than the liquid phase), both water soluble substances (^{99m}Tc-DTPA) and particulate matter in chyme (^{131}I-fibrin) travel at the same speed within the small bowel.[307] The liquid phase marker reaches the colon first, due solely to the differential rate of gastric emptying. Particulate matter in chyme spreads out over a considerable length of

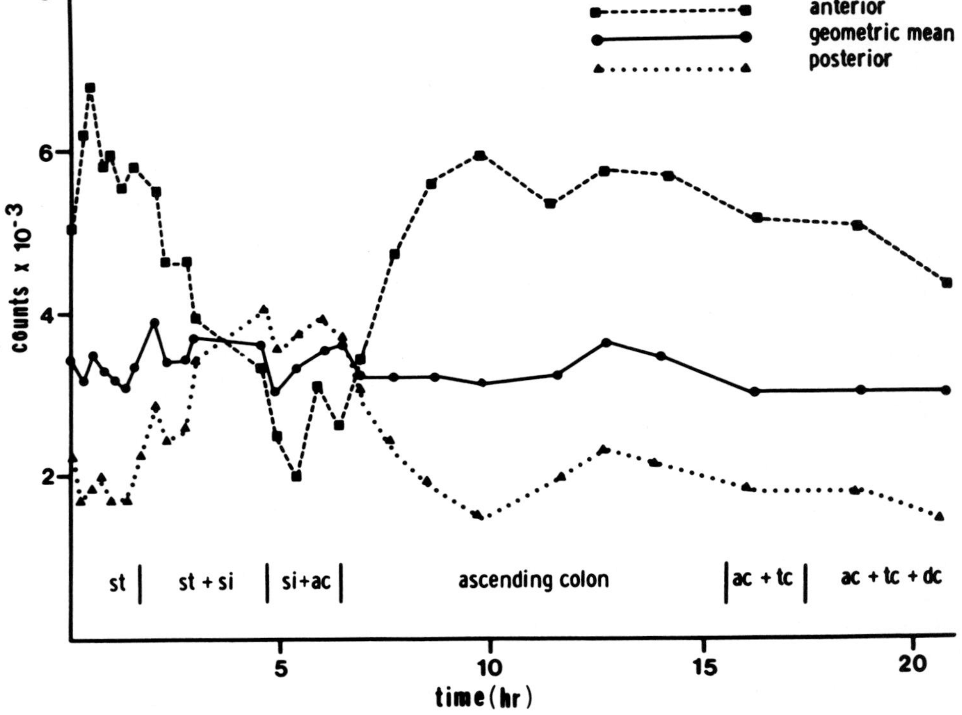

Figure 45. Geometric mean correction of intestinal transit. Anterior, posterior, and geometric mean count rates recorded during transit of ^{111}In-cation exchange resin particles through the small and large intestine of one subject. The locations of the tracer are indicated, st (stomach), si (small intestine), ac (ascending colon), tc (transverse colon), and dc (descending colon). (With permission, Hardy JG and Perkins AC: Validity of the geometric mean correction in the quantification of whole bowel transit. *Nucl Med Commun* 1985;6:217–224.[316])

the small bowel during transit due to the combined effects of slow emptying from the stomach and variable rates of transit between the pylorus and ileocecal valve. It has been suggested that this "spreading out" of chyme along the small intestine serves the physiological purpose of increasing the total absorptive surface.[307] Both liquid and solid phases enter the colon in a linear manner.

^{99m}Tc-labeled cellulose fiber[309] is another nondigestible fiber marker that has potential clinical use. In vitro and in vivo stability is high in gastric and intestinal juice, and in stool. Normal mean gastric emptying time was found to be 1.1 ± 0.2 hours and the small bowel transit time, 3.9 ± 0.6 hours.

^{111}Indium-labeled plastic particles have been investigated as a nondigestible marker of intestinal transit.[309] Mean gastric emptying, small intestinal, and large intestinal transit times were 1.9 ± 20.8, 4.0 ± 0.3, and 23 ± 11 hours, respectively, in a limited number of volunteers. Although this agent has almost complete stability and a suitable half-life for measuring transit within all gastrointestinal segments, it is not a physiological marker.

^{111}Indium-resin pellets (Amberlite 120-IRP cation exchange resin pellets, Sigma Chemical, St. Louis, MO) have also been investigated as a solid phase marker of intestinal transit.[314] The labeling efficiency and in vivo stability is high. The resin pellets are retained within the solid phase of chyme throughout gut transit.[308] Comparison of ^{111}In-resin pellets with ^{131}I-fiber has demonstrated similar rates of gastric emptying (mean 164 ± 12 and 177 ± 13 min) and mean half-times of small bowel transit (168 ± 22 and 150 ± 11 min, respectively). The times for 5, 50, and 75% colonic filling were also similar, approximately 245, 330, and 400 minutes, respectively. This study confirmed previous work showing that colonic filling was generally linear, except for periodic pauses (plateaus) in transit. The radiolabeled solid was noted to accumulate just proximal to the cecum, followed by bolus transfers of chyme. This suggests a reservoir function for the distal ileum, with relatively large volumes transferred periodically into the colon, perhaps as part of the gastrocolic reflex.

Methods. Methods vary considerably; however, all use a large field of view scintillation camera so that the entire abdomen can be imaged. Computer acquisition is mandatory. Radioactive markers are useful to realign images and are used as anatomical reference points. The frequency of image acquisition varies depending on specific protocols, from 1-minute frames continuously for 2 hours for a water soluble ^{99m}Tc-DTPA tracer[302] to longer intermittent acquisitions for solid tracers (e.g., every 10 minutes × 1 hour, then every 20 minutes × 1 hour, every 30 minutes × 2 hours and, finally hourly until 80% of the radiotracer enters the colon.[307]

Quantification of small bowel motility poses a number of problems. Because intestinal input depends on the rate of gastric emptying, time zero is not a compact bolus in the proximal small bowel, but a slow and variable input over time. Gastrointestinal intubation with infusion of the meal directly to the site of interest can get around this problem, but it is unpleasant for the patient, time consuming, and not physiological. Intubation has been shown to delay gastric emptying, decrease small bowel residence time, and accelerate colonic filling.[315] Because a meal normally spreads out in the intestine as it moves aborally, there is no single transit time but, rather, a spectrum of transit times. Pulse methods (e.g., intubation) only measure transit over relatively short periods of time. Multiple injections are necessary; however, this would lead to overlapping time-activity curves.

Movement of chyme along the gastrointestinal tract is not always continuous; therefore, scans obtained intermittently do not always provide exact characterization of intestinal movement. Region delineation is subjective. A small bowel region of interest (ROI) can be hard to define with certainty, often overlapping with the stomach and colon. Technical problems to be considered and corrected for are radioactive decay and the effect of scatter from adjacent bowel.

Anterior and posterior motion of intestinal contents results in varying soft-tissue attenuation. Most intestinal transit studies to date have been performed with a single-headed scintillation camera in the anterior projection, not taking into account the effect of attenuation. However, attempts have been made to correct for this potential problem.[303] Anterior and posterior acquisition with geometric mean correction (square root of the product) at each time interval has been used (Fig. 45).[309,315] An underlying assumption of the geometric mean correction method is that the entire radioactivity remains within the region of interest. Unlike gastric emptying studies, this is not the case for measuring regional intestinal transit.

QUANTIFICATION

A variety of quantitative methods have been used to measure small bowel transit. Caride et al.[302] defined small bowel transit as the time required for radioactivity to move from the stomach to its first appearance in the cecum. However, this is more accurately the gastrocecal time. Read et al.[315] used a curve-fitting sequence to correct for overlap of the small bowel with the stomach and colon. In that study, ROIs were drawn for the stomach from the early images and for the colon from the late images. The small-bowel ROI was generated from counts outside these regions. Time-activity profiles were generated for each region (Fig. 46). The time that the labeled meal first entered the cecum and the time that 50%, 80%, and 100% of the meal had entered the colon was determined from profiles of colonic filling. However, this method yields an estimate of the actual small bowel transit time only if gastric emptying were instantaneous and could be predicted. In a subsequent modification, small bowel transit was calculated by subtracting the half-time for gastric emptying from the half-time for colonic filling.[303,308]

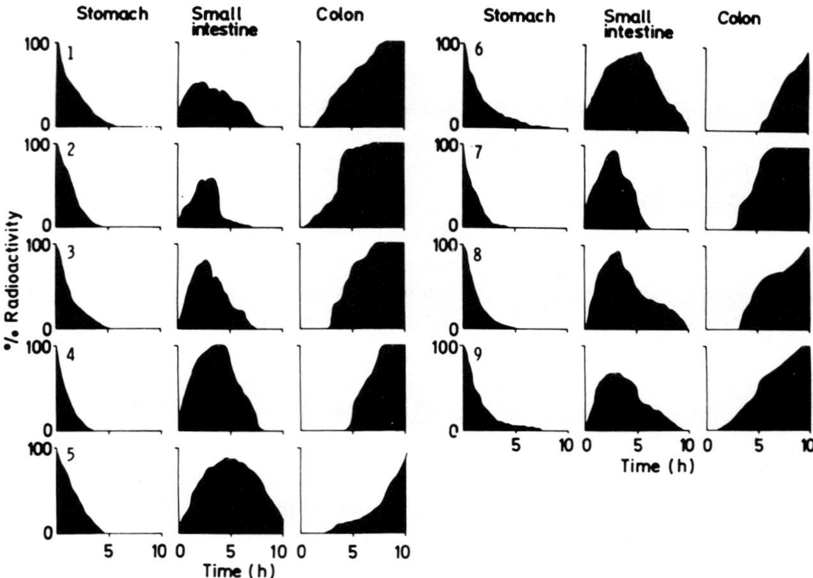

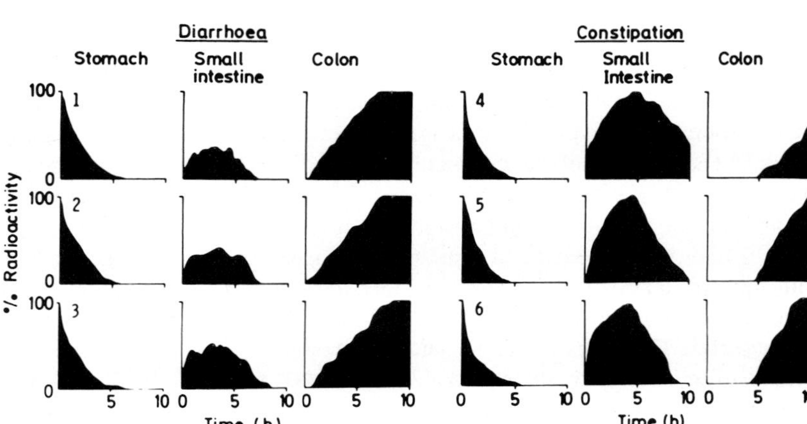

Figure 46. Profiles for gastric emptying, small bowel residence, and colonic filling in 9 normal volunteers (above), and 6 patients with the irritable bowel syndrome (below), of whom 3 had diarrhea and 3 constipation. The initial steep rise in the profiles is dominated by gastric emptying. After rising to a peak, it falls as the rate of exit of residues into the cecum exceeds the rate of entry of food from the stomach. The rate of decline increases as the curve becomes more and more dominated by cecal filling with little or no entry of food from the stomach. The average value for intestinal residence was 3.5 ± 1.4 hours. (With permission, Read NW, AL-Janabi MN, Holgaste AM, et al.: Simultaneous measurement of gastric emptying, small bowel residence and colon meal by the use of a gamma camera. *Gut* 1986;27:300–308.[303])

Malagelada et al.[307] noted that the rate at which material enters the colon involves a convolution of the rate of emptying of the stomach and the rate of transit through the small bowel. Therefore, the small bowel transit spectrum was obtained by deconvolution, a mathematical technique that corrects for the slow input and produces a time-activity curve that would result if a perfect bolus had been injected directly into the small bowel. A mean transit time is then calculated from the corrected intestinal time-activity curve. Others have used variations of this same method.[309]

Table 24. Radiopharmaceuticals and Meals: Large Intestinal Transit

RADIOPHARMACEUTICAL	CARRIER MEAL	REFERENCE
^{99m}Tc-DTPA	Similulated ileal electrolyte solution	Krevsky et al. 1986[317]
^{99m}Tc-cellulose	Cheese, butter	Madsen et al. 1989[309]
^{111}In-plastic particles	Yogurt, bread	
^{111}In-resin pellets in gelatin capsule	Standard meal after capsule empties from stomach	Proano et al. 1990[319]
^{131}I-cellulose	Crackers, cheese, water	McLean et al. 1990[320]
^{131}I-cellulose	Ingested fasting alone	Smart et al. 1991[321]
^{99m}Tc-DTPA	Normal diet	
^{111}In-chloride encapsulated	Standard diet	Stubbs et al. 1991[322]

CLINICAL RESULTS OF INTESTINAL TRANSIT STUDIES

To date, most studies have focused on normal physiology. Considerable variation in small bowel transit times among normal subjects has been observed. Few clinical studies have been performed. Generally, patients with diarrhea have rapid mean transit times whereas patients with constipation have longer transit times, but most patients have values within the normal range.[303] Some of the methods described above will likely lead to a better understanding of the physiology and pathophysiology of diseases of the small intestine.

Large Intestinal Transit

RADIOGRAPHIC METHODS

Various radiographic techniques have been described to evaluate colonic motility. These include cineradiography, fluoroscopy to estimate transit times, and the use of radiopaque plastic cuttings. However, these methods result in a relatively large radiation dose to the patient and are not physiological. Barium is hypertonic, provides a large volume load, and may not transit the colon as does food; contrast radiography is not quantifiable. Orally ingested radiopaque material does not arrive at the colon as a bolus, so there is no precise starting point for the study.

RADIONUCLIDE SCINTIGRAPHY

Radiopharmaceuticals. Various radiopharmaceuticals have been used to study colonic transit (Table 24). Colonic transit scintigraphy was first described by Krevsky et al. in 1986.[317] The method involved cecal instillation of *^{99m}Tc-DTPA* in a small volume of ileal-like electrolyte solution via a tube placed orally by fluoroscopy; serial images were acquired for 48 hours (Fig. 47). In addition to a weighted tube, a liquid diet was required for several days. Kaufman et al.[318] used a similar technique but allowed subjects a regular diet. The solid diet slowed transit in the cecum and ascending colon compared to a liquid diet. They then investigated the possibility of eliminating the cumbersome cecal intubation by simply instilling the radiopharmaceutical into the jejunum. The calculated transit times were similar on both the liquid and solid diets.

To make colon transit scintigraphy a totally noninvasive method, an original approach has been described[323] and validated by Proano et al.[319] Approximately 1000 ^{111}In–labeled polystyrene Amberlite IR-120 PLUS *cation exchange resin pellets*, measuring 0.5 to 1.8 mm in diameter, are placed in a gelatin capsule. The capsule is coated with a pH-sensitive polymer (methacrylate) which is resistant to disrupts at the pH levels found in the stomach and proximal bowel, but disrupts at the ileocecal valve due to the increasing pH gradient along the small bowel and proximal colon. Labeling efficiency is high and in vitro studies demonstrate that the free pellets are very stable in simulated intestinal secretions. Once

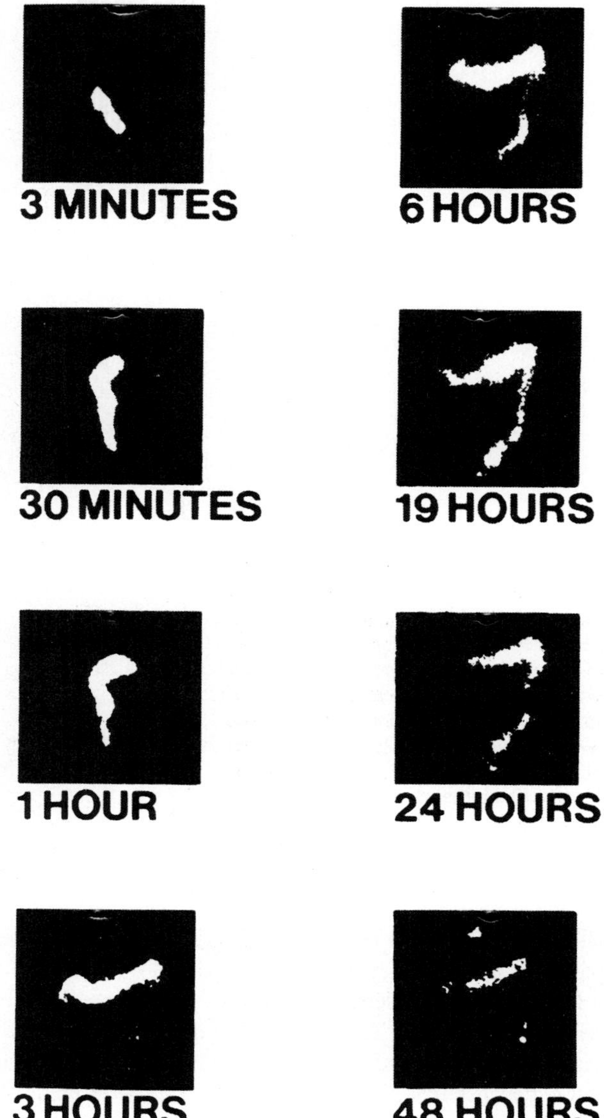

Figure 47. Serial colonic scintigrams in a study subject acquired at intervals after cecal instillation of ^{99m}Tc-DTPA. The serial images demonstrate progression of the radionuclide with time. The predominant activity at 6 hours is in the transverse colon. At 48 hours the image is faint, indicating that most of the activity has been excreted. (With permission, Krevsky B, Malmud LS, D'Ercole F, et al.: Colonic Transit Scintigraphy. *Gastroenterology* 1986; 91:1102–12.[317])

released in the proximal colon, the segmental transit of solids through the colon can be imaged and quantified (Fig. 48).

^{131}I-fiber cellulose, similar to that described under small bowel transit scintigraphy,[313] has also be investigated for use in colon transit scintigraphy.[309,320] This has been fed orally together with a small meal of crackers, cheese, and water and images made intermittently for up to 96 hours. Minimal ($<$3%) dissociation of ^{131}I from cellulose was detected in urine collections. Clear differences were noted in total and segmen-

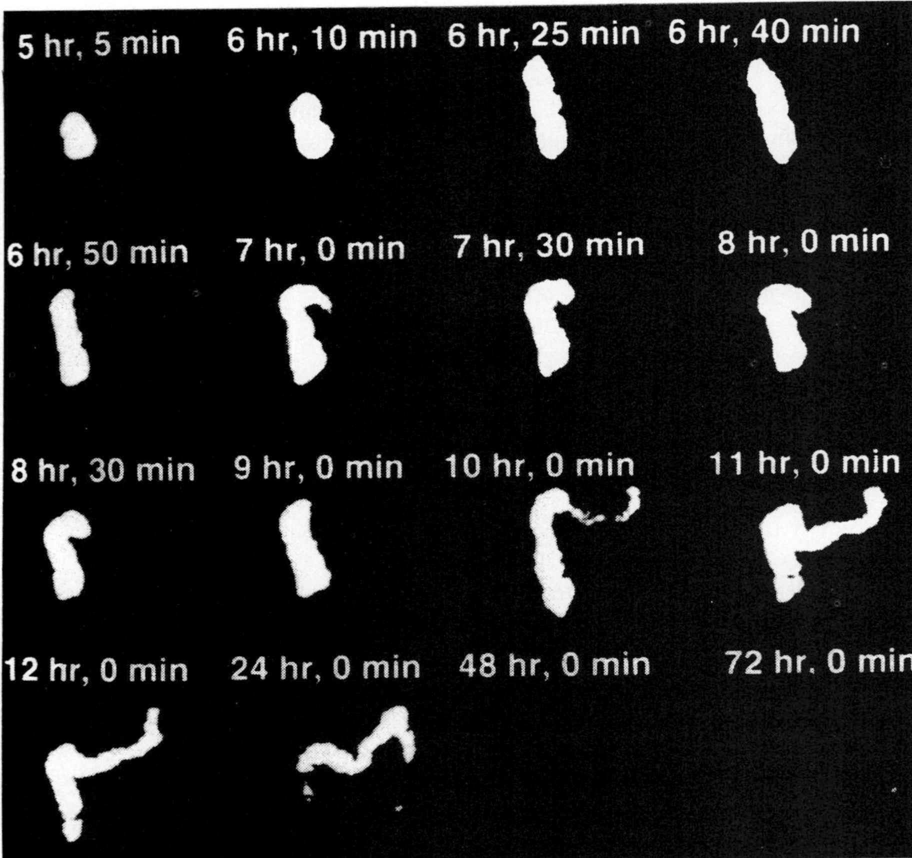

Figure 48. Sequence of colonic images at the designated time intervals after ingestion of the capsule containing ^{111}In-labeled resin pellets. The radioactivity remains in the ascending colon for a prolonged period before subsequent movement into the more distal colon. (With permission, Proano M, Camilleri M, Phillips SF, et al.: Transit of solids through the human colon: regional quantification in the unprepared bowel. *Am J Physiol* 1990;258:G856–862.[319])

tal colonic retention between healthy subjects and patients with constipation. A recent study compared ^{131}I-cellulose and ^{111}In-DTPA simultaneously in normal persons and patients with constipation.[321] The 2 tracers produced nearly identical results. They concluded that ^{111}In-DTPA was the preferable tracer because it avoids the labeling problems and relatively high radiation absorbed dose of ^{131}I-fiber.

^{111}Indium-DTPA encapsulated in 2-cm nondigestible capsules (ten 10-μCi capsules) made of 18 French nasogastric heat-sealed tubing has been used to study large bowel transit.[322] ^{99m}Tc-SC in 150 mL water was administered simultaneously with the capsules to outline the gastrointestinal tract. In vivo testing demonstrated no leakage. Images were acquired at 4-hour intervals until all the capsules were excreted. Segmental transit times were calculated. The technique showed good reproducibility.

QUANTIFICATION

Krevsky et al.[317] defined ROIs based on anatomic subdivisions (e.g., the cecum and ascending colon, hepatic flexure, transverse colon, splenic flexure, descending colon, rectosigmoid colon), and excreted feces. The number of counts in each ROI was determined for each time interval and expressed as a percentage of the original bolus after correction for decay and attenuation. This yielded the fraction of originally instilled activity that was present in a given ROI at a given time. This fraction was graphed as a series of histograms showing the distribution of radionuclide for each time interval. Time-activity curves were generated for each rectangular ROI, showing a percentage of the original bolus plotted as a function of time for each ROI. Finally, geometric center analysis was performed. This technique uses the data from the time distribution analysis to generate a number that reflects the *centroid of activity* or overall progression of fecal material. Each ROI is assigned a number. To calculate the geometric center, the number of counts in a given region is divided by the corrected number of total counts from the start of the study and multiplied by the region number. This calculation is performed for each ROI and the sum of the calculations is performed for each ROI and represents the geometric center for a given time (Fig. 49). Other quantification methods have been reported by Proano et al.[319] and Smart et al.[321]

PHYSIOLOGICAL AND CLINICAL RESULTS

The clinical role of colon scintigraphy is still being defined, although some preliminary physiological and clinical studies have been reported. In their initial study, Krevsky et al.[317] found that the transverse colon, not the cecum and ascending colon, as the primary site for fecal storage. Previous studies using manometric techniques and radiopaque

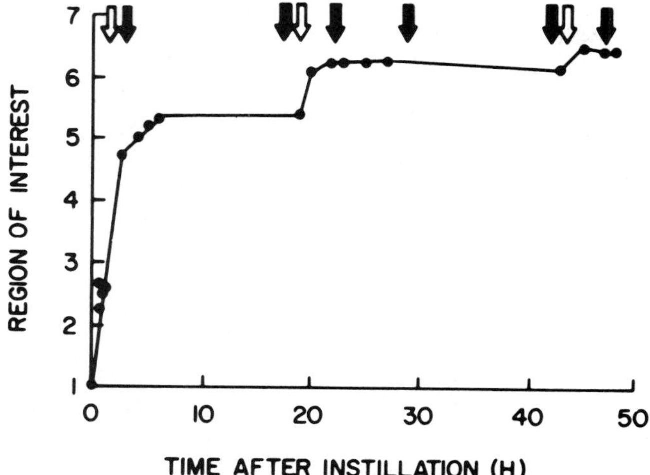

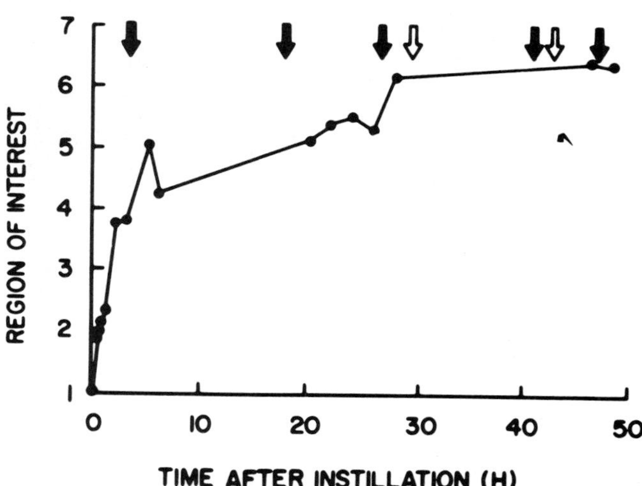

Figure 49. Geometric center analysis for colonic transit in 2 study subjects. The curves show the geometric center plotted against time in hrs. Region 1 is the cecum and ascending colon, where all activity is located at the start of the study. Region 7 is the excreted feces. Open arrows represent bowel movements, and solid arrows represent meals. The top panel shows a stepwise antegrade progression of the geometric center. Although some meals were associated with progression, others were not. Bowel movements seem to have been temporally associated with progression of the geometric center in this subject. The bottom panel shows the geometric center for another subject; in this individual, there was no consistent correlation between either meals or bowel movements and the progression of the geometric center. Net retrograde flow of colonic content was demonstrated in this individual at both 6 hr and 24 hr, when the value of the geometric center decreased. (With permission, Krevsky B, Maurer AH, Fisher RS: Patterns of colonic transit in chronic idiopathic constipation. *Am J Gastroenterol* 1989;84:127–132.[324])

marker studies have defined different patterns of colonic transit (e.g., normal, colonic inertia, and distal slowing). In a subsequent study they found that colonic transit was essentially normal in patients with functional rectosigmoid obstruction.[324] Stivland et al.,[325] using ^{111}In-labeled resin particles, characterized idiopathic constipation by either exaggerated reservoir function of the ascending and transverse colons and/or impairment of propulsive function in the descending colon. Kamm et al.[326] used bisacodyl to initiate colonic motor activity and monitored colonic transit using ^{99m}Tc-DTPA instilled in the colon. In healthy people, there was rapid movement from the right colon to the rectum. In patients with severe idiopathic constipation, a spectrum of colonic abnormalities was observed from slow transit involving the rectum and sigmoid only to slow transit involving the entire colon.

In a study of functional diarrhea, patients had a pattern of transit different from that of normal people: the intraluminal radiotracer moved in and out of the transverse and signoid colon regions during fasting, unlike healthy subjects, in whom the marker remained in the splenic flexure.[327] After eating, radioactivity immediately increased in both the transverse and sigmoid colons in healthy subjects but, in patients with diarrhea, eating did not alter the radiotracer movement into the different regions of the colon compared to fasting. Within 100 minutes of eating, the intraluminal marker almost disappeared from the regions of interest in patients with diarrhea.

The time required to perform intestinal transit studies is a problem from a clinical imaging standpoint. Physiologically, the more frequent the image acquisition, the more accurate the data. However, in a busy clinic, tieing up a camera for many hours poses serious logistic problems. Interestingly, preliminary data suggests that scanning limited to images acquired at 2-, 4-, and 6-hour scans may be adequate to diagnose clinically important gastric and intestinal motility disorders.[328]

PROTEIN-LOSING ENTEROPATHY

Introduction

Excessive protein loss through the gastrointestinal tract has been associated with a variety of gastrointestinal and nongastrointestinal diseases.[329] The resulting hypoproteinemia can become a serious clinical problem.

NonRadionuclide Methods

Alpha$_1$-antitrypsin is an endogenously produced macromolecule that has been used as a fecal marker of malabsorption.[330] It has been found to be as accurate and reproducible as ^{51}Cr-labeled albumin, the generally accepted "gold standard".[331] The disadvantage of this method is that it requires fecal collection.

Nonimaging Radionuclide Methods

In 1957, Citrin et al.[332] first used gastric intubation and aspiration to demonstrate excessive albumin loss into the gastric juice in a patient with gastric hypertrophy using ^{131}I-labeled

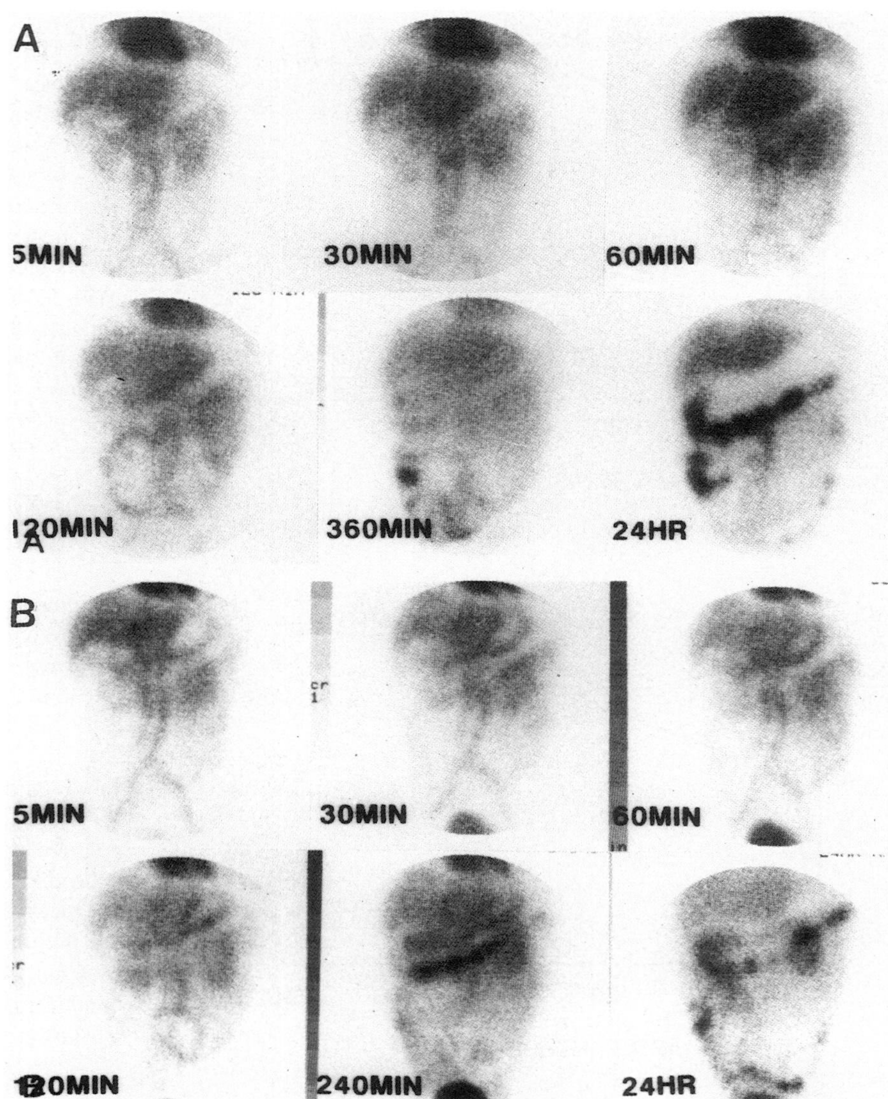

Figure 50. Protein Losing Enteropathy: ^{111}In-transferrin **(A)** and ^{99m}Tc-HSA **(B)** images in a patient with Menetrier's disease. Both show definite activity demonstrating protein loss from the stomach. Appreciable activity in the kidney and urinary bladder are noted on the ^{99m}Tc-HSA images, but not on the ^{111}In-transferrin images. (With permission, Aburano T, Yokoyama K, Kinuya S, et al.: Indium 111 transferrin imaging for the diagnosis of protein-losing enteropathy. *Clin Nucl Med* 1989;14:681–685.[338])

albumin. In 1959 ^{131}I labeled *polyvinyl pyrrolidine* was introduced for the detection of protein-losing enteropathy.[333] A number of other radiolabeled serum proteins or macromolecules have been used to make the diagnosis (e.g., ^{125}I-albumin, ^{95}Nb-albumin, ^{59}Fe-dextran, and ^{67}Cu-ceruloplasmin); however, most have had limited clinical use and are not commercially available.

Measurement of the fecal ^{51}Cr-albumin has generally been considered the most accurate and sensitive test for detecting protein-losing enteropathy.[334] However, since daily stool collection for 48 to 72 hours and fecal quantification is required, it has not been well accepted by the patients or laboratory personnel.

Radionuclide Imaging

Two radiopharmaceuticals have been used to make this diagnosis scintigraphically, ^{99m}Tc-human serum albumin (^{99m}Tc-HSA) and ^{111}In-transferrin. ^{99m}Tc-HSA was first used for qualitative assessment of protein loss in a patient with primary lymphangiectasia.[335] Serial abdominal images for 30 minutes after intravenous injection revealed radiotracer collection in the small bowel, which increased in amount over 24 hours. When the diagnosis is uncertain scintigraphically, gastric secretions can be aspirated via a nasogastric tube and imaged.[336]

Scintigraphy with *^{111}In-transferrin* was first described in a patient with intestinal lymphangiectasia.[337] When injected intravenously, ^{111}In-chloride binds in vivo to serum proteins; most notably to transferrin, and abdominal imaging can be used to visualize the protein leak. However, better binding and imaging may be obtained with in vitro labeling. A recent study of 7 patients with the protein-losing enteropathy syndrome (2 with Menetrier's disease, and 1 patient each with gastric ulcer, intestinal lymphangiectasia, amyloidosis,

Table 25. Validated Clinical Breath Analysis Tests*

CLINICAL APPLICATION	SUBSTRATE	METABOLIC END PRODUCT MEASURED
1. Bacterial overgrowth	^{14}C-glycocholate	$^{14}CO_2$
	^{14}C-xylose	$^{14}CO_2$
	glycose	H_2
2. Ileal dysfunction	^{14}C-glycocholate	$^{14}CO_2$
3. Steatorrhea	^{14}C-triolein	$^{14}CO_2$
4. Lactase deficiency	^{14}C-lactose	$^{14}CO_2$
	lactose	H_2
5. Sucrase-isomaltase deficiency	sucrose	H_2
6. Small bowel transit time	^{14}C-lactulose	$^{14}CO_2$
	lactulose	H_2

*With permission, Reba RC and Salkeld J: In-vitro studies of malabsorption and other GI disorders. *Semin Nucl Med* 1982; 12:147–155.[339]

Crohn's disease, and intestinal fistula) compared the results of scintigraphy with the *alpha₁-antitrypsin clearance* test.[338] Serial scintigraphy for up to 24 hours was positive in 4 patients with greater than 20 ml/day alpha-antitrypsin clearance, but not in 3 patients with less than 20 mL/day (Fig. 50).

Acknowledgement: The author expresses appreciation for John C. Harbert's contribution to "Breath Tests in Gastrointestinal Disease."

REFERENCES

1. Kazem I: A new scintigraphic technique for the study of the esophagus. *AJR* 1972;115:681–688.
2. Taillefer R, Jadliwall M, Pellerin E, et al.: Radionuclide esophageal transit study in detection of esophageal motor dysfunction:comparison with motility studies (Manometry). *J Nucl Med* 1990;312:1921–1926.
3. Ham HR, Piepsz A, Georges B, et al.: Quantitation of esophageal transit by means of 81mKr. *Eur J Nucl Med* 1984; 9:362–365.
4. Castronovo FP: Gastroesophageal scintiscanning in a pediatric population: Dosimetry. *J Nucl Med* 1986;27:1212–1214.
5. Siegel JA, Wu RK, Knight LC, et al.: Radiation dose estimates for oral agents used in upper gastrointestinal disease. *J Nucl Med* 1983;24:835–837.
6. Tatsch K, Schroettle, Kirsch C-M: Multiple swallow test for the quantitative and qualitative evaluation of esophageal motility disorders. *J Nucl Med* 1991;32:1365–1370.
7. Steffey DL, Wahl RL, Shapiro B: Diabetic oesophagoparesis: assessment by solid phase radionuclide scintigraphy. *Nucl Med Commun* 1986;7:165–171.
8. Kjellen G, Svedberg JB, Tibbling L: Solid bolus transit by esophageal scintigraphy in patients with dysphagia and normal manometry and radiography. *Dig Dis Sci* 1984;29:1–5.
9. Holloway RH, Krosin G, Lange RC, et al.: Radionuclide esophageal emptying of a solid meal to quantitate results of therapy in achalasia. *Gastroenterology* 1983;84:771–776.
10. Fisher RS, Malmud LS, Applegate G, et al.: Effect of bolus composition on esophageal transit: concise communication. *J Nucl Med* 1982;32:878–882.
11. Tolin RD, Malmud LS, Reilly J, Fisher RS: Esophageal scintigraphy to quantitate esophageal transit (Quantitation of esophageal transit). *Gastroenterology* 1979;76:1402–1408.
12. Lamki L: Radionuclide esophageal transit (RET) study. The effect of body posture. *Clin Nucl Med* 1985;10:108–110.
13. Styles CB, Holt S, Bowles KL, Hopper R: Esophageal transit scintigraphy—a cautionary note. *J Can Assoc Radiol* 1984; 35:31–33.
14. Carrette S, Lacourciere Y, Lavoie S, Halle P: Radionuclide esophageal transit in progressive systemic sclerosis. *J Rheum* 1985;12:478–481.
15. Bartlett RJV, Parkin A, Ware FW, et al.: Reproducibility of oesophageal transit studies: several 'single swallows' must be performed. *Nucl Med Communic* 1987;8:317–326.
16. Russell COH, Hill LD, Holmes ER, et al.: Radionuclide transit: a sensitive screening test for esophageal dysfunction. *Gastroenterology* 1981;80:887–892.
17. Taillefer R, Beauchamp G, Duranceau A: Radionuclide esophageal transit studies, in Van Nostrand D and Baum S (eds.): *Atlas of Nuclear Medicine*. Philadelphia, J.B. Lippincott Company, 1988: pp 1–40.
18. Blackwell J, Haannan WWJ, Adam RD, Heading RC: Radionuclide transit studies in the detection of esophageal dysmotility. *Gut* 1983;24:421–426.
19. Klein HA and Wald A: Esophageal Transit Scintigraphy, in Freeman LM (ed.): *Nuclear Medicine Annual 1988*. New York, Raven Press, 1988: pp 79–124.
20. Klein HA and Wald A: Normal variation in radionuclide esophageal transit studies. *Eur J Nucl Med* 1987;13:115–120.
21. Klein HA and Wald A: Computer analysis of radionuclide esophageal transit studies. *J Nucl Med* 25:957–964, 1984.
22. Klein HA: Editorial. Improving esophageal transit scintigraphy. *J Nucl Med* 1991;32:1371–1374.
23. DeVincentis N, Lenti R, Pona C, et al.: Scintigraphic evaluation of the esophageal transit time for the noninvasive assessment of esophageal motor disorders. *J Nucl Med Allied Sci* 1984;28:137–142.
24. Llamas-Elvira JM, Martinez-Paredes M, Sopena-Monforte M, et al.: Value of radionuclide oesophageal transit in studies of function dysphagia. *Br J Rad* 1986;59:1073–1078.
25. Netscher D, Larson GM, Polk HC: Radionuclide esophageal transit. *Arch Surg* 1986;121:843–848.
26. Svedberg JB: The bolus transport diagram: a functional display method applied to oesophageal studies. *Clin Phys Physiol Meas* 1982:3:267–272.
27. Rozen P, Gelfond M, Zaltzman S, Baron J, Gilat T: Dynamic, diagnostic, and pharmacological radionuclide studies of the esophagus in achalasia. *Radiology* 1982;144:587–590.
28. DeCaesteker JS, Blackwell JN, Adam RD, et al.: Clinical value of radionuclide esophageal transit measurement. *Gut* 1986;27:659–666.
29. Gross R, Johns LF, Kaminski RJ: Esophageal emptying in achalasia quantitated by a radioisotope technique. *Dig Dis Sci* 1979;24:945–949.
30. Richter JE, Castell DO: Diffuse esophageal spasm: a reappraisal. *Ann Intern Med* 1984;100:242–245.
31. Richter JE, Wu WC, Cowan RJ, Ott DJ, Blackwell JN: Letter to the editor: Nutcracker esophagus. *Dig Dis Sci* 1985; 30:188–190.
32. Richter JE, Wu WC, Ott DJ, Chen YM: Letter to Editor: "Nutcracker" esophagus: diagnosis with radionuclide esophageal scintigraphy versus manometry. *Radiology* 1987; 164:877–880.
33. Cohen S. Esophageal motility disorders and their response to calcium channel antagonists. *Gastroenterology* 1987; 97:201–203.
34. Benjamin SB, Gerhardt DC, Casttell DO: High amplitude,

peristaltic esophageal contractions associated with chest pain and/or dysphagia. *Gastroenterology* 1979;77:478–483.

35. Richter JE, Blackwell JN, Wu WC, et al.: Relationship of radionuclide liquid bolus transport and esophageal manometry. *J Lab Clin Med* 1987;109:217–224.
36. Benjamin SB, O'Donnell JK, Hancock J, et al.: Prolonged radionuclide transit in "nutcracker esophagus". *Dig Dis Sci* 1983;28:775–779.
37. Drane WE, Johnson DA, Hagan DP, Cattau EL: "Nutcracker" esophagus: Diagnosis with radionuclide esophageal scintigraphy versus manometry. *Radiology* 1987;163:33–37.
38. Mughal MM, Marples M, Bancewicz J: Scintigraphic assessment of esophageal motility: what does it show and how reliable is it? *Gut* 1986;27:946–953.
39. Drane WE, Karvelis K, Johnson DA, et al.: Progressive systemic sclerosis: radionuclide esophageal scintigraphy and manometry. *Radiology* 1986;160:73–76.
40. Horowitz M, McNeil JD, Maddern GJ, et al.: Abnormalities of gastric and esophageal emptying in polymyositis and dermatomyositis. *Gastroenterology* 1986;90:434–439.
41. Eckert VF, Nix W, Kraus W, Bohl J: Esophageal motor function in patients with muscular dystrophy. *Gastroenterology* 1986;90:628–630.
42. Russell COH, Gannan FR, Coatsworth J, et al.: Relationship among esophageal dysfunction, diabetic gastroenteropathy and peripheral neuropathy. *Dig Dis Sci* 1983;28:289–293.
43. Hollis JB, Castell DO, Braddom RL: Esophageal function in diabetes mellitus and its relation to peripheral neuropathy. *Gastroenterology* 1977;73:1098–1102.
44. Gelfond M, Rozen P, Gilat T: Isorsorbide dinitrate and nifedipine treatment of achalasia: A clinical, manometric and radionuclide evaluation. *Gastroenterology* 1982;83:963–969.
45. Hogan WJ, Dodds WJ: Gastroesophageal reflux disease (reflux esophagitis), in Sleisenger MH, Fordtran JS (eds.): *Gastrointestinal Disease*. 4th edition. Philadelphia, W.B. Saunders Co, 1989: pp 594–616.
46. Jenkins AF, Cowan RJ, Richter JE: Gastroesophageal scintigraphy: Is it a sensitive screening test for gastroesophageal reflux disease? *J Clin Gastroenterol* 1985;7:127–131.
47. Richter JE: Gastroesophageal reflux: diagnosis and management. *Hospital Pract* 1992;59–66.
48. Wu WC: Ancillary test in the diagnosis of gastroesophageal reflux disease, in McCallum RW, Mittal RK (eds.): *Gastroenterology Clinics of North America*. Philadelphia, W.B. Saunders, vol. 19, 1990: pp 671–682.
49. Sondheimer JM: Gastroesophageal reflux; update on pathogenesis and diagnosis. *Ped Clin N Amer* 1988;35:103–453.
50. Fisher RS, Malmud LS, Roberts GS, Lobis IF: Gastroesophageal (GE) scintiscanning to detect and quantitate GE reflux. *Gastroenterology* 1976;70:301–308.
51. Kaul B, Petersen H, Grette K, Erichsen H, Myrvold HE: Scintigraphy, pH measurement, and radiography in the evaluation of gastroesophageal reflux. *Scand J Gastroenterol* 1985;20:289–294.
52. Velasco N, Pope CE, Gannan RM, et al.: Measurement of esophageal reflux by scintigraphy. *Dig Dis Sci* 1984; 11:977–982.
53. Styles CB, Holt S, Bowes KL, et al.: Gastroesophageal reflux and transit scintigraphy: a comparison with esophageal biopsy in patients with heartburn. *J Canad Assoc Radiol* 1984; 35:124–127.
54. Fung W-P, Van der Schaaf A, Grieve JC: Gastroesophageal scintigraphy and endoscopy in the diagnosis of esophageal reflux and esophagitis. *Am J Gastroenterol* 1985;80:245–247.
55. Hoffman GC, Vansant JH: The gastroesophageal scintiscan. *Arch Surg* 1979;114:727–728.
56. Rudd TG, Christie DL: Demonstration of gastroesophageal reflux in children by radionuclide gastroesophagography. *Radiology* 1979;131:483–486.
57. Heyman S, Kirkpatrick JA, Winter HS, Treves S: An improved radionuclide method for the diagnosis of gastroesophageal reflux and aspiration in children (milk scan). *Radiology* 1979;131:479–482.
58. Blumhagen JD, Rudd TG, Christie DL: Gastroesophageal reflux in children: radionuclide gastroesophagography. *Am J Roentgenol* 1980;135:1001–1004.
59. Arasu TS, Wyllie R, Fitzgerald JF, et al.: Gastroesophageal reflux in infants and children—comparative accuracy of diagnostic methods. *J Pediatr* 1980;96:798–803.
60. Seibert JJ, Byrne WJ, Euler AR, et al.: Gastroesophageal reflux—the acid test:scintigraphy or the pH probe? *Am J Roentgenol* 1983;140:1087–1090.
61. Malmud LS, Fisher RS: Radionuclide studies of esophageal transit and gastroesophageal reflux. *Semin Nucl Med* 1982;12:104–115.
62. Malmud LA, Vitti RA, Fisher RS: Gastroesophageal Reflux, in Freeman LM (ed.): *Freeman and Johnson's Clinical Radionuclide Imaging*, Vol 3, Third Ed. Orlando, FL, Grune & Stratton, 1986, pp 1669–1779.
63. Malmud LS, Fisher RS: Scintigraphic evaluation of esophageal transit, gastroesophageal reflux, and gastric emptying, in Gottschalk A, Hoffer PB, Potchen EJ (eds.): *Diagnostic Nuclear Medicine*. Second Ed. Baltimore, William & Wilkins, 1988, pp 663–686.
64. Fisher RS, Malmud LS: Functional scintigraphy: diagnostic applications in gastroenterology, in Berk JE (ed.): *Developments in Digestive Diseases*. Philadelphia, Lea & Febiger, 1980, pp 139–164.
65. Kaul B, Halvorsen T, Petersen H, Grette K, Myrvold HE: Gastroesophageal reflux disease. *Scand J Gastroenterol* 1986;21:134–138.
66. Von Leisner B, Witte J, Kiefhaber P, et al.: Nucklearmedizinische Diagnostik des gastroesophagealen refluxes. *Zeitsch Gastroenterol* 1978;16:235–241.
67. Sherbaniuk RW, Wensel R, Trautman A, Grace M, et al.: Gastrin, gastric emptying and gastroesophageal reflux after ranitidine. *J Clin Gastroenterol* 1983;5:239–244.
68. Shay SS, Eggli D, Johnson L: Simultaneous esophageal pH monitoring and scintigraphy during the postprandial period in patients with severe reflux esophagitis. *Dig Dis Sci* 1991;36:558–564.
69. Kahrilas PJ, Dodds WWJ, Hogan WWJ, et al.: Esophageal peristaltic dysfunction in peptic esophagitis. *Gastroenterology* 1986;91:897–904.
70. Carre IJ: The natural history of the partial thoracic stomach ("hiatal hernia") in children. *Arch Dis Child* 1959;34: 344–353.
71. Miller J: Editorial: Upper gastrointestinal tract evaluation with radionuclides in infants. *Radiology* 1991;178:326–327.
72. Rosen P, Treves ST: Gastroesophageal reflux and gastric emptying, in Treves ST (ed.): *Pediatric Nuclear Medicine*. New York, Springer-Verlag, 1985, pp 171–177.
73. Swanson MA, Cox KL, Cannon RA: Gastroesophageal scintigraphy with and without compression. *Clin Nucl Med* 1981;6:62–66.
74. Heyman S: Pediatric nuclear gastroenterology: evaluation of gastroesophageal reflux and gastrointestinal bleeding, in Freeman LM, Weissmann, HS (eds.): *Nuclear Medicine Annual 1985*. New York, Raven Press, 1985: pp 133–153.
75. Piepsz A, Georges B, Rodeschj P, Cadranel S: Gastroesophageal scintiscanning in children. *J Nucl Med* 1982;23: 631–632.
76. Boonyaprapa S, Alderson PO, Garfinkel DJ, et al.: Detection of pulmonary aspiration in infants and children with respira-

tory disease: concise communication. *J Nucl Med* 1980;21:314–318.
77. Jona JZ, Sty JR, Glicklich M: Simplified radioisotope technique for assessing gastroesophageal reflux in children. *J Pediatr Surg* 1981;16:114–117.
78. MacFayden UM, Hendry GMA, Simpson H: Gastro-esophageal reflux in near-miss sudden infant death syndrome or suspected recurrent aspiration. *Arch Dis Child* 1983;58:87–91.
79. Berger D, Bischof-Delaloye A, Reinberg O, et al.: Esophageal and pulmonary scintiscanning in gastroesophageal reflux in children. *Prog Pediatr Surg* 1985;18:69–77.
80. McVeagh P, Howman-Giles R, Kempt A: Pulmonary aspiration studied by radionuclide milk scanning and barium swallow roentgenography. *AJDC* 1987a;141:917–921.
81. Heyman S, Respondek M: Detection of pulmonary aspiration in children by radionuclide "salivagram". *J Nucl Med* 1989;30:697–699.
82. Tolia V, Calhoun JA, Kuhns LR, Kauffman RE: Lack of correlation between extended pH monitoring and scintigraphy in the evaluation of infants with gastroesophageal reflux. *J Lab Clin Med* 1990;115:559–63.
83. Devos PG, Forgert P, DeRoo M, et al.: Scintigraphic evaluation of gastrointestinal reflux (GER) in children (Abstr). *J Nucl Med* 1979;30:636.
84. Piepsz A, Georges B, Perlmutter N: Gastro-oesophageal scintiscanning in children. *Pediatr Radiol* 1981;11:71–74.
85. Cavell B: Gastric emptying in preterm infants. *Acta Paediatr Scand* 1979;68:725–730.
86. Cavell B: Reservoir and emptying function of the stomach of the premature infant. *Acta Paediatr Scand* (suppl) 1982;296:60–61.
87. Gelfand MJ, Wagner GG: Gastric emptying in infants and children: limited utility of 1-hour measurement. *Radiology* 1991;178:379–181.
88. McCallum RW, Berkowitz DM, Lerner E: Gastric emptying in patients with gastroesophageal reflux. *Gastroenterology* 1981;80:285–291.
89. Maddern GJ, Chatterton BE, Collins PJ, et al.: Solid and liquid emptying in patients with gastro-oesophageal reflux. *Br J Surg* 1985;72:344–347.
90. Shay SS, Eggli D, McDonald C, Johnson LF: Gastric emptying of solid food in patients with gastroesophageal reflux. *Gastroenterology* 1987;92:459–465.
91. Johnson DA, Winters C, Drane WE, et al.: Solid-phase gastric emptying in patients with Barrett's esophagus. *Dig Dis Sci* 1986;31:1217–1220.
92. Hillemeier AC, Lange R, McCallum R, Gryboski J: Delayed gastric emptying in infants with gastroesophageal reflux. *J Pediatr* 1981;98:190–193.
93. Rosen PR, Treves S: The relationship between gastroesophageal reflux and gastric emptying in infants and children. *J Nucl Med* 1984;25:571–574.
94. Di Lorenzo C, Piepsz A, Ham H, Cadranel S: Gastric emptying with gastro-esophageal reflux. *Arch Dis Child* 1987; 62:449–453.
95. Howman-Giles R, Trochei M: Radionuclide "milk" scan for detection of pulmonary aspiration in infants and children. *J Nucl Med* 1980;21:9.
96. Griffith GA, Owen GM, Kirkman S, et al.: Measurement of the rate of gastric emptying using chromium-51. *Lancet* 1966;1:1244–1245.
97. Kelly KA: Motility of the stomach and gastroduodenal junction, in Johnson LR (ed.): *Physiology of the gastrointestinal tract*. New York, Raven Press, 1981: pp 393–410.
98. Itoh Z, Honda R, Hitwatashi K: Motilin-induced mechanical activity in the canine alimentary tract. *Scand J Gastroenterol* 1976;11(suppl 39):933–110.
99. Gelsrud PO, Taylor IL, Watts HD, et al.: How gastric emptying of carbohydrate affects glucose tolerance and symptoms after truncal vagotomy with pyloroplasty. *Gastroenterology* 1980;78:1463–1497.
100. Mayer EA, Thomson JB, Jehn D, et al.: Gastric emptying and sieving of solid food and pancreatic and biliary secretion after solid meals in patients with truncal vagotomy and antrectomy. *Gastroenterology* 1982;83:184–192.
101. MacGregor IL, Gueller R, Watts HD, Meyer JH: The effect of acute hyperglycemia on gastric emptying in man. *Gastroenterology* 1976;70:190–196.
102. Campbell IW, Heading RC, Tothill P, et al.: Gastric emptying in diabetic autonomic neuropathy. *Gut* 1977;18:462–467.
103. Buysschaert M, Moulart M, Urbain JL, et al.: Impaired gastric emptying in diabetic patients with cardiac autonomic neuropathy. *Diabetes Care* 1987;10:448–452.
104. Keshavarzian A, Iber FL, Vaeth J: Gastric emptying in patients with insulin-requiring diabetes mellitus. *Am J Gastroenterol* 1987;82:29–35.
105. Feldman M, Smith HJ, Simon TR: Gastric emptying and solid radiopague markers: studies in healthy subjects and diabetic patients. *Gastroenterology* 1984;87:895–902.
106. Ziessman HA, Fahey FH, Collen MJ: Biphasic solid and liquid gastric emptying in normal controls and diabetics using continuous acquisition in the LAO view. *Dig Dis Sci* 1992;37:744–750.
107. Muller-Lissner SA: Bile reflux is increased in cigarette smokers. *Gastroenterology* 1986;90:1205–1209.
108. Barboriak JJ, Meade RC: Effect of alcohol on gastric emptying in man. *Am J Clin Nutr* 1970;23:1151–1153.
109. Moore JG, Christian PE, Datz FL: Effect of wine on gastric emptying in humans. *Gastroenterology* 1981;81:1072–1075.
110. Chaudhuri TK, Fink S: Update: Pharmaceuticals and gastric emptying. *Am J Gastroenterol* 1990;85:223–230.
111. Albibi R, McCallum RW: Metoclopramide: pharmacology and clinical application. *Ann Intern Med* 1983;98:86–95.
112. Brodgen RN, Carmine AA, Heel RC, et al.: Domperidone: a review of its pharmacological activity, pharmacokinetics and therapeutic efficacy in the treatment of chronic dyspepsia and as an antiemetic. *Drugs* 1982;24:360–400.
113. McCallum RW, Prakash C, Campoli-Richards DM, Goa K: Cispramide. A preliminary review in pharmacodynamic and pharmaco-kinetic properties and therapeutic use as a prokinetic agent in gastrointestinal motility disorders. *Drugs* 1988;36:652–681.
114. Loo FD, Palmer DW, Soergel KH, et al.: Gastric emptying in patients with diabetes mellitus. *Gastroenterology* 1984; 86:485–494.
115. Snape WJ, Battle WS, Schwartz S, et al.: Metoclopramide to treat gastroparesis due to diabetes mellitus, *Ann Intern Med* 1982;96:444–446.
116. Schade RR, Dugas M, Lhotsky D, et al.: Effect of metoclopramide on gastric liquid emptying in patients with diabetic gastroparesis. *Dig Dis Sci* 1985;30:10–15.
117. Horowitz M, Harding PE, Chatterton BE, et al.: Acute and chronic effects of domperidone on gastric emptying in diabetic autonomic neuropathy. *Dig Dis Sci* 1985;30:1–9.
118. Horowitz M, Maddox A, Harding PE, et al.: Effect of cisapride on gastric and esophageal emptying in insulin-dependent diabetes mellitus. *Gastroenterology* 1987;92:1899–1907.
119. Janssens J, Peeters TL, Vantrappen G, et al.: Improvement in gastric emptying in diabetic gastroparesis by erthromycin. *N Engl J Med* 1990;322:1028–1031.
120. Urbain JLC, Vantrappen G, Janssens J, et al.: Intravenous erythromycin dramatically accelerates gastric emptying in gastroparesis diabeticorum and normals and abolishes the

emptying discrimination between solids and liquids. *J Nucl Med* 1990;31:1490–1493.

121. McCallum RW, Ricci P, Rakantansky H, et al.: A multicenter placebo controlled clinical trial of oral metoclopramide in diabetic gastroparesis. *Diabet Care* 1983;6:643.

122. Maurer AH, Heyman S, Vitti RA, Winzelberg GG: Gastrointestinal nuclear medicine, in Siegel BA, Kirchner PT (eds.): *Nuclear Medicine Self Study Program* I. New York Soc Nuclear Med, 1988: pp 59–86.

123. Meyer JH, MacGregor IL, Gueller R, et al.: Tc-99m tagged chicken liver as a marker of solid food in the human stomach. *Dig Dis* 1976;21:296–304.

124. McCallum RC, Saldino T, Lange R: Comparison of gastric emptying rates of intracellular and surface-labeled chicken liver in normal subjects. *J Nucl Med* 1980;21:67.

125. Christian PE, Moore JG, Datz FL: In vitro comparison of solid food radiotracers for gastric emptying studies. *J Nucl Med Technol* 1981;9:116–117.

126. Christian PE, Moore JG, Datz FL: Comparison of Tc-99m labeled liver and liver paté as markers for solid phase gastric emptying. *J Nucl Med* 1984;25:364–366.

127. Knight LC, Malmud LS: Tc-99m ovalbumin labeled eggs: Comparison with other solid food and markers in vitro. *J Nucl Med* 1981;22:28.

128. Kroop HS, Long WB, Alavi A, et al.: Effect of water and fat on gastric emptying of solid meals. *Gastroenterology* 1979;77:997–1000.

129. Knight LC, Fisher RS, Malmud LS: Comparison of solid food marker in gastric emptying studies, In: *Nuclear Medicine & Biology: Proceedings of the Third World Congress of Nuclear Medicine and Biology*, Paris Vol III New York, Pergamon Press, 1982, pp 2407–2410.

130. Dworkin JH, Gutkowski RF: Rapid closed-system production of Tc-99m albumin using electrolysis. *J Nucl Med* 1971;12:562–565.

131. Shivshanker K, Bennett RW, Haynie TP: Tumor associated gastroparesis correction with metoclopramide. *Am J Surg* 1983;145:221–225.

132. Wirth N, Swanson D, Nakajo M, et al.: A conventiently prepared Tc-99m resin for semsolid gastric emptying studies. *J Nucl Med* 1983;24:511–514.

133. Schulze-Delrieu K: Metoclopramide. *N Engl J Med* 1981; 305:28–33.

134. Carryer PW, Brown ML, Malagelada J-R, et al.: Quantification of the fate of dietary fiber in humans in a newly developed radiolabeled fiber marker. *Gastroenterology* 1982;82: 1389–1394.

135. Cunningham KM, Baker RJ, Horowitz M, et al.: Use of Technetium-99m(V)Thiocyanate to measure gastric emptying of fat. *J Nucl Med* 1991;32:878–881.

136. Christian PE, Moore JG, Sorenson JA, et al.: Effects of meal size and correction technique on gastric emptying time: Studies with two tracers and opposed detectors. *J Nucl Med* 1980;21:883–885.

137. Malmud LS, Fisher RS, Knight LC, et al.: Scintigraphic evaluation of gastric emptying. *Semin Nucl Med* 1982; 12:116–125.

138. Urbaine J-L, Siegel JA, Charkes ND, et al.: The two-component stomach: effects of meal particle size on fundal and antral emptying. *Eur J Nucl Med* 1989;15:254–259.

139. Christian PE, Datz FL, Moore JG: Gastric emptying in the morbidly obese before and after gastroplasty. *J Nucl Med* 1986;27:1686–1690.

140. Moore JG, Datz FL, Christian PE, et al.: Effect of body posture on radionuclide measurements of gastric emptying. *Dig Dis Sci* 1988;33:1592–1595.

141. Tothill P, McLoughlin GP, Holt S, et al.: The effect of posture on errors in gastric emptying measurements. *Phys Med Biol* 1980;25:1071–1077.

142. Moore JG, Datz FL, Christian PE, et al.: Exercise increases solid meal gastric emptying rates in men. *Dig Dis Sci* 1990;35:428–432.

143. Tothill P, McLoughlin GP, Heading RC: Techniques and errors in scintigraphic measurements of gastric emptying. *J Nucl Med* 1978;19:256–261.

144. VanDeventer G, Thomson J, Graham LS, et al.: Validation of corrections for errors in collimation on measuring gastric emptying of nuclide labeled meals. *J Nucl Med* 1982; 24:187–196.

145. Collins PJ, Horowitz MB, Shearman DJC, Chatterton BE: Correction for tissue attenuation in radionuclide gastric emptying studies: A comparison of a lateral image method and a geometric mean method. *Br J Radiol* 1984;57: 689–695.

146. Fahey FH, Ziessman HA, Collen MJ, Eggli DF: Left anterior oblique projection and peak-to-scatter ratio for attenuation compensation of gastric emptying studies. *J Nucl Med* 1989;30:233–239.

147. Collins PJ, Horowitz MB, Cook DJ, et al.: Gastric emptying in normal subjects—a reproducible technique using a single scintillation camera and computer system. *Gut* 1983; 24:1117–1125.

148. Meyer JH, VanDeventer G, Graham LS, et al.: Error and corrections with scintigraphic measurement of gastric emptying of solid foods. *J Nucl Med* 1983;24:197–203.

149. Maurer AH, Knight LC, Charkes ND, et al.: Comparison of left anterior oblique and geometric mean gastric emptying. *J Nucl Med* 1991;32:2176–2180.

150. Ford PV, Kennedy RL, Vogel JM: Comparison of left anterior oblique, anterior, and geometric mean methods for determining gastric emptying times. *J Nucl Med* 1992;33:127–130.

151. Christian PE, Datz FL, Moore JG: Confirmation of short solid-food lag phase by continuous monitoring of gastric emptying. *J Nucl Med* 1991;32:1349–1352.

152. Glowniak JV, Wahl RL: Patient motion artifacts on scintigraphic gastric emptying studies. *Radiology* 1983; 154:537–538.

153. Brophy CM, Moore JG, Christian PE, et al.: Variability of gastric emptying measurements in man employing standardized radiolabeled meals. *Dig Dis Sci* 1986;31:799–806.

154. Roland J, Dobbeleir A, Vandevivere J, Ham HR: Evaluation of reproducibility of solid-phase gastric emptying in healthy subjects. *Eur J Nucl Med* 1990;17:130–133.

155. Goo RH, Moore JG, Greenbert A, et al.: Circadian variation in gastric emptying of meals in humans. *Gastroenterology* 1987;93:515–518.

156. Datz FL, Christian PE, Moore JG: Gender related differences in gastric emptying. *JNM* 1987;208:604–605.

157. Elasoff JD, Reedy TJ, Meyer JH: Analysis of gastric emptying data. *Gastroenterology* 1982;83:1306–1312.

158. Meyer JH, Ohashi H, John D, Thomson JB: Size of liver particles emptied from the human stomach. *Gastroenterology* 1981;80:1489–1496.

159. Weiner K, Graham LS, Reedy T, et al.: Simultaneous gastric emptying of two solid foods. *Gastroenterology* 1981; 81:257–266.

160. Moore JG, Christian PE, Taylor AT, Alazraki N: Gastric emptying measurements: delayed and complex emptying patterns without appropriate correction. *J Nucl Med* 1985;26:1206–1210.

161. Jian R, Vigneron N, Najean Y, et al.: Gastric emptying and intragastric distribution of lipids in man. A new scintigraphic method of study. *Dig Dis Sci* 1982;27:705–711.

162. Moore JG, Tweedy C, Christian PE, et al.: Effect of age

on gastric emptying of liquid-solid meals in man. *Dig Dis Sci* 1983;28:340–344.

163. Siegel JA, Urbain J-L, Adler LP: Biphasic nature of gastric emptying. *Gut* 1988;29:85–89.
164. Moore JG, Christian PE, Coleman RE: Gastric emptying of varying meal weight and composition in man. *Dig Dis Sci* 1981;26:16–22.
165. Moore JG, Christian PE, Brown JA, et al.: Influence of meal weight and caloric content on gastric emptying of meals in man. *Dig Dis Sci* 1984;29:513–519.
166. Horowitz M, Collins PJ, Cook DJ, et al.: Abnormalities of gastric emptying in obese patients. *Int J Obesity* 1983; 7:415–421.
167. Camilleri M, Colemont LJ, Phillips SF, et al.: Human gastric emptying and colonic filling of solids characterized by a new method. *Am J Physiol* 1989;257:G284–G290.
168. Paraskevopoulos JA, Houghton LA, Eyre-Brooke I, et al.: Effect of composition of gastric contents on resistance to emptying of liquids from stomach in humans. *Dig Dis Sci* 1988;33:914–918.
169. Siegel JA, Krevsky B, Maurer AH: Scintigraphic evaluation of gastric emptying: are radiolabeled solids necessary? *Clin Nucl Med* 1989;14:40–46.
170. Choe AI, Ziessman HA, Fleischer DE: Tumor-associated gastroparesis with esophageal carcinoma. *Dig Dis Sci* 1989; 34:1132–1134.
171. Reddy AB, Wright RA, Wheeler GE, et al.: Nonobstructive gastroparesis in amyloidosis improved with metoclopramide. *Arch Intern Med* 1983;134:237–248.
172. Ziessman HA, Argoff CE, Barton NW: Delayed gastric emptying in Fabry's disease. *Eur J Nucl Med* 1989;15:538.
173. Perkel MS, Moore C, Hersh T, et al.: Metoclopramide therapy in patients with delayed gastric emptying: A randomized, double blind study. *Am J Dig Dis Sci* 1979;24:662–666.
174. Domstad PA, Kim EE, Beihn R, et al.: Biologic gastric emptying time in diabetic patients, using Tc-99m-labeled resin-oatmeal with and without metoclopramide. *J Nucl Med* 1980;21:1098–1100.
175. Arnstein NB, Shapiro B, Eckhauser FE, et al.: Morbid obesity treated by gastroplasty: radionuclide gastric emptying studies. *Radiology* 1985;156:501–504.
176. Vezina WC, Grace DM, Chamberlain MJ, et al.: Gastric emptying before and after transverse gastroplasty for morbid obesity. *Clin Nucl Med* 1986;11:308–312.
177. Ziessman HA, Collen MJ, Fahey FH, et al.: The effect of the Garren-Edwards Gastric Bubble on solid and liquid gastric emptying. *Clin Nucl Med* 1988;13:586–588.
178. McCallum RW, Polepalle SC, Schirmer B: Completion gastrectomy for refractory gastroparesis following surgery for peptic ulcer disease. *Dig Dis Sci* 1991;36:1556–1561.
179. Metz G, Gassull MA, Drasar BS, et al.: Breath hydrogen test for small-intestinal bacterial colonization. *Lancet* 1976; 1:668.
180. Newcomer AD, McGill DB, Thomas PJ, Hofmann AF: Prospective comparison of indirect methods for detecting lactase deficiency. *N Engl J Med* 1975;293:1232.
181. Sherr HP, Sasaki Y, Newman A, Banwell JG, et al.: Detection of bacterial deconjugation of bile salts by a convenient breath-analysis technique. *N Engl J Med* 1971;285:656.
182. Pederson NT, Marqverson J: Metabolism of ingested ^{14}C-triolein. Estimation of radiation dose in tests of lipid assimilation using ^{14}C- and ^{3}H-labeled fatty acids. *Eur J Nucl Med* 1981;6:327.
183. Landau BR, Shreeve WW: Radiation exposure from long-lived beta emitters in clinical investigation. *Am J Physiol* 1991;261:E415.
184. Shreeve WW, et al.: C-14 studies in carbohydrate metabolism. II. The oxidation of glucose in diabetic human subjects. *Metabolism* 1956;5:22.
185. Shreeve WW, Hennes AR, Schwartz R: Production of $^{14}CO_2$ from 1- and 2-C^{14} acetate by human subjects in various metabolic states. *Metabolism* 1959;8:741.
186. LeRoy GV, et al.: Continuous measurement of specific activity of ^{14}C-labeled carbon dioxide in expired air. *Int J Appl Radiat* 1960;7:273.
187. Tolbert BM, Kirk M, Upham F: Carbon-14 respiration pattern analyzer for clinical studies. *J Appl Physiol* 1959;30:116.
188. Abt AF, von Schuching SL: Fat utilization test in disorders of fat metabolism. *Bull Johns Hopkins Hosp* 1966;119:316.
189. Schoeller DA, et al.: Clinical diagnosis with the stable isotope ^{13}C in CO_2 breath tests: methodology and fundamental considerations. *J Lab Clin Med* 1977;90:412.
190. Hirano S, et al.: A simple infrared spectroscopic method for the measurement of expired $^{13}CO_2$. *Anal Biochem* 1979;96:64.
191. McDowell RS: Determination of carbon-13 by infrared spectrophotometry of carbon monoxide. *Anal Chem* 1970; 42:1192.
192. Schwabe AD, et al.: Estimation of fat absorption by monitoring of expired radioactive carbon dioxide after feeding a radioactive fat. *Gastroenterology* 1962;42:285.
193. Kaihara S, Wagner HN, Jr: Measurement of intestinal fat absorption with carbon-14 labeled tracers. *J Lab Clin Med* 1968;71:400.
194. Chen IW, et al.: ^{14}C-tripalmitin breath test as a diagnostic aid for fat malabsorption due to pancreatic insufficiency. *J Nucl Med* 1974;15:1125.
195. Watkins JB, et al.: ^{13}C-trioctanoin: a nonradioactive breath test to detect fat malabsorption. *J Lab Clin Med* 1977;90:422.
196. Caspary WF: Breath tests. *Clin Gastroenterol* 1978;7:351.
197. Fish MB, Pollycove M, Wallerstein RO: In vivo oxidative metabolism of propionic acid in human vitamin B_{12} deficiency. *J Lab Clin Med* 1968;72:767.
198. Sasaki Y, et al.: Measurement of ^{14}C-lactose absorption in the diagnosis of lactate deficiency. *J Lab Clin Med* 1970;76:824.
199. King CE, Toskes PP, Guilarte TR, et al.: Comparison of the one-gram d-[^{14}C] xylose breath test to the [^{14}C] bile acid breath test in patients with small-intestine bacterial overgrowth. *Dig Dis Sci* 1980;25:53.
200. McNulty CAM: The treatment of Campylobacter associated gastritis. *Am J Gastroenterol* 1987;82:245.
201. Marshall BJ, Francis G, Langton S, et al.: Rapid urease test in the management of Campylobacter pyloridis associated gastritis. *Am J Gastroenterol* 1987;3:200.
202. Marshall BJ, Plankey MW, Hoffman SR, et al.: A 20-minute breath test for *Helicobacter pylori*, *Am J Gastroenterol* 1991;86:438.
203. Debongnie JC, Pauwels S, Raat A, et al.: Quantification of *Helicobacter pylori* infection in gastritis and ulcer disease using a simple and rapid carbon-14-urea breath test. *J Nucl Med* 1991;32:1192.
204. Henze E, Malfertheiner P, Clauxen M, et al.: Validation of a simplified carbon-14-urea breath test for routine use for detecting *Helicobacter pylori* noninvasively. *J Nucl Med* 1990;31:1940.
205. Baker AL, Kotake AH, Schoeller DA: Clinical utility of breath tests for the assessment of hepatic function. *Semin Liver Dis* 1983;3:318.
206. Schneider JF, Baker AL, Haines NW, et al.: Aminopyrine N-demethylation: a prognostic test of liver function in patients with alcoholic liver disease. *Gastroenterology* 1980;79:1145.
207. Monroe PS, Baker AL, Schneider JF, et al.: The aminopyrine breath test and serum bile acids reflect histologic severity in chronic hepatitis. *Hepatology* 1982;2:317.
208. Miotti T, Bircher J, Preisig R: The 30-minute aminopyrine

breath test: optimization of sampling times after intravenous administration of ^{14}C-aminopyrine. *Digestion* 1988;39:241.

209. Shreeve WW, et al.: Test for alcoholic cirrhosis by conversion of [^{14}C]-; or [^{13}C]-galactose to expired CO_2. *Gastroenterology* 1976;71:98.
210. Caspary WF, Schaeffer J: ^{14}C-D-galactose breath test for evaluation of liver function in patients with chronic liver disease. *Digestion* 1978;17:410.
211. Shreeve WW: Impaired oxidation of carbon-labeled galactose by alcoholic or diabetic liver in vivo. *Nuklearmedizin* 1987;26:159.
212. Shreeve WW, et al.: Evaluation of diabetes by oxidation of ^{14}C- or ^{13}C-labeled glucose to CO_2 in vivo, in *Radiopharmaceuticals and Labeled Compounds*. Copenhagen, Symposium International Atomic Energy Agency, 1973, p 281.
213. Lefebvre P, et al.: Naturally labeled ^{13}C-glucose. Metabolic studies in human diabetes and obesity. *Diabetes* 1975;24:185.
214. Ravussin E, et al.: Carbohydrate utilization in obese subjects after an oral load of 100 g. naturally-labelled ^{13}C-glucose. *Br J Nutr* 1980;43:281.
215. Sweetman L, et al.: Glycine-1-^{13}C in the investigation of children with inborn errors of metabolism, in Klein, Paterson (eds.): *Proceedings of the First International Conference on Stable Isotopes*. Argonne, IL, Argonne National Laboratories, 1973, p 404.
216. Coppen C, et al.: Changes in 5-hydroxytryptophan metabolism in depression. *Br J Psychiat* 1965;111:105.
217. Chaudhuri TK, Winchell HS: Diminished oxidation of ^{14}C-UL-L-asparagine to $^{14}CO_2$ in mice and humans with tumors: a possible means for assessing efficacy of therapy? *J Nucl Med* 1970;11:597.
218. Fish MB, et al.: Effect of route and load of administered phenylalanine on human in vivo phenylalanine catabolism. *J Nucl Med* 1968;9:317.
219. Owen CA Jr, Cooper M, Grindlay JH, et al.: Quantitative measurement of bleeding from alimentary tract by use of radiochromium-labeled erythrocytes. *Surg Forum* 1955; 5:663–667.
220. Alavi A, Dann RW, Baum S, Biery DN: Scintigraphic detection of acute gastrointestinal bleeding. *Radiology* 1977; 124:753–756.
221. Winzelberg GG, McKusick KA, Strauss HW, et al.: Evaluation of gastrointestinal bleeding by red blood cells labeled in vivo with technetium-99m. *J Nucl Med* 1979;20:1080–1086.
222. Alavi A, Ring EJ: Localization of gastrointestinal bleeding: superiority of 99mTc sulfur colloid compared with angiography. *AJR* 1981;137:741–748.
223. Alavi A: Detection of gastrointestinal bleeding with 99mTc-sulfur colloid. *Semin Nucl Med* 1982;XII:126–138.
224. Winn M, Weissman HS, Sprayregen S, et al.: The radionuclide detection of lower gastrointestinal bleeding sites. *Clin Nucl Med* 1983;8:389–395.
225. Simpson AJ, Previti FW: Tc-99m sulfur colloid scintigraphy in the detection of lower gastrointestinal tract bleeding. *Surg Gynecol Obstet* 1982;155(1):33–36.
226. Barry JW, Engle CV: Detection of hemorrhage in a patient with cecal varices using Tc-99m sulfur colloid. *Radiology* 1978;129:489–490.
227. Berger RB, Seman RK, Gottschalk A: The technetium-99m sulfur colloid angiogram in suspected gastrointestinal bleeding. *Radiology* 1983;147:555–558.
228. DeWangee MK: Binding Tc-99m ion to hemoglobin. *J Nucl Med* 1974;15:703–706.
229. Pavel DG, Zimmer AM, Patterson VN: In vivo labeling of red blood cells with 99mTc: a new approach to blood pool visualization. *J Nucl Med* 1977;18:170–174.
230. Srivastava SC, Chervu LR: Radionuclide-labeled red blood cells: current status and future projects. *Semin Nucl Med* 1984;14:68–82.
231. Callahan RJ, Froelich JW, McKusick KA, et al.: A modified method from the in vivo labeling of red blood cells with Tc-99m. Concise communication. *J Nucl Med* 1982;23:315–318.
232. Landry A, Hartshorne MF, Bunker SR, et al.: Optimal technetium-99m RBC labeling for gastrointestinal hemorrhage study. *Clin Nucl Med* 1985;10:491–493.
233. Benedetto AR, Nusynovwitz ML: A technique for the preparation of Tc-99m red blood cells for evaluation of gastrointestinal hemorrhage. *Clin Nucl Med* 1983;8:160–162.
234. Smith TD, Richard P: A simple kit for the preparation of Tc-99m labeled red blood cells. *J Nucl Med* 1974;15:03–706.
235. Wahl RL, Lee ME: Pelvic radionuclide angiography in the diagnosis of gastrointestinal bleeding. *Radiology* 1984; 151:793–794.
236. Froelich JW: Gastrointestinal bleeding, in Thrall JH, Swanson DP (eds.): *Diagnostic Interventions in Nuclear Medicine*. Chicago, Yearbook Medical Publishers, 1985: pp 195–203.
237. Miskowiak J, Nielsen SL, Munck O: Scintigraphic diagnosis of gastrointestinal bleeding with 99mTc-labeled blood-pool agents. *Radiology* 1981;141:499–504.
238. Johnson DG, Coleman RE: Gastrointestinal bleeding. *Radiol Clin North Am* 1982;20:644–651.
239. Smith RK, Arterburn G: Detection and localization of gastrointestinal bleeding using Tc-99m-pyrophosphate in vivo labeled red blood cells. *Clin Nucl Med* 1980;5:55–60.
240. Jacobson AF: Delayed positive gastrointestinal bleeding studies with technetium-99m red blood cells: utility of a second injection. *J Nucl Med* 1991;32:330–332.
241. Jacobson AF, Cerqueira MD: Prognostic significance of late imaging results in technetium-99m-labeled red blood cell gastrointestinal bleeding studies with early negative images. *J Nucl Med* 1992;33:202–207.
242. Winzelberg GG, Froelich JW, McKusick KA, et al.: Radionuclide localization of lower gastrointestinal hemorrhage. *Radiology* 1981;139:465–469.
243. McKusick KA, Foelich, Callahan RJ, Winzelberg GG, Strauss HW: 99mTc red blood cells for detection of gastrointestinal bleeding: experience with 80 patients. *AJR* 1981;137: 1113–1118.
244. Winzelberg GG, McKusick KA, Froelich JW, et al.: Detection of gastrointestinal bleeding with 99mTc-labeled red blood cells. *Semin Nucl Med* 1982;XII:139–146.
245. Markisz JA, Front D, Royal HD, et al.: An evaluation of 99mTc-labeled red blood cell scintigraphy for the detection and localization of gastrointestinal bleeding sites. *Gastroenterology* 1982;83:394–398.
246. Bunker SR, Brown JM, McAuley RJ, et al.: Detection of gastrointestinal bleeding sites. Use of in vitro technetium Tc99m-labeled RBCs. *JAMA* 1982;247:789–792.
247. Gupta S, Luna E, Kingsley S, et al.: Detection of gastrointestinal bleeding by radionuclide scintigraphy. *Am J Gastroenterol* 1984;79:26–31.
248. Thorne DA, Datz FL, Remley K, Christian PE: Bleeding rates necessary for detecting acute gastrointestinal bleeding with technetium-99m-labeled red blood cells in an experimental model. *J Nucl Med* 1987;28:514–520.
249. Smith R, Copely DJ, Bolen FH: 99Tc RBC scintigraphy: Correlation of gastrointestinal bleeding rates with scintigraphic findings. *AJR* 1987;148:869–874.
250. Bunker SR, Lull RJ, Hattner RS, Brown JM: Letter to the editor: The ideal radiotracer in gastrointestinal bleeding detection. *AJR* 1982;138:982–983.
251. McKusick KA, Froelich J, Callahan RJ, et al.: Reply: Letter to the editor: The ideal radiotracer in gastrointestinal bleeding detection. *AJR* 1982;138:983.

252. Alavi A: Reply: Letter to the editor: The ideal radiotracer in gastrointestinal bleeding detection. *AJR* 1982;138:983–984.
253. Tanasescu P, Rigby J, Brachman M, et al.: Comparison of Tc-99m red blood cells with Tc-99m sulfur colloid in the detection of gastrointestinal hemorrhage. *J Nucl Med* 1984;24:48 (abstr).
254. Siddiqui AR, Schauwecker DS, Wellman HN, Mock BH: Comparison of technetium-99m sulfur colloid and in vitro labeled technetium-99m RBCs in the detection of gastrointestinal bleeding. *Clin Nucl Med* 1985;10:546–549.
255. Bunker SR, Lull RJ, Tanasescu DE, et al.: Scintigraphy of gastrointestinal hemorrhage: superiority of 99mTc red blood cells over 99m Tc sulfur colloid. *AJR* 1984;143:543–548.
256. Thrall JH, Freitas JE, Swanson D, et al.: Clinical comparison of cardiac blood pool visualization with technetium-99m red blood cells labeled in vivo and with technetium-99m human serum albumin. *J Nucl Med* 1978;19:796–803.
257. Som P, Oster ZH, Atkins HL, et al.: Detection of gastrointestinal blood loss with 99mTc-labeled heat-treated red blood cells. *Radiology* 1981;138:207–209.
258. Ferrant A, Dahasque N, Leners N, et al.: Scintigraphy with 111-Ind labeled red cells in intermittent gastrointestinal bleeding. *J Nucl Med* 1980;21:844–845.
259. Schmidt KG, Rasmussen JW, Strate M: Scintigraphic localization of occult gastrointestinal bleeding using a combination of ^{111}In-labeled platelets and ^{99}mTc sulfur colloid. *Eur J Nucl Med* 1985;11:94–95.
260. Harden RM, Alexander WD, Kennedy I: Isotope uptake and scanning of stomach in man with 99mTc-pertechnetate. *Lancet* 1967;1:1305–1307.
261. Bickel JG, Witten TA, Killian MK: Use of pertechnetate clearance in the study of gastric physiology. *Gastroenterology* 1972;63:60–66.
262. Taylor TV, Pullen BR, Elder JB, et al.: Observations of gastric mucosal blood flow using 99mTc in rat and man. *Br J Surg* 1975;62:788–791.
263. Irvine WWJ, Stewart AG, McLoughlin GP, et al.: Appraisal of the application of 99mTc in the assessment of gastric function. *Lancet* 1967;2:648–653.
264. Meier-Ruge W, Fridich R: Die Verteilung von Technetium-99m and Jod-131 in der Magenschleimhaut. *Histochemie* 1969;19:147–150.
265. Chaudhuri TK, Polak JJ: Autoradiographic studies of distribution in the stomach of 99mTc-pertechnetate. *Radiology* 1977;123:223–224.
266. Chaudhuri TK, Chaudhuri TK, Shirazi SS, et al.: Radioisotope scan—a possible aid in differentiating retained gastric antrum from Zollinger-Ellison in patients with recurrent peptic ulcer. *Gastroenterology* 1973;65:697–698.
267. Berquist TH, Nolan NG, Carlson HC, et al.: Diagnosis of Barrett's esophagus by pertechnetate scintigraphy. *Mayo Clin Proc* 1973;48:276–279.
268. Marsden DS, Alexander C, Yeung P, et al.: Autoradiographic explanation for the uses of 99mTc in gastric scintiphotography. (abstr) *J Nucl Med* 1973;14:632.
269. Pecora DV, Sagar V, Piccone J: Technetium-99m pertechnetate as an indicator of gastric mucosal proliferation. *AJR* 1978;131:1041–1042.
270. Williams JG: Pertechnetate and the stomach—a continuing controversy. *J Nucl Med* 1983;24:633–636.
271. Spiro HM: Congenital lesions, in *Clinical Gastroenterology*, 3rd Ed. New York, Macmillan, 1983: pp 520–541.
272. Endlich HL, Kafka HL, Powsner LG: Giant Meckel's diverticulum. *JAMA* 1965;191:1084–1085.
273. Rutherford RB, Akers DR: Meckel's diverticulum: a review of 148 pediatric patients, with special reference to the pattern of bleeding and to mesodiverticular vascular bands. *Surgery* 1966;59:618–626.
274. Meguid MM, Wilkinson RH, Canty T, et al.: Futility of barium sulfate in diagnosis of bleeding Meckel's diverticulum. *Arch Surg* 1974;108:361–362.
275. Maglinte DDT, Elmore MF, Isenberg M, Dolan PA: Meckel diverticulum: radiologic demonstration by enteroclysis. *Am J Radiol* 1980;34:925–932.
276. Bree RL, Reuter SR: Angiographic demonstration of a bleeding Meckel's diverticulum. *Radiology* 1973;108:287–288.
277. Jewett TC, Duszynski DO, Allen JE: Visualization of Meckel's diverticulum with 99mTc-pertechnetate. *Surgery* 1970; 68:567–570.
278. Treves S, Grand RJ, Eraklis AJ: Pentagastrin stimulation of technetium-99m uptake by ectopic gastric mucosa in a meckel's diverticulum. *Radiology* 1978;128:711–712.
279. Sfakianakis GN, Anderson GF, King DR, Boles ET, Jr: The effect of gastrointestinal hormones on the pertechnetate imaging of ectopic gastric mucosa in experimental Meckel's diverticulum. *J Nucl Med* 1981;22:678–683.
280. Petrokubi RJ, Baum S, Rohrer GV: Cimetidine administration resulting in improved pertechnetate imaging of Meckel's diverticulum. *Clin Nucl Med* 1978;3:385–388.
281. Diamond RH, Rothstein RD, Alavi A: The role of cimetidine-enhanced technetium-99m pertechnetate imaging for visualizing Meckel's diverticulum. *J Nucl Med* 1991;32:1422–1424.
282. Priebe CJ, Marsden DS, Lazarevic B: The use of ^{99m}technetium pertechnetate to detect transplated gastric mucosa in the dog. *J Pediatr Surg* 1974;9:605–613.
283. Conway JJ: Radionuclide diagnosis of Meckel's diverticulum. *Gastrointest Radiol* 1980;5:209–212.
284. Sfakianakis GN, Conway JJ: Detection of ectopic gastric mucosa in Meckel's diverticulum and in other aberrations by scintigraphy: I. Pathophysiology and 10-year clinical experience. *J Nucl Med* 1981;22:647–654.
285. Sfakianakis GN, Conway JJ: Detection of ectopic gastric mucosa in Meckel's diverticulum and in other aberrations by scintigraphy: Indications and methods—a 10 year experience. *J Nucl Med* 1981;22:732–738.
286. Conway JJ, Pediatric Nuclear Club of the Society of Nuclear Medicine: The sensitivity, specificity and accuracy of radionuclide imaging of Meckel's diverticulum. (Abstr) *J Nucl Med* 1976;17:553.
287. Schwartz MJ, Lewis JH: Meckel's diverticulum: pitfalls in scintigraphic detection in the adult. *Am J Gastroenterol* 1984;79:611–618.
288. Winter PF: Sodium pertechnetate Tc-99m scanning of the abdomen. Diagnosis of an ileal duplication cyst. *JAMA* 1977;237:1352–1353.
289. Schwesinger WH, Croom RD, Habibian MR: Diagnosis of an enteric duplication with pertechnetate 99mTc scanning. *Ann Surg* 1975;181:428.
290. Rose JS, Gribetz D, Krasna IH: Ileal duplication cyst: the importance of sodium pertechnetate Tc99m scanning. *Pediatr Radiol* 1978;6:244–245.
291. Ohba S, Fukuda A, Kohno S, et al.: Ileal duplication and multiple intraluminal diverticula:scintigraphy and barium meal. *AJR* 1981;136:992–994.
292. Mark R, Young L, Ferguson C, et al.: Diagnosis of an intrathoracic gastrogenic cyst using 99mTc-pertechnetate. *Radiology* 1973;109:137–138.
293. Kamoi I, Nishitani H, Oshiumi Y, et al.: Intrathoracic gastric cyst demonstrated by 99mTc pertechnetate scintigraphy. *AJR* 1980;134:1080–1081.
294. Sciarretta G, Malaguti P, Turba E, et al.: Retained gastric antrum syndrome diagnosed by [99mTc] pertechnetate scinti-

photography in man: hormonal and radioisotopic study of two cases. *J Nucl Med* 1978;19:377–389.
295. Dunlap JA, McLane RC, Roper TJ: The retained gastric antrum. A case report. *Radiology* 1975;117:371–372.
296. Lee C, P'eng F, Yeh PH: Sodium pertechnetate Tc-99m antral scan in the diagnosis of retained gastric antrum. *Arch Surg* 1984;119:309–311.
297. Naef AP, Savary M, Ozzello L: Columnar-lined lower esophagus. An acquired lesion with malignant predisposition. A report on 140 cases of Barrett's esophagus with 12 adenocarcinomas. *J Thorac Cardiovasc Surg* 1975;70: 826–835.
298. Mangla JC, Brown M: Diagnosis of Barrett's esophagus by pertechnetate radionuclide. *Am J Dig Dis* 1976;21: 324–328.
299. Bond JH, Levitt MD: Investigation of small bowel transit time in man utilizing pulmonary hydrogen(H2) measurements. *J Lab Clin Med* 1975;85:546–555.
300. Read NW, Al-Janabi MN, Bates TE, et al.: Interpretation of the breath hydrogen profile obtained after ingesting a solid meal containing unabsorbable carbohydrate. *Gut* 1985; 26:834–842.
301. Kellow JE, Borody TJ, Phillips SF, et al.: Sulfapyridine appearance in plasma after salicylsulfapyridine: another simple measure of intestinal transit. *Gastroenterology* 91:396–420, 1986.
302. Caride VJ, Prokop EK, Troncale FJ, et al.: Scintigraphic determination of small intestinal transit time: comparison with the hydrogen breath technique. *Gastroenterology* 1984; 86:714–720.
303. Read NW, Al-Janabi, Holgate AM, et al.: Simultaneous measurement of gastric emptying, small bowel residence and colonic filling of a solid meal by the use of the gamma camera. *Gut* 1986;27:300–308.
304. Jian R, Najeah Y, Bernier JJ: Measurement of intestinal progression of a meal and its residues in normal subjects and patients with functional diarrhea by a dual isotope technique. *Gut* 1984;25:728–731.
305. Meyer JH, Ohashi H, Jehn D, Thompson JB: Size of liver particles emptied from the human stomach. *Gastroenterology* 1981;80:1489–1496.
306. Read NW, Cammack J, Edwards CE, et al.: Is the transit time of a meal through the small intestine related to the rate at which it leaves the stomach? *Gut* 1982;23:824–828.
307. Malagelada JR, Robertson JS, Brown ML, et al.: Intestinal transit of solid and liquid components of a meal in health. *Gastroenterol* 1984;87:1255–63.
308. Camilleri M, Colemont LJ, Phillips SF, et al.: Human gastric emptying and colonic filling of solids characterized by a new method. *Am J Physiol* 1989;257:G284–G290.
309. Madsen JL, Jensen M: Gastrointestinal transit of technetium-99m-labeled cellulose fiber and indium-111-labeled plastic particles. *J Nucl Med* 1989;30:402–406.
310. Madsen JL, Larsen NE, Hilsted J, Worning H: Scintigraphic determination of gastrointestinal transit times. A comparison with breth hydrogen and radiologic methods. *Scand J Gastroenterol* 1991;26:1263–1271.
311. Cummings J: Cellulose and the human gut. *Gut* 1984; 25:805–810.
312. Carryer PW, Brown ML, Malagelada J-R, et al.: Quantification of the fate of dietary fiber in humans by a newly developed radiolabeled fiber marker. *Gastroenterology* 1982; 82:1389–1394.
313. Malagelada JR, Carter SE, Brown ML, Carlson GL: Radiolabeled fiber. A physiological marker for gastric emptying and intestinal transit of solids. *Dig Dis Sci* 1980;25:81–87.
314. Hardy JG, Wood E, Clark AG, Reynolds JR: Whole-bowel transit in patients with the irritable bowel syndrome. *Eur J Nucl Med* 1986;11:393–396.
315. Read NW, Al-Janabi MN, Bates TE, Barber DC: Effect of gastrointestinal intubation on the passage of a solid meal through the stomach and small intestine in humans. *Gastroenterol* 1983;84:1586–1572.
316. Hardy JG, Perkins AC: Validity of the geometric mean correction in the quantification of whole bowel transit. *Nucl Med Commun* 1985;6:217–224.
317. Krevsky B, Malmud LS, D'ErcoleF, et al.: Colonic transit scintigraphy. A physiologic approach to the measurement of colonic transit in humans. *Gastroenterology* 1986;91: 1102–1112.
318. Kaufman PN, Richter JE, Chilton HM, et al.: Effects of liquid versus solid diet on colonic transit in humans. *Gastroenterology* 1990;98:73–81.
319. Proano M, Camilleri M, Phillips SF, et al.: Transit of solids through the human colon: Regional quantification in the unprepared bowel. *Am J Physiol* 1990;258:G856–G862.
320. McLean RG, Smart RC, Gastron-Parry, et al.: Colon transit scintigraphy in health and constipation using I-131 cellulose. *J Nucl Med* 1990;31:985–989.
321. Smart RC, McLean RG, Gaston-Parry D, et al.: Comparison of oral iodine-131 cellulose and Indium-111-DTPA as tracers for colon transit scintigraphy: Analysis by colon activity profiles. *J Nucl Med* 1991;32:1668–1674.
322. Stubbs JB, Valenzuela GA, Stubbs CC: A noninvasive scintigraphic assessment of the colonic transit of nondigestible solids in man. *J Nucl Med* 1991;32:1375–1381. *Gastroenterol* 1991;101:107–115.
323. Hardy JG, Wilson CG, Wood E: Drug delivery to the proximal colon. *J Pharm Pharmacol* 1985;37:874–877.
324. Krevsky B, Maurer AH, Fisher RS: Patterns of colonic transit in chronic idiopathic constipation. *Am J Gastroenterol* 1989;84:127–132.
325. Stivland T, Camilleri M, Vassalo M, et al.: Scintigraphic measurement of regional gut transit in idiopathic constipation. *Gastroenterology* 1991;101:107–115.
326. Kamm MA, Lennard-Jones JE, Thompson DG, et al.: Dynamic scanning defines a colonic defect in severe idiopathic constipation. *Gut* 1988;29:1085–1092.
327. Bazzocchi G, Ellis J, Villaneuva-Meyer J, et al.: Effect of eating on colonic motility and transit in patients with functional diarrhea. *Gastroenterology* 1991;101:1298–1306.
328. Camilleri M, Zinsmeister A, Greydanus MP, et al.: Towards a less costly but accurate test of gastric emptying and small bowel transit. *Dig Dis Sci* 1991;36:609–615.
329. Waldmann TA: Protein-losing enteropathy and kinetic studies of plasma protein metabolism. *Semin Nucl Med* 1972; 2:251–263.
330. Crossley JR, Elliot RB: Simple method for diagnosing protein-losing enteropathy. *Br Med J* 1977;2:428–429.
331. Florent C, L'Hirondel C, Desmazure SC, et al.: Intestinal clearance of alpha$_1$-antitrypsin. *Gastroenterology* 81;81: 777–780.
332. Citrin Y, Sterlin K, Halsted JA: The mechanism of hypoproteinemia associated with giant hypertrophy of the gastric mucosa. *N Engl J Med* 1957;257:906–912.
333. Gordon RC, Jr: Exudative enteropathy: abnormal permeability of the gastrointestinal tract demonstrated with radiolabeled poly-vinyl pyrrolidine. *Lancet* 1959;1:325–326.
334. Waldman TA: Gastrointestinal protein loss demonstrated by Cr-51 labeled albumin. *Lancet* 1961;2:1221–1223.
335. Divgi CR, Lisann NM, Yeh S, Benua RS: Technetium-99m albumin scintigraphy in the diagnosis of protein-losing enteropathy. *J Nucl Med* 1986;27:1710–1712.
336. Yoshida T, Toshihiko II, Sakamoto H, et al.: Technetium-99m

serum albumin measurement of gastrointestinal protein loss in a subtotal gastrectomy patient with giant hypertrophic gastritis. *Clin Nucl Med* 1987;12:773–776.

337. Saverymuttu SH, Peters AM, Lavender JP, Hodgson HJF: Detection of protein-losing enteropathy by ^{111}In-transferrin scanning. *Eur J Nucl Med* 1983;8:40–41.

338. Aburano T, Yokoyama K, Kinuya S, et al.: Indium-111 transferrin imaging for the diagnosis of protein-losing enteropathy. *Clin Nucl Med* 1989;14:681–685.

339. Reba RC, Salkeld J: In-vitro studies of malabsorption and other GI disorders. *Semin Nucl Med* 1982;12:147–155.

27 The Liver

John C. Harbert

The liver is the largest abdominal organ; it weighs 1400 to 1600 g in the adult and occupies most of the right upper quadrant. The superior surface is attached and fixed to the diaphragm by the peritoneal ligaments and hepatic veins. The shape of the liver is highly variable and changes with both position and respiration when fibrosis, infiltration, or mass lesions do not reduce its elasticity.

ANATOMY AND PHYSIOLOGY

Conventionally, the liver has been divided into left and right lobes by the insertion of the falciform ligament (Fig. 1). The right lobe is larger, incorporating two smaller lobes (the caudate and quadrate lobes) projecting from the posteroinferior surface. The anatomic lobes, however, coincide with neither the hepatic venous nor the biliary drainage systems, all of which overlap to some extent. Thus, the liver is one parenchymal mass without true anatomic division. Each anatomic lobe has its own vascular supply and biliary tree, but there are extensive intercommunications.

The liver has a dual blood supply. Like the remainder of the gut of which it is an outgrowth, the liver is perfused by anastomosing arteries arising from the celiac axis and superior mesenteric artery, which supplies approximately 300 mL of blood per minute. The portal vein, formed by the confluence of the splenic and superior mesenteric veins, enters the liver at the inferior margin through the porta hepatis, and supplies approximately 1200 mL/minute. Both supply oxygen and nutrients to the hepatic cells. Xenon washout studies suggest that regional hepatic blood flow varies from one individual to another.[1]

Histologically, the liver is organized into lobules surrounded by hepatic venous sinusoids. The polygonal cells or hepatocytes are aligned radially and converge toward the central lobular vein. These cells make up about 85% of the liver parenchyma and perform all of the metabolic functions of the liver. In the portal spaces are found the supporting elements of the lobe, including the *portal triad*: branches of the hepatic artery, portal vein, and bile collecting ducts.

The walls of the sinusoids are lined with reticuloendothelial cells, called Kupffer cells. These make up about 15% of the liver cells and 80 to 90% of the reticuloendothelial population of the body.

The liver is responsible for an extraordinary variety of physiological functions, two of which figure most prominently in radionuclide studies: phagocytosis of circulating foreign particles and bile formation. Phagocytosis is an activity of the Kupffer cells. Normally, they extract approximately 95% of colloid particles in a single pass; this fact forms the basis for measuring hepatic blood flow and for radiocolloid imaging.[2,3] Bile formation is a function of the hepatocytes, which clear and metabolize a large number of substances that are then excreted into the bile and drained by the biliary system.

Most diseases that alter hepatic structure affect both hepatocyte and reticuloendothelial cell populations, so that measures of one population usually reflect changes in the other.[4] Imaging techniques may reveal dissociation of the two distribution patterns, however, in hepatic adenomas, hepatocellular carcinoma, cirrhosis, chemotherapy, and obstructive jaundice.[5–8]

The Reticuloendothelial System

The reticuloendothelial system (RES) consists of both fixed macrophages and a small number of "wandering" macrophages, but does not include the polymorphonuclear leukocytes.[9] Most of the fixed macrophages line the blood sinuses of the liver, spleen, bone marrow, and lung. The macrophages' clear the bloodstream of unwanted particulate matter. Clearance efficiency depends on (1) certain host factors, including organ blood flow, reticuloendothelial cell integrity, and the presence of serum *opsonins* and, (2) particle factors such as size, number, and surface characteristics. The parallel relationships between bone marrow erythropoietic activity, RES activity, and blood flow are illustrated in Figure 2, which charts the regional distribution of erythropoietic activity in the rabbit femur as measured by ^{59}Fe uptake, the RES population as measured by ^{99m}Tc-sulfur colloid uptake, and blood flow as measured by the capillary embolization of ^{131}I-macroaggregated albumin (15 to 50 μm particles) injected into the aorta.

RADIOCOLLOIDS

Colloids are suspended particles ranging in size from 1 nm to 5 μm. The chemical and physical properties of colloids are determined by charge-mediated interactions at the surface of the particles.[10] The biological distribution of a colloid is determined by the size, surface charge, antigenic properties,

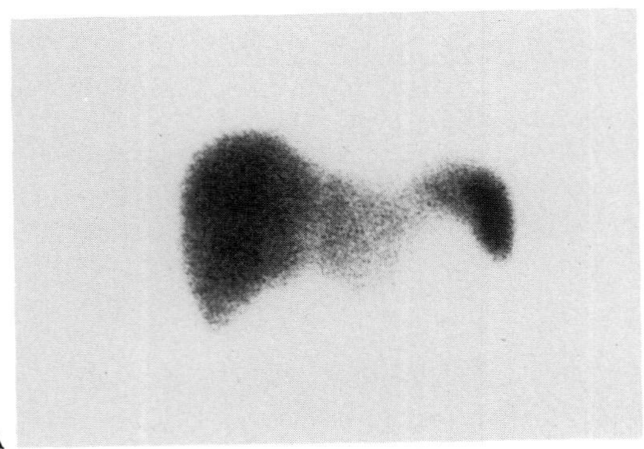

A

Figure 1. **(A).** Anterior planar ^{99m}Tc-sulfur colloid liver/spleen scintiphoto; **(B).** the pertinent correlative anatomy.

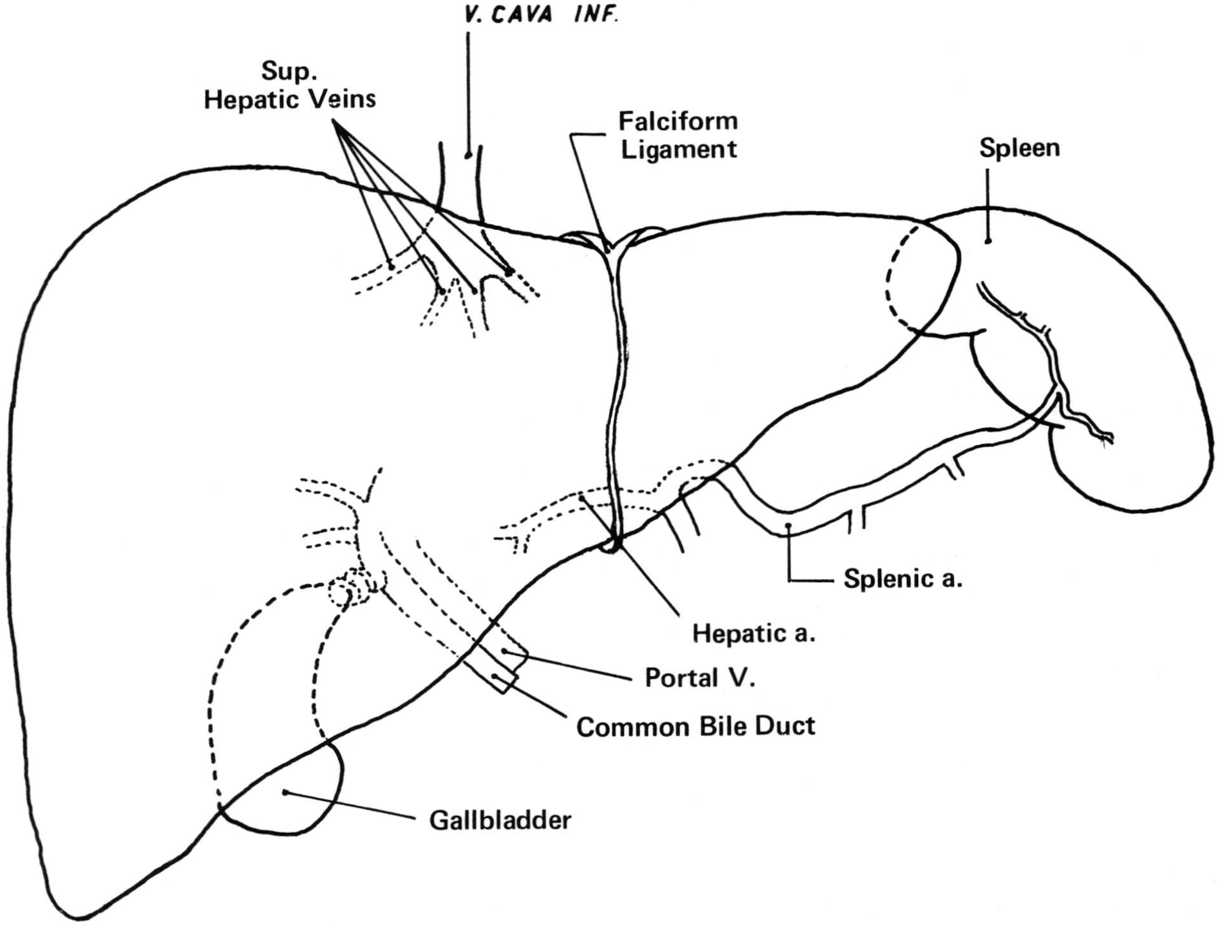

V. CAVA INF.
Sup. Hepatic Veins
Falciform Ligament
Spleen
Splenic a.
Hepatic a.
Portal V.
Common Bile Duct
Gallbladder

B

and the number of particles injected.[4] Colloids foreign to the body are bound by the plasma protein opsonin and phagocytized by macrophages in the RES. Colloids are useful in imaging organs with large populations of reticuloendothelial cells, such as the liver, spleen, and bone marrow. The relative distribution of colloids between these organs can be altered by changing particle size.[11] Particles less than 100 nm are concentrated to a greater extent by the marrow RES elements than by those in the liver and spleen. Particles ranging from 300 to 1000 nm localize mostly in the liver, whereas particles in the 1 to 5 μm range are deposited mostly in the spleen. Saba found that the rate of phagocytosis increases with increasing particle size.[9] Particles larger than 5 μm are not true colloids, and they tend to settle out of solution in the absence of continuous mixing. Very small particles may be excreted by the kidneys.[11]

The colloids of interest in liver-spleen scintigraphy are solid particles (usually smaller than 1 to 2 μm), dispersed in an aqueous phase. These particles are thought to be coated with antibody-like opsonins, which interact with cell membranes of the RES elements to stimulate phagocytosis.

Since diagnostic conclusions are drawn from changing

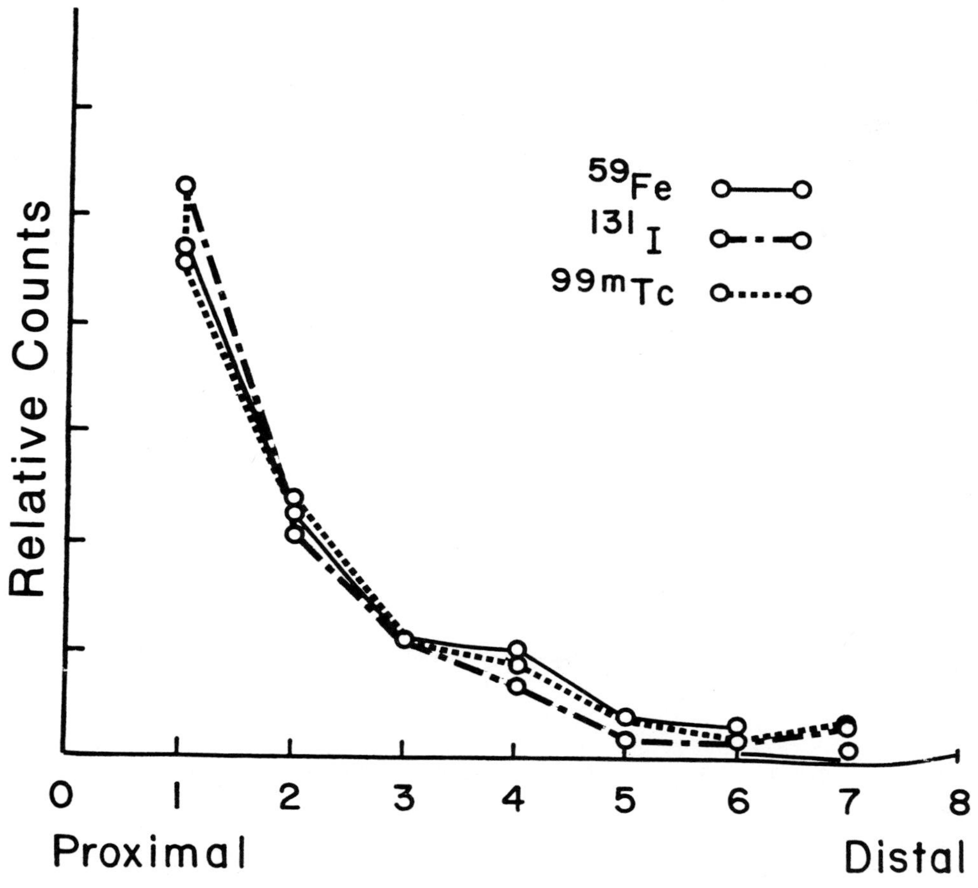

Figure 2. Study in rabbit bone marrow showing similar distribution of blood flow (^{131}I-MAA), RES distribution (^{99m}Tc-sulfur colloid) and erythropoiesis (^{59}Fe-transferrin) in femoral bone marrow. Numbers on the x axis refer to sequential segments from proximal to distal femur. (From reference 10.)

particle distribution, care must be exercised in the preparation and quality control of colloids. For example, ^{99m}Tc-sulfur colloid is normally distributed between liver, spleen, and bone marrow approximately according to their weight, or 85:10:5.[12] ^{99m}Tc-stannous phytate distribution generally is more disposed toward the liver, with relatively little spleen and bone marrow uptake. However, varying the calcium content of the stannous phytate colloid preparation increases splenic uptake, presumably by increasing colloid size.[13] It is also known that varying the boiling time in the preparation of ^{99m}Tc-sulfur colloid affects particle size; prolonged heating reduces particle size.

The exact mechanism of colloid particle localization in the liver is not known. Particles larger than 100 nm are apparently taken up exclusively by the Kupffer cells. Autoradiographic studies show that extracted particles are attached in groups to the Kupffer cell membranes without evidence of endocytosis.[14,15] Frier et al. showed that sulfur colloid particles labeled with ^{99m}Tc and ^{35}S are broken down rapidly with elution of the ^{35}S, but not the ^{99m}Tc.[16] Although these facts do not affect the utility of ^{99m}Tc-sulfur colloid as an imaging agent of the liver and spleen, they may have broad implications about the relevance of sulfur colloid for defining the distribution of the RES. The chemistry of radiocolloids is discussed in detail in Chapter 11.

Functional Tests

For many years, attempts have been made to assess global hepatic function by measuring the blood clearance of radioactive tracers extracted by the liver. Because the liver contains approximately 85% of the cells of the RES, colloid clearance may be considered essentially an hepatic function. According to this concept, a reduction in the rate of colloid clearance reflects either a reduction in hepatic blood flow, a reduction in the effective hepatic RES mass, or both. Such reduced clearance may occur with the development of intrahepatic shunting or parenchymal replacement, especially in cirrhosis.

Several techniques for estimating hepatic blood flow or perfusion have been described. Early studies measured blood clearance of intravenously injected radiocolloids.[3,17] Rate constants can be derived from serial blood activity measurements (Fig. 3). Clearance is then calculated from:

$$\text{Clearance (mL/min)} = \lambda V$$

where λ is the rate constant, $0.693/T_{1/2}$ min^{-1}, and V is the circulating blood volume in mL. Clearance values vary with the type of colloid used because of varying extraction efficiency. ^{99m}Technetium-sulfur colloid is extracted with about 85% efficiency and yields values of approximately 750 mL/

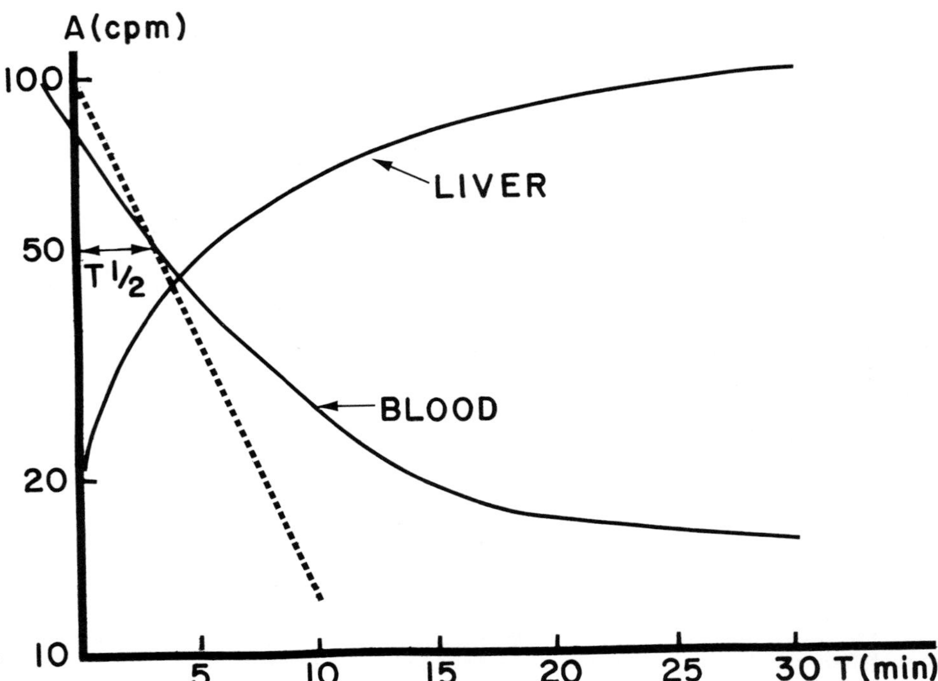

Figure 3. Blood clearance and liver uptake of ^{99m}Tc-sulfur colloid.

minute.[18] The slope of the uptake derived between 2 and 5 minutes is used to determine the rate constant.[19]

These studies show decreased perfusion in cirrhosis, increased perfusion in acute injury, and normal values in alcoholic liver disease without cirrhosis. In addition, most investigators believe that clearance measurements serve as an index of hepatic perfusion rather than RES function.[15]

HEPATIC ARTERY VS. PORTAL VENOUS BLOOD FLOW

Several investigators have used radionuclide tracers to estimate the relative contributions of the hepatic artery and portal vein to total hepatic blood flow.[20–23] Such studies have been used in the evaluation and management of patients with portal hypertension,[24–26] in the follow-up of liver transplantation,[27] and in the early detection of metastatic liver disease.[28,29] It is tempting to use ^{99m}Tc-sulfur colloid for this purpose, because the estimation of blood flow can be conveniently combined with standard scintigraphy.[22,23] However, this technique assumes that both the liver and spleen have equal extraction efficiencies for colloidal particles and that the extraction efficiency is close to 100%. While these assumptions may be valid with normal hepatic function, they are probably not true for patients with significant liver disease.[22]

Normally, the portal circulation contributes 60 to 70% of total hepatic blood flow. In portal hypertension, collateral communications between the portal vein and the inferior vena cava develop so that this value may fall to as low as 20 to 30%.[21] It is for this reason that hepatic insufficiency and encephalopathy develop. Noninvasive estimates of portal flow are useful in evaluating portal hypertension, liver transplant function, and providing the indications for and prognosis after surgical portacaval shunting.

Estimates of portal blood flow can be derived by integrating beneath the time-activity curve that is recorded from the liver after an intravenous bolus of ^{99m}Tc-labeled red blood cells. The hepatic artery and portal circulation components are sufficiently well separated in time to allow the relative contributions to be distinguished (Fig. 4).

The arterial and portal contributions to hepatic perfusion can be quantified by integrating the activity during the hepatic arterial (h) and portal (p) phases of the recording. Integration of the two phases can be determined by several algorithms.[22] At least one study suggests that measurement of the portal contribution to total hepatic blood flow may be a useful means of evaluating acute rejection in liver transplants.[30] A recent comparison of various algorithms for determining hepatic artery/portal blood flow using first-pass techniques found that methods using deconvolution analysis and peak liver-curve activity both correlate well with (invasive) flow probe techniques for determining flow ratios.[31]

A number of other imaginative techniques have been explored. The injection of intrasplenic ^{131}I-HSA[32] or ^{133}Xe[33] obviously suffer from the invasive nature of tracer administration. Better tolerated have been rectally administered tracers: ^{133}Xe,[34] ^{201}T1,[35] ^{123}I-iodoamphetamine,[36] and ^{99m}Tc-pertechnetate.[37,38] Figure 5 shows scintigrams and heart-liver curves derived following the per-rectal administration of ^{99m}Tc-pertechnetate.[38] A portal shunt index, SI, was calculated by taking the ratio of counts integrated over the heart

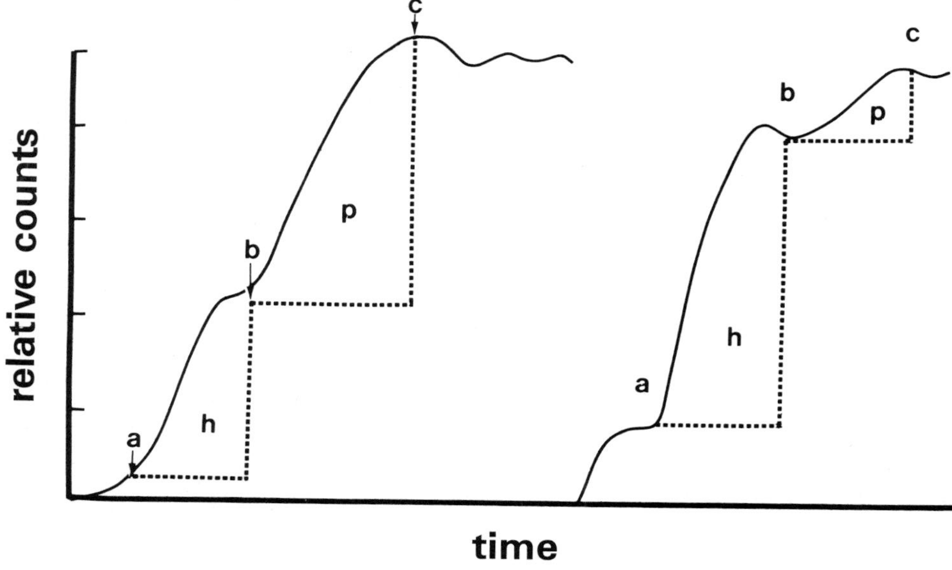

Figure 4. Hepatic blood pool activity following intravenous injection of 555 MBq (15 mCi) of ^{99m}Tc-red blood cells. At left is a normal curve; right curve is from a patient with portal hypertension. The vertical axis represents relative activity. h = hepatic artery contribution; p = portal vein contribution. (Adapted from reference 21.)

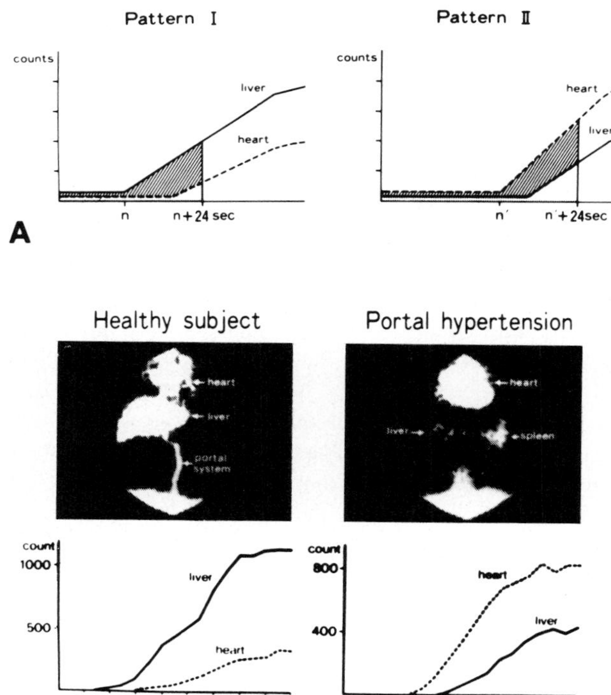

Figure 5. Method of determining the portacaval shunt index by per-rectal administration of ^{99m}Tc-pertechnetate. **(A).** The shunt index is determined by dividing the area under the heart curve by the area under the sum of the liver and heart areas. **(B).** The summed images are integrated over 5 minutes following the per-rectal instillation of 75 MBq of ^{99m}Tc-pertechnetate. The raw counts are shown at the bottom. (Reproduced from reference 38 by permission.)

and liver. Good separation was found between the SI values in normals and cirrhotic patients.

FUNCTIONAL TESTING WITH RECEPTOR-BINDING TESTS

The functioning hepatic mass can also be estimated using specific hepatocyte receptors to bind radiolabeled ligands in vivo. Receptors are special binding sites on cell membranes and within cells that recognize and bind to specific circulating ligands prior to transmembrane transport or the elicitation of some physiological or pharmacological effect.[39] The best-known hepatocyte receptor is the *hepatic binding protein* (HBP), which is specific for asialoglycoproteins.[40] These receptors also recognize a synthetic glycoprotein that has been developed as a radiopharmaceutical, ^{99m}Tc-galactosyl-neoglycoalbumin (NGA).[41,42]

Since NGA binds specifically to the hepatocyte membrane, the tracer can be used not only as an imaging agent, but also as an indicator of total functioning hepatic mass. To do this, the precise quantity of NGA must be known because the receptor sites are capable of becoming saturated.[43,44] Recently, compartmental models have been developed to derive hepatic blood flow estimates without blood sampling.[45] The uses of such a tracer are expected to be primarily (1) in following the course of chronic liver disease and to gauge the effects of therapy, (2) in estimating hepatic functional capacity to determine the safe limit of hepatectomy for hepatocellular carcinoma and, (3) in the differential diagnosis of hepatic tumors, especially in distinguishing focal nodular hyperplasia, macro-regenerating nodules, and adenomatous hyperplastic nodules, all of which contain normal functioning hepatocytes, from hepatocellular carcinoma.[46,47]

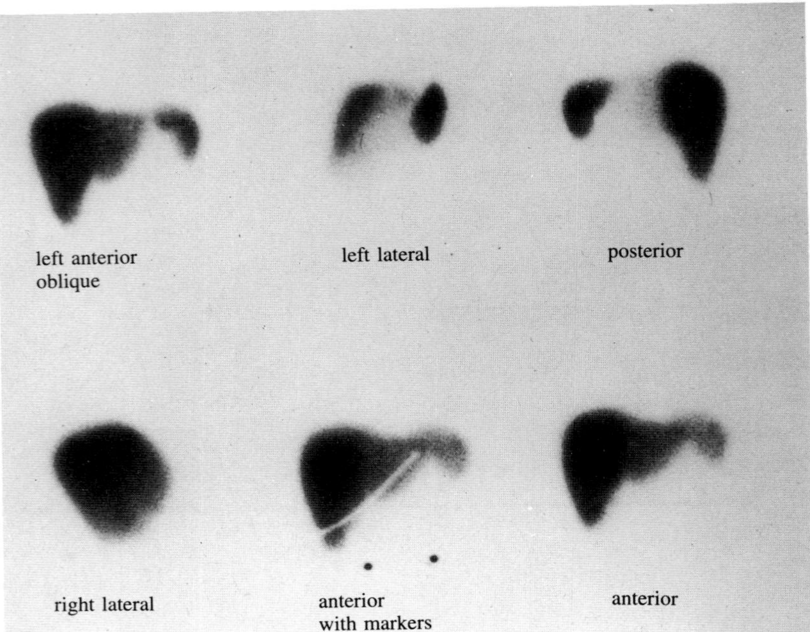

Figure 6. Normal 6-view planar liver-spleen scintigraphy using ^{99m}Tc-sulfur colloid. The lead bar marks the inferior costal margin in the anterior view. The two radioactive markers are placed 10 cm apart to aid measurement of liver and spleen size.

LIVER AND SPLEEN SCINTIGRAPHY

Most laboratories use a large-field-of-view scintillation camera fitted with an all-purpose parallel-hole collimator to obtain planar images of the liver and spleen. Careful quality control of the imaging instrumentation is essential, particularly in assuring a uniform field. In such a large organ as the liver, small areas of increased or decreased sensitivity may easily create artifactual "lesions," which result in serious diagnostic misinterpretations. A good description of scintigraphic pitfalls as well as normal variants has been published by Ryo and colleagues.[48]

When using radioactive colloids, sufficient time for localization in the liver and spleen must be allowed. In general, 30 minutes is adequate although, in hepatic insufficiency, longer times are advised.

Because the liver is a flexible organ, it changes shape easily with different positions. This factor is especially important to recognize with serial scans, during which patients should be imaged in the same position.

External landmarks should be carefully marked. A lead strip may be placed on the costal margin as a useful reference and calibration markers can provide an estimate of liver size (Fig. 6). Multiple views are essential. A minimum study includes the anterior, posterior, and right and left lateral views. Various oblique views may elucidate unusual features and help separate left lobe from spleen in splenomegaly. It is common practice to collect 5 to 10 $\times$ 10^5 total counts in the anterior view, using 150 to 250 MBq (4 to 6 mCi) ^{99m}Tc-colloid. To assess the relative uptake of activity by the liver and spleen, which often provides an early indication of changing hepatic function, the time is noted, and the remaining views are taken for the same time.

Dynamic scintiphotos are frequently obtained with the patient supine in the anterior view. Serial 3-second images are collected for approximately 1 minute following intravenous injection of the radiocolloid. Ruppert et al. estimated that these dynamic studies can provide useful additional diagnostic information in as many as 20% of studies.[49]

Normal Scintigraphy

The shape of the liver is highly variable. Mould has listed 38 variations in the anterior view alone.[50] With experience, however, this variability becomes less confusing. Figure 6 shows the four standard views of a normal liver, along with a left anterior oblique view that better separates the spleen from the left lobe of the liver. In the anterior view, the liver is roughly triangular with smooth borders. Because the liver is nonrigid, it assumes the shape of the cavity that contains it: smoothly convex over the diaphragmatic surface, proceeding to a concavity between the right and left lobes as the liver follows the crura of the diaphragm. The small left lobe may be thin and is frequently quite truncated. The right lobe margin may contain a slight indentation due to the *costal impression* of the lower rib margin (Fig. 7 **A**). Occasionally, the right lobe is greatly elongated, forming a Riedel's lobe (Fig. 7 **B**). The inferior margin is frequently irregular, with projections caused by the caudate lobe and impressions caused by insertion of the ligamentum teres (Fig. 7 **C**). The division between the left and right lobes is often thinned by the entry through the inferior margin of structures of the porta hepatis and especially by dilated biliary ducts (Fig. 7 **D**). Eventration of the diaphragm causes superior bulging of the right lobe (Fig. 7 **E**).

The right lateral view is ovoid or triangular. Often, an

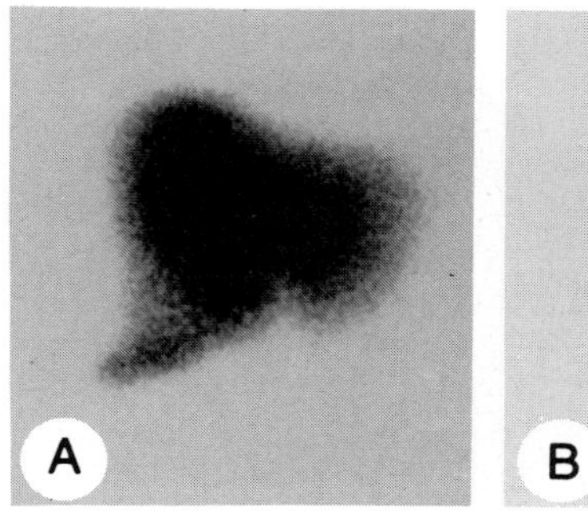

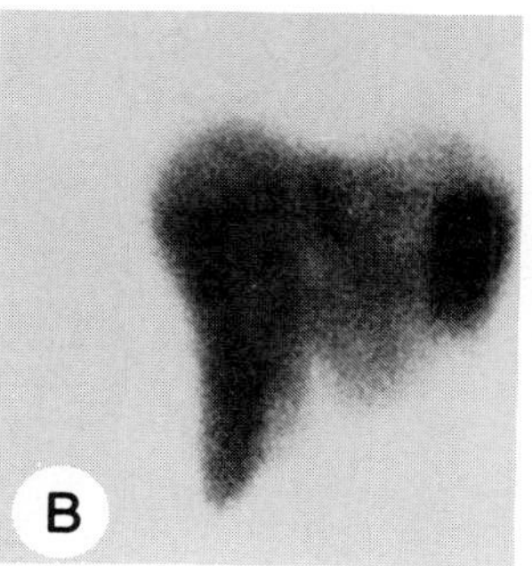

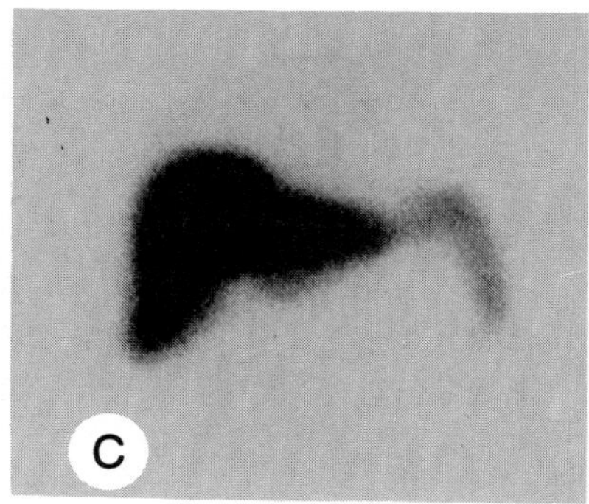

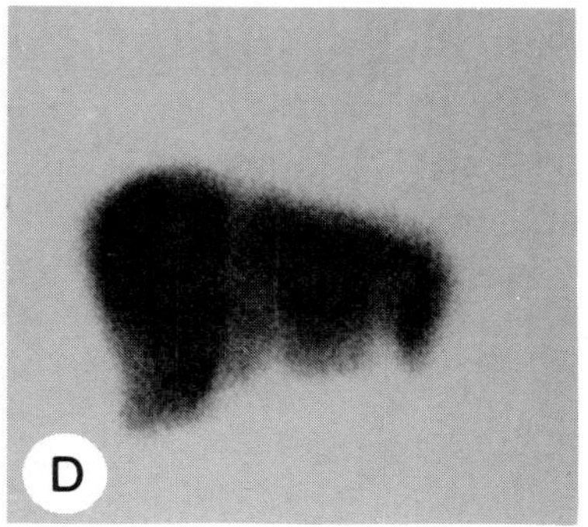

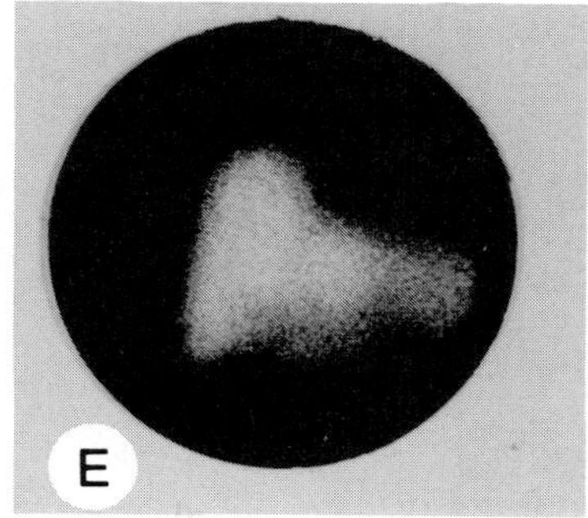

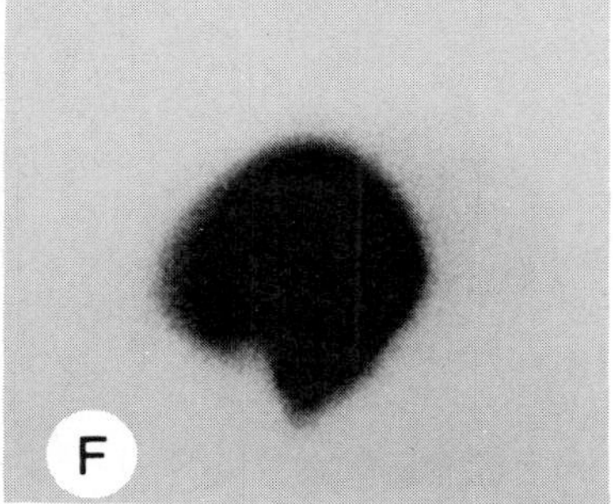

Figure 7. Variations in hepatic configuration. **(A).** Anterior view demonstrating costal impression along the right inferior margin of the liver. **(B).** Riedel's lobe. **(C).** Indentation produced by insertion of the ligamentum teres. **(D).** Prominent separation of the left and right lobes. **(E).** Eventration of the diaphragm creating a high, domed liver. **(F).** Right lateral view showing prominent lobulation.

acute accentuation is seen between the anterior and posterior positions of the right lobe (Fig. 7 **F**). In the posterior view, the renal fossa is a more or less constant feature. The left and right lobes are separated from one another by the spine, which absorbs most of the photons originating from the overlying liver. The spleen is prominent in the posterior view, lying posterior to the left lobe. The splenic density is normally the same or decreased in comparison with the right posterior liver activity.

In the left lateral view, the left lobe lies anterior to the spleen. With splenomegaly, a left anterior oblique view may be required to separate the spleen and left lobe.

Several formulas have been advocated for determining liver size.[51–53] Perhaps the most commonly employed is a measure of the maximum cephalocaudal dimension, which Spencer and Antar found to be 17 ± 2 cm in adults.[54] Drum and Beard consider an adult liver more than 17 cm in height and more than 18 cm in width to be evidence of hepatomegaly.[55]

Eikman et al. described a computer-assisted method of estimating liver mass in which an edge detection algorithm is used for the right lateral projection.[56] The correlation between computer-estimated and autopsy weights was found to be 0.83.

SPECT techniques for estimating liver size have been published and appear to correlate well with estimates determined by computed tomography (CT).[57,58] Most studies have shown that radionuclide imaging is superior to estimates of liver and spleen size by physical examination, probably because of the difficulty in determining the upper borders by percussion.[59–61]

Volumetric formulas to determine splenic mass have also been published.[59,62,63] Most clinicians, however, use the greatest dimension in either the lateral or posterior view, with 12 cm considered the upper limit of normal.[59,64]

Several factors may produce unusual variations and artifacts in liver images. The most commonly encountered arti-

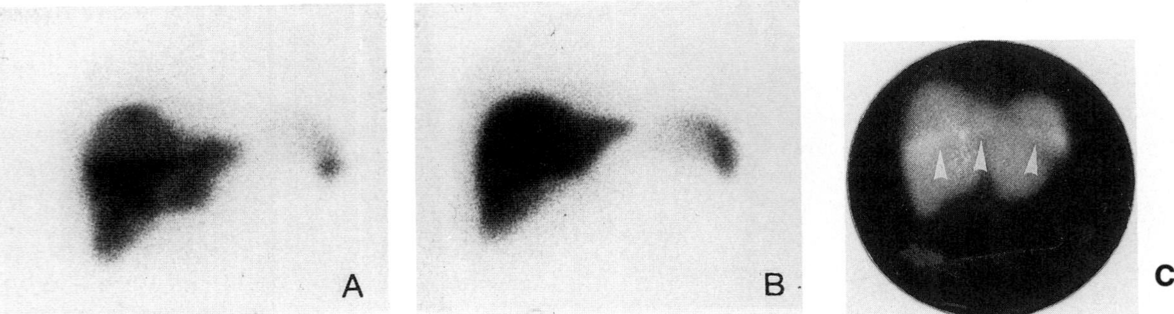

Figure 8. **(A).** Normal liver with the breasts obscuring the upper portions of the liver and spleen. **(B).** Breasts retracted. **(C).** Compton scatter from the breasts.

facts are caused by absorption of the weak gamma energy of ^{99m}Tc by overlying structures—the female breast is an example (Fig. 8). The tissue half-value layer for the 140-keV gamma ray of ^{99m}Tc is only 4.6 cm, so that a breast shadow frequently appears in patients with ample breasts. This shadow disappears with manual retraction of the breast upward. Occasionally, overlying fat produces similar artifacts, which disappear when scintigraphy is repeated in the supine position. Compton-scattered photons from the breast may also produce artifacts (Fig. 8 **C**).

Residual barium in the bowel has been reported to produce a cold "lesion" in the anterior view only when the bowel overlies the liver.[65] However, this occurs infrequently because the bowel is not easily interposed between the liver and the anterior chest wall. Such artifacts should disappear by rescanning the patient in the upright position. More often, ornaments and articles of clothing cause sharply demarcated, discrete defects in one view only.

Another common finding is pulmonary uptake of colloid (Fig. 9). This phenomenon has been associated with a variety of conditions (Table 1). A cause is aluminum breakthrough from a ^{99}Mo-^{99m}Tc generator, resulting in flocculation of sulfur colloid particles. Proper quality control for aluminum breakthrough in the generator eluate should eliminate this problem. Patients on high daily doses of aluminum hydroxide antacids may have sufficiently high plasma Al^{3+} levels to produce flocculation in vivo.[66] Klingensmith and Ryerson attributed pulmonary uptake of colloids to phagocytosis by the pulmonary RES rather than flocculation of the colloid into macroaggregates.[67] This theory is supported by the slow uptake of colloid by the lungs. If the phenomenon were caused by macroaggregates of sulfur colloid, pulmonary activity would plateau in the first pass; however, the pulmonary accumulation is gradual. Why this is seen in some patients and not others is not yet understood. Mikhael and Evans demonstrated migration of RES cells into the lungs under the influence of estrogen (which is elevated in some liver diseases).[68] Klingensmith et al. found that intraperitoneal injections of endotoxins into animals induced uptake of colloid in both lungs and kidneys.[69] Because this effect could be blocked by administration of heparin, they postu-

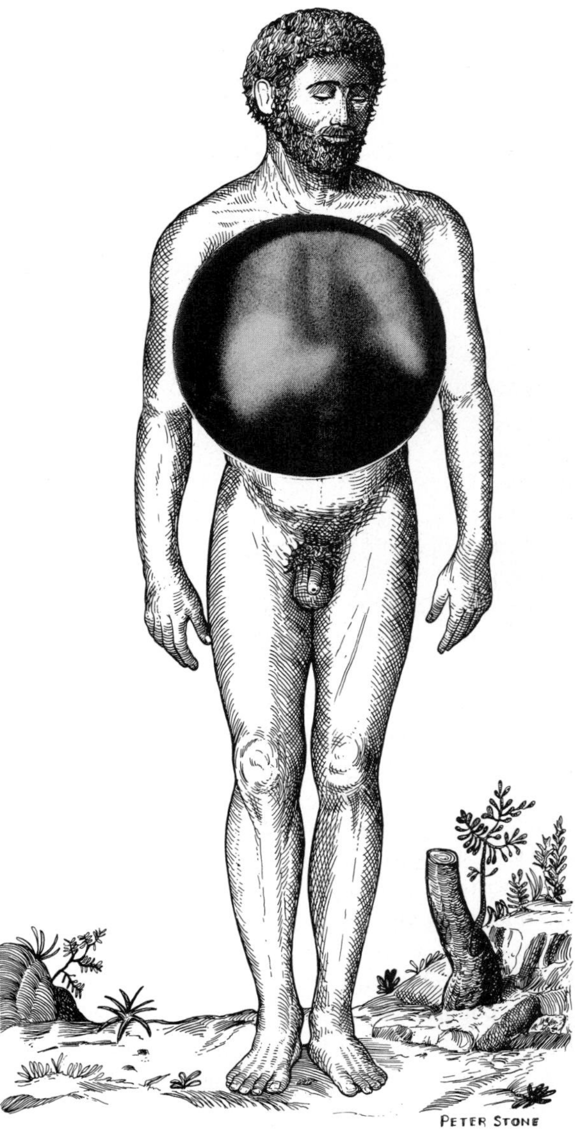

Figure 9. Obvious pulmonary and bone marrow uptake of ^{99m}Tc-sulfur colloid in a patient with jaundice and gram-negative septicemia. There was no scintigraphic evidence of liver abscess. Note uptake in sternum, spine, and ribs, caused by activation of marrow RES.

Table 1. Conditions Associated with Pulmonary Uptake of ^{99m}Tc-Sulfur Colloid

CONDITION	REFERENCE
Normal variant in children	Winter et al.[70]
Increased serum Al^{3+}	Bobinet et al.[66]
Bacterial endotoxemia	Klingensmith and Lovett[71]
Histiocytosis X	Bowen et al.[72]
Advanced breast cancer	Gillespie et al.[73]
Mucopolysaccharidosis	Klingensmith et al.[74]
Organ transplants	Klingensmith et al.[75]
Abdominal abscess	Imarisio[76]
Atelectasis	Mettler and Christie[77]
Heparin administration	Mikhael and Evans[68]
Blunt trauma	Johnson and Hladik[78]
Collagen vascular disease	Klingensmith et al.[79]
General anesthesia	Lentle et al.[80]
Severe liver dysfunction	Keyes et al.[81], Turner et al.[82], Stadalnick[83]
Malaria	Leclerc et al.[84]

lated that colloid uptake may be related to fibrin deposits secondary to intravascular coagulation.

Although lung uptake is usually diffuse, transient focal uptake occurs occasionally at sites of inflammation and in regions of atelectasis.[76,77] The mechanism in these cases may be increased local phagocytic activity.

Several reports have documented an association between congestive heart failure and colloid uptake by the kidneys.[85–88] The mechanism for this association is not yet understood. Occasionally, renal uptake of colloid has been observed when colloid is prepared from the eluate of first-day generators.[89] This uptake probably results from residual reducing substances that form chelates or other soluble compounds with pertechnetate.

Renal uptake of colloid also occurs in renal transplants.[90–92] Two mechanisms have been suggested: (1) entrapment of colloid in renal fibrin deposits, and (2) increased phagocytic activity. No simple mechanism explains renal colloid uptake in all of the conditions reported.

Increased spleen and bone-marrow uptake is associated with cirrhosis, diabetes, malignancy, melanoma, mucopolysaccharidosis, and hepatitis.[93–97] With decreasing hepatic sequestration, the blood concentration of colloid perfusing these organs remains higher, which increases their relative uptake of colloid.

Transient changes in colloid distribution occur frequently during the course of systemic chemotherapy. Usually these changes are manifested by slightly increased bone marrow and splenic uptake.[98] This effect has also been reported following general anesthesia.[80]

The apparent spleen-liver activity ratio (S/L) may change with the position in which the patient is imaged. Mackler et al. found that the median S/L ratio determined by area-of-interest counting in the posterior view was 20% greater when determined in the erect than in the supine position.[93] Normal S/L ratio varies between 0.77 ± 0.2 and 0.84 ± 0.3.[93,99,100]

Several imaging techniques have been devised to increase hepatic image resolution by eliminating the effects of respiratory motion.[101–103] Most employ a feedback mechanism whereby images are taken only during inspiration or expiration. Most of these measures are ineffective because the level of respiration is not the same from breath to breath. There is little question, however, that respiration does degrade the image slightly.

In general, the liver is displaced downward and medially, and the dome is flattened in pleural effusion, emphysema, and subphrenic abscess. Marked displacement also occurs (Fig. 10). In congenital asplenia, the liver is situated in its embryonic position in the midline. In situs inversus, the liver and spleen are reversed in location.

Liver-lung scintigraphy is a technique that was once employed to detect subdiaphragmatic abscesses.[104–108] The liver is first imaged using ^{99m}Tc-sulfur colloid to detect any focal disease. ^{99m}Tc-macroaggregate albumin (75 MBq) is then injected to image the lungs. Any separation between liver and the right lung may be attributed to an interposing substance: abscess, ascites, tumor, or bowel (Fig. 11). The test is quite nonspecific and insensitive and has been replaced by ultrasound (US) and CT.

SPECT Imaging of the Liver

Single-photon emission computed tomography (SPECT) imaging of the liver is usually performed with a rotating gamma camera with one to three heads. The camera must have good intrinsic uniformity characteristics, and all images should be attenuation and uniformity corrected with a high-count field flood (at least 3×10^7 counts). The correct center-of-rotation should be determined daily to prevent image distortion.[109] The usual acquisition procedure consists of obtaining 120 projections of 10 to 20 seconds per view over a full 360° (3° per view) circular or elliptical rotation orbit.[110] The patient is centered with the arms out of the field of view. A standard dose of 150 to 225 MBq (4 to 6 mCi) ^{99m}Tc-sulfur colloid is sufficient activity. The resultant data are reconstructed with appropriate filtering into 6 to 12 mm contiguous slices and displayed in transaxial, coronal, and sagittal planes (Fig. 12). The display of hepatic SPECT is enhanced using rotating cine displays (Fig. 12D).[111] It may also be appropriate to generate a *sinogram* display to detect patient motion, assess proper patient position, and detect data loss from dropped frames.[112,113]

The most widely used reconstruction algorithms currently use backprojection to derive transaxial images. This Fourier-based reconstruction is fast and relatively easy. However, it may impose limitations for correcting for attenuation, scatter, and collimator resolution. Several other algorithms have been developed that may provide greater resolution and con-

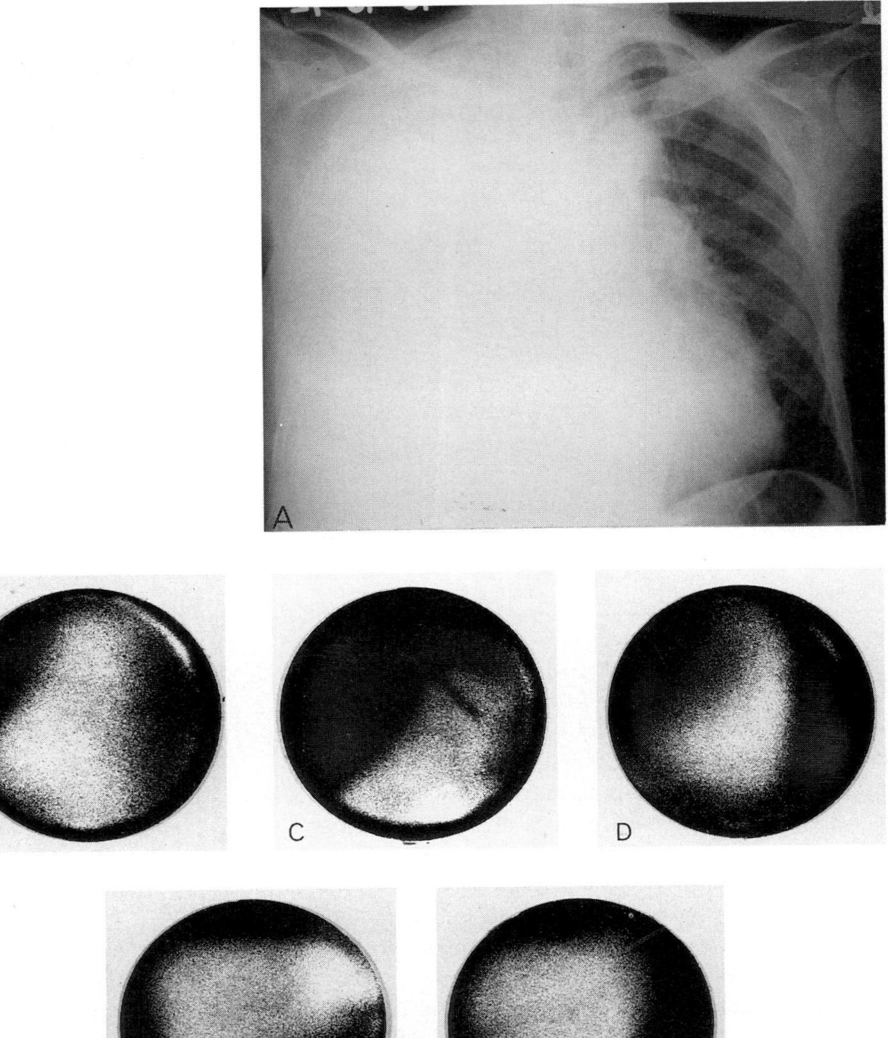

Figure 10. **(A).** Chest roentgenogram showing massive right pleural effusion, **(B).** Right anterior view showing liver on end; **(C).** Left anterior with lead marker on left costal margin; **(D).** Right lateral view demonstrating diaphragmatic impression on the right lobe; **(E).** Normal position of the liver in the right anterior view after removal of 10 liters of pleural fluid. Note the "hot" left lobe caused by superficial venous shunting secondary to superior vena cava obstruction; **(F).** Right lateral view after thoracentesis.

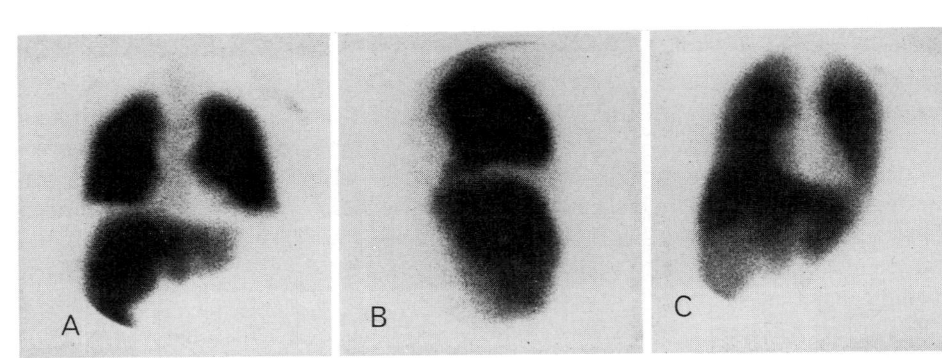

Figure 11. Subdiaphragmatic abscess. Anterior **(A)** and right lateral **(B)** lung-liver images demonstrate abnormal separation between right lung and dome of the right lobe of the liver; **(C).** Normal anterior lung-liver study in same patient following surgical drainage.

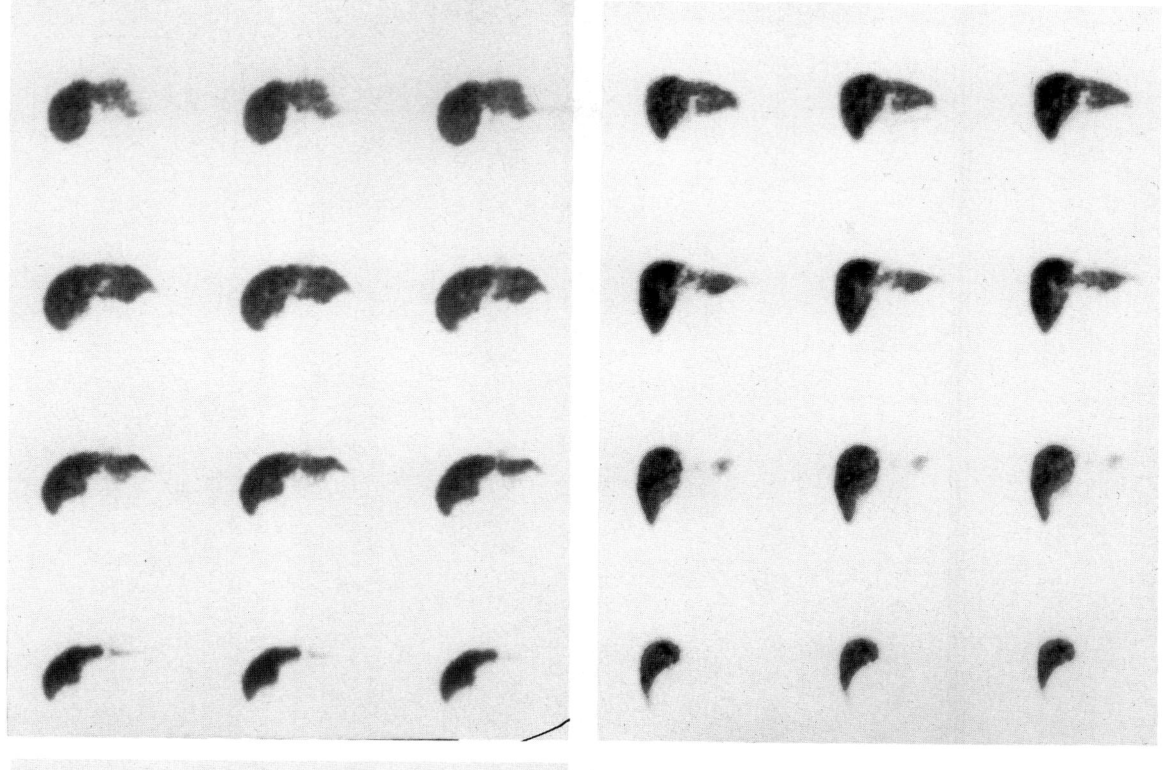

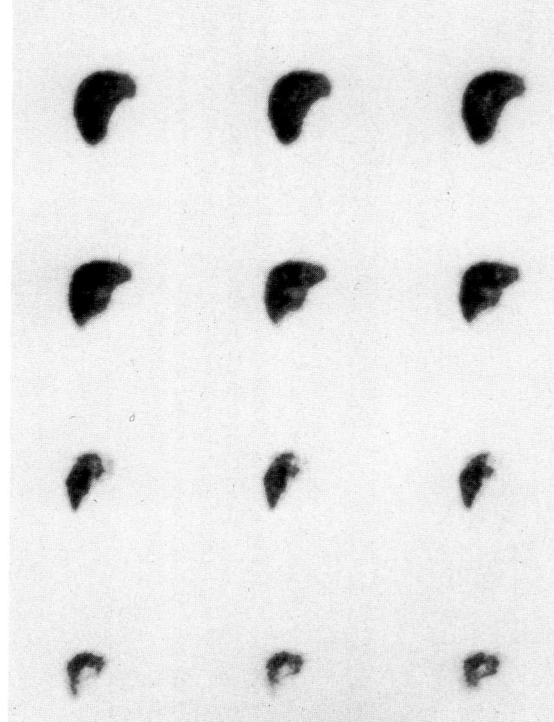

Figure 12. Normal liver SPECT taken with a dual-headed scintillation camera with 360° contour rotation, 3° per step. Each slice is 3 mm thick with Hamming filter (cutoff at 1.1 cycle/cm). The patient is a 39-year-old with sickle cell disease and functional asplenia. **(A).** Selected transaxial sections (12 of 48) proceeding cephalad to caudad as the images progress from top to bottom. The images are viewed as CT images would be viewed, viz. from below. Note the highly irregular left lobe and narrow connection between left and right lobe at the porta hepatis. Photopenic regions within the parenchyma represent blood and bile vessels; **(B).** Selected (12 of 48) coronal sections. The order progresses anterior to posterior as the images proceed from top to bottom; **(C).** Selected sagittal sections. The order progresses from right lobe to left lobe as the images proceed from top to bottom. Anterior is on the reader's left. The rotational image set for this patient is shown in **D**. (Figure continued on next page.)

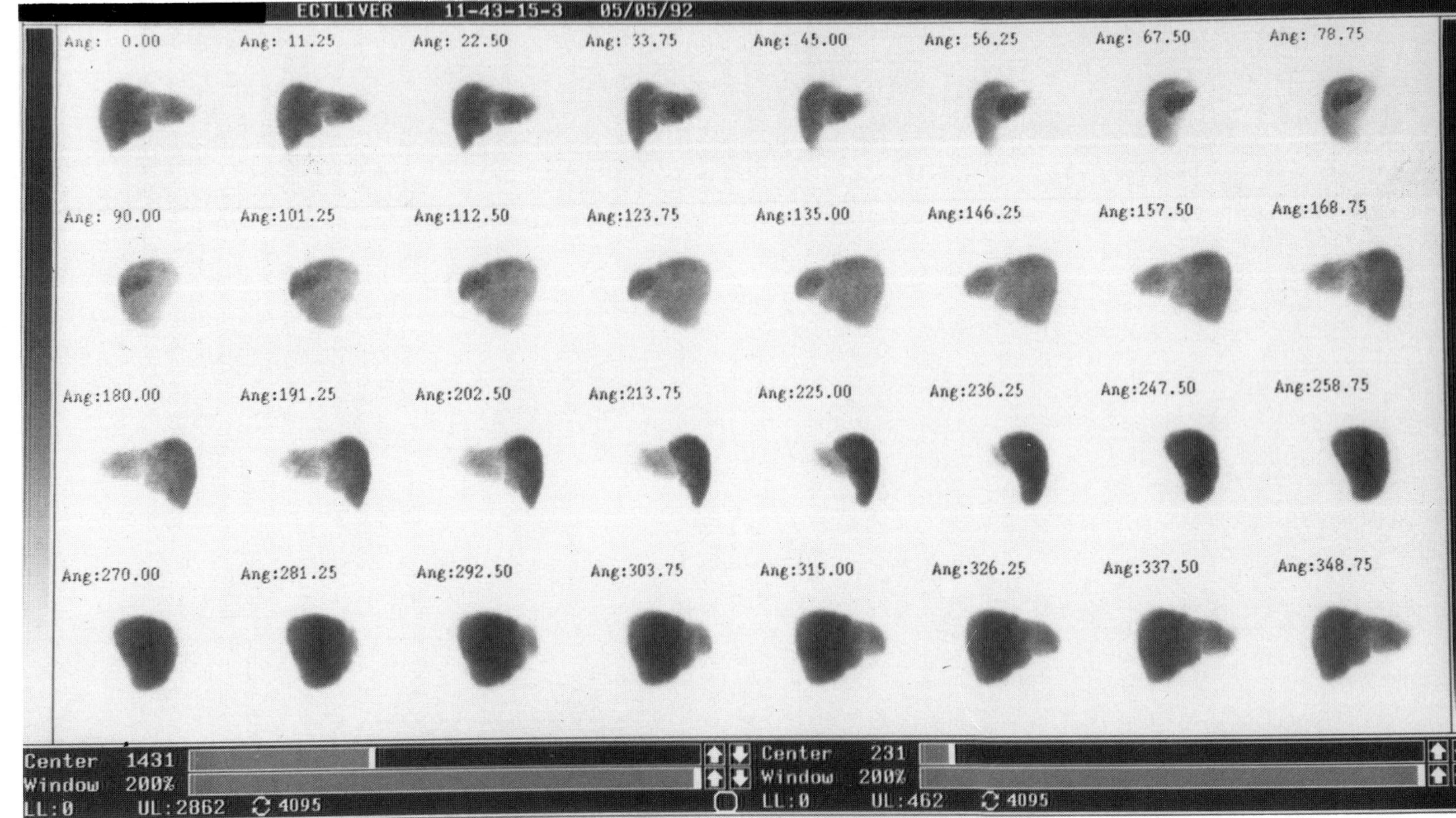

Figure 12. Continued. (D). SPECT rotational display of a normal liver (postsplenectomy) which when projected on a CRT in a cine mode provides a pseudo-three-4-dimensional effect. The standard anterior, left lateral, posterior, and right lateral planar views are presented in the 0.00°, 90°, 180°, and 270° images. The SPECT images were obtained with a dual-headed scintillation camera with contoured rotation of 180°, 3° per step, 25 s/step, 3.3 mm pixels, Hamming filter, and 1.1 cycle/cm cutoff.

trast for intrahepatic lesions, including maximum-likelihood and inverse Monte Carlo reconstruction algorithms.[114,115] SPECT considerably improves lesion resolution in colloid liver scans; lesions as small as 1 cm should be detectable in cooperative patients, as opposed to 3 cm in the deep liver parenchyma by planar imaging.[110] Quantification of lesion and organ size is also possible using thresholding or gradient techniques.[116,117] Several different filters may be applied. Perhaps the most common is the two-dimensional Butterworth filter.[110]

The limits of resolution of "cold" lesions in colloid liver imaging depend greatly upon the resolution and quality control of the system. Most modern systems can resolve cold lesions 15 to 18 mm in diameter. However, thus far liver scintigraphy with single-headed SPECT units has been beset with a large number of artifacts that have rendered overall accuracy of the tomographic images little better than planar imaging.[118,119] Numerous studies have compared SPECT and planar imaging. These have been well summarized by Oppenheim et al.[120] Most of these studies are difficult to compare because of different criteria of patient selection and widely varying imaging instrumentation. It is probably not merely banal to suggest that newer instrumentation will doubtless reduce artifacts and improve resolution, and clinicians should be encouraged to use SPECT for all routine liver imaging, with both colloid and blood pool tracers, especially using multidetector SPECT units. In most instances, interpretation of the SPECT tomographic slices is greatly aided by comparison with the rotating cine image.[119]

INDICATIONS FOR LIVER-SPLEEN SPECT

Although some would say that most or all liver scintigraphy should be SPECT, there are certain clinical problems for which tomography is especially useful. These have been summarized by Van Heertum[110]:

1. detect focal liver disease, including primary and metastatic tumors, abscess, granuloma, focal nodular hyperplasia, and focal fatty liver,
2. improve specificity of equivocal US and CT studies,
3. detect trauma to liver and spleen,
4. assess extent of tumor involvement prior to hepatic resection,
5. detect focal and diffuse splenic disease, including primary and metastatic tumors, cyst, abscesses, infarction, and hematological disorders,
6. determine liver and spleen volumes,
7. follow-up known hepatic and splenic disease,
8. detect accessory spleens.

Most comparative studies have found SPECT to be both more sensitive and specific than planar imaging[121–125]; however, others have found the advantages marginal.[118] Clearly, SPECT images require more experience to interpret. As experience increases and as SPECT technology improves, so does accuracy.[110]

CLINICAL APPLICATIONS

The great technological strides that mark the recent advances in US, CT, and MR imaging, including increased resolution, more accurate tissue signature recognition, and increased imaging speed, have greatly decreased the demand for radiocolloid liver scintigraphy. These studies have always been of relatively low resolution, and are neither very sensitive nor specific. Nevertheless, these studies are encountered in older literature and they are still ordered to determine liver size when comparing to previous scintiphotos, to confirm diffuse liver disease, to help differentiate focal fatty infiltration, and to search for accessory spleens.

Much more commonly ordered are hepatic blood pool studies to search for such vascular lesions as hemangiomas. As already discussed, advances in receptor imaging may lead to an increase in hepatic functional imaging. Table 2 lists several of the numerous conditions that can create patterns of focal or diffusely decreased colloid uptake in liver scintigraphy.

Diffuse Disease

Diffuse liver diseases produce a wide variety of scintigraphic manifestations, from no perceptible change to hepatomegaly (the most common finding) with patchy distribution of the tracer throughout the organ. These changes are entirely nonspecific and do not permit differentiation between one disease and another. The most common diseases affecting the liver diffusely are alcoholic cirrhosis, hepatitis, and chronic passive congestion.

Cirrhosis is a generic term that encompasses many forms of chronic diffuse liver disease, and is characterized by widespread loss of liver cells, collapse and fibrosis of the supporting reticulin network, distortion of the vascular structures, and nodular regeneration of the remaining liver cell mass. The most common causes of cirrhosis are (1) alcoholic (Laennec's), (2) postnecrotic, (3) biliary, (4) hemochromatosis and, (5) cardiac or congestive cirrhosis. Common scintigraphic features in the early stages of the disease include hepatosplenomegaly, decreased hepatic uptake of radiocolloid, and increased bone marrow and splenic uptake (Fig. 13).

As cirrhosis advances, atrophy of the right lobe with compensatory hypertrophy of the left lobe may develop.[126] The irregular tracer pattern and focal hypertrophy may create a pattern indistinguishable from that produced by multiple metastases, although the latter is less often associated with increased splenic uptake (Fig. 14). The increased bone marrow and splenic uptake is caused by several anatomic and physiological factors, including increased intrahepatic resistance (portal hypertension) and intrahepatic and portacaval anastomoses. These result in prolonged elevation of blood colloid concentration.[127] Often, the right lobe decreases in size, and left lobe activity increases relative to the right, in intermediate and advanced cirrhosis (Fig. 15). Shreiner and Barlai-Kovach found that quantitative measurements of

Table 2. Etiology of Focal and Diffuse Liver Disease

	FOCAL	DIFFUSE
Malignant neoplasms	hepatoma lymphoma metastasis	leukemia lymphoma miliary metastases
Benign cysts and tumors	adenoma hemangioma polycystic disease solitary cyst	polycystic disease
Infections	abscess echinococcosis fascioliasis granuloma hydatid cyst	acute and chronic hepatitis leishmaniasis malaria mononucleosis schistosomiasis sickle cell disease syphilis Weil's disease histoplasmosis
Trauma	hematoma surgical resection radiation	
Metabolic	amyloidosis fatty infiltration	amyloidosis collagen vascular disease diabetes fatty infiltration galactosemia Gaucher's disease hemochromatosis Niemann-Pick disease von Gierke's disease Wilson's disease
Others	biliary duct ectasia cirrhosis (pseudomass) hepatic vein thrombosis choledochal cyst hypereosinophilic syndrome infarction intrahepatic gallbladder radiation hepatitis vascular malformation Caroli's disease	biliary obstruction Budd-Chiari syndrome cirrhosis congestive failure drug toxicity (lead poisoning) extramedullary hematopoiesis Dubin-Johnson syndrome hypergammaglobulinemia polyarteritis nodosa sarcoidosis ulcerative colitis Waldenström's macroglobulinemia

right/left hepatic lobe ratios of ^{99m}Tc-sulfur colloid uptake by region-of-interest (ROI) analysis provided a good discriminator for alcoholic cirrhosis.[128] The mean right/left ratio for cirrhotic patients was 1.08 ± 0.33, versus 2.85 ± 0.65 in healthy people.

The hypothesis advanced to explain these findings is based on portal "blood streaming." The authors suggest that low-alcohol blood from the spleen, stomach, and large bowel (inferior mesenteric vein) enters and tends to stream along the left side of the portal vein and thus flow preferentially to the left lobe, sparing that region the drug's toxic effects. High-alcohol blood from the small intestine (superior mesenteric vein) tends to flow to the right lobe. There are animal data corroborating this hypothesis, but no independent verification in man.

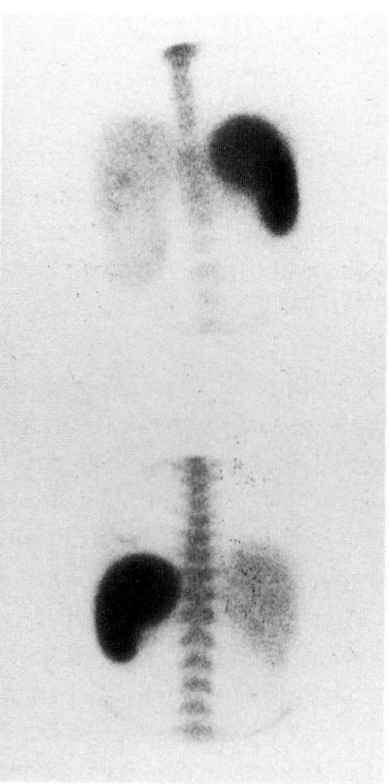

Figure 13. Moderately severe cirrhosis showing hepatosplenomegaly, decreased hepatic uptake, and markedly increased splenic and bone marrow uptake of ^{99m}Tc-sulfur colloid in the anterior (top) and posterior (bottom) views.

With intermediate stages of cirrhosis, the picture is not so dramatic or characteristic. Extrahepatic colloid localization rises with aggravation of the disease and diminishes with clinical improvement. The same pattern is found in chronic hepatitis. The primary usefulness of radiocolloid liver-spleen imaging is to follow the course of disease.

Several investigators have correlated spleen/liver ratios of colloid distribution with various hepatic disease parameters. In general, increased splenic uptake correlates with disease severity.[99,100] Splenomegaly and heterogeneous colloid distribution within the liver also correlate with disease severity.[96] The usual criterion for judging increased splenic uptake is if splenic activity on the posterior view is as or more intense than activity in the posterior right hepatic lobe (Fig. 13).

BUDD-CHIARI SYNDROME

The Budd-Chiari syndrome is caused by obstruction of hepatic venous outflow, in either the major hepatic veins or the inferior vena cava. Clinically, this gives rise to hepatomegaly, ascites, and sometimes abdominal pain. It is associated with hepatic malignancy, infections, and thrombotic

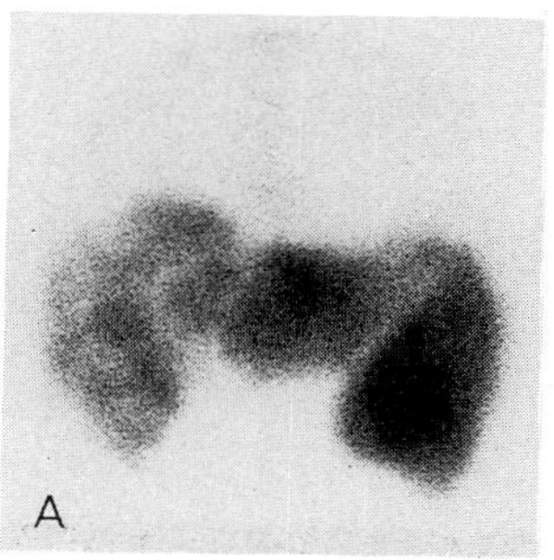

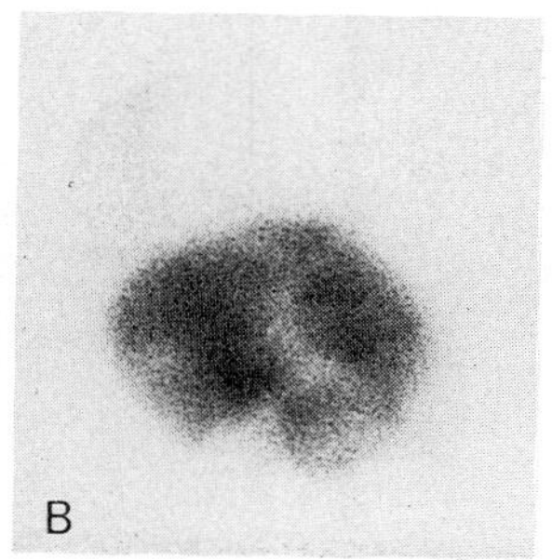

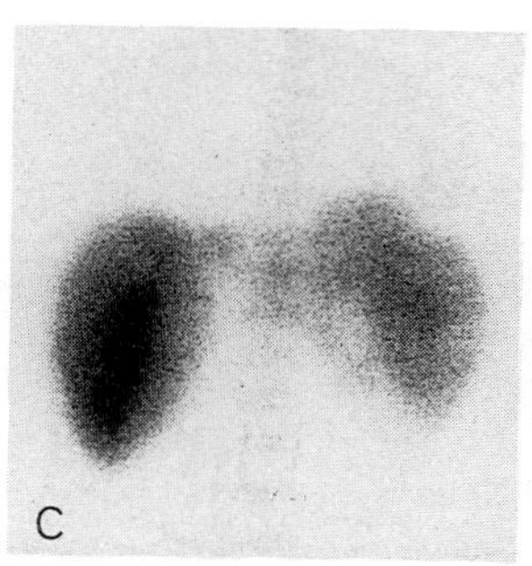

Figure 14. Advanced cirrhosis with multiple cold lesions, splenomegaly, and increased bone marrow activity; **(A).** Anterior; **(B).** Right lateral; **(C).** Posterior views.

disorders. If only a few hepatic veins are involved, radiocolloid uptake may be decreased in these segments. If most of the veins or the inferior vena cava is involved, uptake is generally decreased. However, the caudate lobe in the central posterior portion of the liver is often spared, giving rise to a triangular area of relatively increased activity (Fig. 16).[129] Injection of radiocolloid into the pedal veins while imaging over the heart and upper abdomen clearly demonstrates the inferior vena cava obstruction and the collateral circulation.[130]

OTHER DIFFUSE LIVER DISEASES

Such metabolic diseases as von Gierke's disease (glycogen storage disease type I), amyloidosis, galactosemia, and diabetes are all diseases to which the liver characteristically responds with variable degrees of fatty infiltration. The usual scintigraphic findings are hepatomegaly with or without heterogeneous colloid uptake.

Various tropical diseases produce serious morphological alterations in the liver. Schistosomiasis caused by *S. mansoni* does not attack the liver initially. Later, in the hepatosplenic stage, the liver becomes small and globular in shape with increased extrahepatic uptake. In malaria, uptake greatly increases in the spleen, and in visceral leishmaniasis a truly enormous spleen size may be attained.

Although the patterns of colloid distribution are not specific for a particular disease, scintigraphy is sensitive for the *presence* of disease. One study compared ^{99m}Tc-sulfur colloid scintigraphy with CT as a means of screening for the presence of diffuse liver disease.[132] Scintigraphy had a sensitivity of 87% versus 67% for CT. The predictive values for a positive and negative test were 67 and 91%, respectively, versus 76 and 73%, respectively for CT.

Focal Liver Disease

As noted earlier, advances in other noninvasive imaging technologies have greatly decreased the indications for radiocolloid scintigraphy. This is especially true in the detection of focal diseases, where US, CT, and MR imaging are generally more sensitive and specific. Table 2 lists the most common conditions giving rise to focal hepatic disease; the lesions may be solitary or multiple. In either case, radiocolloid scintigraphy is nonspecific, being manifested only by solitary or multifocal defects of the colloid distribution. Normal variants that can create the appearance of focal defects include intrahepatic gallbladder, prominent porta hepatis, prominent hepatic veins, costal margin impressions, thin left lobe, and prominent renal fossa (Fig. 7).

METASTASES

The search for metastases either in staging known malignancy or in patients suspected of occult malignancy once accounted for a large percentage of all liver scintigraphy. CT and MRI now account for most of these studies because (1) lesion resolution is superior, (2) specificity is greater, (3) the sensitivity for detecting focal lesions is not greatly reduced by the presence of diffuse liver disease as is the case with radiocolloid imaging and, (4) extrahepatic alterations in abdominal morphology resulting from metastases are readily appreciated. In a recent comparison of CT, MRI, and US, all three modalities were 100% sensitive for detecting hepatic metastases ≥ 2 cm; this is the practical limit of in vivo resolution with most scintigraphic techniques.[133]

Nevertheless, there may be certain clinical situations in which colloid scintigraphy may be useful in detecting metastases. These include mostly cases in which other imaging modalities cannot render technically adequate studies. For example, CT scanning may be difficult or even prohibited in patients who will not fit within the gantry, who have surgical clips in the region of interest, or who are allergic to contrast media. US may be insensitive to lesions in the dome of the liver, and may yield unsatisfactory studies in patients who have excessive bowel gas, or who are obese. MRI may also be unsatisfactory in patients who cannot remain still, or who become claustrophobic. Thus, radionuclide imaging may be appropriate in selected patients, or where cost and availability exclude more sensitive imaging procedures.

Liver metastases characteristically create solitary or multifocal lesions on radiocolloid scintigrams (Figs. 17 and 18). When multifocal liver lesions are encountered in patients with known primaries, the probability of metastases is high, although this pattern may be found with multiple cysts, hemangiomas, and abscesses. Lymphomas and leuke-

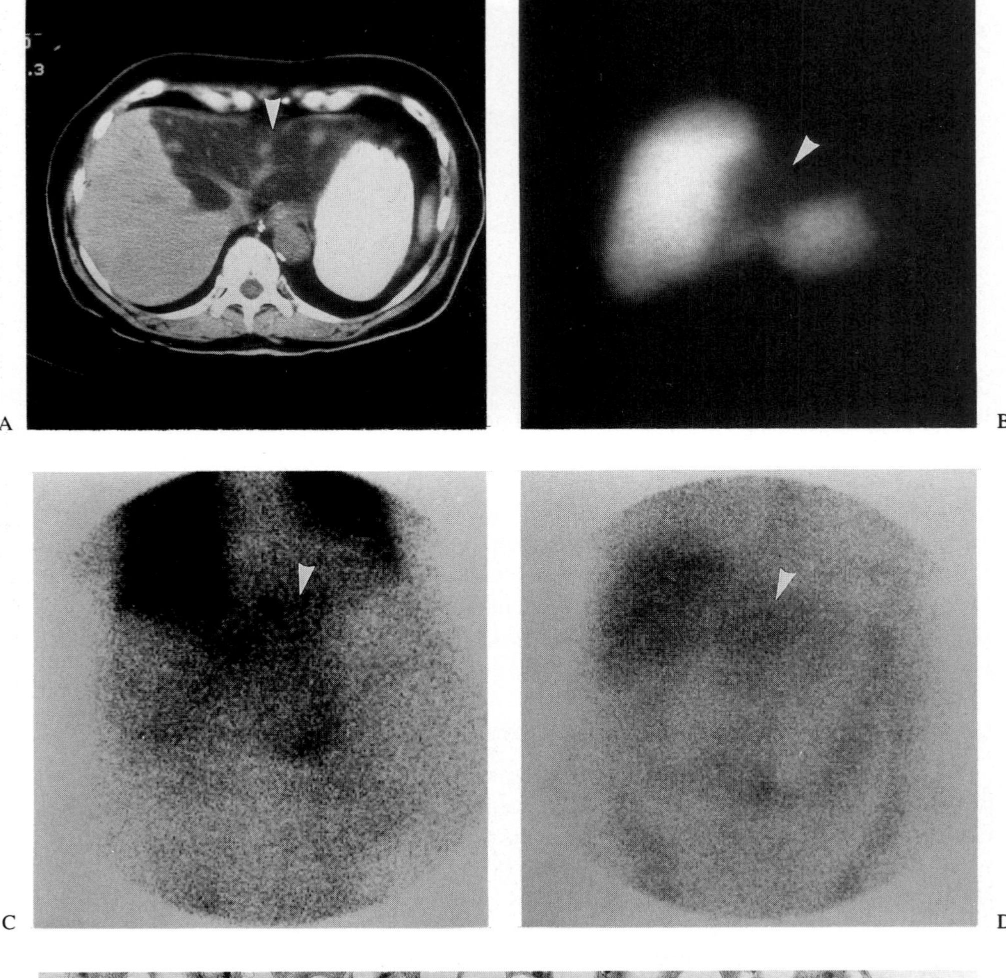

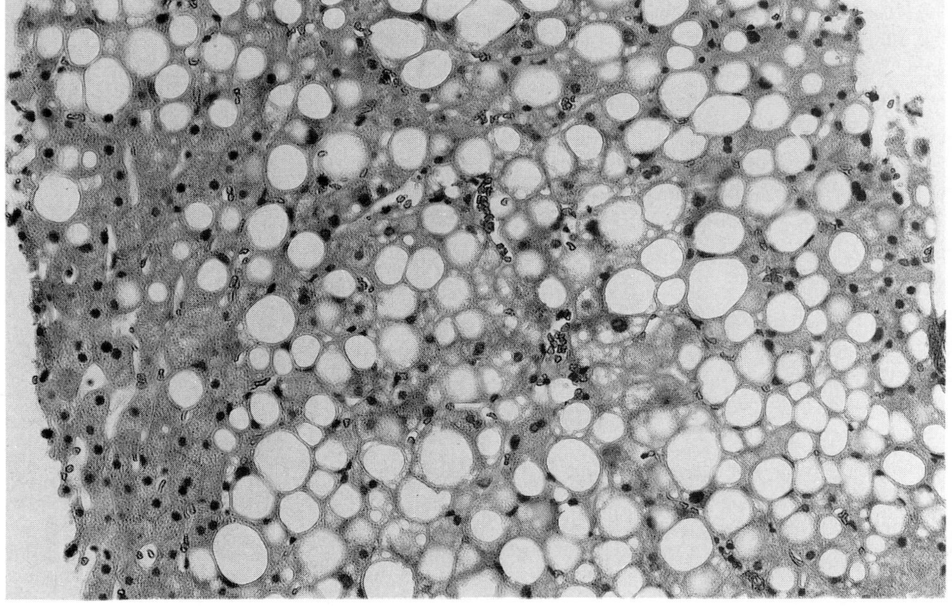

Figure 15. A 60-year-old woman with diabetes mellitus and hypercholestrolemia whose workup revealed elevated serum liver enzymes. **(A).** CT of the liver shows a large low-density lesion (arrowhead) in the left lobe and adjacent right lobe; **(B).** Anterior view with ^{99m}Tc-sulfur colloid shows a large defect in the corresponding region; **(C).** Anterior image of lungs and liver taken after rebreathing 740 MBq ^{133}Xe gas shows concentration within the lesion (arrowhead); **(D).** ^{67}Ga scintigraphy at 72 hours reveals normal activity within the lesion (arrowhead); **(E).** Photomicrograph from liver biopsy reveals marked fatty change and hyperplastic Kupffer cells. Reproduced with permission from reference 131.

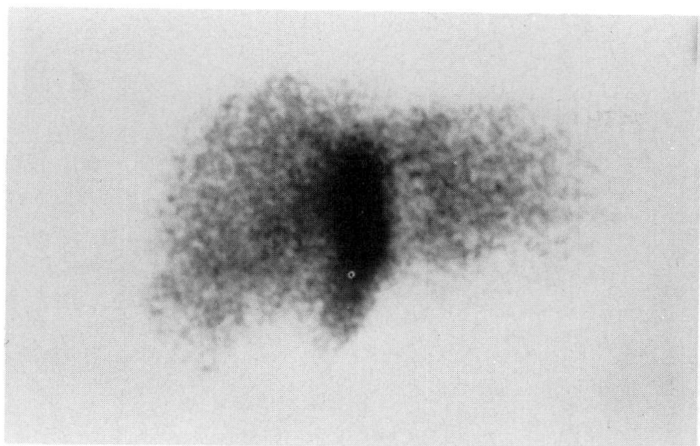

Figure 16. Hepatic venous thrombosis with Budd-Chiari syndrome in a 32-year-old male with disseminated intravascular coagulation. Anterior scintiphoto demonstrates decreased ^{99m}Tc-sulfur colloid hepatic uptake except in the quadrate lobe.

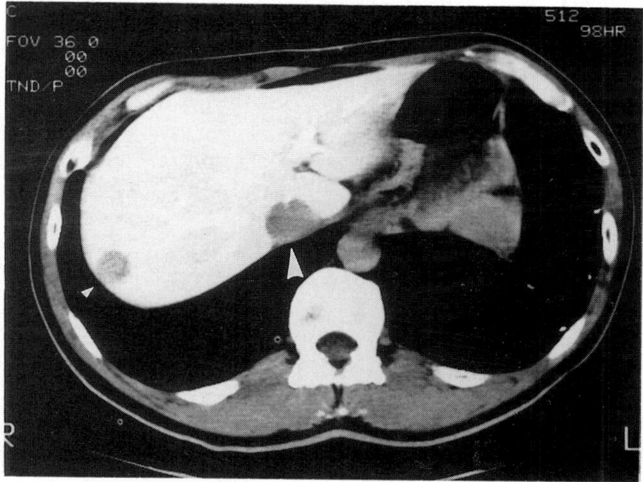

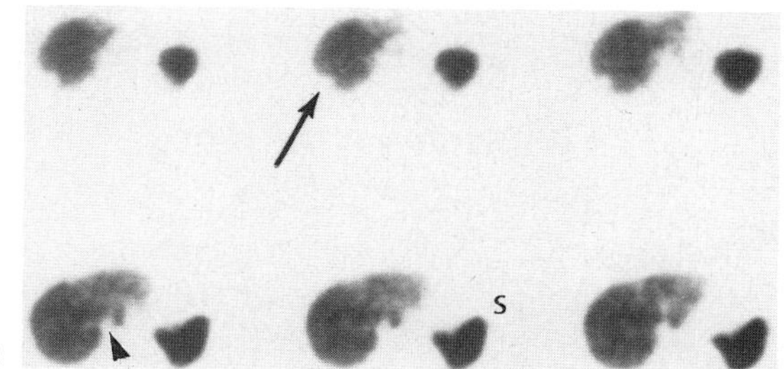

Figure 17. Solitary liver metastasis from renal cell carcinoma in a 54-year-old patient. **(A).** CT demonstrates a low-density subcapsular lesion measuring 1.5 cm in the right lobe (small arrowhead). Note the superior vena cava (large arrowhead); **(B).** Selected transverse SPECT sections showing absent ^{99m}Tc-sulfur colloid uptake in the metastasis (arrow). Planar images (not shown) were normal. Note the well-defined superior vena cava (arrowhead) in the lower sections. S = spleen.

mias often create a pattern of diffuse inhomogeneity that is indistinguishable from diffuse liver disease. When focal defects are found in the spleen as well as in the liver, lymphoma and melanoma are the first considerations.[134]

Most older reports of a high yield of positive liver scintigraphy described images made late in the disease. In fact, one should be concerned with the efficacy of any screening test in early disease stages, when therapy selection is crucial. Table 3 is a summary of several efficacy studies for most malignancies that commonly metastasize to the liver.[135] These figures give the true-positive (TP) yield at the time of initial cancer staging. The "true-positive yield" is simply the ratio of true-positive (TP) studies to all studies performed. This measure is less useful than the "true-positive fraction," but must suffice when there is no indication of the number of false-negative (FN) studies, a figure that is not often reported. Nevertheless, the data presented in this table are useful.

Nearly all efficacy studies report a much higher TP yield in patients with other clinical evidence of liver disease, including abnormal liver function tests (especially, elevated alkaline phosphatase) and hepatomegaly. For example, in preoperative bronchogenic carcinoma, Hooper et al. and Ramsdell et al. reported no TP scans in 109 patients who had no evidence of liver disease.[136,137] Among 154 patients who had at least one clinical finding supporting liver disease, 15% had TP scans. Because of the high number of false-positive (FP) results, biopsy is essential if the presence of metastases will alter patient management.

Drum and Beard have shown the effect of *strict* versus *liberal* scintigraphic criteria for diagnosing metastases.[55] In patients with breast cancer, for example, the percentage of TP liver scans rose from 67%, when only scintigrams demonstrating focal defects were interpreted as positive, to 87% when the criteria included either hepatomegaly, heterogeneity, *or* focal defects. As expected, the percentage of false-positive (FP) liver scans rose by an equal amount, from 9 to 27%. Drum and Beard found quite different results when they applied strict and liberal criteria to liver scintigrams of patients with colorectal cancer. In this condition, the TP yield remained high at 88%, and the percentage of FP scans again rose: from 6 to 27%. The difference between the two tumors is probably that, in general, breast cancer metastases are smaller than colorectal metastases at the time of clinical presentation. As a result, breast cancer metastases are manifested not as clearly focal lesions, but as a pattern of inhomogeneity.

PRIMARY MALIGNANT TUMORS

Hepatoma is the most common primary liver cancer. It is frequently associated with cirrhosis and is more common in males than in females. About 5% of patients with cirrhosis and as many as 20% of patients with chronic active hepatitis eventually develop hepatoma.[138] Hepatoma is also associated with androgen therapy.[139] The tumor grows rapidly and is often quite large by the time the patient is evaluated (Fig. 19).

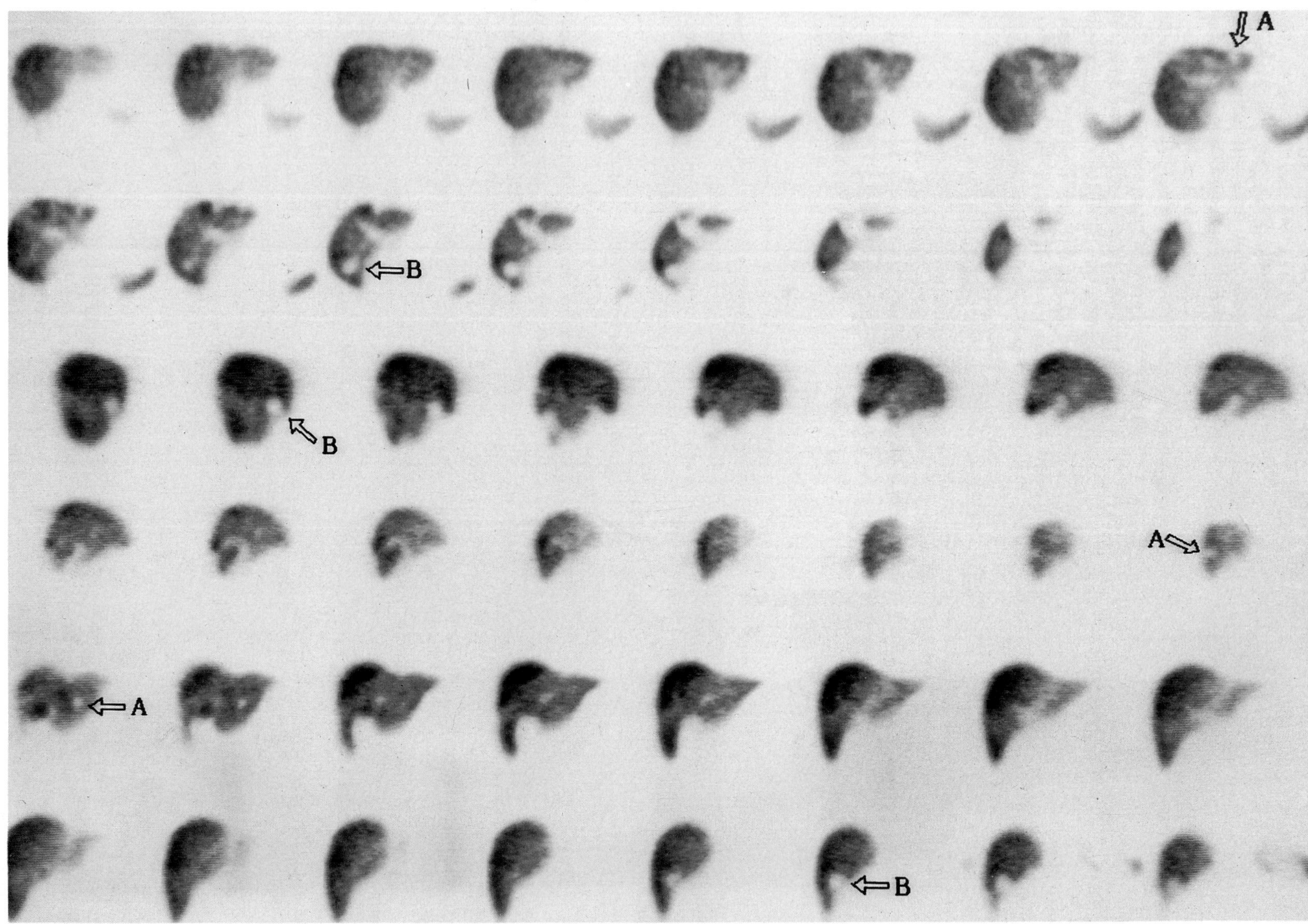

Figure 18. Breast carcinoma metastatic to the liver. Two lesions (**A** and **B**) are evident in transverse (top 2 rows), sagittal (middle 2 rows) and coronal (bottom 2 rows) projections. Courtesy of Mr. Ray Witulich.

Table 3. Efficacy of Liver Scintigraphy in Staging Metastatic Disease*

	TRUE-POSITIVE YIELD (%)	FALSE-POSITIVE YIELD (%)
Breast		
Perioperative	1.5	3
Recurrent tumor	8	2
Colorectal (preoperative)	15	7
Head and neck (preoperative)	0	1
Lung (preoperative)		
Bronchogenic	0	7
Small cell	12	–
Malignant melanoma		
Stages I and II	0	1
Stage III	20	1.5
Urogenital		
Bladder	1	5
Prostatic	6	5
Testicular	4	–

*From Harbert JC: The efficacy of bone and liver scanning in malignant disease—Facts and opinion, *in* Freeman LM, Weissmann HS (eds.): *Nuclear Medicine Annual, 1982.* New York, Raven Press.

There are no particular scintigraphic features that distinguish hepatoma from metastasis. The presence of a large solitary mass lesion in a patient with clinical cirrhosis or chronic liver disease should raise the suspicion of hepatoma. The serum α-fetoprotein should always be measured whenever hepatoma is suspected, because this test is quite specific and is elevated in about half of all cases.[140,141]

In patients with cirrhosis, it is important to distinguish hepatoma from pseudotumor. To this end, dynamic blood pool imaging may be useful. Hepatomas receive their blood supply from the hepatic artery and, thus, are seen to be perfused earlier than the remainder of the liver, which is perfused predominantly by the portal circulation. Pseudotumors have normal or slightly decreased perfusion.

Gallium imaging has also been helpful in distinguishing hepatoma from pseudotumor. In about 90% of hepatomas, gallium uptake is increased, uptake in pseudotumor is diminished, and the defects observed in colloid images persist on gallium images.[142,143]

Several radiopharmaceuticals are taken up by hepatomas (Table 4), including ^{67}Ga-citrate,[144,145] ^{75}Se-methionine,[146] radiolabeled bleomycin,[147] ^{99m}Tc-HIDA,[148] and ^{99m}Tc-PMT (pyridoxyl-5-methyltryptophan).[149,150] None of these is sufficiently specific to warrant routine use at this time; however, a recent study suggests that the intensity of ^{99m}Tc-PMT uptake in hepatoma may be positively related to survival.[149] Some reports suggest that uptake of biliary agents is related to degree of tumor differentiation: well-differentiated tumors retain hepatocyte function, while poorly differentiated tumors do not.[151] Distant metastases of hepatoma have also been imaged with a variety of agents, including ^{99m}Tc-HIDA,[152] ^{99m}Tc-PMT,[153] ^{99m}Tc-PIPIDA,[154] and possibly ^{123}I-IMP.[155]

Cholangiocarcinoma and Kupffer cell sarcomas are rare and have no particular distinguishing features scintigraphically.

PET Imaging of Liver Tumors. A few preliminary studies that measured the glucose metabolism of hepatic metastases and primary tumors have been reported.[156,157] Okazumi et al.[157] used a three-compartment model in which plasma ^{18}F-FDG enters tumor tissue by facilitated diffusion and is then phosphorylated by hexokinase and trapped intracellularly as FDG-6-PO_4. Because dephosphorylation is very slow, most positron emissions emanating from tissues after 40 minutes come from FDG-6-PO_4 within the cells. In these delayed views, images can be evaluated qualitatively for the presence of local tissue uptake. Input functions were derived from arterial sampling. In some cases, the input function might be derived directly from rapid dynamic imaging of the heart, if that organ is in the field of view, or possibly from the images of the aorta.[158]

In the studies of Okazumi and colleagues, malignant tumors could easily be distinguished from benign lesions by comparing the phosphorylation rate constant, k_3. Utilizing both the phosphorylation and dephosphorylation rate constants, the degree of differentiation of hepatocellular carcinomas was possible. After treatment, k_3 decreased according to the effectiveness of therapy; these investigators suggest this as a means of assessing the efficacy of treatment.

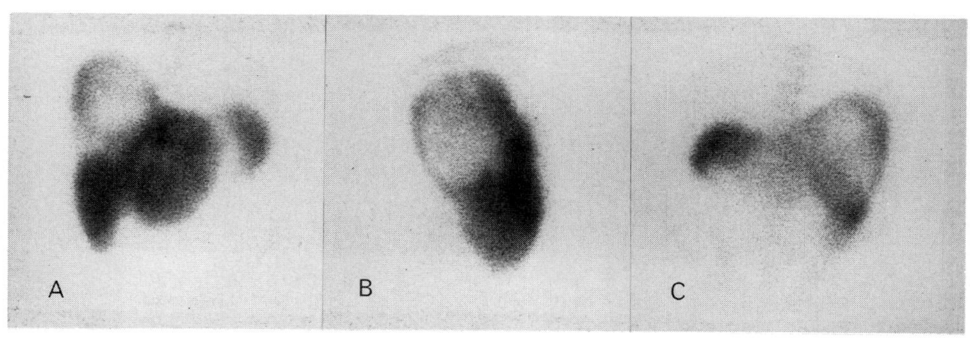

Figure 19. ^{99m}Tc-sulfur colloid scintigraphy in a 54-year-old male with long-standing cirrhosis demonstrates a large expansile mass lesion in the right upper lobe proven by biopsy to be a hepatoma. **(A).** anterior; **(B).** right lateral; **(C).** posterior.

Table 4. Comparative Imaging in Lesions of the Liver

LESION	COLLOID	GALLIUM	BILIARY	RBC	COMMENTS
Hepatoma	cold	↑	Early = ↓ Late = ? ↑	↑ Flow	Vascular; lack Kupffer cells
Hemangioma	cold	cold	cold	Early = ↓ Late = ↑	Vascular
Adenoma	cold	variable usually ↓	normal or ↓	usually ↑	Lack Kupffer cells and bile ducts
FNH*	normal or ↑	normal or ↑	Early-normal Late-↑	normal or ↑	Hepatocytes, but no Kupffer cells
Metastasis	cold	↑ in 50%	cold	normal or ↓	Depends on vasc.
Fatty infiltration	normal	normal	normal	normal or ↓	Kupffer cells if no mass effect
Abscess	cold	hot	cold	may show "rim effect"	

*FNH = Focal nodular hyperplasia

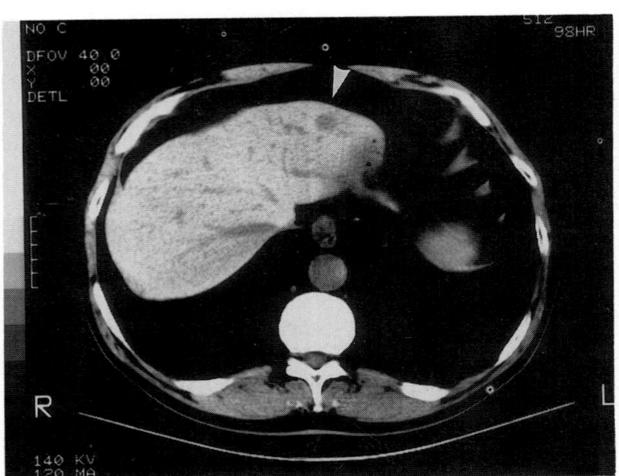

A

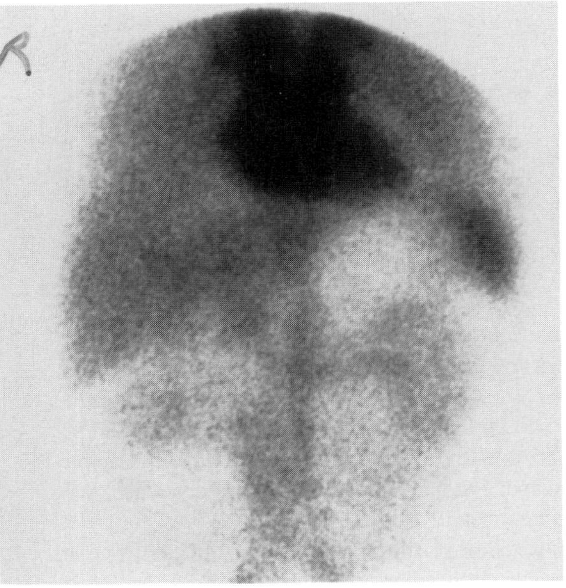

B

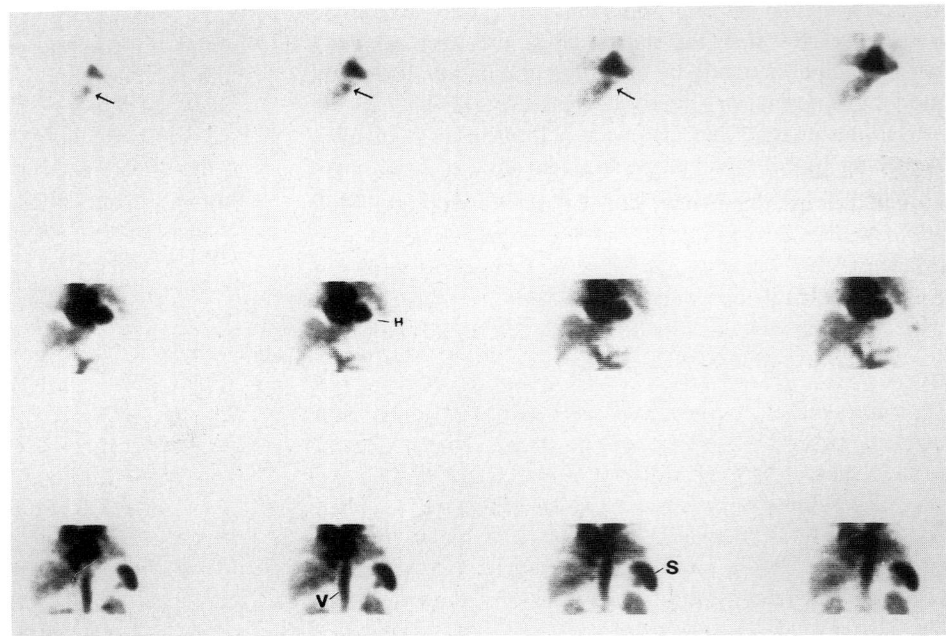

C

Figure 20. Small hepatic hemangioma found incidentally in a 46-year-old male with renal cell carcinoma. **(A).** Contrast CT demonstrates a 1-cm low-density lesion in the anterior left lobe (arrow head); **(B).** Static anterior blood pool image acquired 45 min following intravenous injection of 925 MBq (25 mCi) ^{99m}Tc-RBCs is normal. Radionuclide angiogram (not shown) was normal as well; **(C).** Selected (12 of 48 sections @ 3 mm per section) coronal SPECT sections (dual detector) show a subtle vascular focus (arrows) in the far anterior sections that would be missed without additional SPECT projections.

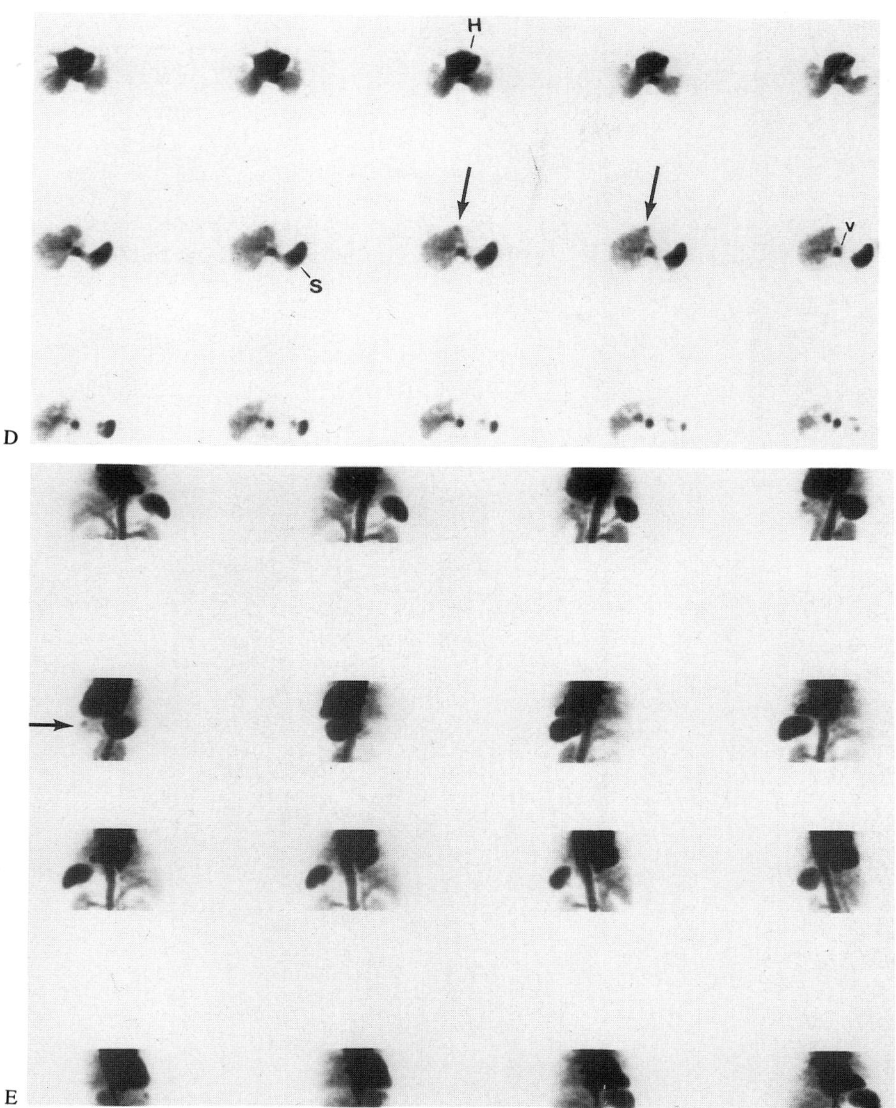

Figure 20. Continued. (D). Selected transverse sections clearly outline the hemangioma (arrows); **(E).** Selected angular projections from the rotational images again show the extreme anterior hemangioma (arrow). These images proceed from upper left to bottom right as the body rotates from left to right. Notations: H = heart; S = spleen; V = inferior vena cava.

NONMALIGNANT TUMORS

Benign tumors of the liver are relatively common, although they usually do not cause symptoms. Most often they are encountered as incidental findings in the pursuit of other disease. If they become very large, they may create discomfort and a palpable upper abdominal mass. The most common histological types are *hemangiomas, focal nodular hyperplasia*, and *liver cell adenoma.*

Hemangiomas. Cavernous hemangiomas are the most common benign tumor of the liver, found in from 1 to 7% of autopsies.[159,160] They are more prevalent in women and are most often found in subcapsular regions of the liver, predominantly in the right lobe. Multiple hemangiomas occur in about 20% of cases.[161] Hepatic hemangiomas are typically less than 3 cm in diameter; when they are larger than 4 cm, they are classified as "giant hemangiomas."[162] Histologically, cavernous hemangiomas consist of interconnected blood-filled spaces, lined by a single layer of endothelium. They are being encountered with increasing frequency because of the burgeoning use of abdominal US, CT, and MRI, where they are detected incidentally in as many as 2 to 3% of cases, often when they are of very small size.[163] These small tumors usually are asymptomatic and require no therapy. However, they must be distinguished from more serious metastatic disease and, thus, present a common clinical dilemma. Of particular concern is the possibility of fatal hemorrhage if they are biopsied,[159] particularly if they are subcapsular masses without a cuff of normal hepatic parenchyma. They occasionally rupture spontaneously, but prophylactic resection is not generally recommended.[164]

The usual US appearance of cavernous hemangiomas is that of a homogeneous, hyperechoic mass with well-defined margins and posterior acoustical enhancement; however,

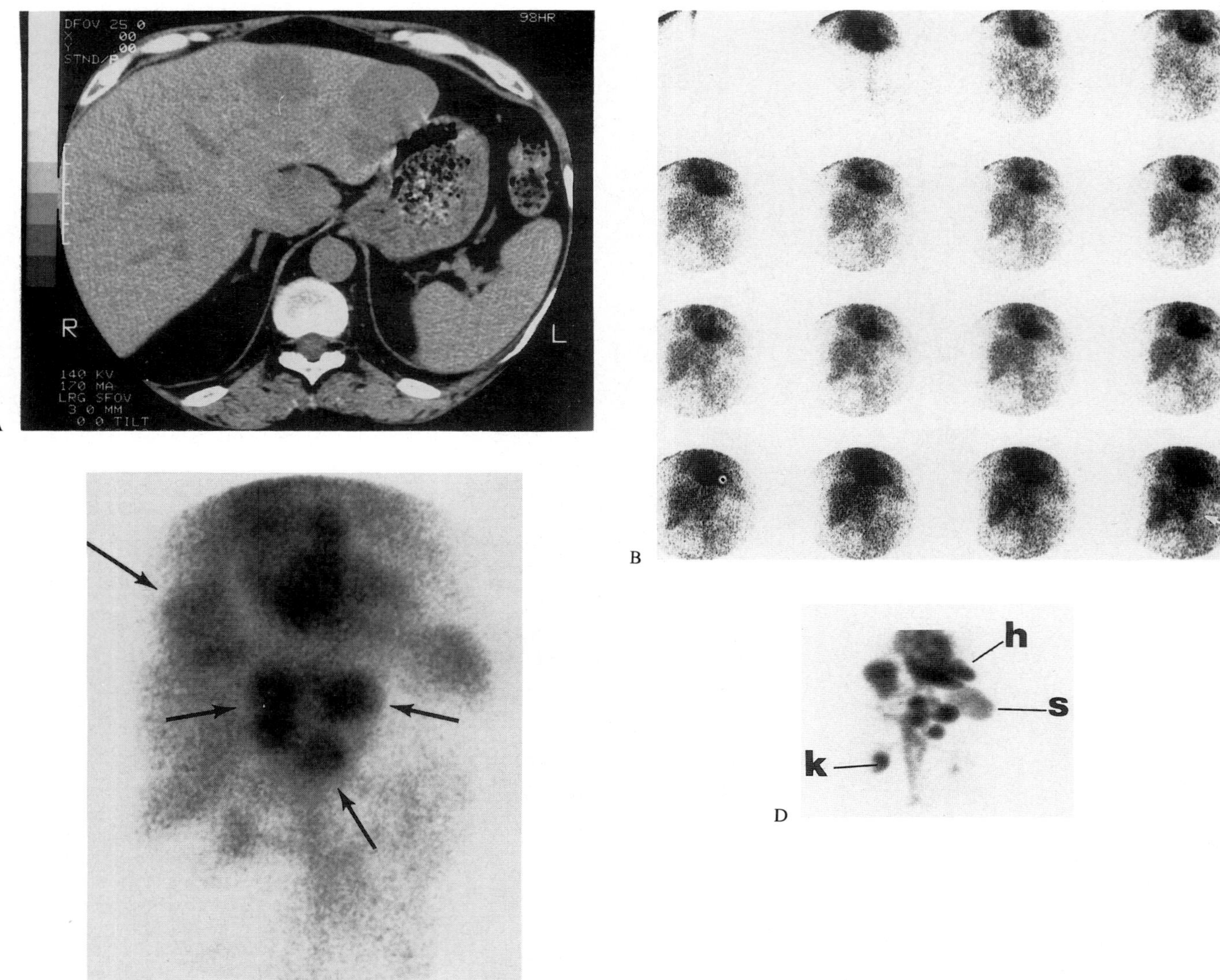

Figure 21. **(A).** Noncontrast CT scan demonstrates four low-density lesions in the left hepatic lobe of a 45-year-old woman being staged for breast cancer. The largest lesion measures 4 cm; **(B).** Radionuclide angiogram obtained at 3 s per image following the intravenous injection of 925 MBq (25 mCi) ^{99m}Tc-RBCs demonstrate two possible vascular lesions in the late images (arrow); **(C).** Planar blood pool image obtained 30 min later demonstrates three vascular lesions in the left lobe and a fourth in the upper right lobe (arrows); **(D).** The rotational image from the SPECT study, shown here from the anterior projection (0.0° rotation), clearly reveal 5 discrete vascular lesions. Notations are: h = heart; k = kidney (free pertechnetate); and s = spleen. These findings are characteristic of multiple hemangiomas.

they may be hypoechoic, isoechoic, or of mixed echogenicity.[165] Although US is sensitive for detecting hepatic hemangiomas, it is not specific.

CT is quite specific for the diagnosis of hemangiomas when strict criteria are applied. These are: (a) relative hypoattenuation compared with normal liver on precontrast images, (b) early peripheral enhancement with contrast administration, (c) progressive opacification toward the center of the lesion and, (d) complete isoattenuating fill-in occurring not less than 3 minutes nor more than 60 minutes after contrast administration.[166] However, the diagnosis can be made with certainty in only 50 to 75% of cases.[167,168] Small hemangiomas, in particular, fail to meet these criteria.

MRI has both high sensitivity and specificity for detecting hemangiomas. They most often demonstrate marked hyperintensity on T2-weighted images, the so-called "lightbulb" sign. Stark et al. found that MRI had a sensitivity of 90%, a specificity of 92%, and an accuracy of 90%.[169] However, the lightbulb sign and other patterns associated with the morphology of hemangiomas has been observed in islet cell tumors, carcinoids, and pancreatic tumors.[166]

^{99m}Tc-red blood cell (RBC) scintigraphy is the most spe-

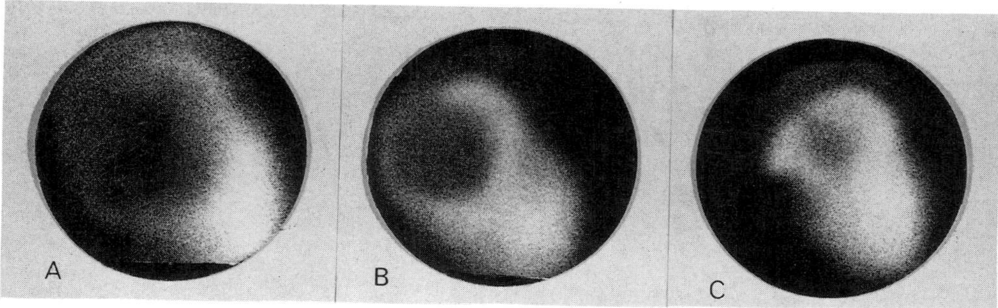

Figure 22. Amebic abscess. Right lateral scintiphoto at start of metronidazole therapy **(A)**, 7 days later **(B)**, and 30 days later **(C)**.

cific study available for the noninvasive diagnosis of cavernous hemangioma.[170–172] In larger hemangiomas (≥4 cm) radionuclide angiography demonstrates normal or even diminished flow at the site of the lesion, while delayed (5-min to 2-hour) images reveal increased vascularity.[170,159,173] This perfusion-blood pool mismatch is caused by the slow-mixing of the labeled RBCs with the relatively stagnant nonlabeled blood within the tumors. The rate of mixing depends on the size of the tumor; small lesions "fill in" more rapidly than large tumors.[161] This appearance was described by Engel et al. using planar imaging, in which they found sensitivity, specificity, and accuracy of 89%, 100%, and 95%, respectively.[174] Although some hypervascular lesions, such as hepatic adenomas, focal nodular hyperplasia, hepatomas, and some endocrine tumors may demonstrate progressive enhancement with RBCs on delayed blood-pool images, these lesions would be expected to demonstrate increased activity on early dynamic images as well. Some very large hemangiomas undergo infarction, in which case a nonperfused defect results, but these lesions usually retain a hypervascular rim.[161]

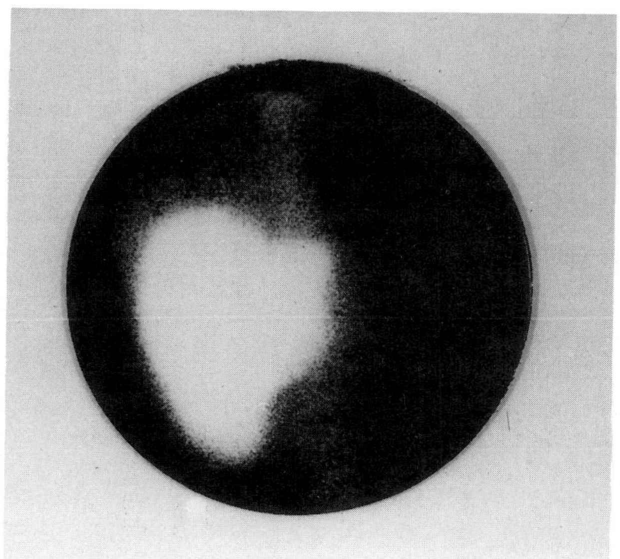

Figure 23. Anterior planar image demonstrating absent left lobe secondary to external irradiation.

The use of SPECT greatly enhances the sensitivity of scintigraphy for small lesions, those located centrally and those located near large blood vessels[171,172,175] (Fig. 20). Ziessman showed that high-resolution, multi-detector SPECT is much more sensitive than planar imaging[172] and this has been the experience at the NIH, where multi-detector SPECT instruments have been much more sensitive than rotating single-head instruments (Fig. 20). In Ziessman's study, lesions larger than 1.4 cm in diameter were detected with 100% sensitivity and lesions as small as 0.5 cm could be detected in some cases. The criteria for a positive lesion was any focus of activity that correlated with CT or US in location, with greater than hepatic parenchymal vascularity. Lesions that are positive by planar imaging, however, are not better identified by SPECT[175] (Fig. 21).

The diagnostic workup will vary between institutions, with the sophistication of the physicians, and with the equipment they have available. The recommendations of Nelson and Chezmar seem appropriate at this time.[166] Generally, a combination of two confirmatory studies can be considered diagnostic. If a lesion has a classic or near-classic appearance on either CT or US, a ^{99m}Tc-RBC study with SPECT is recommended if the lesion is larger than 2.5 cm (1 cm if high-resolution SPECT is available). Otherwise, MRI with T2 weighting is recommended as the complementary test.

If MRI is the initial imaging study with which a lesion with a classic or near-classic appearance is detected, a ^{99m}Tc-RBC study with SPECT is recommended. If the lesion is smaller than the likely resolution of the SPECT unit, follow-up contrast-enhanced CT or, less preferably, US is recommended. If these studies cannot reconcile the nature of the lesion in a high-risk patient, CT-guided percutaneous needle biopsy is recommended.

Focal Nodular Hyperplasia. These tumors are found usually in women, are solitary, and of unknown cause. These tumors are quite vascular and give rise to a vascular blush with radionuclide angiography. Often, they contain Kupffer cells and take up colloid; in such instances, the scintiscan is virtually diagnostic.[176,177] In some cases, hepatobiliary scin-

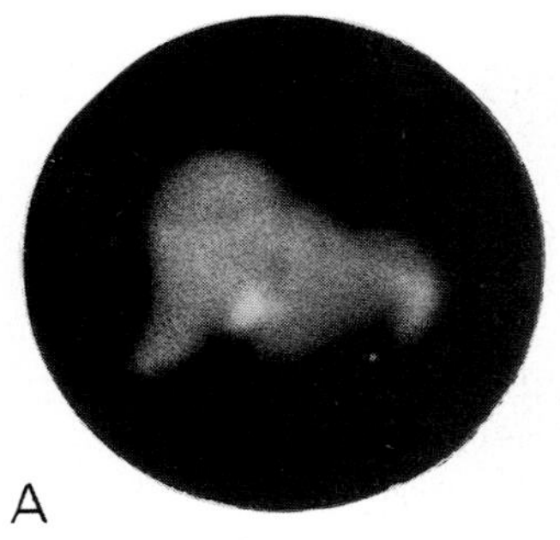

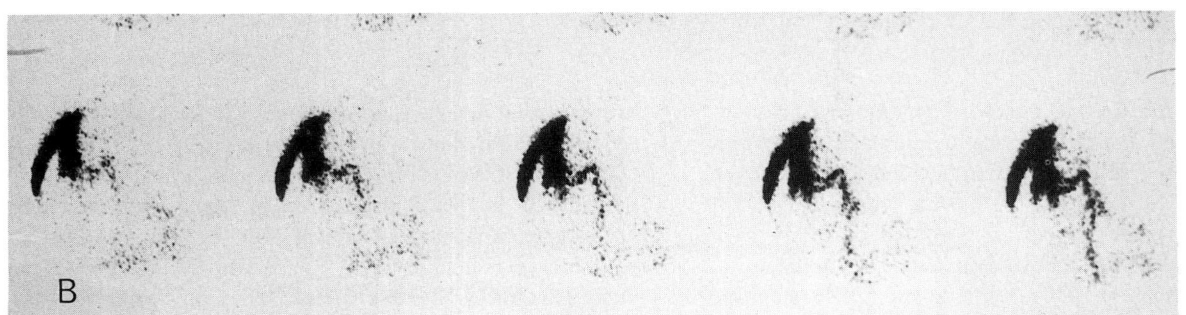

Figure 24. Superior vena cava obstruction resulting in focal hot spot in the caudate lobe **(A).** Obstruction in this case is demonstrated by sequential 1-s dynamic views of the thorax following right antecubital injection of ^{99m}Tc-sulfur colloid **(B).** Compare with the normal blood flow pattern demonstrated in Figure 21 (B).

tigraphy demonstrates hepatocyte function within the intrahepatic lesion, again a strong indication of focal nodular hyperplasia.[177] In other cases, colloid uptake is decreased and the scan is nonspecific or normal.

Liver Cell Adenoma. These benign tumors are commonly associated with oral contraceptive use and are usually encountered after they hemorrhage. They have the appearance of a solitary cold lesion because they do not take up colloid.[178]

Liver cell adenomas associated with glycogen storage disease are multiple in about 50% of patients. The glycogen storage disease affects primarily hepatocytes, but colloids are taken up by Kupffer cells. Splenomegaly and colloid shift are also frequently observed. Hepatic tumors appear as cold defects within the liver.

Cirrhosis. Focal defects may be found in advanced stages of cirrhosis. They are caused by areas of fibrosis and hypovascularity rather than by regenerating nodules. Their scintigraphic appearance may be indistinguishable from that of metastases. Unfortunately, the history of alcoholism is of little help, because these patients may have hepatoma or metastases also.

Focal Fatty Infiltration. Fatty infiltration of the liver is associated with a variety of disorders, including alcohol abuse, obesity, diabetes mellitus, malnutrition, i.v. hyperalimentation, hepatitis, intestinal bypass, glycogen storage disease, and cystic fibrosis. Fatty infiltration itself is relatively benign and may be reversible, especially when induced by drugs such as steroids. More often, however, it progresses to cirrhosis.[180,181] Usually the diagnosis of fatty liver can be confirmed by CT if the mean CT number (Hounsfield unit) for the liver is lower than that for the spleen. A diagnostic dilemma occurs when fatty infiltration appears on CT images as a low-density mass lesion, or on US as a hypoechoic mass.

Several studies have shown that radiocolloid scintigraphy is not affected by the presence of fat droplets in the hepatocytes because the reticuloendothelial cells are spared.[182–184] Consequently, both planar and SPECT imaging are normal. Furthermore, planar imaging with radioxenon, a lipophilic inert gas (Fig. 15), demonstrates accumulation within the lesions.[182,185] Biliary function may also be preserved within regions of fatty infiltration and gallium uptake may be normal (Table 4). Yeh and colleagues showed that the hepatic retention of ^{133}Xe following a period of rebreathing correlates well with the percentage of fat on biopsy specimens.[186]

When focal fatty infiltration is suspected and SPECT liver images reveal focal defects, blood-pool imaging is useful to rule out hemangioma or metastases.[182]

Abscess. Pyogenic abscesses of the liver are relatively uncommon. Clinically, they are characterized by fever, liver tenderness, pain in the right upper quadrant, leukocytosis, and elevated alkaline phosphatase. Scintigraphy with ^{99m}Tc-sulfur colloid may be negative in early stages of disease when only inflammation exists. When infection consolidates and pus forms, one or more focal defects develops. ^{67}Gallium and ^{111}In-labeled leukocyte scintigraphy may be useful to distinguish abscess from noninflammatory lesions.

Amebic abscesses are usually solitary and occur predominantly in the right lobe as a complication of colonic amebiasis. The differential diagnosis from pyogenic abscess is usually made by needle aspiration. The liver scan is useful in following the course of therapy (Fig. 22).

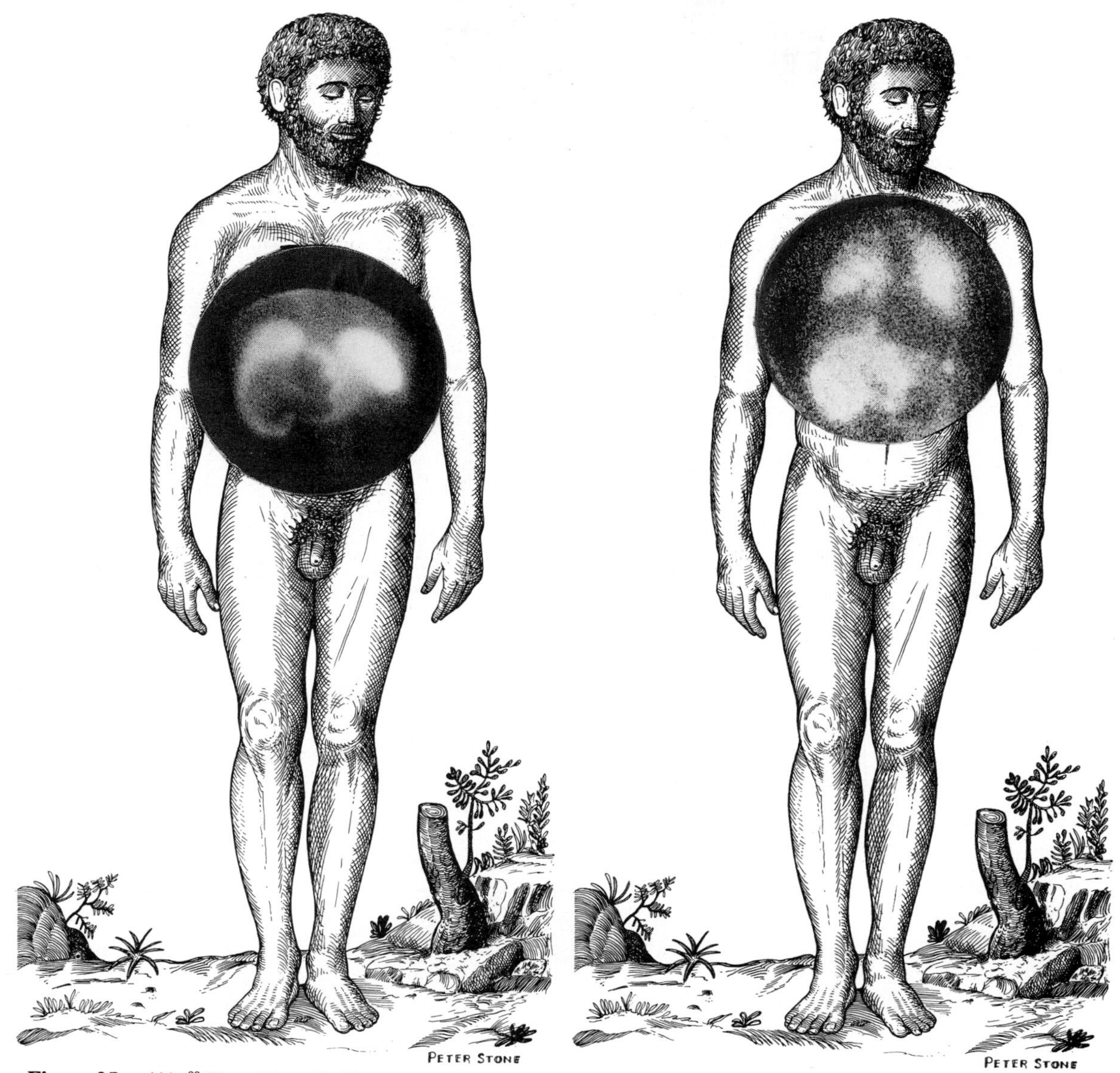

Figure 25. **(A).** ^{99m}Tc-sulfur colloid scan demonstrating large, irregular metastasis; **(B).** Anterior scintiphoto following intra-arterial infusion of 37 MBq of ^{99m}Tc-MAA at a rate of 100 mL/hr. The tumor and right hepatic lobe are well perfused. A small amount of central tumor necrosis and significant lung activity secondary to A-V shunting are apparent.

Schistosomiasis may also produce focal scintigraphic lesions although, in its early stages, the pattern is diffuse with irregular colloid distribution.

Cysts. Single and multiple cysts are often found in patients with renal polycystic disease, which is manifested earlier. Cysts may produce hepatomegaly, displacing the liver from its normal position. They are identified easily with US as well-circumscribed, echo-free regions.

In cattle- and sheep-rearing countries, hydatid disease (*echinococcosis*), caused by the larvae of the tapeworms *Echinococcus granulosus* or *E. multilocularis,* is frequently manifested by hepatomegaly and liver cysts. These cysts enlarge slowly and are usually single and found in the right lobe. Liver scintigraphy has been useful as a screening test in endemic regions.[187]

Trauma. Liver scintigraphy may be useful in detecting lacerations of the liver that require immediate surgical intervention.[188–190] The lesion produced is highly variable and is often indistinguishable from a mass lesion. Focal defects reduce in size gradually with time, but may leave a permanent scar. Subcapsular hematomas usually cause displacement of the liver, rather than an intrinsic lesion. Ultrasound and CT are generally more useful than scintigraphy in confirming or ruling out subcapsular hemorrhage, and also permit examination of such adjacent structures as kidneys and pancreas.

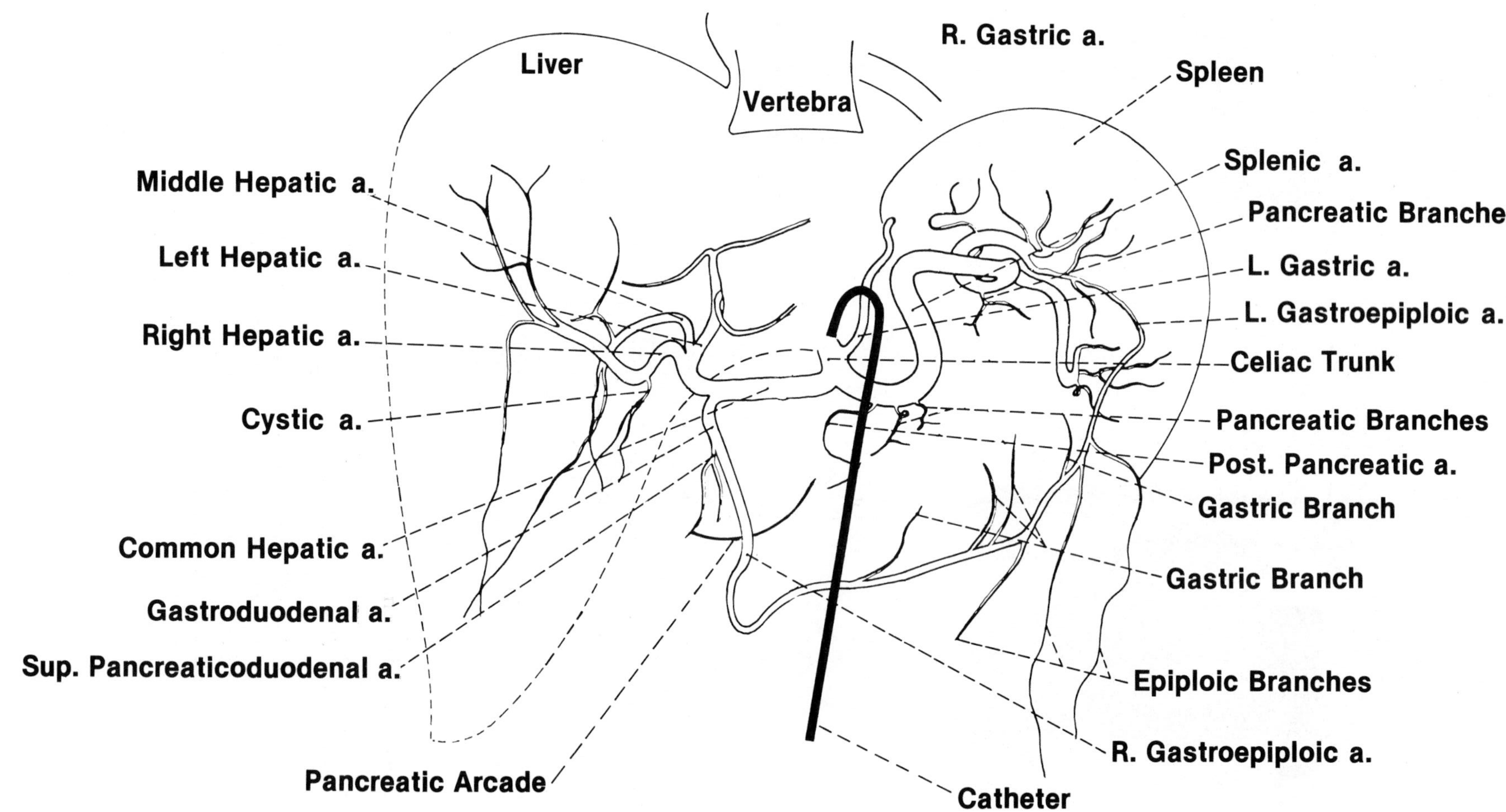

Figure 26. **(A).** The principal arterial branches of the celiac axis.

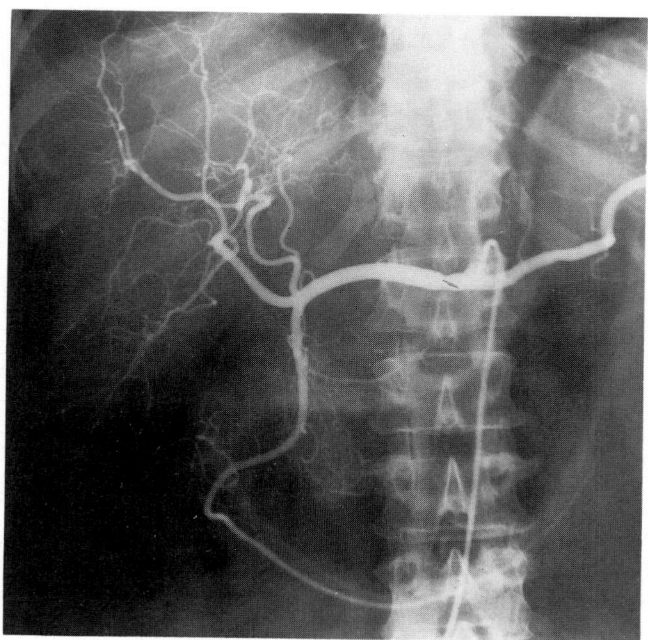

Figure 26. Continued. (B). Hepatic arteriogram.

Partial hepatectomy for tumors or cystic lesions create unusual remnants. Sequential scans over several months document the remarkable regenerative capacity of the liver.[191] The regenerated liver is usually globular in shape.

OTHER LESIONS

Distinctive defects are created by radiation therapy to the liver (Fig. 23). Often, a linear edge is created by the radiation ports. The threshold dose is 3000 to 4000 rad.[192,193] In many cases, Kupffer cell function recovers after several months. In children, compensatory hypertrophy of the nonirradiated lobe of the liver may occur.[194]

Biliary duct obstruction and dilatation may appear as a central lesion in the region of the porta hepatis. Such a lesion may be difficult to recognize by radiocolloid scintigraphy because this region may be thinned normally. In general, however, the cause is easily diagnosed by ultrasound or hepatobiliary imaging.

Caroli's disease (communicating cavernous ectasia of the intrahepatic bile ducts) may be associated with multiple focal hepatic defects on colloid scintigraphy.[195] When a biliary agent such as ^{99m}Tc-IDA is administered, these defects fill with tracer.

Intrahepatic lithiasis is uncommon in this country, but is more frequently encountered in the Orient. It is caused by concretion of stones within the bile ducts, which causes blockage and dilatation resulting in Charcot's triad: upper abdominal pain, fever, and jaundice. The disease may produce large cold lesions on colloid scintigrams. The nature of the defects can be discovered by hepatobiliary scintigraphy, wherein tracer accumulates in the dilated biliary ducts and produces hot areas corresponding to the colloid defects.[196]

Focal "Hot Spots." Occasionally, focal areas of increased colloid concentration have been described.[197–204] Examples are shown in Figures 16 and 24. This phenomenon might occur by one of three mechanisms: (1) local increase in the number of phagocytic cells, (2) local increase in perfusion and, (3) regions of normal parenchyma surrounded by areas of decreased function.

Most reported cases have involved superior vena cava obstruction with associated cavoportal shunting, which supports the concept of increased regional perfusion. After injection of colloid into an upper extremity, dynamic flow studies show that activity descends through the paraumbilical veins (especially the internal mammary and lateral thoracic veins), enters the portal circulation, and passes through the liver before entering the heart. Focal hot spots occur where a high concentration of colloid enters the liver through the shunting vessels—usually in the caudate lobe. Repeat injections into the dorsal pedal veins show a normal distribution. In the case of inferior vena cava obstruction, the cavoportal shunting is demonstrated by leg injections of colloid.[205]

Increased local vascularity may also be responsible, since hot spots have been associated with hemangiomas,[205] liver abscess,[206] hamartoma, adenoma,[207] and focal nodular hyperplasia.[208] Nevertheless, the occurrence of these hot spots is rare.

HEPATIC ARTERY INFUSION STUDIES

Direct hepatic artery infusion of chemotherapeutic agents has been used for many years for the treatment of nonresectable intrahepatic tumors.[209,210] Naturally, correct placement of the infusion catheter is essential to perfuse all of the tumor and to spare adjacent vital structures from the toxic effects of the chemotherapeutic drugs. Contrast angiography does not predict the flow distribution at the flow rates used for drug infusion.[211] Rather, a more accurate method of imaging the distribution of perfusion is achieved by slow injection of 37 MBq (1 mCi) ^{99m}Tc-MAA through the infusion pump line. When these images are compared with a baseline colloid scintigraphy, the adequacy of the catheter placement can be judged. Dynamic studies should be obtained during the first few minutes of tracer infusion.[210]

Figure 25 **A** demonstrates a large irregular solitary metastasis by colloid scintigraphy. Figure 25 **B** illustrates the distribution of perfusion distal to the hepatic artery catheter using ^{99m}Tc-MAA. Note the considerable lung activity caused by arteriovenous shunting within the tumor. Note also the small area of central tumor necrosis seen in Figure 25 **B.** These imaging techniques are especially useful for determining optimum catheter placement at the time of surgery.[212]

Figure 26 depicts the major arterial divisions of the celiac axis. This diagram is useful in determining the distribution of chemotherapeutic infusions. Note that the three branches of the hepatic artery lie very near the junction of the gastroduodenal artery. With optimum catheter placement, all three

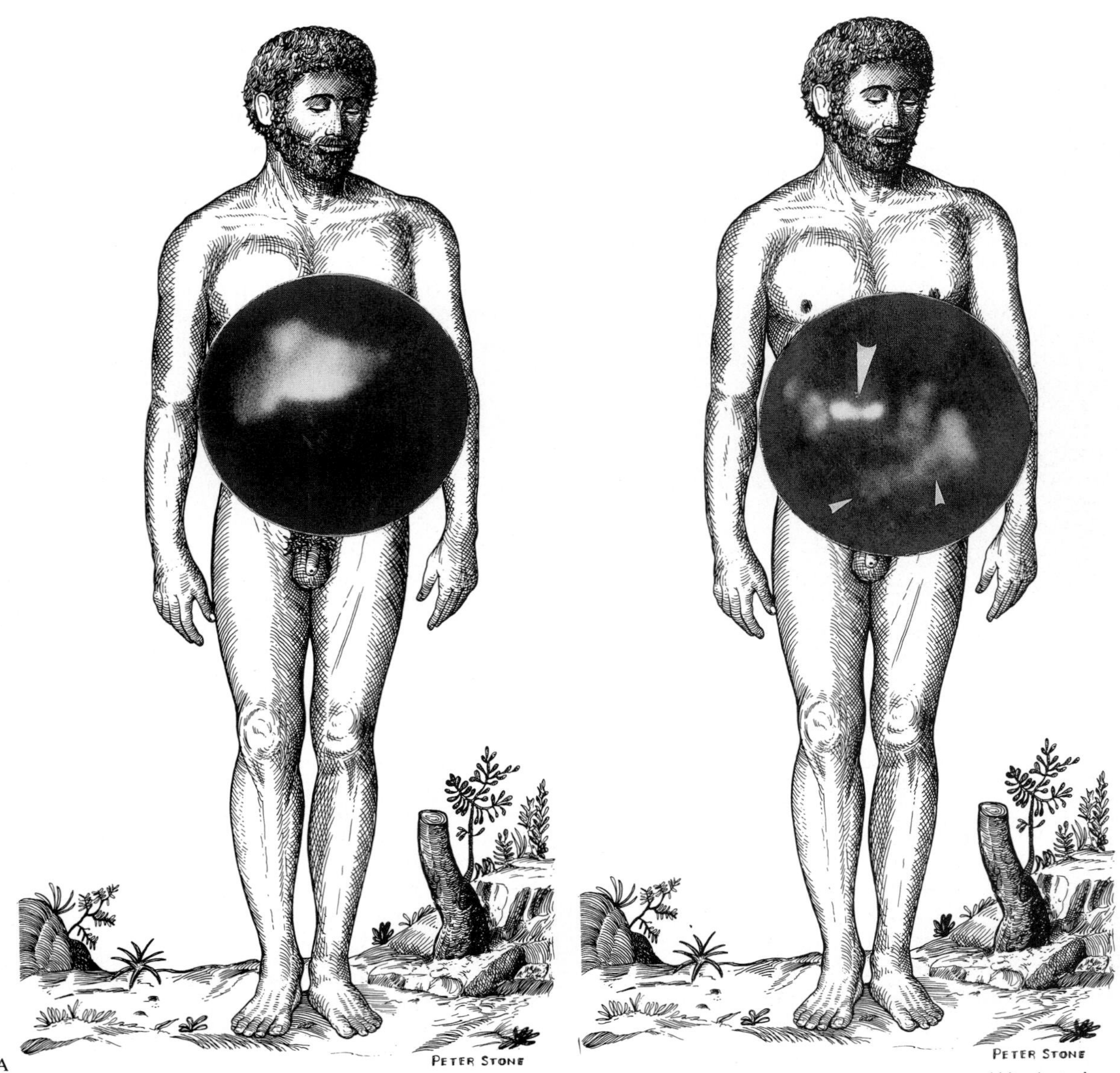

Figure 27. Hepatic artery perfusion study in a patient with nonresectable colon cancer metastases. **(A).** Anterior scintiphoto following slow infusion of 37 MBq ^{99m}Tc-MAA shows good initial perfusion to the liver with no apparent A-V shunting; **(B).** Several days later, the patient complained of abdominal pain. The tracer study now shows most of the MAA adhering to a clot at the catheter tip (large arrowhead) and widespread distribution to branches of the gastroduodenal and gastroepiploic arteries (small arrowheads). Administration of streptokinase failed to restore hepatic artery perfusion and the catheter was withdrawn.

hepatic artery branches are perfused, and there is no flow to the gastroduodenal. Cytotoxic drugs delivered to the gastroduodenal artery result in severe abdominal pain and a risk of stomach necrosis. The distribution of catheter perfusion should be determined periodically because the catheter can move, the perfused artery may thrombose, and the tip may become occluded by blood clots. All of these complications require corrective action and are best diagnosed by radionuclide imaging. Thrombosis and catheter movement result in altered distribution of perfusion (Fig. 27). Clotting of the catheter tip usually results in agglomerations of macroaggregates. Figure 27 demonstrates several problems associated with hepatic artery catheters and indicates the usefulness of these studies in defining the problems.

Recently, hepatic artery infusion has been combined with hepatic artery embolization to increase the effectiveness of treatment.[213] Theoretically, embolization of the arteries supplying the tumor produces tumor ischemia and cell death, increases the antitumor activity in an hypoxic environment, and slows the flow of chemotherapeutic drugs to increase regional concentrations. However, embolization itself may alter the distribution. Hall et al. suggest that such flow reversal is often temporary and tracer studies 24 hours later may demonstrate adequate tumor perfusion.[214]

REFERENCES

1. Kashiwagi T, et al.: Heterogeneous intrahepatic distribution of blood flow in humans. *Eur J Nucl Med* 1981;6:545.
2. Dobson EL, Jones HB: The behaviour of intravenously injected particulate material: Its rate of disappearance from the blood stream as a measure of liver blood flow. *Acta Med Scand* (Suppl) 1952;144:273.
3. Vetter H, Falkner R, Neumayer A: The disappearance rate of colloidal and radiogold from the circulation and its application to the estimation of liver blood flow in normal and cirrhotic subjects. *J Clin Invest* 1954;33:1594.
4. Bergqvist L, Sundberg R, Ryden S, Strand S-E: The "critical colloid dose" in studies of reticuloendothelial function. *J Nucl Med* 1987;28:1424.
5. Klingensmith WC, Fritzberg AB, Zerbe GO, et al.: Relative role of Tc-99m sulfur colloid in the evaluation of liver function. *Clin Nucl Med* 1980;5:341.
6. Ueno K, Haseda K: Concentration and clearance of Tc-99m-pyridoxylidene isoleucine by a hepatoma. *Clin Nucl Med* 1980;5:196.
7. Utz JA, Lull RJ, Anderson JH, et al.: Hepatoma visualization with Tc-99m pyridoxylidene glutamate. *J Nucl Med* 1980; 21:747.
8. Antar MA, Sziklas JJ, Spencer RP: Liver imaging during reticuloendothelial failure. *Clin Nucl Med* 1977;2:294.
9. Saba TM: Physiology and physiopathology of the reticuloendothelial system. *Arch Intern Med* 1970;126:1031.
10. Bell EG, McAfee JG: Concepts of colloid chemistry, in Gilson AJ et al. (eds.): *Hematopoietic and Gastrointestinal Investigations with Radionuclides.* Springfield, Charles C. Thomas, 1972.
11. Atkins HL, Hauser W, Richards P: Factors affecting distribution of technetium-sulfur colloid. *J Reticuloendothel Soc* 1970;8:176.
12. Nelp WB: Distribution and radiobiological behavior of colloids and macroaggregates, in Cloutier RJ et al. (eds.): *Medical Radionuclides: Radiation Dose and Effects.* Springfield, VA, USAEC Symposium Series 20, 1970.
13. Arzoumanian A, Rosenthall L, Sato H: Clinical comparison of ^{99m}Tc-labeled preformed phytate colloid and sulfur colloid: concise communication. *J Nucl Med* 1977;18:118.
14. Chaudhuri TK, Evans TC, Chaudhuri TK: Autoradiographic studies of distribution in the liver of ^{198}Au and ^{99m}Tc-sulfur colloids. *Radiology* 1973;109:633.
15. George EA, Hendershott LR, Klos DJ, et al.: Mechanism of hepatic extraction of gelatinized 99mtechnetium sulfur colloid. *Eur J Nucl Med* 1980;5:241.
16. Frier M, Griffiths P, Ramsey A: The biological fate of sulfur colloid. *Eur J Nucl Med* 1981;6:371.
17. Dobson EL, Warner GF, Finney GR, et al.: The measurement of liver circulation by means of the colloid disappearance rate. *Circulation* 1953;7:690.
18. DeNardo SJ, Bell GB, DeNardo GL: Diagnosis of cirrhosis and hepatitis by quantitative hepatic and other reticuloendothelial clearance rates. *J Nucl Med* 1976;17:449.
19. Miller J, Diffey BL, Fleming JS: Measurement of colloid clearance rate as an adjunct to static liver imaging. *Eur J Nucl Med* 1979;4:1.
20. Boyd RO, Stadalnik RC, Barnett CA, et al.: Quantitative hepatic scintiangiography. *Clin Nucl Med* 1978;3:478.
21. Biersack HJ, Torres J, Thelen M, et al.: Determination of liver and spleen perfusion by quantitative sequential scintigraphy: Results in normal subjects and in patients with portal hypertension. *Clin Nucl Med* 1981;6:218.
22. O'Connor MK, MacMathuna P, Keeling PWN: Hepatic arterial and portal venous components of liver blood flow: a dynamic scintigraphic study. *J Nucl Med* 1988;29:466.
23. Fleming JS, Ackeryu DM, Walmsley BH, Karran SJ: Scintigraphic estimation of arterial and portal blood supplies to the liver. *J Nucl Med* 1983;24:1108.
24. Biersack HJ, Torres J, Thelan M, et al.: Determination of liver and spleen perfusion by quantitative sequential scintigraphy: results in normals and in patients with portal hypertension. *Clin Nucl Med* 1981;6:218.
25. Rypins EB, Fajman W, Sarper R, et al.: Radionuclide angiography of the liver and spleen. *Am J Surg* 1981;142:574.
26. Hesdorffer CS, Bezwoda WR, Danilewitz MD, et al.: Radioisotopic flow scanning for portal blood flow and portal hypertension. *Clin Nucl Med* 1987;12:610.
27. Juni JE, Merion RM, Campbell DA, Warber-Matich SL: Diagnosis of liver transplant rejection by scintigraphy with deconvolutional analysis. *J Nucl Med* 1988;29:790.
28. Sarper R, Fajman WA, Tarcan YA, Nixon DW: Enhanced detection of metastatic liver disease by computerized flow scintigrams: concise communication. *J Nucl Med* 1981;22:318.
29. Leveson SH, Wiggins PA, Giles GR, et al.: Deranged liver blood flow patterns in the detection of liver metastases. *Br J Surg* 1985;72:128.
30. Martin-Comin J, Mora J, Figueras H, et al.: Calculation of portal contribution to hepatic blood flow with ^{99m}Tc-microcolloids. A noninvasive method to diagnose liver graft rejection. *J Nucl Med* 1988;29:1776.
31. O'Connor MK, Krom RF, Carton EG, et al.: Ratio of hepatic arterial-to-portal venous blood flow—validation of radionuclide techniques in an animal model. *J Nucl Med* 1992;33:239.
32. Reichman S, Davis WD, Storaasli JP, et al.: Measurement of hepatic blood flow by indicator dilution techniques. *J Clin Invest* 1958;37:1848.
33. Nakamura T, Nakamura S, Kaneko T, et al.: Measurement of extrahepatic shunted blood flow in liver cirrhosis. *J Lab Clin Med* 1962;60:889.
34. Castell DI, Grace ND, Wennar MH, et al.: Evaluation of portal circulation in hepatic cirrhosis: a new method using xenon-133. 1969;57:533.
35. Tonami N, Nakajima K, Hisada K, et al.: A noninvasive method for evaluating portal circulation by administration of T1-201 per rectum. *J Nucl Med* 1982;23:965.
36. Yen C-K, Pollycove M, Crass R, et al.: Portasystemic shunt fraction quantification with colonic iodine-123 iodoamphetamine. *J Nucl Med* 1986;27:1321.
37. Kuroki T, Minowa T, Kawa M, et al.: Evaluation of perrectal portal scintigraphy in hepatic cirrhosis. *Acta Hepatol Jap* 1978;19:669.
38. Shiomi S, Kuroki T, Kurai O: Portal circulation by technetium-99m pertechnetate per-rectal portal scintigraphy. *J Nucl Med* 1988;29:460.
39. Eckelman WC, Reba RC: The classification of radiotracers. *J Nucl Med* 1978;19:1179.
40. Poralły T, Treichel U, Lohr H, Fleischer B: The asialoglycoprotein receptor as target structure in autoimmune liver diseases. *Semin Liver Dis* 1991;11:215.
41. Stadalnik RC, Vera DR, Woodle ES, et al.: Technetium-99m-NGA functional hepatic imaging: Preliminary clinical experience. *J Nucl Med* 1985;26:1233.
42. Kudo M, Vera DR, Stadalnik RC, et al.: In vivo estimates of hepatic binding protein concentration: correlation with classical indicators of hepatic functional reserve. *Am J Gastroenterol* 1990;85:1142.
43. Vera DR, Stadalnik RC, Trudeau WL, et al: Measurement of receptor concentration and forward-binding constant via radiopharmacokinetic modeling of ^{99m}Tc-galactosyl-neoglycoalbumin. *J Nucl Med* 1991;32:1169.

44. Kudo M, Vera DR, Trudeau WL, Stadalnik RC: Validation of in vivo receptor measurements via in vitro radioassay: technetium-99m-galactosyl-neoglycoalbumin as a prototype model. *J Nucl Med* 1991;32:1177.
45. Ha-Kawa SK, Tanaka Y: A quantitative model of Technetium-99m-DTPA-galactosyl-HSA for the assessment of hepatic blood flow and hepatic binding receptor. *J Nucl Med* 1991;32:2233.
46. Kudo M, Todo A, Ikekubo K: Nuclear medicine imaging of hepatocellular carcinoma. *Clin Imag* 1990;6:70.
47. Kudo M, Tomita S, Tochio H, et al.: Imaging diagnosis of hepatic nodules associated with liver cirrhosis. *Diagn Imag Abdomen* 1990;10:968.
48. Ryo UY, Alavi A, Collier BD, et al.: *Atlas of Nuclear Medicine Artifacts and Variants,* Chicago, Year Book Medical Publisher, 1990, p 74.
49. Ruppert D, Shirkhoda A, McCartney WH: Anterior dynamic imaging of the liver and spleen. *Clin Nucl Med* 1988; 13:402.
50. Mould RF: An investigation of variations in normal liver shape. *Br J Radiol* 1972;45:586.
51. Naftalis J, Leevy CM: Clinical estimation of liver size. *Am J Dig Dis* 1963;8:236.
52. Rollo FD, DeLand FH: The determination of liver mass from radionuclide images. *Radiology* 1968;91:1191.
53. Rosenfield AT, Schneider PB: Rapid evaluation of hepatic size on radioisotope scan. *J Nucl Med* 1974;15:237.
54. Spencer RP, Antar MA: Radionuclides in the investigation of liver disease, in Progress in Liver Disease. Vol 4, Edited by Popper H, Schaffner F (eds). New York, Grune and Stratton, 1972.
55. Drum DE, Beard JM: Scintigraphic criteria for hepatic metastases from cancer of the colon and breast. *J Nucl Med* 1976;17:677.
56. Eikman EA, et al.: Computer-assisted liver mass estimation from gamma camera images. *J Nucl Med* 1979;20:144.
57. Kan MK, Hopkins GB: Measurement of liver volume by emission computed tomography. *J Nucl Med* 1979;20:514.
58. Strauss LG, Clorius JH, Frank T, VanKaich G: Single photon emission computerized tomography (SPECT) for estimates of liver and spleen volume. *J Nucl Med* 1984;25:81.
59. Angeberg S, Stockel M, Sorenson PJ: Prediction of spleen size by routine radioisotope scintigraphy. *Acta Haematol (Basel)* 1983;69:243.
60. Rosenfield AT, Laufer I, Schneider PB: The significance of a palpable liver. A correlation of clinical and radioisotope studies. *AJR* 1974;122:313.
61. Halpern S, Coel M, Ashburn W, et al.: Correlation of liver and spleen size. Determinations by nuclear medicine studies and physical examination. *Arch Intern Med* 1974;134:123.
62. Rollo FD, DeLand FH: The determination of spleen mass from radionuclide images. *Radiology* 1970;97:583.
63. Mattsson O: Scintigraphic spleen volume calculation. *Acta Radiol [Diagn] (Stockh)* 1982;23:471.
64. Larson SM, Tuell SH, Moores KD, Nelp WB: Dimensions of the normal adult spleen scan and prediction of spleen weight. *J Nucl Med* 1971;12:123.
65. Seymour EQ, Puckette SE, Edwards J: Pseudoabnormal liver scans secondary to residual barium in the bowel. *Am J Roentgenol* 1969;107:54.
66. Bobinet DD, et al.: Lung uptake of ^{99m}Tc-sulfur colloid in patients exhibiting presence of Al^{3+} in plasma. *J Nucl Med* 1974;15:1220.
67. Klingensmith WC, Ryerson TW: Lung uptake of ^{99m}Tc-sulfur colloid. *J Nucl Med* 1973;14:201.
68. Mikhael MA, Evans RG: Migration and embolization of macrophages to the lung—A possible mechanism for colloid uptake in the lung during liver scanning. *J Nucl Med* 1975; 16:22.
69. Klingensmith WC, Tsan MF, Wagner HN: Factors affecting the uptake of ^{99m}Tc-sulfur colloid by the lung and the kidney. *J Nucl Med* 1976;17:681.
70. Winter PF, Perl LJ, Johnson PM: Lung uptake of colloid during liver-spleen scanning: a normal finding in children. *Nucl Med (Stuttg)* 1976;15:294.
71. Klingensmith WC, Lovett VJ: Lung uptake of ^{99m}Tc-sulfur colloid secondary to intraperitoneal endotoxin. *J Nucl Med* 1974;15:1028.
72. Bowen BM, Coates G, Garnett ES: Technetium-99m-sulfur colloid lung scan in patients with histiocytosis X. *J Nucl Med* 1975;16:332.
73. Gillespie PJ, Alexander JL, Edelstyn GA: High concentration of ^{99m}Tc-sulfur colloid found during routine liver scan in lungs of patients with advanced breast cancer. *J Nucl Med* 1973;14:711.
74. Klingensmith WC, Eikman EA, Maumenee I, et al.: Widespread abnormalities of radiocolloid distribution in patients with mucopolysaccaridoses. *J Nucl Med* 1975;16:1002.
75. Klingensmith WC, et al: Lung uptake of ^{99m}Tc-sulfur colloid in organ transplantation. *J Nucl Med* 1973;14:757.
76. Imarisio JJ: Liver scan showing intense lung uptake in neoplasia and infection. *J Nucl Med* 1975;16:188.
77. Mettler FA, Christie JH: Focal lung uptake of Tc-99m sulfur colloid. *Clin Nucl Med* 1981;6:322.
78. Johnson RA, Hladik WB: Post-traumatic pulmonary accumulation of Tc-99m sulfur colloid. *J Nucl Med* 1982;23:147.
79. Klingensmith WC, Yang SL, Wagner HN: Lung uptake of Tc-99m sulfur colloid in liver and spleen imaging. *J Nucl Med* 1978;19:31.
80. Lentle BC, Scott JR, Noujaim AA, et al.: Iatrogenic alterations in radionuclide biodistributions. *Semin Nucl Med* 1979;9:131.
81. Keyes JW, Wilson GA, Quinones JD: An evaluation of lung uptake of colloid during liver imaging. *J Nucl Med* 1973;14:687.
82. Turner JW, Syed IB, Hanc RP: Lung uptake of ^{99m}Tc-sulfur colloid during liver scanning. *J Nucl Med* 1974;15:460.
83. Stadalnick RC: Diffuse lung uptake of Tc-99m-sulfur colloid. *Semin Nucl Med* 1980;10:106.
84. Leclerc Y, Verreault J, Bisson G: Diffuse lung uptake of Technetium-99m sulfur colloid in malaria. *J Nucl Med* 1989;30:117.
85. Coleman RE: Renal colloid localization. *J Nucl Med* 1974;15:367.
86. Higgins CB, Taketa RM, Taylor A, et al.: Renal uptake of ^{99m}Tc-sulfur colloid. *J Nucl Med* 1974;15:564.
87. Shook DR, Shafer RB: Renal uptake of ^{99m}Tc-sulfur colloid. *Clin Nucl Med* 1975;1:223.
88. Klingensmith WC, Datu JA, Burdick DC: Renal uptake of ^{99m}Tc-sulfur colloid in congestive heart failure. *Radiology* 1975;127:185.
89. Jackson GL: Renal accumulation of ^{99m}Tc-SC. *Clin Nucl Med* 1977;2:176.
90. George EA, Codd JE, Newton WT, et al.: Further evaluation of ^{99m}Tc-sulfur colloid accumulation in rejecting renal transplants in man and a canine model. *Radiology* 1975;116: 121.
91. Frick MP, Loken MK, Goldberg ME, et al.: Use of ^{99m}Tc-sulfur colloid in evaluation of renal transplant complications. *J Nucl Med* 1976;17:181.
92. Kim YC, Massari PU, Brown ML, et al.: Clinical significance of ^{99m}Tc-sulfur colloid accumulation in renal transplant patients. *Radiology* 1977;124:745.
93. Mackler PT, Goldstein HA, Velchik MG, et al.: Variation of

spleen-liver activity ratio due to a change in position. *Clin Nucl Med* 1984;9:85.
94. Millette B, et al.: The extrahepatic uptake of radioactive colloidal gold in cirrhotic patients as an index of liver function and portal hypertension. *Am J Dig Dis* 1973;18:719.
95. Fernandez SP, et al.: The extrahepatic uptake of ^{198}Au as an index of portal hypertension. *Dig Dis* 1970;11:883.
96. Simon TR, Neumann RL, Gorelick F, et al.: Scintigraphic diagnosis of cirrhosis: A receiver operator characteristic analysis of the common interpretive criteria. *Radiology* 1981; 138:723.
97. Wilson GA, Keyes JW: The significance of the liver-spleen uptake ratio in liver scanning. *J Nucl Med* 1974;15:593.
98. Kaplan WD, Drum DE, Likich JJ: The effect of cancer chemotherapeutic agents on the liver-spleen scan. *J Nucl Med* 1980;21:84.
99. Geslein GE, Pinsky SM, Poth RK, et al.: The sensitivity and specificity of ^{99m}Tc-sulfur colloid liver imaging in diffuse hepatocellular disease. *Radiology* 1976;118:115.
100. Wasnich R, Glober G, Hayashi T, et al.: Simple computer quantitation of spleen-to-liver ratios in the diagnosis of hepatocellular disease. *J Nucl Med* 1979;20:149.
101. Gottschalk A, Harper PV, Jiminez FF, et al.: Quantification of the respiratory motion artifact in radioisotope scanning with the rectilinear focused collimator scanner and the gamma scintillation camera. *J Nucl Med* 1966;7:243.
102. Smoak WM, Smith EM, Kenny PJ: Reduction of physiologic degradation in imaging of the liver. *J Nucl Med* 1971;12:119.
103. Turner DA, Fordham EW, Ali A, et al.: Motion-corrected hepatic scintigraphy: An objective clinical evaluation. *J Nucl Med* 1978;19:142.
104. Brown DW: Combined lung-liver radioisotope scan in the diagnosis of subdiaphragmatic abscess. *Am J Surg* 1965; 109:521.
105. Karlsen RL, Nerdrum HJ, Froyen J, et al.: Combined scintigraphy of the liver, spleen and lung in the diagnosis of subphrenic abscess. *Scand J Gastroenterol* 1982;17:11.
106. Brown DW: Combined lung-liver radioisotope scan in the diagnosis of subdiaphragmatic abscess. *Am J Surg* 1965; 109:521.
107. Brown DW: Lung-liver radiosiotope scans in the diagnosis of subdiaphragmatic abscess. *JAMA* 1966;197:728.
108. Briggs RC: Combined liver-lung scanning in detecting subdiaphragmatic abscess, in Freeman LM, Blaufox MD (eds.): *Radionuclide Studies of the Gastrointestinal System.* New York, Grune and Stratton, 1972.
109. Jaszczak RJ, Greer KL, Coleman RE, SPECT system misalignment: Comparison of phantom and patient images, in Esser PE (ed.): *Emission Computed Tomography: Current Trends.* New York, Society of Nuclear Medicine, 1983, p 57.
110. Van Heertum RL, Brunetti JC, Yudd AP: Abdominal SPECT Imaging. *Semin Nucl Med* 1987;17:230.
111. Kalff V, Satterlee W, Harkness BA, et al.: Liver-spleen studies with the rotating gamma camera. I. Utility of the rotating display. *Radiology* 1984;153:533.
112. Van Heertum RL, Brunetti JC, Yudd AP, et al.: Liver SPECT. *J Nucl Med Technol* 1985;13:236.
113. Gerson MC, Thomas SR, Van Heertum RL: Tomographic myocardial perfusion imaging, in Gerson MC (ed): *Cardiac Nuclear Medicine.* New York, McGraw-Hill, 1987, p 25.
114. Floyd CE, Jaszczak RJ, Coleman RE, Convergence of the maximum likelihood reconstruction algorithm for emission computed tomography. *Phys Med Biol* 1987;32:463.
115. Floyd CE, Jaszczak RJ, Greer KL, et al.: Inverse Monte Carlo as a unified reconstruction algorithm for ECT. *J Nucl Med* 1986;27:1577.
116. Kircos LT, Carey JE, Keyes JW: Quantitative organ visualization using SPECT. *J Nucl Med* 1987;28:334.
117. Strauss LG, Clorius JH, Frank T, et al.: Single photon emission computerized tomography (SPECT) for estimates of liver and spleen volume. *J Nucl Med* 1984;25:81.
118. Fawcett HD, Sayle BA: SPECT versus planar liver scintigraphy: Is SPECT worth it? *J Nucl Med* 1989;30:57.
119. Keyes JW, Singer D, Satterlee W, et al.: Liver-spleen studies with the rotating gamma camera. II: Utility of tomography. *Radiology* 1984;153:537.
120. Oppenheim BE, Wellman HN, Hoffer PB: Liver Imaging, in Gottschalk A, Hoffer PB, Potchen EJ (eds.): *Diagnostic Nuclear Medicine.* Baltimore, Williams & Wilkins, 1988, p 538.
121. Berche C, Aubry F, Langlais C, et al.: Diagnostic value of transverse axial tomoscintigraphy for the detection of hepatic metastases: Results on 53 examinations and comparison with other diagnostic techniques. *Eur J Nucl Med* 1981; 6:435.
122. Khan O, Ell PJ, Jarritt PH, et al.: Comparison between emission and transmission computed tomography of the liver. *Br Med J* 1981;283:1212.
123. Strauss L, Bostel F, Clorius JH, et al.: Single-photon emission computed tomography (SPECT) for assessment of hepatic lesions. *J Nucl Med* 1982;23:1059.
124. Yamamoto K, Nukai T, Dodo Y, et al.: Clinical usefulness of emission computed tomography for liver scintigraphy, in Raynaud C (ed.): *Nuclear Medicine and Biology.* Paris, Pergamon Press, 1982, p 2866.
125. Biersack HJ, Reichman K, Reske SN, et al.: Improvement of scintigraphic liver imaging by SPECT—A review of 797 cases (Abs). *J Nucl Med* 1983;24:P29.
126. Christie JH, et al.: The correlation of clearance and distribution of colloidal gold in the liver as an index of hepatic cirrhosis. *Radiology* 1967;88:334.
127. Carter JH, Welch CS, Barron RE: Changes in hepatic blood vessels in cirrhosis of the liver. *Surg Gynecol Obstet* 1961;113:133.
128. Shreiner DP, Barlai-Kovach M: Diagnosis of alcoholic cirrhosis with right-to-left hepatic lobe ratio. *J Nucl Med* 1981;22:116.
129. Meindok M, Langer B: Liver scan in Budd-Chiari syndrome. *J Nucl Med* 1976;17:365.
130. Huang M-J, Liaw J-F, Tzen K-Y: Radionuclide venography in Budd-Chiari syndrome with intrahepatic venacaval obstruction. *J Nucl Med* 1985;26:145.
131. Khedkar N, Pestika B, Rosenblate H, Martinez C: Large focal defect on liver/spleen scan caused by fatty liver and masquerading as neoplasm. *J Nucl Med* 1992;33:258.
132. McClees EC, Gedgaudas-McClees RK: Screening for diffuse and focal liver disease: the case for hepatic scintigraphy. *J Clin Ultrasound* 1984;12:75.
133. Wernecke K, Rummeny E, Bongartz G, et al.: Detection of hepatic masses in patients with carcinoma: comparative sensitivities of sonography, CT, and MRI. *AJR* 1991,157:731.
134. Gould HR, Clemmett AR, Rossi P: Radiologic diagnosis of splenic metastasis. *Am J Roentgenol* 1970;109:775.
135. Harbert JC: The efficacy of bone and liver scanning in malignant disease—Facts and opinion, in Freeman LM, Weissman HS (eds.): *Nuclear Medicine Annual,* New York, Raven Press, 1982.
136. Hooper RG, Beechler CR, Johnson MC: Radioisotope scanning in the initial staging of bronchogenic carcinoma. *Am Rev Resp Dis* 1978;118:272.
137. Ramsdell JW, Peters RM, Taylor AT, et al.: Multiorgan scans for staging lung cancer. *J Thorac Cardiovasc Surg* 1977; 73:653.

138. Schiff L: Hepatic neoplasia: selected clinical aspects. *Semin Roentgenol* 1983;18:71.
139. Westaby D, Portmann B, Williams R: Androgen related primary hepatic tumors in non-Fanconi patients. *Cancer* 1983;51:1947.
140. Alpert E, Hershberg R, Schur PH, Isselbacher KJ: α-Fetoprotein in human hepatoma; improved detection in serum, and quantitative studies using a new sensitive technique. *Gastroenterology* 1971;61:137.
141. Kew M: Alpha-fetoprotein in primary liver cancer and other diseases. *Gut* 1974;15:814.
142. Levin J, Kew MC: Gallium-67 citrate scanning in primary cancer of the liver: diagnostic value in the presence of cirrhosis and relation to alpha-fetoprotein. *J Nucl Med* 1975;16:949.
143. Lomas F, Dibos PE, Wagner HN: Increased specificity of liver scanning with the use of gallium-67 citrate. *N Engl J Med* 1972;286:1323.
144. Langhammer H: ^{67}Ga for tumor scanning. *J Nucl Med* 1972;13:25.
145. Turner DA, Pinsky SM, Gottschalk A: The use of ^{67}Ga scanning in the staging of Hodgkin's disease. *Radiology* 1972;104:97.
146. Ben-Porath M, Clayton G, Kaplan E: Modification of a multi-isotope color scanner for multipurpose scanning. *J Nucl Med* 1967;8:411.
147. Goodwin DA, et al.: ^{111}In labeled bleomycin for tumor localization by scintiscanning. *J Nucl Med* 1973;14:401.
148. Lee VW, Shapiro JH: Specific diagnosis of hepatoma using ^{99m}Tc-HIDA and other radionuclides. *Eur J Nucl Med* 1983;8:191.
149. Hasegawa Y, Nakano S, Hiyama T, et al.: Relationship of uptake of technetium-99m(Sn)-N-Pyridoxyl-5-methyltryptophan by hepatocellular carcinoma to prognosis. *J Nucl Med* 1991;32:228.
150. Hasegawa Y, Nakano S, Ibuka K, et al.: Specific diagnosis of hepatocellular carcinoma by delayed hepatobiliary imaging. *Cancer* 1986;57:230.
151. Calvert X, Pons F, Bruix J, et al.: Technetium-99m DISIDA hepatobiliary agent in diagnosis of hepatocellular carcinoma: Relationship between detectability and tumor differentiation. *J Nucl Med* 1988;29:1916.
152. Lee VW, O'Brien MJ, Devereux DF, et al.: Hepatocellular carcinoma: uptake of Tc-99m-IDA in primary tumor and metastasis. *Am J Roentgenol* 1984;143:57.
153. Hasegawa Y, Nakano S, Ibuka K, et al.: Concentration of ^{99m}Tc-Sn-N-pyridoxyl-5-methyltryptophan, a biliary agent, in distant metastases of hepatomas. *Eur J Nucl Med* 1985;10:255.
154. Cannon JR, Long RF, Berens SV, et al.: Uptake of c-PIPIDA in pulmonary metastases from a hepatoma. *Clin Nucl Med* 1980;5:22.
155. Morita K, Ono S, Fukunaga M, et al.: Accumulation of N-Isopropyl-p-(^{123}) Iodoamphetamine and (^{99m})Hexamethyl-propyleneamine oxime in metastatic hepatocellular carcinoma. Letter *J Nucl Med* 1988;29:1460.
156. Yonekura Y, Benua RS, Brill AB, et al.: Increased accumulation of 2-deoxy-2[^{18}F]fluoro-D-glucose in liver metastases from colon cancer. *J Nucl Med* 1982;23:1133.
157. Okazumi S, Isono K, Enomoto K, et al.: Evaluation of liver tumors using fluorine-18-fluorodeoxyflucose PET: Characterization of tumor and assessment of effect of treatment. *J Nucl Med* 1992;33:333.
158. Hawkins RA, Choi Y, Huang S-C, et al.: Quantitating tumor glucose metabolism with FDG and PET (Editorial). *J Nucl Med* 1992;33:339.
159. Engel MA, Marks DS, Sandler MA, Shetty P: Differentiation of focal intrahepatic lesions with ^{99m}Tc-red blood cell imaging. *Radiology* 1983;146:777.
160. Edmondson HA: Tumors of the liver and intrahepatic bile ducts, in: *Atlas of tumor Pathology.* Sect VII, fasc. 25, Washington, DC: Armed Forces Institute of Pathology, 1958, p 113.
161. Groshar D, Ben-Haim S, Gips S, et al.: Spectrum of scintigraphic appearance of liver hemangiomas. *Clin Nucl Med* 1992;17:294.
162. Adam YG, Huvos AG, Fortner JG: Giant hemangiomas of the liver. *Ann Surg* 1970;172:230.
163. Personal communication with Dr. John L. Doppman, the National Institutes of Health, and Dr. A. Everette James, Vanderbilt University, 1994
164. Sewell JH, Weiss K: Spontaneous rupture of hemangioma of the liver. *Arch Surg* 1961;83:729.
165. Freeny PC, Vimont TR, Barnett DC: Cavernous hemangioma of the liver: ultrasonography, arteriography and computed tomography. *Radiology* 1979;132:143.
166. Nelson RC, Chezmar JL: Diagnostic approach to hepatic hemangiomas. *Radiology,* 1990;176:11.
167. Freeny PC, Marks WM: Patterns of contrast enhancement of benign and malignant hepatic neoplasms during bolus dynamic and delayed CT. *Radiology* 1986;160:613.
168. Ashida C, Fishman EK, Zerhouni EA, et al.: Computed tomography of hepatic cavernous hemangioma. *J Comput Assist Tomogr* 1987;11:455.
169. Stark DD, Felder RC, Wittenberg J, et al.: Magnetic resonance imaging of cavernous hemangioma of the liver: tissue-specific characterization. *AJR* 1988;145:213.
170. Rabinowitz SA, McKusick KA, Strauss KW: ^{99m}Tc-red blood cell scintigraphy in evaluating focal liver lesions. *Am J Roentgenol* 1984;143:63.
171. Itenzo C, Kim S, Madsen M, et al.: Planar and SPECT Tc-99m-red blood cell imaging in hepatic cavernous hemangiomas and other hepatic lesions. *Clin Nucl Med* 1988;13:237.
172. Ziessman HA, Silverman PM, Patterson J, et al.: Improved detection of small cavernous hemangiomas of the liver with high-resolution three-headed SPECT. *J Nucl Med* 1991;32:2086.
173. Moinuddin M, Allison JR, Montgomery JH, et al.: Scintigraphic diagnosis of hepatic hemangioma: its role in the management of hepatic mass lesions. *Am J Roentgenol* 1985;145:223.
174. Engel MA, Marks DS, Sandler MA, Shetty P: Differentiation of focal intrahepatic lesions with ^{99m}Tc-red blood cell imaging. *Radiology* 1983;146:777.
175. Brodsky RI, Friedman AC, Maurer AH, et al.: Hepatic cavernous hemangiomas: diagnosis with ^{99m}Tc-labeled red cells and single-photon emission CT. *Am J Roentgenol* 1987;148:1251.
176. Salvo AF, Schiller A, Athanasoulis C, et al.: Hepatoadenoma and focal nodular hyperplasia; pitfalls in radiocolloid imaging. *Radiology* 1977;125:451.
177. Sandler MA, Petrocelli RD, Marks DS, Lopez R: Ultrasonic features and radionuclide correlation in liver cell adenoma and focal nodular hyperplasia. *Radiology* 1980;135:393.
178. Sandler MA, Petrocelli RD, Marks DS, Lopez R: Ultrasonic features and radionuclide correlation in liver cell adenoma and focal nodular hyperplasia. *Radiology* 1980;135:393.
179. Miller JH, Gates GF, Landing BH, Kogut MD, Roe TF: Scintigraphic abnormalities in glycogen storage disease. *J Nucl Med* 1978;19:354.
180. Massarrar S, Jordan GM, Sahrhage G, et al.: Follow-up study on patients with non-alcoholic and non-diabetic fatty liver. *Acta-Hepato Gastroenterol* 1979;26:296.
181. Thaler IdI: Relation of steatosis to cirrhosis. *Clin Gastroenterol* 1975;4:273.

182. Lisbona R, Mishkin S, Derbekyan V, et al.: Role of scintigraphy in focally abnormal sonograms of fatty livers. *J Nucl Med* 1988;29:1050.
183. Baker MK, Schauwecker DS, Wenker JC, Kopecky KK: Nuclear medicine evaluation of focal fatty infiltration of the liver. *Clin Nucl Med* 1986;11:503.
184. Bashist B, Hecht HL, Harley WD: Computed tomographic demonstration of rapid changes in fatty infiltration of the liver. *Radiology* 1982;142:691.
185. Scott W, Sanders R, Siegelman S: Irregular fatty infiltration of the liver. Diagnostic dilemmas. *AJR* 1980;135:67.
186. Yeh S-H, Wu L-C, Wang S-J, et al.: Xenon-133 hepatic retention ration: A useful index for fatty liver quantification. *J Nucl Med* 1989;30:1708.
187. Morris J, Doust B, Hanks T: Roentgenologic and radioisotopic assessment of hydatid disease of the liver. *AJR* 1967;101:519.
188. Gelfand MJ: Scintigraphy in upper abdominal trauma. *Semin Roentgenol* 1984;19:296.
189. Kaufman RA, Towbin R, Babcock DS, et al.: Upper abdominal trauma in children: imaging evaluation. *AJR* 1984; 142:449.
190. Froelick JW, Simeone JF, McKusick KA, et al.: Radionuclide imaging and ultrasound in liver/spleen trauma: a prospective comparison. *Radiology* 1982;145:457.
191. Aronsen KF, et al.: Evaluation of hepatic regeneration by scintillation scanning, cholangiography and angiography in man. *Ann Surg* 1970;171:567.
192. Johnson PM, Grossman FM, Atkis HL: Radiation-induced hepatic injury: its detection by scintillation scanning. *AJR* 1967;99:453.
193. Kurohara SS, Swensson NL, Usselman JA, George FW: Response and recovery of liver to radiation as demonstrated by photoscans. *Radiology* 1967;89:129.
194. Samuels LD, Grosfeld JL, Kartha M: Reversal of liver scan image after right-sided renal radiotherapy. *JAMA* 1971; 215:1816.
195. Sty JR, et al.: Hepatic scintigraphy in Caroli's disease. *Radiology* 1978;126:732.
196. Yeh SH, Liu OK, Huang MJ: Sequential scintiphotography with ^{99m}Tc-pyridoxylidene glutamate for the detection of intraheptic lithiasis. *J Nucl Med* 1980;21:17.
197. Coel M, Halpern S, Alazraki N, et al.: Intrahepatic lesion presenting as an area of increased radiocolloid uptake on a liver scan. *J Nucl Med* 1972;13:221.
198. Joyner JT: Abnormal liver scan (radiocolloid "hot spot") associated with superior vena cava obstruction. *J Nucl Med* 1972;13:849.
199. Holmques D, Burdine JA: Caval-portal shunting as a cause of a focal increase in radiocolloid uptake in normal livers. *J Nucl Med* 1973;14:348.
200. Morita ET, McCormack KR, Weisberg RL: Further information on a "hot spot" in the liver. *J Nucl Med* 1973;14:606.
201. Kumar B, Coleman RE, McKnight R: Asymptomatic superior vena cava obstruction. *J Nucl Med* 1976;17:853.
202. Lee KR, Preston DF, Martin NL, et al.: Angiographic documentation of systemic-portal venous shunting as a cause of a liver scan "hot spot" in superior vena caval obstruction. *Am J Roentgenol* 1976;127:637.
203. Lin MS, Fletcher JW, Donati RM: Local colloid trapping in the liver in the inferior vena cava syndrome. *J Nucl Med* 1981;22:344.
204. Suneja SK, Teal JS: Discrepant sulfur colloid and radioparticle liver uptake in superior vena cava obstruction: Case report. *J Nucl Med* 1989;30:113.
205. Volpe JA, McRae J, Johnston GS: Transmission scintigraphy in the evaluation of subphrenic abscess. *Am J Roentgenol* 1970;109:733.
206. Chayes Z, Koenigsberg M, Freeman LM: The "hot" hepatic abscess. *J Nucl Med* 1974;15:305.
207. Sackett JF, Mosenthal WT, House RK, Jeffery RF: Scintillation scanning of liver cell adenoma. *Am J Roentgenol* 1971;113:56.
208. Rogers JV, Mack LA, Freeny PC, et al.: Hepatic focal nodular hyperplasia: angiography, CT sonography and scintigraphy. *Am J Roentgenol* 1981;137:983.
209. Ansfield FJ, Ramirez G, David HL, et al.: Further clinical studies with intrahepatic arterial infusion with 5-fluorouracil. *Cancer* 1975;36:2413.
210. Thrall JH, Gyves JW, Ziessman HA, Ensminger WD: Hepatic arterial chemotherapy: Pharmacokinetic rationale and radionuclide perfusion imaging, in Freeman LF, Weissmann HS (eds.): *Nuclear Medicine Annual 1984.* Raven Press, New York 1984.
211. Kaplan WD, Ensminger WD, Come SE, et al.: Radionuclide angiography to predict patient response to hepatic artery chemotherapy. *Cancer Treat Rep* 1980;64:1217.
212. Yang PJ, Thrall, Ensminger WD, et al.: Perfusion scintigraphy (Tc-99m MAA) during surgery for placement of chemotherapy catheter in hepatic artery. *J Nucl Med* 1982;23:1066.
213. Chuang VP, Wallace S: Arterial infusion and occlusion in cancer patients. *Semin Roentgenol* 1981;16:13.
214. Hall JT, Kim EE, Charnsangavej C, et al.: Variable patterns of technetium-99m MAA perfusion in the therapeutically embolized liver. *J Nucl Med* 1989;30:1012.

28 The Biliary System

Clara C. Chen

Hepatobiliary scintigraphy is used to noninvasively assess the patency of the biliary system, particularly in suspected acute cholecystitis and following biliary surgery. It is also used to evaluate the biliary system in non-acute settings and to assess hepatocyte function.

RADIOPHARMACEUTICALS

Modern hepatobiliary scintigraphy has been made possible by the development of ^{99m}Tc-labeled iminodiacetic acid (IDA) agents, in which the nitrogen of iminodiacetic acid is substituted by various acetanilide analogues.[1,2] One of the first of these ^{99m}Tc-IDA agents was ^{99m}Tc-N(2,6-dimethylphenylcarbamoylmethyl)-iminodiacetic acid (^{99m}Tc-HIDA).[3,4] Following this, numerous other ^{99m}Tc-IDA compounds were developed. As a group, these agents rapidly replaced ^{131}I-rose bengal, an earlier radiopharmaceutical that had been used with moderate success.

Like bilirubin, bile acids, bromosulfonphthalein (BSP), and other organic anions handled by the liver, ^{99m}Tc-IDA agents bind loosely to serum proteins, such as albumin, while in circulation. A small percentage of an injected dose is excreted in the urine, but most is rapidly taken up by hepatocytes and excreted into bile. The exact uptake mechanism(s) are unknown but are probably similar, if not identical, to those used by other organic anions such as bilirubin. In vitro and animal studies have shown that compounds such as BSP and bilirubin competitively inhibit ^{99m}Tc-IDA uptake and clearance.[5,6] This is reflected in studies of animals and humans with hyperbilirubinemia, in whom prolonged blood pool activity, decreased liver uptake, and increased urinary excretion of ^{99m}Tc-IDA is demonstrated.[4,7–9]

Of the numerous ^{99m}Tc-IDA compounds developed, 2,6-diisopropyl-iminodiacetic acid (DISIDA) and 2,4,6-trimethyl-3 bromo-iminodiacetic acid (mebrofenin) are the most widely used for clinical hepatobiliary imaging. Compared to other ^{99m}Tc-IDA agents, both have high specificity for the hepatobiliary system, exhibit high liver:kidney excretion ratios, rapid hepatic transit times, and are efficiently cleared in patients with elevated serum bilirubin levels.[1,8,10–12] Of the two, mebrofenin appears to have several advantages over DISIDA. In rats, hepatic extraction of mebrofenin and DISIDA were 95 and 90%, respectively, while total urinary excretion 30 minutes after injection was 1.2 and 7.4%, respectively.[7] In normal patients, 1.1% of an injected dose of mebrofenin is excreted in the urine by 3 hours, vs. 7.1% for DISIDA.[8,9] And, although urinary excretion of both agents increases as serum bilirubin levels rise, this effect is more marked with DISIDA. Excretion of DISIDA increases to approximately 30% of the injected dose in 3 hours at a bilirubin level of 25 mg/dl, compared to <10% for mebrofenin.[9] However, despite these differences and apparent superiority of mebrofenin over DISIDA, both agents provide excellent studies in most clinical situations; the exception being severely jaundiced patients for whom mebrofenin is the radiopharmaceutical of choice. If not available, however, higher doses of DISIDA can improve image quality in hyperbilirubinemia.

Another radiopharmaceutical—^{99m}Tc-pyridoxyl-5-methyltryptophan (PMT[13])—has been developed for hepatobiliary scintigraphy in Japan. A ^{99m}Tc-labeled N-pyridoxylaminate, PMT is characterized by rapid uptake and excretion by hepatocytes, minimal urinary excretion, and resistance to the effects of hyperbilirubinemia.[13] PMT has been used in acute cholecystitis,[14] and in the workup of intrahepatic masses.[15,16]

THE BILIARY SYSTEM

In humans, bile is produced at a rate of approximately 0.4 cc/min. or 600 cc/d.[17] After excretion by hepatocytes into bile canaliculi, bile flow continues into ductules, right and left hepatic ducts, the common hepatic duct, the common bile duct (CBD) and, finally into the gallbladder or second part of the duodenum through the sphincter of Oddi.[18] Bile flow is a passive process and follows the path of least resistance. Therefore, the amount of bile entering the gallbladder relative to the duodenum is determined by the particular physiological and anatomic conditions that exist at any given time. Under normal fasting conditions (when the gallbladder is at rest), approximately 70% of the bile flows into the gallbladder.[19]

Control of gallbladder emptying is both neurologic and hormonal, with the latter playing the dominant role. Patients who have undergone vagotomy[20] or who have autonomic nervous dysfunction secondary to diabetes[21] often have decreased gallbladder contractility.

Of the hormonal factors, cholecystokinin (CCK) is the primary substance regulating gallbladder and sphincter of Oddi contractility. CCK is a 33-amino acid polypeptide with an active 8-amino acid C-terminal end. Released by the duodenal mucosa in response to lipids and amino acids, it causes gallbladder contraction, relaxation of the sphincter of Oddi, and subsequent direction of bile flow into the duodenum. Bile in the small intestine acts in turn to inhibit further CCK release, and eventually flow ceases. Thus, eating results in a sustained but limited increase in CCK levels, depending mainly on the fat content of the meal.

Recently, sincalide (Kinevac)—a synthetic CCK consisting of the 8-amino acid C-terminal end—has been used to mimic the effects of CCK on the biliary system. Narcotic analgesics, such as morphine, can also be used to alter biliary dynamics by constricting the sphincter of Oddi.[22] This effect can be reversed by naloxone.[23] Both sincalide and morphine are employed diagnostically during hepatobiliary scintigraphy.

NORMAL HEPATOBILIARY SCINTIGRAPHY

In general, patients should have fasted for 4 hours prior to hepatobiliary scintigraphy. This is not necessary if the clinical question does not pertain to gallbladder function (e.g., studies to assess biliary obstruction, bile leaks, patent anastomoses). Patients should be asked if they have recently received any opiate medications (e.g., morphine), as these can cause constriction of the sphincter of Oddi and delayed bowel visualization.[22]

Patients are positioned supine with the scintillation camera (peaked to 140 keV, 20% window) over the upper abdomen, so that the entire liver, proximal small bowel, and cardiac blood pool lie in the field of view. After ^{99m}Tc-IDA (5 mCi, 185 MBq, adult dose; 0.05 mCi/kg, 1.85 MBq/kg, pediatric dose, minimum 1 mCi, 37 MBq) is administered as an intravenous bolus, a flow study (2-3 seconds/frame) is acquired. This is followed by sequential imaging for up to 1 hour with delayed views as needed for up to 24 hours. Anterior oblique and lateral images are sometimes obtained to estimate the depth of visualized structures. If needed, the study should be acquired on computer (1 minute/frame) for quantitative analysis; analog images obtained every 10 minutes for the first hour with delayed images as required (first image: 500,000 to 1,000,000 counts, subsequent images for time) suffice for visual interpretation.

Review of the flow images should include a search for areas of abnormal vascularity, as well as a general assessment of liver perfusion. Subsequent images are examined for liver size, shape, and homogeneity of parenchymal uptake and excretion of ^{99m}Tc-IDA. In healthy patients, flow to the liver is uniform and delayed when compared to structures such as the spleen and kidneys, consistent with the fact that the liver derives most of its blood flow from the portal circulation. Liver uptake of IDA is rapid, with little if any tracer visible in the cardiac blood pool by 5 minutes.[24] With DISIDA, early transient renal activity is not unusual, but this is almost never seen with mebrofenin.[9,24]

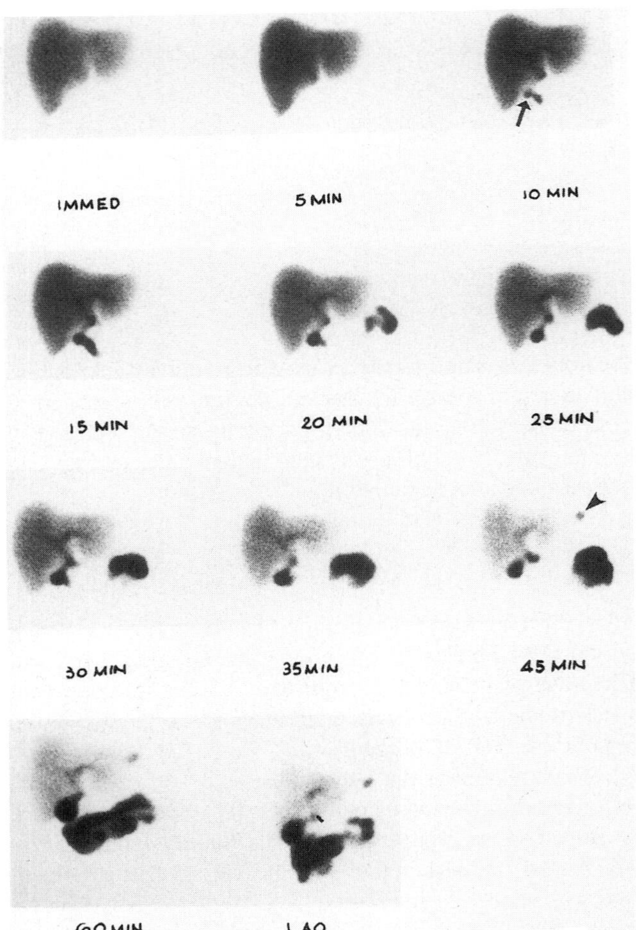

Figure 1. Normal mebrofenin hepatobiliary study. Anterior views demonstrate left hepatic duct, common bile duct, and duodenal visualization by 10–15 minutes. The right hepatic duct is seen in later images as hepatic activity clears. Gallbladder is seen beginning as early as 10 minutes (arrow), as confirmed by later images. A small amount of duodenogastric reflux is seen at 45 minutes (arrowhead). Left anterior oblique (LAO) view at 60 minutes shows that the gallbladder moves as an anterior structure.

In most normal fasting subjects, radioactive bile appears in the gallbladder and small bowel by 1 hour (Fig. 1). In a series of 115 such patients, Williams et al.[25] found that the gallbladder visualized by 15 minutes in 50% of cases, by 30 minutes in 90%, and by 1 hour in 100%. Visualization of hepatic ducts was variable, but the left duct tended to be more prominent than the right. In 22% of patients neither hepatic duct was visualized, and this seemed to correlate with earlier small bowel visualization. Excretion into duodenum occurred by 1 hour in 81% of cases, and in 48% both gallbladder and duodenum were visualized by 30 minutes. In the 19% of patients without bowel activity at 1 hour, all had prompt bowel visualization after CCK administration.

The occasional failure to visualize small bowel by 1 hour in normal fasting patients is generally thought to be due to a tight sphincter of Oddi.[1] A similar observation has been

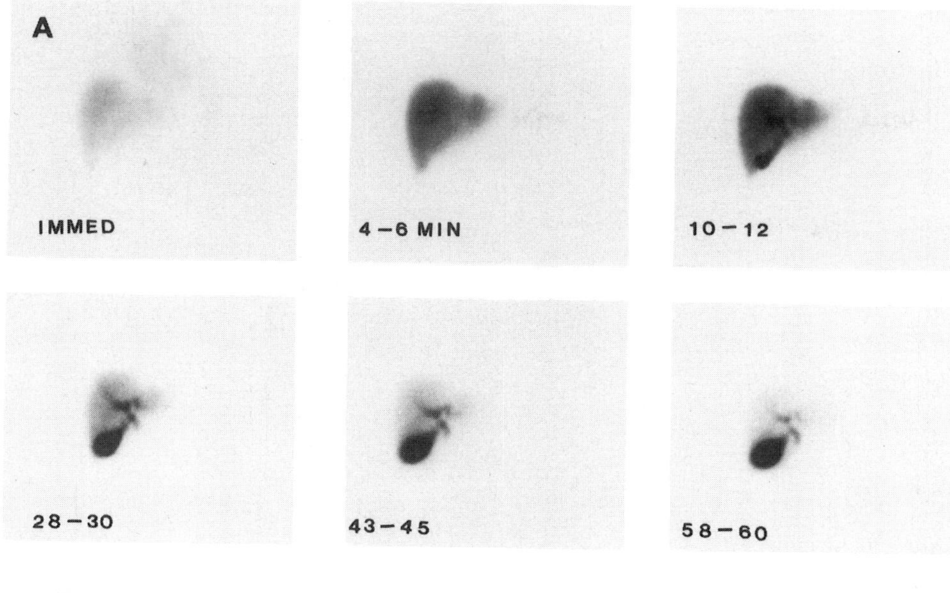

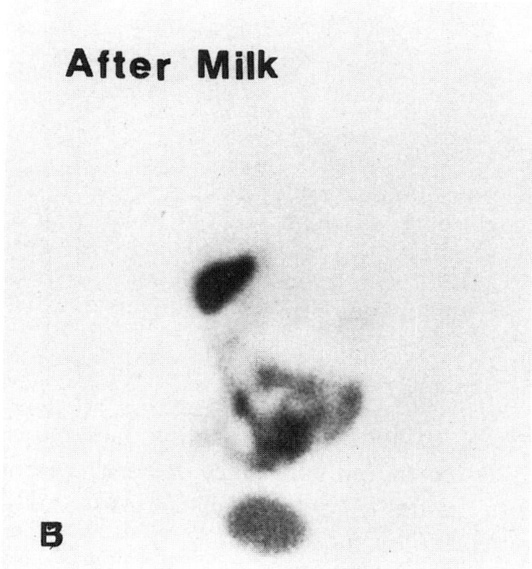

Figure 2. DISIDA study in a normal volunteer showing normal uptake and excretion of activity into the biliary system, but no bowel activity at 1 hr **(A).** Shortly after the subject drank some milk, rapid gallbladder emptying into the bowel occurred **(B).**

made in normal subjects pretreated with CCK 20 minutes before a study,[26] presumably because these patients' gallbladders are in a "filling phase" following initial emptying by CCK. These patients can be distinguished from those with true biliary obstruction by their otherwise normal study results, and the rapid appearance of bowel upon stimulation. Stimulation can be accomplished by an injection of CCK or with a drink of milk, both of which should result in gallbladder contraction, relaxation of the sphincter, and rapid bowel visualization, proving that no obstruction is present (Fig. 2).

Occasionally, it is difficult to determine if a focus of activity is located within the gallbladder or in overlapping bowel. Oblique and lateral images are often useful in these cases, as are delayed images. Other useful interventions include having the patient drink a glass of water to "flush" activity from the duodenum (Fig. 3), or to ambulate the patient between images. In difficult cases, the area in question can be marked and the patient sent to ultrasound for confirmation.

ACUTE CHOLECYSTITIS

The most common indication for hepatobiliary scintigraphy is to assess the patency of the cystic duct in patients with suspected acute cholecystitis (cystic duct obstruction). These patients classically present with right upper quadrant pain, fever, nausea, vomiting, elevated white blood cell counts, and possibly elevated liver function studies. They may or may not have a history of gallstones. However, the majority

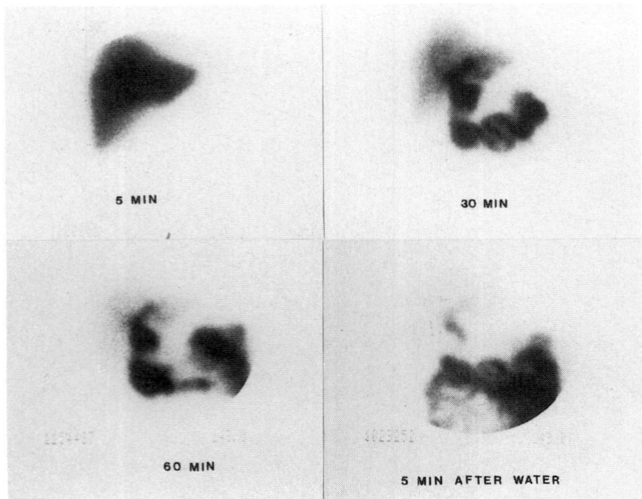

Figure 3. Anterior DISIDA images show activity in the duodenum with questionable gallbladder visualization at 30 and 60 min. Immediately after drinking water, however, a repeat image shows washout of duodenal activity and absence of true gallbladder visualization.

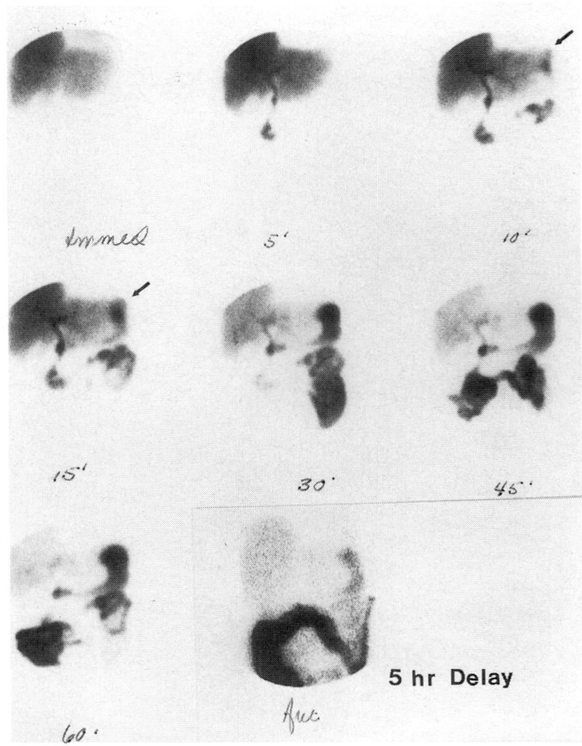

Figure 4. Acute cholecystitis. Anterior DISIDA images in a patient with fever, right upper quadrant pain and tenderness, and acute cholecystitis at surgery. No gallbladder activity is seen up to 5 hours. Gastric reflux is seen beginning at 10 minutes (arrow). Corresponding ultrasound images are shown in Figure 5.

of cases are associated with gallstones; only 5 to 15% are of the acalculous variety.[27]

Hepatobiliary scintigraphy is highly sensitive and specific for acute cholecystitis. Using the criteria of nonvisualization of the gallbladder by 4 hours, Weissmann et al.[28] reported a sensitivity of 95% and specificity of 99% in 296 patients referred with possible acute cholecystitis (Figs. 4, 5). Delayed gallbladder visualization (between 1 to 4 hours) was predictive of chronic cholecystitis (Figs. 6, 7). In a similar study of 211 patients, Freitas et al.[29] found that as the cutoff for nonvisualization was extended from 1 to 4 hours, the sensitivity for acute cholecystitis decreased from 100 to 98%, whereas the specificity increased from 90 to 96.5%. Thus, the longer a gallbladder fails to visualize, the greater the likelihood of acute cholecystitis.

The Rim Sign

In addition to gallbladder nonvisualization, a finding known as the "rim sign" has been described in association with acute cholecystitis. This consists of a pericholecystic band of relatively increased activity, usually appearing between 30 and 60 minutes as activity clears from the rest of the liver[30] (Fig. 8). The rim sign is thought to be due to localized tracer retention and bile stasis in inflamed, edematous hepatic parenchyma surrounding the gallbladder in acute cholecystitis. Rim signs are associated with a high incidence of complicated cholecystitis.[31,32] In 334 studies performed for possible acute cholecystitis, Smith et al.[31] found that 114 demonstrated gallbladder nonvisualization. Of these, 24 (21%) had rim signs and 13 of these underwent surgery; 11 patients were found to have acute cholecystitis and 2 chronic cholecystitis. Of these 13, 4 (31%) patients had gangrenous cholecystitis and 5 (39%) a perforated gallbladder. No rim signs were seen in association with other imaging patterns, including those suggesting chronic gallbladder disease, obstruction, or normal biliary function.

False-positive Results

The specificity of hepatobiliary scintigraphy for acute cholecystitis depends in large part on the patient population studied. Delayed or absent gallbladder visualization is seen in a variety of circumstances in the absence of acute cholecystitis. For instance, patients who have not fasted adequately before a study often exhibit false-positive results for physiological reasons.[24,33] Patients with chronic cholecystitis also often exhibit gallbladder nonvisualization, although the majority have normal studies.[29,34]

The small number of false-positive ^{99m}Tc-IDA studies in suspected acute cholecystitis is usually due to chronic cholecystitis.[29] In certain subgroups, however, the incidence of false-positive studies is significantly increased. These include patients who: are critically ill,[35–37] are postsurgical,[37] have sustained trauma,[36] are chronic alcoholics with alcoholic hepatitis or cirrhosis,[38] are on total parenteral nutrition (TPN),[38,39] or have undergone prolonged (>24 hours) fasting.[40–42] In many of these situations, thickened, viscous bile

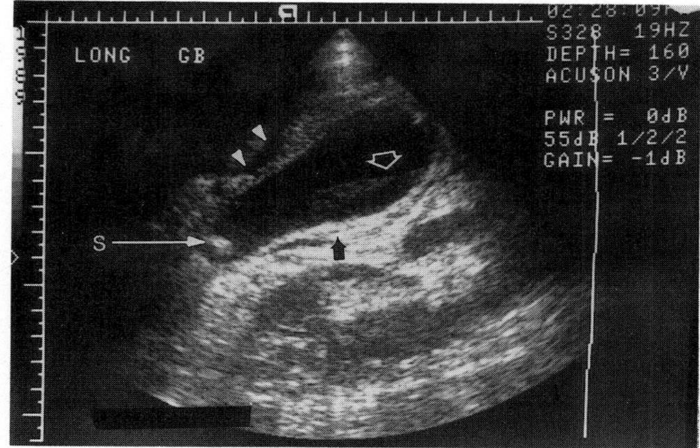

A

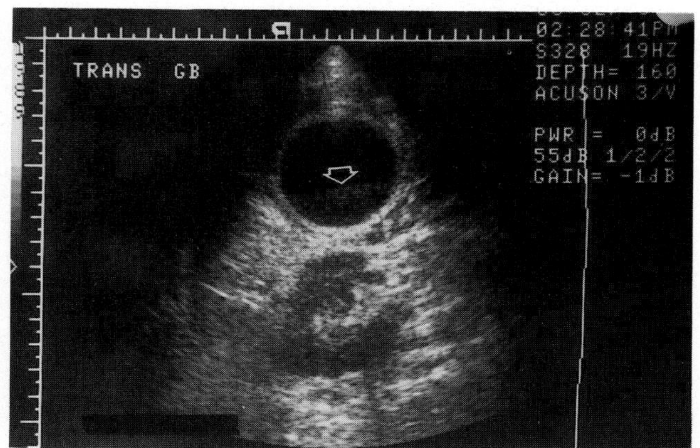

B

Figure 5. Acute cholecystitis. **(A).** Longitudinal ultrasound image of the gallbladder in a patient with acute cholecystitis (see Fig. 4). Findings include gallstone (S), gallbladder sludge (open arrow), thickened gallbladder wall (black arrow), and pericholecystic fluid (arrowheads). **(B).** Transverse ultrasound image of the gallbladder showing sludge (open arrow).

or sludge is thought to accumulate in the gallbladder, altering bile flow and shunting it toward the bowel.[35,38] In these patients, CCK (sincalide—0.02 to 0.04 μg/kg i.v. over 3 minutes) can be administered 20 to 30 minutes prior to the study. This should cause gallbladder contraction and emptying of the thickened bile, increasing the likelihood of gallbladder visualization.[43] The success of this intervention depends, of course, on an adequate gallbladder response to CCK.

Two other situations in which false-positive nonvisualization of the gallbladder is commonly seen are complete CBD obstruction and hepatocellular dysfunction. Both conditions are easily recognized with hepatobiliary scintigraphy although, in their advanced stages, they may be confused with each other. In complete CBD obstruction, no tracer excretion into bowel is seen, even with delayed imaging (see below). In most cases, the bile ducts and gallbladder also fail to visualize, while hepatic function and uptake of radiotracer remain relatively preserved until late in the process. On the other hand, the major findings in patients with hepatocellular dysfunction are decreased tracer uptake by the liver with slow blood pool clearance and increased urinary excretion (Fig. 9). In these patients, the rate and amount of bile formation is decreased, often causing delayed or absent visualization of biliary structures. However, contrary to what occurs in complete CBD obstruction, the bile that is formed is excreted into bowel, as no obstruction to flow exists.

False-positive studies have also been reported in patients with pancreatitis (see below)[44] and in those with congenital abnormalities of the biliary system, including gallbladder ectopia.[45]

False-negative Results

False-negative studies (gallbladder visualization despite the presence of acute cholecystitis) occur infrequently, although the incidence is probably underestimated because surgical intervention is much less likely in these patients. Causes include acalculous cholecystitis, acute passage of a gallstone prior to the study, or the presence of localized gallbladder inflammation that spares the cystic duct and leaves it patent. Occasionally, prominent cystic duct activity is seen adjacent to the CBD and is mistaken for gallbladder visualization. This is known as the "dilated cystic duct sign" (Fig. 10).[46]

At times, a bile leak localizes in the gallbladder fossa, mimicking gallbladder filling (Fig. 11).[47–49] In these cases, delayed images usually demonstrate dispersion of the leak and free bile accumulation elsewhere in the abdomen. A more rare cause of false gallbladder visualization is accumulation of activity within a choledochal cyst.[50] Correlation with ultrasound, CT, or cholangiography is generally required to clarify these findings.[51]

Last, focal accumulation of activity in the right renal collecting system can be mistaken for the gallbladder early in a study, but will fluctuate and decrease in intensity during the course of the study as the renal pelvis fills and empties (assuming no renal obstruction exists). The gallbladder should not empty during the course of a normal study unless stimulated (eating, CCK). Lateral images can also be used for confirmation.

MORPHINE-AUGMENTED CHOLESCINTIGRAPHY

Recently, the traditional 4-hour hepatobiliary study for acute cholecystitis has been replaced in many centers by a shorter 90-minute procedure in which morphine sulfate is administered during the study. Since bile flow is a passive process, constriction of the sphincter of Oddi increases the "back-pressure" of the system, directing bile into the gallbladder. Low doses of intravenous morphine cause the sphincter of Oddi to contract, and can result in up to a 10-fold increase in resting CBD pressures.[22] Thus, if patency of the CBD has already been demonstrated by visualization of bowel activity, and if the gallbladder has not appeared by 60 minutes, morphine can be administered (0.04 mg/kg

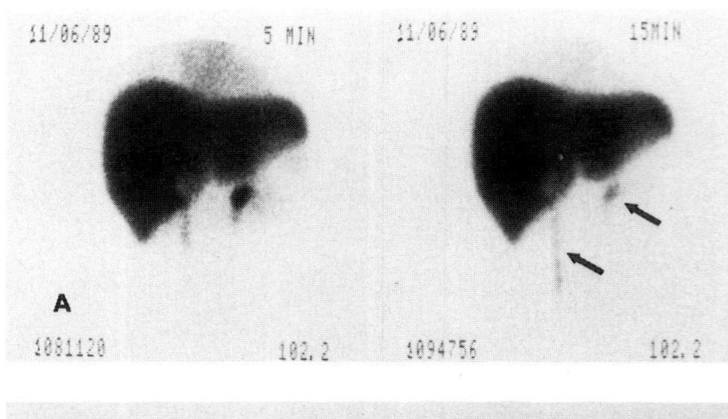

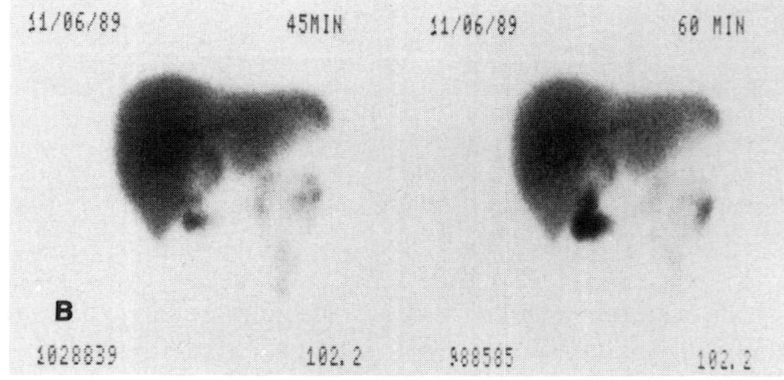

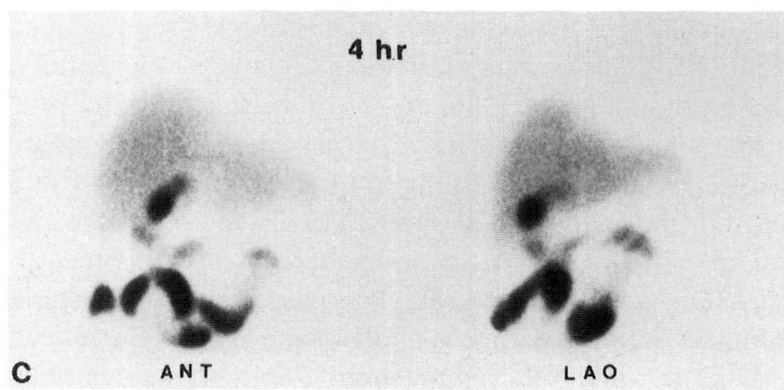

Figure 6. Chronic cholecystitis. DISIDA study in a patient with sepsis, right upper quadrant pain, and rising bilirubin levels. Anterior images show absence of gallbladder visualization by 60 minutes (**A** + **B**). At 4 hours (**C**) the gallbladder has filled, consistent with chronic cholecystitis. Renal excretion and ureteral visualization are seen in the early images (arrows). See Fig. 7 for corresponding gallbladder ultrasound.

over 2 to 3 minutes iv) and imaging continued. Nonvisualization of the gallbladder 30 minutes after morphine administration indicates cystic duct obstruction, whereas gallbladder visualization is interpreted as consistent with chronic cholecystitis, as in conventional imaging. In some cases, the amount of activity remaining in the liver at the time of morphine administration may be too low for clear-cut gallbladder visualization to occur, despite cystic duct patency. In such cases, the patient should receive an additional dose of 3 to 5 mCi (111 to 185 MGq) ^{99m}Tc-IDA several minutes before the morphine is given.

Depending on the clinical question and setting, it may be appropriate to administer morphine as early as 30 to 45 minutes, once bowel visualization has occurred. However, the ability to diagnose chronic cholecystitis will be lost, and morphine will be given to some patients who would have

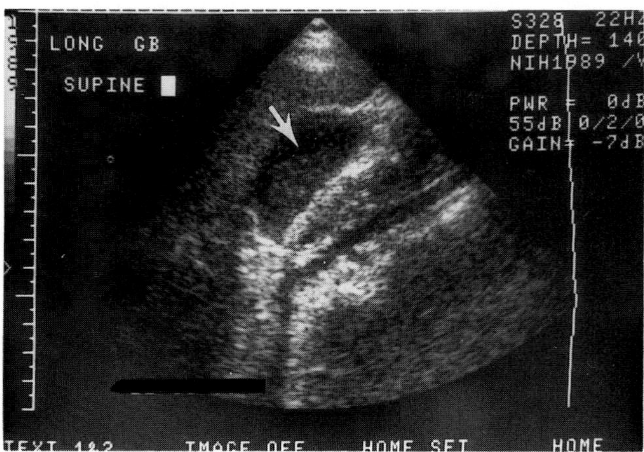

Figure 7. Chronic cholecystitis. Longitudinal image of the gallbladder in a patient with chronic cholecystitis (see Fig. 6). Gallbladder sludge (arrow) is seen.

had normal gallbladder visualization within the hour without the use of morphine.

In a study by Fink-Bennett et al.[52] morphine-augmented cholescintigraphy was performed in 61 patients suspected of having acute cholecystitis. Patients who had fasted >48

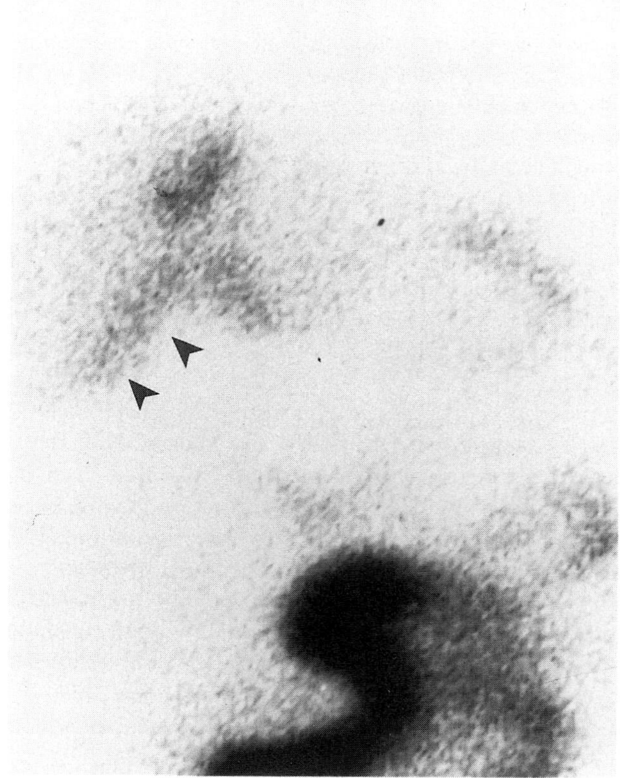

Figure 8. Rim sign; 2-hour anterior DISIDA image demonstrating a "rim sign" of retained pericholecystic activity (arrowheads). At surgery the patient was found to have gangrenous cholecystitis. (Courtesy of R. K. Zeman.)

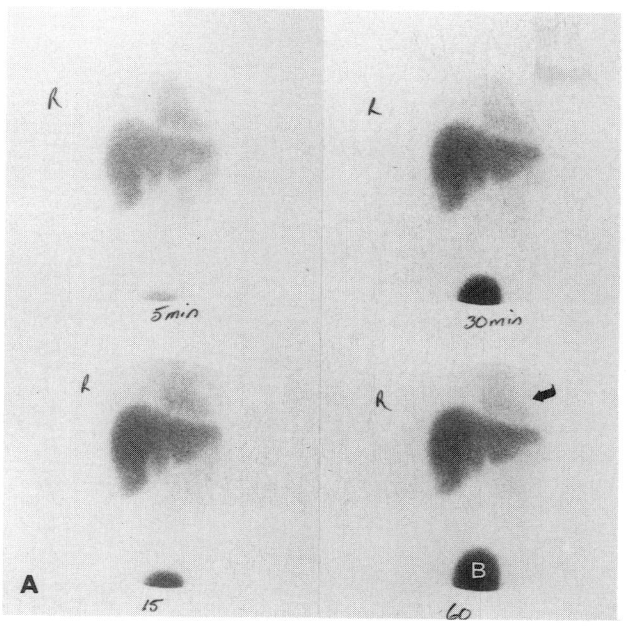

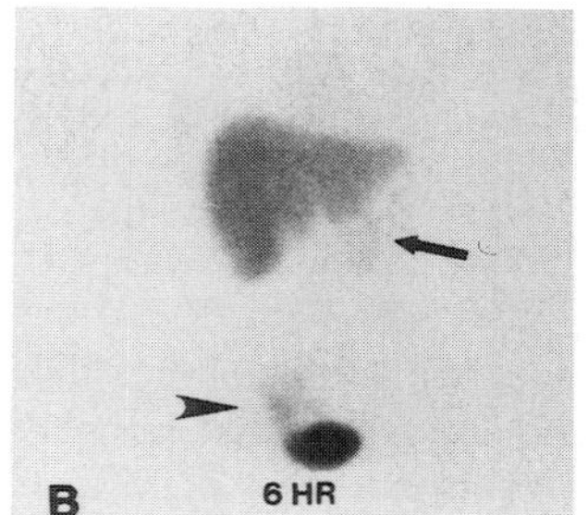

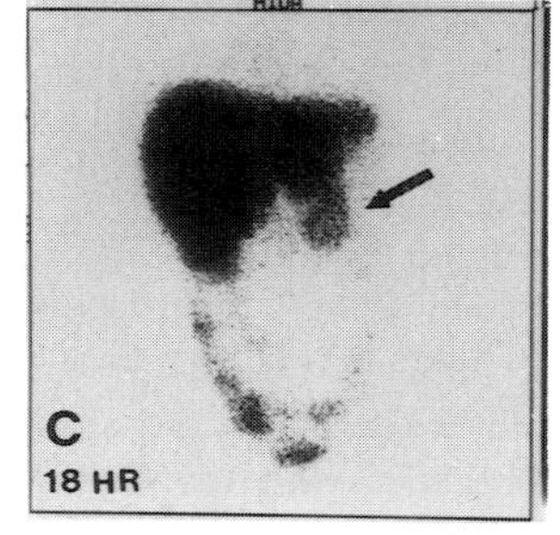

Figure 9. Severe hepatocellular dysfunction. DISIDA study in a patient with sepsis, rising liver enzymes, and a total bilirubin of 12.3 following an autologous bone marrow transplant. Anterior images **(A)** at 5, 15, 30, and 60 mins show decreased hepatic uptake, prolonged cardiac blood pool (curved arrow), liver retention of tracer, and absence of biliary or bowel activity. Bladder **(B)** is seen inferiorly. At 6 hrs **(B)** minimal bowel activity is seen (arrowhead). At 18 hrs **(C)** definite intestinal activity excludes complete common bile duct obstruction. Liver retention and kidney visualization persist in these late images (arrows). Failure to visualize the gallbladder in this patient was due to poor hepatic function and not acute cholecystitis. Ultrasound, CT, and MRI of the gallbladder were normal.

hours were pretreated with CCK (0.02 μg/kg) 30 minutes before the study. In these patients, the sensitivity and specificity of the study were 95 and 99%, respectively, for acute cholecystitis. Thus, morphine administration enabled the authors to shorten hepatobiliary scintigraphy from 4 hours to 90 minutes without compromising accuracy. More recently, Kim et al.[53] have made the case that morphine-augmented cholescintigraphy is actually superior to delayed imaging at 3 to 24 hours, having higher specificity and positive predictive value for acute cholecystitis in their experience.

Morphine-augmented cholescintigraphy in severely ill patients (in whom shortened studies are even more important) has met with varying success. Flancbaum and Alden[54] performed morphine-augmented scintigraphy in 25 critically ill patients with suspected acute cholecystitis and found a sensitivity of 100% and specificity of 92%. These authors administered 0.05 to 0.1 mg/kg morphine at 35 to 60 minutes, and continued imaging to 150 minutes. One of 25 patients had acute cholecystitis, and there were 2 false-positive results, yielding a false-positive rate of 67% (FP/(FP + TP)). On the other hand, Fig et al.[55] found morphine-augmented cholescintigraphy to have a sensitivity of only 80% and a specificity of 54% in 18 severely ill patients. In this study, morphine was administered at 60 minutes at a dose of 0.04 mg/kg, and imaging continued to 90 minutes. There were 4 true-positive, 7 true-negative, 6 false-positive, and 1 false-negative studies, for a false-positive rate of 60%. The discrepancy in sensitivity and specificity between these two reports is due in part to the differences in prevalence of acute cholecystitis in their patients. In the former, only 1 (4%) of 25 patients was eventually found to have acute cholecystitis, compared to 5 (27.7%) of 18 in the latter. As in conventional hepatobiliary imaging of severely ill patients (see above), the false-positive rates in both reports were higher in these patients than in those who were not critically ill.

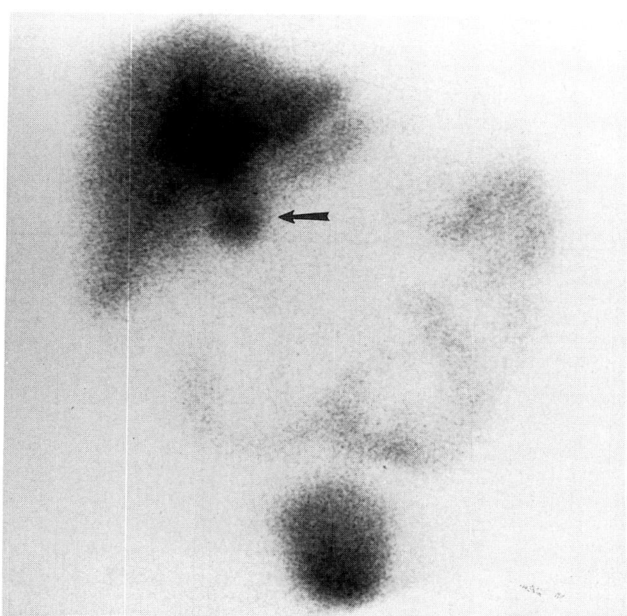

Figure 10. Cystic duct sign. Anterior hepatobiliary image shows accumulation of activity in a dilated cystic duct (arrow), mimicking gallbladder visualization.

Contraindications to the use of morphine include a history of allergy to the drug, respiratory insufficiency, and pancreatitis. In addition, the possibility of an increased false-negative rate must be considered, as might occur in patients with acalculous cholecystitis. Morphine administration may occasionally cause a cystic duct stone to dislodge acutely[52] or a dilated cystic duct sign to appear (Fig. 10).[56] If such a sign is seen, morphine should not be given. There is also concern that morphine administration may actually cause

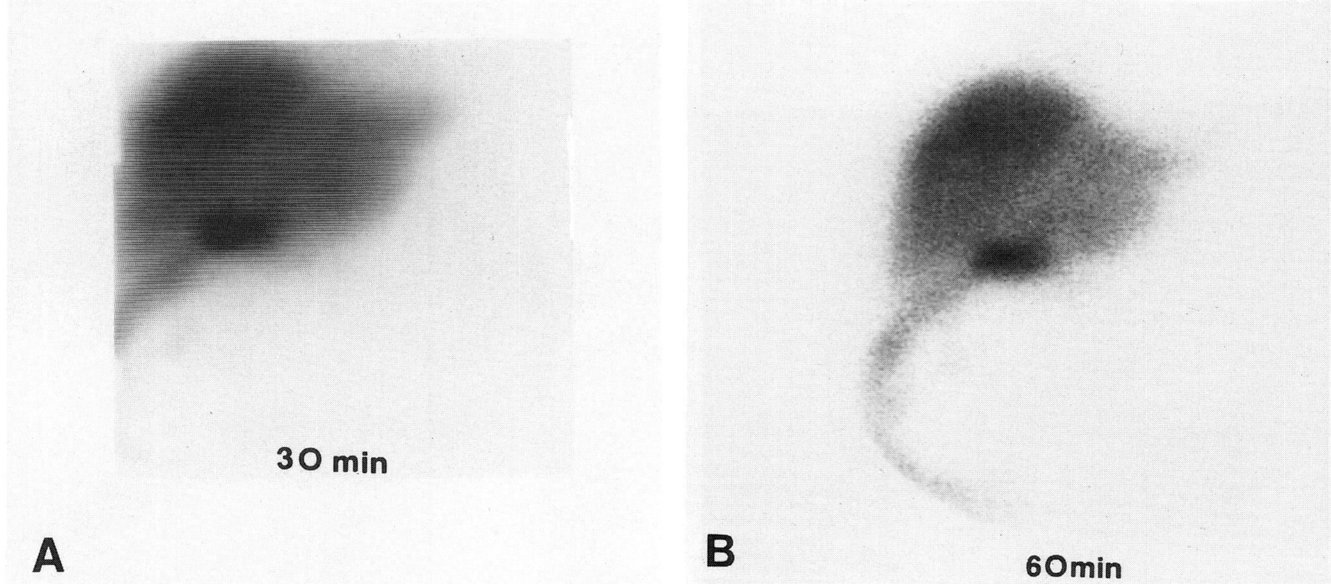

Figure 11. Bile leak. Anterior DISIDA images showing bile leakage from the cystic duct stump 2 days after elective laparoscopic cholecystectomy. At 30 min **(A)** activity is seen pooling in the gallbladder fossa. At 60 min **(B)** free bile is seen along the right lateral peritoneal cavity. (Figure reprinted with permission from Estrada et al., *J Nucl Med* 1991;32:1910.)

gallbladder perforation, as there have been several reports of studies demonstrating bile leaks after morphine was given.[57–59]

Acute Acalculous Cholecystitis

Acute acalculous cholecystitis accounts for 5 to 15% of cases of acute cholecystitis, and occurs predominantly in patients with serious concomitant conditions, such as trauma, burns, and sepsis, and in postoperative patients.[27,60] In the postoperative setting, up to 90% of cases of acute cholecystitis may be acalculous.[61]

Acute acalculous cholecystitis is associated with a significantly higher morbidity and mortality than the calculous variety.[27,61] In a study by Swayne,[62] 20 of 41 patients with acute acalculous cholecystitis had gangrenous or perforated gallbladders at surgery. Hepatobiliary scintigraphy demonstrated a rim sign (Fig. 8) or leakage of activity into the abdomen in 7 (35%) of 20. Swayne also reviewed 7 published studies and reported that the sensitivity of hepatobiliary scintigraphy in patients with acute acalculous cholecystitis approximates 91%.

Other Imaging Modalities in Acute Cholecystitis

Despite the high sensitivity and specificity of hepatobiliary scintigraphy for acute cholecystitis, ultrasound is still preferred by some as the screening study of choice.[63,64] Advantages of ultrasonography include its availability, its independence from patients' fasting states and medication history, and its ability to provide information about other abdominal structures. Disadvantages include its nonspecificity. Sonographic evidence of acute cholecystitis include findings such as gallstones, sludge, thickening of the gallbladder wall, and a "sonographic" Murphy's sign (pain upon palpation of the gallbladder) (Fig. 5).[64] In the clinical setting of possible acute cholecystitis, the combination of either gallstones plus gallbladder wall thickening or gallstones plus a positive sonographic Murphy's sign are reported to have positive predictive values >92%.[63] Evidence of gangrenous cholecystitis and gallbladder perforation (including visualization of sloughed gallbladder mucosa and pericholecystic fluid) are even more specific.

Whether ultrasound or scintigraphy is performed in acute cholecystitis will depend primarily on the experience and preference of individual clinicians and institutions. In most cases, scintigraphy is more sensitive and specific than ultrasound. However, in clinical situations where scintigraphy is known to have a high false-positive rate (see above), ultrasound may be more useful.

Occasionally, neither scintigraphy nor ultrasound is conclusive, and further information is desired. ^{111}Indium-WBC imaging has been used in these situations.[65] One problem, however, is the high activity normally present in the liver in WBC studies, so that foreknowledge of the exact location of the gallbladder is often necessary for accurate interpretation of the study.

CHRONIC CHOLECYSTITIS

Of all biliary disorders, chronic cholecystitis is the most common. Most cases are associated with gallstones, which are estimated to occur in 10 to 15% of adults in the US[66]

Diagnosis is most readily made by ultrasound, with scintigraphy playing a minor role.

The diagnosis of chronic cholecystitis is made by hepatobiliary scintigraphy when there is delayed (>1 hour) gallbladder visualization (Fig. 6). However, most patients with chronic cholecystitis have normal hepatobiliary studies. In a study of 101 patients with known chronic cholecystitis, 81% had normal gallbladder visualization within the first hour.[34] Even among patients with acute biliary symptoms, Freitas et al.[29] found that 69% of 64 patients eventually diagnosed as having chronic cholecystitis had normal hepatobiliary scintigraphy.

CHRONIC ACALCULOUS DISORDERS

Entities that cause chronic biliary symptoms in the absence of gallstones include chronic acalculous cholecystitis, the cystic duct syndrome (acalculous partial obstruction of the cystic duct due to kinking, fibrosis, etc.), sphincter of Oddi dysfunction, and gallbladder dyskinesia.[43] These disorders are often difficult to diagnose, and efforts have been made to increase the usefulness of hepatobiliary scintigraphy in these conditions. In particular, quantitative scintigraphy using CCK and measurements of gallbladder ejection fractions and rates have been studied.

Gallbladder Ejection Fractions

One common scintigraphic method of measuring gallbladder ejection fractions (EF) is to place regions of interest (ROI) over the gallbladder and background (usually placed lateral and adjacent to gallbladder), calculating the amount of emptying 20 minutes after an infusion of CCK (0.02 μg/kg i.v. over 3 minutes).[67] Others advocate using lower doses of CCK[2,68] and slower rates (over 30 minutes) of infusion, claiming that this results in better gallbladder emptying, increased specificity, and fewer adverse effects such as nausea and biliary colic. In a study of 23 healthy subjects, Ziessman et al.[69] compared infusion of 0.02 μg/kg over 3 minutes vs. 30 minutes and found that the slower rate yielded higher EFs. Using an EF > 35% as "normal," only 74% of their subjects had normal EFs after the 3-minute protocol versus 91% with the 30-minute method. With the 3-minute method, patients also had a high frequency (11 of 23) of CCK-induced side effects compared to none with the 30-minute infusion.

Numerous other techniques for measuring gallbladder EFs exist, including substituting a fatty meal for CCK.[34,70–73] It has become clear that the EFs obtained and their significance depend on the details of the procedure used. Therefore, it is important for each laboratory to establish its own protocol and its own database of "normal" gallbladder EFs to interpret the results of this procedure properly.

In general, abnormal gallbladders have lower EFs than normal gallbladders.[19,74,75] With the 0.02 μg/kg 3-minute infusion protocol, Fink-Bennett et al.[67] found that an EF < 35% at 20 minutes was 94% sensitive for identifying patients with confirmed chronic acalculous cholecystitis and/or the cystic duct syndrome. However, other studies show that a considerable degree of overlap in EF values often exists,[34,70,73,76] making reliance upon gallbladder EFs controversial. Among other things, patient selection is probably an important factor in determining the accuracy of gallbladder EFs for differentiating between normal and abnormal gallbladders.

The Cystic Duct Syndrome

The cystic duct syndrome is defined as partial acalculous obstruction of the cystic duct by fibrosis, kinking etc., and is one of the chronic acalculous disorders known to cause chronic biliary pain. Using CCK stimulation, Fink-Bennett et al.[77] found that the gallbladder EFs of 14 of 14 patients with this syndrome were < 22%. However, these patients could not be separated from those with chronic cholecystitis.

Sphincter of Oddi Dysfunction

Sphincter of Oddi dysfunction (SOD) is a term used to encompass the structural (strictures, fibrosis, muscular hypertrophy) and functional (spasm, abnormal propagation of contractions, paradoxical response to CCK) disorders of the sphincter of Oddi.[78] These can occur in conjunction with gallbladder disease, but are usually identified in postcholecystectomy patients. Also known as the *postcholecystectomy syndrome, biliary dyskinesia,* and *papillary stenosis,* SOD is characterized by abnormal sphincter pressures and contractile function, resulting in obstruction to normal bile flow.

Normally, the sphincter of Oddi acts in concert with the gallbladder to regulate biliary flow into the duodenum. Relaxation of the sphincter is induced by substances such as CCK, glucagon, and amyl nitrate, and constriction by morphine.[20,22] With SOD, structural problems and functional abnormalities disrupt normal bile flow, leading to increased biliary system pressures which, in turn, cause dilatation, stasis, and biliary colic. Treatment generally involves sphincterotomy to relieve the obstruction.

The diagnosis of SOD must be considered in patients with postcholecystectomy symptoms after problems such as retained stones and structural abnormalities of the biliary tree have been excluded. No "gold standard" for the diagnosis of SOD exists, but it usually rests on the demonstration of increased CBD and sphincter pressures by manometry. Endoscopic retrograde cholangiopancreatography (ERCP) findings, such as contrast drainage delayed >45 minutes and CBD dilatation also suggest SOD.[20,78] However, both these studies are invasive, cannot be performed successfully in all patients, are not yet fully validated, and can yield disparate results.[78–80] Therefore, a need for alternative noninvasive studies exists, and diagnostic criteria for hepatobiliary scintigraphy have been developed.

Both visual[81,82] and quantitative[70,79] scintigraphic criteria have been used to evaluate patients for SOD, and are generally the same as those seen with partial CBD obstruction from other causes.[81–83] Sostre et al.[79] have developed a system for scoring hepatobiliary scan findings, including delayed hepatic uptake, delayed bile duct visualization, prominent bile ducts, delayed bowel visualization, decreased CBD emptying, and ratio of CBD to liver activity at 60 minutes. Manometry and ERCP were used in these patients as well. Using this system, normal and SOD patients could be separated with 100% sensitivity and specificity. However, the patient population in this small study included a high proportion of SOD patients as well as patients with nonbiliary pain or no symptoms at all, and the sensitivity and specificity of the technique in a more general population remains to be determined.

BILIARY OBSTRUCTION

Hepatobiliary scintigraphy provides information about the patency of the entire biliary system. Obstruction to bile flow may be partial or complete, functional or structural, and calculous or acalculous. Common bile duct stones are found in approximately 15% of patients undergoing cholecystectomy in the US,[84] and acalculous processes include problems such as strictures and extrinsic compression. Opiates, such as morphine, increase sphincter of Oddi tone,[22] and may transiently obstruct drainage. Depending on the etiology, acuteness, and degree of obstruction, patients present with symptoms such as jaundice, pain, pruritus, and abnormal liver function tests.

Complete Common Bile Duct Obstruction

In biliary obstruction, scintigraphic abnormalities are often detectable before ductal dilatation occurs and before the diagnosis can be made by ultrasound.[85] Scintigraphy can also assist in differentiating dilated, obstructed systems from dilated, but patent, systems. In complete CBD obstruction, findings vary depending on the time elapsed between the onset of obstruction and imaging. If performed in the acute stage (<24 hours), there is absent bowel activity despite normal liver uptake and visualization of the biliary tree, including the gallbladder.[86–88] At this stage, the gallbladder is still able to act as a bile reservoir, preventing significant increases in biliary system pressure. After approximately 24 hours, rising biliary pressures slow further bile production, and the bile ducts and gallbladder are no longer visualized. Mildly decreased hepatic uptake may also be observed. By 96 hours, a definite decrease in hepatic uptake is usually evident.[88]

When both the biliary system and bowel activity fail to appear by 4 hours despite adequate liver uptake, the probability of complete CBD obstruction is very high (Fig. 12). Both Egbert et al.[89] and Lecklitner et al.[90] found this pattern to be 100% sensitive for total CBD obstruction. Specificity was also very high, with only a few false-positive results encountered in patients with severe hepatocellular disease with elevated bilirubin levels and decreased tracer uptake by the liver (Fig. 9). In the former study, this pattern was found to have a 100% positive predictive value for obstruction in patients with serum bilirubin < 10mg/dL, whereas in patients with bilirubin > 20 mg/dL the positive predictive value was only 88%. False-positive studies for obstruction have also been found in patients with intrahepatic cholestasis, sepsis, peritonitis, the Dubin-Johnson syndrome, and portal vein thrombosis.[91]

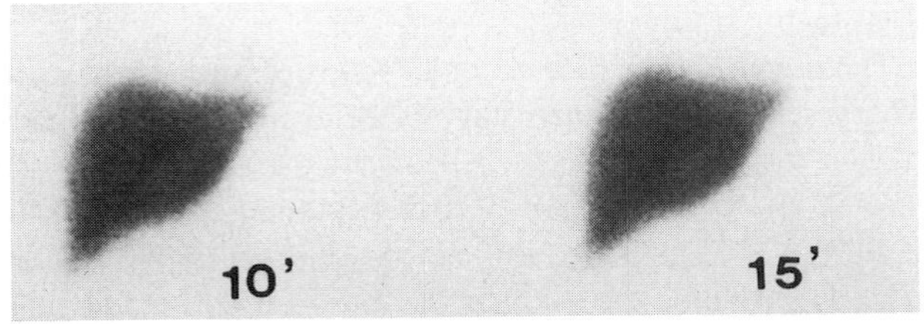

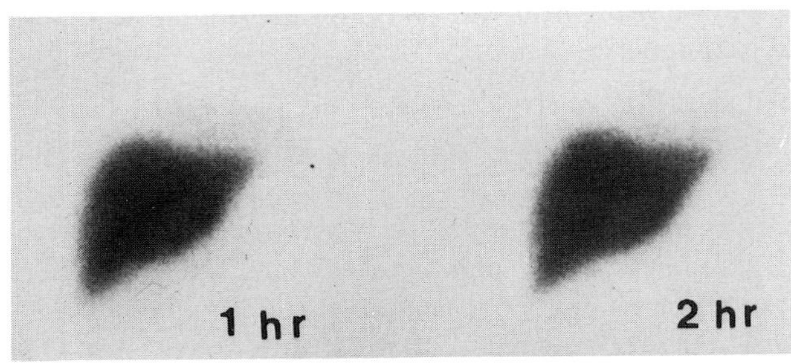

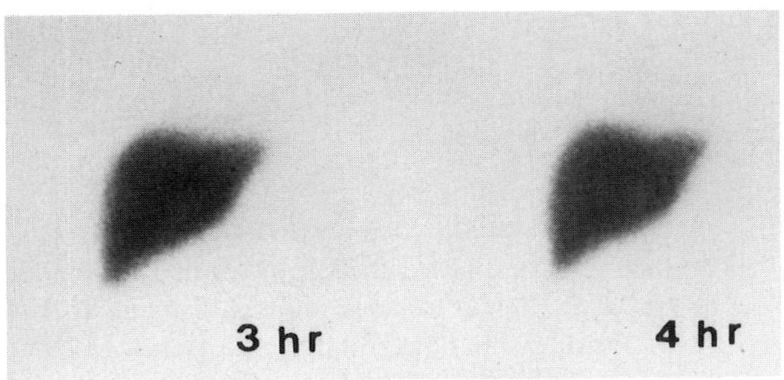

Figure 12. Complete common bile duct obstruction. Anterior hepatobiliary images show prompt hepatic uptake with nonvisualization of biliary structures and bowel by 4 hours. (Figure reprinted with permission from Lecklitner et al., *J Nucl Med* 1986;27:1403.)

Partial Common Bile Duct Obstruction

The scintigraphic diagnosis of partial CBD obstruction is suggested by (1) delayed biliary to bowel transit >1 hour, (2) delayed emptying of bile ducts with abnormal ductal time-activity curves and, occasionally, (3) apparent ductal dilatation.[83,85] Abnormal ductal time-activity curves showing greater activity at 2 hours compared to 1 hour suggest obstruction, even with visualization of bowel before 1 hour.[82,83] Filling defects caused by stones or strictures are also occasionally seen, especially on early images.[92] With partial CBD obstruction, gallbladder filling is normal unless concomitant gallbladder or cystic duct disease exists.

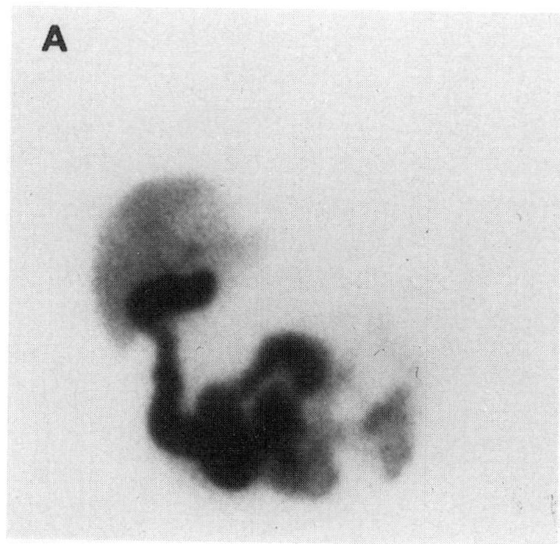

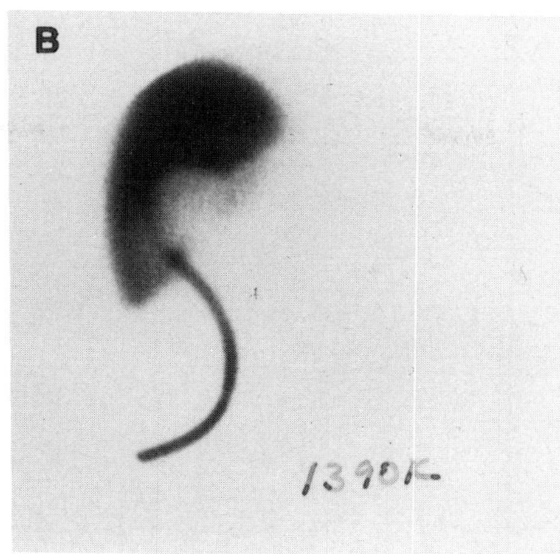

Figure 13. Postsurgical hepatobiliary scintigraphy. **(A).** Anterior DISIDA image at 45 minutes demonstrating patency of a choledochojejunostomy. The gallbladder and left hepatic lobe have been surgically removed. **(B).** Anterior DISIDA image at 15 minutes showing bile excretion through an external drain in the hepatic bed. The patient is 4 days post-resection of the left hepatic lobe and also has a T-tube in place. No T-tube or bowel activity is seen, suggesting obstruction.

The extent to which the above abnormalities are found in partial biliary obstruction depends on the degree and constancy of obstruction present. Patients with early mild or intermittent partial obstruction often have normal-appearing studies. In these "normal" cases, CCK is sometimes successful in eliciting signs that suggest obstruction, including decreased gallbladder EFs and rates[92] and prolonged increased CBD activity after CCK administration (as gallbladder contraction occurs and obstruction of flow into bowel is encountered).[75]

EVALUATION OF POSTOPERATIVE PATIENTS

Hepatobiliary scintigraphy is useful in evaluating patients following cholecystectomy, during which complications such as bile duct injury, bile leaks, obstruction, and retained stones may occur.[93] Damage to the biliary tree during surgery occurs in 0.1 to 0.2% and 0.2 to 0.6% of cases during open and laparoscopic cholecystectomy, respectively.[66] This latter procedure is being performed with increasing frequency, and accurate data on its relative merits/problems compared to open cholecystectomy is not available. Scintigraphy can also be used to assess patients after gallstone lithotripsy.[94] Long-term, hepatobiliary scintigraphy frequently plays a role in the workup of patients with persistent or recurrent biliary pain after cholecystectomy.[83] Studies can help identify patients with retained stones, cystic duct remnants, biliary obstruction, or SOD. The patency of biliary anastomoses can also be evaluated (Fig. 13).[95]

Bile Leaks

Bile leaks occur in a variety of situations, the most common being postsurgical. Most leaks are clinically unimportant and do not require intervention.[96,97] Leaks have been demonstrated in up to 44% of patients after cholecystectomy.[96] Other settings in which leaks occur include gallbladder perforation and trauma. The incidence of gallbladder perforation is estimated to be between 2 to 11%[98] in acute cholecystitis. It is even higher in acute acalculous cholecystitis.[62]

Scintigraphic signs of bile leakage include visualization of free bile in the abdomen and pericholecystic hepatic activity. When a leak is suspected, the entire liver should be included within the field of view during imaging. Delayed imaging—even up to 24 hours—is often required to detect slow, small leaks. Free bile may pool in the gallbladder fossa, and can mimic normal structures early on.[47–49] The true nature of the leak in these cases usually becomes clear on delayed images, as activity in the liver and biliary tree decreases and as free bile spills into other areas (Fig. 11). Free bile can accumulate perihepatically, over the dome of the liver in the subdiaphragmatic space (Fig. 14), and in the colonic gutters. If abdominoperitoneal drains are present, imaging of the drain or its reservoir should also be performed.

Evaluation of Liver Transplants

Hepatobiliary scintigraphy is used to evaluate several problems arising after liver transplantation. As in other postoperative patients, post-transplant biliary complications, such as bile leaks and extrahepatic obstruction, are readily assessable scintigraphically. More difficult to evaluate, however, are the complications of ischemia, rejection, intrahepatic cholestasis, and diffuse infection.[99]

Total loss of graft perfusion due to vascular compromise is demonstrated by absent liver activity in the flow and static phases of hepatobiliary scintigraphy. Images in patients with subtotal liver infarction or localized ischemia secondary to vascular stenosis or thrombosis demonstrate photopenia in the areas involved. Global ischemia, on the other hand, results in the less specific findings of globally decreased hepatic uptake and blood pool clearance of IDA, similar to the pattern seen with hepatocyte dysfunction of other etiologies.

After liver transplantation, hyperacute rejection with total loss of graft perfusion and function is not known to occur,[100] unlike that observed in renal transplantation. Acute and

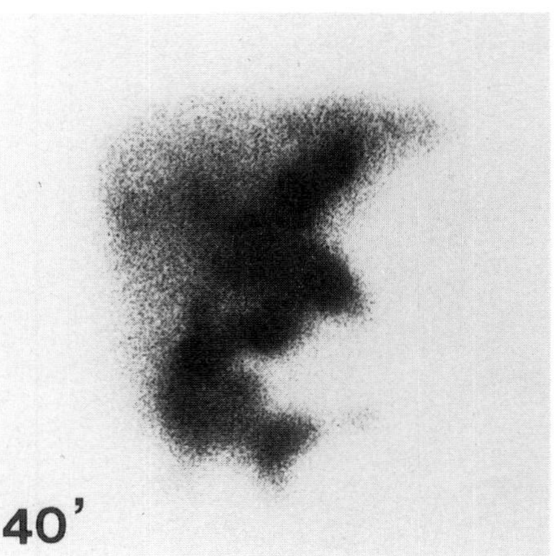

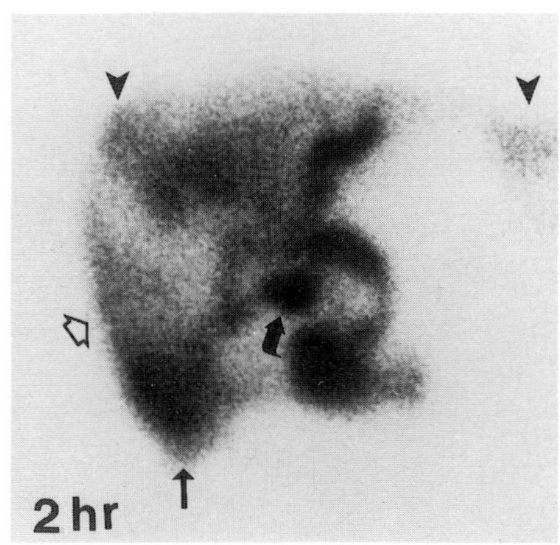

Figure 14. Bile leak in a patient with acute acalculous cholecystitis and a perforated gallbladder at surgery. Images at 40 min. and 2 hrs show gallbladder activity (curved arrow) and leakage of bile into the subhepatic (arrow), perihepatic (open arrow) and subdiaphragmatic (arrowheads) spaces. (Figure reprinted with permission from Swayne et al., *J Nucl Med* 1990; 31:1915.)

chronic rejection are of concern, though, and just as with renal transplants, are diagnoses of exclusion. Hepatobiliary scintigraphy in patients with rejection demonstrates a nonspecific pattern of decreased liver uptake and blood pool clearance and prolonged tracer retention in the liver.[99,100] Similar findings are seen in patients with intrahepatic cholestasis, which itself has multiple causes including hepatitis, obstruction, sepsis, and ischemia.

Infectious processes of the liver may be localized or diffuse. Focal abscesses are manifested by photopenic areas if the lesions are large enough, as with any space-occupying lesion of the liver. With diffuse liver involvement, hepatobiliary scintigraphy again demonstrates the nonspecific findings of decreased blood pool clearance, decreased liver uptake, and prolonged retention of radiotracer.

It is clear that hepatobiliary scintigraphy often provides nonspecific information after transplantation, and that clinical information and other noninvasive and invasive (biopsy) techniques must be employed in evaluating these patients. In many of these situations, scintigraphy's most useful role may be in monitoring a patient's response to therapy. Scintigraphy can also be used for following patients over time, as it can detect changes in hepatic function before they become apparent biochemically or can be detected by other imaging modalities.[99,101]

HEPATIC ABNORMALITIES AND HEPATOBILIARY SCINTIGRAPHY

Aside from providing information about the biliary system, hepatobiliary scintigraphy also reveals abnormalities of hepatic function and configuration. Focal as well as diffuse disease can be detected, particularly in the "liver phase" of the study. Not only is information derived from the pattern of uptake and excretion, but methods of quantitative analysis of hepatocyte function using parameters such as hepatic extraction fractions have recently been described.[102–104]

Although most of the hepatic abnormalities detected by scintigraphy are nonspecific, these findings sometimes provide useful diagnostic information in patients being studied for other reasons. In others, the study can be used as a noninvasive means of confirming or following certain diseases. Diffuse hepatic processes include those in which the primary insult is to the hepatocytes (congenital defects, hepatitis, and cirrhosis), and those in which the primary problem involves the intrahepatic biliary system (drug-induced cholestasis, primary biliary cirrhosis, and sclerosing cholangitis) (Fig. 15).[102] Examples of focal liver disease include space-occupying lesions of both hepatic and extrahepatic origin.

Diseases Causing Diffuse Hepatic Dysfunction

HEPATOCYTE DYSFUNCTION

Diseases primarily affecting hepatocyte function include the various forms of hepatitis and cirrhosis. In these patients, the major abnormality seen with hepatobiliary scintigraphy is decreased hepatic uptake of the radiotracer. Associated findings include decreased blood pool clearance and increased renal excretion (Fig. 9). Depending on the severity of disease, visualization of biliary structures and bowel may be delayed or even absent when hepatocyte function is severely compromised. This does not necessarily indicate true biliary pathology, and other diagnostic modalities must be used in these patients if coexistent cholecystitis or biliary obstruction is suspected.

CHOLESTASIS

As with other processes, the scintigraphic findings in patients with diffuse intrahepatic cholestasis vary depending on the severity and duration of disease. Commonly caused by drugs, infection, TPN, or found in conjunction with other diffuse liver diseases, the major scintigraphic findings are delayed and decreased excretion into bile ducts and bowel with prolonged retention of tracer in the liver (Fig. 9).[102] Decreased blood pool clearance and hepatic uptake of tracer is also observed.

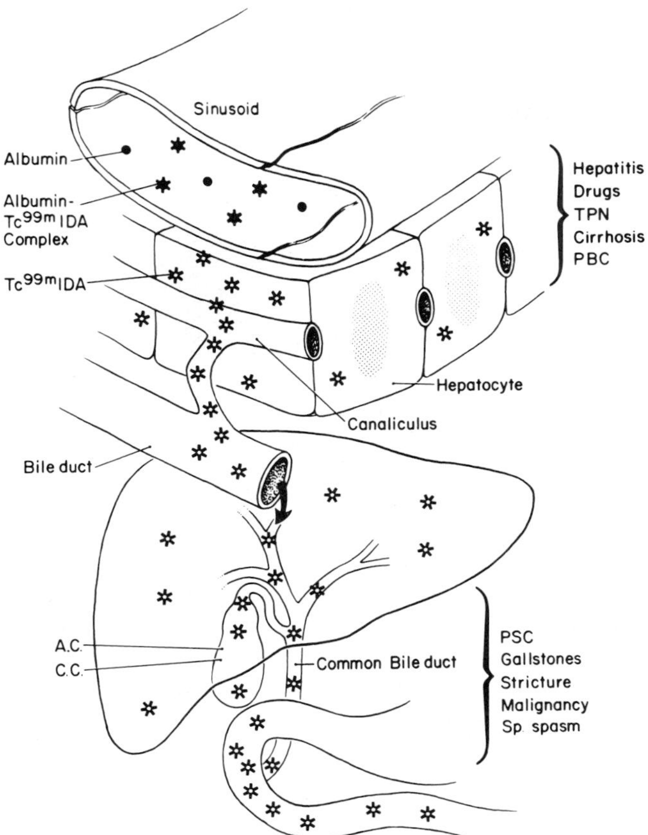

Figure 15. Schematic diagram of ^{99m}Tc-IDA transit through the hepatobiliary system and the disease categories affecting each level. ^{99m}Technetium-IDA is carried to the liver loosely bound to albumin and enters the bile canaliculi without undergoing conjugation during transit through the hepatocyte. Diseases that affect the hepatocyte and canaliculi are shown on the upper right and those that affect the major ducts are shown in the lower right. (Abbreviations: AC = acute cholecystitis, CC = chronic cholecystitis, PSC = primary sclerosing cholangitis, Sp = Sphincter, PBC = primary biliary cirrhosis, and TPN = total parenteral nutrition). (Figure reprinted with permission from Krishnamurthy et al., *J Nucl Med* 1988;29:1144.)

SCLEROSING CHOLANGITIS

While the diagnosis of sclerosing cholangitis should be made radiologically with cholangiography or ERCP, characteristic findings on hepatobiliary scintigraphy have been described. The etiology of this disease is unknown. Patients present with a variety of symptoms, including progressive jaundice, pruritus, pain, fever, and loss of weight.[105] Pathologically, inflammation of the biliary system leads to progressive fibrosis of both intrahepatic and extrahepatic ducts. Radiographically, multiple strictures and tortuous biliary ducts are seen. The disease often has a patchy distribution, and may affect some areas more than others.[105,106]

Hepatobiliary studies in sclerosing cholangitis may show retained activity proximal to the multiple strictures present.[107] Overall, hepatic clearance of radiotracer is decreased significantly, with regional variations corresponding to the patchy nature of the disease. In addition, gallbladder filling is often absent due to involvement of the cystic duct or gallbladder itself. If the gallbladder does fill, EFs and ejection rates are decreased compared to normals.[108]

PRIMARY BILIARY CIRRHOSIS

In primary biliary cirrhosis, diffuse inflammation and destruction causes progressive obliteration of small intrahepatic bile ducts. This disease is of unknown etiology, and usually affects middle-aged women. Antimitochondrial antibodies are present in >95% of patients.[109] Patients often present with progressive jaundice and pruritus. Diagnosis requires a positive liver biopsy and the exclusion of an obstructive process of the larger bile ducts.

As in sclerosing cholangitis, hepatobiliary scintigraphy in these patients reveals prolonged hepatic retention of radiotracer. However, unlike sclerosing cholangitis where the degree of hepatic retention often varies from region to region, the findings in primary biliary cirrhosis are much more uniform.[107,108] In addition, the biliary tree appears normal in primary biliary cirrhosis, as larger bile ducts, including the cystic duct and CBD, are spared. Despite this, gallbladder EFs and ejection rates are reduced in primary biliary cirrhosis (as in sclerosing cholangitis), although the reasons for this are not clear.[108]

FOCAL LESIONS OF THE LIVER

Space-occupying lesions of the liver, such as cysts, hemangiomas, and metastatic disease from other primaries, appear as photon-deficient areas on hepatobiliary scintigraphy and are best appreciated during the "liver phase" of the study, before significant excretion into the biliary system and bowel occurs (Fig. 16). Mass lesions of hepatocyte origin, on the other hand, can demonstrate varying degrees of IDA uptake. These lesions, which include adenomas, focal nodular hyperplasia (FNH), and hepatomas, often contain functioning hepatocytes, and attention to the different phases of the study—flow, early, and late—often aids in the differential diagnosis.

HEPATIC ADENOMAS

Benign hepatic adenomas occur primarily in women and are frequently associated with the use of oral contraceptives. These lesions are composed mainly of hepatocytes and are classically described as demonstrating a centripetal perfusion pattern—from the periphery inward.[110] Adenomas have variably been reported to take up decreased, normal, and increased amounts of IDA relative to surrounding liver parenchyma, and the majority are not hyperperfused on radionuclide flow studies.[111,112] Correlation with other radiologic studies such as ultrasound (US), computed tomography (CT), and angiography is useful in clarifying the diagnosis.[113,114]

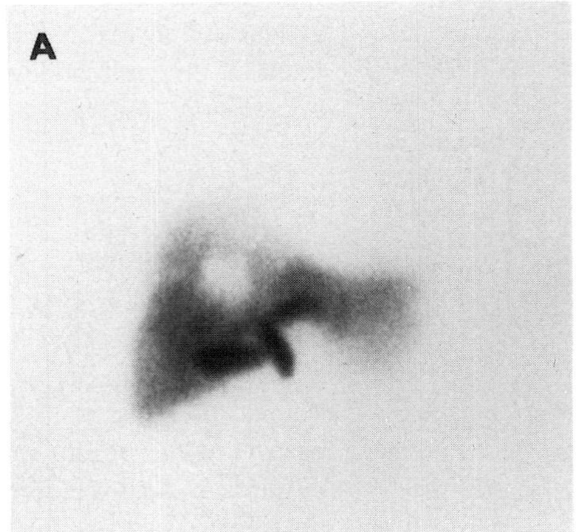

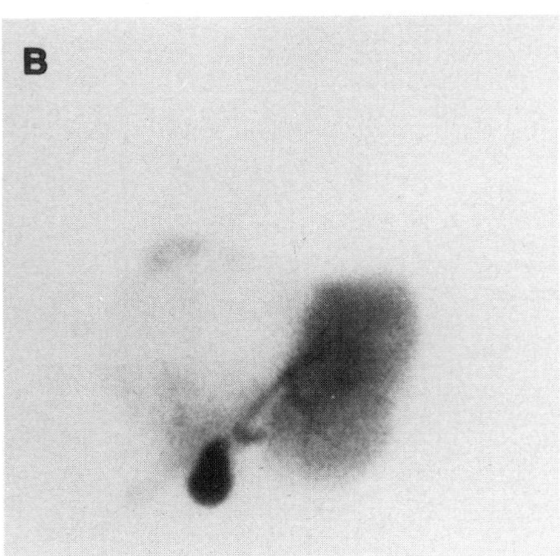

Figure 16. Ten-minute anterior DISIDA images in 2 patients with space-occupying lesions of the liver. Photopenic areas correspond to **(A)** colon cancer metastasis and **(B)** a large hepatoma.

FOCAL NODULAR HYPERPLASIA

Focal nodular hyperplasia (FNH), in which there is benign proliferation of hepatocytes, reticuloendothelial (RE) cells, and biliary ductules, can also have a variable appearance on hepatobiliary scintigraphy. These, too, occur mostly in women and may be associated with oral contraceptive use, and are usually described as being fed by a large central artery with centrifugal blood flow.[110] Scintigraphically, most (76 to 86%) FNH lesions are hyperperfused on the flow phase, with subsequent normal or increased early IDA uptake (5 to 10 minutes) and late retention of tracer (1 to 3 hours).[111,115] This pattern was found to be 98% specific for FNH in one study.[111]

HEPATOCELLULAR CARCINOMA

As opposed to FNH lesions, hepatocellular carcinomas only rarely appear hyperperfused during hepatobiliary imaging.[116] Of the 67 hepatomas included in the series of Kotzerke et al.[111], only one demonstrated the characteristic pattern associated with FNH (see above). This and other studies[15,117] have shown that over 40% of hepatomas are able to take up IDA agents, appearing as "hot spots" on delayed imaging (Fig. 17). Some also exhibit early uptake (5 to 20 minutes), while in others, uptake is seen only on delayed images (2 to 3 hours). Occasionally, uptake of tracer by extrahepatic hepatoma metastases also occurs.[117,118] Calvert et al.[117] found that the ability to take up IDA correlated with the degree of differentiation of a hepatoma. Of their 34 patients in whom histological correlation was available, 70% of well-differentiated lesions took up IDA, compared to 30% of moderately differentiated, and 0% of poorly differentiated lesions.

PEDIATRIC HEPATOBILIARY SCINTIGRAPHY

Hepatobiliary scintigraphy has several applications in the pediatric population. As in adults, scintigraphy can be used to detect acute cholecystitis, although this is a rare problem in children.[119] More common indications in this age group include the evaluation of jaundice in neonates and the investigation of choledochal cysts.

Evaluation of Neonatal Jaundice—Biliary Atresia vs. Cholestasis/Hepatitis

Biliary atresia is a disease in which inflammation of extrahepatic bile ducts causes ductal obliteration and interruption

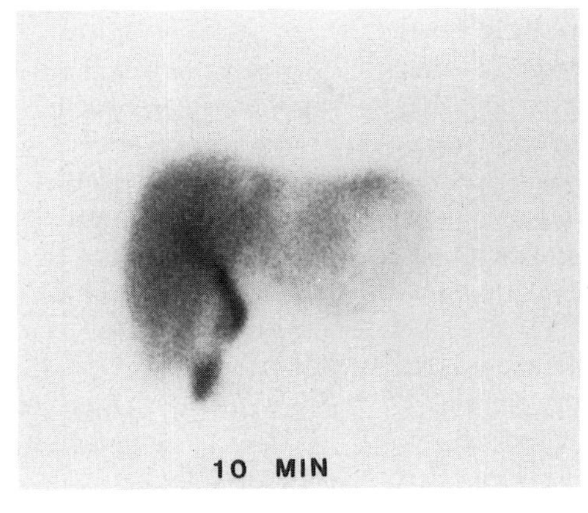

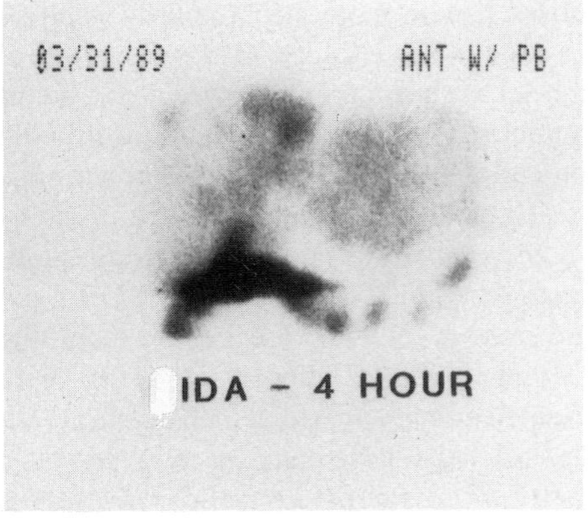

Figure 17. Hepatoma. Anterior DISIDA images in a patient with multifocal hepatoma. Areas of tumor are photopenic at 10 min. but appear as "hot spots" at 4 hrs.

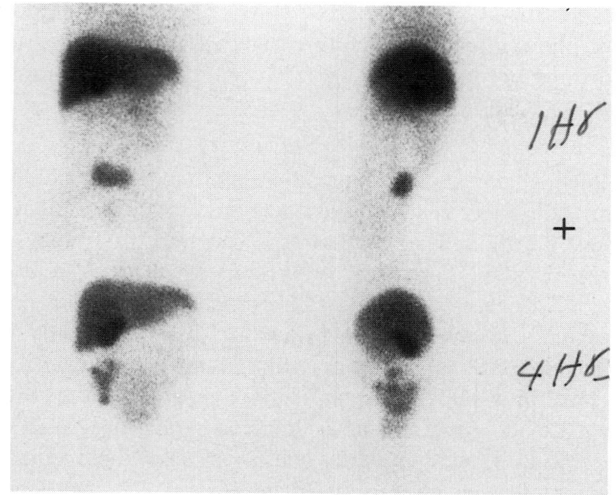

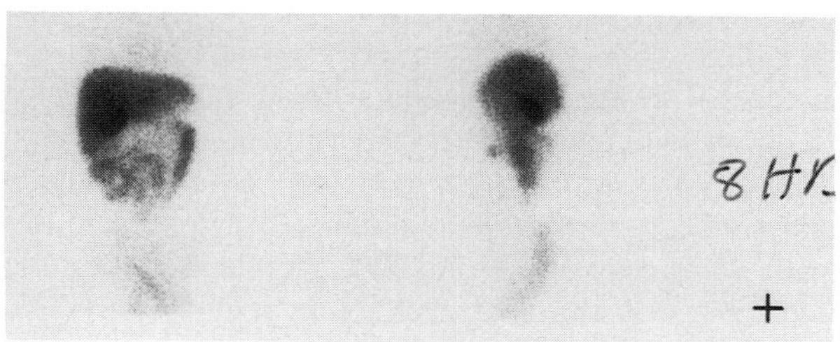

Figure 18. Neonatal hepatitis. Hepatobiliary study in an infant with neonatal jaundice and hepatitis, pretreated with phenobarbital. Anterior and right lateral views at 1, 4, and 8 hrs demonstrate gallbladder and bowel visualization by 1 hr. Note prolonged cardiac blood pool. (Courtesy of M. Majd.)

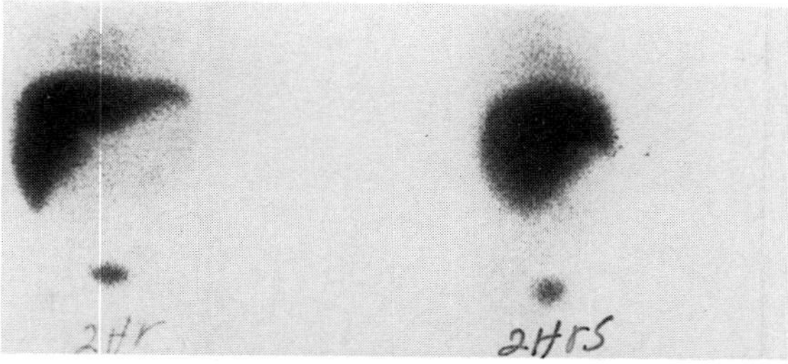

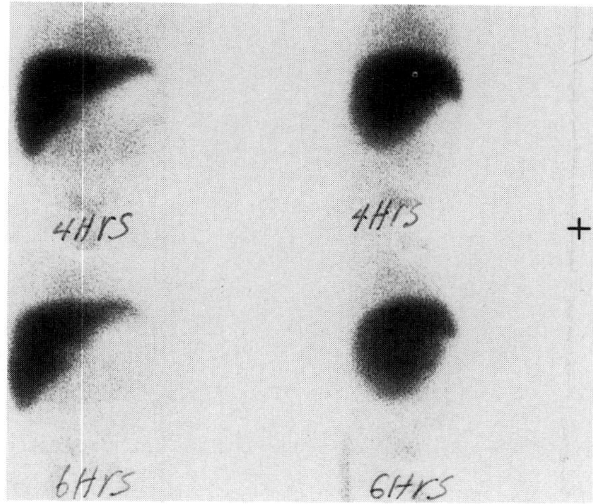

Figure 19. Biliary atresia. Hepatobiliary study in an infant with neonatal jaundice and biliary atresia, pretreated with phenobarbital. Anterior and right lateral views at 2, 4, and 6 hrs demonstrate total absence of biliary and bowel visualization. A prolonged cardiac blood pool is seen throughout the study. (Courtesy of M. Majd.)

of bile drainage. This disease is curable only with corrective surgery, the timing of which is crucial. Over 90% of infants have a good outcome if a portoenterostomy (Kasai procedure) is performed within the first 60 days of life; after this the success rate declines significantly.[120] Therefore, differentiation between biliary atresia and processes such as cholestasis or hepatitis (for which treatment is generally conservative) is critical in infants with neonatal jaundice. Fortunately, hepatobiliary scintigraphy provides a reliable means of making these distinctions.

In infants with biliary atresia, hepatobiliary scintigraphy fails to demonstrate any gallbladder or bowel activity, even on delayed 24-hour images. Visualization of any bowel activity during scintigraphy effectively rules out biliary atresia, and delayed imaging is therefore essential. Infants with hepatitis or cholestasis are still able to excrete bile into the bowel, although this may only be detectable with delayed imaging. As opposed to atresia, bile ducts in these patients are patent, allowing drainage to occur (Figs. 18 to 20). Only in extremely severe cases of hepatitis and cholestasis (when hepatic function becomes so compromised that bile production essentially ceases) may bowel activity fail to appear, leading to a false-positive study for atresia. One way of minimizing the likelihood of this type of false-positive study is to stimulate bile production prior to imaging. This can be accomplished by pretreating patients with phenobarbital (2.5 mg/kg orally twice daily for 5 days).[121] This drug increases hepatic conjugation and excretion of bile, thereby maximizing the likelihood of visualizing bowel in cases of cholestasis and hepatitis, and is reported to improve the specificity of hepatobiliary scanning for biliary atresia from 63 to 94%.[122]

HEREDITARY DISORDERS

Rotor's and Dubin-Johnson Syndromes

Rotor's syndrome is an inherited disorder in which abnormalities of hepatic uptake and storage of organic anions results in hyperbilirubinemia. Hepatobiliary scintigraphy in these patients reflects these abnormalities, demonstrating markedly decreased to absent liver uptake and extremely delayed blood pool clearance (Fig. 21).[123,124]

The Dubin-Johnson syndrome is a hereditary hyperbilirubinemia in which the primary defect is in excretion of conjugated bilirubin from the hepatocytes.[17] Unlike Rotor's, hepatobiliary scintigraphy in these patients demonstrates prompt, intense visualization of the liver with rapid blood pool clearance, followed by prolonged hepatic retention of

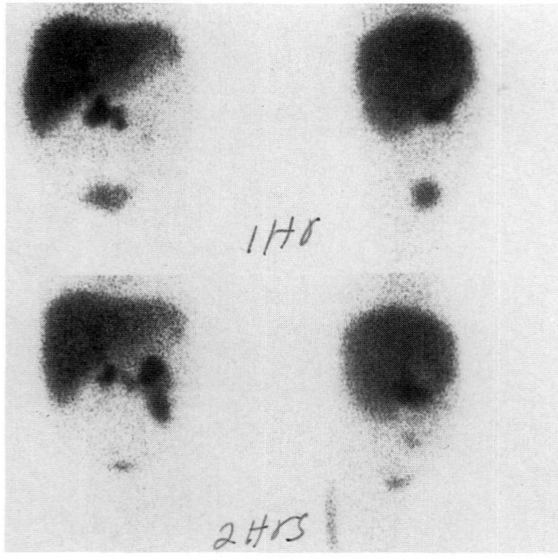

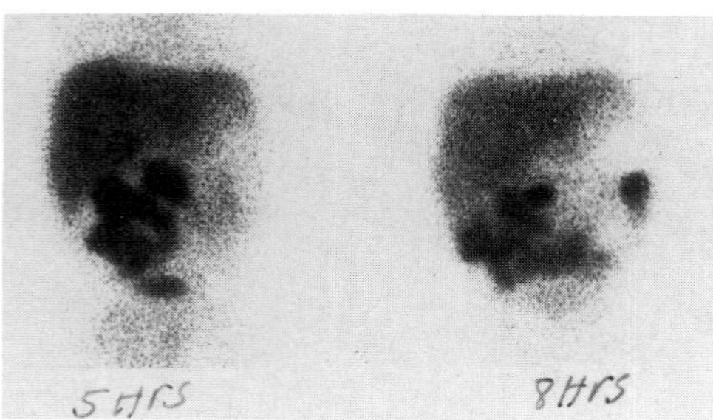

Figure 20. Surgical correction of biliary atresia. Repeat hepatobiliary study in the infant seen in Fig. 19 following surgical correction of biliary atresia (Kasai procedure). Anterior and right lateral views at 1 and 2 hours, and anterior views at 5 and 8 hrs now demonstrate biliary and bowel visualization by 1 hr. (Courtesy of M. Majd.)

the radiotracer.[123] Nonetheless, slow excretion of bile does take place, allowing variable visualization of biliary structures and bowel.

Choledochal Cysts

Choledochal cysts are congenital abnormalities of extrahepatic bile ducts in which the ducts are abnormally dilated. These are thought to be part of a spectrum of fibrocystic diseases of the hepatobiliary system, which also includes Caroli's disease (see below). Choledochal cysts occur more frequently in females than males, and most frequently involve the CBD. Hepatobiliary scintigraphy is used primarily to confirm the biliary origin of these cystic structures after they are identified by other imaging modalities, such as ultrasound. Findings usually consist of early photopenia of the region(s) in question with late filling (>1 hour) and retention of radiotracer for a prolonged period of time. The variability of these findings is demonstrated by Campanovo et al.[51] in a series of 12 surgically documented cases of choledochal cysts. These authors found that filling of the cyst occurred before 1 hour in over 50% of patients, and in 17% the cyst never filled. (In these latter cases the diagnosis could not be confirmed scintigraphically.) Prominent intrahepatic ducts were detected in 42% of patients and gallbladder visualization was delayed or absent in the majority of patients.

Caroli's Disease

Caroli's disease is another congenital fibrocystic abnormality of the hepatobiliary system in which both intrahepatic and extrahepatic bile ducts are dilated; associated findings can include hepatic fibrosis and cirrhosis. Hepatobiliary scintigraphy in these patients again serves to confirm the biliary

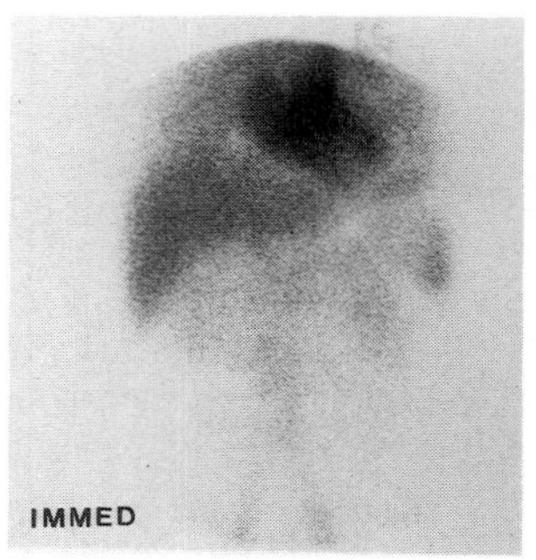

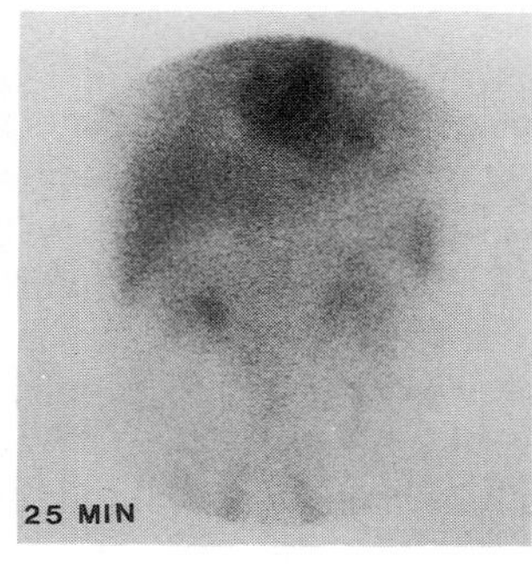

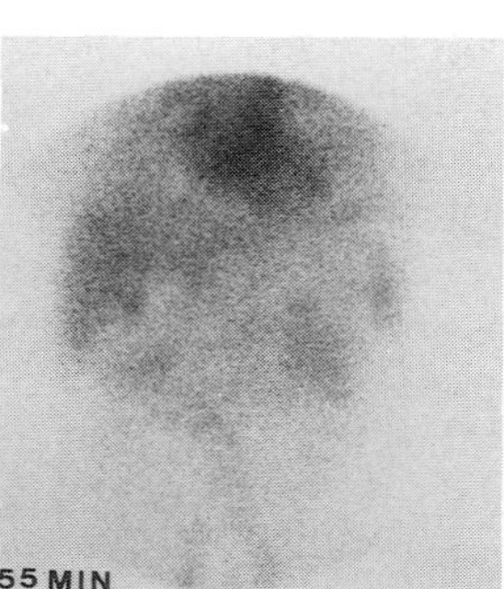

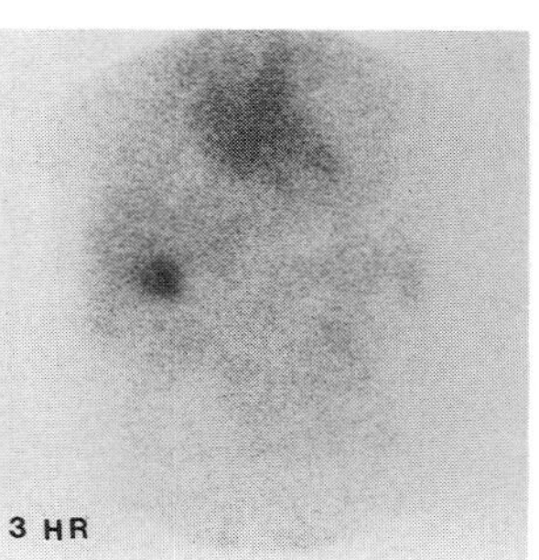

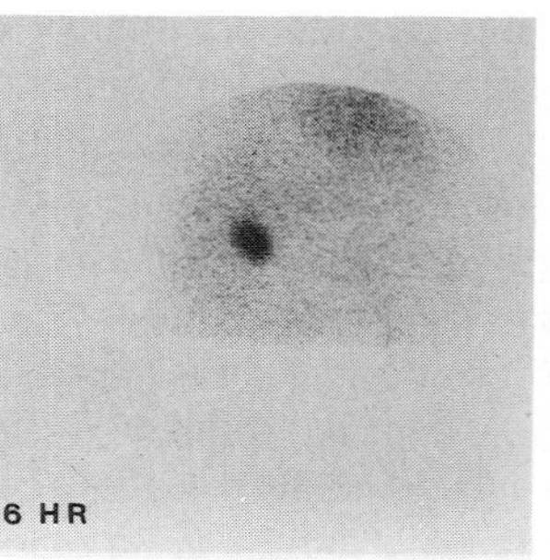

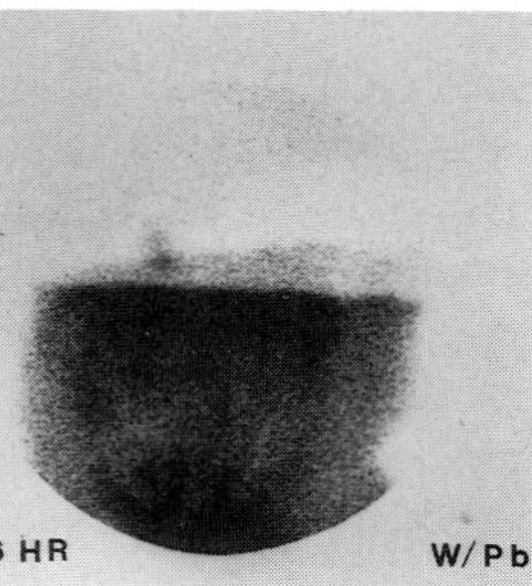

Figure 21. Rotor's disease. ^{99m}Tc-mebrofenin study shows slow liver uptake, persistent cardiac blood pool, and prominent urinary tract visualization. The gallbladder was seen at 55 minutes. Intestinal activity is seen at 6 hours (bottom right, with lead shield over liver). (Figure reprinted with permission from LeBouthillier et al., *J Nucl Med* 1992;33:1550.)

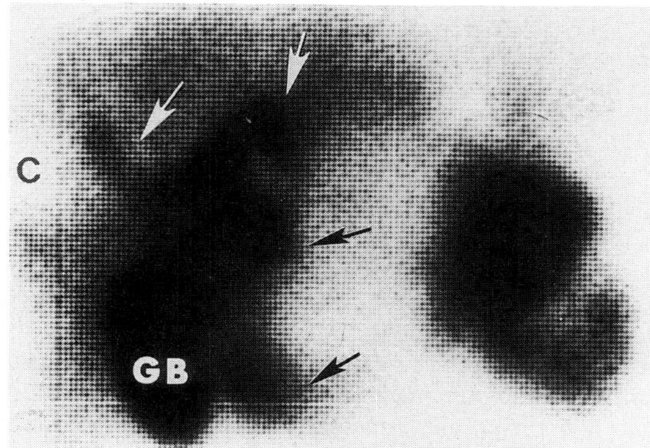

Figure 22. Caroli's disease. Anterior PIPIDA image at 70 minutes shows dilated intrahepatic and common bile ducts with retained radiotracer (arrows). Also note gallbladder (GB) and hepatic cyst (C). (Figure reprinted with permission from Moreno et al., *Am J Gastroenterol* 1984;79:299.)

nature of abnormalities detected with other imaging modalities. As with extrahepatic choledochal cysts (see above), scintigraphy usually reveals prominence and dilatation of the affected bile ducts, which often also demonstrate prolonged tracer retention (Fig. 22).[125] Invasive procedures, such as ERCP, cholangiography, or surgery, are generally needed to make a definitive diagnosis (Fig. 23).

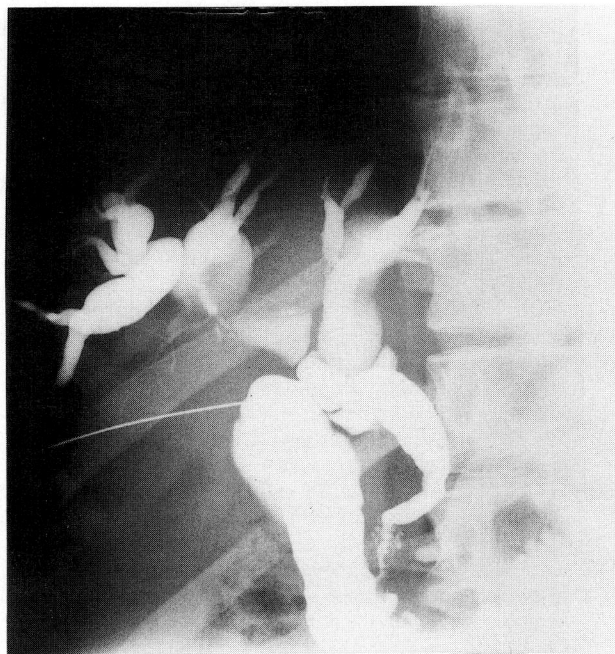

Figure 23. Caroli's disease. Percutaneous transhepatic cholangiography shows dilated intrahepatic and extrahepatic bile ducts. (Figure reprinted with permission from Moreno et al., *Am J Gastroenterol* 1984;79:299.)

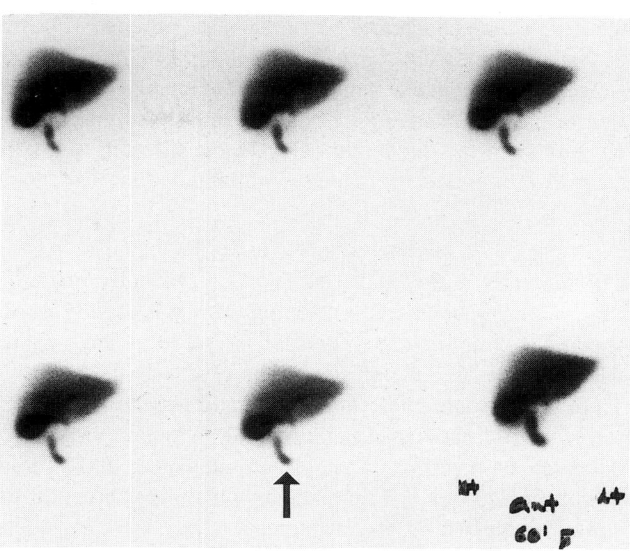

Figure 24. Pancreatitis: The duodenal cutoff sign. Note abrupt termination of activity in the third part of the duodenum (arrow) secondary to acute pancreatitis and local inflammation of the duodenum. (Figure reprinted with permission from Shanley et al., *Clin Nucl Med* 1991;16:223.)

MISCELLANEOUS DISORDERS

Pancreatitis

Abnormal findings are frequently seen during hepatobiliary scintigraphy in patients with acute pancreatitis, including delayed or absent gallbladder visualization (suggesting coexistent cholecystitis) and delayed or absent bowel visualization (suggesting coexistent biliary obstruction). In many cases, these findings truly represent coexistent biliary pathology whereas, in others, no such pathology is ever confirmed.[44] Pancreatitis may be biliary or nonbiliary in etiology. One literature review of 5019 reported cases of acute pancreatitis calculated that approximately 27% were related to cholelithiasis (biliary pancreatitis), and 55% were associated with excessive alcohol ingestion (an example of nonbiliary pancreatitis).[126] In biliary pancreatitis, it is thought that the passage of a gallstone into the Ampulla of Vater is the initiating event and leads to bile reflux into the pancreatic duct.[127] Perhaps not surprisingly, Serafini et al.[128] found that 31 (78%) of 40 patients with biliary pancreatitis had abnormal hepatobiliary studies compared to 1 (5%) of 20 patients with nonbiliary pancreatitis.

Several scintigraphic findings can alert physicians to a possible diagnosis of acute pancreatitis. The "duodenal cutoff sign" consists of the abrupt termination of bowel activity, usually in the third portion of the duodenum (Fig. 24).[129] This pattern of activity can persist for a prolonged length of time and is presumably due to localized, abnormal bowel function and motility secondary to inflammation and thickening in the area adjacent to the pancreatitis.

Other scintigraphic signs that suggest pancreatic disease include widening of the duodenal loop as it sweeps around the head of the pancreas,[130] or a persistent absence of bowel activity in localized areas of the sweep.[131] These findings suggest the presence of pancreatic enlargement by inflammation or a mass, causing local displacement and interruption of activity in the duodenum. Duodenogastric reflux is also frequently reported in patients with pancreatitis.[130,132]

Duodenogastric Reflux

Duodenogastric reflux of bile is often clinically insignificant.[133] During hepatobiliary scintigraphy it is usually a nonspecific, asymptomatic finding observed in patients with a wide variety of clinical conditions (Figs. 1, 4) including acute and chronic cholecystitis[134,135] and pancreatitis.[130] In a series of 198 patients, Elgazzar et al.[136] found evidence of duodenogastric reflux in 36 (18%), occurring with similar frequencies (23 to 38%) in patients with acute cholecystitis, chronic cholecystitis, acute pancreatitis, and duodenal ulcers. Reflux is also observed in normal subjects, after gallbladder or upper gastrointestinal tract surgery, and in those with hepatitis, abscesses, bowel inflammation, bowel ileus, and sepsis, as listed by Shih and Fockele.[137]

In symptomatic patients, hepatobiliary scintigraphy can be used as a noninvasive tool for detection and evaluation of reflux. Not only can scintigraphy define the level to which reflux occurs (gastric or esophageal), it can also be used for quantitation.[138] Unfortunately, accurate quantitation is often limited by overlap of activity in the liver or bowel with that in the stomach.

References

1. Bobba VR, Krishnamurthy GT, Kingston E, et al.: Comparison of biokinetics and biliary imaging parameters of four Tc-99m iminodiacetic acid derivatives in normal subjects. *Clin Nucl Med* 1983;8:70.
2. Krishnamurthy S, Krishnamurthy GT: Quantitative assessment of hepatobiliary diseases with Tc-99m-IDA scintigraphy, in Freeman LM, Weissmann HS, (eds.): *Nuclear Medicine Annual.* New York, Raven Press 1988, p 309.
3. Harvey E, Loberg MD, Cooper M: Tc-99m-HIDA: A new radiopharmaceutical for hepato-biliary imaging. *J Nucl Med* 1975;16:533.
4. Ryan J, Cooper M, Loberg M, Harvey E, Sikorski S: Technetium-99m-labeled n-(2,6-dimethylphenylcarbamoylmethyl) iminodiacetic acid (Tc-99m HIDA): A new radiopharmaceutical for hepatobiliary imaging studies. *J Nucl Med* 1977; 18:997.
5. Harvey E, Loberg M, Ryan J, Sikorski S, et al.: Hepatic clearance mechanism of Tc-99m-HIDA and its effect on quantitation of hepatobiliary function: Concise communication. *J Nucl Med* 1979;20:310.
6. Okuda H, Nunes R, Vallabhajosula S, et al.: Studies of the hepatocellular uptake of the hepatobiliary scintiscanning agent, Tc-99m-DISIDA. *J Hepatol* 1986;3:251.
7. Nunn AD, Loberg MD, Conley RA: A structure-distribution-relationship approach leading to the development of Tc-99m mebrofenin: An improved cholescintigraphic agent. *J Nucl Med* 1983;24:423.
8. Klingensmith III WC, Fritzberg AR, Spitzer VM, et al.: Clinical comparison of diisopropyl-IDA Tc-99m and diethyl-IDA Tc-99m for evaluation of the hepatobiliary system. *Radiology* 1981;140:791.
9. Klingensmith III WC, Fritzberg AR, Spitzer VM, et al.: Work in progress: Clinical evaluation of Tc-99m-trimethylbromo-IDA and Tc-99m-diisopropyl-IDA for hepatobiliary imaging. *Radiology* 1983;146:181.
10. Hernandez M, Rosenthall L: A crossover study comparing the kinetics of Tc-99m-labelled diethyl- and diisopropyl-IDA. *Clin Nucl Med* 1980;5:352.
11. Hernandez M, Rosenthall L: A crossover study comparing the kinetics of Tc-99m-labelled diisopropyl and P-butyl IDA analogs in patients. *Clin Nucl Med* 1980;5:159.
12. van Aswegen A, van Wyk AJ, Roodt JP, et al.: Radionuclide cholescintigraphic imaging: An evaluation of several Tc-99m labelled hepatobiliary radiopharmaceuticals. *Nucl Med Biol* 1986;13:509.
13. Kato-Azuma M: Tc-99m(Sn)-N-pyridoxylaminates: A new series of hepatobiliary imaging agents. *J Nucl Med* 1982; 23:517.
14. Takada T, Yasuda H, Uchiyama K, et al.: Diagnostic evaluation of hepatobiliary scintigraphy using Tc-99m-N-pyridoxyl-5-methyltryptophan in acute cholecystitis. *Gastroenterol Japon* 1988;23:553.
15. Hasegawa Y, Nakano S, Hashizume T, et al.: Comparison of delayed imaging with Tc-99m PMT and Tc-99m DEIDA for visualization of hepatoma. *Clin Nucl Med* 1989;14: 526.
16. Oyamada H, Yamazaki S, Makuuchi M, Hasegawa H: Clinical significance of Tc-99m-N-pyridoxyl-5-methyltryptophan (Tc-99m-PMT) in the diagnosis of intrahepatic masses. *Radioisotopes* 1989;38:244.
17. Billing B: Bilirubin metabolism, in Schiff L, Schiff ER (eds.): *Diseases of the Liver.* Philadelphia, J.B. Lippincott, 6th, 1987, p 103.
18. Rappaport AM: Physioanatomic considerations, in Schiff L, Schiff ER, (eds.): *Diseases of the Liver.* Philadelphia, J.B. Lippincott, 6th, 1987, p 1.
19. Krishnamurthy GT, Bobba VR, McConnell D, et al.: Quantitative biliary dynamics: Introduction of a new noninvasive scintigraphic technique. *J Nucl Med* 1983;24:217.
20. Hogan WJ, Geenen JE, Dodds WJ: Dysmotility disturbances of the biliary tract: Classification, diagnosis, and treatment. *Semin Liver Dis* 1987;7:302.
21. Stone BG, Gavaler JS, Belle SH, et al.: Impairment of gallbladder emptying in diabetes mellitus. *Gastroenterology* 1988;95:170.
22. Murphy P, Salomon J, Roseman DL: Narcotic anesthetic drugs. Their effect on biliary dynamics. *Arch Surg* 1980; 115:710.
23. Patch GG, Morton KA, Arias JM, Datz FL: Naloxone reverses pattern of obstruction of the distal common bile duct induced by analgesic narcotics in hepatobiliary imaging. *J Nucl Med* 1991;32:1270.
24. Klingensmith III WC, Spitzer VM, Fritzberg AR, Kuni CC: The normal fasting and postprandial diisopropyl-IDA Tc-99m hepatobilary study. *Radiology* 1981;141:771.
25. Williams W, Krishnamurthy GT, Brar HS, Bobba VR: Scintigraphic variations of normal biliary physiology. *J Nucl Med* 1984;25:160.
26. Kim CK, Palestro CJ, Solomon RW, et al.: Delayed biliary to bowel transit in cholescintigraphy after cholecystokinin treatment. *Radiology* 1990;176:553.
27. Frazee RC, Nagorney DM, Mucha P: Acute acalculous cholecystitis. Mayo Clin Proc 1989;64:163.
28. Weissman HS, Badia J, Sugarman LA, et al.: Spectrum of 99m-Tc-IDA cholescintigraphic patterns in acute cholecystitis. *Radiology* 1981;138:167.

29. Freitas JE, Coleman RE, Nagle CE, et al.: Influence of scan and pathologic criteria on the specificity of cholescintigraphy: Concise communication. *J Nucl Med* 1983;24:876.
30. Bushnell DL, Perlman SB, Wilson MA, Polcyn RE: The rim sign: Association with acute cholecystitis. *J Nucl Med* 1986;27:353.
31. Smith R, Rosen JM, Gallo LN, Alderson PO: Pericholecystic hepatic activity in cholescintigraphy. *Radiology* 1985; 156:797.
32. Meekin GK, Ziessman HA, Klappenbach RS: Prognostic value and pathophysiologic significance of the rim sign in cholescintigraphy. *J Nucl Med* 1987;28:1679.
33. Qvist N, Oster-Jorgensen E, Rasmussen L, et al.: Postprandial gallbladder filling: Relation to gastrointestinal motility. *Scand J Gastroenterol* 1989;24:969.
34. Raymond F, Lepanto L, Rosenthall L, Fried GM: Tc-99m-IDA gallbladder kinetics and response to CCK in chronic cholecystitis. *Eur J Nucl Med* 1988;14:378.
35. Kalff V, Froelich JW, Lloyd R, Thrall JH: Predictive value of an abnormal hepatobiliary scan in patients with severe intercurrent illness. *Radiology* 1983;146:191.
36. Mirvis SE, Vainright JR, Nelson AW, et al.: The diagnosis of acute acalculous cholecystitis. A comparison of sonography, scintigraphy, and CT. *AJR* 1986;147:1171.
37. Garner WL, Marx MV, Fabri PJ: Cholescintigraphy in the critically ill. *Am J Surg* 1988;155:727.
38. Shuman WP, Gibbs P, Rudd TG, Mack LA: PIPIDA scintigraphy for cholecystitis: False positives in alcoholism and total parenteral nutrition. *AJR* 1982;138:1.
39. Warner BW, Hamilton FN, Silberstein EB, et al.: The value of hepatobiliary scans in fasted patients receiving total parenteral nutrition. *Surgery* 1987;102:595.
40. Larsen MJ, Klingensmith III WC, Kuni CC: Radionuclide hepatobiliary imaging: nonvisualization of the gallbladder secondary to prolonged fasting. J Nucl Med 1982;23:1003.
41. Sippo WC, Moreno AJ, Cabellon S, Turnbull GL: The effect of prolonged fasting and total parenteral nutrition on hepatobiliary imaging with technetium 99m DISIDA. *Clin Nucl Med* 1987;12:169.
42. Kistler AM, Ziessman HA, Gooch D, Bitterman P: Morphine-augmented cholescintigraphy in acute cholecystitis. A satisfactory alternative to delayed imaging. *Clin Nucl Med* 1991;16:404.
43. Fink-Bennett D: The role of cholecystogogues in the evaluation of biliary tract disorders, in Freeman LM, Weissman HS (eds.): *Nuclear Medicine Annual*. New York, Raven Press, 1985, p 107.
44. Edlund G, Kempi V, van der Linden W: Transient nonvisualization of the gallbladder by Tc-99m HIDA cholescintigraphy in acute pancreatitis: Concise communication. *J Nucl Med* 1982;23:117.
45. Gad MA, Krishnamurthy GT, Glowniak JV: Identification and differentiation of congenital gallbladder abnormality by quantitative technetium-99m IDA cholescintigraphy. *J Nucl Med* 1992;33:431.
46. Coleman RE, Freitas JE, Fink-Bennett DM, Bree RL: The dilated cystic duct sign. A potential cause of false negative cholescintigraphy. *Clin Nucl Med* 1984;9:134.
47. Shih WJ, Duff D, Mostowycz L: Bile leakage accumulating in the gallbladder bed mimicking normal visualization of gallbladder in technetium-99m Disida hepatobiliary imaging. *Clin Nucl Med* 1989;14:222.
48. Singh A, Valle G: Pseudonormal hepatobiliary scintigraphy in a patient with a bile leak. *Clin Nucl Med* 1990;15:843.
49. Estrada WN, Zanzi I, Ward R, et al.: Scintigraphic evaluation of postoperative complications of laparoscopic cholecystectomy. *J Nucl Med* 1991;32:1910.
50. Wang PW, Chen HY, Wan YL: Choledochal cyst mimicking gallbladder in Tc-99m Disofenin radionuclide cholescintigraphy. *Clin Nucl Med* 1990;15:811.
51. Campanovo E, Buck JL, Drane WE: Scintigraphic features of choledochal cyst. *J Nucl Med* 1989;30:622.
52. Fink-Bennett D, Balon H, Robbins T, Tsai D: Morphine-augmented cholescintigraphy: Its efficacy in detecting acute cholecystitis. *J Nucl Med* 1991;32:1231.
53. Kim CK, Tse KKM, Juweid M, Mozley PD, et al.: Cholescintigraphy in the diagnosis of acute cholecystitis: Morphine-augmetation is superior to delayed imaging. *J Nucl Med* 1993;34:1866.
54. Flancbaum L, Alden SM: Morphine cholescintigraphy. *Surg Gynecol Obstet* 1990;171:227.
55. Fig LM, Wahl RL, Stewart RE, Shapiro B: Morphine-augmented hepatobiliary scintigraphy in the severely ill: Caution is in order. *Radiology* 1990;175:467.
56. Achong DM, Oates E: The cystic duct sign during morphine-augmented cholescintigraphy. *Clin Nucl Med* 1991;16:627.
57. Achong DM, Newman JS, Oates E: False-negative morphine-augmented cholescintigraphy: A case of subacute gallbladder perforation. *J Nucl Med* 1992;33:256.
58. Moreno AJ, Ortenzo CA, Rodriguez AA, et al.: Gallbladder perforation seen on hepatobiliary imaging following morphine sulfate injection. *Clin Nucl Med* 1989;14:651.
59. Mack JM, Slavin JD, Spencer RP: Two false negative results using morphine sulfate in hepatobiliary imaging. *Clin Nucl Med* 1989;14:87.
60. Glenn F: Acute acalculous cholecystitis. *Ann Surg* 1979; 189:458.
61. Inoue T, Mishima Y: Postoperative acute cholecystitis: A collective review of 494 cases in Japan. *Jpn J Surg* 1988; 18:35.
62. Swayne LC: Acute acalculous cholecystitis: Sensitivity and detection using technetium-99m iminodiacetic acid cholescintigraphy. *Radiology* 1986;160:33.
63. Ralls PW, Colletti PM, Lapin SA, et al.: Real-time sonography in suspected acute cholecystitis. Prospective evaluation of primary and secondary signs. *Radiology* 1985;155: 767.
64. Cooperberg PL, Gibney RG: Imaging of the gallbladder, 1987. *Radiology* 1987;163:605.
65. Fink-Bennett D, Clarke K, Tsai D, et al.: Indium-111-leukocyte imaging in acute cholecystitis. *J Nucl Med* 1991;32:803.
66. NIH Consensus Panel (1992): Gallstones and Laparoscopic Cholecystectomy, *NIH Consensus Statement.* 1992 Sep 14–16; 10(3):1.
67. Fink-Bennett D, De Ridder P, Kolozsi WZ, et al.: Cholecystokinin and cholescintigraphy: Detection of abnormal gallbladder motor function in patients with chronic acalculous gallbladder disease. *J Nucl Med* 1991;32:1695.
68. Krishnamurthy GT, Bobba VR, Kingston E, Turner F: Measurement of gallbladder emptying sequentially using a single dose of Tc-99m-labelled hepatobiliary agent. *Gastroenterology* 1982;83:773.
69. Ziessman HA, Fahey FH, Hixson DJ: Calculation of a gallbladder ejection fraction: Advantage of continuous Sincalide infusion over the three-minute infusion method. *J Nucl Med* 1992;33:537.
70. Drane WE, Johnson DA: Sincalide-augmented quantitative hepatobiliary scintigraphy (QHBS): Definition of normal parameters and preliminary relationship between QHBS and sphincter of Oddi (SO) manometry in patients suspected of having SO dysfunction. *J Nucl Med* 1990;31:1462.
71. Mackie CR, Baxter JN, Grime JS, et al.: Gallbladder emptying in normal subjects—a database for clinical cholescintigraphy. *Gut* 1987;28:137.

72. Masclee AAM, Hopman WPM, Corstens FHM, et al.: Simultaneous measurement of gallbladder emptying with cholescintigraphy and US during infusion of physiologic doses of cholecystokinin: A comparison. *Radiology* 1989;173:407.
73. Pickleman J, Peiss RL, Henkin R, et al.: The role of sincalide cholescintigraphy in the evaluation of patients with acalculous gallbladder disease. *Arch Surg* 1985;120:693.
74. Bobba VR, Krishnamurthy GT, Kingston E, et al.: Gallbladder dynamics induced by a fatty meal in normal subjects and patients with gallstones: Concise communication. *J Nucl Med* 1984;25:21.
75. Fink-Bennett D: Augmented cholescintigraphy: Its role in detecting acute and chronic disorders of the hepatobiliary tree. *Semin Nucl Med* 1991;21:128.
76. Kronert K, Gotz V, Reuland P, et al.: Gallbladder emptying in diabetic patients and control subjects assessed by real-time ultrasonography and cholescintigraphy: A methodological comparison. *Ultrasound Med Biol* 1989;15:535.
77. Fink-Bennett D, DeRidder P, Kolozsi W, et al.: Cholecystokinin cholescintigraphic findings in the cystic duct syndrome. *J Nucl Med* 1985;26:1123.
78. Steinberg WM: Sphincter of Oddi dysfunction: A clinical controversy. *Gastroenterology* 1988;95:1409.
79. Sostre S, Kalloo AN, Spiegler EJ, et al.: A noninvasive test of sphincter of Oddi dysfunction in postcholecystectomy patients. The scintigraphic score. *J Nucl Med* 1992;33:1216.
80. Meshkinpour H, Mollot M: Sphincter of Oddi dysfunction and unexplained abdominal pain: Clinical and manometric study. *Dig Dis Sci* 1992;37:257.
81. Zeman RK, Burrell MI, Dibbins J, et al.: Postcholecystectomy syndrome. Evaluation using biliary scintigraphy and endoscopic retrograde cholangiopancreatography. *Radiology* 1985;156:787.
82. Lee RGL, Gregg JA, Koroshetz AM, et al.: Sphincter of Oddi stenosis: Diagnosis using hepatobiliary scintigraphy and endoscopic manometry. *Radiology* 1985;156:793.
83. Weissmann HS, Gliedman ML, Wilk PJ, et al.: Evaluation of the postoperative patient with Tc-99m-IDA cholescintigraphy. *Semin Nucl Med* 1982;12:27.
84. Silfen D, Long WB, Alavi A: The role of hepatobiliary imaging in the evaluation and management of patients with common bile duct gallstones. *J Nucl Med* 1991;32:1261.
85. Zeman RK, Lee C, Jaffe MH, Burrell MI: Hepatobiliary scintigraphy and sonography in early biliary obstruction. *Radiology* 1984;153:793.
86. Blue PW: Hyperacute complete common bile duct obstruction demonstrated with Tc-99m-IDA cholescintigraphy. *Nucl Med Commun* 1985;6:275.
87. Floyd JL, Collins TL: Discordance of sonography and cholescintigraphy in acute biliary obstruction. *AJR* 1983;140:501.
88. Klingensmith III WC, Whitney WP, Spitzer VM, et al.: Effect of complete biliary-tract obstruction on serial hepatobiliary imaging in an experimental model: Concise communication. *J Nucl Med* 1981;22:866.
89. Egbert RN, Braunstein P, Lyons KP, Miller DR: Total bile duct obstruction—prompt diagnosis by hepatobiliary imaging. *Arch Surg* 1983;118:709.
90. Lecklitner ML, Austin AR, Benedetto AR, Growcock GW: Positive predictive value of cholescintigraphy in common bile duct obstruction. *J Nucl Med* 1986;27:1403.
91. Hughes KS, Marrangoni AG, Turbiner E: Etiology of the obstructive pattern in hepatobiliary imaging. *Clin Nucl Med* 1984;9:222.
92. Krishnamurthy GT, Lieberman DA, Brar HS: Detection, localization, and quantitation of degree of common bile duct obstruction by scintigraphy. *J Nucl Med* 1985;26:726.
93. Henry ML, Carey LC: Complications of cholecystectomy. *Surg Clin North Am* 1983;63:1191.
94. St George JK, Velchik MG: Biliary complications of gallstone lithotripsy detected by Tc-99m DISIDA scintigraphy. *Clin Nucl Med* 1991;16:157.
95. Belli G, Romano G, Monaco A, Santangelo ML: HIDA scan in the followup of biliary enteric anastomoses. *HPB Surg* 1988;1:29.
96. Gilsdorf JR, Phillips M, McLeod MK, et al.: Radionuclide evaluation of bile leakage and the use of subhepatic drains after cholecystectomy. *Am J Surg* 1986;151:259.
97. Rosenberg DJ, Brugge WR, Alavi A: Bile leak following an elective laparoscopic cholecystectomy: Role of hepatobiliary imaging in the diagnosis and management of bile leaks. *J Nucl Med* 1991;32:1777.
98. Swayne LC, Filippone A: Gallbladder perforation: Correlation of cholescintigraphic and sonographic findings with the Niemeier classification. *J Nucl Med* 1990;31:1915.
99. Hawkins RA, Hall T, Gambhir SS, Busuttil RW, et al.: Radionuclide evaluation of liver transplants. *Semin Nucl Med* 1988;18:199.
100. Busuttil RW, Goldstein LI, Danovitch GM, et al.: Liver transplantation today. *Ann Intern Med* 1986;104:377.
101. de Jonge MWC, Pauwels EKJ, Hennis PJ, et al.: Cholescintigraphy and Tc-99m diethyl IDA for the detection of rejection of auxiliary liver transplants in pigs. *Eur J Nucl Med* 1983;8:485.
102. Krishnamurthy S, Krishnamurthy GT: Nuclear hepatology: Where is it heading now? *J Nucl Med* 1988;29:1144.
103. Brown PH, Juni JE, Lieberman DA, Krishnamurthy GT: Hepatocyte versus biliary disease: A distinction by deconvolutional analysis of technetium-99m IDA time-activity curves. *J Nucl Med* 1988;29:623.
104. Gambhir SS, Hawkins RA, Huang SC, Hall TR, et al.: Tracer kinetic modeling approaches for the quantification of hepatic function with technetium-99m DISIDA and scintigraphy. *J Nucl Med* 1989;30:1507.
105. Wiesner RH, LaRusso NF: Clinicopathologic features of the syndrome of primary sclerosing cholangitis. *Gastroenterology* 1980;79:200.
106. LaRusso NF, Wiesner RH, Ludwig J, MacCarty RL: Primary sclerosing cholangitis. *N Engl J Med* 1984;310:899.
107. Rodman CA, Keeffe EB, Lieberman DA, et al.: Diagnosis of sclerosing cholangitis with technetium 99m-labelled iminodiacetic acid planar and single photon emission computed tomographic scintigraphy. *Gastroenterology* 1987;92:777.
108. Keeffe EB, Lieberman DA, Krishnamurthy S, et al.: Primary biliary cirrhosis: Tc-99m IDA planar and SPECT scanning. *Radiology* 1988;166:143.
109. Sherlock S: Primary biliary cirrhosis, in Schiff L, Schiff ER, (eds.): *Diseases of the Liver.* Philadelphia, J.B. Lippincott 6th, 1987, p. 979.
110. Edmundson HA, Craig JR: Neoplasms of the liver, in Schiff L, Schiff ER, (eds.): *Diseases of the Liver.* Philadelphia, J.B. Lippincott 6th, 1987, p 1109.
111. Kotzerke J, Schwarzrock R, Krischek O, et al.: Technetium-99m DISIDA hepatobiliary agent in diagnosis of hepatocellular carcinoma, adenoma and focal nodular hyperplasia. *J Nucl Med* 1989;30:1278.
112. Kipper MS, Reed KR, Contardo M: Visualization of hepatic adenoma with Tc-99m diisopropyl IDA. *J Nucl Med* 1984;25:986.
113. Drane WE, Krasicky GA, Johnson DA: Radionuclide imaging of primary tumors and tumor-like conditions of the liver. *Clin Nucl Med* 1987;12:569.
114. Welch TJ, Sheedy PF, Johnson CM, et al.: Focal nodular hyperplasia and hepatic adenoma: Comparison of angiography, CT, US, and scintigraphy. *Radiology* 1985;156:593.

115. Boulahdour H, Cherqui D, Charlotte F, Rahmouni A, et al.: The hot spot hepatobiliary scan in focal nodular hyperplasia. *J Nucl Med* 1993;34:2105.
116. Intenzo CM, Hendricks P, Kim S, Park CH: Dynamic hepatobiliary scan appearance of hepatocellular carcinoma. *Clin Nucl Med* 1988;13:325.
117. Calvert X, Pons F, Bruix J, et al.: Technetium-99m DISIDA hepatobiliary agent in diagnosis of hepatocellular carcinoma: Relationship between detectability and tumor differentiation. *J Nucl Med* 1988;29:1916.
118. Wang P, Tai D, Chen H: Tc-99m HIDA hepatobiliary agent in the diagnosis of pulmonary metastasis from hepatocellular carcinoma. *Clin Nucl Med* 1991;16:120.
119. Coughlin JR, Mann DA: Detection of acute cholecystitis in children. *Can Assoc Radiol J* 1990;41:213.
120. Kasai M, Suzuki H, Ohashi E, et al. Technique and result of operative management of biliary atresia. *World J Surg* 1978;2:571.
121. Majd M, Reba RC, Altman RP: Hepatobiliary scintigraphy with 99mTc-PIPIDA in the evaluation of neonatal jaundice. *Pediatrics* 1981;67:140.
122. Majd M: Tc 99m-IDA scintigraphy in the evaluation of neonatal jaundice. *RadioGraphics* 1983;3:88.
123. Bar-Meir S, Baron J, Seligson U, et al.: Tc-99m-Hida cholescintigraphy in Dubin-Johnson and Rotor syndromes. *Radiology* 1982;142:743.
124. LeBouthillier G, Morais J, Picard M, et al.: Scintigraphic aspect of Rotor's disease with technetium 99m-mebrofenin. *J Nucl Med* 1992;33:1550.
125. Moreno AJ, Parker AL, Spicer MJ, Brown TJ: Scintigraphic and radiographic findings in Caroli's disease. *Am J Gastroenterol* 1984;79:299.
126. Ranson JHC: Etiological and prognostic factors in human acute pancreatitis: A review. *Am J Gastroenterol* 1982; 77:633.
127. Balart LA, Ferrante WA: Pathophysiology of acute and chronic pancreatitis. *Arch Intern Med* 1982;142:113.
128. Serafini AN, AL-Sheikh W, Barkin JS, et al.: Biliary scintigraphy in acute pancreatitis. *Radiology* 1982;144:591.
129. Shanley DJ, Buckner AB, Alexander HG: The scintigraphic "duodenal cut off sign" in acute pancreatitis. *Clin Nucl Med* 1991;16:223.
130. Kupfer M, Coletti P, Ralls P: Acute pancreatitis: Secondary findings on hepatobiliary scintigraphy. *Eur J Nucl Med* 1988;13:511.
131. Weissmann HS, Sugarman LA, Frank MS, Freeman LM: Serendipity in technetium-99m dimethyl iminodiacetic acid cholescintigraphy. *Radiology* 1980;135:449.
132. Slavin JD, Skarzynski JJ, Spencer RP: High incidence of gastric reflux during hepatobiliary imaging in pancreatitis. *Clin Nucl Med* 1985;10:5.
133. Nasrallah SM, Johnston GS, Gadacz TR, Kim KM: The significance of gastric bile reflux seen at endoscopy. *J Clin Gastroenterol* 1987;9:514.
134. Colletti PM, Barakos JA, Siegel ME, Ralls PW, Halls JM: Enterogastric reflux in suspected acute cholecystitis. *Clin Nucl Med* 1987;12:533.
135. Oates E, Achong DM: Incidence and significance of enterogastric reflux during morphine-augmented cholescintigraphy. *Clin Nucl Med* 1992;17:926.
136. Elgazzar AH, Fernandez-Ulloa M, Ryan JR, et al.: Significance of duodenogastric reflux (DGR) in the diagnosis of acute cholecystitis. *J Nucl Med* 1992;33:898.
137. Shih WJ, Fockele DS: Enterogastric reflux demonstrated by radionuclide hepatobiliary scintigraphy. *Semin Nucl Med* 1990;20:367.
138. Drane WE, Karvelis K, Johnson DA, Silverman ED: Scintigraphic evaluation of duodenogastric reflux: Problems, pitfalls, and technical review. *Clin Nucl Med* 1987;12:377.

29 The Pancreas

John C. Harbert

The pancreas is a mixed exocrine-endocrine gland, lying in the midline retroperitoneally below the liver. Carcinoma of the pancreas is the fourth leading cause of cancer deaths in men and the fifth in women, with fewer than 3% of patients surviving 5 years after diagnosis.[1] Unfortunately, the earliest clinical manifestations of pancreatic carcinoma, pain and jaundice, occur relatively late in the course of disease development; they also mimic the symptoms of pancreatitis. Such imaging procedures as computerized tomography (CT) and ultrasound (US), which are sensitive for visualizing pancreatic carcinomas, do not reliably distinguish tumor from inflammation. The principal thrust in developing radiopharmaceuticals to image the pancreas has been toward making this differentiation.

Other areas of clinical interest include the localization of pancreatic endocrine tumors and identifying pancreatic transplant complications.

PANCREATIC CARCINOMA VS. PANCREATITIS

Historical Background

The first attempts at pancreas imaging with radioactive zinc, manganese, and pancreatic antibodies were generally unsuccessful.[2,3] Later, analogs of natural amino acids were tested as potential imaging agents because of the high rate of protein synthesis in the pancreas. Scintigraphy with iodinated tyrosine, tryptophan, and phenylalanine, and with ^{18}F-fluorinated phenylalanine and tryptophan, was tried without success.[4–7] In 1961, Blau observed that ^{75}Se-selenomethionine was incorporated into proteins in a manner similar to ^{35}S-methionine.[8–10] Selenomethionine is produced by chemical synthesis or biosynthetically, using microorganisms grown on sulfur-deficient media. The analog retains the biological properties of the sulfur-containing amino acid.

An example of a ^{75}Se-selenomethionine scan taken with a planar scintillation camera is shown in Figure 1. Abnormal patterns (varying degrees of organ nonvisualization) are associated with pancreatitis,[11–14] pseudocyst,[15,16] diabetes,[17,18] and pancreatic neoplasms.[19–21] A normal pattern usually rules out pancreatic carcinoma, but an abnormal pattern is entirely nonspecific. The clinical usefulness of this tracer is further limited by its long effective half-life, which restricts the injectable dose to about 10 MBq (370 μCi), and many of the high-energy gamma rays of ^{75}Se are suboptimum for most scintillation cameras. As a screening test for pancreatic cancer, scanning with selenomethionine has had both low sensitivity and specificity.[22,23] This, and the fact that CT and magnetic resonance imaging (MRI) are much more sensitive are the reasons that these scans are seldom performed.

Other Developments

In a search for better pancreatic imaging agents, several amino acids labeled with ^{11}C have been tested, including ^{11}C-valine, ^{11}C-tryptophan and ^{11}C-aminocyclobutanecarboxylic acid.[24–26] Of these, ^{11}C-tryptophan appeared most promising because pancreas/liver ratios reach as high as 4 to 6.[27] Still, few studies with this tracer have been performed.

More recently, the use of ^{123}I-HIPDM to image the pancreas has assumed interest.[28,29] Yamamoto et al. found pancreas/liver ratios calculated from SPECT images in normal subjects were 1.26 $\pm$ 0.22 by 20 hours after injection (Fig. 2). The uptake of ^{123}I-HIPDM was reduced in pancreatitis (pancreas/liver = 0.74 $\pm$ $-$.15) but still visible. Uptake within pancreatic carcinoma was not detected (Fig. 3), leading these investigators to believe that the distinction between pancreatitis and pancreatic carcinoma may be made with this tracer.

Another approach to differentiating pancreatitis from pancreatic carcinoma has been reported by Yamamoto et al., using ^{18}F-FDG.[30] In this preliminary report, FDG was found to concentrate well in pancreatic carcinoma, but very little in normal glands or in pancreatitis. These results appear somewhat more promising than the use of ^{131}I-labeled CEA.[31]

Acute pancreatitis can be imaged with ^{67}Ga-citrate.[32] This is entirely a nonspecific labeling technique and the possibility of differentiating pancreatitis from pancreatic carcinoma is doubtful.

PANCREATIC ENDOCRINE TUMORS

Pancreatic endocrine tumors (also known as *islet cell* tumors) secrete several substances, including insulin, gastrin, somatostatin, glucagon, etc. Early attempts to image these tumors with ^{131}I-diphenylhydantoin were unsuccessful.[33] Recently, many of these tumors have been shown to have large numbers of somatostatin binding sites.[34,35] Early studies have demonstrated that these tumors can be imaged with ^{123}I-Tyr–3-

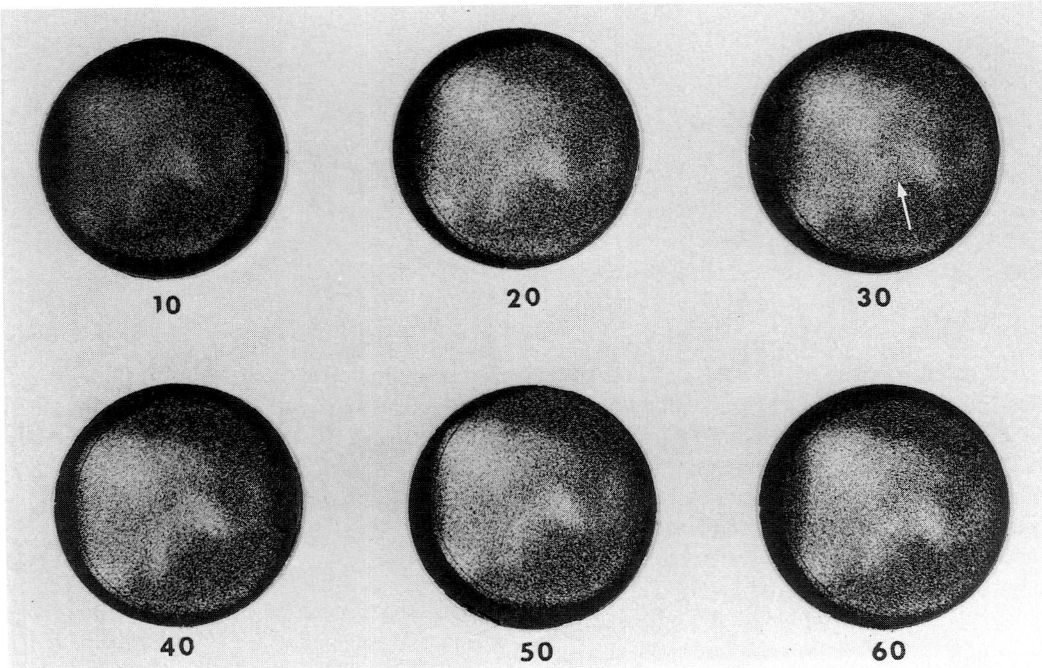

Figure 1. Normal planar images of the pancreas, integrated every 10 min following intravenous injection of 10 MBq (370 μCi) ^{75}Se-selenomethionine. Thinning of the pancreas over the aorta seen at 30 min (arrow) is a normal feature of planar images.

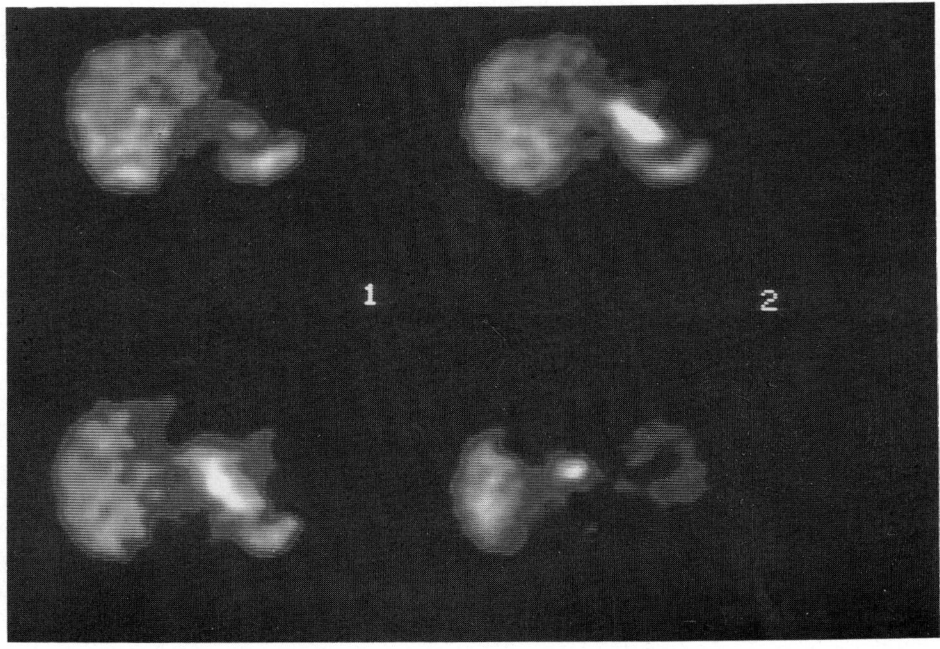

Figure 2. Transverse SPECT images in a normal adult obtained 3 hr following administration of 111 MBq (3 mCi) ^{123}I-HIPDM. The pancreatic tail, body, and head are clearly imaged without overlap of radioactivity in the liver and spleen (Reproduced with permission of Yamamoto et al.[29]). (See Plate 31.)

A

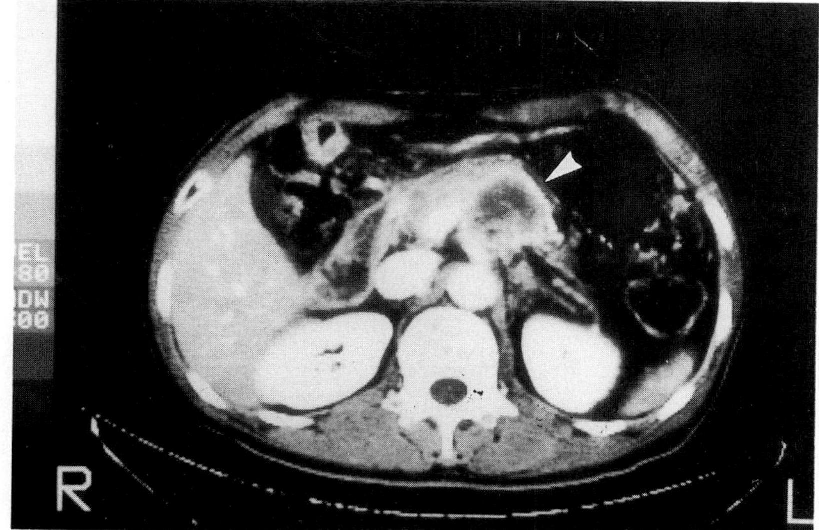

B

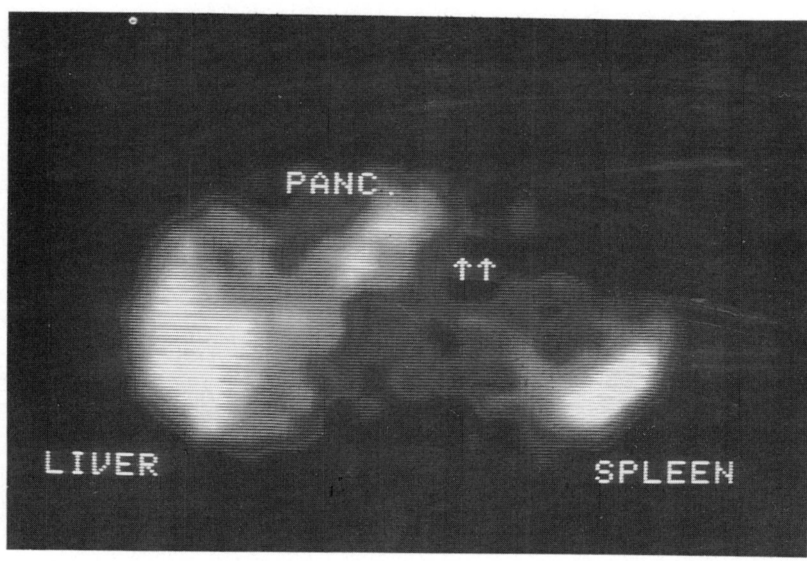

Figure 3. **(A).** Transverse CT scan showing low-density carcinoma in body of the pancreas (arrow head). **(B).** Transverse SPECT image showing absent uptake of ^{123}I-HIPDM in the tumor (double arrows) (Reproduced with permission of Yamamoto et al.[29]). (See Plate 32.)

octreotide, an analog of the neuropeptide somatostatin.[36,37] Because of the high density of receptors, some tumors as small as 1 cm can be imaged. The entire body can be surveyed in total body scans, while this is not easily accomplished with CT and MR imaging. Somatostatin-receptor imaging is further discussed in Chapter 36.

PANCREATIC TRANSPLANT IMAGING

Pancreatic transplants have primarily been reserved for those with severe insulin-dependent diabetes. Because these patients often have concomitant renal disease, simultaneous renal allografts are common. In some cases, the spleen and a portion of the duodenum are included in the transplant to increase the blood supply and assist the exocrine drainage functions, respectively. Pancreatic transplants share many of the complications of renal transplants: ischemia, rejection, anastomotic leaks, infections, and vascular thrombosis. Pancreatitis and anastomotic leaks, with activation of the exocrine drainage causing ascites and parapancreatic fluid collection around extraperitoneal transplants, are unique complications of pancreatic grafts.[38]

The diagnosis of transplant failure is often difficult because biopsies are usually contraindicated and measures of serum glucose, C-peptide, and urine amylase are often unreliable indicators. On the other hand, early identification of complications is essential in initiating prompt therapy that will preserve the transplant. The three principal imaging procedures employed to evaluate pancreatic transplants have

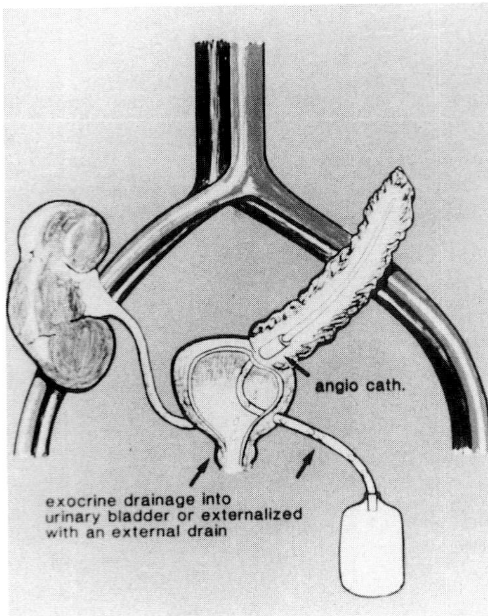

Figure 4. Diagram showing combined renal and pancreatic transplants in the iliac fossae; note the angiographic catheter within the pancreas to aid exocrine drainage. (Reproduced with permission of A. Erica George, M.D., St. Louis University Medical Center.)

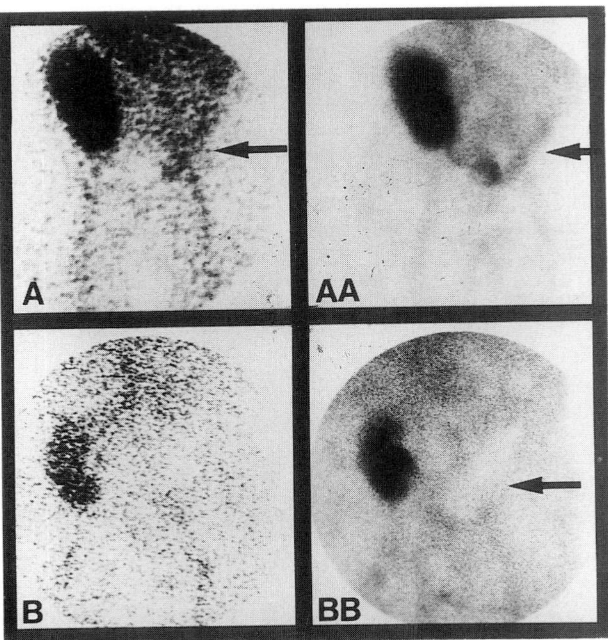

Figure 5. Dynamic and blood pool images following injection of 555 MBq (15 mCi) ^{99m}Tc-glucoheptonate. **(A).** Normal transplant perfusion; arrow points to the pancreas allograft. **(AA).** Blood pool image in same patient. **(B).** Patient with infarcted, nonviable pancreatic transplant demonstrating absent perfusion. **(BB).** Same patient showing large photopenic defect in the blood pool image (arrow). (Reproduced with permission of A. Erica George, M.D.)

been ultrasound, MRI, and radionuclide imaging. Radionuclide imaging procedures have focused on assessing (1) transplant function, (2) perfusion and, (3) cell-mediated rejection.

Transplant Function

The uptake of ^{75}Se-selenomethionine by the graft has been measured to assess overall graft function.[39,40] Unfortunately, nearly 90% of islet-cell function must be compromised before gross reduction of the tracer is apparent and this coincides with an increase in serum glucose levels. Therefore, this is not a useful method for the early detection of transplant rejection.

Transplant Perfusion

Most investigators have sought to evaluate pancreatic transplants using radionuclide perfusion studies to assess transplant blood flow in combination with urine amylase and serum creatinine.[41] Dynamic and equilibrium blood flow studies with ^{99m}Tc-DTPA (740 MBq) are used to assess both pancreatic and renal allografts.[42,43] ^{99m}Tc-glucoheptonate,[38] a combination of ^{99m}Tc-glucoheptonate and ^{99m}Tc-sulfur colloid[44] and ^{201}Th scintigraphy[45] have also been used. These studies have been quite sensitive in detecting rejection and vascular thrombosis, although they cannot distinguish between the two (Fig. 4, 5). This is not so important because that distinction can easily be made by color doppler US.

Cell-Mediated Rejection

Because the earliest phase of organ rejection consists of interstitial cellular infiltrates and thrombotic vasculitis, it is reasonable to suppose that labeled platelets might accumulate in the rejected pancreas.[46–49] Not only do platelets accumulate early in the rejecting pancreas, there also appears to be the possibility of distinguishing rejection from thrombosis and even parapancreatic hematomas.[49]

Catafau et al. labeled platelets with ^{111}In and imaged repeatedly over several days.[49] Using area-of-interest analysis, they calculated allograft/adjacent tissues ratios. Clinically rejecting kidneys had diffuse uptake of platelets with ratios greater than 1.4, while ratios in unaffected transplants were generally less than 1.1.

Monitoring pancreatic grafts with duplex ultrasound increases the ability to differentiate between pancreatitis and rejection.[50] Blood flow is reduced in rejection and often normal in cases of acute pancreatitis. Correlative imaging with ultrasound and scintigraphic techniques promises improved specificity of posttransplant complications.

REFERENCES

1. Ries LAG, Hankey BF, Miller BA, et al. *Cancer Statistics Review 1973-88*. Washington, DC: National Cancer Institute, NIH Pub. No. 91-2789, 1991.

2. Meschan I, et al. The utilization of radioactive zinc and manganese in an effort to visualize the pancreas. *Radiology* 1959;73:62.
3. Shapiro R. Radiopacification of the pancreas: a review of experimental efforts. *Semin Roentgenol* 1968;3:318.
4. Taylor DM, Cottrall MF. *Radiopharmaceuticals and Labeled Compounds*. Vol. I. Vienna, I.A.E.A., 1973, p 433.
5. Ullberg S, Blomquist L. Selective localization to pancreas of radioiodinated phenylalanine analogues. *Acta Pharm Suec* 1968;5:45.
6. Varma VM, et al. Pancreatic concentration of ^{125}I-labeled phenylalanine in mice. *J Nucl Med* 1969;10:219.
7. Cottrall MF, Taylor DM, McElwain TJ. Investigations of ^{18}F–p–fluorophenylalanine for pancreas scanning. *Br J Radiol* 1973;46: 277.
8. Blau M. Biosynthesis of [^{75}Se]-selenomethionine and [^{75}Se]-selenocystine. *Biochem Biophys Acta* 1968;49:389.
9. Blau M, Manske RF. The pancreas specificity of ^{75}Se-methionine. *J Nucl Med* 1961;2:102.
10. Blau M, Bender MA. ^{75}Se-methionine for visualization of the pancreas by isotope scanning. *Radiology* 1962;78:874.
11. Blanquet PC, et al. Intérêt et limites de la scintigraphie du pancréas. *Acta Gastroenterol Belg* 1970;33:409.
12. Leger L, Roucayrol JC, Leuriot JP. Scintigraphie dans les pancréatitis aigues. *Presse Med* 1970;78:1441.
13. Bouchier IAD. Radiologic and isotopic investigation of the pancreas. *Proc R Soc Med* 1970;63:434.
14. Desgrez A, et al. Pancréas, scintigraphie et soustraction électronique. *Nouv Presse Med* 1972;1:1003.
15. Mattar AG, Prezio JA. Visualization of pancreatic pseudocyst. *J Nucl Med* 1975;16:326.
16. Melmed RN, Agnew JE, Bouchier IAD. The normal and abnormal pancreatic scan. *Q J Med* 1968;37:607.
17. Espiritu CR, Rolfs HE. Diagnostic accuracy of pancreatic scanning. *Surg J Dig Dis* 1972;17:539.
18. Spencer AM, et al. Pancreatic scanning as a diagnostic tool in the district general hospital. *Br Med J* 1974;4:153.
19. Blanquet PC, et al. Scintigraphie pancréatique par soustraction électronique. A propos de 200 examens. *Presse Med* 1969;77:1237.
20. Fink S, et al. Current status of dual-channel pancreas scanning. *J Nucl Med* 1969;10:78.
21. McCarthy DM, et al. ^{75}Se-selenomethionine scanning in the diagnosis of tumors of the pancreas and adjacent viscera: the use of the test and its impact on survival. *Gut* 1972;13:75.
22. Hall FJ, Cooper M, Hughes RG, et al. Pancreatic cancer screening: Analysis of the problem and the role of radionuclide imaging. *Am J Surg* 1977;134:543.
23. Barkin J, et al. Computerized tomography, diagnostic ultrasound, and radionuclide scanning. Comparison of efficacy in diagnosis of pancreatic carcinoma. *JAMA* 1977;238:2040.
24. Washburn LC, et al. (1-^{11}C)DL-valine, a potential pancreas-imaging agent. *J Nucl Med* 1978;19:77.
25. Hayes RL, et al. Synthesis and purification of ^{11}C-carboxyl-labeled amino acids. *Int J Appl Radiat Isotop* 1978;29:186.
26. Buonocore E, Hübner KF. Positron-emission computed tomography of the pancreas: A preliminary study. *Radiology* 1979;133:195.
27. Hübner KF, Andrews GA, Buonocore E, et al. Carbon-11-labeled amino acids for the rectilinear and positron tomographic imaging of the human pancreas. *J Nucl Med* 1979;20:507.
28. Kubota K, Som P, Brill AB, et al. Comparative dual-tracer studies of carbon-14-tryptophan and iodine-131 HIPDM in animal models of pancreatic diseases. *J Nucl Med* 1989;30:1848.
29. Yamamoto K, Shibata T, Saji H, et al. Human pancreas scintigraphy using iodine-123-labeled HIPDM and SPECT. *J Nucl Med* 1990;31:1015.
30. Yamamoto K, Kubo S, Mukai T, et al. Differential diagnosis of pancreas cancer from chronic pancreatitis with F-18 FDG PET study (abs). *J Nucl Med* 1989;30:887.
31. Goldenberg DM, Goldenbert H, Lee RE, Ford EH. Imaging of pancreatic cancer with radiolabeled antibodies to CEA (abs). *J Nucl Med* 1988;29:833.
32. Aburano T, Yokoyama K, Hisada K, et al. The role of Ga-67 citrate imaging in pancreatitis. *Clin Nucl Med* 1988;13:808.
33. Balachandran S, et al. Tissue distribution of ^{14}C-, ^{124}I- and ^{131}I-diphenylhydantoin in the toadfish, rat and human with insulinomas. *J Nucl Med* 1975;16:775.
34. Reubi J-C, Hacki WH, Lamberts SW. Hormone-producing gastrointestinal tumors contain a high density of somatostatin receptors. *J Clin Endocrinol Metab* 1987;65:1127.
35. Reubi J-C, Maurer R, von Werder K, et al. Somatostatin receptors in human endocrine tumors. *Cancer Res* 1987;47:551.
36. Lamberts SWJ, Bakker WH, Reubi J-C, Krenning EP. Somatostatin-receptor imaging in the localization of endocrine tumors. *Engl J Med* 1990;18:1246.
37. Krenning EP, Bakker WH, Breeman WAP, et al. Localisation of endocrine-related tumours with radioiodinated analogue of somatostatin. *Lancet* 1989;1:242.
38. Patel B, Markivee CR, Mahanta B, et al. Pancreatic transplantation: Scintigraphy, US, and CT. *Radiology* 1988;167:685.
39. Svahn T, Lewander R, Hardstedt C, et al. Angiography and scintigraphy of human pancreatic allografts. *Acta Radiol {Diagn} (Stockh)* 1977;19:297.
40. Toledo-Pereira LH, Kristen KT, Mittal VK. Scintigraphy of pancreatic transplants. *Am J Roentgenol* 1982;138:621.
41. Stratta RJ, Sollinger HW, Perlman SB, D'Allessandro AM. Early detection of rejection in pancreas transplantation. *Diabetes* 1989;38(suppl):63.
42. Shulkin BL, Dafoe DC, Wahl RL. Simultaneous pancreatic-renal transplant scintigraphy. *Am J Roentgenol* 1986;138:1193.
43. Yuh WTC, Wiese JA, Abu-Yousef MM, et al. Pancreatic transplant imaging. *Radiology* 1988;167:679.
44. George EA, Salimi Z, Carney K, et al. Radionuclide surveillance of the allografted pancreas. *Am J Roentgenol* 1988;150:811.
45. Hirsch H, Fernandez-Ulloa M, Munda R, et al. Diagnosis of segmental necrosis in a pancreas transplant by Thallium-201 perfusion scintigraphy. *J Nucl Med* 1991;32:1605.
46. Sollinger HW, Lieberman LM, Kanps D, et al. Diagnosis of early pancreas allograft rejection with indium-111-oxine labeled platelets. *Transplant Proc* 1984;16:785.
47. Jurewicz WA, Buckels JAC, Dykes JGA, et al. 111-Indium platelets in monitoring pancreatic allografts in man. *Br J Surg* 1985;72:228.
48. Jurewicz WA, Buckels JAC, Dykes JGA, et al. Indium 111 labeled platelets in monitoring pancreatic transplants in humans. *Transplant Proc* 1984;16:720.
49. Catafau AM, Lomena FJ, Ricart MJ, et al. Indium-111-labeled platelets in monitoring human pancreatic transplants. *J Nucl Med* 1989;30:1470.
50. Patel B, Wolverson M, Nahanta B. Pancreatic transplant rejection: Assessment with duplex US. *Radiology* 1989;173:131.

30 The Genitourinary System

John C. Harbert, Mary P. Andrich, Patrick J. Peller

The applications of nuclear medicine techniques to nephrologic and urologic problems are more varied than for most other organ systems. Imaging procedures involve the renal cortex, medulla, collecting system, bladder, penis, and testes. Functional studies measure renal plasma flow, glomerular filtration rates, renal transit times, and bladder kinetics (including residual urine). This chapter deals with the selection of radiopharmaceuticals, renal function studies, and imaging of genitourinary organs.

RADIOPHARMACEUTICALS

Agents Cleared by Effective Renal Plasma Flow

In the term *effective renal plasma flow* (ERPF), "effective" means the blood flow to renal parenchyma, excluding flow to capsule and interstitial tissue, and "plasma" indicates that only plasma activity is assayed. The concept derives from plasma clearance studies and indicates the volume of plasma flowing through the kidney each minute that would account for the measured quantity of reagent excreted per minute in the urine.

Orthoiodohippurate (OIH), also known as Hippuran, has been used extensively to measure renal plasma flow. Smith et al. recognized that OIH is an analog of para-aminohippuric acid (PAH).[1] PAH was used only because it could be analyzed chemically more easily than OIH. With the development of radionuclide labeling and counting techniques, however, OIH came to be preferred. Radiolabeled OIH was first synthesized by Tubis et al. using ^{131}I.[2] Nordyke et al. investigated ^{131}I-OIH for renographic studies, employing techniques similar to those previously described by Taplin et al.[3,4] Because it is excreted by both the glomeruli (20%) and the renal tubules (80%), is not secreted significantly by other organs, and has a high extraction efficiency from renal arterialblood (70 to 90%), OIH was for many years the principal radiopharmaceutical used to evaluate many renal functional disorders.

Normal adult OIH clearance values approximate 500 mL of plasma per minute, and 70% of the injected dose appears in the urine 35 minutes after injection. Maximum concentration within the kidney is reached 2.5 to 3.4 minutes after injection, depending on the degree of hydration of the patient.

The principal drawback limiting the use of ^{131}I-OIH was the high-energy (364 keV) gamma photon, which limits image spatial resolution, and the emission of a beta particle, which substantially increases radiation absorbed dose. ^{123}I-OIH has much better imaging properties and lacks beta emission. However, it is much more costly, has a short 13-hour half-life, and is no longer commercially available in the United States.

Because imaging so often forms an integral part of renal functional studies, ^{99m}Tc-labeled renal tubular agents were sought. This goal was realized by Fritzberg et al., who synthesized the triamide mercaptide (N_3S) ligand, benzoyl mercaptoacetyltriglycine (MAG_3).[5] This agent, shown in Figure 1, has largely replaced OIH. The development and comparison with other radiopharmaceuticals has been extensively reviewed elsewhere.[6,7] In comparison with OIH, the plasma clearance of MAG_3 is slower (0.59), protein binding is higher (90 vs 70%), red blood cell uptake is lower (5 vs 15%), and affinity for tubular transport is lower.[8–11] Despite 90% protein binding, more than 50% of MAG_3 is extracted on each pass through the kidneys, compared to only 20% for DTPA.[12] By three hours, almost 90% of the injected dose has been excreted.

MAG_3 combines the favorable imaging properties of ^{99m}Tc with rapid tubular secretion. Renograms are similar to those of OIH, but of much greater count density and better anatomic resolution (Figs. 2 and 3), similar to DTPA (Fig. 4).[13–15] However, MAG_3 has a higher clearance rate than DTPA due to its active tubular secretion, and yields better images than DTPA in patients with decreased renal function.[15–17]

Agents Cleared by Glomerular Filtration

Several radiopharmaceuticals have been used to measure *glomerular filtration rate* (GFR) in man, including ^{131}I-diatrizoate (Hypaque),[18] ^{14}C-inulin,[19] ^{131}I-iothalamate,[20] vitamin B_{12} labeled with various isotopes of cobalt,[21] penicillin, and diethylenetriaminepentaacetic acid (DTPA) chelated to various radionuclides.[22] Of these, only DTPA is commonly used.

The plasma disappearance of ^{99m}Tc-DTPA resolves into three clearance exponents with half-times of approximately 10, 90, and 600 min, respectively. When ^{99m}Tc-DTPA is injected, a small fraction of the activity (presumably an impurity) is bound to plasma proteins. This causes an error in the calculation of glomerular filtration rate from plasma clearance. However, if the fraction is known, it can be corrected. This fraction is usually determined by chromatography or gel filtration.[23]

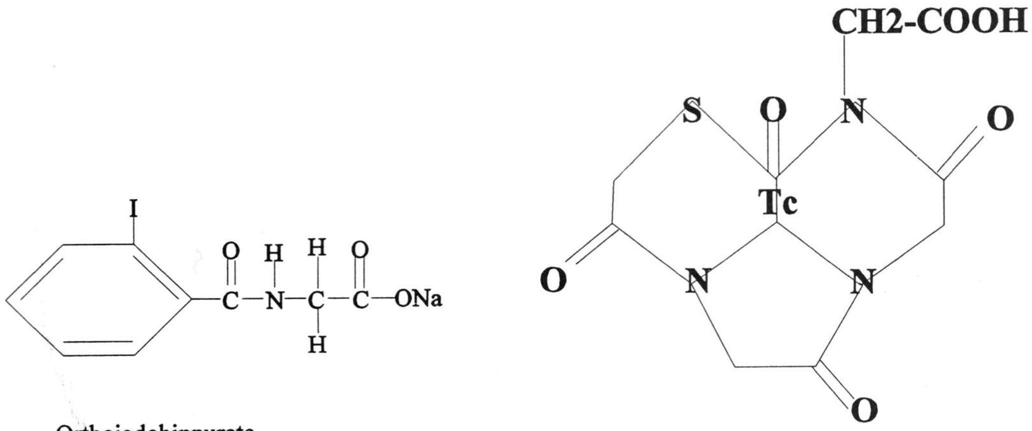

Figure 1. Structures of Orthoiodohippurate (OIH) and ^{99m}Tc-mercaptoacetyltriglycine (MAG_3).

Agents Used for Renal Scintigraphy

Besides DTPA and MAG_3, there are two other commonly used radiopharmaceuticals for renal scintigraphy: glucoheptonate (glucose mono-carboxylic acid, or GHA) and 2,3-dimercaptosuccinic acid (DMSA).[24,25] These radiopharmaceuticals bind to the renal tubular cells.

The distribution of DMSA in the kidney is similar to that of chlormerodrin. It concentrates largely in the renal cortex and to a lesser degree in the liver. Its body retention is considerably longer than that of DTPA or GHA because of its strong binding to plasma proteins. This protein binding may account for its hepatic uptake. About one half of the injected dose binds to sulfhydryl in the renal cortex 6 hours after injection. Renal extraction is slow, 4 to 5% on each pass through the kidneys; only about one third of the dose appears in the urine 24 hours after injection.[26] Using a combination of ^{14}C and ^{99m}Tc labels, Moretti et al. found that the molecule apparently splits upon reaching the kidney; one moiety binds to renal tubular cells and the other is excreted.[27] Consequently, the renal cortex can be imaged (Fig. 5) and urinary excretion can be evaluated in the same study. DMSA can also be used to measure differential renal function, but it is not useful in measuring precise renal function.[28]

GHA is both filtered at the glomerulus and bound by the tubules. About 50% of the injected dose is protein bound, leading to partial glomerular filtration. Early imaging allows assessment of perfusion, excretion, and transit through the collecting system (Fig. 6). At 2 hours, approximately 10% is bound to renal tubules, significantly less than DMSA.[29] Delayed imaging at 2 to 4 hours demonstrates renal parenchyma after collecting system activity has cleared.

Both GHA and DMSA can be easily prepared by injecting sterile pertechnetate into vials containing these reagents. Because some kits of DMSA may deteriorate in vitro it is necessary to check the kit insert for acceptable periods of injection after preparation. GHA is stable up to 6 hours after preparation.

Raynaud et al. observed that ^{201}Tl uptake by the kidney is sufficiently high to be suitable for renal scintigraphy.[30] Although the distribution is pan-parenchymal for the first few hours after injection, it becomes largely medullary thereafter.

Several other radiopharmaceuticals have been used for renal imaging, including: radiomercury-labeled chlormerodrin,[31] mercuric chloride,[32] ^{99m}Tc-iron ascorbate, calcium gluconate,[34] and various chelates of EDTA.[35] None of these radiopharmaceuticals is widely used at this time.

QUANTIFICATION OF RENAL FUNCTION

Historically, nuclear medicine techniques have been employed to quantify renal function since the 1950's.[21] Data from external probes produced time-activity curves to estimate renal function. The introduction of ^{131}I-OIH and agents filtered at the glomerulus allowed measurement of renal blood flow and GFR. Currently, computers interfaced with scintillation cameras are used in a variety of clinically useful methods of renal quantification.

RENAL FUNCTION STUDIES

Continuous Infusion Clearance Techniques

The use of radiolabeled OIH and iothalamate greatly increased the ease and accuracy of renal function studies, which formerly required nearly an entire day to perform. The mathematical analysis is relatively simple:

$$\text{Clearance} = \frac{U \times V}{P}$$

where:

Clearance = mL of plasma cleared per min, U = urine concentration, V = mL of urine excreted per min, and P = plasma concentration.

To avoid the problem of continuously changing plasma con-

A

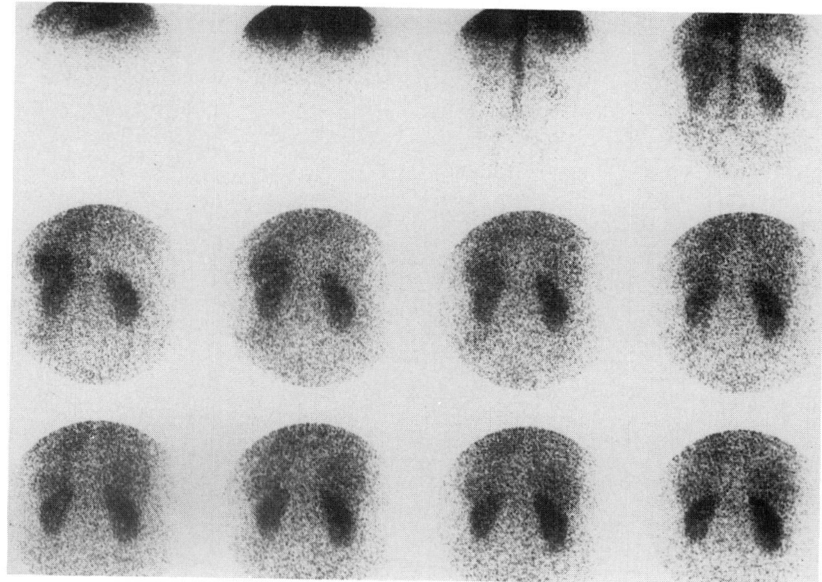

B

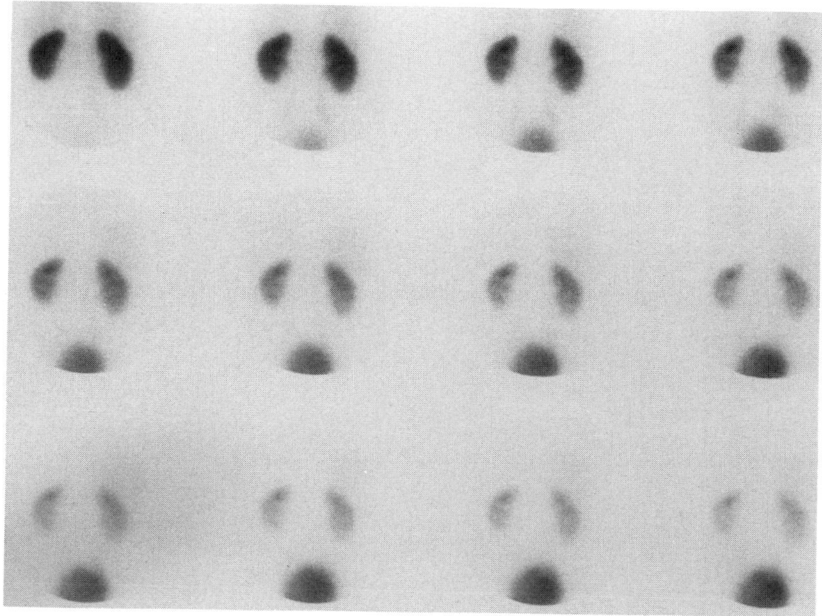

Figure 2. Normal ^{99m}Tc-MAG_3 study. **(A).** Sequential 3-sec images in the posterior projection showing symmetric blood flow to the kidneys and early activity in the spleen above the left kidney. Hepatic flow is seen in frame 7, because perfusion is primarily venous in origin. **(B).** Peak MAG_3 extraction occurs at 3 min (first frame). Ureteral transit of excreted tracer is rapid and excellent cortical detail are characteristic of this radiopharmaceutical.

centration, clearance studies were most commonly performed by continuous intravenous infusion of the test substance (OIH or iothalamate) until a steady concentration in the plasma was reached. At that point, 3 sequential 20-minute total collections of urine were obtained from the catheterized bladder or, if differential studies were required, ureteral catheters. Two or more timed plasma samples were taken to determine the plasma concentration. The values of ERPF or GFR were then determined by the foregoing equation.

Although they were once the standard for ERPF and GFR techniques, continuous infusion studies are now performed infrequently; single-injection techniques have become the standard. These 2 methods do not always yield the same results, because they do not necessarily measure the same aspects of renal function. Continuous infusion clearances of PAH measure the transit time from plasma to bladder without regard for possible fixation of the tracer to the renal parenchyma, as occurs in acute tubular necrosis. Plasma disappearance curves, on the other hand, measure the passage of tracer from plasma to the point of kidney extraction only.

SINGLE-INJECTION TECHNIQUE

ERPF and GFR determinations are greatly simplified by the use of single-injection techniques based on compartmen-

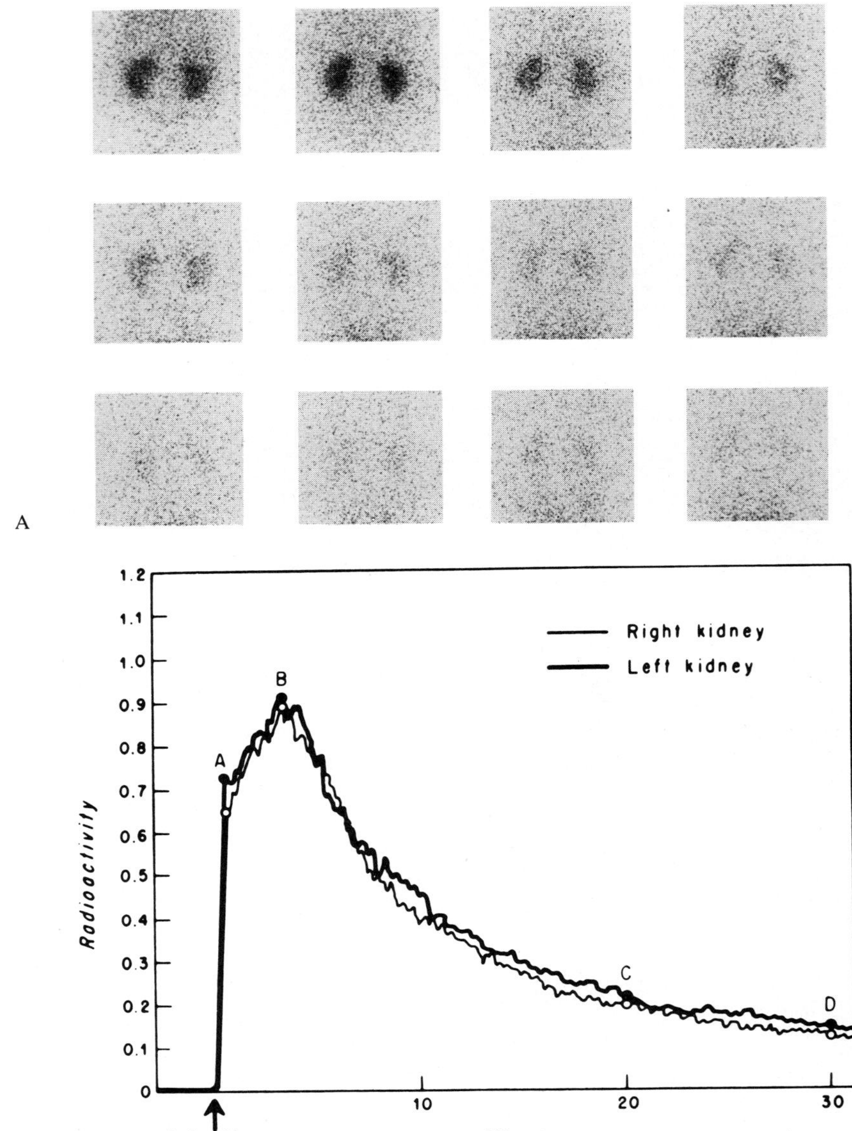

Figure 3. (A). Normal ^{131}I-OIH study. Sequential two-minute images in the posterior projection reveal peak tracer extraction in the second frame with symmetric renal activity. **(B).** Normal OIH time-activity curve, or renogram. A is the initial deflection, B is the point of maximum intensity and C and D are the 20- and 30-min activities, respectively.

tal analysis. The use of external detectors obviates the need for urine collections. The model shown in Figure 7 reflects the interchange between the plasma compartment V_1 and a second pool. There is a continuous one-way clearance pathway (the kidneys) from the plasma to the urine. The plasma clearance is described by a biexponential curve illustrated in Figure 8.

The flow ($F_{1\text{-}3}$) from the injected volume (V_1) to the kidneys (V_3) can be calculated from the disappearance rates derived from the formula of Sapirstein[36]:

$$F_{1\text{-}3}(\text{Clearance}) \frac{I \times \lambda_a \times \lambda_b}{(A \times \lambda_b) + (B \times \lambda_b)} \tag{1}$$

where I represents the total injected dose in cpm, A and B represent Y intercepts, and λ_a and λ_b represent the respective rate constants. Alternatively, the following relationship can be used:

$$\text{Clearance} = \frac{0.693\, I}{(A \times T_{1/2}A) + (B \times T_{1/2}B)} \tag{2}$$

where I, A, and B are defined as in formula (1), $T_{1/2}\,A$ and $T_{1/2}\,B$ are the respective half-times of the two disappearance rates.

Estimations of ERPF and GFR have been further simplified by the introduction of a single-sample technique by Tauxe et al.[37] A high degree of correlation has been found between ERPF as determined by the continuous infusion of PAH and OIH clearances and the reciprocal of the concentration in the plasma at 44 min after injection of radioiodine-labeled OIH.[38,39] The usefulness of the single-sample tech-

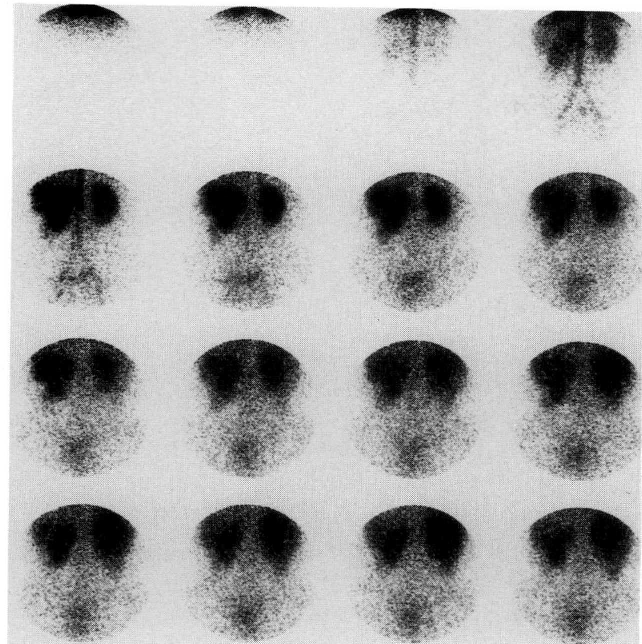

A

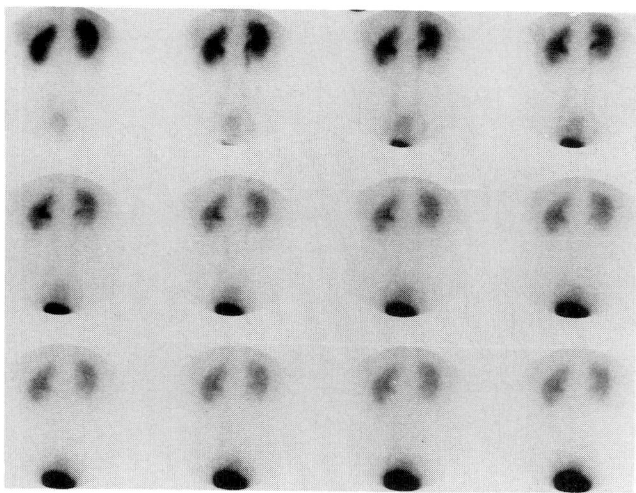

B

Figure 4. Normal ^{99m}Tc-DTPA study. **(A).** Sequential 3-sec images in the posterior position; renal activity is observed one frame after initial aortic activity. **(B).** Serial 2-min images show rapid extraction, with high renal:background ratio in frame one with prompt excretion evident in frame two. An incidental finding is the persistent blood pool activity seen in the patient's uterine tumor located cephalad to the bladder. A gravid uterus has a similar appearance.

nique for measuring ERPF has been confirmed by other investigators. Botsch et al. found that the best sampling time was 45 min with the following regression equation:[40]

$$\mathrm{ERPF} = 10 + 6.81\,X - 0.0165\,X^2$$

where X equals the theoretical volume of distribution in liters:

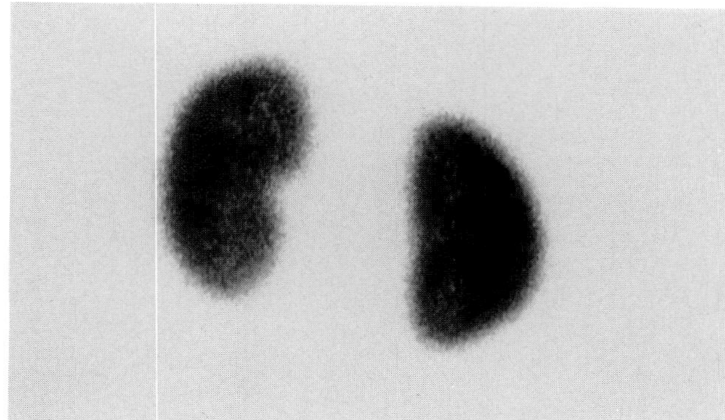

Figure 5. Normal DMSA scintigraphy, 3-hr image, posterior projection.

$$V_{45} = \frac{\text{injected dose cps}}{\text{plasma cps/mL}} \div 1000$$

These formulas have been validated only in individuals over 13 years of age and apply to OIH kinetics. Single-sample regression equations have been derived for use in pediatric nephrologic patients using height-weight scaling, so that adult data can be applied to pediatric patients. Scaled times will, thus, vary approximately as the cube root of the body weight, so that 60 min for a 70-kg adult corresponds to 28 min for a 7-kg child.[41]

In adults, the normal ERPF as derived from kidney donors can best be expressed as a function of age:[42]
Males: $534 + 10.01\,(\text{age}) - 0.19\,(\text{age})^2$

$$S_{y..x} = 88.3\ \text{mL/min}$$

where $S_{y.x}$ = standard error of estimate.
Females: $636 + 0.57\,(\text{age}) - 0.07\,(\text{age})^2$;

$$S_{y.x} = 88.4\ \text{mL/min}$$

Within the first postoperative week after nephrectomy, the ERPF of the remaining kidney usually increases by one third, after which time it is usually stable:
Males: $502 + 0.10\,(\text{age}) - 0.06\,(\text{age})^2$;

$$S_{y.x} = 70.1\ \text{mL/min}$$

Females: $368 + 4.44\,(\text{age}) - 0.11\,(\text{age})^2$;

$$S_{y.x} = 70.5\ \text{mL/min}$$

Often such values are useful in determining, in a patient with one diseased kidney, whether the healthy kidney has undergone full compensation. Also, the preceding formulas are useful in predicting the ERPF of a healthy kidney when a diseased kidney is to be removed.

Prediction of Function in the Residual Kidney after Unilateral Nephrectomy

Downing et al. observed that if global ERPF and differential function are within normal limits prior to unilateral nephrectomy, a normal compensatory increase in ERPF in the re-

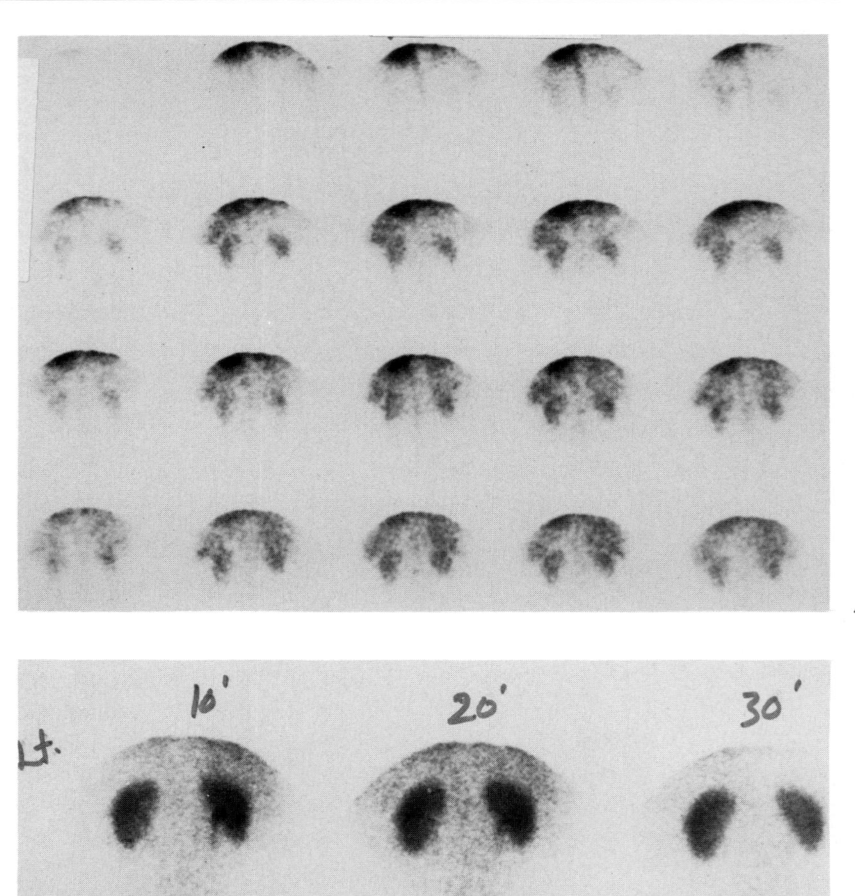

A

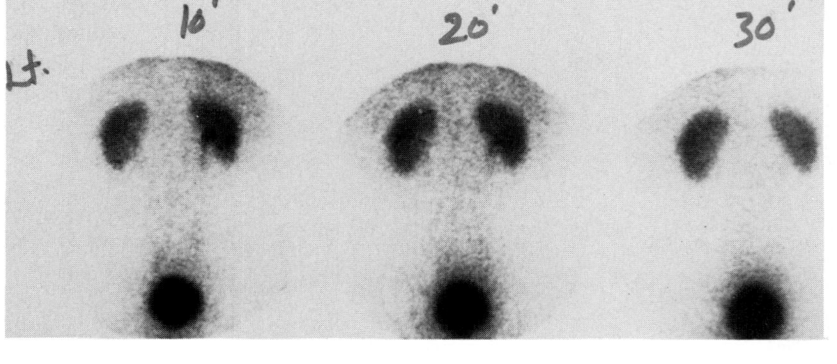

B

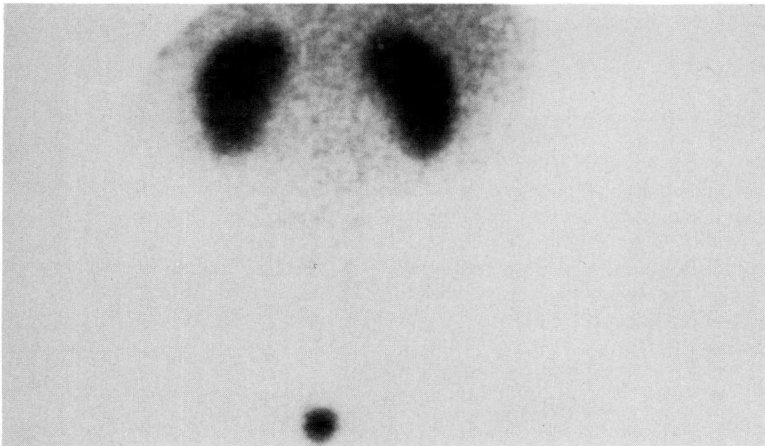

Figure 6. Normal ^{99m}Tc-GHA study. **(A).** Sequential 2-sec images demonstrate symmetric perfusion with renal activity seen 5–6 sec after aortic activity. **(B).** Static posterior images at 10, 20, 30, and 40 min show excretion by glomerular filtration in the earlier images and normal cortical retention at 40 min (postvoid image).

maining kidney can be expected.[43] This clinical problem might arise in a patient with a kidney containing a small tumor that has not significantly altered overall function. If global ERPF is somewhat decreased, removal of one of the pair may not result in compensation in the remaining kidney. This lack of compensation may also occur if both kidneys are somewhat diseased (e.g., bilateral nephrolithiasis). If ERPF in the kidney to be removed is greatly decreased, ERPF in the remaining kidney may not increase, because it may already have undergone maximal compensation. A

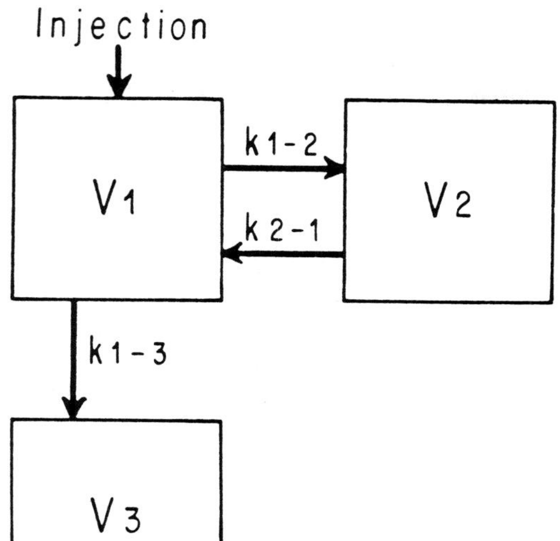

Figure 7. Compartment model of OIH kinetics. The first volume V_1, exchanges with a theoretic volume V_2. The injected OIH is excreted into an end volume, V_3. The product ($k_{1\text{-}3} \times V_1$) represents effective renal plasma flow.

decrease in ERPF—often to azotemic levels—may be expected if a unilaterally diseased kidney is removed from a hypertensive patient whose blood pressure returns to normal postoperatively.

The filtration fraction (GFR/ERPF) is calculated easily by using simultaneous estimates of each factor (e.g., ^{99m}Tc-DTPA and ^{131}I-OIH). The usefulness of the filtration fraction in discriminating various clinical entities remains to be explored, however.

Bianchi et al. have found the filtration fraction to be useful in certain aspects of renovascular hypertension.[44] This parameter is also useful in differentiating certain glomerulopathies and transplant rejection processes, and is fairly constant throughout a wide spectrum of clinical problems. These findings suggest that GFR and ERPF are of equal diagnostic use. When the two are discordant, however, the ERPF is more discriminating because it is usually more diminished than the GFR. Also, the ERPF is more easily and accurately measured.

Differential blood flow to the kidneys can be calculated from the integrated counts over the first 1 to 2 min of the OIH time-activity curve, using appropriate background subtraction.[45]

Quantification of Renal Function with ^{99m}Tc-MAG$_3$
There has been a great deal of interest in using the clearance of ^{99m}Tc-MAG$_3$ to quantify renal function, because simultaneous blood flow and highly resolved functional imaging can be accomplished at the same time that function parameters are obtained. The clearance kinetics of MAG$_3$ are quite different from those of OIH (a measure of ERPF) and ^{99m}Tc-DTPA (a measure of GFR). However the clearance of MAG$_3$ is proportional to both in most patients.[6] One approach to derive useful clinical measurements that would preserve the traditional concept of ERPF would be to convert MAG$_3$ clearance to estimated ERPF. In a large number of patients, ERPF calculated from a single sample of OIH at 44 minutes correlated well (r = 0.96) with values obtained from MAG$_3$ plasma levels corrected by the proportionality constant 0.563.[46] Corrected MAG$_3$ plasma activity can then be used with published formulas for calculations of ERPF.[46–48] Others have obtained nearly identical values for the constant.[49]

Probably the most meaningful functional measurement, however, is merely to express renal function in terms of "MAG$_3$ clearance" without the need for corrections, particularly in patients who have not had prior measurements that require comparisons to follow the course of disease. For

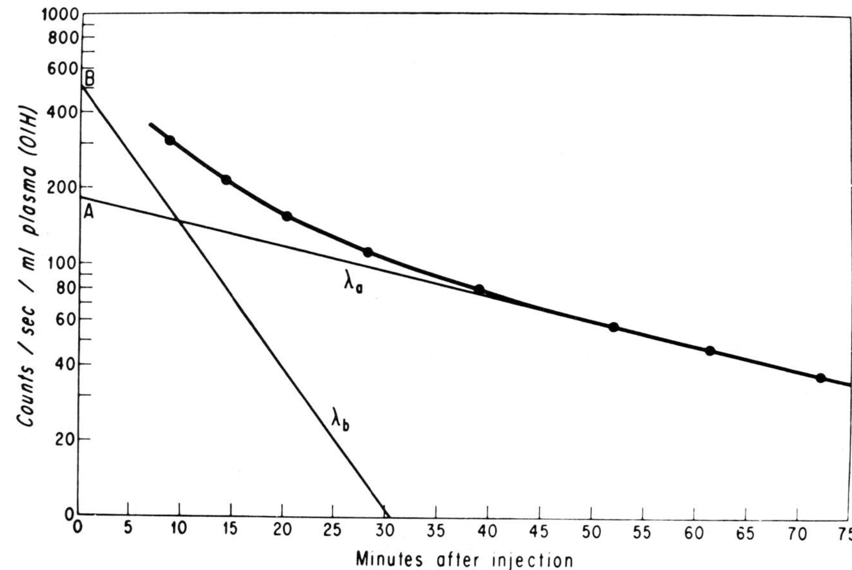

Figure 8. The plasma disappearance of injected ^{131}I-OIH. The fractional disappearance rates ($0.693/T_{1/2}$) are designated λ_a and λ_b with intercepts *A* and *B*.

such purposes, each laboratory would need to establish its own range of normal values. This is necessary, in any event, because of the differing radiochemical purities associated with different kit preparations of MAG_3.[50–53]

Claessens and Corstens[54] found excellent correlation between a multiple plasma sampling method and an analysis of time-activity curves derived from external counting over the heart as recommended by Blaufox et al.[55] Using the volume distribution method of Tauxe et al.,[37] the lowest error in estimates of MAG_3 clearance was obtained with plasma samples drawn at 41 minutes (SEE = 15.9 mL). The external counting method slightly overestimated MAG_3 clearance with an error of 18 mL. The authors concluded that the single-sample method is more accurate and more convenient for clinical purposes but that, when renal function is markedly impaired, external counting is preferred. The *percentage* error may be large when renal function is poor (below 25 mL/min for GFR or 125 mL/min for ERPF); however, the absolute error is not great. It should be noted that the single-sample method may be unreliable in the presence of ascites or edema.[6]

The calculation of MAG_3 clearance using a single sample has been presented by Russell and Dubovsky.[6,56] These authors have recently updated their methods of calculation using a computer program to solve the non-linear model equations.[57]

From a single ^{99m}Tc-MAG_3 plasma sample at some time (t) between 35 and 55 min and in the absence of edema or ascites:

$$\text{MAG}_3 \text{ clearance} = F_{max}[1 - \exp(-\alpha(1/c - V_{lag}))]$$

where

c = fraction of dose per liter of plasma, liter^{-1}
t = time between injection and withdrawing of sample in min (between 35 and 55 min)
$F_{max} = 0.040t^2 - 8.20t + 915$ mL/min
$\alpha = 6.50 \times 10^{-6}t^2 - 8.60 \times 10^{-4}t + 3.91 \times 10^{-2}$ liter^{-1}
$V_{lag} = -0.0015t^2 + 0.01t + 8.79$ liter

The result is in mL/min.

EXCRETORY FUNCTION

Excretory function can be evaluated by estimating the fraction of excreted activity in the urine at 30 min. The fractional excretion of MAG_3 and OIH are essentially the same.[46] An excretory index (EI) can be derived from external counting and urine flow rates[46] that compares the amount of activity that appears in the urine with that disappearing from the blood. With normally functioning kidneys, this ratio is 1.0 and is a measure of transit time. Low values indicate cortical or pelvic retention; high values usually indicate a laboratory error. When low values are determined, the site of the missing activity must then be identified from the images: either in the collecting system (obstruction, dehydration) or parenchyma (acute rejection, acute tubular necrosis). The EI is an adjunct to the imaging study, and requires both imaging and ERPF measurements. The EI is used mainly for the diagnosis of acute rejection in renal transplants. Examples of EI determinations are detailed in reference 56.

Renal Time-Activity Curves

A *renogram* curve is a time-activity plot of the passage of a radiopharmaceutical (usually OIH or MAG_3) through the kidney. Originally, curves were derived from the output of external scintillation probes placed over the kidneys; however, some correction for extrarenal radioactivity is necessary. This correction is most easily accomplished by computer processing of selected regions-of-interest (ROI) from scintillation camera data.

The normal ^{131}I-OIH tracing usually has three components: an initial deflection phase (O—A in Figure 3**b**), an accumulation phase (A—B), and a washout phase (B—C—D). A difference in OIH transit may be observed between the hydrated and dehydrated states (Fig. 9). Normal values for these parameters, normalized to the peak, have proved useful in the analysis of these curves. The slope A—B closely correlates with differential ERPF values. The terminal slope correlates positively with the urine volume and negatively with urine osmolality, sodium reabsorption, and other factors.[58]

KIDNEY-AORTA RATIO

The kidney-aorta (K/A) ratio is used as a quantitative index of renal perfusion. On flow images, a region-of-interest (ROI) is placed over each kidney and the aorta cephalad to the renal arteries. Time-activity curves encompassing the first minute after intravenous bolus injection of a ^{99m}Tc-labeled radiopharmaceutical (DTPA or MAG_3) are plotted for each ROI. The initial rise in activity is compared by dividing the slope of each renal curve by the slope of the aortic curve. This gives a quantitative index of relative kidney perfusion, with normal values ranging from 0.6 to 1.15.[59]

DIFFERENTIAL RENAL FUNCTION

Differential renal function (DRF) may be calculated semiquantitatively during studies using DTPA, MAG_3, OIH, GHA, or DMSA. Relative percentages for differential and segmental function are obtained based on the amount of radiopharmaceutical extracted by each kidney. Regions-of-interest are drawn around the kidneys or the specific renal segments, on images obtained between 1 and 3 minutes after administration of tracer for DTPA, MAG_3, OIH, and GHA, and on the delayed images for GHA and DMSA. The total number of counts in each region are summed, and the relative percentages are determined. A quantitative estimate of renal function can be obtained by multiplying the glomerular filtration rate by the relative percentage from the DRF.

With DTPA, the DRF is determined during the period of

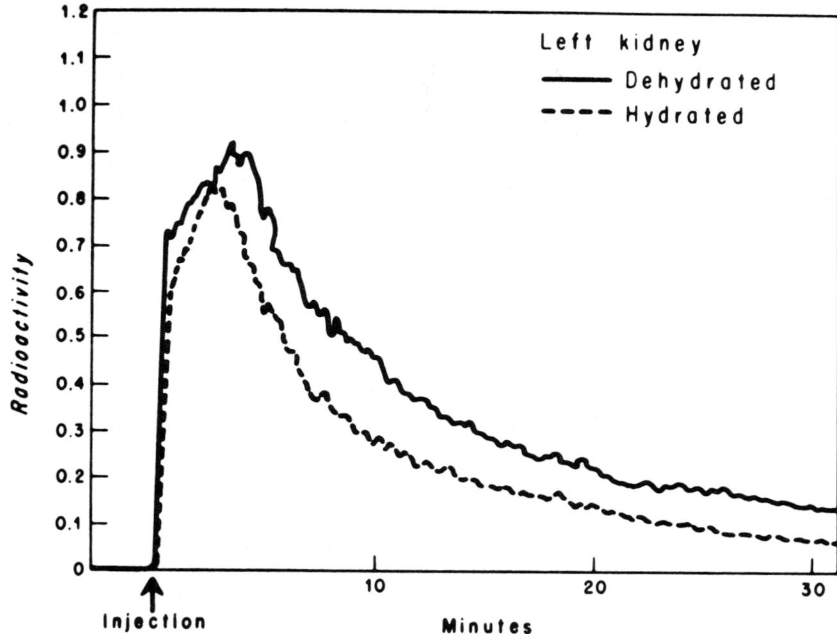

Figure 9. Left renogram curves from a single normal kidney show the effects of relative hydration and dehydration.

glomerular filtration just prior to the appearance of tracer in the collecting systems. The differential uptake of MAG_3 and OIH, is also quantified prior to passage into the collecting systems. During delayed imaging with either GHA or DMSA, the DRF represents the amount of tracer bound to the tubular cells in the renal cortex. Thus, the DRF reflects glomerular and/or tubular function, depending on the choice of imaging agent.

The DRF helps to guide therapy for patients with unilaterally decreased function. If function is severely decreased on one side with normal function on the contralateral side, nephrectomy may be indicated. However, when disease exists in both kidneys, a partial nephrectomy may avoid renal insufficiency. Among renal transplant donors, the effective renal plasma flow (ERPF) of the remaining kidney may increase by one third, with an even greater increase in the GFR.[60,61] In patients with chronic disease in one kidney, a compensatory increase in function usually occurs in the contralateral kidney, which does not improve further after nephrectomy. For those with bilateral disease, contralateral compensatory increase in function will be limited by the type of disease present.[60,62] DRF may also be used to assess the degree of improved function after angioplasty or surgery for renovascular hypertension.

CLINICAL APPLICATIONS

Diuretic Renography

Patients found to have hydronephrosis or hydroureteronephrosis by ultrasonography are candidates for diuretic renography to determine if obstruction is present. Causes of dilatation include vesicoureteral reflux, urinary tract infection, previous obstruction (posterior urethral valves), congenital malformations (prune belly syndrome, megacalyces/megaureter), noncompliant bladder, and urinary tract obstruction (congenital stenosis, tumor, lithiasis).[63] Several radiopharmaceuticals can be used for this procedure. The one most commonly chosen has been ^{99m}Tc-DTPA. ^{99m}Tc-MAG_3 is currently replacing OIH, because of the improved imaging characteristics.

Prior to the study, the nuclear medicine physician should review renal ultrasound results if they are available. This will show whether the hydronephrosis is unilateral or bilateral, if there is concomitant dilatation of the ureters, and if other anomalies, such as duplication, are present. It is imperative that the patient be well hydrated with good urine output, because poor hydration may result in images with apparent decreased renal function and delayed excretion.

For pediatric patients who cannot void on command, a bladder catheter should be inserted into the bladder to insure adequate drainage. If dilatation is at the level of the ureteropelvic junction, a catheter with an inflatable balloon may be used to drain the bladder. On the other hand, if there is hydroureteronephrosis and ureterovesical junction obstruction is suspected, the catheter should be a feeding tube, because even a small balloon may compress the bladder at the insertion of the ureters, giving the false impression of obstruction.

After intravenous injection of tracer, serial posterior images are obtained. Flow images are acquired every 2 to 3 seconds for the first minute; then static images are obtained every 2 to 3 minutes for 30 minutes. In a normal study, the tracer starts to be excreted into the urine within 3 to 5 minutes, and then drains from the renal pelvis and ureters into the bladder. By 20 to 30 minutes, tracer should have cleared from the renal parenchyma and collecting systems.

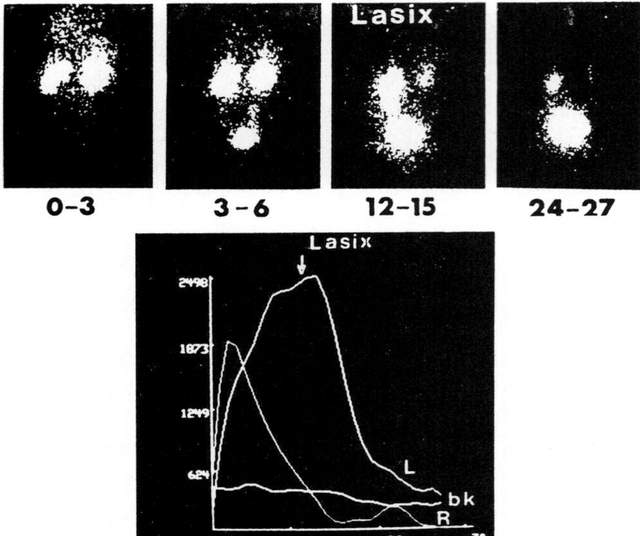

Figure 10. ^{131}I-OIH renogram in a child with congenitally enlarged left renal pelvis. The images at normal urine flow rates are essentially indistinguishable from those seen in ureteropelvic junction obstruction. Intravenous injection of furosemide, however, accelerates elimination of radioactivity in contrast to its effect in postrenal obstruction. These are background-subtracted time-activity curves.

When renal function is significantly diminished, the procedure does not accurately assess the diuretic response. Results are also unreliable if accumulation of tracer in the collecting system is delayed. The results of diuretic renography are not reliable when the affected kidney has less than 20% of the total renal function or when the collecting system is not completely filled within 60 minutes of injection of tracer.[64,65]

When the collecting system is dilated, retention of tracer is often seen, and furosemide (40 mg for adults, 1 mg/kg up to a maximum of 40 mg for children) should be given to increase urine output. The diuretic is administered at the point when the collecting systems are full, usually occuring about 20 minutes (F + 20) after injection (Fig. 10). Regions of interest are drawn over the collecting systems, and should also include the ureters if they contain retained tracer. Time-activity curves are generated, and a single exponential clearance curve is fitted to determine the clearance half-time. Clearance half-times of less than 10 minutes indicate that the system is probably not obstructed, while half-times over 20 minutes are suspicious for obstruction (Fig. 11). Between 10 and 20 minutes, results are indeterminate.

Brown et al.[66] measured urine flow rates at 3 to 6 minutes and 15 to 18 minutes after injection of furosemide, and found that the flow rates were higher at the later time. This led them to inject the diuretic 15 minutes before (F–15) injection of the radiopharmaceutical so that maximum flow rates coincided with the tracer injection. Using this technique, Upsdell et al.[67] reduced the number of equivocal diuretic renograms from 17 to 3%. Protocols for diuresis renography have been described recently by O'Reilly.[68]

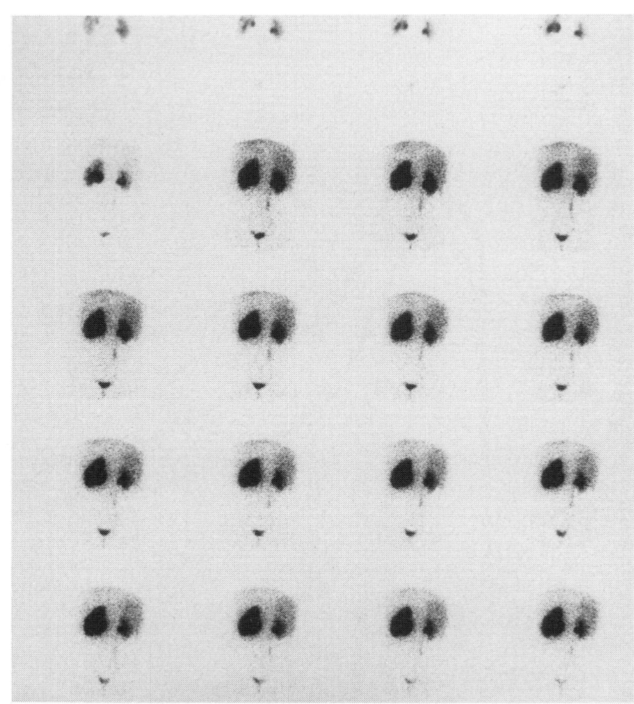

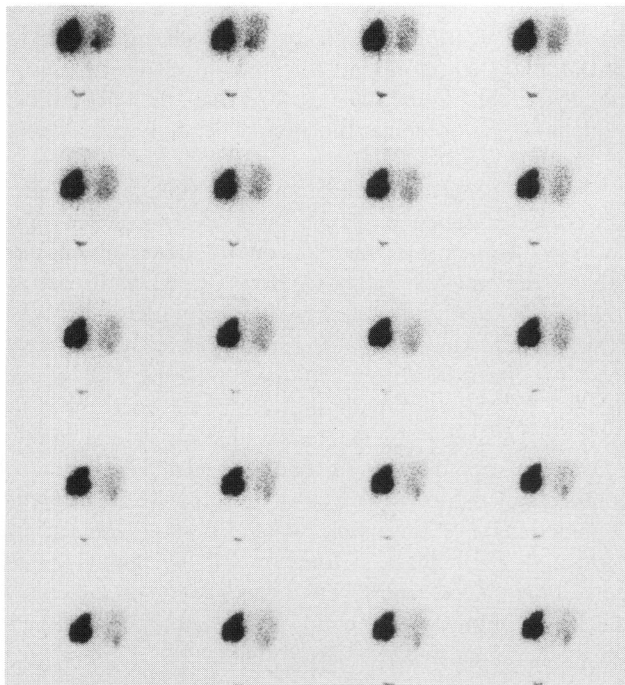

Figure 11. Left hydronephrosis with obstruction: **(A).** Serial 2-min posterior images following injection of ^{99m}Tc-MAG$_3$ demonstrate delayed filling of the left renal pelvis and prolonged retention. **(B).** Following administration of 40 mg furosemide, there is delayed washout of tracer on the left. **(C).** The clearance half-time following furosemide injection is 27 minutes.

Renovascular Hypertension

Most patients with elevated blood pressure have idiopathic or primary hypertension, while relatively few have secondary hypertension with a treatable cause. Renovascular abnormalities, the most common cause of secondary hypertension, are responsible for less than 5% of all cases of hypertension.[69,70] However, this subset of disorders is clinically important because surgical correction may be possible. Renovascular hypertension may be caused by unilateral or bilateral stenosis of the main renal artery, branch arterial stenosis, whole kidney or focal renal infarction, aneurysms, arteriovenous malformations, iliac artery stenosis in renal transplant patients, and renal artery or aortic thrombosis in neonates.[71] In the past, the "gold standard" for the diagnosis of renal artery stenosis was arteriography. Now, however, renal scintigraphy utilizing captopril, an angiotensin-converting enzyme (ACE) inhibitor, is recognized as more sensitive and specific in selecting those patients who might benefit from therapy.[72]

The most common cause of renal artery stenosis is atherosclerosis. With a false-positive rate of 10% for captopril renal scintigraphy, it is not cost-effective to screen all patients presenting with hypertension. However, certain clinical findings help identify the subset of patients at risk for atherosclerotic disease who might benefit from captopril scintigraphy. These findings include: (1) hypertension initially presenting in patients under 20 years of age or those over 60; (2) drug-resistant, severe, or accelerated hypertension; (3) previously well-controlled hypertension that has become difficult to control; (4) unexplained renal dysfunction in patients with recent onset of hypertension; (5) target organ damage (renal, retinal, cardiac); (6) other vascular disease (coronary artery disease, cerebral vascular disease, peripheral vascular disease); (7) abdominal bruits; (8) history of heavy cigarette smoking (>25 pack-years); and (9) Caucasian race.[73,74]

Atherosclerosis of the renal artery is often progressive and, if untreated, can lead to worsening hypertension. The average rate of decrease of the renal arterial transluminal diameter was estimated to be 1.5% per month in one study.[75] Atheromatous lesions are often bilateral. In one autopsy series, 60% of patients with severe stenosis of one renal artery also had severe stenosis on the contralateral side, and only 10% had a normal contralateral renal artery.[76] When lesions are bilateral, renal failure may result. Thus, surgical intervention may be indicated for some patients, even when the hypertension can be controlled with medication.

The second most common cause of renal artery stenosis is fibromuscular dysplasia, seen mainly in young women under 35 years of age. The stenosis tends to be slowly progressive, but rarely leads to complete occlusion or renal failure.[77] Stenosis caused by fibromuscular dysplasia can also be corrected by angioplasty. Other more rare causes of renal artery stenosis or occlusion of the renal artery include Takayasu's arteritis, polyarteritis, aneurysm, radiation-induced fibrosis, emboli, and tumors, including pheochromocytoma and neurofibromatosis.[78]

When renal perfusion pressure decreases, the kidneys attempt to maintain GFR through autoregulatory mechanisms. Cells in the juxtaglomerular apparatus, located in the walls of the afferent arterioles immediately proximal to the glomeruli, respond to reduced renal blood flow by releasing renin, an enzyme that catalyzes the conversion of angiotensinogen, made in the liver, to angiotensinogen I. This, in turn, is converted into angiotensin II by angiotensin-converting enzyme (ACE) located in the lungs. Angiotensin II, the most potent vasoconstrictor known, causes constriction of the renal efferent arterioles, thus increasing renal perfusion pressure and systemic blood pressure. ACE inhibitors, such as captopril and enalaprilat, block this compensatory response and decrease the level of angiotensin II, thus decreasing renal efferent arteriolar pressure.[79]

In patients with significant renal artery stenosis and decreased perfusion pressure, the transcapillary forces driving glomerular filtration are sustained by a preferential increase in efferent arteriolar resistance behind the glomerulus. The renogram may appear to be normal in such cases because the GFR is maintained. Administration of an ACE inhibitor blocks the efferent renal arteriolar constriction, and decreases function in the affected kidney. This technique was first described in pediatric patients,[80] and has also been validated in adults.[81,82]

Generally, the renogram with ACE inhibition is compared to a similar renal study without pretreatment. The baseline study can be performed first, followed by the ACE-inhibitor study on the same day. Administration of therapeutic ACE inhibitors should be discontinued for 48 hours prior to the study. No food should be taken for 4 hours prior to the captopril study, to facilitate absorption of the oral medication.

A single oral dose of captopril 60 minutes before administration of the radiopharmaceutical produces characteristic scintigraphic changes in patients with renal artery stenosis[83] (Fig. 12). Alternatively, enalaprilat can be given intravenously 15 minutes before radiopharmaceutical injection. In patients with uncertain gastrointestinal (GI) absorption of oral medications, this may be preferred. Prior to administering ACE inhibitors, patients should have stable blood pressure readings; blood pressure and pulse are recorded serially throughout the course of the study. Before beginning the study, intravenous access is recommended to insure adequate hydration and good urine output. Occasionally, patients who are volume-depleted become hypotensive after receiving captopril, requiring a bolus of normal saline to normalize the blood pressure.

Scintigraphic findings after an ACE inhibitor depend on the radiopharmaceutical used and the degree of stenosis. If DTPA is used, there is decreased tracer accumulation in the affected kidney during the first 5 minutes of imaging and a delay in time to peak activity. MAG_3 and OIH demonstrate prolonged cortical retention. There is uptake by the renal tubular cells because they retain some function due to preservation of renal blood flow, even when GFR is reduced. Cortical activity persists because of decreased urine production.

A

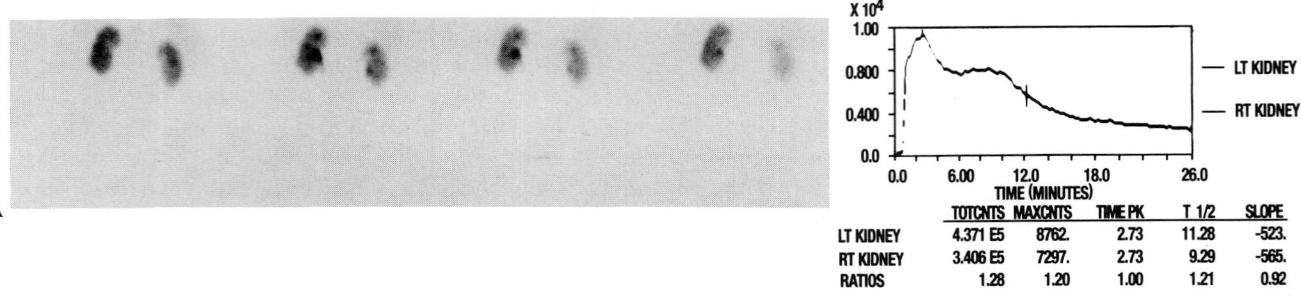

B

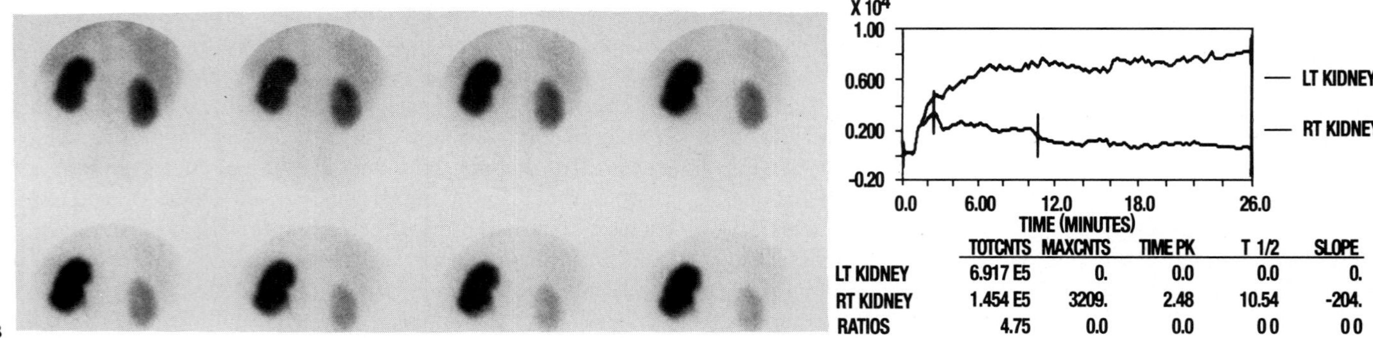

Figure 12. Renovascular hypertension and ^{99m}Tc-MAG$_3$ captopril scintigraphy. Following these studies, arteriography demonstrated severe left and moderate right renal artery stenosis. Renal angioplasty markedly decreased patient's requirement for antihypertensive medications. **(A).** Baseline study shows normal extraction and excretion of MAG$_3$. **(B).** Thirty minutes after oral administration of 50 mg captopril, there is marked retention of MAG$_3$ in the left kidney.

These scintigraphic changes are usually seen in patients with occlusions of 60 to 90% of the lumen. If less than 60% stenosis is present, scintigraphy may not demonstrate an abnormality. When the stenosis is greater than 90% with a concomitant decrease in renal function, the renin-angiotensin system may not be effective in restoring perfusion pressure. In this last case, the baseline pre-captopril inhibitor study may be abnormal, and the post-captopril study may not show a significant change in GFR on the affected side.[71]

Segmental renal artery stenosis has also been demonstrated by captopril renography.[84–87] If the stenosis is bilateral, the GFR for both kidneys may be decreased. With bilateral stenosis, unilaterally decreased function has been reported, with subsequent contralaterally decreased function following correction with angioplasty on the initial side.[88] This case emphasizes the need for careful follow-up of these patients. Captopril scintigraphy may also be used with patients who are hypertensive following renal transplantation.[89]

Renal Transplant Evaluation

Scintigraphic evaluation of renal transplants has been performed routinely for more than fifteen years.[90] Functional assessment of the transplanted kidney during the early postoperative period and the detection of complications is often difficult. Clinical and laboratory parameters are frequently nonspecific and, at times, even misleading. Renal scintigraphy provides a noninvasive and quantitative method of evaluating renal graft function (Fig. 13). DTPA, MAG$_3$, and OIH are the most commonly used radiopharmaceuticals for serial renal transplant evaluations. Imaging is similar to that performed in standard renal scintigraphy, except that the patient is in the supine position and anterior images over the transplanted kidney are obtained.

The combined use of the excretion index (EI) and ERPF has been used to identify patterns of acute tubular necrosis, rejection, or vascular compromise.[91,92] For quantitative data, regions-of-interest may be drawn over the kidney and either the aorta or iliac artery. Time-activity curves are then generated to determine indices of perfusion that may help differentiate between acute rejection and acute tabular necrosis.[93,94] Using DTPA, the mean transit time is significantly prolonged in obstruction, moderately prolonged in both acute rejection and acute tubular necrosis, and normal in chronic rejection.[92]

Early vascular complications of transplantation are rare but serious causes of anuria. Renal artery or vein compression or thrombosis may interrupt graft perfusion. Renal scintigraphy then demonstrates a photopenic region corresponding to the transplant. Renal artery stenosis is a later complication, heralded by accelerating hypertension and/or progressive renal insufficiency. Renal scintigraphy demon-

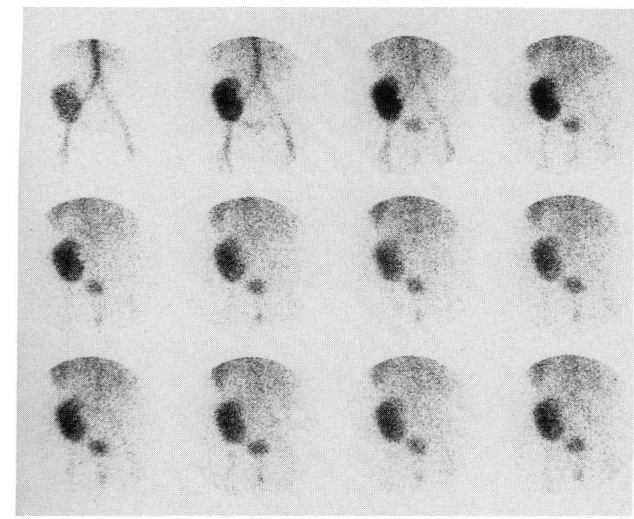
A

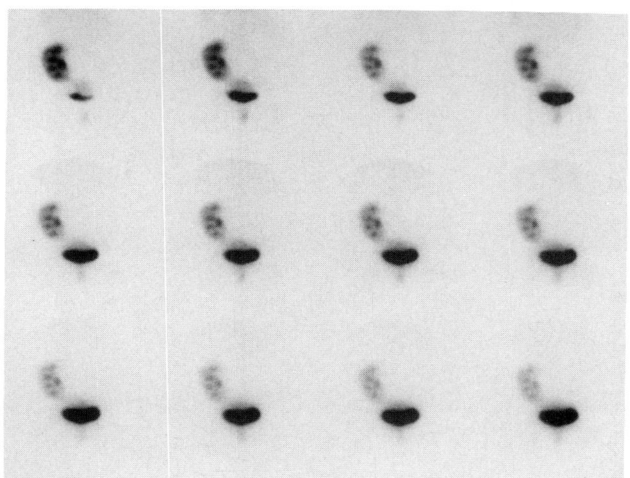
B

Figure 13. Good renal transplant function: **(A).** Anterior ^{99m}Tc-DTPA flow study (3 sec/frame) shows good graft perfusion. **(B).** Serial static anterior images (2 min/frame) show prompt parenchymal tracer uptake and clearance with mild caliectasis, but without obstruction.

strates parallel decrements in flow and function, similar to that seen with rejection. Captopril renography can be helpful in differentiating renal arterial stenosis from rejection.

Transplant rejection may occur at three different times: hyperacute (0 to 24 hours), acute (5 to 90 days), and chronic (after 6 months).[92] In hyperacute rejection, preformed antibodies lead to rapid vascular thrombosis. Acute rejection is cell-mediated, with lymphocytic infiltration into the graft, producing fever, tenderness over the graft, and renal swelling. EI is decreased (0.4 to 0.6), while ERPF is generally preserved. Chronic rejection is humorally mediated, resulting in slowly progressive narrowing of the vascular bed due to antibody attachment to endothelial and interstitial cells. In this case, EI may be normal or decreased, while ERPF is low or only moderately decreased. In all 3 types of rejection, scintigraphic images demonstrate markedly diminished perfusion (Fig. 14). Residual function depends on the acuteness of rejection. Generally, function deteriorates less than perfusion. Other radiopharmaceuticals used to diagnose rejection include ^{67}Ga-citrate,[95] ^{125}I-fibrinogen,[96–98] ^{99m}Tc-sulfur colloid,[95,98,99] and ^{111}In-labeled white blood cells or platelets.[100–104] All are associated with increased uptake following rejection.

Two other complications that occur after transplantation are obstruction and extravasation of urine.[105] The most common cause is ischemia of the ureter or renal pelvis. Urinomas, or collections of extravasated urine, are seen as photopenic regions adjacent to the transplant that have increased activity at 2 to 4 hours after filling with "hot" urine (Fig. 15). Lymphoceles and hematomas produce similar photopenic areas, but do not become "hot" on delayed views.

Acute tubular necrosis (ATN) results from ischemia just prior, during, and after graft harvesting (Fig. 16). It usually occurs during the first 24 hours, reaching its maximum after 48 to 72 hours of reperfusion. The tubular dysfunction of ATN slowly resolves over the next month. The renal flow study demonstrates only mildly decreased perfusion, with DTPA extraction. MAG_3 and OIH are also extracted poorly, but there is progressive accumulation of the tracer. Excretion is delayed or even absent. Cyclosporin nephrotoxicity produces a similar scintigraphic pattern as ATN, but cyclosporin effects are seen after the first few weeks when ATN has resolved.

Renal Cortical Scintigraphy

Renal cortical scintigraphy (RCS) may be performed with either ^{99m}Tc-DMSA or ^{99m}Tc-GHA. DMSA binds to renal tubular cells and accumulates in the functioning renal cortex. Cortical uptake of this tracer is determined by intrarenal blood flow and proximal tubular cell membrane transport function. Any pathologic process that alters these parameters results in areas of diminished uptake. GHA is both taken up by the renal cortex and filtered by the glomeruli, with excretion of the filtered portion into the pelvicalyceal collecting systems. The absorbed radiation dose is similar for both agents. If information about drainage of urine as well as cortical function is desired, GHA is the radiopharmaceutical of choice. At some institutions, DMSA is the preferred radiopharmaceutical because better quality images are obtained.

Applications of RCS include the diagnosis of pyelonephritis, definition of renal anomalies such as horseshoe kidney (Fig. 17), location of an ectopic kidney, and determining whether a space-occupying lesion contains functioning renal tissue. Flow images may be obtained immediately after injection. Delayed imaging is performed 2 to 3 hours later in the posterior and posterior oblique projections. Anterior views are used when the patient has had a renal transplant or has

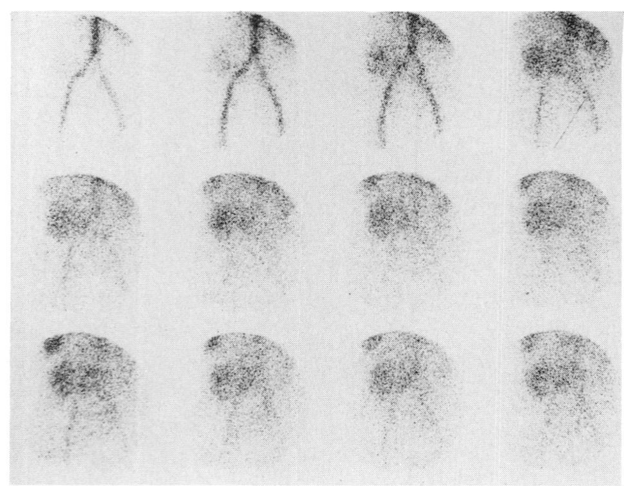

A

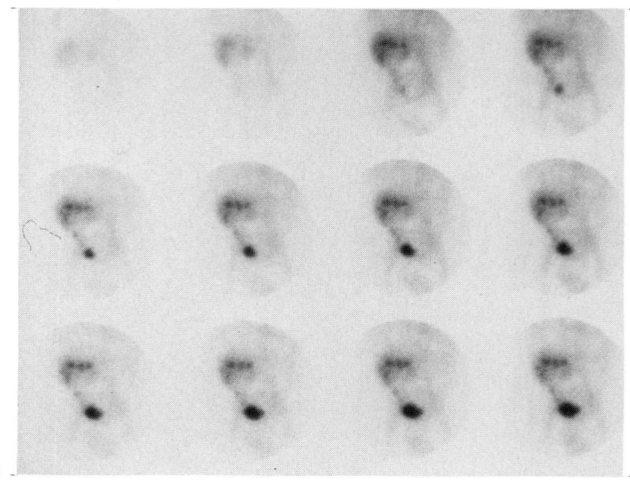

B

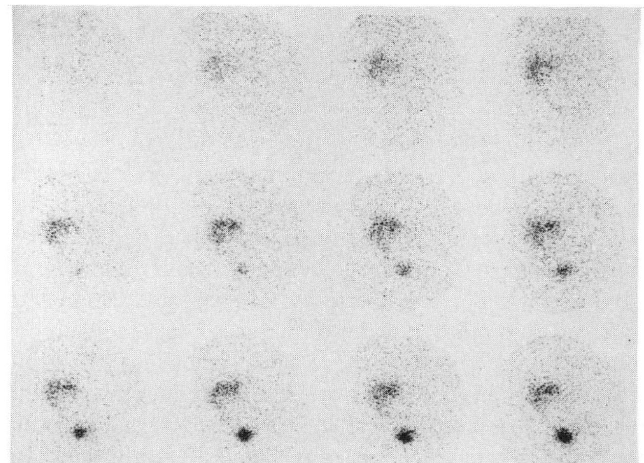

C

Figure 14. Acute rejection of a renal transplant: **(A).** Anterior ^{99m}Tc-DTPA study (3 min/frame) shows decreased transplant perfusion. **(B).** Serial anterior images (2 min/frame) show reduced extraction, and delayed excretion. **(C).** ^{131}I-OIH study (3 min/frame) demonstrates reduced uptake and excretion.

a horseshoe kidney. In the latter case, this is avoids attenuation by the vertebral bodies in the posterior projection.

The use of SPECT techniques as an adjunct to renal scintigraphy has been reviewed by Williams.[106] At this time, it seems to be useful principally in assessing renal scarring in renal infectious disease.

PYELONEPHRITIS

RCS is the current "gold standard" for the diagnosis of pyelonephritis. Animal experiments have demonstrated a high sensitivity and specificity for DMSA scintigraphy when correlated with histopathology.[107–109] Studies have shown RCS to be more sensitive and specific than either sonography or intravenous urography in identifying renal parenchymal infection, because both of these modalities underestimate the degree of involvement, and have a high false-negative rate.[110–117] Neither clinical parameters nor standard laboratory tests, such as a complete blood count or sedimentation rate, are reliable in identifying children with renal parenchymal infection.[110,111] RCS may also be helpful in adult patients to confirm the presence and extent of renal parenchymal involvement.

Imaging is performed in the posterior and posterior oblique projections. With acute infection, 3 patterns are seen: focal, multifocal, or diffusely decreased activity (Figs. 18, 19, 20). These occur without loss of volume, and may have associated edema. An area of decreased uptake, along with volume contraction of the affected region, indicates scarring from previous infection (Fig. 21). When a photopenic area is identified, correlation with renal sonography should be performed, to insure that the area of decreased activity represents infection rather than a cyst or other space-occupying lesion.

HORSESHOE KIDNEY

Horseshoe kidney is a congenital fusion anomaly characterized by distal conversion of the longitudinal axes with an isthmus of functioning renal tissue passing anterior to the aorta and inferior vena cava that connects the two kidneys (Fig. 17). Children with this condition have an increased

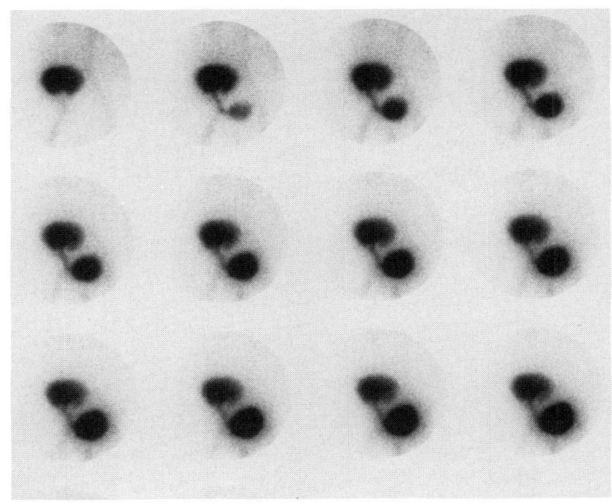

A

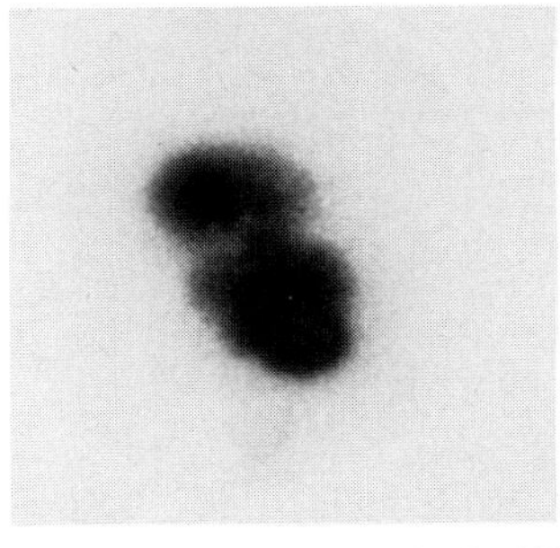

B

Figure 15. Renal transplant with urine leak: **(A).** Sequential ^{99m}Tc-MAG$_3$ images (2 min/frame) show normal uptake and excretion. Moderate MAG$_3$ retention is seen in this kidney 3 weeks after transplantation due to residual ATN and cyclosporin effect. **(B).** Anterior postvoid view demonstrates a large urine collection outside and superior to the bladder; urine leakage was occurring at the site of ureteral anastomosis to the bladder.

incidence of urinary tract infections. Obstruction may be seen in association with a horseshoe kidney, especially at the ureteropelvic junction. Adults complain of episodic abdominal pain that may be related to obstruction. RCS defines the anatomy of the horseshoe kidney and also helps to rule out other congenital variants. Imaging with DTPA or MAG$_3$ may be utilized if obstruction is suspected.

ECTOPIC KIDNEY

Renal ectopia is a congenital malposition of one or both kidneys. The most common location of unilateral ectopia is within the pelvis. The ectopic kidney may have a small or dysplastic renal mass, and anomalies of ureteral origin or insertion may be present. Crossed fused renal ectopia is another congenital anomaly, in which the ectopic kidney is usually caudal to and fused with the normal kidney. RCS is the best imaging modality to locate the ectopic kidney, which may be difficult to visualize by intravenous urography.

SPACE-OCCUPYING LESIONS

When space-occupying renal lesions are identified, those comprised of nonfunctioning renal tissue should be differentiated from those with demonstrable function. Photopenic areas caused by nonfunctioning parenchyma may represent tumors, cysts, abscesses, or infarcts. Infarcts usually appear as wedge-shaped defects. Solid lesions, such as tumors, may be differentiated from fluid-filled collections, such as cysts and abscesses, by the use of renal sonography, CT, or MRI. A functioning, space-occupying mass may represent a pseudotumor, which is defined as "a real or simulated mass in the kidney roentgenologically resembling neoplasm but consisting histologically of normal renal parenchyma."[118] Causes include columns of Bertin, focal regenerating nodules, fetal lobulation, dromedary kidney, and distortion of normal renal architecture by ectopic renal arteries.[119] Columns of Bertin represent normal cortical tissue extending centrally between the papillae of the medullary pyramids. They are usually located at the junction of the upper and middle thirds of the kidney, in association with a duplication anomaly.[120] The appearance of normally functioning tissue in a renal mass lesion essentially rules out malignancy. On the other hand, an area of absent function indicates the need for further imaging studies.

TRAUMA

During the evaluation of abdominal trauma, renal lesions may be seen on CT, renal sonography, or intravenous urography. Nuclear imaging can then provide additional information and address three main issues. First, is blood flow through one of the renal arteries or its branches interrupted? Failure to visualize a kidney on images obtained immediately after injection of tracer suggests this possibility. Second, renal cortical scintigraphy defines the renal function when suspected contusion or hematoma is identified by other imaging modalities. Finally, renal cortical scintigraphy can be used to identify extravasated urine. ^{99m}Tc-GHA is the radiopharmaceutical of choice. Early views of renal excretion and delayed images of renal cortical architecture provide information about all three concerns.

TESTICULAR SCINTIGRAPHY

The chief clinical indication for testicular scintigraphy is to differentiate acute testicular torsion from acute epididymoorchitis. In the years prior to scintigraphy and ultrasound, surgical exploration was generally recommended in most cases of acute scrotum (inflammation, swelling, and exquisite tenderness), because the two conditions were difficult to distinguish clinically with reliability. Consequently, up to two thirds of patients presenting with acute scrotum were found at surgery to have some condition other than torsion.[121] With the development of scintigraphy and Doppler ultrasound, many operations can be avoided because these

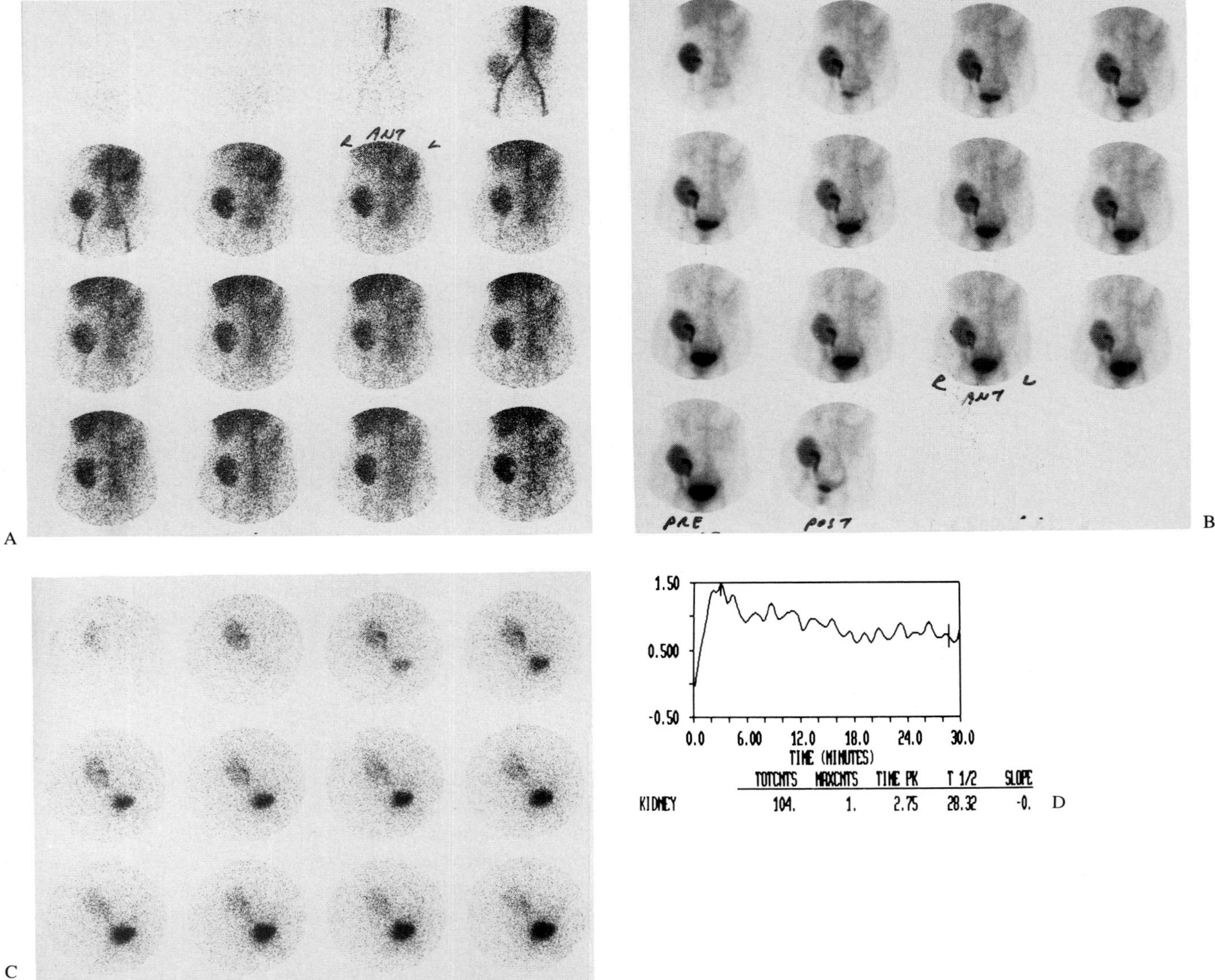

Figure 16. Moderate ATN in a renal transplant patient who received a cadaver kidney 5 days prior to imaging: **(A).** ^{99m}Tc-DTPA flow study (anterior, 3 sec/frame) shows good transplant perfusion. **(B).** Sequential images (2 min/frame) show decreased extraction and persistent high background activity. **(C).** After initial upslope, the renogram curve is flat, indicative of moderate tubular dysfunction of ATN.

examinations are rapidly performed, sensitive, and quite specific.

Anatomy of the Testis and Scrotum

The essential features of the normal testis and hemiscrotum are shown in Figure 22. The testis forms embryologically from the urogenital ridge and descends into the scrotum during intrafetal or neonatal life. As it descends it carries its blood supply, nerves, lymphatics, and spermatic duct, all enclosed within the spermatic cord, into the scrotum. In the process, an extension of the peritoneum, the *tunica vaginalis,* is carried along and covers the anterior and inferior margins of the testis. The posterior testis is connected to the epididymis, a tortuous system of collecting tubules that lead to the spermatic duct. The epididymis is, in turn, connected closely to the scrotal wall. The epididymis and testis are connected by a broad-based condensation of the mesentery, the *mesorchium.*

Torsion of the testis can come about in two ways: (1) in the so-called "bell-clapper" anomaly, the testis is completely invested by the tunica vaginalis and the fixation of the posterior epididymis to the scrotal wall is missing (Fig. 23). This permits the testis to twist and strangulate its arterial blood supply through the spermatic cord. (2) A less frequent abnormality occurs in which the mesorchium forms a narrow or weak connection between the testis and the epididymis (Fig. 24). This attachment allows the testis to twist, while the epididymis remains fixed.

There are also various vestigial remnants of other struc-

A

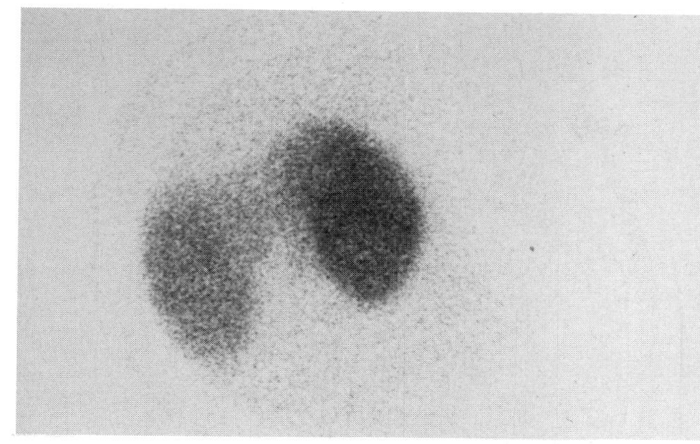

B

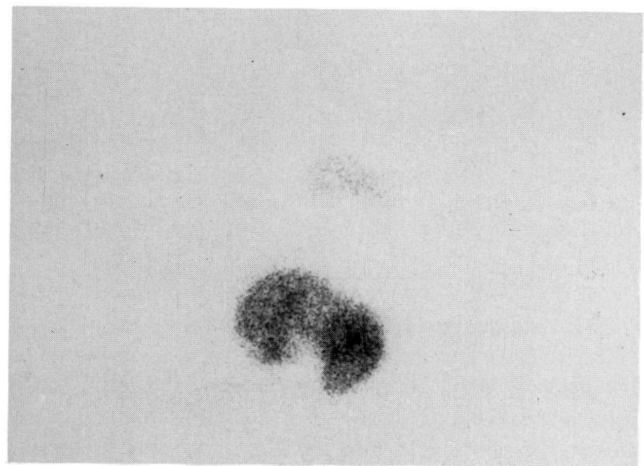

Figure 17. Horseshoe kidney in a five-year-old boy presenting with asymptomatic hematuria: **(A).** Posterior image demonstrates uniform distribution of ^{99m}Tc-DMSA in both kidneys. Apparent decreased uptake in the left kidney is due only to a more anterior location. **(B).** Anterior image shows a band of functioning tissue connecting the kidneys.

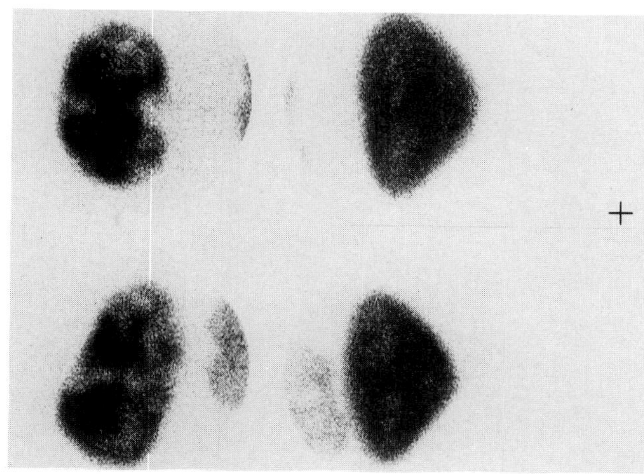

Figure 19. Multifocal left pyelonephritis (posterior and posterior oblique) pinhole images with ^{99m}Tc-DMSA.

tures that remain attached to the testis and are known as *testicular appendages*. These may also twist and become strangulated, causing milder forms of clinical torsion.

Clinical Presentation of Acute Scrotum

The incidence of testicular torsion peaks around puberty, although the condition may occur in childhood and even the elderly.[122,123] There is also a neonatal form of testicular torsion that may occur in late intrauterine life or early postnatally, accompanied by swelling and discoloration of the scrotum. Scintigraphy does not play a part in this condition, because the testes are too small to be accurately resolved and there is almost no other condition with which to confuse it.[124]

Typically, testicular torsion is accompanied by sudden onset of exquisite testicular or lower abdominal pain, swelling of the hemiscrotum, and often nausea and vomiting.

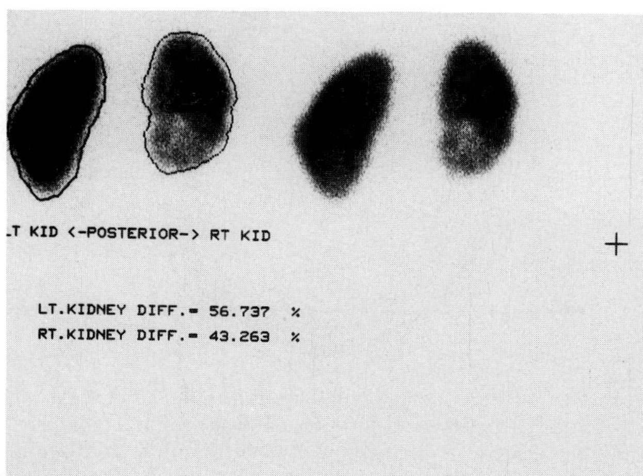

Figure 18. Posterior ^{99m}Tc-DMSA demonstrates a right lower pole defect, caused by old pyelonephritis.

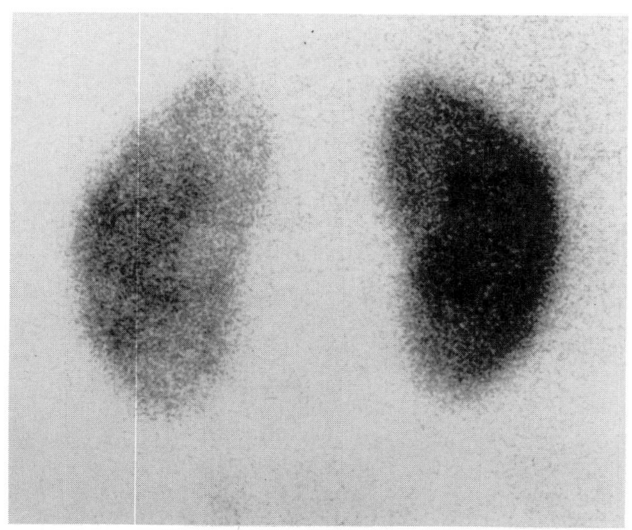

Figure 20. Diffuse left pyelonephritis (posterior image).

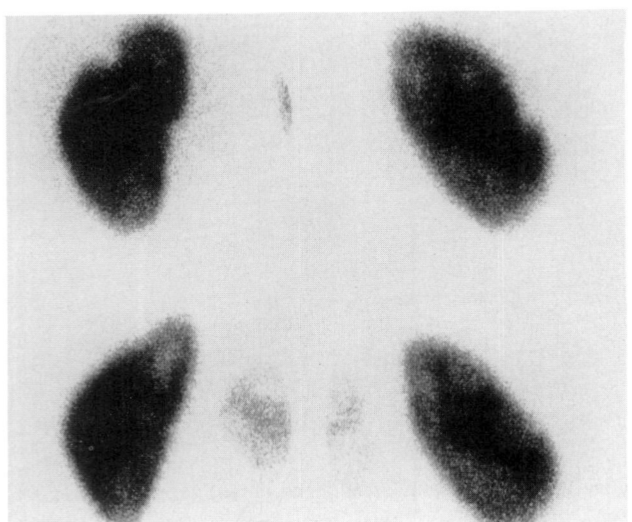

Figure 21. Scarring from previous infection, left upper pole and right midpole (posterior and posterior oblique pinhole images).

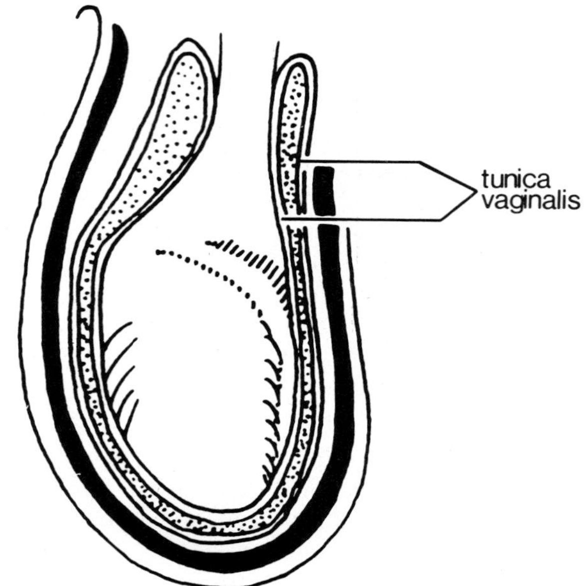

Figure 23. "Bell clapper" anomaly: complete investment of the testis and epididymis by the tunica vaginalis permits the cord to twist. (Reproduced from Reference 121 with permission.)

The temperature may or may not be elevated. Urinalysis is usually unremarkable with fewer than 5 white blood cells per high-power field. Occasionally, the unaffected testis may assume a transverse position when the patient stands.[1] A history of recent trauma is a frequent precursor of testicular torsion.

In "late phase torsion" (the term "missed torsion" has largely been replaced because of unfortunate legal connotations[125]), the presence of torsion has gone unrecognized, or has been incorrectly treated as orchitis or epididymitis. Such patients may present with chronic pain, atrophy of the involved testicle, or with persistent swelling.

Acute epididymitis is the most common cause of acute scrotum and the peak incidence is also in young adulthood. However, with the increase in early sexual experience, more young adolescents are presenting with this disease, often following or associated with a sexually transmitted urethritis. Pediatric cases unrelated to sexual activity also occur. The onset of acute epididymitis is usually more gradual; there may be a history of frequency and dysuria, and urinalysis

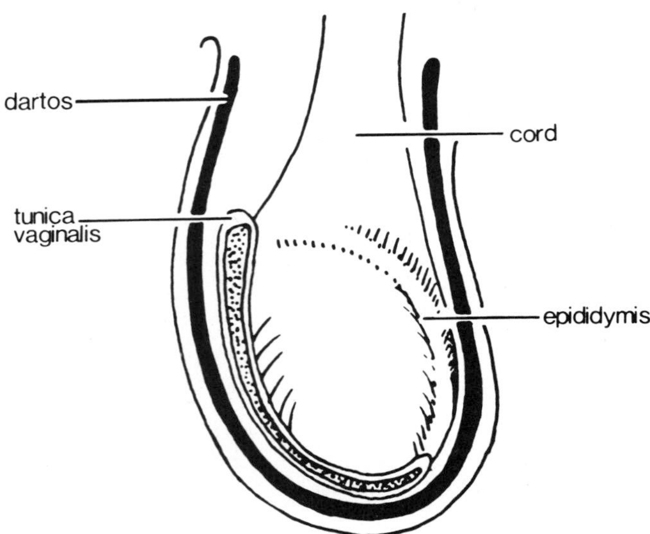

Figure 22. Normal scrotal anatomy: tunica vaginalis invests the testis on three sides only. Posterolateral fixation of the testis to the epididymis and scrotal wall make twisting of the spermatic cord impossible. (Reproduced from Reference 121 with permission.)

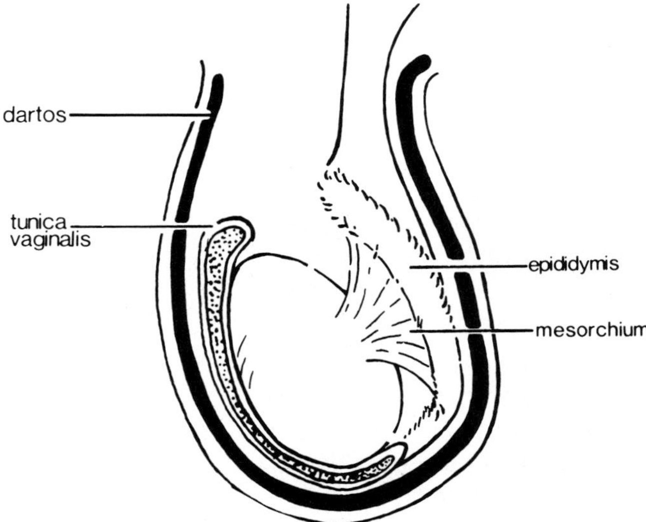

Figure 24. Anomalous mesorchium: elongation of the mesorchium or a narrow area of fixation of testis to the epididymis permits the testis to rotate without cord torsion. The epididymis remains in its normal position and is uncompromised. (Reproduced from Reference 121 with permission.)

often shows more than 10 white blood cells per high-power field. Urine cultures, while frequently positive, are of little help in the differential diagnosis acutely, because the decision to operate must be made before the results are obtained. There is a good probability of salvaging the testis if surgical detorsion occurs within about 4 hours of onset of symptoms and declines to less than 50% after 24 hours.[126]

Other, albeit uncommon, causes of acute scrotum include mumps orchitis (with or without parotid swelling), strangulated hernia, inflammatory type of testicular tumor, and traumatic hemorrhage. These can usually be distinquished by careful history, physical examination, and by scintigraphic and radiographic findings.

Scintigraphy

With the patient in the supine position and thighs slightly abducted, the testes are supported by a folded towel so that they are separated as much as possible, are equidistant from, and as close to the detector as possible. The penis is taped to the lower abdomen so its vascularity does not interfere with the scrotal images. It is also useful to place a lead shield beneath the scrotum to reduce background from the thighs during the static images.

A standard or large-field camera may be used. If available, a converging collimator should be used to increase resolution of these small structures. Otherwise, computer magnification can be employed. When children are studied, a pinhole camera should be used because of the very small prepubertal testes. Since dynamic acquisition is not feasible with a pinhole collimator, static images are begun as soon as the child is injected.[1]

Adults are injected with 550 to 750 MBq (15 to 20 mCi)^{99m}Tc-pertechnetate. Children are administered 7.5 MBq/kg (200 μCi/kg). Sequential 5-second dynamic images are obtained for 1 minute following injection. The intensity is lowered, and a static blood pool image of 500,000 to 1,000,000 counts is obtained. Subsequent images should be timed to the initial static image to offset the gradual accumulation of activity in the bladder. A thin lead strip may be used as a marker to define the median raphe of the scrotum. Hot markers may be confusing upon later review of the images. The entire procedure should consume no more than 15 minutes.

INTERPRETATION

^{99m}Tc-pertechnetate has no affinity for testicular tissue; what is imaged is the current vascularity of the scrotal contents. A systematic evaluation of the findings of both the dynamic and static images, beginning with the normal side, aids in the interpretation of the study. The quantity of blood received by the scrotum and its contents is small in relation to surrounding structures. Consequently, in normal patients, the early dynamic images reveal little else than prominent activity within the iliac vessels as shown in Figure 25. The skin-dartos perfusion (from the pudendal vessels lying out-

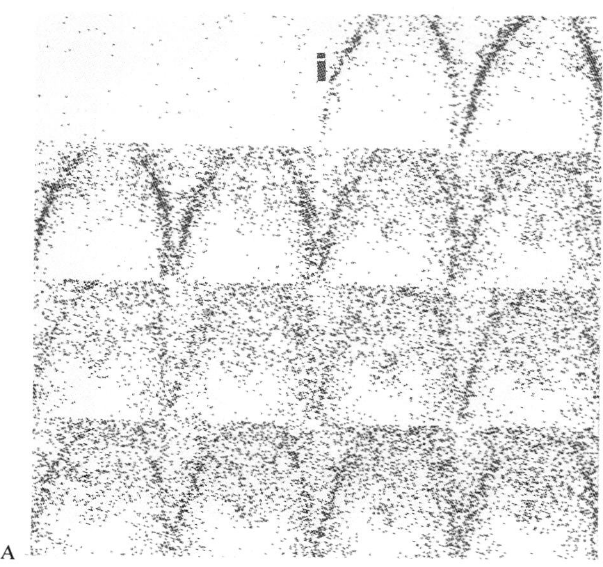

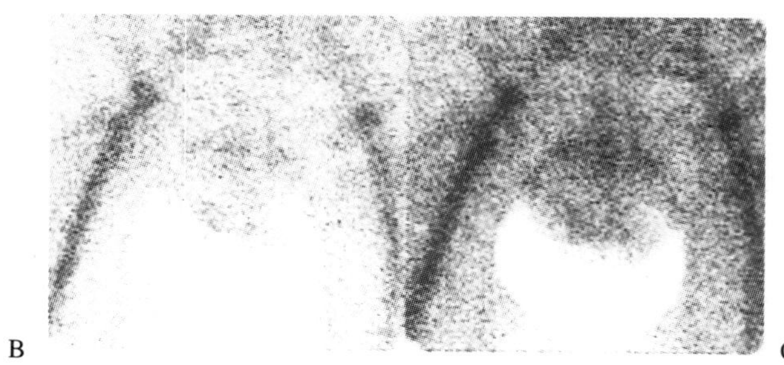

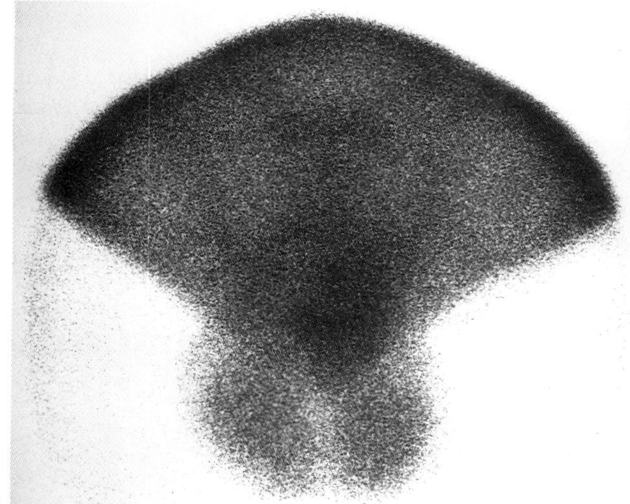

Figure 25. Normal testicular scintgraphy: **(A).** Radionuclide angiogram of the anterior pelvis shows prominent outline of the iliac vessels (i). Neither the testicular nor the deferens vessels passing through the cord nor the pudendal vessels outside the cord are well defined. No significant scrotal perfusion is normally seen. These are 2-s images following intravenous injection of 740 MBq $^{99m}TcO_4$. **(B).** Early static image shows minimal scrotal activity. Minimal activity is seen in the region of the spermatic cord. **(C).** Scrotal image with lead shielding which eliminates thigh background (this image has been computer enhanced). **(D).** Pinhole view with lead shield. (Panel **D** is reproduced by kind permission of Dr. Lawrence Holder.)

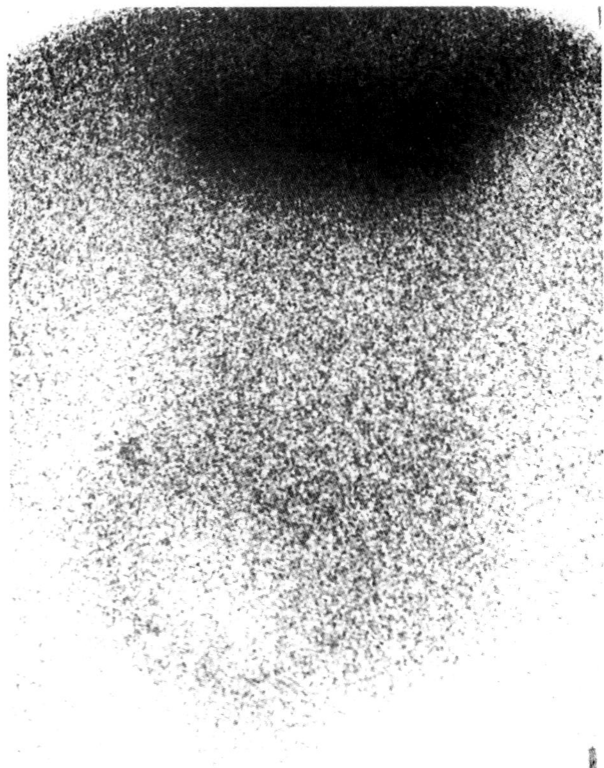

Figure 26. Static image of early torsion: note that the scrotal rim about the ischemic right testis is unaccentuated. The radionuclide angiogram was normal. (Reproduced by kind permission of Dr. Lawrence Holder.)

side the cord) is evaluated towards the end of the dynamic sequence and on the static blood pool images.[121] This contribution is apparent only when hyperemic, so that vascularity of the normal scrotum is largely unremarkable. In later images, the bladder activity appears above the scrotum and high activity at the base of the penis often is seen as a midline hot spot. If the glans is in the field of view, it may also appear as an area of increased activity.

TORSION

Following the onset of torsion, the vascular pattern revealed by scintigraphy changes with time and relates both to the severity of testicular ischemia and to the likelihood of viability after surgical detorsion.[125, 127–137] In the *early* phase of testicular torsion, perfusion in the radionuclide angiogram is usually normal, or there may be a so-called "nubbin sign," an obvious projection from the iliac artery representing reactive increased blood flow in the spermatic cord vessels that terminates abruptly at the site of the twist.[127] This feature may be seen at all stages of torsion as shown in Figures 26 and 27 and is thought to be pathognomonic of torsion. On the static images, testicular activity is decreased and the scrotal halo around the ischemic testis is unaccentuated (Fig. 26). Surgical salvage of the testis is probable, given prompt intervention at this stage.

In the *midphase* of torsion, scrotal dartos perfusion increases by way of the pudendal vessels in response to testicular ischemia. This causes a halo or "rim sign" around the testis (Fig. 27).

In the *late* phase of torsion, the radionuclide angiogram often shows the "nubbin sign" and dartos perfusion around the infarcted testis becomes pronounced (Fig. 28). The probability of salvage by surgical detorsion is low; however, surgery should still be undertaken as soon as possible.[125]

Torsion of an appendage of the testis usually results in a normal study, or a variable sized focal area of increased activity.[18] Figure 29 illustrates appendix torsion of the right testicle.

Inflammatory Disease

In epididymitis, testicular perfusion through the cord vessels is increased in both early and late phases of the radionuclide angiogram (Fig. 30). This increased perfusion usually persists in the static images, which demonstrate intense perfusion laterally, corresponding to the swollen, inflamed epididymis. A photopenic center and hyperactive rim can be seen in inflammatory disease, trauma, and some tumors.[137–141] However, these conditions are seldom confused with torsion, because the dynamic flow studies usually demonstrate *increased* perfusion (Fig. 31) and the hyperactive rim is usually inhomogenious.

Accuracy of Testicular Scintigraphy

In 4 large series totaling 1184 patients studied with suspected torsion of the testis, 223 cases of acute or missed torsion were found.[142–145] Of these, 208 demonstrated a photopenic area in the hemiscrotum by scintigraphy, giving a sensitivity of 93%. If one eliminates those false-negative studies that were either technically inadequate or temporally inappropriate, sensitivity approaches 96%.[121]

Although a photopenic hemiscrotum is a sensitive indicator of torsion, it is by itself nonspecific. In the above series, of 326 cold lesions reported, only 208 (63%) were found to have torsion. Other causes of cold lesions include orchitis, epididymitis, abscess, trauma, hydrocele, inguinal hernia, spermatocele, and tumors. In most of these cases, careful interpretation of testicular blood flow and the clinical presentation along with physical examination, transillumination, and ultrasonography suggested a diagnosis other than torsion. Considering that the purpose of any test in the setting of acute testicular pain is to avoid unnecessary surgery, scintigraphic findings alone can avoid approximately 90% of nonproductive explorations.

COMPARISON WITH ULTRASOUND

Gray-scale ultrasonography yields high-resolution images of the scrotal contents. However, the morphological abnormalities in torsion and epididymo-orchitis are practically

A

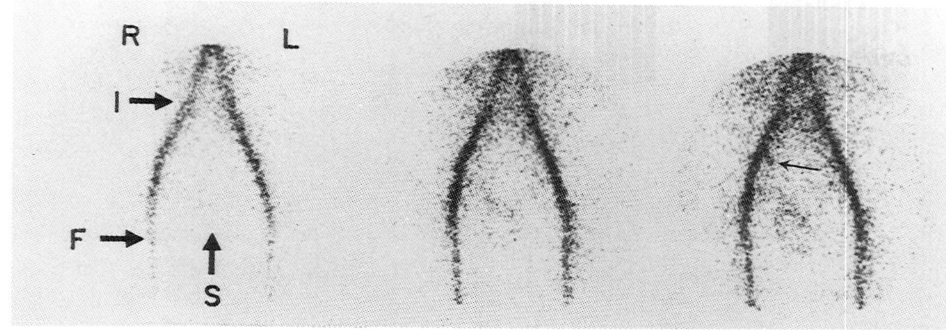

B

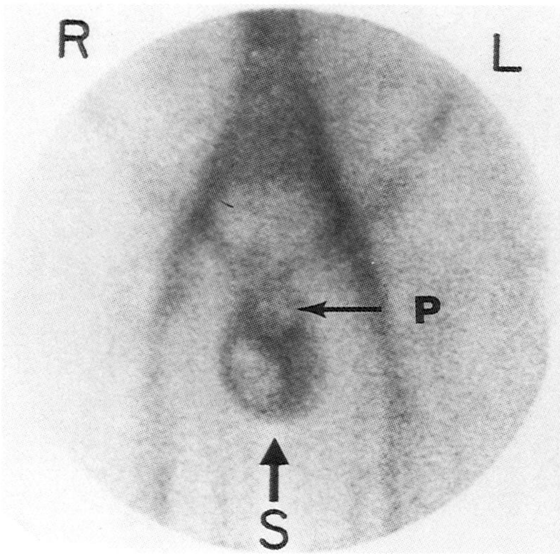

Figure 27. **(A)**. Midphase torsion: the radionuclide angiogram demonstrates prompt filling of the iliac (I) and femoral (F) vessels as well as slightly increased perfusion of the scrotal dartos (s) from the pudendal vessels. Note the "nubbin sign" (small arrow) caused by torsion of the cord vessels. **(B).** The ischemic testis is surrounded by increased perfusion of the dartos. The base of the penis (P) is identified as a phonopenic area above the scrotum.

identical and, thus, it is not an adequate means of evaluating acute scrotal disorders.[145] Color Doppler ultrasound, on the other hand, is capable of simultaneous real-time display of tissue morphology in gray scale and blood flow in color.[146] Recent studies on limited numbers of patients have shown high sensitivity (86 to 100%) and very high specificity (100%).[147–149] These preliminary studies suggest that color Doppler is sensitive to absent or reduced testicular blood flow and correctly identifies the hyperemia associated with inflammatory disease. Color Doppler may be more sensitive in identifying 180° torsion, in which cases scintigraphy may miss the reduced blood flow in a compromised testis.[147]At this time, the 2 tests appear to be complimentary and surgery is probably advised if either test suggests torsion in the acute scrotum. A very real problem with any ultrasound procedure in patients with acute scrotal pain is getting the patient to submit to the examination.

At least one early report of magnetic resonance (MR) imaging in subacute scrotal pain suggests that this modality may also have promise for differentiating torsion from acute epididymitis.[150]

Conclusions

The value of testicular scintigraphy has been summarized by Lutzker and Zuckier[151] as follows:

1. In patients with acute hemiscrotal symptoms, the proper use of testicular scintigraphy is to exclude the possibility of torsion masquerading clinically as an inflammatory or other nonemergent condition, and to detect unsuspected devascularization caused by inflammation, trauma, tumor, etc. Patients who most urgently need scintigraphy are those whose physicians believe that a condition other than torsion exists and who will, therefore, be treated conservatively.
2. A photon-deficient testis with no other findings is most likely to represent early acute torsion. In the case of a cold lesion with a vascular rim, other image findings help differentiate between late torsion and other causes of testicular ischemia. Nevertheless, the avascular testis is in jeopardy and surgery is most likely required to salvage the testis, either through detorsion and orchiopexy or by epididymotomy and decompression.
3. Normal or increased testicular perfusion may exist in the presence of incomplete torsion or of spontaneously resolved torsion, unless epididymitis is obvious by scintigraphy. If a cause other than torsion cannot be proven to explain the symptoms, surgical exploration may be indicated.
4. Testicular scintigraphy is of value postsurgically to confirm restoration of vascularity after detorsion or decom-

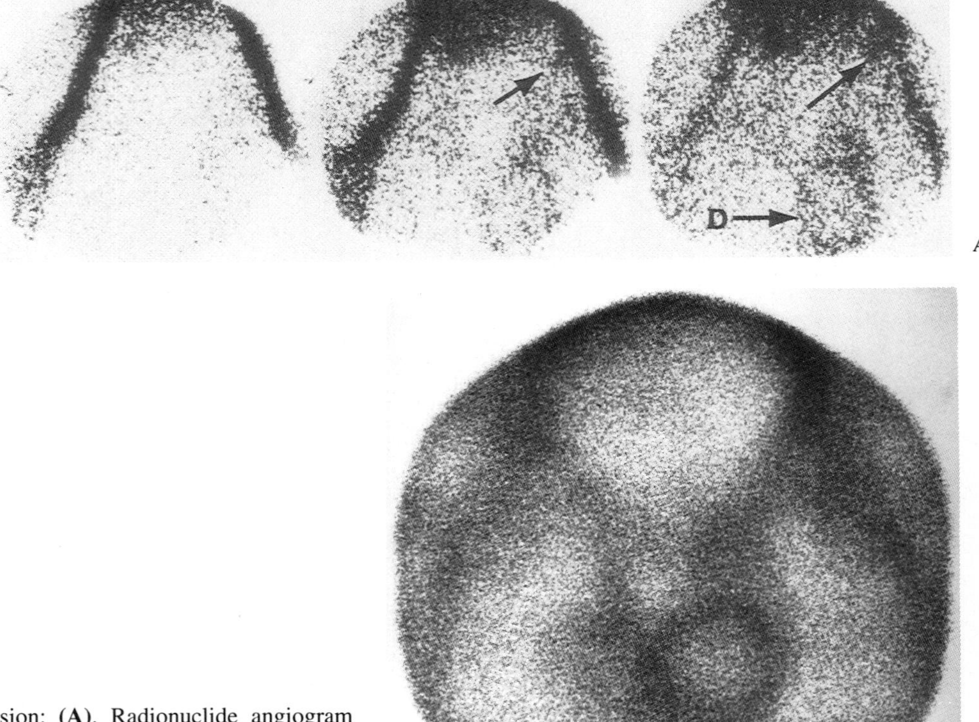

Figure 28. Late-phase testicular torsion: **(A)**. Radionuclide angiogram taken at 5 s/frame shows a "nubbin" sign (arrow) and increased perfusion to the dartos (D) causes a pronounced halo of activity around the infarcted testis. **(B)**. Static image shows an avascular left testicle surrounded by intense vascularity in the dartos. (Reproduced with permission of Dr. Lawrence Holder.)

pression. By the same reasoning, repeat imaging following diagnosis of acute epididymitis may be useful to rule out the development of ischemia that may require surgical decompression.

5. Testicular scintigraphy is of no value in evaluating neonatal torsion, because the structures of interest are beyond the limits of scintillation camera resolution and because there are virtually no other conditions causing scrotal swelling at this age.
6. Ultrasound rather than scintigraphy is the preferred imaging procedure in the evaluation of painless scrotal masses, because of the superior definition of fluid and solid tissues signatures.

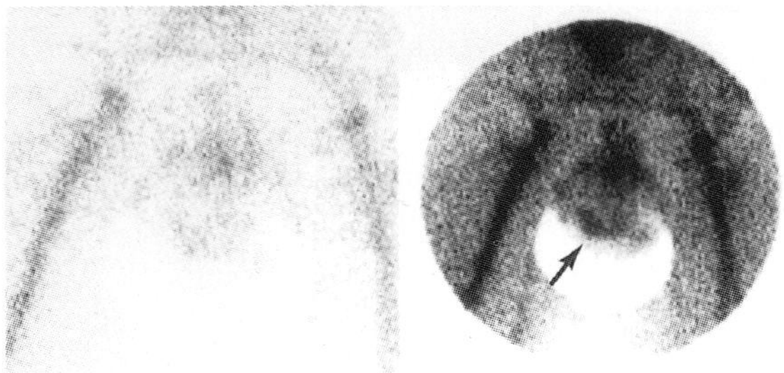

To this list we would add a seventh use, suggested by McConnell et al., who found a high predictability for determining scrotal rupture by testicular scintigraphy in trauma patients.[125]

Figure 29. Appendix torsion of the right testicle in a 40-year-old man with acute right testicular pain, but without fever, redness, or swelling of the testicle. The radionuclide angiogram was normal. The blood pool image **(A)** demonstrates minimally increased perfusion to the right testicle. Computer enhancement **(B)** demonstrates a linear area of increased activity in the lower right testicle (arrow).

Scintigraphy in the Detection of Varicocele

Varicocele is a varicosity of the pampiniform plexus, thought to be caused by blood refluxed from the internal spermatic vein, possibly due to absent or incompetent venous valves.[152] Most varicoceles occur on the left side; they occur bilaterally in about 20% of cases. They rarely occur only on the right.[153]

Varicoceles are often palpable and have been staged as Grades 1 to 3, according to the classification of Dublin and Amelar, which is based upon the degree of reflux into the scrotal vessels.[154] However, subclinical varicocele, which is

A 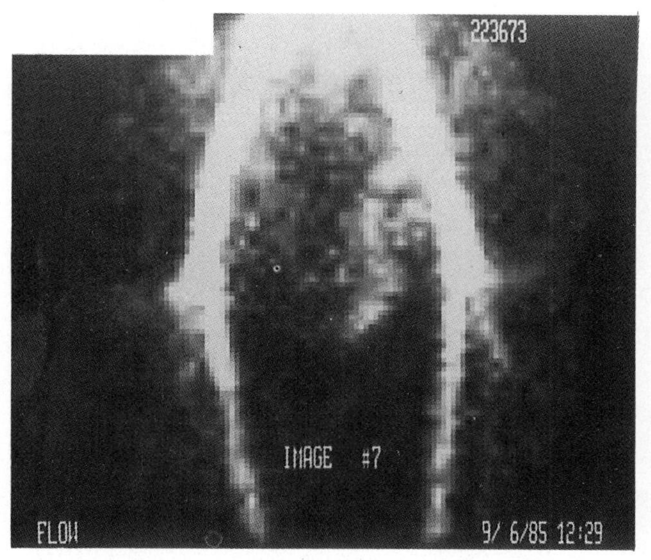

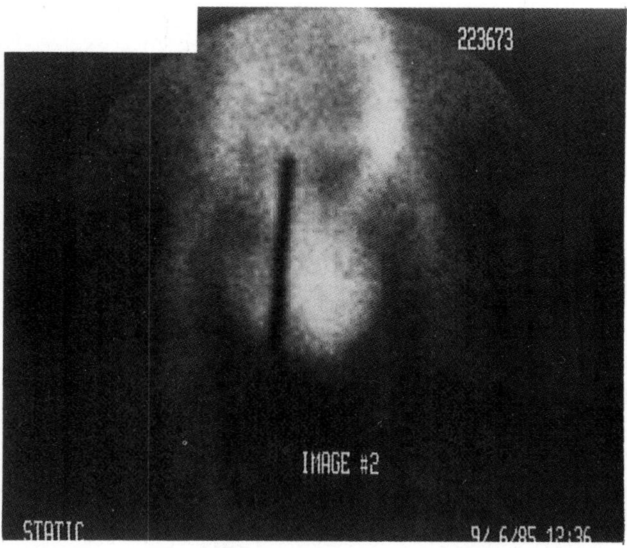 B

Figure 30. Acute epididymitis in a 45-year-old male with a four-day history of acute left scrotal pain: **(A)**. Radionuclide angiogram demonstrates the classic comma-shaped increased perfusion laterally in the epididymis in this early 5-s frame. **(B)**. Static image demonstrates intense perfusion in entire left hemiscrotum. (Reproduced with kind permission of Dr. Letty Lutzker.)

reflux in the absence of palpable enlargement, is also thought to figure as a cause of infertility.[155,156]

Contrast phlebography is generally considered the definitive test in the diagnosis of varicocele.[157] However, this is an invasive procedure which is uncomfortable for the patient and is not without risks.[158] Other diagnostic tests include thermography,[156,159] ultrasound,[160,161] Doppler ultrasound,[162] and scintigraphy.[127, 163–167] All of these tests are reasonably sensitive and are probably more appropriate for postsurgical evaluation to judge the effectiveness of treatment.

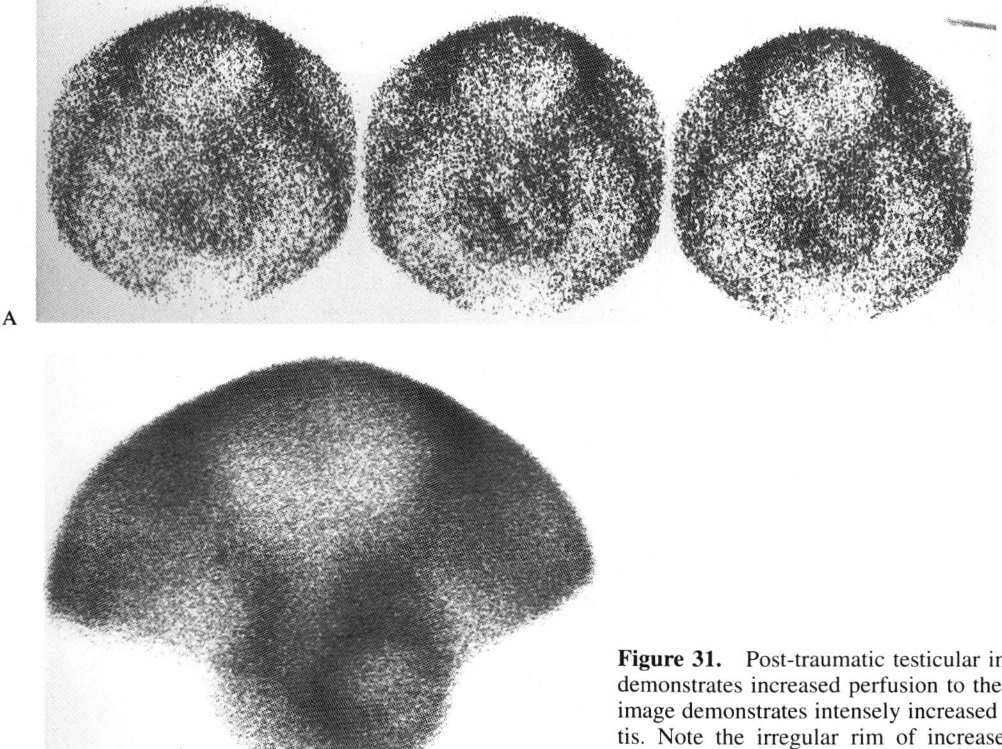
A
B

Figure 31. Post-traumatic testicular infarct: **(A)**. Radionuclide angiogram demonstrates increased perfusion to the cord vessels on the left. **(B)**. Static image demonstrates intensely increased perfusion surrounding infarcted testis. Note the irregular rim of increased activity. (Reproduced with kind permission of Dr. Lawrence Holder.)

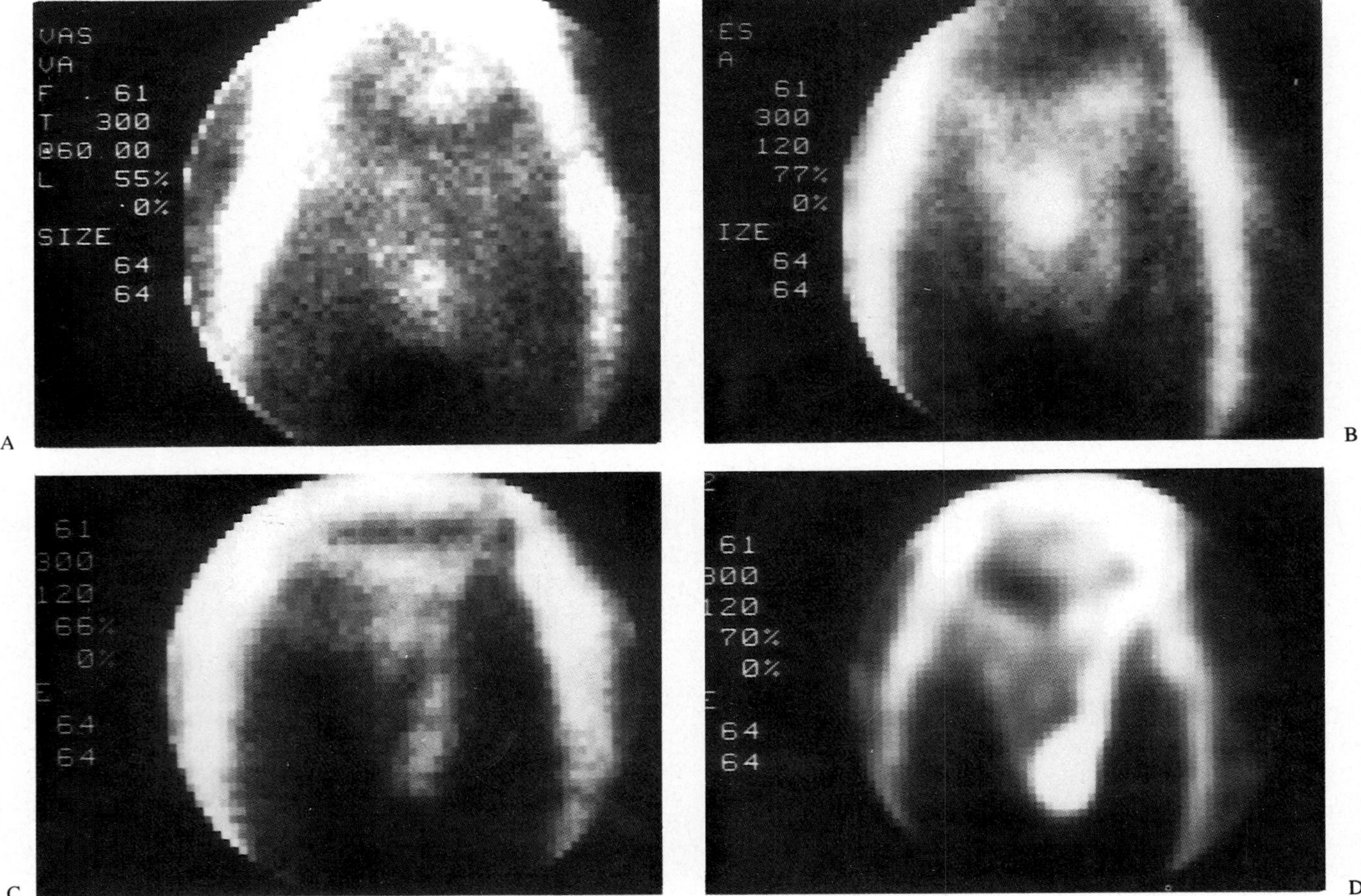

Figure 32. Scintigraphic studies in evaluating varicocele. Examples of blood-pool scintigraphy demonstrating: (**A**) Grade O (normal study), (**B**) Grade 1 (minimal reflux), (**C**) Grade 2 (moderate reflux), and (**D**) Grade 3 (severe reflux). (Reproduced from Reference 138 with permission.)

TECHNIQUE

The radionuclide method described by Geatti et al. provides a useful means of diagnosing and grading varicocele.[165] The patient is prepared as for scrotal scintigraphy described above. In vivo thinning of red blood cells with 0.15 μg/kg of stannous chloride is followed by intravenous administration of 370 MBq (10 mCi) ^{99m}Tc-pertechnetate. Dynamic frames are collected at 5-second intervals, followed by static blood pool images of 500K counts. Figure 32 shows various grades of reflux. Figure 33 demonstrates an example of the dynamic flow study in Grade 3 reflux.

EFFICACY

Most studies have shown a reasonably good correlation between the size of blood pool activity and clinical estimates of varicocele size.[127, 163–167] Geatti et al. found that scintigraphy was as accurate as ultrasound and thermography and had a slightly greater concordance with estimation of varicocele grade by contrast phlebography. Preliminary studies suggest that scintigraphy may be useful in detecting subclinical varicocele. Wheatley et al. found positive blood-pool images in several patients who had stress patterns by semen analysis, yet who had no clinical evidence of varicocele. This may prove to be the most useful type of case to study with scintigraphy. Scintigraphy is also a logical test to assess the results of surgery on scrotal reflux, because quantitative images of reasonable resolution can be obtained noninvasively in minutes.

PENILE SCINTIGRAPHY IN THE EVALUATION OF IMPOTENCE

For many years the only practical approach to impotence due to organic causes was the implantation of prosthetic devices.[168] However, advances in the treatment of vascular impotence by penile revascularization procedures have spurred an interest in diagnostic procedures that can provide the basis for specific therapeutic approaches.[169] Perhaps with

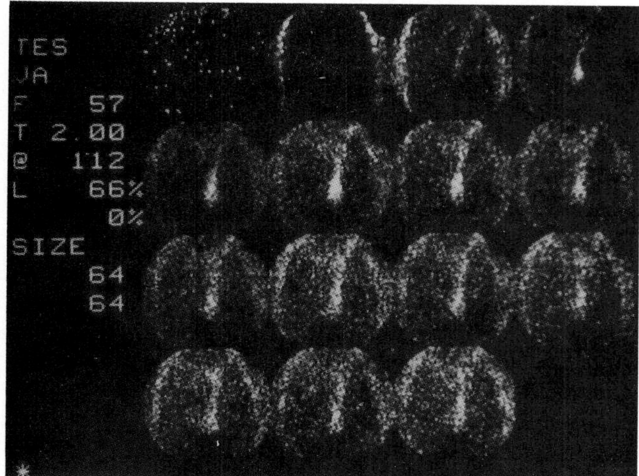

A

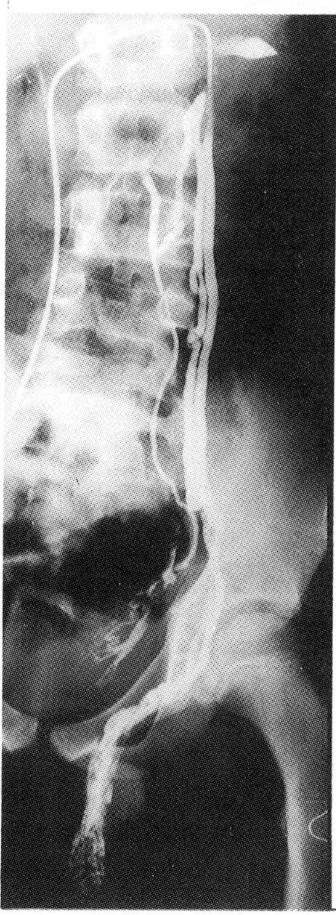

B

Figure 33. **(A)**. Radionuclide angiogram demonstrating Grade 3 varicocele reflux via the left internal spermatic vein (Series of 8-s frames added from 2-s per frame acquisition. **(B)**. Left internal spermatic vein phlebography demonstrating a moderate (Grade 2) varicocele. (Reproduced from Reference 138 with permission.)

no other organ is there a greater need for the type of noninvasive means of evaluating arterial and venous vascular integrity that nuclear diagnostic procedures offer.

Vascular Anatomy and Erectile Dynamics

The penis is supplied by branches of the internal pudendal artery which, after giving off branches to the perineum and scrotum, becomes the penile artery. The penile artery, in turn, divides into branches that supply the skin and glans (*dorsal* artery), spongiosum (*urethral* a.), the urethral bulb (*bulbar* a.), and the erectile tissues of the corpora cavernosa (*cavernous* a.). Venous blood drains through three groups of veins at varying depths: the *superficial dorsal v.* drains the skin and superficial structures; the *deep dorsal v.* drains the glans penis; and the *cavernous veins* drain the three corpora. All of these veins converge into the external pudendal vein and, thence, to the external iliac vein.

Normal erection takes place through a series of neurovascular and neuromuscular processes, all mediated by the autonomic nervous system. In simplest terms, the erectile response begins by relaxation of the smooth muscles of the cavernous arterioles and sinusoids, resulting in arterial dilatation and increased corporal blood flow. During tumescence, there is an increase in intracavernosal pressure which, secondarily, decreases arterial flow and closes venous outflow. When the intracorporal pressure nears the systolic pressure of the cavernosal artery, both arterial inflow and venous outflow approach zero. This results in a sustained, rigid erection. Detumescence follows relaxation of smooth muscles and opening of the venous channels.[170]

Types of Impotence

It was once believed that most cases of impotence were psychogenic in nature. Recent evidence suggests that 50 to 70% of cases have an underlying organic cause: neurogenic, hormonal dysfunction, drug-induced impairment, and anatomic and vascular abnormalities.[168,169,171] The initial history, physical examination, and laboratory workup exclude most neurological, drug-related, hormonal (e.g. hypoprolactinemia), and metabolic causes. In many centers nocturnal penile tumescence monitoring is performed to distinguish psychogenic from a neurogenic or vascular etiology of impotence. More often, the initial screening examination is the intracavernosal injection of such vasoactive agents as papaverine, phentolamine or prostaglandin E1.[171,172] Papaverine is the most commonly used. It acts by relaxing the smooth muscle of the cavernous sinusoids and arterioles. This bypasses neurogenic factors and simulates the hemodynamic changes that occur in normal physiological erection. A normal response generally rules out vascular insufficiency as the cause of impotence, and a less than full response suggests the need for further examinations of vascular competence.[172,173]

Vasculogenic impotence is of 2 general types: arterial and venous. Arterial impotence is usually due to occlusive disease resulting from atherosclerosis, and is predominantly a disease of older men. The diagnosis of arterial occlusion is made by penile plethysmography (comparing penile systolic pressure with that in the arm), by pulsed Doppler ultrasound, and by contrast arteriography.[174] The latter procedure is often reserved for patients who are reasonable candidates for angioplasty or bypass surgery. Occlusions of the proximal internal iliac and hypogastric arteries can often be corrected by reconstructive surgery or angioplasy, but occlusions of more distal arteries are more difficult to correct.[175]

Venous impotence is caused by incomplete closure and leakage through the venous outflow vessels. Traditionally, the diagnosis of venous disease has been made by dynamic infusion cavernosometry, in which the rate of infused saline required to sustain tumescence is measured and a determination made as to whether or not the rate of inflow is normal. Often, the incompetent vessels can be specifically localized by cavernosography, a procedure in which contrast media is injected into the tumescent cavernosa and the drainage assessed.[174,176]

Radionuclide Studies

Early studies using radionuclide techniques to evaluate impotence were conducted by Shirai and Nakamura, using ^{131}I-labeled human serum albumen,[177] ^{113m}In-microcolloid,[178] and ^{99m}Tc-pertechnetate to evaluate penile blood flow.[179] Kim et al. have shown reasonably good separation of arterial and venous impotence using time/activity curves before and after intracavernosal injection of papaverine.[180]

Several studies have used the washout of ^{133}Xe-injected into the penis to assess penile vascularity.[181–184] Typically, 3 to 4 MBq ^{133}Xe in saline is injected into one corpora cavernosum in the midshaft using a 25- or 26-gauge needle.[183] The washout of activity is measured with a scintillation camera and the clearance half-time determined. The calculation of blood flow is then determined according to the method defined by Lassen[185]:

$$\text{Flow (mL/min/100g)} = K \times \lambda \times 100$$

where K is the disappearance constant = 0.693/T1/2 (mL/min − 1) and λ is the partition coefficient of muscle/blood for xenon = ~0.7 mL/g. Hayden found penile blood flow in the flaccid state in normal people ranged from 0.1 to 1.7 mL/min/100 g with a mean of 0.7 0.6 mL/min/100 g.[183] In these flaccid state measurements, there was no difference between normal and impotent patients.

Yeh et al. measured ^{133}Xe washout before and 20 minutes after intracavernosal injection of prostaglandin E1, a smooth muscle relaxant, to induce erection.[186] They showed, as expected, that clearance is reduced by erection in normal subjects but, in patients with venous leakage without arterial disease, clearance is increased.

To evaluate both arterial and venous integrity in the same setting, Schwartz et al. have combined penile plethysmography with ^{127}Xe washout studies.[187] In the plethysmography portion of the study, circulating red cells are labeled with ^{99m}Tc-pertechnetate and the penile blood *inflow* and volume changes are measured during papavarine-induced erection (Fig. 34). Flow rates are determined by deriving time/activity curves over the penis during tumescence and comparing with a standard syringe of the patient's own labeled red cells (Fig. 35). Normal inflow rates were 20 mL/min.

In the xenon washout studies, ^{127}Xe in saline was used

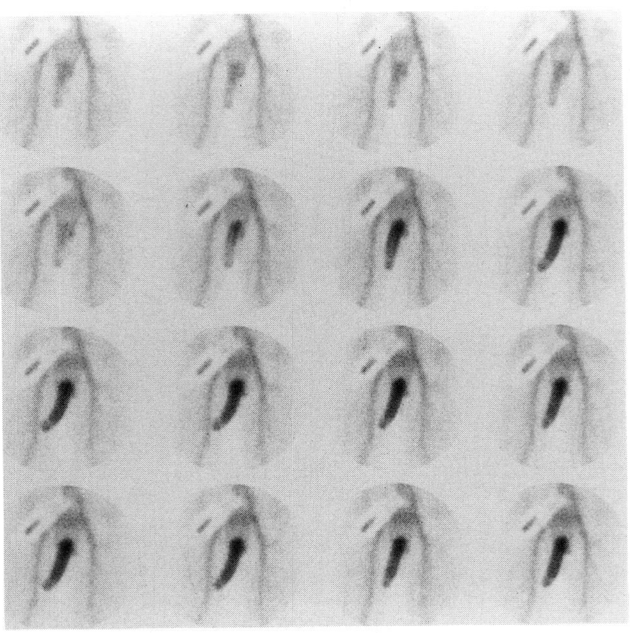

Figure 34. Serial 15–sec images from a radionuclide penile plethysmography study. Intracorporal papaverine was injected after 30 seconds (top row). Increased inflow is visible 45 seconds later as tumescence begins. (Reproduced with kind permission of Alan Schwartz and Michael Graham.)

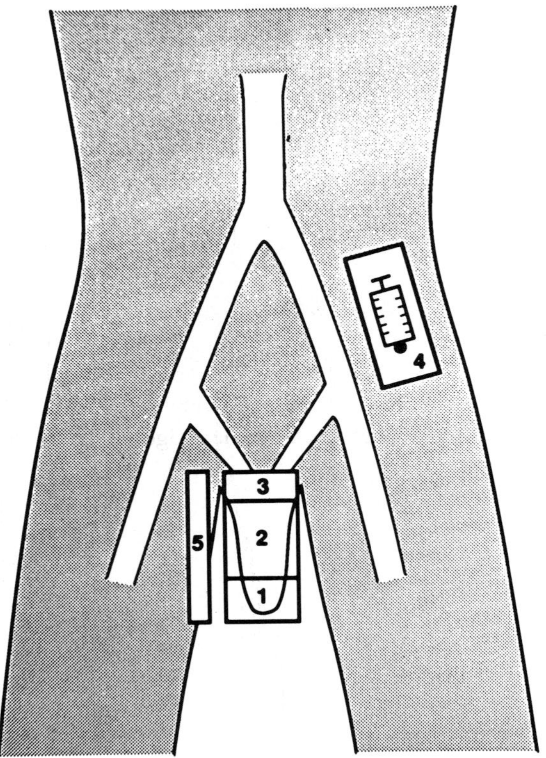

Figure 35. Regions of interest from which time-activity curves and background corrections are derived in radionuclide penile plethysmography. (Reproduced from Reference 187 with permission.)

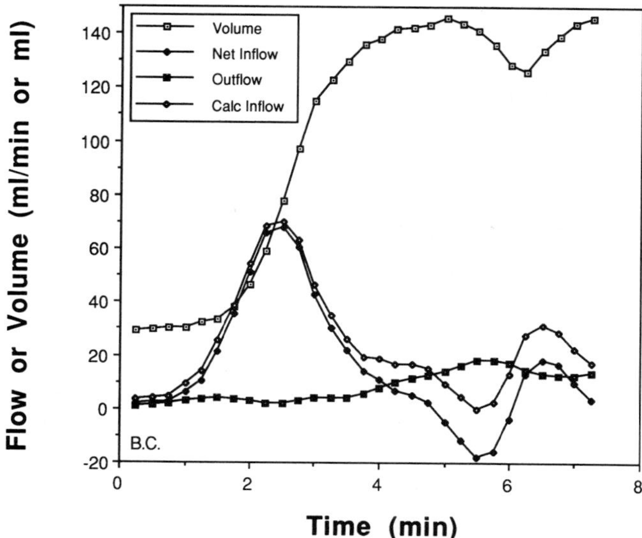

Figure 36. Time-activity curves from a normal volunteer representing total penile blood volume, net inflow, and net outflow. Note that outflow remains low during the period of tumescence and that total blood volume rises steeply during onset of tumescence. (Reproduced from Reference 187 by permission.)

because of its higher energy principle gamma ray (68% 203 keV). Scatter into the lower energy ^{99m}Tc window is corrected, using dual channel recording and computer subtractions. By this technique, penile inflow and outflow rates can be assessed simultaneously (Fig. 36). In arterial insufficiency, reduced inflow is recorded, but outflow rates increase in venous vascular leakage.[187]

Miraldi and colleagues have confirmed the results of Schwartz et al. and have shown that patients with venous leak and arterial insufficiency can be separated from healthy patients by the dual-radioisotope technique using vasoactive drugs to induce tumescence, and a relatively simple compartmental model.[192]

Relation to Other Imaging Tests

We have aready described the most common radiographic and sonographic techniques used to evaluate arterial and venous integrity. Recent advances in duplex and color Doppler ultrasound appear to give a decided edge to these noninvasive procedures when combined with drug-induced erection.[188–191] Measurements of peak blood flow velocities can be measured, even in small penile arteries, and analysis of peak systolic and dyastolic velocities reliably separates arterial insufficiency from venous incompetency. Nevertheless, the ability to measure blood flow per unit tissue mass is an important contribution toward understanding physiological mechanisms, especially when studying the effect of drugs that alter blood flow and erectile response.

Acknowledgments. Figures 6, 13–16 courtesy of Dr. Massoud Majd, Department of Diagnostic Imaging, Children's National Medical Center, Washington, D.C.

REFERENCES

1. Smith HW, Goldring W, Chasis H. The measurement of the tubular excretory mass, effective blood flow and filtration rate in the normal human kidney. *J Clin Invest* 1938;17:263.
2. Tubis M, Posnick E, Nordyke RA. Preparation and use of I-131 labelled sodium iodohippurate in kidney function tests. *Proc Soc Exp Biol Med* 1960;103:497.
3. Nordyke RA, Tubis M, Blahd WH. Use of radioiodinated hippuran for individual kidney function tests. *J Lab Clin Med* 1960;56:438.
4. Taplin GV, et al. *The radioisotope renogram: An external test for individual kidney function and upper tract patency.* UCLA School of Medicine Atomic Energy Project No. 366, 1956.
5. Fritzberg AR, Klingensmith WC, Whitney WP, et al. Chemical and biological studies of Tc-99m N,N′-bis(mercaptoacetamide)ethylenediamine: a potential replacement for I-131 iodohippurate. *J Nucl Med* 1981;22:258.
6. Dubovsky EV, Russel CD. ^{99m}Tc-MAG$_3$: The multipurpose renal radiopharmaceutical, in Freeman, LM (ed): *Nuclear Medicine Annual.* New York, Raven Press, 1991, p 1.
7. Eshima D, Taylor A Jr. Technetium-99m (^{99m}Tc) Mercaptoacetyltriglycine: Update on the new ^{99m}Tc renal tubular function agent. *Semin Nucl Med* 1992;22:61.
8. Eshima D, Taylor A, Fritzberg AR, et al. Animal evaluation of Tc-99m triamide mercaptide complexes as potential renal imaging agents. *J Nucl Med* 1987;28:1180.
9. Taylor A, Eshima D. Effects of altered physiologic states on clearance and biodistribution of technetium-99m MAG$_3$, iodine-131 OIH and iodine-125 iothalamate. *J Nucl Med* 1988;29:616–622.
10. Muller-Suur R, Muller-Suur C. Renal and extrarenal handling of a new imaging compound (99m-Tc-MAG-3) in the rat. *Eur J Nucl Med* 1986;12:438–442.
11. Muller-Suur R, Muller-Suur C. Glomerular filtration and tubular secretion of MAG-3 in the rat kidney. *J Nucl Med* 1989;30:1986–1991.
12. Bubeck B, Brandau W, Weber E, Kalble T, Parekh N, Georgi P. Pharmacokinetics of Technetium-99m-MAG3 in humans. *J Nucl Med* 1990;31:1285–1293.
13. Taylor A, Ziffer JA, Steves A, Eshima D, Delaney VB, and Welchel JD. Clinical Comparison of I-131 Orthoiodohippurate and the Kit Formulation of Tc-99m Mercaptoacetyltriglycine. *Radiology* 1989;170:721–725.
14. Russell CD, Thorstad B, Yester MV, Stutzman M, Baker T, Dubovsky EV. Comparison of Technetium-99m MAG3 with Iodine-131 Hippuran by a Simultaneous Dual Channel Technique. *J Nucl Med* 1988;29:1189–1193.
15. Al-Nahhas AA, Jafri RA, Britton KE, et al. Clinical experience with 99mTc-Mag3, mercaptoacetyltriglycine, and a comparison with 99mTc-DTPA. *Eur J Nucl Med* 1988; 14:453.
16. Bannister KM, Penglis S, Bellen JC, Baker RJ, Chatterton BE. Kit preparation of technetium-99m-mercaptoacetyltriglycine: Analysis, biodistribution and comparison with technetium-99m-DTPA in patients with impaired renal function. *J Nucl Med* 1990;31:1568–1573.
17. Fraille M, Castell J, Buxeda M, et al. Transplant renography: 99m-Tc-DTPA versus 99m-Tc-MAG3. A preliminary note. *Eur J Nucl Med* 1989;15:776–779.
18. Farmer CD, et al. Measurement of renal function with radioiodinated diatrizoate and omicron hippurate. *Am J Clin Pathol* 1967;47:9.
19. Cotlove E. ^{14}C-carboxyl-labeled inulin as tracer for inulin (abst.). *Fed Proc* 1955;14:32.
20. Sigman EM, Elmwood CM, Knox F. The measurement of

glomerular filtration rate in man with sodium iothalamate ^{131}I (Conray). *J Nucl Med* 1966;7:60.
21. Watkin DM, et al. Renal clearance of intravenously administered vitamin B-12. *Proc Soc Exp Biol Med* 1961;107:219.
22. Funck-Brentan JL, et al. Nouvelle methode de mesure de la filtration glomerulaire sans prelevement d'urine. Mesure de la clearance du DTPA lanthane 140 par enregistrment de la decroissance de la radioactivite receueillie par detection externe. *Rev Fr Etud Clin Biol* 1967;12:790.
23. Russell CD, Rowell K, Scott JW. Quality control of Tc-99m-DTPA: Correlation of analytic tests with in vivo protein binding in man. *J Nucl Med* 1986;23:560.
24. Boyd RE, Robson J, Hunt FC. 99mTc-gluconate complexes for renal scintigraphy. *Br J Radiol* 1973;46:604.
25. Handmaker H, Young B, Lowenstein J. Clinical experience with ^{99m}Tc-DMSA (dimercaptosuccinic acid). A new renal imaging agent. *J Nucl Med* 1975;16:28.
26. deLange MJ, Piers DA, Kosterink JGW, van Luijk WHJ, Meijer S, de Zeeuw D, van der Hem GK. Renal Handling of Technetium-99m DMSA: Evidence for Glomerular Filtration and Peritubular Uptake. *J Nucl Med* 1989;30:1219–1223.
27. Moretti JL, et al. Dimercapto-succinic acid complexes: Their structure, biological behavior and renal localization, in Joekes AM et al. (eds): *Radionuclides in Nephrology.* London, Academic Press, 1982.
28. Bingham JB, et al. Use of ^{99m}Tc-DMSA as a static renal imaging agent. *Contrib Nephrol* 1978;11:95.
29. Lee H-B, Blaufox MD. Mechanism of renal concentration of Technetium-99m glucoheptonate. *J Nucl Med* 1985;26:1308.
30. Raynaud C, et al. Radioactive thallium: A new agent for scans of the renal medulla, in Blaufox MD, Funck-Brentano I (eds.): *Radionuclides in Nephrology.* New York, Grune and Stratton, 1972.
31. McAfee JG, Wagner HN Jr. Visualization of the renal parenchyma by scinti-scanning with ^{203}Hg-Neohydrin. *Radiology* 1960;75:820.
32. Raynaud C, Desgrez A, Kellershohn C. Exploration renale a l'aide de la neohydrine et du bichlorure de Hg, marque aux mercure radioactive ^{197}Hg, in *Radioaktive Isotopes in Klinic und Forschung*. Vol 5 Munich/Berline, Urgan und Schwartzenberg, 1963.
33. Harper PV, et al. Technetium-99m as scanning agent. *Radiology* 1965;85:101.
34. Charamza O, Budikova M. Herstellungsmethode eines ^{99m}Tc-Zink-Komplexes fur die Nierenszintigraphie. *Nuclearmedizin* 1969;8:301.
35. Stacy BD, Torburn GD. Chromium-51 ethylenediamine tetraacetate for estimation of glomerular filtration rate. *Science* 1966;152:1076.
36. Sapirstein LA. Volume of distribution and clearance of intravenously injected creatinine in the dog. *Am J Physiol* 1955;181:330.
37. Tauxe WN, Maher FT, Taylor WF. Effective renal plasma flow—estimation from theoretical volumes of distribution of intravenously injected ^{131}I-orthoiodohippurate. *Mayo Clin Proc* 1971;46:524.
38. Tauxe WN. Use of radioactive media in assessment of renal function: A review. *Br J Urol* 1969;41:64.
39. Tauxe WN, Dubovsky EV, Kidd T, et al. Parameters of renal function in normal subjects before and after kidney donation, in *Proceedings of the Third World Congress, World Federation of Nuclear Medicine and Biology*, Vol II. Paris, Pergamon, 1982, p 51.
40. Botsch H, et al. Estimation of effective renal plasma flow by a simplified method using a single plasma sample. Comparison with the 2-compartment analysis and other simplified methods, in Hollenberg NK, Lunge S (eds.): *Radionuclides in Nephrology.* Stuttgart, Georg Thieme, 1980.
41. Russell CD, Dubovsky EV, Scott JW. Simplified methods for renal clearance in children: scaling for patient size. *J Nucl Med* 1991;32:1821.
42. Tauxe WN et al. Prediction of urinary excretion of ^{131}I-orthoiodohippurate. *Eur J Nucl Med* 1982;7:102.
43. Downing M, et al. Prediction of renal function after unilateral nephrectomy in patients with various nephrourological problems (abst.). *J Nucl Med* 1982;23:110.
44. Bianchi C, et al. Filtration fraction in unilateral hypertensive renal disease and a new noninvasive method for its measurement. *Contrib Nephrol* 1978;11:29.
45. Dubovsky EV, et al. Dynamic renal studies in the early post-transplant period, in *Dynamic Studies with Radioisotopes in Medicine*. Vol I. Vienna, IAEA, 1975.
46. Russell CD, Thorstad BL, Yester MV, et al. Quantitation of renal function with Tc-99m mercaptoacetyltriglycine, a technetium-labeled analog of iodohippurate. *Radiology* 1989; 172:427.
47. Tauxe WN, Dubovsky EV, Kidd T, et al. New formulae for the calculation of effective renal plasma flow. *Eur J Nucl Med* 1982;7:52.
48. Dubovsky EV, Gates GF, Russell CD. Three approaches to computer-assisted function studies of the kidney and evaluation of scintigraphic methods, in Tauxe WN, Dubovsky EV (eds.): *Nuclear Medicine in Clinical Urology and Nephrology.* Norwalk, Appleton-Century-Crofts, 1985, p 157.
49. Schaap GH, Alferink THR, de Jong RBJ, et al. ^{99m}Tc-MAG$_3$: dynamic studies in patients with renal disease. *Eur J Nucl Med* 1988;14:28.
50. Jafri RA, Britton KE, Nimmon CC, et al. Technetium-99m MAG$_3$, a comparison with iodine-123 and iodine-131 orthoiodohippurate in patients with renal disorders. *J Nucl Med* 1988;29:147.
51. Al-Nahhas A, Jafri RA, Britton KE, et al. Clinical experience with ^{99m}Tc-MAG$_3$, mercaptoacetyltriglycine, and a comparison with ^{99m}Tc-DTPA. *Eur J Nucl Med* 1988;14:453.
52. Maini CL, Antonacci P, Sargiotto A, et al. Dynamic renal scanning using ^{99m}Tc-MAG$_3$ in man. *Eur J Nucl Med* 1989; 15:635.
53. Bannister KM, Penglis S, Bellen JC, et al. Kit preparation of technetium-99m-mercaptoacetyltriglycine: analysis, biodistribution and comparison with technetium-99m-DTPA in patients with impaired renal function. *J Nucl Med* 1990;31:1568.
54. Claessens RAMJ, Corstens FHM. Tc-99m-MAG$_3$ clearance determined in patients by simplified methods. *J Nucl Med* 1989;30:943.
55. Blaufox MD, Potchen EJ, Merrill JP. Measurement of effective renal plasma flow in man by external methods. *J Nucl Med* 1967;8:77.
56. Russell CD, Yound D, Billinglsey JD, Dubovsky EV. Technical procedures for use of the new kidney agent technetium-99m MAG$_3$. *J Nucl Med Technol* 1991;19:147.
57. Russell CD, Taylor AT Jr, Dubovsky EV, Eshima D. A single-injection, two-sample method for measuring renal ^{99m}Tc-MAG$_3$ clearance in both children and adults. *Nucl Med Biol* 1995;22:55.
58. Tauxe WN, Hunt JC, Burbank MK. The radioisotope renogram (orthoiodohippurate-I-131): Standardization of technique and expression of data. *Am J Clin Pathol* 1962;37:367.
59. Kirchner P, Goldman MH, Leapman SAB, Keipfer RF. Clinical application of the kidney to aortic blood flow index (K/A ratio). *Contrib Nephrol* 1978;11:120.
60. Larsson I, Lindstedt E, Ohlin P, et al. A scintillation camera technique for quantitative estimation of separate kidney func-

tion and its use before nephrectomy. *Scan J Clin Lab Invest* 1975;35:517.

61. Skov PE, Hansen HE. Glomerular filtration rate, renal plasma flow and filtration fraction in living donors before and after nephrectomy. *Acta Med Scand* 1974;195:97.
62. Dubovsky EV, Russell CD. Quantitation of renal function with glomerular and tubular agents. *Semin Nucl Med* 1982; 12:308.
63. Conway JJ. "Well-tempered" diuresis renoghraphy: Its historical development, physiological and technical pitfalls and standardized technique protocol. *Semin Nucl Med* 1992; 22:74.
64. Thrall JH, Koff SA, Keyes JW. Diuretic radionuclide renography and scintigraphy in the differential diagnosis of hydroureteronephrosis. *Semin Nucl Med* 1981;11:89.
65. Majd M. Avoiding Pitfalls in Pediatric Uroradiology—Diuretic Renography in Shortliffe LMD (ed): *Dialogues in Pediatric Urology.* vol. 12. William J. Miller Associates, Inc. 1989, pp 6–8.
66. Brown SCW, Upsdell SM, O'Reilly PH. The importance of renal function in the interpretation of duresis renography. *Br J Urol* 1992;69:121.
67. Upsdell SM, Testa HJ, Lawson RS. The F-15 diuresis renogram in suspected obstruction of the upper urinary tract. *Br J Urol* 1992;69:126.
68. O'Reilly PH. Diuresis renography. Recent advances and recommended protocols. *Br J Urol* 1992;69:113.
69. Gifford RW. Evaluation of the hypertensive patient with emphasis on detecting curable causes. *Milbank Mem Fund Q* 1969;47:170–186.
70. Berglund C, Andersson O, Wihelmsen L. Prevalence of primary and secondary hypertension: Studies in a random population sample. *Br Med J* 1976;2:554–556.
71. Sfakianakis GN, Sfakianaki E, and Bourgoignie J. Renal Scintigraphy Following Angiotensin-Converting Enzyme Inhibition in the Diagnosis of Renovascular Hypertension (Captopril Scintigraphy). *Nuclear Medicine Annual* 1988;125–170.
72. Fommei E, Ghione S, Hilson AJW, et al. Captopril radionuclide test in renovascular hypertension: a European multicentre study. *Europ J Nucl Med* 1993;20:617.
73. Saddler MC and Black HR. Captopril renal scintigraphy; a clinician's perspective, in *Yearbook of Nuclear Medicine.* Baltimore, Md, Williams and Wilkins Co, 1990, pp xiii–xxxiv.
74. Wilcox CS. ACE Inhibitors in the Diagnosis of Renovascular Hypertension. *Hosp Practice*; January, 1992:117–126.
75. Schreiber MJ, Pohl MA, Novick AC. The natural history of atherosclerotic and fibrous renal artery disease. *Urol Clin North Am* 1984;11:383–392.
76. Schwartz CJ, White TA. Stenosis of renal artery: An unselected necropsy study. *Br Med J* 1964;2:1415–1421.
77. Luscher TF, Lie JT, Stanson AW, Houser OW, Hollier LH, Sheps SG. Arterial fibromuscular dysplasia. *Mayo Clin Proc* 1987;62:931–952.
78. Pickering TG. Renovascular Hypertension: Etiology and Pathophysiology. *Semin Nucl Med* 1989;XIX:79–88.
79. Nally JV, Black HR. State-of-the-art review: Captopril renography—pathophysiological considerations and clinical observations. *Semin Nucl Med* 1992;XXII:85–97.
80. Majd M, Potter BM, Guzzetta PC, Ruley EJ. Effect of captopril on efficacy of renal scintigraphy in detection of renal artery stenosis. *J Nucl Med* 1983;24:23.
81. Hovinga TKK, de Jong PE, Piers A, Beekhuis H, van der Hem GK, de Zeeuw D. Diagnostic use of angiotensin converting enzyme inhibitors in radioisotope evaluation of unilateral renal artery stenosis. *J Nucl Med* 1989;30:605–614.
82. Dondi M, Franchi R, Levorato M, Zuccala' A, Gaggi R, Mirelli M, Stella A, Marchetta F, Losinno F, Monetti N. Evaluation of hypertensive patients by means of captopril enhanced renal scintigraphy with technetium-99m DTPA. *J Nucl Med* 1989;30:615–621.
83. Sfakianakis GN, Bourgoignie JJ, Jaffe D, Kyriakides G, Perez-Stable E, Duncan RC. Single dose captopril scintigraphy in the diagnosis of renovascular hypertension. *J Nucl Med* 1987;28:1383–1392.
84. Bajnok L, Varga J, Kurta G. Technetium-99m diethylene triamine penta-acetic acid and dimercaptosuccinic acid in the detection of a segmental branch stenosis of the renal artery by captopril renography. *Eur J Nucl Med* 1992;19:62–64.
85. Katial R, Ziessman HA. Segmental branch renal artery stenosis diagnosed with captopril renography. *J Nucl Med* 1992; 33:266–268.
86. Morton KA, Rose SC, Haakenstad AO, Handy JE, Scuderi AJ, Datz FL. Diagnostic use of angiotensin converting enzyme (ACE)-inhibited renal scintigraphy in the identification of selective renal artery stenosis in the presence of multiple renal arteries: a case report. *J Nucl Med* 1990;31: 1847–1850.
87. Simon T, Cuocolo A, Sandrock D, Miller DL. Renal scintigraphy in renovascular hypertension secondary to stenosis of a supplemental renal artery. *J Nucl Med* 1990;31:674–678.
88. Itoh K, Shinohara M, Togashi M, Koyanagi T. Captopril renal scintigraphy in a patient with bilateral renal artery stenosis. *J Nucl Med* 1989;30:2042–2045.
89. Miach PJ, Ernest D, McKay J, Dawborn JK. Renography with captopril in renal transplant recipients. *Transplant Proc* 1989;21:1953–1954.
90. Dubovsky EV, Diethelm AG, Tobin M, Tauxe WN. Early recognition of chronic humoral rejection in long-term followup of kidney recipients by a comprehensive renal radionuclide study. *Transplant Proc* 1977;9:43–47.
91. Manier SM, Van Nostrand D, Kyle RW. Primer and atlas for renal transplant scintigraphy: flow, Tc-99m DTPA, I-131 Hippuran. *Clin Nucl Med* 1985;10:118–133.
92. Dubovsky EV, Russell CD. Radionuclide evaluation of renal transplants. *Semin Nucl Med* 1988;18:181–198.
93. Jackson SA, Erlich L, Martin RH. The renal washout parameter as an indicator of transplant rejection. *Eur J Nucl Med* 1986;12:86–90.
94. Rutland MD. A comprehensive analysis of renal DTPA studies. II. Renal transplant evaluation. *Nucl Med Commun* 1985;6:21–30.
95. George EA, Codd JE, Newton WT, Haibach H, Donati RM. Comparative evaluation of renal transplant rejection with radioiodinated fibrinogen, ^{99m}Tc-sulfur colloid, and ^{67}Ga-citrate. *J Nucl Med* 1976;17:175–80.
96. Salaman JR. Renal transplant rejection detected with 125I-fibrinogen. *Proc R Soc Med* 1972;65:34.
97. Yeboah ED, Chisholm GD, Short MD, Petrie A. The detection and prediction of acute rejection episodes in human renal transplants using radioactive fibrinogen. *Br J Urol* 1973; 45:273–280.
98. George EA, Meyerovitz M, Codd JE, Fletcher JW, Donati RM. Renal allograft accumulation of Tc-99m sulfur colloid: Temporal quantitation and scintigraphic assessment. *Radiology* 1983;148:547–551.
99. Sundram FX, Edmondson RPS, Ang ES, Goh ASW, Toh HJ. ^{99}Tc^{m}-(tin) colloid scans in the evaluation of renal transplant rejection. *Nucl Med Commun* 1986;7:897–906.
100. Chandler ST, Buckels J, Hawker RJ, Smith N, Barnes AD, McCollum CN. Indium-labeled platelet uptake in rejecting renal transplants. *Surg Gynecol Obstet* 1983;157:242–246.
101. Collier BD, Isitman AT, Kaufman HM, Rao SA, Knobel J, Hellman RS, Zielonka JS, Pelc L. Concentration of In-111-oxime-labeled autologous leukocytes in noninfected and non-

rejecting renal allografts: concise communication *J Nucl Med* 1984;25:156–159.

102. Forstrom LA, Loken MK, Cook A, Chandler R, McCullough J. In-111-labeled leukocytes in the diagnosis of rejection and cytomegalovirus infection in renal transplant patients. *Clin Nucl Med* 1981;6:146–149.
103. Martin-Comin J. Kidney graft rejection studies with labeled platelets and lymphocytes. *Nucl Med Biol Int J Radiat Appl Instrum Part B* 1986;13:173–181.
104. Tisdale PL, Collier BD, Kauffman HM, Adams MB, Isitman AT, Hellman RS, Hoffmann RG, Rao SA, Joestgen T, Krohn L. Early diagnosis of acute postoperative renal transplant rejection by Indium-111-labeled platelet scintigraphy. *J Nucl Med* 1986;27:1266–1272.
105. Alavi A, Grossman R, Siegel A. Intraperitoneal urine leak following renal transplant. The role of radionuclide imaging. *J Nucl Med* 1990;31:1206–1210.
106. Williams ED. Renal single photon emission computed tomography: Should we do it? *Semin Nucl Med* 1992;22:112.
107. Majd M, Rushton HG. Renal cortical scintigraphy in the diagnosis of acute pyelonephritis. *Semin Nucl Med* 1992; 22:98–111.
108. Arnold AJ, Brownless SM, Carty HM, Rickwood AMK. Detection of renal scarring by DMSA scanning—an experimental study. *J Pediatr Surg* 1990;25:391–393.
109. Parkhouse HF, Godley ML, Cooper J, Risdon RA, Ransley PG. Renal imaging with 99Tcm-labelled DMSA in the detection of acute pyelonephritis: an experimental study in the pig. *Nucl Med Commun* 1989;10:63–70.
110. Majd M, Rushton HG, Jantausch B, Wiedermann BL. Relationship among vesicoureteral reflux, P-fimbriated Escherichia coli, and acute pyelonephritis in children with febrile urinary tract infection. *J Pediatr* 1991;119:578–585.
111. Bjorgvinsson E, Majd M, Eggli KD. Diagnosis of acute pyelonephritis in children: comparison of sonography and 99mTc-DMSA scintigraphy. *A J R* 1991;157:539–543.
112. Farnsworth RH, Rossleigh MA, Leighton DM, Bass SJ, Rosenberg AR. The detection of reflux nephropathy in infants by 99m Technetium dimercaptosuccinic acid studies. *J Urol* 1991;145:542–546.
113. Verber IG, Strudley MR, Meller ST. 99mTc dimercaptosuccinic acid (DMSA) scan as first investigation of urinary tract infection. *Arch Dis Child* 1988;63:1320–1325.
114. Monsour M, Azmy AF, MacKenzie JR. Renal scarring secondary to vesicoureteric reflux. Critical assessment and new grading. *Br J Urol* 1987;60:320–324.
115. Sty JR, Wells RG, Starshak RJ, Schroeder BA. Imaging in acute renal infection in children. *A J R* 1987;148:471–477.
116. Stoller ML, Kogan BA. Sensitivity of 99m Technetium-dimercaptosuccinic acid for the diagnosis of chronic pyelonephritis: Clinical and theoretical considerations. *J Urol* 1986; 135:977–980.
117. Traisman ES, Conway JJ, Traisman HS, Yogev R, Firlit C, Shkolnik A, Weiss S. The localization of urinary tract infection with 99m Tc glucoheptonate scintigraphy. *Pediatr Radiol* 1986;16:403.
118. Felson BE, Moskowitz M. Renal pseudotumors: The regenerated nodule and other lumps, bumps, and dromedary humps. *A J R* 1969;107:720–729.
119. Kyaw MM, Newman H. Renal pseudotumors due to ectopic accessory renal arteries: The angiographic diagnosis. *A J R* 1971;113:443–446.
120. Green WG, Pressman BD, McClennan BL, Casarella WJ. "Column of Bertin": diagnosis by nephrotomography. *AJR* 1972;116:715–723.
121. Lutzker LG, Zucker LS. Testicular scanning and other applications of radionuclide imaging of the genital tract. *Semin Nucl Med* 1990;20:159.
122. Skoglund RW, McRoberts JW, Magda H. Torsion of the spermatic cord: A review of literature and an analysis of 70 new cases. *J Urol* 1970;104:604.
123. Haynes BE, Bessen HA, Haynes VE. The diagnosis of testicular torsion. JAMA 1983;249:2522.
124. Hitch DC, Shandling B, Lilly JR. Recognition of bilateral neonatal testicular torsion. *Arch Dis Child* 1980;55:153.
125. Chen DCP, Holder LE, Melloul M. Radionuclide scrotal imaging: Further experience with 210 new patients. Part 2: Results and discussion. *J Nucl Med* 1983;24:841.
126. Atallah MW, Mazzarino AF, Horton BF. Testicular scan, diagnosis and follow-up for torsion of testis. *J Urol* 1977; 118:120.
127. Wheatley JK, Fajman WA, Witten FR. Clinical experience with the radioisotope varicocele scan as a screening method for the detection of varicocele. *Urology* 1982;128:57.
128. Heck LL, Coles JL, Van Hove ED, et al. Value of Tc-99m pertechnetate imaging in evaluation of testicular torsion. *J Nucl Med* 1974;15:501.
129. Mukerjee MG, Vollers RA, Mittemeyer BT, et al. Diagnostic value of Tc-99m in scrotal scan. *Urology* 1975;6:453.
130. Riley TW, Mosbaugh PG, Coles JL, et al. Use of radioisotope scan in evaluation of intrascrotal lesion. *J Urol* 1976;116:472.
131. Abu-Sleiman R, Ho JE, Gregory. Scrotal scanning: Present value and limits of interpretation. *Urology* 1979;13:326.
132. Boedecker RA, Sty JR, Jona JZ. Testicular scanning as a diagnostic aid in evaluating scrotal pain. *J Pediatr* 1979; 94:760.
133. Wasnick RJ, Pohutsky KR, Macchia RJ: Testicular torsion and usefulness of radionuclide scanning. *Urology* 1980;15:318.
134. Stage KH, Schoenvogel R, Lewis S: Testicular scanning: Clinical experience with 72 patients. *J Urol* 1980;125:334.
135. Fink-Bennett D, Uppal TK, Conway GF. Redux testis: A potential pitfall in testicular imaging. *J Urol* 1978;121: 821.
136. Dunn EK, Macchia RJ, Solomon NA. Scintigraphic pattern in missed testicular torsion. *Radiology* 1981;139:175.
137. Holder LE, Melloul M, Chen D: Current status of radionuclide scrotal imaging. *Semin Nucl Med* 1981;11:232.
138. Gilday DL, Ash JM, Savage JP, et al. The differentiation of testicular appendage, recent testicular and old testicular torsions in children. *J Nucl Med* 1978;19:719.
139. Boedecker RA, Glicklich M, Sty JR. Rim sign in endodermal sinus tumor. *Clin Nucl Med* 1979;4:130.
140. Vieras F, Kuhn CR. Nonspecificity of the "rim sign" in the scintigraphic diagnosis of missed testicular torsion. *Radiology* 1983;146:519.
141. Mishkin FS. Differential diagnostic features of the radionuclide scrotal image. *AJR* 1977;128:127.
142. Lutzker LG. Scrotal scintigraphy, in Tauxe WN, Dubovsky EV (eds.): *Nuclear Medicine in Clinical Urology and Nephrology.* Norwalk, Appleton-Century-Crofts, 1985, p321.
143. Mueller DL, Amundson GM, Rubin SZ, et al. Acute scrotal abnormalities in children: Diagnosis by combined sonography and scintigraphy. *AJR* 1988;150:643.
144. Mendel JB, Taylor GA, Treves S, et al. Testicular torsion in children: Scintigraphic assessment. *Pediatr Radiol* 1985; 15:110.
145. Chen DCP, Holder LE, Kaplan GN. Correlation of radionuclide imaging and diagnostic ultrasound in scrotal diseases. *J Nucl Med* 1986;27:1774.
146. Middleton WD, Melson GL. Testicular ischemia: color Doppler sonographic findings in five patients. *AJR* 1989; 1521:1237.
147. Middleton WD, Siegel BA, Melson GL, et al.: Acute scrotal

disorders: Prospective comparison of color doppler US and testicular scintigraphy. *Radiology* 1990;177:177.
148. Burks DD, Markey BJ, Burkhard TK, et al. Suspected testicular torsion and ischemia: evaluation with color Doppler sonography. *Radiology* 1990;175:815.
149. Lerner RM, Mevorach RA, Hulbert WC, Rabinowitz R. Color Doppler US in the evaluation of acute scrotal disease. *Radiology* 1990;176:355.
150. Trambert MA, Mattrey RF, Levine D, Berthoty DP: Subacute scrotal pain: Evaluation of torsion versus epididymitis with MR imaging. *Radiology* 1990;175:53.
151. Lutzker LG, Zuckier LS: Testicular scanning and other applications of radionuclide imaging of the genital tract. *Semin Nucl Med* 1990;20:159.
152. Ivanissevich O: Left varicocele due to reflux. Experience with 4470 operative cases in forty-two years. *J Int Coll Surg* 1960;34:742.
153. Dubin C, Amelar RD. Varicocelectomy as therapy in male infertility: a study of 504 cases. *J Urol* 1975;113:640.
154. Dublin L, Amelar RD. Varicocele size and results of varicocelectomy in selected subfertile men with varicocele. *Fertil Steril* 1970;21:606.
155. Task Force on the Diagnosis and Treatment of Infertility, Special Program of Research, Development and Research Training in Human Reproduction, World Health Organization. Comparison among different methods for the diagnosis of varicocele. *Fertil Steril* 1985;43:575.
156. Comhaire F, Monteyne R, Kunnen M. The value of scrotal thermography as compared with selective retrograde venography of the internal spermatic vein for the diagnosis of "subclinical varicocele." *Fertil Steril* 1976;27:694.
157. Comhaire F, Kunnen M. Selective retrograde venography of the internal spermatic vein: a conclusive approach to the diagnosis of varicocele. *Andrologia* 1976;8:11.
158. Gonda RL, Karo JJ, Forte RA, O'Donnell KT. Diagnosis of subclinical varicocele in infertility. *AJR* 1987;148:71.
159. Kormano M, Kahanpaa K, Svinhufvud V, Tanti E. Thermography of varicocele. *Fertil Steril* 1970;21:558.
160. Wolverson MD, Houttuin E, Heiber E, Sundaran M, Gregory J. High resolution real-time sonography of scrotal varicocele. *AJR* 1983;141:775.
161. Rifkin MD, Foy PM, Kurtz AB, et al. The role of diagnostic ultrasonography in varicocele evaluation. *J Ultrasound Med* 1983;2:271.
162. Hirsh AV, Cameron KM, Tyler JP, et al. The Doppler assessment of varicoceles and internal spermatic vein reflux in infertile men. *Br J Urol* 1980;51:50.
163. Freund J, Handelsman DJ, Bautovich GJ, et al. Detection of a varicocele by radionuclide blood-pool scanning. *Radiology* 1980;137:227.
164. Harris JD, Lipshultz LI, Conoley PH, et al. Radioisotope angiography in diagnosis of varicocele. *Urology* 1980;16:69.
165. Geatti O, Gasparini D, Shapiro B. A comparison of scintigraphy, thermography, ultrasound and phlebography in grading of clinical varicocele. *J Nucl Med* 1991;32:2092.
166. Coolsaet BLRA. The varicocele syndrome: venography determining the optimal level for surgical management. *J Urol* 1980;124:883.
167. Mali WPTM, Dei HY, Arndt JW, et al. Hemodynamics of the varicocele. Part I. Correlation among the clinical phlebographic and scintigraphic findings. *J Urol* 1986;135:483.
168. Padma-Nathan H, Goldstein I, Krane RJ. Evaluation of the impotent patient. *Semin Urol* 1986;4:225.
169. Baum N. Treatment of impotence. 1. Non-surgical methods. 2. Surgical methods. *Postgrad Med* 1987;81:133.
170. Aboseif SR, Lue TF. Hemodynamics of penile erection. *Urol Clin North Am* 1988;15:1.
171. Mueller SC, Lue TF. Evaluation of vasculogenic impotence. *Urol Clin North Am* 1988;15:65.
172. Lue RF, Tanagho CA. Physiology of erection and pharmacological management of impotence. *J Urol* 1987;137:829.
173. Abber JC, Lue TF, Orvis BR, et al. Diagnostic tests for impotence: a comparison of papaverine injection with penile-brachial index and nocturnal penile tumescence monitoring. *J Urol* 1986;135:923.
174. Krysiewicz S, Mellinger BC. The role of imaging in the diagnostic evaluation of impotence. *AJR* 1989;153:1133.
175. Orvis BR, Lue TF. New therapy of impotence, in Lytton B, Catalonia WJ, Lipshultz LI, et al. (eds.). *Advances in Urology.* Chicago, Year Book Medical, 1988, pp 173.
176. Mueller SC, Lue TF. Evaluation of vasculogenic impotence. *Urol Clin North Am* 1988;15:65.
177. Shirai M, Nakamura M. Differential diagnosis of organic and functional impotence by use of I131 human serum albumen. *Tohoku J Exp Med* 1970;101:317.
178. Shirai M, Nakamura M. Radioisotope penogram by means of 113m-In-microcolloid. *Tohoku J Exp Med* 1971;105:137.
179. Shirai M, Nakamura M. Diagnostic discrimination between organic and functional impotence by radioisotope penogram with 99m-Tc04. *Tohoku J Exp Med* 1975;116:9.
180. Kim SC, Kim KB, Oh CH. Diagnostic value of the radioisotope erection penogram for vasculogenic impotence. *J Urol* 1990;144:888.
181. Shirai M, Ishii N, Mitsukawa N, et al. Hemodynamic mechanism of erection in the human penis. *Arch Andrology* 1978;1:345.
182. Nseyo UO, Wilbur HJ, Kang SC, et al. Penile xenon-133 washout: a rapid method of screening for vasculogenic impotence. *Urology* 1984;23:31.
183. Haden HT, Katz PG, Mulligan T, Zasler ND. Penile blood flow by xenon-133 washout. *J Nucl Med* 1989;30:1032.
184. Wagner G. Differential diagnosis of erectile failure, in Wagner G, Green R (eds.). *Impotence: physiological, psychological, surgical diagnosis and treatment.* New York, Plenum Press, 1981, pp 109.
185. Lassen NA, Lindbjerg J, Munck O. Measurement of blood-flow through skeletal muscle by intramuscular injection of xenon-133. *Lancet* 1964;1:686.
186. Yeh SH, Liu RS, Ng MN, et al. Diagnosis of venous leakage by Xe-133 corporeal clearance after intracavernous injection of Prostaglandin E1 (PGE-1) in poor response patients (abst). *J Nucl Med* 1990;31:762.
187. Schwartz AN, Graham MM. Combined technetium radioisotope penile plethysmography and xenon washout: a technique for evaluating corpora cavernosal inflow and outflow during early tumescence. *J Nucl Med* 1991;32:404.
188. Schwartz AN, Wang KY, Mack LA, et al. Evaluation of normal erectile function with color flow Doppler sonography. *AJR* 1989;153:1141.
189. Quam JP, King BF, James EM, et al. Duplex and color Doppler sonographic evaluation of vasculogenic impotence. *AJR* 1989;153:1141.
190. Benson CB, Vickers MA. Sexual impotence caused by vascular disease: diagnosis with duplex sonography. *AJR* 1989; 153:1149.
191. Mellinger BC, Fried JJ, Vaughan ED. Papaverine-induced penile blood flow acceleration in impotent men measured by duplex scanning. *J Urol* 1990;144:897.
192. Miraldi F, Nelson AD, Jones WT, et al. A dual-radioisotope technique for the evaluation of penile blood flow during tumescence. *J Nucl Med* 1992;33:41.

31 The Adrenal Glands and Neural Crest Tumors

John C. Harbert

The adrenal glands are two small retroperitoneal organs, slightly superior and medial to the upper poles of the kidneys. They lie next to the vertebral column at approximately the level of the eleventh rib. The right adrenal is positioned somewhat higher than the left. The glands measure 2 to 3 cm in width and 4 to 6 cm in length, and they weigh 4 to 6 g, although their size and weight are quite variable in adults. Often, the left adrenal is larger and somewhat crescentic in shape; the right is smaller and triangular. In adrenal scintigraphy, however, the right adrenal usually appears slightly more active in posterior views because of its more posterior position. Both glands are fixed, and in the upright position, they do not descend with the kidneys.[1]

The adrenal cortex and medulla are composed of entirely different tissues histologically, embryologically, and functionally. The cortex constitutes approximately 90% of the gland volume and is, in turn, functionally and anatomically divided into 3 histologic zones. Each zone is responsible for the synthesis and excretion of a principal adrenal steroid. The outermost zone, the *zona glomerulosa*, produces aldosterone, the principal mineralocorticoid. The large central *zona fasciculata* produces primarily cortisol, a glucocorticoid hormone. The inner *zona reticularis* produces the androgenic steroids, chiefly androstenedione and dihydroepiandrosterone. The adrenal medulla secretes the catecholamines epinephrine and norepinephrine.

The growth and secretory functions of the adrenal cortex are controlled by the anterior pituitary adrenocorticotropic hormone (ACTH). Aldosterone secretion is controlled by angiotensin II, blood volume, and electrolyte concentration. Cholesterol is stored in abundance in the adrenal cortex and is the principal metabolic precursor in the synthesis of adrenocortical steroids, which include aldosterone.[2] This process forms the basis for successful adrenal scintigraphy with cholesterol analogs, particularly ^{131}I-6β-iodomethyl-19-norcholesterol, often referred to as NP-59.[3–6]

ADRENOCORTICAL IMAGING

Radiobiology and Radiochemistry of Iodocholesterols

Studies with ^{125}I- and ^{131}I-iodocholesterol, the first radiopharmaceuticals produced, by Beierwaltes et al. have demonstrated adrenal-to-liver ratios as high as 168:1 and adrenal-to-kidney ratios of 300:1.[7,8] Furthermore, a progressive increase of activity occurs over several days. Although cholesterol is a metabolic precursor in steroid synthesis, radiolabeled metabolic end products are not recovered with either 19-iodocholesterol or 6β-iodomethyl-19-norcholesterol. Their behavior more closely resembles enzyme inhibitors than metabolic precursors.

For adrenal imaging, ^{131}I-6β-iodomethyl-19-norcholesterol (NP-59) has replaced 19-iodocholesterol. As a marker of adrenocortical cholesterol uptake, it appears to be bound to plasma low-density lipoproteins. Using a Leydig tumor cell model, Freeman and Counsell[9] found that NP-59 enters the cell by binding to the plasma membrane and becomes internalized along with plasma membrane cholesterol. Membrane transport is under the control of cyclic adenosine monophosphate (cAMP), as is cholesterol. Internalized NP-59 is readily esterified, but does not enter mitochondria, nor is it converted into progesterone. Esterified NP-59 is metabolically inert and can not be converted back to free NP-59 and free fatty acid. Thus, it appears to be trapped irreversibly within the cell. Adrenal uptake appears to be controlled by ACTH: increased plasma ACTH levels result in increased uptake in NP-59.[8]

Thin-layer chromatographic silica gel with 100% chloroform as the solvent is used for assaying radiochemical purity. In this system NP-59 moves with an Rf of approximately 0.4, and free iodine remains at the origin. Unbound ^{131}I greater than 10% is considered unacceptable. If another chromatographic system is used, the migration patterns of free and bound iodine must be established.

The approximate radiation absorbed dose in adults in rad/mCi is: total body = 1.2; adrenals = 25; ovaries = 8; testes = 2.3; and liver = 2.4. Carey et al.[10] have estimated the adrenal dose in patients with Cushing's disease to be 57 ± 25 rad/mCi (1.54 ± 0.67 cGy/MBq).

Imaging Techniques

Prior to intravenous administration of NP-59, patients are given either Lugol's solution or saturated solution of potassium iodide (SSKI) equivalent to 100 mg iodine or 130 mg potassium iodide daily. This treatment is continued for 2 weeks thereafter to block uptake of free radioiodine by

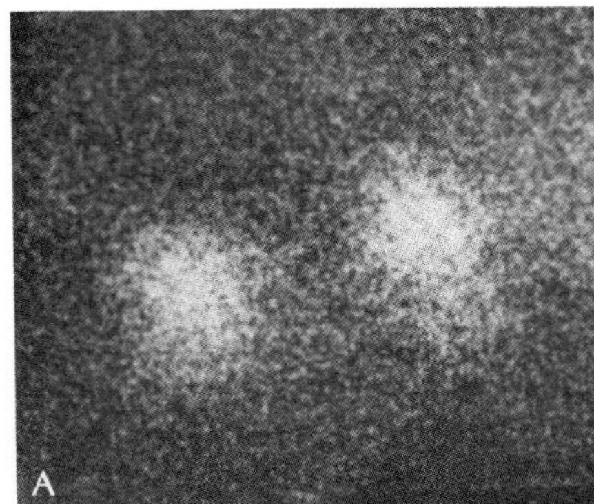

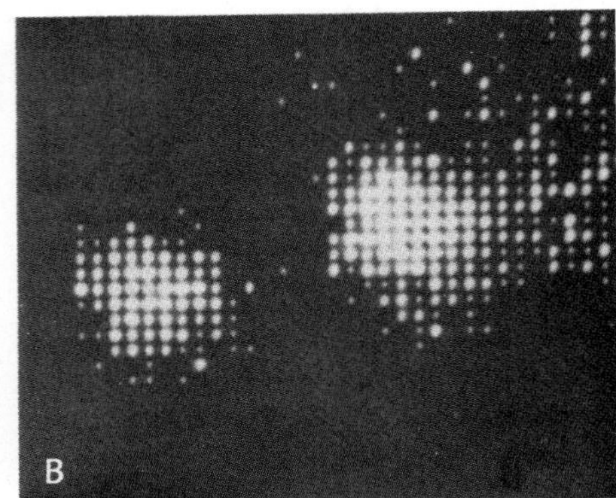

Figure 1. **(A).** Normal posterior adrenal image 7 days after injection of 1 mCi (37 MBq) ^{131}I-NP-59. **(B).** Right adrenal appears more active in this computer-enhanced image because of its more posterior position.

the thyroid. In cases of iodine sensitivity, 200 mg of oral potassium perchlorate q.i.d. may be substituted. In addition, all patients studied for hyperaldosteronism and hyperandrogenism receive 5 mg of oral dexamethasone daily starting 7 days prior to injection and ending on the last day of imaging, to suppress normal corticosteroid synthesizing tissue.

The usual imaging dose is 1 mCi (37 MBq) of ^{131}I-NP-59. The injection is given slowly because, with rapid injections, histamine release reactions, possibly caused by the Tween buffer, have been reported. At the University of Michigan adverse reactions were reported for 8 injections out of a total of 729 (~1%).[11] Only one of these was severe, in a 21-year-old female with a history of adverse reactions to multiple procedures. This reaction included nausea and dizziness, followed by flushing, headache, difficulty breathing, chest and back pain, 20-second loss of consciousness, tachycardia, and hypertension. Symptoms cleared within 1 hour following oral administration of 25 mg diphenhydramine hydrochloride.

Sufficient time must be allowed between injection and imaging for background activity to clear from soft tissues. NP-59 accumulates in the adrenal with an uptake half-time of almost one day. Therefore, uptake is not complete for several days. The usual imaging interval is 5 to 7 days after injection, except in cases of hyperaldosteronism, where imaging at 3 to 5 days following injection is designed to detect the earliest appearance of adrenal activity. Bisacodyl or other suitable laxative should be given the night before imaging to clear colonic activity.

The standard view for baseline imaging is the posterior view (Fig. 1) using a scintillation camera with high-energy parallel-hole collimator. Images are obtained for 20 minutes or for 50,000 counts. Simultaneous computer acquisition of data facilitates simple processing to optimize images for the activity levels in the adrenal.

Interpretation of adrenal images can be made by determining the percent uptake in each adrenal, correcting for tissue scatter and depth.[12] By this method, the normal range of uptake is 0.07 to 0.26% with a mean of 0.16% for both adrenal glands. The right-to-left ratio ranges from 0.9 to 1.2. ACTH increases adrenal uptake, and dexamethasone decreases uptake in healthy glands.[13] The adrenal uptake test was originally developed to confirm the diagnosis of Cushing's disease in patients with borderline biochemical findings. Just as with the thyroid uptake test, some overlap occurs between high normal and low abnormal values, although uptake higher than 0.3% per gland has invariably been associated with adrenal disease. Most clinicians rely on visual symmetry or asymmetry of the glands, as well as noting the earliest day after injection when concentration can be discerned.[11]

CLINICAL APPLICATIONS

Cushing's Syndrome

Patients with Cushing's syndrome exhibit biochemical and clinical evidence of excess glucocorticoids, usually cortisol. The clinical criteria are listed in Table 1.[11] The hypercortisolism results from excessive ACTH secretion from the pituitary, from ectopic sources stimulating adrenal cortisol secretion (ACTH-dependent), or directly from an adrenal adenoma or bilateral nodular adrenal hyperplasia (ACTH-independent).

The laboratory diagnosis of Cushing's syndrome is based on findings of elevated plasma cortisol, the absence of the normal diurnal variation of cortisol, and elevated urinary metabolites of cortisol and its precursors. Previously, the separation of pituitary, or ACTH-dependent, from ACTH-independent disease rested on the demonstration of suppressed urinary and plasma glucocorticoids induced by either low or high doses of dexamethasone. Usually, pituitary adenomas producing ACTH are suppressed by administration of high doses of dexamethasone. Increased urinary glucocorticoid metabolites appearing after administration of metapyrone in patients with ACTH-dependent disease result in increased urinary oxycorticoids. This change is caused by decreased pituitary feedback from cortisol and by an increase in ACTH, as differentiated from an absent response in ectopic, or ACTH-independent disease.

Without reliable ACTH measurements or, in the case of

Table 1. Criteria for the Diagnosis of Cushing's Disease

A. Diagnosis of Cushing's syndrome
  1. Clinical
    a. Hypertension
    b. Obesity: centripetal, facial
    c. Stria: purple
    d. Virilization in the syndrome
    Should have *at least one* of the clinical features, *and*
  2. Laboratory
    a. Evidence of cortisol excess
      1. High normal or high plasma cortisol (>25 μg/dL in a.m.) *or*
      2. Lack of diurnal variation in plasma cortisol *or*
      3. Elevated rate of excretion of free cortisol (>125 μg/24 hr) *or*
      4. Elevated rate of excretion of 17-hydroxysteroids (>10 mg/24 hr), *and*
    b. Evidence of altered control of cortisol secretion
      1. Failure to suppress plasma cortisol to <15 μg/dL, preferably failure to suppress to <5 μg/dL by
        a. 1 mg dexamethasone in evening *or*
        b. 4 (or 16) mg of dexamethasone over 48 hr, *or*
      2. Failure to suppress urine 17-hydroxysteroids to less than half of basal by 4 (or 16) mg of dexamethasone over 48 hr.

B. Location of primary abnormality in Cushing's syndrome
  1. Pituitary
    a. Plasma ACTH >90 pg/mL (in a.m.), *and*
    b. Either
      1. Evidence of pituitary adenoma by CT or by removal *or*
      2. Presumptive by absence of evidence of ectopic source of ACTH (by chest x-ray or other means), *or*
    c. Suppression urine (or plasma) cortisol by 16 mg/d but not by 4 mg/d of dexamethasone over 2 days.
  2. Ectopic ACTH or CRH
    a. Plasma ACTH >90 pg/mL, *and*
    b. Tumor secreting ACTH or CRH from
      1. Measurement of ACTH or CRH in blood of vein from tumor, *or*
      2. Measurement of hormones in tumor *or*
      3. Relief of clinical and laboratory abnormalities of the syndrome upon removal of the tumor, *and*
    c. Lack of suppression of plasma cortisol by 16 mg/d of dexamethasone over 2 days.
  3. Adenoma
    a. Biochemical-image
      1. Lack of ACTH dependence by
        a. Plasma ACTH <60 pg/mL (in a.m.), *or*
        b. Failure of plasma cortisol or urine 17-hydroxysteroids to suppress with 10 mg of dexamethasone over 48 hr; *and*
      2. Enlargement of one adrenal gland on CT or other image of anatomy, *or*
    b. Relief of clinical and laboratory abnormalities by removal of adenoma.
  4. Bilateral nodular hyperplasia
    a. Lack of ACTH dependence as described under B-2 c, *and*
    b. Bilateral morphologic abnormalities by
      1. CT or other image of anatomy, *or*
      2. Histologically.
  5. Carcinoma

the ectopic ACTH syndrome which involves secretion of excess ACTH, these distinctions are more difficult to recognize. Further localization of the disease process requires demonstration of a pituitary tumor, or occult neoplasm, with ectopic ACTH production.

In the absence of obvious pituitary disease, distinguishing between an adrenal tumor producing cortisol and a hyperfunctioning pituitary microadenoma may be difficult without adrenal scintigraphy. Adrenal scintigraphy is helpful in determining whether the excessive hormone production is due to hyperplasia, to adenoma, or to carcinoma.[3,11,14] The specific diagnosis is inferred from the pattern of adrenal NP-59 uptake.

SYMMETRICAL UPTAKE

In patients with confirmed Cushing's syndrome, symmetrical visualization invariably represents bilateral hyperplasia (Fig. 2). Usually, adrenal uptake is markedly increased and the adrenals are well visualized because of increased target-to-background ratios. They may also appear somewhat larger than normal.

ASYMMETRIC UPTAKE

Slight depth-dependent asymmetry may be seen in patients with Cushing's syndrome, just as in healthy patients. In some patients with Cushing's syndrome, however, nodular

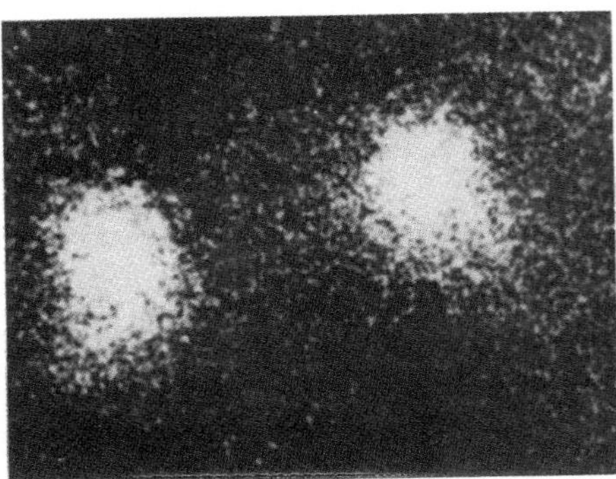

Figure 2. Posterior image (3 days) of patient with ACTH-excess Cushing's disease; note bilaterally increased activity from bilateral hyperplasia.

hyperplasia is distinctly asymmetric and, in a few of these patients, the asymmetry is caused by the coexistence of a Cushing's adenoma with hyperplasia. Uptake percentages differing by over 50% suggest this combination. Moreover, if an adenoma is removed in a patient with Cushing's syndrome in whom both glands were visualized by scintigraphy, continued hypercortisolism should be anticipated because of probable hyperplasia of the contralateral gland.

UNILATERAL UPTAKE

The classic pattern of glucocorticoid-producing adrenal adenoma involves increased radiocholesterol uptake in the affected gland and absent uptake in the contralateral gland (Fig. 3). The suppression of ACTH results in absent or decreased NP-59 uptake in normal tissue. Unilateral uptake can also be present with a unilateral carcinoma imaged without suppression.[11] Usually, corollary imaging procedures such as computed tomography (CT) and magnetic resonance imaging (MRI) make this diagnosis apparent.

ECTOPIC UPTAKE

Carpenter et al. have reported two cases of steroid-producing gonadal tumors.[15] One case was of a male with Cushing's syndrome who had no NP-59 uptake in the abdomen but intense uptake in both testes, which were found to contain Leydig cell tumors. The second patient who had adrenal virilism also had elevated uptake at the site of a Leydig cell ovarian tumor. In cases of steroid excess and normal adrenal scintigraphy, it is prudent to search for ectopic functioning tissue.

NO UPTAKE

Except for technical problems or the administration of exogenous hormone, the only documented cause of bilateral nonvisualization in the face of hypercortisolism is adrenal cortical carcinoma. Carcinomas function poorly but, if sufficiently large, they can cause Cushing's syndrome and suppress ACTH and NP-59 uptake. Several case reports have demonstrated NP-59 uptake in adrenal carcinoma metastases.[16,17] In some patients with large adenomas, focal areas of carcinomatous degeneration occur. These areas are usually not recognized because of avid uptake in the adenoma. Occasionally, carcinomas cause a distortion of the adrenal pattern, as shown in Figure 4.

Accuracy. In the University of Michigan experience, which reviewed NP-59 studies in 108 patients, all 18 patients with unequivocal Cushing's syndrome clinically were correctly identified and classified.[11] Accuracy was, thus, deemed to be 100%. Among these 18 patients, 7 had pituitary adenomas, 5 had nodular hyperplasia, 3 had adrenal adenoma, and 3 had adrenal carcinoma.

Primary Aldosteronism

The clinical criteria for primary aldosteronism are listed in Table 2.[11] The scintigraphic patterns in patients with primary aldosteronism are significantly different from those described in Cushing's syndrome, because aldosterone does not suppress ACTH production. On standard NP-59 images, aldosteronomas result in an asymmetrical appearance of the two adrenals, but this asymmetry cannot be distinguished from asymmetrical hyperplasia.

Dexamethasone-suppression imaging is used to enhance

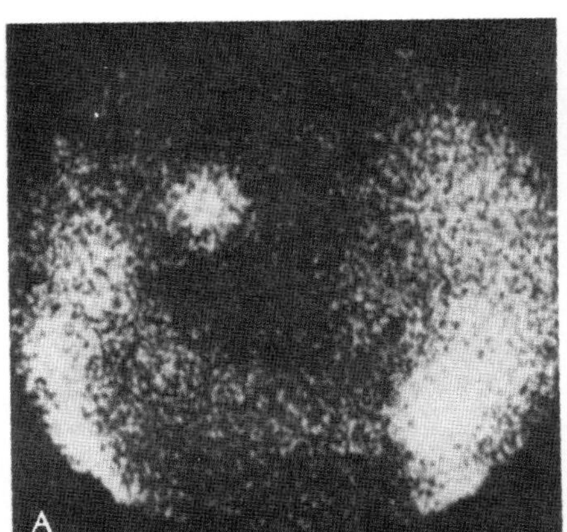

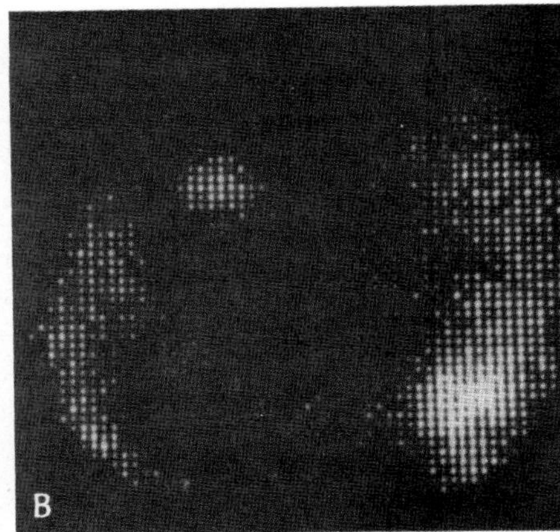

Figure 3. Left adrenal adenoma: activity at far left and far right is within bowel. There is decreased uptake and downward displacement of the right adrenal. **(A).** Unprocessed image. **(B).** Computer-enhanced image.

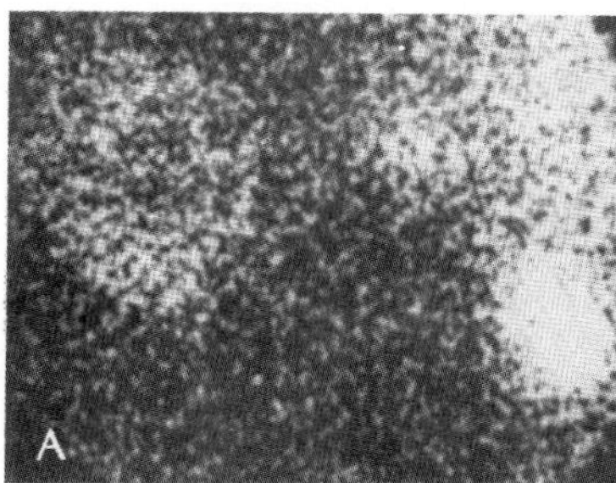

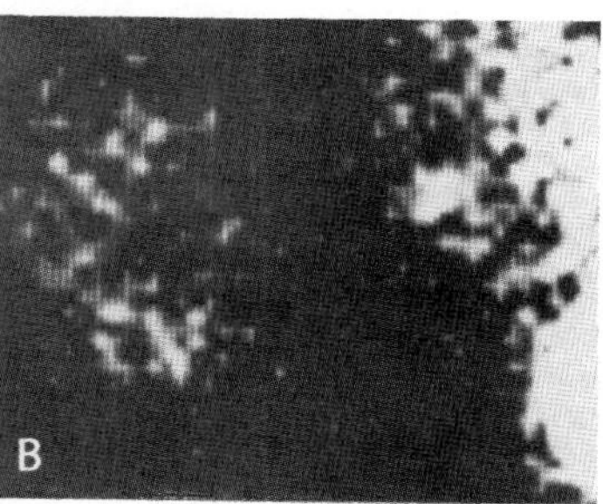

Figure 4. Left adrenal carcinoma producing androgen: unprocessed image **(A)** and computer-enhanced image **(B)** demonstrate distorted left and normal right adrenal glands.

aldosteronomas result in an asymmetrical appearance of the two adrenals, but this asymmetry cannot be distinguished from asymmetrical hyperplasia.

Dexamethasone-suppression imaging is used to enhance detection and lateralization of aldosterone-producing adenomas. For this purpose, 1.25 mg is given orally q.i.d. for 7 days prior to injection and continued throughout the study. This regimen suppresses tracer uptake in normal tissue, but uptake in the adenoma is unaffected. Adenomas are typically visualized early, with absent or poor visualization in the opposite adrenal (Fig. 5 and Table 3).

In patients with hyperplasia, uptake is usually symmetrical

Table 2. Criteria for the Diagnosis of Primary Aldosteronism

A. Diagnosis of primary Aldosteronism
  1. Clinical
    a. Hypertension (usually without edema)
  2. Laboratory
    a. Usual entry evidence
      Hypokalemia
      —spontaneous (i.e., in absence of diuretics) *or*
      —difficult to repair by oral potassium with diuretics.
    b. More definitive criteria
      1. Plasma renin value is low and cannot be elevated by upright posture (walking) for 3 hr plus and/or injection of furosemide.
      2. Urinary aldosterone level is elevated and is not suppressed by
        —oral sodium, 200 mEq/d for 3 days, *or*
        —desoxycorticosterone injections.
  3. Interpretation
    —b (1) plus b (2) make the diagnosis definite.
    —Hypertension, hypokalemia, and a low renin value in upright position make the diagnosis probable.
    —Hypertension and hypokalemia make the diagnosis possible.

B. For confirmation of the type of primary aldosteronism, the following are required:
  1. Adenoma
    a. Definitive evidence
      1. Resection of an adenoma (by histology), *and*
        a. no evidence of abnormality in the contralateral adrenal gland on CT, *and*
        b. disappearance of hypertension *or* at least disappearance of hypokalemia.
      2. Levels of aldosterone in blood from one adrenal vein that are twenty or more times higher than those in blood from the contralateral vein.
    b. As presumptive evidence: tumor in one adrenal gland <2.5 cm in diameter when no operation has been performed.
  2. Bilateral hyperplasia
    a. Definite
      1. Either no abnormality or bilateral enlargement of adrenal glands on CT *and* decline in blood pressure and repair of hypokalemia by spironolactone treatment, *or*
      2. Equal (less than two-fold difference) *and* substantial concentrations of aldosterone in blood from the adrenal veins *and* decline in blood pressure and repair of hypokalemia by spironolactone treatment.
    b. Possible or probable: no nodule or tumor or more than borderline and equal enlargement of adrenal glands by CT.
  3. Carcinoma (rare); invasion of tissue by tumor as seen
    a. by surgeon *or*
    b. by pathologist *or*
    c. by angiography *or*
    d. by CT (which may show metastases).

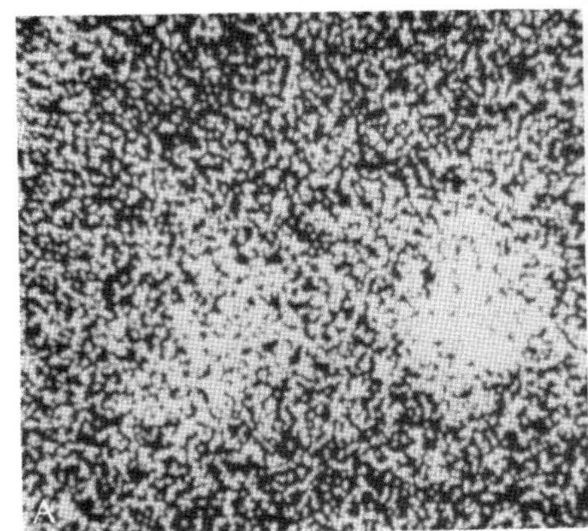

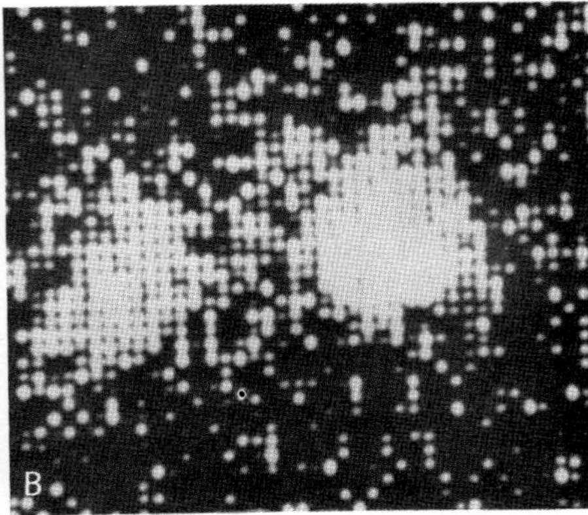

Figure 5. Discrete aldosteronoma on the right: **(A).** Unprocessed image. **(B).** Computer-enhanced image.

or irregularly symmetrical and is visualized before 5 days. In patients with well-documented primary aldosteronism (Table 2), unilateral uptake is highly specific for adenoma and should obviate the need for radiographic procedures or venous hormone sampling. The distinction between these patterns is important because the usual treatment of bilateral hyperplasia is medical, and adrenalectomy is indicated for aldosteronoma.

Accuracy. In the University of Michigan review,[11] 10 of 14 patients with clinical primary hyperaldosteronism were correctly identified (71%). In 3 patients, images were of poor quality and were deemed indeterminate. In another patient, bilateral uptake occurred in the presence of a unilateral adenoma; fortunately, CT scanning clarified the diagnosis in this patient. Although the specificity of lateralization is high, the sensitivity appears low: Lund et al. found lateralization in only 6 of 12 patients with proven adenoma.[19] The low sensitivity is probably due to the small size of many aldosteronomas.

Hyperandrogenism

Adrenal virilism secondary to hyperandrogenism is a common endocrine problem in women. The clinical criteria are listed in Table 4. Excess androgens may originate from the ovaries, the adrenals, and through peripheral conversion of androstenedione to testosterone.[20,21] Androgen secretion by the adrenal gland is controlled by ACTH; androgen secretion by the ovaries is controlled by pituitary luteinizing hormone (LH). Studies in women with hyperandrogenism indicate that the usual suppression and stimulation tests of the adrenals and ovaries do not reliably identify the origin of excessive androgen production.[21] Both adrenal and ovarian androgens are suppressed by dexamethasone, estrogens, and/or progesterone. Adrenal scintigraphy using NP-59 and dexamethasone suppression are useful in defining the proper cause.[11,22–24] The same 3 patterns found in hyperaldosteronism are found in hyperandrogenism (Table 3).

Accuracy. Several studies[11,22–26] of women with hirsutism and virilism have described the same 3 patterns found in hyperaldosteronism. The first pattern, bilateral early visualization (<5 days postinjection) was seen in 15 of 39 patients (38%). In all patients who received confirmatory adrenal vein sampling, elevated androgen concentrations were found, consistent with bilateral hyperplasia. The second pattern, unilateral visualization (<5 days postinjection), was observed in 5 of 39 patients (13%). Four of these 5 patients had adrenal adenomas at surgery. Bilateral visualization >5 days postinjection was observed in 17 of 39 patients (44%), and is considered the normal response. Two other patients showed no visualization,[11] one in a patient with a 12-cm adrenal mass on CT, consistent with the adrenal cortical carcinoma subsequently confirmed at adrenalectomy. In the second case, there was NP-59 concentration in the pelvis corresponding to the 3-cm left ovarian mass on ultrasound and CT. At surgery, the mass proved to be a benign lipoid cell ovarian tumor, known to be associated with virilization.

Table 3. Interpretation of Dexamethasone-Suppression Scans of the Adrenals

SCAN APPEARANCE	TIME OF VISUALIZATION	INTERPRETATION
Bilateral uptake	<5 days	Bilateral hyperplasia
Unilateral uptake	<5 days	Adenoma
Bilateral uptake or nonvisualization	>5 days	Nondiagnostic

Euadrenal Tumors

In the University of Michigan experience, 36 patients were evaluated for euadrenal tumors (i.e., patients discovered to have adrenal tumors incidentally on CT, who have normal serum and urinary hormone levels). Of the 36, 27 (75%) were correctly identified by adrenal scintigraphy. These cases are described in detail by Kazerooni et al.[11]; most proved to be nonsecreting tumors, carcinomas, or clinically nonsignificant adenomas.

Table 4. Criteria for Hyperandrogenism

A. Diagnosis of virilization (adult women)
  1. Clinical
    a. Not specific but almost
      1. Hirsutism, more specific if florid and of few months duration
      2. Acne
    b. More specific of virilization (at least one feature should be present)
      1. Cliteromegaly
      2. Frontal balding
      3. Deepening voice
    c. Onset over weeks or few months.
  2. Laboratory
    a. Ovary
      1. Plasma total testosterone: >1 ng/mL usually >2 ng/mL; *or*
      2. Free testosterone elevation if total testosterone is not elevated *and*
    b. Adrenal (the tumors are usually large)
      1. 17-ketosteroids (urine) elevation, *and/or*
      2. DHEA-S (plasma) elevation, *and*
    c. LH and FSH (plasma) low levels.
    d. Caution
      1. Many patients with hirsutism do not have an endocrine cause for hair growth, and few have androgen-secreting tumors. For example, the polycystic ovarian syndrome usually is associated with hirsutism, amenorrhea, and modest elevation in plasma testosterone (<2 ng/mL); high LH and low FSH are also commonly seen in women afflicted with this disorder.
      2. Adrenal genital hyperplasia in adult cases typically will be associated with clinical virilization and increased 17-ketosteroid excretion. The diagnosis is supported by elevation in serum 17-hydroxyprogesterone levels.
      3. Cushing's syndrome may be associated with clinical virilization; usually there are other clinical manifestations of Cushing's syndrome and the criteria of Cushing's syndrome would be fulfilled.

B. Criteria for determining site(s) of androgen production (tumor in the ovary may be small).
  1. Probable:
    a. CT or MRI or ultrasound evidence of tumor in ovary or adrenal, *or*
    b. Excised tumor appearing morphologically typical of an androgen-secreting tumor.
  2. Definition
    a. Levels of androgen in adrenal or ovarian venous effluent are much higher (>5-fold) than those from the contralateral gland, *or*
    b. Disappearance of clinical and biochemical abnormalities upon removal of the tumor.

Postadrenalectomy Remnants

Adrenal imaging is a sensitive means of identifying functioning residual tissue following adrenalectomy. In one series of 11 patients with recurrent or persistent Cushing's syndrome after surgery, adrenal imaging with NP-59 successfully visualized functioning remnants in 9.[27] In none of these patients could the remnants be localized by radiographic means or by hormone sampling.

ADRENOMEDULLARY SCINTIGRAPHY OF NEUROENDOCRINE TUMORS

Pathology

In the 1960s, Pearse[28] came to realize that a miscellaneous group of cells, arranged diffusely and distributed widely throughout the body, had certain histological and histochemical features in common. All of these cells he regarded as neuroendocrine, with some derived from neuroectoderm, others from neural crest, and still others from more primitive cells of the ectoblast. Ultimately, more than 40 such cell types have been recognized and given the acronym APUD, derived from their amine handling properties: they have high *amine* content (A), a capacity for amine *precursor uptake* (PU), and the function of carrying out *decarboxylation* (D) of these precursors to form potent amine substances (Table 1, chapter 42). These cells are divided into 2 principal groups: a central division of glandular structures that includes the pituitary, pineal, and hypothalamus; and a peripheral division, that consists of cells in the gastrointestinal tract, pancreas, the C cells of the thyroid, the sympathetic nervous system, adrenal medulla, dermal melanocytes, Merkel cells, and certain cells in the lungs, carotid body, and urogenital tract.[28]

The APUD cells have similar immunofluorescent properties; they are labeled with peroxidase and other histochemical methods, and they contain the enzyme, neuron-specific enolase (NSE), previously thought to be unique to neurons.[29] All of these observations have led to the concept of a single neuroendocrine system that pervades nearly every tissue of the body.[30] Its cells synthesize amines and regulatory peptides which act through 3 different modes of action: *endocrine*, secreted systemically (e.g., ACTH and calcitonin); *paracrine*, secreted locally and acting on adjacent cells (e.g., somatostatin and 5-hydroxytryptamine); and *neurocrine*, secreted at synapses and acting as neurotransmitters (e.g., norepinephrine and vasoactive intestinal peptide). For this reason the term "APUD system" is giving way to the term "neuroendocrine system" which connotes the common physiologic rather than histochemical characteristics of the system.[31] Tumors derived from these cells are APUDomas, or more often *neuroendocrine*, and sometimes "neural crest" tumors, indicating their embryologic precursor. Often, these tumors occur in well-defined pluriglandular endocrinopathies, giving rise to several syndromes known as *multiple endocrine neoplasia*, MEN I and MEN II.

MIBG

Early work by Morales et al.[32] showed that radiolabeled epinephrine and epinephrine precursors, such as ^{14}C-dopamine, concentrate in the adrenal medulla. However, in vivo imaging studies with such agents were not successful. Later, Wieland and colleagues[33,34] developed radioiodinated analogs of bretylium, which concentrate in the myocardium and adrenal medulla. They combined the benzyl portion of bretylium with the guanidine groups of guanethidine to form ortho-, para-, and metaiodobenzylguanidine. The meta-isomer (MIBG) was the most stable and most subsequent work has concentrated on this tracer.

The mechanism of MIBG uptake by sympathoadrenal tissues is not completely understood. However, the prevailing model suggests that the majority of MIBG enters the cytoplasm of these tissues by an active sodium and energy-dependent (uptake-one) mechanism.[35,36] A smaller fraction enters by passive diffusion. Once in the cytoplasm, MIBG then enters the intracellular hormone storage vesicles by means of an active uptake mechanism.[35] Thus, MIBG acts as a tracer of catecholamine uptake and storage capacity by the sympathoadrenal system. The primary sites of normal uptake are the adrenal medulla, and in the sympathetic neuronal innervation of the heart, spleen, and salivary glands. Uptake in neuroendocrine tumors is based upon the same mechanisms.[37]

Pharmacological intervention studies in animals and clinical observations in humans show that MIBG uptake is blocked by such uptake-one inhibitors as tricyclic antidepressants, cocaine, reserpine, and phenylpropanolamine.[33,38] Most alpha- and beta-blocking drugs are without effect. MIBG is discharged from the adrenal medulla in response to insulin hypoglycemia.[39] Uptake is also decreased in the heart and salivary glands by denervation.[39]

METABOLISM AND DOSIMETRY OF MIBG

The usual scintigraphic distribution of MIBG includes uptake in the salivary glands, nasopharynx, heart, liver, and bladder. The adrenal medulla may be imaged, particularly if ^{123}I-MIBG is used.[37] Colon activity also may be observed, as well as the thyroid gland, if inadequately blocked with iodide. In rare instances, the lacrimal glands, lungs, brain, menstruating uterus, and dilated kidneys may be visualized.[40]

Most radioactivity is excreted as unchanged MIBG. From 2 to 16% of the activity is excreted in the form of free iodide, metaiodobenzoic acid, and as 4-hydroxy-3-iodobenzylguanidine.[41] The prominent liver uptake appears to be due to metabolism and not type-one uptake. Within 24 hours, 55% of the injected radioactivity is excreted in the urine; about 90% is excreted in 4 days. Thus, it is not surprising that in renal failure the image quality is severely impaired by high tissue background and increased colon excretion.[42] It is prudent to check the plasma creatinine level prior to administration of MIBG; if elevated, delayed imaging may be useful to allow background levels to decline.

Only about 2% of the injected dose of MIBG is taken up in tumor in patients with malignant pheochromocytoma.[43] In 8 patients studied by Lindberg et al., tumor uptake ranged from 0.0033 to 0.038% ID/g of tumor tissue.[44] Radioactivity exracted from excised tumors shows most in the form of MIBG.[41] The dosimetry of ^{131}I-MIBG is described by Lindberg et al.[44]

Interfering Drugs. Numerous drugs interfere with MIBG uptake in neuroendocrine tissues and tumors. These are reviewed by Khafagi et al.[45] and listed in Table 3, chapter 42. The interference mechanisms in most cases are uptake-one inhibition and/or storage vesicle depletion. Related drugs that have *no* significant effect on MIBG uptake are listed in Table 4, chapter 42. A careful review of potentially interfering medications should be made prior to diagnostic and therapeutic administration of MIBG.

IMAGING TECHNIQUES

Once a careful history, physical examination, and biochemical evaluation support the diagnosis of neuroendocrine tumor with a reasonable level of certainty, and any interfering drugs (Table 6) have been stopped, thyroid uptake of free radioiodine is blocked with oral iodide (1 drop SSKI t.i.d.) begun 1 day prior and continued for 1 week after imaging. MIBG is administered by slow intravenous injection of 0.5 to 1.0 mCi (18 to 37 MBq) ^{131}I-MIBG or 3 to 10 mCi (111 to 370 MBq) ^{123}I-MIBG in adults with appropriate downscaling for children. Multiple overlapping images are obtained with a scintillation camera from the skull to the upper femurs in adults and to the feet in children. Imaging is performed at 1 and 2 days with ^{123}I-MIBG and at 1, 2, and 3 days with ^{131}I-MIBG. If ^{123}I-MIBG is used, appropriate SPECT images may be taken of sites of focal uptake.

IMAGING OF PHEOCHROMOCYTOMAS

Pathophysiology. During early fetal life, primitive ectodermal stem cells migrate down from the neural crest to form the sympathetic nervous chain and ganglia and invade the developing mesodermal adrenal cortex to form the adrenal medulla. The mesodermal cells give rise to pheochromoblasts and catecholamine-producing chromaffin cells. Chromaffin cells are distributed not only within the adrenal medulla, but all along the sympathetic nerve chain and in the organ of Zukerkandl at the lower end of the aorta (Fig.

6). The distribution accounts for the wide dispersal of extra-adrenal sites; chromaffin tissue may even be drawn into the scrotum during descent of the testes. At birth, the adrenal medulla is small and medullary tissue function is due largely to the paraganglionic masses. During early childhood, the extramedullary sites normally undergo involution, but there is always the potential for stimulation and tumor development.

Pheochromocytomas are rare; they occur in from 0.01 to 0.001% of the population and it has long been believed that 10 to 13% of these exhibit malignancy.[46,47] However, with extended follow-up and with the introduction of MIBG scintigraphy, which localizes chromaffin tissue with high accuracy, this proportion has increased in recent years, and may reach as high as 50% with prolonged follow-up.[47–50] Bilateral tumors occur in about 10% of adults and 20% of children. Extramedullary pheochromocytomas occur in about 13% of patients.[51] In adults, about 90% of malignant pheochromocytomas occur within the adrenal gland.[52] In children, extra-adrenal tumors account for about 30% of pheochromocytomas and as many as 40% of these are malignant.[52] Malignancy cannot be distinguished in pheochromocytomas by histological criteria; the sole criteria for malignancy is the presence of metastases in anatomic sites where chromaffin tissue is normally not present. The most frequent sites are bone (55%), lymph nodes and liver (37%), and lung (27%).[53]

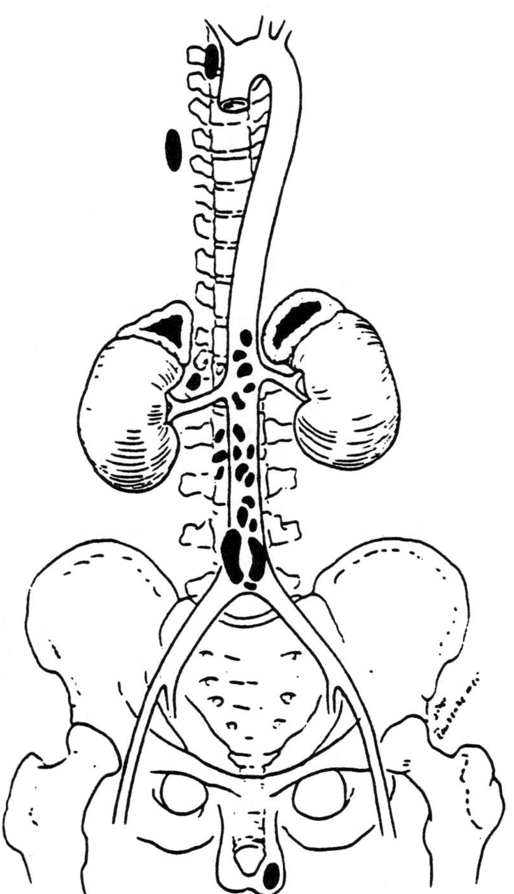
Figure 6. Extraadrenal sites of medullary tissue.

The signs and symptoms of pheochromocytoma include headache, palpitations, hyperhidrosis, and hypertension. Paroxysms may be triggered by emotional stress and physical exertion, as well as palpation of the tumor itself. The sudden release of catecholamines may precipitate very high blood pressure, ventricular fibrillation, cerebral hemorrhage, and pulmonary edema. The onset of symptoms may occur at any time from childhood to advanced years, although most tumors are diagnosed in the fourth or fifth decades of life. Tumor size varies from as small as 1 cm up to several kilograms, but averages 5 to 6 cm in diameter. The spectrum of malignancy also varies, from relatively static with only local invasion to highly aggressive tumors that behave as neuroblastomas with rapid dissemination.

Pheochromocytomas are part of the MEN type II (Sipple's syndrome), in which they may be associated with medullary thyroid carcinoma and parathyroid adenomas. They may also be associated with neurofibromatosis (von Recklinghausen's disease) or with cerebral hemangioblastomas, as in von Hippel-Lindau disease.

Diagnosis. The diagnosis of pheochromocytoma is based on the demonstration of elevated and/or nonsuppressible concentrations of the plasma catecholamines norepinephrine and epinephrine, and of elevated rates of catecholamine and catecholamine metabolite excretion in the urine.[54] In the majority of patients, urine levels of the metabolites vanillylmandellic acid (VMA), metanephrine, and normetanephrine are elevated and additional testing is not necessary. Clonidine, a centrally acting agent which inhibits catecholamine secretion from the nervous system, can be given to differentiate between pheochromocytoma and other nonpheochromocytoma causes of elevated concentrations of catecholamine, such as essential hypertension and stress.[54] Failure of plasma catecholamine concentrations to decrease by 50% of the initial value after clonidine administration is strong (though not conclusive) evidence for the presence of pheochromocytoma.

The 3 imaging techniques, MRI, CT, and MIBG scintigraphy, are all about equal in sensitivity (85 to 95%).[55] CT is less specific, as pheochromocytomas cannot be differentiated from adenomas and metastases. Both CT and MRI are less sensitive for extra-adrenal tumors. The sensitivity of scintigraphy with either ^{123}I- or ^{131}I-MIBG is 85 to 90% and the specificity is over 95% in the correct clinical setting.[56] Thus, the fact that MIBG does not distinguish between pheochromocytoma and such other neuroendocrine tumors as carcinoid or neuroblastoma is of little clinical relevance.

The advantages of ^{123}I-MIBG over ^{131}I-MIBG, of course, lie in the characteristics of ^{123}I, which permit sharper images and reduce radiation absorbed dose. A real clinical advantage, however, has yet to be proven and, in any event, ^{123}I-MIBG is not available commercially.[56] With both tracers, it

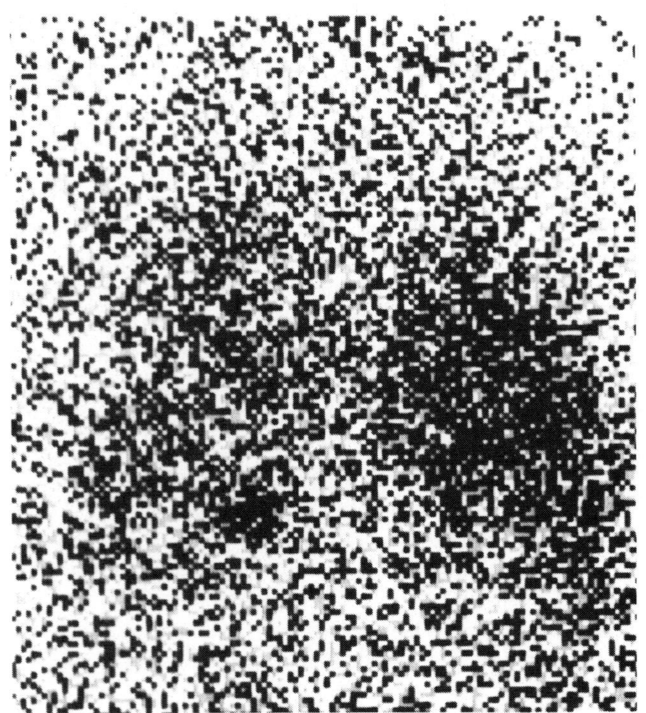

Figure 7. Left pheochromocytoma imaged 48 hours following the injection of 1 mCi (37 MBq) of ^{131}I-MIBG.

is essential to discontinue all interfering medications (Table 6) at least 7 days before injection. Figure 7 shows a large pheochromocytoma in the left adrenal gland imaged 48 hours after intravenous injection of 0.5 mCi (18.5 MBq) of ^{131}I-MIBG.

Venography with venous sampling of catecholamine levels provides accurate functional location of pheochromocytomas, but is invasive and technically demanding, particularly in patients who have been previously operated. The use of contrast injections also risks catecholamine crisis, tumor infarction, and rupture.[57]

The results from 7 published reports of ^{131}I-MIBG scintigraphy are shown in Table 5. Because of its high sensitivity, MIBG scintigraphy is the screening procedure of choice in suspected pheochromocytoma. If MIBG scintigraphy is suspected of being falsely negative, CT, MRI, and venous sampling may then be used for tumor localization.[58]

Imaging of the adrenal region with CT reveals about 80% of tumors, including almost all intra-adrenal lesions. However, even if CT locates a tumor, the lesion may not be due to a pheochromocytoma and, in up to 10% of patients, there may be occult metastatic or second primary tumors. Thus, MIBG scintigraphy is still useful as a confirmatory study.[59]

IMAGING OF NEUROBLASTOMAS

Neuroblastoma is the third most frequent malignant disease of childhood and the most common solid tumor found in infants under 1 year of age.[60] Most primary tumors arise in the adrenal gland, although they can arise anywhere along the extra-adrenal sympathetic chain; 15 to 20% arise in the thorax. Neuroectodermal tissue can even enter the scrotum during testicular descent, from which neuroblastomas can arise.[61] About one third of tumors found in children over one year of age are disseminated at the time of discovery, most commonly to liver, lung, and bone (Fig. 8). Therefore, the earlier the tumor is diagnosed, the better is the prognosis. Even so, only 10 to 20% of children are alive 2 years after diagnosis.[62] The most common presenting signs and symptoms include a palpable mass or the secondary conditions associated with bone-marrow involvement: anemia, thrombocytopenia, and leukopenia.

The staging procedures and staging classification of neuroblastomas is detailed in chapter 42. Imaging with MIBG is recommended because it is most sensitive in assessing the extent of metastatic disease and in distinguishing residual active tumor from masses composed of scar tissue, and it is more sensitive in detecting response of tumor involving cortical bone.[63] Approximately 90% of neuroblastomas concentrate MIBG,[64] although because most neural crest tumors do also, it is much more sensitive than specific. In general, MIBG uptake correlates well with elevated tumor markers, especially increased urinary VMA and dopamine and high serum neuron-specific enolase (NSE).[65] As with all neural crest tumors, the number of lesions identified by scintigraphy is dose dependent; nearly twice as many lesions are identified when imaged after therapeutic doses (150 + mCi) as imaged following diagnostic doses (0.5 to 1.0 mCi).[66] MIBG

Table 5. Results of ^{131}I-MIBG Scintigraphy for Suspected Pheochromocytoma*

REFERENCE	NO. OF PATIENTS	PREVALENCE (%)	SENSITIVITY (%)	SPECIFICITY (%)
59	927	20	88	99
60	64	47	88	88
61	191	34	88	99
62	99	46	91	96
63	46	52	88	95
64	42	45	79	96
65	27	33	89	94

*Data from reference 40

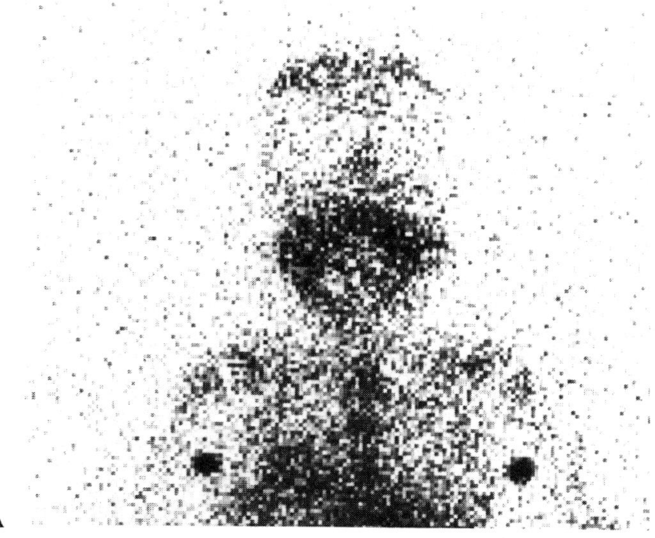
A

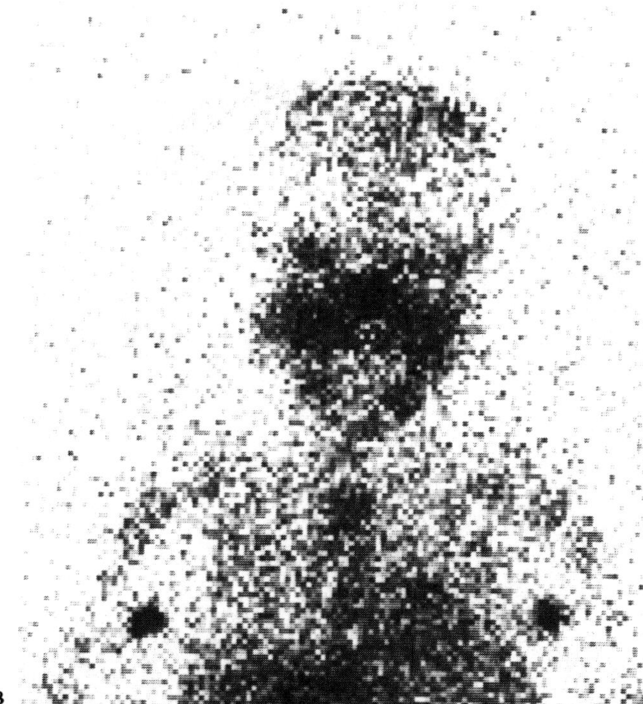
B

Figure 8. Metastatic neuroblastoma in a 3-year-old girl imaged with ^{131}I-MIBG: note focal lesions in the skull, about the orbits, in the maxillary sinus and left mandible, sternum, and left humerus. The cardiac activity is normal. **(A).** Anterior; **(B).** posterior.

scintigraphy does not relieve the necessity of bone scintigraphy, because small bone lesions are missed in infants using MIBG, especially those adjacent to epiphyses.[67]

The results of several studies reporting MIBG scintigraphy in patients with neuroblastoma are shown in Table 6. Scintigraphy may be useful in occasional patients with such tumors, in which histology is nondiagnostic, because MIBG is only taken up by neuroblastoma and not by other small, round-cell tumors of childhood.[40] The chief utility of MIBG imaging is in the staging of neuroblastoma at presentation and for monitoring the extent of disease during and following therapy. The therapy of neuroblastomas with ^{131}I-MIBG is described in chapter 42.

Radioimmunoscintigraphy in Neuroblastoma. Several monoclonal antibodies against neuroblastoma have been tested for diagnosis and therapy.[72–78] One of these, ^{131}I-3F8, a murine IgG_3 monoclonal antibody specific for ganglioside G_{D2} has appeared promising. The antigen is expressed in high concentrations in human neuroblastomas.[79] Preliminary imaging studies have shown a relatively high uptake in neuroblastoma (0.08% ID/g) compared with ^{131}I-MIBG (0.002% ID/g), which may account for uptake in more neuroblastoma lesions in some patients.[78]

IMAGING OF OTHER NEUROENDOCRINE TUMORS

Paragangliomas. Paragangliomas are tumors that arise from extra-adrenal paraganglion tissue, a multicentric system of histologically similar organs known as paraganglia. Paragangliomas contain small amounts of catecholamines and may be "functional" or "nonfunctional," according to whether or not they secrete catecholamines in sufficient quantities to produce the clinical syndrome of a pheochromocytoma: hypertension, headache, and flushing.[80] Other names for these tumors include "chemodectoma" and "glomus tumor." As with pheochromocytomas (the same tumor arising in the adrenal medulla), malignancy is defined by either local invasion, spread to regional lymph nodes, or metastases to distant sites not associated with neuroendocrine tissue. Multicentric tumors occur in about 10% of cases.[81]

The mechanism of uptake of MIBG in paragangliomas is presumed to be the same as that in pheochromocytomas. Interestingly, the uptake of MIBG is unrelated to the secretory activity of the tumor because "nonfunctional" paragangliomas take up MIBG in sufficient quantities to effectively treat them.[82,83] Imaging procedures are the same as described for pheochromocytomas.

Octreotide analogs have recently been used to image neuroendocrine tumors; see below under Carcinoid tumors.

Carcinoid Tumors. Carcinoid tumors are slow-growing neoplasms of enterochromaffin cells. They occur widely throughout the gastrointestinal tract from the larynx to anus, including the pancreas and biliary tract, and many that obstruct the appendix.[84] Their tendency to metastasize to the liver and to cause hepatic failure is well recognized. The carcinoid syndrome with clinical features of diarrhea, flushing, dyspnea, and bronchospasm, occurs in only about 10% of carcinoid tumors.[85] Many of these tumors secrete 5-hydroxytryptamine (serotonin), which causes elevated urinary levels of its metabolite, 5-hydroxyindolacetic acid (5-HIAA). Other tumors secrete the serotonin precursor 5-hy-

Table 6. Results of MIBG Scintigraphy in Patients with Neuroblastoma*

REFERENCE	NO. OF PATIENTS	PREVALENCE (%)	SENSITIVITY (%)	SPECIFICITY (%)
59	36	92	85	100
74	24	83	70	100
75	16	100	75	–
76	19	74	57	60
77	5	80	100	100

*Data from reference 40

droxytryptophan, which gives rise to normal urinary 5-HIAA excretion, despite the occurrence of carcinoid syndrome.

Uptake of MIBG is documented in about 60% of carcinoid tumors.[86] Therefore, MIBG scintigraphy is not a useful diagnostic screening procedure but, once carcinoid has been diagnosed, total body MIBG scintigraphy is useful to document the extent of disease and to evaluate the potential for therapeutic application. In general, the uptake of MIBG within these tumors is less than is found with neuroblastoma and pheochromocytoma.[87]

Carcinoid tumors frequently possess binding sites for somatostatin and therapy with the somatostatin analog, octreotide, has been used to control carcinoid symptoms.[88] Radiolabeled octreotide has also been used to image carcinoids.[89–91] Bomanji et al.[91] compared ^{123}I-MIBG and ^{123}I-octreotide and found great variability of uptake between the two tracers; this is not surprising, considering their different mechanisms of uptake. An advantage of octreotide is that optimum imaging time is 10 to 30 minutes compared with 24 to 48 hours for MIBG. This subject is duscussed in detail in chapter 36.

REFERENCES

1. Soffer LJ, Dorfman RI, Gabrilove JL. *The Human Adrenal Gland.* Philadelphia, Lea & Febiger, 1961.
2. Samuels LT, Uchikawa T. Biosynthesis of adrenal steroids, in Eisenstein AB (ed): *The Adrenal Cortex*, Boston, Little Brown, 1967, p 61.
3. Beierwaltes WH, Lieberman LM, Ansari AN, Nishiyama H. Visualization of human adrenal glands in vivo by scintillation scanning. *JAMA* 1971;216:275.
4. Lieberman LM, Beierwaltes WH, Conn JW, et al. Diagnosis of adrenal disease by visualization of human adrenal glands with ^{131}I-19-iodocholesterol. *N Engl J Med* 1971;285:1387.
5. Sarkar SD, Beierwaltes WH, Ice RO, et al. A new and superior adrenal scanning agent: NP-59. *J Nucl Med* 1975;16:1038.
6. Basmadjian GP, Hetzel KR, Ice RD, Beierwaltes WH. Synthesis of a new adrenal cortex scanning agent 6β-I-131-iodomethyl-19-norcholest-5(10)en-3β-ol (NP-19). *J Label Comp Radiopharm* 1975;11:427.
7. Counsell RE, Ranade VV, Blair RJ et al. Tumor localizing agents. IX. Radioiodinated cholesterol. *Steroids* 1970;16:317.
8. Blair RS, Beierwaltes WH, Lieberman LM, et al. Radiolabeled cholesterol as an adrenal scanning agent. *J Nucl Med* 1971; 12:176.
9. Freeman DA, Counsell RE. Cellular internalization, transport, and esterification of Iodine-125-NP59 by MA-10 Leydig tumor cells. *J Nucl Med* 1991;32:495.
10. Carey JE, Thrall JH, Freitas JE, Beierwaltes WH. Absorbed dose to the human adrenals from iodomethyl-norcholesterol (I-131) "NP-59". *J Nucl Med* 1979;20:60.
11. Kazerooni EA, Sisson JC, Shapiro B, et al. Diagnostic accuracy and pitfalls of [Iodine-131]6-beta-iodomethyl-19-norcholesterol (NP-59) imaging. *J Nucl Med* 1990;31:526.
12. Morita R, Leiberman LM, Beierwaltes WH, et al. Percent uptake of I-131 radioactivity in the adrenal from radioiodinated cholesterol. *J Clin Endocrinol Metab* 1972;34:36.
13. Rizza RA, Wahner HW, Spelsberg TC, et al. Visualization of non-functioning adrenal adenomas with iodocholesterol: Possible relationship to subcellular distribution of tracer. *J Nucl Med* 1978;19:458.
14. Moses DC, Schteingart DE, Sturman MF, et al. Efficacy of radiocholesterol imaging of the adrenal glands in Cushing's syndrome. *Surg Gynecol Obstet* 1974;139:1.
15. Carpenter PC, Wahner HW, Salassa RM, Dierch DG. Demonstration of steroid-producing gonadal tumors by external scanning with the use of NP-59. *Mayo Clin Proc* 1979;54:322.
16. Mitty HA, Nicholis GL, Gabrilove JL. Adrenal venography: Clinical roentgenographic correlation in 80 patients. *Am J Roentgenol* 1973;119:564.
17. Forman BH, Antar MA, Toulovkian RJ, et al. Localization of a metastatic adrenal carcinoma using I-131-19-iodocholesterol. *J Nucl Med* 1973;15:332.
18. Seabold JE, Cohen EL, Beierwaltes WH, et al. Adrenal imaging with ^{131}I-19-iodocholesterol in the diagnostic evaluation of patients with aldosteronism. *J Clin Endocrinol Metab* 1976;42:41.
19. Lund JO, Elmgreen J, Gammelgaard PA, Hasner E. Adrenal scintigraphy in primary aldosteronism caused by an aldosterone producing adenoma. *Scand J Urol Nephrol* 1980;14:292.
20. Givens JR. Hirsutism and hyperandrogenism. *Adv Intern Med* 1976;21:222.
21. James VHT, Rippon AF, Jacobs JS. Plasma androgens in patients with hirsutism, in James VHT, et al. (eds.): *The Endocrine Function of the Human Ovary.* New York, Academic Press, 1976.
22. Gross MD, Freitas JE, Swanson DP, et al. Dexamethasone suppression adrenal scintigraphy in hyperandrogenism. *J Nucl Med* 1981;22:12.
23. Schteingart DE, Woodbury MC, Taos HS, et al. Virilizing syndrome associated with an adrenal cortical adenoma secreting predominantly testosterone. *Am J Med* 1979;67:140.
24. Freitas JE, Beierwaltes WH, Nishiyama R. Adrenal hyperandrogenism: Detection by adrenal scintigraphy. *J Endocrinol Invest* 1978;1:59.
25. Kirschner MA, Zucker IR, Jespersen DL. Ovarian and adrenal vein catheterization studies in women with idiopathic hirsutism, in James VHT et al. (eds.): *The Endocrine Function of the Human Ovary.* New York, Academic Press, 1976.
26. Chatal JF, Charbonnel B, Guihard D. Radionuclide imaging of the adrenal glands. *Clin Nucl Med* 1978;3:71.

27. Freitas JE, Grekin RJ, Thrall JH, et al. Adrenal imaging with iodomethyl-norcholesterol (I-131) in primary aldosteronism. *J Nucl Med* 1979;20:7.
28. Pearse AGE. Common cytochemical and ultrastructural characteristics of cells producing polypeptide hormones (the APUD series) and their relevance to thyroid and ultimobranchial C cells and calcitonin. *Proc R Soc Lond* [Biol] 1968;170:71.
29. Schmechel D, Marangos PJ, Brightman M. Neurone-specific enolase is a molecular marker for peripheral and central neuroendocrine cells. *Nature* 1978;276:834.
30. Welbourn RB, Manolas KJ, Khan O, et al. Tumors of the neuroendocrine system (APUD-cell tumors—APUDOMAS). *Curr Prob Surg* 1984;21:7.
31. Andrew A. The APUD concept: Where has it led us? *Br Med Bull* 1982;38:221.
32. Morales JO, Beierwaltes WH, Counsell RE, et al. The concentration of radioactivity from labeled epinephrine and its precursors in the dog adrenal medulla. *J Nucl Med* 1967;8:800.
33. Wieland DM, Swanson DP, Brown LE, et al. Imaging the adrenal medulla with an I-131-labeled antiadrenergic agent. *J Nucl Med* 1979;20:155.
34. Wieland DM, Brown LE, Tobes MC. Imaging the primate adrenal medulla with ^{123}I- and ^{131}I-meta-iodobenzylguanidine. *J Nucl Med* 1981;22:358.
35. Sisson JC, Wieland DM, Sherman P, et al. Metaiodobenzylguanidine as an index of the adrenergic nervous system integrity and function. *J Nucl Med* 1987;28:1625.
36. Tobes MC, Jaques S, Wieland DM, et al. Effect of uptake-one inhibitors on the uptake of nerepinephrine and metaiodobenzylguanidine. *J Nucl Med* 1985;16:897.
37. Nakajo M, Shapiro B, Copp J, et al. The normal and abnormal distribution of the adrenomedullary imaging agent metal[I-131] iodobenzylguanidine (131-I-MIBG) in man: Evaluation by scintigraphy. *J Nucl Med* 1983;24:672.
38. Wieland DM, Wu JL, Brown LE, et al. Radiolabeled adrenergic neuron blocking agents: adrenomedullary imaging with [^{131}I]iodobenzylguanidine. *J Nucl Med* 1981;22:358.
39. Shapiro B, Wieland DM, Brown LE, et al. ^{131}I-metaiodobenzylguanidine (MIBG) adrenal medullary scintigraphy: Interventional studies, in Spencer RP (ed.): *Interventional Nuclear Medicine*. New York, Grune and Stratton, 1984, p 451.
40. Shapiro B. Imaging of catecholamine-secreting tumours: uses of MIBG in diagnosis and treatment. *Baillière's Clin Endocrinol Metab* 1993;7:491.
41. Mangner TJ, Tobes MC, Wieland DW, et al. Metabolism of Iodine-131 metaiodobenzylguanidine in patients with metastatic pheochromocytoma. *J Nucl Med* 1986;27:37.
42. Tobes MC, Fig LM, Carey J, et al. Alterations of Iodine-131-MIBG biodistribution in an anephric patient: Comparison to normal and impaired renal function. *J Nucl Med* 1989;30:1476.
43. Sisson JC, Frager MS, Val TW, et al. Scintigraphic localization of pheochromocytoma. *N Engl J Med* 1981;305:12.
44. Lindberg S, Fjalling M, Jacobsson L, et al. Methodology and dosimetry in adrenal medullary imaging with Iodine-131 MIBG. *J Nucl Med* 1988;29:1638.
45. Khafagi FA, Shapiro B, Fig LM, et al. Labetalol reduces iodine-131 MIBG uptake by pheochromocytoma and normal tissues. *J Nucl Med* 1989;30:481.
46. Scott WH, Reynolds V, Green N, et al. Clinical experience with malignant pheochromocytomas. *Surg Gynecol Obstet* 1982;154:801.
47. Scott WH, Halter SA. Oncologic aspects of pheochromocytoma: The importance of follow-up. *Surgery* 1984;96:1061.
48. Pheochromocytoma: current status and changing trends. *Surgery* 1982;91:367.
49. Shapiro B, Copp JE, Sisson JC, et al. Iodine-131 metaiodobenzylguanidine for the locating of suspected pheochromocytoma. Experience in 400 cases. *J Nucl Med* 1985;26:576.
50. Beierwaltes WH. Update on basic research and clinical experience with metaiodobenzylguanidine. *Med Ped Oncol* 1987; 15:163.
51. Schonebe CK. Malignant pheochromocytoma. *Scan J Urol Nephrol* 1969;3:64.
52. Mangner WM, Gifford RW. *Pheochromocytoma*. New York, Springer-Verlag, 1972.
53. Shapiro B, Fig LM. Management of pheochromocytoma. *Endocrinol Metab Clin North Am* 1989;18:443.
54. Bravo EL, Tarazi RC, Fouad FM, et al. Clonidine-suppression test: A useful aid in the diagnosis of pheochromocytoma. *N Engl J Med* 1981;305:623.
55. Velchik MG, Alavi A, Kressel HY, Engelman K. Localization of pheochromocytoma: MIBG, CT MRI Correlation. *J Nucl Med* 1989;30:328.
56. Shapiro B. Summary, conclusions, and future direction of [^{131}I]metaiodobenzylguanidine therapy in the treatment of neural crest tumors. *J Nucl Biol Med* 1991;35:357.
57. Jones DH, Allison DJ, Hamilton CA, et al. Selective venous sampling in the diagnosis and localization of pheochromocytoma. *Clin Endocrinol* 1979;10:179.
58. Francis IR, Glazer G, Shapiro B, et al. Complementary roles of CT scanning and ^{131}I-MIBG scintigraphy in the diagnosis of pheochromocytoma. *Am J Roentgenol* 1983;141:719.
59. Chatal JF, Charbonnel B. Comparison of iodobenzylguanidine imaging with computed tomography in locating pheochromocytoma. *J Clin Endocrinol Metab* 1985;61:769.
60. Matthay KK. Congenital malignant disorders, in Taeusch HF, Ballard RA, Avery ME (eds.): *Schaeffer and Avery's Diseases of the Newborn*. 6th ed. Philadelphia, Saunders, 1991, p 1025.
61. Shulkin BL, Beatti O, Hattner RS, et al. Bilateral testicular neuroblastoma. Scintigraphic depiction and therapy with I-131 MIBG. *Clin Nucl Med* 1992;17:638.
62. Breslow N, McCann B. Statistical estimation of prognosis for children with neuroblastoma. *Cancer Res* 1971;31:2098.
63. Voute PA, Hoefnagel CA, Marcuse HR, et al. Detection of neuroblastoma with ^{131}I-meta-iodobenzylguanidine, in Evans AE, D'Angio GJ, Seeger RC (eds.): *Advances in Neuroblastoma Research*. New York, Liss. 1985, pp 389–398.
64. Moyes JSE, Babich JW, Carter R, et al. Quantitative study of radioiodinated metaiodobenzylguanidine uptake in children with neuroblastoma: correlation with tumor histopathology. *J Nucl Med* 1989;30:474.
65. Yeh SDJ, Helson L, Benua RS. Correlation between iodine-131 MIBG imaging and biological markers in advanced neuroblastoma. *Clin Nucl Med* 1988;13:46.
66. Parisi MT, Matthay KK, Hubety JP, Hattner RS. Neuroblastoma: dose-related sensitivity of MIBG scanning in detection. *Radiology* 1992;184:463.
67. Gordon AM, Peters M, Morony S, et al. Skeletal assessment in neuroblastoma—the pitfalls of Iodine-123-MIBG scans. *J Nucl Med* 1990;31:129.
68. Lumbroso J, Hartmann O, Lemerle J, et al. Scintigraphic detection of neuroblastoma using ^{131}I- and ^{123}I-labeled metaiodobenzylguanidine (abst). *Eur J Nucl Med* 1985;11:A16.
69. Munkner T. I-131 meta-iodobenzylguanidine scintigraphy of neuroblastomas. *Semin Nucl Med* 1985;15:154.
70. Heyman S, Evans AE. I-131-meta-iodobenzylguanidine (I-131-MIBG) in the diagnosis of neuroblastoma (abst). *J Nucl Med* 1986;27:931.
71. Feine U, Muler-Schauenburg W, Treuner J, Klingebiel TH. Meta-iodobenzylguanidine (MIBG) labeled with I-123/I-131 in neuroblastoma. *Med Ped Oncol* 1984;15:181.
72. Goldman A, Vivian G, Gordon I, et al. Immunolocalization

of neuroblastoma using radiolabeled monoclonal antibody UJ 13A. *J Pediatr* 1984;105:252.

73. Baum RP, Maul FD, Schwarz A, et al. Diagnosis and treatment of stage IV neuroblastoma with Tc-99m- and I-131-labeled monoclonal antibody BW 575/9. *J Nucl Med* 1989;30:904.
74. Cheung NKV, Saarinen UM, Neely JE, et al. Monoclonal antibodies to a glycolipid antigen on human neuroblastoma cells. *Cancer Res* 1985;45:2642.
75. Cheung NKV, Neely JE, Landmeier B, et al. Targeting of ganglioside G_{D2} monoclonal antibody to neuroblastoma. *J Nucl Med* 1987;28:1577.
76. Cheung NKV, Landmeier B, Neely J, et al. Complete tumor ablation with iodine-131 radiolabeled disialoganglioside G_{D2} monoclonal antibody to neuroblastoma. *J Nucl Med* 1987; 28:1577.
77. Miraldi FD, Nelson AD, Kraly C, et al. Diagnostic imaging of human neuroblastoma with radiolabeled antibody. *Radiology* 1986;161:413.
78. Yeh SDJ, Larson SM, Burch L, et al. Radioimmunodetection of neuroblastoma with Iodine-131-3F8: Correlation with biopsy, iodine-131-metaiodobenzylguanidine and standard diagnostic modalities. *J Nucl Med* 1991;32:769.
79. Wu ZL, Schwartz E, Seeger R, et al. Expression of G_{D2} ganglioside by untreated primary human neuroblastomas. *Cancer Res* 1986;46:440.
80. Glenner GG, Grimley PM. Tumors of the extra-adrenal paraganglion system (including chemoreceptor), in *Atlas of Tumor Pathology*, Second Series, Fascicle 9. Washington, DC: Armed Forces Institute of Pathology, 1974.
81. Irons GB, Wieland LH, Brown WL. Paragangliomas of the neck: Clinical and pathological analysis of 116 cases. *Surg Clin North Am* 1977;15:897.
82. Khafagi F, Egerton-Vernon J, van Doorn T, et al. Localization and treatment of familial malignant nonfunctional paraganglioma with Iodine-131 MIBG: Report of two cases. *J Nucl Med* 1987;28:528.
83. Baulieu JL, Guilloteau D, Baulieu F, et al. Therapeutic effectiveness of Iodine-131 MIBG metastases of a nonsecreting paraganglioma. *J Nucl Med* 1988;29:2008.
84. Berge T, Linell F. Carcinoid tumors. *Acta Pathol Microbiol Immunol Scand* (A), 1976;84:322.
85. Davis Z, Moertel CG, McJirath DC. The malignant carcinoid syndrome. *Surg Gynecol Obstet* 1973;137:637.
86. Hoefnagel CA. Radionuclide therapy revisited. *Eur J Nucl Med* 1991;18:408.
87. Hoefnagel CA, Taal BG, Valdes Olmos RA. Role of [^{131}I]Metaiodobenzylguanidine treatment in metastatic carcinoid. *J Nucl Biol Med* 1991;35:346.
88. Kvols LK, Moertel CG, O'Connell J, et al. Treatment of the malignant carcinoid syndrome: evaluation of a long-acting somatostatin analogue. *N Engl J Med* 1988;315:663.
89. Lamberts SWJ, Bakker WH, Rubi JC, Krenning EP. Somatostatin-receptor imaging in the localization of endocrine tumors. *N Engl J Med* 1990;323:1246.
90. Krenning EP, Bakker WH, Breeman WAP, et al. Localization of endocrine-related tumors with radio-iodinated analogue of somatostatin. *Lancet* 1990;1:246.
91. Bomanji J, Ur E, Mather S, et al. A scintigraphic comparison of Iodine-123-metaiodobenzylguanidine and an Iodine-labeled somatostatin analog (Tyr-3-octreotide) in metastatic carcinoid tumors. *J Nucl Med* 1992;33:1121.

32 The Hematopoietic System

David C. Price

PERIPHERAL BLOOD

The use of radionuclides in clinical hematology began in 1938 when John Lawrence first utilized ^{32}P, produced by his brother Ernest in the Berkeley cyclotron, to treat a young man with chronic myelogenous leukemia.[1] In 1939, Hevesy introduced ^{32}P-labeled red blood cells to measure blood volume.[2] Since these beginnings, nuclear hematology has continued to figure importantly in the development of nuclear medicine. This chapter reviews the hematologic procedures in current use and, in most instances, their clinical applications and the characteristic findings in both normal and hematologic disease states. The use of radiolabeled white blood cells (leukocytes) in the clinical assessment of infection, the use of labeled platelets in the clinical evaluation of thrombosis, and the use of radionuclides in hematologic therapy are topics discussed in other chapters.

Cell Labeling—General Principles

An ideal isotopic label for the formed elements of the blood should have certain general properties:

1. Incorporation of the label should alter neither cell function nor cell life span.
2. The label should neither elute from the cell nor be reutilized after destruction of the cell.
3. The label should incorporate a gamma-emitting radionuclide with energy characteristics appropriate to current counting and imaging instruments and with a half-life appropriate to the parameter (life span, volume of distribution, etc.) being measured.
4. Uptake of the label should be uniform throughout the targeted cell population, and unique to that cell population.

Such cellular labels are of two general types: *cohort* labels and *random* labels.

COHORT LABELS

Ideally, a cohort (or *pulse*) label of hematopoietic cells is available only to the marrow precursors of a given cell type for a brief period of time, and is not taken up directly by circulating cells. Incorporation of the cohort label into marrow precursors then leads to its appearance in the youngest circulating cells, and to its persistence throughout the life span of the labeled cells. A label that meets these criteria and those listed previously permits the study of the rate of production of the given cell type, its kinetics, longevity, manner of death, and ultimate fate within the body. None of the radiopharmaceuticals currently available for cohort labeling of blood cellular elements satisfies all of these requirements for clinical usefulness. Indeed, most cohort labels are so limited by their properties that, with the exception of radioiron, none is currently used in routine clinical studies.

RANDOM LABELS

These radiopharmaceuticals label cells of all ages in the peripheral blood and, thus, provide a measure of mean cell survival. Labeling the different morphological types of circulating cells generally requires physical separation of the cells prior to labeling, usually by differential centrifugation of anticoagulated autologous peripheral blood. Table 1 lists the radiopharmaceuticals that have been used most frequently to label blood cells. These labels and labeling techniques have been described in various reports.[3–20]

REVIEW OF CELL LABELS

Erythrocytes. The various radioisotopes of iron are the oldest, and still the most useful, cohort labels for determining the rate of erythrocyte production. However, the body has a great ability to conserve hemoglobin iron. When labeled red cells are removed from circulation, the heme is degraded, and the label returns to the plasma iron pool to reappear in new cells. This continued reutilization makes radioiron less than ideal for directly measuring red cell survival. It is best used to determine the rate and sites of production of labeled erythrocytes.

The three radioisotopes of iron used for in vivo studies are ^{52}Fe, ^{55}Fe, and ^{59}Fe (Table 2). Although ^{59}Fe is easy to quantify in blood samples and to detect by probes over localization sites in vivo, its gamma emissions are too energetic for good spatial resolution with existing imaging instruments. At the other extreme, measurement of ^{55}Fe by external detection is almost impossible. Even in vitro quantification is difficult because of the low energies of the 5.8 keV X-rays emitted by the manganese daughter. ^{52}Fe can be imaged by positron (PET) scanners but, because of its 8.3-hr half-life, it is unsuitable for full ferrokinetic studies, which extend over 10 to 14 days. Also, the cost of cyclotron production

Table 1. Radioisotopic Labels of the Blood Cellular Elements

	COHORT*	RANDOM*
Erythrocytes	^{15}N-, ^{3}H-, or ^{14}C-glycine (^{75}Se-methionine) ^{59}Fe-, ^{55}Fe-, or ^{52}Fe-sulfate/chloride	^{11}CO (PET) (^{32}P-orthophosphate) ^{32}P-, ^{3}H-, and ^{14}C-diisopropyl fluorophosphate (DFP) ^{51}Cr-sodium chromate ^{68}Ga-oxine (PET) ^{99m}Tc-pertechnetate ^{111}In-oxine, -tropolone, -acetylacetone, or -merc (2-mercaptopyridine-N-oxide)
Platelets	$Na^{35}SO4$ (^{75}Se-methionine)	(^{14}C-serotonin) (^{32}P-orthophosphate) (^{32}P-, ^{3}H-, or ^{14}C-DFP) ^{51}Cr-sodium chromate ^{68}Ga-oxine (PET) ^{111}In-oxine, -tropolone, -acetylacetone, or -merc Labeled anti-platelet antibodies (^{111}In, ^{99m}Tc)
Granulocytes	^{3}H-thymidine (^{32}P-orthophosphate)	(^{75}Se-selenomethionine) (^{99m}Tc-pyrophosphate) ^{32}P-, ^{3}H-, or ^{14}C-DFP ^{99m}Tc-albumin colloid ^{111}In-oxine, -tropolone, -acetylacetone, or -merc Labeled anti-granulocyte antibodies (^{111}In, ^{99m}Tc) Labeled chemotactic peptides and their analogs (^{111}In, ^{99m}Tc)

*The radiopharmaceuticals in parentheses have been described for this use, but subsequently have been demonstrated to be unsatisfactory, generally because of excessively rapid elution, exchange, or reutilization. Radiocolloids and labeled particles are judged to be unsatisfactory labels for granulocytes because of the difficulty inherent in separating unbound particles from the labeled cells prior to re-infusion.

of ^{52}Fe is prohibitive for routine clinical use. ^{59}Iron, therefore, remains the radioisotope of choice for evaluating ferrokinetics. There are no other routine cohort labels for the study of erythrocytes, although labeled glycine has been used for research studies (Table 1).

A widely used random label for erythrocytes is ^{51}Cr as sodium chromate. The detailed procedure is given later. When Cr(VI) is incubated with anticoagulated whole blood at room temperature, it promptly crosses the red cell membrane and enters the cells. Within the red cell, chromate is promptly reduced to the chromic (3+) ion, the majority of which binds to the beta chain of hemoglobin. After 10 to 15 minutes of incubation, the red cells can be washed free

Table 2. Physical Characteristics of the Medically Useful Radioisotopes of Iron*

ISOTOPE	PHYSICAL HALF-LIFE	RADIATION	PRINCIPAL PHOTON ENERGIES (MeV)
^{52}Fe	8.3 hr	γ, β^+	0.169 (99%) β+ (56%)
^{55}Fe	2.7 yr	Mn x-rays	0.0058
^{59}Fe	45.0 day	γ, β^-	1.10 (55%) 1.29 (44%)

*See Appendix for dosimetry

of excess chromate. Alternatively, ascorbic acid can be added to reduce the residual free chromate to chromic ion, which is then unable to enter the red cell. When ascorbate reduction is used, preparation of both a red cell standard and a plasma standard is necessary for proper calculation of the red cell volume.

Labeling efficiency with ^{51}Cr chromate is approximately 90%, and the label resists cell washing and dialysis. Causes of reduced labeling efficiency include: (1) prolonged incubation of ^{51}Cr chromate with the ACD solution; (2) presence of stannous ions; (3) presence of excess calcium ions; (4) high pH of the ACD solution; (5) low specific activity of the ^{51}Cr.

Whole blood is used routinely for ^{51}Cr labeling, but if the white blood cell count exceeds 25,000/mm^3, or if the platelet count exceeds 500,000/mm^3, a significant fraction of the ^{51}Cr attaches to these cells and is unavailable to the red cells. In these cases, a buffy-coat-free red cell suspension must be prepared prior to labeling to study the distribution and fate of the erythrocytes alone.

^{51}Cr-labeled erythrocytes are used for several clinical purposes:

1. Measurement of red cell volume (and from this, estimation of the total blood volume).
2. Calculation of red cell survival and splenic sequestration.
3. Quantification of occult blood loss.
4. In vivo cross matching.

There are four important limitations to the use of ^{51}Cr to label erythrocytes:

1. Only 9% of ^{51}Cr disintegrations yield gamma emissions, with a relatively high energy of 320 keV. The remainder contribute to the radiation absorbed dose without providing useful information.
2. ^{51}Cr elutes from normal red cells at the rate of about 1% per day, and this elution rate varies in different diseases.
3. The 28-day half-life is very long for such short-term measurements as red cell volume.
4. Because of its high gamma energy and low photon yield, ^{51}Cr is ineffective for gamma scintigraphy at acceptable doses.

Diisopropyl fluorophosphate (DFP) labeled with ^{32}P, ^{3}H, or ^{14}C binds to the red cell membrane, does not elute after the first 24 hours, and causes no detectable damage to the cells. These radionuclides are pure beta emitters, however, and determining organ localization of the labeled cells by external detection is not possible.

Radiolabeled DFP can also serve as a cohort label. A sufficient amount of nonradioactive DFP must first be injected to block the binding sites on circulating cells, so that only marrow precursors are able to incorporate the label.

^{99m}TECHNETIUM-RED BLOOD CELL LABELING

^{99m}Technetium-labeling of erythrocytes (^{99m}Tc-RBC) has come into wide use in clinical nuclear medicine for several important applications: imaging of the cardiovascular system, particularly gated wall-motion studies; detection and localization of gastrointestinal hemorrhage; measurement of red cell volume; and selective splenic imaging. Erythrocyte labeling with ^{99m}Tc can be done by a completely in vitro technique, by in vivo methods, or by a combination of these two, sometimes called "in vivtro" labeling.

Fischer et al.[21] first labeled RBCs with ^{99m}Tc in 1967, but high labeling efficiency was not achieved until the importance of stannous reduction of technetium was recognized.[22–25] In 1976, Smith and Richards described a simple kit technique for red cell labeling, now known as the Brookhaven National Laboratories or BNL kit, which has gained wide usage because of its simplicity.[26,27] Other techniques have been published by Gutkowski et al. and Ansari et al.[28,29] The steps of the BNL kit labeling procedure are as follows:

1. Draw 4 mL of the patient's whole blood into a heparinized syringe, and transfer to the kit Vacutainer® containing a lyophilized stannous citrate mixture containing 2 μg of tin$^{(II)}$. The blood is incubated with these reagents for 5 minutes.
2. Add 1 mL of 4.4% EDTA (disodium or calcium disodium salt), mix, and centrifuge the tube upside down at 1300 g for 5 minutes.
3. Withdraw 1.25 mL of the packed RBCs, transfer to a vial containing 1 to 3 mL ^{99m}Tc-pertechnetate, and incubate with gentle mixing for 10 minutes.

The red cells are now ready for injection. Alternatively, they can be heated at 49°C for 15 minutes and used to image the spleen. The labeling efficiency of the BNL kit method is approximately 98%. There is close agreement between blood volume measurements made with ^{51}Cr-RBCs and ^{99m}Tc-RBCs.[30] A different commercial kit now available avoids the problems of multiple transfers and centrifugation by using NaClO to oxidize extracellular Sn$^{(II)}$ to Sn$^{(IV)}$ prior to the addition of the ^{99m}Tc-pertechnetate.[30] Thus, the only Sn$^{(II)}$ available to reduce the ^{99m}Tc is red-cell-bound, and labeling yields of approximately 100% are achieved with a simple 4-step procedure:

1. draw anticoagulated blood from the patient;
2. add stannous ion (5 minutes);
3. add sodium hypochlorite preparation; and
4. add ^{99m}Tc pertechnetate (20 minutes), followed by patient injection.

In vivo methods for ^{99m}Tc-RBC labeling are based on McCrae's observation that the in vivo distribution of pertechnetate is greatly altered by prior injection of stannous ion.[31,32] Pavel et al. found that stannous pyrophosphate was the most effective agent for "tinning" the red cells in vivo.[33] Several variations of in vivo labeling have been reported. The following method yields a labeling efficiency that varies from 60 to 90%:

1. Reconstitute commercial stannous pyrophosphate containing 2 to 4 mg of stannous ion with normal saline, and inject into the patient an aliquot containing 10 to 20 μg of tin per kg body weight.
2. After 30 min, inject the required quantity of ^{99m}Tc pertechnetate (usually 20 to 30 mCi, or 740 to 1110 MBq). RBC labeling occurs immediately.

It is important to inject the stannous pyrophosphate shortly after reconstitution to minimize spontaneous oxidation of the tin. This method results in stable binding of tin to the RBC, even with stannous pyrophosphate kits that are up to 2 months old.[34] In vivo labeling is less efficient and less reproducible than the in vitro and even the in vivo/in vitro (in vivtro) method, but it is much more convenient for procedures such as cardiac wall motion or first-pass cardiac studies.

The following combined in vivtro method is recommended by Callahan et al.[35]

1. Inject 0.5 mg stannous ion intravenously from a reconstituted commercial stannous pyrophosphate kit.
2. Insert a 19-gauge butterfly infusion set into an appropriate vein. Attach a four-way stopcock, and flush with saline containing ACD.[36]
3. Approximately 20 minutes following injection of the tin, withdraw 3 mL of blood into a 5-mL shielded syringe

containing 20 to 30 mCi (740 to 1110 MBq) ^{99m}Tc-pertechnetate.

4. Flush the tubing with ACD solution. After 10 minutes of incubation with gentle agitation at room temperature, the labeled RBCs are reinjected through the infusion set.

This method has gained wide use because it is relatively simple, is well tolerated by patients, and results in about 95% labeling efficiency.[35]

Mechanism of Pertechnetate Labeling. The mechanism of ^{99m}Tc-RBC labeling has been summarized in general terms by Srivastava and Chervu[30] and by Callahan et al.[37] as follows:

1. The stannous ion, held in solution by its chelation to pyrophosphate, diffuses or is transported into the red cell and binds to some cellular component. There is evidence that this is, in fact, a specific energy-dependent transport process.[38]
2. Pertechnetate ion is transported across the red cell membrane by the anion transport system band-3 protein, the system responsible for chloride/bicarbonate exchange (Hamburger shift).[37] This energy-dependent transport system can be blocked by such compounds as stilbene sulfonates (e.g., SITS) and dipyridamole.
3. In the presence of intracellular tin$^{(II)}$ the ^{99m}Tc is reduced and bound firmly to large molecules, predominantly the β-chain of hemoglobin.[39,40]
4. Neither stannic ion ($Sn^{(IV)}$) nor reduced forms of technetium cross the cell membrane. Any tin$^{(II)}$ remaining outside the cell reduces pertechnetate before it enters the red cell, and results in its binding to circulating proteins.
5. The purpose of adding EDTA in the in vitro method is to chelate and inactivate any tin$^{(II)}$ not bound to the red cells, thus increasing labeling efficiency. The purpose of hypochlorite added before pertechnetate is to oxidize any tin not bound to red cells so that it cannot reduce the ^{99m}Tc outside the cell.

In addition to dipyridamole and SITS as mentioned above, there are other medications that can interfere with ^{99m}Tc labeling of RBCs, including certain antimicrobial agents, anticonvulsants, antihypertensive drugs, cardiac glycosides, tranquilizers, heparin, and anti-inflammatory agents.[41,42] Diseases and medications associated with RBC antibody formation also reduce labeling efficiency.[43]

PLATELETS

When ^{35}S-sodium sulfate is injected intravenously, a significant fraction enters the megakaryocytes and acts as a partial cohort label for platelets. ^{35}Sulfur is a beta emitter, however, associated with an unacceptably high radiation absorbed dose to the patient. ^{32}P-DFP (diisopropyl fluorophosphate) labels platelets as it does red cells by binding to enzymes in the cell membrane, but it is used only investigatively to study platelet survival. ^{14}C-5-hydroxytryptamine binds rapidly to platelets and mixes with the nonradioactive platelet serotonin in the dense bodies. However, it is released upon platelet stimulation and therefore is unsatisfactory for in vivo studies.

Until recently, ^{51}Cr-sodium chromate has been the most widely used random label for estimating platelet survival and localizing sites of destruction or thrombus formation by external probe counting. However, as mentioned previously, ^{51}Cr does not have good physical characteristics for in vivo scintigraphy. Furthermore, the efficiency of human platelet labeling with ^{51}Cr is low. Even when the harvesting procedure and labeling yield are optimum, only some 10 to 30 μCi (0.370 to 1.11 MBq) of the starting ^{51}Cr are bound to platelets by the standard labeling technique. Finally, ^{51}Cr-platelet sequestration studies have been shown to have limited clinical value. For example, external counting over the liver and spleen, to determine the rates at which platelets accumulate in these organs, does not always correlate well with the subsequent clinical response to splenectomy in patients with idiopathic thrombocytopenic purpura.[44] Thus, the main usefulness for ^{51}Cr platelet labeling in routine studies has been to document shortened survival and, from survival and calculation of the circulating platelet pool, to estimate the platelet production rate.

During the past two decades, platelets have been labeled with ^{111}In-8-hydroxyquinoline (^{111}In-oxine) for study of platelet kinetics and in vivo organ localization.[45–52] ^{111}Indium has the advantages over ^{51}Cr of a 2.8-day half-life for studies lasting up to several days, no beta emission, and gamma emissions of 173 keV (89%) and 247 keV (94%), which are well suited for scintillation camera imaging. Oxine acts as a lipophilic carrier of the ^{111}In in a triple clathrate which crosses the bilipid membrane of blood cells and leaves the ^{111}In bound to intracellular proteins. Other lipophilic carriers, such as tropolone, acetylacetone, and 2-mercaptopyridine-N-oxide (merc), have also been used, but only ^{111}In-oxine is U.S. Food and Drug Administration (FDA)-approved and commercially available. Detailed separation and labeling techniques have been reviewed by Mathias and Welch[10] and Datz,[17] among others.

There has been great interest in the possibility of being able to use radiolabeled platelet antibodies as the tracer for platelets in studies of survival and in vivo thrombus formation. Availability of an ideal platelet antibody should permit comprehensive in vivo studies, without the need to draw the patient's blood and separate the platelets prior to labeling, a process which significantly injures the platelets and alters their function and biokinetics following reinfusion. In addition, with platelets as with white blood cells, eliminating the need to remove and reinject labeled autologous cells will eliminate the small, but real, risk of transmission of disease (hepatitis, HIV, etc.) when there is an error in patient injection.

Several platelet markers have been explored as potential antigens for the production of platelet-specific antibodies:[12,13,19]

1. The platelet glycoprotein membrane receptor complex IIb/IIIa, a stable membrane receptor for fibrinogen that

remains present on the cell membrane throughout the circulating life of the platelet. Antibodies produced against this receptor have included P256, 7E3, B59.2, and 50H.19.[18] Whole IgG MoAbs have been labeled with ^{123}I, ^{131}I, and ^{111}In. Improved scintigraphy will be more likely with the F(ab′) and F(ab′)$_2$ fragments labeled with ^{99m}Tc or ^{111}In because of more rapid blood clearance and improved target-to-background ratios.

2. The platelet activation-dependent granule-external membrane protein GMP 140 (PADGEM). This molecule is a protein expressed on the platelet membrane only during activation-dependent degranulation. Whereas the anti-IIb/IIIa antibodies will bind to all platelets, including those in circulation, anti-GMP-140 antibodies will only bind to those platelets already activated, including those in the process of deposition at a site of thrombus formation. Antibodies currently under evaluation include S12 and KC4.
3. Thrombospondin (TSP), which is a platelet protein secreted by the alpha granules during activation. TSP binds to the IIb/IIIa complex in particularly high concentrations after platelet activation. Consequently, anti-TSP antibodies also have highest affinity for activated platelets.

Each of the latter 2 categories of antiplatelet antibody would have great potential for scintigraphy of thrombosis, but only the first (anti-IIb/IIIa) might be useful as an in vivo label for platelet kinetics.

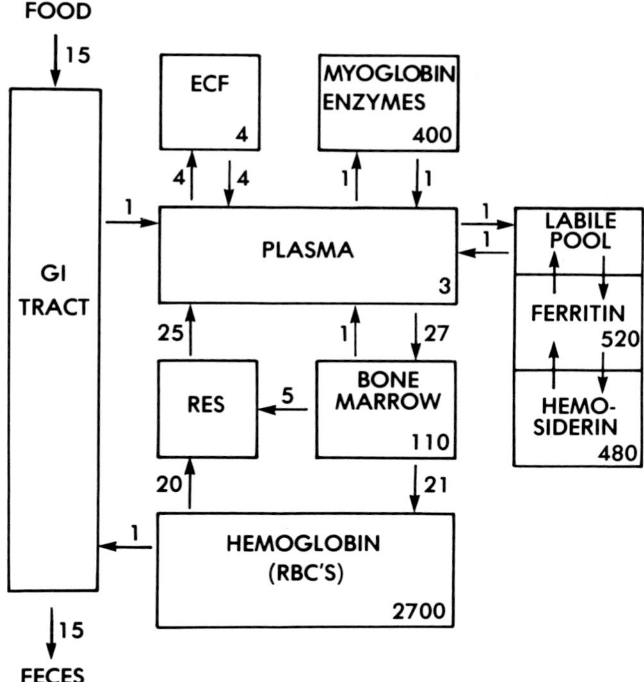

Figure 1. Simplified diagram of iron metabolism in normal adult males. The figures in the boxes represent total iron (in mg) in that compartment. The figures beside arrows represent daily iron exchange (in mg). ECF, extracellular fluid; RES, reticuloendothelial system.

LEUKOCYTES

^{3}H-thymidine is a true cohort label of leukocytes. It is taken up by the myeloid precursors in the bone marrow and appears 1 to 3 days later in the youngest circulating granulocytes. The use of ^{3}H-thymidine has provided important kinetic data on the physiological and pathophysiological characteristics of human granulocytes. This tracer is incorporated into DNA, however, and can potentially cause genetic damage. The lack of gamma emission precludes in vivo localization. Thus, it is not used for routine clinical studies.

Random labels are used experimentally to study granulocyte kinetics. Radioactive DF^{32}P is a random label when incubated with a pure granulocyte preparation in vitro, and predominantly a random label when injected intravenously without a prior "cold" DFP loading dose. ^{51}Cr as sodium chromate is also an effective in vitro random label. The granulocytes must be isolated prior to incubation because ^{51}Cr labels all blood cells indiscriminately in a heterogeneous preparation of cells. A single injection of ^{75}Se-methionine results in a prompt and simultaneous cohort label of all 3 formed elements of the blood, which then can be separated for kinetic studies by in vitro counting. ^{75}Se-methionine is extensively reutilized, however, which makes it unsatisfactory as a cohort label for leukocytes, and it is inferior to radioiron for studying the early phases of erythrokinetics. Despite these problems, it remains a useful research label for studying platelet production.

A great deal of effort has been devoted recently to developing new granulocyte labels.[53,54] Some of these labels rely upon cell phagocytosis (e.g., radioactive colloids and human serum albumin microspheres). A major problem with this approach is difficulty in separating the granulocytes from the uningested labeled particles. ^{111}In-oxine can also be used to label granulocytes, especially to image abscesses and focal inflammation.[53,55–57] There are associated problems, however, in isolating and labeling cells under sterile and pyrogen-free conditions, and in the extreme sensitivity of granulocytes to the physical and chemical trauma of ex vivo separation and labeling, which may result in cell aggregates or nonfunctional cells.

Erythrocyte Studies

FERROKINETICS AND THE STUDY OF ERYTHROPOIESIS

Normal Iron Metabolism. Ferrokinetic studies are useful in evaluating iron metabolism, particularly as it reflects erythrocyte production and the relative contributions of bone marrow and extramedullary sites to total erythropoiesis. The complexities of ferrokinetic studies are best appreciated through an understanding of the metabolic pools of iron being traced.

Figure 1 summarizes iron metabolism in normal adult

males. The total body iron content is 4.5 to 6.0 g in men, and 3.5 to 4.0 g in women.[58] Approximately 3 mg of iron circulates in plasma bound to transferrin, an 80,000 dalton protein having 2 iron-binding sites per molecule. The iron binding sites of circulating transferrin are normally one third saturated with iron. Metabolically active iron moves predominantly from plasma to the bone marrow, where transferrin goes to the erythroid precursors and makes the iron available for hemoglobin synthesis. Upon release into circulation, mature erythrocytes retain their full complement of hemoglobin-bound iron for the 120-day life span. Upon death of the erythrocyte, almost all hemoglobin iron is recycled through the RES, and then, by way of plasma transferrin, back to the marrow for reutilization in erythropoiesis. Under normal conditions, 10 to 20% of the plasma iron pool goes to storage sites in the liver, spleen, and bone marrow RE cells. First, it is stored in a small labile pool. Then, it is incorporated into ferritin and subsequently into hemosiderin for long-term storage. Only a small fraction of the plasma pool is used to synthesize other iron-containing molecules, such as myoglobin and certain iron-containing enzymes (e.g., cytochrome P450). With the exceptions of late fetal life and possibly the immediate postpartum period, erythropoiesis does not normally occur in the liver or spleen.

The largest single iron compartment in the body is the circulating red blood cell mass, which contains 2.5 to 3.0 g of iron incorporated in hemoglobin (3.33 mg of iron per gram of hemoglobin). Iron stores in the normal adult male are 1.0 to 1.5 g. Adult females stores are considerably lower because of regular red cell iron loss with menses and pregnancies. In normal adults approximately 1 mg of iron is absorbed per day from a diet containing 10 to 20 mg. This amount represents only a small fraction of the normal daily plasma iron turnover of 25 to 40 mg because of the high reutilization of hemoglobin iron. Approximately 1 mg of iron is excreted per day through normal sloughing of intestinal mucosal cells. The normal daily loss in sweat and urine is negligible.

FERROKINETICS: PROCEDURE AND NORMAL RESULTS

^{59}Fe is the only radioisotope of iron suitable for a complete in vivo ferrokinetic study. To assess metabolic iron pathways properly in patients, the radioiron must be completely bound to circulating transferrin, preferably by prior incubation with plasma. If non-transferrin-bound radiotracer iron is injected into a patient whose iron-binding capacity is saturated, this excess iron is cleared rapidly from circulation to the RES and is unavailable for tracing iron metabolism. Patients with significantly reduced unsaturated iron-binding capacity include those with hemochromatosis, hemosiderosis, hemolytic anemia, aplastic anemia, and patients who have recently been treated with parenteral iron or transfusions (Fig. 2). In such patients, prior incubation of the tracer with normal donor plasma is necessary.

The determination of serum iron (SI) and unsaturated iron-binding capacity (UIBC) are obligatory first steps in any ferrokinetic study. If the UIBC is less than 40% of the total iron-binding capacity (TIBC), fresh plasma from heparinized blood should be obtained from a healthy ABO-compatible donor. The tracer iron is preincubated with the donor plasma for 15 minutes at room temperature, prior to preparing the injectate and standard. The customary ^{59}Fe dose varies from 5 to 20 μCi (0.185 to 0.740 MBq). The higher doses are necessary when surface counting is performed.

A ferrokinetic study has 3 major parts: the plasma radioiron disappearance curve (PID), the red cell radioiron incorporation (RCI), and surface counting for organ kinetics.

The plasma radioiron disappearance curve involves frequent blood sampling that begins 5 minutes after injection and continues at widening intervals for 4 hours (Fig. 3). When the plasma is separated and its radioactivity is plotted on semilogarithmic paper as a function of time, a straight line is usually obtained (at least from the earlier points), and the T1/2 of the initial rate of plasma iron clearance can be determined from the graph. If the tracer iron is fully bound to transferrin, the initial straight line portion of this curve can be extrapolated to zero time, thereby providing a measure of plasma volume by the dilutional assay technique (see below).

This initial single-exponential clearance curve *does not* fully reflect the overall turnover of plasma iron. If plasma activity is followed for longer periods of time, clearance of the remaining iron slows, adding one or more additional exponential components to the curve.[6] The initial clearance constant, however, does reflect the majority of metabolic iron turnover from plasma. To calculate with precision the true plasma iron turnover and such other parameters as erythrocyte iron turnover, it is necessary to perform a more complex and precise study of plasma radioactive iron disappearance, taking multiple samples over 14 days.[6] Because of the low concentration of radioactive iron in the later samples, even minor amounts of hemolysis cause significant errors. This elaborate long-term study is, therefore, rarely performed other than as a research procedure.

The daily plasma iron turnover (*PIT*) can be calculated from the *PID*, the serum iron, and the plasma volume (*PV*) determined with ^{125}I human serum albumin (HSA). The following formula is used:

$$PIT\ (\text{mg/day}) = \frac{SI(\mu\text{g/mL}) \times PV(\text{mL}) \times 0.693 \times 60 \times 24}{1000 \times \text{Plasma } ^{59}\text{Fe } T_{1/2}(\text{min})} = \frac{SI(\mu\text{g/mL}) \times PV(\text{mL}) \times 0.998}{\text{Plasma } ^{59}\text{Fe } T_{1/2}(\text{min})}$$

The normal plasma radioiron disappearance half-time is 60 to 140 minutes, and the normal *PIT* is 27 to 42 mg/day (0.46 to 0.78 mg/kg/day).

The red cell radioiron incorporation (*RCI*) is determined by counting whole blood samples on days 1, 4, 7, 10, and 14 along with a standard of the injected dose. On day 14, the

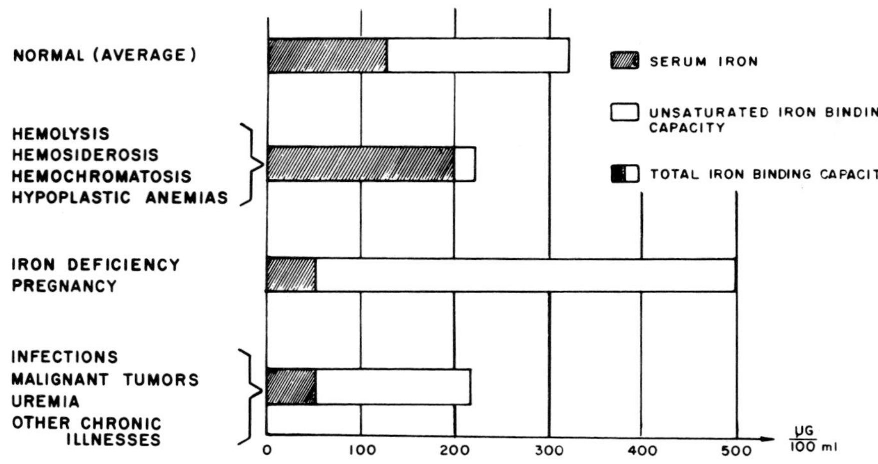

Figure 2. Serum iron, unsaturated iron-binding capacity, and total iron-binding capacity in normals and in several disease states.

total blood volume (*TBV*) is determined using ^{51}Cr-labeled autologous red blood cells, with appropriate corrections made for ^{59}Fe Compton scatter in the ^{51}Cr counting window.

$$RCI\ (\%) = \frac{^{59}\text{Fe cpm/mL blood} \times TBV\ (\text{mL}) \times 100}{\text{Total } ^{59}\text{Fe cpm injected}}$$

The normal *RCI* is 75 to 95% (Fig. 4).

Because 1 g of hemoglobin (Hgb) contains 3.3 mg iron, the daily rate of Hgb synthesis can be calculated from the *PIT* and the *RCI*:

Daily Hgb Synthesis (g) =

$$PIT\ (\text{mg/d}) \times \frac{RCI\ (\%)}{100} \times \frac{1}{3.3\ \text{mg Fe/g Hgb}}$$

The estimated mean red cell survival can then be calculated from *TBV* and blood Hgb concentration:

Mean RBC Survival (days) =

$$TBV\ (\text{mL}) \times \frac{\text{Hgb(g/dL)}}{100} \times \frac{1}{\text{Hgb Synthesis (g/day)}}$$

Organ counts are obtained immediately after radioiron injection to document the initial blood (plasma) distribution. The probe should be a 2-in. or preferably a 3-in. NaI(Tl) detector with adequate shielding for ^{59}Fe and a flat-field collimator. The detector is positioned over the precordium, anterior liver, posterior or lateral spleen, and sacrum (bone marrow). Counts are obtained at several times during the

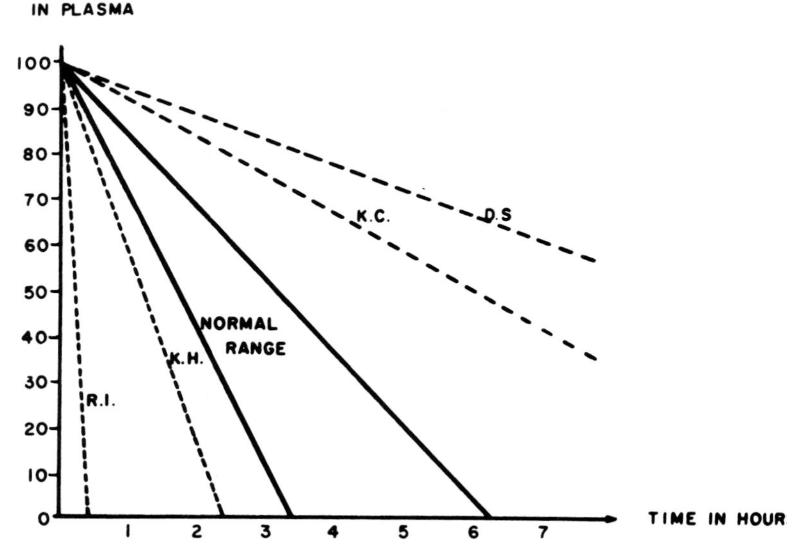

Figure 3. Representative patterns of plasma iron disappearance in certain abnormal conditions. Patient R.I. has refractory sideroblastic anemia with a completely saturated iron-binding capacity. Patients D.S. and K.C. have severe iron overload with markedly delayed clearance of transferrin-bound ^{59}Fe. Patient K.H. has chronic iron deficiency anemia. (Reprinted by permission from McIntyre PA: *Prog Haematol* 1977;10:361.)

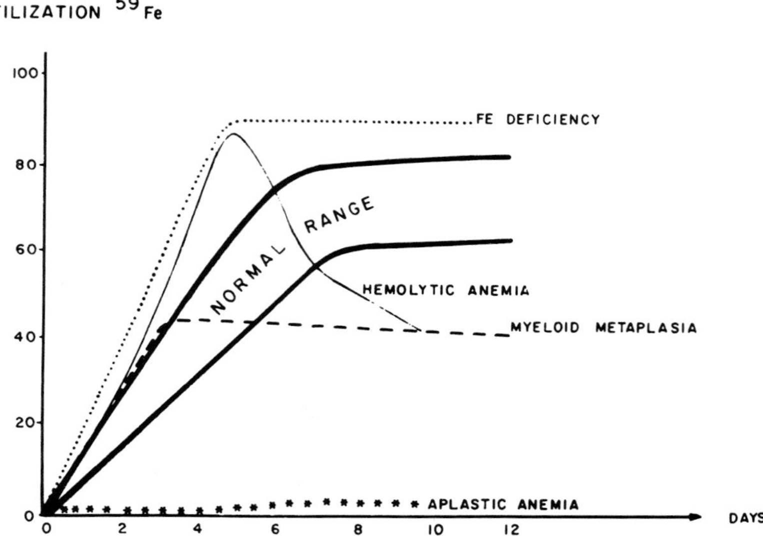

Figure 4. Curves comparing red cell incorporation (RCI) of radioiron in various disease states with normal. A more rapid plasma iron disappearance (PID) and greater RCI occurs in patients with iron deficiency and hemolytic anemias. Note that with concomitant removal or destruction of the labeled cells (as shown here in a patient with autoimmune hemolytic anemia), a single sample taken at the eighth to tenth day would indicate the ^{59}Fe utilization to be lower than it really is. In aplastic anemia, ^{59}Fe incorporation is reduced. (From McIntyre, PA, et al.[28])

first 4 hours, and again on days 2, 3, 4, 7, 10, and 14. All counts are corrected for decay and then divided by the initial count over that organ to normalize to unity at T_0. Initially, blood activity falls over the heart, liver, and spleen to a nadir at 24 hours, then rises toward unity as the ^{59}Fe reappears in circulating erythrocytes. At the same time, sacral bone marrow activity rises progressively over the first 24 hours, then falls to unity thereafter, as the labeled erythroid precursors in the marrow are released into circulation (Fig. 5). These patterns reflect the fact that 75 to 95% of the radioiron is taken up by the marrow during the first day, then reappears in circulating erythrocytes as the marrow red cell precursors mature and enter the circulation.

In general, the *PID* predominantly reflects erythropoiesis; a short half-time indicates accelerated erythrocyte production and a long half-time indicates depressed production. This relationship exists only if the radioiron has been properly bound to transferrin; it does not hold in hemochromatosis, in which nonhematopoietic organs have high iron avidity. The *RCI* is a measure of effective erythropoiesis, indicating the true peripheral release of newly formed red cells. Rapid peripheral destruction may result in a falling *RCI* curve during days 7 to 14. Finally, surface counting indicates the major organ sites involved both in red cell production (seen as sites with an early rise and then subsequent fall in activity as the radioiron is released in RBCs into the circulation), and in iron storage (progressive rise in liver, and to a variable extent in spleen activity).

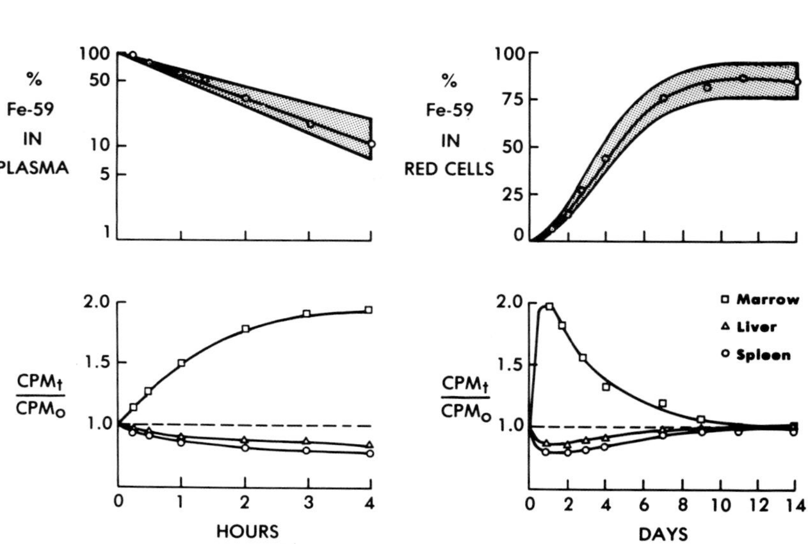

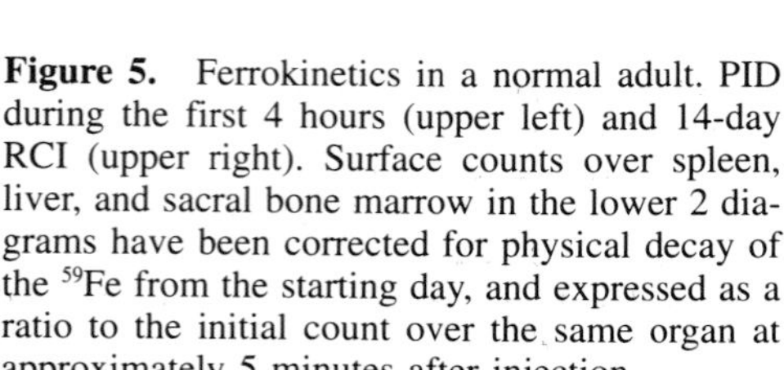
Figure 5. Ferrokinetics in a normal adult. PID during the first 4 hours (upper left) and 14-day RCI (upper right). Surface counts over spleen, liver, and sacral bone marrow in the lower 2 diagrams have been corrected for physical decay of the ^{59}Fe from the starting day, and expressed as a ratio to the initial count over the same organ at approximately 5 minutes after injection.

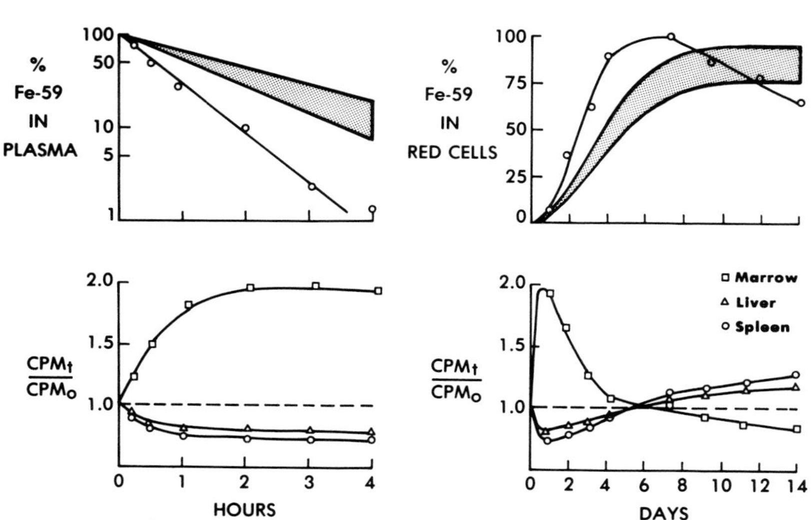

Figure 6. Ferrokinetic study in a patient with hemolytic anemia demonstrates rapid PID caused by the hyperactive bone marrow. RCI is initially normal and then falls off because of peripheral red cell destruction. Organ counts reflect active marrow hematopoiesis, but only minimal late rise over liver and spleen because active red cell sequestration does not occur to a significant degree in either organ.

ABNORMAL FERROKINETIC PATTERNS

Most clinical disorders of iron metabolism (e.g., iron deficiency, hemochromatosis) and of altered erythrokinetics (e.g., autoimmune hemolytic anemias) are best diagnosed by methods other than ferrokinetic studies, which are longer and more complex than other diagnostic tests. The ferrokinetic pattern in iron deficiency is similar to the normal pattern, but *PID* and *RCI* are accelerated, *PIT* is usually reduced because of the depleted plasma iron pool, and *RCI* approaches 100% with little or no iron going to stores. In hemochromatosis, the pattern is reversed. The *PID* is normal or slow, and *RCI* is reduced because of increased iron stored in liver and spleen. Nevertheless, the *PIT* is normal because the level of erythropoiesis in this disorder is normal. In hemolytic anemias, erythropoiesis is increased, so that the *PID* is rapid. The *PIT* is high, and *RCI* is normal or decreased, but there is a progressive late fall in circulating red cell radioiron after the labeled cells are released into circulation and begin to be destroyed. This loss is associated with a rise in liver or spleen activity if these organs are selectively sequestering circulating cells (Fig. 6).

In a few clinical situations, ferrokinetic studies provide essential and otherwise unobtainable information:

Ineffective Erythropoiesis. Patients with ineffective erythropoiesis (intramedullary hemolysis) have severe anemia with a low reticulocyte count, but they also have a hypercellular marrow. This pattern may be found with some hemoglobinopathies such as thalassemia, with certain intrinsic red cell defects such as occur in pernicious anemia and G6PD deficiency, and in some severe autoimmune states. Only ferrokinetic studies can directly demonstrate the fact that, although iron delivery to erythroid precursors in the marrow is increased, release of mature erythrocytes is impaired because of intramedullary hemolysis and radioiron retention (Fig. 7).

Extramedullary Hematopoiesis with Splenomegaly and Concomitant Splenic Red Cell Sequestration. In myelofibrosis, either idiopathic or postpolycythemic, progressive replacement of the central marrow by fibrous tissue may occur, with consequent extramedullary hematopoiesis that involves spleen, liver, and occasionally other sites. With progression of the disease, increasing splenomegaly may result in a degree of red cell destruction that outstrips production, leading to an increasing transfusion requirement. Even without splenic sequestration, massive splenomegaly may cause serious symptoms in the patient, and documentation of the extent of splenic erythropoiesis compared to splenic red cell sequestration may be essential prior to deciding upon splenectomy. Only a ferrokinetic study can demonstrate the degree of effective erythropoiesis in the spleen in such patients, and provide a qualitative indication of the relative roles of the spleen, liver, and central marrow in hematopoiesis (Fig. 8). A ^{51}Cr-red cell survival study with surface counting may also be necessary to document shortened red cell survival and splenic sequestration. This study is customarily performed prior to the ferrokinetic study for counting simplicity.

Severe Peripheral Red Cell Destruction. In certain hemolytic states, destruction of newly formed red cells may be so rapid that only a select population of long-lived cells survives and circulates. The labeling of such autologous red cells with ^{51}Cr then results in an erroneously long estimate of the disappearance half-time. In this situation, only a ferrokinetic study can demonstrate that there is effective red cell production with rapid peripheral destruction. Aggressive

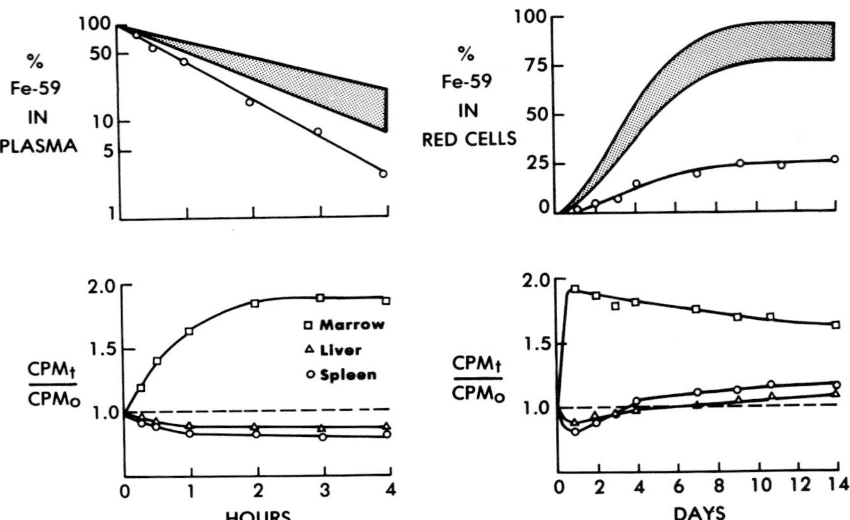

Figure 7. Ferrokinetic pattern in a patient with ineffective erythropoiesis, showing rapid PID, persistently high marrow activity, and low RCI due to impaired erythrocyte maturation and release (i.e., intramedullary hemolysis).

splenic sequestration also is better characterized in this circumstance by the ferrokinetic study, which clearly demonstrates progressive late splenic uptake of ^{59}Fe after labeled cell release into circulation (Fig. 9).

RED CELL SURVIVAL AND SEQUESTRATION STUDIES

In the red cell labeling procedure recommended by the International Committee for Standardization in Haematology (ICSH) in 1980,[9] 10 mL of the patient's blood is collected in a sterile tube that contains 1.5 mL of ACD (NIH A) solution. The blood is then centrifuged, the plasma withdrawn, and 0.5 μCi/kg (18.5 kBq/kg) of high-specific activity ^{51}Cr-sodium chromate is added. The blood is incubated at room temperature for 30 to 40 min with occasional gentle mixing. The cells are washed 3 times with isotonic saline to remove unbound ^{51}Cr. After the third centrifugation and decantation, the original volume is restored with isotonic saline. A measured aliquot of the ^{51}Cr-labeled RBCs is injected into the patient, and a portion is saved to prepare a standard if the red cell mass is to be measured. Blood samples are drawn at 10 and 40 minutes to calculate red cell volume. Twenty-four hours later and every other day for the next 3 weeks, a 5-mL sample of blood is drawn in heparin or EDTA, the hematocrit is determined, and 1 or 2 precisely measured

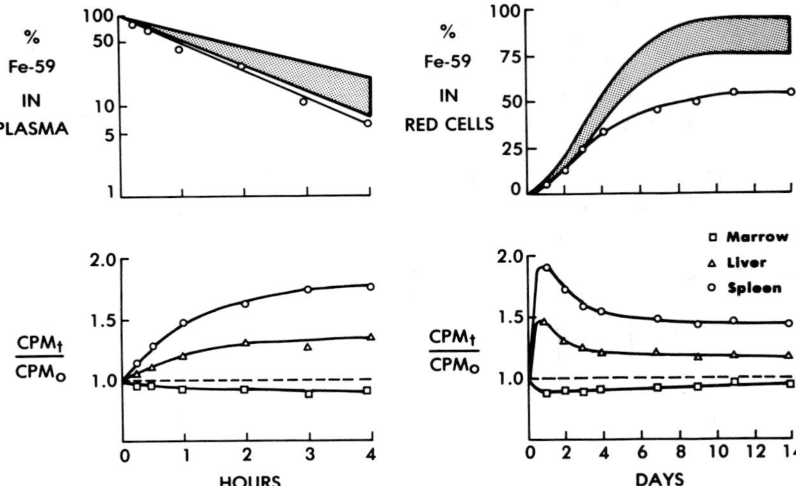

Figure 8. Ferrokinetic pattern in a patient with moderately advanced myelofibrosis including hepatosplenomegaly, demonstrating a somewhat reduced RCI, absent marrow radioiron uptake, and a marrow-like rise over liver and spleen. This rise does not fall back to baseline because the extramedullary hematopoiesis is partially ineffective.

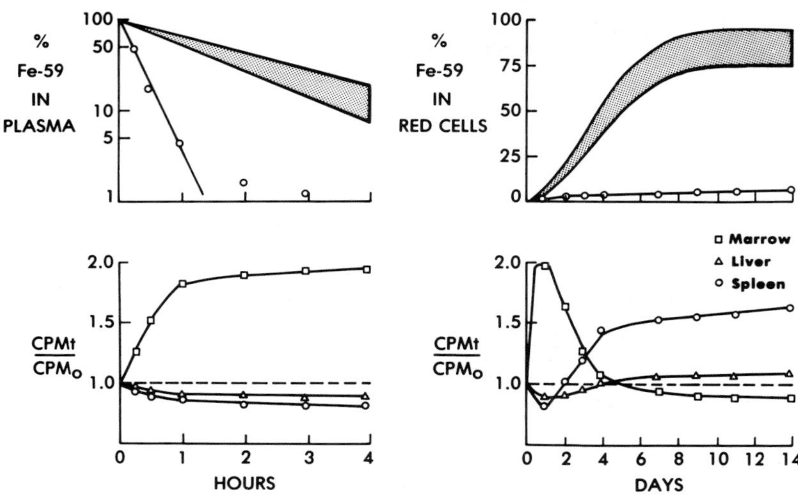

Figure 9. Ferrokinetic pattern in a patient with hemolytic anemia demonstrating substantial splenic sequestration. The hyperactive marrow causes a rapid PID and increased marrow uptake. The aggressive splenic sequestration of newly formed and released erythrocytes results in a low net RCI and a progressive rise in splenic activity after 24 to 48 hours. Minimal hepatic sequestration is also present.

2-mL samples are prepared for counting and are stored at 4°C. On the last day of the study, all samples are counted in a well counter with the spectrometer window set at 280 to 360 keV. The survival half-time is then determined by plotting the background-corrected blood counts on semilogarithmic paper, or by using a suitably programmed small computer to determine the single exponential slope and half-time by least-squares fit. In patients with a stable hematocrit (i.e., under steady-state conditions) the data points scatter least when each sample count has been divided by its own hematocrit, which compensates for normal daily hematocrit fluctuations. The normal disappearance half-time is 25 to 35 days.

There is some loss of chromium label from the erythrocytes during the first 24 hours, averaging 9%. Whether it is caused by early elution of the label or by erythrocyte damage during labeling is not known. As a result, however, the determination of disappearance half-time should begin with the 24-hour sample.

Because red cells have a normal life span of 120 days, the fractional daily loss of erythrocytes by senescence is approximately 0.8%. The expected survival half-time in a ^{51}Cr-RBC study, therefore, would be expected to be 55 to 65 days. In addition to loss by cell senescence, however, ^{51}Cr elutes from the red cells at a rate averaging approximately 1% per day. This shortens the measured normal survival half-time range to 25 to 35 days.

Although this unphysiologically short half-time means that the ^{51}Cr study (unlike the DF^{32}P survival study) is not a true measure of cell survival, it is still clinically useful. Because the ^{51}Cr elution rate is similar to the normal senescence rate, variations in elution rate may significantly affect nearly normal survival values, but their effect is relatively smaller in patients with shortened survivals, in whom the information is of greatest clinical importance.

The red cell life span determined with random labels is meaningful only in patients who are in a steady state of red cell production and destruction (Fig. 10). If either process changes, the measured value of survival changes also, even though the longevity of the individual erythrocyte has not been altered. A constant hematocrit throughout the study is the best index of a steady state. Obviously, inaccurate estimates occur in patients who are being transfused. In the absence of steady-state conditions, the closest approximation to the true erythrocyte survival half-time is obtained by plotting whole blood ^{51}Cr counts without hematocrit correction. The use of sequential whole-body counting has been proposed for estimating the disappearance rate of ^{51}Cr-labeled erythrocytes. Although ^{51}Cr does not relabel new blood cells, it does diffuse into other tissues and is only slowly excreted, so that this approach to measuring red-cell survival is not physiologically accurate.

Splenic sequestration using external probe counting is frequently measured in ^{51}Cr-red cell survival studies. Three sites are counted on each day that the patient returns for a blood sample: precordium, anterior liver, and posterior or lateral spleen. Each area is counted for 2 to 5 minutes (or to 3% statistical precision). For the precordium, the detector is placed over the left third intercostal interspace at the sternal border with the patient supine. For the liver, the detector is placed over the right ninth and tenth ribs at the midclavicular line. For the spleen, the detector is placed between the left ninth and tenth ribs posteriorly, two thirds of the distance from the midline to the lateral edge of the trunk with the patient prone. In elderly subjects or in patients with chronic lung disease, lower-than-normal diaphragm position may require proportionate downward adjustment of the liver and spleen points.

The optimum counting location at each site can be determined during the first hour by taking several 1-minute counts

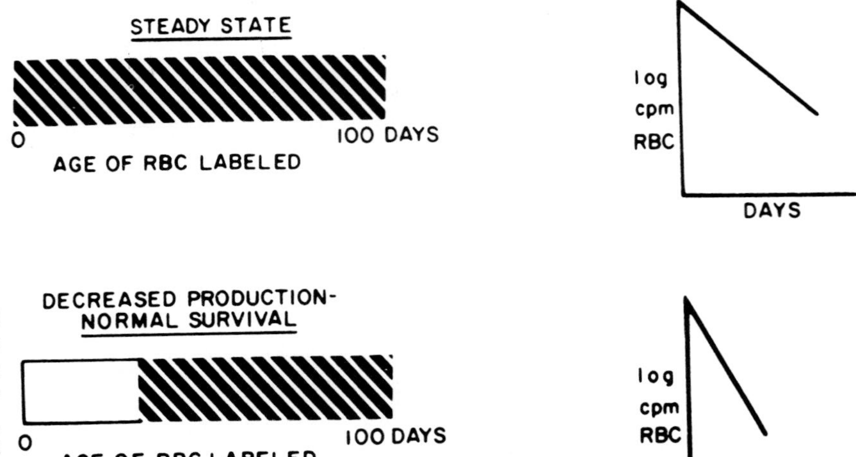

Figure 10. Random red cell labels should bind to relatively equal proportions of cells of all ages when erythrocyte production and destruction is in a steady state. With decreased production of new red cells, predominantly older cells will be labeled, which results in shortened mean cell survival, even though survival of individual cells is not altered. (Reprinted by permission from McIntyre PA: *Prog Haematol* 1977;10:361.)

in the appropriate region to determine the point of maximum counting rate for each organ, reflecting circulating blood activity. Even more accurate localization of spleen activity can be achieved by injecting heat-damaged ^{99m}Tc-labeled autologous red cells.[59,60] The skin is then marked with indelible ink, and the marks are covered with transparent tape, to ensure the same placement of the detector from one day to the next.

Surface counting in normal red cell sequestration studies yields a spleen-to-liver ratio of approximately 1:1 (Fig. 11). In patients with splenomegaly, the starting spleen-to-liver ratio may range from 2:1 to 4:1 (Fig. 12). The most significant finding in pathologic splenic sequestration is not the absolute spleen-to-liver ratio, but a rising ratio as blood activity decreases through one half-life. The spleen-to-precordium ratio may also provide a useful index of the degree of splenic sequestration when compared with the liver-to-precordium ratio; however, a rising spleen-to-liver ratio best reflects predominance of splenic sequestration when a decision regarding splenectomy is to be made (Fig. 13). The accuracy of localizing spleen and liver counting sites should be checked if survival is shortened and the spleen-to-liver

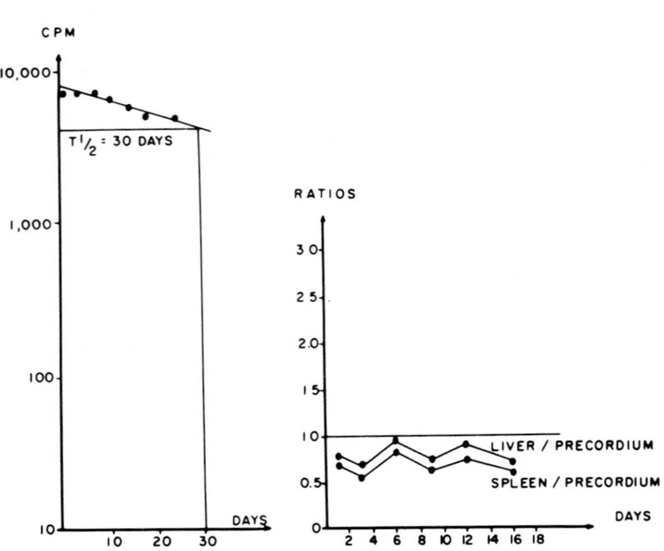

Figure 11. Normal ^{51}Cr-red cell survival and splenic sequestration study. In vitro blood counts are on the left; in vivo organ counts are on the right (From McIntyre PA[131]).

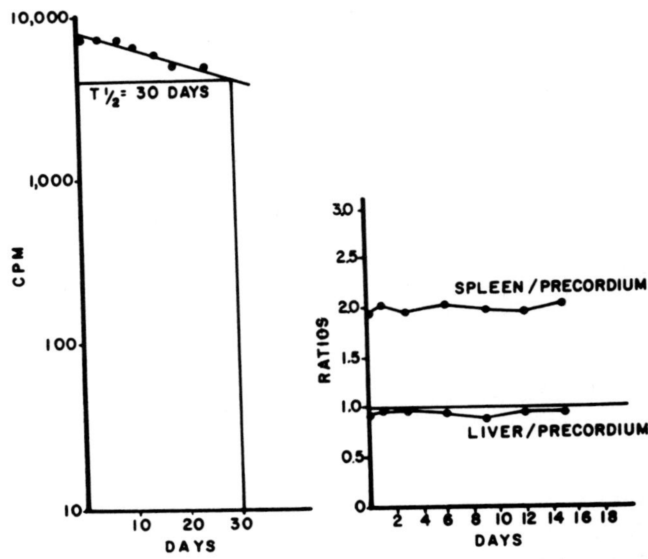

Figure 12. Normal red cell survival in a patient with splenomegaly. A high initial spleen-to-precordium ratio is present, but no further rise occurs throughout the study.

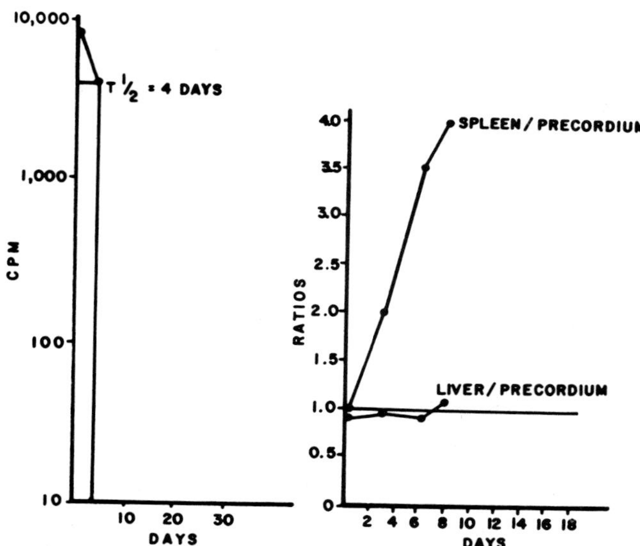

Figure 13. Red cell survival and splenic sequestration study in a patient with severe Coombs'-positive autoimmune hemolytic anemia. There is markedly shortened red cell survival with rapid, progressively increasing splenic sequestration. Splenectomy resulted in a prompt rise to normal hematocrit (From McIntyre PA[131]).

ratio does not rise (i.e., recheck for the highest count rate location over each organ).

Progressive splenic localization of ^{51}Cr-RBCs correlates well with beneficial response to splenectomy. On the other hand, a patient may show no evidence of splenic sequestration, yet still respond to splenectomy. This situation probably results from antierythrocyte antibody synthesis in the spleen, a process that would not be demonstrated by the ^{51}Cr-red cell survival study alone.

Although it is possible to perform a ferrokinetic study and a red cell survival study simultaneously in the same patient, correcting for scatter from ^{59}Fe into the ^{51}Cr energy window is complex and reduces precision of the ^{51}Cr counting. Completion of the ^{51}Cr-red cell survival study prior to the ferrokinetic evaluation is preferable.

In Vivo Cross-Match

In rare instances, even the most modern blood blanks may be unable to identify a satisfactory donor for a patient requiring transfusion.[5,31,61] In vivo cross-match tests using ^{51}Cr-or ^{99m}Tc-labeled donor red cells may be useful when:

1. Serological tests suggest that all donors are incompatible,
2. "cold" antibodies are present and active in vitro at 30°C or higher, and a nonreacting donor cannot be found,
3. the recipient has had a previous unexplained transfusion reaction and requires additional transfusions.

After careful selection of the donor candidate's blood by the transfusion service, 0.5 mL of donor cells are labeled with 20 μCi (740 kBq) ^{51}Cr-sodium chromate or 1 mCi (37 MBq) ^{99m}Tc in vitro as previously described, washed three times with saline, and injected into the patient after retaining a calibration standard. Blood samples are then taken from the recipient at 3, 10, and 60 min, and both whole blood and plasma radioactivity are measured in the samples. Ideally, the recipient's red cell volume (*RCV*) should be measured using ^{99m}Tc-RBCs just prior to ^{51}Cr-labeled donor cell injection or vice versa. Alternatively, the *RCV* can be estimated from standard tables according to height and weight.

No significant incompatibility exists if the *RCV* as determined by the 10-min sample of the labeled donor cells is ±10% of the measured or predicted *RCV*, if the count of the 60-minute whole blood sample does not deviate significantly from the 3-minute sample (94 to 104%), and if no significant radioactivity is present in any plasma sample withdrawn after the infusion of the labeled donor cells. In urgent cases, if the red cell survival at 60 minutes is at least 70% of the administered labeled donor red cells, and if no more than 3% of the injected radioactivity is present in the plasma at 10 and 60 minutes, then reasonably good compatibility can be assumed, and a unit of packed red cells from that donor can be cautiously infused.[5] If incompatibility is found in the first study, 5.0 mL of blood from the next most suitable donor is labeled with double the initial tracer dose, and the procedure is repeated.

The principle of this test is that if rapid destruction of 0.5 mL of donor erythrocytes does not occur, the amount of antibody in circulation is certainly too small to react with a whole unit of packed red cells and cause an immediate, potentially fatal, transfusion reaction. Compatibility as judged by this in vivo cross-match test, however, provides no assurance that the recipient will not have an anamnestic response with delayed hemolysis of donor red cells after one or more days. Delayed hemolysis can occur even in patients with perfect serological matches who have had multiple transfusions or pregnancies in the past.

When survival is significantly lower at 10 minutes than at 3 minutes but shows little or no further fall at 60 minutes, which indicates a two-component curve, the presence of IgM antibody is implied. On the other hand, when survival at 10 minutes is only slightly less than at 3 minutes but is substantially less at 60 minutes, indicating an exponentially falling curve, the most likely interpretation is that the antibody is IgG. This distinction is of some importance because with cold IgM alloantibodies, immune clinical responses are uncommon, whereas with IgG antibodies they are the rule. Although in both cases the survival of a whole unit of red cells may be virtually normal during the 24 hours or so following transfusion, a delayed hemolytic reaction must be expected when the antibody is IgG.[5]

Pineda et al. recommend taking an additional blood sample at 18 to 24 hours to exclude the possibility of delayed hemolytic reactions.[62] It may not always be possible to wait that long. Nevertheless, it is likely that sampling at periods longer than one hour increases the accuracy of the prediction of compatibility.

Figure 14 illustrates a donor survival curve from an abnormal in vivo cross-match in a patient with multiple alloanti-

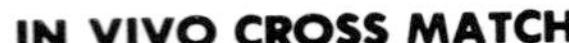

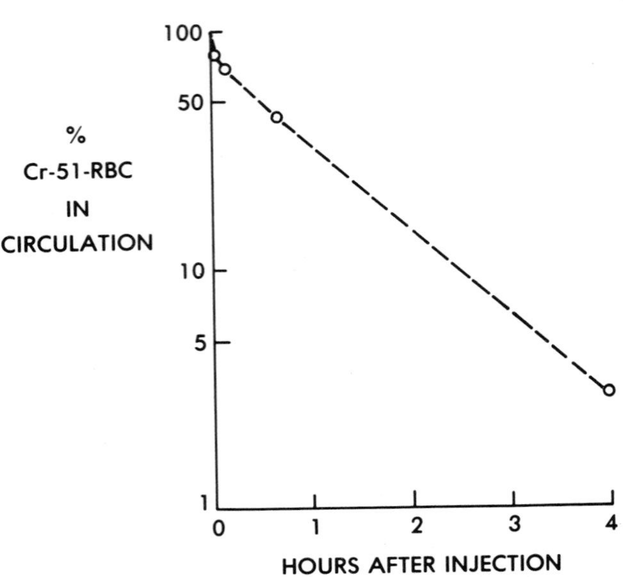

Figure 14. Abnormal in vivo cross-match study in a patient with several red cell alloantibodies; in this case survival is unacceptably short, and transfusion of the donor unit was not considered.

bodies (including anti-Cartwright antibodies) that made adequate in vitro cross-match impossible.

Granulocyte Studies

The leukocytes found in the peripheral blood include polymorphonuclear leukocytes of the neutrophilic, basophilic, and eosinophilic series; monocytes; and lymphocytes of varying sizes, functions, and life spans. Despite the current interest in the pathophysiology of monocytes and lymphocytes, most work on white cell labeling has been directed toward neutrophils (hereafter referred to as granulocytes) for the localization of occult infection. There is no clinical need for routine measurement of leukocyte survival half-times. Although cell labeling techniques are reviewed here, the clinical application of labeled leukocytes to the assessment of infection are discussed in the chapter on Inflammation.

RADIOPHARMACEUTICALS

Much of our knowledge of granulocyte production in the bone marrow and of peripheral cell kinetics has been gained from the pioneering work of Cronkite et al. in the 1950s and 1960s using tritiated thymidine (^{3}H-TdR).[63] This cohort label is incorporated into marrow precursors during DNA synthesis and is evaluated by autoradiography of marrow and peripheral blood cells at appropriate times after intravenous injection. Because of its high radiation absorbed dose, difficulties of beta counting, and impossibility of imaging, ^{3}H-TdR remains a research label for leukocytes.

DF^{32}P is an anticholinesterase that binds to cholinesterase and other enzymes in circulating blood cell membranes. Because it does not elute in circulation, DF^{32}P is customarily used as a random label for granulocyte kinetics. Injected intravenously, it labels marrow precursors as well as circulating cells, so that it also can be employed as a combined cohort and random label for the study of blood cell kinetics. The early work of Athens, Boggs, Cartwright, and Wintrobe with DF^{32}P has provided much of our present understanding of peripheral granulocyte kinetics and the dynamics of granulocyte migration into inflammatory sites.[64–67]

^{51}Cr-sodium chromate crosses the granulocyte membrane and binds to cytoplasmic proteins.[3,68] The labeling technique requires the isolation of granulocytes from 500 mL of ACD-anticoagulated blood. Thus, ^{51}Cr-labeled granulocytes have been used mainly for research studies of granulocyte survival.

Recently, there has been considerable interest in labeling granulocytes in vitro with ^{99m}Tc. Incubation with pertechnetate results in less than 1% uptake even with tin reduction,[53] but 30 to 40% of ^{99m}Tc-sulfur colloid or ^{99m}Tc-albumin colloid[69] is phagocytosed by granulocytes in vitro.[54] Routine use of the latter method has been hampered by indications that the labeling process damages the granulocytes, and by the technical difficulties in separating the ^{99m}Tc-labeled granulocytes from unbound radiocolloid and from radiocolloid bound loosely to cell membranes.

^{67}Gallium has been used extensively for localizing abscesses, partly because there is some active gallium uptake by circulating granulocytes. The clinical applications of ^{67}Ga scintigraphy for infection are discussed in the chapter on Inflammation.

During the past several years, the use of oxine (8-hydroxyquinoline) as a carrier to label granulocytes with ^{111}In has become the preferred scintigraphic approach to abscess localization and evaluation of patients with FUO.[53,54] Water-soluble carriers for ^{111}In, including oxine sulfate,[70] acetylacetone,[71] tropolone,[72] and merc[73] have also been described.

McAfee et al.[74] and Becker et al.,[19] among others, have reviewed the potential utility of monoclonal antibodies (MoAbs) and antibody fragments to label leukocytes. Use of the Kohler-Milstein hybridoma technique has produced over 300 murine monoclonal antibodies that bind to specific cell surface antigens on human leukocytes. They include IgG and IgM immunoglobulins and F(ab′) and F(ab′)$_2$ fragments labeled with ^{99m}Tc, ^{111}In, and ^{123}I. Use of the proper antibody allows great selectivity in labeling specific cell types. In addition, the high specificity of the antibody may obviate the need for laborious differential cell separations. Most earlier work with MoAb labeling for scintigraphy has involved ^{131}I and ^{123}I, but both ^{111}In and ^{99m}Tc can be firmly attached to antibodies using bifunctional chelates.

NORMAL GRANULOCYTE KINETICS

The granulocytes in the vascular system are divided approximately equally into two compartments: the circulating granulocyte pool (CGP) and the marginal granulocyte pool (MGP). The MGP probably represents a reservoir of cells in the spleen and bone marrow, along the endothelial surfaces of some blood vessels, and possibly in the liver. These cells are readily available to circulate and to localize in areas of infection. After production by and release from the bone marrow, granulocytes have a short residence time in the circulation ($T_{1/2}$ = 6 to 10 hours) before migrating into the interstitial spaces of many peripheral tissues. Although the survival time in tissue is not well documented, it may be as much as several days.

INDIUM-111 OXINE LABELING

Granulocytes can be effectively labeled with ^{111}In complexed to the lipophilic carrier 8-hydroxyquinoline (oxine).[53] ^{111}In-oxine is the only radiopharmaceutical currently approved in the US by the FDA for indium labeling of white cells (and platelets). The complexities of granulocyte separation and labeling, however, still represent a deterrent to routine cell labeling with ^{111}In-oxine by smaller laboratories. Some commercial companies now provide granulocyte-labeling services if sterile anticoagulated blood is drawn by the requesting laboratory. With the labeling technique described by Thakur et al.,[57] 75% of the labeled whole-blood granulocytes are viable. Where available, the sulfate form of oxine is preferred because its water solubility leads to a simpler labeling procedure along with high labeling yields of 90 to 95%.[70] After granulocyte labeling, a process taking 1 to 2 hours, the cells are injected intravenously and the patient is imaged the next morning (20 to 24 hours). Because of the short granulocyte survival in circulation, blood background is very low by the next day. In contrast to ^{67}Ga, little is gained by taking additional scintiphotos after 24 hours because there is no further uptake of labeled cells in inflammatory foci nor further decline in blood activity. On rare occasions, a 48-hour image may be helpful to differentiate a fixed abdominal-pelvic focus of uptake from activity moving in the GI tract. Immediately after injection, the recovery of ^{111}In-labeled granulocytes in circulating blood varies from 20 to 50%. At 24 hours, about 40% of injected activity is divided between the liver and spleen; the remainder is mostly in bone marrow.

Granulocytes labeled with ^{111}In-oxine localize in abscesses with a sensitivity similar to that of ^{67}Ga (85 to 95%), but there is much less interference from abdominal and pelvic activity.[75] There is, therefore, a higher specificity than is found with ^{67}Ga.[76]

Figure 15 illustrates normal ^{111}In-WBC images at 24 hours. There is intense splenic activity, lesser hepatic activity, and some marrow activity, which partly represents a granulocyte pool but may also represent free ^{111}In transported to the erythroid marrow via transferrin.[77]

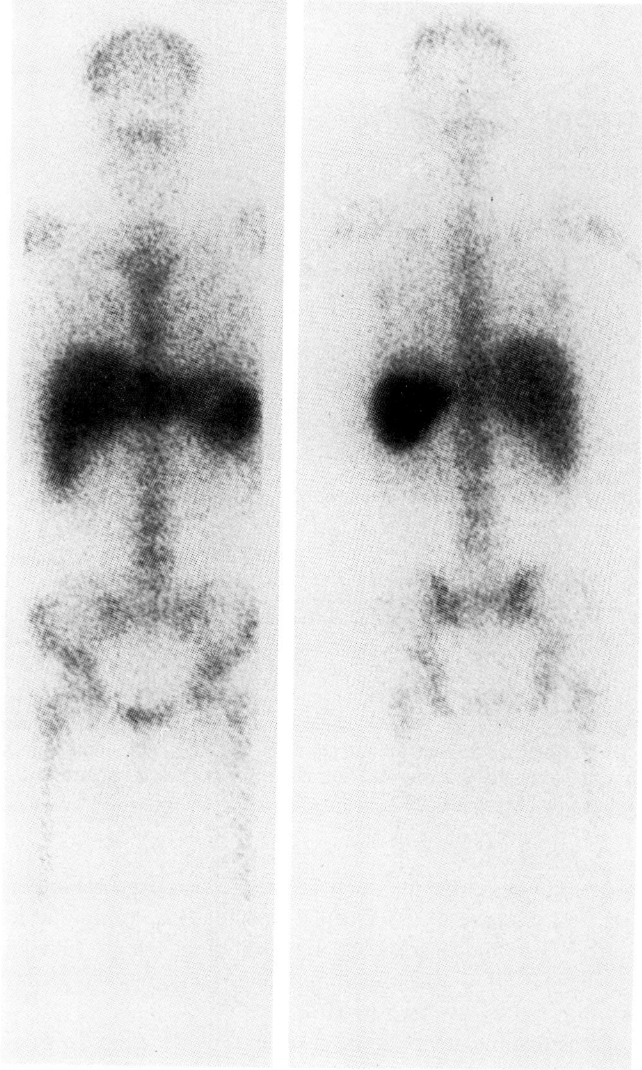

Figure 15. Normal anterior (left) and posterior (right) 20-hr ^{111}In-WBC whole body images.

Platelet Studies

Circulating platelets play a primary role in thrombosis, under both physiological conditions (e.g., trauma) and pathophysiological conditions (e.g., atherosclerosis). Characterization of in vivo platelet kinetics is diagnostically useful in evaluating primary platelet disorders (thrombocytopenia, thrombocytosis), hypercoagulable states (TTP), and such vascular disorders as atherosclerosis, in which the extent of disease may correlate with shortened platelet survival. With the recent availability of ^{111}In-oxine labeled platelets, sites of active thrombus formation can be localized in vivo with good sensitivity.

PLATELET KINETICS

Platelets are non-nucleated fragments of megakaryocyte cytoplasm 1.0 to 1.5 micrometers in diameter. Their normal human life span ranges from 8 to 12 days, with an average of 9.5 days.[78] The normal disappearance half-time of ^{51}Cr-labeled platelets is 4.5 to 5.5 days (Fig. 16). Following intravenous injection, one quarter to one third of labeled platelets pool in the spleen, a process that appears to be physiological rather than pathologic. Platelet recovery at 15

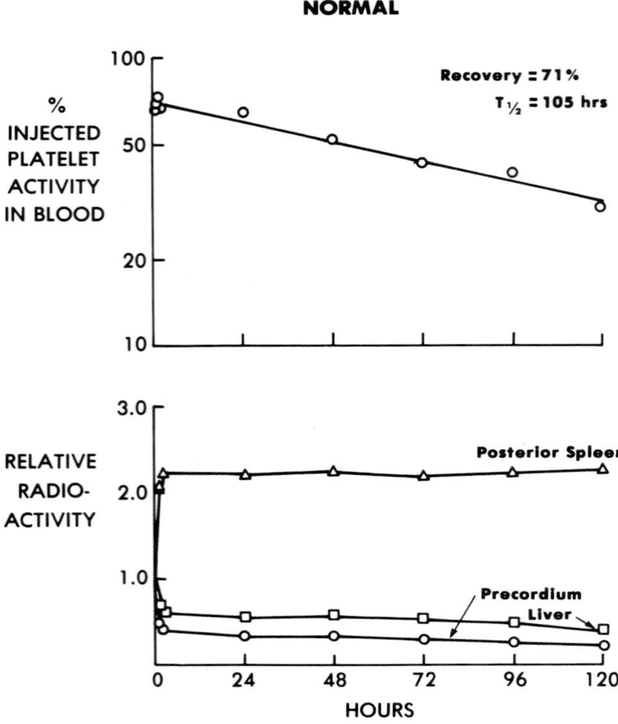

Figure 16. Normal platelet kinetics and surface counting with ^{51}Cr-labeled autologous platelets; note the high but unchanging activity over the spleen. The normal platelet disappearance half-time is 100 hr or greater.

to 30 minutes after injection is inversely related to spleen size and is normally 65% of the injected dose (range 50 to 80%).[78,79] In the absence of a functioning spleen, platelet recovery is 90 to 100%; with massive splenomegaly, recovery may be as low as 5 to 10%.

Considerable uncertainty surrounds the mechanisms of peripheral platelet disappearance in a normal individual and how these mechanisms affect the shape of the platelet disappearance curve. Normal senescence should result in linear disappearance, but there appears to be a curvilinear component to disappearance that suggests some platelet utilization. Both linear and semilogarithmic plots of disappearance seem to be oversimplifications. Several mathematical models for expressing platelet life span have been proposed.[80,81] A practical method consists of following survival through one disappearance half-time and fitting the data points to the following semilogarithmic function by least squares fit:

$$A_t = A_0 e^{-kt}$$

where: A_t = blood (or platelet) activity (cpm/mL) at time t; and k = fractional disappearance per unit time. The result is then expressed as a half-time:

$$T_{1/2} = \frac{0.693}{k}$$

The International Committee on Standardization in Hematology (ICSH) has recommended that both a linear and a logarithmic estimate of survival be calculated by least-squares fit, and that a weighted mean of the two be used.[8] If the shape of the disappearance curve is entirely linear or exponential, then the irrelevant portion of the combined calculation simply drops out of the expression. In a detailed mathematical analysis of ^{111}In-platelet kinetic studies in 15 normal subjects and 54 patients, Lotter et al.[81] recommended that, for greatest accuracy, the platelet survival data be fitted to at least 2 mathematical models, the 2 best for normal individuals being the *modified weighted mean* and the *multiple hit* models. For patients with very short platelet survivals, the *alpha order* model fitted the data best. The same group has further extended compartmental analysis of normal platelet survival to include in vivo scintigraphy throughout the period of study, thus incorporating organ biodistribution into the analysis.[82]

There is no human disease in which platelet life span is prolonged. This is true even with anticoagulation, indicating that the dominant process in normal platelet disappearance is, in fact, senescence, and not platelet consumption in the maintenance of vascular endothelial integrity. On the other hand, many diseases are associated with shortened platelet survival. Idiopathic thrombocytopenic purpura (ITP), a disease in which platelet autoantibodies are probably largely synthesized by the spleen, results in platelet disappearance half-times as short as 30 to 60 minutes (Fig. 17).[83] Other autoimmune diseases, such as lupus erythematosus, may present in the same manner, with or without demonstrable platelet-specific antibodies, but with variably shortened platelet survival. In such diseases, platelet survival studies may help to document the degree of peripheral platelet destruction involved and to rule out reduced platelet production as a significant process. Drug-associated peripheral platelet consumption has been reported, most frequently with quinine administration and, less, frequently, with quinidine, digitoxin, novobiocin, stibophen, and Sedormid® administration.

Increased peripheral platelet utilization with shortened survival and thrombocytopenia is seen in several thrombotic states. Most striking of these is disseminated intravascular coagulation, which is frequently associated with severe thrombocytopenia and which, once diagnosed, may respond dramatically to anticoagulation. Thrombotic thrombocytopenic purpura (TTP) is another thrombotic disorder in which markedly shortened platelet survival with thrombocytopenia is seen. Less severe shortening of platelet survival is found in patients with atherosclerosis, in which peripheral platelet consumption may be a part of the primary atherosclerotic process itself or, more likely, the result of associated intravascular thrombosis.[84,85] Shortened platelet survival also occurs in deep vein thrombophlebitis, with or without pulmonary embolism;[78,85,86] valvular heart disease, especially with embolization; chronic renal disease; Kasabach-Merritt syndrome; during the early postoperative period; and in several other acute and chronic illnesses.[85]

As in labeled erythrocyte studies, surface probe counting

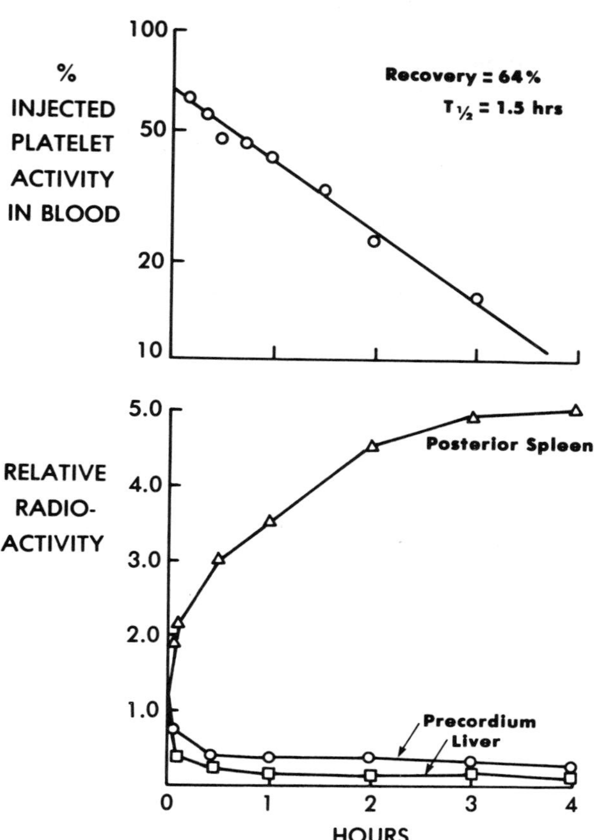

Figure 17. ^{51}Cr-labeled platelet study in a patient with ITP showing shortened platelet survival and progressive rise in splenic activity as platelets are destroyed (splenic sequestration).

has been used widely in platelet survival studies to identify active splenic sequestration. With the advent of ^{111}In-labeled platelets, use of probe counting has given way to camera scintigraphy with computer data storage and region-of-interest (ROI) analysis. Early clinical studies suggested that patients with ITP were likely to have a similar response to splenectomy, whether or not surface counting demonstrated splenic uptake.[44] Recent studies, however, have confirmed that there is a significantly higher clinical response to splenectomy in patients demonstrating active splenic ^{111}In-platelet sequestration (85 to 95% improvement) than in those demonstrating a mixed or an hepatic pattern (15 to 25% improvement).[87–89]

^{111}In-OXINE LABELED PLATELETS

Routine platelet labeling with ^{111}In-oxine was introduced by Thakur et al. in 1976.[45] There appears to be no significant platelet relabeling by the released ^{111}In when labeled platelets are destroyed, although ^{111}In does bind to circulating transferrin and this accounts for 5 to 15% of circulating blood activity during platelet survival studies. Scintigraphy of ^{111}In-platelet deposition in thrombi permits in vivo localization of the active process when it might not otherwise be identifiable clinically, and when it involves too few platelets to shorten overall platelet survival.

The ^{111}In-oxine labeling procedure has been described by Thakur et al.,[45,51] Scheffel et al.,[46] and Heaton et al.,[50] and the ICSH has published its recommended procedure for platelet labeling with [111]In.[90] Labeling efficiencies range from 40 to 70% in plasma, and are higher if the ligand used is oxine sulfate, tropolone, or merc, or if the platelets are labeled in a balanced salt solution such as HEPES. After labeling, exactly 1.0 of the labeled platelets is withdrawn for preparation of a counting standard, and 300 μCi (11.1 MBq) of platelets are injected intravenously. The exact volume of the injection is noted. Calibration of the standard is most accurate if the dose syringe is weighed initially, after standard removal, and after patient injection. Care is taken to avoid drawing blood back into the syringe at the time of injection. The 1-mL platelet aliquot is diluted in 1000 mL distilled water for a counting standard. Whole-blood samples of 3 mL are drawn from the patient into EDTA at 15, 30, 60, and 120 minutes and at 1, 2, 3, and 4 days. Aliquots of 2 mL are pipetted for gamma counting with the diluted standard. Platelet recovery is calculated from the 15-minute sample as follows:

$$\text{Recovery (\%)} = \frac{\text{cpm/mL (blood)} \times TBV \text{ (mL)} \times 100 \times \text{Std dose (gm)}}{\text{cpm/mL (std)} \times 1000 \times \text{inj dose (gm)}}$$

The total blood volume (*TBV*) is estimated from the patient's height and weight. Because platelets circulate in the plasma fraction of blood, the *TBV* can also be estimated from the *PV* as measured with ^{125}I-albumin just prior to labeled platelet injection. Platelet survival is most practically expressed as a disappearance half-time by plotting the blood sample counts against time on semilogarithmic paper. Normal disappearance half-time is greater than 100 hours.

Whole-body imaging is performed at 24 hours and at 48 to 96 hours to identify sites of positive uptake. Most sites of active thrombus formation are positive within 24 hours but, in some instances, sensitivity is increased by later scans, particularly in such areas as the heart, where blood pool activity may reduce the target-to-background ratio. Optimum imaging is obtained by summing the 173- and 247-keV peaks of ^{111}In, using a medium energy collimator on the camera, and obtaining 5- to 10-minute images. In the assessment of splenic sequestration, initial and then daily anterior and posterior thoracic/upper abdominal images are obtained and computer-stored, and the ROI counts over the anterior heart, anterior liver, and posterior spleen are decay-corrected and plotted as percent of initial counts, and as spleen/liver, spleen/heart, and liver/heart ratios. A rising spleen/liver ratio associated with shortened platelet survival is the significant finding regarding consideration of splenectomy.

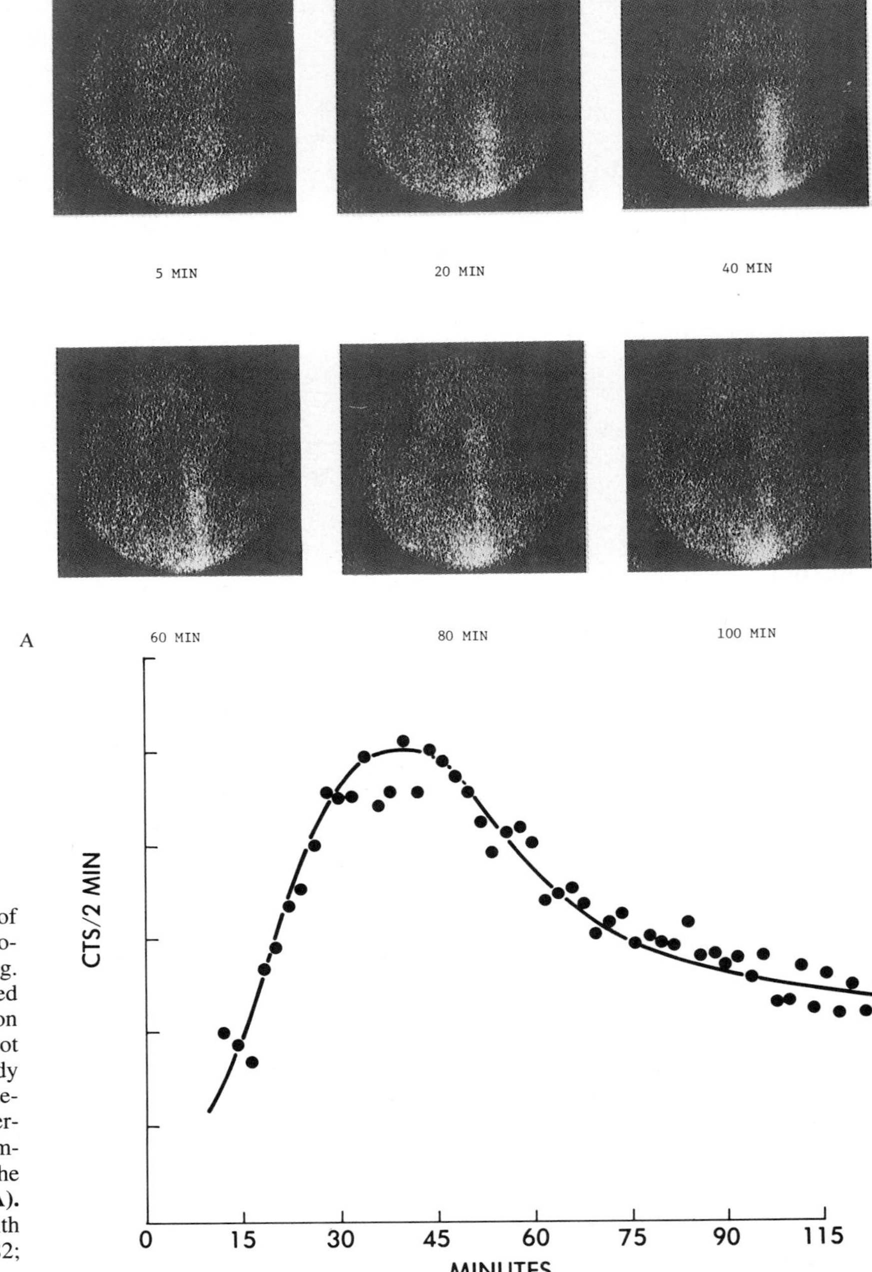

Figure 18. **(A).** Experimental kinetic study of ^{111}In-platelet uptake on a polyethylene angiographic catheter in the carotid artery of a dog. Peak uptake occurs at 40–60 minutes, followed by a fall in ^{111}In activity due to in vivo activation of the fibrinolytic system, and consequent clot lysis. This thrombogenic model is useful to study the relative thrombogenicity of different biomaterials, and to study the relative advantages of different antiplatelet management regimens. **(B).** Computer-derived region-of-interest curve of the catheter thrombus kinetics visualized in **(A).** (From Price DC: In vivo detection of thrombi with ^{111}In-labeled platelets. IEEE *Trans Nucl Sci* 1982; 29:1191. Copyright 1982, IEEE)

EXPERIMENTAL STUDIES

Experimental studies have confirmed the sensitivity of ^{111}In-platelets for identifying new thrombus formation. Figure 18 illustrates the scintigraphic sequence and computer-derived kinetic pattern of labeled platelet deposition on a polyethylene angiographic catheter introduced into the carotid artery of a dog following injection of labeled autologous platelets. A linear correlation is found between ^{111}In uptake and thrombus mass, which confirms that the in vivo technique reliably measures new thrombus formation.[22] Established thrombi (24 hours or more) were found to have little platelet uptake, however, and do not prove to be imageable in vivo. Thus, the imaging applications are limited because most clinical problems present after thrombi have already formed (e.g., vessel occlusion or embolization). Nevertheless, ^{111}In-platelet scintigraphy has found clinical usefulness in the evaluation of deep venous thrombosis, in the search for intracardiac thrombi, and in the assessment of organ transplants (particularly renal transplants) for evidence of early rejection.[11,91]

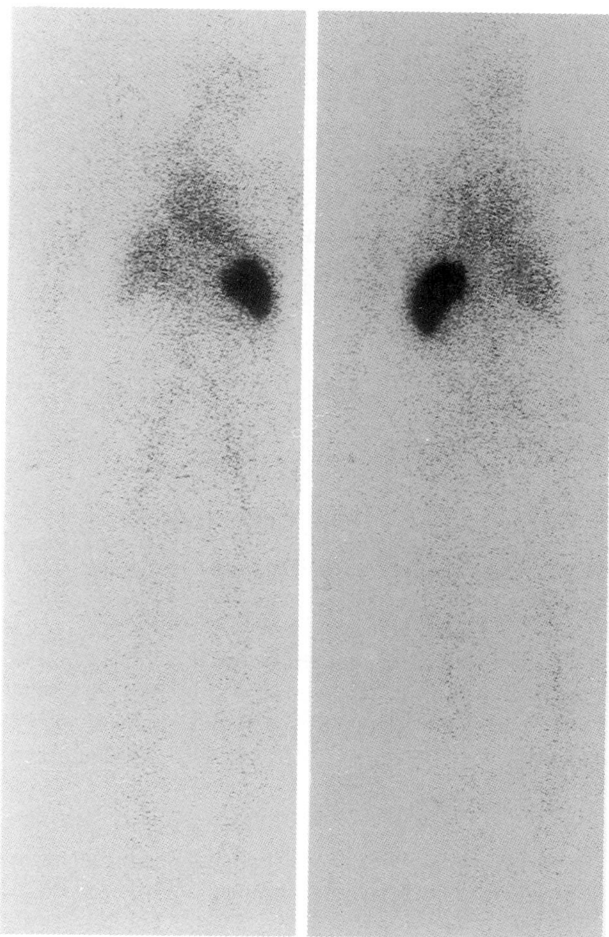

Figure 19. Normal anterior (left) and posterior (right) whole-body ^{111}In-platelet images 24-hours after injection of labeled autologous platelets. These images show greater spleen and blood pool activity but less liver activity than a normal ^{111}In-WBC pattern at 24 hours (see Fig. 15). Later ^{111}In-platelet images demonstrate some uptake in the bone marrow.

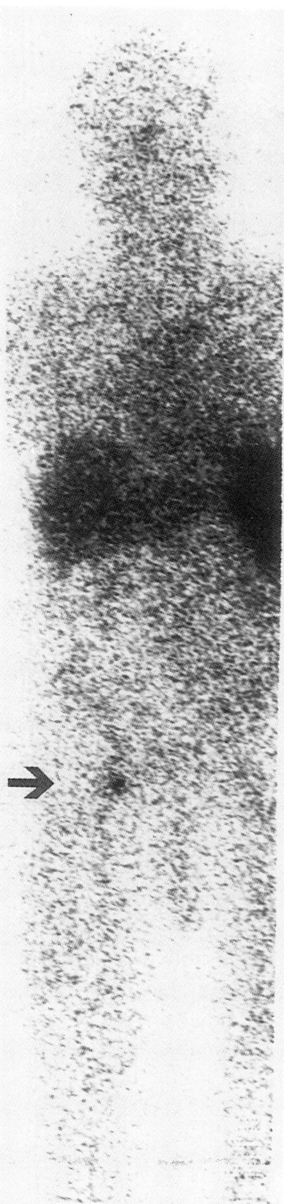

Figure 20. Positive anterior 48-hour ^{111}In-platelet study. The patient had undergone cardiac catheterization one day prior to labeled platelet injection. Note the thrombus formation at the catheter insertion site in the right femoral artery (arrow), which was healing without complication.

CLINICAL STUDIES

Figure 19 illustrates normal 24-hour whole-body images of ^{111}In-platelets. The greatest uptake is in the spleen with less uptake in the liver, bone marrow, and intravascular blood pool. Figure 20 demonstrates positive platelet localization at a recent right femoral artery catheterization site. Davis et al. have described a 61% sensitivity for ^{111}In-platelets in the arterial lesions of carotid atherosclerosis,[92] although, in a smaller series, Price et al. did not find the technique sufficiently sensitive to be clinically useful for this purpose.[93] Further studies will be important to establish the clinical role in atherosclerosis.

Ezekowitz et al.[94] and Stratton et al.[95] studied the use of ^{111}In-platelets in detecting left ventricular thrombi. Among 27 patients, the sensitivity was 67% and the specificity was 98%, with no apparent reduction in sensitivity among patients receiving aspirin.[96] Other diseases associated with abnormal ^{111}In-platelet uptake include coronary artery thrombosis,[97] abdominal aortic aneurysms,[97] prosthetic arterial grafts,[98,99] acute venous thrombosis in patients not receiving heparin,[100] and rejecting renal transplants.[91,101]

Experimental and clinical studies have indicated an 86 to 92% sensitivity of ^{111}In-platelet imaging in detecting venous thrombosis.[48,100,102–106] Although it has not been well characterized, platelet imaging for pulmonary embolism is not likely to be as sensitive as imaging for venous thrombophlebitis.[103,107,108]

Blood Volume

The blood accounts for 6.5 to 7.0% of human body weight. Blood volume is measured using the dilutional assay principle, which can be expressed mathematically as follows:

$$BV = \frac{Q}{C}$$

where Q represents the quantity of tracer injected and C represents the concentration of diluted tracer at equilibrium.

Several requirements must be met for such a tracer technique to be valid:

1. The tracer must mix uniformly in the compartment to be measured;
2. There must be no significant tracer loss during the mixing time, unless such losses can be accurately quantified;
3. There must be no change in the tracer distribution during equilibration;
4. The tracer must have no effect on the compartment being measured;
5. The tracer must not be toxic to the patient;
6. The tracer must be easily measurable.

The total blood volume (*TBV*) is a heterogenous compartment consisting of the plasma volume (*PV*) and a cellular fraction that is predominantly the red cell volume (*RCV*). These 2 volumes are related through the whole-body hematocrit (Hct_b), provided that the platelets and leukocytes are not significantly increased above normal values. Because some organs have relatively higher or lower red cell content than large central vessels, however, the peripheral venous hematocrit (Hct_v) differs from the whole-body hematocrit by a factor termed the F_{cell} ratio, defined such that:

$$F_{cell} \text{ ratio} = \frac{Hct_b}{Hct_v}$$

The F_{cell} ratio can vary from 0.82 to 1.0 or more, and is particularly altered (increased) in the presence of splenomegaly. An average value widely used in blood volume measurements is 0.91. Because the F_{cell} ratio varies so widely, accurate estimation of *TBV* requires independent measurement of *PV* and *RCV*. An additional correction factor arises from the fact that the microhematocrit measured by centrifugation of peripheral blood has an average error of 2% attributable to plasma trapping in the red cell fraction. Consequently:

$$Hct_v = Hct \text{ (measured)} \times 0.98$$

This correction factor is not applied when the *Hct* has been determined by electronic cell counting and sizing, because no plasma trapping occurs by that method of hematocrit determination.

Total blood volume can be estimated from measurement of PV alone, by the formula:

Table 3. Normal Blood Volume Values (mL/kg)

	MALES	FEMALES
Total blood volume	70 (55–80)	65 (50–75)
Red cell volume*	30 (25–35)	25 (20–30)
Plasma volume**	40 (30–45)	40 (30–45)

*95% confidence limits

**Because of the many variables that may influence normal plasma volume, it is not possible to place confidence limits on these values.

$$TBV = \frac{PV}{1 - (Hct \times 0.91 \times 0.98)}$$

and from measurement of *RCV* alone, by the formula:

$$TBV = \frac{RCV}{Hct \times 0.91 \times 0.98}$$

Normal blood volume varies according to height, weight, sex, and age.[109–113]

Although blood volume correlates rather poorly with weight alone, especially in obesity, the ICSH has suggested a normal range of values shown in Table 3. The most accurate correlation is between blood volume and body surface area, constituting a complex function of height and weight.

RED CELL VOLUME

The *RCV* is reliably measured by labeling autologous red blood cells with ^{51}Cr-sodium chromate.[9] The procedure is as follows:

1. Draw 10 mL blood under sterile conditions. Add 6 mL blood to 2 mL ACD in a sterile tube, and mix well. Anticoagulate the remaining 4 mL with EDTA, and pipette a 2-mL aliquot for background count.
2. Inject 35 μCi (1.3 MBq) ^{51}Cr-sodium chromate into the ACD-blood tube, and incubate 45 minutes at room temperature with continuous gentle rotation or agitation.
3. After incubation, centrifuge at 1000 g for 10 min. Remove the supernatant with a spinal needle, and discard as radioactive waste. Usually, 85 to 90% of the tracer remains labeled to the red cells.
4. Resuspend red cells gently in sterile normal saline, almost filling the incubation tube.
5. Recentrifuge and wash twice more with normal saline, then resuspend in normal saline to approximately the original volume.
6. Measure exactly 1.0 mL of the labeled cells, dilute to 1000 ml with distilled water, then pipette 2 2.0-mL aliquots for gamma counting.
7. With the patient in a basal resting state for 30 to 60 minutes, inject exactly 5.0 ml of labeled cells intravenously. With the patient still supine, draw a 5-ml EDTA blood sample at 10 and at 40 minutes from the opposite arm. Obtain the patient's height and weight on the same day.

8. Check the injection site with a hand radiation monitor to be sure that there is no extravasated radioactivity compared with the opposite arm.
9. From each blood sample, pipette 2.0 mL for gamma counting and perform a microhematocrit measurement on the remainder.
10. Calculate *RCV* (mL) for each blood sample as follows:

$$RCV = \frac{\text{net cpm/mL std} \times (Hct \times 0.98) \times 1000 \times 5}{\text{net cpm/mL in 10- or 40-min blood sample}}$$

Then, as indicated above:

$$TBV\ (\text{mL}) = \frac{RCV}{Hct_v \times 0.91 \times 0.98}$$

And:

$$PV = TBV - RCV$$

11. If the 10- and 40-minute calculations are similar, utilize the 10-minute *RCV* value and compare with standard tables for accuracy. If the 40-minute *RCV* value is significantly larger, and if the patient does not have an aggressive hemolytic process or bleeding, which would result in significant loss of RBCs over a 30-minute period, the 40-minute value is considered to be more accurate. This is particularly appropriate if the patient has marked splenomegaly, which causes delayed equilibration.
12. When autologous red blood cells are difficult to obtain (e.g., with severe cold hemagglutinins or hemolysins), type-O Rh-negative donor cells can be labeled for the study.
13. If time or facilities do not permit washing the red cells to remove the unbound ^{51}Cr, add 50 mg of sterile, pyrogen-free ascorbic acid to the labeling vial at the end of the incubation period. This procedure reduces the unbound chromate to the chromic ion and thereby prevents further labeling of erythrocytes, particularly in vivo. The whole blood is then injected. Also, a standard of the plasma from the labeled blood to be injected must be prepared if ascorbate reduction has been carried out, and a plasma sample must be counted from each of the patient's blood samples to correct for free circulating radioactivity. Washing the labeled cells prior to injection is the preferred method, however, and it eliminates the need for ascorbic acid.

Labeling red cells with ^{99m}Tc by the in vitro method described earlier is a useful alternative to using ^{51}Cr.[14,22,26,28,59,114–116] The in vivo labeling methods cannot be used for measuring red cell volume because the cell labeling efficiencies are considerably less than 100%.

Holt et al. have cautioned that circulating stannous ion interferes with ^{51}Cr binding to red cells.[117] In developing a dual RBC labeling technique, they discovered strong inhibition of ^{51}Cr binding to the red cells following in vivo administration of 1.7 mg of nonradioactive stannous chloride in a solution containing 6 mg sodium pyrophosphate. Washing the red cells and anticoagulating the red cells with heparin reversed the interference effect. It is uncertain how long the interference remains after such in vivo labeling but, judging from the effect that a bone scan has on the distribution of other radiopharmaceuticals, it may persist for several weeks.

Plasma Volume

^{125}Iodine-labeled human serum albumin (^{125}I-HSA) is the radiopharmaceutical of choice for determining *PV*.[9] Albumin diffuses slowly into the extravascular space: approximately 10% disappears from plasma in the first hour.[4] However, this slow diffusion results in an error of only 1 to 3% in the plasma volume calculated from a 10-minute blood sample. In diseases with increased protein loss or increased vascular permeability, however, substantial tracer loss can occur in the first 10 minutes. These situations include severe burns, shock, nephrotic syndrome, and protein-losing enteropathy. In such instances, it is best to obtain plasma samples at 10, 20, and 30 minutes and to extrapolate to the zero-time value from the disappearance curve.

The procedure for *PV* determination is as follows:

1. The patient must be in a basal metabolic state (recumbent) for 30 to 60 minutes prior to the study. Determine height and weight that day, and draw 5 mL of blood in EDTA prior to the study for a 2.0-mL plasma background counting sample.
2. Inject intravenously 5 μCi (185 kBq) ^{125}I-HSA that has been carefully measured from a commercial supplier's vial.
3. Monitor the injection site with a hand radiation monitor and compare with the opposite arm for any evidence of isotope extravasation.
4. At exactly 10 min, draw 5 mL blood (EDTA) from a vein other than that injected. Centrifuge, and pipette 2.0 mL plasma for gamma counting.
5. If there is reason to suspect accelerated plasma albumin clearance as discussed previously, draw additional blood samples at 20, 30 and, if appropriate, 60 minutes. In such a case, the zero-time plasma ^{125}I count is determined by extrapolation from the several timed samples plotted on semilogarithmic graph paper.
6. Pipette 5 μCi (185 kBq) ^{125}I-HSA into a 1000-mL volumetric flask almost filled with normal saline. Fill to exactly 1000 mL, mix well, and immediately pipette two 2.0-mL counting standards. Because albumin can adhere to glass, siliconized glassware is recommended, or carrier albumin or a detergent can be added to the diluent.
7. *PV* is calculated from the 10-minute blood sample count as follows:

$$PV\ (\text{mL}) = \frac{\text{net cpm/mL in std} \times 1000}{(\text{net cpm/mL in plasma sample})}$$

The *TBV* and *RCV* are estimated from *PV* using the equations given earlier in this section.

One of the most important clinical applications of blood

volume determination is confirming the diagnosis of polycythemia rubra vera. In this disease, there is an absolute increase in *RCV*, with the *PV* normal or slightly increased (occasionally, slightly reduced). In relative polycythemia, the hematocrit is increased because of decreased *PV* and normal *RCV*, the most notable example being so-called "stress polycythemia." Accurate diagnosis of polycythemia vera is essential because of the implications for therapy. Because of the wide variability of the F_{cell} ratio and the importance of ruling out diminished *PV* as the cause of elevated hematocrit, *PV* and *RCV* must be measured independently, with *PV* determined first because of the lower energy of ^{125}I.

The preoperative, intraoperative, and postoperative measurements of *TBV* have been used extensively in the past for more effective management of patients undergoing surgical procedures associated with major blood loss (e.g., open heart surgery or major orthopedic procedures). *TBV* measurements have also been helpful in patients hospitalized after major trauma, in patients with severe congestive heart disease, and in patients with severe chronic renal disease, which can affect all body fluid compartments. In the past 2 decades, however, such uses of *TBV* measurements have diminished markedly.[7]

BONE MARROW

With 1500 g of red marrow and 1500 g of yellow marrow in normal adults, the bone marrow is one of the largest organs in the body. During fetal growth, hematopoiesis takes place in all bony cavities (axial and appendicular skeleton) as well as in liver and spleen. Prior to birth, splenic and hepatic hematopoiesis disappear, and gradually thereafter hematopoietic tissue in the long bones is replaced by fat. The normal adult distribution of active marrow is then achieved by the middle to late teens (Fig. 21).[118]

Histologically, the bone marrow is composed of many different cellular elements: erythroid and myeloid (leukocytic) precursors, megakaryocytes, reticuloendothelial cells, fixed stromal cells providing a reticulin network on which the marrow precursors proliferate, occasional lymphocytes, and even lymph follicles, bony trabeculae, and scattered immature stem cells. All are surrounded by normal peripheral blood cells. The reticuloendothelial cells and the erythroid precursors provide functional mechanisms for scintigraphic radiopharmaceutical localization. The 2 general applications of marrow scintigraphy are (1) mapping the distribution of hematopoietic marrow, which may be expanded at times of hematopoietic stress (e.g., chronic anemia, infection, and such primary hematological malignancies as leukemia and polycythemia vera)[119] and, (2) defining focal or generalized marrow loss to document extent of disease or to identify sites for biopsy (e.g., in some solid malignancies). Diffuse loss of central marrow as demonstrated by scintigraphy is seen in aplastic anemia, in high-dose radiotherapy (more than 3000 cGy), and in certain myelophthisic processes such as myelofibrosis or widespread skeletal carcinomatosis.

Radiopharmaceuticals

Table 4 summarizes the radiopharmaceuticals used for bone-marrow evaluation. There are no radiopharmaceuticals that permit imaging of the myeloid or megakaryocytic precursors in the marrow. ^{111}In-oxine platelets and granulocytes image the red-marrow distribution because of pooling of mature cells in the marrow, but such images do not necessarily reflect the functional distribution of precursors. Excellent functional images of the erythroid marrow are possible with ^{52}Fe, although its use is limited by high cost, limited availability, and specific instrumentation requirements (PET). Bone-marrow scans with ^{52}Fe and ^{99m}Tc-sulfur colloid show identical marrow distribution patterns in most clinical conditions. The exceptions occur in a few predictable situations: pure red cell aplasia, acute radiation injury, myelosuppressive chemotherapy, and in one reported case of polycythemia vera.[119–123] Thus, it appears that radiocolloid imaging of the marrow is a practical alternative to ^{52}Fe imaging.

The use of ^{111}In-chloride for erythroid marrow scintigraphy has attracted much interest.[77] ^{111}Indium binds to transferrin and is carried, in part, to erythyroid precursors in the marrow. Several studies have confirmed its clinical utility in marrow scintigraphy, particularly in seeking appropriate sites for marrow biopsy.[124–130] Good correlation between ^{111}In uptake and marrow cellularity has been documented.[127] Nevertheless, there is significant non-erythyroid ^{111}In uptake in the skeleton, either by cortical bone or by reticuloendothelial tissues, so that ^{111}In marrow images must be interpreted with caution in patients with hypoplastic marrow.[120,131,132] Other disadvantages of ^{111}In as compared with ^{99m}Tc-sulfur colloid include substantially higher radiopharmaceutical cost, lower data density images, and a 48- to 72-hour wait before imaging.

Radiocolloid marrow scanning has been of demonstrated clinical use since the early experience with ^{198}Au-colloid reported by Edwards et al. and Kniseley et al.[133–135] In recent years, ^{99m}Tc-sulfur colloid (TcSC) has been the agent of choice because of its lower radiation absorbed dose and excellent camera images. Approximately 80 to 85% of the injected TcSC localizes in the liver, 10 to 15% in the spleen, and 2 to 5% in the reticuloendothelial marrow.[136] The procedure consists of injecting 8 to 10 mCi (~300 to 370 MBq) TcSC intravenously, waiting 15 to 20 minutes for blood clearance, and imaging the whole body (or taking selected spot scintiphotos) at a significantly higher photographic intensity than would be used for liver-spleen imaging. Two-minute scintiphotos are adequate for spot views. The radiocolloid technique has the disadvantage of masking the spinal marrow in the region between the liver and spleen, although frequently these vertebral bodies can be visualized at an intensity intermediate between marrow and liver.

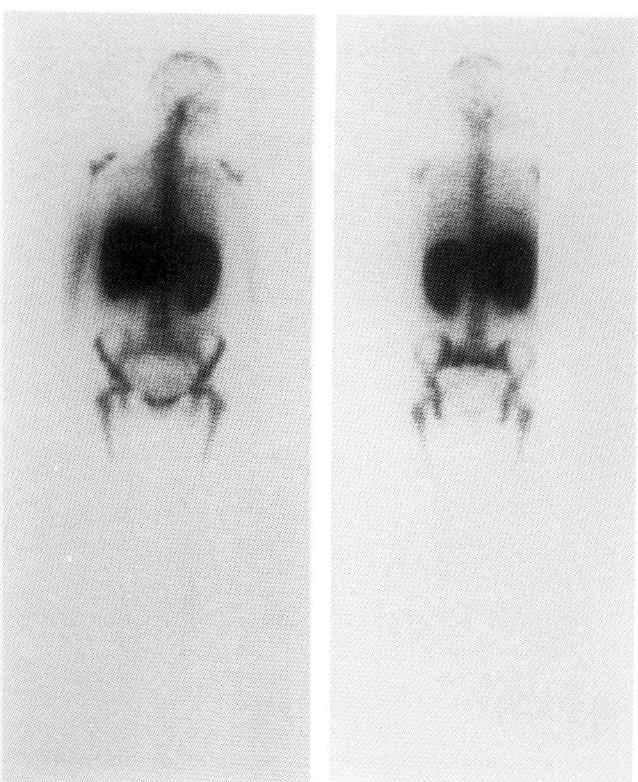

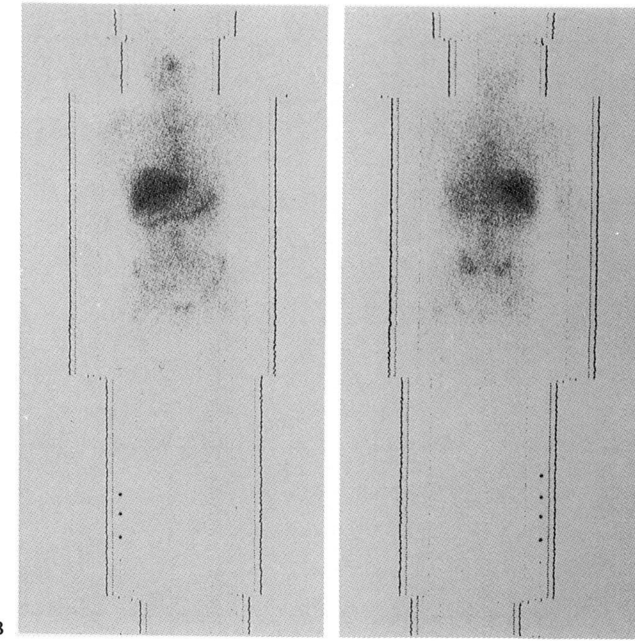

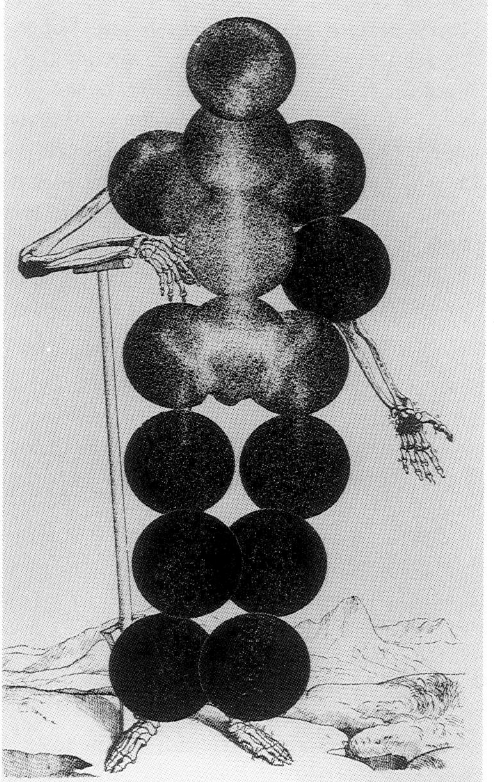

Figure 21. Normal adult red marrow distribution as imaged with ^{99m}Tc-sulfur colloid (**A**), ^{111}In-chloride (**B**), and ^{52}Fe-chloride (**C**). A small amount of bowel activity is evident in the ^{111}In image, found normally in 6–7% of patients. The ^{52}Fe study was performed at Donner Laboratory, University of California at Berkeley. (C from Van Dyke D et al.[119])

Table 4. Bone Marrow Imaging Radiopharmaceuticals

MARROW CELL TYPE	RADIOPHARMACEUTICAL	$T_{1/2}$	PRINCIPAL γ EMISSION	AVAILABILITY	USUAL ADULT DOSE
Reticuloendothelial	^{99m}Tc-sulfur colloid	6 hr	140 keV	generator	5–8 mCi
	^{198}Au-colloid	2.7 days	412 keV	no commercial source	1 mCi
	^{113m}In-colloid	1.7 hr	393 keV	generator	3 mCi
Erythropoietic	^{52}Fe-citrate	8.2 hr	511 keV	cyclotron	100 μCi
	^{59}Fe-citrate	45.6 days	1.1 MeV 1.3 MeV	reactor	20 μCi
	^{111}In-chloride	2.8 days	173 keV 247 keV	cyclotron	2 mCi
Granulopoietic	(^{111}In-oxine WBC*)	2.8 days	173 keV 247 keV	cyclotron	2 mCi
Megakaryopoietic	None				

*The ^{111}In-oxine WBC marrow image consists of partly labeled WBCs pooling in marrow sinusoids and partly free In-111 going to erythroid precursors; granulocytic precursors are not labeled, however.

TcSC prepared by the sodium thiosulfate (kit) technique has particle diameters ranging from 200 to 1000 nm. Prepared by the hydrogen sulfide technique, the particle size is considerably smaller—perhaps 10 to 50 nm in diameter. Because smaller particles tend to be taken up preferentially by bone marrow, the hydrogen sulfide method yields better marrow images. Both ^{99m}Tc-antimony sulfide colloid and ^{99m}Tc-minimicroaggregated albumin colloid are effective marrow radiopharmaceuticals because of their small particle sizes.

Immunoscintigraphy of the bone marrow has been carried out with antibodies to granulocytes (e.g., ^{99m}Tc-labeled antigranulocyte antibody BW 250/183[137,138]) and to platelets. It should be noted, however, that these circulating cell labels provide an image of the marrow to the extent that the labeled cells are pooling in the marrow space, but the pattern seen may not reflect true hematopoietic bone marrow. Other possible radiopharmaceutical approaches to marrow scintigraphy have been reviewed by Desai and Thakur.[139]

Clinical Studies

NORMAL

Figure 21 illustrates normal adult red marrow distribution as imaged with TcSC, ^{52}Fe, and ^{111}In.

HEMATOPOIETIC STRESS

The physiological response of the bone marrow to hematopoietic stress (anemia, infection) is hypertrophy. Initially, hypertrophy is discernible only microscopically, with progressive loss of the 30 to 40% fat content of normal central marrow, but with no change in skeletal distribution. With continued stress over a period of several weeks or even months, activation of peripheral yellow marrow sites to red marrow takes place, and evidence of peripheral marrow extension is demonstrated by scintigraphy (Fig. 22).

LEUKEMIA

The leukemias are malignant proliferative disorders involving the marrow, and with the exception of a few mild cases of early chronic lymphocytic leukemia, they are invariably associated with peripheral marrow extension. Although intense chemotherapy depletes erythroid precursors and affects the ^{52}Fe distribution, the TcSC distribution is usually not altered because reticuloendothelial cells are nonproliferative and are not depleted by chemotherapy. Acute leukemia in blast crisis with pancytopenia due to a packed marrow will generally demonstrate the pattern of a severe myelophthisic process, with little or no visualization of the marrow.

POLYCYTHEMIA VERA

Polycythemia vera, a primary proliferative disorder of the marrow, demonstrates peripheral marrow extension that varies according to how long-standing or aggressive the polycythemia is. Thus, marrow scintigraphy may be of assistance in "staging" the disease. Because 10 to 20% of patients with polycythemia vera progress to central myelofibrosis, the marrow scan may also provide the earliest noninvasive evidence of this developing complication, and indicate the extent of total marrow replacement with the fibrotic process (Fig. 23).

IDIOPATHIC MYELOFIBROSIS

Like postpolycythemic myelofibrosis, idiopathic myelofibrosis (agnogenic myeloid metaplasia) produces progressive central marrow loss and increasing peripheral extension, along with massive splenomegaly, as manifestations of advancing disease. Estimation of the amount of functioning central marrow is readily achieved with bone marrow scin-

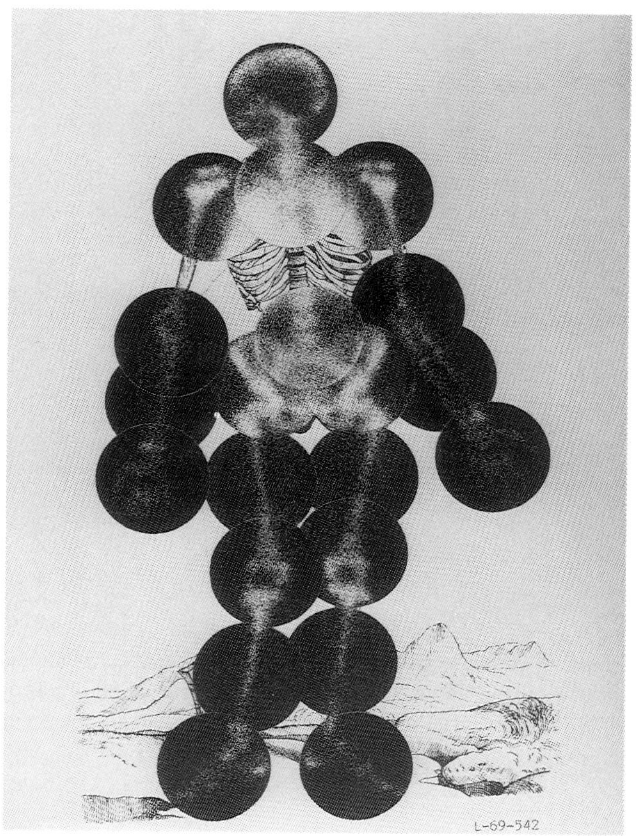

Figure 22. Expanded hematopoietic marrow, visualized with ^{99m}Tc-sulfur colloid throughout the axial skeleton and the long bones in an adult patient with chronic fever and leukocytosis, subsequently proven to have systemic toxoplasmosis.

tigraphy,[140] and this information may be useful when splenectomy for hypersplenism is being considered in the management of the disease. When most of the central marrow has been replaced by fibrous tissue, removal of a massively enlarged spleen generally results in the development or worsening of pancytopenia followed by progressive myeloid metaplasia of the liver.

APLASTIC ANEMIA

Because aplastic anemia is a process that involves loss of all marrow elements, both the reticuloendothelial marrow scan (TcSC) and the erythroid marrow scan (^{52}Fe, ^{111}In) demonstrate little or no central marrow labeling, and no peripheral marrow extension (Fig. 24). In problematic patients with hypoplastic or aplastic anemia, the marrow scan may help to identify a specific marrow biopsy site that is representative of the diffuse marrow process, and not merely a local area of hypoplasia. Uptake of ^{111}In-chloride in cortical bone of patients with pure red cell aplasia may give an erroneous picture of adequate marrow cellularity.[120] The same is occasionally true of reticuloendothelial marrow imaged with TcSC in this disease.[119]

RADIATION EFFECTS ON BONE MARROW

Complete and long-lasting marrow aplasia usually results from therapeutic radiation doses to the marrow above 3000 cGy (Fig. 25).[141,142] There is some ability of locally irradiated marrow to regenerate partially or completely in situations of intense hematopoietic stress, such as anemia or infection. Some marrow recovery may also be seen in response to persistent pancytopenia after extensive skeletal irradia-

A

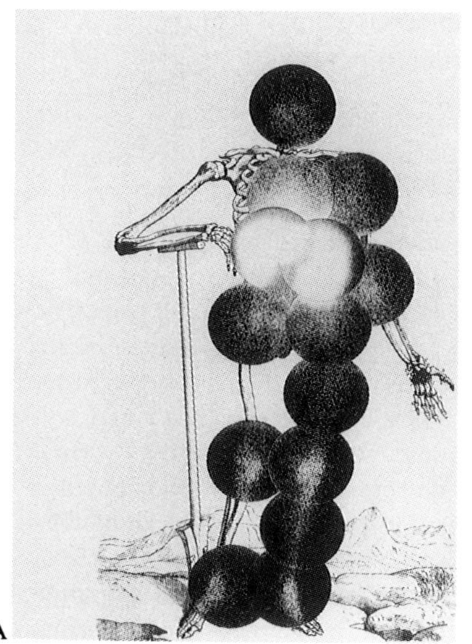

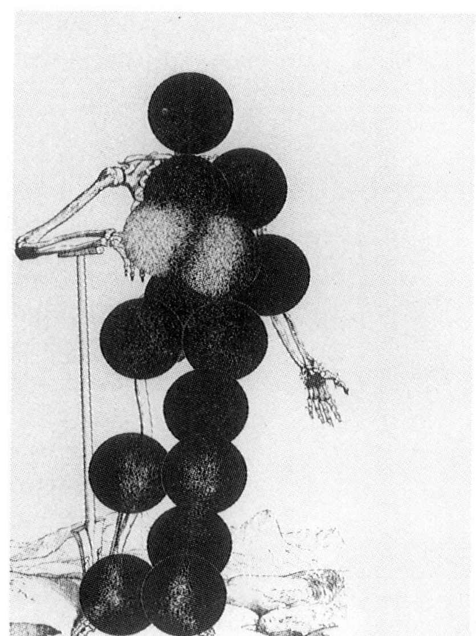

B

Figure 23. ^{99m}Tc-sulfur colloid (**A**) and ^{52}Fe (**B**) studies demonstrate the characteristic marrow distribution pattern of advanced myelofibrosis with myeloid metaplasia (agnogenic myeloid metaplasia). Note the marked splenomegaly and intense spleen (and liver) labeling with ^{52}Fe that result from myeloid metaplasia in those organs. The study was performed at Donner Laboratory, U.C. Berkeley.

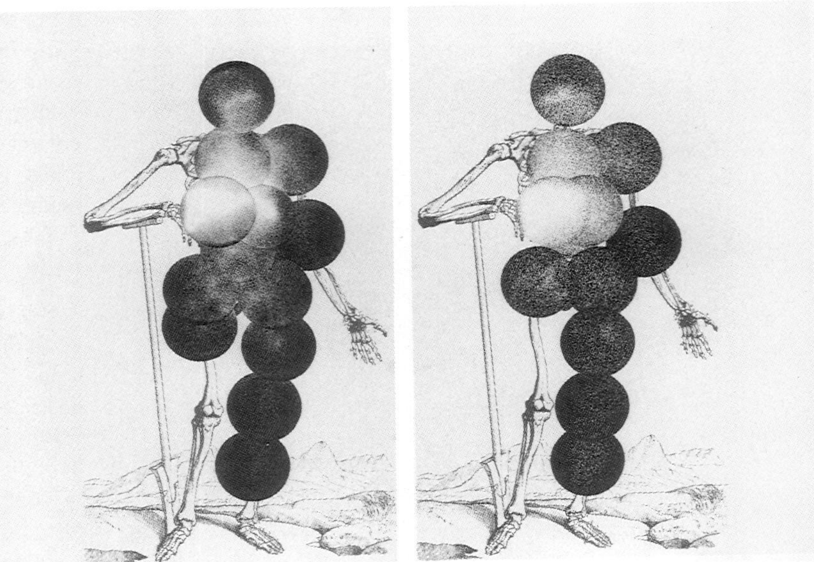

Figure 24. Near total loss of imageable marrow as seen with ^{99m}Tc-sulfur colloid **(A)** and ^{52}Fe **(B)** in a patient with aplastic anemia. The ^{52}Fe study was performed at Donner Laboratory, U.C. Berkeley. (From Van Dyke et al.[119])

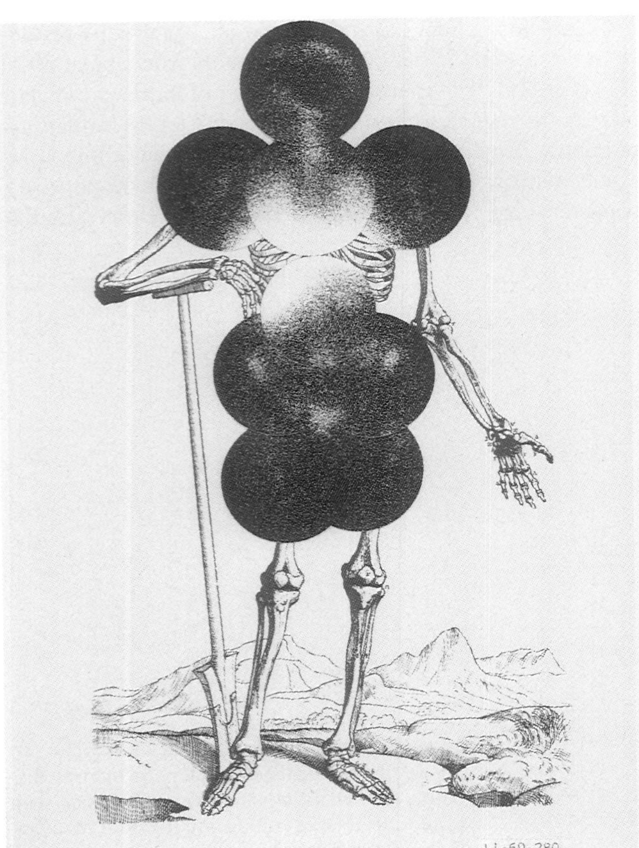

Figure 25. Active radiocolloid marrow distribution several years following total nodal irradiation in a patient with Hodgkin's disease. The permanent radioablation of most of the marrow in the radiation sites is characteristic of high-dose therapy.

tion.[143–147] Because extensive areas of unrecovered irradiated marrow would leave a patient less tolerant to chemotherapy or additional radiotherapy, a marrow scan can be useful in deciding on the best course of further therapy.

METASTATIC MALIGNANCY

Although bone scans are very sensitive for metastatic skeletal disease, some patients with diffuse skeletal involvement, without localized increase in bone blood flow, may have false-negative bone scans. Some of these patients will have tumors that infiltrate the marrow and, consequently, may be seen as cold defects on marrow scintigraphy (Fig. 26).[136,148] In one clinical series, the marrow scan was abnormal in 5% of patients with malignancy who had normal bone scans.[149]

Other potential applications of marrow scintigraphy have been outlined in the literature.[150,151]

THE SPLEEN

The spleen is a reticuloendothelial organ that, along with the liver, is responsible for filtering foreign particulate matter from the circulation. It also has an immunologic role. The spleen is a hematopoietic organ during the third to sixth month of fetal development, a function that is lost thereafter except under specific pathologic conditions (advanced myelofibrosis or severe chronic hemolytic anemia). Normal spleen weight diminishes during adulthood from an average of 146 g at age 20 to 78 g at age 79; it is always somewhat larger in males.[152] The spleen receives approximately 2% of cardiac output and drains via the portal circulation. Impaired portal venous drainage with portal hypertension is often

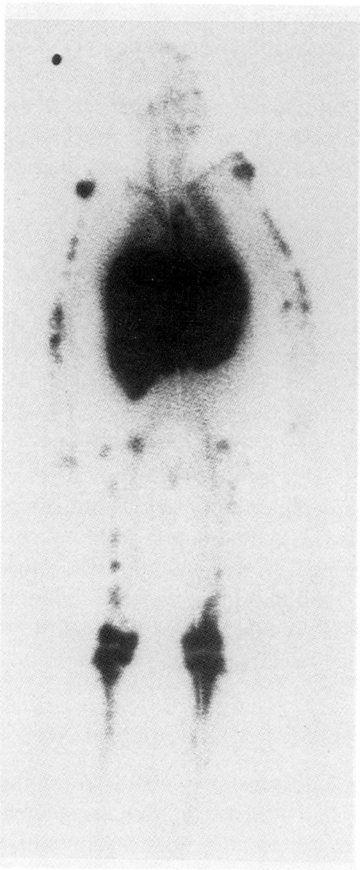

Figure 26. Anterior radiocolloid bone marrow image in a 38-year-old woman with breast cancer and widespread bone metastases. Note the absence of imageable pelvic marrow due to tumor replacement, and multiple cold defects in the long bones (which also show evidence of peripheral extension due to anemia).

associated with some degree of splenomegaly. The normal adult spleen is a posterior organ that lies under the thoracic cage. It is not palpable until it reaches two or three times its normal size.

Radiopharmaceuticals

Spleen scintigraphy is possible with most radiocolloids. As previously mentioned, larger colloidal particles tend to be distributed more to the spleen and less to bone marrow than smaller particles. Initial clinical experience with spleen scintigraphy was gained with ^{198}Au gold colloid. Because of the small particle size (5 to 15 nm), spleen imaging was unsatisfactory. With the introduction of ^{99m}Tc-sulfur colloid prepared by the thiosulfate technique (200 to 1000 nm particles), spleen scintigraphy became a common clinical procedure. Other radiocolloids, such as ^{99m}Tc-antimony colloid (3 to 15 nm), ^{113m}In-colloid (10 to 20 nm), and TcSC prepared by the hydrogen sulfide technique (10 to 50 nm), are smaller in size and more suitable for marrow imaging and lymphoscintigraphy.

The routine procedure for spleen scintigraphy consists of the intravenous injection of 3 to 5 mCi (100 to 200 MBq) of TcSC, followed 15 to 20 minutes later by multiple images of liver and spleen, which include left lateral and left anterior oblique views (the latter particularly in the presence of left hepatic lobe enlargement). All scintiphotos are obtained for the time required for a 1,000,000-count image of the anterior liver.

Several techniques that have been described for spleen imaging utilize damaged red cells, which are preferentially concentrated by the spleen.[153] Early studies were performed with ^{51}Cr-labeled donor erythrocytes that had been sensitized either by incubation with incomplete anti-D antibodies,[154] or by heating to 50°C for 1 hour.[155] Selective splenic scintigraphy is best performed by using ^{99m}Tc-labeled autologous erythrocytes damaged by heating (we heat at 50°C for 15 minutes after labeling), or by labeling in the presence of excess tin.[156,157] These procedures are not in wide use, however, because of the difficulties of having to draw and label the blood, wash the cells, then damage the cells prior to injection. The use of ^{203}Hg- or ^{197}Hg-MHP (1-mercury-2-hydroxypropane) for spleen scintigraphy was proposed in the 1960s, but has never become widely accepted because of the substantial radiation dose to the patient.[158]

Clinical Applications

ESTIMATION OF SPLEEN SIZE

Several studies have established simple formulas for estimating spleen size and weight by scintigraphy.[159–162] Although rectilinear scanning permitted direct measurement of the relevant dimensions on the spleen scan, camera scintigraphy requires calibration of the minification factor with appropriate standards. The normal adult spleen length (*L*) in the posterior projection is 10.7 ± 1.7 cm.[160] The normal spleen size as a function of age (*A*) is:[163]

$$L = 5.7 + 0.31A$$

Adult spleen weight (*W*) in grams can be calculated from the formula:[161]

$$W = 71L - 537$$

In children, Spencer and Pearson found the following relationship:[164]

$$W = 22.6L - 104$$

Such estimates tend to be less accurate for the extremes of spleen sizes. In fact, there are few, if any, clinical situations in which quantification of spleen size is important to diagnosis or management.

Table 5 lists the causes of mild, moderate, and massive splenomegaly. The massive splenomegaly associated with myelofibrosis and chronic myelogenous leukemia may be associated with recurrent splenic infarcts, resulting in marked irregularity in the spleen image.

The most common cause of failure to visualize the spleen

Table 5. Causes of Splenomegaly

MILD SPLENOMEGALY (Up to 500 g)
Infections—acute, subacute, and chronic
Malignant diseases—acute leukemias, malignant melanoma, multiple myeloma
Early stages of moderate or massive splenomegaly, or following response to therapy
Other—ITP, lupus erythematosus, sarcoidosis, acute splenic congestion
MODERATE SPLENOMEGALY (500 to 1000 g)
Acute leukemias
Malignant lymphomas
Chronic lymphatic leukemia
Portal hypertension with congestive splenomegaly
Chronic hemolytic anemias
Polycythemia vera
Subacute bacterial endocarditis
Infectious mononucleosis
MASSIVE SPLENOMEGALY (Greater than 1000 g)
Myelofibrosis with myeloid metaplasia
Chronic myelogenous leukemia
Malaria
Gaucher's disease
Kala-azar, bilharziasis
Thalassemia major (in children)
Splenic cysts and tumors (rarely)

is splenectomy.[165] This information is usually elicited from the patient upon direct questioning. Congenital asplenia, frequently seen in children with situs inversus (Fig. 27), is important to document because of the high risk of life-threatening bacterial infections during childhood, especially pneumococcal and meningococcal infections. Diminished spleen size is found in adults with sickle cell disease, malabsorption syndrome, and prior Thorotrast® injection. Occasionally, no spleen is discernible (see "Functional Asplenia" later in this chapter).

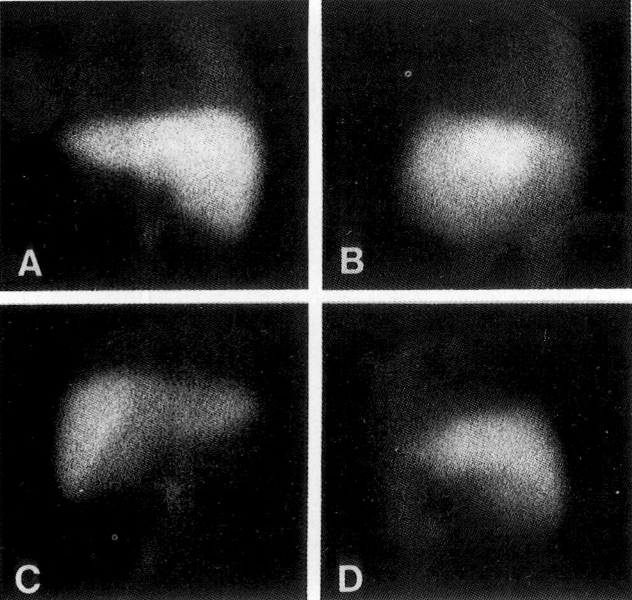

Figure 27. ^{99m}Tc-sulfur colloid liver-spleen scan in a child with situs inversus, confirming the presence of asplenia. **(A).** Anterior. **(B).** Left lateral. **(C).** Posterior. **(D).** Right lateral. (From Price DC: Spleen: Nuclear Medicine, in Margulis AR, Burhenne HJ (eds): *Alimentary Tract Radiology.* 3rd ed. St. Louis, CV Mosby, 1983:1602–1617.)

LEFT UPPER QUADRANT MASS

Spleen scintigraphy is often helpful in distinguishing splenic enlargement, with or without focal disease, from a palpable nonsplenic mass in the left upper quadrant (e.g., gastric, colonic, pancreatic, renal, or adrenal neoplasm, or lymphomatous lymph nodes). The large, firm, irregular spleen of a patient with myelofibrosis, myeloid metaplasia, and recurrent splenic infarcts may be indistinguishable from a hard, irregular LUQ malignancy until radiocolloid scintigraphy is performed. In patients with FUO, the combination of spleen and gallium imaging and abdominal computed tomography (CT) is effective in documenting the presence of an abdominal or subphrenic abscess.[166]

FOCAL SPLENIC PATHOLOGY

Focal splenic lesions may result from metastases, abscesses, cysts, hematomas, infarcts, or splenic neoplasms.

Splenic abscesses are rare, but do occur with such intravascular infections as acute and subacute bacterial endocarditis. Splenic cysts are also uncommon, although chocolate (endometrial) cysts of the spleen have been described, and echinococcal cysts occur in hydatid disease.

Usually, splenic hematomas result from trauma and, occasionally, from minor trauma that the patient himself does not recall, even upon direct questioning. The risk of splenic hematoma is increased in patients with thrombocytopenia and other bleeding diatheses. In one study, Gilday and Alderson found that spleen imaging was highly sensitive for detecting hematomas.[167] There were no false-negative results and only 5 (7%) of 69 cases involved false-positive results. The usual finding is a focal lesion within or adjacent to the spleen.[168] Occasionally, it appears to transect the spleen; sometimes it is just a cold region displacing the spleen medially from the costal wall (Fig. 28).

Suspected hematomas can be confirmed effectively by CT of the spleen.[169] Recent hematomas have a CT number similar to spleen and are not enhanced with contrast, whereas older hematomas have progressively lower CT numbers, and also are not enhanced with contrast. Splenic rupture is a surgical emergency that rarely involves radionuclide scanning.

Splenic infarcts are usually peripheral, wedge-shaped defects (Fig. 29). They occur in association with bacterial endocarditis and are frequently seen with the massive splenomegaly of chronic myelogenous leukemia, and myelofibrosis with myeloid metaplasia. In the latter case, the enlarged

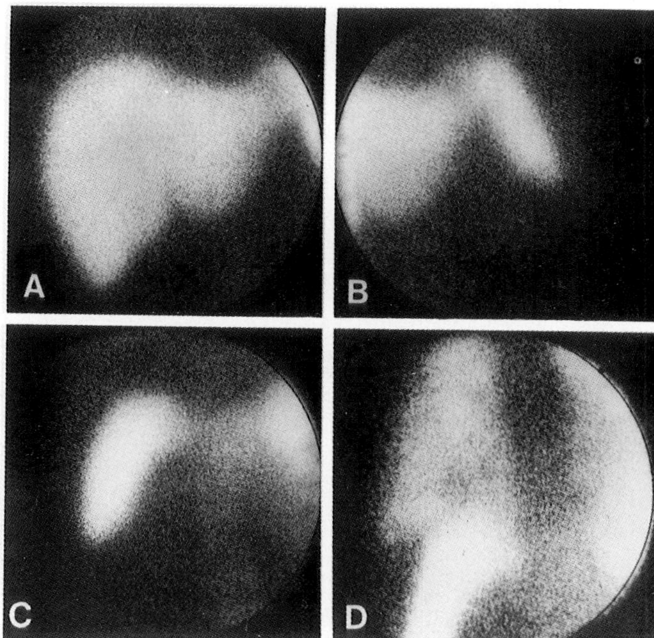

Figure 28. ^{99m}TcSC liver-spleen scintigraphy in a patient with subcapsular hematoma of the spleen. **(A).** Anterior liver image is normal. **(B).** Anterior spleen image demonstrates flattening of the lateral surface of the spleen. **(C).** Posterior spleen image appears unremarkable. **(D).** A posterior lung-liver image after additional IV injection of ^{99m}Tc-MAA demonstrates a space between functioning splenic tissue and the lateral body wall. (From Price DC: Spleen: Nuclear Medicine, in Margulis AR, Burhenne HJ (eds): *Alimentary Tract Radiology.* 3rd ed. St. Louis, CV Mosby, 1983:1602–1617.)

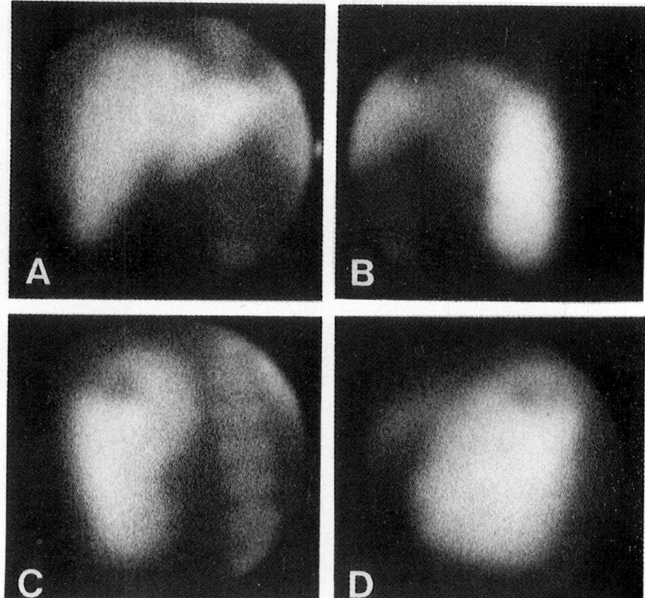

Figure 29. Wedge-shaped peripheral splenic defect in a young drug addict with subacute bacterial endocarditis, left upper quadrant pain, fever, leukocytosis, and a cardiac murmur. Angiography demonstrated a mycotic aneurysm with localized hemorrhage and a splenic infarct. **(A).** Right anterior. **(B).** Left anterior. **(C).** Left posterior. **(D).** Left lateral. The study also demonstrates obvious splenomegaly and increased marrow uptake, manifestations of liver disease. (From Price DC: Spleen: Nuclear Medicine, in Margulis AR, Burhenne HJ (eds): *Alimentary Tract Radiology.* 3rd ed. St. Louis, CV Mosby, 1983:1602–1617.)

spleen usually has numerous irregularities. Splenic infarction in homozygous sickle-cell disease is never visualized because the spleen itself is not imageable in such patients (functional asplenia); however, patients with sickle-cell trait can develop splenic infarcts under such hypoxic conditions as high altitude (Fig. 30). Kuni et al.[170] have described the splenic scan findings, including various degrees of infarction, that follow partial pancreatectomy with splenic artery and vein resection.

Primary splenic neoplasms are rare, except for splenic involvement by lymphomas and leukemias. In such cases, mild to moderate splenomegaly is common, but focal splenic lesions are seldom seen. Even the presence of splenomegaly does not, in itself, correlate well with direct involvement by lymphoma.[171] Hodgkin's disease is the most common lymphoma involving the spleen, although splenic involvement also occurs with lymphosarcoma and reticulum cell sarcoma.

Solid tumor metastases to the spleen are also rare. The most common is malignant melanoma, which can produce cold lesions but which has also been reported in association with diffusely increased splenic uptake of colloid.[172] Koh et al.[173] have noted an interesting association between a scintigraphically bright spleen and poor prognosis in patients with stage 1 and 2 malignant melanoma, but the finding is unexplained and does not appear to be of sufficient relevance to be utilized clinically. Focal splenic lesions can be seen with widely metastatic malignancies, such as breast carcinoma. Occasionally, local primary tumors (stomach, colon, pancreas) may extend to involve the spleen directly.

ACCESSORY SPLEENS

The usual location for accessory spleens is the splenic hilus and along the associated vessels and ligaments. Accessory spleens are rarely found in adults, but occur in as many as 10% of newborns in routine postmortem examinations. In the presence of normal splenic tissue in adults, there is no stimulus for these accessory cell nests to proliferate; thus, they remain too small to detect. Following splenectomy, stimulation and growth of accessory splenic tissue may be sufficient to become scintigraphically detectable. This is particularly true in autoimmune hemolytic anemia, idiopathic thrombocytopenic purpura, and hereditary spherocytosis, in which hypertrophy of accessory spleens may aggravate the primary hematologic disorder (Fig. 31).

Pearson et al. described an unusual splenic recurrence in patients following traumatic splenic rupture and splenectomy.[174] At the time of rupture, spleen cells spread throughout the abdominal cavity. Some of these cells settle and prolifer-

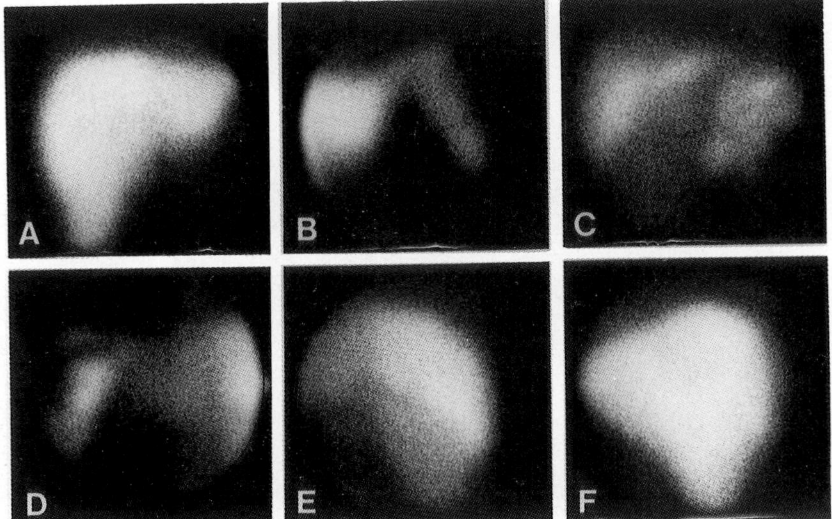

Figure 30. Multiple splenic infarcts in a black adult male with sickle cell trait. Previously in excellent health, the patient had developed left upper quadrant pain while spending several days at 7000 feet altitude in the mountains. (From Price DC: Spleen: Nuclear Medicine, in Margulis AR, Burhenne HJ (eds): *Alimentary Tract Radiology*. 3rd ed. St. Louis, CV Mosby, 1983:1602–1617.)

ate, leading to scattered deposits of splenic tissue (splenosis) that can ultimately become imageable foci throughout the abdomen and pelvis (Fig. 32). These patients do not demonstrate such expected peripheral blood findings of asplenia as nucleated red cells and Howell-Jolly bodies. This condition has been termed "the born-again spleen." Scintigraphic demonstration of such abdominal spleen foci indicates that the patient does not have the same increased risk of infection as a truly asplenic patient.

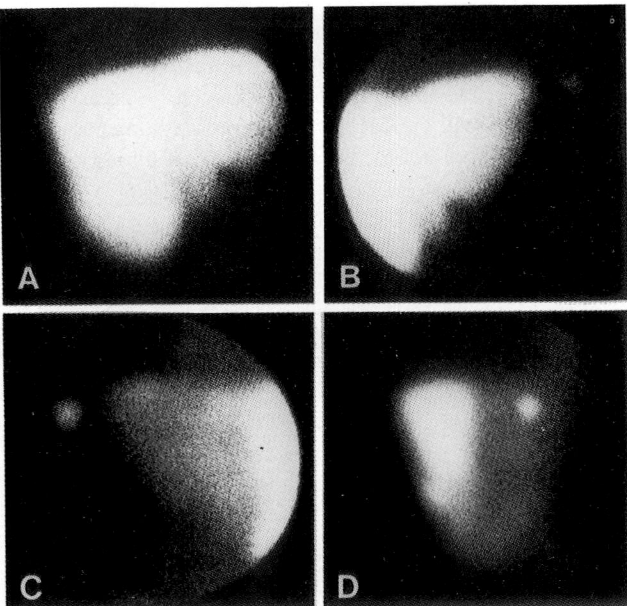

Figure 31. Accessory spleen in a young woman whose autoimmune hemolytic anemia had initially responded well to splenectomy after failure on steroids. Her disease relapsed prior to this study. **(A).** Right anterior. **(B).** Left anterior. **(C).** Left posterior. **(D).** Left lateral. (From Price DC: Spleen: Nuclear Medicine, in Margulis AR, Burhenne HJ (eds): *Alimentary Tract Radiology*. 3rd ed. St. Louis, CV Mosby, 1983:1602–1617.)

FUNCTIONAL ASPLENIA

In 1969, Pearson et al. noted that children with homozygous sickle cell disease have enlarged palpable spleens that fail to label with radiocolloids.[175] This entity was termed *functional asplenia*. The peripheral blood of these patients

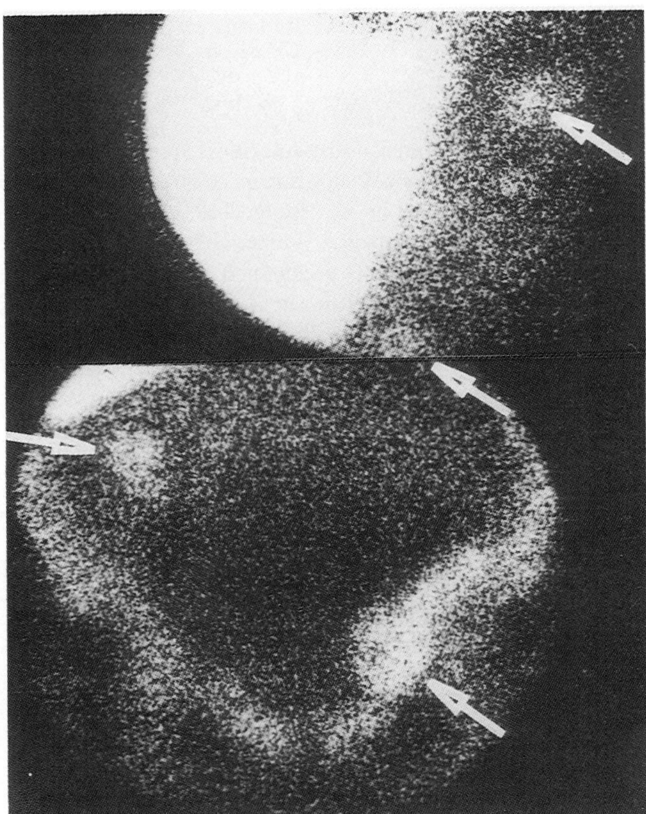

Figure 32. "Born-again spleen" in a 29-year-old man who several years previously had undergone splenectomy for splenic rupture. Several seeded sites of regenerating splenic tissue are indicated by arrows in the LUQ (top) and the pelvis (bottom).

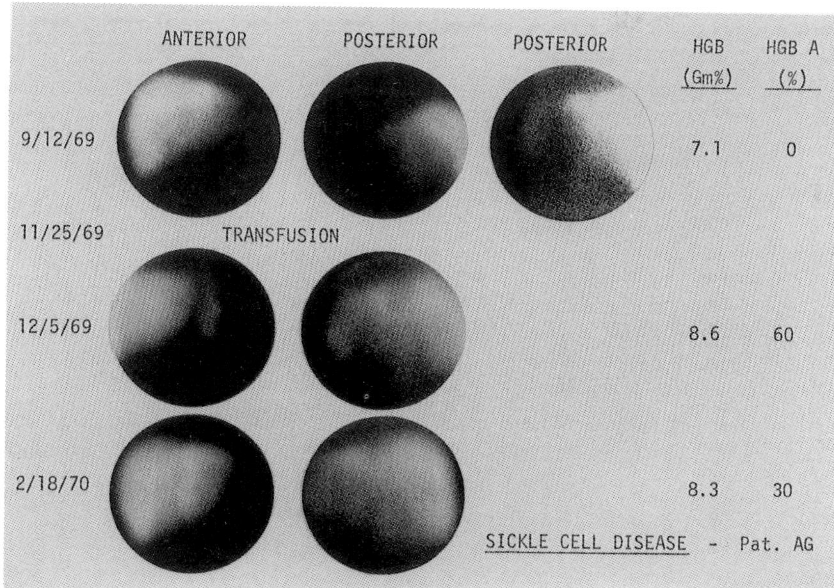

Figure 33. Functional asplenia in a 14-year-old black child with sickle-cell disease. The spleen was slightly enlarged to palpation. Transfusion with normal red cells temporarily stimulates return of some splenic function.

showed the usual erythrocyte pleomorphism, normoblasts, and Howell-Jolly bodies associated with asplenia. Even more interestingly, this failure of splenic labeling is reversible by transfusion of normal red cells (Fig. 33). Thus, it appears to be caused, at least in part, by reduced perfusion of the spleen that results from red cell sickling during splenic transit. This sequence can be interrupted by transfusing sufficient normal erythrocytes to inhibit the sickling process and log-jamming of sickled red cells, and to maintain normal blood flow and oxygen tension in the spleen. Functional asplenia has also been described in chronic Thorotrast® irradiation of the spleen, celiac disease, and beta thalassemia trait,[176,177] as well as a variety of other single case reports with no clear common feature.

Owunwanne et al.[178] have made the interesting observation in 10 patients with sickle cell disease, that functional asplenia defined by failure of spleen visualisation with ^{99m}Tc-tin colloid was associated with excellent spleen visualization using heat-denatured red cells. Because the heat-denatured cells have a much greater uptake in normal spleens than colloids, this observation could also be consistent with reduced, but not absent, blood flow in the functionally asplenic sickle cell patients.

ABSORPTION OF ESSENTIAL HEMATOLOGIC NUTRIENTS

Vitamin B_{12}

The consequences of untreated vitamin B_{12} deficiency include megaloblastic anemia, thrombocytopenia, leukopenia, spinal-cord degeneration (subacute combined degeneration of the cord) and, ultimately, death. Measurement of vitamin B_{12} absorption and serum levels in patients with unexplained macrocytic anemia is important, because anemia is not a disease but only a symptom of a more specific underlying disorder. The onset of vitamin B_{12} deficiency is notoriously insidious, and the initial symptoms are vague; in the early stages, even the classic red cell morphological changes may not occur. Because of the close metabolic relationship between folic acid and vitamin B_{12}, large doses of folic acid given to patients with vitamin B_{12} deficiency may improve the anemia, but may also allow neurological damage to develop or progress. Therefore, casual treatment of anemic patients with multihematinics that contain therapeutic amounts of folic acid is undesirable.

PHYSIOLOGY AND PATHOPHYSIOLOGY OF VITAMIN B_{12} METABOLISM

In 1855, Thomas Addison first described the clinical entity now known as pernicious anemia. Sixty-five years later, Whipple et al. demonstrated the general antianemic effects of increased dietary liver,[179] and shortly thereafter Minot and Murphy identified the specific beneficial effect of oral liver in pernicious anemia.[180] The most important advance in understanding this disease came with the demonstration by Castle in the 1930s that there is an "extrinsic factor" in beef (vitamin B_{12}) that must combine with an "intrinsic factor" (IF) in gastric juice to reproduce the beneficial effects of the antianemic principle in liver.[181]

Vitamin B_{12}, or cyanocobalamin, is actually a family of co-enzymes that are involved biologically in a number of biochemical reactions. In most of these reactions, cobalamins function as donors and acceptors of hydrogen and methyl groups. In humans, the most frequently found cobalamins are methylcobalamin (the predominant form in plasma); adenosylcobalamin or deoxyadenosylcobalamin (the predominant form in tissues); and small amounts of hydroxocobalamin. Because cyanide-activated papain was used in the initial proteolytic isolation and purification of vitamin B_{12} from liver, cyanocobalamin (a stable form of the vitamin)

Table 6. Characteristics of Medically Useful Radioisotopes of Cobalt

RADIONUCLIDE	PHYSICAL HALF-LIFE	EFFECTIVE HALF-LIFE IN LIVER*	DECAY AND EMISSIONS	PRINCIPAL PHOTON ENERGIES (MeV)
^{57}Co	270 days	161 days	EC	0.122 (86%) 0.136 (10%)
^{58}Co	71.3 days	60 days	EC, β^+, γ	0.810 (99%) 0.511 (31%)
^{60}Co	5.2 years	331 days	β^-, γ	1.17 (100%) 1.33 (100%)

*Assuming a biologic half-life of 400 days. See Appendix for radiation dosimetry.

was the first cobalamin identified. It is the form most often utilized in vitamin B_{12} preparations, even though its chemical form is an artifact of the extraction process.

The vitamin B_{12} molecule (1355 daltons) is composed of a planar tetrapyrrole corrin ring with a central cobalt atom and a nucleotide side chain. Radiolabeling of vitamin B_{12} is accomplished by replacement of the central cobalt atom with a radioactive cobalt tracer (Table 6). Cobalamins are essential enzymes in at least two biochemical pathways: the adenosylcobalamin-dependent conversion of methylmalonyl CoA to succinyl CoA; and the methylcobalamin-dependent conversion of homocysteine to methionine, a pathway also intimately associated with folate metabolism. Vitamin B_{12} is essential to the synthesis of DNA, probably through a role in deoxyribosyl synthesis. This pathway has not been fully elucidated, but is clearly related to the megaloblastic changes in the bone marrow that are characteristic of vitamin B_{12} deficiency.

Total body stores of vitamin B_{12} in humans are approximately 5000 μg, of which 1000 to 1500 μg are found in the liver. Daily excretion (largely in stools) is 2 to 5 μg, resulting in a dietary absorption requirement of 5 μg per day. The daily metabolic requirement is considered to be 0.5–1.0 μg per day. The body's needs are readily satisfied by a balanced diet, which normally contains 20 to 30 μg of the vitamin each day. Vitamin B_{12} is synthesized by neither animals nor plants, but only by certain microorganisms in the soil and in the intestines and rumens of animals. As a result, virtually all human dietary B_{12} comes from animal sources, including meat and dairy products. True dietary vitamin B_{12} deficiency is extremely rare, but has been described in strict vegetarians. Because of the large body stores and small daily B_{12} requirement, deficiency does not appear until 3 to 5 years after total exclusion of dietary B_{12} or development of malabsorption.

In humans, dietary B_{12} is dissociated from binding proteins in the food by enzymatic and acidic action of the gastric contents, and is bound to specific B_{12} binding proteins in the stomach (R-proteins). At the same time, IF is secreted into the gastric contents, and moves with the R-protein-bound B_{12} into the proximal small bowel, where pancreatic enzymes separate B_{12} from the R-proteins and allow it to bind to IF. The IF-B_{12} complex then passes on to the distal ileum, where specific mucosal receptors bind the complex in the presence of calcium and an alkaline pH. The vitamin B_{12} separates from IF, diffuses or is transported across the mucosal cell, then binds in the portal circulation to transcobalamin II (TCII), a 36,000-dalton plasma protein that carries the absorbed B_{12} to the liver and other tissues. Over the next several hours, much of this absorbed B_{12} reappears in circulation bound to transcobalamin I (TCI), a 120,000-dalton binding protein that acts as a longer-term transport reservoir for the body's vitamin B_{12} needs. Should the amount of vitamin B_{12} in plasma surpass the carrier protein capability, free vitamin B_{12} is excreted rapidly through the kidneys by glomerular filtration, a process that is central to the effectiveness of the Schilling test.

Vitamin B_{12} deficiency can develop under the following circumstances:

I. Inadequate intake
II. Malabsorption
  A. Due to gastric abnormalities
    1. Absence of intrinsic factor
      a. congenital causes
      b. Addisonian pernicious anemia
      c. total or subtotal gastrectomy
    2. Excessive excretion of hydrochloric acid: Zollinger-Ellison syndrome
  B. Due to intestinal malabsorption
    1. Destruction, removal, or functional incompetence of mucosal absorptive sites in the distal ileum
    2. Competition with host for available dietary vitamin B_{12}
      a. Diphyllobothrium latum (fish tapeworm)
      b. small bowel lesions associated with stagnation and bacterial overgrowth (e.g., jejunal diverticula, strictures, blind loops)
    3. Pancreatic insufficiency
    4. Drug therapy
      a. para-aminosalicylic acid (PAS)
      b. neomycin
      c. colchicine
      d. calcium-chelating agents
  C. Due to genetic abnormality in the transport protein

transcobalamin II, characterized by an inability to properly bind and transport B_{12}

Usually, vitamin B_{12} deficiency results from one of these forms of malabsorption. Thus, the ability to measure vitamin B_{12} absorption, with and without IF, is essential for the proper diagnosis of pernicious anemia and its differentiation from other types of impaired vitamin B_{12} absorption.

ABSORPTION TESTS

Schilling Test. The most frequently utilized procedure for diagnosing malabsorption of vitamin B_{12} was described by Robert F. Schilling in 1953 and is based upon the following fact: if the body is flooded with parenteral vitamin B_{12} shortly after oral administration of a tracer dose of radiolabeled vitamin B_{12}, much of the labeled B_{12} that is absorbed is excreted (by glomerular filtration) because the circulating binding proteins are saturated.[182,183] Thus, in normal individuals, a 24-hour urine collection started at the time of the tracer dose administration contains greater than 10% of the tracer. In IF deficiency, less than 6% of vitamin B_{12} is excreted in the 24-hour urine, and normal excretion is found on a repeat study (usually 2 to 5 days later) if IF is added to the oral tracer. A 24-hour value of 6 to 10% is considered suspicious, but not diagnostic. Most pernicious anemia patients fall well below 6%. Because the procedure depends upon glomerular filtration of the absorbed tracer, false-positive results can occur in the presence of renal failure or urinary retention. This potential problem can be minimized by extending the urine collection over 48 hours.

The total amount of oral vitamin B_{12} administered must be no more than 2.0 μg, because higher doses result in lower fractional absorptions and may surpass the specific IF binding mechanism that is being tested. Also, meticulous collection of the entire 24-hour urine output is essential. Maximum renal excretion of tracer occurs 8 to 12 hours after the oral dose administration, so that a urine sample missed during this time can introduce a substantial error in the direction of abnormality. Urine creatinine, measured on a 24-hour collection, may help evaluate completeness of the urine collection. Excretion of less than 1 g per 24 hours should call the completeness of collection into question.

Chronic vitamin B_{12} deficiency can produce atrophic changes in the intestinal mucosa itself, which result in impaired absorptive capability. In such cases, there may only be minor correction of Schilling test results at the first administration of IF. A repeat study following 2 to 3 months of vitamin B_{12} therapy, after recovery of the mucosa from vitamin B_{12} deficiency, would demonstrate full correction into the normal range of B_{12} excretion with added IF.

The presence and mechanism of vitamin B_{12} malabsorption can also be determined by a modified Schilling test, in which vitamin B_{12} labeled with 2 different isotopes of cobalt (^{57}Co and ^{58}Co) is administered in a single oral dose. One form is already bound to IF by prior incubation with normal human gastric juice, and the other is "free." Normal patients excrete equivalent amounts of both isotopes, while patients lacking intrinsic factor excrete subnormal amounts of the "free" B_{12} but greater quantities of IF-bound B_{12}. Patients with lesions of the small bowel that result in B_{12} malabsorption excrete both isotopes in subnormal quantities. Appropriate corrections for scatter contributions in the 2 gamma counting channels must be made. The chief concern with this combined test is the possibility of unbound isotope exchanging with the IF-bound activity. Appreciable exchange might cause false-negative results. This is of particular concern because such an outcome might prevent effective treatment and lead to irreversible nerve damage.

The availability of ^{57}Co vitamin B_{12} bound to normal human gastric juice offers an alternative to the hog intrinsic factor which is used routinely in many countries and, at times, demonstrates variable potency. Inactive hog IF preparations fail to correct vitamin B_{12} malabsorption caused by IF deficiency, which leads to erroneous conclusions. In addition, some patients with vitamin B_{12} malabsorption that results from IF deficiency (e.g., patients with pernicious anemia) may in the past have taken oral preparations that contained hog intrinsic factor; thus, they may have developed antibodies to this protein. These patients cannot absorb radiolabeled vitamin B_{12} bound to hog IF, but can normally absorb B_{12} bound to human gastric juice.

In patients with vitamin B_{12} malabsorption due to bacterial overgrowth (small intestinal diverticula or blind loops), the malabsorption is not corrected by the addition of IF. In these subjects, treatment with broad-spectrum antibiotics restores normal vitamin B_{12} absorption, as a normal Schilling test without IF after therapy will demonstrate (this is sometimes referred to as a Schilling test part 3).

The usual procedure for the Schilling test is as follows:[184]

1. After an overnight fast, the patient is given 0.5 μCi (18.5 kBq) ^{57}Co-labeled vitamin B_{12} orally in 0.5 μg total vitamin B_{12}. A diluted standard is made, and two 2.0-mL samples are pipetted into counting tubes for dose standards. If there is any possibility of prior tracers in the patient, a 12-hour baseline urine is collected prior to the test (we do this routinely). Immediately after the oral B_{12} tracer dose has been given, the patient begins a complete 24-hour urine collection. If renal failure is present or suspected, 2 24-hour collections are made and pooled prior to assay.
2. One to 2 hours after the oral tracer, 1.0 mg of nonradioactive vitamin B_{12} is injected intramuscularly.
3. At the end of the 24-hour collection, the total volume is measured, and 2 2.0-mL aliquots are counted in a properly calibrated well counter with the 2 standard tubes.
4. The percentage of injected dose excreted over the 24-hour period is calculated. Normal patients excrete greater than 10%, and patients with malabsorption excrete less than 6%. Excretion of 6 to 10% is considered suspicious, but not diagnostic.
5. If the result is low or suspicious, the test is repeated a

few days later, using 0.5 μCi ^{57}Co-labeled B_{12} precomplexed to human IF. Both oral preparations are available in standard commercial kits.

Whole-Body Retention. The most sensitive and accurate method of measuring vitamin B_{12} absorption utilizes ^{60}Co- (or ^{58}Co) labeled vitamin B_{12} and whole-body counting. The oral dose is again administered in 0.5 μg of vitamin B_{12}, a whole-body count is obtained during the next several hours, and the whole-body count is repeated 7 days later. Correcting for decay if ^{58}Co is used, the ratio of the seventh-day count to the first-day count represents the fractional absorption. Normal individuals absorb 45 to 80% of the tracer; malabsorption results in a value well below 45%. Once again, correction of the abnormal absorption with IF confirms the diagnosis of pernicious anemia. Unlike the Schilling test, this procedure does not require administration of a loading dose of cold vitamin B_{12}. The major disadvantage of this procedure is the general unavailability of whole-body counters. A simplified technique for whole-body counting using a scintillation camera and ^{57}Co-B_{12} has been described by Cardarelli et al.[185]

Whole-body retention of the tracer can also be calculated by a quantitative 7- to 10-day stool collection and stool radiocobalt measurement, but the risk of sample loss and the need for stool homogenization and aliquoting discourage this method.

Other Methods. Because radiolabeled vitamin B_{12} is progressively absorbed and bound to TC II over an 8- to 12-hour period, one technique for measuring absorption requires only a single blood sample 8 hours after tracer administration. With a correction for the size of the plasma volume, this procedure permits a reasonably accurate measure of absorption. Both "free" and IF-bound vitamin B_{12} labeled with 2 cobalt radioisotopes can be measured in a single 8-hour blood sample. False-negative results have been reported, however, in patients with Addisonian pernicious anemia. The risk of an occasional false-positive result from an incomplete urine collection in a Schilling test is more acceptable medically than the risk of an occasional false-negative result by the plasma-counting technique.

Finally, Glass et al. noted in 1954 that the substantial hepatic uptake of absorbed vitamin B_{12} could be used to estimate absorption by hepatic probe counting after oral tracer administration, with or without IF.[186] Because unabsorbed bowel activity may be present for several days, however, the hepatic count is best obtained 1 week later, which makes this a lengthy procedure. In addition, radiocobalt from previous studies may persist in the liver for months or years, which introduces a background correction problem. The in vivo probe count does not give a quantitative measure of absorption, nor even of hepatic uptake, so that quantitation and comparisons are inaccurate. The presence of liver disease also would further reduce the accuracy of this method. Consequently, the Glass hepatic uptake test cannot be recommended.

SERUM VITAMIN B_{12} DETERMINATION BY RADIOLIGAND ASSAY

A common procedure for measuring serum vitamin B_{12} is a competitive binding radioligand assay that uses ^{57}Co-labeled B_{12} as the tracer and IF or cobinamide-blocked R-proteins as the ligand.[187] Normal serum vitamin B_{12} levels are 180 to 900 pg/mL, with abnormally low values falling below 130 pg/mL. The 130 to 180 pg/mL range is considered suspicious, but not diagnostic of vitamin B_{12} deficiency. Because it requires 3 to 5 years to deplete body B_{12} stores through malabsorption, the Schilling test becomes positive long before the serum vitamin B_{12} falls below normal. In a patient suspected of having vitamin B_{12} deficiency, collection of the blood sample for serum vitamin B_{12} level prior to the Schilling test is essential because the loading dose of vitamin B_{12} immediately elevates serum levels into or above the normal range. Elevated serum B_{12} values may be found in chronic myelogenous leukemia, apparently because of the release of large amounts of R-proteins (nonspecific B_{12}-binding proteins) from the increased numbers of granulocytes. Elevated values also may be found in polycythemia vera because of increased circulating R-proteins.

Several authors have reported falsely normal serum B_{12} concentrations in patients with pernicious anemia in relapse.[188–195] Cooper and Whitehead noted that 5 out of 43 patients with pernicious anemia had normal serum B_{12} levels by radioligand assay, but low levels by microbiological assay.[196] They ascribed this discrepancy to the fact that cobalamin analogs in plasma might falsely elevate the serum B_{12} determination when unblocked R-proteins are used as the ligand. Kolhouse et al. confirmed this theory in a study of 21 patients.[197] False-negative results occurred for 8 patients when R-proteins were used as the ligand, but no false-negative results occurred when IF was used as the ligand.

In a prospective survey of 919 laboratories that used 13 commercial B_{12} radioligand assay kits, Reynoso and MacKenzie found that the addition of 400 pg/ml cobinamide (a cobalamin analog) did not interfere with the accuracy of the cyanocobalamin assay when purified IF or cobinamide-blocked R-protein was used, but that cobinamide did introduce an error in 2 of the 13 kits when unblocked R-protein was used.[198] Thus, there is the potential for error in using unblocked R-protein as the cobalamin binder, and most kits have been modified to correct for this.[199] Clearly, the optimum ligand is purified IF.

Radioactive vitamin B_{12} can be used in vitro to test gastric juice for IF content.[200] It is especially useful in following some childhood endocrinopathies and prepernicious anemia states. This assay is based on the fact that, unlike IF-bound B_{12}, free B_{12} is absorbed by charcoal-coated protein. The patient's gastric juice is titrated with tracer B_{12} with and without charcoal, and the binding that occurs is compared with that in a similar titration to which antibody to intrinsic factor has been added. The amount of binding inhibited by the antibody reflects the IF level present. With a pool of normal human gastric juice, the same method can be used to detect and measure antibody to intrinsic factor.

Folic Acid

Like cyanocobalamin, folic acid is a vitamin of the B complex that is essential for normal cellular proliferation in many biologic systems. A deficiency in either folic acid or vitamin B_{12} may result in megaloblastic anemia, so that proper evaluation of the absorptive ability and the body stores of both coenzymes is essential in patients with a megaloblastic marrow. As indicated previously, the management of megaloblastic anemia is associated with the risk that treating vitamin B_{12} deficiency with folic acid may ameliorate the anemia, but permit permanent neurological damage to develop or progress. For this reason, the physiology and pathophysiology of both compounds and their relative roles in nutritional anemias must be understood.

PHYSIOLOGY AND PATHOPHYSIOLOGY OF FOLATE METABOLISM

The term *folic acid* is applied to the compound pteroylmonoglutamic acid, the parent compound of a group of related structures referred to as "folates." There are three segments to the pteroylmonoglutamate molecule: a pteridene residue, a para-aminobenzoic acid residue, and an L-glutamic acid residue. The first two segments constitute the pteroyl structure; at its gamma-carboxyl group, the L-glutamic acid residue may link to other glutamic acid residues to form the large family of pteroylpolyglutamates (Fig. 34).

Folic acid participates in many biochemical reactions in vivo as a one-carbon donor and acceptor (largely in methyl, hydroxymethyl, and formyl groups). For this role, it must first be reduced to dihydrofolic acid and then to 5,6,7,8-tetrahydrofolic acid, the metabolically active form. Its essential role in pyrimidine (thymidylate) synthesis is apparently responsible for the impairment of DNA synthesis and the resultant megaloblastic anemia in folate deficiency. Folic acid also plays an essential role in purine synthesis, methionine synthesis, histidine catabolism, and the interconversion of serine and glycine.

The average adult diet contains 400 to 600 μg of folates. Following ingestion, folates are absorbed predominantly in the proximal jejunum by a process that appears to be partly active transport and, at higher doses, partly passive diffusion. Because the human small bowel absorbs predominantly the monoglutamates, and only to a lesser extent the diglutamates and triglutamates, gastrointestinal conjugates, which probably reside on the mucosal cell border, are necessary to permit breakdown and absorption of most dietary folates. There are high folate levels in many vegetables and some fruits, as well as in such animal sources as liver and kidney. Body

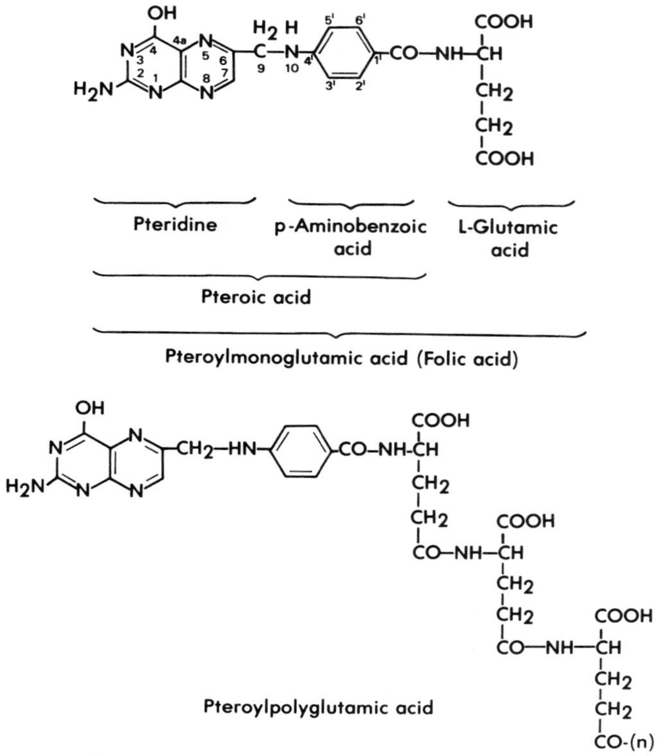

Pteridine — p-Aminobenzoic acid — L-Glutamic acid

Pteroic acid

Pteroylmonoglutamic acid (Folic acid)

Pteroylpolyglutamic acid

Figure 34. Molecular structure of folate residues.

stores of folates are approximately 5 mg, and the minimum daily requirement is 50 μg. Because body stores are proportionately smaller than those of vitamin B_{12}, loss of folate intake due to dietary change or malabsorption produces the deficiency state much sooner, as early as 4 months.[201,202]

The most common cause of folate deficiency in humans is dietary insufficiency. Because folates are both water-soluble and heat-labile, they are almost totally lost in the cooking process. Fresh fruits and uncooked or lightly cooked vegetables are the most important sources of folate in the diet.

The causes of folate deficiency in humans are outlined as follows:

- I. Inadequate intake
  - A. Primary
    - 1. poverty
    - 2. dietary faddism
  - B. Improper food preparation
  - C. Alcoholism
- II. Defective absorption
  - A. Nontropical and tropical sprue
  - B. Other malabsorption syndromes (e.g., blind loop)
  - C. Phenytoin and oral contraceptives
- III. Impaired utilization
  - A. Alcohol
  - B. Vitamin B_{12} deficiency
  - C. Folic acid antagonists
- IV. Increased requirement
  - A. Pregnancy

B. Neoplasms
C. Myeloproliferative diseases
D. Hemolytic anemias
E. Refractory anemias

In contrast with vitamin B_{12}, there are no practical techniques available for measuring folate absorption in humans on a routine basis, although ^{14}C- and tritium-labeled folic acid have been utilized in research studies.

BLOOD FOLATE DETERMINATION BY RADIOLIGAND ASSAY

For many years, the only procedure available for measuring serum and red cell folate levels was a microbiological assay that utilized the folate dependence of bacterial growth as the indicator (*Lactobacillus casei, Streptococcus faecalis,* or *Pediococcus cervisiae*).[203–205] Although the microbiological assay is accurate for pteroylmonoglutamic acid in biologic samples, it is lengthy and complex, and antibiotic therapy can interfere with the procedure; for this reason, a simpler and more reliable method has been sought.

Following discovery that cow's milk contains specific folate-binding proteins,[206] milk-derived folate binders were incorporated into several commercially available competitive radioligand assays for folic acid. These assays use tritiated folic acid or an ^{125}I-labeled pteroylglutamic acid derivative as the quantifiable indicator.[207] Because folate-binding proteins are also present in human serum, these assay procedures require a 15-minute boiling step for inactivation of the serum folate binders and liberation of the folate prior to measurement. In the radioassay technique, pteroylpolyglutamates produce somewhat variable results, whereas the microbiological assay produces a linear response following sample treatment with folate conjugase. Consequently, the microbiological assay remains the preferred procedure for measuring folates in foods and in body tissues, where polyglutamates predominate.[208]

Folic acid turns over rapidly in plasma. In one study, the blood disappearance half-time of tritiated folic acid was reported to be less than 1 minute.[209] As a result, the serum folate level is a complex and rapidly changeable reflection of recent dietary intake, body stores, and ongoing exchange between blood and body tissues. Because the red cell folate content is more stable and more representative of body stores, it is thought to reflect the body's nutritional folate status better. It is the recommended measurement for evaluation of folate deficiency.

Normal serum folate levels by radioassay are approximately 1.9 to 14.0 ng/mL, and normal red cell folate levels are 120 to 674 ng/mL. These ranges vary slightly from one laboratory and commercial kit to another. As can be suspected from the high red-cell values, avoidance of any hemolysis of the test blood is essential when performing the serum assay.

Chen et al. have described a radiometric microbiological assay technique in which the production of $^{14}CO_2$ from D-1-^{14}C-gluconate by *Lactobacillus casei* indicates functional folate present in biologic samples.[210] This method combines the advantages of radioisotopic tracer measurement with the relevance of a true functional assay for folate.

Iron Absorption and Serum Ferritin

The general features of iron metabolism in humans have been reviewed in the section "Ferrokinetics and the Study of Erythropoiesis." Additional background will be presented, however, for the following discussion on measurement of iron absorption and the evaluation of body iron stores.

Iron in humans is absorbed as the ferrous ion by a process of active transport, predominantly in the proximal small bowel. Because the rate of iron excretion is relatively fixed and is beyond direct physiological control, the body's nutritional iron status is modulated primarily by absorption. Daily iron loss averages 1 mg in adult males. As a result of menstruation and pregnancies, the dietary iron needs of adult females can be substantially greater. Normal daily iron absorption is approximately 1 mg per day from the 10 to 20 mg present in an average daily diet (Fig. 1). In the presence of iron deficiency, this can increase substantially, possibly mediated by the ferritin-apoferritin content of the mucosal cells.

Routine measurement of iron absorption is not of practical assistance in diagnosing iron deficiency. Diagnosis of this common hematologic disorder is best made by determining the serum iron, the serum total and unsaturated iron binding capacity, the serum ferritin, and the marrow iron stores. Iron absorption is measured only occasionally in physiological studies, and in characterizing the pathophysiological aspects of such diseases as hemochromatosis and sideroachrestic anemias.

Several representative articles have summarized our current understanding of ferritin.[211–214] Excess iron is stored in the body in ferritin and in hemosiderin, which appears to be a partially denatured and partially deproteinized form of ferritin. Ferritin is a large, complex protein consisting of a central core of iron in the form of ferric oxyhydroxide crystals, and an outer protein shell called *apoferritin* (441,000 daltons). The apoferritin shell consists of 24 similar subunits (*monomers*) of 163 amino acids each, which form a sort of cube with rounded corners. There are 4 monomers lying in the plane of each face of the cube. Iron diffuses into the center of the cube through the interstices between the monomers and is reduced to the divalent form and complexed with oxygen and hydroxyl groups. Then, it is deposited in a ferric oxyhydroxide crystalline matrix that is trapped inside the apoferritin. As many as 4300 iron atoms can be stored inside an apoferritin molecule although, under normal physiological circumstances, the average is approximately 2000.

Much of the body's ferritin is stored in the reticuloendothelial system as a reservoir form of this trace element, but ferritin also circulates freely in plasma in equilibrium with body stores. Consequently, serum ferritin levels usually reflect the body stores of ferritin and, thus, iron. Serum ferritin is low in iron deficiency and is elevated in such iron-loaded states as hemochromatosis, thalassemia, and sideroachrestic anemias. Falsely elevated levels of serum ferritin are found in acute inflammatory diseases, liver disease, chronic renal disease, and some malignancies (especially lymphomas, chronic granulocytic leukemia, and acute leukemias). Such neoplasms as hepatoma and breast carcinoma may have locally increased tissue ferritin levels, with or without increased blood levels. Because some of these nonspecific factors alter circulating ferritin concentrations, serum ferritin is of only moderate usefulness in evaluating body iron stores. It has been of some current interest as a tumor marker for radioimmunoscintigraphy and possibly for radionuclide therapy.[215]

MEASUREMENT OF IRON ABSORPTION

There are several methods for quantifying iron absorption. Because the information obtained is rarely important to patient diagnosis or management, however, these methods are not used routinely. The most accurate technique utilizes whole-body counting after the oral administration of 1 to 10 μCi (37 to 370 kBq) ^{59}Fe in 0.25 to 5 mg carrier iron as ferrous sulfate.[216–218] Whole-body counts are obtained 4 hours after ingestion (100% value) and 7 to 10 days later to determine the retained activity.[219] The amount of carrier iron must lie within the range of 0.25 to 5 mg, which simulates the iron content of a single meal and results in a normal absorption range of 5 to 25%. Sargent et al. combined the reticulocyte count with iron absorption values as a better reflection of erythropoiesis.[218] This approach results in a tighter range for normals.

Total body retention of an oral ^{59}Fe tracer dose can be estimated also by quantitative stool collections over 7 days and counting of a mixed stool aliquot against a precalibrated standard. This procedure incorporates all of the difficulties of obtaining and sampling a complete 7-day stool collection. Saylor and Finch devised a dual-isotope technique in which a tracer dose of ^{55}Fe is given intravenously along with the oral dose of ^{59}Fe.[220] The relative percentage of incorporation of the 2 isotopes in the circulating erythrocytes 7 to 10 days later gives a fairly accurate measurement of the percentage of ^{59}Fe that was absorbed. In such diseases as hemochromatosis, however, which involve high hepatic iron extraction during first passage through the portal blood, this method may result in a substantial error in calculating iron absorption.

Elevated iron absorption is seen most often in iron deficiency. Any type of anemia, however, increases iron absorption; the increase varies according to the degree of anemia.[221] Iron absorption is increased in hemochromatosis, whether or not an excessive iron load is present.[218] Decreased iron absorption occurs in the various forms of sprue and small bowel malabsorption. In fact, in a patient with sprue, high iron absorption may indicate that iron deficiency is more likely the result of blood loss than of malabsorption.

SERUM FERRITIN ASSAY

Serum ferritin can be measured with high accuracy and sensitivity by 1 of 4 immunometric techniques:[211,222]

One-Site Immunoradiometric Assay (IRMA-1). With this procedure, a radioisotopic label is attached to an antiferritin antibody, which is in excess relative to the ferritin present. After equilibrium with serum ferritin, the unbound radiolabeled antibody is adsorbed to an immunoadsorbent and removed by centrifugation, so that the supernatant radioactivity is proportional to the original amount of ferritin.

Two-Site Immunoradiometric Assay (IRMA-2). A "sandwich" technique is used in this assay. Unlabeled antiferritin antibody is attached in excess to the incubation tube or to glass beads. Then the test serum is added so that the ferritin binds to the fixed antibody present, and an additional radiolabeled antiferritin antibody is added in excess. The labeled antibody binds to the ferritin already attached to the first antibody. After rinsing off the unbound radiolabeled antibody, the remaining radioactivity is directly related to the original ferritin concentration.

Radioimmunoassay (RIA). This is a traditional RIA in which the test plasma ferritin competes with a predetermined amount of radiolabeled ferritin for a limited number of available antibody binding sites. The resulting ferritin-antiferritin complex is then precipitated by a second antibody, centrifuged down, and counted.

Enzyme-Labeled Immunosorbent Assay (EIA, ELISA). This procedure is identical to the IRMA-2 procedure, except that the second-stage antibody is conjugated to an enzyme, such as alkaline phosphatase or peroxidase. After removal of the unbound second antibody at the end of the incubation, a substrate indicator is added, and the remaining enzyme is quantified spectrophotometrically or fluorometrically by the enzyme action on the indicator.

Normal Serum Ferritin Level. The normal serum ferritin level is 14 to 250 ng/mL in adult males (mean: 69 ng/mL), 10 to 155 ng/mL in premenopausal adult females (mean: 34 ng/mL), and 6 to 333 ng/mL in postmenopausal adult females.

REFERENCES

1. Lawrence JH. Nuclear physics and therapy: Preliminary report on a new method for the treatment of leukemia and polycythemia. *Radiology* 1940;35:51.
2. Hahn L, Hevesy G. A method of blood volume determination. *Acta Physiol Scand* 1940;1:3.
3. Gray SJ, Sterling K. The tagging of red cells and plasma proteins with radioactive chromium. *J Clin Invest* 1950; 29:1604.
4. Gregersen MI, Rawson RA. Blood volume. *Physiol Rev* 1959;39:307.
5. International Committee for Standardization in Haematology

(ICSH): Recommended methods for radioisotope red-cell survival studies. *Br J Haematol* 1980;45:659.
6. Pollycove M, Tono M. Studies of the erythron. *Semin Nucl Med* 1975;5:11.
7. Wright RR, Tono M, Pollycove M. Blood volume. *Semin Nucl Med* 1975;5:63.
8. International Committee for Standardization in Haematology (ICSH): Recommended methods for radioisotope platelet survival studies. *Blood* 1977;50:1137.
9. International Committee for Standardization in Haematology (ICSH): Recommended methods for measurement of red-cell and plasma volume. *J Nucl Med* 1980;21:793.
10. Mathias CJ, Welch MJ. Radiolabeling of platelets. *Semin Nucl Med* 1984;14:118.
11. Pope CF, Sostman HD. Radioisotope labeled platelets in medical diagnosis. *Invest Radiol* 1986;21:611.
12. Koblik PD, De Nardo GL, Berger HJ. Current status of immunoscintigraphy in the detection of thrombosis and thromboembolism. *Semin Nucl Med* 1989;19:221.
13. Knight LC. Radiopharmaceuticals for thrombus detection. *Semin Nucl Med* 1990;20:52.
14. Srivastava SC, Straub RF. Blood cell labeling with ^{99m}Tc: Progress and perspectives. *Semin Nucl Med* 1990;20:41.
15. Thakur ML. Radiolabeled blood cells: Perspectives and directions. *Nucl Med Biol* 1990;17:41.
16. De Vries RA, De Bruin M, Marx JJM, Van De Wiel A. Radioisotopic labels for blood cell survival studies: a review. *Nucl Med Biol* 1993;20:809.
17. Datz FL. Indium-111-labeled leukocytes for the detection of infection: Current status. *Semin Nucl Med* 1994;24:92.
18. Peters AM. The utility of [^{99m}Tc]HMPAO-leukocytes for imaging infection. *Semin Nucl Med* 1994;24:110.
19. Becker W, Goldenberg DM, Wolf F. The use of monoclonal antibodies and antibody fragments in the imaging of infectious lesions. *Semin Nucl Med* 1994;24:142.
20. Fischman AJ, Babich JW, Rubin RH. Infection imaging with technetium-99m-labeled chemotactic peptide analogs. *Semin Nucl Med* 1994;24:154.
21. Fischer J, Wolf R, Leon A. Technetium-99m as a label for erythrocytes. *J Nucl Med* 1967;8:229.
22. Korubin V, Maisey MN, and McIntyre PA. Evaluation of technetium-labeled red cells for determination of red cell volume in man. *J Nucl Med* 1972;13:760.
23. Eckelman W, Richards P, Hauser W, et al. Technetium labeled red blood cells. *J Nucl Med* 1971;12:22.
24. Eckelman WC, Reba RC, Albert SN. A rapid simple improved method for the preparation of Tc^{99m} red blood cells for the determination of red cell volume. *Am J Roentgenol Radium Ther Nucl Med* 1973;118:861.
25. Ferrant A, Lewis SM, Szur L. The elution of ^{99m}Tc from red cells and its effect on red-cell volume measurement. *J Clin Pathol* 1974;27:983.
26. Smith TD, Richards P. A simple kit for the preparation of Tc-99m-labeled red blood cells. *J Nucl Med* 1976;17:126.
27. Eckelman WC, Smith TD, Richards P, et al. Labeling blood cells with ^{99m}Tc, in Subramanian G et al. (eds): *Radiopharmaceuticals*. New York, Society of Nuclear Medicine, 1975:49–54.
28. Gutkowski RF, Dworkln HJ. Kit-produced Tc-99m-labeled red cells for spleen imaging. *J Nucl Med* 1974;15:1187.
29. Ansari AN, Atkins HL, Smith T, et al. Clinical application of BNL ^{99m}Tc RBC labeling kit. *J Nucl Med* 1975;16:512.
30. Srivastava SC, Chervu LR. Radionuclide-labeled red blood cells: Current status and future prospects. *Semin Nucl Med* 1984;14:68.
31. McRae J, Valk PE. Alteration of ^{99m}Tc red blood cells. *J Nucl Med* 1972;13:399.
32. McRae J, Sugar RM, Shipley BA, et al. Alterations in tissue distribution of ^{99m}Tc pertechnetate in rats given stannous tin. *J Nucl Med* 1974;15:151.
33. Pavel DG, Zimmer AM, Patterson VN. In vivo labeling of red blood cells with Tc: A new approach to blood pool visualization. *J Nucl Med* 1977;18:305.
34. Srivastava SC, Richards P, Yonekura Y, et al. Long-term retention of tin following in vivo RBC labeling. *J Nucl Med* 1982;23:P91.
35. Callahan RJ, Froelich JW, McKusick KA, et al. A modified method for the in vivo labeling of red blood cells with Tc-99m. Concise communication. *J Nucl Med* 1982;23:315.
36. Porter WC, Dees SM, Freitas JE, Dworkin HJ. Acid-citrate-dextrose compared with heparin in the preparation of in vivo/in vitro Technetium-99m red blood cells. *J Nucl Med* 1983;24:383.
37. Callahan RJ, Rabito CA. Radiolabeling of erythrocytes with technetium-99m: Role of band-3 protein in the transport of pertechnetate across the cell membrane. *J Nucl Med* 1990; 31:2004.
38. Dewanjee MK, Rao SA, Penniston GT. Mechanisms of red blood cell labeling with ^{99m}Tc-pertechnetate. The role of the cation pump at RBC membrane on the distribution and binding of Sn^{2+} and ^{99m}Tc with the membrane proteins and hemoglobin. *J Label Comp Radiopharm* 1982;19:1464.
39. Dewanjee MK. Binding of ^{99m}Tc ion to hemoglobin. *J Nucl Med* 1974;15:703.
40. Rehani MM, Sharma SK. Site of Tc-99m binding to the red blood cell: Concise communication. *J Nucl Med* 1980;21:676.
41. Hladik III WB, Nigg KK, Rhodes BA. Drug-induced changes in the biologic distribution of radiopharmaceuticals. *Semin Nucl Med* 1982;12:184.
42. Lee HB, Wexler JP, Scharf SC, et al. Pharmacologic alterations in Tc-99m binding by red blood cells. Concise communication. *J Nucl Med* 1983;24:397.
43. Leitl GP, Drew HM, Kelly ME, et al. Interference with Tc-99m labeling of red blood cells (RBCs) by RBC antibodies. *J Nucl Med* 1980;21:44.
44. Ries C. Platelet kinetics in autoimmune thrombocytopenia: Relation between splenic platelet sequestration and response to splenectomy. (Letter to the editor). *Ann Intern Med* 1977;86:194.
45. Thakur ML, Welch MJ, Joist JG, Coleman RE. Indium-111 labeled platelets: Studies on preparation and evaluation of in vitro and in vivo functions. *Thromb Res* 1976;9:345.
46. Scheffel U, McIntyre PA, Evatt B, et al. Evaluation of Indium-111 as a new high photon yield gamma-emitting "physiological" platelet label. *Johns Hopkins Med J* 1977;140:285.
47. Wistow BW, Grossman ZD, McAfee JG, et al. Labeling of platelets with oxine complexes of Tc-99m and In-111. Pt. 1. In vitro studies and survival in the rabbit. *J Nucl Med* 1978;19:482.
48. Goodwin DA. Cell labeling with oxine chelates of radioactive metal ions: Techniques and clinical implications. *J Nucl Med* 1978;19:557.
49. Scheffel U, Tsan M-F, McIntyre PA. Labeling of human platelets with (^{111}In) 8-hydroxyquinoline. *J Nucl Med* 1979;20: 524.
50. Heaton WA, Davis HH, Welch MJ, et al. Indium-111: A new radionuclide label for studying human platelet kinetics. *Br J Haematol* 1979;42:613.
51. Thakur ML, Walsh L, Malech HL, Gottschalk A. Indium-111-labeled human platelets: Improved method, efficacy, and evaluation. *J Nucl Med* 1981;22:381.
52. Scheffel U, Tsan M-F, Mitchell TG, et al. Human platelets labeled with In-111 8-hydroxyquinoline: Kinetics, distribution and estimates of radiation dose. *J Nucl Med* 1982;23:149.

53. McAfee JG, Thakur ML. Survey of radioactive agents for in vitro labeling of phagocytic leukocytes. I. Soluble agents. *J Nucl Med* 1976;17:480.
54. McAfee JG, Thakur ML. Survey of radioactive agents for in vitro labeling of phagocytic leukocytes. II. Particles. *J Nucl Med* 1976;17:488.
55. Coleman RE, Welch MJ, Thakur ML. Preparation and evaluation of leukocytes labeled with Indium-111, in *Medical Radionuclide Imaging*. Vol. 11. Vienna, International Atomic Energy Agency, 1977, p 47.
56. Segal AW, Thakur ML, Arnot RN, Lavender JP. Indium-111 labeled leukocytes for localization of abscesses. *Lancet* 1976; 2:1056.
57. Thakur ML, Lavender JP, Arnot RN, et al. Indium-111 labeled autologous leukocytes in man. *J Nucl Med* 1977;18:1014.
58. Bothwell TH, Charlton RW, Cook JD, Finch CA. *Iron Metabolism in Man*. Oxford, Blackwell Scientific Publications, 1979.
59. Eckelman W, Richards P, Hauser W, Atkins H. Technetium-labeled red blood cells. *J Nucl Med* 1971;12:22.
60. Hegde UM, Williams ED, Lewis SM, et al. Measurement of splenic red cell volume and visualization of the spleen with Tc-99m. *J Nucl Med* 1973;14:769.
61. Silvergleid AJ, Wells RF, Hafleigh EB, et al. Compatibility test using Cr-51-labeled red blood cells in crossmatch positive patients. *Transfusion* 1978;18:8.
62. Pineda AA, Dharkar DD, Wahner HW. Clinical evaluation of a ^{51}Cr-labeled red blood cell survival test for in vivo blood compatibility testing. *Mayo Clin Proc* 1984;59:25.
63. Cronkite EP, Bond VP, Fliedner TM, Killmann SA. The use of tritiated thymidine in the study of hemopoietic cell proliferation. Ciba Found. Sympos. *Haemopoiesis*. London, Churchill Livingstone, 1960, p 70.
64. Athens JW, Mauer AM, Ashenbrucker H, et al. Leukokinetic studies. I. A method for labeling leukocytes with diisopropylfluorophosphate (DFP^{32}). *Blood* 1959;14:303.
65. Cartwright GE, Athens JW, Boggs DR, Wintrobe MM. The kinetics of granulopoiesis in normal man. *Series Haemat* 1965;1:1.
66. Athens JW, Raab SO, Haab OP, et al. Leukokinetic studies. III. The distribution of granulocytes in the blood of normal subjects. *J Clin Invest* 1961;40:159.
67. Athens JW, Haab OP, Raab SO, et al. Leukokinetic studies. IV. The total blood, circulating and marginal granulocyte pools and the granulocyte turnover rate in normal subjects. *J Clin Invest* 1961;40:989.
68. McMillan K, Scott JL, Marino IV. Leukocyte labeling with Cr-51. 1. Technique and results in normal subjects. *Blood* 1968;32:738.
69. Marcus CS, Kuperus JH, Butler JA, et al. Phagocytic labeling of leukocytes with ^{99m}Tc-albumin colloid for nuclear imaging. *Nucl Med Biol* 1988;15:673.
70. McAfee JG, Gagne GM, Subramanian G, et al. Distribution of leukocytes labeled with In-111 oxine in dogs with acute inflammatory lesions. *J Nucl Med* 1980;21:1059.
71. Sino H, Silvester DJ. Simplified cell labeling with Indium-111 acetylacetone. *Br J Radiol* 1979;52:758.
72. Dewanjee MK, Rao SA, Didisheim P. Indium-111 tropolone, a new high-affinity platelet label: Preparation and evaluation of labeling parameters. *J Nucl Med* 1981;22:981.
73. Thakur ML, Seifert CL, Madsen MT, et al. Neutrophil labeling: Problems and pitfalls. *Semin Nucl Med* 1984;14:107.
74. McAfee JR, Subramanian G, Gagne G. Technique of leukocyte harvesting and labeling: Problems and perspectives. *Semin Nucl Med* 1984;14:83.
75. McDougall IR, Baumert JE, Lantieri RL. Evaluation of In-111 leukocyte whole body scanning. *Am J Radiol* 1979;133:849.
76. Sfakianakis GN, Al-Sheikh W, Heal A, et al. Comparisons of scintigraphy with In-111 leukocytes and Ga-67 in the diagnosis of occult sepsis. *J Nucl Med* 1982;23:618.
77. Lilien DL, Berger HG, Anderson DP, Bennett LR. In-111-chloride: A new agent for bone marrow imaging. *J Nucl Med* 1973;14:184.
78. Marker LA, Slichter SJ. Platelet and fibrinogen consumption in man. *N Engl J Med* 1972;287:999.
79. Aster RH. Pooling of platelets in the spleen: Role in the pathogenesis of "hypersplenic" thrombocytopenia. *J Clin Invest* 1966;45:645.
80. Murphy EA, Robinson GA, Rowsell HC, Mustard JF. The pattern of platelet disappearance. *Blood* 1967;30:26.
81. Lotter MG, Heyns AD, Badenhorst PN, et al. Evaluation of mathematical models to assess platelet kinetics. *J Nucl Med* 1986;27:1192.
82. Sweetlove MA, Lotter MG, Roodt JP, et al. Blood platelet kinetics in normal subjects modelled by compartmental analysis. *Eur J Nucl Med* 1992;19:1023.
83. Ries CA, Price DC. (^{51}Cr) Platelet kinetics in thrombocytopenia: Correlation between splenic sequestration of platelets and response to splenectomy. *Ann Intern Med* 1974;80:702.
84. Murphy EA, Mustard JF. Coagulation tests and platelet economy in atherosclerotic and control subjects. *Circulation* 1962;25:114.
85. Abrahamsen AF. Platelet survival studies in man. *Scand J Haematol* (Suppl)1968;3:1.
86. Mustard JF, Murphy EA, Robinson GA, et al. Blood platelet survival. *Thromb Diath Haemorrh* (Stuttg.) (Suppl)1964; 13:245.
87. Gietz M, Mempel W, Clemm C, et al. Value of preoperative thrombocyte marking in patients with idiopathic thrombocytopenic purpura. *Klin Wochenschr* 1988;66:633.
88. Naouri A, Feghali B, Chabal J, et al. Results of splenectomy for idiopathic thrombocytopenic purpura. Review of 72 cases. *Acta Haematol* 1993;89:200.
89. Lamy T, Moisan A, Dauriac C, et al. Splenectomy in idiopathic thrombocytopenic purpura: its correlation with the sequestration of autologous indium-111-labeled platelets. *J Nucl Med* 1993;34:182.
90. International Committee for Standardization in Hematology. Panel on Diagnostic Applications of Radionuclides: Recommended method for indium-111 platelet survival studies. *J Nucl Med* 1988;29:564.
91. Tisdale PL, Collier BD, Kauffman HM, et al. Early diagnosis of acute postoperative renal transplant rejection by indium-111-labeled platelet scintigraphy. *J Nucl Med* 1986;27:1266.
92. Davis HH, Siegel BA, Sherman LA, et al. Scintigraphic detection of carotid atherosclerosis with Indium-111-labeled autologous platelets. *Circulation* 1980;61:982.
93. Price DC, Lipton MJ, Lusby RJ, et al. In vivo detection of thrombi with indium-111-labeled platelets. *IEEE NS* 1982; 29:1191.
94. Ezekowitz MD, Leonard JC, Smith EO, et al. Identification of left ventricular thrombi in man using Indium-111-labeled autologous platelets. A preliminary report. *Circulation* 1981;63:803.
95. Stratton JR, Ritchie JL, Hamilton GW, et al. Left ventricular thrombi: In vivo detection by Indium-111 platelet imaging and two dimensional echocardiography. *Am J Cardiol* 1981;47:874.
96. Ezekowitz MD, Cox AC, Smith EO, Taylor FB. Failure of aspirin to prevent incorporation of Indium-111 labeled platelets into cardiac thrombi in man. *Lancet* 1981;2:440.
97. Riba AL, Thakur ML, Gottschalk A, Zaret BL. Imaging experimental coronary artery thrombosis with Indium-111 platelets. *Circulation* 1979;60:767.

98. Ritchie JL, Stratton JR, Thiele B, et al. Indium-111-platelet imaging for detection of platelet deposition in abdominal aneurysms and prosthetic arterial grafts. *Am J Cardiol* 1981;47:882.
99. Fuster V, Dewanjee MK, Kaye MP, et al. Non-invasive radioisotopic technique for detection of platelet deposition in coronary artery bypass grafts in dogs and its reduction with platelet inhibitors. *Circulation* 1979;60:1508.
100. Ezekowitz MD, Pope CF, Sostman HD, et al. Indium-111 platelet scintigraphy for the diagnosis of acute venous thrombosis. *Circulation* 1986;73:668.
101. Smith N, Chandler S, Hawker RJ, et al. Indium-labeled autologous platelets as diagnostic aid after renal transplantation. *Lancet* 1979;2:1241.
102. Knight LC, Primeau JL, Siegel BA, Welch MJ. Comparison of In-111-labeled platelets and iodinated fibrinogen for the detection of deep vein thrombosis. *J Nucl Med* 1978;19:891.
103. Moser KM, Spragg RG, Bender F, et al. Study of factors that may condition scintigraphic detection of venous thrombi and pulmonary emboli with Indium-111-labeled platelets. *J Nucl Med* 1980;21:1051.
104. Davis HH, Siegel BA, Sherman LA, et al. Scintigraphy with In-111-labeled autologous platelets in venous thromboembolism. *Radiology* 1980;136:203.
105. Fenech A, Hussey JK, Smith FW, et al. Diagnosis of deep vein thrombosis using autologous Indium-111-labeled platelets. *Br Med J* 1981;282:1020.
106. Grimley RP, Rafigqui E, Hawker RJ, Drolc Z. Imaging of In-111-labeled platelets—A new method for the diagnosis of deep vein thrombosis. *Br J Surg* 1981;68:714.
107. McIlmoyle G, Davis HH, Welch MJ, et al. Scintigraphic diagnosis of experimental pulmonary embolism with In-111-labeled platelets. *J Nucl Med* 1977;18:910.
108. Goodwin DA, Bushberg JT, Doherty PW, et al. Indium-111-labeled autologous platelets for location of vascular thrombi in humans. *J Nucl Med* 1978;19:626.
109. Hidalgo JU, Nadler SB, Bloch T. The use of the electronic digital computer to determine best fit of blood volume formulas. *J Nucl Med* 1962;3:94.
110. Nadler SB, Hidalgo JU, Bloch T. Prediction of blood volume in normal human adults. *Surgery* 1962;51:224.
111. Wennesland R, Brown E, Hopper J, et al. Red cell, plasma and blood volume in healthy men measured by radiochromium (Cr-51) cell tagging and hematocrit: Influence of age, somatotype and habits of physical activity on the variance after regression of volumes to height and weight combined. *J Clin Invest* 1959;38:1065.
112. Brown E, Hopper J, Hodges JL, et al. Red cell, plasma, and blood volume in healthy women measured by radiochromium cell-labeling and hematocrit. *J Clin Invest* 1962;41:2182.
113. Frenkel EP, McCall MS, Reisch JS, Minton PO. An analysis of methods for the prediction of normal erythrocyte mass. *J Clin Pathol* 1972;58:260.
114. Lohrmann HP, Heimpel H. The use of Tc-99m-pertechnetate for the determination of red cell volume. *Klin Wochenschr* 1973;51:141.
115. Ferrant A, Lewis SM, Szur L. The elution of Tc-99m from red cells and its effect on red-cell volume measurement. *J Clin Pathol* 1974;27:983.
116. Ducassou D, Arnaud D, Bardy A, et al. A new stannous agent kit for labeling red blood cells with Tc-99m and its clinical application. *Br J Radiol* 1976;49:344.
117. Holt JT, Spitalnik SL, Wilson G. Inhibition of chromium-51 RBC labeling by stannous pyrophosphate. *J Nucl Med* 1982;23:934.
118. Ellis RE. The distribution of active bone marrow in the adult. *Phys Med Biol* 1961;5:255.
119. Van Dyke D, Shkurkin C, Price D, et al. Differences in distribution of erythropoietic and reticuloendothelial marrow in hematologic disease. *Blood* 1967;30:364.
120. Merrick MV, Gordon-Smith EG, Lavender JP, Szur L. A comparison of In-111 with Fe-52 and Tc-99m-sulfur colloid for bone marrow scanning. *J Nucl Med* 1975;16:66.
121. Nelp WB, Larson SM, Lewis RJ. Distribution of the erythron and the RES in the bone marrow organ. *J Nucl Med* 1967;8:430.
122. Nelp WB, Bower RE. The quantitative distribution of the erythron and the RE cell in the bone marrow organ of man. *Blood* 1969;34:276.
123. Anger HO, Van Dyke DC. Human bone marrow distribution shown in vivo by Iron-52 and the positron scintillation camera. *Science* 1964;144:1587.
124. McNeil BJ, Holman BL, Button LN, Rosenthal DS. Use of indium chloride scintigraphy in patients with myelofibrosis. *J Nucl Med* 1974;15:647.
125. McNeil BJ, Rappoport JM, Nathan DG. Indium chloride scintigraphy: An index of severity in patients with aplastic anemia. *Br J Haematol* 1976;34:599.
126. Gilbert EH, Earle JD, Glatstein E, et al. In-111 bone marrow scintigraphy as an aid in selecting marrow biopsy sites for the evaluation of marrow elements in patients with lymphoma. *Cancer* 1976;38:1560.
127. Gilbert EH, Earle JD, Goris MD, et al. The accuracy of indium-111-chloride as a bone marrow scanning agent. *Radiology* 1976;119:167.
128. Gilbert EH, Glatstein E, Goris ML, Earle JD. Value of In-111-chloride bone marrow scanning in the differential diagnosisof blood count depression in lymphoma. *Cancer* 1978;41:143.
129. Beamish MR, Brown EB. The metabolism of transferrin-bound In-111 and Fe-59 in the rat. *Blood* 1974;43:693.
130. Beamish MR, Brown EB. A comparison of the behavior of In-111 and Fe-59-labeled transferrin on incubation with human and rat reticulocytes. *Blood* 1974;43:703.
131. McIntyre PA, Larson SM, Eikman EA, et al. Comparison of the metabolism of iron-labeled transferrin (Fe-TF) and indium-labeled transferrin (In-TF) by the erythropoietic marrow. *J Nucl Med* 1974;15:856.
132. Rayudu GVS, Shirazi SP, Fordham EW. Comparison of the use of Fe-52 and In-111 for hemopoietic marrow scanning. *Int J Appl Radiat Isot* 1973;24:451.
133. Edwards CL, Andrews GA, Sitterson BW, Kniseley RM. Clinical bone marrow scanning with radioisotopes. *Blood* 1964;23:741.
134. Kniseley RM, Andrews GA, Tanida R, et al. Delineation of active marrow by whole-body scanning with radioactive colloids. *J Nucl Med* 1966;7:575.
135. Kniseley RM. Marrow studies with radiocolloids. *Semin Nucl Med* 1972;2:71.
136. McAfee JG, Subramanian G, Aburano T, et al. A new formulation of Tc-99m minimicroaggregated albumin for marrow imaging: Comparison with other colloids, In-111 and Fe-59. *J Nucl Med* 1982;23:21.
137. Duncker CM, Carrio I, Berna L, et al. Radioimmune imaging of bone marrow in patients with suspected bone metastases from primary breast cancer. *J Nucl Med* 1990;31:1450.
138. Berna L, Germa JR, Estorch M, et al. Bone marrow regeneration after hormonal therapy in patients with bone metastases from prostate carcinoma. *J Nucl Med* 1991;32:2295.
139. Desai AG, Thakur ML. Radiopharmaceuticals for spleen and bone marrow studies. *Semin Nucl Med* 1985;15:229.
140. Arrago JP, Rain JD, Vigneron N, et al. Diagnostic value of bone marrow imaging with ^{111}indium-transferrin and ^{99m}technetium colloids in myelofibrosis. *Am J Hematol* 1985;18:275.

141. Sykes MP, Chu FCH, Savel H, et al. The effects of varying dosages of irradiation upon sternal marrow regeneration. *Radiology* 1964;83:1084.
142. Nelp WB, Gohil MN, Larson SM, Mower RF. Long term effects of local irradiation of the marrow on erythron and red cell function. *Blood* 1970;36:617.
143. Rubin P, Landman S, Meyer E, et al. Bone marrow regeneration and extension after extended field irradiation in Hodgkin's disease. *Cancer* 1973;32:699.
144. Sacks EL, Goris ML, Glatstein E, et al. Bone marrow regeneration following large field radiation. *Cancer* 1978;42:1057.
145. Hill DR, Benak SB, Phillips TL, Price DC. Bone marrow regeneration following fractionated radiation therapy. *Int J Radiat Oncol Biol Phys* 1980;6:1149.
146. Knospe WH, Rayudu VMS, Cardello M, et al. Bone marrow scanning with iron-52. Regeneration and extension of marrow after ablative doses of radiotherapy. *Cancer* 1976;37:1432.
147. Rubin P. Regeneration of bone marrow in rabbits following local fractionated irradiation. *Cancer* 1973;32:847.
148. Judisch JM, McIntyre PA. Recognition of metastatic neuroblastoma by scanning the reticuloendothelial system (RES). *Johns Hopkins Med J* 1972;130:83.
149. Price DC, Hattner RS. Comparison of bone and bone marrow scintigraphy in the evaluation of malignant disease. (Abstr) *J Nucl Med* 1975;16:559.
150. Datz FL, Taylor A Jr. The clinical use of radionuclide bone marrow imaging. *Semin Nucl Med* 1985;15:239.
151. Reske SN. Recent advances in bone marrow scanning. *Eur J Nucl Med* 1991;18:203.
152. DeLand FH. Normal spleen size. *Radiology* 1970;97:589.
153. Hamilton RG, Alderson PO, Harwig JF, Siegel BA. Splenic imaging with Tc-99-labeled erythrocytes: A comparative study of cell damaging methods. *J Nucl Med* 1976;17:1038.
154. Johnson PM, Herion JC, Mooring SL. Scintillation scanning of the normal human spleen utilizing sensitized radioactive erythrocytes. *Radiology* 1960;74:99.
155. Winkelman JW, Wagner HN Jr, McAfee JG, Mozley JM. Visualization of the spleen in man by radioisotope scanning. *Radiology* 1960;75:465.
156. Eckelman W, Richards P, Atkins HL, et al. Visualization of the human spleen with Tc99m-labeled red blood cells. *J Nucl Med* 1971;12:310.
157. McIntyre PA, Wagner HN Jr. Current procedures for scanning of the spleen. *Ann Int Med* 1970;73:995.
158. Wagner HN Jr, Weiner IM, McAfee IG, Martinez J. 1-mercuri-2-hydroxy-propane (MHP). A new radiopharmaceutical for visualization of the spleen by radioisotope scanning. *Arch Intern Med* 1964;113:696.
159. Rollo FD, DeLand FH. The determination of spleen mass from radionuclide images. *Radiology* 1970;97:583.
160. Sigel RM, Becker DV, Hurley JR. Evaluation of spleen size during routine liver imaging with Tc-99m and the scintillation camera. *J Nucl Med* 1970;11:689.
161. Larson SM, Tuell SH, Moores KD, Nelp WB. Dimensions of the normal adult spleen scan and prediction of spleen weight. *J Nucl Med* 1971;12:123.
162. Hegde UM, Williams ED, Lewis SM, et al. Measurement of splenic red cell volume and visualization of the spleen with Tc-99m. *J Nucl Med* 1973;14:769.
163. Spencer RP, Pearson HA, Lange RC. Human spleen: Scan studies on growth and response to medications. *J Nucl Med* 1971;12:466.
164. Spencer RP, Pearson HA. *Radionuclide Studies of the Spleen.* Cleveland, CRC Press, 1975, p 37.
165. McIntyre PA. Diagnostic significance of the spleen scan. *Semin Nucl Med* 1972;2:278.
166. Shimshak RR, Korobkin M, Hoffer PB, et al. The complementary role of gallium citrate imaging and computed tomography in the evaluation of suspected abdominal infection. *J Nucl Med* 1978;19:262.
167. Gilday DL, Alderson PO. Scintigraphic evaluation of liver and spleen injury. *Semin Nucl Med* 1974;4:357.
168. Lutzker L, Koenigsberg M, Meng C-H, Freeman LM. The role of radionuclide imaging in spleen trauma. *Radiology* 1974;110:419.
169. Federle M, Moss AA. Computed tomography of the spleen. *CRC Crit Rev Diagn Imaging* 1983;19:1.
170. Kuni CC, Crass JR, duCret RP, et al. Technetium-99m sulfur colloid spleen imaging following partial pancreatectomy and splenic artery and vein resection. *J Nucl Med* 1989;30:1881.
171. Silverman S, DeNardo GL, Glatstein E, Lipton MJ. Evaluation of the liver and spleen in Hodgkin's disease. II. The value of splenic scintigraphy. *Am J Med* 1972;52:362.
172. Wagstaff J, Phadke K, Adam N, et al. The "hot spleen" phenomenon in metastatic malignant melanoma. *Cancer* 1982; 49:439.
173. Koh HK, Sober AJ, Kopf A, et al. Prognosis in stage 1 malignant melanoma: seven-year follow-up study of splenic radiocolloid uptake as predictor of death. *J Nucl Med* 1984;25:1183.
174. Pearson HA, Johnston D, Smith KA, Touloukian RJ. The born-again spleen. Return of splenic function after splenectomy for trauma. *N Engl J Med* 1978;298:1389.
175. Pearson HA, Spencer RP, Cornelius EA. Functional asplenia in sickle-cell anemia. *N Engl J Med* 1969;281:923.
176. Spencer RP, Dhawan V, Suresh K, et al. Causes and temporal sequence of onset of functional asplenia in adults. *Clin Nucl Med* 1978;3:17.
177. Engelstad B. Functional asplenia in hemoglobin SE disease. *Clin Nucl Med* 1982;7:100.
178. Owunwanne A, Halkar R, Al-Rasheed A, et al. Radionuclide imaging of the spleen with heat denatured technetium-99m RBC when the splenic reticuloendothelial system seems impaired. *J Nucl Med* 1988;29:320.
179. Whipple GH, Hopper GW, Robscheit FS. Blood regeneration following simple anemia. *Am J Physiol* 1920;53:151.
180. Minot GR, Murphy WP. Treatment of pernicious anemia by a special diet. *JAMA* 1926;87:470.
181. Castle WB. Observations on the etiologic relationship of achylia gastrica to pernicious anemia. *Am J Med Sci* 1929; 178:748.
182. Schilling RF. Intrinsic factor studies. II. The effect of gastric juice on the urinary excretion of radioactivity after the oral administration of radioactive B_{12}. *J Lab Clin Med* 1953; 42:860.
183. Schilling RF. Recent studies of intrinsic factor and utilization of radioactive vitamin B_{12}. *Fed Proc* 1954;13:769.
184. International Committee for Standardization in Hematology (ICSH): Recommended methods for the measurement of vitamin B_{12} absorption. *J Nucl Med* 1981;22:1091.
185. Carderelli JA, Slingerland DW, Burrows BA, Miller A. Measurement of total-body cobalt-57 vitamin B_{12} absorption with a gamma camera. *J Nucl Med* 1985;26:941.
186. Glass GBJ, Boyd LJ, Gellin GA, Stephanson L. Uptake for radioactive vitamin B_{12} and intrinsic factor activity. *Arch Biochem* 1954;51:251.
187. Pratt JJ, Woldring MG. Radioassay of vitamin B_{12} and other corrinoids. *Methods Enzymol* 1982;84:369.
188. Wide L, Killander A. A radiosorbent technique for the assay of serum vitamin B_{12}. *Scand J Clin Lab Invest* 1971;27:151.
189. Puutula L, Stenman U-H. Comparison of serum vitamin B_{12} determination by two isotope dilution methods and by Euglena assay, with special reference to low values. *Clin Chim Acta* 1974;55:263.

190. Raven JL, Robson MB, Morgan JO, Hoffbrand AV. Comparison of three methods for measuring vitamin B_{12} in serum: Radioisotopic, *Euglena gracilis* and *Lactobacillus leichmannii. Br J Haematol* 1972;22:21.
191. Van de Wiel DFM, Koster-Otte LJ, Goedemans WTH, Woldring MG. Competitive protein binding analysis of vitamin B_{12} using vitamin B_{12}-free serum as a standard diluent. *Clin Chim Acta* 1974;56:131.
192. Voogd GE, Mantel MJ. Experience with a commercial radioassay for vitamin B_{12}. *Clin Chim Acta* 1974;54:369.
193. Raven JL, Robson MB. Experience with a commercial kit for the radioisotopic assay of vitamin B_{12} in serum: The Phadebas B_{12} test. *J Clin Pathol* 1974;27:59.
194. Green R, Golman N, Metz J. Comparison of results of microbiologic and radioisotopic assays for serum vitamin B_{12} during pregnancy. *Am J Obstet Gynecol* 1975;122:21.
195. Raven JL, Robson MB. Extraction of serum vitamin B_{12} for radioisotopic and *Lactobacillus Leichmannii* assay. *J Clin Pathol* 1975;28:531.
196. Cooper BA, Whitehead VM. Evidence that some patients with pernicious anemia are not recognized by radiodilution assay for cobalamin in serum. *N Engl J Med* 1978;299:816.
197. Kolhouse FJ, Kondo H, Allen NC, et al. Cobalamin analogues are present in human plasma and can mask cobalamin deficiency because current radioisotope dilution assays are not specific for true cobalamin. *N Engl J Med* 1978;299:785.
198. Reynoso G, MacKenzie JR. Are ligand assay methods specific for cobalamin? *Am J Clin Pathol* 1982;78:621.
199. Chen IW, Silberstein EB, Maxon HR, et al. Clinical significance of serum vitamin B_{12} measured by radioassay using pure intrinsic factor. *J Nucl Med* 1981;22:447.
200. Jacob E, Baker SJ, Herbert V. Vitamin B_{12}-binding proteins. *Physiol Rev* 1980;60:918.
201. Herbert V. Minimum daily adult folate requirement. *Arch Int Med* 1962;110:649.
202. Halsted CH. Intestinal absorption and malabsorption of folates. *Ann Rev Med* 1980;31:79.
203. Baker H, Herbert V, Frank O, et al. A microbiologic method for detecting folic acid deficiency in man. *Clin Chem* 1959;5:275.
204. Herbert V. Aseptic addition method for *Lactobacillus casei* assay of folate activity in human serum. *J Clin Pathol* 1966;19:12.
205. Herbert V, Das KC. The role of vitamin B_{12} and folic acid in hemato-and other cell-poiesis. *Vitamins Horm* 1976;34:1.
206. Ghitis J. The folate binding in milk. *Am J Clin Nutr* 1967; 20:1.
207. Waxman S, Schreiber C, Herbert V. Radioisotopic assay for measurement of serum folate levels. *Blood* 1971;38:219.
208. Shane B, Tamura T, Stokstad ELR. Folate assay: A comparison of radioassay and microbiological methods. *Clin Chim Acta* 1980;100:13.
209. Johns DG, Sperti S, Burgen ASV. The metabolism of tritiated folic acid in man. *J Clin Invest* 1961;40:1684.
210. Chen MF, McIntyre PA, Kertchen JA. Measurement of folates in human plasma and erythrocytes by a radiometric microbiologic method. *J Nucl Med* 1978;19:906.
211. Fairbanks VF, Klee GG. Ferritin. *Prog Clin Pathol* 1981;8:175.
212. Aisen P, Listowsky I. Iron transport and storage proteins. *Ann Rev Biochem* 1980;49:357.
213. Halliday JW, Powell LW. Serum ferritin and isoferritins in clinical medicine. *Prog Hematol* 1979;11:229.
214. Worwood M. Serum ferritin. *CRC Crit Rev Clin Lab Sci* 1979;10:171.
215. Order SE. Monoclonal antibodies: Potential role in radiation therapy and oncology. *Int J Radiat Oncol Biol Phys* 1982; 8:1193.
216. Price DC, Cohn SH, Wasserman LR, et al. The determination of iron absorption and loss by whole body counting. *Blood* 1962;20:517.
217. Cook JD, Layrisse M, Finch CA. The measurement of iron absorption. *Blood* 1969;33:421.
218. Sargent T, Saito H, Winchell HS. Iron absorption in hemochromatosis before and after phlebotomy therapy. *J Nucl Med* 1971;12:660.
219. Schiffer LM, Price DC, Cuttner J, et al. A note concerning the "100 percent value" in iron absorption studies by whole body counting. *Blood* 1964;23:757.
220. Saylor L, Finch CA. Determination of iron absorption using two isotopes of iron. *Am J Physiol* 1953;172:372.
221. Schiffer LM, Price DC, Cronkite EP. Iron absorption and anemia. *J Lab Clin Med* 1965;65:316.
222. Halliday JW. Immunoassay of ferritin in plasma. *Methods Enzymol* 1982;84(pt D):148.

Plates

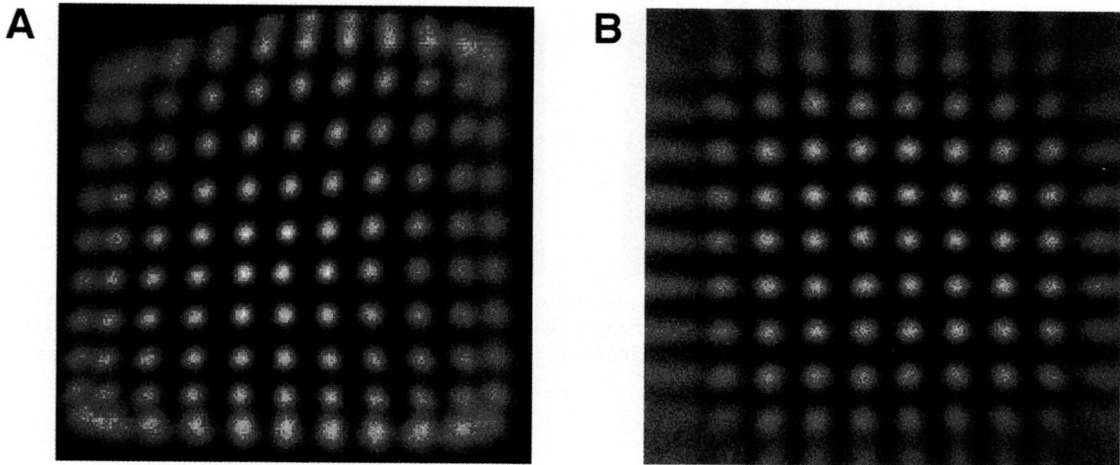

Plate 1 (Figure 5–6, p. 98). Orthogonal hole plate image before (**A**) and after (**B**) correction for spatial nonlinearities.

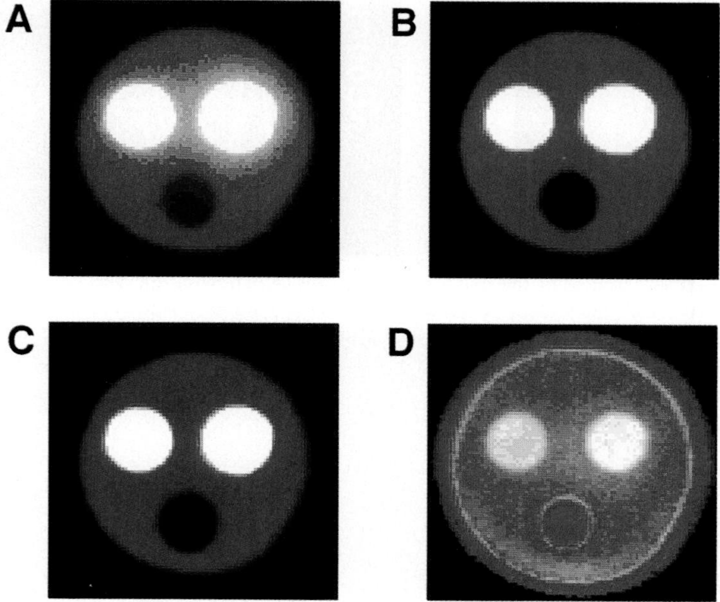

Plate 2 (Figure 5–9, p. 102). Planar, end-on images of a 20-cm diameter water-filled cylindrical "phantom" test object without scatter correction (**A**), with photopeak curve-fitting scatter correction (**B**), and with dual-window scatter correction ($K = 0.5$) (**C**). Panel (**D**) portrays spatial variations in the factor K assuming the photopeak correction method is exact.

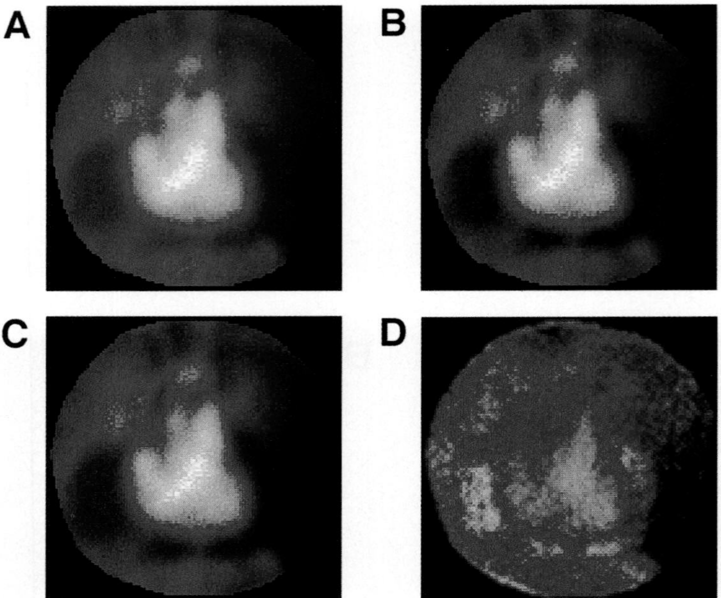

Plate 3 (Figure 5–10, p. 103). Anterior view of a patient's cardiac blood pool before scatter correction **(A)**, after scatter correction with the photopeak curve-fitting method **(B)** and after correction with the dual-window method ($K = 0.05$), **(C)**. Panel **(D)** portrays spatial variations in the factor K assuming the photopeak curve-fitting method is exact.

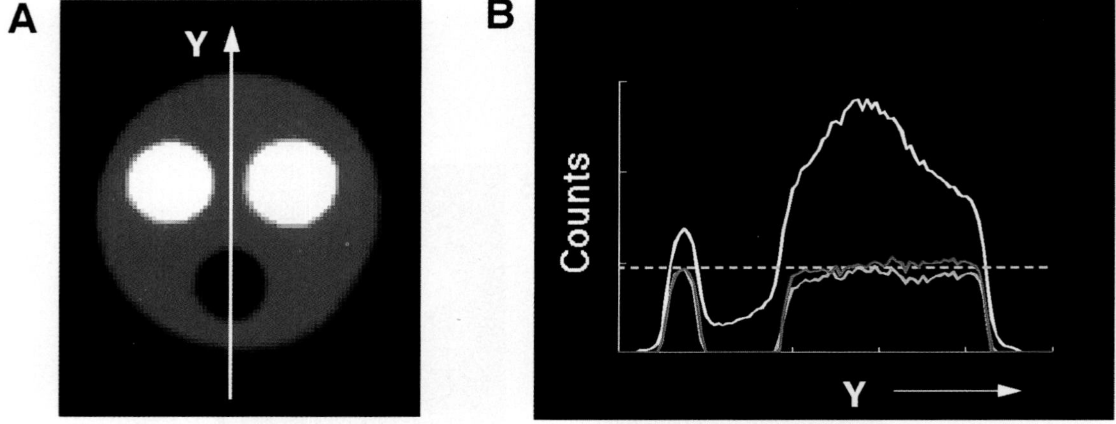

Plate 4 (Figure 5–11, p. 104). Image of the cylindrical phantom **(A)** showing the vertical path (Y) along which the count profiles shown in **(B)** were generated. White curve in **(B)** is without correction, red curve is with photopeak curve-fitting scatter correction, and blue curve is with dual-window scatter correction. Dashed horizontal line indicates true count level in warm background region.

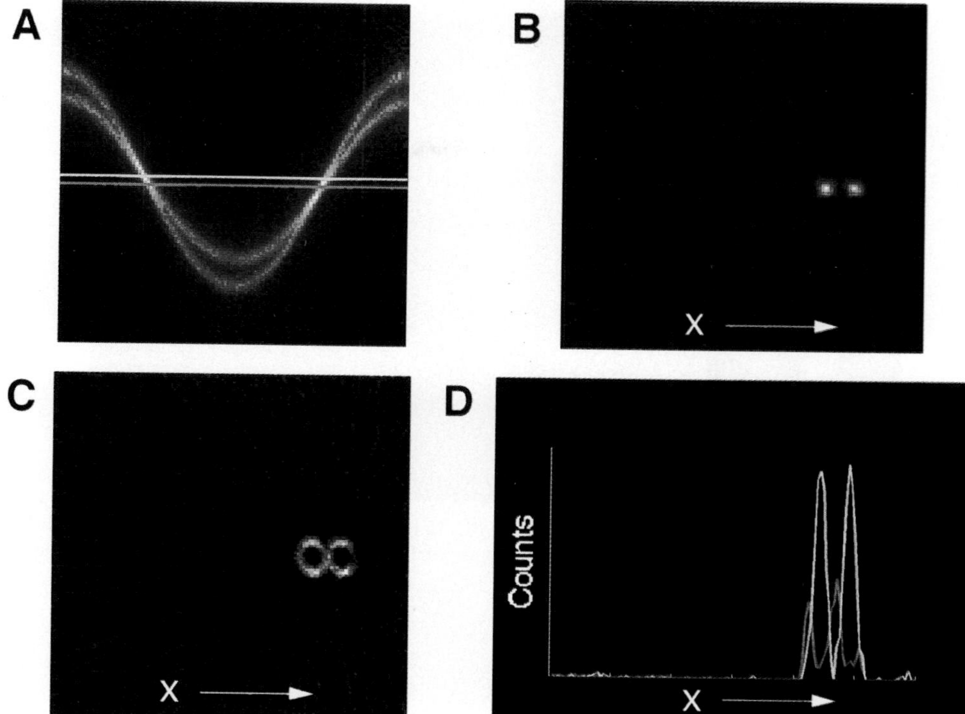

Plate 5 (Figure 5–19, p. 115). **(A).** 360° single-slice sinogram through two capillary tube sources parallel to the axis of rotation. **(B).** Transverse section image computed using the true center of rotation. **(C).** Transverse section image computed using the wrong center of rotation. **(D).** Comparison of count profiles through points in B (yellow) and C (red).

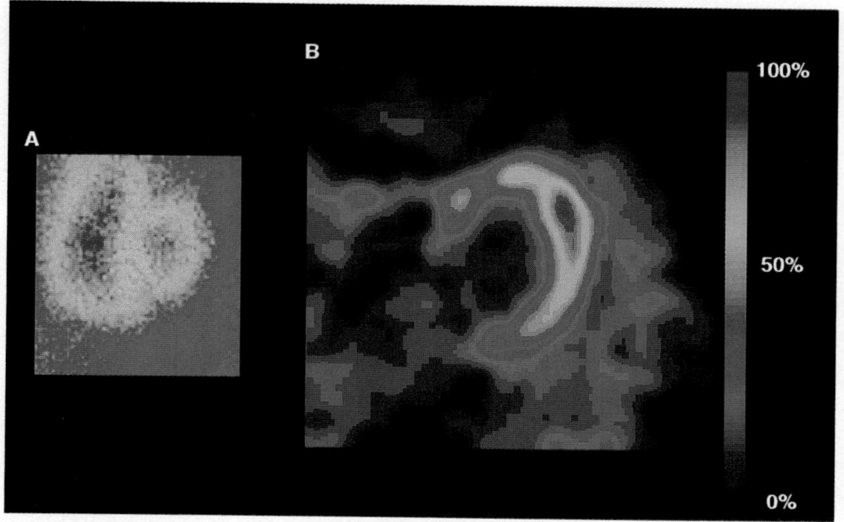

Plate 6 (Figure 7–6, p. 155). **(A).** Same image as Figure 3A, but with three (red, green, blue) LUTs rather than just one. Yellow seems to define the borders of the LV—or does it? **(B).** Same image as Figure 5B but in color. Here a color bar is shown to allow the user to translate colors into pixel values. The numbers to the right indicate percentage of maximum pixel value.

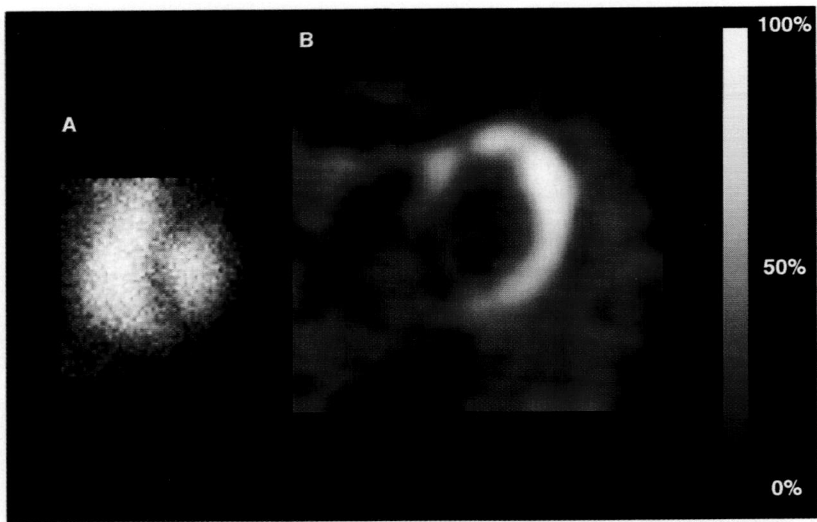

Plate 7 (Figure 7–7, p. 155). **(A).** Same image as Figure 3C, but using "hot-body" color spectrum. **(B).** Same image as Figure 5B but using "hot-body" spectrum. Artificial edges of Figure 6 are for the most part eliminated with this color LUT.

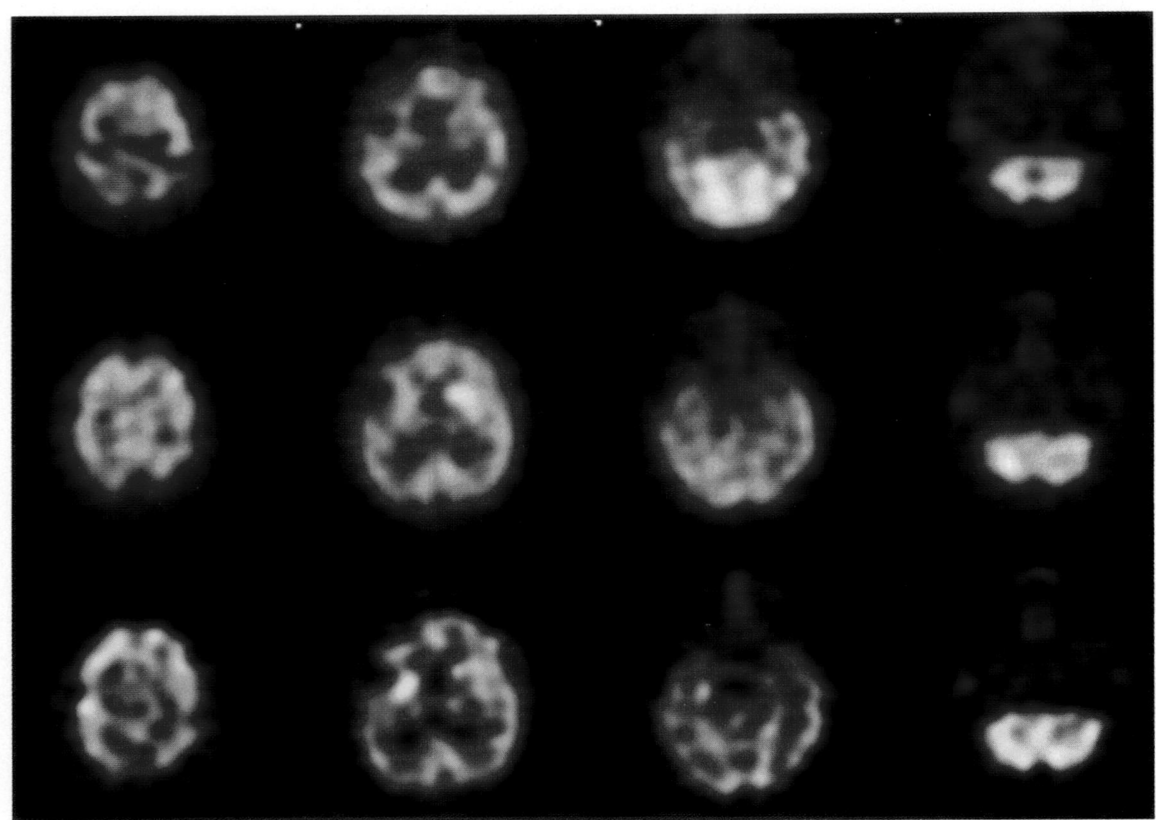

Plate 8 (Figure 17–1, p. 362). Representative HMPAO SPECT images of a 28-year-old woman with systemic lupus erythematous studied on 3 different occasions with single-head (top row), dual-head (middle row), and triple-headed (bottom) SPECT devices. Images show improved image quality with the multi-head devices, with better depiction of deep nuclei and better grey-to-white-matter contrast. (Note for this and all subsequent neurological studies, the patient's right side is on the readers' left.)

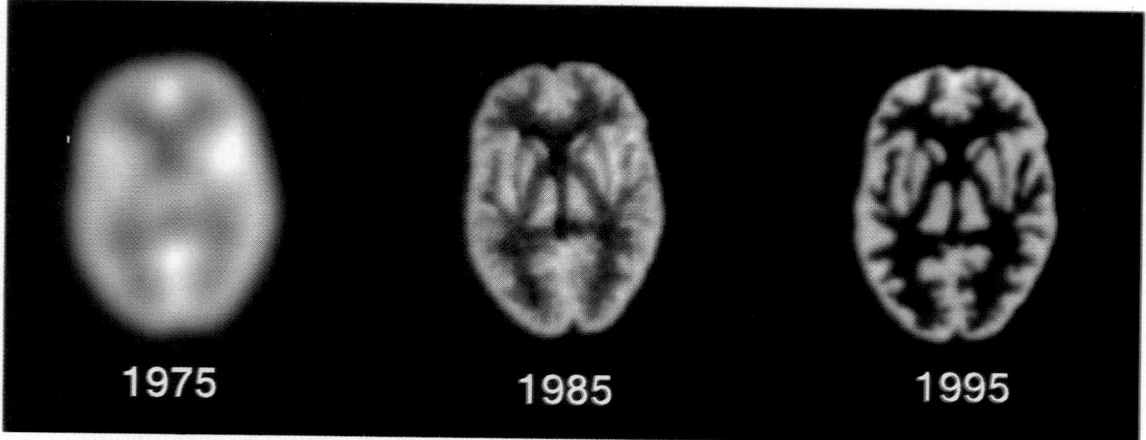

Plate 9 (Figure 17–2, p. 362). Hoffman brain phantom simulations, at level of the deep nuclei and insula, show the improvements in PET resolution over 2 decades.

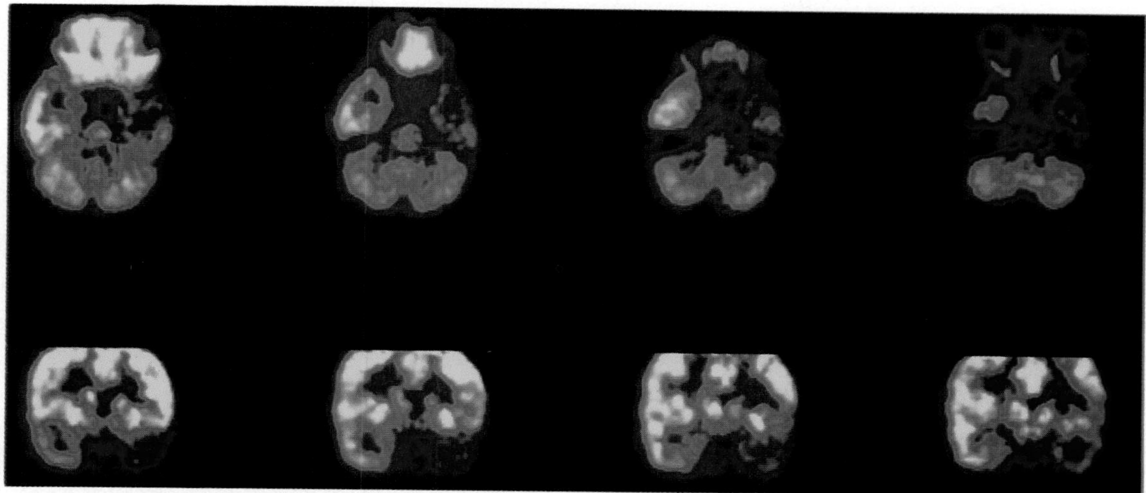

Plate 10 (Figure 17–3, p. 365). A 16-year-old boy with refractory complex partial seizures. Transaxial (top row) and coronal (bottom) FDG PET images show marked left temporal lobe glucose hypometabolism involving mesial and lateral temporal neocortex consistent with an interictal epileptic focus.

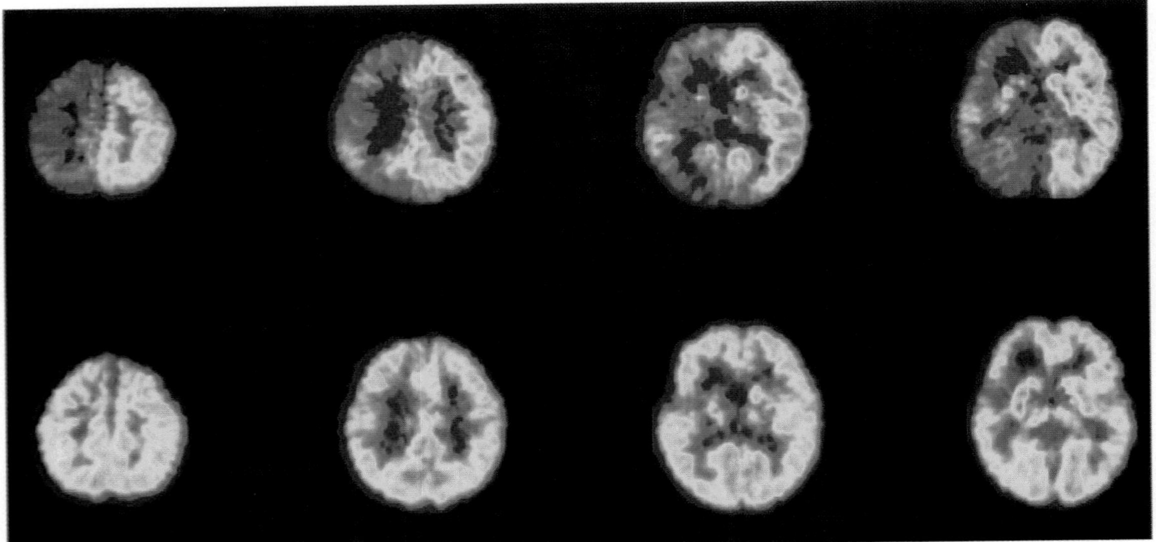

Plate 11 (Figure 17–4, p. 365). A 32-month-old child with refractory epilepsy. First FDG PET (top row) shows right hemispheric glucose hypometabolism suggesting an extensive interictal abnormality. Second study (bottom row) shows almost complete reversal of previous hemispheric hypometabolism except for reduced glucose utilization in right mid frontal lobe, indicating that most of the hypometabolism on first study was postictal.

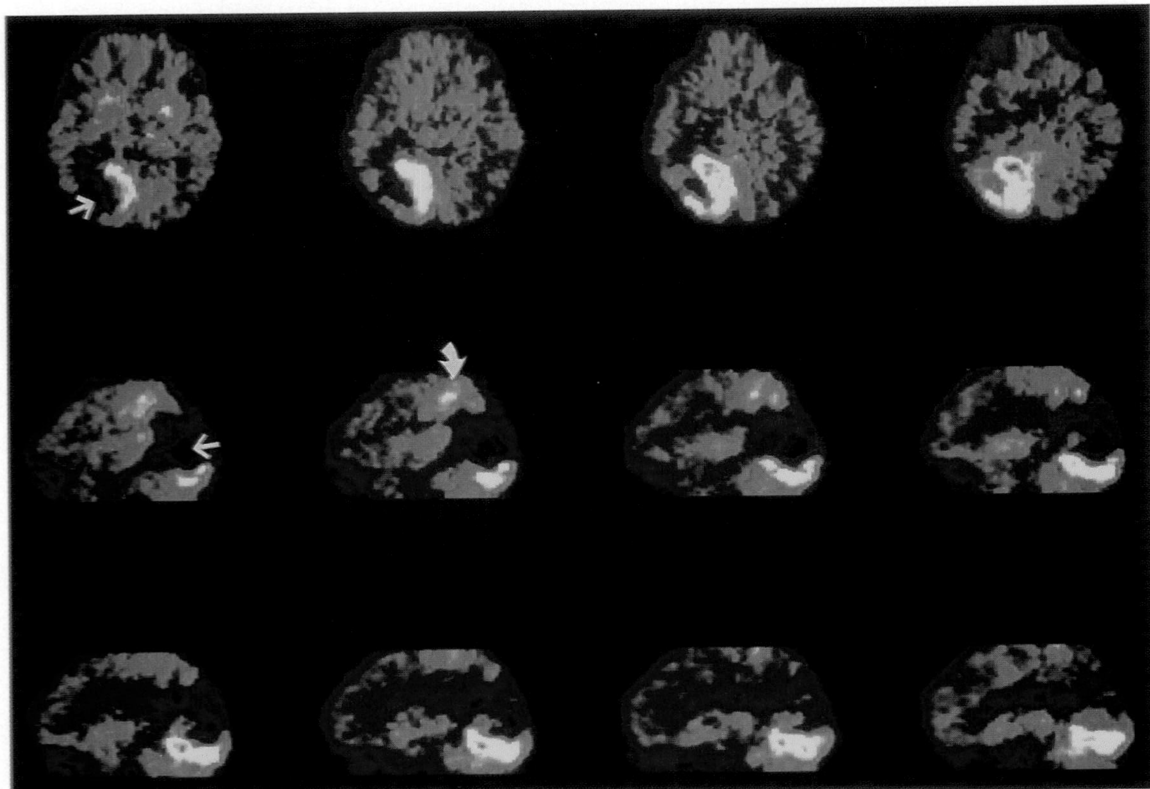

Plate 12 (Figure 17–5, p. 366). A 54-year-old man with complex partial status epilepticus. Transaxial (top row) and sagittal (middle and bottom rows) FDG PET images reveal glucose hypermetabolism in right mesial and inferolateral occipital cortex. Glucose hypermetabolism is posterior and inferior to large ametabolic region (straight arrows) in right parieto-occipital lobe, the site of previous trauma and brain abscess. Increased glucose metabolism (curved arrow) is also seen anterior to porencephalic cyst, but is much less marked than in occipital lobe. Note: there is also a marked reduction in glucose metabolism throughout rest of the brain.

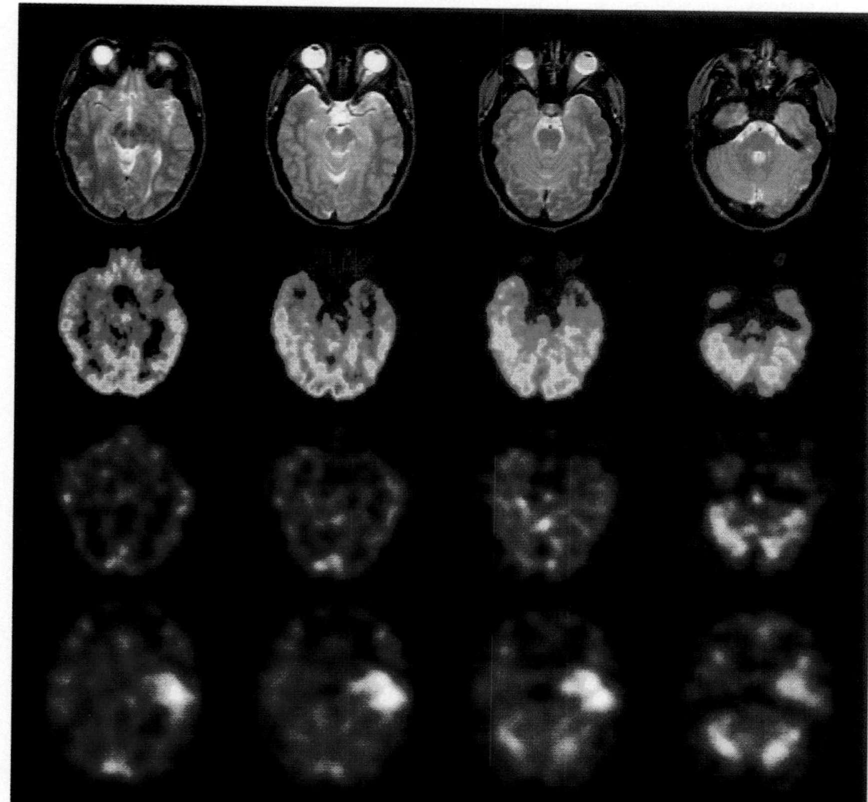

(A)

Plate 13 (Figure 17–6A, p. 367). A 31-year-old woman with complex partial seizures. Multimodality registration of **(A)** transaxial and **(B)** coronal anatomical and functional images. Functional images are registered to MR dataset performed at 1.5 Tesla. **(A).** Transaxial T2-weighted MR images (top row) show slight left temporal lobe atrophy with prominence of left sylvian fissure; left hippocampal atrophy is not evident. FDG PET (second row) reveals glucose hypometabolism of left temporal lobe affecting mesial and lateral temporal neocortex. Interictal HMPAO SPECT (third row) shows mild left temporal lobe hypoperfusion. Ictal SPECT (fourth row) shows a marked increase in left temporal (mesial and lateral) perfusion maximal in inferior and mid temporal lobe. (See below for part **B**.)

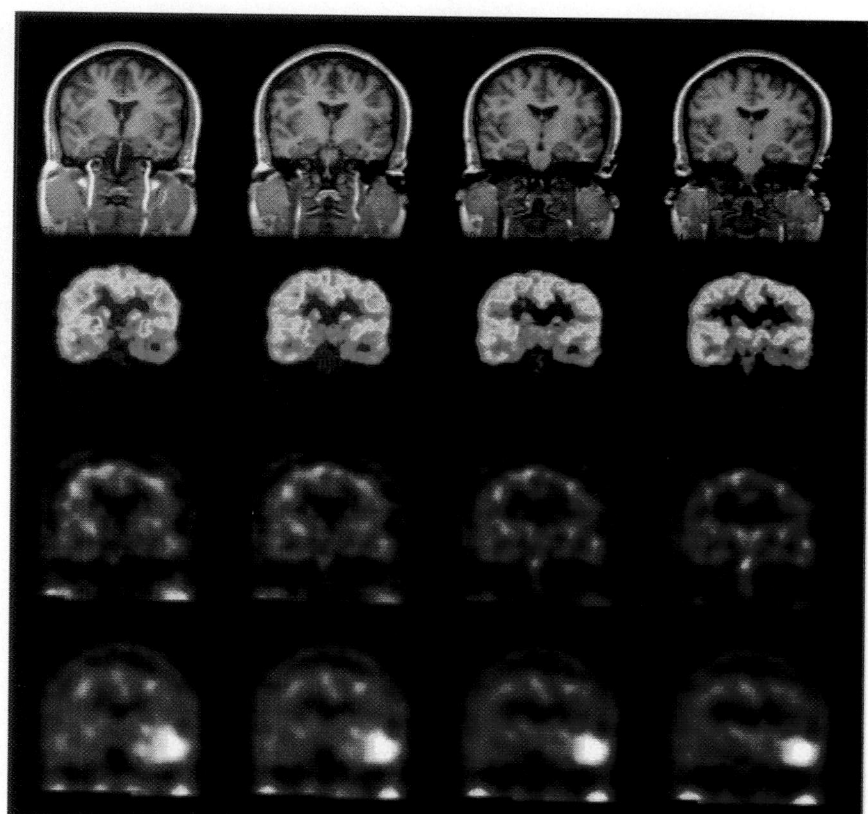

(B)

Plate 13 (cont.) (Figure 17–6B, p. 367). (B). Coronal images. T1-weighted MR images show subtle left to right temporal lobe asymmetry. On FDG PET hypometabolism affects inferomedial temporal lobe maximally. Asymmetric perfusion is difficult to appreciate on interictal SPECT but is clearly evident on ictal SPECT study, with markedly increased perfusion (lateral temporal neocortex > mesial).

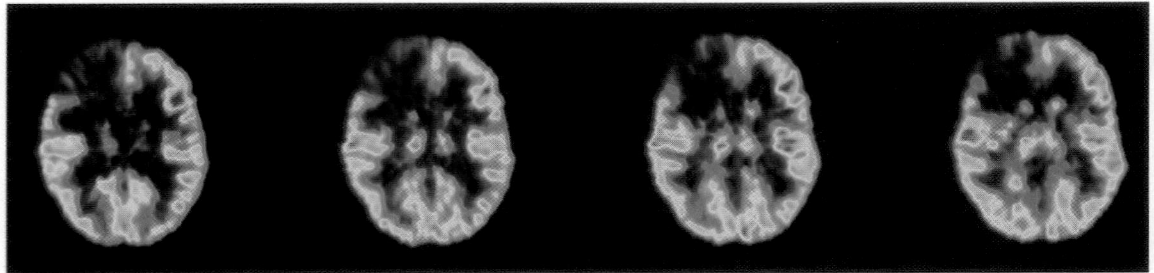

Plate 14 (Figure 17–7, p. 369). A 47-year-old woman with a low-grade glioma. Transaxial FDG PET scan shows an extensive area of glucose hypometabolism in right frontal lobe that affects white and gray matter. There are no foci of increased glucose metabolism to suggest a high-grade tumor.

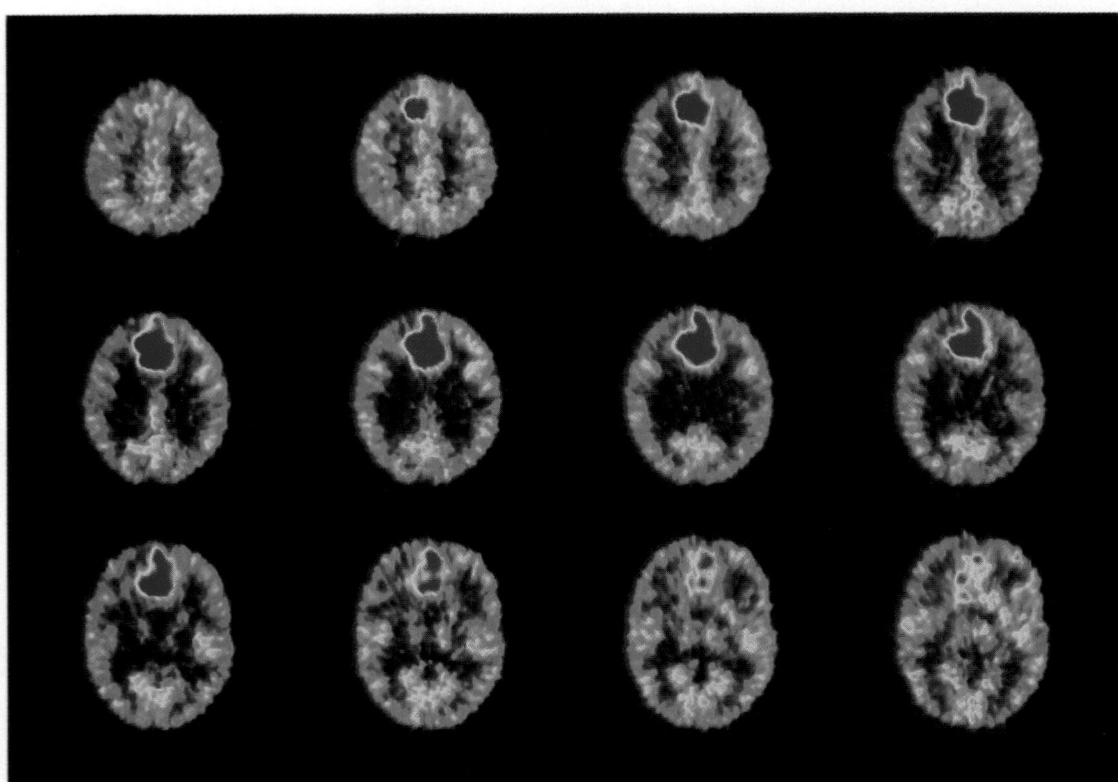

Plate 15 (Figure 17–8, p. 369). A 44-year-old man with a high-grade glioma. On transaxial FDG PET images, the tumor is markedly hypermetabolic and involves the corpus callosum and cortex and white matter of both mesia frontal lobes.

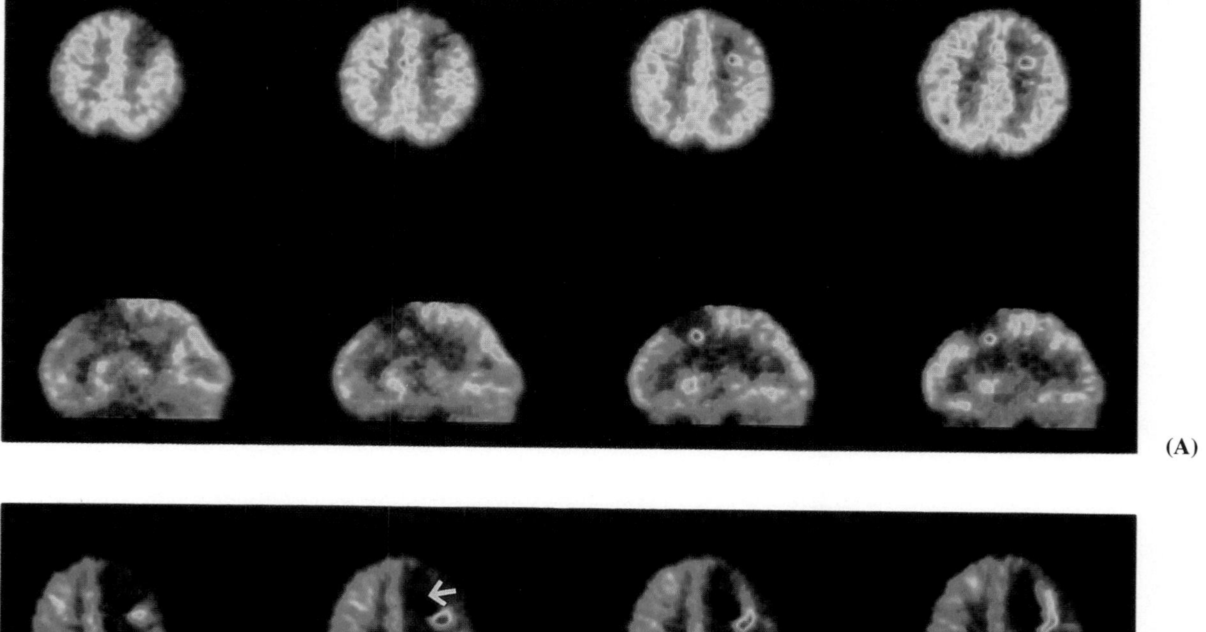

(A)

(B)

Plate 16 (Figure 17–9, p. 370). A 51-year-old man with malignant degeneration of a low-grade glioma. **(A).** Transaxial (top) and sagittal (bottom) FDG PET scans show a large area of hypometabolism in the left sensorimotor cortex with a deep focus (best seen on sagittal images) of markedly increased glucose metabolism consistent with malignant degeneration. **(B).** Transaxial FDG PET images 12 months later show the hypermetabolic lesion is more extensive and curves around a hypometabolic necrotic center (arrow) typical of a glioblastoma multiforme.

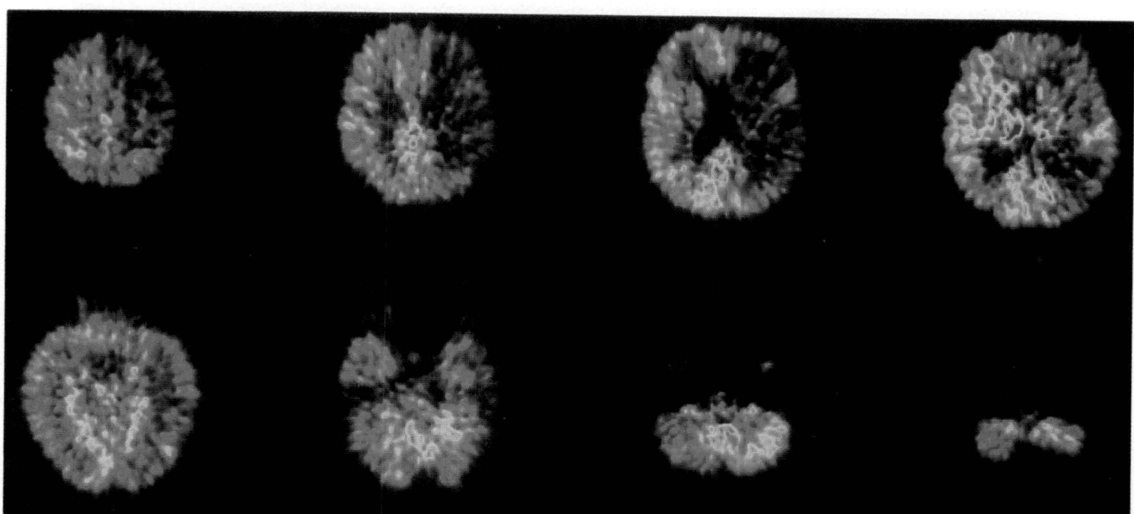

Plate 17 (Figure 17–10, p. 370). A 48-year-old man with an anaplastic astrocytoma of the left parietal lobe. Transaxial FDG PET scan shows extensive left fronto-parietal glucose hypometabolism without foci of glucose hypermetabolism to suggest recurrent tumor. In addition, there is a generalized reduction in cerebral glucose metabolism due to the effects of steroids. Left basal ganglia are hypometabolic and there is right crossed cerebellar diaschisis.

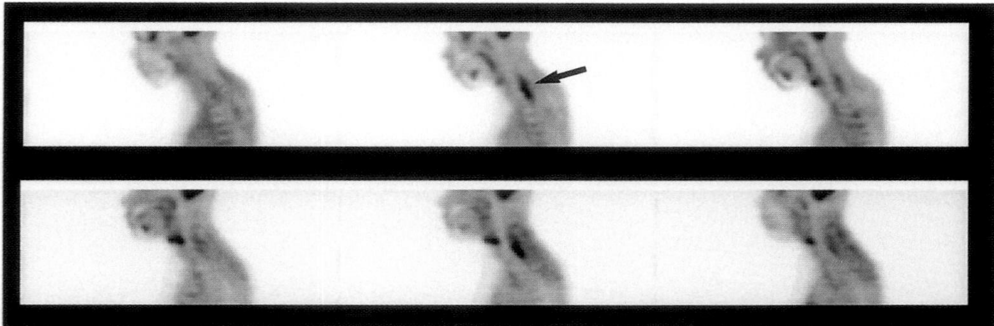

Plate 18 (Figure 17–11, p. 371). A 17-year-old girl with a primitive neuroectodermal tumor of the cervical cord. Prechemotherapy and biopsy sagittal FDG whole-body PET images (top row) show a hypermetabolic focus in mid cervical cord (black arrow). After chemotherapy (bottom row), there is little change in glucose utilization in cervical cord lesion, consistent with poor response.

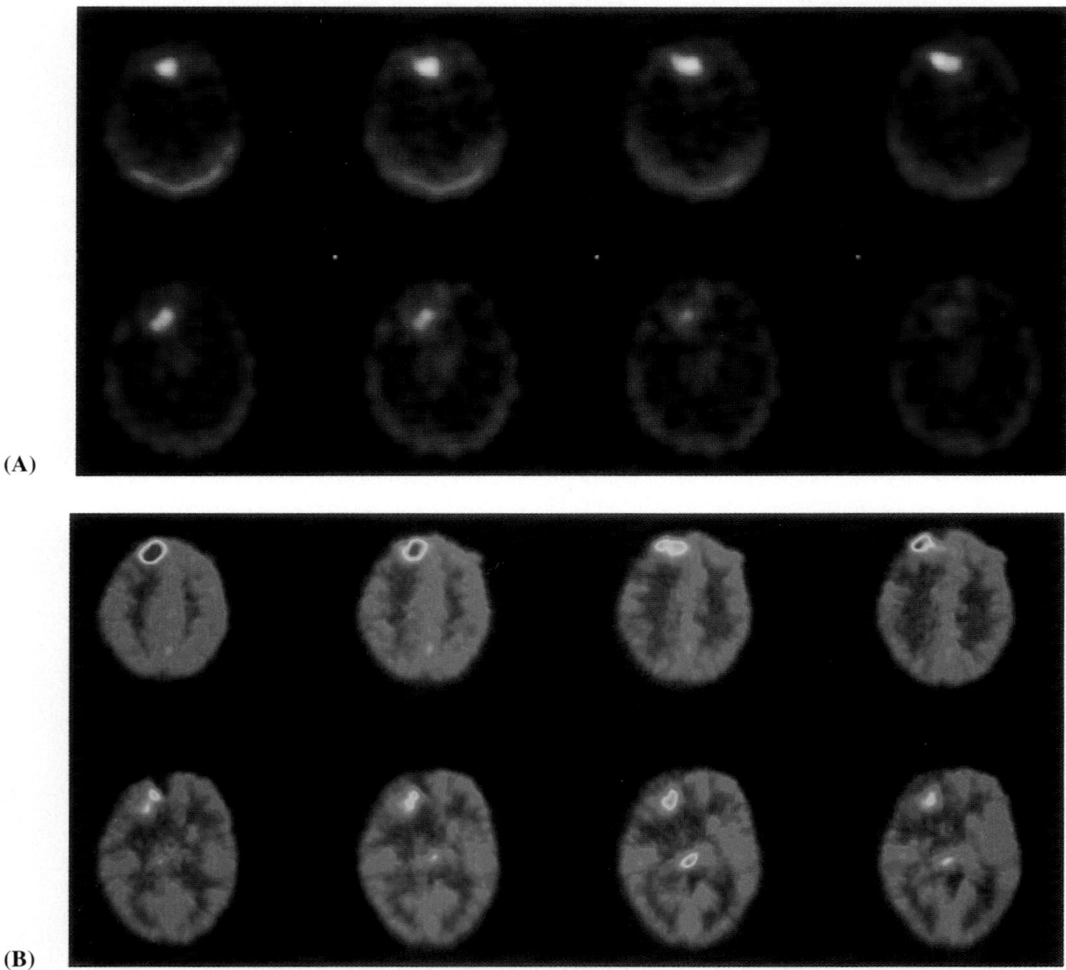

Plate 19 (Figure 17–12, p. 372). A 35-year-old woman with a right frontal anaplastic astrocytoma. **(A).** Thallium SPECT images show a large superficial focus of increased tracer uptake in the right frontal lobe. **(B).** Transaxial FDG PET images show the right frontal lesion is markedly hypermetabolic, consistent with recurrent tumor. Another focus in the right thalamus was not detected with thallium SPECT.

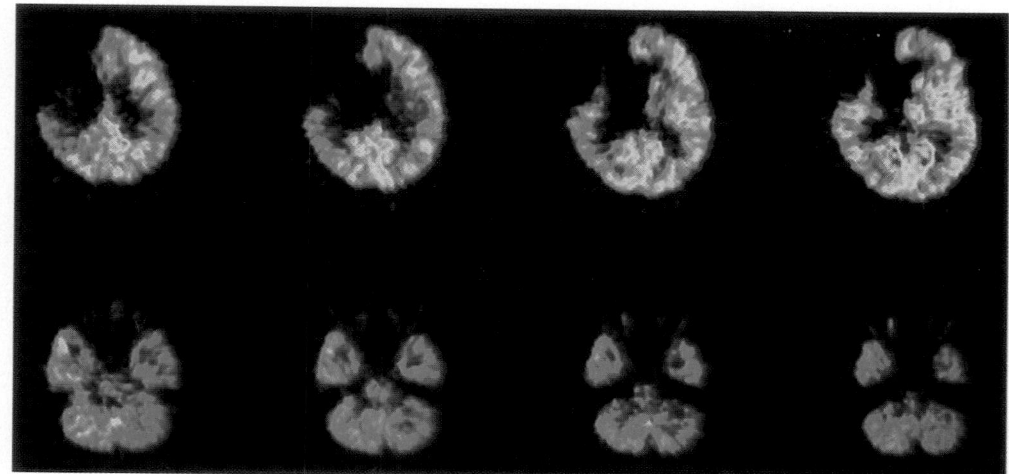

Plate 20 (Figure 17–13, p. 373). A 35-year-old man with unsuccessful right frontal lobectomy for refractory complex partial seizures. Transaxial FDG PET images show a large ametabolic right frontal lobe defect consistent with a frontal lobectomy. Left cerebellar hemisphere is relatively hypometabolic when compared to right. In addition, there is left temporal lobe glucose hypometabolism.

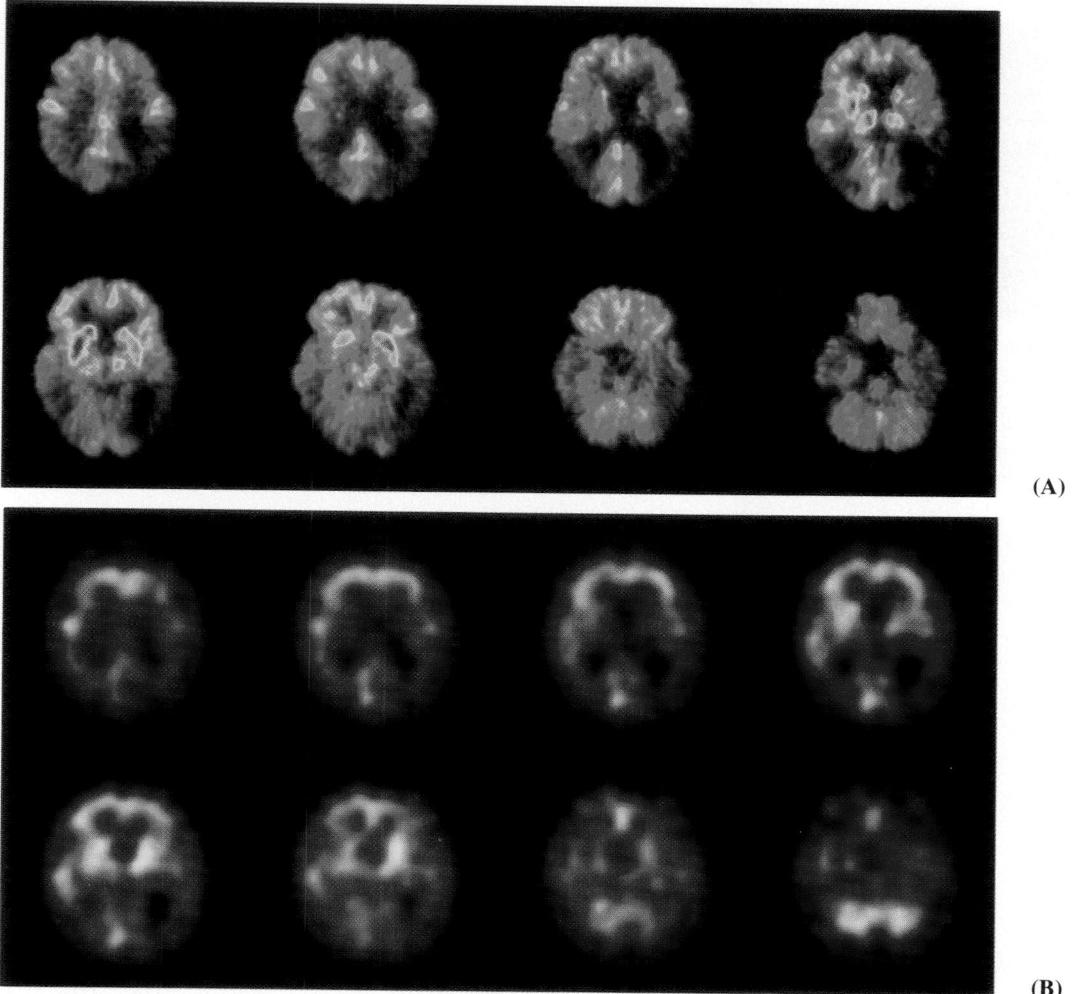

(A)

(B)

Plate 21 (Figure 17–14, p. 374). A 70-year-old woman with a 5-year history of progressive cognitive decline. **(A).** Transaxial FDG PET images show a marked bilateral reduction in parieto-temporal glucose metabolism. Occipital lobes, particularly association cortex, are also affected. Deep nuclei, inferior frontal lobes, sensorimotor cortices (top left images), and cerebellar hemispheres are relatively spared. **(B).** There is close correspondence between reduced perfusion with HMPAO SPECT and FDG PET findings.

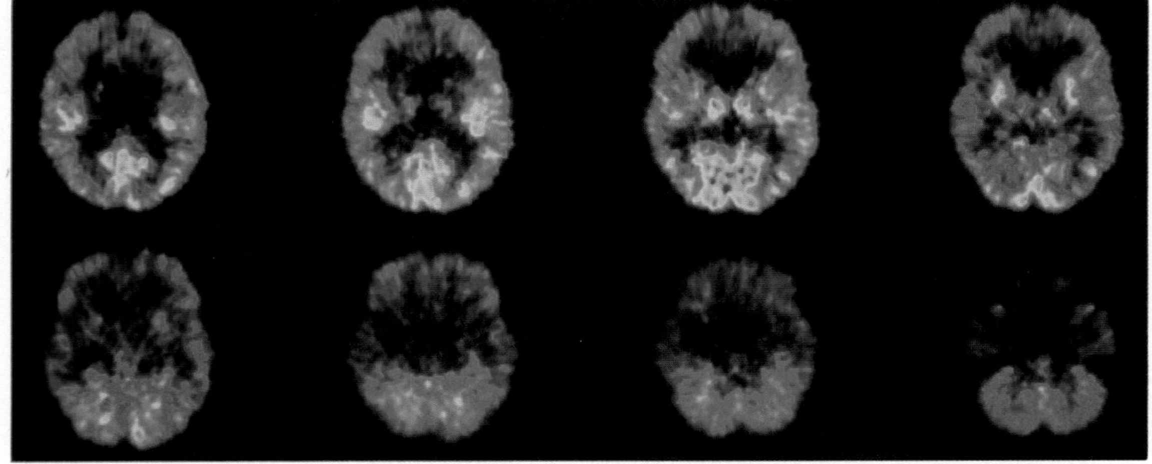
(A)

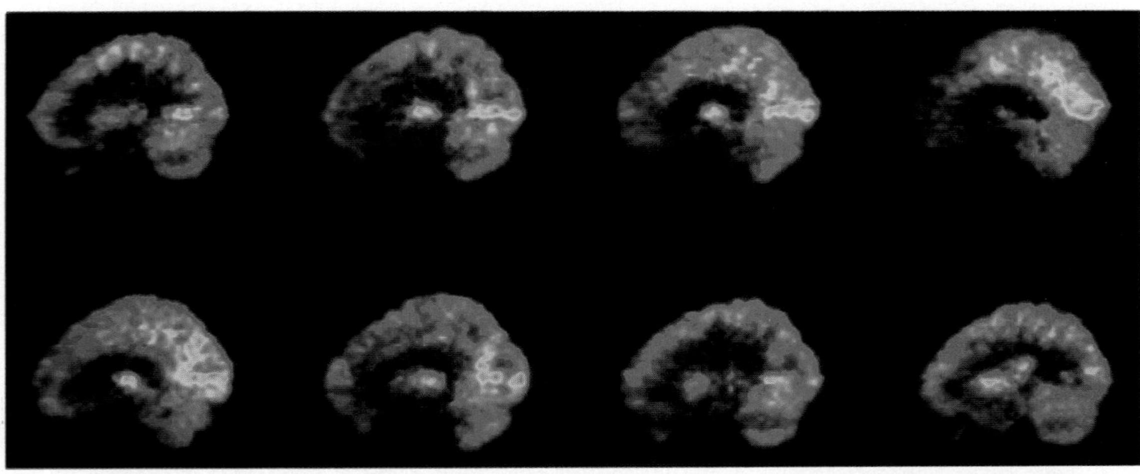
(B)

Plate 22 (Figure 17–15, p. 375). A 44-year-old man with frontal dementia. **(A).** Transaxial FDG PET images show marked glucose hypometabolism affecting both temporal and inferior frontal lobes with less severe involvement of superior frontal lobes. Basal ganglia are splayed laterally consistent with frontal lobe atrophy and caudate nuclei are markedly hypometabolic. There is relative sparing of primary visual cortex, precuneus, and posterior fossa structures. **(B).** Sagittal FDG PET emphasizes severe involvement of fronto-temporal lobes.

18F-6-Fluorodopa

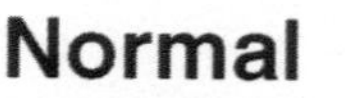

Parkinson's Disease

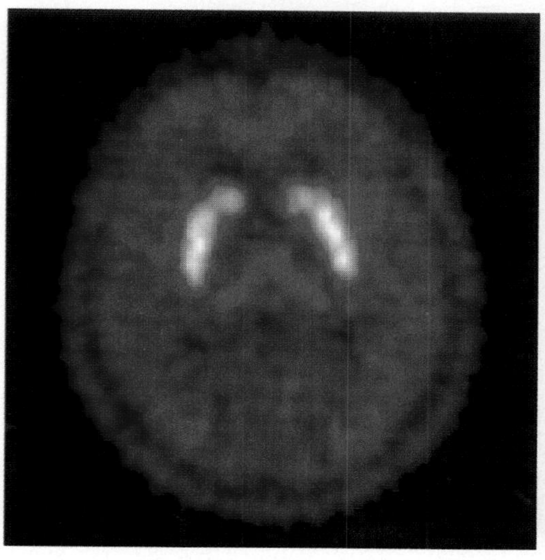

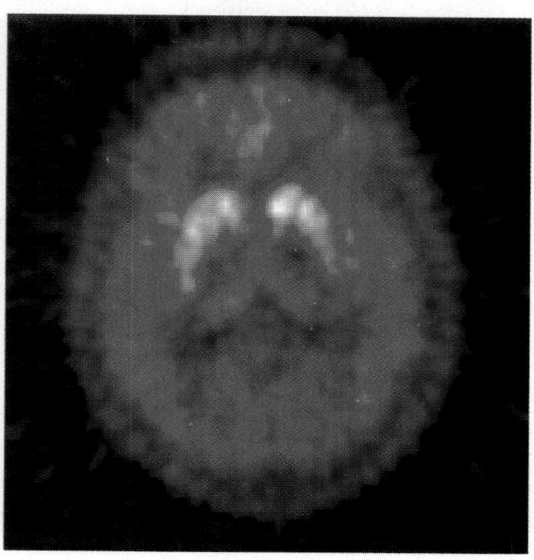

11C-Raclopride

Normal

Parkinson's Disease

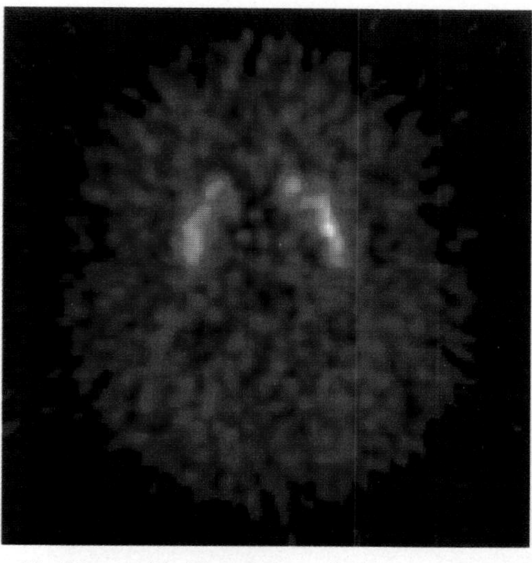

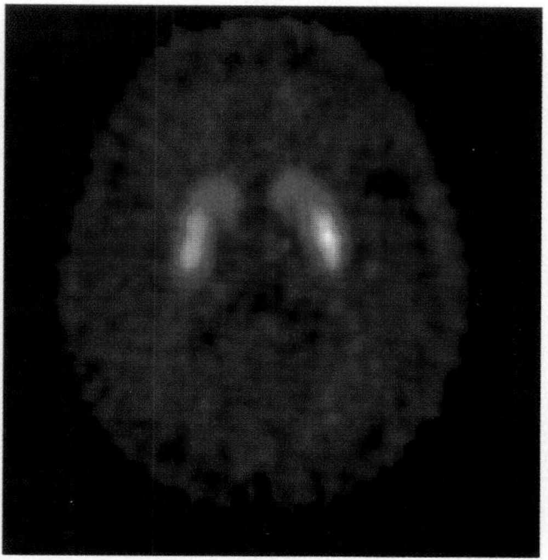

Plate 23 (Figure 17–16, p. 376). ^{18}F-6-fluorodopa (top) and ^{11}C-raclopride (bottom) PET scans in a normal volunteer (on left) and in a patient with Parkinson's disease (on right). Reduced putaminal F-dopa uptake and increased ^{11}C-raclopride uptake are seen in patient when compared to normal volunteer.

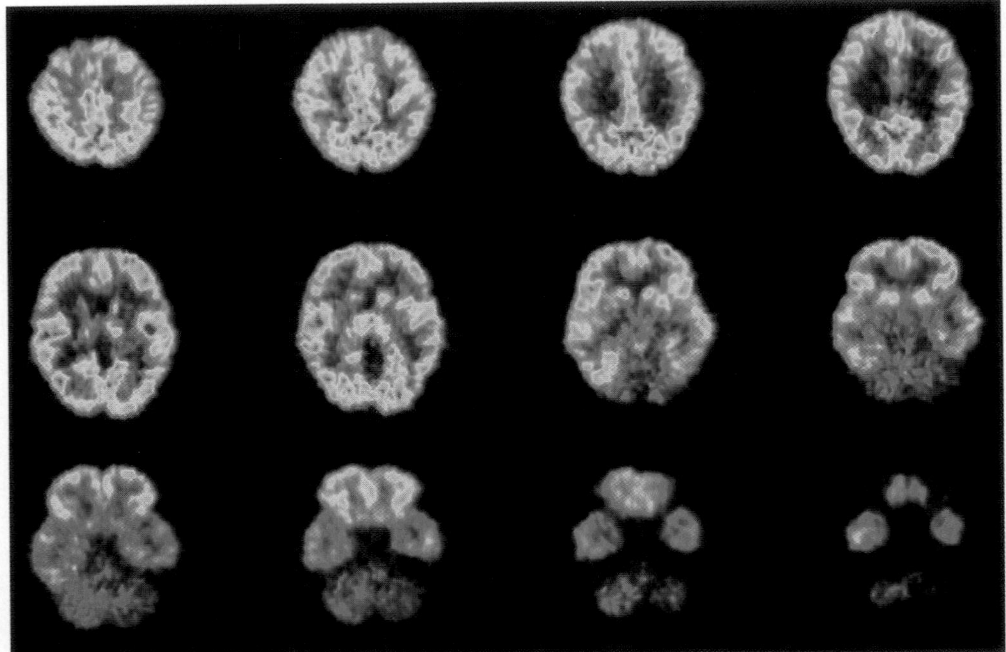

Plate 24 (Figure 17–17, p. 377). A 43-year-old woman with multiple system atrophy. Transaxial FDG PET images show marked glucose hypometabolism in the cerebellum (left > right), brainstem, both putamen (right > left), and a subtle but definite reduction in glucose metabolism in both superior frontal and parietal lobes.

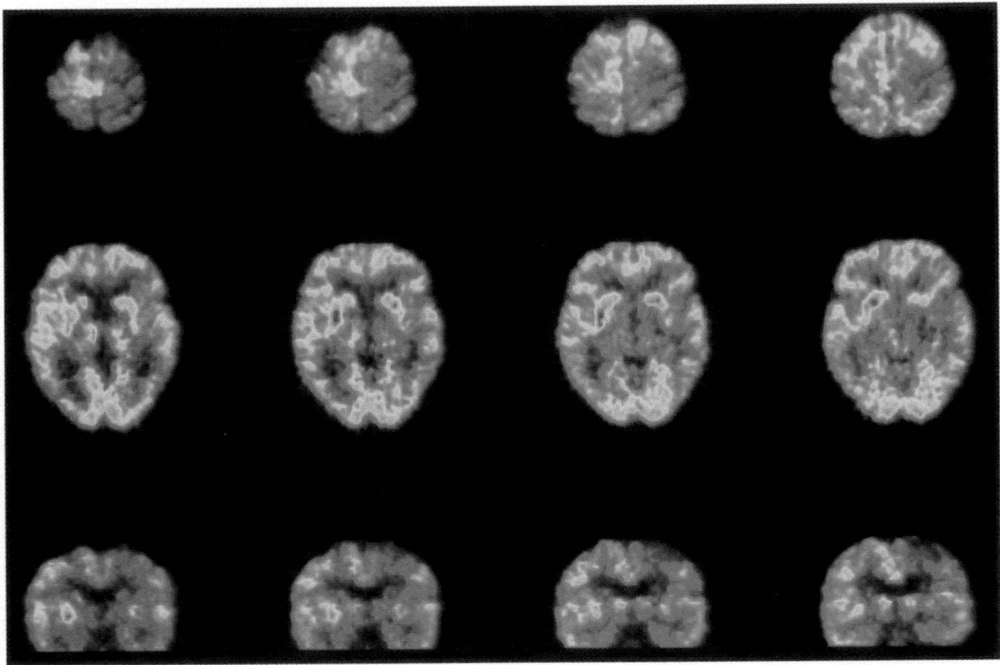

Plate 25 (Figure 17–18, p. 377). An 80-year-old man with suspected corticobasal degeneration. Transaxial (top and middle rows) FDG PET images reveal glucose hypometabolism involving the left Rolandic region together with hypometabolism of the ipsilateral putamen, particularly the posterolateral two thirds, and left thalamus. Sagittal images (bottom) illustrate marked glucose hypometabolism in the postero-superior frontal and antero-superior parietal lobes.

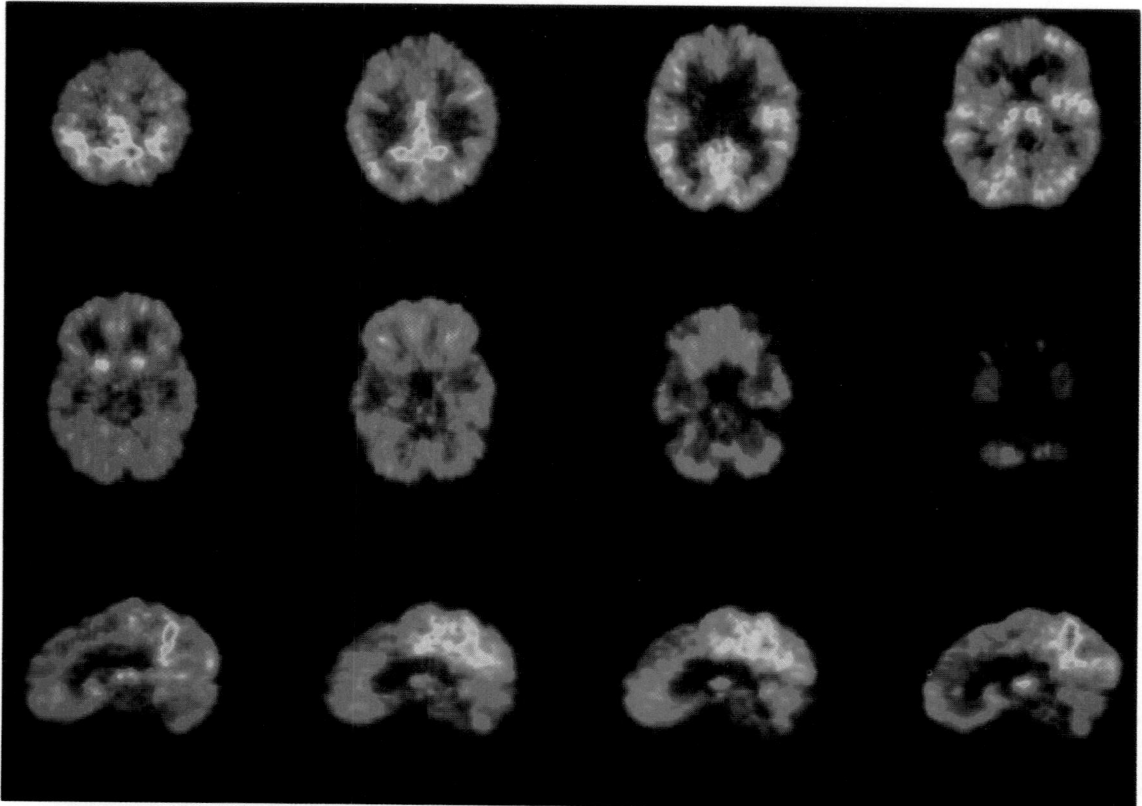

Plate 26 (Figure 17–19, p. 378). A 58-year-old woman with clinical PSP. Transaxial (top and middle rows) and sagittal (bottom row) FDG PET images show reduced glucose metabolism in mid-frontal, superior frontal, and temporal cortices, putamina, and mid-brain with relative sparing of parieto-occipital lobes and cerebellum.

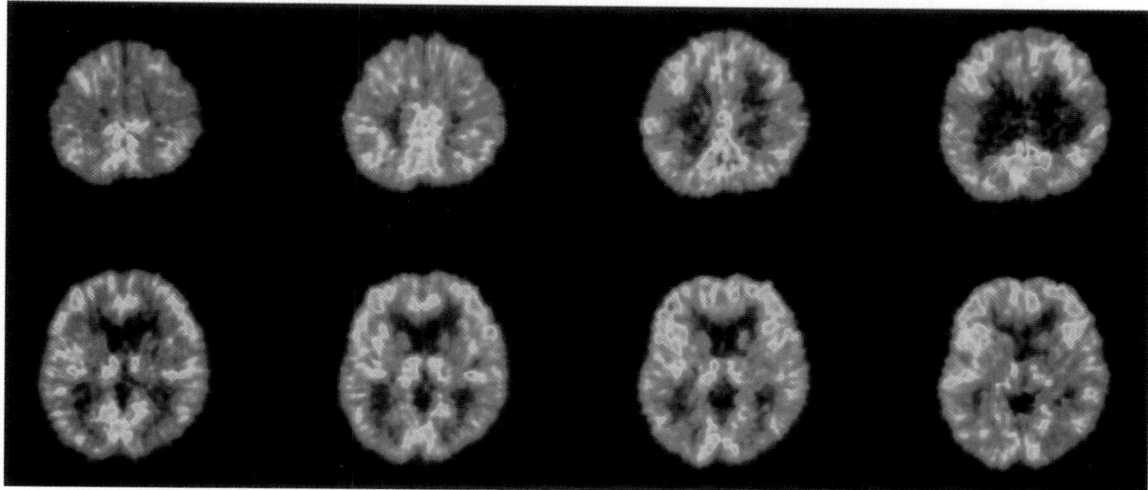

Plate 27 (Figure 17–20, p. 378). A 22-year-old woman with Wilson's disease and tremor and bradykinesia. Transaxial FDG PET scans show reduced cerebral cortical glucose metabolism together with a marked reduction in glucose utilization in the striatum.

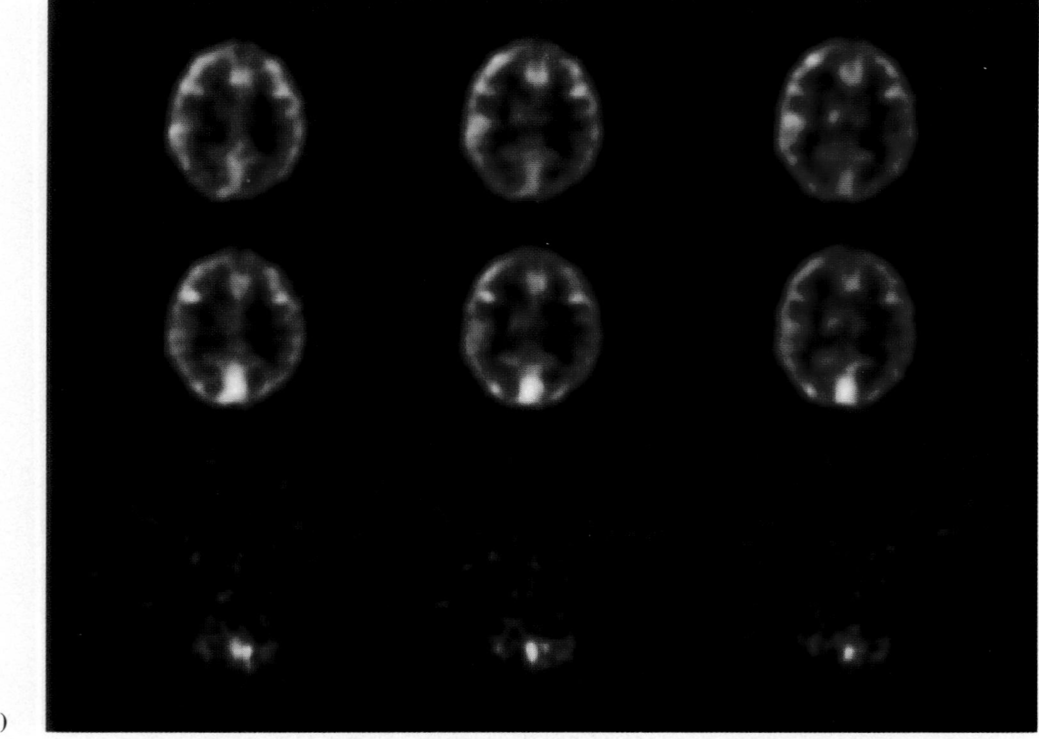

(A)

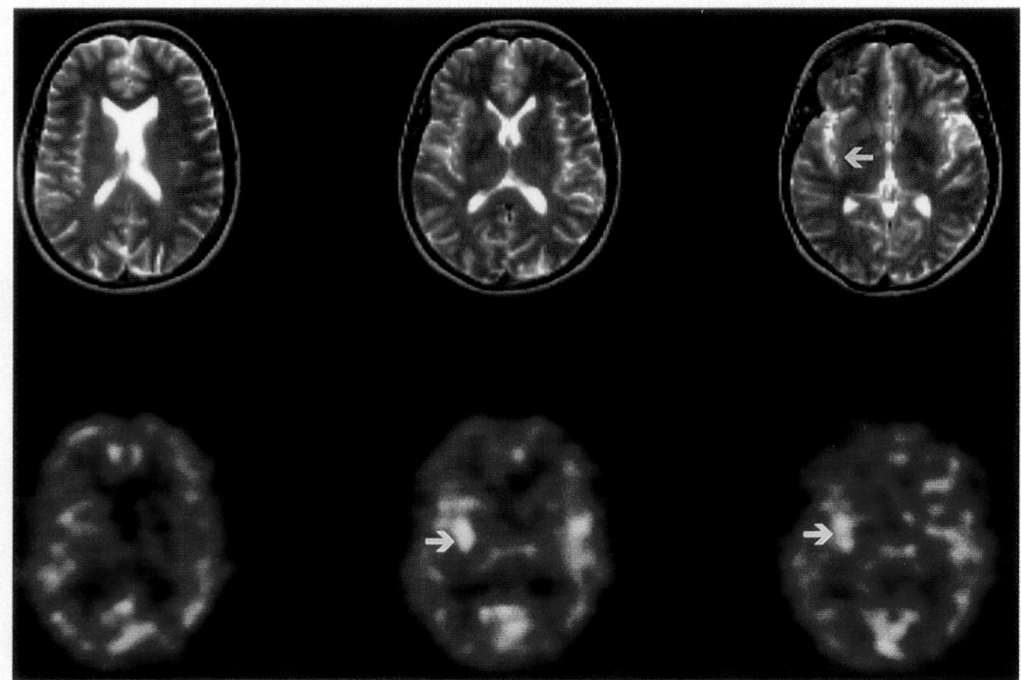

(B)

Plate 28 (Figure 17–21, p. 379). **(A).** ^{15}O-PET activation studies in a 24-year-old normal volunteer. Transaxial images demonstrate increased blood flow to primary visual cortex in response to a simple visual paradigm. Top row is control task with eyes staring at a fixed object, middle row is normal volunteer viewing a complex visual scene, and bottom row is subtraction images of activated minus control state. **(B).** HMPAO SPECT activation and MR studies in a 40-year-old normal volunteer. T2-weighted MR images (top) and registered HMPAO SPECT (bottom) studies are shown. Increased perfusion is seen in right insula (arrows on both MR and SPECT studies) during a strong rotational stimulus.

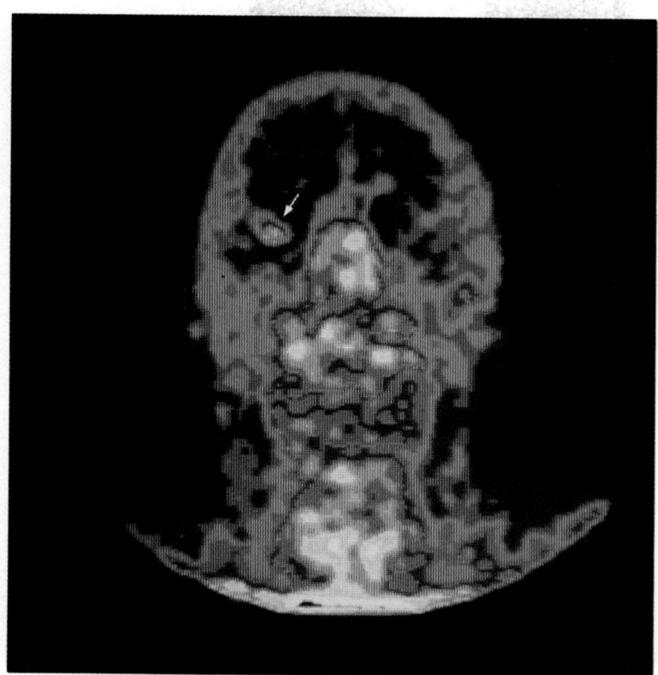

Plate 29 (Figure 19–1, p. 402). Anterior image of the head 7 hours following intravenous injection of 370 MBq (10 mCi) ^{99m}Tc labeled MoAb (Fab′)$_2$ against cutaneous melanoma. The image is positive for a right choroidal melanoma. (Reproduced from Reference 28 with permission.)

(C)

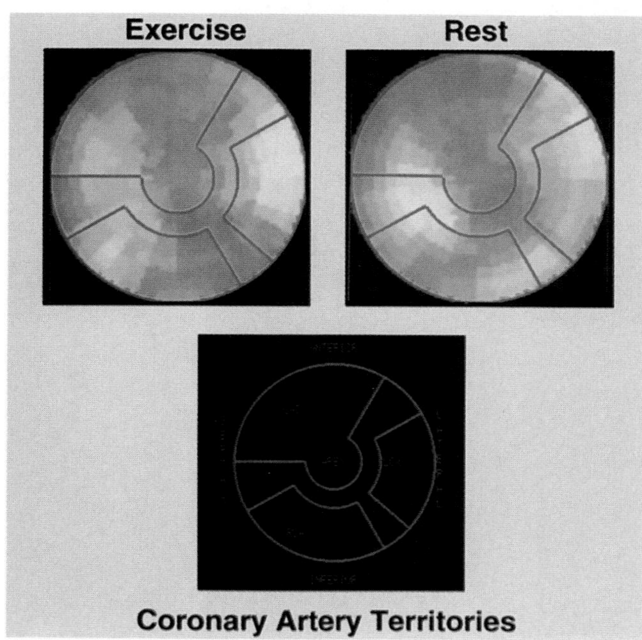

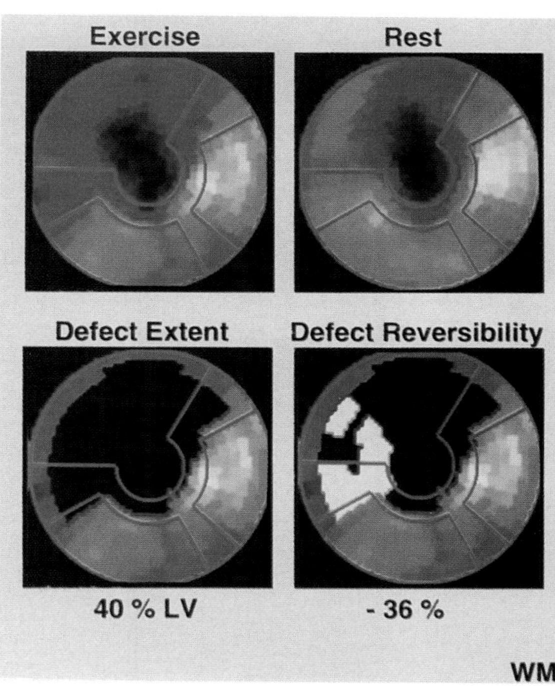

(F)

Plate 30 (Figure 23–7, C and F, p. 450). **(C).** Bull's eye or polar map display of normal SPECT images in **(A)** and **(B).** The coronary artery territories are shown. **(F).** Polar map display of exercise and rest images. The defect is in shades of blue and red. Defect extent (40% LV) is indicated in black; defect reversibility (36%) in white. (From Reference 11.)

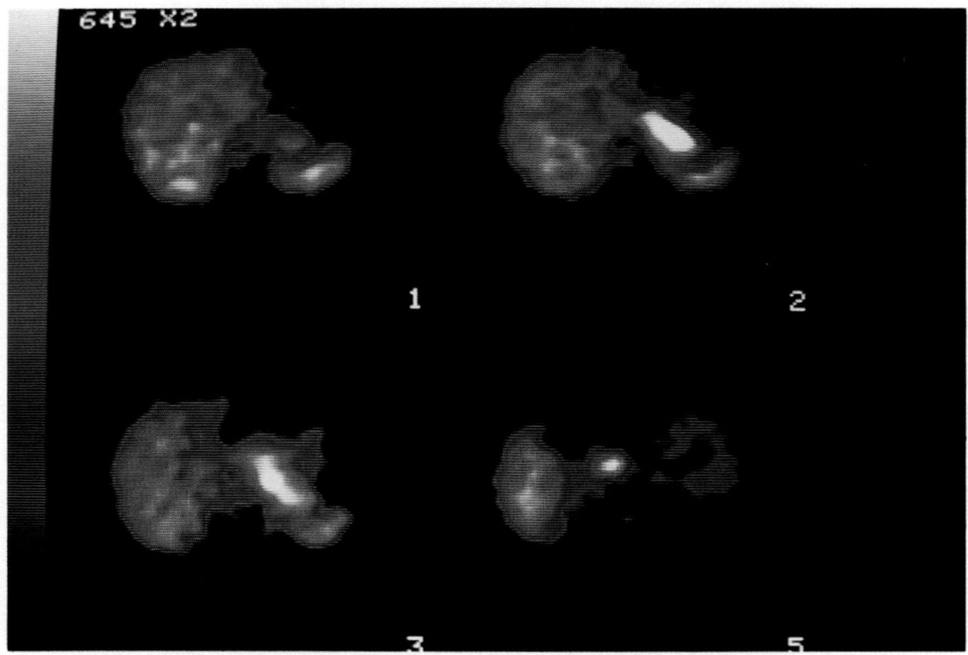

Plate 31 (Figure 29–2, p. 708). Transverse SPECT images in a normal adult obtained 3 hours following administration of 111 MBq (3 mCi) ^{123}I-HIPDM. The pancreatic tail, body, and head are clearly imaged without overlap of radioactivity in the liver and spleen (Reproduced with permission of Yamamoto et al.[29]).

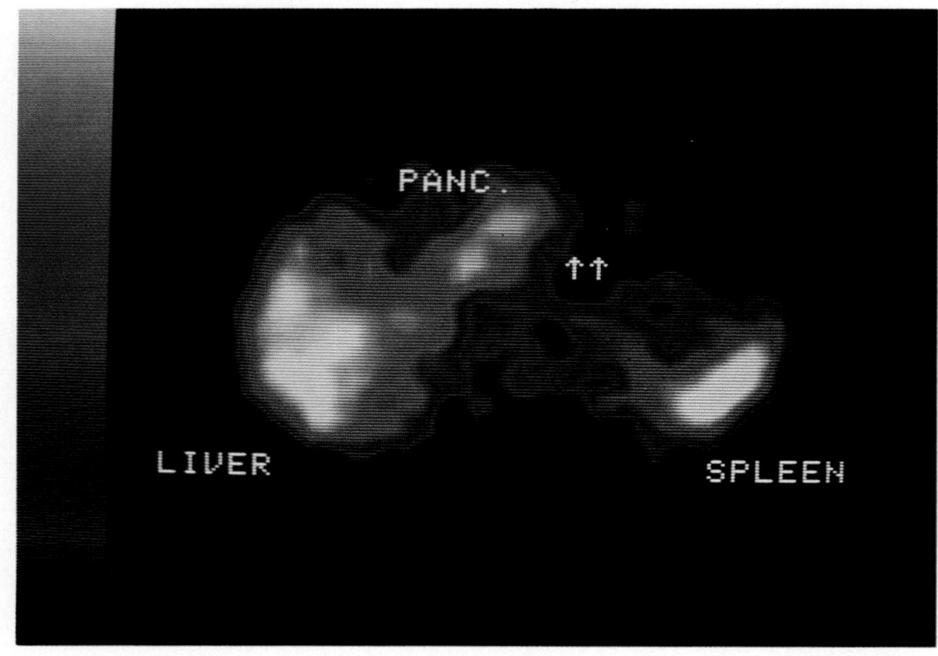

Plate 32 (Figure 29–3B, p. 709). (B). Transverse SPECT image showing absent uptake of ^{123}I-HIPDM in the tumor (double arrows) (Reproduced with permission of Yamamoto et al.[29]).

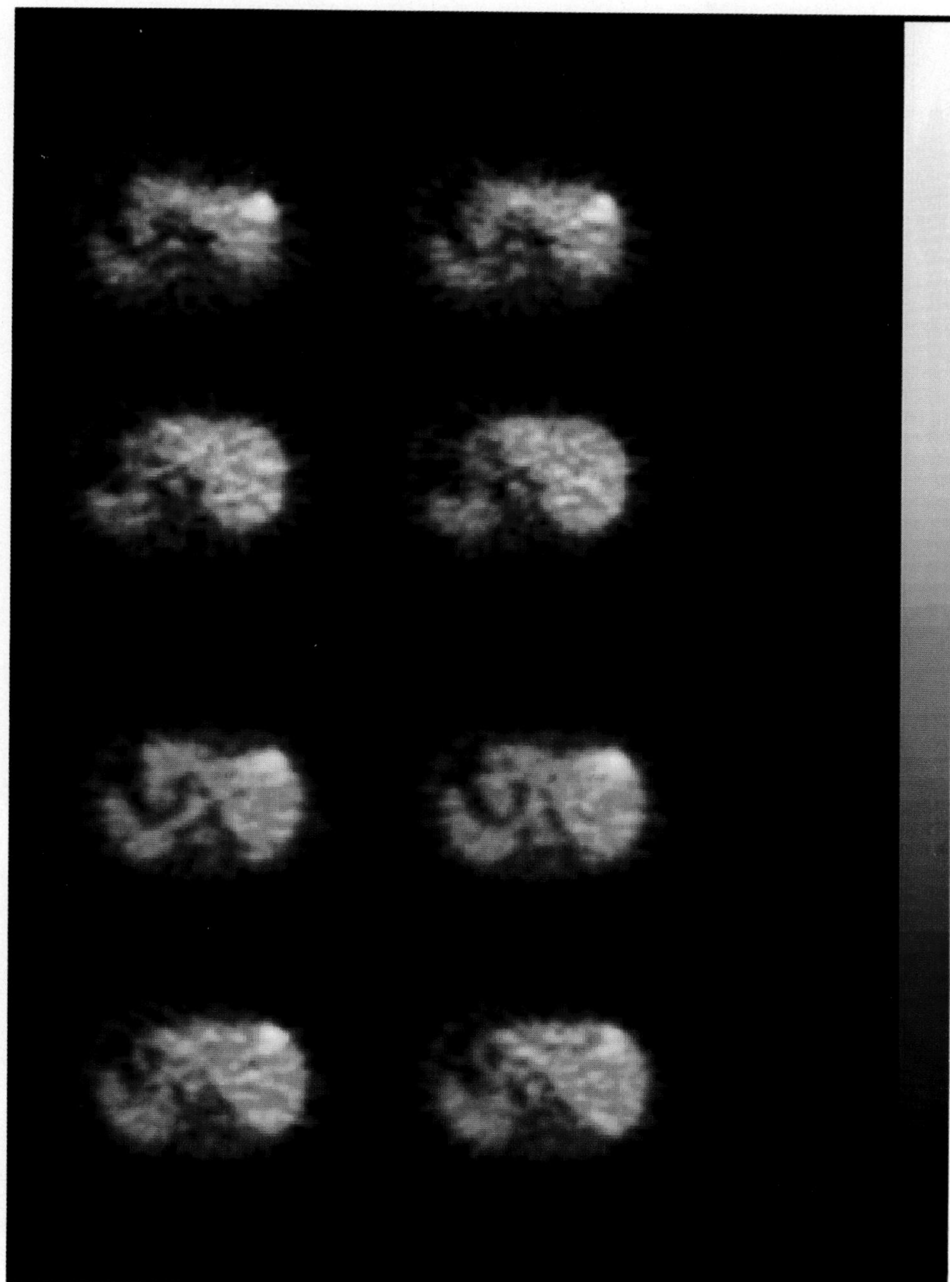

Plate 33 (Figure 36–5, p. 915). Selected transverse abdominal PET images from an ^{18}F-FDG study show increased focal uptake in a liver metastasis from an ocular melanoma primary tumor in this patient. The color intensity bar at the edge of this picture shows the quantitation scale for this study, with white representing the greatest activity and black the least activity.

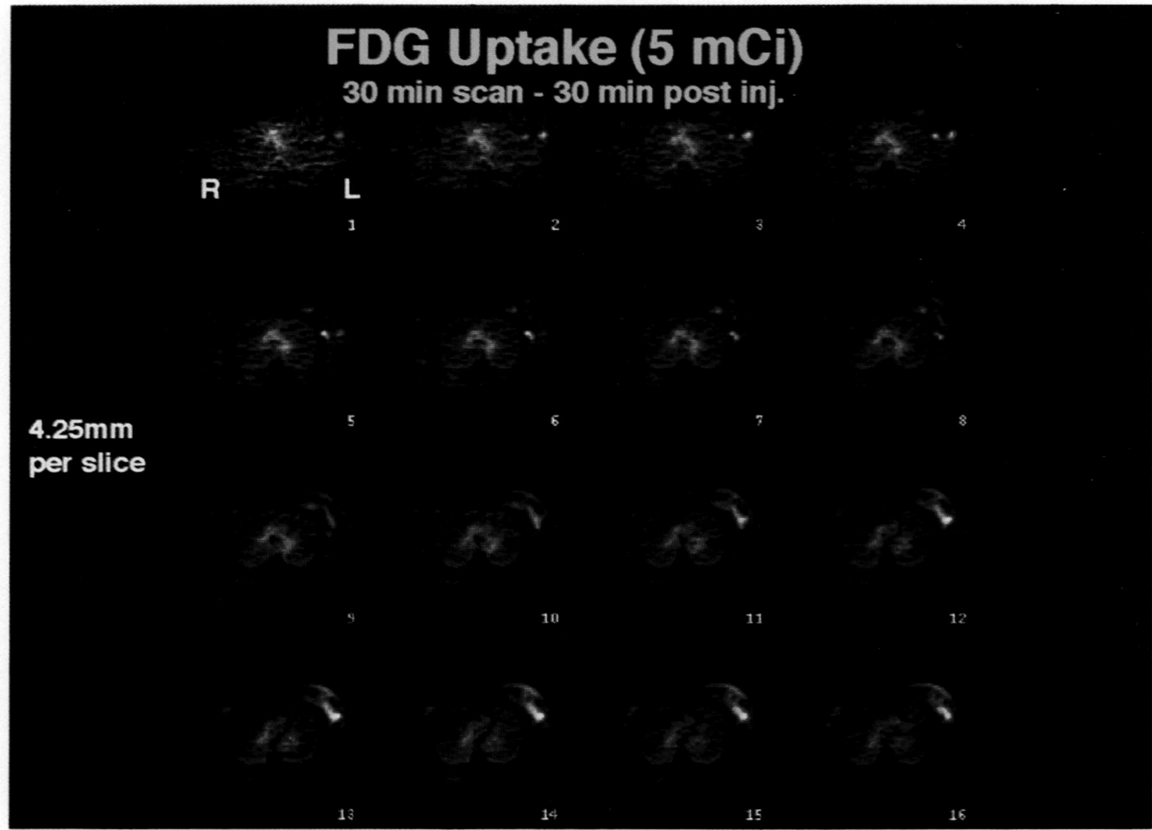

(A)

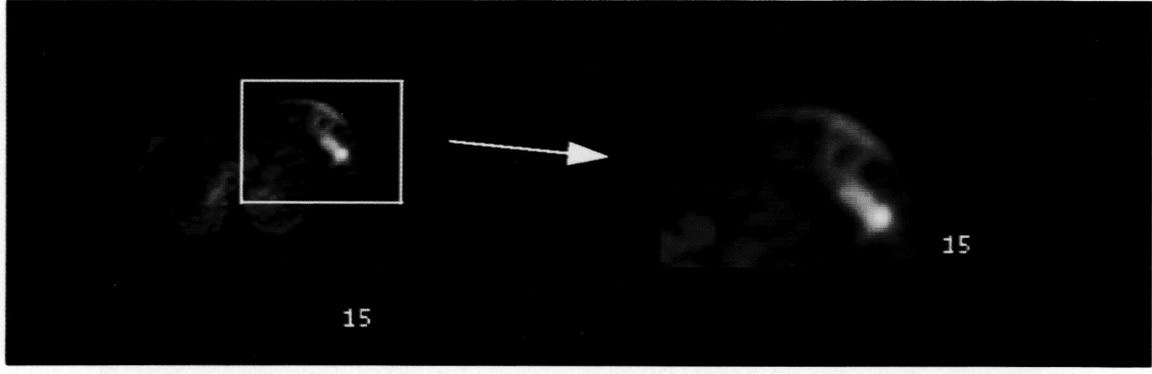

(B)

Plate 34 (Figure 36–6, p. 917). **(A)**. These are transverse scans of the thorax in a female patient with an inflammatory carcinoma of the left breast. The first row of images show focal ^{18}F-FDG uptake in axillary node metastases. Images in the third and fourth row show enhanced uptake in the breast primary and the tumor extension into the skin. **(B).** An enlarged section of the left breast ^{18}F-FDG image shows the increased uptake of this radiopharmaceutical in the primary tumor, as well as in its extensions toward the skin surface and infiltrates in the skin. Such tumor invasion of the skin is responsible for the classic "peau d'orange" sign associated with these cancers.

33 The Musculoskeletal System

John C. Harbert

Bone scintigraphy is the most frequent diagnostic study performed in most nuclear medicine laboratories, often accounting for half of all routine examinations. This chapter will discuss the radiopharmaceuticals, pharmacokinetics, and instrumentation that form the basis of bone scintigraphy, followed by a discussion of clinical applications. The therapy of bone pain with radiopharmaceuticals is discussed in Chapter 49.

Bone Scintigraphy

Radiopharmaceuticals

The introduction of ^{99m}Tc-labeled polyphosphates in 1971 by Subramanian and McAfee marked a major step in the development of bone imaging tracers.[1] These compounds contain P—O—P bonds, of which pyrophosphate is the simplest molecule (Fig. 1). Soon thereafter, the diphosphonates were introduced. These are organic analogs of pyrophosphate that contain P—C—P bonds and are more stable than polyphosphates, in that they resist enzymatic hydrolysis.[2,3] Currently, ^{99m}Tc-methylene diphosphonate (MDP) and ^{99m}Tc-hydroxymethylene diphosphonate (HMDP) stabilized by gentistic acid are the agents of choice for bone scintigraphy. The radiochemistry of these compounds is discussed in Chapter 11.

Interestingly, the use of ionic ^{18}F ($T_{1/2}$ = 110 min), which was introduced in 1962[4] and was completely eclipsed by the ^{99m}Tc-phosphonate complexes, may again find a place in positron emission tomography (PET) studies because of the high resolution possible (Fig. 2) and the ability to quantify tracer concentration.

Mechanisms of Phosphonate Uptake in Bone

The mechanism whereby labeled phosphonates are incorporated into bone is not well understood. Phosphate compounds are thought to *chemisorb* (to absorb by chemical bonding) to amorphous bone and at kink and dislocation sites on the surface of the hydroxyapatite crystal, with the release of the tin reducing agent as well as the bound ^{99m}Tc label. The latter are then hydrolyzed and bound to bone, either separately or together as hydrated tin oxide and technetium dioxide.[5] The large surfaces available for exchange by chemisorption of the technetium-tin-phosphate complex at growth centers and reactive bone lesions result in high tracer concentrations at such sites. The exchange primarily involves the ions of Ca^{+2}, PO_4^{-3}, and OH^- found in the loosely bound outer *hydration shell,* where rapid exchange with serum ions can occur. The tracer uptake is proportional to regional blood flow, as evidenced by the markedly increased tracer bound at sites of inflammation and in reflex sympathetic dystrophy.[6]

Following intravenous injection of diphosphonate, the half-time clearance from the vascular to the extravascular space is 2 to 4 minutes. By 3 hours in normally hydrated individuals, 30 to 40% is bound to bone, approximately 35% of the injected dose has been excreted by the kidneys, 10 to 15% is associated with other tissues and 5 to 10% remains in the blood.[7] The residual blood activity is largely protein-bound and the weaker protein binding of ^{99m}Tc-MDP favors more rapid blood clearance than other phosphonates.[8,9]

The movement of tracer can be followed clinically by "three-phase" bone imaging. During radionuclide angiography (phase 1) the tracer is largely intravascular. During early (1 to 2 min.) static imaging of the blood pool (phase 2) the tracer is both intravascular and extravascular, but predominantly intravascular. In delayed or metabolic imaging (phase 3), the tracer is largely associated with bone (Fig. 3). Parenthetically, the renal route of excretion permits a gross evaluation of the genitourinary tract in a manner analogous to intravenous urography.[7,10] In patients undergoing renal dialysis, injection of tracer should be made prior to dialysis and imaging performed afterward,[11] to achieve the highest bone:tissue contrast.

Maximum bone uptake of ^{99m}Tc-MDP occurs at about 65 min. in well-hydrated individuals, whereas the optimum contrast, or target-to-background, ratio occurs at about 6 hours.[12] Although the most important criterion for determining the interval between injection and imaging is target-to-background contrast, the practical limitations imposed by isotope decay and patient convenience dictates imaging at between 2 and 3 hours.

Two other factors determine the quantity and distribution of radiopharmaceutical uptake by bone; these are the rate of bone turnover and the blood supply. If blood flow to a region of bone is reduced, as in osteonecrosis or radiation injury, a photon-deficient, or "cold" lesion usually results.[13] In regions of hyperemia, increased bone uptake occurs (Fig. 3).

Several investigators have addressed the role of bone blood flow in determining radiopharmaceutical distribu-

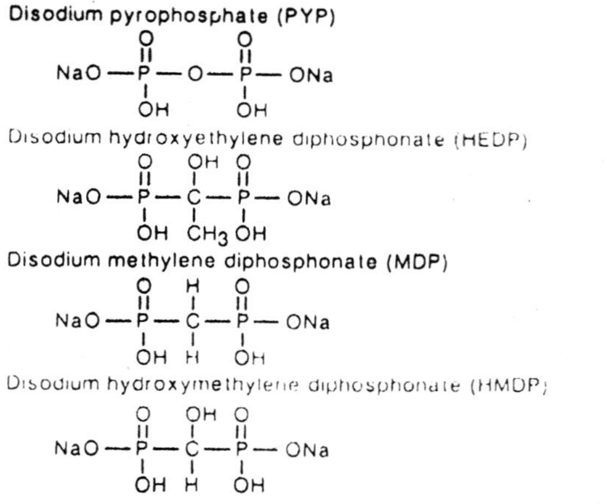

Disodium pyrophosphate (PYP)

$NaO-P(=O)(OH)-O-P(=O)(OH)-ONa$

Disodium hydroxyethylene diphosphonate (HEDP)

$NaO-P(=O)(OH)-C(OH)(CH_3)-P(=O)(OH)-ONa$

Disodium methylene diphosphonate (MDP)

$NaO-P(=O)(OH)-C(H)(H)-P(=O)(OH)-ONa$

Disodium hydroxymethylene diphosphonate (HMDP)

$NaO-P(=O)(OH)-C(OH)(H)-P(=O)(OH)-ONa$

Figure 1. The structure of common ^{99m}Tc-labeled bone tracers.

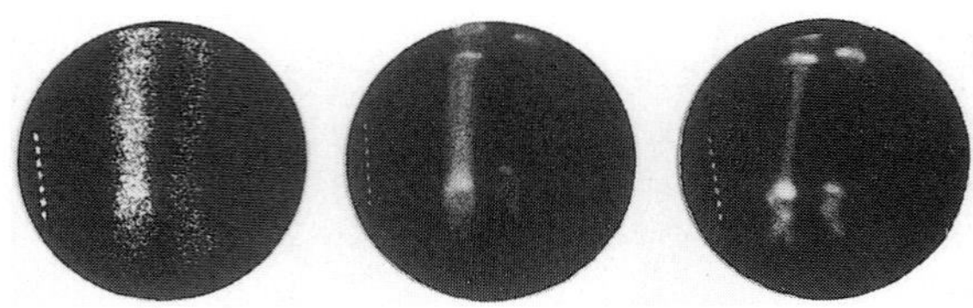

Figure 3. Three-phase bone scintigraphy in a 5-year-old child with osteomyelitis of the distal right tibia. At left is a 5-second blood flow image in the anterior view taken from a series following the intravenous injection of 370 MBq (10mCi) ^{99m}Tc-MDP. It demonstrates diffusely increased perfusion to the right leg. In the center, the blood pool image taken 5 minutes after injection shows diffusely increased perfusion to the right leg, with especially increased blood surrounding the distal right tibia. At right is the 3-hour delayed image demonstrating highly increased bone metabolism at the site of infection. The increased bone uptake in the unaffected right tibial diaphysis and proximal metaphysis is caused by the increased regional perfusion.

tion.[14,15] Following femoral artery ligation, uptake in bones of the affected limb decreases even in the presence of healing fractures.[16] Jones et al. described a nonlinear relationship between variations in blood flow and the degree of ^{99m}Tc-MDP uptake.[5] They postulate a "diffusion-limited" response of the tracer to changes in bone blood flow. For example, a fourfold increase in tibial blood flow results in only about 33% increase in bone uptake of tracer. At lower levels of blood flow alteration, however, uptake is proportional to blood flow. Following sympathectomy, the diffusion-limitation effect persists, but at a higher flow rate.[16]

Charkes showed that sympathetic tone controls the closing and opening of some bone arterioles.[17] With sympathectomy, the normally closed vessels open, permitting locally increased blood flow, known as "recruitment." Both epinephrine and sympathetic stimulation decrease bone blood flow.[18] The effect of sympathectomy is to increase regional blood flow which, in turn, increases tracer accumulation in the affected extremity. The same phenomenon is observed following a stroke that results in hemiplegia.

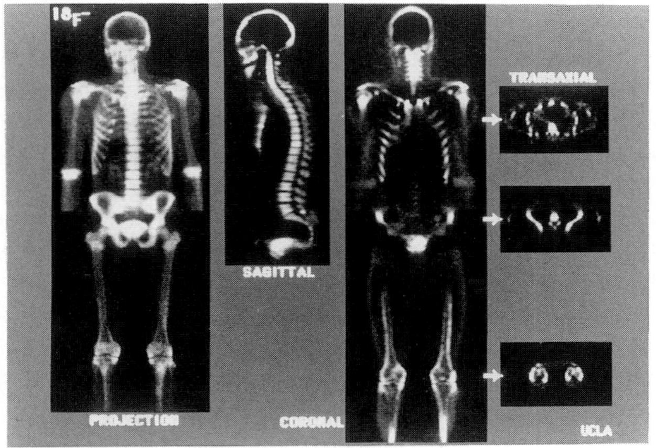

Figure 2. Planar and PET bone images using ^{18}F. Note the extraordinary detail obtainable with this technique. Reproduced with permission of Dr. C.K. Hoh and colleagues, UCLA School of Medicine.

Areas of normally exuberant blood flow (e.g., the metaphyses of long bones) are also sites of high bone turnover. The osteogenic process provides a large surface for ionic exchange and increased alkaline phosphatase and pyrophosphatase activity. The affinity of bone-imaging radiopharmaceuticals for hydroxyapatite, enzymatic systems, and immature collagen all favor osteogenesis and the blood flow associated with it as determining radiopharmaceutical uptake and distribution in bone.[19–21]

Planar and Whole-Body Bone Imaging

In bone imaging, as in all areas of nuclear imaging, use of the proper collimator, patient positioning, count density, and scatter reduction techniques can make the difference between visualizing an abnormality and missing it. In general, the best resolved bone images are obtained with a high-resolution collimator, 10^6 counts/image or greater, no separation between patient and collimator, and the use of scatter reduction techniques, particularly in obese patients.[22]

The usual choice of collimators for planar and whole-body bone imaging include ultra high-resolution, high-resolution, and all-purpose collimators. Naturally, the ultra high-resolution collimators offer the highest resolution ($\approx$6.5 mm at 10 cm in air), but the long acquisition times, about half the sensitivity of high-resolution collimators, generally make this an impractical choice for routine scintigraphy. The high-resolution collimator ($\approx$8 mm at 10 cm in air) usually offers the best compromise between resolution and imaging time.

Scatter reduction techniques include the use of asymmetrical energy window settings[23,24] and preferential weighting of the energy spectrum.[25,26] Each of these parameters taken alone will have marginal effect on image quality, but taken together, the improvement is often unmistakable.

It should go without saying that the highest resolutions

with any collimator is achieved with the patient in direct contact with the collimator. If whole-body surveys are recorded, they should be accompanied by spot views of regions of concern, based on the survey images, patient complaint, and history. Special views may be of assistance[27]:

1. Questionable abnormalities of the upper ribs can be delineated better with apical lordotic projections, as shown in Figure 4.
2. Lesions in the pelvis that are obscured by residual activity in the bladder may require the "tail-on-detector" view, in which the image is taken with the patient sitting on the camera head (Fig. 5).
3. The pinhole collimator is often used to provide greater detail of the hip joints.
4. Postvoiding views help determine the integrity of the pubis and sacrum.
5. Vertex views of the skull help resolve high skull lesions (Fig. 6).
6. Views with the arms abducted and adducted help determine whether a lesion in the scapular region lies within rib or scapula (Fig. 7).
7. Before concluding that a kidney is obstructed, it is essential to repeat the view with the patient standing (Fig. 8), because pooling of tracer in the recumbent position may occur in completely normal kidneys.
8. Superficial activity in the pelvic and upper thigh regions is often due to urine contamination that disappears after removal of underwear and washing.

For imaging the axial skeleton, it is usually recommended that between 8×10^5 and 1.5×10^6 counts be acquired per spot view for a 40-cm LFOV scintillation camera and 4 to 5×10^5 counts for the extremities.[28] This count density translates to about 2.5 to 3.5×10^6 counts per view for whole-body surveys (Fig. 9). When digital images are acquired, a 256×256 matrix should be used.

In such conditions as osteomyelitis, occult fractures, tissue trauma, and joint diseases, the status of bone and active processes involving soft tissue vascularity is evaluated by means of three-phase bone imaging described above.

SPECT Bone Imaging

Single photon emission computed tomography (SPECT) imaging of bone is most useful in evaluating such complex structures as the skull,[29,30] spine,[31,32] hips,[33,34] and knees.[35,36] As with all SPECT imaging, careful attention to quality control is essential (Chapter 5). Currently the most commonly recommended acquisition parameters include use of high-resolution collimators, 128×128 acquisition matrix and 360-degree elliptical orbit with 60 to 70 angular views.[22,37] When imaging the lumbar spine, a 180-degree orbit with the patient in the prone position and using an elliptical orbit may provide better contrast of lesions.[22] The selection of reconstruction filters depends somewhat on patient habitus, the type of SPECT instrumentation, and operator experience.[38–40] Figure 10 illustrates how SPECT can characterize soft-tissue structures in a case of toxic pericarditis.

Normal Scintigraphic Patterns and Variations

Figure 9 illustrates most of the essential scintigraphic features in a young adult. There is variably increased activity in the epiphyses of most joints. This is especially pronounced in children before growth plate closure. Diffusely increased activity may be encountered in such conditions as renal osteodystrophy and hyperparathyroidism.[41,42] Diffusely decreased activity is commonly observed in congestive heart failure, with inadequate radiopharmaceutical quality control, and with the administration of several drugs (Table 1).

CLINICAL APPLICATIONS

Malignant Bone Diseases

BONE METASTASES

In most laboratories, the search for metastatic disease is the principal indication for bone scintigraphy. Bone scintigraphy is a highly sensitive test for detecting metastases to bone and the simplest means of surveying the entire skeleton. Comparisons with plain radiography reveal the obvious superiority of scintigraphy.[59] For example, fewer than 5% of bone scans are normal with radiographically apparent lesions, while 10 to 40% of skeletal metastases have normal radiographs and abnormal scans.[60] Moreover, in approximately 30% of patients with known malignancy who have pain and normal radiographs, bone scintigraphy demonstrates metastatic lesions.[61]

While bone scintigraphy is a sensitive test for the presence of bone metastases, it is not specific. In some studies, false-positives exceed the true-positives.[62] In most cases, therefore, radiographs or other correlative imaging studies should be obtained to corroborate the scintigraphic presence of a lesion. In sites, particularly vertebrae, magnetic resonance imaging (MRI) may be the most sensitive modality for confirming the presence of bone metastases. A commonly followed decision tree is shown in Figure 11.

Scintigraphic Characteristics. The most frequently encountered scintigraphic pattern in metastatic disease to bone is one of multiple, randomly distributed foci of intensely increased tracer accumulation (Figs. 12, 13). Typical lesions include asymmetric lesions in the vertebral bodies; large, rounded skull lesions outside the suture lines; elongated lesions in the ribs; and irregular pelvic lesions. Small, round, solitary rib lesions, pinpoint skull lesions appearing in the suture lines,[63] periarticular lesions, and those involving the vertebral end plates and facet joints, are more likely to be benign.[64]

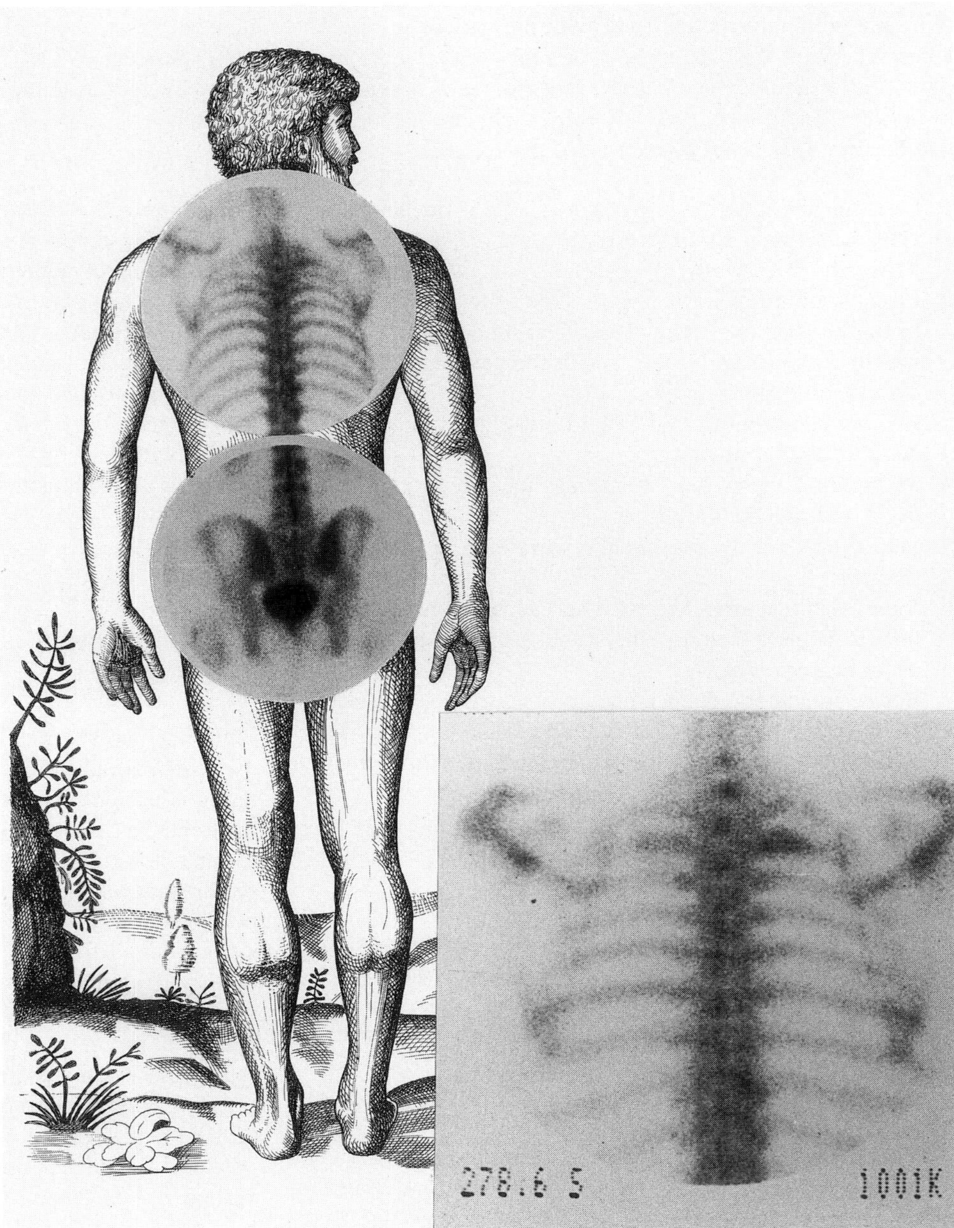

Figure 4. Posterior spine images in a patient with prostatic carcinoma. There are questionable abnormalities involving the upper posterior ribs. Inset, lower right: apical lordotic view taken with a parallel-hole collimator clearly demonstrates lesions of both posterior third ribs, consistent with bone metastases.

It is generally believed that when metastatic tumors enter bone, factors secreted by the neoplastic cells stimulate osteoclasts causing bone lysis.[65–67] This stimulates osteoblastic activity that, in turn, accounts for abnormal uptake on bone scintigraphy. In approximately 5% of metastases, bone scintigraphy is negative or else reveals a cold (photon-deficient) lesion (Fig. 14), while radiographs demonstrate a lytic lesion. Bone metastases from anaplastic tumors, thyroid carcinomas, renal cell carcinoma, and multiple myeloma are frequently cited examples that may fail to stimulate sufficient osteoblastic reaction to increase tracer uptake. Some patients treated with etidronate may also have false-negative bone images.[68] Nevertheless, most cold bone lesions are benign, such as benign tumors, avascular necrosis, surgical or radiation defects (Fig. 14), or artifacts caused by such overlying objects as buttons, pacemakers, or breast prostheses. Tumors with necrotic centers usually have a hyperactive rim in cancellous bone (Fig. 15).

Some tumors spread by regional extension rather than by the hematogenous spread. Common examples are soft-tissue sarcomas and breast cancer. When solitary lesions in the sternum are found in patients with breast cancer, they are most likely caused by direct lymphatic spread and are often found on the same side as the original tumor (Fig. 16).

In some cases, very widespread, diffuse metastatic disease to bone can produce an image with very high bone-to-soft

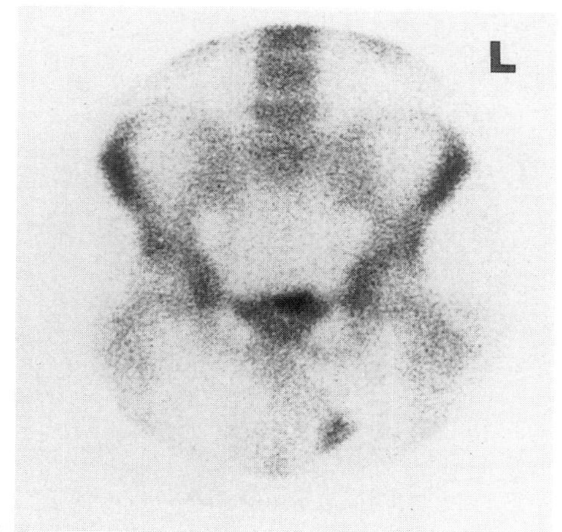

A

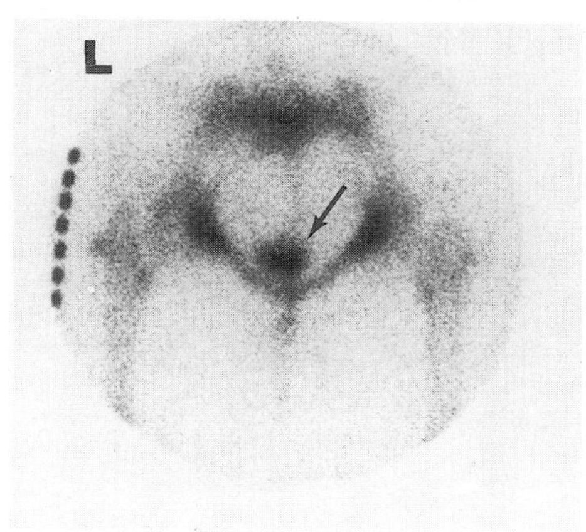

B

Figure 5. **(A).** Anterior view of the pelvis shows a questionable area of activity in the left medial pubic ramus. **(B).** The "tail-on-detector" view demonstrates this to be bladder activity (arrow) and the pubic rami are normal.

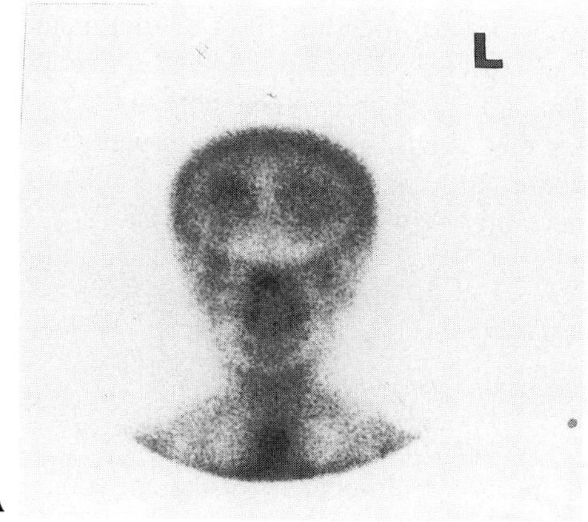

A

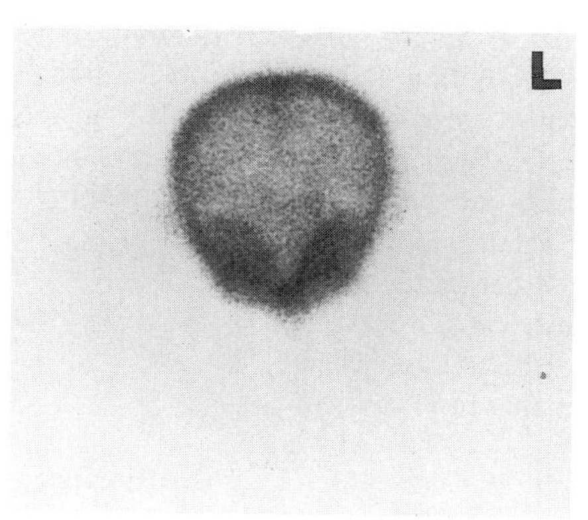

B

Figure 6. Anterior **(A)** and vertex **(B)** views in a patient with hyperostosis frontalis interna.

tissue contrast, known as a "super scan." Frequently individual metastases will not be recognizable, because virtually the entire medullary portion of the bone is involved. In such cases, the kidneys, which are normally visible on delayed bone images, will not be visible at all (Fig. 17). However, faint or absent kidney shadows should not be interpreted as a sign of widespread metastases, since this finding is much more commonly associated with renal insufficiency.[69]

Because most bone metastases are spread hematogenously, their distribution reflects the distribution of red marrow. Approximately 90% are found in the axial skeleton and 10% in the appendicular skeleton.[70] Although most bone metastases are medullary in location, cortical bone metastases also occur. It was once thought that these occurred solely with metastases from bronchogenic carcinoma[71]; however, cortical metastases are found in breast cancer, renal cell cancer, and other primaries.[72]

While most bone metastases are multiple, approximately 15% of patients with malignant disease have solitary scintigraphic abnormalities,[73,74] and between 25 and 65% of these

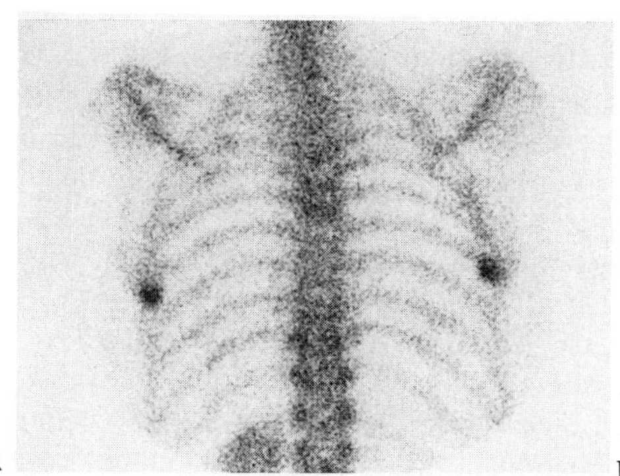

A

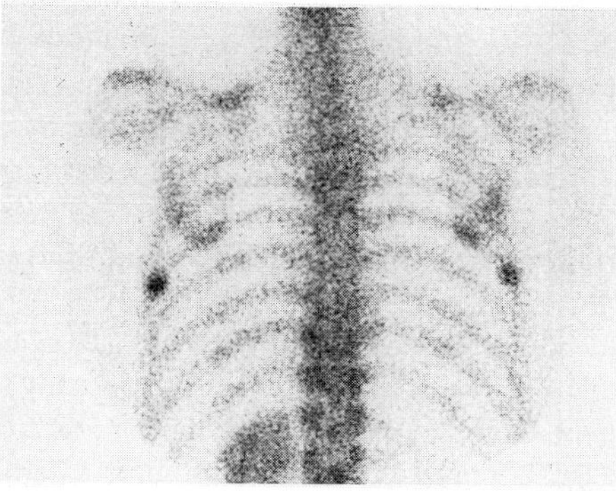

B

Figure 7. **(A).** Posterior view of the thorax with arms abducted demonstrate unusually intense activity at the tips of both scapulae. **(B).** View with the arms adducted to move the scapulae medially reveal two focal rib lesions. Reproduced with permission from Reference 534.

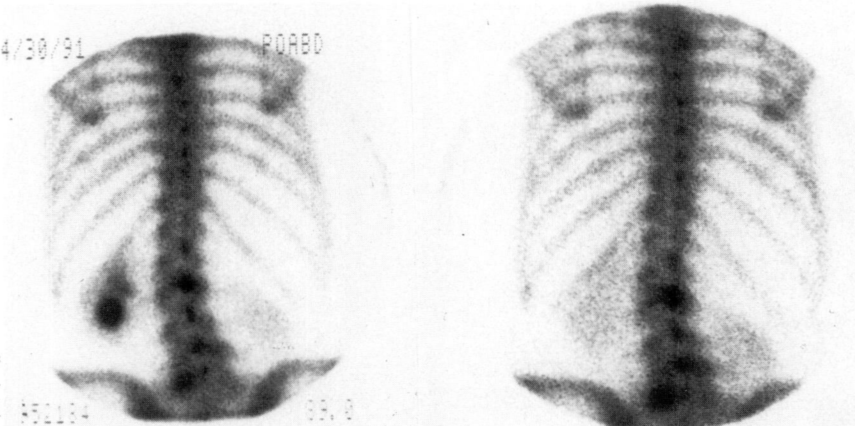

Figure 8. **(A).** Supine view of the lumbar spine showing unusual prominence of the left renal collecting system. **(B).** Standing view shows normal postural drainage.

are found to be malignant.[74,75] Boxer et al. found that 21% of patients with breast cancer relapsed with a solitary bone metastasis.[76] Many of such patients will have normal radiographs, so that MRI, follow-up scintigraphy, or follow-up radiographs should be obtained. In some cases, surgical biopsies of the bone lesion are required, in which case the biopsy should be guided by intraoperative bone scintigraphy.[77]

In general, malignant lesions become larger or more intense with follow-up scintigraphy, while benign processes remain the same or resolve.[78] Correlative radiographs that reveal a benign process are generally reliable in excluding metastases.[79]

The differentiation of rib fractures from metastases is a common diagnostic problem. In a review of 471 cancer patients who had bone scintigraphy, we found that 22% had one or more rib lesions.[62] On the basis of their intensity and appearance in serial scintigraphy, rib lesions could generally be characterized as fractures if they were focal as opposed to linear, with their intensity decreasing within 3 to 6 months, or if they were aligned so that two or more ribs in the same location were involved (Fig. 18).

Another finding that is occasionally found in views of the skull are small, discrete foci as shown in Figure 19 **A** and **B,** which are most commonly encountered in the suture lines and are thought to represent small cartilaginous rest bodies that incompletely calcify.[80] They are most commonly found in the lambdoidal suture, followed by the temporal and coronal sutures. They are entirely benign and do not change on serial scintigrams, while metastases usually increase in size and intensity. These small foci are beyond the limits of skull radiographs. Follow-up scintigraphy is the best means of distinguishing benign from malignant lesions.

In patients who have received chemotherapy, serial bone scintigraphy may often demonstrate a "flare" phenomenon, in which bone metastases demonstrate increased tracer uptake in response to reactive new bone formation associated with the healing (Fig. 20).[81,82] In general, such bone flares are associated with transient rises in osteocalcin and serum alkaline phosphatase bone isoenzyme.[82] The phenomenon is most apparent 1 to 3 months after initiation of treatment, although it may persist longer. Often previously unrecognized lesions will be rendered visible by the increased accumulation, a finding that should not be misinterpreted as progression of disease. New lesions that occur 6 months after therapy are generally evidence of new disease.[82]

SPECIFIC METASTASES

Breast Cancer

Breast cancer is the most common cancer affecting women in all developed countries of the world (except Japan, where gastric cancer is more common).[83] Approximately one in 15 women will develop the disease, of whom more than half will ultimately die from metastatic disease. From 60 to 70% of women who die with breast cancer have bone metastases.[84,85] A large discrepancy exists, however, between the incidence of bone metastases detected at the time of initial therapy or at follow-up and the incidence detected at autopsy, most likely due to occult bone metastases that are undetected at the time of surgery and early follow-up. The reported incidence of positive bone scintigraphy in patients with stage I or II breast cancer at the time of initial staging has ranged from 2 to 38%.[86–88] In stage III disease, the incidence of true-positive scintigraphy is much less variable, approximately 25%. Bone metastases become apparent on follow-up scintigraphy 3 to 4 years after surgery in 20 to 30% of patients who have had negative studies and no evidence of bone metastases at the time of surgery.

The distribution of bone metastases in breast carcinoma favors the vertebrae, a phenomenon thought to be due to the venous drainage of the breast which communicates with the valveless vertebral venous plexus (Batson's plexus).[89] Regional bone metastases also occur in the sternum (Fig. 16), probably by direct extension, in about 3% of cases.[90] Patients with such regional metastases have a much better prognosis than patients with disseminated bone metastases,

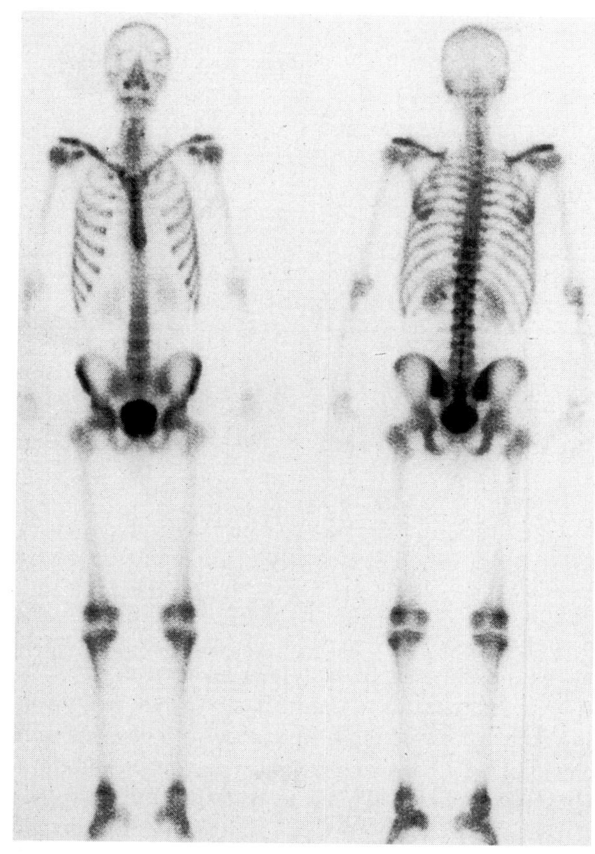

A

Figure 9. (A). Anterior (left) and posterior (right) whole-body surveys obtained simultaneously with a dual-headed scintillation camera. (B). SPECT rotational view (each image rotated 11.25°) that, when projected on a CRT, gives an impression of three-dimensional projection. This is a 22-year-old male with a history of previous fracture of the right clavicle.

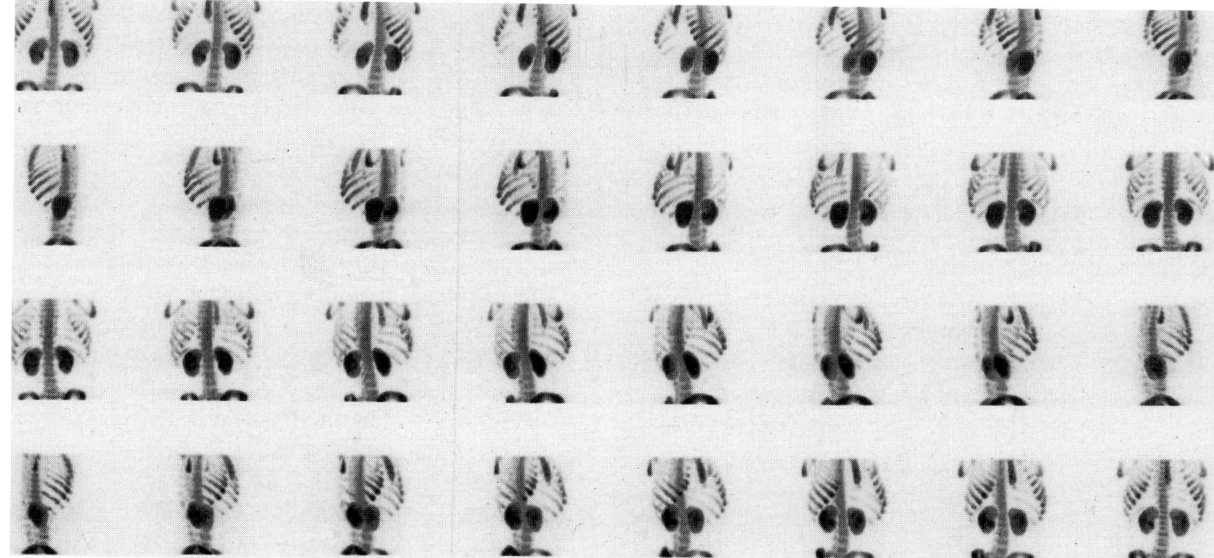

B

and the most effective therapy is aggressive localized treatment.

A second, less common pattern of regional bone involvement is a cluster of lesions that involve two or more contiguous posterior ribs adjacent to the spine.[91] These lesions usually occur between the third and ninth ribs, always on the same side as the mastectomy. The mechanism for this unusual distribution has not been explained.

Occasionally, diffuse bone-marrow infiltration may occur, sometimes in association with a leukoerythroblastic anemia. In such cases, there may be little or no radiographic evidence of bone involvement. The principal scintigraphic features are increased tracer uptake at the ends of long bones with a characteristic globular appearance.[83] Bone-marrow scintigraphy in such patients reveals photopenic lesions corresponding to regions of tumor replacement.

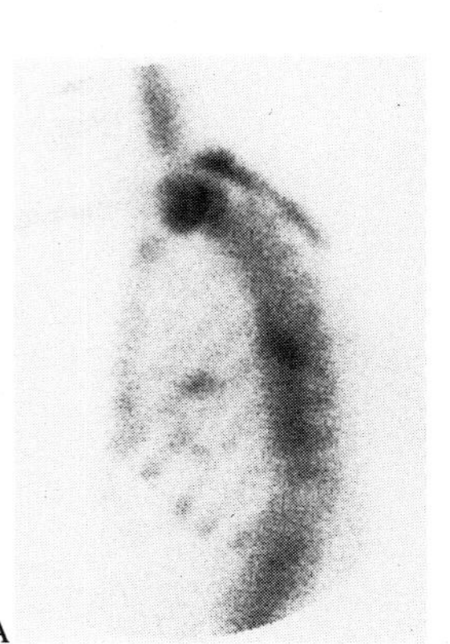

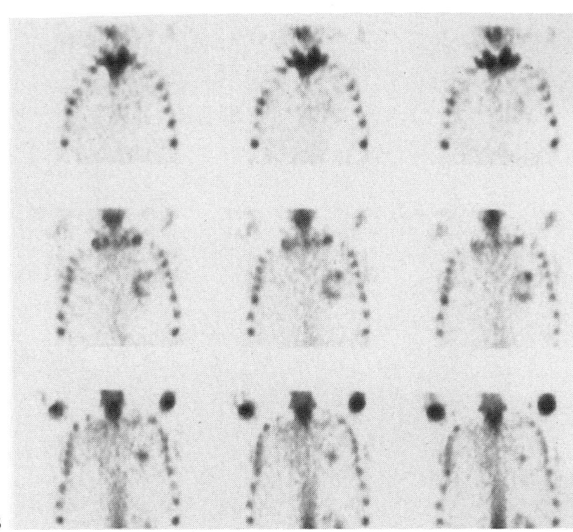

Figure 10. (**A**). Left lateral planar scintiphoto in a patient with malignant melanoma undergoing chemotherapy with Interleukin-2. The ^{99m}Tc-MDP image shows a poorly defined soft-tissue structure in the left thorax. (**B**). Selected coronal SPECT slices through the heart showing the pericardial uptake of the tracer with a particularly intense focus near the left atrium. (Slices = 3.8 mm; Hamming filter; 1.2 cycle cutoff). A B

Uptake of bone radiopharmaceuticals in breast tissue is frequently observed, but is entirely nonspecific. Table 2 lists several reported causes of breast uptake.

BASELINE SCINTIGRAPHY

Considerable controversy exists with regard to the proper use of bone scintigraphy in breast cancer. Many have suggested that the low incidence of true-positive and the relatively large number of false-positive results in stages I and II disease renders bone scintigraphy a poor return on diagnostic investment, and recommend that baseline scintigraphy be reserved for stages III and IV disease.[87,236–239] Others consider bone scintigraphy an important baseline for comparison with future studies, especially in view of the large number of patients who eventually develop bone metastases.[88,240,241]

The recommendations of Coleman et al.[242] are worth considering. They reviewed their experience with baseline scintigraphy in 1155 patients with breast cancer. If they had eliminated baseline studies in all patients with stage I disease, they would have missed only one of 308 patients (0.3%) who presented with bone metastases. They recommend, accordingly, that only patients with preoperative stages II, III, and IV disease receive baseline bone scintigraphy. Of those patients, only 4% had positive baseline studies; however, the authors concluded that the value to those patients in whom needless

Table 1. Drugs that Alter the Biodistribution of Tc-99m-Labeled Phosphates and Phosphonates

INTERFERING DRUG	OBSERVED EFFECTS	MECHANISM	REFS.
Iron dextran	↓bone; ↑renal uptake; ↑uptake at injection site	?transchelation or complex formation; local hyperemia	43,44,45,46
Diphosphonate (Didronel)	↓bone; ↑renal uptake	?alter bone binding sites	47,48
Amphotericin B	↑renal retention	probable nephrotoxicity	49
Gentamycin	"	"	50
Cyclophosphamide	"	"	51
Vincristine	"	"	2
Doxorubicin	"	"	2
"	↑skull uptake (scimitar sign)	??	
Aluminum (antacids)	↑liver uptake	?colloid formation	52,53
Sodium diatrizoate	↑renal uptake ↑liver uptake	?osmotic effect; ?altered pH	54
Estrogens	↑breast uptake	?↑phosphatase receptor sites	55,56
ϵ-aminocaproic acid	↑muscle uptake	drug induced myopathy (rare)	57
Corticosteroids	↓bone uptake	?bone ischemia	58
GMCSF and GCSF	↑bone uptake in long bones	?bone marrow stimulation	NIH exp

GMCSF = Granulocyte myelocyte colony stimulating factor

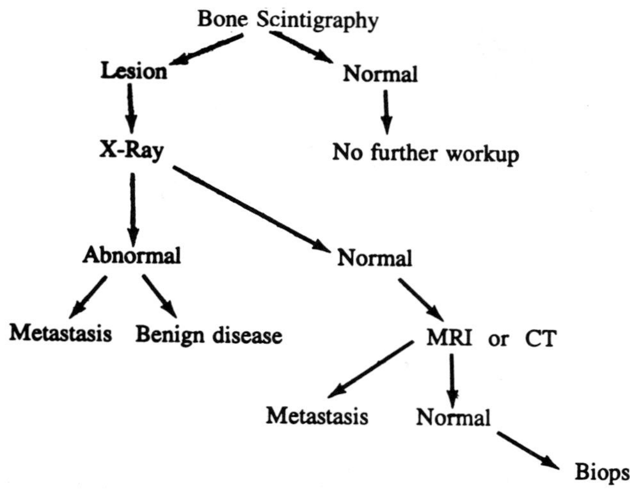

Figure 11. Decision tree for the diagnosis of bone metastases. Modified from Reference 8.

mastectomy was avoided justifies the large number of negative studies. This strategy avoids also a false-positive rate of about 1.6% among patients with stage I disease.

Follow-up Scintigraphy. The diversity of opinion as regards the value of serial bone scintigraphy following surgery in patients with breast cancer is even greater. In recognition of the high incidence of bone metastases in breast cancer, many centers routinely include bone scintigraphy as a part of postsurgical follow-up, usually at intervals of 6 months for the first 2 years and yearly thereafter. Several of these studies have been reviewed by Fogelman and Coleman.[83] Most investigators have concluded that routine follow-up scintigraphy cannot be recommended, because of the high cost and the low percentage (≈3%) of positive studies in the absence of other clinical indications of disease progression. Others point out, however, that a good case can be made for serial follow-up scintigraphy in patients with stage II and III disease, as well as in any patient with bone pain or elevated alkaline phosphatase, or with previous cancer in the opposite breast.[83]

Bone Scintigraphy to Assess Treatment. The use of scintigraphy to assess response to therapy is complicated by the fact that tracer uptake within lesions may increase, decrease, or stay the same following regression of nonosseous lesions elsewhere.[83] The flare phenomenon has been regarded as a positive indication of response to therapy.[243,244] However, this phenomenon probably occurs in a small percentage of patients who have other evidence of response. The use of SPECT quantification to provide objective criteria of lesion response has been suggested,[245] but has not gained wide acceptance.

At the National Institutes of Health (NIH), patients are followed with serial scintigraphy to monitor therapy. Decreases in lesion intensity are corroborated by bone radiographs for radiological evidence of healing (sclerosis), which is usually not apparent for 4 to 6 months (Fig. 20). If new bone lesions are detected scintigraphically after 6 months, therapy is reevaluated for possible modifications.

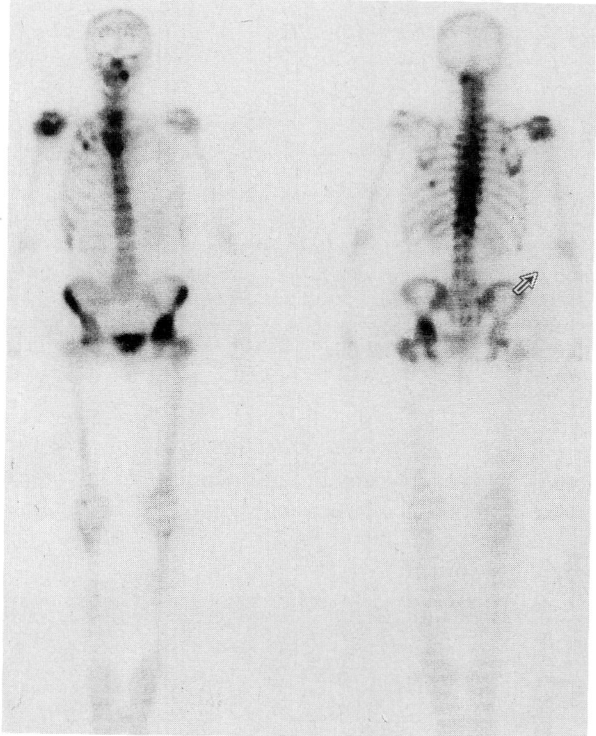

Figure 12. ^{99m}Tc-MDP scintigraphy in a 54-year-old female with breast carcinoma (the arrow points to the injection site). Intense focal lesions in the right shoulder, sternum, cervical and thoracic spine, ribs, left ilium, left acetabulum and ischium, left proximal femur, and right femoral neck suggest metastases. The lumbar spine is difficult to evaluate because prior radiation greatly reduces tracer uptake in this region. Spot films showed a left C1 lesion rather than a maxillary dental lesion and normal activity in the left anterior iliac crest. The diffuse activity in the skull is consistent with hyperostosis frontalis interna. The right patellar lesion is most likely arthritic.

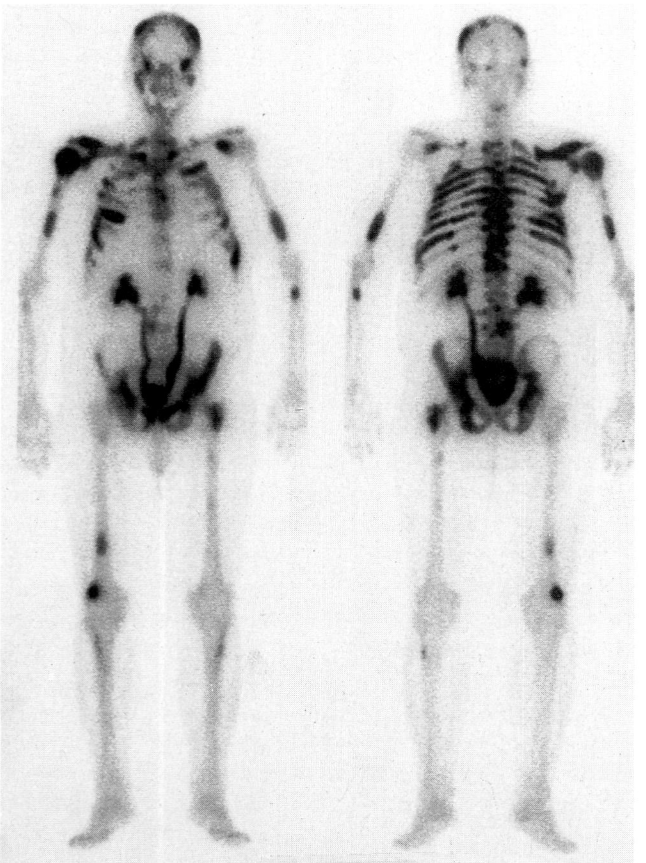

Figure 13. This 62-year-old man has the typical appearance of widely disseminated prostatic carcinoma metastases to bone. Note dilated ureters and renal collecting system, a complication of prostatectomy. In this type of display format, the images are usually reproduced at two intensity settings to highlight fainter lesions. The low-intensity image (not shown) would not visualize the faint lesions in the left femoral diaphysis.

Prostate Carcinoma

There is far greater unanimity of opinion as to the efficacy of bone scintigraphy in patients with prostate carcinoma

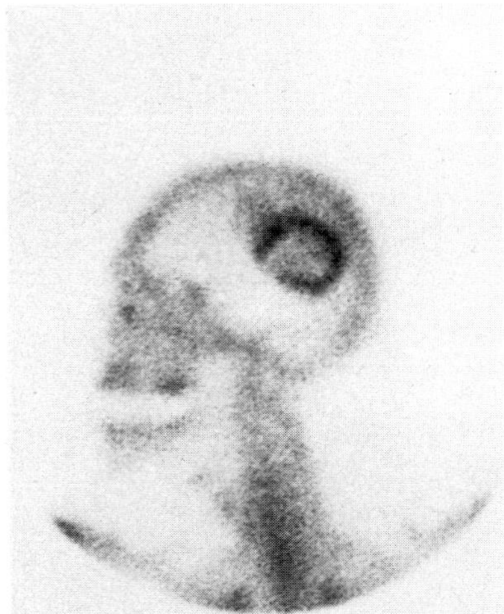

Figure 15. Angiosarcoma metastatic to the skull, showing large expansile lesion with necrotic center in left parietum.

than exists for breast cancer. The incidence of eventual bone metastatic involvement in patients with prostate carcinoma approaches 80%. Early bone metastases are also common; Johansson et al. reported that bone scintigraphy detected skeletal metastases in 24% of patients at the time of presentation.[246] Of these patients, 27% had negative radiographs and 29% had normal serum acid phosphatase. Only 26% of the patients with skeletal metastases had bone pain at the time of presentation. In cases in which scintigraphy was negative, no other tests for bone metastases were positive. Thus, when bone scintigraphy is negative at the time of diagnosis, skeletal radiographs can be considered superfluous. These investigators found, however, that bone scintigraphy was unreliable in evaluating the therapeutic response before 6 months of treatment.

There are no unique scintigraphic characteristics of prostate carcinoma, although two features are commonly encountered: (1) multiple, wide-spread, extremely intense uptake in lesions is a common pattern of distribution (Fig. 13) and

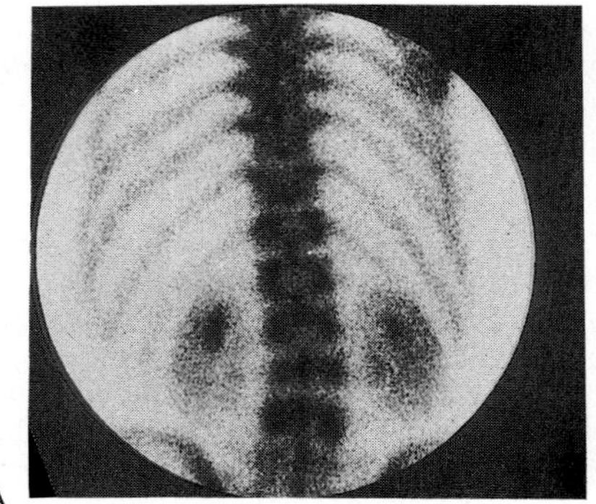

A

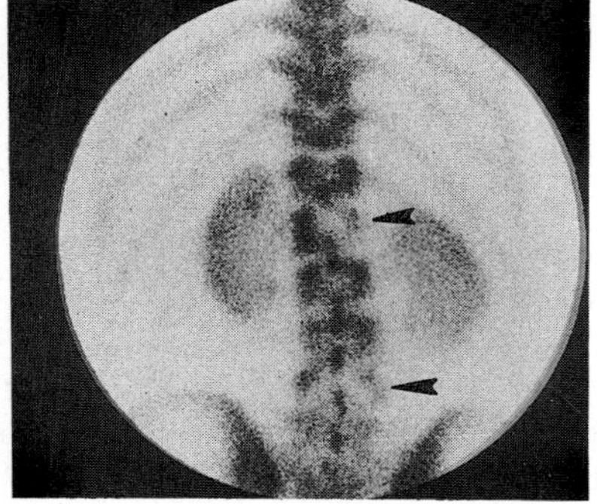

B

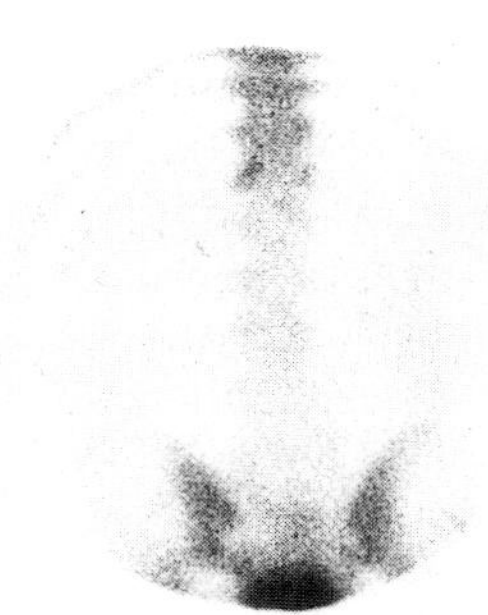

C

Figure 14. ^{99m}Tc-MDP bone scintigraphy in a patient with anaplastic lung carcinoma. **(A).** The initial study was interpreted as negative for metastatic disease. In retrospect, L4 may demonstrate increased intensity. **(B).** Two months later, L1 and L4 (arrows) reveal definite cold lesions that correlated with lytic lesions radiographically. **(C).** Following external beam radiation to the lumbar spine for bone pain, there is markedly decreased uptake in the entire lumbar spine.

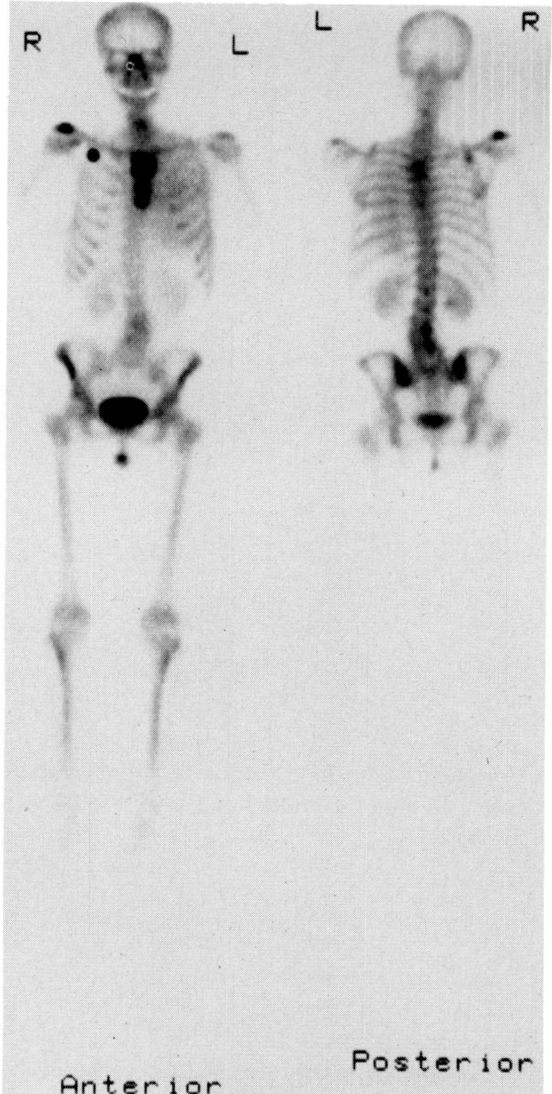

Figure 16. This 48-year-old woman has breast cancer invading the sternum by direct extension, rather than by hematogenous spread. The right acromioclavicular intensity is due to arthritis (radiographs negative) and the intense focus of activity over the right lateral second rib represents the Portacath injection site.

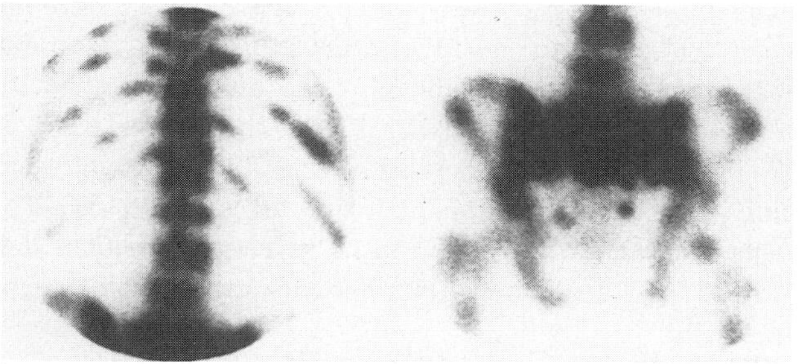

Figure 17. Posterior spine (left) and pelvis (right) in a 60-year-old patient with prostatic carcinoma with extensive metastases and nonvisualization of the kidneys, a pattern known as a "super scan."

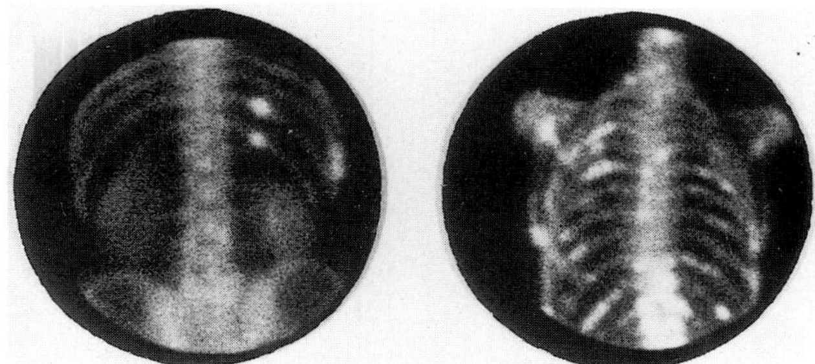

Figure 18. Posterior rib images demonstrating fractures (left) and multiple metastases (right). Rib fractures are focal, are often aligned, decrease in intensity with time, and are frequently found at the costochondral junction. Rib metastases are often linear along the rib shaft and increase in intensity with time.

is rather like the appearance of breast carcinoma metastases in women; (2) widespread involvement of the pelvis or hemipelvis is also commonly encountered, which suggests regional rather than hematogenous spread. At times, this pattern resembles that seen in Paget's disease.

Attempts have been made to use serum markers to predict the need for bone scintigraphy, the two most promising being alkaline phosphatase bone isoenzyme (B-ALP) and prostate specific antigen (PSA).[247–249] Freitas and colleagues found that a PSA value of $\leq$8 ng/ml excluded bone metastases with a predictive value of a negative test of 98.5%.[248] By receiver operating curve (ROC) analysis, B-ALP appears to be the most sensitive marker; a normal serum value indicates a very low probability of bone metastases.[247] Others have shown that patients with normal acid phosphatase, normal alkaline phosphatase, and no bone pain will have positive scintigrams in fewer than 1% of cases.[249]

Serial bone scintigraphy has been the preferred technique for following the course of bone metastases during and following chemotherapy. Pollen et al. found that with carefully standardized methodology, tumor regression could be reliably judged by changes in the number of lesions, changes in the size or extent of lesions, and changes in the intensity of tracer uptake.[250] Lesion stability could be inferred when no significant change occurred in these parameters. Scintigraphic improvement was associated with a mean survival time of 12.3 months. Patients with stable lesions had a mean survival time of 15.7 months. Patients showing progressive lesions had a mean survival of approximately 6 months. The authors reported that only 1% of studies varied from the clinical judgment. They found that the so-called "flare reaction," or apparent lesion deterioration in the face of clinical improvement, was rare. There appears to be little disagreement about the value of bone scintigraphy in staging patients with prostate carcinoma and as a technique to follow response to therapy. The frequency of follow-up will vary with physician experience and reliance on serum markers. At the NIH, patients with proven bone metastases are studied at 3-month intervals during courses of chemotherapy and at

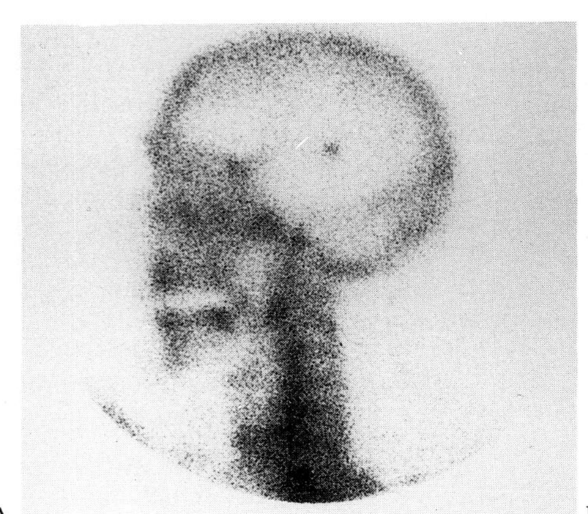

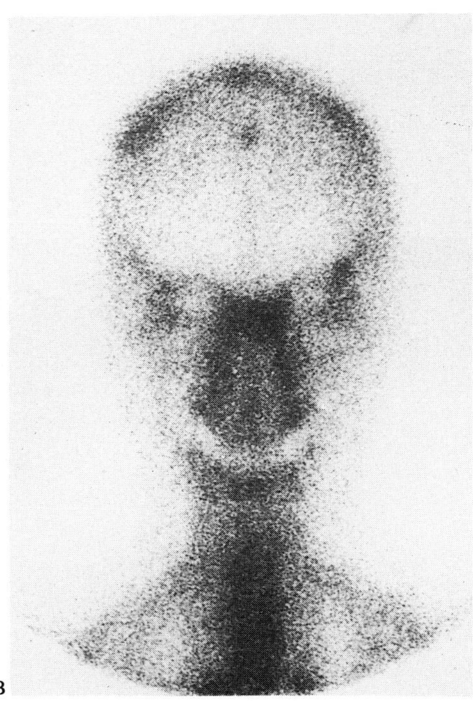

Figure 19 A,B. Small, discrete foci in the skull as shown in these two scintigrams are benign findings, probably cartilaginous rest bodies within cranial sutures.

6-month or 12-month intervals during periods of clinical stability.

Lung Cancer

The incidence of bone metastases at autopsy in patients with primary lung cancer ranges from 30 to 50%. Furthermore, the presence of bone metastases gravely affects prognosis; in one study, 40 of 46 patients with positive scintigraphy died within 6 months of examination.[251] Indeed, there is general agreement that bone scintigraphy at the initial staging is essential when: (1) the histology is small cell (oat cell) type; (2) the patient has bone pain or elevated serum alkaline phosphatase or calcium; or (3) the primary lesion is extensive, regardless of symptoms.[252–256]

The chief unresolved question is the role of bone scintigraphy in asymptomatic patients with stages I or II non-small cell carcinoma. Hooper et al. reported that, although 8% of patients with no clinical evidence of metastases had positive bone scintigraphy, true-positive results occurred in fewer than 4%, and there were about the same number of false-positive results.[254] Others[253] have argued that while the incidence of true-positive scintigraphy in this class of asymptomatic patients is small, the implications for therapy (e.g., 10% operative mortality) are so great that identification of the small number with preoperative metastatic disease makes clinical and economic sense.

No reliable studies exist to guide the clinician in selecting the appropriate interval for follow-up bone scans. At NIH, patients are studied yearly in the absence of clinical findings suggesting worsening disease.

Hypertrophic osteoarthropathy is found in as many as 10% of patients with lung cancer.[257] This condition may disappear with removal of the tumor and reappear with tumor recurrence.

Renal Carcinoma

Cole et al.[258] and Parthasarathy et al.[259] reported 42% and 50% true-positive scintigrams in patients with renal cell carcinoma. Both groups concluded that bone scintigraphy is a useful staging procedure, especially considering the high morbidity associated with nephrectomy, from which patients with disseminated disease may be spared. On the other hand, Rosen and Murphy[260] found only 3 of 40 (7.5%) true-positive results. Only one of these patients was asymptomatic, with bone metastases as the only evidence of metastatic disease. They concluded that bone scintigraphy is not warranted as a routine staging procedure; however, the latter judgment should probably be reserved until more studies have been analyzed. This is especially true because bone scintigraphy appears to be more sensitive in detecting renal carcinoma metastases to bone than either elevated alkaline phosphatase or skeletal roentgenograms.[261,262] Kim et al. found that 7 of 62 (11%) lesions in patients with renal cell carcinoma were "cold," a fact that may increase the true-positive yield if generally recognized.[262] The same investigators noted that fully 45% of "cold" metastases were not apparent roentgenographically.

At the NIH, it is customary to obtain bone scintigrams annually on patients with renal cell carcinoma without evidence of bone metastases. Clyne et al.[263] found that 8 of 23

Table 2. Soft-Tissue Lesions Associated with Uptake of Tc-99m Phosphate Compounds

CONDITION	REFERENCE
BREAST	
BENIGN	
Lactation	O'Connell MEA, Sutton H[92]
Fat necrosis	Schmitt GH, et al.[93]
Mazoplasia	Schmitt GH, et al.[93]
Gynecomastia	Brill DR[94]
Postmastectomy	Isitman AT, et al.[95]
Breast prosthesis	Jayabalan V, Berry S[96]
Fibrocystic disease and mammary dysplasia	McDougall IR, Pistenma OA[97]
	Holmes RA, et al.[98]
MALIGNANT	
Primary breast cancer	Chaudhuri TK, et al.[99]
	Schmitt GH, et al.[93]
Metastatic breast carcinoma	Costello P, et al.[100]
	Berg GR, et al.[101]
	Chaudhuri TK, et al.[99]
CARDIOVASCULAR SYSTEM	
BENIGN	
Acute or chronic myocardial infarction	Bonte FJ, et al.[102]
	Buja LM, et al.[103]
Unstable angina	Willerson JT, et al.[104]
	Perez LA, et al.[105]
Left ventricular aneurysm	Ahmad M, et al.[106]
	Ahmad M, et al.[107]
Aortic aneurysm	Campeau RJ, et al.[108]
Myocardial contusion	Ahmad M, et al.[107]
	Go RT, et al.[109]
	Doty DB, et al.[110]
Mönckeberg's sclerosis	Thrall JH, et al.[111]
Calcified valves	Ahmad M, et al.[106]
	Wald RW, et al.[112]
	Jengo JA, et al.[113]
Calcified coronary arteries	Wald RW, et al.[112]
Prosthetic valves	Seo I, Donoghue G[114]
Chemotherapy	Chacko AK, et al.[115]
Radiotherapy	Ahmad M, et al.[107]
	Soin JS, et al.[116]
Amyloidosis	Braun SD, et al.[117]
Pericarditis and endocarditis	Singh A, et al.[118]
	Riba AL, et al.[119]
	Janowitz WR, Serafini AN[120]
Chagas' disease	Da Rocha AFG, et al.[121]
Cardioversion	Palestro, et al.[122]
MALIGNANT	
Metastatic calcification	Arbona GL, et al.[123]
Malignant pericardial effusions	Quaife MA, et al.[124]
Metastases to heart	Ahmad M, et al.[107]
Hemangiopericytoma	Chew FS, Hudson TM[125]
GASTROINTESTINAL SYSTEM	
BENIGN	
Milk-alkali syndrome	Delcourt E, et al.[126]
	Desai A, et al.[127]
Intestinal infarction	Schimmel DH, et al.[128]
	Ortiz VN, et al.[129]
	Moss AA, Kressel HY[130]
Abdominal aneurysm	Campeau RJ, et al.[108]
Gastric calcification	Jayabalan V, DeWitt B[131]
Necrotizing enterocolitis	Caride V, et al.[132]
Trauma from nasogastric tube	Goldfarb CR, et al.[133]
MALIGNANT	
Metastatic calcification	Richards AG[134]

(Table continued on next page.)

Table 2. Continued

CONDITION	REFERENCE
GASTROINTESTINAL SYSTEM	
MALIGNANT	
Metastases from rectal adenocarcinoma	Shultz MM, et al.[135]
Mucinous adenocarcinoma of the stomach	Singh BN, et al.[136]
Malignant ascites	Gordon L, et al.[137]
Colorectal metastases	Chaudhuri TK, et al.[99]
GENITOURINARY SYSTEM	
BENIGN	
Acute tubular necrosis	Lavelle KJ, et al.[138]
Chemotherapy	Lutrin CL, et al.[139]
	Trackler TR, Chinn RYW[140]
Radiotherapy	Lutrin CL, Goris ML[141]
Kidney (following radiographic contrast)	Lantieri RL, et al.[142]
	Crawford JA, Gummerman LW[54]
Iron excess	Parker JA, et al.[46]
Thalassemia major	Valdez DA, Jacobstein JG[143]
Nephrocalcinosis	Bossuyt A, et al.[144]
Phimosis	Glassman AB, Selby JB[145]
Orchitis	Sty JR, et al.[146]
Wolman's disease	Sty JR, Starshak RJ[147]
Leiomyoma of uterus	Manoli RS, Soin JS[148]
Chronic renal failure	Desai A, et al.[127]
Kidney in sickle cell anemia	Sty JR, et al.[146]
Urinoma	Sham R, et al.[149]
Transplant ischemia	Thomsen HS, et al.[150]
Myoglobinuria	Sty JR, Starshak RJ[151]
MALIGNANT	
Erythroleukemia	
Metastatic calcification	Arbona GL, et al.[123]
Hypernephroma	Dhawan VM, et al.[152]
Primary renal tumors	Sham R, et al.[149]
Lymphatic lymphosarcoma	Richman LS, et al.[153]
Ovarian carcinoma	Gates GF[154]
Metastatic seminoma	Hardy JG, et al.[155]
HEAD, NECK, AND NEUROLOGICAL SYSTEM	
BENIGN	
Cerebrovascular accident	Grames GM, et al.[156]
Brain abscess	Grames GM, et al.[156]
Thyroid nodule	Grames GM, et al.[156]
Arteriovenous malformation	Kim TC[157]
Cerebritis	Grames GM, et al.[156]
Chronic subdural hematoma	Grames GM, et al.[156]
Cerebral infarction	Grames GM, Jansen C[158]
Toxic goiter	Norbash AM and DeLong SR[159]
MALIGNANT	
Metastatic calcification (thyroid)	Arbona GL, et al.[123]
Cerebral tumors	Chaudhuri TK, et al.[99]
	Grames GM, et al.[156]
Calcified thyroid carcinoma	Tonami T, et al.[160]
Brain metastases	Berg GR, et al.[101]
	Chaudhuri TK, et al.[99]
Medullary carcinoma	Van der Vis-Melsen MJE, et al.[161]
Schwannoma	Chew FS, Hudson TM[125]
Neurolemmoma	Chew FS, Hudson TM[125]
Primary neuroblastoma	Fitzer PM[162]
	Smith FW, et al.[163]
LIVER	
BENIGN	
Amyloidosis	Vanek JA, et al.[164]
Postarteriography (sodium diatrizoate)	Crawford JA, Gummerman LW[54]
Necrosis	Lyons KP, et al.[165]

Table 2. Continued

CONDITION	REFERENCE
LIVER	
BENIGN	
Aluminum excess	Jaresko GS, et al.[166]
Cocaine hepatotoxicity	Whitten CG, Luke BA[167]
MALIGNANT	
Cholangiocarcinoma	Guiberteau MJ, et al.[168]
Metastases from colon carcinoma	Poulose KP, et al.[169]
	Garcia AC, et al.[170]
Malignant melanoma	DeLong JF, et al.[171]
Metastases from oat cell carcinoma of lung	
Neuroblastoma, soft-tissue uptake	Rosenfield N, Treves S[172]
Metastases from osteosarcoma	Teates CD, et al.[172]
	Wilkinson RH, Gaede JT[174]
LUNG	
BENIGN	
Radiotherapy	Sarreck R, et al.[175]
	Lowenthal IS, et al.[176]
	Vieras F[179]
Fibrothorax	Ravin CE, et al.[178]
Sarcoidosis	Poulose KP, et al.[169]
Interstitial pulmonary calcification	Grames GM, et al.[179]
	De Graaf P, et al.[180]
	Herry JY, et al.[181]
Berylliosis	Palmer PES, et al.[182]
Lung nodules in chronic hemodialysis	Faubert PF, et al.[183]
Hyperparathyroidism	"
Aspergillosis	"
Tuberculosis	"
Hypervitaminosis D	"
Therapy with phosphates	"
Calcium infusions	"
MALIGNANT	
Metastatic calcification	Richards AG[134]
Bronchogenic carcinoma	Poulose KP, et al.[169]
	Lowenthal IS, et al.[176]
Metastases from osteogenic sarcoma	Brower AC, Teates CD[184]
Malignant pleural effusion	Siegel ME, et al.[185]
MUSCLE AND PERIARTICULAR TISSUES	
BENIGN	
Iron dextran injection	Byun HH, et al.[186]
Rhabdomyolysis	Silberstein EB, Bove KE[187]
Polymyositis	Spies SM, et al.[188]
Muscle trauma	Blair RJ, et al.[189]
Overexertion	Lentle BC, et al.[190]
McArdle syndrome and disorders of glycogenolysis	Swift TR, Brown M[191]
Muscular dystrophy	Bellina CR, et al.[192]
Postrevascularization	Floyd JL, Prather JL[193]
Myositis ossificans	Suzuki Y, et al.[194]
Precordial electrostimulation	Slutsky LT, et al.[195]
	Pugh BR, et al.[196]
	Ahmad M, et al.[107]
Electric burns	Lewis SE, et al.[197]
Sickle cell disease	Gelfand MJ, Planitz MK[198]
Ischemia	Simpson AJ[199]
Chemoperfusion	Sorkin SJ, et al.[200]
Radiotherapy	Bekier A[201]
Amyloidosis	Van Antwerp JD, et al.[203]
Synovitis	Heerfordt J, et al.[203]
Calcific tendinitis	O'Mara RE, Charkes ND[204]
Gouty tophi	Alarcón-Segovia D, et al.[205]
Calcified myoma	Ell PJ, et al.[206]

(Table continued on next page.)

Table 2. Continued

CONDITION	REFERENCE
MUSCLE AND PERIARTICULAR TISSUES	
BENIGN	
Ipsilateral uptake following lumbar sympathectomy	Lentle BC, et al.[207]
Fibromatosis	Sty JR, et al.[208]
Cartilaginous exostosis	Sty JR, et al.[146]
Migratory osteolysis	Strashun A, Chayes Z[209]
Calcinosis universalis	Desai A, et al.[127]
Dystrophic calcifications	Desai A, et al.[127]
Extravasated calcium gluconate	
Chronic dialysis	Tattler, et al.[210]
MALIGNANT	
Rhabdomyosarcoma	Chew FS, Hudson TM[125]
Synovioma	Chew FS, Hudson TM[125]
SKIN AND SUBCUTANEOUS TISSUES	
BENIGN	
Electrical burns	Lewis SE, et al.[197]
Precordial electrostimulation	Pugh BR, et al.[196]
Filariasis	Oster Z[211]
Inflamed breast implant	Jayabalan V, Berry S[96]
Pseudoxanthoma elasticum	Bossuyt A, Verbeelen D[212]
Amyloidosis	Heerfordt J, et al.[203]
	Van Antwerp JD, et al.[202]
	Bada L, et al.[213]
	Vanek JA, et al.[164]
Calcinosis universalis	Pendergrass HP, et al.[214]
Tumoral calcinosis	Eugenidis N, Locher JT[215]
	Desai A, et al.[129]
Infiltrated calcium solution	Balsam D, et al.[216]
Soft-tissue inflammation	Bautovich G, et al.[217]
Abscess	Chaudhuri TK, et al.[99]
	Berg GR, et al.[101]
Surgical incision	Thrall JH, et al.[111]
	Poulose KP, et al.[169]
Radiotherapy	Vieras F[177]
Hyperhydrosis	Ajmani SK, et al.[218]
Fat necrosis	Williams JL, et al.[219]
Spinal cord injury	Prakash V, et al.[220]
Drug injection	Brill DR[221]
Urinary contamination	
Dermatomyositis	Brown M, et al.[222]
	Sarminento AH, et al.[223]
Soft-tissue abscess	Chaudhuri TK, et al.[99]
Healing wound	Poulose KP, et al.[169]
Transcutaneous nitroglycerin patch	Gallini, et al.[224]
Chemoperfusion	Sorkin SJ, et al.[200]
Soft-tissue irradiation	Bekier A[201]
	Lutrin CL, Goris ML[141]
Folds of fat	
Neurofibroma	Nolan NG[225]
Metastatic calcification	McLaughlin AF[226]
	Richards AG[134]
	Lowenthal IS, et al.[176]
Angiolipoma	Chew FS, Hudson TM[227]
Lipoma	Chew FS, Hudson TM[227]
Hematoma	Chew FS, Hudson TM[227]
Fibromatosis	
MALIGNANT	
Soft-tissue sarcoma	Nakajima H, et al.[228]
	Chew FS, Hudson TM[125]
Liposarcoma	Pearlman AW[229]
Malignant fibrous hystiocytoma	Chew FS, Hudson TM[125]

Table 2. Continued

CONDITION	REFERENCE
SKIN AND SUBCUTANEOUS TISSUES	
MALIGNANT	
Ewing's sarcoma of soft parts	Chew FS, Hudson TM[125]
Osteosarcoma	Chew FS, Hudson TM[125]
SPLEEN AND HEMATOLOGIC SYSTEM	
BENIGN	
G6PD deficiency	Lieberman CM, Hemingway DL[230]
Hemosiderosis	Winter PF[231]
Infarction (sickle cell anemia)	Goy W, Crowe WJ[232]
Thalassemia major	Howman-Giles RB, et al.[233]
MALIGNANT	
Splenic lymphoma	Winter PF[231]
Reticulum cell sarcoma	Richman LS, et al.[153]
Lymphosarcoma	Gilday DL, et al.[234]
OTHER	
BENIGN	
Filarial infestation	Oster Z[211]
Christmas disease	Forbes CD, et al.[235]
Lymphoma	Chaudhuri TK, et al.[99]
Uterine fibroid	Ell PJ, et al.[206]
Neuroblastoma	Fitzer PM[162]
Ganglioneuroblastoma	Fitzer PM[162]
"Glove phenomenon" due to arterial injection	

such patients developed true-positive bone scintigrams, 6 of whom had bone pain at the time scintigraphy became positive.

Bladder Carcinoma

Approximately 25% of patients with bladder carcinoma have bone metastases at autopsy.[264] In a retrospective study of unselected patients, Parthasarathy et al. found positive bone scintigrams in 50% of patients studied.[259] However, several studies have shown a much lower incidence (2 to 4.5%) of true positive scintigrams at the time of initial staging.[265–267] Brismar and Gustafson found no true-positive scintigrams in 68 patients and, in reviewing the literature, could find only 4 of 458 patients (0.9%) for whom surgery was avoided by positive bone scintigraphy.[268] It thus appears that bone scintigraphy in bladder carcinoma should be reserved for patients with clinical evidence of bone metastases, both at presentation and during follow-up.

Cervical Carcinoma

Most studies have shown that there is a low incidence of positive bone scintigraphy in patients with stages 0, I, and II carcinoma of the cervix.[269,270] In a large retrospective study, Du Toit and Grove found that none of 210 patients with stage I or II disease had true-positive scintigrams and 11 of 340 (3.2%) with stages III and IV disease had true-positive scans.[271] Of these, only 6 patients were moved from stage III to stage IV on the basis of scintigraphy. Interestingly, Bassan and Glaser found that the degree of tumor differentiation was more important than tumor stage in determining the utility of bone scintigraphy.[270] Of 19 (out of a total of 88 patients) with poorly differentiated tumors or locally advanced tumors, 13 (68%) had true-positive scintigrams. Thus, it appears that there is little utility in routine bone scintigraphy in asymptomatic patients with clinically early and well-differentiated cervical carcinoma. Rather, scintigraphy should be reserved for patients with clinical evidence of bone metastases or who have advanced regional or histologically poorly differentiated tumors.

Endometrial Carcinoma

Fewer than 1% of patients with endometrial carcinoma have positive bone scintigraphy at presentation.[272–274] In patients with recurrent disease, the incidence may be higher.[273]

Ovarian Carcinoma

The incidence of positive scintigrams is also low in ovarian carcinoma.[273,274] Mettler found the incidence was 3 of 40 in stage III ovarian carcinoma.[274] In these gynecologic tumors, bone scintigraphy should be reserved for patients with clinical evidence of bone metastases.

Testicular Cancer

Merrick reported an incidence of 5% positive scintigraphy (3 of 61) in patients with testicular cancer: 2 of 26 patients (8%) with seminoma and 1 of 29 patients (3%) with teratoma.[275] Three additional patients developed positive scintigrams during early follow-up. Merrick concluded that bone scintigraphy is probably not useful in the evaluation of pa-

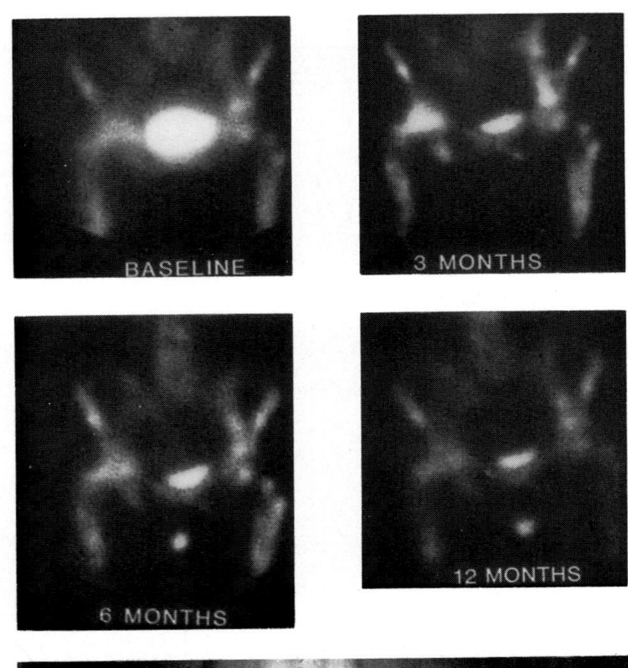

A

Figure 20. **(A).** Serial bone scintigraphy in a patient with breast carcinoma responding to tamoxifen and prednisolone. Increased activity in baseline lesions and new lesions are seen at 3 months, followed by resolution at 6 and 12 months. **(B).** Radiograph of the pelvis before therapy shows primarily lytic lesions. **(C).** Radiograph 6 months later confirms response by sclerosis of the lytic disease. Reproduced by permission from Reference 82.

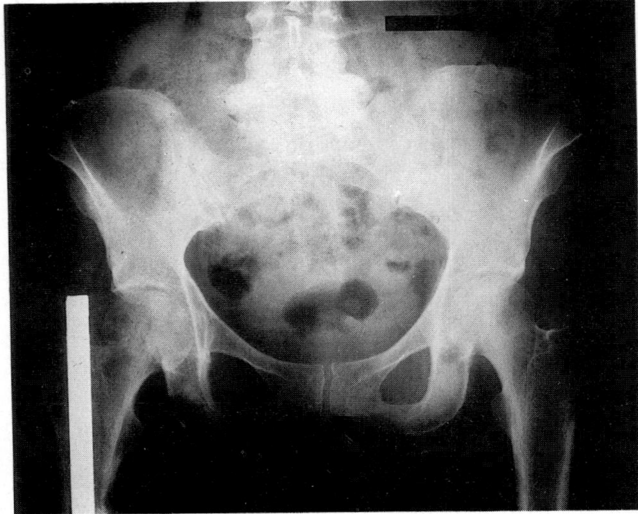

B

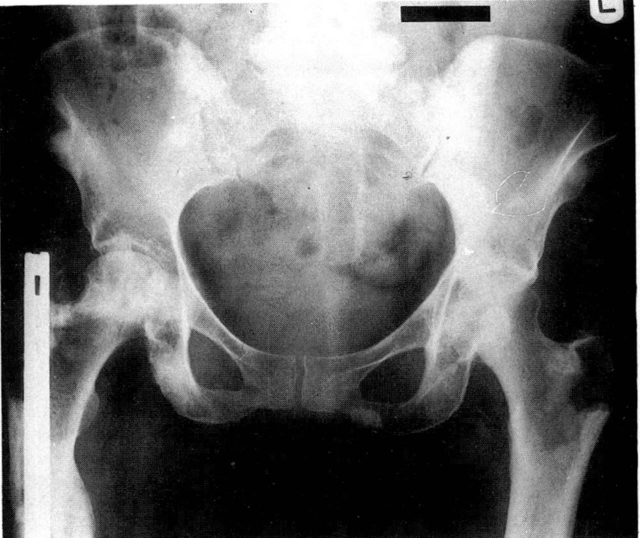

C

tients presenting with early testicular tumors, but that it may be of value in patients with stage IV seminoma, in patients with recurrence, and after radical surgery for seminoma.

Neuroblastoma

Gilday et al. have recommended bone scintigraphy as the screening procedure of choice in children suspected of having skeletal metastases from neuroblastoma.[234] Furthermore, they recommend that roentgenograms be obtained only if bone scintigraphy shows a positive lesion. They found no false-negative scintigrams among 30 patients with neuroblastoma. However, Podrasky et al. reported a false-negative rate of 5%,[276] and Kaufman et al. found that bone scintigraphy detected only 4 of 18 lesions, while roentgenograms detected 14.[279] Most of these false-positives were caused by symmetrical lesions in the metaphyses of long bones. Here, detection of abnormalities is difficult because of the intense uptake of the radiopharmaceutical in the child's adjacent epiphyses.

There are four methods for avoiding this pitfall: (1) three-phase bone scintigraphy (see above), (2) adjust the film exposure so that the epiphyses and metaphyses are not overexposed, (3) perform SPECT on any questionable limb joint, (4) the full assessment of patients with neuroblastoma should include MIBG scintigraphy; whole-body imaging will likely reveal bone metastases. In fact, ^{131}I- or ^{123}I-MIBG scintigraphy is generally reported to be more sensitive than bone scintigraphy for detecting bone metastases from neuroblastoma.[278,279] Bone scintigraphy should be obtained, nevertheless, because some metastases are too small to be visualized with the poor resolution of ^{131}I images. Frequently, the primary tumor is visualized by bone scintigraphy, although this is of no practical value.

Gastrointestinal Tract Carcinomas

In general, bone scintigraphy has little role in the routine staging of gastrointestinal tumors, since they tend to metastasize to bone only late in their course. Most investigators recommend bone scintigraphy only in those patients with other clinical evidence of bone metastases.[280,281] The same recommendation can be made for head and neck tumors.[282,283]

Thyroid Cancer

Bone metastases are a grave sign in the evolution of well-differentiated thyroid carcinoma, which generally has a long and indolent course. Only two studies have evaluated bone scintigraphy in well-differentiated thyroid carcinoma. Both deal with small numbers of patients, but have quite different findings.[284,285] Castillo et al. found bone scintigraphy to be far less sensitive than ^{131}I metastatic surveys in detecting bone metastases, particularly in the spine.[284] Approximately 60% of the bone metastases identified by ^{131}I scintigraphy and by radiography were negative by bone scintigraphy. Another 19% showed only slight increase in the uptake of ^{99m}Tc-phosphonate. One patient with multiple bone metastases would have been missed relying upon bone scintigraphy alone.

In Dewan's study,[285] there was much closer correspondence between bone and ^{131}I scintigraphic findings, although ^{131}I better identified bone metastases. There was a significant difference between the two populations, which may account for the different sensitivities found. In the Castillo study, the average interval between scintigraphy and diagnosis was 6 years, presumably after various forms of treatment including ^{131}I therapy. In the second study, bone scintigraphy was obtained at the time of initial therapy. Since ^{131}I therapy is known to change the metabolic activity of metastases, they may become inactive and, hence, scintigraphically (but not radiographically) negative. Castillo et al. concluded that bone scintigraphy has little utility in the workup of well-differentiated thyroid carcinoma. In neither study did bone scintigraphy contribute to therapeutic decision making.

One study has suggested that ^{201}Tl scintigraphy may be as, or more, sensitive than ^{131}I in detecting thyroid metastases.[286]

In medullary carcinoma of the thyroid, Johnson et al. found that bone scintigraphy may be useful in patients who have elevated serum calcium.[287]

Multiple Myeloma

Bone scintigraphy has consistently been found to be less sensitive than radiography in detecting myeloma bone lesions.[288–291] The same is true for both multiple and solitary plasmacytomas and both early and late disease. Neither type of tumor nor treatment status appears to alter the scintigram:radiograph sensitivity ratio.[288] Bone scintigraphy, however, is more sensitive in detecting lesions in ribs and pelvis, areas that are difficult to evaluate for small lesions radiographically. Woolfenden et al.[288] have shown that lesion detectability changes during the course of the disease. They found typically the following transitions: (a) abnormal scintigraphy and normal radiograph → (b) abnormal scintigraphy and abnormal radiograph → (c) normal scintigraphy and abnormal radiograph. They speculate that early in the genesis of a lesion, before the radiograph becomes positive, metabolic activity is high and, thus, scintigraphy is positive. Later, as calcium is lost, the lesion becomes radiographically apparent. Finally, some transition occurs to reduce metabolic activity within the lesions. The most frequently encountered lesions that are scintigraphically negative and radiographically positive are well advanced, entirely lytic lesions. Preliminary studies suggest that MRI is highly sensitive for myeloma bone lesions.[292]

The utility of scintigraphy in following the course of therapy has not been determined. Bataille et al. found that scintigraphically active disease correlated well with clinically active disease, and that regression of scintigraphic lesions correlated well with disease remission.[293] These authors concluded, therefore, that scintigraphy may have prognostic value.

Lymphoma and Leukemia

Bone metastases account for approximately 5% of extranodal involvement in Hodgkin's lymphoma.[294] False-negative scintigraphy is not uncommon; however, it is still more sensitive than radiography, serum alkaline phosphatase, or even marrow biopsy.[295] This is one of the few tumors in which the long bones are as or more frequently involved than the axial skeleton.

Routine bone scintigraphy appears to have little utility in leukemia. However, it may be useful to explain bone pain. In a study of 32 pediatric patients with acute lymphocytic leukemia (ALL) reported by Kuntz et al., scintigraphy was more sensitive than radiography in locating bone metastases.[296] Here, too, the appendicular skeleton may be more frequently involved. In rare instances, photopenic lesions have been associated with bone metastases in childhood leukemia.[297,298]

Malignant Melanoma

Most studies have shown that the incidence of true-positive scintigrams in stages I and II melanoma is low and does not exceed the false-positive rate.[299–304] However, the incidence rises dramatically with advanced disease and scintigraphy is always more sensitive than radiography. In the series of Muss et al.,[305] 57% of patients studied had bone pain, including half of the patients who had normal scintigraphy. This is perhaps explained by the fact that many patients with advanced tumor have soft tissue metastases that produce

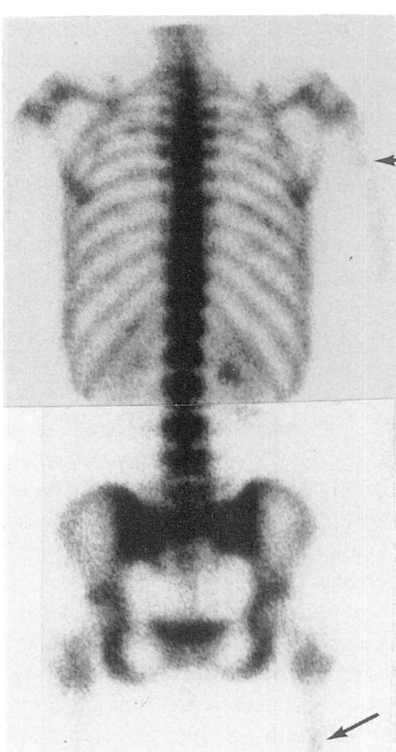

Figure 21. Diffuse abnormalities through the spine, ribs, and pelvis in a 41-year-old patient with systemic mastocytosis. Typical long bone lesions are also seen in the right humerus and femur (arrows).

symptoms resembling bone pain. In a recent review of 200 patients with metastatic malignant melanoma at the NIH (unpublished data), lesions in the lower limb bones accounted for more than 10% of bone metastases. Thus, skeletal surveys that omit the arms and legs will miss substantial numbers of lesions.

Systemic Mastocytosis

Mastocytosis is an uncommon disease of mast cell proliferation that infiltrates bone marrow, spleen, liver, skin, and lymph nodes. Systemic manifestations are caused by release of histamine, serotonin, and other hypersensitivity mediators. They include fever, flushing, diarrhea, peptic ulcer disease, and a characteristic skin rash, *urticaria pigmentosa.*

Bone scintigraphy may reveal a variety of patterns, from normal to diffusely increased uptake resembling a "superscan" (Fig. 21) to unifocal or multifocal distribution.[306–308] Bone radiographs may reveal focal or diffuse sclerotic lesions. Bone-marrow scintigraphy may also show a pattern of expanded marrow.[309]

COMPARISON OF SCINTIGRAPHY WITH MRI

Relatively few prospective studies have yet been published that address the sensitivity of MRI imaging for detecting bone metastases. However, several large retrospective studies suggest that MRI is sensitive for detecting the high-proton content of bone metastases.[293,310–312] In a study by Daffner et al.[292] 50 patients with known primary tumors and abnormal scintigrams were examined by MRI. Plain radiographs showed evidence of metastases in 33 patients, all of whom also had MRI evidence of metastases. An additional 7 patients with normal radiographs were positive by MRI. In the remaining 10 patients, plain radiographs showed benign disease and MRI was negative for bone-marrow involvement. The authors concluded that there were no false-positive and no false-negative MRI examinations in this study.

Avrahami et al.[312] studied 36 patients with a variety of solid primary tumors, all of whom had back pain. CT and bone scintigraphy were normal in all patients. Of these, 17 patients had abnormalities in either T1-weighted or T2-weighted images. All of these patients had positive needle biopsies. The authors concluded that MRI is the most sensitive imaging procedure for demonstrating bone metastases in the spine and that both T1- and T2-weighted sequences are required for maximum sensitivity.

Frank et al.[310] compared MRI with bone scintigraphy in 106 patients with either primary or metastatic bone tumors confirmed histologically by biopsy. In 32 patients, both MRI and scintigraphy were positive and in 41 patients both studies were negative. In 30 patients (28%) MRI was positive, while bone scintigraphy was negative. In 3 patients (3%) MRI was normal and scintigraphy was positive; 2 of these 3 had benign disease by biopsy. Thus, MRI in this study was significantly more sensitive and specific.

Jones et al.[313] studied 84 patients with "high risk," early breast cancer (primary tumor larger than 5 cm or positive axillary nodes). In this study, all patients with definitely positive scintigraphy were excluded. In the presence of normal scintigraphy and negative plain radiographs, 7% of patients were found to have positive MRI images. In patients with equivocal bone scintigraphy, 50% had positive MRI.

In summary, it appears that MRI is both more sensitive and specific for detecting bone metastases and, in patients with high-risk tumors and those who have clinical evidence of bone disease with negative or equivocal scintigraphy, MRI should be obtained. At this writing, however, bone scintigraphy remains the most efficient and cost-effective survey procedure for detecting metastases in most patients with tumors that have a high predilection for metastasizing to bone.

Intraoperative Bone Scintigraphy

Intraoperative bone scintigraphy was developed by Rinsky et al., who were prompted by an unsuccessful attempt to remove an osteoid osteoma, located in a vertebral pedicle.[310] Other conditions in which this technique is useful include biopsy of bone metastases, enchondroma curettement, abscess drainage, and removal of osteoblastoma. Klonecke et al. have described a technique of imaging immediately before and after surgery to help localize the lesion and determine its removal.[315] In their description, patients are injected approximately 3 hours prior to surgery. A portable scintillation camera is taken to the operating room and the detector head covered with a sterile plastic liner. The patient is then positioned for surgery and the area prepped and draped. An image of the lesion site is obtained and the focal abnormality is localized with a fine radioactive marker. The skin at that site is marked by sterile pen or with a needle to direct the surgeon's approach. Immediately afterward, a second scintiscan is made to determine complete removal. This method is obviously superior to the use of a scintillation probe, because of the certainty of localization using an image and the lack of concern for background structures.

PRIMARY BONE TUMORS

Bone scintigraphy is a useful diagnostic study in evaluating primary bone tumors. In the initial evaluation, scintigraphy is more sensitive and more efficient than radiography in determining monostotic from polyostotic involvement. In the follow-up of primary sarcomas that metastasize to bone (osteosarcoma, Ewing's sarcoma), scintigraphy is useful in following the course of disease during the time the patient is principally at risk of developing metastases.

Osteogenic Sarcoma

The peak incidence of osteogenic sarcomas, which account for approximately 20% of all sarcomas, occurs in the second decade, although they may occur at any age.[316] Half of all osteogenic sarcomas are located in the region of the knees. Other common sites include the long bone metaphyses, skull, mandible, ilium, spine, and scapula. Polyostotic involvement occurs at the time of presentation in about 2% of cases (Fig. 22). Bone scintigraphy is not useful in determining the malignant nature of primary bone tumors. Conventional radiography, CT, and MRI are more specific.

When sarcomas develop in bones that have been irradiated, the average latency period is 15 years, with a range of 3 to 55 years.[316] Although osteogenic sarcomas occur with increased frequency in foci of Paget's disease and at sites exposed to radiation therapy, only a minority of patients with primary osteogenic sarcoma have these preexisting conditions.

Bone scintigraphy demonstrates intensely increased uptake at the site of primary and metastatic lesions. Three-phase scintigraphy reflects the increased vascularity in these tumors (Fig. 23). Dissemination of osteogenic sarcoma is usually hematogenous. Rarely, distant metastases follow lymphatic routes.[317]

Soft-tissue metastases also concentrate bone radiotracers in many cases. Extraosseous metastases occur in lungs, kidney, mediastinum, pericardium, and brain. CT and plain radiographs are more sensitive than bone scintigraphy, but the high specificity of scintigraphy for metastases makes this a logical test for their detection.[318]

At autopsy, 25% of patients with primary osteogenic sarcoma have skeletal metastases. Pulmonary metastases occur most frequently, however. Before the introduction of adjuvant chemotherapy, pulmonary metastases were *always* detected prior to bone metastases.[319] Goldstein et al. found that, in patients on adjuvant therapy, 16% of those who developed pulmonary metastases previously had bone metastases.[320] On the basis of those findings, it is now generally recommended that bone scintigraphy be performed at regular intervals in all patients with osteogenic sarcoma, particularly during the first 2 years, to identify metastatic disease early. The yield of identifying metastatic disease is small, but the potential impact on therapy is substantial. In another study, McKillop et al. evaluated 55 patients with osteogenic sarcoma proven by biopsy; they performed serial bone scintigraphy at the time of presentation and during follow-up.[321] Only one patient (2%) had bone metastases at the time of presentation. During follow-up, 20 (36%) developed bone metastases and 11 (20%) of these were asymptomatic by the time scintigraphy become abnormal.

It is generally recognized that ^{99m}Tc-phosphonate scintigraphy is not a sensitive means of following the response to chemotherapy; changes in lesion uptake are quite slow to become manifest. Ramanna et al. showed that both ^{210}Tl and ^{67}Ga-citrate are more sensitive, with ^{201}Tl being superior.[322] Recently Caner et al.[323] have reported that ^{99m}Tc-MIBI may be a sensitive means of following the therapy of osteogenic sarcoma and other malignant bone tumors, and that the changes of uptake reflect the histopathologic evaluation.

Ewing's Sarcoma

Ewing's sarcoma arises from bone-marrow elements and has a peak incidence between the first and second decades. The clinical features of pain, fever, swelling, and leukocytosis may initially suggest osteomyelitis. The long bones of the extremities, especially the femur and tibia, are most often involved; ribs are involved in about 8% of cases.[316]

The typical roentgenographic appearance of Ewing's sarcoma is that of a lesion involving a long bone characterized by lytic destruction and periosteal elevation. However, these features can be seen in a variety of other primary osseous malignancies, including malignant lymphoma, osteogenic sarcoma, and in acute and chronic osteomyelitis. Histological evaluation is required to make the diagnosis.

Bone scintigraphy demonstrates intense uptake of bone-seeking tracers. In a study by Nair[324] 25 of 53 patients were found to have bone metastases at the time of presentation. Unsuspected metastases were identified in 28 of 72 patients. Thus, bone scintigraphy is an essential part of the workup of these patients. In another study by Goldstein et al.,[325] 10 of 22 patients who were initially free of metastases subsequently developed bone metastases. In 6 of these, bone scintigraphy provided the earliest evidence of metastatic disease, suggesting its value during follow-up.

Estes et al.[326] studied 30 patients with Ewing's sarcoma following chemotherapy using ^{99m}Tc-MDP and ^{67}Ga-citrate scintigraphy. They found that all 30 patients showed less primary site ^{67}Ga uptake following therapy. The decrease in ^{99m}Tc-MDP was less and not so consistent. These authors

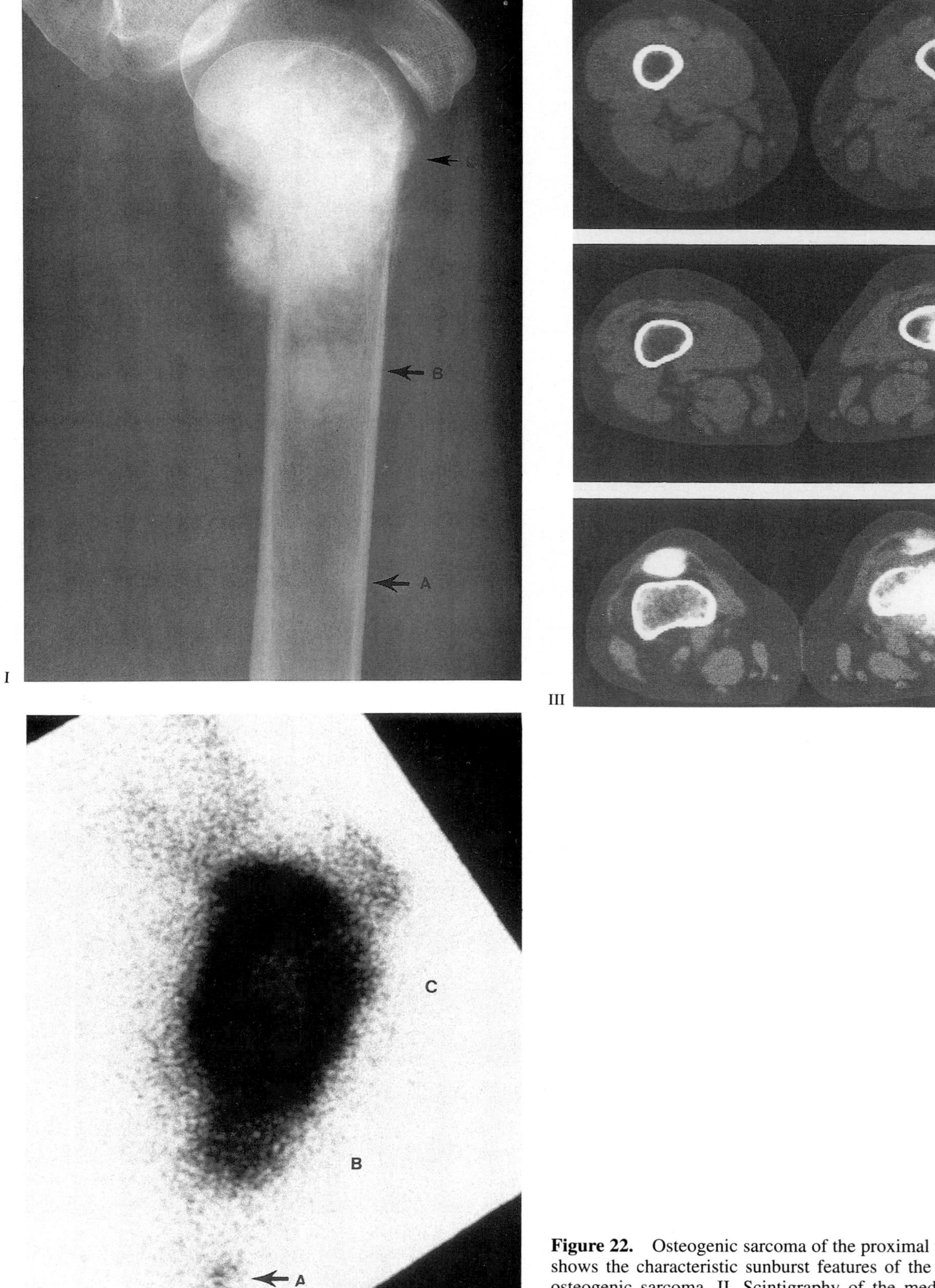

Figure 22. Osteogenic sarcoma of the proximal tibia. I. Radiograph shows the characteristic sunburst features of the sclerosing form of osteogenic sarcoma. II. Scintigraphy of the medial left knee using ^{99m}Tc-MDP shows intense uptake in proximal tibia with smaller lesion (arrow) inferiorly representing either a "skip" metastasis or a second primary. III. Serial CT scans demonstrate intramedullary and soft-tissue extension of the tumor. (Courtesy of Dr. Henry Goodgold.)

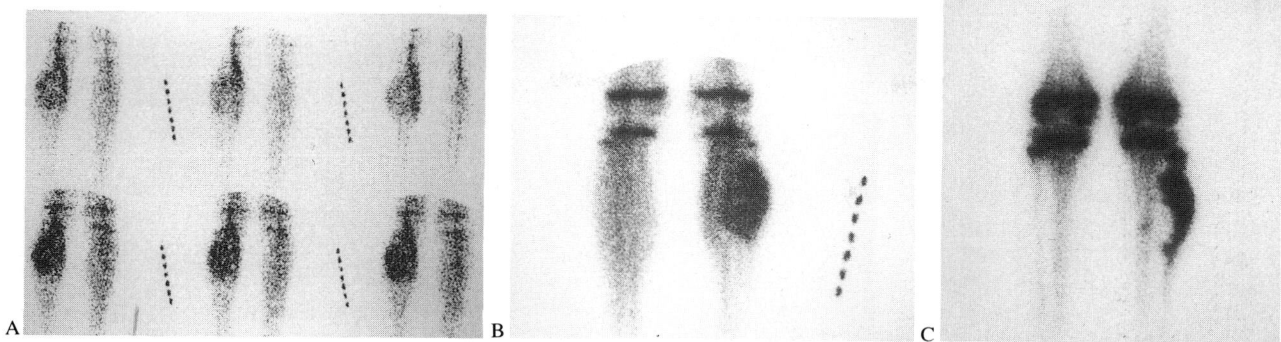

Figure 23. Three-phase bone scintigraphy in a 13-year-old boy with osteogenic sarcoma of the right proximal fibula. **(A).** Radionuclide angiogram using 740 MBq ^{99m}Tc-MDP. Posterior view shows markedly increased perfusion to the right upper fibula. **(B).** Blood pool image. **(C).** Static image shows distortion of the cortex and tumor uptake of tracer.

suggested that ^{67}Ga scintigraphy may be more useful in evaluating therapeutic response.

Chondrosarcoma

Chondrosarcoma rarely occurs in children; more than half of those affected are over 40 years of age.[316] Bone scintigraphy shows intense uptake (Fig. 24), the extent of uptake usually correlating well with roentgenographic extent.[327] The tumors appear in the epiphyseal ossification centers of long bones, adjacent to the enchondral plate, prior to epiphyseal-metaphyseal fusion. The scintigraphic appearance consists of increased bone blood flow and increased uptake at the tumor site. The increased uptake of technetium phosphonates is thought to result from increased blood supply, rather than osteoblastic activity.[328] In peripheral chondrosarcomas, however, intense soft-tissue uptake occurs in the tumoral calcifications. These lesions cannot be differentiated scintigraphically from osteogenic sarcomas.

BENIGN BONE TUMORS

Benign bone tumors, including chondroblastoma, enchondroma, osteoblastoma, giant cell tumors, eosinophilic granuloma, fibrous dysplasia, brown tumors of hyperparathyroidism, osteoid osteoma, and aneurysmal bone cysts all concentrate bone tracers and cannot be reliably differentiated

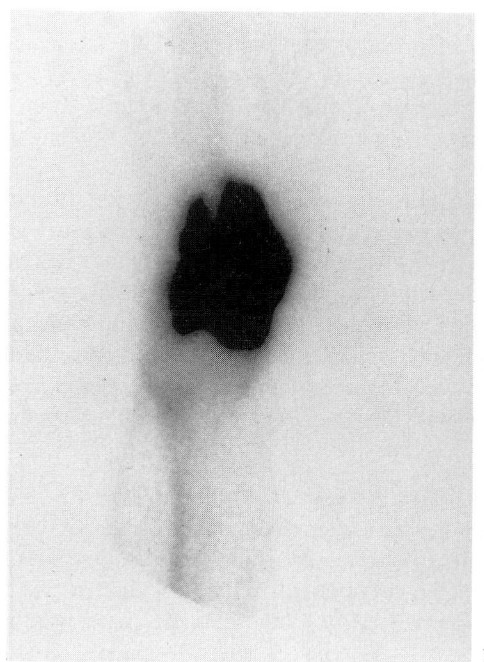

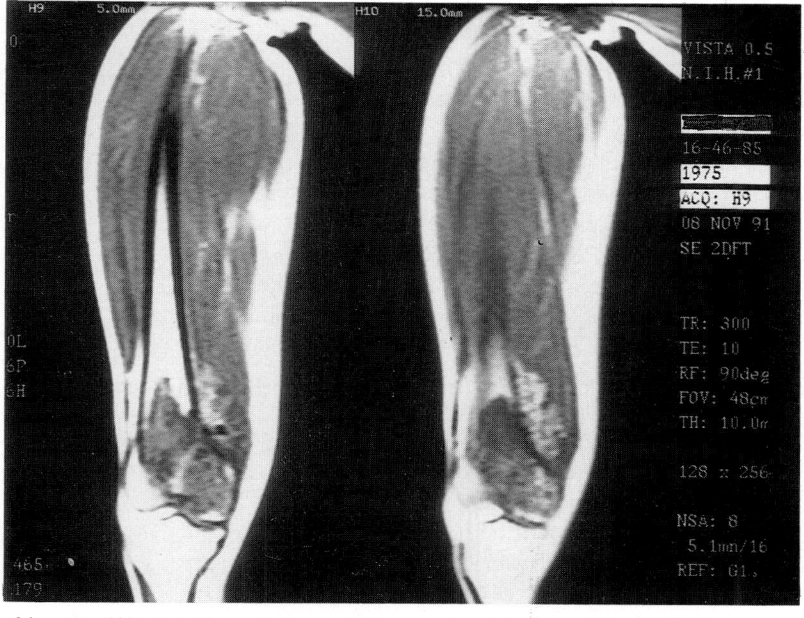

Figure 24. Chondrosarcoma in a 43-year-old male. **(A).** Anterior scintigram demonstrates intense uptake of ^{99m}Tc-MDP in the distal right femur. **(B).** T-1 weighted (S/E = 300/10) MR image showing erosion of tumor into soft tissues.

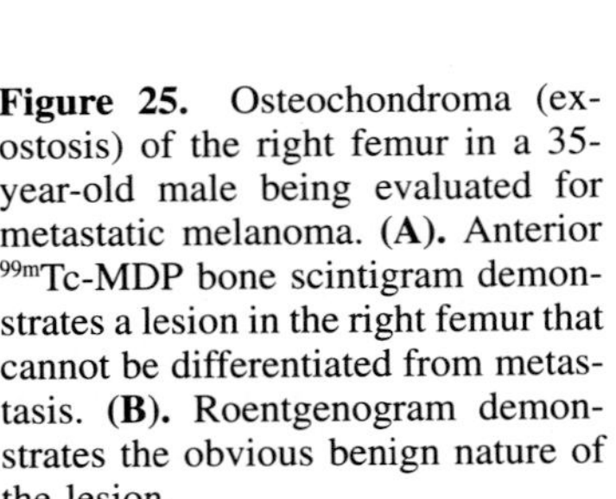

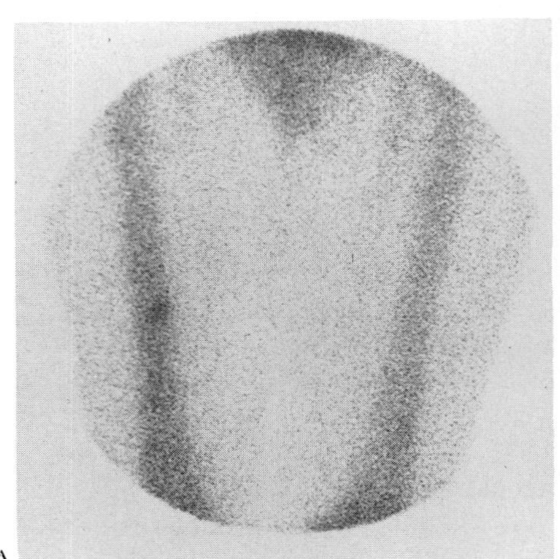

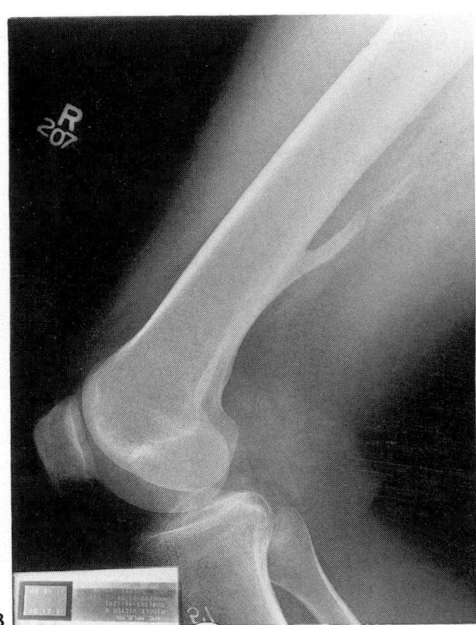

Figure 25. Osteochondroma (exostosis) of the right femur in a 35-year-old male being evaluated for metastatic melanoma. **(A).** Anterior ^{99m}Tc-MDP bone scintigram demonstrates a lesion in the right femur that cannot be differentiated from metastasis. **(B).** Roentgenogram demonstrates the obvious benign nature of the lesion.

from malignant tumors. Bone scintigraphy is useful when demonstrating normal uptake in a lesion that radiographically shows nonspecific sclerosis or lucency. In such cases, a benign lesion is highly likely, and can usually be followed for potential radiographic changes. In most cases, these radiographic findings are incidental and not related to the patient's principal complaint. The value of ^{67}Ga scintigraphy is questionable in these cases.

Benign osteochondroma (exostosis), which is one of the more common primary bone tumors, also cannot be reliably differentiated scintigraphically from chondrosarcomas.[329,330] While exostoses generally reveal less uptake (Fig. 25), considerable overlap exists with that exhibited by chondrosarcomas.

Osteoid Osteoma. Bone scintigraphy may be particularly useful in patients who present with bone pain, but in whom radiographic examination shows no abnormality. Occasionally, such benign bone tumors as osteoid osteomas fail to visualize radiographically, but produce an intense focal scintigraphic lesion (Fig. 26). These are benign osteoid-forming tumors and occur often in children and young adults. Most of these tumors develop in the femur (40%). About 10% involve the posterior elements of the spine, especially the lumbar spine.[331] Pain is a common symptom associated with osteoid osteomas, possibly because they form prostaglandins.[332]

Helms et al. described a "double-density" pattern, in which the smaller, more intense focus corresponds to the tumor nidus.[333] In the series of 42 patients with osteoid osteoma reported by Smith and Gilday,[334] blood pool images showed a small, localized hyperemic lesion in all cases. This finding was useful in differentiating osteoid osteoma from a healing stress fracture or metastasis. These lesions have a typical CT appearance, usually a small, rounded lesion with a lytic inner region and a densely sclerotic central nidus.[331]

Bone scintigraphy is also useful in the postoperative follow-up of osteoid osteomas. Recurrent pain associated with persistently increased activity suggests incomplete surgical resection and the need for reoperation.[335]

Such benign lesions as bone cysts, bone islands, and fibrous cortical defects (nonosteogenic fibroma) typically demonstrate little or no increased uptake scintigraphically. Dynamic flow studies demonstrate no increased blood flow to these lesions.

The appearance of bone islands varies. They are usually not vascular and, apparently, they are not detected as focal lesions with increased uptake until they become 3 cm or greater in diameter. Growth rate and lesion location are also factors that determine visualization.[336]

Other benign bone tumors, such as ossifying fibroma, enchondroma, osteochondroma, and chondroblastoma produce lesions with intense uptake. Scintigraphy may be clinically helpful in identifying multiple sites of involvement in these diseases; however, the ability to differentiate benign from malignant bone lesions is questionable.[337] A change in a lesion's appearance, together with progressively augmented uptake, nevertheless increases the probability of malignancy.

Grading Musculoskeletal Tumors Using PET

Preliminary studies have suggested that PET metabolic studies may be useful in grading malignant tumors and separating benign from malignant tumors, similar to its use in grading cerebral gliomas.[338–340] Most of these studies have used the glucose analog ^{18}F–2–deoxy–2–fluoro-D-glucose (FDG), which is taken up by the cell as FDG–6 phosphate and retained there, because it does not enter the glycolytic path-

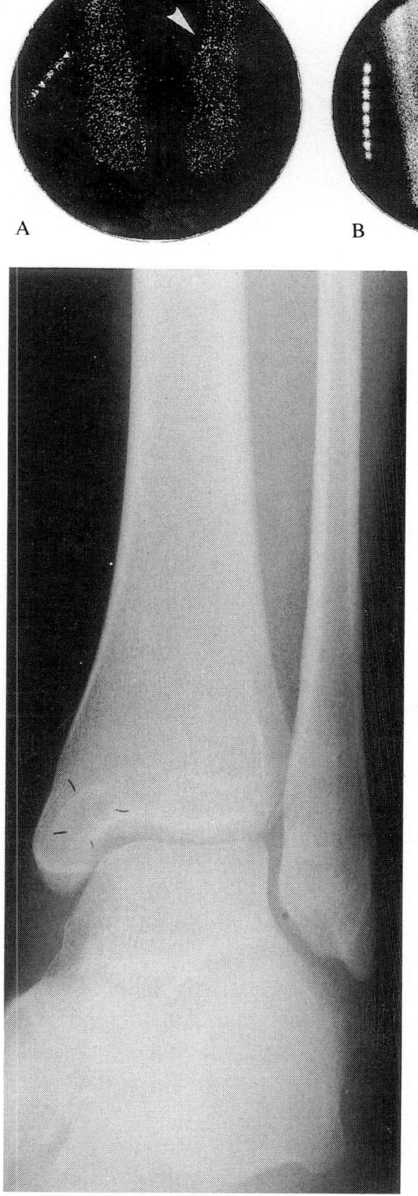

Figure 26. Osteoid osteoma of the left tibial epiphysis. **(A).** Perfusion study at 5 sec. demonstrates increased perfusion (arrow). **(B).** Blood pool image. **(C).** Anterior 2-hour delayed image demonstrates well-defined nidus. **(D).** Medial view of left ankle shows the eccentrically located nidus and surrounding reactive uptake. **(E).** Roentgenogram showing radiolucent tibial lesion.

way. The uptake of FDG is greater in cells with a high metabolic rate, which characterize malignancy; hence its utility.

In a study by Adler et al., all lesions with a normalized FDG uptake value of 1.6 or greater were high-grade, while all lesions less than 1.6 represented either benign tumors or low-grade malignancies. There is a strong relationship between FDG uptake and grade among neoplasms from a wide variety of cell types, including osteo-, angio-, fibro-, and liposarcomas and others. This suggests that PET may provide useful information about neoplasm grade noninvasively, even when the cell type is unknown. An obvious problem exists for tumors with necrotic centers which decreases FDG uptake.

BENIGN BONE DISEASE

Traumatic Injury

After malignant diseases, traumatic injuries to bone caused by accidents, surgical procedures, sports activities, and stress, constitute the next largest clinical indication for bone scintigraphy. Radiographic procedures are generally more useful than scintigraphy in evaluating skeletal injury, since radiography is much more sensitive in detecting altered bony architecture. However, scintigraphy is useful for imaging bones that are difficult to image radiographically because of their variable shape or because of overlying structures: the carpal and tarsal bones, scapula, vertebrae, proximal femur, sternum, and ilium. Examples include stress fractures

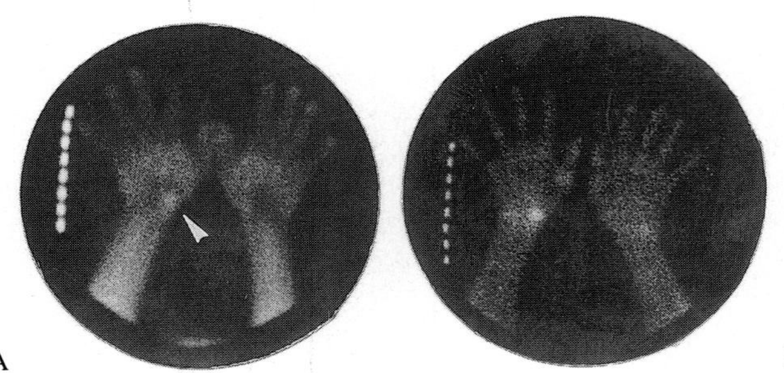

Figure 27. Occult navicular fracture demonstrates increased blood pool activity 24 hours after injury (arrow), **(A)** and focal lesion in the delayed ^{99m}Tc-MDP image, **(B)**. The radiograph was normal.

that are too small to observe radiographically, but that are characterized by intense tracer uptake. Bursal and tendinous injuries create intense scintigraphic lesions, often without radiographic signs. Scintigraphy is also useful in distinguishing small chip fractures from accessory ossicles.

HEALING FRACTURES

Within 24 hours of trauma, repair of bone fractures usually begins, and by 24 hours, healing is reflected on bone scintigraphy as increased focal activity (Figs. 27, 28, 29).[341] Activity peaks several weeks later, then begins to decrease, eventually approaching normal months later.[342] Matin found that 80% of patients with fractures had abnormal bone scintigraphy within 24 hours of injury, and 95% showed abnormal bone uptake by 72 hours.[343] Older patients take longer to develop positive scintigrams and longer to return to normal.[343–345] In the healing process, the radionuclide angiogram normalizes in 3 to 4 weeks, while the blood-pool phase normalizes in 8 to 12 weeks.[346] In older patients with suspected hip fractures that are scintigraphically and radiographically negative at presentation, repeat scintigraphy at 72 hours may demonstrate the lesion.[347] However, in a large series reported by Holder et al., 92 patients were imaged at presentation less than 72 hours following injury.[348] For diagnosis of hip fracture in an individual patient, the overall sensitivity was 0.93; specificity, 0.95; positive predictive value, 0.92; and negative predictive value, 0.96. In the clinically important subgroup of 145 patients with normal or equivocal radiographs, the sensitivity was 0.98. Thus, scintigraphy appears to be exceptionally reliable in detecting occult fractures of the hip.

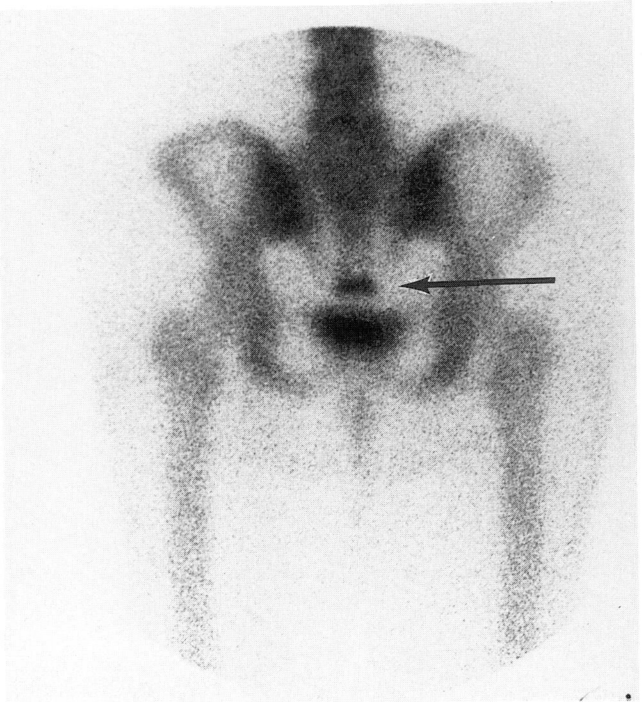

Figure 29. Coccygeal fracture.

In rare cases, fractures remain scintigraphically positive for several years, without clinical evidence of nonunion. These are generally long-bone fractures with callus formation in which the apparent increase in bone uptake is caused by increased bone mass.

In general, recent fractures show intense uptake, and older fractures have normal or slightly increased uptake. This fact is useful in distinguishing between acute and old vertebral compression fractures, which radiographs do not differentiate well.

Bone scintigraphy may be useful in the treatment planning of nonunited fractures.[349–351] Desai et al. reported 77 patients with nonunited fractures who were treated with percutaneous low-grade, direct-current stimulation.[351] Patients who had intense activity at the fracture site responded well to electrostimulation, whereas patients who had a line of decreased

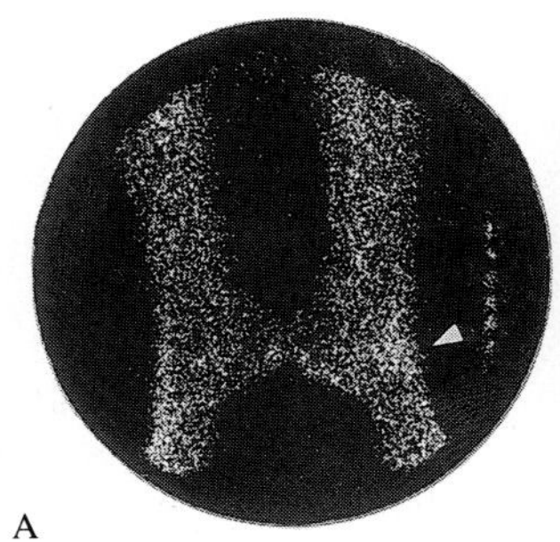

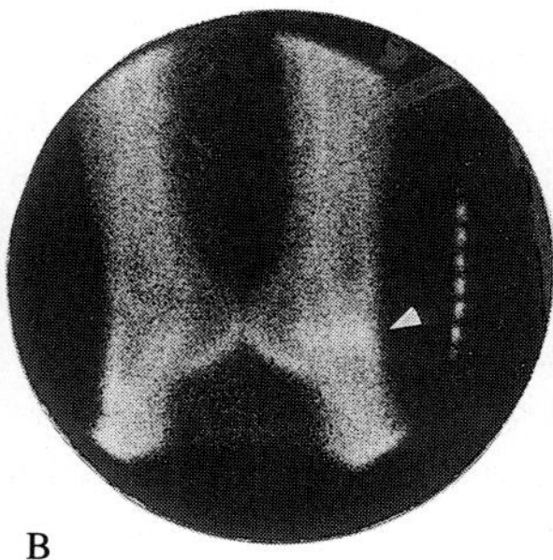

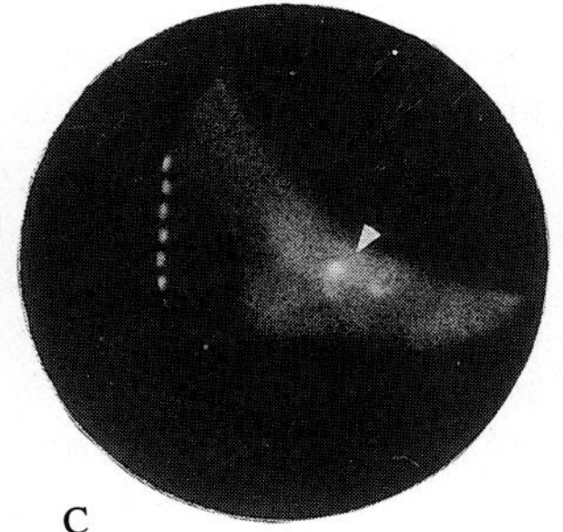

Figure 28. Three-phase scintigraphy demonstrating increased blood flow, **(A)** blood pool, **(B)** and delayed uptake, **(C)** in the tarsal navicular bone (arrows) of a patient with acute ankle pain.

activity surrounded by increased uptake on both sides (fibrous nonunion) failed to heal.

Increased bone uptake occurs at sites of osteotomy. Typically, within 6 to 9 months following surgery, the scintigram returns to nearly normal uptake around a prosthetic joint. Craniotomies and orthopedic surgical interventions cause scintigraphic lesions for varying periods of time, but usually not longer than 6 to 9 months. Bone biopsies may or may not result in scintigraphic lesions. Tyler and Powers reported that bone-marrow biopsies of the iliac crest did not result in scintigraphic abnormalities in 24 patients imaged from several hours to many weeks following biopsy.[352]

STRESS FRACTURES AND OVERUSE INJURIES

Stress fractures result from repetitive, prolonged muscular action on bone that is unaccustomed to such stress. The usual symptoms include bone pain, with or without local swelling, that is relieved by discontinuing the precipitating exercise.[353] Stress fractures are particularly common in young people whose bones are actively remodeling, and especially among soldiers and endurance athletes, such as runners, skaters, and aerobic exercise enthusiasts.

Two types of stress fractures have been described: *fatigue fractures,* which are caused by abnormal muscular stress or torque on normal bone; and *insufficiency fractures,* which result from normal stresses on abnormal bone. Such conditions as osteoporosis, osteomalacia, Paget's disease, osteopetrosis, rheumatoid arthritis, fibrous dysplasia, hyperparathyroidism, bone infarction, and bone irradiation predispose to insufficiency fractures. A fine review of the pathophysiology of many types of stress and overuse injuries is found in reference 353.

Bone scintigraphy has proved to be highly sensitive in the early detection of stress-related bone and tendinous injuries.[354–357] Zwas et al. have graded stress fractures according to their severity and progression continuum.[358] Grade I is a small, thin, localized, mild activity lesion confined to the bone cortex (Fig. 30). Grade II is a continuation of Grade I that extends further along the cortical bone. Further progress leads to a Grade III lesion, which extends into the medullary bone, becomes wider, fusiform, ovally elongated in shape and occupying about half the width of the shaft with intense uptake. Grade IV occupies the full bone shaft width and appears as a transcortico-medullary fusiform lesion. As healing occurs, these grades regress in reverse order. Common sites of stress fractures include the proximal femur, tibia, fibula (Fig. 31), metatarsal, calcaneus (especially in military recruits), and pubic ramus.

Bone radiographs are often negative during the early phases of stress fractures. If the precipitating condition is not treated, late radiographic changes include medullary sclerosis, periosteal thickening, and eventually callus formation.

Shin splints are musculotendinous injuries associated with pain along the muscular insertions into the tibia or fibula (Fig. 32). The scintigraphic pattern is usually a superficial, linear lesion along the anterolateral or posterior tibial surface.[359] The scintigraphic appearance suggests a periosteal injury, in contrast to a stress fracture which is usually more localized and extends into the medullary portions of the bone as the lesion advances. Three-phase bone scintigraphy reveals normal blood flow to shin splints, whereas flow is increased in stress fractures.[346] Total-body bone scintigraphy is essential in examining stress injuries in athletes, because pain denial is common and stress injuries are often multiple.

Le Jeune et al. have described scintigraphic changes in pubic pain syndrome, common among soccer players and swimmers.[360] They found that scintigraphy was useful in differentiating between dynamic pubic arthropathy and abductor and rectus insertion tendinitis. Differentiating the two is important for therapy; the former requires prolonged rest, while the latter responds to anti-inflammatory drugs and physiotherapy. Increased pubic uptake preceded radiographic changes and resolved before radiographs returned to normal. Scintigraphy, thus, serves as a guide to therapy.

Common sites of arthritis among athletes are the tibiofibular joints (Fig. 33), both proximal and distal, and tarsal and carpal joints, especially the navicular bones.

Benign hypertrophy of overuse results in bone remodeling and cortical thickening as shown in Figure 34. Although the scintigraphic appearance may resemble the pattern associated with stress fractures, correlations with radiographic changes help to make this differential diagnosis.

The use of bone scintigraphy to detect occult fractures has obvious merit. Scintigrams become positive as early as 7 to 24 hours following a fracture and,[345] within 2 days, the sensitivity approaches 100%. The specificity, however, is much lower, because tenosynovitis, traumatic arthritis, and other injuries less severe than frank fracture result in positive scintigraphy. Occult fractures of the carpal scaphoid bone (Fig. 27) have been studied by several investigators.[361–363] In these studies, bone scintigraphy was 100% sensitive in detecting carpal scaphoid fractures among 200 patients. The low specificity, however, suggests the best use of bone scintigraphy is as follows:

1. Bone scintigraphy is most useful to exclude scaphoid or other wrist fractures when radiographs are negative or equivocal. A negative scintigram reliably excludes fracture.
2. In the event of a positive scintigram, the injury should be casted and reimaged 10 days later. Removal of the cast before scanning is not necessary.
3. If repeat scintigraphy is negative, the cast can be removed and the patient treated further according to symptoms. If scintigraphy remains positive, casting for the full healing period is recommended. By this strategy, unnecessary scintigraphy and cast-days are minimized.

Scintigraphy is also used to determine the need for further imaging procedures, as in the evaluation of ankle pain for the presence of talar dome fractures.[364] Although CT is re-

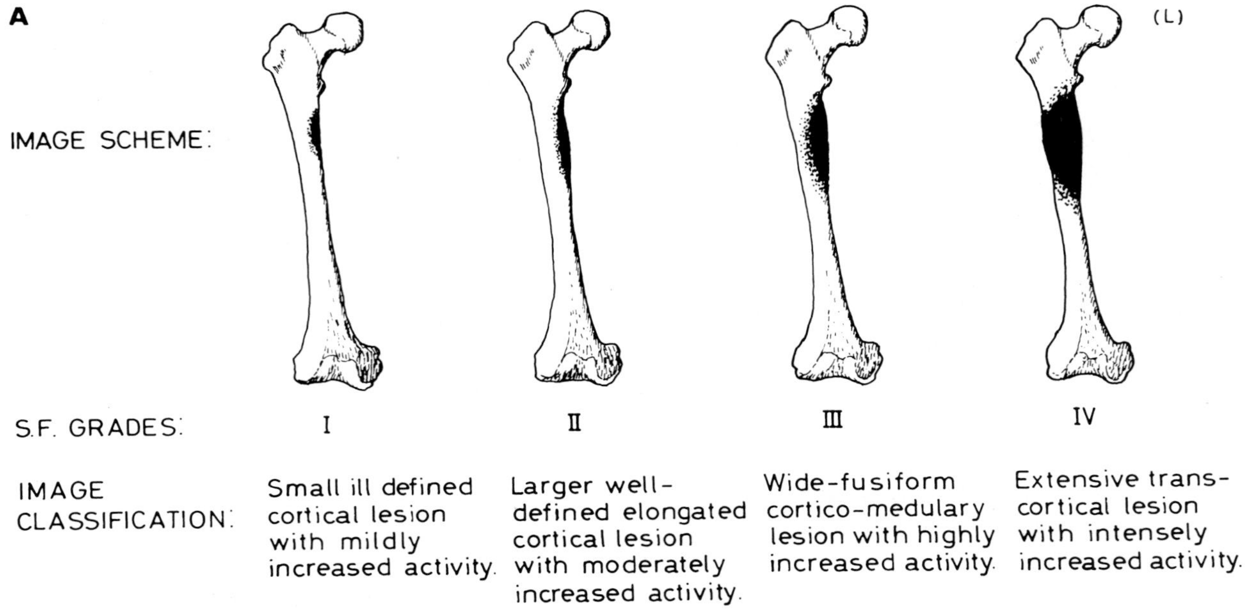

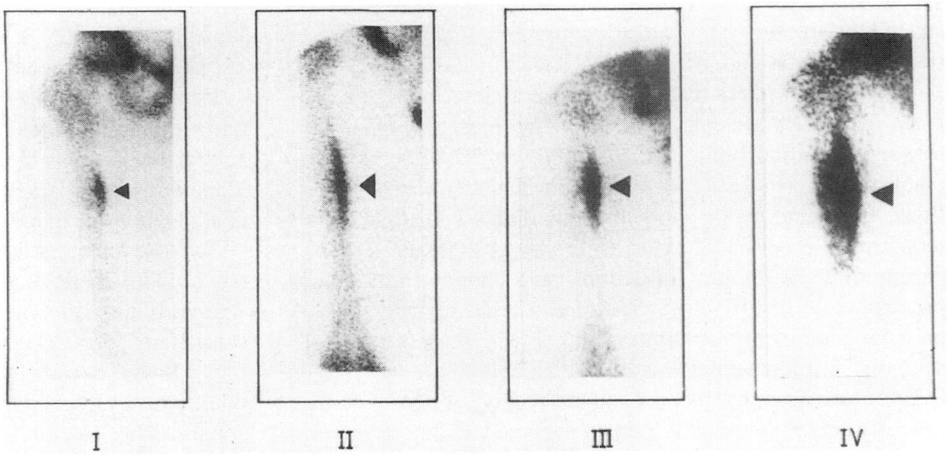

A (L)

IMAGE SCHEME:

S.F. GRADES:	I	II	III	IV
IMAGE CLASSIFICATION:	Small ill defined cortical lesion with mildly increased activity.	Larger well-defined elongated cortical lesion with moderately increased activity.	Wide-fusiform cortico-medulary lesion with highly increased activity.	Extensive trans-cortical lesion with intensely increased activity.

B

I II III IV

Figure 30. Four grades (I-IV) of stress fracture evolution, determined by scintigraphy. Reproduced with permission from Reference 358.

quired in making the diagnosis of talar dome fractures when radiographs are negative, CT is not indicated in the presence of normal scintigraphy.

Child Abuse. Haase et al. reported 44 children who were suspected victims of abuse and who had bone scintigraphy at the time of initial presentation.[365] Of these, 26 children had negative scintigrams and radiographs. Two radiographically apparent skull fractures were missed by scintigraphy. Five of 7 patients with positive scintigrams and normal radiographs later developed bone or periosteal lesions radiographically. In fact, most studies have shown that scintigraphy is more sensitive than radiography in detecting fractures sustained through abuse.[366,367] However, since both modalities have a high number of false-negative results, a patient with a negative study and evidence strongly suggestive of battering should probably have both studies.

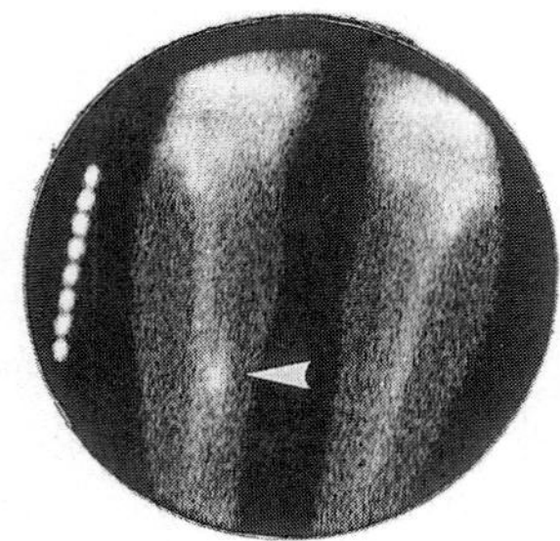

Figure 31. Stress fracture of the right fibula (arrow) in a basketball player.

Although some authors[366] recommend scintigraphy as the initial screening procedure, others advocate plain radiographs, particularly in infants younger than two years of age.[368] There are two problems associated with interpreting radionuclide bone surveys in abused children: healed fractures are not usually detected, and epiphyseal-metaphyseal fractures are difficult or impossible to detect scintigraphically because of the normally intense activity in these areas.

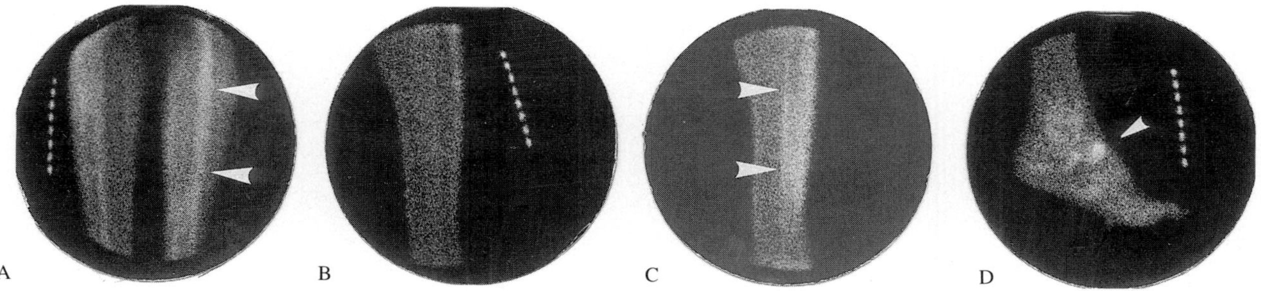

Figure 32. Tc-99m-MDP bone scintigraphy in an exceptionally tall basketball player complaining of left leg pain. **(A).** Anterior view shows increased activity in left midtibia. **(B).** Lateral view of right leg shows normal tibial activity. **(C).** Medial view of left leg shows the increased activity in the tibia corresponding to the insertion of the flexor digitorum longus. **(D).** focal increased activity at the insertion of the talonavicular ligament (arrow) was asymptomatic at the time of this study, but had previously caused right foot tenderness.

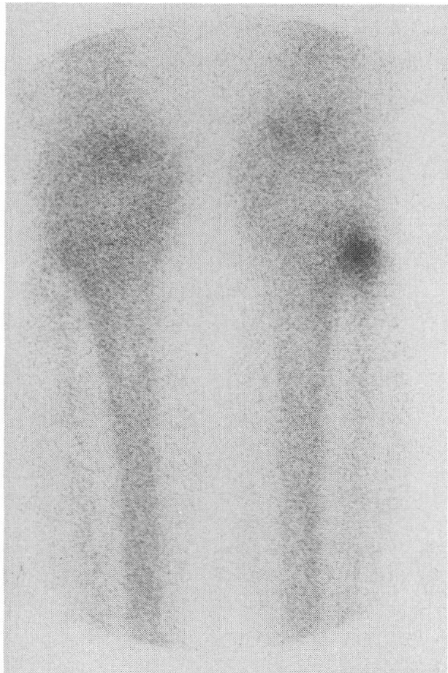

Figure 33. Left proximal tibiofibular tendinitis in a 20-year-old soccer player.

Plantar Fasciitis and Achilles Tendinitis. Plantar fasciitis refers to the clinical condition characterized by pain and tenderness localized to the plantar surface of the heel and to the tendinous insertion of the plantar fascia (aponeurosis) on the tuberosity of the calcaneus. Achilles tendinitis refers to inflammation of the insertion of the Achilles tendon on the superior margin of the calcaneus. Both of these are typical overuse syndromes and are common in soldiers and athletes, those with flat feet, and those who wear high-heeled shoes that limit dorsiflexion of the heel and create a tight gastrocnemius-soleus complex. Radiographs are often negative, unless a stress fracture of the calcaneus has occurred. Scintigraphy reveals increased blood flow to the heel and markedly increased uptake of tracer in superficial calcaneus[369] (Fig. 35). Isolated Achilles tendinitis can be diagnosed when the lesion only involves the upper margin of the calcaneus.

Osteitis Pubis. This overuse syndrome is characterized by pain in the pubis, common in runners and soccer players.[353] It is thought to be caused by stress on the symphysis pubis acting through the gracilis-adductor groups of muscles, adducting the pelvis against the foot in external rotation and abduction. This occurs, for instance when a ball is kicked, or when runners suddenly increase their level of exercise.

The scintigraphic appearance is bilaterally increased tracer uptake, mostly at the pubic rami (Fig. 36).[370,371] Radiographic findings include widening of the symphysis pubis with irregularity of its margins and the adjacent pubis with local sclerosis. These findings occur only in long-standing chronic afflictions.

Other Injuries. The knees are subject to a variety of injuries and stress. Often markedly obvious scintigraphic lesions, with or without increased regional blood flow, are entirely

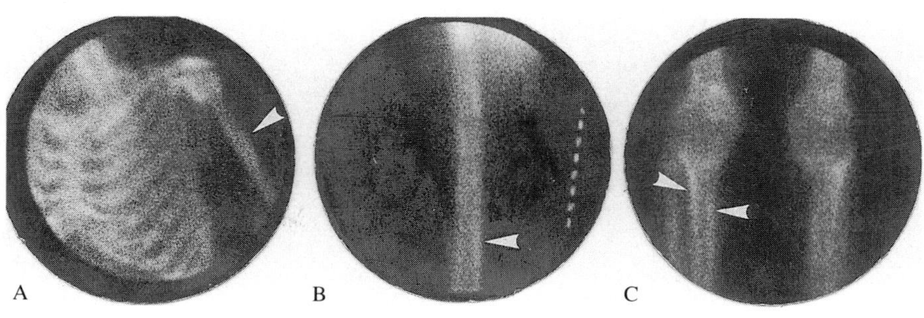

Figure 34. Examples of overuse bone hypertrophy. **(A).** midhumeral thickening in a laborer. **(B).** Femoral cortical hypertrophy in a basketball player. **(C).** Fibular cortical hypertrophy (double stripe sign) in a runner.

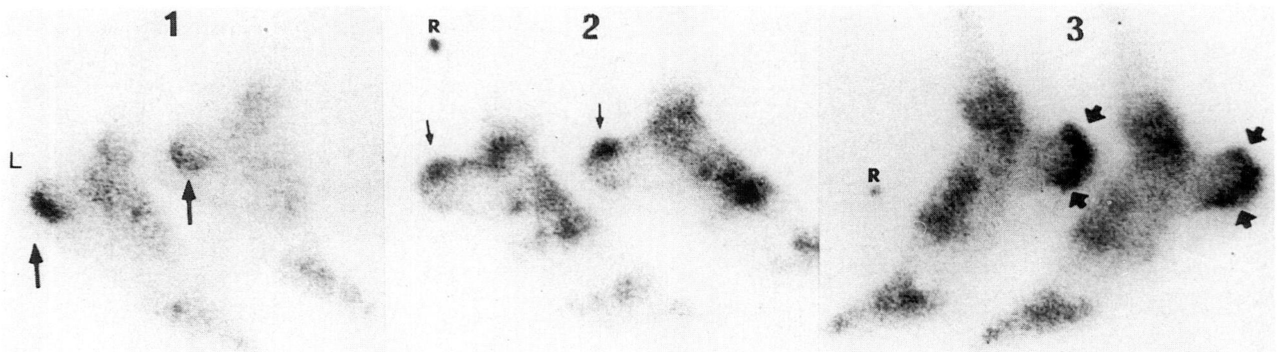

Figure 35. Calcaneal plantar fasciitis and Achilles tendinitis. (1). Lateral scintiphotos in a 19-year-old soldier with swelling in the left heel. Increased bilateral tracer accumulation in both calcaneal inferior borders (arrows) corresponding to the plantar fascia insertion, more pronounced in the left foot, characteristic of bilateral plantar fasciitis. (2). Lateral scintiphotos in an 18-year-old soldier suffering 2 weeks from pain and tenderness in the left heel and ankle. There is increased activity in the upper calcaneal tuberosity (arrows) at the Achilles tendon insertion in both feet, more pronounced on the left, consistent with Achilles tendinitis. There is a grade III stress fracture in the left tarsal region (arrowhead) and a grade II stress fracture in the right talus (arrowhead). (3). Young soldier with bilateral pes-cavus suffering 4 weeks from right heel pain. Note the markedly increased bilateral tracer uptake in the calcaneus, more prominent on the right, distributed diffusely along the posterior calcaneus (arrows). These findings indicate combined Achilles and plantar insertional disorders with extensive involvement of both calcanei. Reproduced with permission from Reference 358.

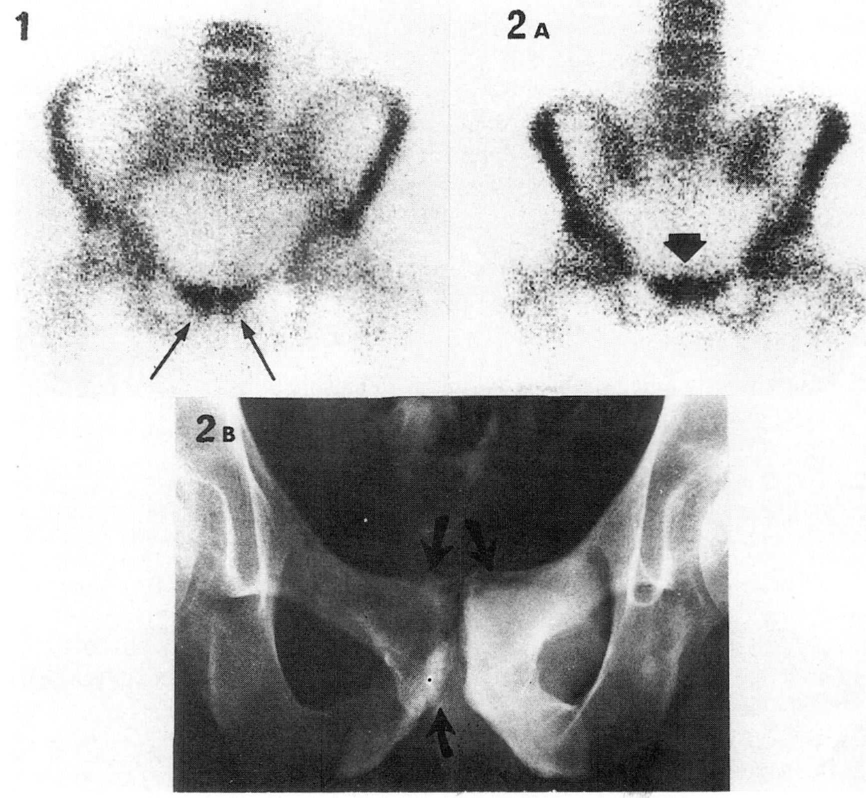

Figure 36. Osteitis pubis. (1). Anterior pelvic scintiphoto in an 18-year-old recruit suffering 2 weeks from groin pain; radiograph negative. Symmetrical bilateral tracer uptake in the superior pubic rami (arrows). (2A). A 19-year-old basketball player suffering 3 months from groin pain demonstrates increased tracer uptake in both superior pubic rami and the symphysis pubis (arrow). (2B). Radiograph of pubic bones demonstrate irregularities and widening of the symphysis pubis margins with adjacent upper and lower periosteal reactive changes, irregularities, and osteophytes on the pubic margin, and bilateral local sclerosis (arrows). These changes indicate chronic, advanced osteitis and symphysitis pubis. Reproduced with permission from Reference 358.

asymptomatic.[353] SPECT of the knees may be useful in delineating the compartments involved.[372]

Patellar tendinitis ("jumper's knee") is an inflammation of the patellar tendon or the quadriceps tendon with involvement at the inferior or superior aspect of the patella. Scintigraphy demonstrates characteristic abnormal radiotracer localization at the inferior pole of the patella or tibial tuberosity on early and delayed images.[373]

Trochanteric bursitis is common among overweight, middle-aged females and demonstrates localized tracer uptake along the outer margin of the greater trochanter, often found incidentally in the metastatic workup.[374]

Bone scintigraphy has been useful in evaluating children with lower extremity pain of unknown origin. Small children frequently cannot describe the precise location of their pain. Englaro et al. found frequent pathology in such patients.[375] Abnormalities included hip synovitis, femoral head avascularity, knee synovitis, toddler's fracture (spiral fracture of the tibia), and various femoral, tibial, and fibular lesions. Over half of such painful bone lesions were accounted for by tarsal bone abnormalities, especially the cuboid bone.

Bone Graft Viability

Bone grafts are used in the repair of trauma, to replace bone infiltrated by tumor, to repair congenital defects and, of course, for cosmetic reasons. Most bone grafts are either allografts (banked human bone) or autografts, harvested from elsewhere in the patient's own skeleton. The latter are either transplanted free of their vascular supply, or else *vascularized*, in which the bone is transferred attached to a nutrient artery which is then anastomosed microsurgically to an artery at the recipient site. In the case of allografts, the entire grafted segment serves as a nonviable support that is replaced with viable bone tissue by progressive substitution from adjacent viable bone. This is known as "creeping substitution" and must take place from the ends to the center, and the practical graft size limit is 5 to 6 cm. In many cases, especially where surrounding tissues have been irradiated to eradicate tumor, the recipient site may be a hostile environment for revascularization of the grafted bone.

Bone scintigraphy is a useful method of determining bone-graft vascularity and, hence, viability at relatively early stages following grafting when estimating vascularity is important to therapeutic decision making.[376–381] This is especially true of en bloc grafts in which the donor site blood supply is maintained intact as it is transplanted to the recipient site.[378] Scintigraphy provides a means of predicting graft failure before radiographic or clinical changes become apparent and helps avoid loss of surrounding tissues from graft necrosis and infection.

One method of assessing the viability of bone allografts has been by repeated scintigraphy, each time using a computer-generated profile slice along the axis of the graft.[382] Successive profiles show two peaks of activity corresponding to the junctures of the recipient and grafted bone. As the "creeping substitution" progresses, the two peaks approach one another, meeting at or near the center upon completion of the substitution. The same procedure can be undertaken with nonvascularized autografts, since the substitution process is essentially the same. This imaging process takes several weeks, but is an effective means of following the healing process.

Vascularized autografts have been assessed by three-phase bone scintigraphy, a procedure that permits evaluation of vascular integrity within the first week.[378] Viable grafts demonstrate intact blood flow and increased uptake within the grafted bone on delayed images. A photopenic region usually signifies vascular insufficiency of the whole graft, or nonunion in a part of the graft, depending upon extent. However three-phase scintigraphy may not be possible in maxillofacial grafts, because underlying vascular structures in the neck may confuse the interpretation of vascularization of overlying structures.[378] In such instances, SPECT has been used to assess local bone uptake.[378,381]

The timing of scintigraphy following surgery is important. Ramsay et al. found that the success of calvarial or ileal grafts in augmentation rhinoplasty could be predicted by as early as 2 to 4 weeks following surgery.[381] If the nasal graft bone was as or more intense as frontal bone on lateral planar images, no grafts failed. Moskowitz and Lukash found that en bloc pedicle grafts into the mandible could be evaluated 3 to 7 days following surgery. Increased activity was demonstrated in the graft in all patients that were later proven to have successful grafts.[378] In another study, revascularized grafts using microvascular anastomoses showed uptake of ^{99m}Tc-MDP within the first week, while conventional grafts and unsuccessful vascularized grafts reflected neither scintigraphic uptake nor viable bone by histological study.[383] Thus, timing of the postoperative scintigraphy may be important to interpretation of vascularity; both radionuclide angiography and SPECT are useful to this end.

Bone Scintigraphy in Low-Back Pain

The increased sensitivity of SPECT bone imaging compared with planar imaging in axial skeletal structures is well recognized. Nowhere is this more true than in the spine in identifying causes of low-back pain. In several studies SPECT demonstrated focal lesions in 25 to 45% of patients with normal planar images.[384–388] In a recent series of 34 patients with chronic low-back pain, 27 patients had lesions imaged by SPECT, of whom 24 (89%) had CT abnormalities and 18 (67%) had radiographic abnormalities.[389] Thus, SPECT provides a sensitive means of localizing spinal lesions that can be then further characterized by CT and radiography. Typical lesions responsible for low-back pain that are identified by SPECT include diskitis, spondylolisthesis, osteoarthritis, spondylolysis, and fractures of the vertebral body, pars interarticularis, and transverse process (Figs. 37 and 38).

A common situation in which spinal scintigraphy is useful is in patients with chronic low-back pain in which the clinical

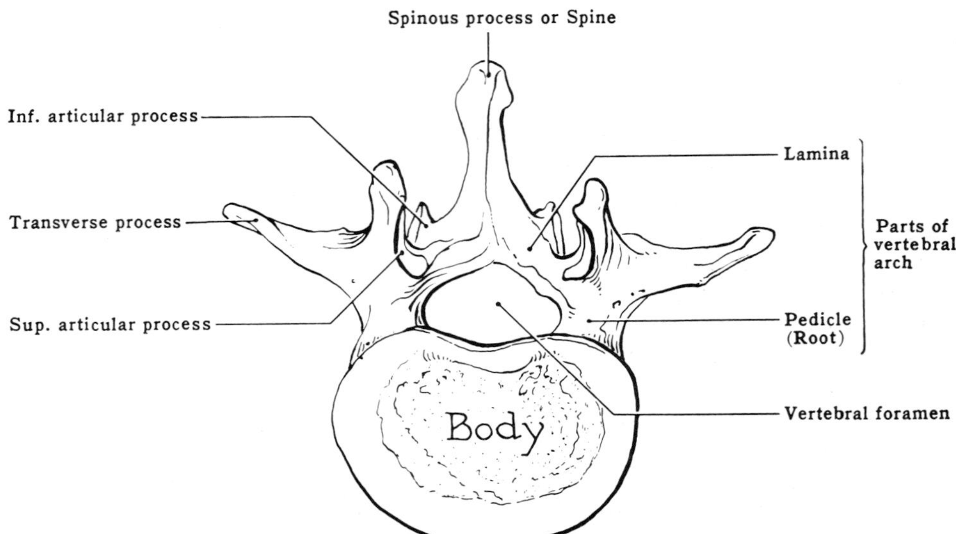

Figure 37. Anatomic features of the L-2 vertebra.

evaluation and plain radiographs have not yielded a diagnosis. The use of SPECT is particularly useful in abnormalities of the neural arch, where lesions of low intensity are frequently not visualized by planar images.[389]

The role of bone scintigraphy in the evaluation of persistent back pain after laminectomy for removal of herniated intervertebral disk (the "failed back syndrome") has been investigated by Lusins et al.[390] One cause of persistent pain is increased stress on the posterior facets as a result of lumbar decompression. The probability of this occurring increases considerably when more than one laminectomy has been performed and greater stress on the facets results. The exact area of stress can often be identified by SPECT, whereas planar images are of little use because of superimposition of the posterior vertebral elements on the vertebral body. Such findings may indicate the need for spinal fusion to reduce facet movement.

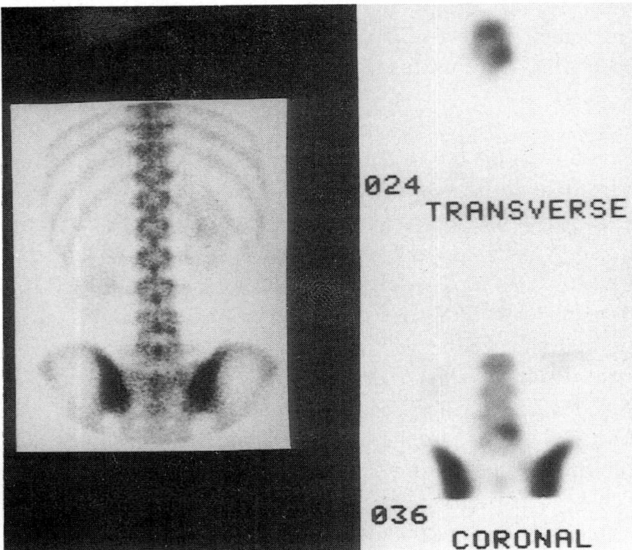

Figure 38. The planar skeletal scintigram in a patient with low-back pain is normal. SPECT images at right show a focal area of increased radiotracer uptake in L-4 on the left, representing stress injury to the pars interarticularis. Reproduced with permission from Reference 388.

Avascular Necrosis

Bone blood supply is compromised by several pathologic processes, including fractures, slipped capital femoral epiphysis, acute septic synovitis, metabolic disorders, fat embolization, corticosteroid therapy, sickle cell anemia, lupus erythematosus, and frostbite, all of which can result in aseptic necrosis. With the possible exception of steroid-induced avascular necrosis, all of these conditions are thought to begin with an initial ischemic episode, followed by bony repair, and usually sclerosis. Bone scintigraphy reflects the pathophysiological processes.[391] Scintigraphy initially demonstrates an area of decreased uptake (Fig. 39), followed gradually by a bone reactive zone of increased uptake and ultimately normal or slightly decreased uptake, depending upon the degree of bone destruction. SPECT images are useful during acute stages of the disease, because they may clearly outline the area of bone that is avascular from surrounding reactive bone (Fig. 40).

The difference exhibited by steroid-induced avascular necrosis is that the initial photopenic lesion is usually not observed. Rather, there is increased uptake from the outset (Fig. 41). This supports the hypothesis that the underlying pathology is osteoporosis and microfractures rather than ischemia.

Bone-marrow scintigraphy reveals decreased marrow uptake in the region of avascular necrosis (Fig. 42) because of loss of reticuloendothelial elements.[392] Because of the superior sensitivity and possibility of tissue characterization

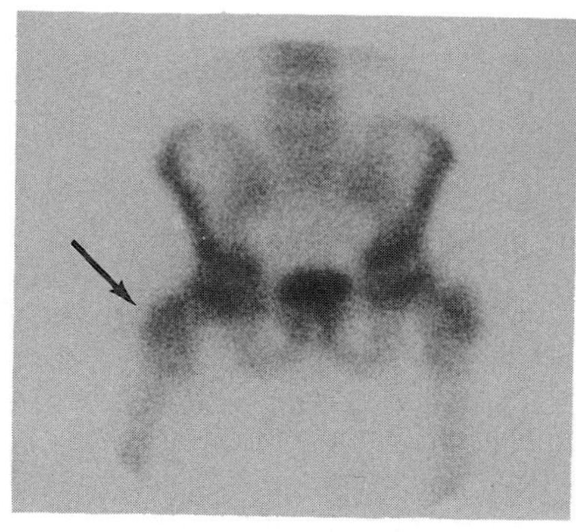

A

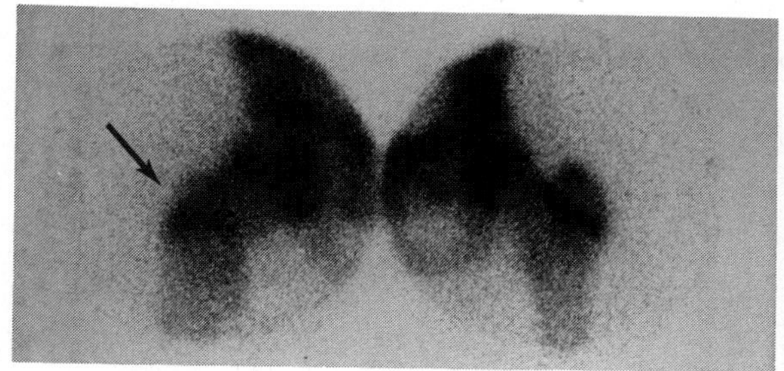

B

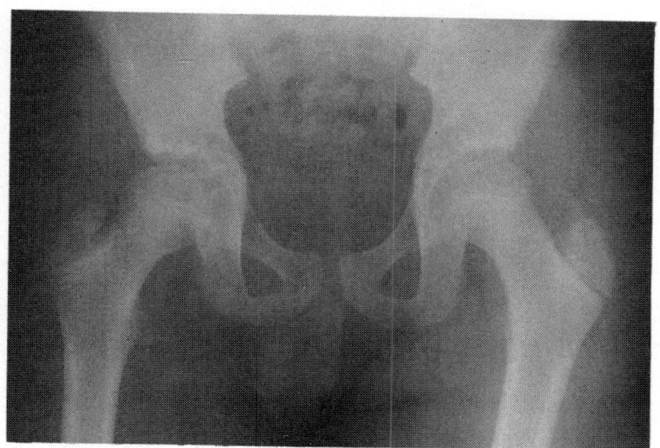

C

Figure 39. Avascular necrosis of the greater trochanter in an 8-year-old boy with leukemia and right hip pain. **(A).** Anterior scintiphoto showing decreased activity in the right greater trochanter (arrow). **(B).** Pinhole views demonstrate the necrosis (arrow) as well as the normal ossification centers on the left. **(C).** Plain radiograph demonstrates epiphyseal sclerosis.

of MRI, these studies are seldom performed. MRI demonstrates increased signal intensity on T2 weighted images, suggesting increased water content of the marrow from edema or vascular congestion in regions that show increased radionuclide tracer uptake.[393,394] Recent studies suggest that careful analysis of T1 and T2 weighting of nonenhanced and gadolinium-enhanced images can differentiate between regions of hypervascularized viable tissue and fat-rich necrotic tissue of the sequestrum.[394]

Scintigraphy is a sensitive means of detecting spontaneous osteonecrosis of the femoral condyle. This is a relatively common syndrome in elderly patients who develop intense pain in the medial femoral condyle, with normal radiographs at the time of presentation.[395] Three-phase bone scintigraphy demonstrates increased blood flow to the medial femoral condyle and markedly increased focal activity on delayed images. As healing progresses, the scintigraphic pattern reverts to normal and the radiographic findings of focal sclerosis appear.

Bone infarcts are common in patients with sickle-cell disease and can be observed in virtually all patients who have developed bone pain. Bone and bone-marrow scintigraphy are useful in distinguishing between bone infarction and osteomyelitis in these cases.[396,397] In most cases, bone scintigraphy demonstrates increased activity in both conditions; however, bone-marrow scintigraphy nearly always demonstrates *decreased* activity in the case of infarction and normal activity in cases of infection.[396] Of the two studies, bone-marrow scintigraphy is probably more useful as an initial study.[397]

Legg-Calvé-Perthe's Disease

Many studies have documented the reliability of bone scintigraphy in the diagnosis and management of Legg-Calvé-Perthe's disease.[398–402] In this disease, necrosis of the femoral capital epiphysis affects children between ages four and eight, usually boys, and it is believed to be of vascular origin. Sutherland et al. reported bone scintigraphy to have a sensitivity of 0.98 and specificity of 0.95 for identifying this disease.[398] Comparable figures for radiographic sensitivity and specificity are 0.92 and 0.78, respectively. The characteristic scintigraphic finding is decreased activity in the femoral capital epiphysis on the involved side (Fig. 43) often with increased uptake in the acetabulum, caused by the associated synovitis. These changes are best appreciated by pinhole imaging of the hip joint. The scintigraphic changes precede radiographic changes by several months. With revascularization and healing, activity in the femoral head and adjacent femoral neck increases.[402]

In children with joint effusions, femoral head activity may be either normal or diminished. Decreased activity is found in patients in whom elevated joint pressure is sufficient to impair vascularity. The femoral head receives its blood supply from a single capsular branch of the medial circumflex artery, which is easily compromised. In severe joint effu-

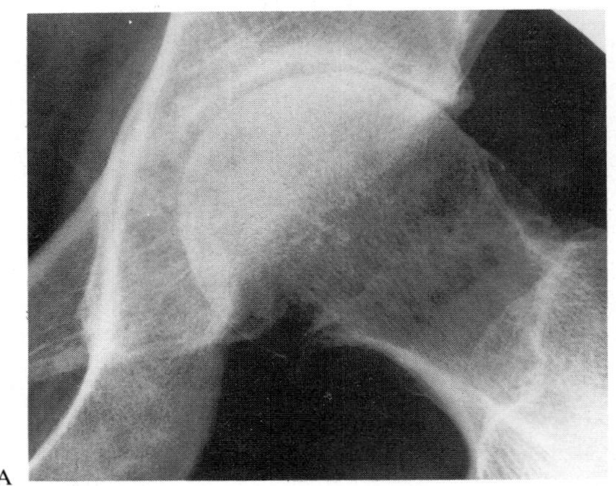
A

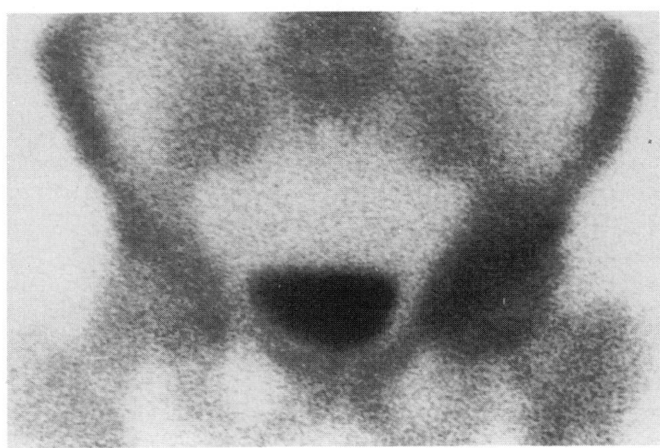
B

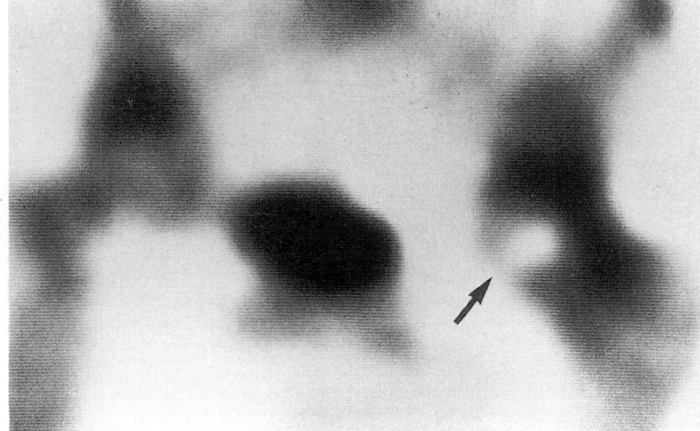
C

Figure 40. 57-year-old man with onset of severe left hip pain 3 months prior. Left hip radiograph, **(A)** shows sclerosis, joint space narrowing and osteophyte formation. Planar bone scintigram, **(B)** shows increased activity over left femoral head and left acetabulum with no evidence of photopenic defect within femoral head. Coronal SPECT image, **(C)** shows photopenic defect in left femoral head located inferior to activity associated with the acetabulum and medial to activity associated with osteophytes and femoral neck (arrow). Reproduced with permission from Reference 34.

sions, the femoral head may undergo infarction. Kloiber et al. found bone scintigraphy useful in predicting viability of the femoral head.[403] Before fluid aspiration, many children had decreased femoral head uptake. Following aspiration, all of these reverted to normal except those found to have undergone infarction.

In a large series of patients with diminished perfusion to the hip joint, in children with "irritable hip," Uren et al. found 22% had septic arthritis at surgery.[404] They recommend that children with decreased perfusion to the hip on three-phase bone scintigraphy undergo drainage of the joint. These authors suggest that, even if the joint effusion is not septic, relieving joint fluid pressure may prevent Legg-Perthe's disease.

The differential diagnosis of irritable hip and the scintigraphic findings in several pediatric hip abnormalities are listed in Table 3.

Frostbite and Ischemic Injuries

Bone scintigraphy can aid the surgeon in selecting amputation levels following frostbite, electrical injuries, diabetes, and other ischemic conditions. In such instances, the level of amputation must be above regions of nonviable bone. Since the bone ends may be quite irregular on planar images, SPECT images may be useful to ensure that the full diameter of the bone at the level of amputation is perfused. Skin markings are made using the persistence oscilloscope and radioactive sources when imaging the patient.

Reflex Sympathetic Dystrophy

Reflex sympathetic dystrophy syndrome (RSDS) consists of pain and tenderness, vasomotor instability (flushing, vasoconstriction), swelling, and often dystrophic skin changes. This syndrome has been known by several names, including causalgia, Sudeck's atrophy, traumatic angiospasm, and posttraumatic sympathalgia. The upper extremities are most frequently involved. Changes in the lower extremities are somewhat less defined. Several different diseases, drugs, and other factors have been associated with RSDS, although in approximately 35% of cases, no specific cause is identified. Radiographic osteopenia is evident in 69% of cases.[405] Pathophysiological mechanisms for the disease have not been determined. Previous trauma is often associated with this syndrome, as are a host of other related entities, including osteoarthritis, tumor, tendinitis, infection, myocardial infarction, herpes zoster, and herniated disc.[406] Bone scintigraphy is helpful in evaluating patients with RSDS. The characteristic pattern in these patients is increased periarticular

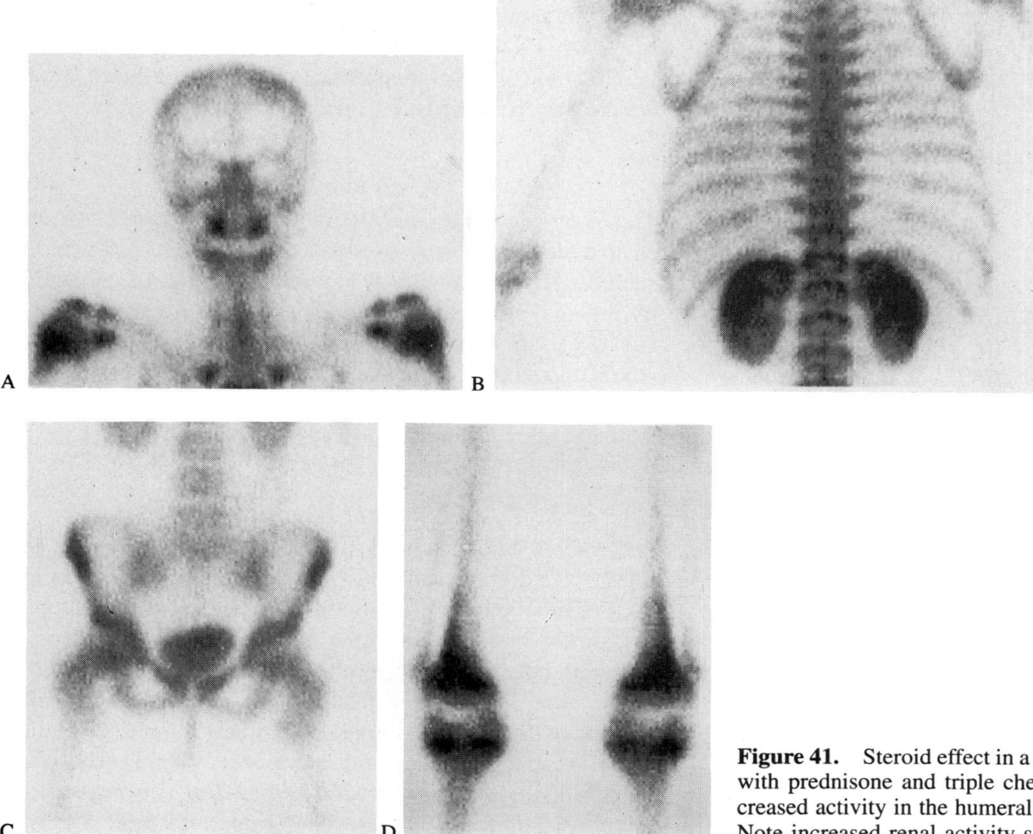

Figure 41. Steroid effect in a 14-year-old boy with ALL treated with prednisone and triple chemotherapy showing diffusely increased activity in the humeral heads, femoral heads, and knees. Note increased renal activity secondary to the chemotherapy.

activity that involves multiple joints on the affected extremity (Fig. 44). Radionuclide angiograms demonstrate increased perfusion to the involved side.[406,407]

Kozin et al. studied 64 patients with suspected RSDS.[405] Scintigraphic abnormalities were demonstrated in 38 (60%). These included increased bone blood flow and augmented periarticular radionuclide activity in the affected extremity. Of 11 patients with serial scintigraphy, 6 (55%) demonstrated a return to normal symmetric patterns following successful therapy. The authors concluded that bone scintigraphy may be useful in establishing the diagnosis and in identifying patients likely to respond to oral steroid therapy. Ninety percent of the patients with positive studies treated with corticosteroids had a good or excellent response, whereas

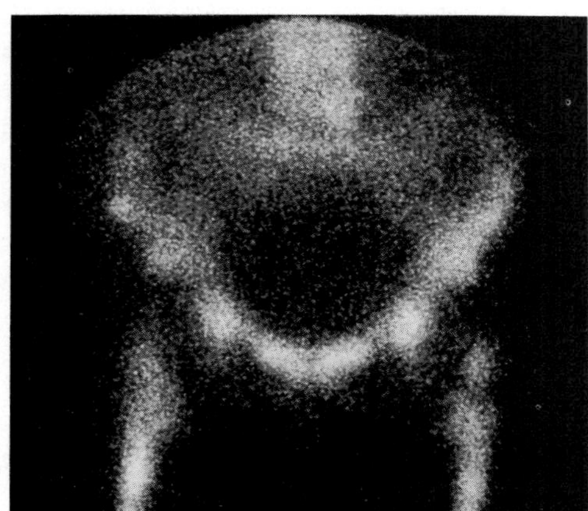

Figure 42. Bone marrow scintigraphy using ^{99m}Tc-sulfur colloid in a patient with bilateral avascular necrosis of the femoral heads shows decreased activity bilaterally.

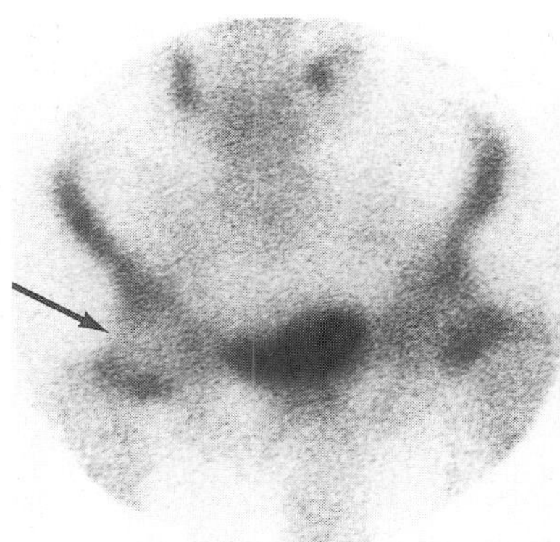

Figure 43. Legg-Calvé-Perthe's disease of the right hip in a 6-year-old boy showing decreased activity in the right femoral head (arrow).

Table 3. Bone-Scan Patterns in Pediatric Hip Diseases

CONDITION	PERFUSION PATTERN	DELAYED IMAGES
Legg-Calvé-Perthes disease	Normal	femoral head ↓
Synovitis	Normal	femoral head N or ↓ acetabulum ↑
Osteomyelitis or septic arthritis	↑	↑
Acute infarction	↓	↓
Healing infarction	↓	↑

64% of patients without scintigraphic abnormalities had a poor or fair response.

Holder and Mackinnon reported high sensitivity (96%) and specificity (97%) for the diagnosis of RSDS when three-phase scintigraphy was performed and strict criteria applied.[407] Their criteria were as follows: (1) The radionuclide angiogram must show diffusely increased blood flow to the entire wrist and hand. Increased perfusion usually appears on the involved side at least one frame before the normal side; (2) There must be diffusely increased activity on the involved side in the blood-pool image; (3) Diffusely increased activity must involve the radiocarpal, intercarpal, carpometacarpal, metacarpophalangeal, and interphalangeal joints; in children, a variable pattern of tracer distribution has been described.[408]

In a large series of patients studied over many months, Demangeat et al. described three stages in the scintigraphic evolution of RSDS.[409] In stage I (0 to 20 weeks from onset) three-phase scintigraphy demonstrated increased blood flow, blood pool, and increased uptake on early and late scintigraphy on the involved side. At stage II (20 to 60 weeks) blood velocity and blood pool were normalized, but early and delayed scintigraphy demonstrated increased tracer uptake.

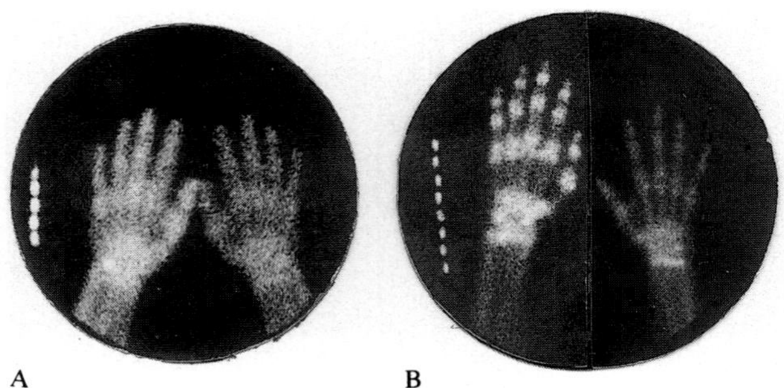

Figure 44. Reflex sympathetic dystrophy. **(A).** The blood-pool image shows markedly increased perfusion to the right hand and wrist 1 min after injection of ^{99m}Tc-MDP. Radioactive markers are used for distance calibration and indicate the right extremity. **(B).** Static 2-hour image demonstrates symmetrically increased joint activity in the right hand.

During stage III (60 to 100 weeks) blood flow and blood pool were reduced on the affected side and early and delayed tracer uptake were normalized. These findings may be related to late vasospasticity and, ultimately, reduced bone uptake may be observed on delayed images.

Rhabdomyolysis

This is an acute muscular injury caused by extensive unaccustomed exercise and overuse, or by a toxic reaction to such drugs as cocaine.[410] It is usually recognized clinically by regional tenderness over distinct muscle groups, occasionally accompanied by swelling.[411,412] Scintigraphy demonstrates moderately increased uptake in the affected muscle groups (Fig. 45). The mechanism of uptake is probably similar to that encountered in myocardial injury.

Heterotopic Ossification

Heterotopic ossification, also called *paraosteoarthropathy*, is associated with neuromuscular disorders and is seen in 20 to 30% of patients (up to 50% in some series) following spinal cord injury.[413] Heterotopic ossification is also associated with other forms of paraplegia and quadriplegia, hemophilia, severe burns, and tetanus. The mechanism for this soft-tissue ossification is not known, but it is a serious clinical problem that can lead to joint ankylosis and nearly total immobility. Ectopic ossification begins 2 to 10 weeks after spinal cord injury and progresses for approximately 6 to 14 months, eventually forming hard, bony masses palpable in the soft tissues (Fig. 46). Radiographs may be normal in early stages. Later, soft-tissue swelling is followed by flocculent densities that later progress to soft-tissue bone with a trabecular pattern 2 to 3 months after injury. By 12 to 18 months, the calcified mass usually becomes radiographically stable. Bone scintigraphy is abnormal before radiographic changes are evident. Serial scintigrams show increased tracer uptake in regions of soft-tissue ossification, until a maximum is reached; uptake then decreases over time as the ossification matures. Surgical removal is most appropriate when the ossification process ceases, to avoid recurrence. Most authors believe that heterotopic-to-normal bone ratio is the best index of maturity.[414,415] Maturity occurs when these ratios, determined by serial bone scintigraphy, decrease and become stable. The older literature suggests that combined bone and bone-marrow scintigraphy may be useful in determining the optimum time for surgical removal of soft-tissue calcifications. However, the latter studies are seldom performed.

Gaucher's Disease

Gaucher's disease is an inborn error of lipid metabolism with an underlying deficiency of glucosyl ceremide B glucoxidase. This results in accumulation of glucocerebroside in reticuloendothelial cells. The disease has a variety of phenotypic expressions; Type I is the most common form,

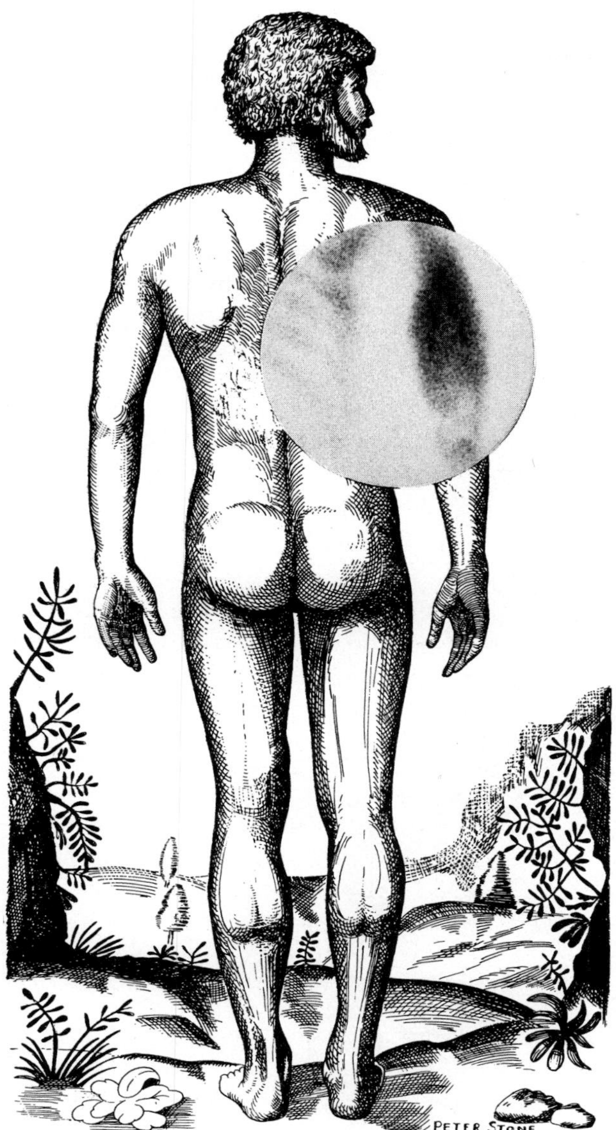

Figure 45. Posterior scintiphoto of right arm and shoulder using ^{99m}Tc-MDP in a young weight lifter complaining of pain and swelling 48 hours following unaccustomed weight lifting. The intense muscle uptake of tracer is characteristic of rhabdomyolysis.

occurring at any age and characterized by hypersplenism, anemia, thrombocytopenia, bone pain, joint swelling, pathologic fractures, and osteomyelitis. The bone pain is thought to be due to increased intramedullary pressure associated with marrow infiltration. This interferes with bone blood supply, causing infarction and aseptic necrosis.[416] The frequent association of osteomyelitis in this disease suggests the need for bone scintigraphy.

The most frequently reported findings are photopenic lesions at the site of pain, probably due to avascular necrosis.[417–419] Gallium scintigraphy is negative in these instances. These patients also may exhibit the classic "Erlenmeyer flask deformity of the distal femurs (Fig. 47).

Radiation Effects

Increased uptake of bone tracers is observed within hours following external irradiation. The uptake intensity appears to depend upon the radiation dose and probably results from increased blood flow and vascular permeability in the irradiated tissues. Later, bone images show decreased uptake as the microvascular injury (*endarteritis obliterans*) affects new bone formation (Fig. 48). Hattner et al. found that decreased uptake occurs 4 to 6 months following radiation, and then only with doses exceeding 20 Gy (2000 rad).[420]

SOFT-TISSUE UPTAKE OF BONE TRACERS

Bone tracers concentrate in many organs and soft-tissue lesions (Fig. 49 and Table 2). Soft-tissue calcification and heterotopic ossification may be identifiable radiographically, but its absence does not exclude microscopic calcification or early heterotopic ossification below the limits of radiographic resolution.

The mechanism for localization of bone tracers in noncalcified muscle may be related to movement of calcium from plasma into damaged muscle cells through abnormally permeable sarcolemma.[422] This mechanism is thought to be responsible for uptake in acute myocardial infarcts. Curiously, such concentration only occurs between approximately one and seven days following the acute injury.[423] Other possible mechanisms of soft-tissue uptake include binding to immature collagen and atypical binding of the ^{99m}Tc-phosphate to phosphatase enzymes.[5,19]

OSTEOMYELITIS

Osteomyelitis is a serious infection that requires prolonged antibiotic therapy and results each year in numerous limb amputations. The scintigraphic diagnosis of osteomyelitis rests upon three seminal articles: that of Duszynski et al.[424] who observed that routine bone scintigraphy could detect osteomyelitis weeks before plain radiographs became positive; of Gilday et al.,[425] who added blood-pool imaging to show increased vascularity accompanying bone infections; and Deysine et al.,[426] who showed that combining ^{67}Ga-citrate with bone scintigraphy increases the specificity for osteomyelitis.

Bone scintigraphy in the diagnosis of osteomyelitis always includes three-phase imaging, to demonstrate increased vascularity as an essential feature of the pathologic process, and to aid in the differentiation from cellulitis. Classically, cellulitis is associated with increased regional blood flow and expanded blood pool, but normal or only minimally increased bone activity on delayed images (Figs. 50 and 51).

Some have proposed a four-phase imaging sequence that includes a 24-hour image.[427,428] In osteomyelitis, the ratio of activity between the lesion and normal bone should increase in the 24-hour image. The reason is that uptake of ^{99m}Tc-MDP stops at 4 hours in normal trabecular bone but continues over 24 hours in woven bone, the abnormal type of bone that is found surrounding osteomyelitis and bone tumors.[428] Four-

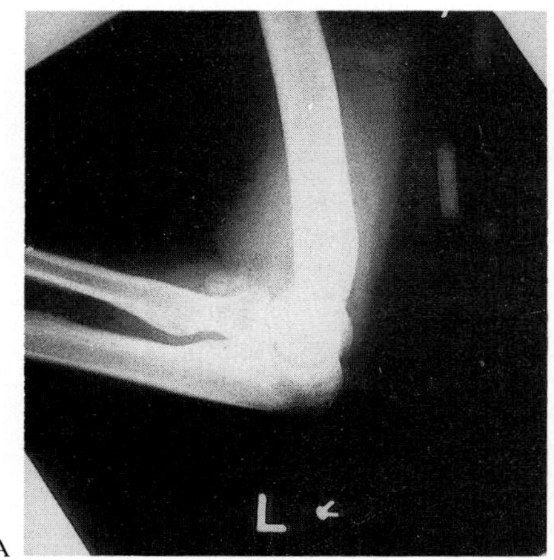

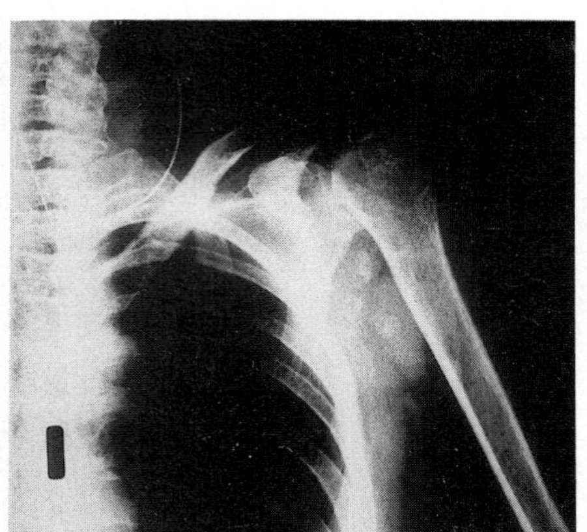

A

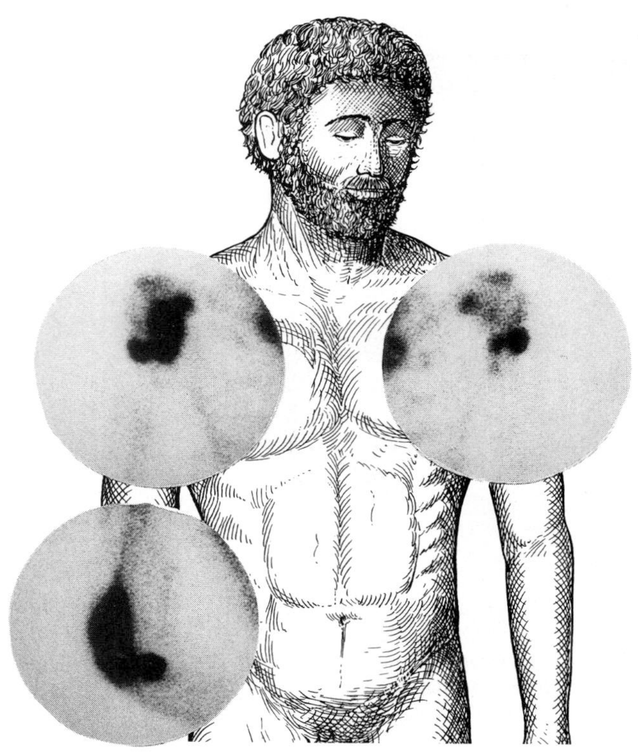

Figure 46. (A). Radiographs of left elbow and right shoulder in a paraplegic patient with extensive soft-tissue ossification. **(B).** ^{99m}Tc-MDP scintigraphy showing intense tracer uptake at sites of heterotopic ossification in both shoulders and right elbow. B

phase bone scintigraphy has been useful in lower extremity lesions in patients with peripheral vascular disease. Obviously, this criterion could not be used to differentiate osteomyelitis from bone tumor, but usually this is not the question.

Bone infections stimulate intense osteoblastic activity in uncompromised bone, and bone scintigraphy is very sensitive to these changes. A negative scintigraphic study essentially rules out osteomyelitis and no other study is usually necessary. The reported sensitivity and specificity of three-phase scintigraphy in patients with osteomyelitis and normal radiographs are 94% and 95%, respectively (the sum of 6 published reports).[429] In children, this figure is somewhat less because osteomyelitis frequently occurs in and about the epiphyses. The greatly increased perfusion and bone turnover in these areas create intense labeling with bone tracers, disguising the presence of infection.[430,431] In subperiosteal abscess, increased pressure may interrupt the blood supply, creating cold lesions. It is important in bone scintigraphy to obtain computer images so that image intensity can be adjusted to avoid film overexposure, and to highlight small differences between opposite extremities. When osteomyelitis is strongly suspected and bone scintigraphy is normal, additional imaging with ^{67}Ga-citrate or radiolabeled leukocytes is essential.[432]

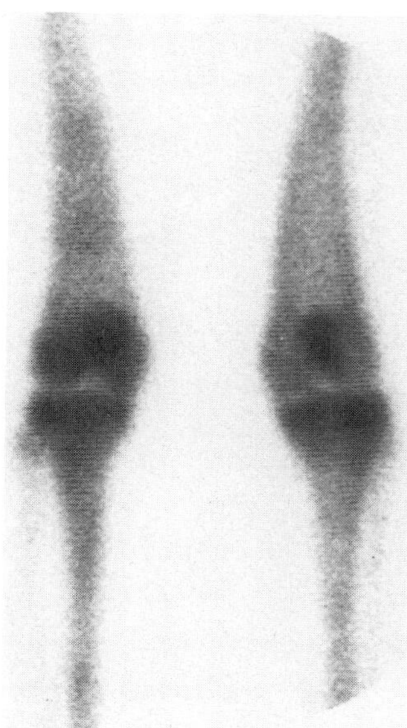

Figure 47. Anterior scintiphoto of the lower extremities in a 24-year-old female with type I Gaucher's disease showing typical appearance of "Erlenmeyer flask" femurs. Tracer distribution is often irregular due to uneven marrow involvement.

The presence of multiple focal lesions does not rule out osteomyelitis, which is common in brucellosis.[433] This pattern is also found in disseminated tuberculosis in about 1% of patients.[434]

In patients who have osteomyelitis superimposed upon another bone complication, three-phase bone imaging alone is much less specific. Such complications include previous or chronic osteomyelitis, surrounding soft tissue infection, fractures, surgery, prostheses, hypertrophic and neuropathic osteoarthropathy, arthritis, bone infarcts, and bone tumors, all of which are associated with bone remodeling and increased tracer uptake. Giant cell tumor, synovial cell sarcoma, gouty arthritis, and Reiter's syndrome all give a pattern on three-phase bone scintigraphy mimicking osteomyelitis.[435] When the above conditions complicate osteomyelitis, the reported sensitivity and specificity of three-phase bone scintigraphy alone (the sum of 14 published reports reviewed by Schauwecker[429]) are 95% and 33%, respectively. In such cases, combination imaging is essential to increase specificity. Additional imaging techniques include the use of ^{67}Ga-citrate, ^{111}In- or ^{99m}Tc-labeled leukocytes, ^{99m}Tc-sulfur colloid marrow imaging, radiolabeled immunoglobulins, MRI to detect inflammatory changes in bone marrow and soft tissues, plain radiographs, and aspiration cultures.

^{111}In-Labeled Leukocytes

Currently, imaging with radiolabeled leukocytes is the preferred imaging procedure in patients with osteomyelitis affecting the non-marrow-containing skeleton, who have abnormal three-phase bone scintigraphy and a coexisting bone complication. Non-marrow-containing bone is mentioned specifically, because labeled leukocytes normally concentrate in bone marrow and their numbers may be only minimally increased by the presence of infection. In osteomyelitis affecting marrow-containing skeleton, ^{99m}Tc-sulfur colloid is combined with bone scintigraphy because radiocolloid labels the reticuloendothelial elements of marrow that are displaced by infection, causing *incongruent* patterns between the marrow and bone scintigraphy.[429,436,437]

Most experience has been obtained with ^{111}In-labeled leukocytes, which accumulate at sites of infection (Fig. 52). The procedure can be carried out immediately after bone scintigraphy, since the lower-energy ^{99m}Tc can be effectively excluded by pulse-height analysis. Scintigraphy is usually performed 24 hours following injection of 18.5 MBq (500 μCi) of labeled autologous leukocytes.

In the 16 studies reviewed by Schauwecker,[429] the overall sensitivity and specificity of ^{111}In-labeled leukocyte imaging were 88 and 85%, respectively. It is particularly difficult to distinguish between osteomyelitis from surrounding cellulitis in diabetic osteoarthropathy, because of the close proximity of structures and the low resolution of the scintillation camera. Cold defects on leukocyte scintigraphy are also difficult to distinguish from metastases, healing fractures, and rheumatoid arthritis.[438] Infections that have recently been treated with antibiotics may also be a source of false-negative results.[439] Chronic osteomyelitis may be difficult to detect

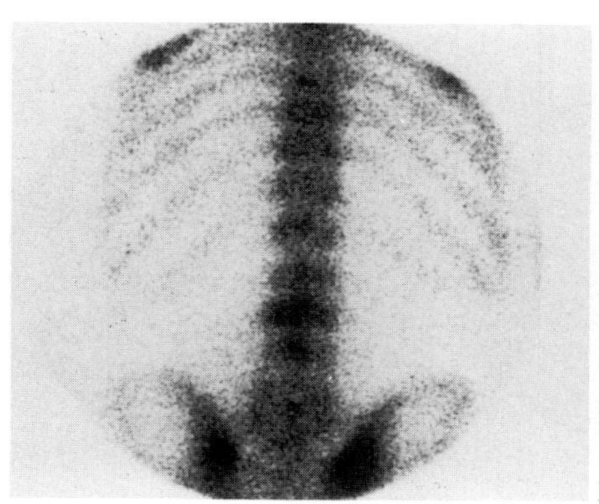

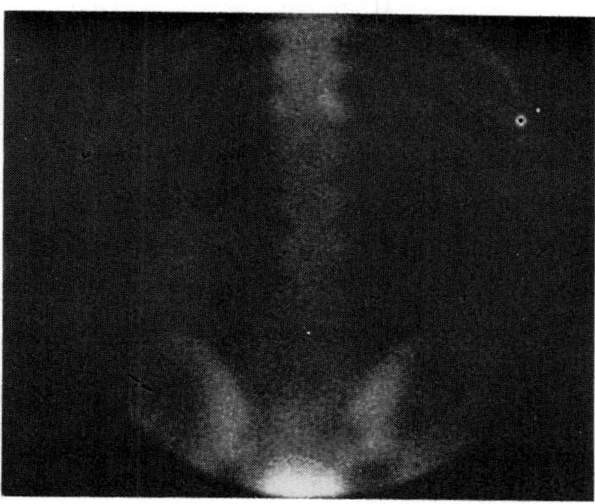

Figure 48. **(A).** Preradiation scintiphoto. **(B).** Six months after lumbar irradiation, scintigram shows markedly reduced uptake in the lumbar vertebrae.

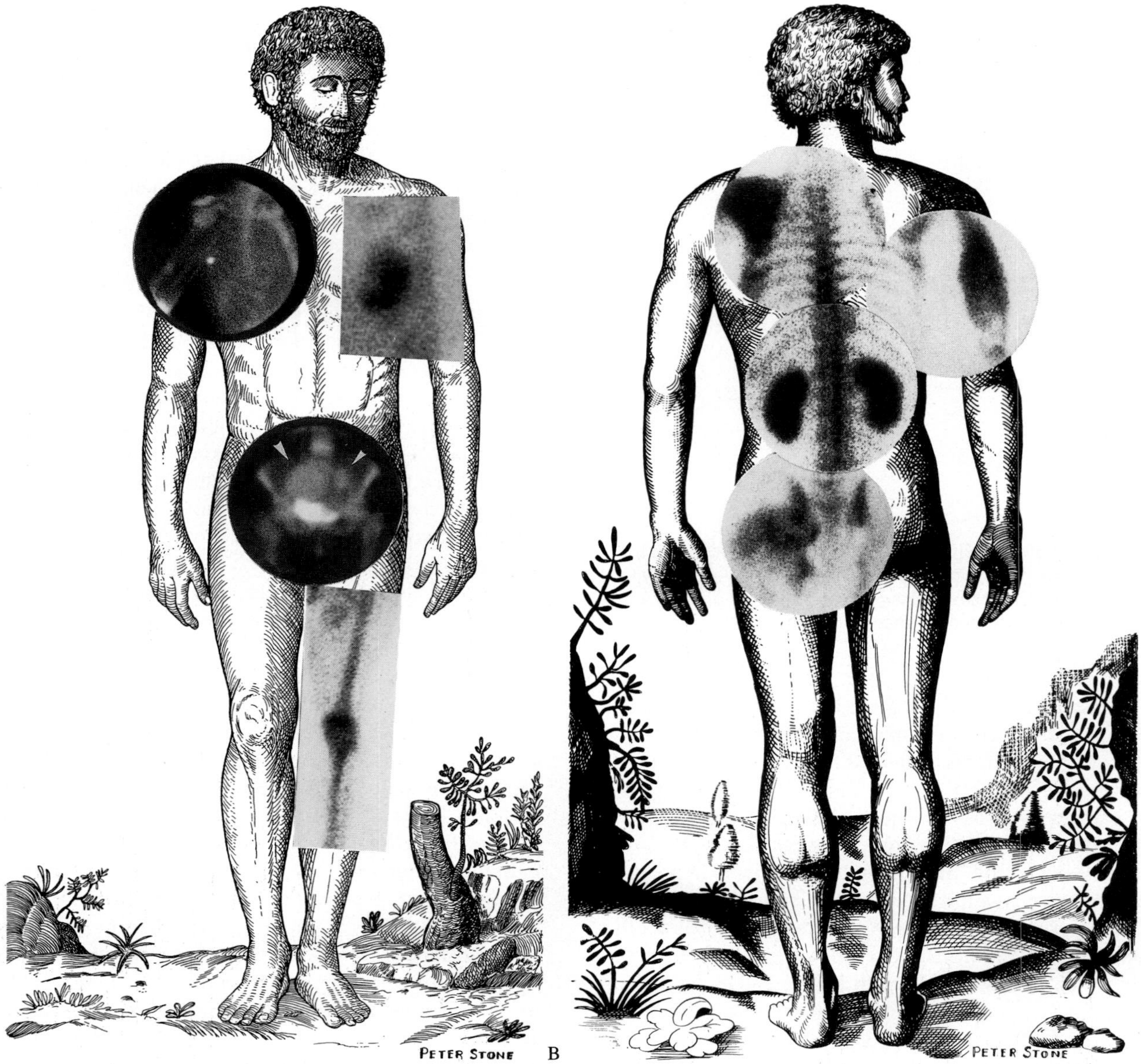

Figure 49. Composites showing various soft tissue lesions. **(A).** Anterior views showing axillary lymph node from extravasation at the injection site, myocardial uptake following direct current cardioversion, uterine fibroids, soft tissue sarcoma of left thigh with lymphedema. **(B).** Posterior views showing myositis ossificans of left shoulder and right arm, radiation nephritis, iron dextran injection of the left buttock.

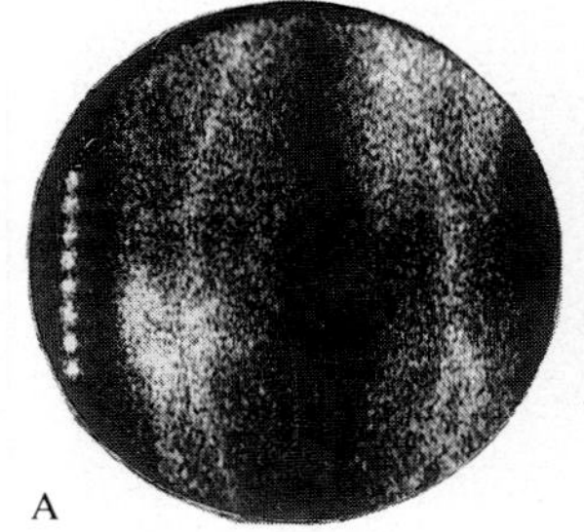

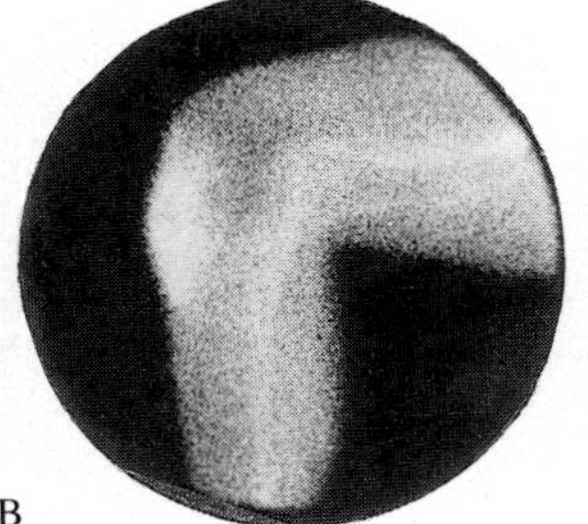

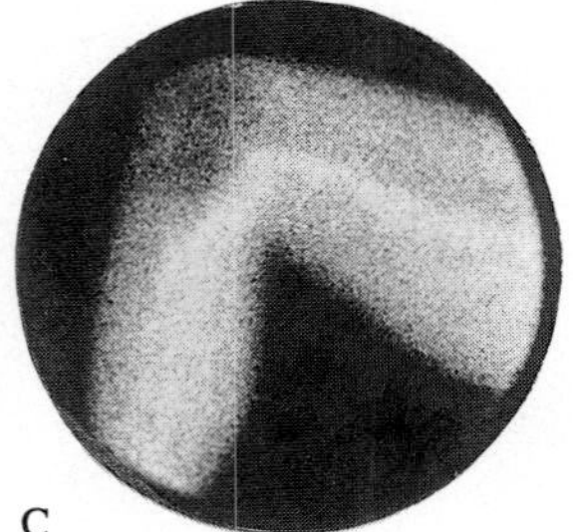

Figure 50. Three-phase bone scintigraphy in a young man with cellulitis of right knee. **(A).** Perfusion image demonstrates increased blood flow to right knee. **(B).** Medial view of right knee shows increased blood pool. **(C).** Medial delayed image shows decreased uptake in area of skin edema and no increased bone activity.

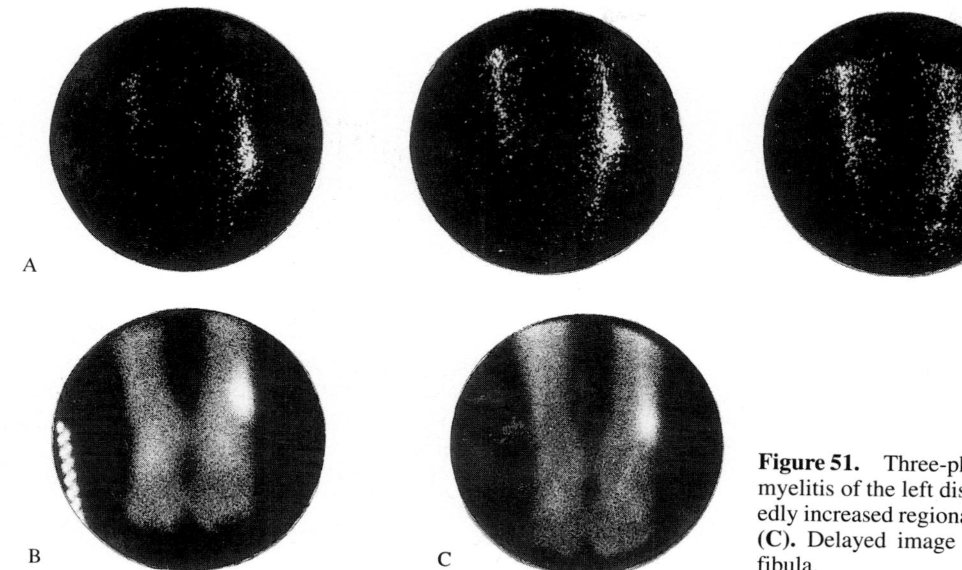

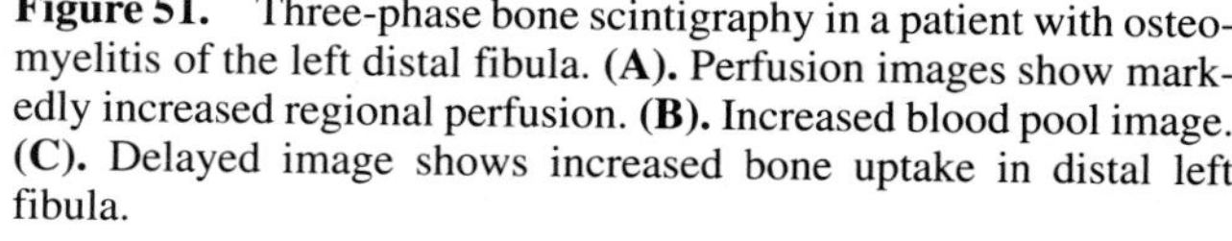

Figure 51. Three-phase bone scintigraphy in a patient with osteomyelitis of the left distal fibula. **(A).** Perfusion images show markedly increased regional perfusion. **(B).** Increased blood pool image. **(C).** Delayed image shows increased bone uptake in distal left fibula.

because of the small numbers of leukocytes found at such sites. This is more problematic in the central than the peripheral skeleton.

^{99m}Tc-Labeled Leukocytes

^{99m}Tc-Hexamethylpropyleneamine oxime (HMPAO) is a lipophilic complex that predominately labels granulocytes. It has the principal advantage that the short-lived ^{99m}Tc permits greatly increased injectable activity (300 MBq vs. 18 MBq of ^{111}In). Therefore, image quality is improved, SPECT can be performed to better localize the precise focus of activity, and chronic osteomyelitis may be more specifically detected. HMPAO comes in a kit form, making it more readily available to the nuclear medicine laboratory. The reported sensitivity and specificity (6 published reports[429]) are 87 and 81%, respectively. These results are similar to those found with ^{111}In-labeled leukocytes, which is logical because the mechanism of localization is the same. Labeling with both radiopharmaceuticals requires careful and time-consuming cell separations (Chapter 32).

^{99m}Tc-HMPAO labeled leukocytes may have an advantage for use in children with suspected osteomyelitis, because of reduced radiation absorbed dose, the ability to image at 3 hours, and a higher epiphysis:diaphysis ratio in infection than experienced with ^{99m}Tc-MDP.[440]

^{67}Ga-Citrate

Gallium binds to serum transferrin, leukocyte lactoferrin, bacterial siderophores, and inflammatory proteins.[441] Gallium uptake parallels the intensity of the inflammatory process more closely than does ^{99m}Tc-MDP. Because the uptake of gallium decreases as the inflammatory process resolves, it may be useful in following the response of osteomyelitis to treatment. The disadvantages of ^{67}Ga-citrate are its relatively high radiation dose compared with bone scintigraphy, its high energy which yields images with poor spatial resolution, and its excretion into bowel often requiring 48 to 72 hours of imaging to differentiate normal bowel activity from an infectious process.

In 15 published reports summarized by Schauwecker,[429]

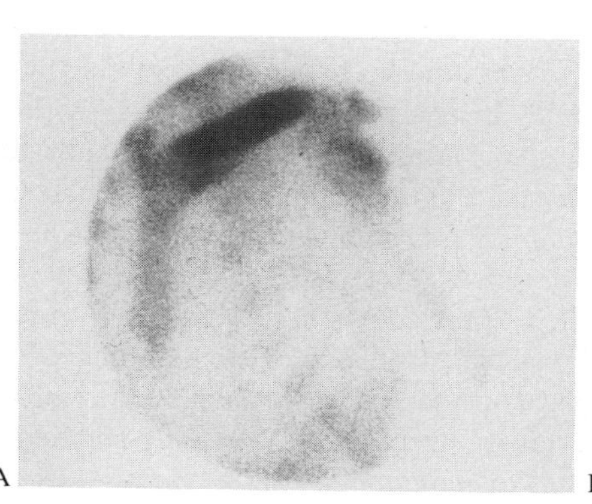

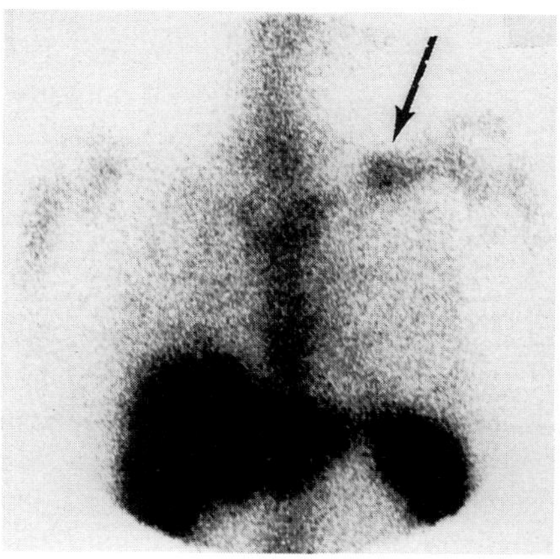

Figure 52. **(A).** Bone scintigraphy in a 26-year-old AIDs patient with osteomyelitis of the left clavicle. **(B).** Scintigraphy using ^{111}In-labeled autologous leukocytes showing intense focus of activity in left clavicular region (arrow). The activity in the liver and spleen is normal.

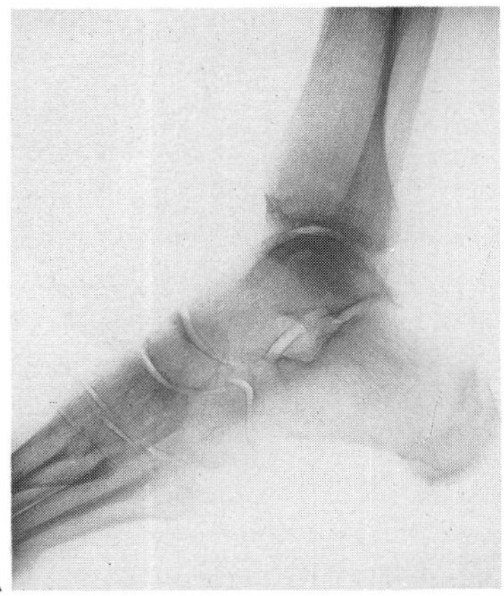

A

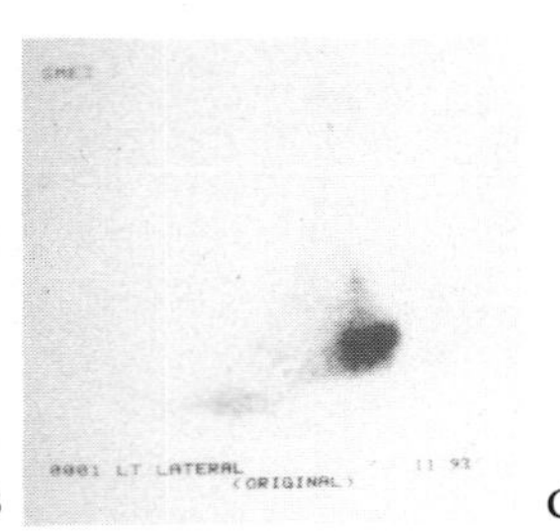

B

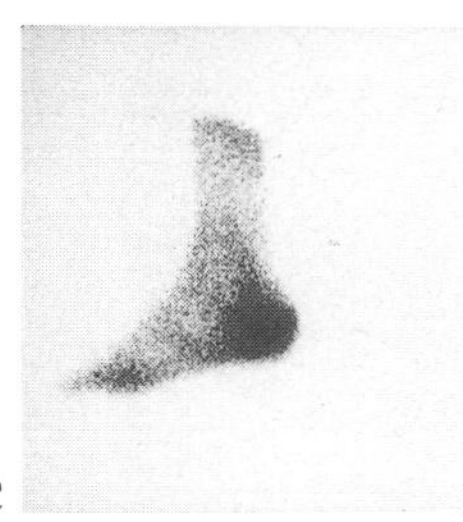

C

Figure 53. Bone scintigraphy in a patient with diabetes and an ulcer on the left heel. **(A).** The radiograph demonstrates minimal change in the calcaneus. **(B).** Bone scintigraphy demonstrates intense activity in the distal calcaneus. **(C).** ^{67}Ga-citrate scintigraphy demonstrates even more intense activity, suggesting osteomyelitis.

the overall sensitivity and specificity of ^{67}Ga scintigraphy were 81 and 69%, respectively. The chief cause of reduced specificity is that gallium is a bone-seeking tracer itself and localizes in bone, whether infection is present or not. Some observers have proposed that gallium scintigraphy is more specific when the pattern of distribution is incongruent with that of MDP.[442,443] When the uptake of gallium exceeds the uptake of ^{99m}Tc-MCP, the probability of active osteomyelitis is very high (Fig. 53); however, this occurs in only about 25% of all patients with osteomyelitis.[444] Most studies that have compared ^{67}Ga-citrate with radiolabeled leukocyte scintigraphy find greater sensitivity and specificity with leukocytes.[445,446] Consequently, ^{67}Ga-citrate is seldom used for the diagnosis of osteomyelitis when leukocytes are available.

Radiolabeled Immunoglobulins

Recently, preparations of both monoclonal (mouse anti-granulocyte antibodies) and nonspecific polyclonal immunoglobulins (IgG) labeled with ^{111}In have been used to diagnose musculoskeletal infections.[447–449] The preparation of labeled IgG is much simpler than labeled leukocytes and also reduces the irradiation of viable leukocytes. Unlike ^{67}Ga-citrate, IgG is not excreted into the bowel, nor is there active bone uptake that can potentially interfere with interpretation. Furthermore, human polyclonal IgG avoids the development of human antimouse antibodies (HAMA) associated with mouse antigranulocyte antibodies. Both sensitivity and specificity have been high in preliminary studies, suggesting the need for further evaluation.[447,449] At least one study that evaluated mouse antigranulocyte antibodies in unselected patients with suspected bone infections has reported both low sensitivity and low specificity.[450]

OTHER RADIOPHARMACEUTICALS

Indium-111 chloride is a 3+ cation that binds transferrin and behaves similarly to gallium, except that it localizes within bone marrow instead of bone. Preliminary studies have shown sensitivity of 92% and specificity of 81% for the detection of osteomyelitis.[451–453] Nevertheless, the use of ^{111}In chloride has not gained wide acceptance.

MRI

MRI is not considered an initial diagnostic test in the detection of osteomyelitis, but with its excellent anatomic resolution it is useful in determining the extent of infection. The sensitivity and specificity of MRI for osteomyelitis are comparable to three-phase bone scintigraphy, but MRI is considerably more expensive.[429,454] Normal bone marrow on MR imaging produces a strong signal intensity on T1-weighted images due to the short T1 of medullary fat.[455] Osteomyelitis results in decreased signal intensity on T1-weighted images and increased signal intensity on short tau inversion recovery (STIR) and T2-weighted images.[456] The decreased signal intensity on T1-weighed images is the result of the exudative changes, hyperemia, ischemia, and edema which lengthen T1 in the replacement of fat with water.[455] Unfortunately, other processes, such as tumors, healing fractures, intramedullary or juxta-medullary inflammations also increase water in the marrow.[457]

MRI is especially valuable in the detection of osteomyelitis of the spine, where the scintigraphic changes caused by infection are difficult to distinguish from postoperative bone healing, metastatic, or degenerative disease. In the spine, there is a decreased signal intensity on T1-weighted images of both the vertebral body and adjacent disc and increased signal intensity of both the body and adjacent disc on T2-weighted images.[457] In one series of 37 patients with suspected vertebral osteomyelitis, comparing radiographs, MRI, bone scintigraphy, and ^{67}Ga-citrate, MRI was found to be equivalent in accuracy and more sensitive than sequential ^{99m}Tc/^{67}Ga scintigraphy.[458]

Berquest studied 42 patients with suspected osteomyelitis and found that ^{111}In-labeled leukocytes had a greater specificity than MRI, but concluded that the combination of MRI and ^{111}In-leukocytes would improve specificity and help determine the extent of infection.[459] The advantages of MRI are its ability to differentiate marrow involvement from inflammation in adjacent soft tissues and its demonstration of sinus tracts and sequestra, because of its fine spatial resolution. Thus, MRI is recommended for evaluating the feet of diabetic patients because of the high false-positive rate associated with bone scintigraphy caused by cellulitis, chronic ulcers, and neuroarthropathy.[460]

CT

The diagnosis of acute osteomyelitis is difficult with radiographs and CT. CT does, however, provide excellent spatial resolution and clear definition of cortical bone. It is superior to MRI in detecting sequestra, foreign bodies, and cloacae, and can also detect intraosseous gas, which is a rare but reliable sign of osteomyelitis.[454] CT can detect bone changes from osteomyelitis earlier than plain radiographs and is useful in detecting abnormalities in the pelvis, sternum, and spine, which are more difficult to detect on plain radiographs.

In many centers, CT has been replaced by MRI in the evaluation of osteomyelitis. In comparison to CT, MRI has more accurate multiplanar reconstruction, better soft tissue resolution, higher definition of sinus tracts and abscesses, and better visualization of infectious foci in chronic osteomyelitis.[454]

EVALUATION OF PROSTHESES

Scintigraphy demonstrates increased uptake of tracer around sites of prostheses, screws, pins, and other orthopedic devices as a part of the healing process. Such nonspecific uptake is observed for up to 2 years, depending upon the type of device, and gradually declines as healing is completed. Complications of prostheses can be detected by bone scintigraphy as an abnormal recurrence or prolonged persistence of a lesion around the prosthesis. Such complications include bone infection, loosening, fractures, and heterotopic bone formation. In the evaluation of a painful prosthesis, loosening and infection are the two most common entities that must be distinguished.

Hip Prostheses. Evaluation of a painful hip prosthesis remains a diagnostic challenge and may require multiple or serial examinations to define. Often, combinations of plain radiographs, scintigraphy, MR imaging, and aspiration arthrography are required to make the diagnosis. Both the femoral and the acetabular components of a total hip prosthesis are evaluated, since either or both may be involved in complications. Several reports have described the scintigraphic findings.[461–466]

In general, if complete three-phase bone scintigraphy is normal, causes of hip pain other than a prosthesis complication should be considered. If three-phase bone scintigraphy demonstrates increased perfusion and the delayed images demonstrate activity significantly greater than surrounding bone, infection must be considered, particularly when images demonstrate increased activity over an extensive area of the prosthetic surface.

The scintigraphic diagnosis of loosening is suggested when perfusion and blood pool images are normal and delayed images demonstrate increased activity beyond the usual healing period (Fig. 54). In a prospective study of *cemented* hip prostheses, Utz et al. found that increased activity in the tip, greater trochanter, and acetabulum persisted for up to 2 years in about 90% of patients, and longer in about 10%. Activity in the shaft and lesser trochanter generally normalized by 6 months.[463] Recent studies have shown that the newer *porous-coated* prostheses heal somewhat differently.[467,468] Presumably because the tip is uncoated, elastic bone distortion and remodeling about the tip causes increased activity to persist longer, especially at the lateral margin and distal end. A complication must be suspected if activity about the medial margin of the porous coated prosthesis increases with time, while increasing activity at the tip or lateral margin is not necessarily abnormal.[468]

Unfortunately, chronic, low-grade infections may result in minimally increased perfusion and the pattern they evoke may be mistaken for loosening.

It is obvious from the foregoing discussion that a single three-phase bone study taken within a year of arthroplasty is unlikely to reliably differentiate between infection and loosening. To improve specificity, combinations of imaging procedures have been devised. Sequential ^{99m}Tc-MDP/^{67}Ga-citrate scintigraphy can detect prosthesis infection with an accuracy of 70 to 75%. The pattern most consistent with infection is that of ^{67}Ga uptake that is either incongruent or more intense than MDP uptake. However, prosthetic loosening often results in intense ^{67}Ga uptake, and gallium scintigraphy is generally considered unreliable in distinguishing between loosening and infection.

Somewhat greater accuracy for detecting infected prostheses have been reported for sequential ^{99m}Tc-MDP/^{111}In-WBC scintigraphy.[445,469–472] Diagnostic accuracies range from 83 to 93%. Images interpreted as positive for infection include those that demonstrate focally increased uptake in an incongruent pattern or else ^{111}In-WBC uptake $\geq$ ^{99m}Tc-MDP uptake (Fig. 55). Nevertheless, several problems in interpretation may occur:

1. The poor resolution of ^{111}In-leukocyte images make soft-tissue uptake difficult to distinguish from bone uptake;
2. Because ^{111}In-leukocytes normally are found in red bone marrow, the differentiation between infection and normal marrow may be difficult;
3. Uptake of leukocytes in marrow-containing heterotopic bone and in rheumatoid joints occasionally gives rise to false-positive results;
4. Leukocyte uptake in chronic infections and following antibiotic therapy may be so reduced as to miss the presence of infection.

For these reasons, some investigators now consider that sequential ^{111}In-labeled leukocyte/^{99m}Tc-sulfur colloid scin-

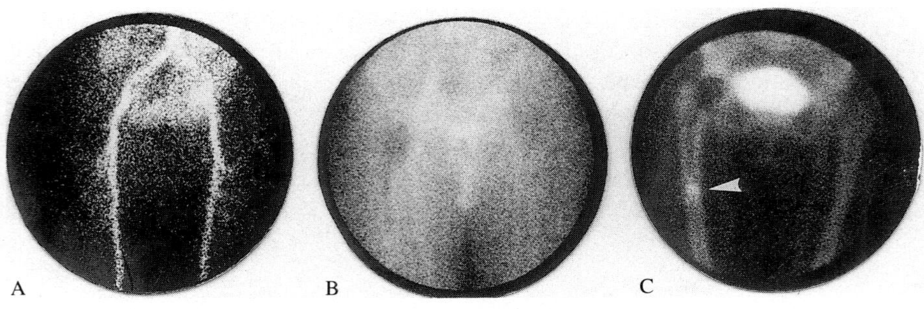

Figure 54. Three-phase bone scintigraphy in a patient with a painful right cemented hip prosthesis, more than two years after insertion. Dynamic frame, **(A)** and early blood-pool image, **(B)** demonstrate normal vascularity. The 2-hour static image, **(C)** demonstrates increased activity at the tip of the prosthesis (arrow). This pattern suggests loosening rather than infection.

tigraphy may provide the most reliable combination scintigraphy for both hip and knee prostheses.[464,469,473,474] The rationale for this combination is as follows: labeled leukocytes normally concentrate both at sites of infection and within normal bone marrow. Sulfur colloid is taken up only by normal marrow, but not in areas of marrow displaced by infection. Therefore, an incongruent pattern in which leukocytes are taken up around the prosthesis but, in which areas sulfur colloid is not taken up, suggests the presence of infection (Fig. 55). When the two patterns are congruent, normal marrow elements are likely (Fig. 56).

In a series of 50 studies reported by Palestro et al.,[473] the sensitivity, specificity, and accuracy for this pattern in infections were 100, 97, and 98%, respectively.

Preliminary reports suggest that sequential ^{99m}Tc-MDP/^{111}In-immunoglobulin scintigraphy may have high sensitivity and acceptable specificity;[448,475] however, further studies are needed to confirm these findings.

Knee Prostheses. Far fewer studies have been reported in the evaluation of total knee arthroplasty. The chief complications following surgery include patellofemoral arthritis, heterotopic bone formation, loosening, and infection.[405] The use of bone scintigraphy alone to evaluate prosthesis complications is limited because of persistent high tracer uptake for several years after prosthetic implantation.[406,407] Probably the greatest success in evaluating painful total knee prostheses has been reported by Palestro et al.[474] The reported accuracy of combined ^{111}In-labeled leukocyte/^{99m}Tc-sulfur colloid (incongruent pattern) was 95%, compared with an accuracy of only 75% for combined ^{111}In-leukocyte/^{99m}Tc-MDP scintigraphy.

Osteomyelitis in the Diabetic Foot

The diagnosis of osteomyelitis of the foot in patients with diabetes mellitus presents a formidable problem, yet early recognition and effective treatment is essential to preventing amputations that have become all too common in this disease. Bone scintigraphy is sensitive in detecting osteomyelitis (>90%), but is quite nonspecific (35–55%).[476–482] Specificity is limited because of the small bones involved; the limited spatial resolution of the scintillation camera; and the superimposition of cellulitis, neuroarthropathy, and trauma, all of which increase regional perfusion and uptake of bone tracers. Plain radiographs are often of limited assistance because of concomitant or preexisting disease and the large

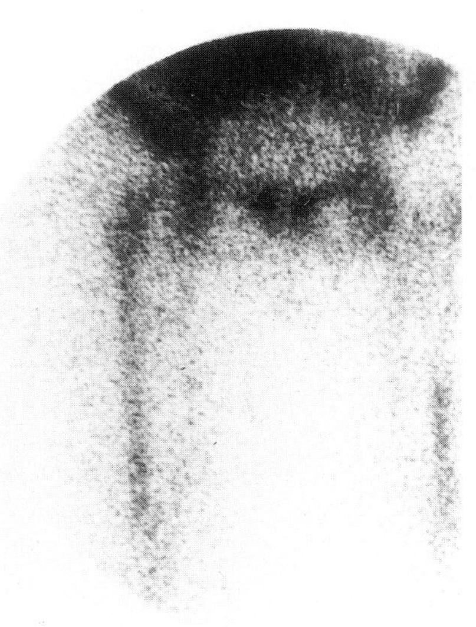

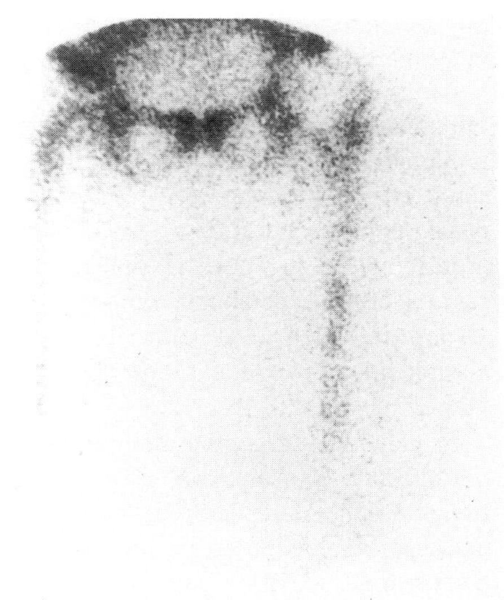

Figure 55. A 60-yr-old female with a left total hip arthroplasty implanted 6 yr prior to imaging. **(A).** Anterior 24-hr labeled leukocyte image demonstrates periprosthetic leukocyte activity in the trochanteric, shaft and tip regions. Although slightly heterogeneous, this activity is approximately the same intensity as surrounding marrow activity and that of the contralateral side. **(B).** Anterior sulfur colloid image performed approximately 1 hr after **(A)** reveals nearly absent marrow activity in the trochanteric and shaft regions. The study was interpreted as incongruent leukocyte/sulfur colloid images, consistent with infection. An infected prosthesis was removed at surgery. Reproduced with permission from Reference 436.

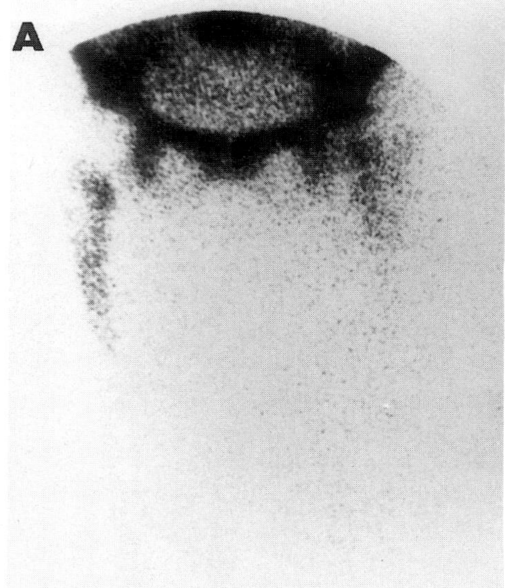

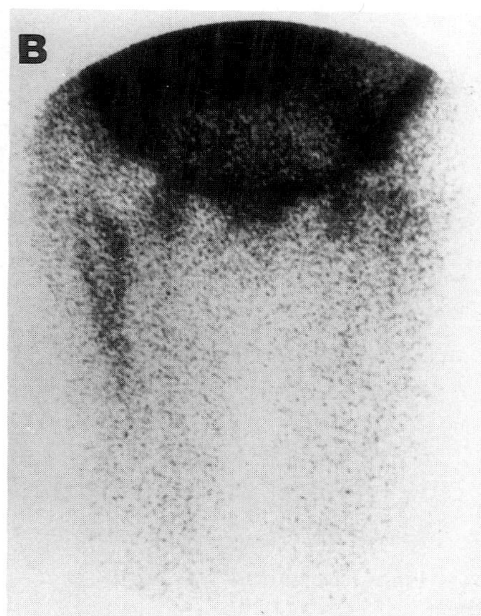

Figure 56. An 81-year-old female with a right total hip arthroplasty inserted 15 yr prior to imaging. **(A).** Anterior 24-hr labeled leukocyte image demonstrates intense periprosthetic activity surrounding the trochanteric shaft and tip zones. This activity is more intense than the corresponding contralateral region. **(B).** Sulfur colloid image reveals distribution of radiotracer similar to that in **(A).** This study was interpreted as congruent leukocyte/sulfur colloid images, without evidence of infection. A loose, but uninfected prosthesis was removed. Reproduced with permission from Reference 436.

amount of bone destroyed before becoming radiographically apparent.[476,477]

Several studies have suggested that ^{111}In-labeled leukocytes are useful for the diagnosis of osteomyelitis in the diabetic foot.[476–484] There is no red marrow in the bones of the feet, so leukocytes do not accumulate there normally. Uninfected neuropathic bones and osteoarthropathy do not concentrate leukocytes. Therefore, any increased activity must be suspicious for infection. The chief source of false-positive results is the presence of infected ulcers that do not extend to bone.

Keenan et al. found leukocyte scintigraphy was 100% sensitive and 79% specific for osteomyelitis.[480] They found that bone scintigraphy added little or nothing to the diagnosis. Schauwecker et al. found a sensitivity of 100% and specificity of 83% for ^{111}In-leukocytes.[482] Bone scintigraphy was used to provide bony landmarks that helped correctly localize foci to bone, the combination of which increased specificity to 89%.

Analysis of the several studies cited above suggest the following:

1. The incidence of osteomyelitis in patients with exposed bone is very high, and such patients should be treated for bone infection regardless of imaging results.[483]
2. Radiolabeled leukocyte scintigraphy is more sensitive and specific than ^{67}Ga scintigraphy, because the latter localizes in both uninfected bone and extraosseus inflammation.[484]
3. Patients with positive three-phase bone and positive leukocyte scintigraphy in which abnormal activity corresponds to bone have approximately 90% chance of having osteomyelitis.[482]
4. Patients with negative radiographs *and* negative leukocyte scintigraphy probably do not have osteomyelitis.
5. The normalization of leukocyte scintigraphy is probably more accurate than bone scintigraphy in judging the effectiveness of therapy, because the resolution of the latter depends upon bone healing, which is a longer process than clearance of infection.
6. The initial experience with MRI suggests that this modality may be both more sensitive and specific than scintigraphy for the presence of osteomyelitis.[459,481]

METABOLIC AND DISSEMINATED BONE DISEASES

Unbalanced bone mineral accretion and reabsorption characterize most metabolic bone diseases. Usually, the entire skeleton is affected; however, particular bones or limbs may be uniquely affected, as in disuse osteoporosis. For the most part, routine skeletal imaging is insensitive to changes in overall skeletal metabolism. Rather, bone scintigraphy is useful in detecting focal complications of metabolic bone disease, including fractures, microfractures, stress fractures, vertebral compression, Milkman-Looser zones, aseptic necrosis, etc.

Osteoporosis

Osteoporosis (osteopenia) is the most common of the metabolic bone diseases. A quantitative reduction in bone mass occurs with cortical thinning and fragmentation, and loss of trabeculae in medullary bone. (This disease is also discussed in Chapter 34. Usually, roentgenograms are normal in early stages of the disease, but later demonstrate characteristic changes, including "codfish vertebrae," vertebral wedging, and vertebral compression fractures.

In osteoporosis, scintigraphic images have no distinguishing features, except for stress and compression fractures that frequently occur. In severe or end-stage disease, osteoblastic

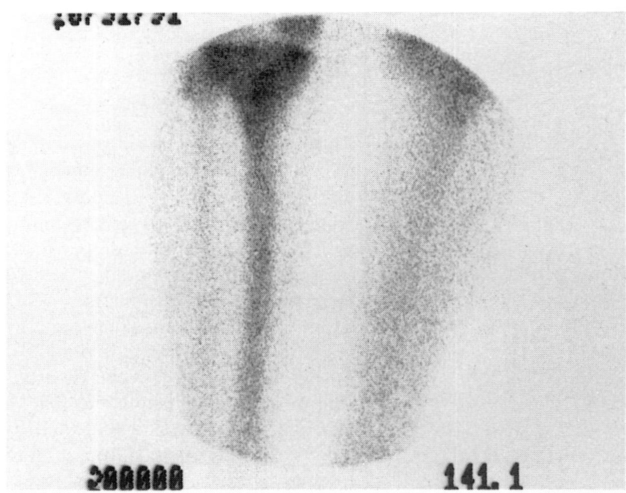

Figure 57. Anterior scintiphotos of the lower limbs in a patient with pain in th right foot that limited weight bearing. Note increased activity in the right tibia and fibula, associated with temporary disuse. The same phenomenon is observed in limb hyperemia.

activity is often reduced and, consequently, tracer uptake within the bones is reduced, particularly within the spine. Special types of osteoporosis (e.g., disuse osteoporosis) are associated with increased bone formation.[485] Increased regional bone blood flow may explain the augmented concentration of bone tracers in paralyzed limbs (Fig. 57). In patients with long-standing disuse, uptake may be normal or decreased.

In *regional migratory osteoporosis,* focal abnormalities may appear on bone scintigraphy before radiographic changes are found.[486] Patients present with severe joint pain and images demonstrate migrating sites of increased periarticular uptake.[487]

Numerous quantitative studies of bone uptake and of urinary excretion of ^{99m}Tc-diphosphonates have been reported. None, however, has demonstrated clinical utility. Many of these methods are summarized in an excellent review by McAfee.[421]

Osteomalacia

Osteomalacia, or rickets, is caused by vitamin D deficiency and results in failure of bone matrix to calcify. The most apparent radiographic effect is widening of the epiphyses of the long bones and the costochondral junctions (rachitic rosary). Bone scintigraphy demonstrates diffusely increased skeletal uptake. The axial skeleton, long bones, mandible, "tie sternum," calvarium, and joints appear especially prominent. Pseudofractures are common in advanced osteomalacia. These are known as Milkman's pseudofractures or Looser's lines, which appear radiographically as ribbon-like lines extending from one cortex through the medullary canal to the opposite cortex, with or without subperiosteal new bone formation. They occur in the scapula, femur, pubic rami, ilium, ribs, and proximal ulna. They may appear on bone

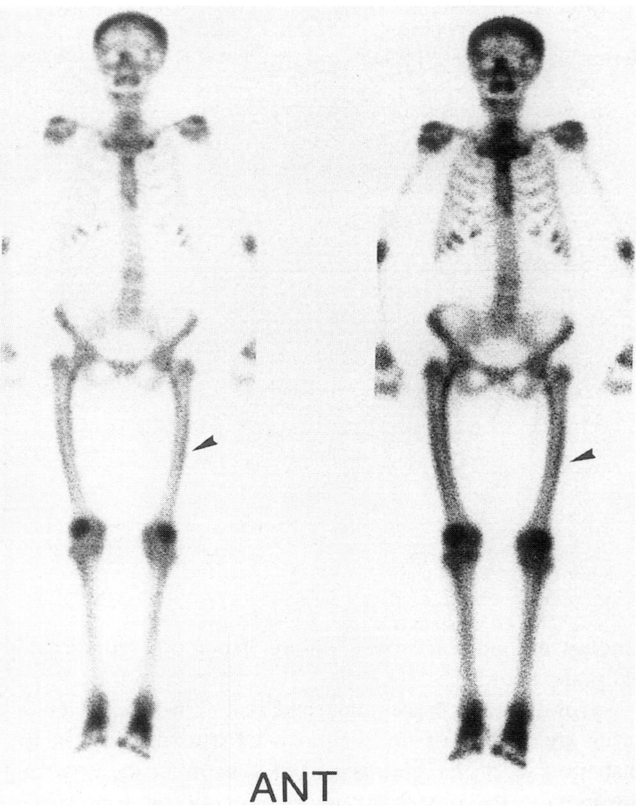

Figure 58. Renal osteodystrophy. Note diffusely increased uptake throughout the skeleton. The kidneys are not visualized and there is pronounced bowing and accentuation of the cortices in the long bones known as the "double stripe" sign. The images differ only in film intensity exposure. Reproduced with permission from Reference 535.

scintigraphy before becoming apparent radiographically.[488] Fogelman et al. found retention of ^{99m}Tc-HEDP to be significantly increased in these patients.[487]

Hyperparathyroidism

Primary hyperparathyroidism may be caused by excessive secretion of parathyroid hormone secondary to parathyroid hyperplasia, adenoma, or carcinoma. The disease is characterized by hypercalcemia, increased bone resorption and, occasionally, soft-tissue calcifications. Roentgenographically, the findings of *osteitis fibrosis cystica* are rarely seen, except in long-standing disease. The characteristics of primary hyperparathyroidism on scintigraphic images range from normal to generalized increased uptake (super scan) found in renal osteodystrophy (Fig. 58). The latter pattern occurs in approximately 50% of patients; roentgenographic evidence of hyperparathyroidism occurs in 25%.[489] Such focal lesions as vertebral collapse, ectopic calcification, and bone cysts are common findings. The so-called "double stripe" sign due to subperiosteal new bone formation is also frequently seen (Fig. 58).

Krishnamurthy et al. measured blood disappearance and

Table 4. Differential Diagnosis of Generalized Increased Skeletal Uptake of ^{99m}Tc-diphosphonates*

COMMON
Renal osteodystrophy (osteomalacia and secondary hyperparathyroidism)
Primary or secondary hyperparathyroidism
Widespread metastatic disease (breast or prostate)
Pulmonary osteoarthropathy
UNCOMMON
Osteomalacia
Renal, vitamin D deficiency
Systemic lupus erythematosus
Scleroderma
Hyperthyroidism
Hypervitaminosis D
Leukemia
Aplastic anemia
Waldenström's macroglobulinemia
Myelofibrosis
Acromegaly
Osteopetrosis
Systemic mastocytosis
Engelmann's disease (diaphyseal dysplasia)
Lipid granulomatosis (Chester-Erdheim disease)
Hyperphosphatasia

*Modified from McAfee.[421]

urinary excretion of ^{99m}Tc-polyphosphate in normal individuals and in patients with primary hyperparathyroidism, pseudohypoparathyroidism, and postsurgical untreated hypoparathyroidism.[490] The blood disappearance curves were identical in all groups; however, significantly increased urinary excretion was recorded in individuals with hyperparathyroidism and pseudohypoparathyroidism. Bone scintigraphy was abnormal in 58% of the hyperparathyroid patients and included focal abnormalities in distal extremities, skull, and mandible. Approximately half of those patients with scintigraphic abnormalities had the radiographic abnormalities of subperiosteal resorption and osteopenia. For the most part, however, biochemical tests are better indications of calcium metabolism in these conditions. The use of SPECT[500] and PET[501] to assess bone metabolism quantitatively has promise, but future studies will be required to define their utility.

Renal Osteodystrophy

Renal osteodystrophy is a combination of osteomalacia and secondary hyperparathyroidism, most commonly a complication of chronic renal failure. It is thought to be caused by impaired renal conversion of vitamin D,[491] but also found in vitamin D deficiency states from other causes, such as starvation or malabsorption. Clinically, osteodystrophy is associated with axial bone pain, muscle weakness, radiographic osteopenia, and fractures of the ribs, vertebrae, pelvis, and hips.

Striking bone images accompany this disease (Fig. 58) marked by generalized increased uptake, the so-called super scan (Table 4). The faint or absent kidney visualization reflect both the poor renal function and the strong competition by the bones for tracer uptake.[492] Focal abnormalities are also seen, including the "double stripe" sign caused by periosteal new bone formation. Increased activity in the ends of long bones and at the costochondral junctions is seen in approximately 80% of these patients.[492]

Renal osteodystrophy may also be caused by aluminum toxicity, in which case the soft tissue activity throughout the body may be abnormally high.[493] Diffusely increased lung uptake may also occur, but usually only after radiographically visible calcifications develop.[494]

Hypertrophic Pulmonary Osteoarthropathy

This is a condition usually associated with malignant or inflammatory intrathoracic disease states. Because it is also associated with such nonrespiratory diseases as ulcerative colitis, it is also called *hypertrophic osteoarthropathy.* The clinical syndrome consists of clubbing of the fingers and toes, new periosteal bone formation in the tubular bones, painful swelling of the limbs, arthralgia, arthritis, and autonomic disturbances, which include sweating, flushing, and blanching of the skin. Radiographically, the condition is associated with accentuation and irregularity of bone cortex, especially of the radius, ulna, tibia, and fibula. Bone scintigraphy shows symmetrically increased uptake along the cortical margins of the diaphyses of the long tubular bones (Fig. 58). Other bone involvement includes the skull, mandible, scapulae, patellae, and clavicles.

Paget's Disease

Paget's disease is a common disorder in the elderly. Autopsy studies show that it occurs in approximately 3% of patients over 40 years of age in the United States, although this is a disease of great geographic variation.[495] There is a known familial predilection and recent evidence points to a slow virus infection of the osteoclasts as the probable etiology of Paget's disease.[496] Pathophysiologically, bone resorption increases, as does formation of new, abnormally "soft," highly cellular bone, which contains many vascular spaces and disorganized trabeculae. This abnormal bone becomes deformed from normal weight bearing, and pain is the most common complaint. Most cases are asymptomatic, however, and are discovered only incidentally by radiography, scintigraphy, or the presence of elevated alkaline phosphatase in the work-up of other conditions. Pathologic fractures are common. Late in the disease, there may be neurological symptoms due to impingement of cranial bones or vertebrae on neurological structures. Deafness, carpal and tarsal tunnel syndromes, papilledema, and high output cardiac failure are rare complications. Sarcomatous degeneration is now uncommon.[497]

Paget's disease predominates in the axial skeleton, especially in the pelvis (40%), spine (75%), skull (65%), and proximal long bones (35%).[498] Involvement of ribs, scapula, and clavicle is less common, but no bone is exempt from involvement. Paget's disease usually presents monostotically, involving the entire bone or only part of a bone. In the latter case, the differentiation from malignancy is usually made by CT. Later, polyostotic involvement is common. The scintigraphic appearance consists of dense, sheet-like uptake generally corresponding to the radiographic distribution of the lesion (Fig. 60).

The radiographic lesion of Paget's disease may be either lytic or sclerotic. During the early osteoporotic, or lytic phase often seen in the skull (*osteoporosis circumscripta cranii*), the scintigraphic appearance is one of greatly enhanced tracer concentration that is most intense at the advancing margin of the lesion and more diffuse centrally.[499] Osteolytic and osteoblastic activity equalize with time and radiographs begin to show a mixed sclerotic and lytic pattern, which is followed by a predominantly blastic radiographic appearance. In the late sclerotic phase of the disease, the increased osteoblastic and osteoclastic activity may resolve; healed osteoblastic and osteolytic lesions remain radiographically obvious, however. The scintigraphic appearance in the "burned-out" phase of healed Paget's disease may be normal. Thus, in contrast to radiographs, scintigraphy reflects the true status of the disease activity.[500] In the past, serial scintigraphy has been a favored means of following patients with Paget's disease, and judging the effectiveness of therapy.[501] According to Boudreau, et al., increased perfusion on the first transit images may be a better indicator of active disease than degree of uptake on delayed images.[502] However, it is now more common to follow the serum alkaline phosphatase and urinary hydroxyproline to gauge therapy.

Scintigraphy is more sensitive than radiography in detecting sites of Paget's disease.[497] In a comparison by Fogelman and Carr,[503] scintigraphy identified 95% of 127 sites of Paget's involvement, while radiographs identified only 74%. Most of the missed sites were in scapulae, ribs, and sternum.

Fibrous Dysplasia

In the original description of fibrous dysplasia by Albright, the bone lesions were accompanied by hyperpigmented skin spots, premature skeletal maturation, and precocious puberty in girls.[504] In fact, relatively few patients with the bone lesions have the other elements of the McCune-Albright syndrome, although early skeletal maturation and deformity is common. Pathologic fractures, facial deformity, and a limp due to unequal leg length are common clinical features.

The etiology of fibrous dysplasia is unknown. The diagnosis is usually made radiographically, in which lesions characteristically demonstrate sclerosis, deformation, expansion with cortical thinning, and an over-all ground glass appearance caused by the numerous tiny trabeculations.[505] The most frequently involved bones include the skull, facial bones, femur, tibia, fibula, and vertebrae. The disease is monostotic in 75% of patients and polyostotic in 25%.[506]

The bone lesions are quite vascular, as is apparent on radionuclide angiography. Delayed images demonstrate dense, extensive lesions, not unlike those seen in Paget's disease, except that the margins of lesions are less well defined (Fig. 59). Scintigraphy is primarily useful in defining the extent of bone involvement and documenting the appearance of new lesions.[507]

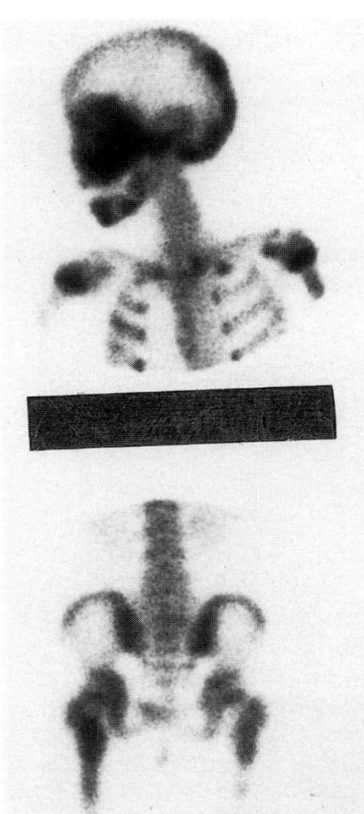

Figure 59. This 6-year-old child with McCune-Albright developed menstrual bleeding at age 3 years. Note the intense, polyostotic bone involvement in the spine, pelvis and femur.

Other Metabolic Disorders

Hemoglobinopathies may be associated with bone scintigraphic abnormalities. Bone and bone-marrow scintigraphy have been used to identify bone infarction in patients with sickle-cell anemia. In the acute stage, both conditions are characterized by focal regions of decreased activity.[508] With healing, bone images change from decreased to *increased* focal activity in the affected region, whereas bone-marrow images may show a return to normal.[509]

The usual differential diagnosis of interest, however, is between infarction and osteomyelitis, which clinically may be indistinguishable. In this case, combined bone-marrow and labeled leukocyte imaging is the preferred imaging sequence. If labeled leukocytes concentrate in a lesion with absent colloid uptake, infection is the probable cause.

In *thalassemia* bone scintigraphy is usually characterized by diffusely *decreased* uptake as a result of marked expansion of the bone-marrow cavities and cortical thinning.[510]

In *hyperostosis frontalis interna* there is diffusely increased frontal skull activity caused by excessive bone formation in the inner table of the frontal squama (Fig. 12). It is more common in women and is usually observed in pa-

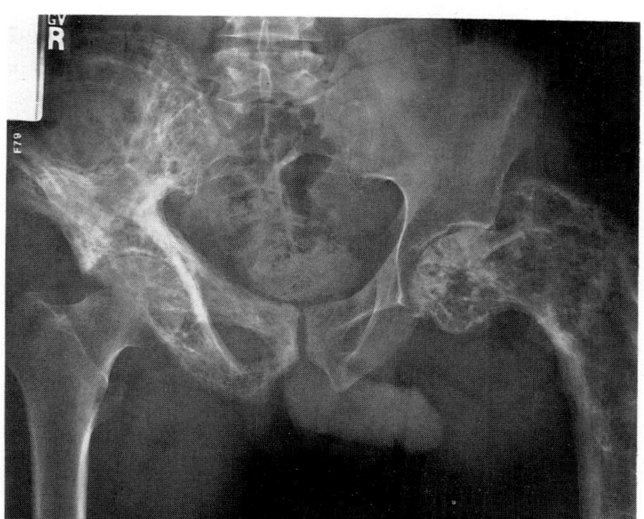

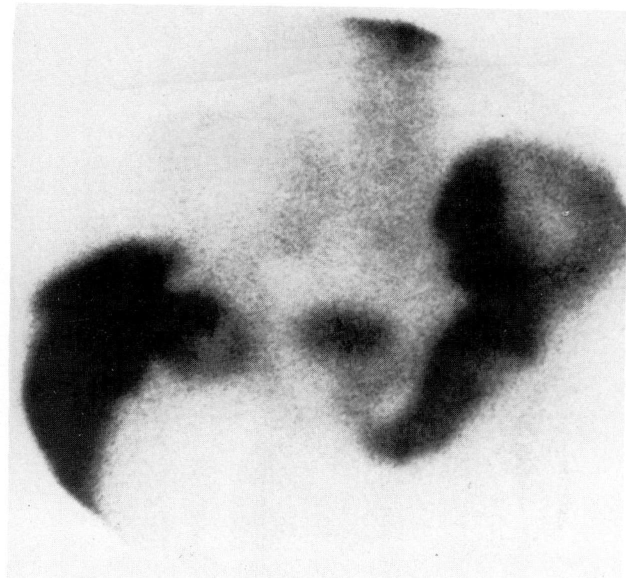

Figure 60. Selected radiographs and scintiphotos from a 60-year-old man with widespread Paget's disease showing the mixed lytic/sclerotic radiographic lesions and the dense, distorted, sharply marginated scintigraphic lesions.

tients over the age of 40 years. Radiographically, some degree of hyperostosis frontalis has been observed in as many as 40% of postmenopausal women.[511]

Melorheostosis is a benign osteosclerotic dysplasia most commonly involving several bones within a single limb and characterized by pain, limb deformity, and muscle atrophy. Scintigraphically, the most common pattern is an asymmetric linear area of increased cortical and medullary uptake that crosses the joint to involve contiguous juxtarticular bone.[512,513] Three-phase bone scintigraphy demonstrates increased perfusion and blood pool in the affected areas that support the dysplastic process.

Scintigraphic abnormalities have also been reported in *pachydermoperiostosis*[514,515]; however, bone scintigraphy is said to be unremarkable in *osteopoikelosis* and *osteopathia striata.*[516]

JOINT DISEASES

As early as 1965, ^{131}I-human serum albumin was used to image joints.[519] Labeled albumin seemed an appropriate tracer because inflammatory joint disease is characterized by increased synovial blood flow and abnormal synovial capillary permeability. Two years later, ^{99m}Tc-pertechnetate was used for joint imaging.[518] In 1971 ^{99m}Tc-phosphate compounds became widely used for joint imaging.[519] The rationale for using bone tracers was that joint diseases are frequently associated with new bone formation, presumably because of increased synovial vascularity. Comparative studies showed that the phosphate compounds are more sensitive than pertechnetate in detecting abnormal joints.[520]

Joint scintigraphy is seldom employed to make a specific diagnosis of arthritis because most patterns of tracer distribution are quite nonspecific. Rather, plain radiographs are much more useful for this purpose, although MR imaging, ultrasound, and arthrography may also be useful in making the diagnosis. Because it is so sensitive, scintigraphy may be useful in establishing the presence of arthritis when radiographs are normal.[521,522] Scintigraphy may also be of value in judging the severity of disease.

Joint scintigraphy is performed in the same manner as bone scintigraphy, except that converging or pinhole collimators should be used to image individual joints. Three-phase bone scintigraphy is useful in evaluating the degree of inflammatory response. Special joint images are integrated for approximately 2.5×10^5 counts per image for peripheral joints and 5.0×10^5 counts for central joints (hips, sacroiliac joints). Frontal and lateral views of the knees should be obtained, because increased activity related to the overlying patella and patellofemoral compartment may be misinterpreted on frontal view as lateral femorotibial compartment disease. For the hips, anterior and posterior views are important and, in children, frog-leg and straight anteroposterior views may be helpful. For the hands, palmar views and, for the feet, plantar views are obtained.

Gallium-67 citrate and ^{111}In-labeled leukocytes have been used to evaluate inflammation. However, attempts to distinguish infectious from noninfectious inflammatory arthritis have not been notably successful.[523]

Normal joints have symmetrical activity, although the shoulder joint on the side of dominant handedness, especially the acromion process, often has greater activity than the opposite shoulder. In the hand, joint activity is usually greatest in the wrist and middle carpophalangeal joints, with

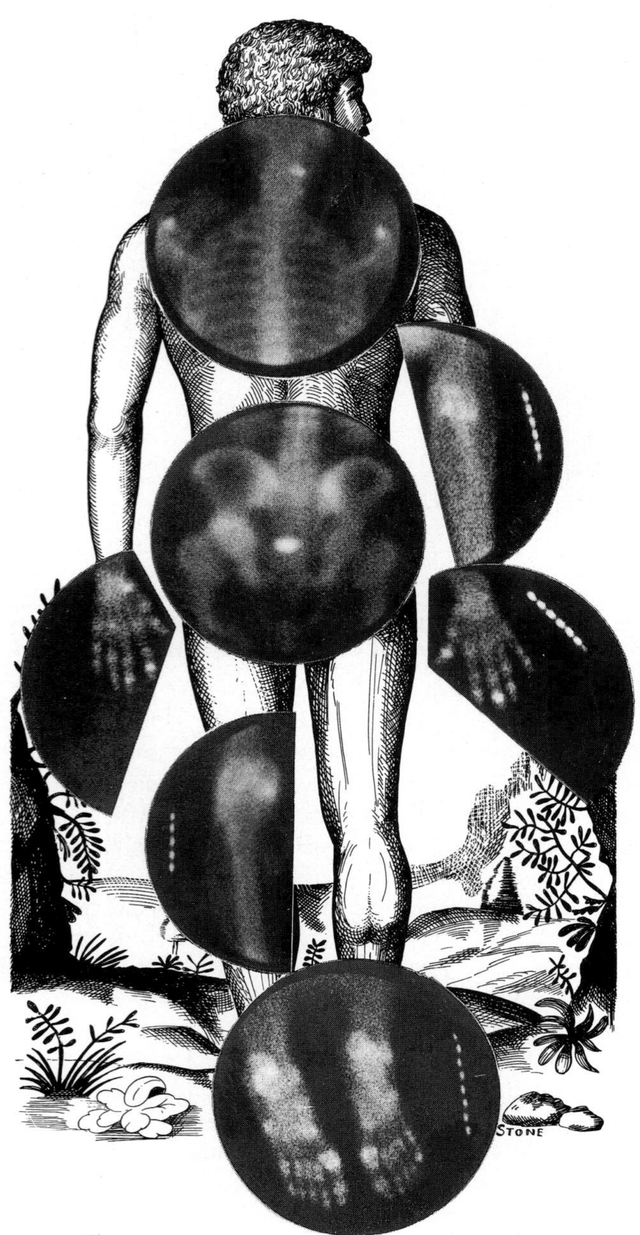

Figure 61. Composite showing degenerative changes in cervical spine, right elbow, left hip, left knee, and both feet and hands.

decreasing activity from the first to the fifth digit and from proximal to distal joints of each finger. The epiphyses in children have greater intensity than periarticular structures in adults.

Degenerative Joint Disease

Degenerative joint disease, or *osteoarthritis* is characterized by gradual destruction of the weight-bearing surfaces of joints with minimal inflammatory response. Pathologic changes include subchondral bone remodeling and cyst formation, erosion of articular cartilage, and osteophytic spur formation at joint margins.

Few bone scintigrams are completely normal in patients more than 40 years of age. Nearly all such patients show some degenerative changes in one or more joints. Often, these joints are asymptomatic and are observed as incidental findings in the evaluation of other diseases. The spectrum of disease is broad. When changes are extensive and activity is markedly increased, correlation with other imaging procedures to differentiate malignancy is essential. The most common locations of osteoarthritis are the spine, hips, knees, hands, feet, sacroiliac joints and shoulders (Fig. 61 and 62).

Thomas et al. used bone scintigraphy to evaluate osteoarthritis of the knee and to guide surgery.[522] Scintigraphy was generally more sensitive that radiography in detecting disease in the lateral femorotibial compartment. Surgical management was altered because moderate lateral compartment abnormalities were detected in 25% of patients.

Rheumatoid Arthritis and Rheumatoid Variant Diseases

Rheumatoid arthritis is characterized by inflammation of the synovial membrane and associated hypervascularity of the joint capsule, tendon sheaths, and bursae. Perfusion to adjacent bone increases. Later in the disease, subchondral and periarticular bone erosion and remodeling occur. The distribution involves the hands, knees, feet, and cervical spine. There is usually symmetrical involvement of the metacarpophalangeal and proximal interphalangeal joints of the hands,[524] and of the metatarsophalangeal joints of the feet.

Bone scintigraphy is sensitive in detecting and estimating the extent of disease in patients with rheumatoid arthritis and such rheumatoid variant diseases as psoriatic arthritis, ankylosing spondylitis, and Reiter's syndrome.[521,525,526] Scintigraphic changes usually occur before radiographic changes. However, most rheumatologists are content to follow patients' progress on the basis of physical examination, and joint scintigraphy has not achieved wide application in these diseases.

Temporomandibular Joint Syndrome

Increased temporomandibular joint (TMJ) activity is observed in approximately 4% of patients presenting for bone scintigraphy for all indications.[527] Furthermore, most of these patients report symptoms suspicious for TMJ pathology: jaw locking, jaw clicking, or preauricular pain with jaw motion. Studies that have used SPECT to examine TMJ activity report higher sensitivity for identifying internal joint derangement than planar imaging.[528,529] Thus, the finding of increased TMJ activity on routine bone scintigraphy merits description in the report.

But, does bone scintigraphy play any useful role in the evaluation of patients presenting with TMJ syndrome? As Epstein et al. point out, patients who present with TMJ disor-

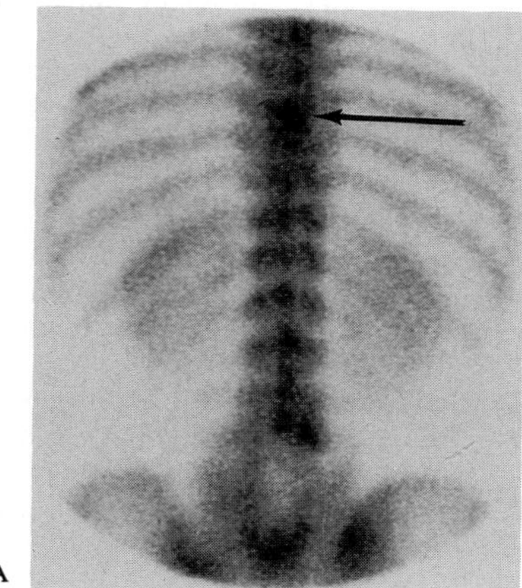

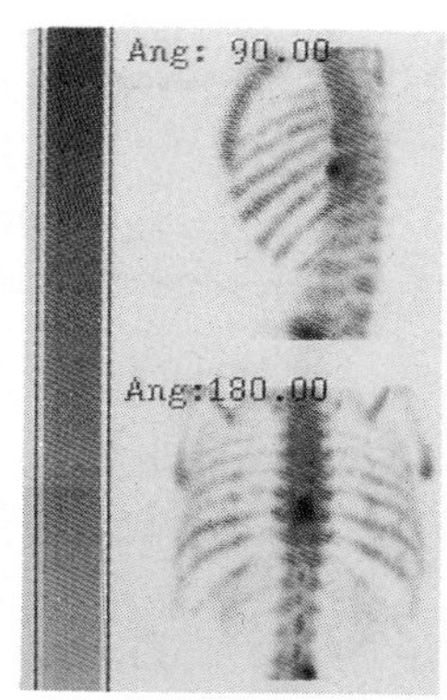

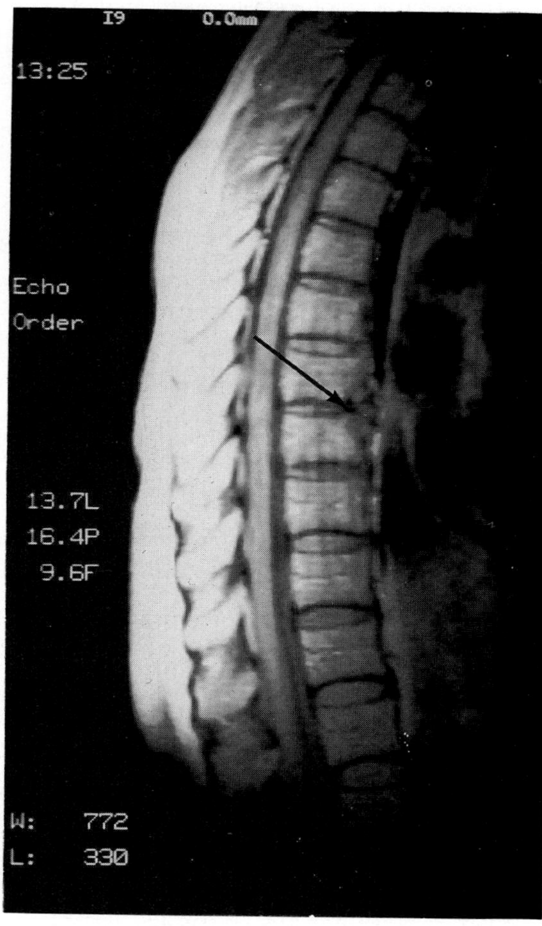

Figure 62. This 48-year-old woman complained of severe midback pain. Planar scintigraphy, **(A)** shows obvious lower lumbar degenerative changes as well as a poorly defined T-8 lesion. SPECT images, **(B)** show a well-defined anterior lesion at T-8, T-9 in the 90° rotational view. The sagittal MRI **(C)** (S/E = 2500/20) shows well-defined degenerative changes and lipping at T-8 and T-9.

ders are "prescreened" (i.e., they present because of specific symptoms). Therefore, they do not require a sensitive test to determine the presence of disease. Even a negative scintigraphic result does not rule out significant pathology because of a substantial number of false-negative scintigrams in patients with arthrographically demonstrated pathology.[529,530] Furthermore, no study has shown that bone scintigraphy obviates other tests, such as arthrography or MRI, in selecting patients for surgery. At this time, scintigraphy appears to be a moderately sensitive test for identifying incidental TMJ disease, but plays no role in the work-up of patients presenting with this diagnosis.

Sports-Related Joint Injuries

Because of the great sensitivity of bone scintigraphy for detecting joint derangement, synovial injury, and ligamentous injuries, it may have a role in athletes and other active individuals who present with acute joint-pain syndromes. Usually, plain radiographs are the initial imaging procedure to be performed. However, if these are normal and pain or swelling persists, bone scintigraphy is useful in locating and defining the extent of injury (Fig. 33).[531–533]

REFERENCES

1. Subramanian G, McAfee JG: A new complex of ^{99m}Tc for skeletal imaging. *Radiology* 1971;99:192.
2. Merrick MV: Bone scanning. *Br J Radiol* 1975;48:327.
3. Davis MA, Jones AG: Comparison of ^{99m}Tc-labeled phosphate and phosphonate agents for skeletal imaging. *Semin Nucl Med* 1976;6:19.
4. Blau M, Nagler W, Bender MA: Fluorine-18. A new isotope for bone scanning. *J Nucl Med* 1962;3:332.
5. Jones AG, Francis MD, Davis MA: Bone scanning: Radionuclide reaction mechanisms. *Semin Nucl Med* 1976;6:3.
6. Siegel B, Donovan RL, Alderson PO, Mack GR: Skeletal uptake of 99m-Tc-diphosphonate in relation to local bone blood flow. *Radiology* 1976;120:121.
7. Krishnamurthy GT, Huebotter RJ, Tubis M, Bladh WH: Pharmacokinetics of current skeletal-seeking radiopharmaceuticals. *AJR* 1976;126:293.
8. Subramanian G, McAfee JG, Blair RJ, et al.: Technetium-99m methylene diphosphonate—A superior agent for skeletal imaging. Comparison with other technetium complexes. *J Nucl Med* 1975;16:744.
9. Saha GB, Boyd CM: A study of protein-binding of ^{99m}Tc-methylene diphosphonate in plasma. *Int J Nucl Med Biol* 1979;6:201.
10. Haden HT, Katz PG, Konerding KF: Detection of obstructive uropathy by bone scintigraphy. *J Nucl Med* 1988;29:1781.

11. Holder LE: Clinical radionuclide bone imaging. *Radiology* 1990;176:607.
12. Makler PT, Charkes ND: Studies of skeletal tracer kinetics IV. Optimum time delay for Tc-99m(Sn) methylene diphosphonate bone imaging. *J Nucl Med* 1980;21:641.
13. Goergen TG, Alazraki N, Halpern SE, et al: "Cold" bone lesions: A newly recognized phenomenon of bone imaging. *J Nucl Med* 1973;15:1120.
14. Genant HK, Bautovich GJ, Singh M, et al: Bone-seeking radionuclides: An in vivo study of factors affecting skeletal uptake. *Radiology* 1974;113:373.
15. Van Dyke D, Anger HO, Yano Y, et al: Bone blood flow shown with ^{18}F and the positron camera. *Am J Physiol* 1965;209:65.
16. Siegel BA, Donovan RL, Alderson PO, et al: Skeletal uptake of ^{99m}Tc-diphosphonate in relation to local bone blood flow. *Radiology* 1976;120:121.
17. Charkes ND: Skeletal blood flow: Implication for bone-scan interpretation. *J Nucl Med* 1980;21:91.
18. Shim SS: Physiology of blood circulation of bone. *J Bone Joint Surg* 1968;50A:812.
19. Rosenthall L, Kaye M: Observations in the mechanism of ^{99m}Tc-labeled phosphate complex uptake in metabolic bone disease. *Semin Nucl Med* 1976;6:59.
20. Francis MD: The inhibition of calcium hydroxyapatite crystal growth by polyphosphonates and poly phosphates. *Calc Tiss Res* 1969;3:151.
21. Zimmer AM, Isitman AT, Holmes RA: Enzymatic inhibition of diphosphonate a proposed mechanism of tissue uptake. *J Nucl Med* 1975;16:352.
22. O'Connor MK, Brown ML, Hung JC, Hayostek RJ: The art of bone scintigraphy—Technical aspects. *J Nucl Med* 1991;32:2332.
23. Collier BD, Palmer DW, Knobel J, et al.: Gamma camera energy windows for Tc-99m bone scintigraphy: effect of asymmetry on contrast resolution. *Radiology* 1984;151:495.
24. LaFontaine R, Stein MA, Graham LS, Winter J: Cold lesions: enhanced contrast using asymmetric photopeak windows. *Radiology* 1986;160:255.
25. Halama JR, Henkin RE, Friend LE: Gamma camera radionuclide images improved contrast with energy-weighted acquisition. *Radiology* 1988;169:533.
26. Wirth V.: Effective energy resolution and scatter rejection in nuclear medicine. *Phys Med Biol* 1989;34:85.
27. Schutte HE: Some special views in bone scanning. *Clin Nucl Med* 1980;5:172.
28. Holder LE: Clinical radionuclide bone imaging. *Radiology* 1990;176:607.
29. Israel O, Jerushalmi J, Frenkel A, et al.: Normal and abnormal single photon emission computed tomography of the skull: comparison with planar scintigraphy. *J Nucl Med* 1988; 29:1341.
30. Collier BD, Carrera GF, Messer EJ, et al.: Internal derangements of the temporomandibular joint: detection by single photon emission computed tomography. *Radiology* 1983; 149:557.
31. Jacobsson H, Larsson SA, Vestersklod L, et al.: The application of single photon emission computed tomography to the diagnosis of ankylosing spondylitis of the spine. *Br J Radiol* 1984;57:133.
32. Lusins JO, Danielski EF, Goldsmith SJ: Bone SPECT in patients with persistent back pain after lumbar spine surgery. *J Nucl Med* 1989;30:490.
33. Stromqvist B, Brismar J, Hansson LI: Emission tomography in femoral neck fracture for evaluation of avascular necrosis. *Acta Orthop Scand* 1983;54:872.
34. Collier BD, Carrera GF, Johnson RP, et al.: Detection of femoral head avascular necrosis in adults by SPECT. *J Nucl Med* 1985;26:979.
35. Gupta SM, Foster CR, Kayani N: usefulness of SPECT in the early detection of avascular necrosis of the knees. *Clin Nucl Med* 1987;12:99.
36. Collier BD, Johnson RP, Carrera GF, et al: Chronic knee pain assessed by SPECT: comparison with other modalities. *Radiology* 1985;157:795.
37. Esser P, Jakimcius A, Foley L: The peanut orbit: a modified elliptical orbit for single-photon emission computed tomography imaging. *Med Phys* 1989;16:114.
38. Madsen MT, Park CH: Enhancement of SPECT images by Fourier filtering the projection image set. *J Nucl Med* 1985;26:395.
39. Nowak DJ, Eisner RL, Fajman WA: Distance-weighted backprojection: a SPECT reconstruction technique. *Radiology* 1986;159:531.
40. Hellman RS, Nowak DJ, Collier BD, et al.: Evaluation of distance weighted SPECT reconstruction for skeletal scintigraphy. *Radiology* 1986;159:473.
41. Cheng TH, Holman BL: Increased skeletal:renal uptake ratio—etiology and characteristics. *Radiology* 1989;136:455.
42. de Graaf P, Schicht IM, Pauwels EKJ, et al.: Bone scintigraphy in renal osteodystrophy. *J Nucl Med* 1978;19:1289.
43. Choy D, Maddalena DJ, Murray IPC: The effect of iron-dextran on the biodistribution of technetium pyrophosphate. *Int J Nucl Med Biol* 1982;9:277–282.
44. McAfee JG, Singh A, Roskopf M, et al: Experimental drug-induced changes in renal function and biodistribution of Tc-99m MDP. *Invest Radiol* 1983;18:470–478.
45. Van Antwerp JD, Hall JN, O'Mara RE, et al: Bone scan abnormality produced by interaction of Tc-99m diphosphonate with iron dextran (Imferon). *J Nucl Med,* 1975;16:577.
46. Parker JA, et al.: Reduced uptake of bone-seeking radiopharmaceuticals related to iron excess. *Clin Nucl Med* 1976;1:267.
47. Espinasse D, Mathieu L, Alexandre C, et al.: The kinetics of Tc-99m labeled EHDP in Paget's disease before and after dichloromethylene-diphosphonate treatment. *Metab Bone Dis Rel Res* 1981;2:321–324.
48. Watt I, Hill P: Effect of acute administration of ethane hydroxydiphosphonate (EHDP) on skeletal scintigraphy with technetium-99m methylene diphosphonic acid (Tc-MDP) in the rat. *Br J Radiol* 1981;54:592–596.
49. Trackler RT, Chinn RYW: Amphotericin B therapy—a cause of increased renal uptake of Tc-99m MDP. *Clin Nucl Med* 1982;7:293.
50. Siddiqui AR: Increased uptake of technetium-99m labeled bone imaging agents in the kidneys. *Semin Nucl Med* 1982;12:101–102.
51. Lutrin CL, McDougall IR, Goris ML: Intense concentration of technetium-99m pyrophosphate in the kidneys of children treated with chemotherapeutic drugs for malignant disease. *Radiology* 1978;128:165–167.
52. Jaresko GS, Zimmer AM, Pavel DG, et al: Effect of circulating aluminum on the biodistribution of Tc-99m-Sn-diphosphonate in rats. *J Nucl Med Technol* 1980;8:160–161.
53. Chaudhuri TK: Liver uptake of Tc-99m-diphosphonate. *Radiology* 1976;119:485–486.
54. Crawford JA, Gumerman LW: Alternation of body distribution of ^{99m}Tc pyrophosphate by radiographic contrast material. *Clin Nucl Med* 1978;3:305.
55. Schmitt GH, Holmes RA, Isitman AT, et al: A proposed mechanism for ^{99m}Tc-labeled polyphosphate and diphosphonate uptake by human breast tissue. *Radiology* 1974; 112:733–735.
56. Ram Singh PS, Pujra S, Logic JR: ^{99m}Tc-pyrophosphate uptake in drug-induced gynecomastia. *Clin Nucl Med* 1977;2:206.

57. Van Renterghem D, De Reuck J, Schelstraete K, et al: Epsilon aminocaproic acid myopathy: additional features. *Clin Neurol Neurosurg* 1984;86:153–157.
58. Conklin JJ, Alderson PO, Zizic TM, et al: Comparison of bone scan and radiograph sensitivity in the detection of steroid-induced ischemic necrosis of bones. *Radiology* 1983; 147:221–226.
59. Schaffer DL, Pendergrass HP: Comparison of enzyme, clinical, radiographic and radionuclide methods of detecting bone metastasis from carcinoma of the prostate. *Radiology* 1976;121:431.
60. DeNardo GL, Jacobson SJ, Raventos A: ^{85}Sr bone scan in neoplastic disease. *Semin Nucl Med* 1972;2:31.
61. O'Mara RE: Bone scanning in osseous metastatic disease. *JAMA* 1988;229:1915.
62. Harbert JC: Efficacy of bone and liver scanning in malignant diseases. Facts and Opinon, in Freeman LM, Weissman HS (eds.): *Nuclear Medicine Annual.* New York, Raven Press, 1982.
63. Harbert JC, Desai R: Small calvarial bone scan foci—normal variation. *J Nucl Med* 1985;26:1144.
64. Holder LE, Clinical radionuclide bone imaging. *Radiology* 176:607, 1990.
65. Citrin DL: The role of the bone scan in the investigation and treatment of breast cancer, in: *CRC Critical Reviews in Diagnostic Imaging.* Boca Raton, CRC Press, 1980, p 39.
66. Parbhoo SP: Serial scintiscans in monitoring patients with bone metastases, in: Stoll BA, Parbhoo SP (eds.): *Bone Metastasis—Monitoring and Treatment.* New York, Raven Press, 1983, p 201.
67. Mundy GR: The hypercalcemia of malignancy. *Kidney Int* 1987;31:142.
68. Krasnow AZ, Collier BD, Isitman AT, et al.: False-negative bone imaging due to etidronate disodium therapy. *Clin Nucl Med* 1988;13:264.
69. Kim SE, Kim DY, Lee DS, et al.: Absent or faint renal uptake on bone scan: Etiology and significance in metastatic bone disease. *Clin Nucl Med* 1991;16:545.
70. McNeil BJ: Rationale for the use of bone scans in selected metastatic and primary bone tumors. *Semin Nucl Med* 1978;8:336.
71. Deutsch A, Resnick D: Eccentric cortical metastases to the skeleton from bronchogenic carcinoma. *Radiology* 1980; 137:49.
72. Hendrix RW, Rogers LF, Davis TM: Cortical bone metastases. *Radiology* 1991;181:409.
73. Corcoran RJ, Thrall JH, Kyle RW, et al.: Solitary abnormalities in bone scans of patients with extraosseous malignancies. *Radiology* 1976;121:663.
74. Galasko CSB: Skeletal metastases. *Clin Orthop Rel Res* 1986;210:18.
75. McNeil BJ: Value of bone scanning in neoplastic disease. *Semin Nucl Med* 1984;14:277.
76. Boxer DI, Todd CEC, Coleman R, Fogelman I: Bone secondaries in breast cancer: the solitary metastasis. *J Nucl Med* 1989;30:1318.
77. Klonecke AS, Licho R, McDougall IR: A technique for intraoperative bone scintigraphy: a report of 17 cases. *Clin Nucl Med* 1991;16:482.
78. Jacobson AF, Cronin EB, Stomper PC, Kaplan WD: Bone scans with one or two new abnormalities in cancer patients with no known metastases: frequency and serial scintigraphic behavior of benign and malignant lesions. *Radiology* 1990;175:229.
79. Jacobson AF, Stomper PC, Cronin EB, Kaplan WD: Bone scans with one or two new abnormalities in cancer patients with no known metastases: reliability of interpretation of initial correlative radiographs. *Radiology* 1990;174:503.
80. Harbert JC, Desai R: Small calvarial bone scan foci—Normal variations. *J Nucl Med* 1985;26:1144.
81. Levenson RM, Sauerbrunn BJL, Bates HR, Eddy JL, Ihde DC: Comparative value of bone scintigraphy and radiography in monitoring tumor response in systemically treated prostate carcinoma. *Radiology* 1983;146:513.
82. Coleman RE, Mashiter G, Whitaker KB, et al.: Bone scan flare predicts successful systemic therapy for bone metastases. *J Nucl Med* 1988;29:1354.
83. Fogelman I, Coleman R: The bone scan and breast cancer, in: *Nuclear Medicine Annual 1988,* New York, Raven Press, 1988, p 1.
84. Galasko CSB: The anatomy and pathways of skeletal metastasis, in Weiss L, Gilbert HA (eds.): *Bone Metastasis.* Boston, G.K. Hall, 1981, p 49.
85. Coleman RE, Rubens RD: The clinical course of bone metastases from breast cancer. *Br J Cancer* 1987;55:61.
86. Citrin DL, Furnival CM, Bessent RG, et al.: Radioactive technetium phosphate bone scanning in preoperative assessment and follow-up study of patients with primary cancer of the breast. *Surg Gynecol Obstet* 1976;143:360.
87. Gerber FH, Goodreau JJ, Kirchner PT: Tc-99m EHDP bone scanning in breast cancer. *J Nucl Med* 1975;16:529.
88. McNeil BJ, Pace PD, Gray EB, et al.: Preoperative and follow-up bone scans in patients with primary carcinoma of the breast. *Surg Gynecol Obstet* 1978;147:745.
89. Batson OV: Role of vertebral veins in metastatic process. *Ann Intern Med* 1942;16:38.
90. Kwai AH, Stomper PC, Kaplan WD: Clinical significance of isolated scintigraphic sternal lesions in patients with breast cancer. *J Nucl Med* 1988;29:324.
91. Fordham EW, Ali A: Skeletal imaging in malignant disease, in Gottschalk A, Hoffer PB, Potchen EJ (eds): *Diagnostic Nuclear Medicine,* Volume 2, Baltimore, Williams & Wilkins, 1988, p 1023.
92. O'Connell MEA, Sutton H: Excretion of radioactivity in breast milk following ^{99m}Tc-(Sn)-polyphosphate. *Br J Radiol* 1976;49:377.
93. Schmitt GH, Holmes RA, Isitman AT, et al.: A proposed mechanism for ^{99m}Tc-labeled polyphosphate and diphosphonate uptake by human breast tissue. *Radiology* 1974; 112:733.
94. Brill DR: Gynecomastia demonstrated on the bone scan. *J Urol* 1977;118:62.
95. Isitman AT, Komaki S, Holmes RA: A benign uptake of ^{99m}Tc-polyphosphate after radical mastectomy. *Radiology* 1974; 110:159.
96. Jayabalan V, Berry S: Accumulation of ^{99m}Tc-pyrophosphate in breast prosthesis. *Clin Nucl Med* 1977;2:452.
97. McDougall IR, Pistenma OA: Concentration of ^{99m}Tc-diphosphonate in breast tissues. *Radiology* 1974;112:655.
98. Holmes RA, Manoli RS, Isitman AT: Tc-99m labeled phosphates as an indication of breast pathology. (Abst) *J Nucl Med* 1976;16:536.
99. Chaudhuri TK, Chaudhuri TK, Gulesserian HP, et al.: Extraosseous noncalcified soft tissue uptake of ^{99m}Tc-polyphosphate. *J Nucl Med* 1974;15:1054.
100. Costello P, Gramm HF, Steinberg D: Simultaneous occurrence of functional asplenia and splenic accumulation of diphosphonate in metastatic breast carcinoma. *J Nucl Med* 1977;18:1237.
101. Berg GR, Kalisher L, Osmand JD, et al.: ^{99m}Tc-diphosphonate concentration in primary breast carcinoma. *Radiology* 1973;109:393.
102. Bonte FJ, Parkey RW, Graham KD, et al.: A new method for

radionuclide imaging of myocardial infacts. *Radiology* 1974;110:473.

103. Buja LM, Poliner LR, Parkey RW, et al.: Clinicopathologic study of persistently positive technetium-99m stannous pyrophosphate myocardial scintograms and myocytolytic degeneration after myocardial infarction. *Circulation* 1977;56: 1016.
104. Willerson JT, Parkey RW, Bonte FJ, et al.: Technetium stannous pyrophosphate myocardial scintigrams in patients with chest pain of varying etiology. *Circulation* 1975;51:1046.
105. Perez LA, Hayt DB, Freeman LM: Localization of myocardial disorders other than infarction with ^{99m}Tc labeled phosphate agents. *J Nucl Med* 1976;17:241.
106. Ahmad M, Dubiel JP, Verdon TA, et al.: Technetium 99m stannous pyrophosphate myocardial imaging in patients with and without left ventricular aneurysm. *Circulation* 1976; 53:833.
107. Ahmad M, et al.: Limited clinical diagnostic specificity of technetium-99m stannous pyrophosphate myocardial imaging in acute myocardial infarction. *Am J Cardiol* 1977;39:50.
108. Campeau RJ, Gottlieb S, Kallos N: Aortic aneurysm detected by ^{99m}Tc-pyrophosphate imaging: Case report. *J Nucl Med* 1977;18:272.
109. Go RT, Doty DB, Chiu CL, et al.: A new method of diagnosing myocardial contusion in man by radionuclide imaging. *Radiology* 1975;116:107.
110. Doty DB, et al.: Cardiac trauma: Clinical and experimental correlations of myocardial contusion. *Am Surg* 1974;180:452.
111. Thrall JH, Ghaed N, Geslien CE, et al.: Pitfalls in Tc99m polyphosphate skeletal imaging. *Am J Roentgenol* 1974; 121:739.
112. Wald RW, Sternberg L, Huckell DF, et al.: Technetium-99m stannous pyrophosphate scintigraphy in patients with calcifications within the cardiac silhouette. *Br Heart J* 1978; 40:547.
113. Jengo JA, Mena I, Joe SH, et al.: The significance of calcifivalvular heart disease in Tc-99m pyrophosphate myocardial infarction scanning: Radiographic, scintigraphic and pathological correlation. *J Nucl Med* 1977;18:776.
114. Seo I, Donoghue G: Tc-99m-pyrophosphate accumulation on prosthetic valves. *Clin Nucl Med* 1980;5:367.
115. Chacko AK, Gordon DH, Bennett JM, et al.: Myocardial imaging with Tc-99m-pyrophosphate in patients on adriamycin treatment for neoplasia. *J Nucl Med* 1977;18:680.
116. Soin JS, Cox JD, Youker JE, et al.: Cardiac localization of ^{99m}Tc-(Sn)-pyrophosphate following irradiation of the chest. *Radiology* 1977;124:165.
117. Braun SD, Lisbona R, Novales-Diaz JA, et al.: Myocardial uptake of ^{99m}Tc-phosphate tracer in amyloidosis. *Clin Nucl Med* 1979;4:244.
118. Singh A, Usher M, Raphael L: Pericardial accumulation of Tc-99m methylene diphosphonate in a case of pericarditis. Letter to editor. *J Nucl Med* 1977;18:1141.
119. Riba AI, Downs J, Thakur ML, et al.: Technetium-99 stannous pyrophosphate imaging of experimental infective endocarditis. *Circulation* 1977;57:111.
120. Janowitz WR, Serafini AN: Intense myocardial uptake of ^{99m}Tc-disphosphonate in a uremic patient with secondary hyperparathyroidism and pericarditis: Case report. *J Nucl Med* 1976;17:896.
121. Da Rocha AFG, Meguerian BA, Harbert JC: Tc-99m pyrophosphate myocardial scanning in Chagas' disease. *J Nucl Med* 1981;22:347.
122. Palestro CJ, Steele MK, Kim CK and Goldsmith SJ: Myocardial uptake of Tc-99m following cardioversion. *Clin Nucl Med* 1991;16:273.
123. Arbona GL, Antonmattei S, Tetalman MR, et al.: Tc-99m diphosphonate distribution in a patient with hypercalcemia and metastatic calcifications. *Clin Nucl Med* 1980;5:422.
124. Quaife MA, et al.: Myocardial accumulation of labeled phosphate in malignant pericardial effusion. *J Nucl Med* 1979;20:392.
125. Chew FS, Hudson TM: Radionuclide imaging of lipoma and liposarcoma. *Radiology* 1980;136:741.
126. Delcourt E, Baudoux M, Neve P: Tc-99m-MDP bone scanning detection of gastric calcification. *Clin Nucl Med* 1980;5:546.
127. Desai A, et al.: ^{99m}Tc-MDP uptake in nonosseous lesions. *Radiology* 1980;135:181.
128. Schimmel DH, Moss AA, Hoffer PB: Radionuclide imaging of intestinal infarctions in dogs. *Invest Radiol* 1976;11:277.
129. Ortiz VN, Sfakianakis G, Haase GM, et al.: The value of radionuclide scanning in early diagnosis of intestinal infarction. *J Pediatr Surg* 1978;13:616.
130. Moss AA, Kressel HY: Intestinal infarction: Current problems and new methods of diagnosis using radionuclide scans. *Appl Radiol* 1976;5:156.
131. Jayabalan V, DeWitt B: Gastric calcification detected in vivo by ^{99m}Tc-pyrophosphate imaging. *Clin Nucl Med* 1978;3:27.
132. Caride VJ, Touloukian RJ, Ablow RC, et al.: Abdominal and hepatic uptake of 99m Tc-pyrophosphate in neonatal necrotizing enterocolitis. *Radiology* 1981;139:205.
133. Goldfarb CR, Shah PJ, Jay M: Extraosseous uptake of bone-seeking tracers: An expected but unsuspected addition to the list. *Clin Nucl Med* 1979;4:194.
134. Richards AG: Metastatic calcification detected through scanning with Tc-polyphosphate. *J Nucl Med* 1974;15:1057.
135. Shultz MM, Morales JO, Fishbein PG, et al.: Bilateral breast uptake of ^{99m}Tc-polyphosphate in a patient with metastic adenocarcinoma. *Radiology* 1976;118:377.
136. Singh BN, Cisternino SJ, Kesala BA: ^{99m}Tc-diphosphonate uptake in mucinous adenocarcinoma of the stomach. *Clin Nucl Med* 1977;2:357.
137. Gordon L, Schabel SI, Holland RD, et al.: ^{99m}Tc-methylene diphosphonate accumulation in ascitic fluid due to neoplasm. *Radiology* 1981;139:699.
138. Lavelle KJ, Park HM, Moseman AM, et al.: Renal hyperconcentration of ^{99m}Tc-HEDP in experimental acute tubular necrosis. *Radiology* 1979;131:491.
139. Lutrin CL, Goris ML: Pyrosphosphate retention by previously irradiated renal tissue. *Radiology* 1979;133:207.
140. Trackler TR, Chinn RYW: Amphotericin B therapy. A cause of increased renal uptake of Tc-99m MDP. *Clin Nucl Med* 1982;7:293.
141. Lutrin CL, Goris ML: Pyrosphosphate retention by previously irradiated renal tissue. *Radiology* 1979;133:207.
142. Lantieri RL, Lin MS, Martin W, et al.: Increased renal accumulation of Tc-99m-MDP in renal artery stenosis. *Clin Nucl Med* 1980;5:305.
143. Valdez DA, Jacobstein JG: Decreased bone uptake of technetium-99m-polyphosphate in thalassemia major. *J Nucl Med* 1980;21:47.
144. Bossuyt A, Verbeelen D, Jonckheer MH, et al.: Usefulness of ^{99m}Tc-methylene diphosphonate scintigraphy in nephrocalcinosis. *Clin Nucl Med* 1979;4:333.
145. Glassman AB, Selby JB: ANother bone imaging agent false-positive: Phimosis. *Clin Nucl Med* 1980;5:34.
146. Sty JR, Chusid MJ, Babbitt DP: Scintigraphic findings of uncommon focal manifestations of Haemophilus influenzae septicemia. *Clin Nucl Med* 1979;4:455.
147. Sty JR, Starshak RJ: Scintigraphy in Woman's disease. *Clin Nucl Med* 1978;3:397.
148. Manoli RS, Soin JS: Concentration of ^{99m}Tc-pyrophosphate in a benign leiomyoma of the uterus. *Clin Nucl Med* 1977;2:60.

149. Sham R, et al.: Localization of ^{99m}Tc-phosphate compounds in renal tumors. *J Nucl Med* 1977;18:311.
150. Thomsen HS, Lokkegaard H, Munck O: Evaluation of kidney grafts with ^{99m}Tc-methylene diphosphonate within 36 hours after transplantation: A marker of ischemic damage. *Eur J Nucl Med* 1984;9:115.
151. Sty JR, Starshak RJ: Abnormal Tc-99m MDP renal images associated with myoglobinuria. *Clin Nucl Med* 1982;7:476.
152. Dhawan VM, Sziklas JJ, Spencer RP, et al.: Surgically related extravasation of urine detected on bone scan. *Clin Nucl Med* 1977;2:411.
153. Richman LS, Gummerman LW, Levine G, et al.: Localization of ^{99m}Tc-polyphosphate in soft tissue malignancies. *Am J Roentgenol* 1975;124:577.
154. Gates GF: Ovarian carcinoma imaged by ^{99m}Tc-pyrophosphate: Case report. *J Nucl Med* 1976;17:29.
155. Hardy JG, Anderson GS, Newble GM: Uptake of Tc-99m pyrophosphate by extragenital seminoma. *J Nucl Med* 1976;17:1105.
156. Grames GM, Jansen C, Carlsen EN, et al.: The abnormal bone scan in intracranial lesions. *Radiology* 1975;115:129.
157. Kim YC: Thyroid uptake in bone scan on a large, multinodular, nontoxic goiter with calcific degeneration. *Clin Nucl Med* 1980;5:561.
158. Grames GM, Jansen C: The abnormal bone scan in cerebral infarction. *J Nucl Med* 1973;14:941.
159. Norbash AM and DeLong SR: Serendipitous diagnosis of hyperthyroidism with Tc-99m bone scan. *Clin Nucl Med* 1991;12:526.
160. Tonami T, Sugihara M, Hisada K: Concentration of ^{99m}Tc-diphosphonate in calcified thyroid carcinoma. *Clin Nucl Med* 1977;2:357.
161. Van der Vis-Melsen MJE, et al.: Autonomously functioning thyroid nodule and medullary carcinoma. *J Nucl Med* 1981;22:929.
162. Fitzer PM: ^{99m}Tc-polyphosphate concentration in a neuroblastoma. *J Nucl Med* 1974;15:904.
163. Smith FW, et al.: Primary neuroblastoma uptake of ^{99m}Technetium methylene disphosphonate. *Radiology* 1980;137:501.
164. Vanek JA, Cook SA, Bukowski RM: Hepatic uptake of Tc-99m-labeled diphosphonate in amyloidosis: Case report. *J Nucl Med* 1977;18:1086.
165. Lyons KP, Kuperus J, Green HW: Localization of Tc-99m-pyrophosphate in the liver due to massive liver necrosis: Case report. *J Nucl Med* 1977;18:550.
166. Jaresko GS, Zimmer AM, Pavel DG, et al.: Effect of circulating aluminum on the biodistribution of Tc-99m-Sn-diphosphonate in rats. *J Nucl Med Technol* 1980;8:160.
167. Whitten CG, Luke BA: Liver uptake of Tc–99m PYP. *Clin Nucl Med* 1991;16:492.
168. Guiberteau MJ, Potsaid MS, McKusick KA: Accumulation of ^{99m}Tc-diphosphonate in four patients with hepatic neoplasm: Case report. *J Nucl Med* 1976;17:1060.
169. Poulose KP, Reba RC, Eckelman WC, et al.: Extraosseous localization of ^{99m}Tc-pyrophosphate. *Br J Radiol* 1975;48:724.
170. Garcia AC, Yeh SDJ, Benua RS: Accumulation of bone seeking radionuclides in liver metastases from colon carcinoma. *Clin Nucl Med* 1977;2:265.
171. DeLong JF, et al.: Case report: ^{99m}Tc-diphosphonate concentration in a malignant melanoma metastatic to liver. *Trans Equilib* 1977;6:1.
172. Rosenfield N, Treves S: Osseous and extraosseous uptake of Fluorine-18 and Technetium-99m polyphosphate in children with neuroblastoma. *Radiology* 1974;111:127.
173. Teates CD, Brower AC, Williamson RJ: Osteosarcoma extraosseous metastases demonstrated on bone scans and radiographs. *Clin Nucl Med* 1977;2:298.
174. Wilkinson RH, Gaede JT: Concentration of Tc-99m methylene-diphosphonate in hepatic metastases from squamous cell carcinoma. *J Nucl Med* 1979;20:303.
175. Sarreck R, Sham R, Alexander LL, et al.: Increased ^{99m}Tc-pyrophosphate uptake with radiation pneumonitis. *Clin Nucl Med* 1979;4:403.
176. Lowenthal IS, Tow DE, Chang YC: Accumulation of ^{99m}Tc-polyphosphate in two squamous cell carcinomas of the lung: Case report. *J Nucl Med* 1975;16:1021.
177. Vieras R: Radiation induced skeletal and soft tissue bone scan changes. *Clin Nucl Med* 1977;2:93.
178. Ravin CE, Hoyt TS, DeBlanc H: Concentration of ^{99m}technetium polyphosphate in fibrothorax following pneumonectomy. *Radiology* 1977;122:405.
179. Grames GM, Sauser DD, Jansen C, et al.: Radionuclide detection of diffuse interstitial pulmonary calcification. *JAMA* 1974;230:992.
180. DeGraaf P, Schicht IM, Pauwels EKJ, et al.: Bone scintigraphy in uremic pulmonary calcification. *J Nucl Med* 1979;20:201.
181. Herry JY, Moisan A, Le Pogamp P, et al.: Pulmonary uptake of Tc-99m-labeled methylene diphosphonate in a patient with a parathyroid adenoma. *J Nucl Med* 1981;22:888.
182. Palmer PES, Stadalnik RC, Khalkhali I: Non-bony uptake of technetium-99m MDP in berylliosis. *Br J Radiol* 1980; 53:1195.
183. Faubert PF, et al.: Pulmonary calcification in hemodialyzed patients detected by technetium-99m diphosphonate scanning. *Kidney Int* 1980;18:95.
184. Brower AC, Teates CD: Positive ^{99m}Tc-polyphosphate scan in case of metastatic osteogenic sarcoma and hypertrophic pulmonary osteoarthropathy. *J Nucl Med* 1974;15:53.
185. Siegel ME, Walker WJ, Campbell JL: Accumulation of ^{99m}Tc-diphosphonate in malignant pleural effusion: Detection and verification. *J Nucl Med* 1975;16:883.
186. Byun HH, Rodman SG, Chung KE: Soft tissue concentration of ^{99m}Tc-phosphates associated with injection of iron dextran complex. *J Nucl Med* 1976;17:374.
187. Silberstein EB, Bove KE: Visualization of alcohol-induced rhabdomyolysis: A correlative radiotracer, histo-chemical, and electron microscopic study. *J Nucl Med* 1979;20:127.
188. Spies SM, Swift TR, Brown M: Increased ^{99m}Tc-polyphosphate muscle uptake in a patient with polymyositis: Case report. *J Nucl Med* 1975;16:1125.
189. Blair RJ, Schoeder ET, McAfee JG, et al.: Skeletal muscle uptake in both traumatic and nontraumatic rhabdomyolysis with acute renal failure. *J Nucl Med* 1975;16:515.
190. Lentle BC, Percy JS, Rigal WM, et al.: Localization of Tc-99m pyrophosphate in muscle after exercise (letter). *J Nucl Med* 1978;19:223.
191. Swift TR, Brown M: Tc-99m pyrophosphate muscle labeling in McArdle syndrome. *J Nucl Med* 1978;18:295.
192. Bellina CR, Bianchi R, Bombardieri R, et al.: Quantitative evaluation of 99m technetium pyrophosphate muscle uptake in patients with inflammatory and noninflammatory muscle disease. *J Nucl Med Allied Sci* 1978;22:89.
193. Floyd JL, Prather JL: ^{99m}Tc-EHDP uptake in ischemic muscle. *Clin Nucl Med* 1977;2:281.
194. Suzuki Y, et al.: Demonstration of myositis ossificans by ^{99m}Technetium-pyrophosphate bone scanning. *Radiology* 1974;111:663.
195. Slutsky LT, et al.: Uptake of ^{99m}Tc-pyrophosphate in chest wall tissue due to defibrillation. *Clin Nucl Med* 1977;2:6.
196. Pugh BR, Buja LM, Parkey RW, et al.: Cardioversion and "false-positive" technetium-99m stannous pyrophosphate myocardial scintigrams. *Circulation* 1976;54:399.
197. Lewis SE, et al.: Identification of muscle damage in acute

electrical burns with technetium 99m pyrophosphate (Tc-99m-PYP) scintigraphy. *J Nucl Med* 1979;20:646.
198. Gelfand MJ, Planitz MK: Uptake of ^{99m}Tc diphosphonate in soft tissue in sickle cell anemia. *Clin Nucl Med* 1977;2:355.
199. Simpson AJ: Localization of ^{99m}Tc pyrophosphate in an ischemic leg. *Clin Nucl Med* 1977;2:400.
200. Sorkin SJ, et al.: Augmented activity on a bone scan following local chemoperfusion. *Clin Nucl Med* 1977;2:451.
201. Bekier A: Extraosseous accumulation of Tc-99m pyrophosphate in soft tissue after radiation therapy. Letter to editor. *J Nucl Med* 1978;19:225.
202. Van Antwerp JD, et al.: ^{99m}Tc-diphosphonate accumulation in amyloid. *J Nucl Med* 1975;16:238.
203. Heerfordt J, Vistisen L, Bohr H: Comparison of ^{18}F and ^{99m}Tc-polyphosphate in orthopedic bone scintigraphy. *J Nucl Med* 1976;17:98.
204. O'Mara RE, Charkes ND: The osseous system, in *Clinical Scintillation Imaging*. New York, Grune and Stratton, 1975.
205. Alarcón-Segovia D, Lazo C, Sepulveda J, et al.: Uptake of ^{99m}Tc-labeled phosphates by gouty tophi. *J Rheumatol* 1974;1:314.
206. Ell PJ, Breitfellner G, Meixner M: Technetium-99m-HEDP concentration in calcified myoma. *J Nucl Med* 1976;17:323.
207. Lentle BC, Glazebrook GA, Peray JS: Sympathetic denervation and the bone scan. *Clin Nucl Med* 1977;2:276.
208. Sty JR, Starshak RJ, Oechler HW: Extraosseous uptake of Tc-99m-MDP in congenital fibromatosis. *Clin Nucl Med* 1981;6:123.
209. Strashun A, Chayes Z: Migratory osteolysis. *J Nucl Med* 1979;20:129.
210. Tattler GLV, Baillod RA, Varghese I, et al.: Evolution of bone disease over 10 years in 135 patients with terminal renal failure. *Br Med J* 1973;4:315.
211. Oster Z: Appearance of filarial infestations on a bone scan. *J Nucl Med* 1976;17:425.
212. Bossuyt A, Verbeelen D: Accumulation of ^{99m}Tc pyrophosphate in the skin lesions of pseudoxanthoma elasticum. *Clin Nucl Med* 1976;1:245.
213. Bada L, Padro L, Cervera C: Scanning for soft tissue amyloid. *Lancet* 1977;1:1012.
214. Pendergrass HP, Potsaid MS, Castronovo FP: The clinical use of ^{99m}Tc diphosphonate (HEDSPA)—A new agent for skeletal imaging. *Radiology* 1973;107:557.
215. Eugenidis N, Locher JT: Tumor calcinosis imaged by bone scanning: Case report. *J Nucl Med* 1977;18:34.
216. Balsam D, Goldfarb CR, Stringer B, et al.: Bone scintigraphy for neonatal osteomyelitis: Simulation by extravasation of intravenous calcium. *Radiology* 1980;135:185.
217. Bautovich G, Genant HK, Hoffer PB, et al.: The in vivo study of the effects of tissue inflammation on the uptake of bone-seeking radionuclides. *J Nucl Med* 1974;15:476.
218. Ajmani SK, Lerner SR, Pircher FJ: Bone scan artifact caused by hyperhidrosis: Case report. *J Nucl Med* 1977;18:801.
219. Williams JL, Capitanio MA, Harcke HT: Bone scanning in neonatal subcutaneous fat necrosis (letter). *J Nucl Med* 1978;19:861.
220. Prakash V, Lin MS, Perkash I: Detection of heterotropic calcification with ^{99m}Tc-pyrophosphate in spinal cord injury patients. *Clin Nucl Med* 1978;3:167.
221. Brill DR: Soft tissue uptake on the bone scan—Exhibit presented at the Society of Nuclear Medicine annual meeting. Dallas, Texas, 1976.
222. Brown M, Swift TR, Spies SM: Radioisotope scanning in inflammatory muscle disease. *Neurology* 1976;26:517.
223. Sarminento AH, Alba J, Lanaro AE, Dietrich R: Evaluation of soft-tissue calcifications in dermatomyositis with Tc-99m phosphate compounds: Case report. *J Nucl Med* 1975;16:467.
224. Gallini C, De Cicco C, Legnaioli M, et al: Potential pitfall in bone scanning by transcutaneous nitroglycerin. *Clin Nucl Med* 1990;15:920.
225. Nolan NG: Intense uptake of ^{99m}Tc-diphosphonate by an extraosseous neurofibroma. *J Nucl Med* 1974;15:1207.
226. McLaughlin AF: Uptake of ^{99m}Tc bone-scanning agent by lungs with metastatic calcification. *J Nucl Med* 1976;16:322.
227. Chew FS, Hudson TM: Radiology of infiltrating angiolipoma. *Am J Roentgenol* 1980;135:781.
228. Nakajima H, et al.: Extra-osseous accumulation of ^{99m}Tc-MDP in 2 cases of soft tissue sarcoma. *Jpn J Clin Radiol* 1981;26:417.
229. Pearlman AW: Preoperative evaluation of liposarcoma by nuclear imaging. *Clin Nucl Med* 1977;2:47.
230. Lieberman CM, Hemingway DL: Splenic visualization in a patient with glucose-6-phosphate dehydrogenase deficiency. *Clin Nucl Med* 1979;4:405.
231. Winter PF: Splenic accumulation of ^{99m}Tc-diphosphonate (letter). *J Nucl Med* 1976;17:850.
232. Goy W, Crowe WJ: Splenic accumulation of ^{99m}Tc-diphosphonate in a patient with sickle cell disease: Case report. *J Nucl Med* 1976;17:108.
233. Howman-Giles RB, et al.: Splenic accumulation of Tc-99m disphosphonate in thalassemia major. Letter to editor. *J Nucl Med* 1978;19:976.
234. Gilday DL, Ash JM, Reilly BJ: Radionuclide skeletal survey for pediatric neoplasms. *Radiology* 1977;123:399.
235. Forbes CD, et al.: Bilateral pseudotumors of the pelvis in a patient with Christmas disease with notes on localization by radioactive scanning and ultrasonography. *Am J Roentgenol* 1974;121:173.
236. Bishop HM, Blamey RW, Morris AH, et al.: Bone scanning: its lack of value in the follow-up of patients with breast cancer. *Br J Surg* 1979;66:752.
237. Moneypenny IJ, Grieve RJ, Howell A, Morrison JM: The value of serial bone scanning in operable breast cancer. *Br J Surg* 1984;71:466.
238. Spencer GR, Khan M, Bird C, et al.: Is bone scanning of value in patients with breast cancer? *Acta Chir Scand* 1981;147:247.
239. Pauwels EKJ, Heslinga JM, Zwaveling A: Value of pre-treatment and follow-up skeletal scintigraphy in operable breast cancer. *Cancer Oncol* 1982;8:25.
240. Furnival CM, Blumgart LH, Citrin DL, et al.: Serial scintiscanning in breast cancer: Indications and prognostic value. *Clin Oncol* 1980;6:25.
241. Wickerham L, Fisher B, Cronin W, et al.: The efficacy of bone scanning in the follow-up of patients with operable breast cancer. *Breast Cancer Res Treat* 1984;4:303.
242. Coleman RE, Rubens RD, Fogelman I: Reappraisal of the baseline bone scan in breast cancer. *J Nucl Med* 1988;29:1045.
243. Gillespie PJ, Alexander JL, Edelstyn GA: Changes in ^{87m}Sr concentrations in skeletal metastases in patients responding to cyclical combination chemotherapy for advanced breast cancer. *J Nucl Med* 1975;16:191.
244. Coleman RE, Mashiter G, Whitaker KB, et al.: Bone scan flare predicts successful systemic therapy for bone metastases. *J Nucl Med* 1988;29:1354.
245. Front D, Israel O, Jerushalmi J, et al.: Quantitative bone scintigraphy (QBS) using SPECT. *J Nucl Med* 1989;29:240.
246. Johansson JE, Beckman KW, Lindell D, et al.: Serial bone scanning in the evaluation of stage and clinical course in carcinoma of the prostate. *Scan J Urol Nephrol* 1980;55:31.
247. Freitas JE, Gilvydas R, Ferry JD, Gonzalez JA: The clinical utility of prostate-specific antigen and bone scintigraphy in prostate cancer follow-up. *J Nucl Med* 1991;32:1387.
248. Amico S, Liehn JC, Desoize B, et al.: Comparison of phospha-

tase isoenzymes PAP and PSA with bone scan in patients with prostate carcinoma. *Clin Nucl Med* 1991;16:643.
249. Gerber G, Chodak GW: Assessment of value of routine bone scans in patients with newly diagnosed prostate cancer. *Urology* 1991;37:418.
250. Pollen JJ, Gerber K, Ashburn WL, et al.: Nuclear bone imaging in metastatic cancer of the prostate. *Cancer* 1981; 47:2585.
251. Gravenstein S, Peltz MA, Pories W: How ominous is an abnormal scan in bronchogenic carcinoma? *JAMA* 1979; 241:2523.
252. Kelly RJ, Cowan RJ, Ferree CB, et al.: Efficacy of radionuclide scanning in patients with lung cancer. *JAMA* 1979;242:2855.
253. McNeil BJ: Value of bone scanning in neoplastic disease. *Semin Nucl Med* 1984;14:277.
254. Hooper RB, Beechler CR, Johnson MC: Radioisotope scanning in the initial staging of bronchogenic carcinoma. *Am Rev Resp Dis* 1978;118:279.
255. Levenson RM, Sauerbrunn BJ, Ihde DC: Small cell lung cancer: radionuclide bone scan for assessment of tumor extent and response. *Am J Radiol* 1981;137:31.
256. Donato AT, Ammerman EG, Sullesta O: Bone scanning in evaluation of patients with lung cancer. *Ann Thorac Surg* 1979;17:300.
257. Ali A, Tetalman MR, Fordham EW, et al.: Distribution of hypertrophic pulmonary osteoarthropathy. *AJR* 1980; 134:771.
258. Cole AT, Mandell J, Fried FA, et al.: The place of bone scans in the diagnosis of renal cell carcinoma. *J Urol* 1975; 114:364.
259. Parthasarathy KL, Landsberg R, Bakshi SP, et al.: Detection of bone metastases in urogenital malignancies utilizing ^{99m}Tc-labeled phosphate compounds. *Urology* 1978;1:99.
260. Rosen PR, Murphy KG: Bone scintigraphy in the initial staging of patients with renal-cell carcinoma. *J Nucl Med* 1984;25:289.
261. Lokich JJ, Harrison JH: Renal cell cancer: natural history and chemotherapeutic experience. *J Urol* 1975;114:371.
262. Kim EE, Bledin AG, Gutierrez C, Haynie TP: Comparison of radionuclide images and radiography for skeletal metastases from renal cell carcinoma. *Oncology* 1983;40:284.
263. Clyne CAC, Frank JW, Jenkins JD, Smart CJ: The place of ^{99m}Tc-polyphosphonate bone scan in renal carcinoma. *Br J Urol* 1983;55:174.
264. Kishi K, Horita T, Matsumoto K, et al.: Carcinoma of bladder: A clinical and pathological analysis of 87 autopsy cases. *Urology* 1981;125:36.
265. Berger GL, Sadlowski RW, Sharpe JR, Finney RP: Lack of value of routine preoperative bone and liver scans in cystectomy candidates. *J Urol* 1981;125:637.
266. Lindner A, Dekernion JB: Cost effectiveness of pre-cystectomy radioisotopic scans. *J Urol* 1982;128:1181.
267. Davey P, Merrick MV, Duncan W, Padpath AT: Bladder cancer: the value of routine bone scintigraphy. *Clin Radiol* 1985;26:77.
268. Brismar J, Gustafson T: Bone scintigraphy in staging of bladder carcinoma. *Acta Radiol* 1988;29:251.
269. Katz RD, Alderson PO, Rosenheim NB, et al.: Utility of bone scanning in detecting occult metastases from cervical carcinoma. *Radiology* 1979;133:469.
270. Bassan JS, Glaser MG: Bony metastases in carcinoma of the uterine cervix. *Clin Radiol* 1982;33:623.
271. Du Toit JP, Grove DV: Radio-isotope bone scanning for the detection of occult bony metastases in invasive cervical carcinoma. *Gynecol Oncol* 1987;28:215.
272. Kamath CRV, Maruyama Y, De Land FH, van Nagell JR: Value of bone scanning in detecting occult skeletal metastases from adenocarcinoma of the endometrium. *Diagn Gynecol Obstet* 1982;4:155.
273. Harbert JC, Rocha L, Smith FO, Delgado G: The efficacy of radionuclide bone scans in the evaluation of gynecological cancers. *Cancer* 1982;49:1040.
274. Mettler FA, Christie JH, Garcia JF, et al.: Radionuclide liver and bone scanning in the evaluation of patients with endometrial carcinoma. *Radiology* 1981;141:777.
275. Merrick MV: Bone scintigraphy in testicular tumours. *Br J Urol* 1987;60:167.
276. Podraskey AE, Stark DD, Hattner RS, et al.: Radionuclide bone scanning in neuroblastoma: skeletal metastases and primary tumor localization of ^{99m}Tc-MDP. *Am J Roentgenol* 1983;141:469.
277. Kaufman RA, Thrall JH, Keyes JW, et al.: False-negative bone scans in neuroblastoma metastatic to the end of long bones. *Am J Roentgenol* 1978;130:131.
278. Lumbroso JD, Guermazi F, Hartmann O, et al.: Meta-iodobenzylguanidine (MIBG) scans in neuroblastoma: sensitivity and specificity, a review of 115 scans. *Prog Clin Biol Res* 1988;271:689.
279. Bouvier JF, Philip T, Chauvot P, et al.: Pitfalls and solutions in neuroblastoma diagnosis using radioiodine MIBG: our experience with 50 cases. *Prog Clin Biol Res* 1988;271:707.
280. Antoniades J, Croll MN, Watner RJ: Bone scanning in carcinoma of the colon and rectum. *Dis. Colon Rectum* 1976; 19:139.
281. Stein JJ: Metastasis to bone from carcinoma of the gastrointestinal tract. *Radiology* 1940;35:486.
282. Wolfe JA, Rowe LD, and Lowry LD: Value of radionuclide scanning in the staging of head and neck carcinoma. *Ann Otol Rhinol Laryngol* 1979;88:832–836.
283. Front D, Hardoff R, and Robinson E: Bone scintigraphy in primary tumors of the head and neck. *Cancer* 1978; 42:111–117.
284. Castillo LA, Yeh SDJ, Leeper RD, Benua RS: Bone scans in bone metastases from functioning thyroid carcinoma. *Clin Nucl Med* 1980;5:200.
285. Dewan SS: The bone scan in thyroid cancer (Letter to Editor). *J Nucl Med* 1979;20:271.
286. Hoefnagel CA, Delprat CC, Marcuse HR, de Viilder JJM: Role of thallium-201 total-body scintigraphy in follow-up of thyroid carcinoma. *Am Rev Resp Dis* 1986;118:279.
287. Johnson DG, Coleman RE, McCook TA, Dale JK, Well SA: Bone and liver images in medullary carcinoma of the thyroid. *J Nucl Med* 1986;27:1854.
288. Woolfenden JM, Pitt MJ, Durie BGM, Moon TE: Comparison of bone scintigraphy and radiography in multiple myeloma. *Radiology* 1980;134:723.
289. Hübner KF, Andres GA, Hayes RL, et al.: The use of rare-earth radionuclides and other bone seekers in the evaluation of bone lesions in patients with multiple myeloma or solitary plasmacytoma. *Radiology* 1977;125:171.
290. Leonard RCF, Owen JP, Proctor SJ, Hamilton PJ: Multiple myeloma: Radiology or bone scanning. *Clin Radiol* 1981;321:291.
291. Wahner HW, Kyle RA, Beabout JW: Scintigraphic evaluation of the skeleton in multiple myeloma. *Mayo Clin Proc* 1980;55:739.
292. Daffner RH, Lupetin AR, Dash N, et al.: MRI in the detection of malignant infiltration of bone marrow. *AJR* 1986;146: 353.
293. Bataille R, Chevalier J, Rossi M, et al.: Bone scintigraphy in plasma-cell myeloma. *Radiology* 1982;145:801.
294. Freeman C, Berg JW, Cutler SJ: Occurrence and prognosis of extranodal lymphomas. *Cancer* 1972;29:252.

295. Ferrant A, Rodhain J, Michaux L, et al.: Detection of skeletal involvement in Hodgkin's disease: a comparison of radiography, bone scanning, and bone marrow biopsy in 38 patients. *Cancer* 1975;35:1346.
296. Kuntz DJ, Leonard JC, Nitschke RM, et al.: An evaluation of diagnostic techniques utilized in the initial workup of pediatric patients with acute lymphocytic leukemia. *Clin Nucl Med* 1984;9:405.
297. Morrison SC, Adler LP: Photopenic areas on bone scanning associated with childhood leukemia. *Clin Nucl Med* 1991; 16:24.
298. Caudle RJ, Crawford AH, Gelfand MJ, et al.: Childhood acute lymphoblastic leukemia presenting as "cold" lesions on bone scan: a report of two cases. *J Pediatr Orthop* 1987;7:93.
299. O'Mara RE: Bone scanning in osseous metastatic disease. *JAMA,* 1974;229:1915.
300. Roth JA, Eilber FR, Bennett LR, Morton DL: Radionuclide photoscanning. Usefulness in preoperative evaluation of melanoma patients. *Arch Surg* 1975;110:1211.
301. Thomas JH, Panoussopoulus D, Liesmann GE, et al.: Scintiscans in the evaluation of patients with malignant melanomas. *Surg Gynaecol Obstet* 1979;149:574.
302. Salwen WA, Krementz ET, Campeau RJ: Bone and liver imaging in regionally advanced melanoma. *J Surg Oncol* 1989;42:225.
303. Aranha GV, Simmons RL, Gunnarsson A, Grage TB, McKhann CF: The value of preoperative screening procedures in stage I and II malignant melanoma. *J Surg Oncol* 1979;11:1.
304. Au FC, Maier WP, Malmud LS, et al.: Preoperative nuclear scans in patients with melanoma. *Cancer* 1984;53:2095.
305. Muss HB, Richards F, Barnes PL, et al.: Radionuclide scanning in patients with advanced malignant melanoma. *Clin Nucl Med* 1979;4:516.
306. Rosenbaum RC, Frieri M, Metcalfe DD: Patterns of skeletal scintigraphy and their relationship to plasma and urinary histamine levels in systemic mastocytosis. *J Nucl Med* 1984;25:859.
307. Malley MJ, Holmes RA: Mastocytosis: Scintigraphic findings with bony involvement. *Clin Nucl Med* 1988;13:673.
308. Arrington ER, Eisenberg B, Hartshorne MF, et al.: Nuclear medicine imaging of systemic mastocytosis. *J Nucl Med* 1989;30:2046.
309. Henry RE, Resnick LH: Bone marrow scanning, in Gottschalk A, Potchen EJ (eds.): *Diagnostic Nuclear Medicine* (Golden's Diagnostic radiology series, section 20). Baltimore, Waverly Press, 1976, p 195.
310. Frank J, Ling A, Patronas N, Carrasquillo J, et al.: Detection of malignant bone tumors: MR Imaging versus scintigraphy. *AJR* 1990;155:1043.
311. Sarpel S, Sarpel G, Yu E, et al.: Early diagnosis of spinal-epidural metastasis by magnetic resonance imaging. *Cancer* 1987;59:1112.
312. Avrahami E, Tadmor R, Dally O, Hadar H: Early MR demonstration of spinal metastases in patients with normal radiographs and CT and radionuclide bone scans. *J Comput Assist Tomogr* 1989;13:598.
313. Jones AL, Williams MP, Powles TJ, et al.: Magnetic resonance imaging in the detection of skeletal metastases in patients with breast cancer. *Br J Cancer* 1990;62:296.
314. Rinsky LA, Goris M, Bleck EE, et al.: Intraoperative skeletal scintigraphy for localization of osteoid osteoma in the spine. *J Bone Joint Surg* 1980;62:143.
315. Klonecke AS, Licho R, McDougall IR: A technique for intraoperative bone scintigraphy. A report of 17 cases. *Clin Nucl Med* 1991;16:482.
316. Dahlin DC, Unni KK: *Bone Tumors. General Aspects and Data on 8542 Cases.* 4th Ed. Springfield, IL, Charles C. Thomas, 1986, p 269.
317. Heyman S: The lymphatic spread of osteosarcoma shown by Tc-99m MDP scintigraphy. *Clin Nucl Med* 1980;5:543.
318. Vanel D, Henry-Amar M, Lumbroso J, et al.: Pulmonary evaluation of patients with osteogenic sarcoma: roles of standard radiography, tomography, CT, scintigraphy, and tomoscintigraphy. *AJR* 1984;143:519.
319. McNeil BJ, Cassady JR, Geiser CF, et al.: Fluorine-18 bone scintigraphy in children with osteosarcoma or Ewing's sarcoma. *Radiology* 1973;109:627.
320. Goldstein H, McNeil BJ, Zufalle E, et al.: Changing indications for bone scintigraphy in patients with osteosarcoma. *Radiology* 1980;135:177.
321. McKillop JH, Etcubanas E, Goris ML: The indications for and limitations of bone scintigraphy in osteogenic sarcoma. A review of 55 patients. *Cancer* 1981;48:1133.
322. Ramann L, Waxman A, Binney G, et al.: Thallium-201 scintigraphy in bone sarcoma: comparison with gallium-67 and technetium-MDP in the evaluation of chemotherapeutic response. *J Nucl Med* 1990;31:567.
323. Caner B, Kitapal M, Unlü M, et al.: Technetium-99m-MIBI uptake in benign and malignant bone lesions: a comparative study with technetium-99m-MDP. *J Nucl Med* 1992;33:319.
324. Nair N: Bone scanning in Ewing's sarcoma. *J Nucl Med* 1985;26:349.
325. Goldstein H, McNeil BJ, Zufalle E, et al.: Is there still a place for bone scanning in Ewing's sarcoma? *J Nucl Med* 1980;21:10.
326. Estes DN, Magill HL, Thompson EI, Hayes FA: Primary ewing sarcoma: follow-up with Ga-67 scintigraphy. *Radiology,* 1990;177:449.
327. Hudson TM, Chew FS, Manaster BJ: Radionuclide bone scanning of medullary chondrosarcoma. *AJR* 1982;139:1071.
328. Humphrey A, Gilday DL, Brown RG: Bone scintigraphy in chondroblastoma. *Radiology* 1980;137:497.
329. Hudson TM, Chew FS, Manaster BJ: Scintigraphy of benign exostoses and exostotic chondrosarcomas. *AJR* 1983; 140:581.
330. Simon MA, Kirchner PT: Scintigraphic evaluation of primary bone tumors: comparison of technetium-99m phosphonate and gallium citrate imaging. *J Bone Joint Surg* 1980;62A:758.
331. Healey JH, Ghelman B: Osteoid osteomas and osteoblastomas: current concepts and recent advances. *Clin Orthop* 1986;204:76.
332. Makely J: Prostaglandins—a mechanism for pain mediation in osteoid osteoma. *Orthop Trans* 1982;6:72.
333. Helms CC, Hattner RS, Vogler JB: Osteoid osteoma: Radionuclide diagnosis. *Radiology* 1984;151:779.
334. Smith FW, Gilday DL: Scintigraphic appearances of osteoid osteoma. *Radiology* 1980;137:191.
335. Janin Y, Epstein JA, Carras R, et al.: Osteoid osteomas and osteoblastomas of the spine. *Neurosurgery* 1981;8:31.
336. Hall FM, Goldberg RP, Davies JAK, et al.: Scintigraphic assessment of bone islands. *Radiology* 1980;135:737.
337. Kirchner PT, Simon MA: Radioisotopic evaluation of bone disease. *J Bone Joint Surg* 1981;63A:673.
338. Kern KA, Brunetti A, Norton JA, et al.: Metabolic imaging of human extremity musculoskeletal tumors by PET. *J Nucl Med* 1988;29:181.
339. Adler LP, Blair H, Makley J, et al.: Noninvasive grading of liposarcomas using PET with FDG. *J Comput Assist Tomogr* 1990;14:960.
340. Adler LP, Blair HF, Makley JT, et al.: Noninvasive grading of musculoskeletal tumors using PET. *J Nucl Med* 1991;32:1508.
341. Marty R, Denney J, McKamey MR, et al.: Bone trauma and

related benign disease: Assessment by bone scanning. *Semin Nucl Med* 1976;6:107.

342. Wendeberg B: Mineral metabolism of fractures of the tibia in man studied with external counting of ^{85}Sr. *Acta Orthop* 1961;52:1.
343. Matin P: The appearance of bone scans following fractures, including immediate and long-term studies. *J Nucl Med* 1979;20:1277.
344. Fordham EW, Ramachandran PC: Radionuclide imaging of osseous trauma. *Semin Nucl Med* 1974;4:411.
345. Rosenthall L, Hill RO, Chuang S: Observation on use of ^{99m}Tc-phosphate imaging in peripheral bone trauma. *Radiology* 1976;119:637.
346. Rupani HK, Holder LW, Espinola DA, Engin SI: Three-phase radionuclide bone imaging in sports medicine. *Radiology* 1985;156:187.
347. McCook BM, Sandler MP, Powers TA, et al.: Correlative bone imaging, in Freeman LM, Weissman HS, (eds): *Nuclear Medicine Annual 1989*, New York, Raven Press, 1989, p 143.
348. Holder LE, Schwarz C, Wernicke PG, Michael RH: Radionuclide bone imaging in the early detection of fractures of the proximal femur (Hip): multifactorial analysis. *Radiology* 1990;174:509.
349. Greiff J: The ^{99m}Tc-Sn-polyphospate scintimetric time course of human tibial fractures with delayed union or pseudoarthrosis. *Injury* 1982;13:279.
350. Basse-Cathalinat B, Arnaud D, Blanquet P, et al.: New radioisotopic method for evaluation of the healing potential of a fracture. *Br J Radiol* 1980;53:863.
351. Desai A, Alavi A, Dalinka M, et al.: Role of bone scintigraphy in the evaluation and treatment of nonunited fractures: Concise communication. *J Nucl Med* 1980;21:931.
352. Tyler JL, Powers TA: Bone scanning after marrow biopsy. Concise communication. *J Nucl Med* 1982;23:1085.
353. Zwas ST, Frank G: The role of bone scintigraphy in stress and overuse injuries, in Freeman LM, Weissman HS, (eds): *Nuclear Medicine Annual 1989.* New York, Raven Press, 1989, p 109.
354. Marty R, Denney JD, McKamey MR, Rowley MJ: Bone trauma and related benign disease: Assessment by bone scanning. *Semin Nucl Med* 1976;6:107.
355. Prather JL, Nusynowitz ML, Snowdy HA, et al.: Scintigraphic findings in stress fractures. *J Bone Joint Surg* 1977;59A:869.
356. Geslin GE, Thrall JH, Espinosa JL, Older RA: Early detection of stress fractures using Tc-99m polyphosphate. *Radiology* 1976;121:683.
357. Wilcox JR, Moniot AL, Green JP: Bone scanning in the evaluation of exercise related stress injuries. *Radiology* 1977;123:699.
358. Zwas ST, Frank G: The role of bone scintigraphy in stress and overuse injuries, in Freeman LM, Weissman HS, (eds): *Nuclear Medicine Annual 1989,* New York, Raven Press, 1989, p 109.
359. Lieberman CM, Hemingway DL: Scintigraphy of shin splints. *Clin Nucl Med* 1982;7:1.
360. Le Jeune JJ, Rochcongar P, Vazelli F, et al.: Pubic pain syndrome in sportsmen: Comparison of radiographic and scintigraphic results. *Eur J Nucl Med* 1984;9:250.
361. Nielsen PT, Hedeboe J, Thommesen P: Bone scintigraphy in the evaluation of fracture of the carpal scaphoid bone. *Acta Orthop Scand* 1983;54:303.
362. Ganel A, Engle J, Oster A, et al.: Bone scanning in the assessment of fractures of the scaphoid. *J Hand Surg* 1979;4:540.
363. Jorgensen TM, Andersen JH, Thommesen P, et al.: Scanning and radiology of the carpal scaphoid bone. *Acta Orthop Scand* 1979;50:663.
364. Urman M, Ammann W, Sisler J, et al.: The role of bone scintigraphy in the evaluation of talar dome fractures. *J Nucl Med* 1991;32:2241.
365. Haase GM, Ortiz VN, Sfakianikis GN, et al.: The value of radionuclide bone scanning in the early recognition of deliberate child abuse. *J Trauma* 1980;20:10.
366. Smith FW, Gilday DL, Ash JM, Green MD: Unsuspected costo-vertebral fractures demonstrated by bone scanning in the child abuse syndrome. *Pediatr Radiol* 1980;10:103.
367. Jaudes PK: Comparison of radiography and radionuclide bone scanning in the detection of child abuse. *Pediatrics* 1984;73:166.
368. Merten DF, Radkowski MA, Leonidas JC: The abused child: A radiological reappraisal. *Radiology* 1983;146:377–381.
369. Intenzo CM, Wapner KL, Park CH, Kim SM: Evaluation of plantar fasciitis by three-phase bone scintigraphy. *Clin Nucl Med* 1991;16:325.
370. Martire JR: The role of nuclear medicine bone scans in evaluating pain in athletic injuries. *Clin Sports Med* 1987; 6:713.
371. Holder LE, Matthews L: The nuclear physician and sports medicine, in Freeman L, Weissman H (eds.): *Nuclear Medicine Annual 1984.* New York, Raven Press, 1984, p 81.
372. Collier D, Johnson RP, Carrera GF, et al.: Chronic knee pain assessed by SPECT: Comparison with other modalities. *Radiology* 1985;157:795.
373. Kahn D, Wilson MA: Bone scintigraphic findings in patellar tendinitis. *J Nucl Med* 1987;28:1768.
374. Allwright SJ, Cooper RA, Nash P: Trochanteric bursitis: Bone scan appearance. *Clin Nucl Med* 1988;13:561.
375. Englaro EE, Gelfand MJ, Paltiel HJ: Bone scintigraphy in preschool children with lower extremity pain of unknown origin. *J Nucl Med* 1992;33:351.
376. Dee P, Lambruschi PG, Heibert JM: The use of Tc-99m-MDP bone scanning in the study of vascularized bone implants: concise communication. *J Nucl Med* 1981;22:522.
377. Kelly JF, Cagle JD, Stevenson JS, et al: Technetium-99m radionuclide bone imaging for evaluating mandibular osseous allografts. *J Oral Surg* 1975;33:11.
378. Moskowitz GW, Lukash F: Evaluation of bone graft viability. *Semin Nucl Med* 1988;28:246.
379. Bergstedt HF, Korlof B, Lind MG, et al.: Scintigraphy of human autologous rib transplants to a partially resected mandible. *Scan J Plast Reconstr Surg* 1978;12:151.
380. Frame JW, Edmondson HD, O'Kane MM: A radioisotope study of the healing mandibular bone graft in patients. *Br J Oral Surg* 1983;21:277.
381. Ramsay SC, Yeates MG, Ho CY: Bone scanning in the early assessment of nasal bone graft viability. *J Nucl Med* 1991;32:33.
382. Taylor GI: Microvascular free bone transfer. *Orthop Clin North Am* 1977;8:425.
383. Berggren A, Weiland AJ, Ostrup LT: Bone scintigraphy in evaluating the viability of composite bone grafts revascularized by microvascular anastomoses, conventional autogenous bone grafts, and free nonrevascularized periosteal grafts. *J Bone Joint Surg* 1982;64A:799.
384. Gates GF: SPECT imaging of the lumbosacral spine and pelvis. *Clin Nucl Med* 1988;13:907.
385. Swanson D, Blecker I, Gahbauer H, Cardie VJ: Diagnosis of discitis by SPECT technetium-99m-MDP scintigram. *Clin Nucl Med* 1986;3:210.
386. Collier BD, Johnson RP, Carrera GF, et al: Painful spondylolysis or spondylolisthesis studied by radiography and single-photon emission computed tomography. *Radiology* 1985; 154:207.
387. Bodner RJ, Heyman S, Drummond DS, Gregg JR: The use of single photon emission computed tomography (SPECT)

in the diagnosis of low back pain in young patients. *Spine* 1988;13:1155.
388. Bellah RD, Summerville DA, Treves ST, Micheli LJ: Low-back pain in adolescent athletes: Detection of stress injury to the pars interarticularis with SPECT. *Radiology* 1991; 180:509.
389. Ryan PJ, Evans PA, Gibson T, Fogelman I: Chronic low back pain: Comparison of bone SPECT with radiography and CT. *Radiology* 1992;182:849.
390. Lusins JO, Danielski EF, Goldsmith SJ: Bone SPECT in patients with persistent back pain after lumbar spine surgery. *J Nucl Med* 1989;30:490.
391. Rosenthall L, Lisbona R: Role of radionuclide imaging in benign bone and joint diseases of orthopedic interest, in Freeman LM, Weissman HS (eds.): *Nuclear Medicine Annual 1980.* New York, Raven Press, 1980, p 267.
392. Meyers MH, Telfer N, Moore TM: Determination of the vascularity of the femoral head with technetium-99m sulfur colloid. *J Bone Joint Surg* 1977;59A:658.
393. Berg BV, Malghem J, Labaisse MA, et al: Avascular necrosis of the hip: comparison of contrast-enhanced and unenhanced MR imaging with histologic correlation. *Radiology* 1992; 182:445.
394. Turner DA, Templeton AC, Selzer PM, et al: Femoral capital osteonecrosis: MR finding of diffuse marrow abnormalities without focal lesions. *Radiology* 1989;171:135.
395. Greyson ND, Lotem MM, Gross AE, Houpt JB: Radionuclide evaluation of spontaneous femoral osteonecrosis. *Radiology* 1982;142:729.
396. Lutzuker LG, Alavi A: Bone and marrow imaging in sickle cell disease: diagnosis of infarction. *Semin Nucl Med* 1976;6:83.
397. Rao S, Solomon N, Miller S, Dunn E: Scintigraphic differentiation of bone infarction from osteomyelitis in children with sickle cell disease. *J Pediat* 1985;107:685.
398. Sutherland AD, Savage JP, Paterson DC, et al.: The nuclide bone-scan in the diagnosis and management of Perthes disease. *J Bone Joint Surg* 1980;62B:3.
399. Calver R, Venugopal V, Dorgan J, et al.: Radionuclide scanning in the early diagnosis of Perthes' disease. *J Bone Joint Surg* 1981;63B.
400. Fisher RL, Roderique JW, Brown DC, et al.: The relationship of isotopic bone imaging findings to prognosis in Legg-Perthes disease. *Clin Orthop* 1980;150:23.
401. Fasting OLJ, Bjerkreim I, Langeland N, et al.: Scintigraphic evaluation of the severity of Perthes' disease in the initial stage. *Acta Orthop Scand* 1980;51:655.
402. Danigelis JA: Pinhole imaging in Legg-Perthes' disease: Further observations. *Semin Nucl Med* 1976;6:69.
403. Kloiber R, Pavlosky W, Portner O, Garke K: Bone scintigraphy of hip joing effusions in children. *Am J Roentgenol* 1983;140:995.
404. Uren RF, Howman-Giles R: The 'cold hip' sign on bone scans. *Clin Nucl Med* 1991;16:553.
405. Kozin F, Soin JS, Ryan LM, et al.: Bone scintigraphy in the reflex sympathetic dystrophy syndrome. *Radiology* 1981; 138:437.
406. Simon H, Carlson DH: The use of bone scanning in the diagnosis of reflex sympathetic dystrophy. *Clin Nucl Med* 1980;3:116.
407. Holder LE, MacKinnon SE: Reflex sympathetic dystrophy in the hand: strict clinical and scintigraphic criteria. *Radiology* 1984;152:517.
408. Laxer RM, Allen RC, Malleson PN, et al.: Technetium 99m methylene diphosphonate bone scans in children with reflex neurovascular dystrophy. *J Pediatr* 1985;106:437.
409. Demangeat J-L, Constantinesco A, Brunot B, et al.: Three-phase bone scanning in reflex sympathetic dystrophy of the hand. *J Nucl Med* 1988;29:26.
410. McCrea MS, Rust RJ, COok DL, Stephens BA: Cocaine-induced rhabdomyolysis. Findings on bone scintigraphy. *Clin Nucl Med* 1992;17:292.
411. Matin P, Lang G, Carretta R, Sinon G: Scintigraphic evaluation of muscle damage following extreme exercise: concise communication. *J Nucl Med* 1983;24:308.
412. Frymoyer PA, Giammarco R, Farrar FM, Schroeder ET: Technetium-99m medronate bone scanning in rhabdomyolysis. *Arch Intern Med* 1985;145:1991.
413. Silver JR: Heterotopic ossification: A clinical study of its possible relationship to trauma. *Paraplegia* 1969;7:220.
414. Muheim G, Donath A, Rossier AB: Serial scintigrams in the course of ectopic bone formation in paraplegic patients. *Am J Roentgenol* 1973;118:865.
415. Tanaka T, Rossier AB, Hussey RW, et al.: Quantitative assessment of para-osteoarthropathy and its maturation on serial radionuclide bone images. *Radiology* 1977;123:217.
416. Sack GH: Clinical diversity in Gaucher's disease. *Johns Hopkins Med J* 1980;146:166.
417. Isreal O, Jerushalmi J, Front D: Scintigraphic findings in Gaucher's disease. *J Nucl Med* 1986;27:1557.
418. Cheng TH, Holman BL: Radionuclide assessment of Gaucher's disease. *J Nucl Med* 1978;19:1333.
419. Bilchik TR, Heyman S: Skeletal scintigraphy of pseudo-osteomyelitis in Gauchers' disease. *Clin Nucl Med* 1992;17:279.
420. Hattner RS, Hartmeyer J, Wara WM: Characterization of radiation-induced photopenic abnormalities on bone scans. *Radiology* 1982;145:161.
421. McAfee JG: Radionuclide imaging in metabolic and systemic skeletal diseases. *Semin Nucl Med* 1987;17:334.
422. Siegel BA, Engel WK, Derrer EC: Localization of technetium-99m diphosphonate in acutely injured muscle. Relationship to muscle calcium deposition. *Neurology* 1977;27:230.
423. Berman DS, Armsterdam EA, Hines HH, et al.: New approach to interpretation of technetium-99m pyrophosphate scintigraphy in detection of acute myocardial infarction. Clinical assessment of diagnostic accuracy. *Am J Cardiol* 1977;39:341.
424. Duszynski DO, Kuhn JP, Afshani E, Riddlesberger MM: Early radionuclide diagnosis of acute osteomyelitis. *Radiology* 1975;117:337.
425. Gilday DL, Paul DJ, Paterson J: Diagnosis of osteomyelitis in children by combined blood pool and bone imaging. *Radiology* 1975;117:331.
426. Deysine M, Rafkin H, Teicher I, et al.: Diagnosis of chronic and postoperative osteomyelitis with gallium-67 citrate scans. *Am J Surg* 1975;129:632.
427. Alazraki N, Dries D, Datz F, et al.: Value of a 24-hour image (four-phase bone scan) in assessing osteomyelitis in patients with peripheral vascular disease. *J Nucl Med* 1985;26:711.
428. Israel OI, Gips S, Jerushalmi J, et al.: Osteomyelitis and soft tissue infection: differential diagnosis with 24 hour/4 hour ratio of Tc99m-MDP uptake. *Radiology* 1987;163:725.
429. Schauwecker DS: The scintigraphy diagnosis of osteomyelitis. *AJR* 1992;158:9.
430. Allwright SJ, Miller JH, Gilsanz V: Subperiosteal abscess in children: scintigraphic appearance. *Radiology* 1991;179:725.
431. Bressler EL, Conway JJ, Weiss SC: Neonatal osteomyelitis examined by bone scintigraphy. *Radiology* 1984;152:685.
432. Handmaker H, Giammona ST: Improved early diagnosis of acute inflammatory skeletal-articular diseases in children: a two radiopharmaceutical approach. *Pediatrics* 1984;73:661.
433. El-Desouki M: Skeletal brucellosis: assessment with bone scintigraphy. *Radiology* 1991;181:415.
434. Boumpas DT, Vieras F, Acio E, Rohatgi PK: Skeletal tubercu-

losis resembling metastatic disease on bone scintigraphy. *J Nucl Med* 1987;28:1507.
435. Delbeke D, Habibian MR: Noninflammatory entities and the differential diagnosis of positive three phase bone imaging. *Clin Nucl Med* 1988;13:844.
436. Palestro CJ, Kim CK, Swyer AJ, et al.: Total hip arthroplasty: periprosthetic indium-111 labeled leukocyte activity and complementary technetium-99m-sulfur colloid imaging in suspected infection. *J Nucl Med* 1990;31:1950.
437. Palestro CJ, Swyer AJ, Kim CK, Goldsmith, SJ: Infected knee prosthesis: diagnosis with In-111 leukocyte, Tc-99m sulfur colloid, and Tc-99m MDP imaging. *Radiology* 1991;179:645.
438. Abreu SH: Skeletal uptake of indium 111-labeled white blood cells. *Semin Nucl Med* 1989;19:152.
439. Whalen JL, Brown ML, McLeod R, et al.: Limitations of indium leukocyte imaging for the diagnosis of spine infections. *Spine* 1991;16:193.
440. Lantto T, Kaukonen J-P, Kokkola A, et al.: Tc-99m HMPAO labeled leukocytes superior to bone scan in the detection of osteomyelitis in children. *Clin Nucl Med* 1992;17:7.
441. Hoffer P: Gallium: mechanisms. *J Nucl Med* 1980;21:282.
442. Rosenthall L, Kloiber R, Damtew B, Al-Majid H: Sequential use of radiophosphate and radiogallium imaging in the differential diagnosis of bone, joint and soft tissue infection: quantitative analysis. *Diagn Imaging* 1982;51:249.
443. Wellman HN, Siddiqui AR, Mail JT, Georgi P: Choice of radiotracer in the study of bone or joint infection in children. *Ann Radiol (Paris)* 1983;26:411.
444. Tumeh SS, Aliabadi P, Weissman BN, McNeil BJ: Chronic osteomyelitis: bone and gallium scan patterns associated with active disease. *Radiology* 1986;158:685.
445. Merkel KD, Brown ML, Fitzgerald RH: Sequential technetium-99m HMDP-gallium-67 citrate imaging for the evaluation of infection in the painful prosthesis. *J Nucl Med* 1986;27:1413.
446. Seabold JE, Nepola JV, Conrad GR, et al.: Detection of osteomyelitis at fracture nonunion sites: comparison of two scintigraphic methods. *AJR* 1989;152:1021.
447. Rubin RH, Fischman AJ, Callahan RJ, et al.: Indium-111 labeled nonspecific immunoglobulin scanning in the detection of focal infection. *N Engl J Med* 1989;321:935.
448. Oyen WJG, Claessens RAMJ, van Horn JR, et al.: Scintigraphic detection of bone and joint infections with indium-111-labeled nonspecific polyclonal human immunoglobulin G. *J Nucl Med* 1990;31:403.
449. Buscombe JR, Lui D, Ensing G, et al.: ^{99m}Tc-human immunoglobulin (HIG): First results of a new agent for the localization of infection and inflammation. *Eur J Nucl Med* 1990;16:649.
450. Hotze AL, Briele B, Overbeck B, et al.: Technetium-99m-labeled anti-granulocyte antibodies in suspected bone infections. *J Nucl Med* 1992;33:526.
451. Sayle BA, Fawcett HD, Wilkey DJ, et al.: Indium-111 chloride imaging in chronic osteomyelitis. *J Nucl Med* 1985;26:225.
452. Sayle BA, Fawcett HD, Wilkey DJ, et al.: Indium-111 chloride imaging in the detection of infected prostheses. *J Nucl Med* 1985;26:718.
453. Iles SE, Ehrich LE, Saliken JC, Martin RH: Indium-111 chloride scintigraphy in adult osteomyelitis. *J Nucl Med* 1987;28:1540.
454. Gold R, Hawkins RA, Katz RD: Bacterial osteomyelitis: findings on plain radiography, CT, MR, and scintigraphy. *AJR* 1991;157:365.
455. Weaver GR, Nance EP: Correlative bone imaging, in Freeman L, Weissman H (eds.): *Nuclear Medicine Annual 1989.* New York, Raven Press, 1989. p 143.
456. Unger E, Moldofsky P, Gatesby R, et al.: Diagnosis of osteomyelitis by MR imaging. *AJR* 1988;150:605.
457. Schauwecker DS, Braunstein EM, Wheat LJ: Diagnostic imaging of osteomyelitis. *Infect Dis Clin N Amer* 1990;4:441.
458. Modic MT, Feiglin DH, Piraino DW, et al.: Vertebral osteomyelitis: assessment using MR. *Radiology* 1985;157:157.
459. Berquist TH, Brown M, Fitzgerald R, May G: Magnetic resonance imaging: application in musculoskeletal infection. *Mag Reson Imaging* 1985;3:219.
460. Yuh WT, Corson JD, Baranlewski HM, et al.: Osteomyelitis of the foot of diabetic patients: evaluation with plain film 99mTc-MDP bone scintigraphy, and MR imaging. *AJR* 1989;152:790.
461. Merkel KD, Brown ML, Fitzgerald RH: Sequential technetium-99m HMDP-gallium-67 citrate imaging for the evaluation of infection in the painful prosthesis. *J Nucl Med* 1983;27:1413.
462. Wellman HN, Schauwecher DS, Capello WN: Evaluation of metallic osseous implants with nuclear medicine. *Semin Nucl Med* 1988;18:126.
463. Utz JA, Lull RJ, Galvin EG: Asymtomatic total hip prosthesis: natural history determined using Tc-99m MDP Bone scans. *Radiology* 1986;161:509.
464. Fink-Bennett D, Stanisavbljevic S, Blake D, et al.: Improved accuracy for detecting an infected hip arthroplasty: sequential technetium-99m sulfur colloid/indium-111 WBC imaging. *J Nucl Med* 1988;29:887.
465. McKillop JH, McKay I, Cuthbert GF, et al.: Scintigraphic evaluation of the painful prosthetic joint: a comparison of gallium-67 citrate and indium-111 labeled leucocyte imaging. *Clin Radiol* 1984;354:239.
466. Johnson JA, Christie MJ, Sandler MP, et al.: Detection of occult infection following total joint arthroplasty using sequential technetium-99m HDP bone scintigraphy and indium-111 WBC imaging. *J Nucl Med* 1988;29:1347.
467. Oswald SG, Van Nostrand D, Savory CG, et al.: The acetabulum: a prospective study of three-phase bone and indium white blood cell scintigraphy following porous-coated hip arthroplasty. *J Nucl Med* 1990;31:274.
468. Oswald SG, Van Nostrand D, Savory CG, Callaghan JJ: Three-phase bone scan and indium white blood cell scintigraphy following porous coated hip arthroplasty: A prospective study of the prosthetic tip. *J Nucl Med* 1989;30:1321.
469. Mulamba L, Ferrant A, Lewers N, et al.: Indium-111 leukocyte scanning in the evaluation of painful hip arthroplasty. *Acta Orthop Scand* 1983;54:695.
470. Capello WN, Wilson NM, Wellman HN: Bone imaging: a means of evaluating hip surface replacement arthroplasty, in Riley LH (ed.): *The Hip.* St. Louis, CV Mosby, 1980 p 165.
471. Forstram L, Hoogland D, Gomez L, et al.: Indium-111-oxime labeled leukocytes in the diagnosis of occult inflammation of abscesses. *J Nucl Med* 1979;20:650.
472. Johnson JA, Christie MJ, Sandler MP, et al.: Detection of occult infection following total joint arthroplasty using sequential technetium-99m HDP bone scintigraphy and indium-111 WBC imaging. *J Nucl Med* 1988;29:1347.
473. Palestro CJ, Kim KCK, Swyer AJ, et al.: Total-hip arthroplasty: periprosthetic indium-111-labeled leukocyte activity and complementary technetium-99m-sulfur colloid imaging in suspected infection. *J Nucl Med* 1990;31:1950.
474. Palestro CJ, Swyer AJ, Kim CK, Goldsmith SJ: Infected knee prosthesis: diagnosis with In-111 leukocyte, Tc-99m sulfur colloid, and Tc-99m MDP imaging. *Radiology* 1991;179:645.
475. Oyen WJG, van Horn JR, Claessens, RAMJ, et al.: Diagnosis of bone, joint, and joint prosthesis infections with In-111-labeled nonspecific human immunoglobulin G scintigraphy. *Radiology* 1992;182:195.

476. Zlatkin MB, Pathria M, Sartoris DJ, Resnick D: The diabetic foot. *Radiol Clin N Am* 1987;25:1095.
477. Zeiger LS, Fox IM: Use of indium-111-labeled white blood cells in the diagnosis of diabetic foot infections. *J Foot Surg* 1990;29:46.
478. Larcos G, Brown ML, Sutton RT: Diagnosis of osteomyelitis of the foot in diabetic patients: value of ^{111}In-leukocyte scintigraphy. *AJR* 1991;157:527.
479. Seabold JE, Flickinger FW, Kao SCS, et al.: Indium-111-leukocyte/technetium-99m-MDP bone and magnetic resonance imaging: difficult of diagnosing osteomyelitis in patients with neuropathic osteoarthropathy. *J Nucl Med* 1990;31:549.
480. Keenan AM, Tindel NL, Alavi A: Diagnosis of pedal osteomyelitis in diabetic patients using current scintigraphic techniques. *Arch Intern Med* 1989;149:2262.
481. Moore TE, Yuh WTC, Kathol MH, et al.: Abnormalities of the foot in patients with diabetes mellitus: findings on MR imaging. *AJR* 1991;157:813.
482. Schauwecker HM, Park RW, Burt BH, et al.: Combined bone scintigraphy and Indium-111 leukocyte scans in neuropathic foot disease. *J Nucl Med* 1988;29:1651.
483. Newman LG, Waller J, Palestro CJ, et al.: Unsuspected osteomyelitis in diabetic foot ulcers: diagnosis and monitoring by leukocyte scanning with indium In-111 oxyquinoline. *JAMA* 1991;266:1246.
484. Segener WA, Alavi A: Diagnostic imaging of musculoskeletal infection. *Orthop Clin N Am* 1991;22:401.
485. Prakash V, Kamel NJ, Lin MS, et al.: Increased skeletal localization of 99mTc-diphosphonate paralyzed limbs. *Clin Nucl Med* 1976;1:48.
486. Bray ST, Parain CL, Teates CD, et al.: The value of the bone scan in idiopathic regional migratory osteoporosis. *J Nucl Med* 1979;20:1268.
487. Fogelman I, Bessent RG, Turner JG, et al.: The use of whole-body retention of Tc-99m diphosphonate in the diagnosis of metabolic bone disease. *J Nucl Med* 1978;19:270.
488. Rai GS, Webster SGP, Wraight EP: Isotopic scanning of bone in the diagnosis of osteomalacia. *J Am Geriatr Soc* 1981;29:45.
489. Fogelman I, Carr D: A comparison of bone scanning and radiology in the evaluation of patients with metabolic bone disease. *Clin Radiol* 1980;31:321.
490. Krishnamurthy GT, Brickman AS, Blahd WH: Technetium 99m Sn-pyrophosphate pharmacokinetics and bone image changes in parathyroid disease. *J Nucl Med* 1977;18:236.
491. Mawer EB, Backhouse J, Taylor CM, et al.: Failure of formation of 1,25-dihydroxy-cholecalciferol in chronic renal insufficiency. *Lancet* 1973;1:625.
492. Sy WM, Mittal AK: Bone scan in chronic dialysis patients with evidence of secondary hyperparathyroidism and renal osteodystrophy. *Br J Radiol* 1975;48:878.
493. Sebes JI, Pinstein ML, Massie JD, et al.: Radiographic manifestations of aluminum-induced bone disease. *AJR* 1984; 142:424.
494. Olgaard K, Heerfordt J, Madsen S: Scintigraphic skeletal changes in uremic patients on regular hemodialysis. *Nephron* 1976;17:325.
495. Hamdy RC: *Paget's Disease of Bone.* Eastbourne, Praeger, 1981, pp 13–21; 37–46.
496. Rebel A, Basle M, Pouplar A, et al.: Towards a viral etiology for Paget's disease of bone. *Metab Bone Dis Re Res* 1981;3:235.
497. Fogelman I, Ignac B: Bone scanning in Paget's disease, in: Freeman LM (ed): *Nuclear Medicine Annual 1991,* New York, Raven Press, 1991, p 99.
498. Resnick D, Niwayama G: *Diagnosis of Bone and Joint Disorders,* Vol 1. Philadelphia, W.B. Saunders, 1981, p 848, 1726.
499. Rausch JM, Resnick D, Goergen TG, Taylor A: Bone scanning in osteolytic Paget's disease: case report. *J Nucl Med* 1977;18:699.
500. Wellman HN, Schauwecker D, Robb JA, et al.: Skeletal scintiimaging and radiography in the diagnosis and management of Paget's disease. *Clin Orthop* 1977;127:55.
501. Serafini AN: Paget's disease of bone. *Semin Nucl Med* 1976;6:47.
502. Boudreau RJ, Lisbona R, Hadjipavlou A: Observations on serial radionuclide blood-flow studies in Paget's disease. *J Nucl Med* 1983;24:880.
503. Fogelman I, Carr D: A comparison of bone scanning and radiology in the assessment of patients with symptomatic Paget's disease. *Eur J Nucl Med* 1980;5:417.
504. Albright F, Butler AM, Hampton AO, Smith P: Syndrome characterized by osteitis fibrosa disseminata, areas of pigmentation and endocrine dysfunction, with precocious puberty in females. Report of five cases. *N Engl J Med* 1937;216:727.
505. Harris WH, Dudley HR, Barry RJ: The natural history of fibrous dysplasia: an orthopaedic, pathological and roentgenographic study. *J Bone Joint Surg* 1962;44A:207.
506. Nance FL, Fonseca RJ, Burkes EJ: Technetium bone imaging as an adjunct in the management of fibrous dysplasia. *Oral Surg Oral Med Oral Path* 1980;50:199.
507. Pfeffer S, Molina E, Feuillan P, Simon TR: McCune-Albright syndrome: the patterns of scintigraphic abnormalities. *J Nucl Med* 1990;31:1474.
508. Lutzker LG, Alavi A: Bone and marrow imaging in sickle cell disease: diagnosis of infarction. *Semin Nucl Med* 1976;6:83.
509. Alavi A, Bond JP, Kuhl DE, et al.: Scan detection of bone marrow infarcts in sickle cell disorders. *J Nucl Med* 1974;15:1003.
510. Valdez VA, Jacobstein JG: Decreased bone uptake of technetium-99m polyphosphate in thalassemia major. *J Nucl Med* 1980;21:47.
511. Resnick D, Niwayama G: *Diagnosis of Bone and Joint Disorders.* Philadelphia, W.B. Saunders, Vol 3, 1981, p 3006.
512. Mahoney J, Achong DM: Demonstration of increased bone metabolism in melorheostosis by multiphase bone scanning. *Clin Nucl Med* 1991;16:847.
513. Drane WE: Detection of melorheostosis on bone scan. *Clin Nucl Med* 1987;12:548.
514. Hattner RS: Skeletal scintigraphy in pachydermoperiostosis. *Eur J Nucl Med* 1981;6:477.
515. Bomanji J, Nagaraj N, Jewkes R, et al.: Pachydermoperiostosis: technetium-99m-methylene diphosphonate scintigraphic pattern. *J Nucl Med* 1991;32:1907.
516. Whyte MP, Murphy WA, Siegel BA: Tc-99m pyrophosphate bone imaging in osteopoikilosis, osteopathia striata, and melorheostosis. *Radiology* 1978;127:439.
517. Weiss TE, Maxfield WS, Murison PJ, et al.: Iodinated human serum albumin (K-131) localization studies of rheumatoid arthritis joints by scintillation scanning. *Arthritis Rheum* 1965;8:976.
518. Alarcón-Segovia D, Trujegue M, Tovaz E, et al.: Scintillation scanning of the joints with technetium-99m. Proceedings of the Annual Meeting of the American Rheumatism Association, New York, 1967.
519. Seaulniers M, Fuks A, Hawkins D, et al.: Radiotechnetium polyphosphate joint imaging. *J Nucl Med* 1974;15:417.
520. Beckerman C, Genant HK, Hoffer PB, et al.: Radionuclide imaging of the bones and joints of the hand: a definition of normal and comparison of sensitivity using ^{99m}-Tc-pertechnetate and ^{99m}Tc-diphosphonate. *Radiology* 1975;118:653.
521. Weissberg DL, Resnick D, Taylor A, et al.: Rheumatoid arthri-

tis and its variants: analysis of scintiphotographic, radiographic, and clinical examinations. *AJR* 1978;131:665.
522. Thomas RH, Resnick D, Alazraki NP, et al.: Compartmental evaluation of osteoarthritis of the knee: a comparative study of available diagnostic modalities. *Radiology* 1975;116:685.
523. Forrester DM, Hensel AL, Brown JC: The use of gallium-67 citrate to distinguish infectious and non-infectious arthritis. *Clin Rheum Dis* 1983;9:333.
524. Sy WM, Bay R, Camera A: Hand images: normal and abnormal. *J Nucl Med* 1977;18:419.
525. McCarty DJ, Polcyn RE, Collins PA: Technetium-99m scintiphotography in arthritis. II. Its nonspecificity and clinical and roentgenographic correlations in rheumatoid arthritis. *Arthritis Rheum* 1970;13:21.
526. Lentle BC, Russell AS, Percy JS, et al.: The scintigraphic investigation of sacroiliac disease. *J Nucl Med* 1977;18:529.
527. Epstein DH, Graves RW, Higgins WL: Clinical significance of increased temporomandibular joint uptake by planar isotope bone scan. *Clin Nucl Med* 1987;12:705.
528. Collier D, Carrera GF, Messer EJ, et al.: Internal derangement of the temporomandibular joint: detection by single-photon emission computed tomography. *Radiology* 1983;149:557.
529. Katzberg RW, O'Mara RE, Tallents RH, et al.: Radionuclide skeletal imaging and single photon emission computed tomography in suspected internal derangements of the temporomandibular joint. *J Maxillofac Surg* 1984;42:782.
530. Craemer TD, Ficara AJ: The value of the nuclear medical scan in the diagnosis of temporomandibular joint disease. *Oral Surg* 1984;58:382.
531. Matin P: Basic principles of nuclear medicine techniques for detection and evaluation of trauma and sports medicine injuries. *Semin Nucl Med* 1988;18:90.
532. Collier BD, Hellman RS, et al.: Bone SPECT. *Semin Nucl Med* 1987;12:247.
533. Kohn HS, Guten GN, Colleir BD, et al.: Chondromalacia of the patella. Bone imaging corelated with arthroscopic findings. *Clin Nucl Med* 1988;13:96.
534. Stewart CA, Fernandez OA: Normal scapulae or rib lesions: Value of arm-abducted and arm-adducted views. *Clin Nucl Med* 1991;16:281.

34 Bone Densitometry

Martin Erlichman, Thomas Holohan

Various medical conditions, such as asymptomatic primary hyperparathyroidism, and treatments, such as long-term steroid therapy and thyroid hormone replacement, can result in premature bone mass loss and osteoporosis, which often go undetected until the person sustains a fracture. About 1.3 million fractures that occur annually in the United States in people over age 45 are ascribed to osteoporosis.[1] Fractures exact an enormous toll on human disability and suffering and greatly increase health-care costs.

Bone densitometry is used to measure bone mass density to determine the degree of osteoporosis and fracture risk. Commonly used techniques are: single-photon absorptiometry (SPA) of the forearm and heel, dual-photon and dual-energy X-ray absorptiometry (DPA and DEXA) of the spine and hip, quantitative computed tomography (QCT) of the spine or forearm, and radiographic absorptiometry (RA) of the hand.

Whether use of bone densitometry to document bone loss effectively alters the medical management of patients, to minimize the development of osteoporosis and fractures, remains controversial. The debate continues over selection of the best measurement sites and the availability of effective treatment to prevent progression of osteoporosis if significant bone loss is detected. Some concern also remains about the accuracy and precision of these techniques. These uncertainties have led to a lack of specific recommendations and protocols for bone mass testing.

In this section we will discuss those techniques that *may* be clinically useful in the medical management of patients with bone loss.

BACKGROUND

Since the 1960s, there has been a gradual development of noninvasive techniques to quantify bone mass density. Bone densitometers (absorptiometers) measure the radiation absorption (electron density) by the skeleton to determine bone mass. The term bone mass indicates the amount of mineralized tissue in bone; the term bone density indicates the mass of bone defined either by length (grams per centimeter, g/cm), area (grams per square centimeter, g/cm^2), or volume (grams per cubic centimeter, g/cm^3).

The geometric distribution of bone tissue, together with its material properties, is critical in determining the structural strength and rigidity of the whole bone. Although a variety of factors may influence bone strength and the probability of fracture, bone mass measurements are currently considered to be the most valuable objective indicator of fracture risk.[2,3]

Bone densitometers can evaluate bone density of the peripheral, axial, and total skeleton. Their clinical use is based on the assumption that bone mass is an important determinant of fractures, and that bone mass measurements may help reduce the number of fractures by identifying high-risk patients, who can then receive effective prophylaxis. Because osteoporosis is generally considered preventable but not reversible, early detection of at-risk individuals is essential.[4,5] Bone densitometry can also be used to document bone mass changes over time, monitoring the course of a disease and response to therapy.

Cortical and Trabecular Bone

Factors that influence bone strength include the amount (mass), type (quality), and architecture (structure) of mineralized bone. Adult bone tissue is primarily arranged either as dense cortical bone (also known as compact bone) or as a latticework of trabecular bone (also known as spongy or cancellous bone).

The combination of a smooth, dense outer layer of compact cortical bone together with spongy trabecular bone provides both structural strength and an extended surface, on which rapid changes in bone formation or resorption can respond to fluctuating metabolic needs. The metabolic responses of the skeleton mainly occur on trabecular bone surfaces.[6] Although the entire skeleton loses bone mass with aging, the distribution of bone loss is not uniform because of the different proportions of trabecular and cortical bone in the various parts of the skeleton.[7]

Osteopenia and Osteoporosis

Osteopenia refers to any condition involving reduced bone mass. Osteoporosis, a form of osteopenia, is decreased bone mass with normal bone mineralization. Bone densitometry generally has been applied to patients with bone loss associated with primary osteoporosis, which occurs mainly in postmenopausal women and the elderly. Secondary osteoporosis, which occurs in fewer than 5% of those with osteoporosis, can be a consequence of such treatment as long-term steroids or such conditions as chronic renal failure, rheumatoid arthritis, and hyperparathyroidism.

Primary osteoporosis is commonly classified as postmenopausal osteoporosis (type I) or age-related osteoporosis (type II).[8] This classification was presented by Riggs and Melton,[9] but not all investigators agree with it, and alternative proposals have been developed.[10] Type I osteoporosis occurs in a subset of postmenopausal women between the ages of 51 and 75 years, affects mainly trabecular bone, and is largely responsible for vertebral crush fractures and Colles' fractures.[11]

Type II osteoporosis is found in a large proportion of women and men over the age of 70 and results from a protracted slow phase of age-related bone loss. This condition affects twice as many women as men and is manifested mainly by hip and vertebral fractures.[9,11]

Historically, osteoporosis was recognized clinically only after fractures occurred. It was considered a syndrome consisting of both substantial bone loss and fractures.[12,13] With the development of techniques that measured bone loss before signs of radiographic change or the occurrence of fractures, osteoporosis was defined as an age-related disorder characterized by decreased bone mass and by increased susceptibility to fractures.[14]

How osteoporosis is defined is not a trivial issue. As a result of the various criteria used to define osteoporosis, estimates of its prevalence differ markedly. For example, if bone mass lower than 2 standard deviations (SD) below the mean of young normal women represents osteoporosis, then 45% of white women aged 50 years and older are osteoporotic.[15] A World Health Organization (WHO) study group recently defined osteoporosis as 2.5 SD below that mean, which identifies 30% of all postmenopausal women as osteoporotic, more than half of whom will have sustained a prior fracture.[16]

There is a growing tendency to define osteoporosis in terms of a continuum of bone density, with greatest fracture risk in those with lowest absolute density values, rather than in considering osteoporosis as a fracture/nonfracture dichotomy.[17] However, so-called "fracture thresholds" have been approximated for various skeletal sites to diagnose osteoporosis based on a level of bone mass above which nontraumatic fractures rarely occur, and below which fractures are more common. For example, 90% of women with vertebral fractures have spinal bone density values less than 0.97 g/cm^2 measured by DPA.[18,19] Although disagreement continues, the definition developed at the Consensus Development Conference,[20] held in Copenhagen in October of 1990, is generally accepted. That conference defined osteoporosis as a disease characterized by low bone mass and microarchitectural deterioration of bone tissue leading to enhanced bone fragility and a consequent increase in fracture risk.

Fractures

Although osteoporosis affects all bones, the most common so-called osteoporotic-related fractures are those involving the spine (thoracic and lumbar vertebral bodies); femur (the neck and intertrochanteric regions); and the wrist (distal radius).[1] In persons over the age of 50, the incidence of these fractures increases markedly. Fractures of the distal radius, common in the middle-aged and elderly, are caused by a fall on the outstretched hand. Approximately 172,000 osteoporotic fractures occurred in the distal radius during 1985.[21] The most severe osteoporotic fracture is that of the hip, a disabling and sometimes fatal event. The prevalence of hip fractures in the United States reaches 15% by age 80 and exceeds 25% by age 90.[1] Between 250,000 and 300,000 hip fractures occur each year in the United States, and the incidence may be increasing.[22–24]

Although the true incidence of vertebral fracture is not known, more than 25% of all women over age 65 may have sustained a crush fracture, most of which are asymptomatic.[1] Fractures occurring at other sites, including the rib, pelvis, humerus, and proximal tibia also may be attributable to osteoporosis.[25]

BONE MASS MEASUREMENT TECHNIQUES

Single-Photon Absorptiometry

SPA is a noninvasive radiologic technique used to assess bone mass in the appendicular skeleton, usually the radius or calcaneus. SPA evaluates the amount of bone mass by measuring the transmission of gamma rays through bone. It is a simple, widely available, and relatively inexpensive measurement technique that involves minimum radiation exposure, with negligible bone-marrow or gonadal radiation.[26,27]

Figure 1 illustrates the principles of single photon bone densitometry described by Cameron and Sorenson.[28] Bone mineral content can be measured by comparing the gamma-ray transmission through bone compared to the transmission through a tissue-dense medium, such as a water bath. If I_O is the intensity of the photon beam through the unobstructed medium (e.g., the water bath) and I_O^* is the intensity as measured through a thickness of T tissue; then:

$$I_O^* = \mathrm{I}_O \exp(-\mu_m T) \qquad (1)$$

where μ_m is the *linear* attenuation coefficient for soft tissue. Then for the measurement through bone,

$$I = I_O \exp(-\mu_m T_m + \mu_b T_b) \qquad (2)$$

where T_m and T_b are unknown thickness of tissue and bone mineral, respectively. If the bone is surrounded by tissue-equivalent material then

$$T = T_m + T_b \qquad (3)$$

The attenuation coefficient for bone, μ_b is found by assuming a standard composition for bone mineral or by measuring a sample of known thickness. Similarly, μ_m can be found either from tabulated values, or from equation (1). From equations

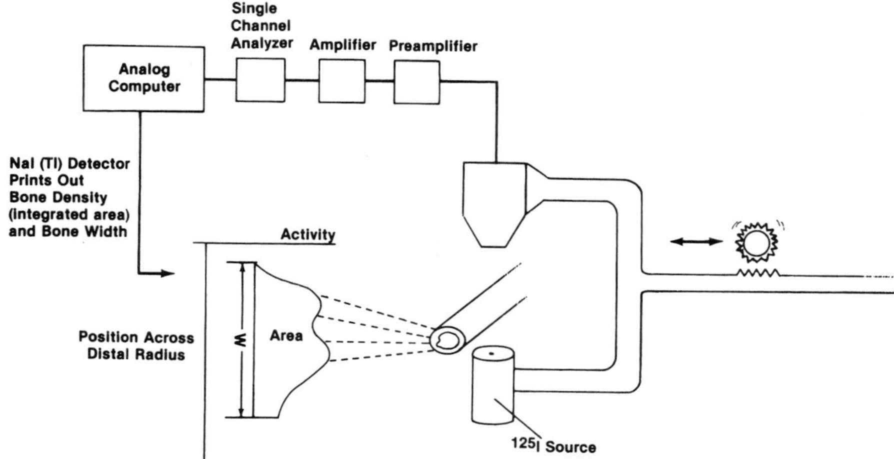

Figure 1. Schematic of bone densitometer and the integration of transmitted counts, which is inversely proportional to bone mineral content.

(2) and (3), with two unknowns, T_m and T_b, T_b, the thickness of bone mineral in the beam path can be calculated. If we assume an average density for bone mineral, say 1.85 g/mL, then multiplying T_b times the density fixes the bone mineral mass in the beam path, M_b, in g/cm^2. Because this varies as the beam moves across the bone, the usual method is to integrate these values across the scan, giving M_b in g/cm. This is generally referred to as bone mineral content.

The earliest SPA measurements were performed at the mid-radius, which is almost all cortical bone (approximately 95%). However, interest in trabecular bone mass, coupled with technical advances in SPA, such as rectilinear scanning and area density measurements, provided the capability of assessing sites with greater proportions of trabecular bone: the calcaneus and distal radius.

The calcaneus is a weight-bearing bone of approximately 90 to 95% trabecular bone by volume. It is very active metabolically and may reflect the effects of age, menopause, exercise, and drugs on axial bone such as the spine.[29] Recent prospective studies show promising results for the value of calcaneus measurements in predicting fractures at peripheral, as well as axial, sites. However, the ability of SPA measurements at the calcaneus and radius to predict spinal bone density remains controversial.[30,31]

A summary of SPA characteristics is presented in Table 1.

The accuracy error of SPA measurements is determined from a calibration of the technique with the ash weight of a dried defatted human radius.[32] Calibration can also be made with standards calibrated against ashed bone sections. SPA can provide highly accurate measurements (1 to 3% error) on phantoms and bone specimens. However, accuracy errors of 3 to 8% are more common in the clinical setting.[30]

The precision error of SPA measurements is determined by repeated measurements of aluminum standards and patient controls. Routine clinical scans of the radius and calcaneus have a precision error of 2 to 5%, largely as a result of repositioning errors and the low, and constantly decreasing, intensity of the photon source.[33] Changes in SPA measurements may also occur as a result of treatment that alters body fat; a measured increase in bone density may reflect a decrease in the subcutaneous forearm fat and not a "real" gain in bone.[34]

The 60-day half-life of the ^{125}I source necessitates source changes several times a year and, thus, has the potential to adversely affect instrument reliability.[33] A similar device that uses an x-ray source (SXA) rather than an isotopic source is also available. The x-ray source, with its significantly greater photon output, improves the precision and the speed of the scans. Because of this and the increasing cost of ^{125}I sources, SPA is being replaced by SXA.

More detailed descriptions of SPA may be found in recent reviews by Lang et al.,[35] Tothill,[36] and Wahner.[37]

Table 1. Comparison of Bone Mass Measurement Techniques

	SITE SCAN TIME (min)	PRECISION ERROR (%)	ACCURACY ERROR (%)	RADIATION EXPOSURE (mrem)
SPA	Radius, calcaneus; 5–15	2–5	3–8	2–5
DPA	Spine, hip; 20–40	2–5	3–10	5–10
QCT	Spine; 5–30	2–6	5–15	100–1000
DEXA	Spine, hip; 5–10	0.5–3	3–9	<5
RA	Hands; 5–10	2–4	5–10	10–100

(Adapted from references 26, 27, 30, 31, 35, 37, 61, 72, 76, 79.)

Dual-Photon Absorptiometry

DPA is usually used to measure bone density in the spine and hip, but can also be used to quantify total body bone mass.[35] It offers no advantage over SPA for measuring appendicular bones. Unlike SPA, its energy source emits photons of two distinct energies, allowing imaging of thicker body parts.

The instrumentation for DPA is similar to that shown schematically in Fig. 1, although the opening is large enough to accommodate the entire body. The most common photon source is ^{153}Gd, which emits photons that average about 45 keV and 100 keV.

The principle of DPA is quite similar to SPA. Equation (2) can be modified, so that if transmission measurements are made at two different energies, 1 and 2, then at each point:

$$I^1 = I_o^2 \exp\left(-\mu_t^1 M_t - \mu_b^1 M_b\right)$$
$$I^2 = I_o^2 \exp\left(-\mu_t^2 M_t - \mu_b^2 M_b\right)$$

where μ_t and μ_b are now the *mass* attenuation coefficients for tissue and bone at the given energies, and M_t and M_b represent the mass of tissue and bone in the photon beam in g/cm^2. Measuring I and I_o, the unattenuated beam, and taking known values of μ, in 2 equations and 2 unknowns, M_t and M_b, yield the value of M_b. Unlike SPA, DPA does not require uniform tissue thickness, so that it is not necessary to know the soft tissue absorption coefficients, because measurements through points containing only soft tissue gives the ratio of μ_t^1 to μ_t^2 so that they can be eliminated from the equation in solving for M_b.

M_b, the mineral mass, is termed the *bone mineral density*, in units of g/cm^2, and represents the total mineral in a column 1 cm in cross-sectional area.

Scanning is somewhat slow (35 minutes), but involves a low radiation dose with negligible gonadal radiation. The 253-days half-life of ^{153}Gd necessitates changing the source every 12 to 18 months. DPA bone density measures reflect the total integrated mineral (cortical and trabecular) content and any extraosseous mineral in the path of the beam.

DPA scan sites and other characteristics are summarized in Table 1 and illustrated in Figs. 2 and 3. Lumbar spine measurements by DPA are usually performed at the L2-L4 region, imaged as a planar area. DPA measurements quantify bone mass of the entire vertebral body, including spinous processes and posterior elements, as well as calcification within surrounding tissues; for example, the aorta.[38] Abnormalities in the spine, including osteophytes, endplate hypertrophy, disc degeneration, calcified aorta, and fractures, are common in patients over 65 years of age.[38,39] These coexisting conditions may result in inaccurate and poorly reproducible vertebral measurements, and have led to a preference for femoral measurements.[38,40]

DPA measurements of the proximal femur are usually performed at the femoral neck but may also include the trochanteric region, as well as a highly trabecular area called Ward's triangle.[38] There are few measurement errors attributable to artifacts in the hip region; however, the results can be affected significantly by patient positioning. DPA computer software that does not compensate adequately for the wide variation in the anatomy of the femoral neck and adjacent soft tissues also contributes to inaccurate measurements.

The accuracy error of DPA measurements is usually determined from calibrations with ashed bone (excised human vertebrae) or equivalent hydroxyapatite in the projected area.[41] DPA can achieve an accuracy error of about 3% on phantoms and bone specimens; however, accuracy errors of 3 to 10% are more common clinically.[42,43]

The precision error of DPA measurements is determined by repeated measurements on phantoms, ashed bones, and patient controls. Routine clinical scans of the spine and femur have precision errors of 2 to 5%. Imprecision largely results from technical factors (as with all radiologic methods), establishment of suitable soft-tissue baselines, and the low and constantly decreasing intensity of the photon source.[44,45] Higher precision measurements (2 to 3% CV) are achieved with careful attention to baselines, bone edges, and quality assurance.

More detailed descriptions of DPA are found in recent reviews by Lang et al.,[35] Tothill,[36] Wahner,[37] and Mazess.[30]

Dual-Energy X-ray Absorptiometry

DEXA is a modification of DPA, using an x-ray, instead of a radionuclide source, to measure bone density. The advantages of DEXA over SPA and DPA, both of which it is rapidly replacing, are scanning speed, low radiation dose, and more precise measurements that make changes in bone density over time easier to assess.[46] Other terms used to describe the dual-energy x-ray technology are quantitative digital radiography, dual-energy radiographic absorptiometry, dual-energy radiography, and dual x-ray absorptiometry. DEXA systems have one x-ray source that produce photons of two distinct energies, a photon detector, and an interface with a computer system for imaging the scanned areas. Table 1 summarizes DEXA characteristics.

DEXA systems have greater photon output (higher photon flux) than radionuclide sources, improved detector configuration, and automated analysis procedures. These developments provide higher spatial resolution, improved precision, shorter scanning times (10 minutes for the lumbar spine and proximal femur and 20 minutes for a total body scan), and reduced radiation dose compared with QCT, DPA, and RA.[48–50] High-resolution imaging facilitates reproducible bone edge detection, improves visualization of the area measured, maximizes the number of bones measurable, and allows artifacts to be recognized and eliminated from the analysis.[51,52] These improvements become particularly important for analyzing spinal bone density in osteoporotics.[35,53] Increased scan speed reduces errors resulting from patient motion and is also more convenient for patients with back pain.

Like DPA, DEXA measurements reflect the total inte-

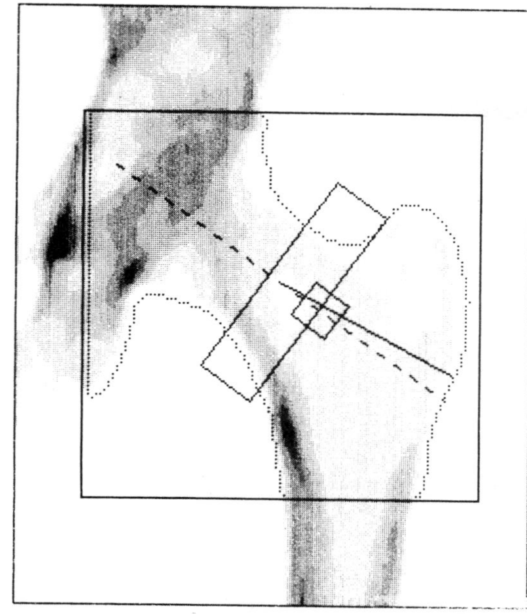

TOTAL BMD CV 1.0%

C.F.	0.988	0.981	1.000
Region	Est.Area (cm2)	Est.BMC (grams)	BMD (gms/cm2)
Neck	5.88	4.15	0.705
Troch	11.06	6.35	0.574
Inter	14.19	13.16	0.927
TOTAL	31.13	23.66	0.760
Ward's	1.12	0.73	0.655

Midline (96,108)-(176, 50)

Neck -58 x 16 at [29, 3]

Troch 8 x 49 at [0, 0]

Ward's -11 x 11 at [6, -7]

Figure 2. DPA scan and BMD measurements of the left hip.

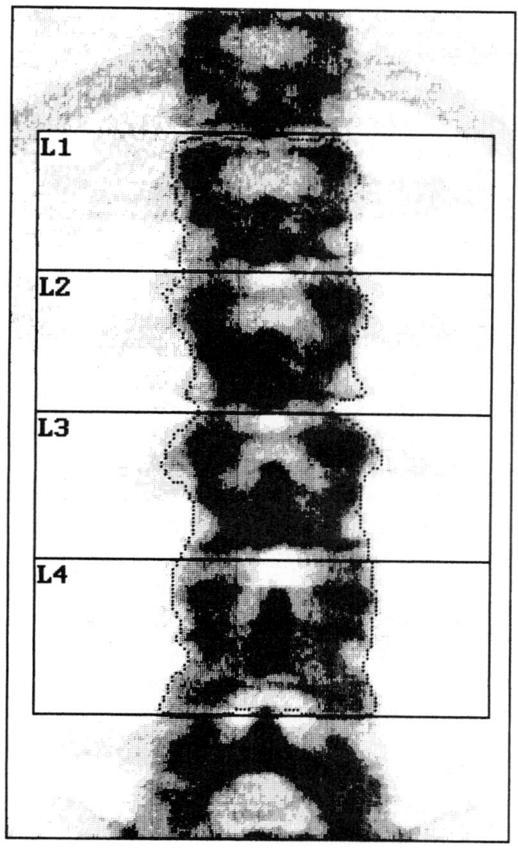

TOTAL BMD CV FOR L1 - L4 1.0%

C.F.	0.988	0.981	1.000
Region	Est.Area (cm2)	Est.BMC (grams)	BMD (gms/cm2)
L1	14.19	12.22	0.861
L2	14.49	13.97	0.964
L3	16.25	16.99	1.046
L4	18.56	18.81	1.013
TOTAL	63.49	61.99	0.976

Figure 3. DPA scan and BMD measurements of the lumbar spine.

grated (cortical and trabecular) mineral and any extraosseous mineral in the path of the beam. These techniques determine the bone density from a conventional anterior-posterior image (AP projection). The sites most commonly measured are the lumbar spine, generally L2-L4 or L1-L4. Other sites include the hip (the femoral neck, the intertrochanteric region, and Ward's triangle) and forearm.[35,54]

DEXA scans of the lumbar spine in the lateral projection were recently developed.[51,55] This may minimize the effect of the posterior arch (cortical bone) on measurements, as well as aortic calcification and posterior osteoarthritis, conditions common in the elderly that can falsely indicate elevated bone density.[38] This modification makes possible a more sensitive, direct approximation of trabecular bone.[51] The clinical value of this scanning technique is currently being evaluated.[56,57]

Although reviews of recent studies report DEXA accuracy errors from 3 to 6%, other data indicate that DEXA accuracy error on ashed bone specimens is about 9%.[58] According to Kelly et al.,[52] systematic errors in DEXA measurements at the spine can alter the apparent normal range for bone density in the population. They found that the mean value of populations measured by various DEXA instruments may differ by as much as 20%.

Routine clinical scans of the spine and femur have a precision error of 0.5 to 3%.[38,49,53] These high-precision measurements are largely the result of increased x-ray flux and improved spatial resolution. Long-term precision depends on technician skill for selecting the correct sequence of vertebrae, correct angulation of the leg (femur measurement), and correct bone area. It is essential that the same area be compared each time or additional errors can result.

More detailed descriptions of DEXA are available in reports by Wahner,[56] Kellie,[48] Wahner et al.,[41] and Kelly et al.[52]

Quantitative Computed Tomography

QCT is the application of conventional CT scanners and commercially available software packages to the quantitative measurement of bone density in the spine. An advantage of QCT, which measures bone in three-dimensional sections (volume), is its ability to separate cortical from trabecular bone with great anatomic detail. QCT precision has improved (2 to 6%), and both scanning time (15 to 20 minutes) and radiation dose (about equal to a chest x-ray, but 200 to 500 times the DEXA dose) have been reduced as a result of new calibration standards, software, and improved scanner design.[46] A summary of QCT characteristics is presented in Table 1. More detailed descriptions are available in recent reviews by Cann,[59] Lang et al.,[35] Mazess,[38] and Genant et al.[60]

Different localization and scanning procedures are used to obtain axial sections at the center of the vertebral body. In principle, total, cortical, or trabecular bone density can be measured centrally or peripherally. In practice, however, the method has been developed to measure the central trabecular portion (the spongiosa) of 2 to 4 adjacent lumbar vertebral bodies.[51,35] These representative volumes of trabecular bone are quantified and averaged, and the results are expressed as mineral equivalents in g/cm^3. This area covers approximately 35% of vertebral trabecular bone and represents a volume of about 3 cm^3 of purely trabecular bone in each of the lumbar vertebrae.

With QCT, the change in vertebral (trabecular) bone during the immediate postmenopausal period was reported as 5 to 7% per year, which is about 2 to 3 times that observed by integral DPA measurements and 3 to 5 times that seen in the cortical radial sites. Recommendations for monitoring postmenopausal bone loss at the spine with QCT are based on these observations of higher estimates of bone loss. However, overestimation of menopausal spinal bone loss due to variable marrow fat, low precision, and higher radiation exposure have limited this use.[36,60,61]

Although QCT can assess the purely trabecular portion of the spine and may, hypothetically, provide a more accurate assessment of fracture risk, there is no evidence that this potential benefit outweighs the problems and limitations of the method. Moreover, the contribution of the cortical compartment to crush fracture is being evaluated, and the concept that only the trabecular bone content is important is being challenged.[62,63] No prospective clinical trials with QCT have been conducted to determine its utility for assessing the risk of spinal fractures.

QCT can be performed with most existing CT units. However, to adapt an existing CT scanner for quantitative measurements of bone density requires software and mineral reference standards (phantoms) with sophisticated calibration and positioning techniques.[40,64] Because CT x-ray output is variable, calibration standards (solutions of varying concentrations of potassium phosphate; K_2HPO_4) should be measured simultaneously with the patient.[39] Even so, some errors remain.

QCT accuracy is also determined with measurements of vertebral specimens correlated with ash weight. The accuracy error of QCT is 1 to 2% for potassium phosphate solutions and 5 to 15% for human vertebral specimens. A variety of technical factors (scattered radiation, beam hardening, position in the beam, slice orientation) contribute to errors in QCT measurements. QCT exhibits an accuracy error of 6 to 9% in healthy younger individuals, but becomes increasingly inaccurate (10 to 15%) with aging and with bone disease because of the variability of marrow fat within the vertebral bodies.[30]

The precision error of QCT measurements is determined by repeated measurements on cadavers, phantoms, and patient controls. Some concern remains about the reproducibility of QCT spinal bone density measurements. Despite procedures that have enhanced the technique, some bone studies still show QCT reproducibility to be relatively poor (>3% precision error).[65] This is usually because of machine drift and repositioning errors.

The precision error of vertebral QCT in research settings providing exact detail to patient positioning and instrument performance is about 1 to 3% and is 2 to 6% in other settings, such as hospitals and clinics.[35,56,59] However, the precision of multipurpose hospital scanners is generally not better than 5 to 10%.[46] In research settings with dedicated CT scanners, quality control for bone density measurements is achieved. However, quality assurance in other clinical settings (for example, hospitals and offices) is frequently lacking.[55,64]

Although most bone mass measurements by QCT use the single-energy scanner, a dual-energy scanner is available that is usually used for research purposes.[66] Although the dual-energy scanner can correct for changes in marrow fat and increase the accuracy of the measurement, it does so at a cost in complexity, precision, and higher radiation exposures.[55,67]

QCT techniques have been applied on a limited basis to the measurement of trabecular bone at the femoral neck.[35,67] Because of the complexity of the anatomy, reproducible bone density measurements will probably be difficult. Moreover, both cortical and trabecular bone loss may predispose to femoral neck fractures. Therefore, identification of individuals at risk may thus be improved by considering both types of bone deficit. An integrated measurement of cortical and trabecular bone may more reliably predict femoral strength and fracture risk than an independent assessment of either component.[68]

Ruegsegger et al.[69] suggest that cortical bone density and trabecular bone density may complement each other in the diagnosis of bone diseases. They believe that trabecular bone density (radius) is highly sensitive to perimenopausal bone loss or iatrogenic effects of drugs such as corticosteroids. However, the disadvantage of trabecular bone density is the broad range of normal values and its considerable age-dependency. In comparison, cortical bone density is limited to a very narrow range and does not show a pronounced age-dependency in healthy subjects. An individual deviation of 5% from the mean is sufficient to be significant.

A specially constructed CT instrument for the separate determination of trabecular and compact bone density in the appendicular skeleton is available.[39,58,68,69] Although much attention has been given to QCT measurements of lumbar vertebral bodies, a number of factors, including poor precision and accuracy and higher levels of radiation exposure, make this location less than ideal for bone density measurements. In comparison to QCT of the spine, measurements at the radius take less time, have improved precision and accuracy, and expose the patient to less radiation.[70]

Radiographic Absorptiometry

RA is a noninvasive radiologic technique primarily used to measure the small bones of the hand (phalanges). It uses a computer-assisted densitometric measurement of the x-ray image of these bones.[71] Similar techniques are referred to as aluminum equivalency, photodensitometry, and radiographic densitometry.[64,72] Measurements of bone density by RA have been used to provide an index for skeletal status in the assessment of renal osteodystrophy,[73] and to assess bone density in studies of bone response to various treatment regimens for osteoporosis and other metabolic bone diseases.[72,74] A summary of RA characteristics is presented in Table 1. More detailed descriptions are available in the 1987 OHTA RA assessment report by Erlichman[75] and elsewhere.[36,72]

RA involves minimal radiation exposure (up to 100 mrem), with negligible bone marrow or gonadal radiation.[27] On average, RA delivers about 40 mrem to the patient.[72] RA bone mass analyses are based on phalangeal scans of pairs of lightly exposed radiographs taken at different kilovoltage and exposure settings. An aluminum alloy reference wedge, which allows the computer to compensate automatically for any between-film differences in exposure, kilovoltage, filtration, film type, or film processing conditions, is included in the image field. A computer-controlled optical densitometer scans the x-ray image with a light beam. The density of the film image over the bone is compared with that over the soft tissue, and the resultant absorption is related to normal values of phalangeal bone obtained from age- and sex-matched controls.[75,76]

Although RA can be used to study the metacarpal, radius, and other appendicular bones, it is most often used to measure the phalanges, a mixture of compact and trabecular bone with minimal overlying soft tissue.[36] X-rays of small bones, with minimal soft tissue cover, only require multiplication of the optical densitometry measurement by a constant and do not demand immersion of the hand in a layer of tissue-equivalent material (water bath), according to some investigators.[71] Other researchers do not find variations in soft-tissue thickness corrected by a constant multiplier.[72,77,78] This issue remains controversial.

RA was developed in an attempt to circumvent some of the inherent limitations and errors in the use of an x-ray image to measure bone mass. The accuracy error of RA measurements is determined by calibrations of ashed bones and an aluminum reference wedge. The wedge serves as a standard, in which its measured optical density is compared to the optical densities for bone. Certain technical problems inherent in this technique, however, reduce the accuracy of the measurement.[79] The accuracy error for excised bones is 3 to 5% and 5 to 10% for bones with a slight tissue cover.[72,80] As with the other bone densitometry techniques, correcting the measurement for variation in the amount of soft tissue and fat overlying the bone is a problem. The precision error of RA measurements, determined by repeated measurements on phantom hands and patient controls, is between 2 and 4%.[81–83]

Comparison of Bone Mass Measurement Techniques

Both SPA and DPA use radioisotopes as their photon source for imaging bones; DEXA, QCT, and RA use x-ray sources. Like SPA and DPA, DEXA cannot separate cortical from trabecular bone. However, it can scan an area much more rapidly and is more precise than DPA, which it is quickly replacing.[84] Although widely available, DPA devices are no longer manufactured.[85]

The advantage of QCT is its ability to separate cortical from trabecular bone with great anatomic detail. On the other hand, it is a much more difficult scan to perform. Although it only exposes the patient to radiation levels equivalent to a chest x-ray, QCT emits 100 times or more the radiation of DEXA. Finally, RA is used to measure bone density in the hand.

As yet, there is no agreement on which method or methods are most clinically effective for diagnosing and monitoring the individual patient or for identifying the high-risk patient for therapeutic intervention.

Table 1 presents a comparison of the technical features of SPA, DPA, DEXA, QCT, and RA. Important differences in the characteristics and performance of these techniques include radiation exposure from the scan, the bone and bone site measured, and the accuracy and precision achieved. All these factors can affect the clinical utility of a given technique for managing specific patients.

SITE SELECTION

Although cost and radiation exposure are considerations that may influence the choice of a measurement site, the most important consideration is the ability to indicate fracture risk. Presently, there are insufficient longitudinal data to determine if any technique or skeletal site is better than others for quantifying bone mass or measuring bone loss rates.[86] Controversy continues regarding the best choice of a bone mass measurement site for determining the extent of osteoporosis and predicting fracture risk. Some studies conclude that to predict fracture risk in a bone, the bone density of that specific bone should be measured, and that measurements made at other parts of the skeleton have less predictive value.[87] Conversely, others conclude that patients with vertebral fractures have generalized osteoporosis. Therefore, the measurement of spinal bone density has no predictive advantage over that of the forearm and the risk of vertebral fracture can be predicted from appendicular sites as well as the spine (axial skeleton).[88–90] This position is supported by the results of several recent prospective studies,[3,91–93] as well as another study[94] that found no convincing evidence that measurements made at the spine and hip are superior to appendicular sites for predicting subsequent fractures at the spine and hip. Yet, another new study[95] concludes that low bone mass is generalized in some women and more regional in others, and that those with the lowest bone mass measurements at any site are more likely to have extensive osteoporosis.

The ability to use a single-site measurement of bone density to evaluate general fracture risk at all sites has practical importance. It could eliminate the rationale for multiple-site measurements performed by some clinicians, and would put less emphasis on a technique's ability to measure a particular site. Techniques not capable of bone mass measurements at the spine and/or the hip would not be eliminated from consideration for that reason. For example, measurement of appendicular sites is considered easier, costs less, and can be done with most techniques. However, vertebral sites must be measured with DEXA or QCT, and these measurements can be difficult to reproduce in patients with spinal deformities and aortic calcification, artifacts that may confound the bone mass measurements. This has led some to recommend the hip, forearm (radius), and heel as alternative sampling sites.[56]

Site selection is also an issue when bone densitometry is used to monitor response to therapy because the cortical/trabecular composition of the measurement site must reflect the effects of particular therapeutic agents.[96] For example, Mazess et al.[97] consider the spine the most appropriate site for bone loss monitoring because it shows larger decreases in bone mass at the menopause than do appendicular sites, and larger increases in bone mass following estrogen-replacement therapy. However, others suggest that such a distinction may be unnecessary and that measurement of bone density by SPA or QCT of the forearm could be used for clinical followup of bone changes.[98,99]

Accuracy and Precision

Measurements obtained by densitometers are compared with an independent standard measurement of bone mass, such as ashed bone sections or phantom standards calibrated against ashed bone sections (phantoms).[72] The accuracy error is determined by how much the measurement varies from this accepted or "true" value. Precision error is the variability in the measurements occurring with repeated measurements of the same object.[42]

Concern has been expressed about the accuracy of various techniques, particularly in the clinical setting. SPA has the greatest accuracy in vivo; DEXA is considered the most precise, followed by SPA. The accuracy and precision of all the techniques can be reduced by improper patient positioning, changes in the strength of the radionuclide sources (SPA, DPA), improper calibration of the equipment, and inadequate quality assurance programs.

A technique's precision is critical for serial measurements that correctly document bone loss over time. A number of factors influence serial measurements, regardless of the technique chosen or site selected to determine bone mass. Attention to patient repositioning is necessary to assure that the exact same bone location is measured each time. If sequential scan locations are not matched, erroneous measurements may result, especially in regions of bone where bone mass is not uniform.

When the bone mass is expressed as an "area" density (SPA, DPA, DEXA), the limb must have the same rotation and axis at each measurement so that the projected area will be the same. When the forearm, spine, hip, or heel are measured, variations in rotation or angulation of the axis will adversely affect measurements.[2]

Changes in soft-tissue composition can also have significant effects on bone mass measurements. A change in soft tissue composition surrounding the bone to be measured changes the baseline reference values against which the bone absorbance values are compared. This is true equally for RA, SPA, DPA, and DEXA. For example, changes in SPA measurements may occur with treatment that alters body fat, such as anabolic steroids, norethindrone, or estrogen.[34] An increase in radial density determined by SPA may reflect a decrease in the subcutaneous forearm fat, rather than an increase in bone mass. Furthermore, the fat content of red marrow in the spine and femur changes with age and can influence absorbance. As a result, errors in QCT measurements of these sites generally increase in older patients.[2]

Changes in the strength of radionuclide sources (SPA, DPA) can significantly affect the precision of serial measurements. Serial DPA measurements can be subject to errors of up to 6% due to age (diminished activity) of the radionuclide source.[33,100,101] The relatively low and constantly decreasing intensity of photon sources leads to problems with long-term stability of these instruments. Instrumental instability and problems with software changes have now been recognized. Yet, it is still unclear how well certain calibration standards are able to correct for changes in radiation source intensity.[102]

The ability of densitometers to measure rates of change in bone mass depends on the magnitude of change, the precision of the method, and the number of measurements taken.[26] All 5 bone densitometry techniques are suitable for assessing rates of bone loss, provided that the interval between assessments is sufficiently long. If a technique has too high a precision error, its clinical utility is limited by the length of time it takes to detect significant bone loss in patients.[16,103]

The requisite minimum intervals between measurements that are necessary to reliably detect a reduction in bone mass are related to the precision attainable with current instruments and the rate of bone mass loss, assuming that the accuracy of the instrument is invariable. Table 2 illustrates the calculation of such intervals based upon published precision data, with assumed annual bone mass losses of 1 to 3%. The requisite intervals range from 1 to 17 years. However, it is unlikely that yearly densitometry would be clinically indicated, given the fact that 1% precision error is rarely attained and that a 3% annual loss in bone mass would be distinctly uncommon. Precision errors in the range of 2 to 3% and annual bone mass losses of 1 to 2% are parameters more representative of published data. In those instances, the minimum interval between densitometry measures necessary to document bone mass loss would be between 3.7 and 6 years.

Past experience with bone density measurements indicates that strict quality control, including calibration and standardization procedures, is required to maintain both precision and accuracy for reliable measurements.[33,101,104] Because differences in operator technique during scan analysis can result in large measurement variations, it is also important that a consensus be reached over procedural methods for positioning. Those who publish normal ranges should accurately describe the technique used.[47]

Even with instruments calibrated according to manufacturers' instructions, bone density values obtained by DPA and DEXA imaging of spine phantoms have differed by as much as 16%, because of differences as great as 8% in bone mass and approximately 8% in bone area.[96] Discrepancies in bone density measurements by different instruments appear to reflect differences in instrument design, computer algorithms, and calibration procedures.[37,96,105] For example, when comparing 3 DEXA instruments, Arai et al.[105] found each of them to be accurate when using their own standard. However, when the same lumbar spine phantom (standard) was used by each of the 3 systems, the bone mass density values measured by one system were 5 to 8% higher than those of the other two systems.

The calibration and standardization of bone densitometers is a complex undertaking that requires more attention because there is little agreement among manufacturers.[51,56] Although all manufacturers provide protocols for reference standards and phantom measurements, there is no industry-wide agreement for 1 specific standard that would provide machine-to-machine comparability. Users and/or manufacturers of bone densitometers need to adopt a uniform procedure for calibrating and standardizing instruments, and carry out quality control measurements using an accepted "gold standard."[96]

A report on bone mineral assessment by the National Health Technology Advisory Panel to the Australian Institute of Health recommends an accreditation policy to establish and identify quality assurance programs.[26] A review of the impact of such programs on the precision of densitometric techniques used in multicenter clinical studies shows that a 1 to 2% improvement in precision is achievable.[106]

ALTERNATIVE TECHNIQUES

Ultrasound

There are those who question whether low bone mass alone is a sufficient explanation for fractures.[7,107,108] Of significance is the discrepancy between bone density and fracture observed in studies where fluoride caused dramatic increases in the bone density of osteoporotic women without an expected decrease in fractures.[109,110]

Although bone mass correlates well with bone strength, other factors that influence the strength of bone cannot be assessed by bone mass measurements.[111,112] Ultrasound techniques, recently introduced to assess bone mass, can provide information that may be relevant to other aspects of bone quality, such as its geometry, architecture, and biomechanical properties.[113–117] These techniques use either ultrasonic veloc-

Table 2. Intervals Required to Reliably Detect Bone Mass Loss Over Time

TECHNIQUE PRECISION ERROR (CV %)	ESTIMATED BONE LOSS (%)	DIFFERENCE IN MEASUREMENTS (%)*	FOLLOWUP MEASUREMENT APPROXIMATELY (yrs)†
1	1	2.77	2.77
1	3	2.77	0.92
2	1	5.54	5.54
2	3	5.54	1.85
3	1	8.32	8.32
3	3	8.32	2.77
4	1	11.08	11.08
4	3	11.08	3.70
5	1	13.30	13.30
5	3	13.30	4.43
6	1	16.63	16.63
6	3	16.63	5.54

*Two scans (measurements) would have to differ by more than this amount to be confident that a real change had occurred, with 95% confidence that the detected losses are real.

†Time frame for a reliable bone mass measurement followup.

Note: This table assumes that accuracy is invariable.

ity or ultrasonic absorption in bone as an index of bone quality. Preliminary studies[113,115,116] of ultrasound bone assessment are promising, and have encouraged interest in the use of ultrasound as a technique to identify women with osteopenia. However, a recent study shows that DEXA measurements of the lumbar spine and femoral neck are significantly better than any of the ultrasound findings for determining osteopenia in the hip and spine.[118]

Ultrasound has clinical potential because of its relative low cost and ease of use, without the need for ionizing radiation. However, data are too limited to verify the usefulness of ultrasound to assess fracture risk, evaluate bone quality and structure, and identify what characteristics referable to bone quality are being measured.[114]

Biochemical Markers of Bone Turnover

Biochemical markers of bone turnover (bone formation and resorption) may help to determine the rate of bone loss.[20] There is considerable interest in the use of serum and urinary markers of bone metabolism to predict the skeletal status of women at risk of developing osteoporosis. These biochemical markers can reflect the enzymatic activity of osteoblasts or osteoclasts (for example, alkaline or acid phosphatase activity); can be proteins synthesized by the bone-forming cells (for example, osteocalcin or procollagen-1 extension peptides); or can be bone matrix components released into the circulation during resorption (for example, hydroxyproline or the pyridinoline crosslinks).[84]

According to Arnaud,[119] the utility of some bone markers may be limited by factors that make them both insensitive and nonspecific. Hansen et al.,[120] however, predicted future bone mass using SPA measurements of peak bone mass and an estimated rate of bone mass loss based on biochemical measurements. They found that the estimated bone loss was almost identical to the actual loss of bone mass measured 12 years later.

Recently, immunoassays have been developed to quantify urinary excretion of pyridinoline and deoxypyridinoline crosslinks. These were shown to measure the degree of collagen degradation and bone resorption. The potential clinical utility of crosslinks measurement will be in the detection of increased bone turnover in the perimenopause, so that osteoporosis prophylaxis can be instituted before appreciable menopausal bone loss occurs.[119] Alone or in combination with bone absorptiometry, bone markers may aid in the identification of patients at high risk for fracture.[121–123]

Bone Mass Measurements in Clinical Practice

There are a number of conditions in which bone mass measurements have been employed; these include asymptomatic primary hyperparathyroidism, long-term steroid therapy, and estrogen deficiency in women. However, it is not yet entirely clear whether the measurement of bone density ultimately improves patient outcome.

ASYMPTOMATIC PRIMARY HYPERPARATHYROIDISM

Primary hyperparathyroidism (PHPT) is a generalized disorder of calcium, phosphate, and bone metabolism caused by excessive parathyroid hormone (PTH) secretion.[124,125] Excess PTH enhances release of calcium from the bones, causing bone loss and hypercalcemia.[126] Approximately 100,000 new cases of primary hyperparathyroidism are diagnosed each year in the United States.[127] The disease occurs in women more than twice as often as in men, and the frequency increases with age. Most new cases are discovered incidentally to an elevated serum calcium detected on routine blood chemistry testing. Half or more of these newly diagnosed cases are asymptomatic, and many others have very mild or subtle symptoms.[124] We employ the term mild PHPT to include both asymptomatic patients and those with minimal symptoms.

Although all patients with PHPT may be considered potential candidates for parathyroidectomy, debate about the proper management of hyperparathyroid patients has intensified with the realization that new cases of PHPT are accompanied by a shift toward clinically milder disease.[127,128] Parathyroidectomy is becoming less frequently performed on patients with mild PHPT, particularly in the elderly.[129]

Because PHPT is primarily associated with cortical bone loss, single-photon absorptiometry (SPA) of the radius has been used to assess bone loss in most studies. Occasionally, quantitative computed tomography (QCT) or dual-photon absorptiometry (DPA) of the spine or hip have been used and, more recently, dual energy x-ray absorptiometry (DEXA). Bone densitometry measurements of the forearm essentially reflect cortical bone at the proximal site. The distal site, although predominantly cortical bone, is considered to have a higher percentage of trabecular bone (approximately 20 to 25%) than other radial sites.

Considerable evidence documents bone loss as diagnosis in patients with mild PHPT;[130–132] however, some studies also suggest that such accelerated osteoporosis may be self-limited, with patients showing little further decline in bone mass density after diagnosis.[133] Moreover, it is not clear as to whether PTH-related bone loss is associated with increased risk of fracture. Studies that have evaluated the risk of fracture in patients with mild PHPT are inconsistent.[134–137] One study,[128] in particular, found these patients were more likely than control subjects (matched by age and gender) to have a history of fractures prior to diagnosis (30% vs 18%, p = .055). Although over the entire pre-diagnosis medical history (median, 30 years) almost twice as many PHPT patients had one or more fractures, this difference did not reach statistical significance. Moreover, when only osteoporotic fractures were considered, 10% of the patients and 7% of the control subjects 35 years and older had experienced a fracture, a difference that was not statistically significant. Additionally, from the time of diagnosis both groups had similar rates of fracture during a follow-up of 12 years (36% vs 31%, p = .61). Fifty-three percent of the PHPT patients were not subject to parathyroidectomy during the 12-year follow-up period. These nonoperated patients had a slightly greater, but not significant excess of fractures than control patients. The only factor significantly related to fracture risk was age; serum calcium levels, surgical intervention, or comorbid conditions (e.g., hypertension, renal failure, peptic ulcer) were unrelated to excess fractures. Whether or not the bone loss associated with mild PHPT increases the risk of forearm, spine, or hip fractures in specific subpopulations of PHPT patients remains to be determined in much larger studies.

Currently, decisions to perform parathyroidectomy are based on signs and symptoms of bone disease, renal stones, decreased renal function, fatigue and/or depression, and high levels of serum calcium. Although the use of bone mass measurements has been advocated to aid clinical decisions regarding the risks and benefits of surgery, specific bone changes that indicate the need for parathyroidectomy have not been clearly established.

There are no prospective studies that evaluate decisions to operate based upon bone mass measurements, nor randomized clinical trials comparing the outcome of surgically treated patients with those who have not had surgery. In the absence of controlled clinical trials, the long-term risk/benefit ratio of decisions to operate based mainly upon bone mass measurements remains unknown.

LONG-TERM STEROID THERAPY

Steroids (glucocorticoids) have broad effects on both immune and inflammatory processes and are used to treat a wide variety of immunologically mediated diseases, such as connective tissue diseases (e.g., systemic lupus erythematosus, rheumatoid arthritis) severe asthma, vasculitides, granulomatous diseases, autoimmune hemolytic anemia, and organ transplant rejection.[138,139] Although steroids should be initiated only after less toxic therapy has been employed, sixteen million prescriptions for steroids are written annually.[140] Osteoporosis and vertebral compression fractures are considered major complications of prolonged steroid use.[138,139]

The true incidence of steroid-induced osteoporotic fracture is unknown. However, the reported incidence of bone fractures in steroid-treated patients ranges from 8 to 20% in some reviews[141,142] and 30 to 50% in others.[143,144] Because bone loss is intrinsically associated with some of the disease conditions treated with steroids, such as rheumatoid arthritis, the relationship between steroid therapy, bone loss, and fractures is complex.[143,145] Nevertheless, it has been established that prolonged exposure to therapeutic doses of steroids causes loss of bone, with the most rapid bone loss believed to occur in the first 2 to 6 months of therapy.[143,146]

Currently, steroid-induced osteoporosis is considered the most common secondary form of osteoporosis.[1] The higher incidence in women with rheumatic diseases that may require steroid therapy, coupled with the relatively compromised skeletal status of the postmenopausal female, may explain why steroid-induced osteoporosis is more common among women.[1]

Single-photon absorptiometry (SPA) and dual-photon absorptiometry (DPA) are bone mass measurement techniques often used to document bone mass loss in patients receiving steroids; use of quantitated computed tomography (QCT) is less common and dual-energy x-ray absorptiometry (DEXA) is replacing DPA. Typically, SPA is performed on the nondominant arm at a diaphyseal site (proximal radius) of primarily compact cortical bone (approximately 90%) and at a metaphyseal site (distal radius) with a larger proportion of trabecular bone (approximately 20 to 25%). In some studies, a diaphyseal mass (DM): metaphyseal mass (MM) ratio is calculated because steroid therapy is considered to be associated with a disproportionate loss of MM, producing elevation of the DM:MM ratio that would identify patients with steroid-induced osteopenia.[147] However, the utility of appendicular site measurements to identify loss of bone mass and predict fractures at vertebral sites remains controversial.

It has been suggested that bone densitometry be used to guide clinical decisions in patients receiving prolonged steroid therapy. Several important issues must be considered in this evaluation: the type and extent of bone loss, risk for fracture, whether steroid dose reduction or alternative therapy is an option, and whether steroid-induced osteoporosis can be prevented or treated. However, predicting the overall effect of steroid treatment on the musculoskeletal system in individual patients is difficult, due to large variations in bone mass, complications of the underlying disease, and susceptibility to the steroid treatment.

Moreover, the relationship between prolonged steroid therapy and osteoporosis in rheumatic and pulmonary diseases is difficult to define. Confounding factors predispose these individuals to osteopenia, and these are difficult to quantify or to separate from the effect of steroid therapy on bone. For example, reduced physical activity, common in patients with chronic lung and arthritic disorders, is itself a potential risk factor for osteoporosis.[143,148]

Clinical data from studies evaluating the efficacy of treatment protocols for steroid-induced osteoporosis are meager[149–152] and need to be obtained from long-term, controlled clinical trials or well-designed prospective cohort studies to allow more definitive conclusions.

ESTROGEN-DEFICIENT WOMEN

Numerous studies have confirmed the cause-and-effect relation between loss of ovarian function and accelerated bone loss,[153] and studies of women with bilateral oophorectomy demonstrated that the rate of bone loss in women appeared to be related to loss of ovarian function rather than age.[154] Cancellous bone of vertebral bodies appears particularly sensitive to declining female sex hormone production, with bone loss beginning earlier and being most rapid.[155]

Near the end of the fourth decade of life there is a gradual, continuous loss of bone mass in both sexes that continues into extreme old age. This process occurs at a rate of approximately 1 to 2% per year and is slightly greater in trabecular than in cortical bone. A relatively small subset of postmenopausal women experience accelerated bone loss[155] due to estrogen deficiency that lasts anywhere from 1 to 10 years.[156–158] Bone loss gradually slows to a basal rate of approximately 1% per year in most individuals and that rate of loss continues into very old age.

Other situations in which there are reductions in the circulating concentrations of ovarian hormones include amenorrhea induced by exercise,[159] anorexia nervosa,[160] and hyperprolactinemia.[161] Estrogen deficiency following menopause, oophorectomy, or prolonged amenorrhea from any cause is associated with bone loss.[159,160,166,163]

Although there is little doubt that bone mass is an important factor in fracture risk,[38,164] the question of just how useful it is for predicting fractures or as a guide to therapy in elderly populations where many have a low bone mass,[91] remains debatable. If bone mass accounts for 75 to 80% of the variance in ultimate strength of bone tissue, bone mineral density should be significantly related to fracture risk in patients.[120,165] However, if variation in density predicts only 50% of the variation in bone strength, as reported by Cooper,[166] then the importance of other aspects of bone structure independent of bone density, but related to age, are more apparent.

Other factors contribute to fracture, such as inadequate skeletal repair of microfractures. Heaney[167] emphasizes that inadequate skeletal repair appears to be a principle factor in hip fracture in the "old elderly," and may be a part of the explanation as to why only some elderly individuals develop hip fracture, although all have low bone mass levels.

Even among individuals with low bone mass the risk of fracture is relatively low. In women with the lowest 5% of femoral bone mass, the incidence of hip fractures is estimated at only about 2% per year.[18] Cummings et al.[91] reported the incidence of hip fractures in a population of 9703 women was 2 per 1000 person-years for women 65 through 69 years old. Although a statistical correlation between bone mass density at various sites and risk of fracture has been demonstrated, Cummings et al.[91,168] proposed that decreased bone density (osteopenia) accounts for only part of the age-related increase in risk of hip fracture among older women. As the authors suggest, other age-related factors, such as increased risk of falling, changes in the mechanics of falls, or qualitative changes in bone, are likely to contribute independently to the increased risk of hip fractures with age.

The clinical utility of routine densitometry in estrogen-deficient women remains unclear. It has not been demonstrated that the use of bone mass measurements to select patients for interventions, such as hormone replacement therapy (HRT), is an efficient strategy. Because the major benefit of HRT relates to diminished risk of cardiovascular disease, this treatment might, thus, be logically recommended irrespective of bone mass.[169,170] Recent reviews provided by the health ministries of Spain, France, Australia, and Great Britain are not supportive of post-menopausal women benefiting from routine bone densitometry.[171,172]

REFERENCES

1. Tohme JF, Silverberg SJ, Lindsay R. Osteoporosis, in Becker KL, Bilezikian JP, Bremner WJ, et al. (eds): *Principles and Practice of Endocrinology and Metabolism.* Philadelphia, J.B. Lippincott, 1990, pp 491–504.
2. Wasnich RD, Ross PD, Vogel JM, Davis JW (eds): *Osteoporosis Critique and Practicum.* Honolulu, Bayan Press, 1989.

3. Black MB, Cummings SR, Genant HK. Axial and appendicular bone density predict fractures in older women. *J Bone Miner Res* 1992;7(6):633–638.
4. Prelevic GM, Adashi EY. Postmenopausal osteoporosis: Prevention and treatment with calcitonin. *Gynecol Endocrinol* 1992;6:141–147.
5. Parfitt AM. Bone remodeling: Relationship to the amount and structure of bone, and the pathogenesis and prevention of fraction of fractures, in Riggs BL, Melton LJ III (eds): *Osteoporosis: Etiology, Diagnosis, and Management*. New York: Raven Press, 1988, pp 45–93.
6. Raisz LG. Physiology of bone, in Becker KL, Bilezikian JP, Bremner WJ, et al. (eds): *Principles and Practice of Endocrinology and Metabolism*. Philadelphia, J.B. Lippincott, 1990, pp 468–475.
7. Heaney RP. Osteoporotic fracture space: An hypothesis. *Bone Miner* 1989;6:1–13.
8. Riggs BL. Osteoporosis, in Wyngaarden JB, Smith LH, Bennett JC (eds): *Cecil Textbook of Medicine*. Vol 2, 19th ed. Philadelphia, W.B. Saunders, 1992, pp 1426–1430.
9. Riggs BL, Melton LJ. Involutional osteoporosis. *N Engl J Med* 1986;413(26):1676–1686.
10. Need AG, Nordin BEC, Horowitz M, Morris HA. Osteoporosis: New insights from bone densitometry. *J Am Geriatr Soc* 1990;38(10):1153–1158.
11. Krane SM, Holick MF. Metabolic bone disease, in Wilson JD, Braunwold E, Isselbacher KJ et al. (eds): *Principles of Internal Medicine*. New York, McGraw-Hill, 1991, pp 1921–1935.
12. Eastell R, Riggs BL. Diagnostic evaluation of osteoporosis. *Endocrinol Metab Clin North Am* 1988;17(3):547–571.
13. Notelovitz M. Osteoporosis: Screening, prevention, and management. *Fertil Steril* 1993;59(4):707–725.
14. NIH Consensus Conference: Osteoporosis, *JAMA* 1984; 252:799–802.
15. Melton LJ. How many women have osteoporosis? *J Bone Miner Res* 1992;9:1005–1010.
16. Assessment of Fracture Risk and its Application to Screening for Postmenopausal Osteoporosis. Report of World Health Organization, Geneva, 1994.
17. Wasnich RD. Fracture prediction with bone mass measurements, in Genant HK (ed): *Osteoporosis Update 1987*. Berkeley, University of California Press, 1987, pp 95–101.
18. Melton LJ, Wahner HW, Richelson LS, et al. Osteoporosis and the risk of hip fracture. *Am J Epidemiol* 1986;124(2): 254–261.
19. Ross PD, Wasnich RD, Heilbrum LK, Vogel JM. Definition of a spine fracture threshold based upon prospective fracture risk. *Bone* 1987;8:271–278.
20. NIH Consensus Development Conference: Diagnosis, prophylaxis and treatment of osteoporosis. *Am J Med* 1993; 94(6):646–650.
21. Alvioli LV. Significance of osteoporosis: A growing international health care problem. *Calcif Tissues Int* 1991; 49(Suppl):s5–s7.
22. Cooper C, Campion G, Melton LJ. Hip fractures in the elderly: A world-wide projection. *Osteoporosis Int* 1992;2:285–289.
23. Obrant KJ, Bengner U, Johnell O, et al. Increasing age-adjusted risk of fragility fractures: A sign of increasing osteoporosis in successive generations? *Calcif Tissue Int* 1989;44:157–167.
24. American Academy of Orthopaedic Surgeons: *Osteoporosis as a National Health Priority: A Joint Position Statement of the American Academy of Orthopaedic Surgeons and the National Osteoporosis Foundation*. Rosemont, IL: American Academy of Orthopaedic Surgeons, 1993.
25. Nottestad SY, Baumel JJ, Kimmel DB, et al. The proportion of trabecular bone in human vertebrae. *J Bone Miner Res* 1987;2(3):221–229.
26. *Bone Mineral Assessment—An Update. A Report by the National Health Technology Advisory Panel*. Australian Institute of Health, Oct 1989.
27. Health and Public Policy Committee, American College of Physicians: Bone mineral densitometry. *Ann Intern Med* 1987;107(6):932–936.
28. Cameron JR, Sorenson J. Measurement of bone mineral in vivo: An improved method. *Science* 1963;142:230.
29. Vogel JM, Wasnich RD, Ross PD. The clinical relevance of calcaneus bone mineral measurements: A review. *Bone Miner* 1988;5:35–58.
30. Mazess RB, Wahner HM. Nuclear medicine and densitometry, in Riggs BL, Melton LJ (eds): *Osteoporosis: Etiology, Diagnosis and Management*. New York, Raven Press, 1988, pp 251–295.
31. Chestnut CH. Bone imaging techniques, in Becker KL, Bilezikian JP, Bremner WJ, et al. (eds): *Principles and Practice of Endocrinology and Metabolism*. Philadelphia, J.B. Lippincott Company, 1990, pp 480–483.
32. Wahner HW, Dunn WL, Thorsen HC, et al. Bone mineral measurements: Review of various techniques, in Wahner HW (ed): *Nuclear Medicine: Quantitative Procedures*. Boston, Little Brown and Company, 1983, pp 107–132.
33. Dunn WL, Kan SH, Wahner HW. Errors in longitudinal measurements of bone mineral: Effect of source strength in single and dual photon absorptiometry. *J Nucl Med* 1987; 28:1751–1757.
34. Weinstein RS, New KD, Sappington LJ. Dual-energy x-ray absorptiometry versus single photon absorptiometry of the radius. *Calcif Tissue Int* 1991;49:313–316.
35. Lang P, Steiger P, Faulkner KF, et al. Current techniques and recent developments in quantitative bone densitometry. *Radiol Clin North Am* 1991;29(1):49–76.
36. Tothill P. Methods of bone mineral measurement. *Phys Med Biol* 1989;34(5):543–572.
37. Wahner HW. Measurements of bone mass and bone density. *Endocrinol Metab Clin North Am* 1989;18(4):994–1012.
38. Mazess RB. Bone densitometry for clinical diagnosis and monitoring, in DeLuca HF, Mazess R (eds): *Osteoporosis: Physiological Basis, Assessment, and Treatment*. New York, Elsevier Science Publishing, 1989, pp 63–85.
39. Alhava EM. Bone density measurements. *Calcif Tissue Int* 1991;49(Suppl)S21–S23.
40. Andresen J, Nielsen HE. Assessment of bone mineral content and bone mass by non-invasive radiologic methods. *Acta Radiol* 1986;27:609–617.
41. Wahner HW, Dunn WL, Brown ML, et al. Comparison of dual-energy x-ray absorptiometry and dual-photon absorptiometry for bone mineral measurements of the lumbar spine. *Mayo Clin Proc* 1988;63:1075–1084.
42. Hassanger C, Jensen B, Gotfredsen A, Christiansen C. The impact of measurement errors on the diagnostic value of bone mass measurements: Theoretical considerations. *Osteoporosis* 1991;1:250–256.
43. Gotfredsen A, Podenphant J, Norgaard H, et al. Accuracy of lumbar spine bone mineral content by dual photon absorptiometry. *J Nucl Med* 1988;29:248–254.
44. LeBlanc AD, Evans HJ, Marsh C, et al. Precision of dual photon absorptiometry measurements. *J Nucl Med* 1986; 27(8):1362–1365.
45. Nilas L, Hassager C, Christiansen C. Long-term precision of dual photon absorptiometry in the lumbar spine in clinical settings. *Bone Miner* 1988;3:305–315.
46. McGowan JA. Osteoporosis: Assessment of bone loss and remodeling. *Aging Clin Exp Res* 1993;5(2):81–93.

47. Blake GM, Tong CM, Fogelman I. Intersite comparison of the Hologic QDR-1000 dual energy x-ray bone densitometer. *Br J Radiol* 1991;64:440–446.
48. Kellie SE. Diagnostic and therapeutic technology assessment (DATTA): Measurement of bone density with dual-energy X-ray absorptiometry (DEXA). *JAMA* 1992;267(2): 286–294.
49. Pacifici R, Rupich R, Vered I, et al. Dual energy radiography (DER): A preliminary comparative study. *Calcif Tissue Int* 1988;43:189–191.
50. Mazess RB, Barden HS: Measurement of bone by dual-photon absorptiometry (DPA) and dual-energy x-ray absorptiometry (DEXA). *Ann Chir Gynaecol* 1988;77:197–203.
51. Mazess RB. Bone densitometry of the axial skeleton. *Orthop Clin North Am* 1990;21(1):51–63.
52. Kelly TL, Slovik DM, Schoenfeld DA, Neer RM. Quantitative digital radiography versus dual photon absorptiometry of the lumbar spine. *J Clin Endocrinol Metab* 1988;67(4):839–844.
53. Gluer C-C, Steiger P, Selvidge R, et al. Comparative assessment of dual-photon absorptiometry and dual-energy radiography. *Radiology* 1990;174(1):223–228.
54. Sievänen H, Kannus P, Oja P, Vuori I. Precision of dual energy x-ray absorptiometry in the upper extremities. *Bone Miner* 1993;20:235–243.
55. Chesnut CH. Noninvasive methods for bone mass measurement, in Avioli LV (ed): *The Osteoporotic Syndrome: Detection, Prevention, and Treatment*. (3rd ed). New York, Wiley-Liss, 1993, pp 77–87.
56. Wahner HW. Clinically useful and readily available techniques for measurements of bone mineral and body composition by photon or x-ray absorptiometry. *Trends Endocrinol Metab* 1990;Nov-Dec:382–387.
57. Reid IR, Evans MC, Stapleton J. Lateral spine densitometry is a more sensitive indicator of glucocorticoid-induced bone. *J Bone Miner Res* 1992;7(10):1221–1225.
58. Ho CP, Kim RW, Schaffler MB, Sartoris DJ. Accuracy of dual-energy radiographic absorptiometry of the lumbar spine: Cadaver study. *Radiology* 1990;176:171–173.
59. Cann CE. Quantitative CT for determination of bone mineral density: A review. *Radiology* 1988;166(2):509–522.
60. Genant HK, Steiger P, Block JE, et al. Quantitative computer tomography: Updated 1987. *Calcif Tissue Int* 1987; 41:179–186.
61. Johnston CC, Melton LJ, Lindsay R, Eddy DM. Clinical indications for bone mass measurements. *J Bone Miner Res* 1989;4(Suppl 2):1–28.
62. Mazess RB. Fracture risk: A role for compact bone. *Calcif Tissue Int* 1990;47:191–193.
63. Ruff CB, Hayes WC. Age changes in geometry and mineral content of the lower limb bones. *Ann Biomed Eng* 1984; 12:573–584.
64. Cann CE. Quantitative CT applications: Comparison of current scanners. *Radiology* 1987;162:257–261.
65. Lavel-Jeantet A-M, Genant HK, Wu C-Y, et al. Factors influencing long-term in vivo reproducibility of QCT (vertebral densitometry). *J Comput Assist Tomogr* 1993;17(6):915–921.
66. Cann CE, Ettiger B, Gennant HK. Normal subjects versus osteoporotics: No evidence using dual energy computed tomography for disproportionate increase in vertebral marrow fat. *J Comput Assist Tomogr* 1985;9(3):617–618.
67. Rao GU, Yaghmai I, Wist AO, Arora G. Systematic errors in bone-mineral measurements by quantitative computed tomography. *Med Phys* 1987;14(1):62–69.
68. Sartoris DJ, Andre M, Resnick C, Resnick D. Trabecular bone density in the proximal femur: Quantitative CT assessment. *Radiology* 1986;160(3):707–712.
69. Ruegsegger P, Durand EP, Dambacher MA. Differential effects of aging and disease on trabecular and compact bone density of the radius. *Bone* 1991;12:99–105.
70. Orphanoudakis SC, Holman H, Jensen PS. Automated processing of computed tomographic images for bone mass determination in the radius, in *Proceedings of the 10th Annual Northeast Bioengineering Conference*, Mar. 1982, pp 304–307.
71. Colbert C, Bachtell RS. *Radiographic absorptiometry: System for measuring mineral chances in patients with bone disease*. Paper presented at the Combined Meeting of the 12th International Conference on Medical and Biological Engineering and 5th International Conference on Medical Physics, Jerusalem, Israel, Aug 19–24, 1979.
72. Huddleston AL (ed). *Quantitative Methods in Bone Densitometry*. Boston, Kluwer Academic Publisher, 1988.
73. Colbert C, Bachtell RS, Sharp R, et al. Bone mineral density in chronic renal failure. *Dialys Transp* 1977; 6:77–83.
74. Aloia JF, Vaswani A, Yeh JK, et al. Calcitriol in the treatment of postmenopausal osteoporosis. *Am J Med* 1988;84: 401–408.
75. Erlichman MS. *Radiographic Absorptiometry for Measuring Bone Mineral Density. Health Technology Assessment Report*, 1987, No. 2. Rockville, MD, National Center for Health Services Research and Health Care Technology Assessment, 1987.
76. Colbert C, Bachtell RS. Radiographic absorptiometry (photodensitometry), in Cohn SH (ed): *Non-Invasive Measurements of Bone Mass and Their Clinical Application*. Boca Raton, FL, CRC Press Inc., 1981, pp 51–84.
77. Wahner HW, Dunn WL, Riggs BL. Assessment of bone mineral. Part 1. *J Nucl Med* 1984;1134–1141.
78. Mazess RB. The noninvasive measurement of skeletal mass, in Peck WA (ed): *Bone and Mineral Research*. Amsterdam, Excerpta Medica, 1983, pp 223–279.
79. Cohn SH. Noninvasive measurements of bone mass, in Avioli LV, Krane SM (eds): *Metabolic Bone Disease and Clinically Related Disorders*. Philadelphia, W.B. Saunders, 1990, pp 264–282.
80. Colbert C, Mazess RB, Schmidt PB. Bone mineral determination in vitro by radiographic photodensitometry and direct photon absorptiometry. *Invest Radiol* 1970;5:336–340.
81. Chestnut CH. *Noninvasive Techniques in the Diagnosis of Osteoporosis*. National Institutes of Health Consensus Development Conference, Apr 2–4, 1994.
82. Bachtell R, Colbert C. Written communication, CRTL Report No. 113, Sept 30, 1983.
83. Bachtell R, Colbert C. Written communication, CRTL Report No. 163, Oct 16, 1986.
84. Baran DT. Osteoporosis: Monitoring techniques and alternate therapies. *Obstet Gynecol Clin North Am* 1994;21(2): 321–335.
85. Wahner HW, Steiger P, Von Stetten E. Instruments and measurement techniques, in Wahner HW, Fogelman I (eds): *The Evaluation of Osteoporosis: Dual Energy X-ray Absorptiometry in Clinical Practice*. Cambridge, University Press, 1994, pp 14–34.
86. Vogel JM, Ross PD, Wasnich RD, Davis JW. *Technologies to Detect Osteoporosis: Final Report* (Hawaii Osteoporosis Center). Washington, Office of Technology Assessment, 1991.
87. Eastell R, Wahner HW, O'Fallon M, et al. Unequal decrease in bone density of lumbar spine and ultradistal radius in Colles' and vertebral fracture syndromes. *J Clin Invest* 1989;83:168–174.
88. Nilas L, Podenphant J, Riis BJ, et al. Usefulness of regional bone measurements in patients with osteoporosis fractures of the spine and distal forearm. *J Nucl Med* 1987;28:960–965.

89. Gardsell P, Johnell O, Nilsson BE. Predicting fractures in women by using forearm bone densitometry. *Calcif Tissue Int* 1989;44:235–242.
90. Ott SM, Kilcoyne RF, Chesnut CH. Ability of four different techniques of measuring bone mass to diagnose vertebral fractures in postmenopausal women. *J Bone Min Res* 1987; 2(3):201–210.
91. Cummings SR, Black DM, Nevitt MC, et al. Bone density at various sites for prediction of hip fractures. *Lancet* 1993;341:72–75.
92. Wasnich RD, Ross PD, Heilbrum LK, Vogel JM. Selection of the optimal site for fracture risk prediction. *Clin Orthop* 1985;216:262–269.
93. Bouillon R, Burckhardt P, Christiansen C, et al. Consensus Development Conference: Prophylaxis and treatment of osteoporosis. *Am J Med* 1991;90:107–110.
94. Melton LJ, Atkinson EJ, Ofallon WM, et al. Long-term fracture prediction by bone mineral assessed at different skeletal sites. *J Bone Miner Res* 1993;8(10):1227–1233.
95. Davis JW, Ross PD, Wasnich RD. Evidence for both generalized and regional low bone mass among elderly women. *J Bone Miner Res* 1994;9(3):305–309.
96. Consensus Development Conference: Prophylaxis and treatment of osteoporosis. *Am J Med* 1991;90(1):107–110.
97. Mazess RB, Gallagher JC, Notelovitz M, et al. Monitoring skeletal response to estrogen. *Am J Obstet Gynecol* 1989; 161(4):843–848.
98. Gotfredsen A, Nilas L, Riis BJ, et al. Bone changes occurring spontaneously and caused by oestrogen in early postmenopausal women: A local or generalized phenomenon? *BMJ* 1986;292:1098–1100.
99. Nordin BEC, Wishart JM, Horowitz M, et al. The relation between forearm and vertebral mineral density and fractures in postmenopausal women. *Bone Miner* 1988;5: 21–33.
100. Erlichman MS. *Dual Photon Absorptiometry for Measuring Bone Mineral Density. Health Technology Assessment Report, 1986*. No. 6. Rockville, MD, National Center for Health Services Research and Health Care Technology Assessment, 1986.
101. Ross PH, Wasnich RD, Vogel JM. Precision error in dual-photon absorptiometry related to source age. *Radiology* 1988;166(2):523–527.
102. Kelly TL, Slovik DM, Neer RM. Calibration and standardization of bone mineral densitometers. *J Bone Miner Res* 1989;4(5):663–669.
103. Heaney RP. En recherche de la difference (P < 0.05). *Bone Miner* 1986;1:99–114.
104. Nilas L, Borg J, Gotfredsen A, Christiansen C. Comparison of single- and dual-photon absorptiometry in postmenopausal bone mineral loss. *J Nucl Med* 1985;26:1257–1262.
105. Arai H, Ito K, Nagao K, Furutachi M. The evaluation of three different bone densitometry systems: XR-26, QDR-1000, and DPX. *Image Technol Info Displ* 1990;22(18):1–6.
106. Gluer C-C, Faulkner KG, Estilo MJ, et al. Quality assurance of bone densitometry research studies: Concept and impact. *Osteopor Int* 1993;3:227–235.
107. Parfitt AM. Trabecular bone architecture in the pathogenesis and prevention of fracture. *Am J Med* 1987;82(Suppl 1B):68–72.
108. Cummings SR. Are patients with hip fractures more osteoporotic? *Am J Med* 1985;78:487–494.
109. Genant HK, Block JE, Steiger P, Gluer C-C. Quantitative computed tomography: Update 1989, in DeLuca HF, Mazess R (eds): *Osteoporosis: Physiological Basis, Assessment, and Treatment*. New York, Elsevier Science Publishing, 1989, pp 87–98.
110. National Institute on Aging: *Workshop on Aging and Bone Quality*. Bethesda, MD, National Institutes of Health, 1992.
111. Kaufman JJ, Einhorn TA. Perspectives: Ultrasound assessment of bone. *J Bone Miner Res* 1993;8(5):517–525.
112. Parfitt AM. Bone remodeling: Relationship to the amount and structure of bone and the pathogenesis and prevention of fractures, in Riggs BL, Melton LJ (eds): *Osteoporosis: Etiology, Diagnosis, and Management*. New York, Raven Press, 1988, pp 45–89.
113. Kaufman JJ, Einhorn TA. Perspectives: Ultrasound assessment of bone. *J Bone Miner Res* 1993;8(5):517–525.
114. Faulkner KG, Glüer C-C, Majumdar S, et al. Noninvasive measurements of bone mass, structure, and strength: Current methods and experimental techniques. *Am J Roentgenol* 1991;157:1229–1237.
115. Massie A, Reid DM, Porter RW. Screening for osteoporosis: Comparison between dual energy x-ray absorptiometry and broadband ultrasound attenuation in 100 perimenopausal women. *Osteopor Int* 1993;3:107–110.
116. Heaney RP, Avioli LV, Chesnut CH, et al. Osteoporosis bone fragility. *JAMA* 1989;261(20):2986–2990.
117. Porter RW, Miller CG, Grainger D, et al. Prediction of hip fracture in elderly women: A prospective study. *BMJ* 1990;301:638–641.
118. Herd RJ, Blake GM, Miller CG, et al. The ultrasonic assessment of osteopenia as defined by dual x-ray absorptiometry. *Br J Radiol* 1994;67:631–635.
119. Arnaud CD. *Biochemical Markers of Bone Turnover*. Program in Osteoporosis and Bone Biology, University of California, San Francisco. Presented at the 45th National AACC meeting, Jul 11–15, 1993, New York.
120. Hansen MA, Overgaard K, Riis BJ, Christiansen C. Role of peak bone mass and bone loss in postmenopausal osteoporosis: 12 year study. *BMJ* 1991;303:961–964.
121. Christiansen C, Riis BJ. New methods for identifying "at risk" patients for osteoporosis. *Clin Rheumatol* 1989;8(Suppl 2):52–55.
122. Christiansen C, Riis BJ, Rodbro P. Screening procedure for women at risk of developing postmenopausal osteoporosis. *Osteoporos Int* 1990;1:35–40.
123. Delmas PD. Biochemical markers of bone turnover for the clinical investigation of osteoporosis. *Osteopor Int* 1993; (Suppl 1):S81–S86.
124. Potts JT. Disorders of parathyroid gland, in Petersdorf RG, Adams RD, Braunwald E, et al. (eds): *Harrison's Principles of Internal Medicine*. 10th ed. New York, McGraw-Hill, 1993, pp 1929–1943.
125. Fitzpatrick LA, Bilezikian JP. Primary hyperparathyroidism, in Becker KL, Bilezikian JP, Bremner WJ, et al. (eds): *Principles and Practice of Endocrinology and Metabolism*. Philadelphia, J.B. Lippincott, 1990, pp 430–437.
126. Mundy GR (ed). Primary hyperparathyroidism, in: *Calcium Homeostasis: Hypercalcemia and Hypocalcemia*. second ed. 1990, pp 137–167.
127. Consensus Development Conference Panel: Diagnosis and management of asymptomatic primary hyperparathyroidism: Consensus development conference statement. *Ann Intern Med* 1991;114(7):593–597.
128. Melton IJ III, Atkinson EJ, O'Fallon WM, Health H III. Risk of age-related fractures in patients with primary hyperparathyroidism. *Arch Intern Med* 1992;152:2269–2273.
129. Barzel US. Primary hyperparathyroidism: Problems in management. *Hosp Pract* 1992;27(7):167–176.
130. Mole PA, Walkinshaw HH, Gunn A, et al. Bone mineral content in patients with primary hyperparathyroidism. A comparison of conservative management with surgical treatment. *Br J Surg* 1992;79:263–265.

131. Warner J, Clifton-Bligh P, Posen S, et al. Longitudinal changes in forearm bone mineral content in primary hyperparathyroidism. *J Bone Miner Res* 1991;6(Suppl 2):S91–S124.
132. Silverberg SJ, Shane E, De La Cruz L, et al. Skeletal disease in primary hyperparathyroidism. *J Bone Miner Res* 1989; 4(3):283–291.
133. Rao DS, Wilson RJ, Kleerekoper M, et al. Lack of biochemical progression or continuation of accelerated bone loss in mild asymptomatic primary hyperparathyroidism: Evidence for biphasic disease course. *J Clin Endocrinol Metab* 1988;67(6):1294–1298.
134. Wilson RJ, Rao DS, Ellis B, et al. Mild asymptomatic primary hyperparathyroidism is not a risk factor for vertebral fractures. *Ann Intern Med* 1988;109:959–962.
135. Peacock M, Horsman A, Aaron JE, et al. The role of parathyroid hormone in bone loss, in Christianson C, Arnaud CD, Nordin BEC, et al. (eds): *Osteoporosis*. Denmark, Aalborgs Stiftsbogstrykkeri, 1984, pp 463–467.
136. Posen S, Clifton-Bligh P, Reeve TS, et al. Is parathyroidectomy of benefit in primary hyperparathyroidism? *Q J Med* 1985; New Series 54(215):241–251.
137. Kochersberger G, Buckley NJ, Leight GS, et al. What is the clinical significance of bone loss in primary hyperparathyroidism? *Arch Intern Med* 1987;147:1951–1953.
138. Axelrod L. Corticosteroid therapy, in Becker KL, Bilezikian JP, Loriaux DL, et al. (eds): *Principles and Practice of Endocrinology and Metabolism* Philadelphia, J.B. Lippincott, 1990, pp 613–623.
139. Department of Drugs, Division of Drugs and Toxicology. Anti-inflammatory agents: Glucocorticoids in American Medical Association: *Drug Evaluations Annual* 1991, (Chapter 74), pp 1619–1651.
140. Eufemio MA. Advances in the therapy of osteoporosis—Part V. *Geriatric Med Today* 1990;9(2):41–56.
141. Hahn BH. Metabolic bone disease, in Schumacher HR, Klippel JH, Robinson DR (eds): *Primer on the Rheumatic Diseases*. 9th ed. Atlanta, GA, Arthritis Foundation, 1988, pp 276–278.
142. Reid IR, Schooler BA, Stewart AW. Prevention of glucocorticoid-induced osteoporosis. *J Bone Min Res* 1990;5(6): 619–623.
143. Lukert BP, Raisz LG. Glucocorticoid-induced osteoporosis: Pathogenesis and management. *Ann Intern Med* 1990; 112(5):352–364.
144. Reid IR, Veale AG, France JT. Glucocorticoid osteoporosis. *J Asthma* 1994;31(1):7–18.
145. Abinoff AD, Hollister JR. Steroid-induced fractures and bone loss in patients with asthma. *N Engl J Med* 1983; 309(5):265–268.
146. Jenkinson T, Bhalla AK. A reappraisal of steroid-induced osteoporosis. *Br J Hosp Med* 1993;50(8):472–476.
147. Dykman TR, Gluck OS, Murphy WA, et al. Evaluation of factors associated with glucocorticoid-induced osteopenia in patients with rheumatic diseases. *Arthritis Rheum* 1985; 28(4):361–368.
148. Reid IR, Evans MC, Wattie DJ, Ames R, Cundy TF. Bone mineral density of the proximal femur and lumbar spine in glucocorticoid-treated asthmatic patients. *Osteoporosis* 1992;2:103–105.
149. Luengo M, Picado C, Del Rio L, et al. Treatment of steroid-induced osteopenia with calcitonin in corticosteroid-dependent asthma: A one-year follow-up study. *Am Rev Respir Dis* 1990;142:104–107.
150. Reid IR, Alexander CJ, King AR, Ibbertson HK. Prevention of steroid-induced osteoporosis with (3-amino-1-hydroxypropylidene)-1, 1-bisphosphonate (APD). *Lancet* 1988;1(8578): 143–146.
151. Sambrook P, Birmingham J, Champion D, et al. Postmenopausal bone loss in rheumatoid arthritis: Effect of estrogens and androgens. *J Rheumatol* 1992;19(3):357–361.
152. Olbricht T, Benker G. Glucocorticoid-induced osteoporosis: pathogenesis, prevention and treatment, with special regard to the rheumatic diseases. *J Intern Med* 1993;234:237–244.
153. Lindsay R. Prevention and treatment of osteoporosis. *Lancet* 1993;3141:801–805.
154. Lindsay R, Cosman F. Primary Osteoporosis, in Coe FL, Favus MJ (eds): *Disorders of Bone and Mineral Metabolism*. New York, Raven Press, 1992, pp 831–888.
155. Riggs LB. Causes of age-related bone loss and fractures, in DeLuca HF, Mazess R (ed): *Osteoporosis Physiological Basis, Assessment, and Treatment*. New York, Elsevier, 1990, pp 7–16.
156. Levin RM. The prevention of osteoporosis. *Hosp Pract* 1991;26:77–97.
157. Heaney RP. Lifelong calcium intake and prevention of bone fragility in the aged. *Calcif Tissue Int* 1991;49(Suppl): s42–s45.
158. Nordin BEC, Polley KJ. Metabolic consequences of the menopause. *Calcif Tissue Int* 1987;41(Suppl 1):s1–s59.
159. Drinkwater BL, Nilson K, Ott S, et al. Bone mineral density after resumption of menses in amenorrheic athletes. *JAMA* 1986;256(3):380–382.
160. Salisbury JJ, Mitchell JE. Bone mineral density and anorexia nervosa in women. *Am J Psychiatry* 1991;148(6):768–774.
161. Klibanski A, Greenspan SL. Increase in bone mass after treatment of hyperprolactinemic amenorrhea. *N Engl J Med* 1986;315(9):542–546.
162. Fabbri G, Petraglia F, Segre A, et al. Reduced spinal bone density in young women with amenorrhoea. *Eur J Obstet Gynecol Repr Biol* 1991;41(2):117–122.
163. Stepan JJ, Pospichal J, Presl J, et al. Bone loss and biochemical indices of bone remodeling in surgically induced postmenopausal women. *Bone* 1987;8:279–284.
164. Melton LJ. Epidemiology of fractures, in Riggs L, Metlon LJ (eds): *Osteoporosis: Etiology, Diagnosis, and Management*. New York, Raven Press, 1988, pp 133–153.
165. Melton LJ III. Fracture Patterns, in DeLuca HF, Mazess R (eds): *Osteoporosis Physiological Basis, Assessment, and Treatment*. New York, Elsevier, 1989, pp 39–44.
166. Cooper C. Who will develop osteoporosis?, in Roger S (ed): *Osteoporosis*. London, Royal College of Physicians, 1990, pp 163–171.
167. Heaney RP. Prevention of osteoporotic fracture in women, in Avioli LV (ed): *The Osteoporotic Syndrome, Detection, Prevention, and Treatment*. New York, Wiley-Liss, 1993; pp 89–107.
168. Cummings SR, Black DM, Nevitt MC, et al. Appendicular bone density and age predict hip fracture in women. *JAMA* 1990;263(5):665–668.
169. *Clinician's Handbook of Preventive Services. Estrogen and Progestin*, U.S. Department of Health and Human Services, Public Health Service, 1994, pp 245–250.
170. The Writing Group for the PEPI Trial. Effects of estrogen or estrogen progestin regimens on heart disease risk factors in postmenopausal women. *JAMA* 1995;273:190–208.
171. National Health Technology Advisory Panel. *Bone mineral assessment—an update*. Australian Institute of Health, Canberra, October 1989.
172. International Network of Agencies for Health Technology Assessment. Second Annual Meeting Evergreen House Baltimore, MD, Saturday June 18, 1994.

35 Inflammatory Disorders of Soft Tissues

John G. McAfee

A failure to diagnose and localize a focus of infection remains a serious medical problem because many lesions are occult, yet the majority are curable if treatment is initiated early. The two common agents used to detect and localize these foci by gamma camera imaging, ^{67}Ga-citrate and ^{111}In-labeled autologous leukocytes, were compared in a literature review up to 1984.[1] The authors concluded that the sensitivity of detection with the 2 radiotracers was about the same, but the specificity of labeled leukocytes was superior. In a comparative study of ^{111}In-leukocytes and ^{67}Ga imaging performed in the same patients for the diagnosis of occult sepsis, the false-negative studies with labeled leukocytes tended to occur in infections more than 2 weeks old, whereas the false-negative gallium images tended to occur in infections less than 1 week in duration.[2] Gallium may be better in chronic granulomatous non-pyogenic infections, particularly viral infections, and in patients with immunosuppression or leukopenia.[3] On the other hand, ^{111}In-leukocytes have a higher target-to-background ratio than ^{67}Ga in acute pyogenic infections. With the labeled cells, there is normally no activity in the bowel or urinary tract so they are preferred for abdominopelvic infections.[3]

As with the experience with ^{67}Ga, imaging with ^{111}In-leukocytes in patients with spontaneous fever of unknown origin (fever of 3 weeks duration reaching 38.3°C more than 3 times) has a very low diagnostic yield for focal infections.[4] A variety of other conditions may be found on follow-up, including connective tissue diseases, amyloidosis, thrombosis, chronic pancreatitis, fictitious fever, or occult malignancies. On the other hand, in patients febrile in the immediate postoperative period, the positive yield of leukocyte imaging is high.[4]

According to some authors,[5] computed tomography (CT) and ultrasound should be the first diagnostic methods in suspected intraabdominal infections, because they can be completed within an hour or two instead of a day for ^{111}In-leukocytes and several days for ^{67}Ga. However, infections without liquefaction (phlegmonous lesions) may be missed by CT or ultrasound, yet well demonstrated with labeled leukocytes. Leukocyte imaging is especially useful in patients without localizing signs, and in comatose and paralyzed patients. Moreover, leukocyte images often show foci in unsuspected locations beyond the areas included in CT and ultrasound examinations. However, leukocyte images are usually negative in tuberculous lesions unless secondary infections are present.[5] Abscesses superimposed on the normal liver or spleen activity may be missed,[6] but sometimes may be detected by subtracting normalized radiocolloid images from the leukocyte images. Labeled leukocytes also may fail in walled-off chronic abscesses, infected cysts, or fungal infections. In another clinical comparison of these imaging modalities,[7] indium leukocyte images had a sensitivity of 85% and a specificity of 95%, ultrasound had a sensitivity of 82% and a specificity of 95%, whereas CT had a sensitivity of 98% and a specificity of 95%. This report concluded that CT and ultrasound should be the first diagnostic methods when clinical manifestations are localized. When these studies are inconclusive, or when there are no localizing signs, leukocyte imaging is indicated. Ultrasound is often not useful in the immediate postoperative period to examine the area of the fresh surgical wound. Leukocyte images may fail to distinguish intrinsic inflammatory bowel disease from intraabdominal sepsis of other structures.[8] This problem may be resolved with the other modalities, which possess better spatial resolution.

None of the modalities, including ^{67}Ga or labeled leukocyte images, CT, or ultrasound have findings that are specific for the diagnosis of abscesses. Intense uptake of labeled leukocytes increases the probability of abscess formation.[6] With CT or ultrasound, it may be difficult to distinguish abscess cavities from other fluid collections. Because a misdiagnosis of abscess may have serious consequences, in doubtful situations multiple modalities should be tried to resolve the diagnosis.

The clinical application of labeled leukocytes in children is much more limited than in adults. In one pediatric series[9] the sensitivity of detection of acute infections was 85% and the specificity was 86%. Autologous leukocytes successfully localized a lesion as early as 5 weeks in an infant. In patients with chronic granulomatous disease, autologous leukocytes may fail to localize in foci of infection.[10] Donor leukocytes should be used in immunosuppressed children.[9]

In another pediatric series,[11] the sensitivity of detecting acute infections was 94%, but the specificity was only 57% because of false-positives in 6 patients. Four of these had unexplained uptake in submandibular glands, 2 had persistent cardiac blood pool activity perhaps due to excessive erythrocyte tagging, 2 had unexplained abdominal foci and 1 had unexplained bladder activity. Four children had persistently high myocardial activity from Kawasaki disease (mucocutaneous lymph node syndrome frequently complicated by coronary arteritis, myocarditis, cardiac dilatation, and aneurysm formation). In yet another series of 42 children and adolescents,[12] the sensitivity of detecting acute inflammatory conditions was 81%, and the specificity was 94%. In children with multiple foci of infection, some lesions were positive, and some negative.[10] Liver abscesses and pericarditis, in particular, were missed.

BRIEF HISTORY OF RADIONUCLIDE IMAGING IN INFLAMMATION

The gallium radionuclides were developed for biomedical applications at the Oak Ridge National Laboratories. Dudley et al.[13] studied the biodistribution of reactor produced ^{72}Ga in both animals and patients, and found fairly high concentrations in proliferating tissues. Bruner, Hayes, and Perkinson[14] found that the distribution of ^{67}Ga was considerably different from that of ^{72}Ga, the bone uptake of ^{67}Ga was much lower. Edwards and Hayes discovered that ^{67}Ga localized in tumors, especially lymphomas.[15] Bell et al.[16] reported in an abstract in 1971 that ^{67}Ga localized in a variety of non-neoplastic lesions in patients, including abscesses. Later that same year, Lavender et al.[17] reported positive ^{67}Ga-citrate images in both neoplastic and inflammatory lesions.

Leukocyte suspensions were first labeled with ^{51}Chromium by McCall et al.[18] for measuring their in vivo survival after reinjection. ^{51}Chromium-labeled leukocytes were successfully used for imaging abscesses in rabbits by Winkelman et al.[19]; however, both the labeling yield and photon yield were so low that the clinical application of this radionuclide was impractical. In a survey of radioactive agents for labeling leukocytes, McAfee and Thakur[20] obtained high labeling yields with ^{111}In-hydroxyquinoline (oxine) and the intracellular labeling appeared irreversible both in vitro and in vivo. Thakur et al.[21] used this agent successfully for imaging abscesses in dogs and compared the distribution of the radiolabeled leukocytes with that of ^{67}Ga. Clinical studies with this agent were first reported by Thakur et al.[22] Another lipophilic chelate, ^{111}In-tropolonate successfully labeled leukocytes, as first reported by Danpure et al.[23] Unlike oxine, the tropolonate chelate could label leukocyte suspensions in the presence of plasma. As a result, this agent has become popular in Europe; however, any clinical application of this agent in the U.S.A. must be performed under an investigational new drug protocol (IND) with the Food and Drug Administration. The lipophilic ^{99m}Tc-chelate, hexamethylpropyleneamine oxime (HMPAO) was originally developed as a brain imaging agent. However, it was discovered that this chelate could label suspensions of leukocytes. The clinical application of this agent for labeling leukocytes and imaging inflammatory lesions was first reported by Peters et al.[24] In recent years, literally hundreds of papers have been published on the application of ^{67}Ga and labeled leukocytes for inflammatory imaging. Later in the chapter, still other agents under development will be briefly summarized.

RADIATION DOSE AND EFFECTS

Some published radiation dose estimates[25–28] for ^{67}Ga and ^{111}In-leukocytes are shown in Table 1. The radiation dose in rad/mCi or cGy/MBq to the spleen is much higher for the labeled leukocytes than for gallium. However, the customary administered activity of ^{67}Ga (5 to 10 mCi or 185 to 370 MBq) is higher than that of ^{111}In [0.5 to 1 mCi or 18 to 37 MBq]; as a result, the radiation dose to the erythropoietic marrow is higher with gallium.

Neutrophils receive a radiation dose of 1480 rads (cGy) while circulating when 10^8 cells are labeled with 1 mCi (37 MBq) of ^{111}In.[29] At a microscopic level, Auger electrons are the major contributors to the radiation dose.[30] These postmitotic cells are considered relatively radioresistant. Their morphology and at least some of their functions remain intact after 50,000 rads (cGy) of irradiation. However their recovery from the circulation is reduced by 5000 rads (cGy) of radiation (Fig. 1).

The possibility of radiation-induced oncogenesis has been raised due to irradiation of lymphocytes that are present in mixed leukocyte suspensions. These cells are exquisitely sensitive to the radiation from Auger electrons when ^{111}In atoms concentrate in the cell nuclei.[30] In in vitro studies, chromatid and chromosomal aberrations have been increased by doses as low as 30 μCi/10^8 cells.[31] However, in in vivo studies in man, lymphocytes with chromosomal aberrations induced by extracorporeal irradiation of blood rapidly disappear.[32] When 10^8 mixed leukocytes are labeled with 0.5 mCi of ^{111}In, lymphocytes receive a radiation dose of 8750 rad (cGy), well in excess of the killing dose.[33]

Gallium-67 Citrate

MECHANISMS OF LOCALIZATION

The mechanisms of uptake of ^{67}Ga at inflammatory sites remain uncertain and continue to be controversial, despite decades of experiments. There is negligible binding of gallium to polymorphs in vivo[34] as was once postulated. Even in patients with marked leukopenia, the localization of gallium at inflammatory sites is usually evident. There is abnormal permeability at inflammatory sites, permitting the passive diffusion of transferrin-bound ^{67}Ga through capillaries and postcapillary venules. Gallium has a higher affinity for lactoferrin than for transferrin at neutral and acidic pHs at the inflammatory sites. Lactoferrin is secreted from the secondary granules of neutrophils, and gallium may transchelate from transferrin to the released lactoferrin. Normal glands secreting lactoferrin, such as the lachrymal glands and lactating breasts, may concentrate gallium intensely.

Table 1. Radiation Dose Estimates

	^{67}Ga-Citrate		^{111}In-WBC	
Author	Cloutier[25]	Thomas[26]	Williams[27]	Gainey[28]
Reference No.	25	26	27	28
Subjects	23 adults	2 children	6 adults	7 children
Age	–	1 year	–	mean 18 mos
Spleen % organ uptake		.7–1.5	25	28
rad/mCi	.53	2.4–5.2	23.4	89
liver % organ uptake		3.4–10.3	27	28
rad/mCi	.46	.52–4.0	3.8	16
marrow % organ uptake			6	15
rad/mCi	.58		.65	9
rest of body % uptake				29
total body rad/mCi	.26		.45	2.9
blood % uptake			34	
lungs % uptake			8	
rad/mCi			1.5	
ovaries rad/mCi	.28		.14	
testes rad/mCi	.24		.029	
stomach wall rad/mCi	.22		1.0	
small bowel rad/mCi	.36			
upper large bowel rad/mCi	.56			
lower large bowel rad/mCi	.90			
kidneys rad/mCi	.41			
bone rad/mCi	.44			
metaphyses rad/mCi		2.9–4.2		

Lower molecular weight siderophores, elaborated by bacteria, and ferritin may also concentrate gallium.

In inflammatory lesions in rats[35] autoradiographs showed negligible ^{67}Ga concentrations in regions with high neutrophil and macrophage infiltration. On the contrary, the gallium was concentrated in the extracellular spaces. Permeability indices, measured with labeled albumin, were much greater in inflammatory than in normal tissues, reaching a maximum at 3 hours. On the other hand, ^{67}Ga concentrations increased progressively up to 6 days. The binding substances in inflammatory tissues thought to retain the gallium were keratin polysulfate or other oversulfated mucopolycaccharide products of fibroblasts.

Planas-Bohne et al. compared concentrations of different radiometals in turpentine induced abscesses up to 29 days old in rats. The radionuclide concentration difference between normal and abscessed tissue was as great with other radiometals as with ^{67}Ga (Fig. 2). Perhaps, as these authors suggested, radionuclides transported in blood by transferrin may achieve better abscess concentrations than other radionuclides. The abscess concentration of these radiotracers appeared to correlate with beta-glucuronidase activity. The nuclide ^{203}Hg had a relatively high abscess/muscle concentration ratio, but this element is not bound at all to transferrin. In a subsequent similar study by the same group of workers[37] in rat abscesses up to 21 days, there was no consistently significant difference in the concentrations between the various radionuclides. These findings suggested a common mechanism for clearance of these elements from normal or inflamed muscle. However, the clearance of ^{203}Hg was faster than that of the other elements and its normal muscle concentration was low, compared to ^{67}Ga. Thus, there was no evidence that gallium possessed unique properties for localizing at inflammatory sites (Fig. 2).

The clinical popularity of ^{67}Ga for imaging inflammatory lesions is probably more determined by its availability, physical characteristics, and extensive past usage. Although many authors have emphasized plasma protein binding of radionuclides for enhanced detection of inflammatory lesions, some have been demonstrated by scintigraphy with ^{201}Tl as free thallous ions (without any plasma protein binding).[38]

NORMAL DISTRIBUTION OF GALLIUM

The content of ^{67}Ga-citrate (cyclotron-produced, without added carrier gallium) in the normal skeleton is variable. In adults, about 9% of the administered activity localizes in bone (assuming a bone mass of 5 kg/70 kg man), and about 4.2% in the erythropoietic marrow (assuming a mass of 1.5 kg/70 kg man).[39] In adolescents, on the other hand, as much as 32% of the administered activity may localize in bone and 9% in the erythropoetic marrow. In children, uptake is accen-

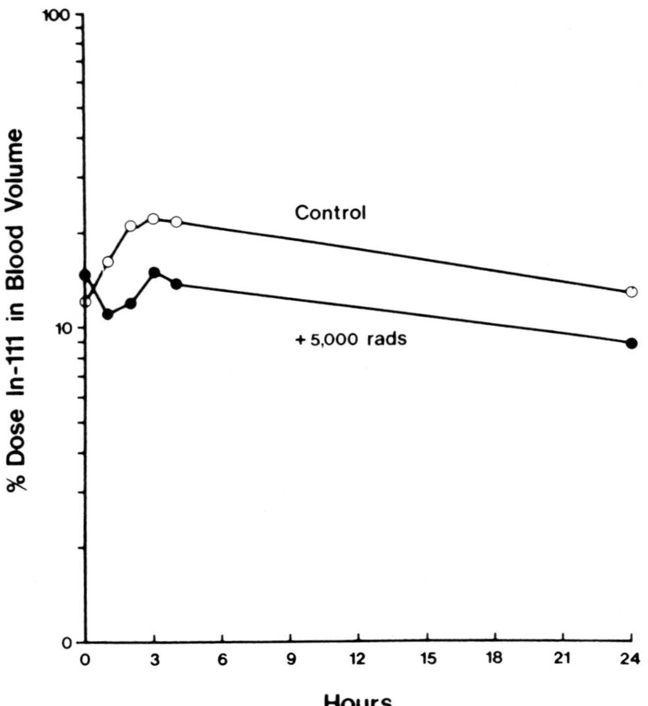

Figure 1. Radiation effects of mixed leukocyte suspensions. Canine leukocytes (~10^8 cells) labeled with 500 μCi ^{111}In-oxine and reinjected had a maximum recovery of 22% of the administered radioactivity in the circulating cell pool. A duplicate study of labeled leukocytes given an additional 5000 rads in a ^{60}Co-irradiator in the same dog showed a marked reduction in cell recovery in the circulation.

tuated in the metaphyseal regions of the long bones, similar to the localization of the ^{99m}Tc-diphosphonates.

The gastrointestinal wall concentration of ^{67}Ga is variable in different individuals, ranging from 2.5 to 15% administered activity/kg wet weight,[40] but does not change much with time, as determined by surgical tissue samples. About 2 to 3% of the administered dose is excreted in the bowel per day, accounting for a sizable fraction in the gastrointestinal contents. The concentrations of gallium in the gastrointestinal wall are often higher than those of the gastrointestinal contents. Bowel preparation is considered to be of little value in eliminating the gastrointestinal activity, which may obscure intraabdominal pathology.[41]

Soon after the intravenous injection of ^{67}Ga-citrate, about 70% of the circulating activity is bound to serum albumin and to globulins to some extent, but is dialysable. By 3 hours, however, 85% of the remaining activity is bound to serum proteins and is not dialysable. Virtually all is plasma protein bound by 24 hours. By cross electroimmunodiffusion, the binding proteins are transferrin and haptoglobin.[42] Oddly, the results of in vitro incubation of ^{67}Ga with plasma or serum are somewhat different than the results obtained from in vivo binding.

NORMAL ^{67}Ga IMAGES

After an administered dose of 5 to 10 mCi (185 to 370 MBq) of ^{67}Ga intravenously, imaging is performed at 24 hours and often repeated at 48 and 72 hours, depending on the time of clearance of the widespread soft-tissue activity. Some authors recommend "early" 6-hour images. Many workers prefer total-body anterior and posterior images, supplemented by regional "static" images. Administered activity up to 9 to 10 mCi (333 to 370 MBq) is necessary to localize lesions by SPECT imaging. Normal images regularly show activity in the liver, spleen, skeleton, and marrow (Fig. 3). Dual isotope imaging with both ^{67}Ga and ^{99m}Tc-sulfur colloid may be successful in unmasking inflammatory lesions that

A
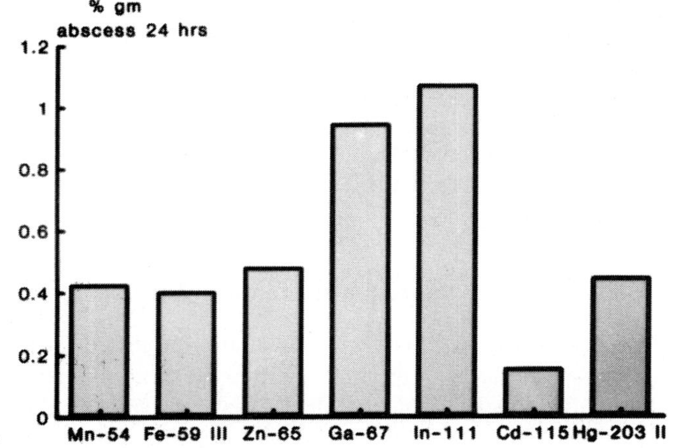

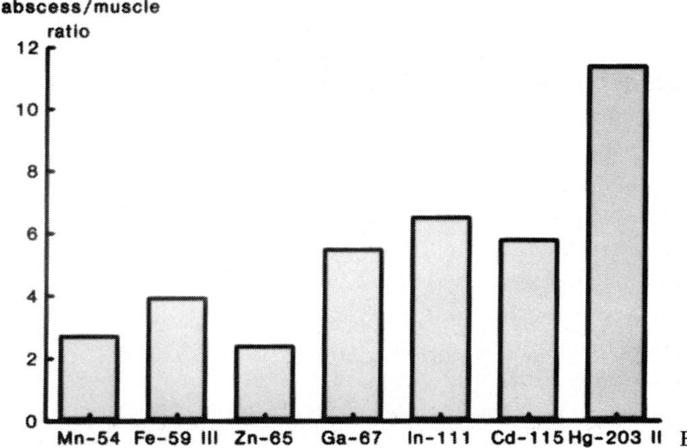

B

Figure 2. Concentration of various radiometals in turpentine abscesses in rats at 24 hours. **(A).** Abscess concentrations in % administered activity/gm. **(B).** Abscess/muscle concentration ratios. The abscess localization of ^{67}Ga is not strikingly different from other radiometals. (Graphs constructed from data by Planas-Bohne F, *Br J Radiol* 55:289, 1982; ref. 36)

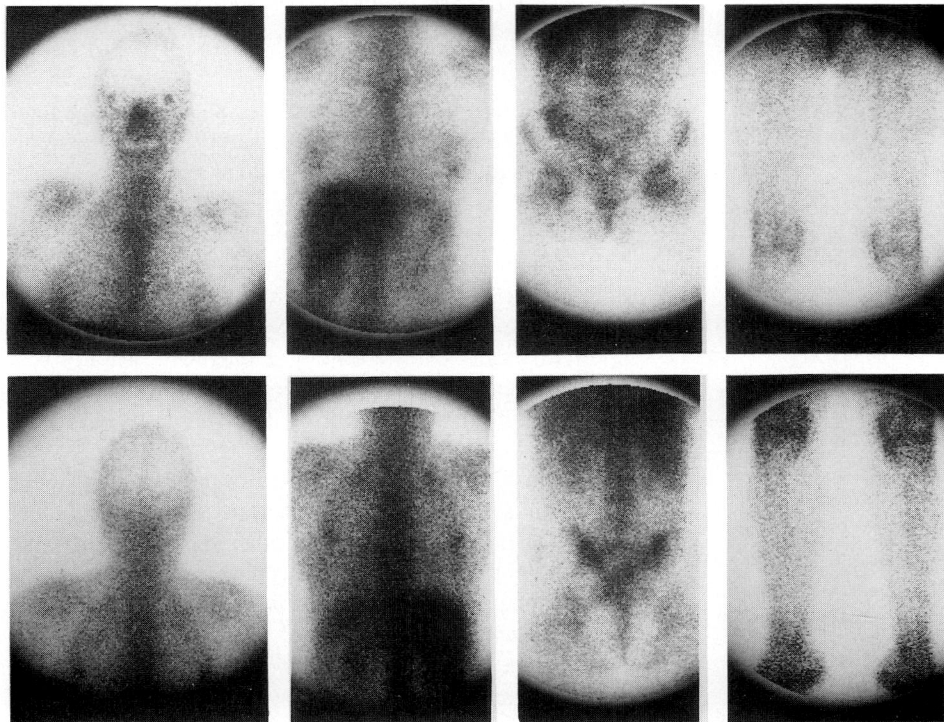

Figure 3 A. Selected normal 48-hour planar ^{67}Ga images. (Upper row) anterior images of the head and neck, chest and upper abdomen, lower abdomen and pelvis, and thighs. (Lower row) corresponding posterior images of the head, chest and abdomen, and anterior view of the legs. Note the activity in the liver, spine, and pelvis, lachrymal glands, nasopharyngeal lymphoid tissue, sternum, inferior angles of the scapulae, juxta-articular regions of the extremities, and bowel contents.

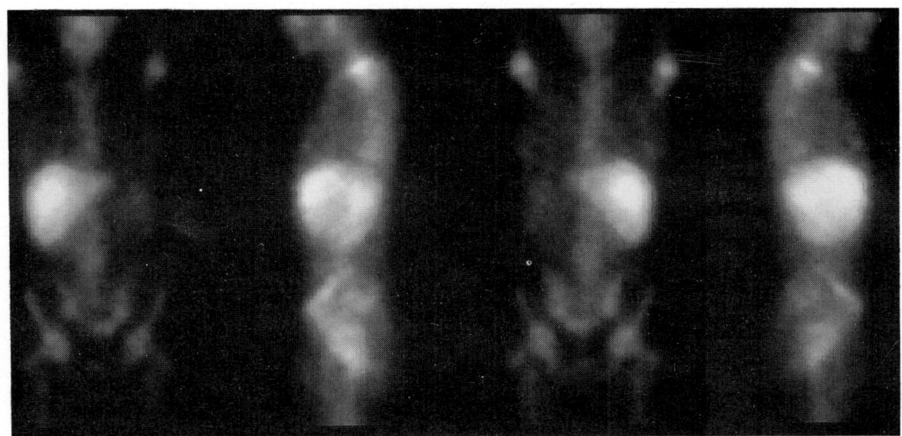

Figure 3 B. Selected 48-hour ^{67}Ga back projection "maximum pixel" torso images from a 3-headed SPECT camera showing anterior, L lateral, posterior, and R lateral projections.

might otherwise be missed within or surrounding the liver or spleen.[43]

In the head and neck, there may be normal uptake of varying degree in the nasopharyngeal lymphoid tissue, lachrymal glands, and faint uptake in the salivary glands. In the thorax, diffuse soft tissue activity is usually visible. Bilateral breast uptake is usually normal; symmetrical breast activity may be seen in as many as 10 to 15% of younger women.[44] The initial lung uptake may be slow in clearing, and may take longer than 72 hours in elderly patients. In posterior images of the abdomen, there may be faint normal renal uptake at 24 hours but normally this is usually not evident by 48 hours. Anteriorly, bladder activity may be seen for several days. Soft-tissue activity is commonly seen in the external genitalia. Thymic and splenic uptake may be prominent in normal young children.

ATYPICAL ^{67}Ga-LOCALIZATION

Atypical predominantly skeletal localization resembling the appearance of diphosphonate bone images is occasionally observed with gallium, usually with low liver, bowel, and soft tissue uptake and increased renal and bladder activity (Fig. 3 **C**). This appearance is associated with chemother-

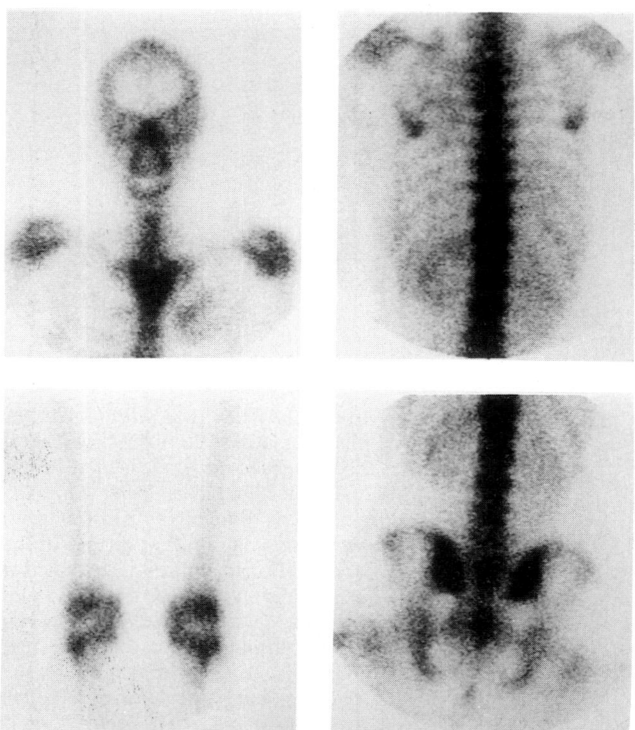

Figure 3 C. Altered distribution of 10 mCi ^{67}Ga in 48-hour images in a 24-year-old female during treatment with many chemotherapy drugs and GM-CSF for Hodgkin's disease. High uptake in the skeleton is seen with minimal uptake in the liver. Months after completion of therapy, the radiogallium distribution reverted to the more normal pattern, with activity in the liver, spleen, and lacrimal glands.

apy, blood transfusions, or iron therapy. With this altered biodistribution, probably due to decreased ^{67}Ga binding to plasma transferrin, inflammatory or neoplastic lesions may be missed. In iron overload conditions, the serum iron levels may be normal, but the iron-binding capacity is reduced and the serum ferritin levels often elevated.[45] The same phenomenon has been observed in chronic anemia, tumor infiltration of the bone marrow, or radiation treatments.[46] Administered with stable carrier (^{70}Ga) or scandium, ^{67}Ga becomes a bone-seeker.[47] This pattern has also occurred when ^{67}Ga is administered within hours after the magnetic resonance imaging (MRI) contrast agent Gd-DTPA (gadopentetate).[48]

In contrast to the pattern of increased skeletal localization, ^{67}Ga administered after desferoxamine treatment for aluminum toxicity has abnormally prolonged retention in the soft tissues without localization in the skeleton or other organs, probably because it becomes firmly bound to the desferoxamine.[49] Increased breast uptake may be seen with drugs inducing gynecomastia and hyperprolactinemia, such as metoclopromide, reserpine, phenothiazines, oral contraceptives, or diethylstilbestrol.[50] Localized muscle uptake has been reported after calcium gluconate intramuscular injections or interstitial extravasation.

RESULTS OF GALLIUM IMAGING

In a review of 36 published reports from 1970 to 1976,[51] comprising 910 patients, the sensitivity of detection of inflammatory lesions with gallium was 80% in 545 patients with the disease. The specificity was 96% in 365 patients without inflammatory disease. However, patients with neoplasms were excluded, because gallium cannot distinguish between neoplastic and inflammatory lesions.

The results of gallium imaging have varied widely in different reports. Ebright et al.[52] reported a sensitivity of 90% but a specificity of only 64%. Gallium was the most important means of establishing a diagnosis in only 6%. Many discrepancies and misinterpretation were encountered and, in 27% of all patients, the gallium studies were considered unnecessary in retrospect.

In contrast, Forgacs et al.[53] found a sensitivity of only 67% for abdominal abscesses but a specificity of 86%, excluding neoplasms. In their review of 8 other reported series, the sensitivity for inflammatory processes varied from 58 to 100% and the specificity from 75 to 100%. In another retrospective review of intraabdominal abscesses, the sensitivity was 73% and the specificity 81%.[54] These values did not vary significantly in different regions of the abdomen or pelvis. The results of gallium imaging were inferior to those of CT and ultrasound.

The common pitfalls in gallium abdominal imaging[55] included paralytic ileus, residual intraluminal activity in hepatic or splenic flexures or the cecum, and bladder activity obscuring pelvic inflammatory disease. At least in one series,[56] immunosuppressive therapy with glucocorticoids, renal, or hepatic failure were not significant factors in influencing the sensitivity of detection of occult infections.

Pulmonary Lesions. For differential diagnoses of increased gallium uptake in various regions of the body, see the review.[57] In a study of over 1100 pulmonary examinations in patients with gallium,[44] the sensitivity of detection of active pulmonary tuberculosis was 97%, untreated sarcoidosis 75%, silicosis or asbestosis 100%, and radiation pneumonitis 50%. Although 91% of acute bacterial pneumonias were demonstrated, only 30% of chronic pneumonias and 30% of interstitial fibrotic lesions were detected. Pulmonary images were rarely positive in bronchitis. Although pulmonary gallium uptake is nonspecific and due to many causes, it is an indicator of active disease. Serial images are often valuable in the follow-up of treatment regimens.

Following thoracotomy for lung cancer resection, a postoperative increase in gallium activity at the incision site or diffuse pleural activity is seen in as many as 30% of patients,[58] usually clearing in 3 to 6 months and almost always by 18 months. There are many causes of diffuse bilateral pulmonary uptake of gallium observed on 48-hour or later images. Active sarcoidosis is the most common cause, but opportunistic infections due to *Pneumocystis carinii* or cytomegalovirus are increasing in prevalence (See AIDS Section, this chapter). Other common causes of diffuse uptake include

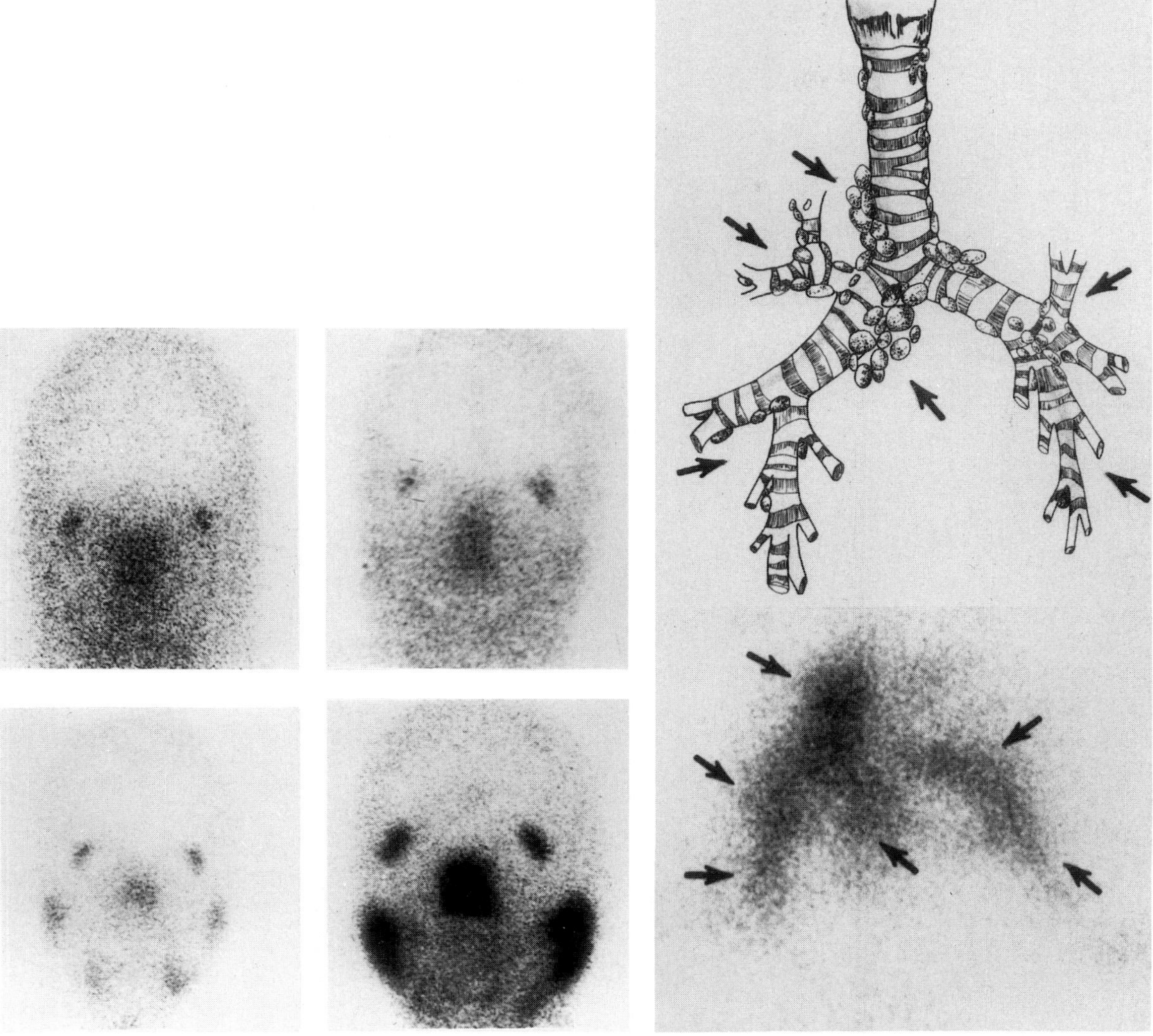

Figure 4. ^{67}Ga uptake. **(A).** (Upper left) normal lachrymal gland uptake, no parotid uptake. (Upper right) lachrymal uptake, mild diffuse parotid uptake (normal variant). (Lower) sarcoidosis (left) diffuse lachrymal and discrete parotid uptake. (right) marked lachrymal and parotid uptake (panda pattern). **(B).** (Upper) intrathoracic lymph node distribution. (Lower) sarcoidosis lymph node uptake distribution (lambda pattern). Arrows—upper right paratracheal, lower right and left parahilar, infrahilar, and central subcarinal nodes. (Reprinted with permission, from Sulavik SB et al, *J Nucl Med* 1990;31:1909–1914, ref 64.)

the pneumoconioses, disseminated lupus, lymphangitic carcinoma, eosinophilic granuloma, radiation, interstitial fibrosis, and lipiodol. Many drugs induce a toxic interstitial pneumonitis, such as bleomycin, busulfan, nitrosoureas, amiodarone,[59] cyclophosphamide, methotrexate, nitrofurantoin, BCG, and talc and other foreign agents in intravenous drug abusers.[50] Drug-induced pulmonary disease has been extensively reviewed.[60] The nitrosoureas, in particular, may cause pulmonary fibrosis after a few years of therapy. Rheumatoid migratory polyarthritis may produce intense diffuse lung activity due to interstitial pneumonia from infiltration of plasmacytes and activated lymphocytes.[61] The recently described tryptophan-induced eosinophilia myalgia syndrome produced diffusely increased pulmonary uptake of gallium associated with myalgia, arthralgia, fever, skin rash, edema, and marked dyspnea.[62] Bronchial biopsies have shown infiltrations of eosinophils, mass cells, and lymphocytes.

Demonstrating diffuse pulmonary uptake of gallium in many of the conditions mentioned above is particularly valuable when chest radiographic changes are minimal or absent. Many authors have generated a semiquantitative "gallium index" to indicate diffusely increased pulmonary uptake by camera-computer techniques. One such index[63] is the average counts/pixel in lung regions of interest divided by the average counts/pixel in the liver area of interest in posterior

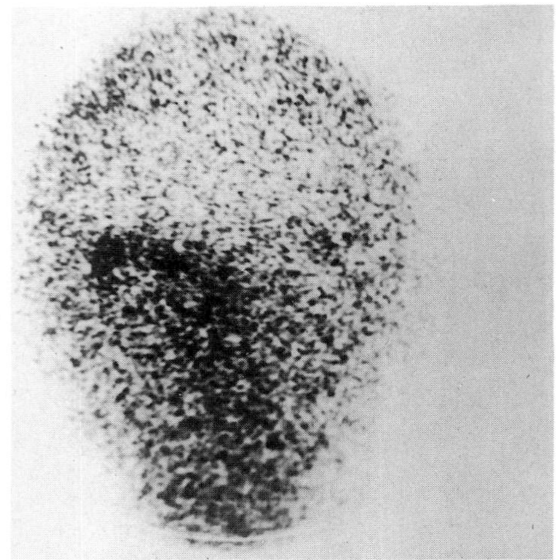

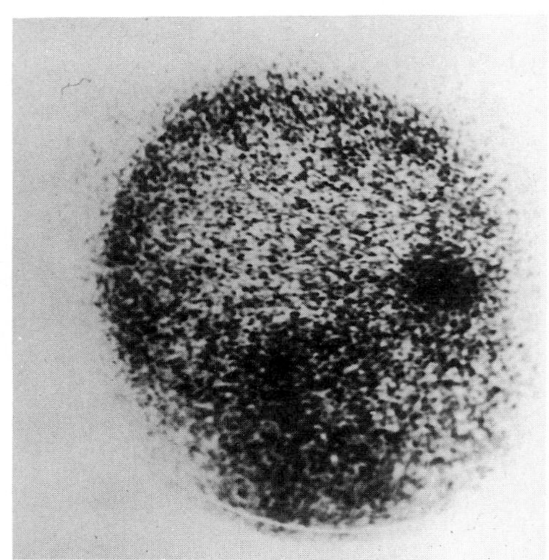

Figure 5. Anterior and right lateral 72-hour gallium images of the head of a 72-year-old woman with fever and swollen right eyelids. The right orbital abscess, best seen in the lateral view, required drainage.

projection images. For this index, the normal range is 28.4 ± S.D. 4.5% of the liver uptake. However, no standardized method of quantitation is widely accepted as yet.

In sarcoidosis, ^{67}Ga uptake in intrathoracic, mediastinal, and bronchopulmonary lymphadenopathy tends to have a distinctive pattern resembling the Greek letter lambda, often with symmetrical parotid uptake (panda appearance) (Fig. 4). This "panda appearance" is commonly associated with radiographic symmetrical hilar adenopathy. In contrast, lymphomas with intrathoracic lymphadenopathy have an asymmetrical, nonuniform, "bulky" appearance. In one series of 40 sarcoid patients,[65] as many as 75% had some increased uptake in the salivary glands. Other causes of this increased uptake included infectious parotitis, alcoholic

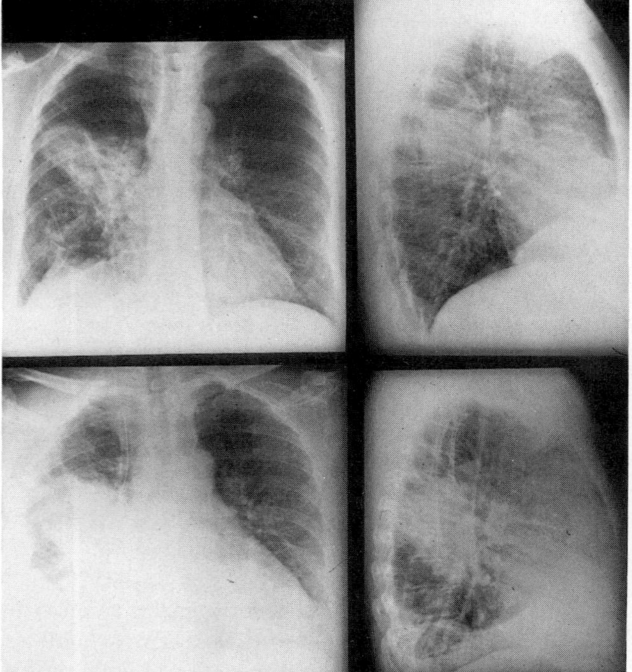
A

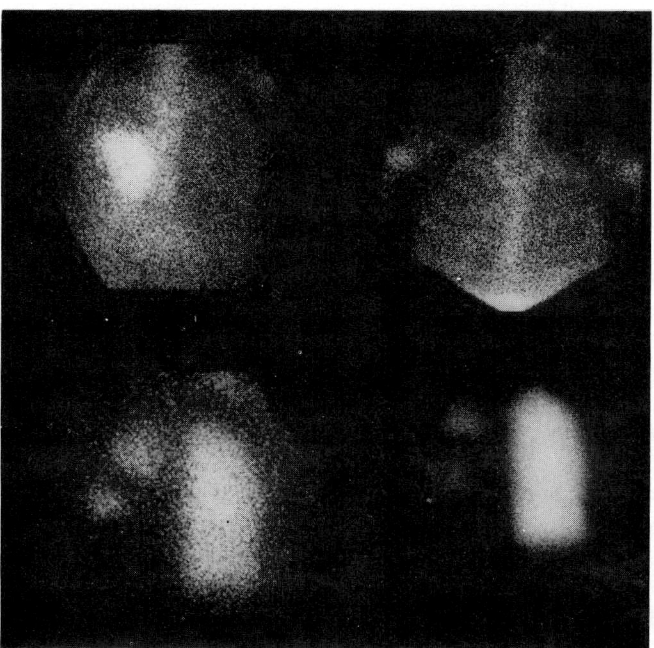
B

Figure 6. Chronic lymphocytic interstitial pneumonitis (by biopsy) in a 60-year-old female **(A).** PA and lateral chest radiographs show a large mass extending from the right hilum into the right lung laterally and posteriorly and a pneumatocele superiorly. Lower films 4 years later show some expansion of the mass. **(B).** Camera images. (Left upper) gallium posterior image shows an intense concentration in the mass whereas the indium-labeled leukocyte image (right upper) is almost negative. Posterior wash-in xenon (lower left) and perfusion (lower right) images show large matching V/Q defects due to the mass.

parotitis, scleroderma, and laceration of the cheek injuring Stensen's duct. A curvilinear rim of increased uptake in the orbits has been observed rarely in sarcoid uveitis[66] and commonly in orbital abscesses (Fig. 5). Increased uptake in calf muscles has been observed in a patient with longstanding fever and muscle tenderness, proven to be sarcoidosis by biopsy.[67] Increased bilateral uptake of gallium in submandibular and parotid salivary glands has been noted in primary but not secondary Sjögrens syndrome.[68] In this condition, there is a high incidence of increased pulmonary parenchymal uptake and sometimes increased mediastinal uptake as well.

Phenytoin administration may cause local or diffuse benign lymph node hyperplasia (pseudolymphoma), especially in mediastinal and hilar nodes.[50] Increased thymic or splenic uptake has been seen rarely in children after antibiotics or chemotherapy.[50] Discrete pulmonary parenchymal foci may be seen, not only in pneumonias, abscesses, and neoplasms, but also in active granulomas and chronic lymphocytic interstitial pneumonitis (Fig. 6).

Precordial Lesions. Patchy or diffusely increased myocardial uptake of gallium may be seen on 48- or 72-hour images in postviral myocarditis weeks after pharyngitis and coryza.[69] There may be chest pain, fever, elevated sedimentation rate, lymphopenia, and a failure to respond to antibiotics. This gallium uptake may disappear in several weeks in response to prednisone therapy, sometimes with azathioprine also. In a series of 68 patients with dilated cardiomyopathy and negative coronary arteriograms,[70] endomyocardial biopsies were compared with gallium precordial images. Five out of 6 patients with positive inflammatory changes on biopsy had dense gallium precordial uptake, whereas 9 of 65 negative biopsy samples had equivocal uptake and the remainder, no uptake. The biopsy positive and negative groups could not be distinguished clinically or by other laboratory techniques. Gallium, therefore, appeared useful in differentiating inflammatory from "idiopathic" cardiomyopathy. An example of increased myocardial gallium uptake is shown in Figure 7.

Gallium imaging is positive in acute bacterial pericarditis. However, it is also sometimes positive in acute nonspecific pericarditis.[71] This may be accompanied by fluid demonstrated by echocardiography, pericardial friction rub, chest pain, ST segment changes on EKG, and serum enzyme evidence of myocardial ischemia. Serial imaging may be useful in monitoring response to treatment with corticosteroids, salicylates, or indomethacin.

Postpericardiotomy syndrome (days or months after initial intrapericardial surgery) often produces chest pain, fever, dyspnea, sweating, malaise, anorexia, myalgias, pericardial friction rub, pericardial effusion, increased sedimentation rate, and leukocytosis. Gallium images are usually negative early, but patients with symptoms persisting 2 weeks or more have focal or diffusely increased pericardial gallium uptake, suggesting an inflammatory etiology.[72] Gallium is of little or no value for the detection of cardiac transplant rejection.[73]

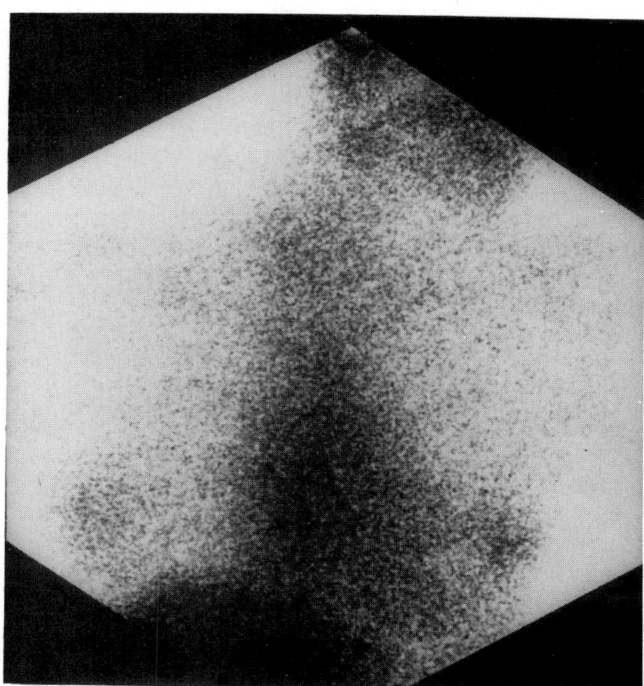

Figure 7. Gallium 48-hour image demonstrates high uptake in the mediastinum due to sarcoid cardiomyopathy (biopsy proven). This 36-year-old woman had symptoms of congestive heart failure. Note increased activity also in the breasts and salivary glands.

However, postcardiac transplant mediastinitis, a fairly common complication, may be detected by increased uptake of gallium retrosternally.[74]

In summary, the differential diagnosis of increased gallium uptake in the precordium includes acute pericarditis, both bacterial and nonspecific, postpericardiotomy syndrome, postcardiac transplant mediastinitis, cardiomyopathy of inflammatory origin, acute myocardial infarction, sarcoidosis, myocardial abscess in infective endocarditis,[75] amyloidosis, mycotic aneurysm, and infected grafts.

Renal Lesions. Gallium activity in the kidneys is normally not visible by 48 hours in planar posterior images, but may still be faintly visible in tomographic images.[76] Although normal gastrointestinal activity may obscure lesions in the peritoneal cavity, it usually does not obscure renal lesions. Focal or unilateral renal lesions include renal abscess, focal pyelonephritis, or acute lobar nephronia. The last condition is a severe form of pyelonephritis with focal uptake and edema, but not liquefaction, as in abscess or carbuncle.[77] A differentiation between these two conditions is best made by computed tomography, which demonstrates liquefaction in abscesses as areas of decreased attenuation. Acute pyelonephritis, particularly in childhood, may resolve with no residual changes on images with gallium or conventional renal radiodiagnostic agents. Gallium imaging has proven valuable in differentiating active lower tract from upper tract infections[78]; the sensitivity of detection was 75% in 43

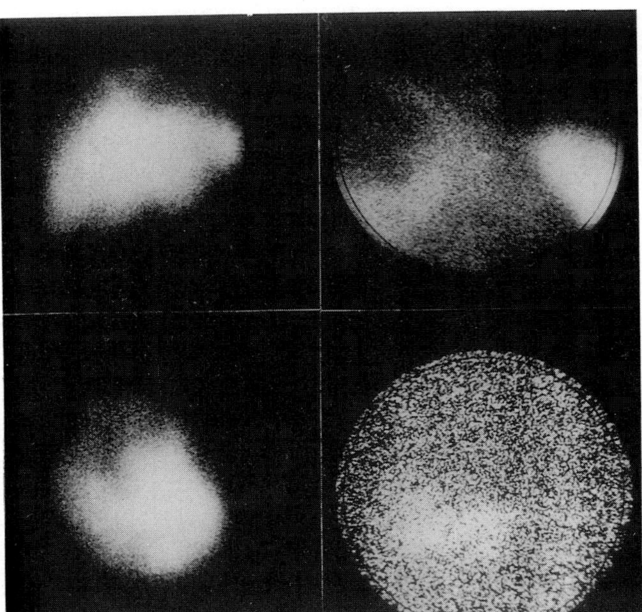

Figure 8 A. This 31-year-old male had a low-grade fever. Anterior and posterior ^{99}Tc-sulphur colloid images (upper row) and right lateral image (left lower) showed a large photopenic defect in the upper right hepatic lobe. A 72-hour posterior ^{67}Ga image (right lower) showed increased concentration in the lesion. A large confluent abscess was found surgically.

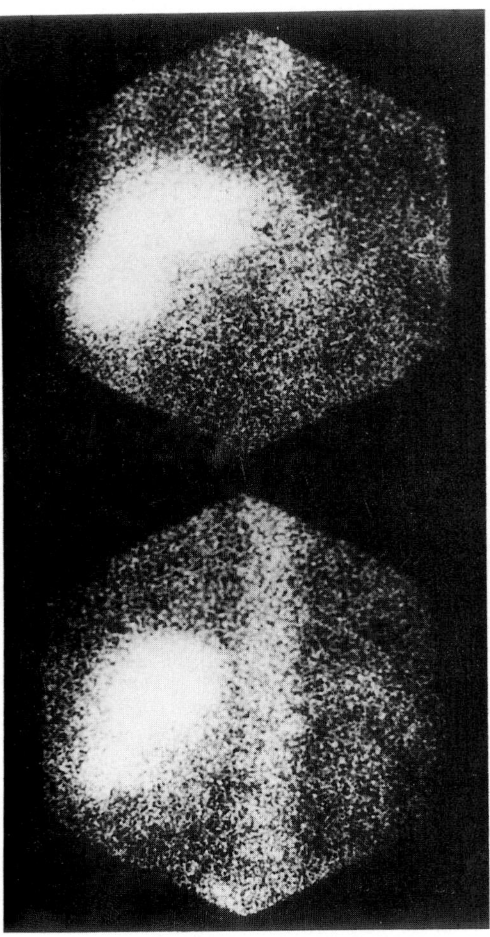

Figure 8 B. Anterior and posterior ^{67}Ga images of the upper abdomen at 48 hours in a febrile 60-year-old male. The intense activity in a large area of the liver was due to innumerable microabscesses. This abnormality was not detected by ultrasonography or CT.

patients who had pyelonephritis and the specificity was 87%. Usually, the increased uptake involved the whole kidney, but some had only focal lesions. Imaging for acute pylonephritis could usually be performed at 24 hours rather than 48 hours. As a rule, gallium images became normal after 2 or more weeks of antibiotic therapy.

In a retrospective review of 500 ^{67}Gallium images,[79] abnormal renal uptake of gallium occurred in 6%. The common causes of this increased accumulation were infection, drug-induced renal damage, urinary stasis, collagen vascular disease, and renal failure.

With bilateral increased gallium uptake, it is important to distinguish between abnormal bilateral parenchymal retention and stasis in the pelvocalyceal systems. For complete differential diagnoses of abnormal renal gallium uptake, see references 57 and 79. Differential diagnosis includes vasculitis, Wegener's granulomatosis, ATN, acute interstitial nephritis, hemochromatosis, lymphomas, advanced hepatocellular disease, and after ureterosigmoidostomy.

Many drugs induce interstitial nephritis,[50] such as ampicillin, methicillin, sulfonamides, sulfinpyrazone, ibuprofin, cephalexin, other cephalosporins, furosemide, hydrochlorothiazide, erythromycin, rifampin, pentamidine, phenylbutazone, gold salts, allopurinol, phenazone, phenobarbital, phenytoin, and phenindione. Some patients with retroperitoneal fibrosis show increased uptake of gallium, whereas others do not.[80]

Other Intra-abdominal Lesions. The differential diagnosis of abnormal hepatic concentrations of gallium include abscess, pyogenic and amoebic, cholecystitis, hepatoma, lymphoma, and metastatic melanoma. The abscesses may be large and confluent (Fig. 8 A) or multiple microabscesses (Fig. 8 B). Metastatic carcinoma is a relatively uncommon cause of focal hepatic uptake of gallium.

Of many intraabdominal inflammatory lesions, gallium imaging is of little or no value in the detection of acute pancreatitis.[56] Infants and young children may have marked diffusely increased intraabdominal gallium uptake due to severe hypoproteinemia from malnutrition[81] resembling the appearance of generalized peritonitis.

RADIOLABELED LEUKOCYTES

Labeling Techniques

Several reports[82–85] provide detailed protocols on harvesting mixed leukocyte suspensions from fresh whole blood and

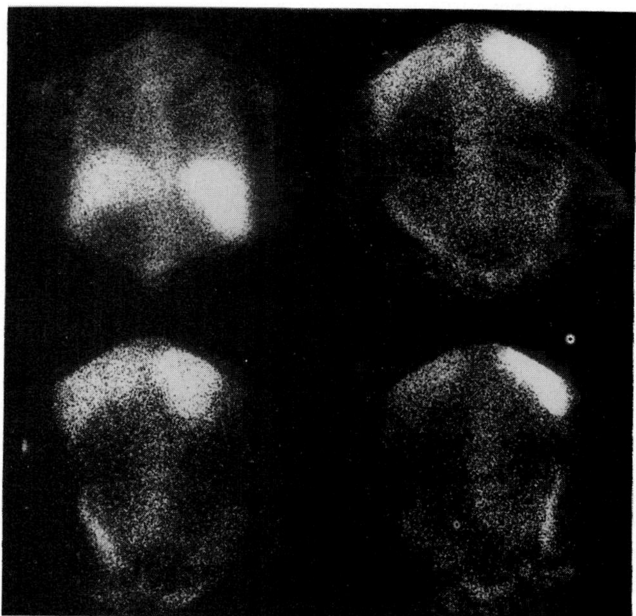

Figure 9. Normal torso images 24 hours after 1 mCi ^{111}In-oxine-labeled mixed leukocytes. (Left upper) anterior, (right upper) posterior, and (lower) anterior oblique images. Activity is seen only in the liver, spleen, and marrow. With satisfactory harvesting and labeling of the leukocytes, splenic activity should be more intense than hepatic uptake.

labeling with ^{111}In-oxine. Similar clinical results were obtained with mixed leukocytes suspensions prepared by simple gravity sedimentation and granulocytes isolated by centrifugation using discontinuous gradients.[86] Similar clinical results were obtained with ^{111}In-tropolone or ^{111}In-oxine. In patients with leukopenia, (2000 leukocytes/mL or less) ABO-matched donor cells must be used from HIV- and hepatitis-negative subjects. Labeled donor leukocytes tend to migrate very rapidly in leukopenic patients.[87]

Leukocyte Images

On 24-hour images, the normal anatomical structures seen are the liver, spleen, and erythropoietic marrow (Fig. 9). When the preparation of the labeled leukocytes is technically satisfactory, there should be a higher concentration of activity in the spleen than the liver. With technically unsatisfactory preparations, the liver concentration is higher than that of the spleen, and there may even be persistent pulmonary activity. When the harvesting and labeling procedures ex vivo consume more than about 3 hours, their migration pattern tends to be abnormal, and inflammatory lesions may be missed. Images within the first hour or two after injection show diffuse pulmonary activity that normally disappears by about 4 hours. This transient diffuse pulmonary activity is less with ^{111}In-tropolone than ^{111}In-oxine because the former agent labels the cells effectively in the presence of plasma.

Intraarterially injected ^{111}In-oxine labeled leukocytes clear from the body more rapidly than intravenously injected leukocytes clear from the lungs. This has suggested to some workers that the lung capillaries may have specific receptors.[88] However, these kinetic differences could be entirely due to other factors[89]—the lung capillaries are smaller than the average systemic capillary, the perfusion pressure is an order of magnitude lower, and the flow is pulsatile.

A sizable fraction of the labeled leukocytes in the spleen is capable of recirculating. Normally, the fall in splenic activity between 3 and 24 hours is less than 10%. In a variety of infections, however, this fall can be as high as 40 to 50%.[90]

Results of Labeled Leukocyte Imaging

In one large series[91] representative of many published reports, 991 leukocyte studies were retrospectively reviewed, including 363 inflammatory sites. The sensitivity of detection was 80%. There were 19 false-positive diagnoses of focal infection, resulting in a specificity of 97%. The sensitivities of detection in the abdomen and chest were similar (88%), but the specificity of chest lesions was poorer.

CLINICAL APPLICATIONS OF RADIOLABELED LEUKOCYTES

Head and Neck. The common lesions producing positive leukocyte images in the head and neck[6,92] are gingivitis, apical and periodontal abscesses, recent tooth extraction or dental surgery, sinusitis, mastoiditis, thrush, pharyngitis, osteomyelitis of the jaws, neck abscesses, and lymphadenopathy. Jugular phlebitis may produce a vertical, linear focus of increased uptake in the neck. In a comparison of labeled leukocytes, ^{67}Ga and ^{99m}Tc-MDP in inflammatory lesions of the head and neck,[92] the sensitivity and specificity of the labeled leukocytes were 94 and 100%, respectively, compared to 56 and 43% for ^{67}Ga, and 86 and 0% for MDP. The labeled leukocyte images became negative in response to successful treatment much sooner than the gallium images, and the MDP images tended to remain positive indefinitely in successfully treated lesions.[92] Both gallium and leukocyte images may be positive in malignant otitis media before radiographic changes are evident.[93]

Intracranial Lesions. In a literature review of 39 positive leukocyte imaging studies of the skull,[94] 18 proved to be abscesses or other infections, 9 were gliomas, 9 were metastases, 2 were attributed to marrow activity associated with hyperostosis, and the remaining lesion was an infarct. Nonetheless, most brain abscesses show an intense localization of labeled leukocytes.[95] In patients on high or moderate doses of corticosteroids, however, the abscesses may go undetected. In epidural abscesses, the leukocyte images may be negative.[5] Gliomas and intracerebral metastases often show weak or moderate infiltration.[95] Positive images have been reported in meningitis[5] and subdural hematomas.[96]

The Lungs. Persistent bilateral diffuse pulmonary uptake of labeled leukocytes is a nonspecific finding seen in a variety of conditions, including severe sepsis, congestive

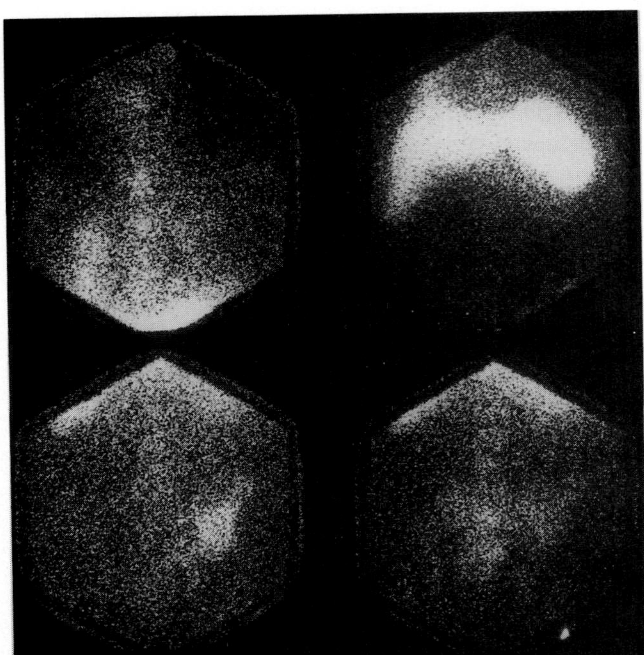

Figure 10. This obtunded 57-year-old female had *Legionella* pneumonitis and required a respirator. Labeled leukocyte images of the chest (upper) show abnormal uptake in both lungs, and midline activity around the tracheostomy tube. The anterior abdominal image (left lower) showed unexpected fixed focal uptake in the left lower quadrant and the posterior image (right lower) showed activity overlying the sacrum. A Gastrografin enema confirmed the presence of a pericolic abscess from a ruptured diverticulum. The abscess was drained. (Reprinted with permission from *Radiology* 1985;155:221–229.)

heart failure, uremia, leukemia, viral pneumonitis, after hemodialysis or peritoneal dialysis, after cardiopulmonary resuscitation, postradiation therapy, and CMV infection complicating renal transplantation.[3] Imaging has not often been performed in adult respiratory distress syndrome (ARDS), but both ^{67}Ga[97] and labeled leukocytes[6] have produced strongly positive images. In systemic vasculitis (Wegener's granulomatous and microscopic polyarteritis),[98] leukocyte images show marked early and diffuse pulmonary activity, often with marked splenic, bowel, and nasal uptake also.

Local or regional areas of increased uptake in the lungs are usually due to such infections as pneumonia (Fig. 10), abscess, atelectatic pneumonia (Fig. 11), empyema, septic embolus (Fig. 12), bronchiectasis, bacterial or fungal mediastinal abscess, or infected catheters.[3] Indwelling tubes, including nasal, gastric, or endotracheal tubes (Fig. 10), drains, or intravascular catheters often produce a focus of faint to moderately increased uptake after they have been in place for several days, even though they do not appear infected clinically. Localized single or multiple intense foci of activity in the lung fields may be artifactual due to leukocytic emboli from clumping in vitro.

Necrotizing tracheobronchitis may produce a distinctive pattern in leukocyte pulmonary images. Increased uptake in the trachea, major bronchi, and perihilar areas may be observed.[99] This condition occurs in newborns and infants and, uncommonly, in adults after several hours of assisted respiration.

In one reported series[100] 16% of patients with intraabdominal infections had extraabdominal foci of infection, frequently unsuspected, and many of these were chest lesions.

The Heart. In subacute bacterial endocarditis, the infected vegetations are generally too small to be visualized by labeled leukocyte or gallium images.[6] However, myocardial abscesses associated with prosthetic or native valvular endocarditis have been detected by leukocyte images when echocardiography is nondiagnostic.[101] Moreover, in CT or MRI examinations, these abscesses may have the same appearance as hematomas, seromas, or noninfected thrombi.[102] Diffusely increased myocardial activity has been seen in viral myocarditis, uremic or bacterial endocarditis, and acute rheumatic carditis.[3]

Silent acute myocardial infarcts may show increased leukocyte accumulation; however, some acute myocardial infarcts have been missed.[3] In one series,[103] 60% of patients with acute myocardial infarction had focal or diffuse cardiac uptake optimally seen 24 to 48 hours after the onset of pain. In another series of 30 patients,[104] leukocyte planar images were positive in 23 (77%) and SPECT images were positive in 6 patients with negative planar images. The lesions were best observed if the labeled leukocytes were reinjected within 18 hours of the onset of symptoms and imaged 24 hours later. Although leukocyte imaging is normally not needed for the diagnosis of acute myocardial infarction, it may shed some light on the mechanism of the reperfusion injury following myocardial ischemia.

Vascular Lesions. Acute aortofemoral or iliofemoral bypass infections in the first 6 postoperative weeks often present as draining groin fistulas. In contrast, late graft infections of this type, and especially intraabdominal graft infections may be difficult to diagnose. Dacron grafts are more susceptible to hematogenous spread of infection because pseudointima formation occurs slowly. In a review of 8 reported series totaling 201 patients,[105] ^{111}In-leukocyte scintigraphy had a sensitivity of 94% in 78 patients with graft infection and a specificity of 87%. False-positives have been due to hematoma, aseptic aneurysms, and pseudoaneurysms, wound infections surrounding or near the graft, or thrombosed grafts. Postoperative uptake may persist for at least a week after graft placement. CT or MRI may demonstrate the extent of the infection better than scintigraphy. Leukocyte imaging is useful in distinguishing active from quiescent graft infections after a course of antibiotic therapy.[106] Leukocyte scintigraphy generally is also diagnostic in mycotic aneurysms.[107]

The sensitivity of detecting infected synthetic vascular grafts for chronic hemodiaylsis is high.[108] This procedure is especially valuable when physical examination of the access site reveals no abnormality.

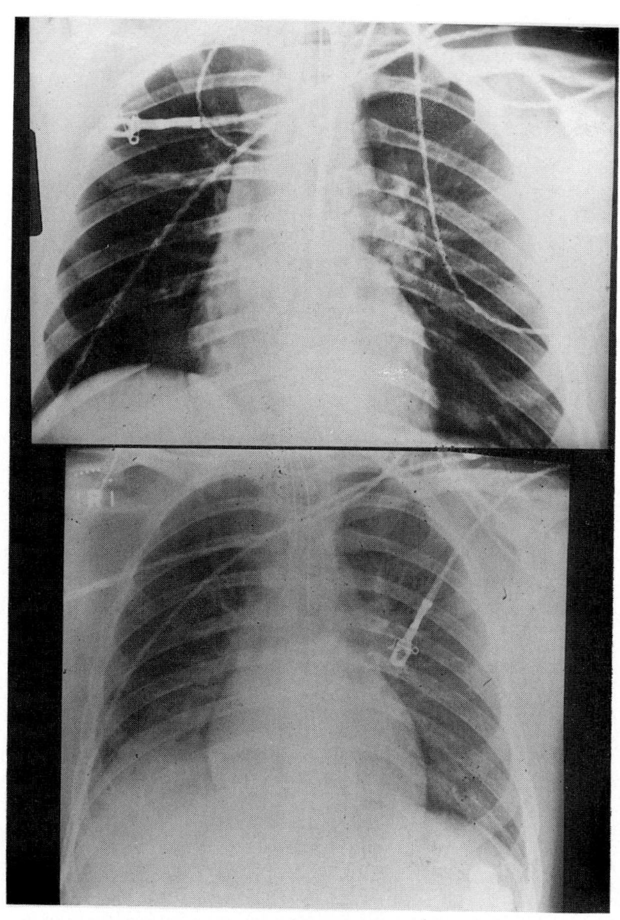

A

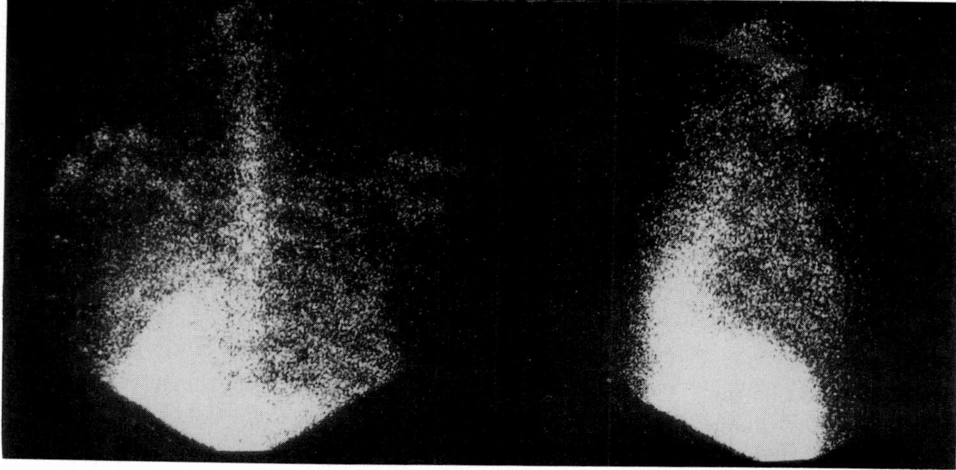

B

Figure 11. This 76-year-old male patient was recovering from surgery following a motor vehicle accident. A routine postoperative chest film (**A**, upper) was clear. However, suddenly he became weak and developed a low-grade fever. The next day, the chest film (**A**, lower) showed atelectasis of the right lower lobe, obscuring the right dome of the diaphragm. ^{111}In-leukocyte posterior and right lateral images **(B)** the next day indicated the diagnosis of atelectatic pneumonia.

Abdomen and Pelvis. A great variety of abdominopelvic lesions produce positive leukocyte images, including infected surgical wounds, pyogenic or amoebic abscesses (Fig. 13), diverticulitis (Fig. 10), peritonitis (Fig. 14), acute appendicitis, and bowel infarction. Larger liver abscesses may be seen as foci of increased activity greater than in the normal hepatic parenchyma (Fig. 15). However, smaller ones may be missed, or detected only by subtraction with ^{99m}Tc-colloid images.

The activity of intrinsic inflammatory bowel diseases such as Crohn's disease, ulcerative colitis, or pseudomembranous colitis is assessed, particularly in Europe, by serial leukocyte imaging.[109] Sometimes this is combined with quantitative radioassays of stools collected over 4 days. When gastrointestinal uptake is observed, follow-up images showing progression through loops of bowel help to distinguish radioactivity in the lumen from intrinsic lesions in the bowel wall.

In Crohn's disease, ^{111}In-leukocyte imaging demonstrates the location, extent, and degree of activity of the inflammatory process.[109] Nonetheless, the images may overestimate

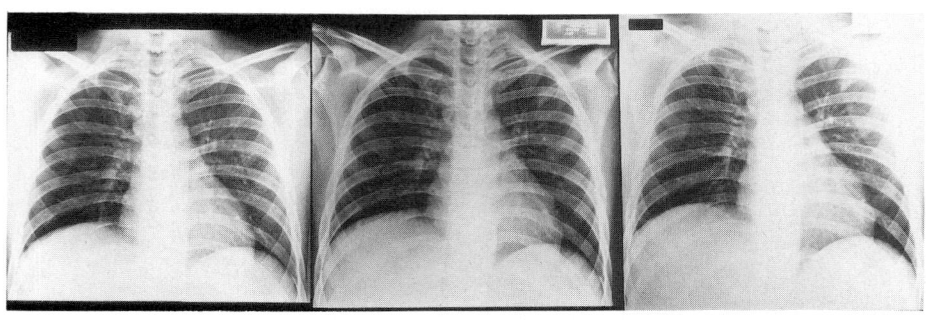

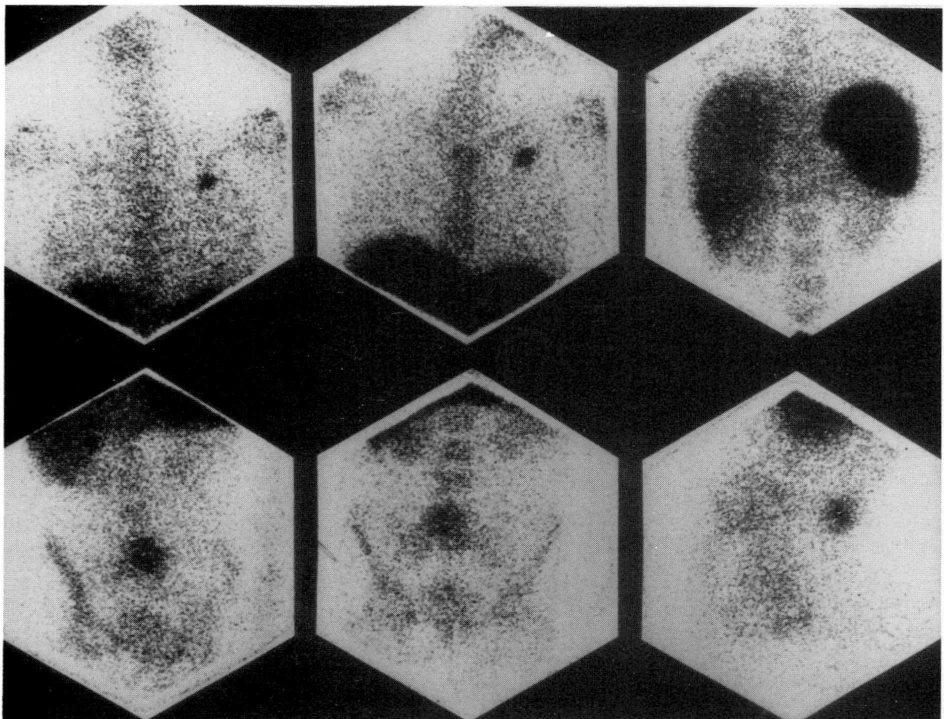

Figure 12. This 16-year-old male was recoverying from surgery for an enterocutaneous fistula, and the initial postoperative chest film was negative. (**A**, left). Eight days later, he became febrile again, and a second chest film (**A**, middle) showed a localized infiltrate in the left upper lobe which persisted three days later (**A**, right). ^{111}In-leukocyte anterior and posterior images of the chest (**B**, upper row) showed high activity in the left upper lobe lesion—presumptive evidence of a septic embolus. (**B**, lower row) anterior, posterior, and right lateral abdominal images show a residual superficial abscess in the region of the umbilicus which ruptured spontaneously a few days later.

the extent of the lesions when the intrinsic bowel and luminal activity are not separated.[110] The images may be particularly helpful when symptoms are of recent onset, and barium studies may still be negative. Lesions of the terminal ileum are not approachable by endoscopy, either.[110] Moreover, with more advanced disease, images may distinguish strictures primarily due to inflammatory edema from inactive fibrotic ones. The intrinsic bowel lesions, as a rule, are best demonstrated on 4- to 6-hour images. By 24 hours, most of the activity tends to be in the distal bowel lumen. Persistent stationary activity raises the suspicion of complications[110]—extraintestinal activity from abscess, sinus, or fistulous tracts.

The differential diagnosis of abnormal activity in the intestinal lumen includes swallowed pus from infected sinuses, upper or lower respiratory tract, thrush of the mouth, pharynx, or esophagus, intrinsic inflammatory bowel diseases, gastrointestinal bleeding,[111] and abdominal fistulae into the gastrointestinal tract (Fig. 16). There may be faint to moderate colonic accumulation from multiple enemas or in patients with "antibiotic colitis." Mucosal infections of the distal large bowel are commonly seen in psychiatric patients with marked constipation (Fig. 17).

A tunnel infection along the tract of a Tenckhoff catheter is a common complication of continuous ambulatory peritoneal dialysis (CAPD). Infections of the external tract in subcutaneous tissue and skin are usually apparent clinically, but infections at the internal cuff that can lead to peritonitis are often occult. However, these "inner tract" infections, as a rule, can be detected by leukocyte imaging.[112] By placing a radioactive marker on the site of external emergence, external and internal tract infections can be distinguished from one another. On 24-hour leukocyte images in the posterior projection, renal activity is normally either not or only faintly visualized. Moderate or marked activity in the urinary system, including the renal parenchyma, pelvocalyceal systems, ureters, or bladder usually indicates a urinary tract infection.[6] This imaging may be helpful in differentiating between upper

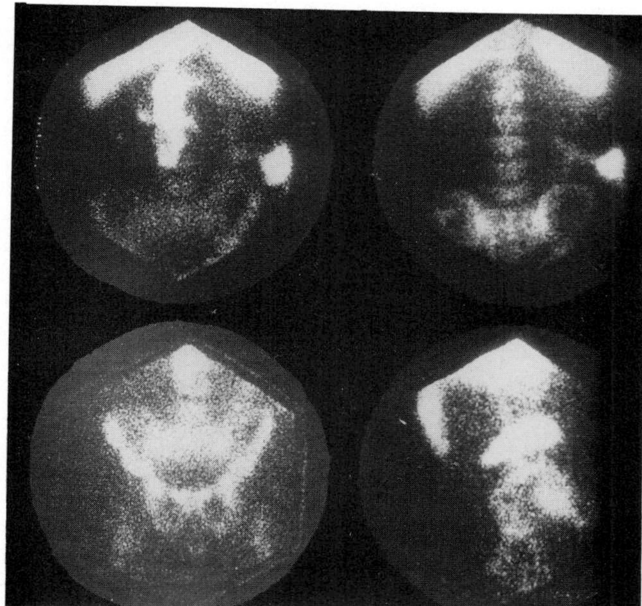

Figure 13. ^{111}In-leukocyte images in a 33-year-old male with postoperative fever after resection of a pseudocyst of the pancreas. (Upper) anterior and posterior abdominal images show intense activity in the midline due to infection of the surgical incision and a second intense focus in the flank. In the left lateral view (right lower) the infected wound is seen anteriorly, and the flank abscess is between the spleen and the iliac crest. The flank abscess was drained.

tract and lower urinary tract infections (Fig. 18). Uncommonly, activity in the urinary system may be due to fistulae from the intestinal tract, other adjacent structures, or malignancies.

Increased leukocyte uptake in renal transplants has been observed in 73% of episodes of acute rejection.[113] In cytomegalovirus (CMV) infections, there is also increased renal uptake usually accompanied by increased diffuse pulmonary uptake. Abnormal transplant infiltration of leukocytes may be produced also by cyclosporine nephrotoxicity or following administration of antilymphocyte (OKT3) monoclonal antibody. Sometimes increased uptake is observed in well-functioning renal transplants for no apparent reason.[114]

LEUKOCYTE INFILTRATION IN NONINFECTIOUS INFLAMMATION AND NONINFLAMMATORY LESIONS

Many noninfectious inflammatory lesions, as well as abscesses and phlegmonous foci of infection, cause focal accumulations of leukocytes, and some noninflammatory lesions will do so as well.[6] Aside from technical failures in cell labeling, however, abnormal foci of activity are rarely seen in the absence of microscopic leukocytic infiltration. Hence, the term "false-positive leukocytes images" can have different meanings. Intense concentrations of labeled leukocytes increase the likelihood of the presence of abscess or recent hematoma (Fig. 19).[115] Recent skin grafts may have striking uptake without evidence of infection.

Photopenic lesions in the erythropoietic marrow may be seen in many conditions[116] such as lymphoma, vertebral osteomyelitis, after radiation therapy, following extensive surgery, metastatic carcinoma, multiple myeloma, avascular necrosis, Paget's disease, myelofibrosis, and fibrous dysplasia.[117] In one review of over 300 leukocyte imaging studies, the incidence of skeletal photopenic areas was 12% and the most common causes were fractures, avascular necrosis, tumors, prostheses, and other orthopedic hardware.[118] Liver metastases also often appear photopenic on leukocyte images.

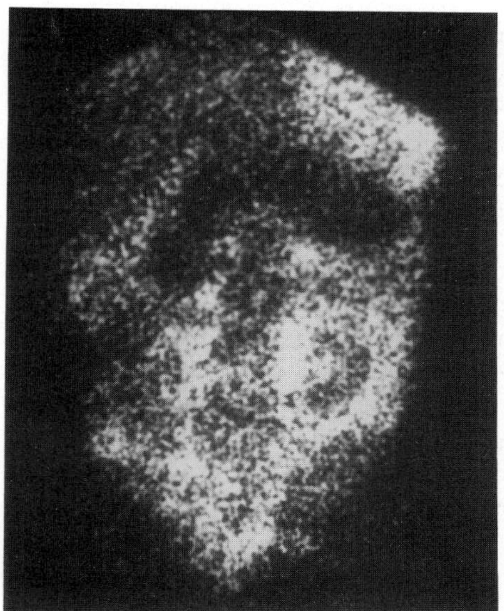

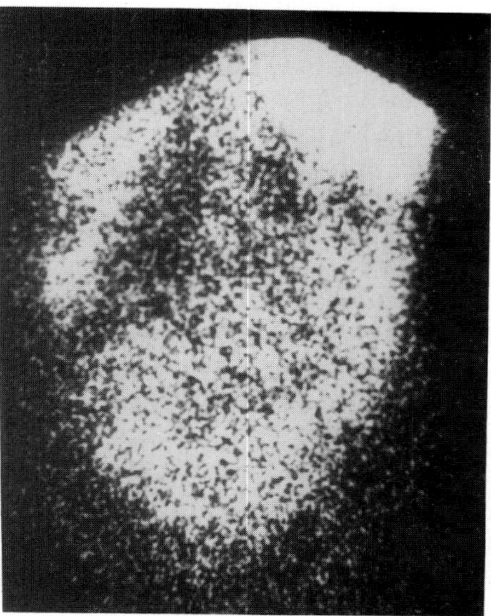

Figure 14. Multiple organ failure from prolonged sepsis in a 30-year-old female following laparotomies for recurrent small bowel necrosis. ^{111}In-leukocyte 24-hour anterior abdominal image (left) shows multiple patches of uptake and vertical stripes corresponding to the edges of the infected dehiscent surgical wound. Posterior image (right) demonstrates diffuse abdominal activity from generalized peritonitis. (Reprinted with permission from *Radiology* 1985; 155:221–229.)

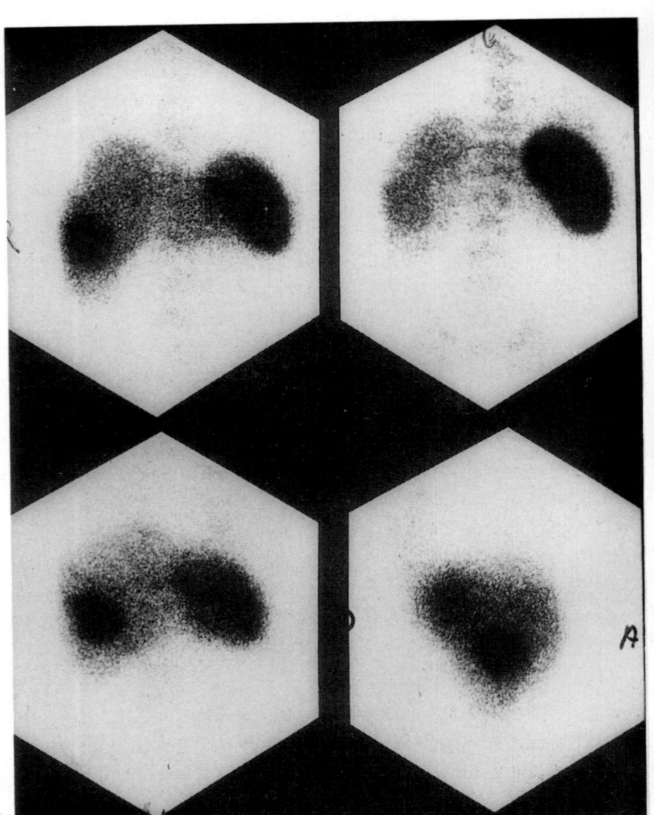

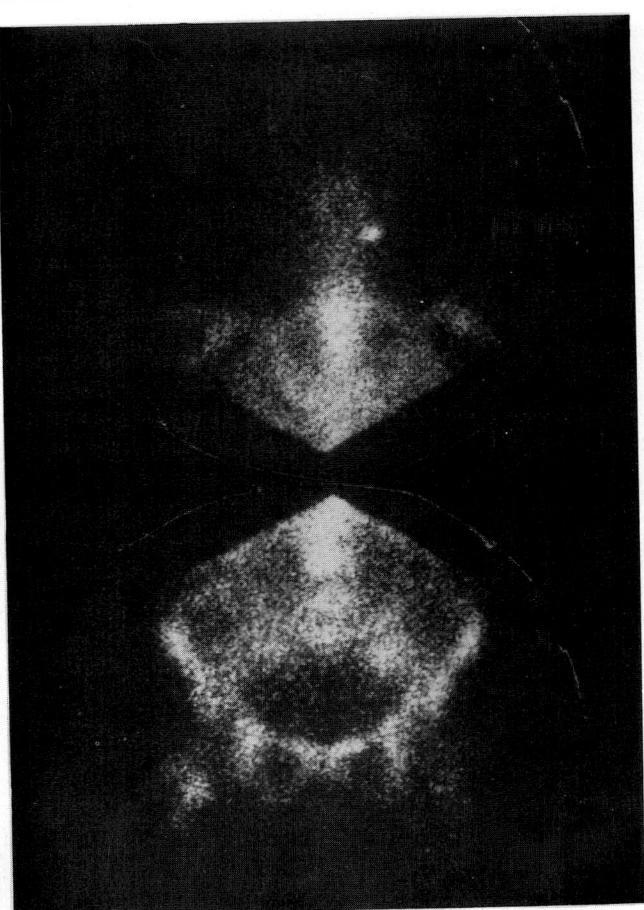

Figure 15. **(A)** (upper) anterior and posterior, and (lower) right anterior oblique and lateral ^{111}In-leukocyte 24-hour images were obtained in a 78-year-old febrile woman. A large area of increased uptake is seen in the anteroinferior right lobe of the liver. This abscess was drained surgically. In searching for the source of the infection, other images of the body **(B)** showed a focus in the left pharynx. The patient remembered that her left tonsil was biopsied several weeks previously. The focus below the right lesser trochanter was attributed to the patient's asymptomatic right hip prosthesis.

The incidence of increased accumulation of labeled leukocytes in uninfected neoplasms varies widely in different reports. In one series of 150 cancer patients,[119] there was only one false-positive study attributable to an osteolytic metastasis of a shoulder from breast carcinoma. In another series,[120] the incidence of false positive uptake of labeled leukocytes due to neoplasms was 2.3%. In 12% of the patients with known malignancies the intensity of uptake was usually faint, mostly in soft tissue neoplasms, but occasionally in bone metastases also.

In another series of 61 patients with fever of unknown origin in a cancer hospital,[121] noninfected neoplasms produced positive images in 34%. These lesions occurred in lymph nodes, soft tissues, and bone neoplasms, either primary or secondary, and in either hematological or solid tumors. In another study of 25 patients with malignancy[122] 10 had positive leukocyte images correlated with granulocytic infiltration histologically. In still another study,[123] leukocyte images were more frequently positive in brain metastases, especially from lung carcinoma. The infiltrating cells were sometimes granulocytes, lymphocytes, macrophages, or mixed leukocyte populations. Intense leukocyte uptake may be more common in lymphomas than in other malignancies.[122]

The marrow at the site of recent radiation portals may show intense activity with labeled leukocytes after about 2000 cGy. This appearance tends to be more striking than is demonstrated on diphosphonate images.[124]

In rheumatoid arthritis, even of long duration, there may be intense uptake in multiple joints. In this disease, there is frequently marked neutrophilic infiltration of the joints daily, extending over many years. Likewise, intense uptake is commonly seen in gouty arthritis.[125] Repeat studies after successful therapy may show marked regression.

False-positive abdominal leukocyte images have been described in thrombosis of the inferior vena cava[8] and probably occur from venous thrombosis at many other sites. Accessory spleens or splenic implants after splenectomy commonly appear as single or multiple foci. However, they are rarely confused with infectious foci unless they are large or ec-

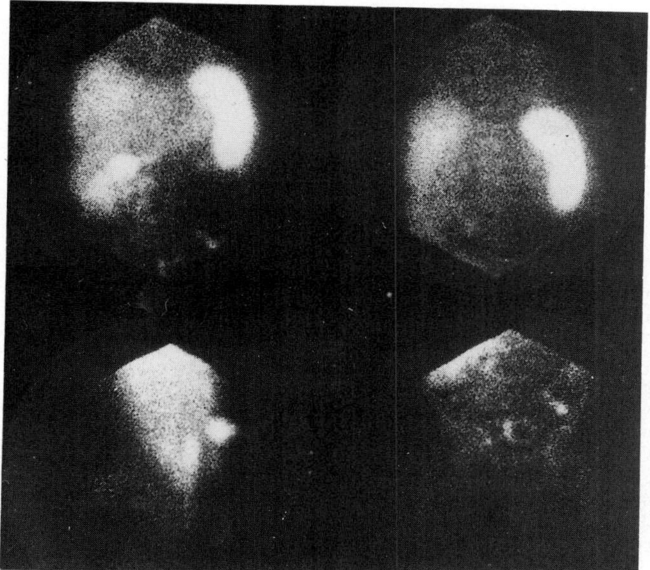

Figure 16. This 80-year-old developed a spiking fever one month after a Whipple's procedure for carcinoma of the ampulla. Blood cultures were positive for *Enterococci*, but the CT exam was negative. (Upper) anterior and posterior images of the upper abdomen. An intense focus is seen anteriorly superimposed on the inferior margin of the right side of the liver. The right lateral view (left lower) shows the focus superficial to the gallbladder bed due to a residual Enterococcal abscess. The anterior view of the pelvis (right lower) shows activity in scattered loops of small bowel from a fistula between the abscess bed and jejunum.

topic.[6] As a rule, recent surgical wounds may appear as faint foci unless they are infected. Decubitus ulcers healing by granulation also have only faint uptake. When they show intense uptake, infection should be suspected. In patients with diarrhea, the skin may be contaminated with labeled leukocytes from feces producing irregular patches of increased activity. Superficial uninfected burns of the abdomen and elsewhere on the body have shown leukocytic infiltration (Fig. 20).

In the lungs of severely ill septic patients, the diffuse bilateral pulmonary increased activity is often triggered by endotoxin. Monocytes secrete Interleukin-1 (IL-1) and tissue necrosis factor alpha (TNF alpha), which activate neutrophils and increase their adherence to pulmonary endothelium. Leukotriene B4[126] and bacterial lipopolysaccharides[127] also play important roles in this response. In the extreme, these interactions give rise to the adult respiratory distress and septic shock syndromes with gross pulmonary sequestration of granulocytes.

Increased uptake in cervical nodes is common in both adults and children. Inguinal node activity is less common, and axillary node activity is more unusual. Often this nodal activity is the consequence of a regional infection but, frequently, there is no apparent clinical explanation.[128]

^{99m}Tc-HMPAO LEUKOCYTE IMAGING

This is the best agent available for labeling leukocytes in vitro with ^{99m}Tc for imaging inflammatory foci. A detailed description of the methods of harvesting and labeling leukocytes with HMPAO in plasma or saline-plasma was provided by Roddie et al.[129] Imaging was performed at 1, 4, and 24 hours. These workers preferred 4-hour over 24-hour images because of the appearance of bowel activity at the later time. Activity is seen also in the kidneys and bladder normally; hence, this agent is of doubtful value in urinary infections. Occasionally, the gallbladder is visualized normally. Reynolds et al.[130] estimated that this occurs in 5 to 10% of patients at and beyond 3 hours. Because of this, the diagnosis of acute cholecystitis with this agent must be made with caution. The biliary excretion into the bowel adds to the gastrointestinal activity normally seen after 4 hours. Localized activity in the right lower quadrant due to normal bowel contents may be confused with acute appendicitis.[130]

In a clinical comparison of ^{99m}Tc-HMPAO and ^{111}In-tropolone for leukocyte labeling, Peters et al.[131] found that the plasma disappearance half-time of the ^{99m}Tc label was 4.4 hours, whereas the half-time clearance of the ^{111}In label was 6.3 hours. It was concluded that the shorter half-time of the ^{99m}Tc-HMPAO was due to some elution of the label.

Using another technique of labeling the leukocyte suspension in small volumes of saline (1 to 2 ml), the cell labeling yields are higher than in plasma.[132] The initial high diffuse lung activity normally falls rapidly during the first hour. Marrow activity in normal images appears more prominent than with the ^{111}In lipophilic agents.

Many inflammatory lesions of the abdomen are visualized within a few minutes, but the activity progressively accumulates up to 4 hours.[133] The mechanism of this early accumulation is not known. However, comparative studies with ^{99m}Tc-labeled erythrocytes show only faint or no uptake in inflammatory lesions. Irritable bowel syndrome may produce positive images by 4 hours.

In a comparative clinical study, ^{99m}Tc-HMPAO labeled leukocytes and ^{67}Ga had the same sensitivity in detecting inflammatory lesions, but the labeled leukocytes had a higher specificity.[134] Furthermore, ^{99m}Tc is more readily available on an emergency basis, and the results with the labeled cells are obtained within a few hours of injection. Because a larger dose of ^{99m}Tc activity can be administered, compared with ^{111}In, SPECT imaging becomes easier.

Four- and 24-hour images were performed with both ^{99m}Tc-HMPAO and ^{111}In-oxine labeled leukocytes in another series of 41 patients.[135] The two radioactive labels had an equal sensitivity of detection. The ^{99m}Tc-HMPAO images were better at 4 hours, and the ^{111}In-oxine images were better at 24 hours. The specificity of the ^{99m}Tc agent was relatively low (62%) at 4 hours, due to physiological bowel activity, compared to 80% for the 24-hour ^{111}In images.

In a comparison of ^{99m}Tc-HMPAO with ^{111}In-oxine labeled leukocytes simultaneously injected in dogs with induced

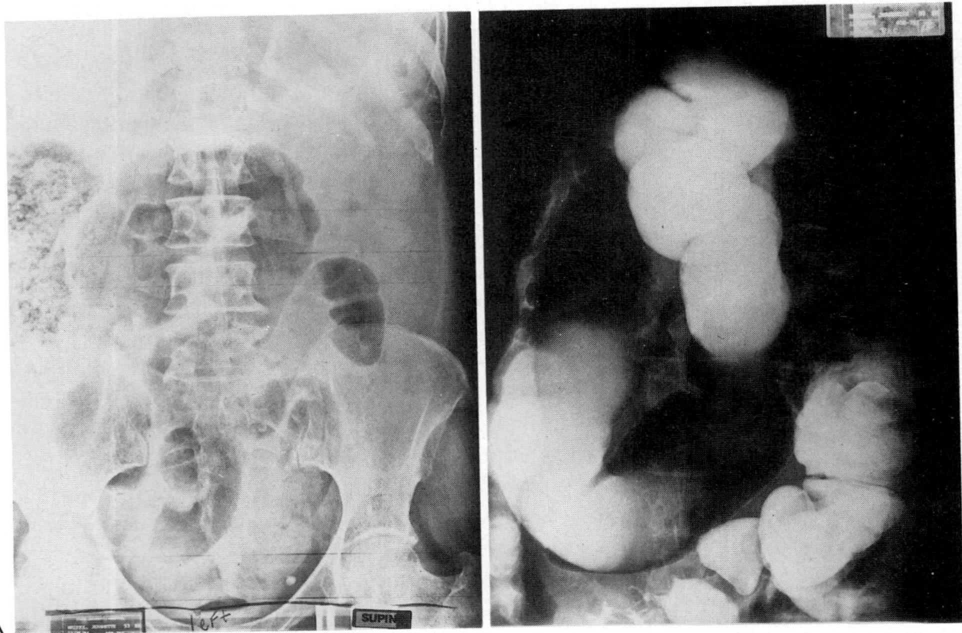

A

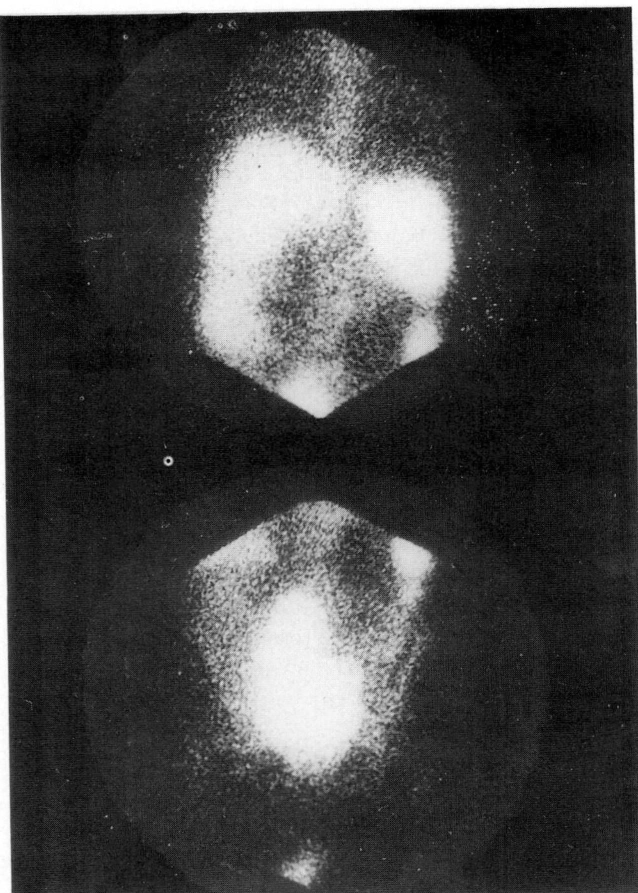

B

Figure 17. This 33-year-old severely retarded female from a psychiatric institution developed fever and abdominal distention. A plain film of the abdomen (**A,** left) shows loops of large bowel distended with gas and feces on the right. The barium enema (**A,** right) proved that the distended large bowel was patent. ^{111}In-leukocyte 24-hour images (**B**) of the abdomen and pelvis showed intense activity in the large bowel. Note the similarity in contour of the sigmoid colon between the image and the barium enema. The colitis was due to a *Clostridial* infection secondary to prolonged constipation and responded well to vancomycin therapy.

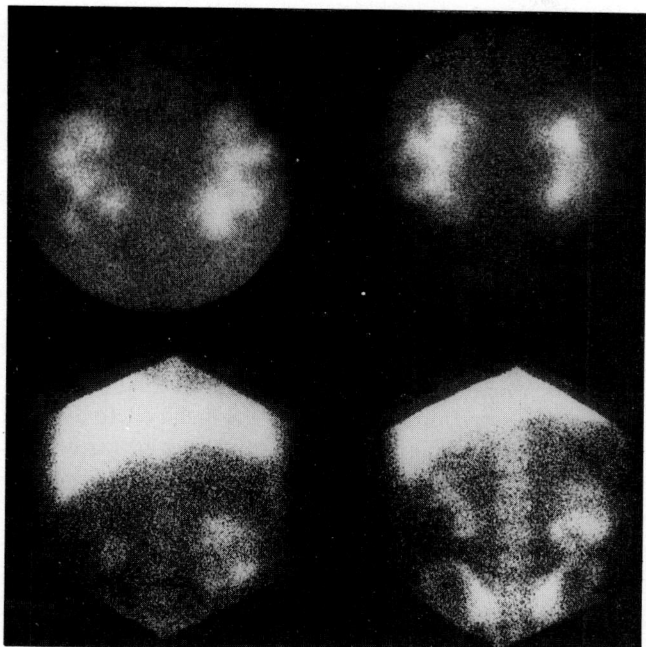

Figure 18. Acutely infected polycystic kidneys in a 31-year-old male diabetic. (Upper) 4-minute and 1-hour images after ^{99m}Tc-glucoheptonate show enlarged kidneys, multiple photopenic defects due to cysts and activity in dilated calyces at 1 hour. (Lower) anterior and posterior 24-hour indium-leukocyte images show activity in the dilated renal collecting systems and ureters due to bilateral pyelonephritis.

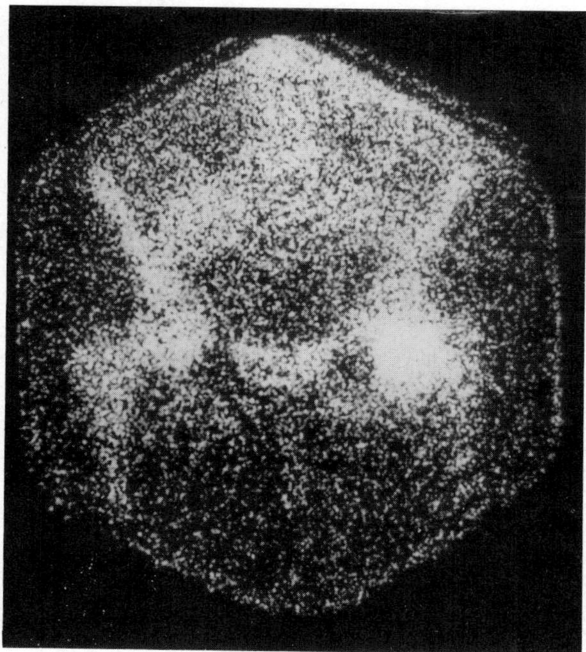

Figure 19. ^{111}In-leukocyte image of anterior pelvis at 24 hours shows localized uptake overlying the left femoral head due to a small hematoma. A percutaneous femoral puncture for cardiac catherization was performed 1 day before the radioactive injection. The patient's fever lasted only a few hours, without evidence of infection. (Reprinted with permission from *Radiology* 1985; 155:221–229.)

E. coli abscesses, the mean abscess concentration, abscess/blood, and abscess/muscle concentration ratios were 3 to 3.5 times higher with ^{111}In-oxine than ^{99m}Tc-HMPAO at 18 hours.[136] The estimated leukocyte radiation dose while circulating from the Auger electrons in cGy/mCi with ^{99m}Tc was greatly reduced (390 vs. 14,080 for ^{111}In).[29] However, if leukocyte suspensions after labeling contained 8 to 10 mCi of ^{99m}Tc to improve image quality, the cell radiation dose would be 3120 to 3900 cGy. Previous experiments (McAfee, unpublished) showed that 5000 cGy or more of added radiation lowers the concentration of activity in *E. coli* abscesses by about 80%, in addition to decreasing the cell recovery in the circulation (Fig. 1). Although some authors have used higher levels of 15 to 20 mCi ^{99m}Tc for cell labeling, this may have an undesirable effect on the migration to inflammatory foci, if the cell labeling efficiency were high. Labeling isolated mixed leukocytes in plasma from 46 ml of blood with 20 mCi ^{99m}Tc-HMPAO (labeling efficiency about 32%) induces nuclear damage to lymphocytes estimated to be equivalent to 2600 cGy of X-radiation.[137] This induces an almost complete impairment of their proliferation capacity.

A single case was reported of anaphylactoid reaction, producing hypotension and collapse immediately after the injection of ^{99m}Tc-HMPAO leukocytes, with complete recovery.[138]

After an extensive clinical experience with ^{111}In and ^{99m}Tc-HMPAO labeled leukocytes, Peters[139] prefers ^{99m}Tc-HMPAO in acute sepsis for which an answer is urgently required. However, he prefers ^{111}In for more chronic processes, such as infected hip prostheses, renal sepsis, or suspected intraabdominal abscesses, when the turnover of granulocytes is slower and 24-hour images are better than earlier ones.

RADIONUCLIDE IMAGING IN AIDS

The diagnosis of human immunodeficiency virus (HIV) infection is confirmed primarily by enzyme immunoassay, Western blot tests, and depression of the T-cell helper/suppressor lymphocyte ratio (CD 4/CD 8 ratio normally 0.8 to 2.9). Radionuclide imaging is invaluable in demonstrating many of the myriad complications of acquired immune deficiency syndrome (AIDS). Excellent reviews on this subject have been published by Vanarthos et al.[140] and Miller.[141]

Gallium Imaging

INTRACRANIAL LESIONS

With CT or MRI, it is frequently difficult to differentiate inflammatory processes, such as toxoplasmosis, from gliomatous or lymphomatous tumors complicating AIDS. However, thallium images are usually positive in neoplasms and negative with inflammatory lesions.[140] In AIDS encephalopa-

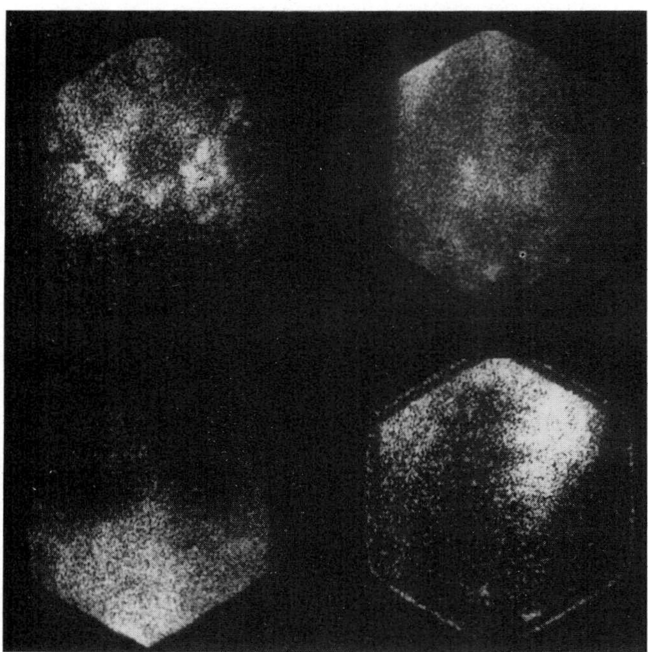

Figure 20. ^{111}In-leukocyte 24-hour images of a 70-year-old psychiatric patient with fever and multiple burns from an overheated electric blanket. (Upper) anterior and posterior pelvic views show irregular patches of increased uptake, chiefly in the groins. (Lower left) a large area of diffuse uptake overlies the lower chest posteriorly. (Lower right) increased uptake in both upper thighs anteriorly, more intense on the left. Only the left thigh burn was infected clinically.

thy, ^{99m}Tc-HMPAO images of the brain often show patchy focal or multifocal areas of hypoperfusion, sometimes when CT and MR images are normal.[142]

THORACIC COMPLICATIONS

The most common complication of AIDS is *Pneumocystis carinii* pneumonia (PCP), which typically causes diffuse bilateral increased uptake of ^{67}Ga (Fig. 21 **A**). There may or may not be associated diffuse pulmonary infiltrates visible radiographically. When this infection is treated by inhalation of such agents such as trimethoprim-sulfamethoxazole (Bactrim, and others), follow-up gallium images may show increased uptake only in the upper lung fields (Fig. 21 **B**), because the gas and aerosol exchange there is not as great as in the lower lung fields. ^{133}Xe ventilation and ^{99m}Tc-MAA images sometimes show pneumatoceles associated with PCP. Some workers have measured the lung clearance half-time of ^{99m}Tc-DTPA aerosol after 4 or 5 minutes as an indicator for PCP. Due to the increased lung capillary permeability, the half-time is very short even compared to that of noninfected smokers or patients with bacterial infections.[143–145] This method has the advantage that the results are available immediately, rather than waiting 48 hours after administering the gallium for pulmonary imaging.

Diffuse pulmonary uptake of ^{67}Ga in children with AIDS is frequently due to lymphocytic interstitial pneumonitis (LIP).[146] This condition usually has an insidious onset with salivary gland swelling, digital clubbing, extensive lymphadenopathy, frequent splenomegaly, and sometimes coarse nodular pulmonary interstitial infiltrates radiographically. Biopsies show nodular peribronchial lymphocytic infiltration. There may be mediastinal widening and prominent hili in addition to the diffuse pulmonary parenchymal uptake of gallium. However, the pulmonary uptake tends to be not as marked as in PCP.[140]

In cytomegalovirus infection, typically there is slight perihilar activity. Eye uptake may be due to retinitis, and adrenal involvement frequently produces increased uptake. In PCP and other diffuse infections, the hepatic uptake is often depressed, accompanied by increased pulmonary activity. As a result, lung-to-liver uptake ratios tend to be abnormally high.

Localized or regional increased lung uptake of gallium may be due to bacterial pneumonia, but sometimes also may occur in PCP.[147] Nodal or perihilar uptake is commonly due to *Mycobacterium avium intracellulare*, but may also be seen in *M. tuberculosis* infections. Generally, these inflammatory nodes can be differentiated from the contiguous more bulky masses of lymphomas complicating AIDS. Typically, in infections associated with AIDS, ^{201}Tl images are negative, ^{67}Ga images are positive; however, in Kaposi's sarcoma, gallium images are typically negative and thallium images positive.[148]

AIDS-related myocarditis or pericarditis may produce increased cardiac gallium uptake. Myocarditis may also result in increased uptake of anticardiac myosin monoclonal antibodies and a decreased ejection fraction of multi-gated imaging (MUGA) studies.[140]

SALIVARY GLANDS

Almost half of all AIDS patients with increased salivary uptake of gallium have diffuse infiltrative lymphocytosis syndrome (DILS).[149] In the remaining patients, the increased uptake may be due to undifferentiated salivary gland disease or to AIDS itself. The increased uptake then is generally not as intense as in DILS. The CD8 cell counts are markedly elevated and the CD4 counts moderately reduced in DILS; in contrast, AIDS patients have normal CD8 counts and markedly reduced CD4 counts.

RENAL COMPLICATIONS

In AIDS nephropathy, bilateral diffusely increased uptake of gallium may be present in some patients[140] but not in others.[150] The kidneys tend to be uniformly enlarged, and renal atrophy and hypertension are conspicuously absent. The increased gallium uptake correlates well with the degree of proteinuria, but not with the BUN or serum creatinine.[151] Twelve to 55% of AIDS patients (average about 30%) develop acute renal failure with a rapid progression of disease.[152] Frequently, there is proteinuria in the nephrotic stage. HIV nephropathy is seen in asysmptomatic HIV individuals and only about half of the patients have AIDS.[153] This com-

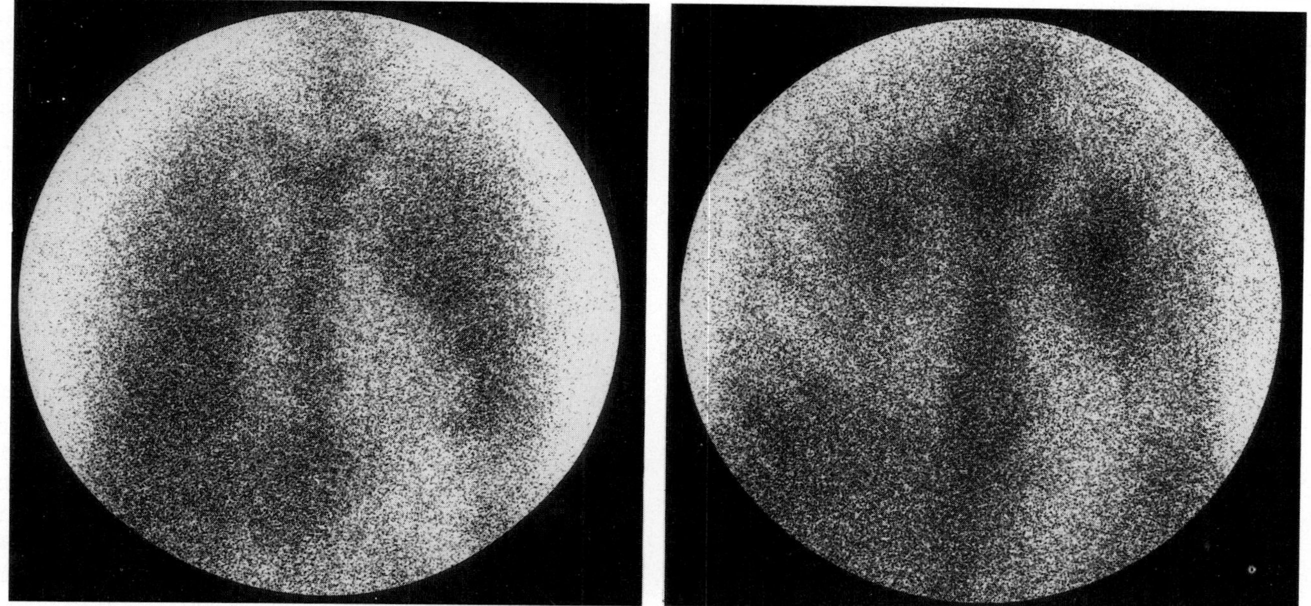

Figure 21. *Pneumocystis carinii* pneumonia in 2 HIV-positive young male patients. Anterior images of the thorax 48 hours after 5 mCi ^{67}Ga-citrate. **(A).** Bilateral diffuse increased lung uptake with an intensity like that of the liver. The mediastinum appears photopenic except for the midline sternal activity **(B).** Bilateral increased uptake is predominantly in the upper lung fields because previous treatment with trimethoprim-sulfamethoxazole [Bactrin] cleared the inflammation disproportionately in the lung bases.

plication occurs predominantly in male, black, intravenous drug users. Other renal complications in AIDS patients[154] include infiltrative lymphoma or leukemia, ATN from drug toxicity, heroin-associated nephropathy (HAN),[155] and similar lesions from other narcotics, CMV, and other incidental urinary infections.

Radiolabeled Leukocyte Imaging in AIDS

In a comparative study of ^{111}In radiolabeled leukocyte images and gallium images performed in the same series of febrile AIDS patients,[156] 56% of foci of infection, chiefly of bacterial origin, were identified only on the labeled leukocyte images. Some of these lesions were pulmonary infections, but many were abdominal. On the other hand, PCP pneumonia and lympadenopathy were detected most frequently on gallium images. Because AIDS patients often have leukopenia, compatible donor leukocytes should be used for ^{111}In radiolabeling. In handling blood specimens from AIDS patients, special precautions must be used, and misadministration of the labeled cells must be scrupulously avoided.

GASTROINTESTINAL COMPLICATIONS

Labeled leukocyte images are much more valuable than gallium images in detecting gastrointestinal (GI) complications of AIDS, because of the absence of normal GI activity with the former. Hence, in such conditions, intense colonic activity with radiolabeled leukocytes may remain undetected with gallium.[157] In immunocompromised patients, candidiasis of multiple regions such as the oral cavity, esophagus, stomach, and vagina is well demonstrated with labeled leukocytes.[158] Many other conditions causing diarrhea and increased intestinal uptake of labeled leukocytes or gallium include infections from: *Cryptosporidium, Giardia, Isospora, Salmonella, Shigella*, or mycobacterial organisms (Fig. 22). Increased uptake may also be caused by antibiotic-induced colitis. A syndrome of AIDS-related sclerosing cholangitis is apparently caused by opportunistic organisms, such as CMV or *Cryptosporidia*. Hepatobiliary imaging may demonstrate dilatation and cholestasis of the bile ducts.[141]

MUSCULOSKELETAL COMPLICATIONS

Reiter's Syndrome, psoriasis, and seronegative polyarthritis-like rheumatoid arthritis have an increased prevalence in AIDS patients, and may be complicated by musculoskeletal infections. The primary lesions may be demonstrated on diphosphonate images, and the secondary infections with gallium or labeled leukocyte images. Bone involvement, especially in the thorax, may be due to actinomycosis or nocardiosis. These lesions may be seen on gallium or diphosphonate images.[140]

NEWER RADIOLABELED AGENTS FOR IMAGING INFLAMMATORY FOCI

In attempting to avoid the time-consuming process of harvesting and labeling leukocytes in vitro, other agents besides ^{67}Ga have been tried that can be directly injected intravenously. A nanometer-sized albumin colloid (Nanocoll TN Solco Basle Ltd., Switzerland) has a mean particle size of

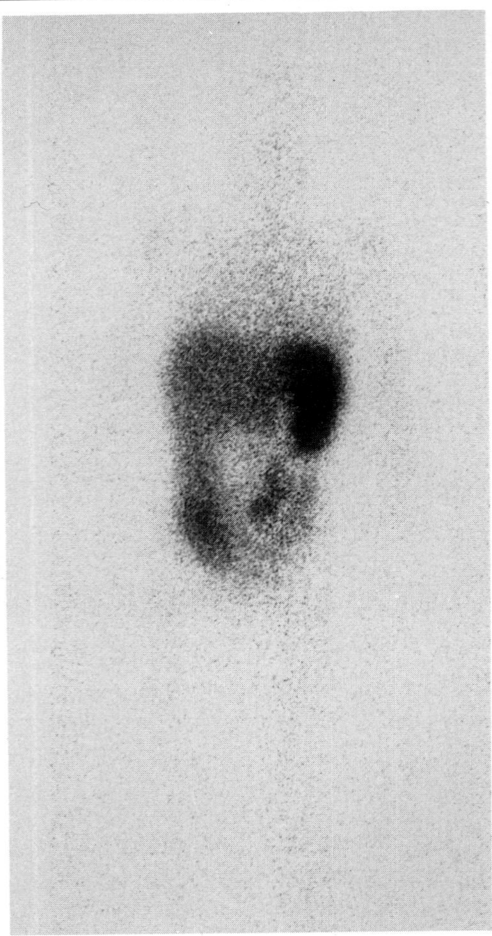

Figure 22. Anterior whole-body 24-hour ^{111}In-leukocyte image in a 29-year-old hemophiliac male with AIDS running high fevers for a few weeks, with left lower quadrant pain. Peripheral leukocyte count 2400/mm^3. Intense pancolic activity consistent with colitis and splenomegaly are shown. Colonoscopy with biopsy confirmed extensive infiltration by *Mycobacterium avium intracellulare*. No evidence of extramural involvement. Absence of marrow activity was probably due to diffuse MAI replacement. (This illustration was kindly provided by Dr. Christopher J. Palestro, Long Island Jewish Medical Center.)

only 30 nm and particles no larger than 80 nm.[159] Its plasma clearance is much more rapid than macromolecules, such as serum albumin or gamma globulin. Images with this ^{99m}Tc-labeled nanocolloid can be obtained from 30 minutes to 2 hours. It has been advocated particularly for osteomyelitis and septic arthritis, but it cannot differentiate septic from sterile lesions or postsurgical trauma.[159,160] In a clinical comparison with ^{99m}Tc-HMPAO, the detection sensitivity of the ^{99m}Tc-nanocolloid was only 59% compared to 97% for ^{99m}Tc-HMPAO labeled leukocytes; it was concluded that the labeled nanocolloid was satisfactory only for bone or joint inflammatory lesions.[161] Anionic phospholipid liposomes labeled with ^{99m}Tc also have been proposed for local inflammatory lesions, including arthritis.[162]

A ^{99m}Tc-labeled synthetic porphyrin, tetraphenylporphyrinsulfonate (TPPS), originally proposed for tumor localization, has been tried for imaging inflammatory foci because it accumulated in sites of histamine injection in mice and is tightly bound to plasma proteins. In a clinical trial of ^{99m}Tc-TPPS in 16 patients, the images at 2 hours were positive, as were 24-hour images with ^{111}In-labeled leukocytes.[163] However, the ^{99m}Tc-label for TPPS proved to be too unstable.

In deep thigh inflammatory lesions in rats, Rubin et al.[164] observed a greater accumulation of ^{125}I- or ^{111}In-labeled polyclonal human IgG than with ^{67}Ga citrate or ^{99m}Tc-albumin at 3 and 24 hours. However, ^{99m}Tc-albumin has been notoriously unstable in vivo. By autoradiography,[165] almost all the ^{111}In-IgG activity was in the extracellular space with minimal association with inflammatory cells. Hence, binding to leukocytes through their Fc receptors was not the mechanism of localization, as was formerly thought. Increased tissue permeability appeared to be the major factor in localization. A hydrazine nictotinamide bifunctional chelate was developed for coupling to polyclonal IgG for labeling with ^{99m}Tc. This proved to be similar to the ^{111}In-labeled IgG in rat experiments.[166]

For clinical studies, human nonspecific polyclonal immunoglobulin (hIgG), prepared commercially for intravenous therapeutic use (Sandoglobulin) was conjugated with diethylenetriamine pentaacetic acid (DTPA) carboxycarbonic anhydride labeled with ^{111}In. This product was administered intravenously (1.75 mg protein, 1.5 mCi ^{111}In). Gamma camera images at 6, 24, and especially 48 hours, successfully demonstrated 58 of 63 focal inflammatory lesions (sensitivity 92%).[167] However, 13 of 16 malignant neoplasms also showed focal localization. Because there was no normal gastrointestinal excretion of this product, it was potentially useful for delineating inflammatory bowel disease. In another clinical series,[168] all 37 known inflammatory lesions were demonstrated by 9 hours, but better demonstrated by 24 hours. These lesions included abscesses, pelvic inflammatory diseases, tuberculosis, sarcoidosis, *Pneumocystis carinii* pneumonia, hematoma, and synovitis.

Since the introduction of radiolabeled polyclonal IgG for imaging focal infections, a large number of clinical studies have been reported, but there are very few comparative studies with labeled leukocytes. In Europe, ^{99m}Tc-labeled polyclonal IgG has been used clinically. In one comparison of ^{111}In-labeled leukocytes with ^{99m}Tc-HIgG in intraabdominal sepsis, 1 of 9 inflammatory lesions was missed with the ^{99m}Tc agent but demonstrated with ^{111}In-leukocytes.[169] The presence of ^{99m}Tc in the kidney and bladder precluded the detection of urinary infections, and the prolonged retention of the ^{99m}Tc activity in the plasma resulted in a high background activity surrounding the inflammatory lesions.

There are practical difficulties in comparing these newer radiodiagnostic agents with "established" agents for demonstrating inflammatory foci in humans. Therefore, different agents were compared with ^{111}In-oxine labeled leucocytes in acute soft tissue abscesses and acute arthritic lesions in 24 dogs.[170] These agents included ^{67}Ga citrate, human polyclonal

A 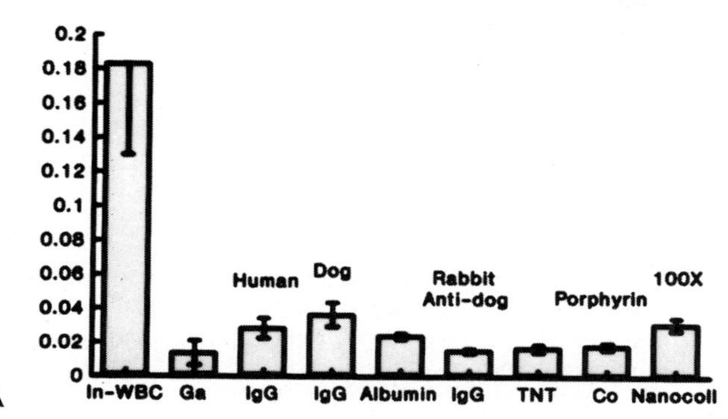

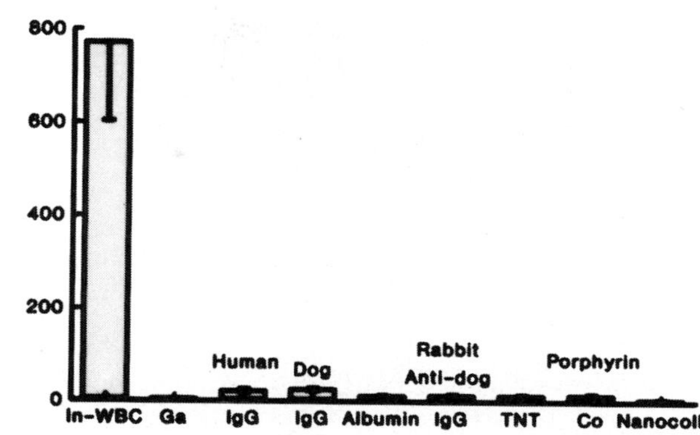 B

Figure 23. 24-hour localization of 8 different radiopharmaceuticals compared with simultaneously injected autologous ^{111}In-oxine labeled leukocytes in *E. coli* canine abscesses. **(A)** Abscess concentration in administered activity/gm and **(B)** abscess/muscle concentration ratios. All of the directly injected agents tested were inferior to the in vitro labeled leukocytes. The localization of labeled polyclonal IgG and serum albumin were not significantly different (data from reference 170).

IgG, canine IgG, canine antigen-antibody complex, human serum albumin, other proteins, ^{57}Co-labeled TPPS, and ^{99m}Tc-nanocolloid. None of these 8 agents exhibited abscess concentrations, abscess/blood, or abscess/muscle concentration ratios in any way comparable to the high values obtained with simultaneously injected ^{111}In-oxine labeled leukocytes (Fig. 23). There was no significant difference between the values of any of the labeled proteins or labeled porphyrin. Hence, there was no significant difference between radioiodinated human serum albumin and radiolabeled polyclonal IgG. The ^{99m}Tc-labeled nanocolloid had a much lower abscess concentration than any of the other agents. The values for the oldest agent, ^{67}Ga-citrate were disappointing in these acute experiments.

In an analogous study of bacterial abscesses in mice,[171] abscess concentrations, abscess/blood, and abscess/muscle ratios at 4 and 24 hours were similar for ^{67}Ga, ^{99m}Tc-labeled serum albumin, polyclonal IgG, and monoclonal antibody TNT-1 against nuclear histone.

Fishman et al.[172] developed 4 analogs of the chemotactic oligopeptide of N-Formyl-methionyl leucyl phenylalanine (N-Formyl-Met-Leu-Phe), coupled with DTPA for ^{111}In-labeling. Neutrophils and monocytes possess specific receptors for these chemoattractants. *E. coli* abscesses in rats are imaged within 5 minutes with these agents and the blood clearance is extremely rapid, compared to the slow clearance of ^{67}Ga and labeled IgG. However, this agent does not sequester in the spleen, as one would expect if the leukocytes were labeled in vitro. Very small microgram quantities of these peptides profoundly activate neutrophils and induce immediate marked neutropenia.[82] Activated neutrophils have greatly increased their adherence to endothelium. Moreover, there is no evidence, as yet, that activated neutrophils will be better for localizing inflammatory foci than inactivated cells with a normal blood biological half-time of 6 hours.

An anticarcinoembryonic antigen (anti-CEA) monoclonal antibody (MAb), originally developed for tumor localization, designated MAb 047[173] is bound to leukocytes in in vitro studies. In clinical studies,[174] this ^{123}I-labeled monoclonal antibody injected intravenously localized inflammatory lesions by binding to the circulating granulocytes in vivo. This became a commercial product available in Europe (Granuloszint, Mallinckrodt).

Another antigranulocyte monoclonal antibody designated BW250/183 and produced by Behringwerk AG (Granulozyt) and originally developed by Bosslet et al.[175] became available in Europe labeled with ^{99m}Tc for imaging inflammatory foci. This antibody binds to an epitope of nonspecific cross-reacting antigen (designated NCA-95). In clinical studies,[176–178] 75 to 150 μg MAb labeled with 8 mCi ^{99m}Tc were injected intravenously and the half-time of disappearance from the blood proved to be approximately 6 hours. The initial uptake in the lungs cleared by about 4 hours. The spleen activity was lower than with leukocytes labeled in vitro and the marrow activity appeared considerably higher. By 90 minutes after injection, only about 15% of the blood activity could be recovered in the circulating granulocytes.[179] Hence, the apparent localization of this agent in inflammatory foci may be largely nonspecific, due to increased capillary permeability. In addition, it is possible that free MAb may migrate to an infectious focus and bind to viable or damaged neutrophils already localized there. With this monoclonal antibody, the incidence of subsequent anti-idiotypic human antimouse antibodies (HAMA) is relatively low compared to other murine monoclonals.[177]

With another ^{99m}Tc-labeled antigranulocyte MAb against lacto-N-fucopentose (alpha-stage specific embryonic antigen or alpha-SSEA-1), an IgM, Thakur et al.[180] obtained a higher level of in vivo binding to circulating neutrophils ranging from 14 to 44% and successfully imaged infectious foci in a limited number of patients (Fig. 24). Although these antigranulocyte MAbs are currently being used clinically in Europe on a limited basis, their future clinical use, at least

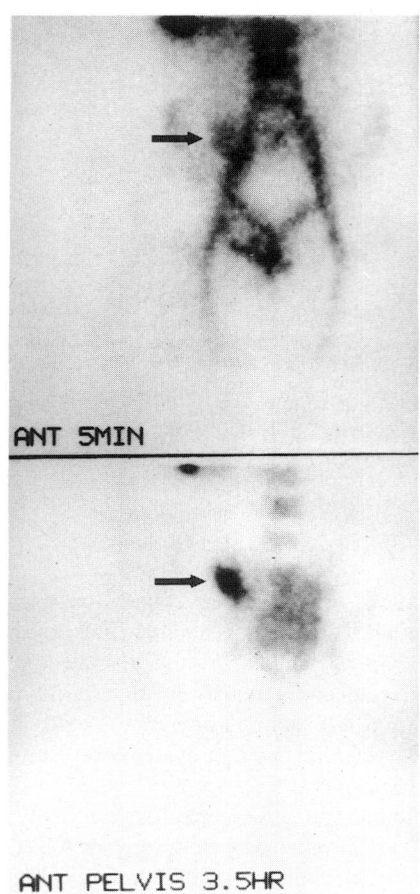

Figure 24. Anterior lower abdominal images after IV injection of 100 μg granulocyte specific monoclonal antibody (MAb) labeled with 8.2 mCi ^{99m}Tc showed a focal uptake in the right lower quadrant increasing in intensity by 3.5 hours as the blood pool activity fell. At 3 hours, 44% of the total blood activity was bound to neutrophils and another 11% to other blood cells. A perforated gangrenous appendix and peritoneal infection were found at surgery. The MAb was a murine IgM against stage specific embryonic antigen (alpha-SSEA-1) on cell line MCA 480, which binds with high affinity to lacto-N-fucopentose on human neutrophils. (Presented with permission of Dr. Matthew Thakur, Thomas Jefferson University Hospital and Dr. Carol Marcus, Harbor-UCLA Medical Center; see reference 180.)

in the US, remains in doubt. Their efficacy for imaging infectious foci cannot be compared with established agents experimentally in animals, because the monoclonal antibodies are highly species specific. Some ethical questions have arisen concerning the use of diagnostic murine monoclonal antibodies for nonmalignant lesions, because of the formation of human antimouse monoclonal antibodies which may preclude the use of other murine monoclonal antibodies for therapeutic purposes. Recently, it has even proposed that well-known agents for conjugating monoclonal antibodies, biotin, followed by ^{111}In-conjugated streptavidin be used without monoclonal antibodies for localizing inflammatory sites.[181]

A critical appraisal of the value of these newer agents for the detection of inflammatory foci suggests that the search for better agents should continue.[182]

REFERENCES

1. Froelich JW, Swanson D. Imaging of inflammatory processes with labeled cells. *Semin Nucl Med* 1982;14:128.
2. Sfakianakis GN, al-Sheik W, Heal A, et al. Comparison of scintigraphy with In-111 leukocytes and Ga-67 in the diagnosis of occult sepsis. *J Nucl Med* 1982;23:618.
3. Oates E, Ramberg K. Imaging of intrathoracic disease with indium 111-labeled leukocytes. *J Thorac Imaging* 1990;5:78.
4. Macsweeney JE, Peters AM, Lavender JP: Indium labelled leukocyte scanning in pyrexia of unknown origin. *Clin Radiol* 1990;42:414.
5. Syrjälä MT, Liewendahl K, Valtonen V, et al. Sensitivity of 111 In-granulocyte scintigraphy in various local infections. *Radiol Acta* 1987;28:549.
6. McAfee JG, Samin A. In-111 labeled leukocytes: A review of problems of image interpretation. *Radiology* 1985;155: 221.
7. Knochel JQ, Koehler PR, Lee TG. Diagnosis of abdominal abscesses with computed tomography, ultrasound, and In-111 leukocyte scans. *Radiology* 1980;137:425.
8. Baldwin JE, Wraight EP. Indium labelled leukocyte scintigraphy in occult infection: A comparison with ultrasound and computed tomography. *Clin Radiol* 1990;42:199.
9. Gordon I, Vivian G. Radiolabeled leukocytes: A new diagnostic tool in occult infection/inflammation. *Arch Dis Child* 1984;59:62.
10. Haentjens M, Piepsz A, Schell-Frederick E, et al. Limitations in the use of indium-111 oxine-labeled leukocytes for the diagnosis of occult infections in children. *Pediatr Radiol* 1987;17:139.
11. Williamson SL, Williamson MR, Seibert JJ, et al. Indium-111 white blood cell scanning in the pediatric populations. *Pediatr Radiol* 1986;16:493.
12. Gainey MA, McDougall IR. Diagnosis of acute inflammatory conditions in children and adolescents using In-111 oxine white blood cells. *Clin Nucl Med* 1984;9:71.
13. Dudley HC, Imirie GW Jr, Istock JT. Deposition of radiogallium (Ga^{72}) in proliferating tissues. *Radiology* 1982;55:571.
14. Bruner HD, Hayes RL, Perkinson JD Jr. Preliminary data on gallium^{67}. *Radiology* 1953;61:602.
15. Edwards CL, Hayes RL. Tumor scanning with ^{67}Ga citrate. *J Nucl Med* 1969;10:103.
16. Bell EG, O'Mara RE, Henry CA, et al. Non-neoplastic localization of ^{67}Ga citrate. (Abst) *J Nucl Med* 1971;12:338.
17. Lavender JP, Lowe J, Barker JR. Gallium-67 citrate scanning in neoplastic and inflammatory lesions. *Br J Radiol* 1971; 44:361.
18. McCall MS, Sutherland DA, Eisentraut AM, et al. The tagging of leukemic leukocytes with radioactive chromium and measurement of their *in vivo* cell survival. *J Lab Clin Med* 1955;45:717.
19. Winkelman J, Collica CJ, Sandler SG. The delineation of abscesses by scintiphotography using Cr-51 labeled leukocytes. *Am J Roentgenol Ther Nucl Med* 1968;103:881.
20. McAfee JG, Thakur ML. Survey of radioactive agents for *in vitro* labeling of phagocytic leukocytes I. Soluble agents. *J Nucl Med* 1976;17:480.
21. Thakur ML, Coleman RE, Welch MJ. Indium-111 labeled

leukocytes for the localization of abscesses: Preparation, analysis, tissue distribution and comparison with gallium-67 citrate in dogs. *J Lab Clin Med* 1977;89:217.
22. Thakur ML, Lavender JP, Arrot RN, et al. Indium-111 labeled autologous leukocytes in man. *J Nucl Med* 1977;18:1014.
23. Danpure HS, Osman S, Brady F. The labelling of blood cells in plasma with ^{111}In-tropolonate. *Br J Radiol* 1982;55:247.
24. Peters AM, Danpure NJ, Osman S, et al. Clinical experience with 99m-Tc hexamethyl propyleneamine oxine for labelling leukocytes and imaging inflammation. *Lancet* 1987;11:946.
25. Cloutier RJ, Watson EE, Hayes RL, et al. Summary of current radiation dose estimates to humans from ^{66}Ga, ^{67}Ga, ^{68}Ga and ^{72}Ga-citrate: MIRD dose estimate report no 2. *J Nucl Med* 1973;14:755.
26. Thomas SR, Gelfand MJ, Burns GS, et al. Radiation dose estimates for the liver, spleen and metaphyseal growth complexes in children undergoing Gallium-67 citrate scanning. *Radiology* 1983;146:817.
27. Williams LE, Forstrum L, Weiblen BJ, et al. Human dosimetry of In-111 granulocytes. (Abst) *J Nucl Med* 1980;21:P86.
28. Gainey MA, Siegel JA, Smergel EM, et al. Indium-111-labeled white blood cells: dosimetry in children. *J Nucl Med* 1988;29:689.
29. Bassano DA, McAfee, JG. Cellular radiation doses of labeled neutrophils and platelets. *J Nucl Med* 1979;20:255.
30. Hofer KG, Harris CR, Smith JM. Radiotoxicity of intracellular 67 Ga. 125 I and 3H. Nuclear *vs* cytoplasmic radiation effects in murine L1210 leukemia. *Int J Radiat Biol* 1975; 28:225.
31. ten Berge RJM, Natarajan AT, Hardeman MR, et al. Labeling with indium-111 has detrimental effects on human lymphocytes: Concise Communication. *J Nucl Med* 1983;24: 615.
32. Field EO, Sharpe HBA, Dawson KB, et al. Turnover rate of normal blood lymphocytes and exchangeable pool size in men, calculated from analysis of chromosomal aberrations sustained during extracorporeal irradiation of the blood. *Blood* 1972;39:39.
33. Thakur ML, McAfee JG. The significance of chromosomal aberrations in indium-111-labeled lymphocytes. *J Nucl Med* 1984;25:922.
34. McAfee JG, Gagne GM, Subramanian G, et al. Distribution of leukocytes labeled with In-111 oxine in dogs with acute inflammatory lesions. *J Nucl Med* 1980;21:1059.
35. Ando A, Nitta K, Ando I, et al. Mechanisms of gallium-67 accumulation in inflammatory tissue. *Eur J Nucl Med* 1990;17:21.
36. Planas-Bohne F, Taylor DM, Lamble G, et al. The localization of metallic radionuclides in abscesses in rats. *Br J Radiol* 1982;55:289.
37. Taylor DM, Planas-Bohne F. The retention of metallic radionuclides in experimental abscesses in rats. *Br J Radiol* 1985;58:655.
38. Krishna L, Slizofski WJ, Katsetos CD, et al. Abnormal intracerebral thallium localization in a bacterial brain abscess. *J Nucl Med* 1992;33:2017.
39. Nelson B, Hayes RL, Edwards CL, et al. Distribution of gallium in human tissues after intravenous administration. *J Nucl Med* 1972;13:92.
40. Newstead G, Taylor GM, McCready VR, et al. Gallium-67 deposition in the human gastrointestinal tract. *Intern J Nucl Med Biol* 1977;4:109.
41. Zeman RK, Ryerson TW. The value of bowel preparation in Ga-67 citrate scanning. Concise Communication. *J Nucl Med* 1977;18:886.
42. Gunasekera SW, King LA, Lavender JP. The behavior of tracer Gallium-67 towards serum proteins. *Clin Chim Acta* 1972;39:401.
43. Malik MH. Simultaneous dual isotope studies in the diagnosis of infection. *J Nucl Med* 1985;26:722.
44. Siemsen JK, Grebe SF, Waxman AD. The use of Ga-67 in pulmonary disorders. *Semin Nucl Med* 1978;8:235.
45. Engelstad B, Luk SS, Hattner RS. Altered 67 Ga citrate distribution in patient with multiple red blood cell transfusions. *AJR* 1982;139:755.
46. Lentle BC, Penney H, Ensslen R. A generalized increase in uptake of Gallium-67 in bone. *Semin Nucl Med* 1984;14: 143.
47. Dudley HC, Maddox GE, La Rue HC. Studies of the metabolism of gallium. *J Pharmacol Exp Ther* 1949;96:135.
48. Hattner RS, White DL. Gallium-67/stable gadolinium antagonism: MRI contrast agent markedly alters the normal biodistribution of gallium-67. *Nucl Med* 1990;31:1844.
49. Brown SJ, Slizofski WJ, Dadparvar S. Altered biodistribution of Gallium-67 in a patient with aluminum toxicity treated with desferoxamine. *J Nucl Med* 1990;31:115.
50. Hladik WB III, Ponte JA, Lentle BC, et al. Iatrogenic alterations in the biodistribution of radiotracers as a result of drug therapy: Reported Instances, in Hladik WB, Saha GB, Study KT (Eds.): *Essentials of Nuclear Medicine Science*. Baltimore: Williams & Wilkins, 1987, p 189.
51. Verma RC, Ramanna L, Webber MM. Comprehensive review of gallium scanning for inflammatory lesions. (Abst) *J Nucl Med* 1978;19:734.
52. Ebright JR, Soin JS, Manoli RS. The gallium scan: Problems and misuse in examination of patient with suspected infection. *Arch Intern Med* 1982;142:246.
53. Forgacs P, Wahner HW, Keys TF, et al. Gallium scanning for the detection of abdominal abscesses. *Am J Med* 1978;65: 949.
54. Dobrin PB, Gully PH, Greenlee HB, et al. Radiologic diagnosis of an intra-abdominal abscess: Do multiple tests help? *Arch Surg* 1986;121:41.
55. Hauser MF, Alderson PO. Gallium-67 imaging in abdominal disease. *Semin Nucl Med* 1978;8:251.
56. Maderazo E, Hickingbotham NB, Woronick CL, et al. The influence of various factors on the accuracy of Gallium-67 imaging for occult infection. *J Nucl Med* 1988;29:608.
57. Silberstein EB, McAfee JG (eds.): *Differential Diagnosis in Nuclear Medicine*. New York, McGraw-Hill 1984, pp 125, 242.
58. Hatfield MR, MacMahon H, Martin WB, et al. The effect of previous thoracic surgery on gallium uptake in the chest. *J Nucl Med* 1987;28:1831.
59. van Rooij WJ, van der Meer SC, van Royen EA, et al. Pulmonary Gallium-67 uptake in amiodarone pneumonitis. *J Nucl Med* 1984;25:211.
60. Rosenow EC, Myers JL, Swensen SJ, et al. Drug-induced pulmonary disease: An update. *Chest* 1992;102:239.
61. Specht HD, Bakke AC, Braziel R, et al. Cellular basis for the elevated Ga-67 computed lung index in a rheumatoid lung patient. *J Nucl Med* 1990;32:2288.
62. Kim SM, Park CH, Intenzo CM, et al. Gallium uptake in tryptophan-related pulmonary disease. *J Nucl Med* 1991; 32:328.
63. Wesselius LJ, Witztum KF, Taylor AT, et al. Computer-assisted *versus* visual lung Ga-67 index in normal subjects and in patients with interstitial lung disorders. *Am Rev Respir Dis* 1983;128:1084.
64. Sulavik SB, Spencer RP, Weed DA, et al. Recognition of distinctive patterns of Gallium-67 distribution in sarcoidosis. *J Nucl Med* 1990;31:1909–1914.
65. Mishkin FS, Tanaka TT, Niden AH. Abnormal gallium scan

patterns of the salivary glands in pulmonary sarcoidosis. *Ann Intern Med* 1978;89:933.

66. Mochizuki T, Ichijo K, Takehara Y, et al. Gallium-67-citrate scanning in patients with sarcoid uveitis. *J Nucl Med* 1992;33:1851.
67. Patel N, Krasnow A, Sebastian JL, et al. Isolated muscular sarcoidosis causing fever of unknown origin. *J Nucl Med* 1991;32:319.
68. Collins RD Jr, Bell GV, Logic JR. Gallium-67 scanning in Sjögren's syndrome: Concise Communication. *J Nucl Med* 1984;25:299.
69. Robinson JA, O'Connell J, Henkin R, et al. Gallium imaging in cardiomyopathy. *Ann Intern Med* 1979;90:198.
70. O'Connell JB, Henkin RE, Robinson JA, et al. Gallium-67 imaging in patients with dilated cardiomyopathy and biopsy proven myocarditis. *Circulation* 1984;70:58.
71. O'Connell JB, Robinson JA, Henkin RE, Gunnar RM. Gallium-67 citrate scanning for non-invasive detection of inflammation in pericardial diseases. *Am J Cardiol* 1980; 46:879.
72. Bufalino VJ, Robinson JA, Henkin R, et al. Gallium-67 scanning: A new diagnostic approach to the post-pericardiotomy syndrome. *Am Heart J* 1983;106:1138.
73. Yamamoto S, Bergsland J, Michalek SM, et al. Uptake of myocardial imaging agents by rejecting and non-rejecting cardiac transplants. A comparative clinical study of Thallium-201, Technetium-99 and Gallium-67. *J Nucl Med* 1989; 30:1464.
74. Quince R, Serano J, Arnal C, et al. Detection of mediastinitis after heart transplantation by Gallium-67 scintigraphy. *J Nucl Med* 1991;32:860.
75. Miller SW, Palmer EL, Dinsmore RE, et al. Gallium-67 and magnetic resonance imaging in aortic root abscess. *J Nucl Med* 1987;28:1616.
76. Mendez G Jr, Morillo G, Alonso M, et al. Gallium-67 radionuclide imaging in acute pyelonephritis. *AJR* 1980;134:17.
77. Rosenfield AT, Glickman MG, Taylor KJW, et al. Acute focal bacterial nephritis (acute lobar nephronia). *Radiology* 1979; 132:553.
78. Hurwitz SR, Kessler WD, Alazraki NP, et al. Gallium-67 imaging to localize urinary-tract infections. *Br J Radiol* 1976;19:156.
79. Lin DS, Sanders JA, Patel Br. Delayed renal localization of Ga-67: Concise Communication. *J Nucl Med* 1983;24:894.
80. Jacobson A. Gallium-67 imaging in retroperitoneal fibrosis: Significance of a negative result. *J Nucl Med* 1991;32: 521.
81. Kim EE, Gobuty A, Gutierrez C. Diffuse abdominal uptake of Ga-67 citrate in a patient with hypoproteinemia. *J Nucl Med* 1983;24:508.
82. McAfee JG, Subramanian G, Gagne G. Technique of leukocyte harvesting and labeling; problems and perspectives. *Semin Nucl Med* 1984;14:83.
83. Thakur ML, Seifert C, Madsen MT, et al. Neutrophil labeling: Problems and pitfalls. *Semin Nucl Med* 1984;14:107.
84. Danpure HL, Osman S. A review of methods of separating and radiolabelling human leukocytes. *Nucl Med Commun* 1988;9:681.
85. Datz FL. Radiolabeled leukocytes and platelets. *Invest Radiol* 1986;21:191.
86. Schauwecker DS, Burt RW, Park H-M, et al. Comparison of purified Indium-111 granulocytes and Indium-111 mixed leukocytes for imaging of infections. *J Nucl Med* 1988;29:23.
87. Dutcher JP, Schiffer CA, Johnston GS. Rapid migration of In-111 Indium labeled granulocytes to sites of infection. *N Engl J Med* 1981;304:586.
88. Williams JH Jr, Wilson AF, Moser KM. Is lung sequestration of Indium-111-labeled granulocytes organ specific? *J Nucl Med* 1989;30:1531.
89. MacNee W, Selby C. Editorial Review: Neutrophil kinetics in the lungs. *Clin Sci* 1990;79:97.
90. Loréal O, Moisan A, Bretagre J-F, et al. Scintigraphic assessment of Indium-111-labeled granulocyte splenic pooling: a new approach to inflammatory bowel disease activity. *J Nucl Med* 1990;31:1470.
91. Forstrum LA, Weiblen BJ, Gomez L, et al. Indium-111-oxine-labeled leukocytes in the diagnosis of occult inflammatory disease, in Thakur ML, Gottschalk A (eds.): *Indium-111 Labeled Neutrophils, Platelets, and Lymphocytes*. New York, Trivirum Publishing, 1980, p 123.
92. Epstein JS, Ganz WI, Lizak M, et al. Indium 111-labeled leukocyte scintigraphy in evaluating head and neck infections. *Ann Otolaryngol* 1992;101:961.
93. Strashun AM, Nejatheim M, Goldsmith SJ. Malignant external otitis, early scintigraphic detection. *Radiology* 1984; 150:541.
94. Spieth ME, Kim HH, Ford PV. Unsuspected meningitis diagnosed by In-111 labeled leukocytes. A case report. *Clin Nucl Med* 1992;17:627.
95. Schmidt KG, Rasmussen JW, Frederiksen PB, et al. Indium-111-granulocyte scintigraphy in brain abscess diagnosis: Limitations and pitfalls. *J Nucl Med* 1990;31:1121.
96. Palestro CJ, Swyer AJ, Kim CK, et al. Role of In-111 leukocyte scintigraphy in the diagnosis of intracerebral lesions. *Clin Nucl Med* 1991;16:305.
97. Passamonte PM, Martinez AJ, Singh A. Pulmonary gallium concentration in the adult respiratory distress syndrome. *Chest* 1984;85:828.
98. Jonker ND, Peters AM, Gaskin G, et al. A retrospective study of radiolabeled granulocyte kinetics in patients with systemic vasculitis. *J Nucl Med* 1992;33:491.
99. Desai SP, Yuille DL: Necrotizing tracheobronchitis identified on an Indium-111 white blood cell scan. *J Nucl Med* 1992; 33:1704.
100. Seabold JE, Wilson DG, Lieberman LM, et al. Unsuspected extra-abdominal sites of infection: Scintigraphic detection with indium-111-labeled leukocytes. *Radiology* 1984; 151:213.
101. Cerqueria MD, Jacobson AF. Indium-111 leukocyte scintigraphic detection of myocardial abscess formation in patients with endocarditis. *J Nucl Med* 1989;30:703.
102. Cequeria MD. Editorial: Detection of cardiovascular infections with radiolabeled leukocytes. *J Nucl Med* 1992;33: 1493.
103. Zaret BL, Davies RE, Thakur ML, et al. Imaging the inflammatory response to acute myocardial infarction, in Thakur ML, Gottschalk A, (eds.): *Indium III labeled Neutrophils, Platelets and Lymphocytes*. New York, Trivirum Publishing, 1981, p 151.
104. Muir AJ, Bell D, Jackson M, et al. The use of ^{111}In-labeled autologous neutrophils in imaging myocardial infarction. *Nucl Med Commun* 1988;9:707.
105. Seabold JE. Imaging of vascular graft infection. In Murray IPC, Ell PV (eds). *Nuclear Medicine in Clinical Diagnosis and Treatment*, Volume 1, Section 1. Edinburgh: Churchill Livingstone, 1994, p 159.
106. Chung CJ, Hicklin OA, Pagan JM, et al. Indium-111-labeled leukocyte scan in detection of synthetic vascular graft infection: The effect of antibiotic treatment. *J Nucl Med* 1991; 32:13.
107. Ben-Haim S, Seabold JE, Hawes DR, et al. Leukocyte scintigraphy in the diagnosis of mycotic aneurysm. *J Nucl Med* 1992;33:1486.
108. Palestro CJ, Vega A, Kim CK, et al. Indium-111-labeled leu-

kocyte scintigraphy in hemodialysis access-site infection. *J Nucl Med* 1990;31:319.
109. Saverymuttu SH, Camilleri M, Rees H, et al. Indium-111 granulocyte scanning in the assessment of disease extent and disease activity in inflammatory bowel disease. *Gastroenterology* 1986;90:1121.
110. Rothstein RD. The role of scintigraphy in the management of inflammatory bowel disease. *J Nucl Med* 1991;37: 856.
111. Wilson DG, Lieberman LM. Gastrointestinal bleeding in leukocyte scintigraphy. *Clin Nucl Med* 1985;10:513.
112. Kipper SL, Steiner RW, Witztum KF, et al. In-111-leukocyte scintigraphy for detection of infection associated with peritoneal dialysis catheters. *Radiology* 1984;151:491.
113. Forstrum LA, Loken MK, Cook A, et al. Indium-111-labeled leukocytes in the diagnosis of rejection and cytomeglaovirus infection in renal transplant patients. *Clin Nucl Med* 1981;6:146.
114. Collier BD, Isitman AT, Kaufman HM, et al. Concentration of In-111-oxine labeled autologous leukocytes in noninfected and nonrejecting renal allografts: Concise Communication. *J Nucl Med* 1984;25:156.
115. Wing VM, von Sonnenberg E, Kipper S, et al. Indium-111 labeled leukocyte localization in hematomas: A pitfall in abscess detection. *Radiology* 1984;152:173.
116. Mok YP, Carney WH, Fernandez-Ulloa M. Skeletal photopenic lesions in In-111 WBC imaging. *J Nucl Med* 1984;25:1322.
117. Swyer A, Palestro CJ, Kim CK, et al. Appearance of fibrous dysplasia on In-111 labeled leukocyte scintigraphy. *Clin Nucl Med* 1991;16:133.
118. Datz FL, Thorne DA. Cause and significance of cold bone defects on Indium-111-labeled leukocyte imaging. *J Nucl Med* 1987;28:820.
119. Schell-Frederick E, Frühling J, Van der Auwera P, et al. ^{111}Indium-oxine-labeled leukocytes in the diagnosis of localized infection in patients with neoplastic disease. *Cancer* 1984;54:817.
120. Fortner A, Datz FL, Taylor A Jr, et al. Uptake of ^{111}In-labeled leukocytes by tumor. *AJR* 1986;146:621.
121. Lamki L, Kasi LP, Haynie TP. Localization of Indium-111 leukocytes in non-infected neoplasms. *J Nucl Med* 1988; 29:1921.
122. Schmidt KG, Rasmussen JW, Wedebye IM, et al. Accumulation of Indium-111 labeled granulocytes in malignant tumors. *J Nucl Med* 1988;29:479.
123. Balachandran S, Boyd CM, Husain MM, et al. Indium-111 leukocyte uptake in neoplasms. *Clin Nucl Med* 1987;12: 930.
124. Palestro CJ, Kim CK, Vega A, et al. Acute effects of radiation therapy on Indium-111-labeled leukocyte uptake in bone marrow. *J Nucl Med* 1989;30:1889.
125. Palestro CJ, Vega A, Kim CK, et al. Appearance of acute gouty arthritis on Indium-111-labeled leukocyte scintigraphy. *J Nucl Med* 1990;31:682.
126. Samuelsson B, Funk CD. Enzymes involved in the biosynthesis of leukotriene B_4. *J Biol Chem* 1989;264:19469.
127. Weinberg JR, Boyle P, Meager A, et al. Lipopolysaccharide, tumor necrosis factor, and interleukin-1 interact to cause hypotension. *J Lab Clin Med* 1992;120:205.
128. Oates E, Staudinger K, Gilbertson V. Significance of nodal uptake on Indium labeled leukocyte scans. *Clin Nucl Med* 1989;14:282.
129. Roddie ME, Peters AM, Danpure HL, et al. Inflammation. Imaging with Tc-99 HMPAO-labeled leukocytes. *Radiology* 1988;166:767.
130. Reynolds JH, Graham D, Smith FW. Imaging inflammation with ^{99}Tc^{m} HMPAO labelled leukocytes. *Clin Radiology* 1990;42:195.
131. Peters AM, Roddie ME, Danpure HJ, et al. ^{99}Tc^{m}-HMPAO labelled leukocytes: comparison with ^{111}In-tropolonate labelled granulocytes. *Nucl Med Comm* 1988;9:449.
132. Mortelmans L, Malbrain S, Stuyck J, et al. *In vitro* and *in vivo* evaluation of granulocyte labeling with [^{99m}Tc] d, I-HM-PAO. *J Nucl Med* 1989;30:2022.
133. Lantto EH, Lantto TJ, Vorne M. Fast diagnosis of abdominal infections and inflammations with Technetium-99m-HMPAO labeled leukocytes. *J Nucl Med* 1991;32:2029.
134. Vorne M, Soini I, Lannto T, et al. Technetion-99m HM-PAO-labeled leukocytes in detection of inflammatory lesions: Comparison with Gallium-67 citrate. *J Nucl Med* 1989;30:1332.
135. Mountford PJ, Kettle AG, O'Doherty MJ, et al. Comparison of Technetium-99m-HM-PAO leukocytes with Indium-111-oxine leukocytes for localizing intraabdominal sepsis. *J Nucl Med* 1990;31:311.
136. McAfee JG, Subramanian G, Gagne G, et al. ^{99m}Tc-HM-PAO for leukocyte labeling—experimental comparison with ^{111}In-oxine in dogs. *Eur J Nucl Med* 1987;13:353.
137. Thierens HMA, Vral AM, Van Haelst JP, et al. Lymphocyte labeling with Technetium-99m-HMPAO: A radiotoxicity study using the micronucleus assay. *J Nucl Med* 1992; 33:1167.
138. Giaffer MH, Tindale WB, Senior S, et al. Anaphylactoid reaction associated with the use ^{99}Tc^{m} hexamethyl propylene amine oxime as a leukocyte labelling agent. *Br J Radiol* 1991; 64:625.
139. Peters AM. Imaging inflammation: Current role of labeled autologous leukocytes (Editorial). *J Nucl Med* 1992;33:65.
140. Vanarthos WJ, Ganz WI, Vanarthos JC, et al. Diagnostic uses of nuclear medicine in AIDS. *Radiographics* 1992;12:731.
141. Miller RF. Nuclear medicine and AIDS. *Eur J Nucl Med* 1990;16:103.
142. Tatsch K, Schielke E, Einhaupl KM, et al. 99mTc-HMPAO-SPECT in patients with HIV infection: a comparison with neurological, CT, and MRI findings. *Eur J Nucl Med* 1989;15:418.
143. Van der Wall H, Murray IPC, Jones PD, et al. Optimizing technetium-99m diethylene triaminepenta-acetate lung clearance in patients with the acquired immunodeficiency syndrome. *Eur J Nucl Med* 1991;18:235.
144. Picard C, Meighan M, Rosso J, et al. Technetium-99m DPTA aerosol and gallium scanning in acquired immune deficiency syndrome. *Clin Nucl Med* 1987;12:501.
145. O'Doherty MJ, Pagen CJ, Nunan TO, et al. Diagnostic values of lung clearance of 99mTc DTPA compared with other noninvasive investigations in *Pneumocystis carinii* pneumonia in AIDS (Letter). *Thorax* 1992;47:138.
146. Zuckier LS, Ongseng F, Goldfarb CR. Lymphocytic interstitial pneumonitis: A cause of pulmonary Gallium-67 uptake in a child with acquired immunodeficiency syndrome. *J Nucl Med* 1988;29:707.
147. Kramer EL, Sanger JJ, Garay SM, et al. Gallium 67 scans of the chest in patients with acquired immunodeficiency syndrome. *J Nucl Med* 1987;28:1107.
148. Lee VW, Fuller JD, O'Brien MJ, et al. Pulmonary Kaposi sarcoma in patients with AIDS; Scintigraphic diagnosis with sequential thallium and gallium scanning. *Radiology* 1991; 180:409.
149. Rosenberg ZS, Joffe SA, Itescu S. Spectrum of salivary gland disease in HIV-infected patients: Characterization with Ga-67 citrate imaging. *Radiology* 1992;184:761.
150. Bourgoignie JJ. Renal complications of human immunodeficiency virus type 1. *Kidney Int* 1990;37:1571.
151. Sfakianakis GN, Fayad F, Fernandez JA, et al. Ga-67 renal

hyperactivity in AIDS patients and its relationship to laboratory renal data (Abst). *J Nucl Med* 1988;29:909.

152. Korbet SM, Schwartz MM. Human immunodeficiency virus infection and nephrotic syndrome. *Am J Kidney Dis* 1992; 20:97.
153. Rao TK, Friedman EA, Nicastri AD. The types of renal disease in acquired immunodeficiency syndrome. *N Engl J Med* 1987;316:1062.
154. Rao TKS. Clinical features of human immunodeficiency virus associated nephropathy. *Kidney Int* 1991;49(suppl 35):S13.
155. Rao TK, Nicastri AD, Friedman EA. Natural history of heroin associated nephropathy, *N Engl J Med* 1974;290:19.
156. Fineman DS, Palestro CJ, Kim CK, et al. Detection of abnormalities in febrile AIDS patients with In-111-labeled leukocyte and Ga-67 scintigraphy. *Radiology* 1989;170:677.
157. Palestro CJ, Kim CK, Needle L et al. In-111 labeled leukocyte and Ga-67 scintigraphy in cytomegalovirus colitis. *Clin Nucl Med* 1990;15:848.
158. Palestro CJ, Vega A, Kim CK, et al. In-111 labeled leukocyte scintigraphy in a case of multifocal candidiasis. *Clin Nucl Med* 1990;15:392.
159. De Schrijver M, Streule K, Senekowitsch R, et al. Scintigraphy of inflammation with nanometer-sized colloidal tracers. *Nucl Med Commun* 1987;8:895.
160. Abramovici J, Rubinstein M. Tc-99m nanocolloids: An alternative approach to diagnosis of inflammatory lesions and bones and joints (Abst). *Eur J Nucl Med* 1988;14:244.
161. Vorne M, Lantto T, Paakkinen S, et al. Clinical comparison of ^{99}Tc^{m}-HMPAO labelled leukocytes and ^{99}Tc^{m}-nanocolloid in the detection of inflammation. *Acta Radiol* 1989;30:633.
162. Morgan JR, Williams LA, Howard CB. Technetium-labelled liposome imaging for deep-seated infection. *Br J Radiol* 1985;58:35.
163. Zanelli GD, Bhjarnason I, Smith T, et al. Technetium-99m labeled porphyrin as an imaging agent for occult infections and inflammation. *Nucl Med Commun* 1986;7:17.
164. Rubin RH, Fischman RH, Neddleman M, et al. Radiolabeled, nonspecific, polyclonal human immunoglobulin in the detection of focal inflammation by scintigraphy: Comparison with Gallium-67 citrate and Technetium-99m labeled albumin. *J Nucl Med* 1989;30:385.
165. Fischman AJ, Rubin RH, White JA, et al. Localization of Fc and Fab fragments at nonspecific polyclonal IgG of focal sites of inflammation. *J Nucl Med* 1990;31:1199.
166. Abrams MJ, Juweid M, ten Kate Cl, et al. Technetium-99m-human polyclonal IgG radiolabeled via the hydrazino nicotinamide derivative for imaging focal sites of infection in rats. *J Nucl Med* 1990;31:2022.
167. Rubin RH, Fischman AJ, Callahan RJ, et al. ^{111}In-labeled nonspecific immunoglobulin scanning in the detection of focal infection. *N Engl J Med* 1989;321:935.
168. Serafini AN, Garty I, Vargas-Cuba R, et al. Clinical evaluation of a scintigraphic method for diagnosing inflammatory infection using Indium-111-labeled nonspecific human IgG. *J Nucl Med* 1991;32:2227.
169. Buscombe J, Lui D, Sargeant I, et al. Tc-99m HIG: A new agent for the identification and localization of active inflammatory bowel disease and intraabdominal sepsis. (Abst) *Radiology* 1989;171:433.
170. McAfee JG, Gagne G, Subramanian G, et al. The localization of indium-111-leukocytes, Gallium-67, polyclonal IgG and other radioactive agents in acute focal inflammatory lesions. *J Nucl Med* 1991;32:2126.
171. Thakur ML, De Folvio J, Park CH, et al. Technetium-99m-labeled proteins for imaging inflammatory foci. *Nucl Med Biol* 1991;18:605.
172. Fischman AJ, Pike MC, Kroon D, et al. Imaging focal sites of bacterial infection in rats with Indium-111-labeled chemotactic peptide analogs. *J Nucl Med* 1991;32:483.
173. Audette M, Buchegger F, Schreyer M, et al. Monoclonal antibody against carcinoembryonic antigen (CEA) identifies two new forms of cross-reacting antigens of molecular weight 90,000 and 160,000 in normal granulocytes. *Mol Immunol* 1987;24:1177.
174. Seybold K, Locher JT, Coosemans C, et al. Immunoscintigraphic localization of inflammatory lesions: clinical experience. *Eur J Nucl Med* 1988;13:589.
175. Bosslet K, Luben G, Schwartz A, et al. Immunohistochemical· localization and molecular characteristics of three monoclonal antibody-defined epitopes detectable on carcinoembryonic antigen (CEA). *Int J Cancer* 1985;36:75.
176. Joseph K, Hoffken H, Bosslet K, et al. Imaging of inflammation with granulocytes labeled *in vivo*. *Nucl Med Commun* 1988;9:763.
177. Lind P, LangstegerW, Koltringer P, et al. Immunoscintigraphy of inflammatory processes with a Tc-99m-labeled monoclonal antigranulocyte antibody (Mab BW 250/183). *J Nucl Med* 1990;31:417.
178. Segarra J, Roca M, Baliellas C, et al. Granulocyte-specific monoclonal antibody technetium-99m-BW 250/183 and In-111-oxine-labeled leukocyte scintigraphy in inflammatory bowel disease. *Eur J Nucl Med* 1991;18:715.
179. Becker W, Borst U, Fishbach W, et al. Kinetic data of in-vivo labeled granulocytes in humans with a murine Tc-99m-labeled monoclonal antibody. *Eur J Nucl Med* 1989;15:361.
180. Thakur ML, Marcus CS, Hennemann P, et al. Imaging inflammatory diseases with neutrophil (PMN)-specific Tc-99m-monoclonal antibody (Abstr). *J Nucl Med* 1991;32:1836.
181. Rusckowski M, Fritz B, Hnatowich D. Improved localization of inflammation with streptavidin-biotin as a substitute for antibody (Abstr). *J Nucl Med* 1991;32:1836.
182. McAfee JG. Editorial: What is the best method for imaging focal infections? *J Nucl Med* 1990;31:413.

36 Nuclear Medicine Tests for Oncology Patients

Ronald D. Neumann, Jorge A. Carrasquillo, Ronald E. Weiner, Clara C. Chen, Mary P. Andrich

The nuclear medicine tests available for staging and post-treatment evaluations of cancer patients are most useful when used to survey patients for unsuspected sites of disease and to evaluate physiological or biochemical parameters to determine whether lesions identified by other imaging tests, such as computed tomography (CT) or magnetic resonance imaging (MRI), represent viable tumor tissue. In general, nuclear medicine tests have high sensitivity for detecting active neoplastic disease, but they often have low specificity. The many possible organ locations for cancers and the wide variety of clinical presentations preclude a simple scheme for using nuclear medicine tests in such patients. We will thus discuss the major tests available, their common applications, and their relative efficacies.

GALLIUM SCINTIGRAPHY

In 1969, Edwards and Hayes[1] reported that ^{67}Ga-citrate localizes in the tumors of Hodgkin's disease. The initial clinical interest was to exploit the bone-localizing characteristics of gallium.[2] To their surprise, investigators found that ^{67}Ga localized both in bone and in tumor tissue.

In the first 10 years following this discovery, ^{67}Ga imaging was attempted in most malignant tumors in which detection and staging was important and otherwise difficult.[3–7] Several mechanisms have been proposed to explain gallium localization in tumors. Although not all investigators agree, gallium probably acts as an analog of ferric ion.

Gallium as an Iron Analog

In the early 1970s, it was shown that ^{67}Ga in serum was bound tightly to the iron-transport protein, transferrin (TF),[8,9] and that TF, due to its iron-binding ability, stimulates ^{67}Ga incorporation into cultured tumor cells.[10,11] Other iron-binding molecules, desferrioxamine,[12,13] lactoferrin (LF),[14] and ferritin,[15,16] also bind ^{67}Ga with high affinity. Subsequent experiments showed that ^{67}Ga binds to the iron-binding site of TF, lactoferrin, and a variety of bacterial iron transport molecules called siderophores; binding causes only slight alterations in the three-dimensional structures of these molecules. This led to the hypothesis that ^{67}Ga was handled as an iron analogue.[17] However, this concept was criticized because animal[18] and human[19] studies showed great disparity in biodistribution between ^{59}Fe and ^{67}Ga. Iron localizes in hematopoietic tissues and red blood cells (RBCs), but not in most tumor tissues. In contrast, ^{67}Ga has a high affinity for tumor tissue but low affinity for marrow, and remains in liver, spleen and other tissues much longer than ^{59}Fe. Hoffer[17] suggested that this difference relates to the unique oxidation-reduction properties of each. For iron to be absorbed in the gastrointestinal (GI) tract and eventually bind to hemoglobin, hematopoietic cells in the marrow, and the cytochrome enzyme system in the mitochondria, requires that iron cycle between its 2 physiological stable states Fe^{2+} and Fe^{3+}.[20–22] In contrast, Ga^{3+} is the only stable state for gallium under physiological conditions.[23] For example, Ga is not incorporated into hemoglobin in RBCs because it is not reduced to Ga^{2+}, nor can it follow metabolic pathways where reduction is necessary.

More recent evidence[24–26] suggests that the aqueous solubility of the 2 metals is as important as the redox properties in determining their biodistributions. In a physiological environment and at trace levels, ^{67}Ga is soluble, whereas iron is not. Therefore, iron, not ^{67}Ga, absolutely requires a chelate of some type (e.g., TF) for in vivo transport.

Transferrin Receptors As ^{67}Ga Transporters

Larson and co-workers[27] extended the iron analog concept to specifically include TF receptors (TfR). Based on both in vivo[28,29] and in vitro[27,28] evidence, they proposed that "a tumor-associated TF receptor is the functional unit responsible for the affinity of gallium for certain neoplasms." Autoradiographic and cell organelle isolation studies demonstrated that ^{67}Ga is incorporated into the lysosomes of viable tumor cells.[30–34] At normal concentrations of Fe*TF in the blood, TfR is saturated with Fe*TF, and cells must upregulate the number of TfR to increase iron uptake.[21] Iron is required for several cellular processes, but TfR is regulated mainly to meet specific iron needs of DNA synthesis.[22] The specific target for this iron is ribonucleotide reductase, a nonheme iron-requiring enzyme that catalyzes the first rate-limiting step in DNA synthesis, conversion of ribonucleotides to deoxyribonucleotides. In rapidly proliferating tumor cells with high DNA synthesis, upregulation of the surface TfR would also lead to increased ^{67}Ga uptake. Increased TfR has been detected in a variety of tumor cells.[35–37]

TfRs are, thus, important in neoplastic cell localization of ^{67}Ga. However, experiments with animals that congenitally lack TF and still permit good tumor ^{67}Ga uptake could not be easily explained.[38] Furthermore, cells in certain circumstances can acquire Fe and possibly ^{67}Ga by TF-independent means. When cells are cultured in a TF-free environment, a non-TF transport system can be demonstrated in some cell lines.[39–41] This alternate iron transport system, however, is regulated quite differently than the TFR system. It is not affected by cellular growth rate, induction of DNA synthesis, cell division, or depletion of cellular iron.[39,40] Moreover, this system has an affinity for iron chelates that is a few orders of magnitude lower than that of Fe for TF. All this suggests that TF-independent systems may enhance clearance of a toxic excess of iron. In circumstances where effective TF concentration is reduced or absent, this alternate system, although slower, may be responsible for ^{67}Ga accumulation. However, in normal circumstances the TF-dependent system would mainly be responsible for ^{67}Ga uptake.

The importance of ^{67}Ga scintigraphy as a diagnostic tool lies in its ability to both identify tumor and to differentiate viable tumor from nonviable tumor and/or nontumor tissues. There is some data to connect cell viability and DNA synthesis to ^{67}Ga utpake. Iosilevsky et al.[42] showed that both ^{67}Ga and deoxyglucose uptake in a tumor model decline in parallel after chemotherapy and radiotherapy. Inhibiting tumor ATP production causes a similar decline in ^{67}Ga incorporation,[43] suggesting that ^{67}Ga uptake correlates with cellular metabolism.

Imaging Technique

^{67}Ga emits a spectrum of photons. The lower energy photons at 91 to 93 keV, 184 keV, and 296 keV are most suitable for use in imaging. The 388 keV emission is usually not useful for imaging, but must be considered in selecting a medium- to high-energy collimator that will minimize high-energy-photon septal penetration. Physical considerations dictate that ^{67}Ga is usually best imaged using separate energy windows around each of the 3 lower energy peaks. A single broad energy window admits excessive scatter radiation and degrades image quality. Although planar gamma cameras are still used for ^{67}Ga imaging, single-photon emission tomography (SPECT) imaging is particularly useful because it helps distinguish ^{67}Ga uptake in normal structures from true tumor uptake. ^{67}Ga uptake in deep tissues is better detected with the 184 keV and 296 keV peaks because of less degradation by scatter.

A dose of 10 mCi (370 mBq) ^{67}Ga-citrate is recommended in adults for tumor imaging. The higher radiation exposure with a 10 mCi dose is usually acceptable in oncology patients who will, in most cases, be at much higher subsequent secondary oncogenic risk from their radiation therapy and/or chemotherapy than from radiation associated with the ^{67}Ga they receive.

Imaging is usually performed 48 to 72 hours following administration of ^{67}Ga to allow time for clearance of background activity. Bowel activity may be reduced by use of cathartics and/or enemas which also serve to decrease radiation dose to the patient. Despite attempts to clear bowel activity, some gallium usually remains—which may necessitate repeat images to determine if abdominal and pelvic activity has moved (bowel) or is stationary (lesion). Repeat images of suspicious areas are often done using a gamma camera, but SPECT images can be particularly useful in this context, again, because of the better anatomic localization possible with tomographic technique. Multihead SPECT cameras provide increased sensitivity to speed acquisition of delayed images.

Patterns of Gallium Localization

^{67}Ga normally localizes in the liver, spleen, bone, and bone marrow. Variable uptake is also noted in female breasts, salivary and lacrimal glands, nasal mucosa, and external genitalia. Activity in salivary glands is usually faint or undetectable, but can become prominent following radiation therapy to the head and neck and, occasionally, following chemotherapy. Prominent salivary gland uptake can persist and should not be mistaken for recurrent tumor. Mediastinal uptake can occur in normal children and is presumed to be due to gallium accumulation in normal thymic tissue. Uptake can also be prominent in normal thymic tissue following infections (Fig. 1). Occasionally, faint hilar activity is seen in patients without known pulmonary disease. Faint gastric activity is sometimes discernible on the 48 to 72-hour images, but usually decreases with time. Renal activity can be moderately prominent on images obtained within the first 24 to 48 hours after injection, but is usually faint or absent by 48 to 72 hours after injection. Several agents or conditions can alter the normal patterns of gallium uptake: stable gallium sometimes given as chemotherapy, gadolinium that is used as an MRI contrast agent, drugs that alter serum iron levels and previous radiation or chemotherapy. The presence of persistent intestinal gallium activity is an obstacle to accurate detection of abdominal disease, and creates the greatest point of dissatisfaction with gallium scintigraphy. In infants, prominent activity is often observed in the base of the skull. Epiphyseal activity is often prominent in children. Surgical wounds can show activity for several weeks following surgery, and localized activity may occur following bone marrow biopsy, fractures, and orthopedic procedures.

Lymphoma

The detectability of lymphoma by gallium scintigraphy depends on several factors: (1) histology: Burkitt's lymphoma,

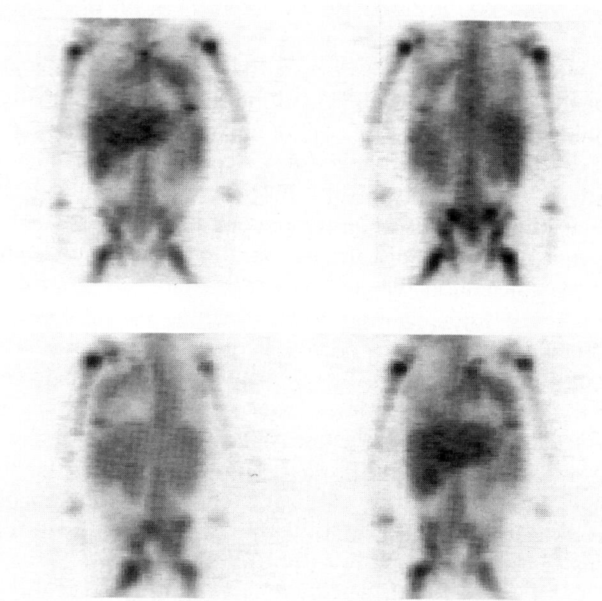

Figure 1. Selected images from a ^{67}Ga SPECT study of a 2-year-old child show abnormal uptake in the thorax and mediastinum. The child was HIV positive and EBV positive. A thymic biopsy showed only follicular hyperplasia, not lymphoma.

Hodgkin's disease, and diffuse "histiocytic" lymphoma have high detectability but, in other histologic types of lymphoma, sensitivity is more variable. (2) Size: tumor masses less than 1 cm in diameter may not be reliably detected in planar images, but larger lesions are detected with reasonable sensitivity. (3) Anatomic location of disease sites can affect the sensitivity of gallium scintigraphy; in part, because of normal organ localization patterns and, in part, because of the characteristics of scintigraphic instruments used for gallium imaging.[44–47] Detection of tumors in the liver or spleen, for example, is complicated by normal uptake of radiogallium by these organs. (4) Technical factors: much of the published data on the sensitivity of radiogallium scintigraphy in patients with lymphoma are based on older imaging methods (i.e., gallium doses of 3 to 5 mCi using rectilinear scanners and using older nomenclature for the types of lymphomas studied).[44–46] Subsequent studies demonstrating good to excellent sensitivity for detecting sites of non-Hodgkin's lymphomas (NHL), using the newer techniques of "high-dose" (10 mCi) gallium injections and modern instrumentation soon appeared.[47–51] Kaplan et al. found 92% sensitivity and nearly 100% specificity in detecting NHL.[49,51]

Recent papers demonstrate the utility of ^{67}Ga scintigraphy including SPECT in detecting NHL sites involving the gastrointestinal tract,[52] pulmonary hila,[53] and in determining recurrence after treatment.[54–61] Their results confirm the high sensitivity of ^{67}Ga in detecting mediastinal involvement, and confirm the prognostic significance of persistent ^{67}Ga uptake after treatment. But, Cooper et al.[61] warn that, after negative images, 20% of their patients relapsed with disease above the diaphragm; thus, negative posttreatment studies may be of more limited value in determining tumor "sterilization" in Hodgkin's disease.

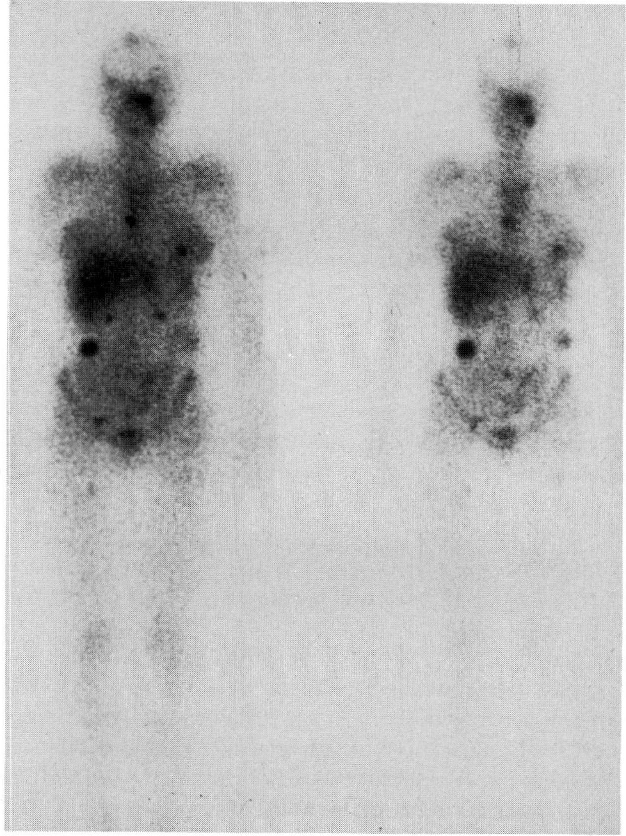

Figure 2. Anterior (left) and posterior (right) whole-body images from a ^{67}Ga study of a young female patient with widespread metastatic melanoma show the utility of these studies in this disease. There is also enhanced gallium uptake in the breasts.

Melanoma

Most malignant melanomas and metastases are sufficiently gallium-avid to be detected when tumor mass exceeds 1 cm in diameter. Of course, the primary lesions of malignant melanoma are usually detected by physical examination. Gallium scintigraphy can be useful in detecting and following metastatic melanoma in patients undergoing various types of chemotherapy and immunotherapy.[62–64] Kirkwood et al.[65] described a prospective study of 67 patients with metastatic melanoma who were imaged with 10 mCi (370 MBq) of ^{67}Ga-citrate using an early tomographic instrument (Pho/Con®). Overall sensitivity and specificity were 82 and 99%, respectively (Fig. 2). A more recent report by Kogan et al.[66] confirmed the accuracy of ^{67}Ga imaging for melanoma detection, but did not find that it added to the routine workup of melanoma patients.

Hepatoma

Most hepatomas are gallium-avid, but "pseudotumors" of cirrhosis, which represent zones of fibrosis and regenerating hepatic tissue, rarely take up gallium.[67–77] Thus, gallium scintigraphy is useful in distinguishing between pseudotumor and hepatoma in patients with known cirrhosis who present with signs of hepatic decompensation and liver masses. Cornelius and Atterbury[78] reviewed the pre-1984 literature on ^{67}Ga scintigraphy of hepatomas. Among 164 patients reported in 9 articles, 63% of hepatomas concentrated more gallium than did host liver tissue, 25% of the hepatomas had ^{67}Ga uptake about equal to surrounding liver tissue, and only 12% of hepatomas had less uptake than host liver. Thus, approximately 88% of hepatomas are "gallium-avid" with reference to "normal" liver. However, exceptional care must be used in interpreting radiogallium hepatic scintigraphy, because many hepatic lesions other than hepatoma (e.g., abscesses and metastases) take up gallium, greatly limiting its specificity.

Lung Carcinoma

Gallium is taken up by primary lung tumors with 85 to 95% sensitivity, depending on tumor histology and size; tumors must be 1 cm or more in diameter to be reliably detected, even with current instruments and techniques.[79] But, gallium scintigraphy is neither more sensitive nor more specific than simple chest radiography for detecting primary lung cancers. Gallium scintigraphy may be useful in evaluating mediastinal metastatic disease because detecting hilar and mediastinal lymph node involvement is critical in determining prognosis and treatment of lung cancers. Small-cell tumors are not usually treated surgically, but other cell types are typically treated by resection of primary lesions. In the absence of hilar or mediastinal node involvement, posttreatment survival approaches 50% at 5 years for patients with squamous cell cancers. However, if lymph nodes of the hilum and mediastinum are involved, the 5-year disease-free survival is less than 10% and thoracotomy is usually not indicated.[80]

Mediastinoscopy has been the procedure of choice for detecting mediastinal metastases, but it is a highly invasive procedure, and fails to detect lesions in a small percentage of cases.[81] Alazraki et al.[82] advocated gallium scintigraphy to screen for mediastinal involvement. Because they found gallium scintigraphy sensitive but nonspecific, they recommended preoperative mediastinoscopy only for patients with mediastinal uptake of gallium. Fosberg et al.,[83] and Lesk et al.,[84] in retrospective series, confirmed these findings. Lunia et al.[85] reported ^{67}Ga imaging was more accurate than chest x-rays in assessing regional node involvement, in a prospective comparison. DeMeester and others,[86] however, found gallium to be relatively insensitive in detecting mediastinal lymph node involvement, with a false-negative rate of about 33% for paramediastinal primary lesions. In our personal experience,[87] nonSPECT gallium imaging was neither sensitive nor specific for detecting of mediastinal involvement in lung carcinoma.

More recently, a prospective study[88] of 75 patients with lung cancer imaged with ^{67}Ga followed by thoracotomy with total mediastinal node dissection reported a very low sensitivity of 23%, specificity of 82%, and overall accuracy of only 63% for ^{67}Ga scintigraphy. The low sensitivity was due to inability to detect microscopic metastases in mediastinal lymph nodes. The specificity was diminished by gallium uptake in enlarged reactive nodes that contained no metastases. These results reinforce earlier findings that gallium scintigraphy is not accurate enough to determine which patients have hilar or mediastinal lymph node metastatic lung carcinoma. A similar report followed from one of the groups who initially were very enthusiastic about ^{67}Ga imaging of the mediastinum.[89] At present, conventional ^{67}Ga nuclear medicine techniques should not be relied upon for preoperative staging of mediastinal lymph node metastases in lung cancer patients.

Gallium is also insensitive for detecting extrathoracic spread of lung carcinoma.[90] In one study of patients with small cell carcinoma, only 7% of extrathoracic metastases were found, although 84% of mediastinal disease was identified.[91] Another study, which included tumors of all cell types, found that 75% of metastatic sites found by all other clinical methods (radionuclide imaging of individual organs, CT scans, and clinical examination) were detected by whole-body gallium imaging.[86] However, the evidence currently available is insufficient to determine the value of whole-body gallium imaging in detecting widespread metastatic lung cancer.

Gallium scintigraphy may be useful in evaluating local extent of disease and distant metastases in patients with pleural mesotheliomas.[92,93] The authors cited found gallium to be more sensitive than chest radiography in defining sites of malignant mesothelioma from benign pleural thickening.

Head and Neck Tumors

The utility of ^{67}Ga scintigraphy in the staging and follow-up of head and neck tumors has been the subject of several reports with varying results. Kashima et al.[94] found positive ^{67}Ga uptake in 86% of patients with primary tumors of the head and neck. All lesions detected were 2 cm or more in diameter, which is inferior to current CT or MR scanning. Teates et al.[95] reported an overall sensitivity of only 56% in patients with head and neck tumors. Of interest, previous surgery and/or irradiation of the primary or metastatic head and neck tumors did not seem to affect the tumor detection rate. Thus, gallium scintigraphy may be of occasional use in these patients in detecting recurrent tumor following therapy, when obscured anatomic planes and landmarks prevent accurate CT exams. Silverstein et al.[96] reported a poor prognosis for head and neck tumor patients whose studies showed uptake in recurrent tumor, as compared to "gallium-negative" residual mass patients.

Abdominal and Pelvic Organ Tumors

Primary and metastatic tumors involving the abdominal and pelvic organs can be detected by ^{67}Ga scintigraphy with varying accuracy, including some histological types of testicular malignancies.[97–100] Pinsky et al.[100] reported 92% accuracy in a series of 36 patients with surgically proven testicular tumors with intra-abdominal lymph node metastases. Patterson et al.[98] found a correlation between gallium uptake and the histological tumor type: all seminomas studied were detectable but only about one fifth of teratomas accumulated sufficient gallium to be detected. Approximate sensitivities determined in these reports are: 75% for metastatic embryonal cell carcinoma, 57 to 90% for metastatic seminoma, about 25% for teratomas of the testes, and 93 to 100% for primary extragonal seminomas.

The poor results of ^{67}Ga scintigraphy for most gynecologic tumors[101–103] are not easily understood because tumors of the ovaries are counterparts to gallium-avid testicular tumors, and one might expect a similar degree of gallium uptake.

Tumors of the gastrointestinal tract and pancreas, chiefly adenocarcinomas, are not usually evaluated by ^{67}Ga scintigraphy, again, because of poor accuracy.[104–106]

Malignant Soft-Tissue Tumors

Schwartz and Jones[107] reported high sensitivity and specificity in detecting soft tissue sarcomas and occult metastases with ^{67}Ga. Their prospective study results were better than previous reports of this use of gallium[108–109] and suggest the need for further study.

SCINTIGRAPHY WITH RADIOLABELED OCTREOTIDE

The presence of somatostatin receptors on a wide variety of tumors has recently led to the development of radiolabeled somatostatin analogues as a means of scintigraphic localization. Somatostatin is a 14-amino acid cyclic peptide that functions primarily to inhibit hormone secretion.[110] As would be expected, target tissues express specific somatostatin receptors,[111] of which there appear to be several subtypes.[112,113] Tumors arising from these tissues frequently express increased numbers of somatostatin receptors.

As reviewed by Reubi et al.,[114] 3 tumor groups express somatostatin receptors with a high incidence: (1) neuroendocrine tumors (including pituitary adenomas, pancreatic islet-cell tumors, pheochromocytomas, carcinoids, medullary thyroid carcinoma, paragangliomas, and small-cell lung carcinomas); (2) nervous system tumors (including neuroblastomas, meningiomas, and astrocytomas); and (3) lymphomas. Other tumors that express somatostatin receptors with a lower incidence include breast,[115] ovarian,[116] and renal[117] carcinomas.

With the introduction of ^{123}I-labeled octreotide in 1989[118] and later of ^{111}In-DTPA octreotide,[119] in vivo detection of somatostatin receptor–positive tissues became practical. Octreotide, an 8-amino acid cyclic peptide, is one of a number of biologically active somatostatin analogs, and is used therapeutically in patients with diseases such as acromegaly and Zollinger-Ellison syndrome.[120]

Initial experience with ^{123}I-Tyr-3-octreotide, identified some problems, including the short half-life of ^{123}I and handling of the agent by the hepatobiliary system, which often obscured abdominal structures.[119] Subsequently, ^{111}In-DTPA-D-Phe-1-octreotide (^{111}In-pentetreotide or Octreoscan®) was developed to overcome these problems. The longer half-life of ^{111}In facilitates delayed imaging and approximately 85% of the injected dose is excreted by the kidneys.[121] Approximately 50% is excreted in the urine in 6 hours. Less than 2% is excreted in the feces, resulting in a modest amount of bowel activity.[121] To facilitate renal clearance and minimize interference from bowel activity, patients should be well hydrated and receive laxatives.

The recommended dose of octreotide for adults is 3 mCi (111 MBq) for planar imaging or 6 mCi for SPECT imaging. Imaging protocols vary with institutions, but generally include imaging at 2 different times, with SPECT performed electively. At NIH, we take planar and selected SPECT images at 4 and 24 hours after injection. Rarely, 48-hour images are obtained. Patients are encouraged to drink fluids and are usually given a laxative between the first and second day of imaging. Because of the theoretical possibility of a paradoxical reaction to octreotide, patients with insulinoma are initially injected during a dextrose infusion, and receive laxatives at the discretion of their physicians.

Uptake of octreotide is normal in the liver, spleen, kidneys, and bladder, with lesser amounts in the pituitary, thyroid, salivary glands, and breasts.[122] Activity excreted through the hepatobiliary system appears in bowel and gallbladder, which can be recognized by their characteristic conformation, position, and variability over time. Because of the presence of somatostatin receptors on many leukocytes,[123] areas of inflammation can be mistaken for tumor.

As for the causes of false-negative studies, not all tumors express somatostatin receptors, and others do so at various densities and with different degrees of uniformity. Several subtypes of somatostatin receptors have been found, some of which demonstrate lower affinities for octreotide than others.[112–113]

Neuroendocrine Disease

Octreotide has been used most extensively in patients with neuroendocrine tumors, and uptake correlates well with in vitro assays of somatostatin receptors,[120,124] many of which are small and difficult to detect by other imaging techniques.

PITUITARY TUMORS

Octreotide as a nonlabeled drug has been used to treat patients with growth hormone (GH)- and thyroid stimulating hormone (TSH)-producing pituitary adenomas.[125] In these patients, octreotide not only suppresses hormone secretion,

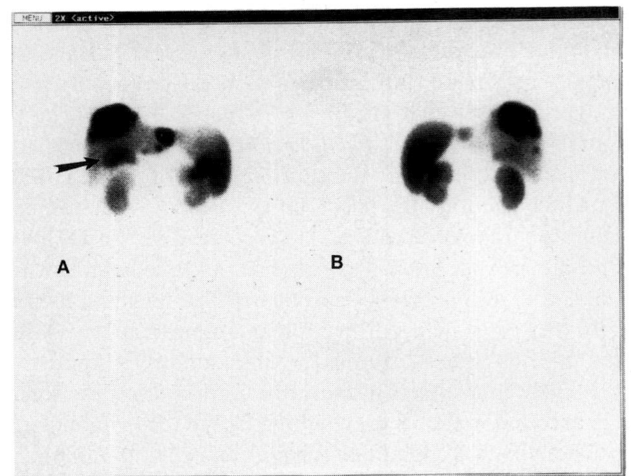

Figure 3. Gastrinoma: **(A)** anterior and **(B)** posterior planar images of the abdomen obtained at 24 hrs after intravenous administration of 3 mCi (111 MBq) ^{111}In-octreotide in a patient with Zollinger-Ellison syndrome and metastatic gastrinoma. A large lesion is seen in the tail of the pancreas between the left kidney and spleen. Multiple metastases are seen in the liver, including a very large mass in the dome of the right lobe. Note normal activity present in the gallbladder (arrow).

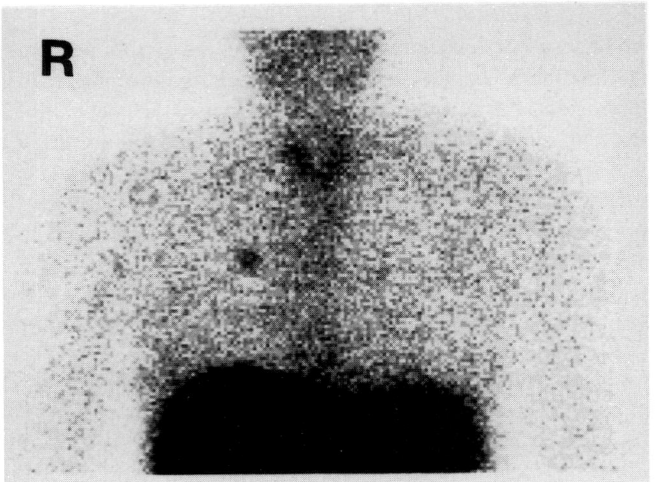

Figure 4. Carcinoid: anterior 24-hour image of the chest in a patient with MEN1 and a bronchial carcinoid; note the normal presence of uptake of octreotide in the thyroid gland.

but also reduces tumor size in many cases. In vivo uptake of radiolabeled octreotide by GH-secreting tumors has been shown to predict a positive response (hormone suppression) to octreotide.[126] As an imaging agent, octreotide is reported to have a sensitivity of 70 to 75% for GH-secreting adenomas,[124,127] and was taken up by 1 of 2 TSH-secreting tumors,[124] corresponding to the high incidence of somatostatin receptors in these tumors.[126,128]

The role of octreotide is less clear for nonfunctioning pituitary adenomas, although some tumors do respond to treatment.[125,126] Somatostatin receptor status in these patients appears to be somewhat variable.[124,126] Nevertheless, octreotide is taken up by approximately 75% of these tumors.[124] Octreotide has been less effective in imaging ACTH-producing adenomas (Cushing's disease) and prolactinomas.[125,126,129]

GASTROENTEROPANCREATIC TUMORS

Other tumors that concentrate octreotide are the gastroenteropancreatic tumors, gastrinomas, VIPomas (vasoactive intestinal polypeptide), glucagonomas, and insulinomas (Fig. 3). Reported sensitivities for gastrinomas range from 81 to 100%[124,130,131] and, in many cases, octreotide identifies lesions undetected by other imaging techniques.[130–132] For insulinomas, however, sensitivity ranges from 50 to 61%[124,133] because many of these tumors lack somatostatin receptors.[134]

OTHER NEUROENDOCRINE TUMORS

Although octreotide does not localize sufficiently to detect pituitary adenomas in patients with Cushing's disease, sites of ectopic ACTH production are often identified. In a series of 9 patients with ectopic ACTH production due to carcinoid (n = 5), medullary thyroid carcinoma (n = 2), gastrinoma (n = 1), and small cell lung cancer (n = 1), de Herder et al.[129] localized 7 lesions with octreotide (sensitivity = 78%), missing 2 bronchial carcinoids. In vivo response to octreotide therapy was assessed in 6 of these patients; responses were seen in 5 patients in whom scintigraphy was also positive, whereas 1 patient with negative scintigraphy had no response to octreotide.

In larger groups of carcinoid patients, other investigators have reported sensitivities of 78 to 96%[124,130,135,136] (Fig. 4). In particular, Westlin et al.[136] showed that octreotide detected 18 sites of previously unknown disease. Octreotide also localizes in medullary thyroid carcinoma; with a sensitivity of 71–90%.[124,137]

In neuroblastomas, pheochromocytomas, and paragangliomas, octreotide has sensitivities of 89%, 86%, and 100%, respectively.[124,138,139] In a study that compares octreotide with meta-iodobenzylguanidine (MIBG) in patients with malignant pheochromocytoma or paraganglioma, Tennenbaum et al.[138] found that the 2 modalities complemented each other, each identifying lesions missed by the other agent. Overall, MIBG imaging was superior to octreotide in these patients.

In 2 studies, octreotide had a sensitivity of 100% for meningiomas, which have a high density of somatostatin receptors.[124,127] This tumor is often classified as a neuroendocrine tumor. Somatostatin receptors are actually found in several brain tissues,[140] and other types of brain tumors are detectable by octreotide. Astrocytomas, which have somatostatin receptors in approximately 82% of cases, were localized in vivo by octreotide in 4 of 6 cases.[124]

In patients with small cell lung cancer, octreotide has an 87 to 100% sensitivity for the primary lesion.[124,141,142] Its sensitivity for metastatic disease, however, appears to be lower.[142]

Non-neuroendocrine Tumors

The use of octreotide imaging is also being explored in various non-neuroendocrine tumors. Approximately 75% of breast tumors,[115] 47% of renal carcinomas,[117] and 77 to 100% of non-small-cell lung carcinomas[124,142] are localized. Whereas localization is presumed to reflect positive somatostatin receptor status in breast and renal carcinoma, somatostatin receptors have not been demonstrated in cases of non-small-cell lung cancer,[143] despite their positive imaging. One explanation for this may be that octreotide localizes in somatostatin receptor-positive inflammatory cells that are closely associated with the tumor.[124]

In 74 patients with non-Hodgkin's lymphoma and 24 patients with Hodgkin's disease, Krenning et al.[124] have reported sensitivities of 80% and 96% for octreotide, respectively. Others have found somewhat lower sensitivities, particularly for non-Hodgkin's lymphoma.[144–146] Closer analysis has also shown that, in some series, sensitivity for extra-abdominal disease appears to be better than for intra-abdominal disease.[144,145] Sensitivity may also depend, in part, on the grade of the lymphoma, being higher in those with high-grade disease.[144,146] See also Chapter 31.

PET IN ONCOLOGY PATIENTS

Positron emission tomography (PET) may be used to localize tumors and to assess tumor viability before, during, and after therapy, both in primary and metastatic sites. Although CT and convential MRI provide anatomic details, they give little functional information about tumor viability. PET, on the other hand, can be used to evaluate blood flow, blood volume, glucose metabolism, protein metabolism, oxygen concentration, nucleic acid metabolism, concentration of receptors, and distributions of cytotoxic agents.[147–149]

Early PET studies in oncology patients evaluated the response to treatment of brain tumors.[150,151] Subsequent studies have demonstrated the utility of ^{18}F-fluorodeoxyglucose (^{18}F-FDG) PET in evaluating response to treatment in tumors of the head and neck,[152,153] breast,[154] lung,[155] liver,[156,157] colon,[158,159] and several other malignancies.[160] Changes in ^{11}C-methionine uptake in response to radiation or chemotherapy have been shown with PET for pituitary tumors,[161] gliomas,[162] lymphoma,[163] lung cancer,[164] and breast cancer.[165] Tumor blood flow in breast cancer has been studied with $^{15}O\text{-}H_2O$.[166] We will review some recent findings in which PET has been used to monitor tumor response to cytotoxic chemical or biologic therapies.

PET measures the absolute regional concentration of radioactive tracers. From such data, physiological parameters such as glucose uptake may be calculated. After computer reconstruction of the data, an image is produced that is coded to represent the amount of radioactivity per unit volume of tissue (Fig. 5). Whole-body PET scans are now possible, which is important for oncology patients because it permits a survey of the entire body for metastatic tumors.[167]

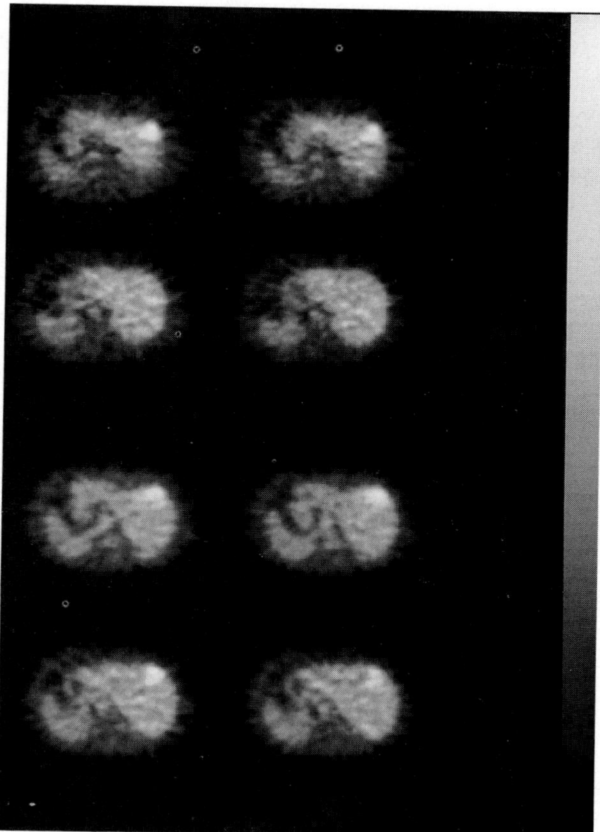

Figure 5. Selected transverse abdominal PET images from an ^{18}F-FDG study show increased focal uptake in a liver metastasis from an ocular melanoma primary tumor in this patient. The color intensity bar at the edge of this picture shows the quantitation scale for this study, with white representing the greatest activity and black the least activity. (See Plate 33.)

Although many radiopharmaceuticals have been labeled with positron emitters, ^{18}F-FDG is presently the most widely used for oncology studies. It is taken up in cells by the same carrier-mediated transport system as glucose. Like glucose, it is phosphorylated by hexokinase. However, FDG-6-phosphate cannot undergo further metabolism in the glycolytic pathway or diffuse back out of cells. In certain cells with low activity of the enzyme glucose-6-phosphatase, there is little conversion back to FDG and, thus, FDG-6-phosphate is trapped within the cell. This occurs in various malignant cells, as well as certain normal tissues such as brain and myocardium. Trapped FDG activity, thus, gives a measure of intracellular FDG. Oncology patients are usually studied in the fasting state because uptake of FDG is somewhat sensitive to variations in blood glucose levels.[168–170]

Malignant cells often have an enhanced rate of glycolysis.[171,172] Because FDG acts as a competitive substrate for both glucose transport and phosphorylation, accumulation of FDG proceeds at a rate approximately proportional to that of local glucose metabolism. In addition to providing images proportional to glucose uptake, quantitative data can be obtained for numerical estimates of glucose utilization. In general, more aggressive tumors have a higher rate of glycolysis and, thus accumulate more FDG. FDG uptake, for example, correlates well with the histological grade of brain tumors.[173,174]

The accumulation of FDG in head and neck tumors[152] and lymphoma[175] correlates histologically with the percentage of proliferative cells in biopsies. The same correlation was shown with flow cytometry.[176] In vitro uptake of FDG in a human ovarian adenocarcinoma cell line was related to the number of viable tumor cells present, but uptake did not correlate with proliferative activity.[177]

Blood flow, which can give an indication of the tumor's general metabolic activity, may be measured with $^{15}O\text{-}H_2O$, a tracer that is freely diffusable. By comparing the concentration of tracer within tumor to an arterial input function, tissue blood flow in mL/min/cc of tissue can be calculated in a reproducible manner.[166] The short half-life of ^{15}O (2.1 minutes) allows studies to be repeated several times in the same visit. Tumor blood flow measurements can be used to study the delivery of chemotherapeutic agents, monoclonal antibodies, or other tumor-targeted agents that depend on blood flow for delivery.

Labeled amino acids, such as ^{11}C-methionine (MET), have been used to study protein metabolism in tumors and changes in MET uptake during therapy have been demonstrated.[171] Consideration has been given to administering MET in the fasting state, because tumor uptake may be decreased after eating.[178] Uptake of ^{11}C-thymidine also relates to tumor proliferative rate as assessed by DNA flow cytometry.[177]

The pharmacokinetics of chemotherapeutic agents such as 5-fluorouracil (FU) can be evaluated with radiotracers such as ^{18}F-FU. Renal excretion, liver uptake, gall bladder transport, and uptake in tumors can be measured directly with PET, whereas such information can only be inferred from plasma data and tissue biopsies. For chemotherapeutic drugs with small therapeutic margins, measuring the actual drug delivery to the tumor is thought to better predict tumor response.

Breast cancer patients have been studied with ^{18}F-fluorinated estrogen, to detect estrogen receptors.[179]

Children with brain tumors—medulloblastoma or primitive neuroectodermal tumor—underwent serial FDG-PET studies prior to and during therapy.[180] This use of FDG-PET was to evaluate early treatment responses, both to modify clinical trials and to reduce treatment-related sequelae.

In patients with glioblastoma who had pre- and post-treatment FDG-PET studies,[181] a tumor metabolic index representing maximum tumor metabolism, normalized to contralateral brain metabolism was found to correlate directly with tumor progression and, inversely, with patient survival. Absolute tumor metabolism, on the other hand, was not as good at predicting progression of disease.

The effectiveness of tumor therapeutic regimens has usually been evaluated retrospectively after several months of treatment, and is based on changes in tumor size. However, changes in tumor metabolic activity may be a better index of response (Fig. 6). Sequential FDG-PET scans performed in women with newly diagnosed breast cancers[182] showed a general decrement in tumor standard uptake values (SUVs) in those patients who benefited from treatment, but changes in tumor size, as measured on serial mammograms, occurred less rapidly.

The response to combined chemotherapy/radiotherapy or radiotherapy alone was evaluated in patients with lung cancer using ^{11}C-MET.[183] Uptake measurements were able to distinguish between those patients who would develop early recurrence of tumor (1 to 4 months) versus those with late recurrence (more than 11 months).

Planar imaging with FDG has also been tested as a less-expensive imaging method for oncology patients.[184] In patients with lymphomas planar imaging with FDG did not add significant information compared to imaging with ^{67}Ga, perhaps because planar imaging is less sensitive than PET.

PET studies have also been performed with ^{18}Fluoride ion, which is taken up in osseous tissues by an exchange process with hydroxyl ions in hydroxyapatite and thus may be used to study skeletal tumors.[185]

RADIOIMMUNOSCINTIGRAPHY OF CANCERS

Radioimmunoscintigraphy (RIS) of cancers is a technique in which radiolabeled antitumor antibodies are administered for tumor detection. This method was made possible by the development of a multitude of antibodies that recognize various tumor-associated antigens. The concept is that after an antibody is administered (usually intravenously) it will circulate and be carried passively throughout the body. However, when the antibody enters a target-antigen-bearing tissue, it will bind and be retained. Because the tumors typically express higher levels of the target antigen, there is greater tumor accumulation of the radiolabeled antibody than in normal tissues. The principles of antibody production and radiolabeling are discussed in Chapter 51 and the interested reader is invited to review those sections.

Patient Preparation

The adverse effects from radiolabeled antibodies administered for diagnostic applications are infrequent, estimated to occur in about 1:1100 cases[186]; this is a lower rate than observed with x-ray contrast agents. Although RIS side effects are infrequent, they can occur and are mainly idiosyncratic, consisting of fever, chills, and rashes.[187] There are some radiolabeled antibodies that more frequently elicit adverse reactions.[186,188] No special premedication of patients is usually necessary, but antihistamines should be immediately available, in particular when doses are repeated. With radioiodine labels, it is necessary to block the patient's thyroid using potassium iodide (~100 mg bid) prior to radioimmunopharmaceutical administration, and continuing for up to 2 weeks when ^{131}I is used. In addition, potassium perchlorate

A

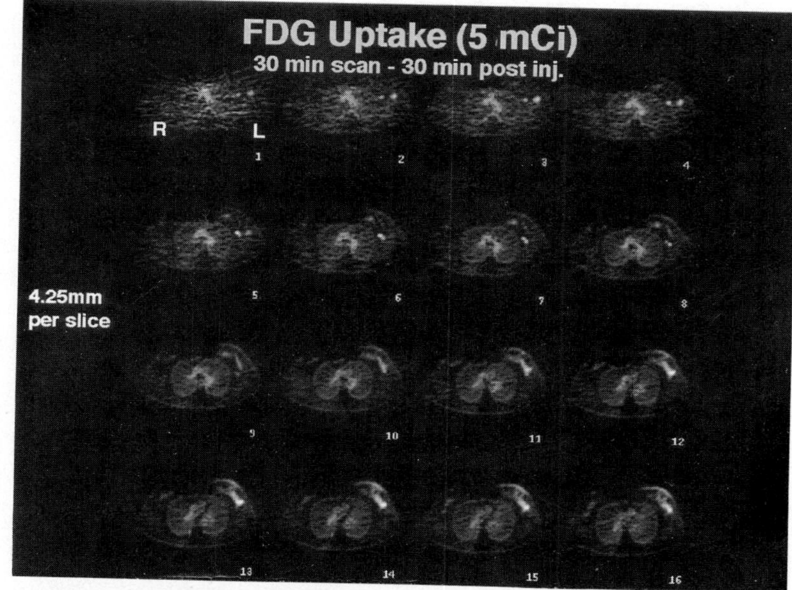

B

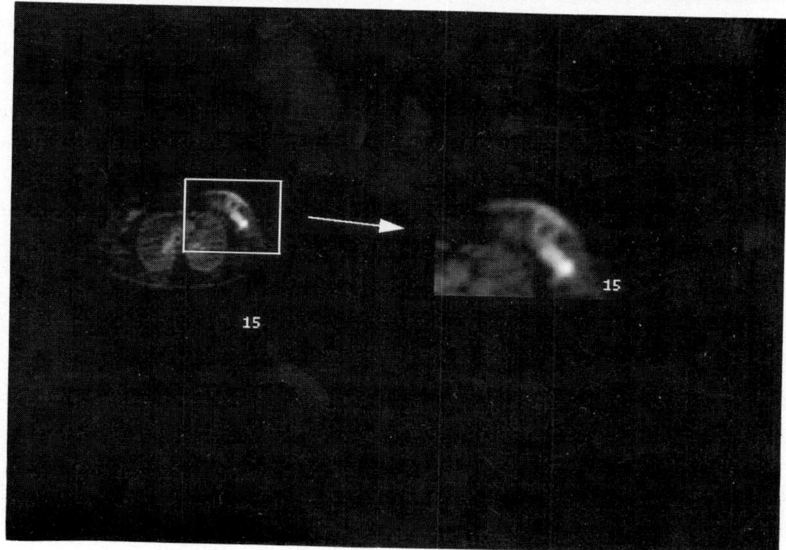

Figure 6 (A). These are transverse scans of the thorax in a female patient with an inflammatory carcinoma of the left breast. The first row of images show focal ^{18}F-FDG uptake in axillary node metastases. Images in the third and fourth row show enhanced uptake in the breast primary and the tumor extension into the skin. **(B).** An enlarged section of the left breast ^{18}F-FDG image shows the increased uptake of this radiopharmaceutical in the primary tumor, as well as in its extensions toward the skin surface and infiltrates in the skin. Such tumor invasion of the skin is responsible for the classic "peau d'orange" sign associated with these cancers. (See Plate 34.)

may be used to additionally block thyroid and stomach uptake. Although serum sickness has been reported after antibody administration, this is an infrequent occurrence.

Imaging Methods

Radioimmunoscintigraphy is acquired in the whole-body mode or by obtaining multiple spot images to cover the body. For a given malignancy the typical patterns of spread are usually known, and special emphasis to selected regions is appropriate. With the availability of multiple-head gamma cameras, SPECT imaging is routinely performed and improves sensitivity of localization.[189] The timing of scintigraphy depends on the biokinetics of the antibody used. For whole IgG preparations, images are typically obtained at approximately 4 to 7 days, but optimal images may be obtained in less than 24 hours with Fab-fragment radioimmunopharmaceuticals.

To better identify the exact anatomic location in which antibody has accumulated, alignment ("fusion") imaging techniques are used.[190–192] Most experience with image fusion techniques has involved neuroimaging where PET or SPECT studies are aligned with MRI or CT scans.[190] Perhaps the most popular method is that developed by Pelizzari et al.[190] adapted for body images.[192]

Antibody Formulation

Initial RIS studies relied mostly on the use of whole IgG for imaging. Although tumor targeting with unmodified IgG can be successful, several limitations became evident. Intact IgG molecules have a slow clearance from the circulation and penetration into solid tumors is hampered by the molecular size.[193,194] In addition, murine IgGs also appear to be more immunogenic than their fragments.[195] Several clinical studies have evaluated chemically generated antibody fragments,

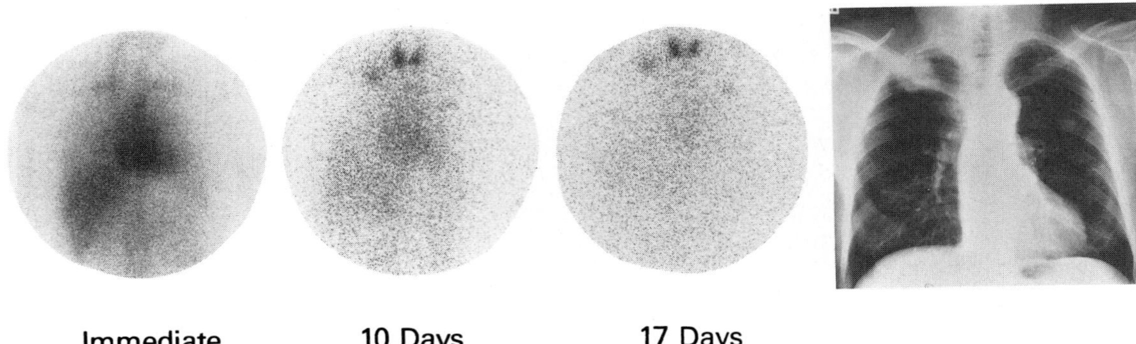

Figure 7. Serial planar images from a 54-year-old man were obtained after intravenous administration of ^{131}I-16.88 human monoclonal antibody (4.9 mCi and 57 mg). Tumor imaging of 2 of the patient's 3 lung lesions was first seen at 72 hours (data not shown) and showed improved contrast with time. Thyroid activity is seen in spite of blocking with saturated solution of potassium iodide.[67]

such as F(ab′)2, Fab, or Fab′.[189] These reagents exhibit faster kinetics and produce higher tumor-to-nontumor ratios, so that imaging results are more favorable.[189] Fab fragments are also usually less immunogenic.[195] With the advent of molecular engineering techniques, "humanized" antibody radiopharmaceuticals are being developed in an attempt to overcome the limitations of murine antibody reagents. Humanized IgGs are currently being evaluated in clinical trials,[196,197] and genetically engineered fragments (Fv fragments) are undergoing preclinical testing.[193,194,198–200]

Human monoclonal antibodies have, thus far, undergone limited evaluation.[201] Initially, IgMs were evaluated because these were the most easily available antibodies from human lymphocyte fusions.[201] Steis et al.[202] reported the use of ^{131}I-labeled 16.88 and 28A32, 2 different human IgMs. The serum kinetics after i.v. injection of the 2 antibodies was significantly different. Antibody 16.88 showed a beta half-life of 56.9 hrs, whereas 28A32 was cleared faster with a mean beta half-life of 40 hours. Twenty-one of 28 cancer patients studied showed positive tumor localization by RIS. These 21 included 13 of 16 patients receiving ^{131}I-28A32 and 8 of 11 patients receiving ^{131}I-16.88. Metastatic disease in liver, lung, lymph node, peritoneum, bone, and brain was detected. Scans obtained immediately after the antibody injection showed predominantly blood pool activity with clear visualization of the heart, liver, and spleen, but no tumor uptake (Fig. 7). Liver metastases were usually seen as photopenic lesions in the early scans. As normal tissue background cleared, contrast improved and lesions were better visualized. The best scintigraphy was at approximately 7 days, but positive results were obtained in some patients as long as 16 days after injection.

More recently, humanized IgG 88BV59 has been evaluated.[203] Similarly to the IgM 16.88, it recognizes an epitope of antigen CTA 16.88 that is homologous with cytokeratins 8, 18, and 19. This antibody was labeled with ^{99m}Tc and used in 36 patients prior to undergoing surgery. The RIS antibody was determined to be more sensitive than the concurrent CT scans (68% vs 40%). These human antibodies were shown to be either nonimmunogenic or only very weakly immunogenic.[202,203]

An approach to decrease the prolonged circulation of radiolabeled antibody in the blood, with the resultant high background, is the use of pretargeting techniques.[204–207] The most popular at present uses avidin-biotin reagents.[204] Such an approach usually has three steps: (1) a biotin-labeled antibody directed against the tumor-associated antigen of interest is administered; time is allowed for tumor concentration; (2) avidin is then injected intravenously; this will remove any nonbound circulating antibody; a second dose of avidin is then injected, which will bind to the biotin on the tumor-bound antibody; (3) ^{111}In or iodine-labeled biotin is then injected intravenously several days later so that it will attach to the avidin on the tumor-bound antibody. This technique has been used successfully in patients: Paganelli et al. reported sucessful scintigraphy of 18 of 19 patients with CEA-positive cancers[204] using biotin-labeled F023C5 murine MoAb. Tumor uptake was seen promptly after injection of the radiolabeled biotin, with little or no background activity.

RADIOIMMUNOSCINTIGRAPHY OF CARCINOMAS

By far, the most studied antibodies are those directed against antigens present on epithelial carcinomas.[208,209] In this section, we will discuss the experience with anti-CEA and anti-TAG 72 RIS.

CEA

Carcinoembryonic antigen (CEA) was initially described by Gold and Freedman in 1965[210] and was the first tumor-associated antigen studied for RIS,[211] and the first to be successfully targeted with monoclonal antibodies (MoAbs).[196] The initial experiments using ^{131}I-polyclonal IgG demonstrated suboptimal tumor targeting, thus requiring background subtraction methods,[211] which made image interpretation difficult. With antiCEA MoAbs improved tumor targeting was observed; in particular, when optimal radionuclide-labeled fragments of antiCEA antibodies have been utilized. Many groups have studied myriad antibodies directed against different CEA epitopes with different affinities against CEA. The majority of studies have clearly documented that RIS is possible without the need for background subtraction techniques. Goldenberg et al. have developed Immu-4 as an antiCEA murine MoAb.[212–214] This antibody has been used both as ^{123}I-F(ab′)2 and ^{99m}Tc-Fab′. Both RIS preparations have approximately 95% sensitivity for lesion detection.[212] A trial using ^{99m}Tc-Immu-4 Fab′ in 109 patients showed that this test has a positive predictive value of 87%.[214] This antibody was also effective in detecting metastatic lesions in the liver, as well as other occult disease. Lesions as small as 0.6 cm were identified by using SPECT. Because this preparation uses a Fab′ antibody fragment, tumor targeting occurs early; thus, imaging can be performed within 4 hours. Other groups have also reported improved targeting results using Fab fragments compared to intact IgG.[189]

Although many reports suggest that the optimum time for imaging after IgG fragments may be longer than 48 hours, Baum et al. imaged tumors earlier with a ^{99m}Tc-labeled BW 431/26 murine MoAb.[215] The combined experience with BW 431/26 is large, but somewhat variable.[215–219] Liver metastases can be seen as "hot," although many times "cold" lesions or "cold" lesions with a rim of "hot" activity occur. The optimal time for imaging with this antibody was found to be in the range of 6 to 12 hours.

An Italian multicenter study that evaluated ^{131}I- or ^{111}In-antiCEA F023C5 murine MoAb found F(ab′)2 radiopharmaceuticals more suitable for imaging than IgG or Fab formulations.[220] They reported an overall sensitivity of 69%, and a specificity of 97% for detecting adenocarcinomas. Although their experience with ^{111}In-labeled MoAb was similar to ^{131}I-MoAb for lesions outside the liver, the sensitivity for detecting liver metastases was lower for ^{111}In (54 vs 13%). As in other RIS studies, a large number of previously unknown tumor sites were detected. A comparison with CT and MRI using this antibody[220] showed that, while MRI had a similar test sensitivity, the CT scan has a lower rate of tumor detection (89 vs 69%). A number of other groups have also reported successful results with ^{111}In labeled antiCEA antibodies.[221–223]

Another antiCEA MoAb that has been extensively studied is ^{111}In-antiCEA ZCE-025.[222,223] Haseman evaluated the ability of this MoAb to detect sites of occult carcinoma in patients with elevated serum CEA levels who had negative or equivocal CT scans.[222] Of 140 patients suspected of having occult cancer, 59% had positive and 41% had negative images. Seventy-five of the 82 patients with positive studies were confirmed to have at least one MoAb-positive lesion (91% positive predictive value). Thirty-eight of the 58 patients with negative studies had a negative follow-up (66% negative predictive value). MoAb correctly identified at least one site of tumor in 79% of the 95 patients with recurrent or metastatic disease, and correctly predicted the absence of disease in 84. Doerr et al. studied 20 patients with rising CEA levels and negative initial workup. Nineteen of the 20 patients had positive scans.[223]

TAG 72

B72.3 is an IgG1 monoclonal antibody that recognizes TAG 72, a tumor-associated glycoprotein expressed in many adenocarcinomas.[224] Previous reports document expression in >80% of colorectal cancers and >90%[224] of epithelial ovarian carcinomas.[225] This is one of the most extensively studied antibodies in the field of RIS.[226] In a series of patients receiving B72.3 specific and, as a control, nonspecific MoAb, the specificity of localization was demonstrated (Fig. 8); localization ratios of greater than 3 were observed in 99 of 142 patient tumor biopsies (70%), whereas of 210 nontumor biopsies, only 12 had ratios of more than 3.[227] These 12 sites included biopsies of spleen and draining lymph nodes, which were likely to harbor circulating tumor antigen. Several other trials using other labeling methods or different radionuclides[228,229] have also been reported.

B72.3 was eventually developed commercially by the Cytogen Corporation. ^{111}In-satumomab pentetide is the only FDA-approved MoAb presently available for tumor imaging in the USA. This antibody is also known as OncoScint® CR/OV and CYT-103 (Cytogen Corporation, Princeton, NJ). The radiopharmaceutical carries ^{111}In using glycyl-tyrosyl-(N,e-diethylenetriaminepentaacetic acid)-lysine (GYK-DTPA) attached to the antibody through oligosaccharide side chains present in the antibody constant region. This radiolabeling method is, therefore, less likely to have a detrimental effect on immunoreactivity.[230]

The antibody preparation comes in a kit form; 1 mg of B72.3 is labeled with 5 mCi (185 MBq) of ^{111}In. The antibody is given intravenously; thus, optimum images are obtained 48 to 72 hours later because of its relatively long plasma half-life (mean ~56 hours). One multicenter trial was conducted where patients with suspected or confirmed colorectal cancer received ^{111}In-satumomab and were imaged twice between 2 and 5 days in planar and SPECT modes.[231] These patients were staged using conventional methods, including CT, and all findings were confirmed histologically after surgery. Patients with primary colorectal (n = 109) or recurrent cancers (n = 83) were studied. Of the 192 patients, 174 had histologically confirmed colorectal cancer. When the RIS was evaluated on a per-patient basis, its sensitivity was 69%, specificity 76%, accuracy 70%, positive predictive value 97%, and negative predictive value 19%. On a per-lesion basis, the sensitivity was 60%. Occult lesions were detected in 19 patients. When compared to CT scanning, the sensitivity for tumor site detection of RIS was similar, ~69%. RIS and CT were found to be complementary because when used together, they detected ~88% of proven cancer lesions. This

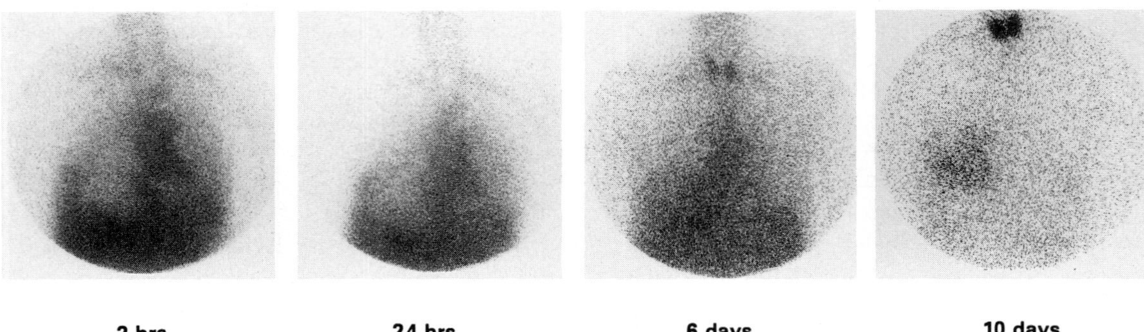

Figure 8. Patient with metastatic colorectal carcinoma to the liver. Initial planar images following intravenous injection of 10 mCi of ^{131}I B72.3 show the liver metastasis as a photopenic lesion compared to the normal liver. At 6 days the activity in the liver has the same intensity as the normal liver. By 10 days when the blood pool has cleared and the radioactivity has cleared from the liver, the tumor is well visualized. Thyroid uptake is noted due to incomplete blocking of the thyroid.

combined test enhancement was due to superior detection of extrahepatic abdominal lesions with antibody (74 vs 57%) when compared to CT. CT was more sensitive than MoAb in finding liver metastases (84 vs 41%).

A second multicenter trial evaluating the utility of ^{111}In-satumomab in detecting ovarian cancers has been performed.[232] Of 103 patients evaluated, 71 had documented ovarian cancer. The sensitivity for RIS in these patients was 59% compared to 29% for CT scanning. RIS detected disease in patients both with elevated CA125 (67%) and normal CA125 (46%); in both instances, the sensitivity for antibody imaging was higher than that of CT scanning. In addition, 28% of patients with a negative presurgical workup, who were found to have disease at surgery, were identified correctly by RIS.

A series of second-generation MoAbs[233] that recognize different epitopes of TAG 72 have been developed. Favorable results in pre-clinical testing[234] led to the use of CC49, one of these second generation products, in various clinical trials.[235,236] Kostakoglu et al. found high sensitivity in detecting colorectal carcinoma when patients were preselected for high TAG 72 antigen expression within tumor biopsies. Using high doses of ^{131}I-labeled CC49, they were able to detect 94% of proven lesions.

Radioimmunoguided Surgery

In radioimmunoguided surgery (RIGS), a radiolabeled antitumor antibody is injected and permitted to localize in tumor sites.[237] At a suitable time after injection when normal tissue background has sufficiently decreased, exploratory laparotomy is performed with the assistance of hand-held gamma detection probes. Tumor tissue is expected to have a higher count rate than normal tissue. A multicenter RIGS trial evaluating ^{125}I-B72.3 MoAb in 104 patients with colorectal cancer showed successful localization of tumor metastases in 78% of patients.[238] Seventy-five percent of primary lesions and 63% of recurrences were localized; clinically occult tumor was localized in 23% of patients. In this study RIGS affected patient management and directed the extent of surgery. Long-term follow-up of these patients showed improved survival in those patients designated as resectable by RIGS as compared to CT.[238] The same group evaluated the use of CC49 (the second-generation, higher-affinity antibody against TAG 72) in a series of 60 patients. RIGS detected the primary tumor in 86% of patients and found 97% of the recurrences.[239] These results represented an improved RIGS sensitivity when compared to RIGS using B72.3. In addition, the surgical treatment plan was altered in one half of the patients due to RIGS findings.

Most hand-held intraoperative probes are optimized for detecting low-energy photons and, therefore, most work has been performed with ^{125}I-labeled MoAbs. The use of ^{111}In-labeled MoAbs for RIGS has been less successful because of its higher energy gamma spectrum.[240]

Other Clinical RIS Trials

There have been several studies with other antibodies directed against tumors, particularly malignant melanoma.[189,209,241] Reviews of RIS for prostate cancer,[242,243] ovarian cancer,[242] head and neck tumors, and lung cancer,[244] have been published.

RADIOIMMUNOSCINTIGRAPHY OF LYMPHOMAS

The detection of lymphomas by RIS preceded the extensive applications of radioimmunotherapy using antitumor antibodies. This subject is discussed in detail in Chapter 51.

REFERENCES

1. Edwards CL, Hayes RL. Tumor scanning with gallium citrate. *J Nucl Med* 1969;10:103–105.
2. Dudley HC, Maddox GE. Deposition of radio-gallium (Ga-67) in skeletal tissues. *J Pharmacol Exp Ther* 1949;96:224.
3. Hoffer PB, Bekerman C, Henkin ER (eds): *Gallium-67 imaging, Part 3. Neoplastic Diseases*. New York, John Wiley & Sons, 1978.
4. Freeman LM, Blaufox MD. Gallium-67 citrate. *Semin Nucl Med* 1978;3:181–270.
5. Halpern S, Hagan P. Gallium-67 citrate imaging in neoplastic and inflammatory disease, in Freeman LM, Weissmann HS (eds): *Nuclear Medicine Annual*. New York, Raven Press, 1980, p 219.
6. Hoffer PB. Status of gallium-67 in tumor detection. *J Nucl Med* 1980;21:394–398.
7. Bekerman C, Hoffer PB, Bitran JD. The role of gallium-67 in the clinical evaluation of cancer. *Semin Nucl Med* 1984;14:296–323.
8. Gunsekera SW, King LJ, Lavender PJ. The behaviour of tracer gallium-67 towards serum proteins. *Clin Chim Acta* 1972;39:401–406.
9. Vallabhajosula SR, Harwig JF, Siemsen JK, Wolf W. Radiogallium localization in tumors: Blood binding, transport and the role of transferrin. *J Nucl Med* 1980;21:650–656.
10. Harris AW, Sephton RG. Transferrin promotion of Ga-67 and Fe-59 uptake and cultured mouse myeloma cells. *Cancer Res* 1977;37:3634–3638.
11. Sephton RG, Harris AW. Gallium-67 citrate uptake by cultured tumor cells, stimulated by serum transferrin. *J Natl Can Inst* 1975;54:1263–1266.
12. Larson SM, Rasey JS, Grunbaum Z, et al. Pharmacologic enhancement of Ga-67 tumors to blood ratios for EMT-6 sarcoma. *Radiology* 1979;130:241–243.
13. Hoffer PB, Samuel A, Bushberg JT, et al. Effect of desferrioxamine on tissue and tumor retention of Ga-67: Concise communication. *J Nucl Med* 1979;20:248–251.
14. Hoffer PB, Huberty J, Khayam-Bashi H. The association of Ga-67 and lactoferrin. *J Nucl Med* 1977;18:713–717.
15. Clausen J, Edeling C-J, Fogh J. Ga-67 binding to human serum proteins and tumor components. *Cancer Res* 1974;34:1931–1937.
16. Hegge FN, Mahler DJ, Larson SM. The incorporation of Ga-67 into the ferritin fraction of rabbit hepatocytes in vivo. *J Nucl Med* 1977;18:937–939.
17. Hoffer PB. Gallium: Mechanisms. *J Nucl Med* 1980; 21:282–284.
18. Sephton RG, Hodgson GS, De Abrew S, et al. Ga-67 and Fe-59 distributions in mice. *J Nucl Med* 1978;19:930–935.
19. Logan KJ, Ng PK, Turner CJ, et al. Comparative pharmacokinetics of Ga-67 and Fe-59 in humans. *Int J Nucl Med Biol* 1981;8:271–276.
20. Aisen P, Listowsky I. Iron transport and storage proteins. *Ann Rev* 1980;49:357–393.
21. Crichton RR, Ward RJ. Iron metabolism—new perspectives in view. *Biochemistry* 1992;31:11255–11264.
22. Taetle R. The role of transferrin receptors in hemopoetic cells growth. *Exp Hematol* 1990;18:360–365.
23. Cotton FA, Wilkinson G. *Advanced Inorganic Chemistry.* 5th ed. New York: Interscience, 1988, p 215–230.
24. Harris WR, Pecoraro VL. Thermodynamic binding constants for gallium transferrin. *Biochemistry* 1983;22:292–299.
25. Weiner RE, Schreiber GJ, Hoffer PB, Bushberg JT. Compounds which mediate Ga-67 transfer from lactoferrin to ferritin. *J Nucl Med* 1985;26:908–916.
26. Weiner RE. The role of phosphate-containing compounds on the transfer of Ga-67 and In-111 from transferrin to ferritin. *J Nucl Med* 1989;30:70–79.
27. Larson SM, Rasey JS, Allen DR, et al. Common pathway for tumor cell uptake of Ga-67 and iron-59 via a transferrin receptor. *J Natl Can Inst* 1980;64:41–53.
28. Larson SM, Rasey JS, Nelson NJ, et al. The kinetics of uptake and macromolecular binding of Ga-67 and Fe-59 by the EMT-6 sarcoma-like tumor of Balb/c mice, in Sorenson JA (ed.): *Radiopharmaceuticals II: Proceedings of the 2nd International Symposium on Radiopharmaceuticals*. New York, Society of Nuclear Medicine, 1979, p 277–308.
29. Larson SM, Rasey JS, Allen DR, et al. A transferrin-mediated uptake of Ga-67 by EMT-6 sarcoma. II. Studies in vivo (BALB/c mice): Concise communication. *J Nucl Med* 1979;20:843–846.
30. Hayes RL, Nelson B, Swartzendruber DC, et al. Gallium-67 localization in rat and mouse tumors. *Science* 1970; 167:289–290.
31. Thesingh CW, Driessen OMJ, Daems W-Th, et al. Accumulation and localization of Ga-67 in various types of primary lung carcinoma. *J Nucl Med* 1978;19:28–30.
32. Swartzendruber DC, Nelson B, Hayes RL. Gallium-67 localization in lysosomal-like granules of leukemic and nonleukemic murine tissues. *J Natl Cancer Inst* 1971;46:941–952.
33. Brown DH, Byrd BL, Carlton JE, et al. A quantitative study of the subcellular localization of Ga-67. *Cancer Res* 1976;36:956–963.
34. Berry JP, Escaig F, Poupon MF, Galle P. Localization of gallium in tumor cells. Electron microscopy, electron probe microanalysis and analytical ion microscopy. *Int J Nucl Med Biol* 1983;10:199–204.
35. Manfredi OL, Weiss LR. Gallium-67 citrate in human tumors. *NY State J Med* 1978;78:884–887.
36. DeAbrew S. Assays for transferrin and transferrin receptors in tumor and other mouse tissues. *Int J Nucl Med Biol* 1981;8:217–221.
37. Enns CA, Shindelman JE, Tonik SE, Sussman HA. Radioimmunochemical measurement of the transferrin receptor in human trophoblast and reticulocyte membranes with a specific anti-receptor antibody. *Proc Natl Acad Sci* 1981; 78:4222–4225.
38. Sohn M-E, Jones BJ, Whiting JH, et al. Distribution of Ga-67 in normal and hypotransferrinemic tumor-bearing mice. *J Nucl Med* 1993;34:2135–2143.
39. Basset P, Quesneau Y, Zwiller J. Iron-induced L1210 cell growth: evidence of a transferrin-independent iron transport. *Cancer Res* 1986;46:1644–1647.
40. Kaplan J, Jordan I, Sturrock A. Regulation of the transferrin-independent iron transport system in cultured cells. *J Biol Chem* 1991;266:2997–3004.
41. Chitambar CR, Zivkovic Z. Uptake of Ga-67 by human leukemic cells: demonstration of transferrin receptor-dependent and transferrin-independent mechanisms. *Cancer Res* 1987;47:3929–3924.
42. Iosilevsky G, Front D, Betman L, et al. Uptake of gallium-67 citrate and (2 H-3) deoxyglucose in the tumor model following chemotherapy and radiotherapy. *J Nucl Med* 1985;26:278–282.
43. Higashi T, Kobayashi M, Wakao H, et al. The relationship between Ga-67 accumulation and ATP metabolism in tumor cells in vitro. *Eur J Nucl Med* 1989;15:152–156.
44. Greenlaw RH, Weinstein MB, Brill AB, et al. Ga-67 citrate imaging in untreated malignant lymphoma: preliminary report of (the) cooperative group. *J Nucl Med* 1974;15: 404–407.
45. Johnston GS, Mae FG, Benua RS, et al. Gallium-67 citrate

imaging in Hodgkin's disease: final report of (The) cooperative group. *J Nucl Med* 1977;18:692–698.

46. Longo DL, Schilsky RL, Bleu L, et al. Gallium-67 scanning: limited usefulness in staging patient with non-Hodgkin's lymphoma. *Am J Med* 1980;68:695–700.
47. McLaughlin AF, Magee MA, Greenough R, et al. Current role of gallium scanning in the management of lymphoma. *Eur J Nucl Med* 1990;16:755–771.
48. McLaughlin AF, Chu J, Howman-Giles R. Whole body gallium scanning in malignant lymphoma—its role in 1980. *Austral NZ J Med* 1980;11:438.
49. Kaplan WD, Anderson KC, Leonard RCF. High dose gallium imaging in the evaluation of lymphoma. *J Nucl Med* 1983;24:50.
50. Anderson KC, Leonard RCF, Cavellos GP. High dose gallium imaging in lymphoma. *Am J Med* 1983;75:327–331.
51. Tumeh SS, Rosenthal DS, Kaplan WD, et al. Lymphoma-evaluation with Ga-67 SPECT. *Radiology* 1987;164:111–114.
52. Kataoka M, Kawamura M, Tsuda T, et al. The role of Ga-67 imaging in non-Hodgkin's lymphoma of the gastrointestinal tract. *Europ J Nucl Med* 1990;17:142–147.
53. Champion PE, Groshar D, Hoper HR, et al. Does gallium uptake in the pulmonary hila predict involvement by non-Hodgkin's lymphoma? *Nucl Med Comm* 1992;13:730–737.
54. Kaplan WD, Jackelson MS, Herman TS, et al. Ga-67 imaging: a predictor of residual tumor viability and clinical outcome in patients with diffuse large-cell lymphoma. *J Clin Oncol* 1990;8:1966–1970.
55. Israel O, Front D, Epelbaum R, et al. Residual mass and negative gallium scintigraphy in treated lymphoma. *J Nucl Med* 1990;31:365–368.
56. Kaplan WD. Residual mass and negative gallium scintigraphy in treated lymphoma—when is the gallium scan really negative? (editorial) *J Nucl Med* 1990;31:369–371.
57. Front D, Ben-Haim S, Israel O, et al. Lymphoma: predictive value of Ga-67 scintigraphy after treatment. *Radiology* 1992;182:359–363.
58. Front D, Bar-Shalom R, Epelbaum R. Early detection of lymphoma recurrence with Ga-67 scintigraphy. *J Nucl Med* 1993;34:2101–2104.
59. Kostakoglu L, Yeh SD, Portlock C, et al. Validation of gallium-67-citrate SPECT in biopsy-confirmed residual Hodgkin's disease in the mediastinum. *J Nucl Med* 1992; 33:345–350.
60. Karimjee S, Brada M, Husband J, et al. A comparison of gallium-67 SPECT and CT in mediastinal Hodgkin's disease. *Europ J Cancer* 1992;28A:1856–1857.
61. Cooper DL, Caride VJ, Zloty M, et al. Gallium scans in patients with mediastinal Hodgkin's disease treated with chemotherapy. *J Clin Oncol* 1993;11:1092–1098.
62. Milder MS, Frankel RS, Bulkey CB, et al. Ga-67 scintigraphy in malignant melanoma. *Cancer* 1973;32:1350–1356.
63. Jackson FI, McPherson TA, Lentle BC. Ga-67 scintigraphy in multisystem malignant melanoma. *Radiology* 1977; 122:163–167.
64. Romolo JL, Fisher SG. Ga-67 scanning compared with physical examination in the pre-operative staging of malignant melanoma. *Cancer* 1979;44:468–472.
65. Kirkwood JM, Myers JE, Vlock DR, et al. Tomographic Ga-67 citrate scanning: useful new surveillance for metastatic melanoma. *Ann Intern Med* 1982;97:694–699.
66. Kogan R, Witt T, Bines S, et al. Ga-67 scanning for malignant melanoma. *Cancer* 1988;61:272–274.
67. Suzuki T, Honjo I, Hamamoto K, et al. Positive scintiphotography of cancer of the liver with Ga-67 citrate. *AJR* 1971;113:92–103.
68. Lomas FR, Dibos PE, Wagner HN. Increased specificity of liver scanning with the use of Ga-67 citrate. *N Engl J Med* 1972;286:1323–1329.
69. James O, Wood J, Maze M, et al. Ga-67 citrate liver scanning: evaluation of its use in 80 patients and evidence of intrahepatic distribution by autoradiography. *Gut* 1974;15:342.
70. Blazek G, Mastnak C, Kahn P, et al. Ga-67 scintigraphy as an auxiliary method for differentiation of mass lesions of the liver. *Wien Klin Wochenschr* 1975;87:77–81.
71. Levin J, Kew MC. Ga-67 citrate scanning in primary cancer of the liver: diagnostic value in the presence of cirrhosis and relation to alpha-fetoprotein. *J Nucl Med* 1975;16:949–951.
72. Buraggi GL, Laurini R, Rodari A, et al. Double-tracer scintigraphy with Ga-67 citrate and 99mTc sulfur colloid in the diagnosis of hepatic tumors. *J Nucl Med* 1976;17:396–373.
73. Moreau R, Soussaline F, Chauvaud S, et al. Detection of hepatoma in liver cirrhosis. *Eur J Nucl Med* 1977;2:183.
74. Yeh S, Leeper R, Benau R. A study of filling defects in the liver and spleen with multiple radionuclides. *Clin Bull* 1977;7:3.
75. Waxman AD, Richmond R, Juttner H, et al. Correlation of contrast angiography and histologic pattern with gallium uptake in primary liver-cell carcinoma: noncorrelation of alpha fetoprotein. *J Nucl Med* 1980;21:324–327.
76. Broderick TW, Gosink B, Menuck L, et al. Echographic and radionuclide detection of hepatoma. *Radiology* 1980; 135:149–151.
77. Negasue N. Gallium scanning in the diagnosis of hepatocellular carcinoma: a clinicopathological study of 45 patients. *Clin Radiol* 1983;34:139–142.
78. Cornelius EA, Atterbury CE. Problems in the imaging diagnosis of hepatoma. *Clin Nucl Med* 1984;9:30–38.
79. Abdel-Dayem HM, Scott A, Macapinlac H, et al. Tracer imaging in lung cancer. *Eur J Nucl Med* 1994;21:57–81.
80. Mountain CF. Biologic, physiologic and technical; determinants in surgical therapy for lung cancer, in Strauss MJ (ed): *Lung cancer—Clinical Diagnosis and Treatment*. New York, Grune & Stratton, 1977, pp 185–198.
81. Goldberg EM. Mediastinoscopy in assessment of lung cancer, in Strauss MJ (ed): *Lung cancer—Clinical Diagnosis and Treatment*. New York, Grune & Stratton, 1977, pp 113–128.
82. Alazraki NP, Ramsdell JW, Taylor A, et al. Reliability of gallium scan, chest radiography compared to mediastinoscopy for evaluating mediastinal spread in lung cancer. *Am Rev Respir Dis* 1978;117:415–420.
83. Fosburg RG, Hopkins GB, Kan MK. Evaluation of the mediastinum by Ga-67 scintigraphy in lung cancer. *J Thorac Cardiovasc Surg* 1979;77:76–82.
84. Lesk DM, Wood TE, Carrol SE, Reese L. The application of Ga-67 scanning in determining the operability of bronchogenic carcinoma. *Radiology* 1978;128:707–709.
85. Lunia SL, Ruckdeschel JC, McKneally MF. Noninvasive evaluation of mediastinal metastases in bronchogenic carcinoma; a prospective comparison of chest radiography and Ga-67 scanning. *Cancer* 1981;47:672–679.
86. DeMeester TR, Golumb HM, Kirchner P, et al. The role of Ga-67 scanning in the clinical staging and preoperative evaluation of patients with carcinoma of the lung. *Ann Thorac Surg* 1979;18:451–464.
87. Neumann RD, Hoffer PB, Merino MJ, et al. Clinical value of Ga-67 in imaging patients with lung carcinoma and melanoma, in *Medical Radionuclide Imaging 1980*. Vol. II, Vienna, I.A.E.A., 1981, pp 475–486.
88. McKenna RJ, Haynie TP, Libshitz HI, et al. Critical evaluation of the Ga-67 scan for surgical patients with lung cancer. *Chest* 1985;87:428–431.
89. Friedman PJ, Feigin DS, Liston SE, et al. Sensitivity of chest radiography, computer tomography and gallium scanning to metastasis of lung carcinoma. *Cancer* 1984;54:1300–1306.

90. Hooper RG, Beechler CR, Johnson MC. Radioisotope scanning in the initial staging of bronchogenic carcinoma. *Am Rev Resp Dis* 1978;118:279–286.
91. Brereton HD, Line BR, Londer HN, et al. Gallium scans for staging small cell lung cancer. *JAMA* 1978;240:666–667.
92. Sorek M, Teirstein AS, Goldsmith SJ, et al. Ga-67 citrate uptake in benign and malignant pleural disease. *Clin Res* 1979;27:491A.
93. Wolk RB. Ga-67 scanning in the evaluation of mesothelioma. *J Nucl Med* 1978;19:808–809.
94. Kashima H, McKusick K, Malmed L, et al. Ga-67 scanning in patients with head and neck cancer. *Laryngoscope* 1974;84:1078–1089.
95. Teates CD, Preston DF, Boyd CM. Ga-67 citrate imaging in head and neck tumors: report of the cooperative group. *J Nucl Med* 1980;21:622–627.
96. Silverstein EG, Kornblut A, Shumrich DA, et al. Ga-67 as a diagnostic agent for, detection of head and neck tumors and lymphoma. *Radiology* 1974;110:605–608.
97. Jackson FI, Dietrich HC, Lentle BC. Ga-67 citrate scintiscanning in testicular neoplasia. *J Canad Assoc Radiol* 1976;27:84–88.
98. Patterson AH, Peckham MJ, McCready VR. Value of gallium scanning in seminoma of the testis. *Br Med J* 1976;1: 1118–1121.
99. Sauerbrunn B, Andrews G, Hubner K. Ga-67 citrate imaging in tumors of the genitourinary tract: report of cooperative study. *J Nucl Med* 1978;19:470–475.
100. Pinsky SM, Bailey TB, Blom, J. et al. Ga-67 citrate in the staging of testicular malignancies. *J Nucl Med* 1973;14:439.
101. Symmonds RE, Tauke WN. Ga-67 scintigraphy of gynecologic tumors. *Am J Obstet Gynecol* 1972;114:356–369.
102. Pelosi MA, D'Amico RJ, Apuzzio J. Combined use of ultrasonography and gallium scanning in the diagnosis of pelvic pathology. *Surg Gynecol Obstet* 1980;150:331.
103. Okamura S. Diagnosis of ovarian tumors by CT and Ga-67 citrate scintigraphy. *Nippon Sanka Fujinka Gakkai Zasshi* 1983;35:805.
104. Langhammer H, Glaubitt G, Grebe SF, et al. Ga-67 for tumor scanning. *J Nucl Med* 1972;13:25–30.
105. Silberstein EB. Cancer diagnosis: the role of tumor imaging radiopharmaceuticals. *Am J Med* 1974;60:226–237.
106. Hauser MF, Alderson PO. Ga-67 imaging in abdominal disease. *Semin Nucl Med* 1978;8:251–270.
107. Schwartz HS, Jones CK. The efficacy of gallium scintigraphy in detecting malignant soft tissue neoplasias. *Ann Surg* 1992;215:78–82.
108. Kaufman JH, Cedermark BJ, Parthasarathy KL, et al. The value of Ga-67 scintigraphy in soft tissue sarcoma and chondrosarcoma. *Radiology* 1977;123:131–134.
109. Bitran JD, Bekerman C, Golomb HM, et al. Scintigraphic evaluation of sarcomata in children and adults by Ga-67 citrate. *Cancer* 1978;42:1760–1765.
110. Reichlin S. Somatostatin (first of two parts). *N Engl J Med* 1983;309:1495.
111. Reubi JC, Kvols L, Krenning E, Lamberts SWJ. Distribution of somatostatin receptors in normal and tumor tissue. *Metabolism* 1990;39:78.
112. Kubota A, Yamada Y, Kagimoto S, Shimatsu A, et al. Identification of somatostatin receptor subtypes and an implication for the efficacy of somatostatin analogue SMS 201-995 in treatment of human endocrine tumors. *J Clin Invest* 1994;93:1321.
113. Reubi JC, Schaer JC, Waser B, Mengod G. Expression and localization of somatostatin receptor SSTR1, SSTR2, and SSTR3 messenger RNAs in primary human tumors using in situ hybridization. *Cancer Res* 1994;54:3455.
114. Reubi JC, Laissue J, Krenning E, Lamberts SW. Somatostatin receptors in human cancer: incidence, characteristics, functional correlates and clinical implications. *J Steroid Biochem Mol Biol* 1992;43:27.
115. van Eijck CH, Krenning EP, Bootsma A, Oei HY, et al. Somatostatin-receptor scintigraphy in primary breast cancer. *Lancet* 1994;343:640.
116. Reubi JC, Horisberger U, Klijn JG, Foekens JA. Somatostatin receptors in differentiated ovarian tumors. *Am J Pathol* 1991;138:1267.
117. Flamen P, Bossuyt A, De Greve J, Pipeleers-Marichal M, et al. Imaging of renal cell cancer with radiolabelled octreotide. *Nucl Med Commun* 1993;14:873.
118. Krenning EP, Bakker WH, Breeman WA, Koper JW, et al. Localisation of endocrine-related tumours with radioiodinated analogue of somatostatin. *Lancet* 1989;1:242.
119. Bakker WH, Albert R, Bruns C, Breeman WA, et al. [111In-DTPA-D-Phe1]-octreotide, a potential radiopharmaceutical for imaging of somatostatin receptor-positive tumors: synthesis, radiolabeling and in vitro validation. *Life Sci* 1991; 49:1583.
120. Lamberts SW, Krenning EP, Reubi JC. The role of somatostatin and its analogs in the diagnosis and treatment of tumors. *Endocr Rev* 1991;12:450.
121. Krenning EP, Bakker WH, Kooij PP, Breeman WA, et al. Somatostatin receptor scintigraphy with indium-111-DTPA-D-Phe-1-octreotide in man: metabolism, dosimetry and comparison with iodine-123-Tyr-3-octreotide. *J Nucl Med* 1992;33:652.
122. Bajc M, Palmer J, Ohlsson T, Edenbrandt L. Distribution and dosimetry of 111In DTPA-D-Phe-octreotide in man assessed by whole body scintigraphy. *Acta Radiol* 1994;35:53.
123. van Hagen PM, Krenning EP, Kwekkeboom DJ, Reubi JC, et al. Somatostatin and the immune and haematopoetic system; a review. *Eur J Clin Invest* 1994;24:91.
124. Krenning EP, Kwekkeboom DJ, Bakker WH, Breeman WA, et al. Somatostatin receptor scintigraphy with [111In-DTPA-D-Phe1]- and [123I-Tyr3]-octreotide: the Rotterdam experience with more than 1000 patients. *Eur J Nucl Med* 1993;20:716.
125. von Werder K. Somatostatin analogues in pituitary adenomas. *Recent Results Cancer Res* 1993;129:25.
126. Lamberts SW, Hofland LJ, de Herder WW, Kwekkeboom DJ, et al. Octreotide and related somatostatin analogs in the diagnosis and treatment of pituitary disease and somatostatin receptor scintigraphy. *Front Neuroendocrinol* 1993;14:27.
127. Scheidhauer K, Hildebrandt G, Luyken C, Schomacker K, et al. Somatostatin receptor scintigraphy in brain tumors and pituitary tumors: first experiences. *Horm Metab Res Suppl* 1993;27:59.
128. Reubi JC, Landolt AM. The growth hormone responses to octreotide in acromegaly correlate with adenoma somatostatin receptor status. *J Clin Endocrinol Metab* 1989;68:844.
129. de Herder WW, Krenning EP, Malchoff CD, Hofland LJ, et al. Somatostatin receptor scintigraphy: its value in tumor localization in patients with Cushing's syndrome caused by ectopic corticotropin or corticotropin-releasing hormone secretion. *Am J Med* 1994;96:305.
130. Joseph K, Stapp J, Reinecke J, Skamel HJ, et al. Receptor scintigraphy with 111In-pentetreotide for endocrine gastroenteropancreatic tumors. *Horm Metab Res Suppl* 1993; 27:28.
131. de Kerviler E, Cadiot G, Lebtahi R, Faraggi M, et al. Somatostatin receptor scintigraphy in forty-eight patients with the Zollinger-Ellison syndrome. *Eur J Nucl Med* 1994;21:1191.
132. Lamberts SW, Chayvialle JA, Krenning EP. The visualization

of gastroenteropancreatic endocrine tumors. *Digestion* 1993;54(Suppl 1):92.
133. Ur E, Bomanji J, Mather SJ, Britton KE, et al. Localization of neuroendocrine tumours and insulinomas using radiolabelled somatostatin analogues, 123I-Tyr3-octreotide and 111In-pentatreotide. *Clin Endocrinol (Oxf)* 1993;38:501.
134. Reubi JC, Hacki WH, Lamberts SW. Hormone-producing gastrointestinal tumors contain a high density of somatostatin receptors. *J Clin Endocrinol Metab* 1987;65:1127.
135. Hammond PJ, Arka A, Peters AM, Bloom SR, Gilbey SG. Localization of metastatic gastroenteropancreatic tumours by somatostatin receptor scintigraphy with [111In-DTPA-D-Phe1]-octreotide. *Q J Med* 1994;87:83.
136. Westlin JE, Janson ET, Arnberg H, Ahlstrom H, et al. Somatostatin receptor scintigraphy of carcinoid tumours using the [111In-DTPA-D-Phe1]-octreotide. *Acta Oncol* 1993;32:783.
137. Krausz Y, Ish-Shalom S, De Jong RBJ, Shibley N, et al. Somatostatin-receptor imaging of medullary thyroid carcinoma. *Clin Nucl Med* 1994;19:416.
138. Tennenbaum F, Lumbroso J, Schlumberger M, Mure A, et al. Comparison of radiolabeled octreotide and meta-iodobenzylguanidine [MIBG] scintigraphy in malignant pheochromocytoma. *J Nucl Med* 1995;36:1.
139. Kwekkeboom DJ, van Urk H, Pauw BKH, Lamberts SW, et al. Octreotide scintigraphy for the detection of paragangliomas. *J Nucl Med* 1993;34:873.
140. Reubi JC, Lang W, Maurer R, Koper JW, Lamberts SWJ. Distribution and biochemical characterization of somatostatin receptors in tumors of the human central nervous system. *Cancer Res* 1987;47:5758.
141. Maini CL, Tofani A, Venturo I, Pigorini F, et al. Somatostatin receptor imaging in small cell lung cancer using 111In-DTPA-octreotide: a preliminary study. *Nucl Med Commun* 1993;14:962.
142. Kirsch CM, von Pawel J, Grau I, Tatsch K. Indium-111 pentetreotide in the diagnostic work-up of patients with bronchogenic carcinoma. *Eur J Nucl Med* 1994;21:1318.
143. Reubi JC, Waser B, Sheppard M, Macaulay V. Somatostatin receptors are present in small-cell but not in non-small-cell primary lung carcinomas: relationship to EGF-receptors. *Int J Cancer* 1990;45:269.
144. Lipp RW, Silly H, Ranner G, Dobnig H, et al. Radiolabeled octreotide for the demonstration of somatostatin receptors in malignant lymphoma and lymphadenopathy. *J Nucl Med* 1995;36:13.
145. Bares R, Galonska P, Dempke W, Handt S, et al. Somatostatin receptor scintigraphy in malignant lymphoma: first results and comparison with glucose metabolism measured by positron-emission tomography. *Horm Metab Res Suppl* 1993;27:56.
146. Bong SB, VanderLaan JG, Louwes H, Schuurman JJ. Clinical experience with somatostatin receptor imaging in lymphoma. *Semin Oncol* 1994;21:46.
147. Strauss LG, Conti PS. The application of PET in clinical oncology. *J Nucl Med* 1991;32:623–48.
148. Hawkins RA, Hoh C, Glaspy J, Choi Y, et al. The role of positron emission tomography in oncology and other whole-body applications. *Semin Nucl Med* 1992;22:268–284.
149. Scott AM, Larson SM. Tumor Imaging and Therapy. A review of the oncologic applications of nuclear medicine including both the staging of tumors and monitoring the response to therapy with tumor-specific radionuclides. Discusses the increasing role for PET and monoclonal antibody studies in oncology. *Radiol Clin North Am* 1993;4:859–879.
150. DiChiro G, Hatazawa J, Katz DA, Rizzoli HV, et al. Glucose utilization by intracranial mengiomas as an index of tumor aggressivity and probability of recurrence: a PET study. *Radiology* 1987;164:521–526.
151. Di Chiro G, Oldfield E, Wright DC, De Michele D, et al. Cerebral necrosis after radiotherapy and/or intraarterial chemotherapy for brain tumors: PET and neuropathologic studies. *Am J Roentgenol* 1988;150:189–97.
152. Minn H, Paul R, Ahonen A. Evaluation of treatment response to radiotherapy in head and neck cancer with fluorine-18 fluorodeoxyglucose. *J Nucl Med* 1988;29:1521–1525.
153. Haberkorn U, Strauss LG, Dimitrakopoulou A, Seiffert E, et al. Fluorodeoxyglucose imaging of advanced head and neck cancer after chemotherapy. *J Nucl Med* 1993;34:12–17.
154. Minn H, Soini I. [18F]fluorodeoxyglucose scintigraphy in diagnosis and follow-up of treatment in advanced breast cancer. *Eur J Nucl Med* 1989;15:61–66.
155. Abe Y, Matsuzawa T, Fujiwara T, Itoh M, et al. Clinical assessment of therapeutic effects on cancer using 18F-2-fluoro-2-deoxy-D-glucose and positron emission tomography: preliminary study of lung cancer. *Int J Radiat Oncol Biol Phys* 1990;19:1005–1010.
156. Nagata Y, Yamamoto K, Hiraoka M, Abe M, et al. Monitoring liver tumor therapy with [18F]FDG positron emission tomography. *J Comput Assist Tomogr* 1990;14:370–374.
157. Okazumi S, Isono K, Enomoto K, Kikuchi T, et al. Evaluation of liver tumors using fluorine-18-fluorodeoxyglucose PET: characterization of tumor and assessment of effect of treatment. *J Nucl Med* 1992;33:333–339.
158. Haberkorn U, Strauss LG, Dimitrakopoulou A, Engenhart R, et al. PET studies of fluorodeoxyglucose metabolism in patients with recurrent colorectal tumors receiving radiotherapy. *J Nucl Med* 1991;32:1485–1490.
159. Engenhart R, Kimmig BN, Strauss LG, Hover K-H, Romahn J, Haberkorn U, van Kaick G, Wannenmacher M. Therapy monitoring of presacral recurrences after high-dose irradiation: value of PET, CT, CEA and pain score. *Strahlenther Onkol* 1992;168:203–212.
160. Ichiya Y, Kuwabara Y, Otsuka M, Tahara T, et al. Assessment of response to cancer therapy using fluorine-18-fluorodeoxyglucose and positron emission tomography. *J Nucl Med* 1991;32:1655–1660.
161. Bergstrom M, Muhr C, Lundberg PO, Bergstrom K, et al. Rapid decrease in amino acid metabolism in prolactin-secreting pituitary adenomas after bromocriptine treatment: a PET study. *J Comput Assist Tomogr* 1987;11:815–819.
162. Derlon J-M, Bourdet C, Bustany P, Chatel M, et al. [11C]L-methionine uptake in gliomas. *Neurosurgery* 1989;25:720–728.
163. Leskinen-Kallio S, Minn H, Joensuu H. PET and [11C]methionine in assessment of response in non-Hodgkin lymphoma. *Lancet* 1990;336:1188.
164. Kubota K, Yamada S, Ishiwata K, Ito M, et al. Positron emission tomography for treatment evaluation and recurrence detection compared to CT in long-term follow-up cases of lung cancer. *Clin Nucl Med* 1992;17:877–881.
165. Huovinen R, Leskinen-Kallio S, Nagren K, Lehikoinen P, et al. Carbon-11-methionine and PET in evaluation of treatment response of breast cancer. *Br J Cancer* 1993;67:787–91.
166. Wilson CBJH, Lammertsma AA, McKenzie CG, Sikora K, et al. Measurements of blood flow and exchanging water space in breast tumors using positron emission tomography: A rapid and noninvasive dynamic method. *Cancer Res* 1992;52:1592–1597.
167. Dahlbom M, Hoffman EJ, Hoh CK, Schiepers C, et al. Whole-body positron emission tomography: Part I. Methods and performance characteristics. *J Nucl Med* 1992;33:1191–1199.
168. Wahl RL, Henry CA, Ethier SP. Serum glucose: effects on tumor and normal tissue accumulation of 2-[F-18]-fluoro-2-deoxy-D-glucose in rodents with mammary carcinoma. *Radiology* 1992;183:643–647.

169. Lindholm P, Minn H, Leskinen-Kallio S, Bergman J, et al. Influence of the blood glucose concentration on FDG uptake in cancer: a PET study. *J Nucl Med* 1993;34:1–6.
170. Langen K-J, Braun U, Rota Kops E, Herzog H, et al. The influence of plasma glucose levels on fluorine-18-fluorodeoxyglucose uptake in bronchial carcinomas. *J Nucl Med* 1993;34:355–359.
171. Warburg O. On the origin of cancer cells. *Science* 1956;123:309–314.
172. Weber G. Enzymology of cancer cells. *N Engl J Med* 1977;296:541–551.
173. DiChiro G, DeLaPaz RL, Brooks RA, Sokoloff L, et al. Glucose utilization of cerebral gliomas measured by [18F]fluorodeoxyglucose and positron emission tomography. *Neurology* 1982;32:1323–1329.
174. Patronas NJ, DiChiro GD, Kufta C, Bairamian D, et al. Prediction of survival in glioma patients by means of positron emission tomography. *J Neurosurg* 1985;62:816–822.
175. Leskinen-Kallio S, Ruotsalainen U, Nagren K, Teras M, et al. Uptake of carbon-11-methionine and fluorodeoxyglucose in non-Hodgkin's lymphoma: a PET study. *J Nucl Med* 1991;32:1211–1218.
176. Haberkorn U, Strauss LG, Reisser CH, Haag D, et al. Glucose uptake, perfusion, and cell proliferation in head and neck tumors: relation of positron emission tomography to flow cytometry. *J Nucl Med* 1991;32:1548–1555.
177. Higashi K, Clavo AC, Wahl RL. Does FDG uptake measure proliferative activity of human cancer cells? In vitro comparison with DNA flow cytometry and tritiated thymidine uptake. *J Nucl Med* 1993;34:414–19.
178. Lindholm P, Leskinen-Kallio S, Kirvela O, Nagren K, et al. Head and neck cancer: Effect of food ingestion on uptake of C-11 methionine. *Radiology* 1994;190:863–867.
179. Mintun WA, Welch MJ, Siegel BA, Mathias CJ, et al. Breast cancer: PET imaging of estrogen receptors. *Radiology* 1988;169:45–48.
180. Holtoff VA, Herholz K, Berthold F, Widemann B, et al. In vivo metabolism of childhood posterior fossa tumors and primitive neuroectodermal tumors before and after treatment. *Cancer* 1993;72:1394–1403.
181. Holzer T, Herhold K, Jeske J, Heiss W-D. FDG-PET as a prognostic indicator in radiochemotherapy of glioblastoma. *J Comp Assist Tomogr* 1993;17:681–687.
182. Wahl RL, Zasadny K, Helvie M, Hutchins GD, et al. Metabolic monitoring of breast cancer chemohormonotherapy using positron emission tomography: Initial evaluation. *J Clin Oncology* 1993;11:2101–2111.
183. Kubota K, Yamada S, Ishiwata K, Ito M, et al. Evaluation of the treatment response of lung cancer with positron emission tomography and I-[methyl-11C]methionine; a preliminary study. *Eur J Nucl Med* 1993;20:495–501.
184. Hoekstra OS, Ossenkoppele GJ, Golding R, van Lingen A, et al. Early treatment response in malignant lymphoma, as determined by planar fluorine-18-fluorodeoxyglucose scintigraphy. *J Nucl Med* 1993;34:1706–1710.
185. Tse N, Hoh C, Hawkins R, Phelps M, et al. Positron emission tomography of pulmonary metastases in osteogenic sarcoma. *Am J Clin Oncol* 1994;17:22–25.
186. Britton KE, Buraggi GL, Bares R, Bichof-Delaloye A, et al. A brief guide to the practice of radioimmunoscintigraphy and radioimmunotherapy in cancer. *Int J Biol Markers* 1989; 4:106–18.
187. Dillman RO, Beauregard JC, Halpern SE, Clutter M. Toxicities and side effects associated with intravenous infusions of murine monoclonal antibodies. *J Biol Resp Mod* 1986; 5:73–84.
188. Carrasquillo JA, Bunn PA, Keenan AM, Reynolds JC, et al. Radioimmunodetection of cutaneous T-cell lymphoma with In-111 T101 monoclonal antibody. *N Engl J Med* 1986; 315:673–680.
189. Delaloye B, Bischof-Delaloye A, Buchegger F, von Fliedner V, et al. Detection of colorectal carcinoma by emission-computerized tomography after injection of ^{123}I-labeled Fab or F(ab$'$)$_2$ fragments from monoclonal anti-carcinoembryonic antigen antibodies. *J Clin Invest* 1986;77:301–311.
190. Pelizzari CA, Chen GTY, Spelbring DR, Weichselbaum RR, et al. Accurate three-dimensional registration of CT, PET, and/or MR images of the brain. *J Comput Assist Tomogr* 1989;13:20–6.
191. Kramer ES, Noz ME. CT-SPECT fusion for analysis of radiolabeled antibodies: applications in gastrointestinal and lung carcinoma. *Int J Radiat Appl Instru* [B] 1991;18:27–42.
192. Scott AM, Divgi CR, McDermott K, et al. Comparative radiolocalization of monoclonal antibodies (MAB) B72.3 and CC49 in patients with colorectal cancer. *Antibody Immunoconjugates Radiopharm* 1992;5:332.
193. Yokota T, Milenic DE, Whitlow M, Schlom J. Rapid tumor penetration of a single-chain Fv and comparison with other immunoglobulin forms. *Cancer Res* 1992;52:3402–3408.
194. Yokota T, Milenic DE, Whitlow M, Wood JF, et al. Microautoradiographic analysis of the normal organ distribution of radioiodinated single-chain Fv and other immunoglobulin forms. *Cancer Res* 1993;53:3776–3783.
195. Reynolds JC, Del Vecchio S, Sakahara H, Lora ME, Carrasquillo JA, Neumann RD, Larson SM. Anti-murine antibody response to mouse monoclonal antibodies: clinical findings and implications. *Nucl Med Biol* 1989;16:121–125.
196. Winter G, Milstein C. Man-made antibodies. *Nature* 1991;349:293–299.
197. LoBuglio AF, Wheeler RH, Trang J, et al. Mouse/human chimeric monoclonal antibody in man: kinetics and immune response. *Proc Natl Acad Sci USA* 1989;86:4220–4.
198. Milenic DE, Yokota T, Fipula DR, Finkelman MAJ, et al. Construction, binding properties, metabolism, and tumor targeting of a single-chain Fv derived from the pancarcinoma monoclonal antibody CC49. *Cancer Res* 1991;51: 6363–6371.
199. Adams GP, McCartney JE, Tai M-S, Oppermann H, et al. Highly specific in vivo tumor targeting by monovalent and divalent forms of 741F8 anti-c-*erb*B-2 single-chain Fv. *Cancer Res* 1993;53:4026–4034.
200. Colcher D, Bird R, Roselli M, Hardman KD, et al. In vivo tumor targeting of a recombinant single-chain antigen-binding protein. *J Natl Cancer Inst* 1990;82:1191–1197.
201. Haspel MV, McCabe RP, Pomato N, et al. Generation of tumor cell-reactive human monoclonal antibodies using peripheral blood lymphocytes from actively immunized colorectal carcinoma patients. *Cancer Res* 1985;45:3951–3961.
202. Steis GS, Carrasquillo JA, McCabe R, Bookman M, et al. An evaluation of the toxicity, immunogenicity, and tumor radioimmunodetection of two human monoclonal antibodies, 18.88 and 28A32, in patients with metastatic colorectal carcinoma. *J Clin Oncol* 1990;8:476–90.
203. De Jager R, Abdel-Nabi H, Serafini A, Pecking A, et al. Current status of cancer immunodetection with radiolabeled human monoclonal antibodies. *Semin Nucl Med* 1993; 23:165–79.
204. Paganelli G, Magnani P, Zito F, Villa E, et al. Three-step monoclonal antibody tumor targeting in carcinoembryonic antigen-positive patients. *Cancer Res* 1991;51:5960–5966.
205. Paganelli G, Malcovati M, Fazio F. Monoclonal antibody pretargetting techniques for tumour localization: the avidin-biotin system. *Nucl Med Commun* 1991;12:211–234.

206. Stickney DR, Anderson LD, Slater JB, Ahlem CN, et al. Bifunctional antibody: a binary radiopharmaceutical delivery system for imaging colorectal carcinoma. *Cancer Res* 1991;51:6650–5.
207. Goodwin DA. Pharmacokinetics and antibodies. *J Nucl Med* 1987;28:1358–1362.
208. Dykes PW, Bradwell AR, Chapman CE, Vaughan TM. Radioimmunotherapy of cancer: clinical studies and limiting factors. *Cancer Treatm Rev* 1987;14:87–106.
209. Sfakianakis GN, Garty II, Serafini AN. Radioantibodies for the diagnosis and treatment of cancer, radioimmunoimaging (RAI) and (RAT). *Cancer Invest* 1990;8:381–405.
210. Gold P, Freedman SE. Demonstration of tumor specific antigen in human colonic carcinomata by immunological tolerance and absorption techniques. *J Exp Med* 1965; 121:439.
211. Goldenberg DM, DeLand F, Kim E, et al. Use of radiolabeled antibodies to carcinoembryonic antigen in the detection and localization of diverse cancers by external photoscanning. *N Engl J Med* 1978;298:1384–8.
212. Goldenberg DM, Goldenberg H, Sharkey RM, et al. Clinical studies of cancer radioimmunodetection with carcinoembryonic antigen monoclonal antibody fragments labeled with 123I or 99mTc. *Cancer Res* 1990;50:909–21.
213. Lind P, Lechner P, Eber O, et al. A prospective study of CEA immunoscintigraphy with a Tc-99m-labeled antibody fragment (IMMU-4 Fab′) in colorectal cancer patients. *J Nucl Med* 1991;32:1051.
214. Pinsky CM, Sasso NL, Mojsiack JZ, et al. Results of a multicenter phase III clinical trial of ImmuRAID-CEA-Tc99m imaging in patients with colorectal cancer. *Proc Am Soc Clin Oncol* 1991;10:136.
215. Baum RP, Hertel A, Lorenz M, et al. 99Tcm-labelled anti-CEA monoclonal antibody for tumour immunoscintigraphy: first clinical results. *Nucl Med Commun* 1989;10:345–52.
216. Hertel A, Baum RP, Lorenz M, et al. Immunoscintigraphy using a technetium-99m labelled monoclonal anti-CEA antibody in the follow-up of colorectal cancer and other tumors producing CEA. *Br J Cancer* 1990;72:34–6.
217. Muxi A, Sola M, Bassa P, et al. Radioimmunoscintigraphy of colorectal carcinoma with a 99Tcm-labelled anti-CEA monoclonal antibody (BW 431/26). *Nucl Med Commun* 1992; 13:261–70.
218. Kairemo KJA. Immunolyphoscintigraphy with 99mTc-labeled monoclonal antibody (BW 431/26) reacting with carcinoembryonic antigen in breast cancer. *Cancer Res* 1990; 50:949s–954s.
219. Lind P, Lechner P, Arian-Schad K, et al. Anti-carcinoembryonic antigen immunoscintigraphy (technetium-99m-monoclonal antibody BW 431/26) and serum CEA levels in patients with suspected primary and recurrent colorectal carcinoma. *J Nucl Med* 1991;32:1319–25.
220. Gasparini M, Crippa F, Regalia E, et al. Role of immunoscintigraphy in local recurrences of colorectal carcinoma: comparison with other diagnostic methods, in: Schmidt H, Buraggi GL (eds): *Nuclear Medicine*. Stuttgart, Schattauer Verlag, 1989, p 519–22.
221. McEwan AJB, MacLean GD, Hooper HR, et al. Mab 170H.82: an evaluation of a novel panadenocarcinoma monoclonal antibody labelled with 99Tcm and with 111In. *Nucl Med Commun* 1992;13:11–19.
222. Haseman MK, Brown DW, Keeling CA, Reed NL. Radioimmunodetection of occult carcinoembryonic antigen-producing cancer. *J Nucl Med* 1992;33:1750–6.
223. Doerr RJ, Abdel-Nabi H, Merchant B. Indium 111 ZCE-025 imunoscintigraphy in occult recurrent colorectal cancer with elevated carcinoembryonic antigen level. *Arch Surg* 1990; 125:226–9.
224. Stramignoni D, Bowen R, Atkinson B, Schlom J. Differential reactivity of monoclonal antibodies with human colon adenocarcinomas and adenomas. *Int J Cancer* 1983;35: 543–552.
225. Thor A, Gortein F, Ohuchi N, Szpak CA, et al. Tumor associated glycoprotein (TAG-72) in ovarian carcinomas defined by monoclonal antibody B72.3. *J Natl Cancer Inst* 1986; 76:995–1003.
226. Application of immunoscintigraphic technology, in Maguire RT, van Nostrand D (eds): *Diagnosis of Colorectal and Ovarian Carcinoma*. New York, Marcel Dekker 1992.
227. Colcher D, Esteban JM, Carrasquillo JA, Sugarbaker P, et al. Quantitative analyses of selective radiolabeled monoclonal antibody localization in metastatic lesions of colorectal cancer patients. *Cancer Res* 1987;47:1185–1189.
228. Yokoyama K, Carrasquillo JA, Chang AE, Colcher D, et al. Differences in biodistribution of Indium-111 and Iodine-131 B72.3 monoclonal antibody in patients with colorectal cancer. *J Nucl Med* 1989;30:320–327.
229. Carrasquillo JA, Mulligan T, Chung Y, Milenic D, et al. Pharmacokinetics and biodistribution of intravenous Lu-177 CC49 murine monoclonal antibody (Mab) in patients with metastatic adenocarcinoma. *J Nucl Med* 1994;35:100P.
230. Rodwell JD, Alvarez VL, Lee C, Lopes AD, et al. Site-specific covalent modification of monoclonal antibodies: in vitro and in vivo evaluation. *Proc Natl Acad Sci USA* 1986;83:2632–6.
231. Doerr RJ, Abdel-Nabi H, Krag D, Mitchell E. Radiolabeled antibody imaging in the management of colorectal cancer: results of a multicenter clinical study. *Ann Surg* 1991; 214:118–24.
232. Surwit EA, Krag DN, Katterhagen JG, Gallion HH, et al. Clinical assessment of 111In-CYT-103 immunoscintigraphy in ovarian cancer. *Gynecol Oncol* 1993;43:285–92.
233. Muraro R, Kuroki M, Wunderlich D, Poole DJ, et al. Generation and characterization of B72.3 second generation monoclonal antibodies reactive with the tumor-associated glycoprotein 72 antigen. *Cancer Res* 1988;48:4588–4596.
234. Colcher D, Minelli MF, Roselli M, Muraro R, et al. Radioimmunolocalization of human carcinoma xenografts with B72.3 second generation monoclonal antibodies. *Cancer Res* 1988;48:4597–4603.
235. Kostakoglu L, Divgi CR, Holton S, Cordon-Cardo C, et al. Preselection of patients with high TAG-72 antigen expression leads to targeting of 94% of known metastatic tumor sites with monoclonal antibody I-131-CC49. *Cancer Invest* 1994;12:551–8.
236. Murray JL, Macey DJ, Kasi LP, et al. Phase II radioimmunotherapy trial with 131I-CC49 in colorectal cancer. *Cancer* 1994;73:1057–66.
237. Kim JA, Triozzi PL, Martin Jr EW. Radioimmunoguided surgery for colorectal cancer. *Oncol* 1993;7(2):55–64.
238. Cohen AM, Martin EW Jr, Lavery I, Daly J, et al. Radioimmunoguided surgery using iodine 125 B72.3 in patients with colorectal cancer. *Arch Surg* 1991;126(3):349–352.
239. Arnold MA, Schneebaum S, Berens A, et al. Intraoperative detection of colorectal cancer with radioimmunoguided surgery and CC49, a second-generation monoclonal antibody. *Ann Surg* 1992;216:11–16.
240. Curtet C, Vuillez JP, Daniel G, Aillet G, et al. Feasibility study of radioimmunoguided surgery of colorectal carcinomas using indium-111 CEA-specific monoclonal antibody. *Eur J Nucl Med* 1990;17:299–304.
242. Neal CE, Swenson LC, Fanning J, Texter JH. Monoclonal

antibodies in ovarian and prostate cancer. *Semin Nucl Med* 1993;23:114–26.

243. Texter JH Jr, Neal CE. Current applications of immunoscintigraphy in prostate cancer. *J Nucl Med* 1993;34:549–53.
244. Balm AJ, Hageman PC, Mulder CL, Hilkens J. Carcinoma-associated monoclonal antibodies in head and neck carcinoma. Immunohistochemistry and biodistribution of monoclonal antibodies 175F4 and 175F11. *Eur Arch Otorhinolaryngol* 1992;249:237–42.

37 Special Problems in Pediatric Nuclear Medicine

Mary P. Andrich

Nuclear medicine imaging techniques have been adapted for use in pediatric patients since the mid-1960s. The majority of these early studies were done in children with cancer. Subsequently, pediatric applications of nuclear medicine have been expanded to include a wide variety of procedures. At the present time, the majority of children who are studied have benign conditions. These studies are safe, relatively noninvasive, usually do not require special preparation, and are tolerated well by patients. The radiation absorbed dose is usually the same or lower than that of comparable radiographic procedures. Nuclear medicine plays an important role in the diagnostic evaluation and therapeutic management of many pediatric problems.

SPECIAL CONSIDERATIONS

Unless children are seen on a regular basis in the nuclear medicine clinic, their evaluation may require some additional preparation. It is crucial that staff have an interest in this area and are patient in dealing with the behavior of young children. When necessary, the use of an appropriate sedative will facilitate obtaining a high-quality study that provides clinically useful information. Chloral hydrate (50 to 80 mg/kg; maximum dose 1.7 g) is the first choice for sedation, because it causes relatively little respiratory depression. In rare cases where chloral hydrate is not effective, the patient's physician should choose the sedative, taking into account the child's condition and current medications.

To ensure patients remain stationary during imaging, it may be necessary to use a restraint device, such as a "papoose" board with velcro straps that wrap across the body. In some cases, it may be difficult to adequately monitor vital signs of a child who is lying beneath a scintillation camera within a darkened room. For this reason, many facilities utilize cardiorespiratory monitors or pulse oximeters. The latter are preferred because they require only one lead attached to the child, and the pulse oximeter can usually be placed on a part of the body outside the field of view. Pulse oximeters work on the principles of optical plethysmography (utilizing absorbed light to recognize the peak and trough of each pulse waveform) and spectrophotometry (performing quantitative measurements of light absorption on reduced and oxidized hemoglobin). Hemoglobin and oxyhemoglobin absorption are measured at the peak and trough of the pulse amplitude. At the trough, there is arterial, capillary, and venous blood present, and at the peak there is additional arterial blood. Arterial oxygen concentration can be determined from differences in absorption at peak and trough.[1] Proper monitoring is essential for infants and small children, as well as for older children who are sick, especially if respiratory function is compromised.

Infants and toddlers may have a high amount of activity in the bladder that obscures the view of the pelvis during bone imaging. A small feeding tube or Foley catheter may be inserted into the bladder under aseptic conditions, by staff who are experienced in performing this procedure. The tube is then connected to a drainage system for the remainder of the study. Before placing the catheter, the referring physician should be consulted to make certain there are no contraindications to catheterization.

Parents should be allowed to remain with their children throughout the study to lend support. A possible exception to this is at the time of injection of the radiopharmaceutical, when the parent may be encouraged to leave for a brief period. The proper dose for the child's weight must be selected, with attention to the minimum recommended dose for adequate imaging. See Table 1 for suggested doses of some commonly used radiopharmaceuticals.

SKELETAL SCINTIGRAPHY

The normal scintigraphic appearance of the skeleton changes throughout childhood, up to the adult years. Proper interpretation of studies requires a familiarity with normal findings. Bone scintigraphy is performed with ^{99m}Tc-methylene diphosphonate (MDP). Figures 1–4 demonstrate the anatomic appearance of MDP bone images from children ages 1, 4, 10, and 15 years, respectively, using a dual-headed camera. Normal physiological activity is seen in the growth plates. Pinhole images may be helpful in evaluating abnormal areas close to or including the growth plates, and are especially useful in examinations of the hips.

Table 1. Pediatric Radiopharmaceutical Dosages*

TYPE OF STUDY	RADIOPHARMACEUTICAL	DOSE average (μCi/kg)	min mCi	max mCi
Bone	^{99m}Tc-methylene diphosphonate (MDP)	250	2	20
Brain	^{99m}Tc-pertechnetate	250	2	20
	^{99m}Tc-hexametazime (HMPAO)	250	2	20
Cisternogram	^{111}In-DTPA	15	0.2	0.5
Cystogram	^{99m}Tc-pertechnetate		0.5	1
Gallium	^{67}Gallium citrate			
infection/inflammation		50	0.5	5
tumor		100	1	8
Gastroesophageal reflux	^{99m}Tc-sulfur colloid	5 μCi/mL		1
Hepatobiliary	^{99m}Tc-iminodiacetic acid (IDA)	50	1	5
Liver-spleen	^{99m}Tc-sulfur colloid	50	0.5	5
Lung perfusion	^{99m}Tc-macroaggregated albumin (MAA)	50	0.3	4
Meckel's	^{99m}Tc-pertechnetate	50	0.3	3
MIBG	^{123}I or ^{131}I-metaiodo-benzylguanidine (MIBG)	25		1
MUGA	pyrophosphate + ^{99m}Tc-pertechnetate	250	2	20
Renal:				
GFR	^{99m}Tc-diethylenetriamine-pentacetic acid (DTPA)		0.2	0.5
Renogram	^{99m}Tc-DTPA	100	1	5
	^{99m}Tc-mercaptoacetyl-triglycine (MAG3)	50	1	3
Renal cortical scintigraphy	^{99m}Tc-dimercaptosuccinic acid (DMSA)	0.05	0.5	3
Renogram/cortical scintigraphy	^{99m}Tc-glucoheptonate (GHA)	0.15	1.5	6
Shunt (*Qp/Qs*)	^{99m}Tc-DTPA	250	2	15
Testicular	^{99m}Tc-pertechnetate	250	2	15
Thallium				
Cardiac/tumor	^{201}Tl-chloride	30	0.3	2
Thyroid	^{99m}Tc-pertechnetate	150	0.5	5
	^{123}I-sodium iodide	5	0.05	0.2

*Dosages courtesy of Massoud Majd, M.D., Department of Diagnostic Imaging, Children's National Medical Center, Washington, D.C.

Osteomyelitis

Early diagnosis of osteomyelitis and prompt institution of therapy are essential. Radiographs obtained when the patient first exhibits symptoms may be normal or have nonspecific changes. Bone scintigraphy, on the other hand, can help differentiate between osteomyelitis, septic arthritis, and cellulitis early in the course of the disease. For further discussion of the typical scintigraphic findings of osteomyelitis, see Chapter 33. Occasionally, normal or decreased activity at the site of osteomyelitis is seen on delayed images at the beginning of the infectious process.[2–4] This may be related to temporary occlusion of small blood vessels, decreased blood flow secondary to edema, or packing of the bone marrow with white blood cells. False-negative studies have also been reported in neonates who had concomitant radiographic changes of osteomyelitis.[5,6]

Tumor

Bone scintigraphy cannot differentiate such malignant primary bone tumors as osteosarcoma or Ewing's sarcoma from benign bone lesions, such as fibrous dysplasia or osteoid osteoma, because all may demonstrate increased activity on all 3 phases of scintigraphy. For patients with malignancies such as osteosarcoma, Ewing's sarcoma, or neuroblastoma, bone scintigraphy is a routine part of the initial staging to assess metastatic disease[7,8] (Fig. 5). Bone scintigraphy is also used to follow these patients, both during and after completion of therapy, to assess therapeutic response, and to look for new lesions. Bone scintigraphy is also helpful in the initial staging and follow-up of children who have other tumors that metastasize to bone, such as rhabdomyosarcoma.

Such benign bone tumors as osteoid osteoma are also identified by scintigraphy. About 10% of osteoid osteomas are in the spine, and these lesions may not be visible on plain films.[9] In addition to localizing the osteoid osteoma, bone scintigraphy can be used intraoperatively to determine if all of the tumor has been removed. Bone scintigraphy is also a useful imaging modality in patients with fibrous dysplasia to assess the number and extent of lesions and to chart progression of disease. Patients with McCune-Albright syndrome (polyostotic fibrous dysplasia, precocious puberty, and cafe-au-lait spots) can be studied with bone scintigraphy[10,11] (Fig. 6).

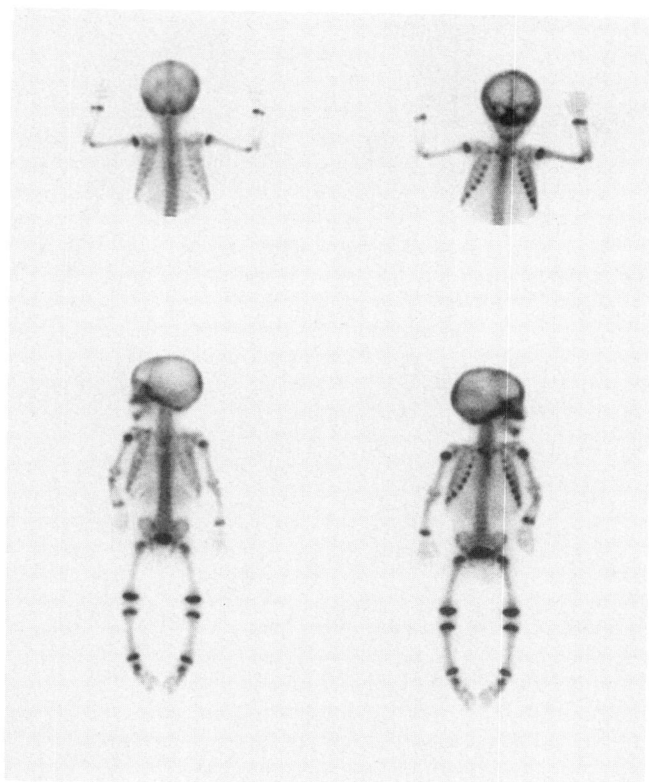

Figure 1. Normal bone scintigraphy, one-year-old child.

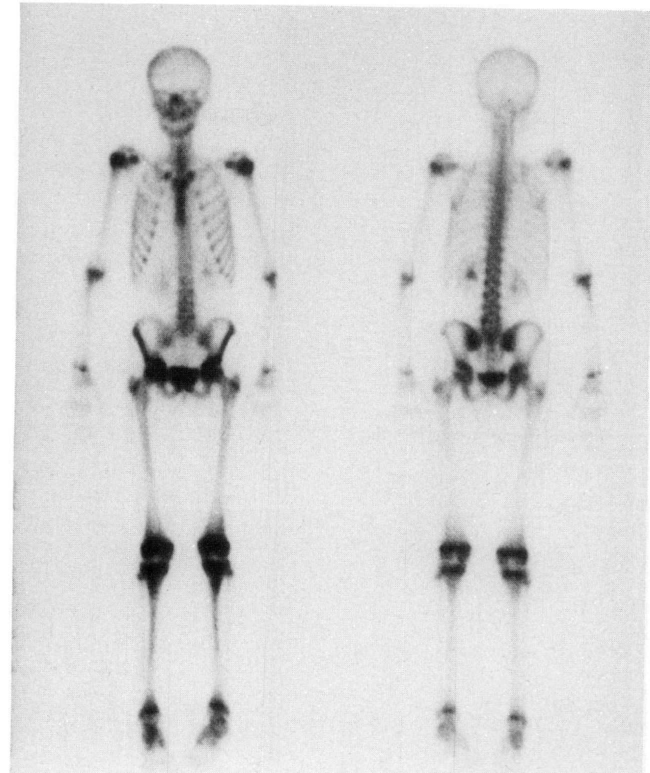

Figure 3. Normal bone scintigraphy, ten-year-old child.

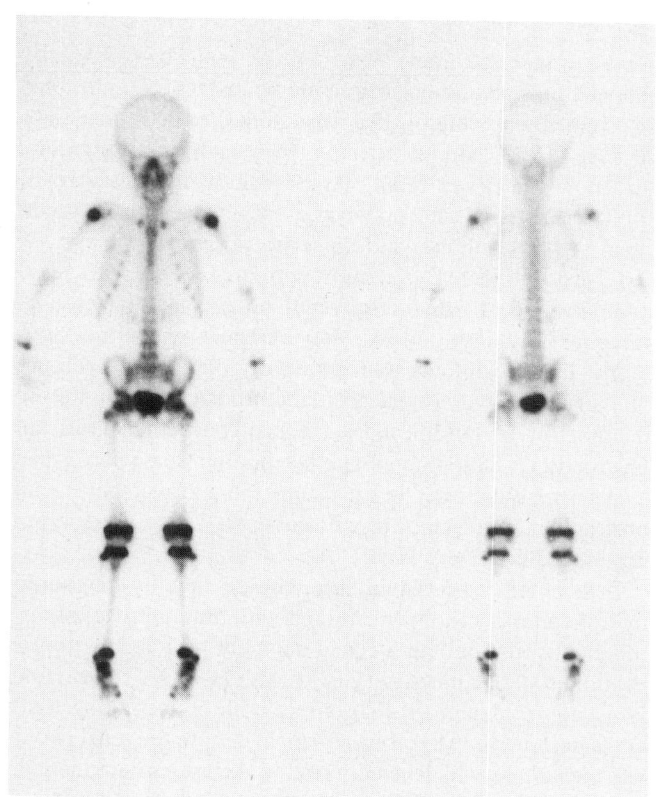

Figure 2. Normal bone scintigraphy, four-year-old child.

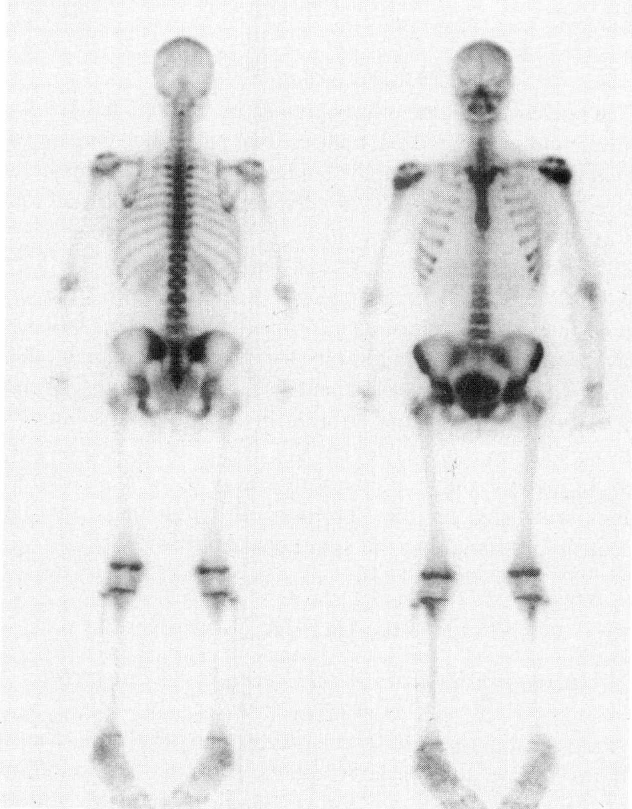

Figure 4. Normal bone scintigraphy, fifteen-year-old female.

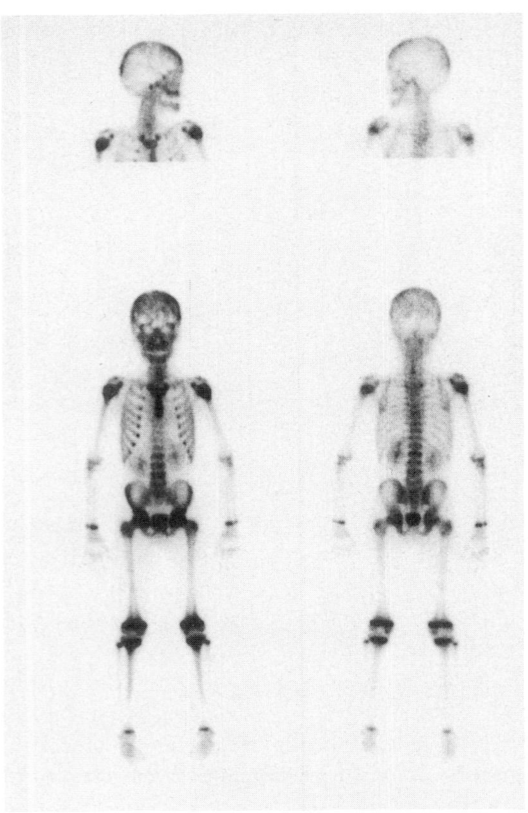

Figure 5. Bone metastases in a 9-year-old child with Stage 4 neuroblastoma.

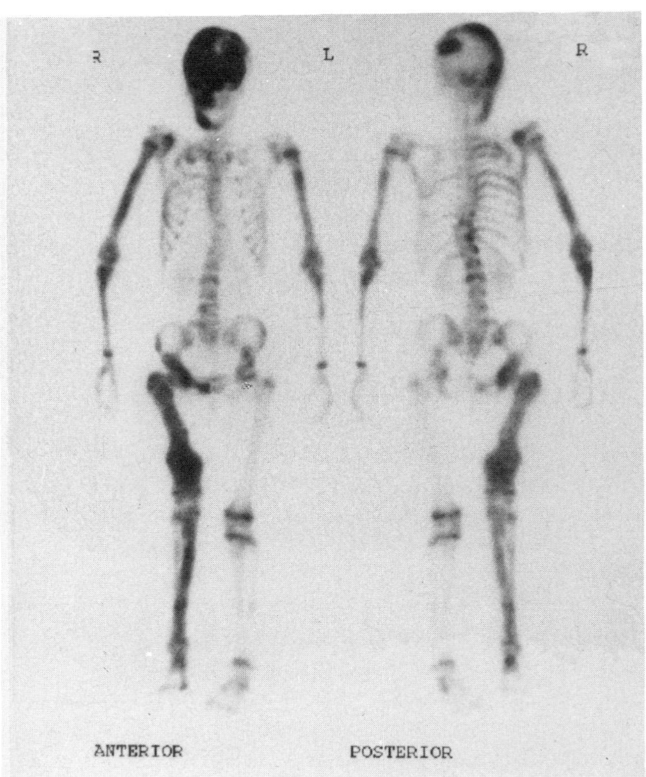

Figure 6. Nine-year-old female child with McCune-Albright syndrome. Bone scintigraphy demonstrating lesions of polyostotic fibrous dysplasia. Deformity and shortening of the right leg secondary to fractures and surgery.

Obscure Skeletal Pain

The nuclear medicine physician may be asked to help evaluate a child with persistent bone or joint pain when the clinical evaluation and radiographic studies are normal or inconclusive. In one series of 358 patients, bone scintigraphy demonstrated evidence of trauma in 12%, inflammatory disease in 20%, neoplasia in 3%, and Legg-Perthes disease in 1%. One half of those with inflammatory disease required therapy with intravenous antibiotics for osteomyelitis, septic arthritis, or sacroiliitis. Scintigraphy was normal for 64% of children with no significant skeletal disease on follow-up, except for juvenile rheumatoid arthritis in 10% of this group. Although scintigraphy is not helpful in confirming the diagnosis of juvenile rheumatoid arthritis early in the disease, findings may suggest the presence of malignancy, such as leukemia, mimicking the symptoms of arthritis.[12]

GENITOURINARY SCINTIGRAPHY

Abdominal Mass in the Neonate—Congenital Hydronephrosis

Abdominal masses are found in approximately 0.5% of newborns.[13–15] Because of the relatively decreased tone and bulk of the anterior abdominal musculature in neonates and infants compared to older children, masses may be more easily palpated. Of abdominal masses in neonates, 65% are renal in origin. The remaining 35% arise from sites in the intestines or liver (15%), adrenal glands (10%), and female genitalia (10%).[16,17] Causes of renal masses include: hydronephrosis, multicystic dysplasia, polycystic kidneys, ectopia, tumor, renal vein thrombosis, and horseshoe kidney.[18–20]

Hydronephrosis is the most common congenital renal anomaly and is often discovered on prenatal ultrasound. Imaging should not consist solely of repeat renal ultrasonography, because infants with prenatally diagnosed hydronephrosis may have normal postnatal ultrasonography during the first few days of life and subsequently develop significant obstruction.[21] Diuretic renography should also be performed to determine the relative renal function and whether or not obstruction is present. For a discussion of diuretic renography, see Chapter 30.

In one series of 134 infants with antenatally diagnosed hydronephrosis who were studied with diuretic renography, the most commonly associated anomaly was obstruction at the ureteropelvic junction (UPJ).[22] Although UPJ obstruction is usually unilateral, it may affect both collecting systems and can result in marked enlargement of both the renal pelvis and the kidney, which usually retains at least partial function. Surgical correction of obstruction may not result in improved function.[23] The diagnosis of UPJ obstruction remains a topic of debate; it can be defined retrospectively, when there is deterioration of function in an untreated hydronephrotic kidney. However, predicting which kidneys are at risk for loss of function is not always possible on the basis of a single diuretic renogram.[22,23] Serial diuretic renograms and renal ultrasound examinations, along with careful clinical follow-up, are required to evaluate renal function and urine flow as the urinary tract system develops.

Urinary Tract Infection

It has been estimated that 3 to 4% of girls and 1% of boys will have a symptomatic urinary tract infection (UTI) during the first decade of life.[24–26] All pediatric patients with a first UTI should be evaluated for vesicoureteral reflux (VUR), the most common anomaly of the urinary tract seen in childhood. Approximately one third of children with symptomatic UTI will have VUR, compared to less than 1% in the general population.[27–30] VUR is usually managed conservatively, because reflux tends to resolve spontaneously in one third of cases with each year of follow-up.[31]

To evaluate patients for VUR, there are 2 different methods of performing cystography—the isotope cystogram (IC), either direct or indirect, and the voiding cystourethrogram (VCUG). The VCUG is graded according to the International Study Classification, where Grade I is reflux into the ureter only; II involves the ureter, pelvis, and calices, without dilatation and with normal caliceal fornices; III has mild or moderate dilatation and/or tortuosity of the ureter and mild or moderate dilatation of the renal pelvis, but no, or slight, blunting of fornices; IV shows moderate dilatation and/or tortuosity of the ureter and moderate dilatation of the renal pelvis and calices, with complete obliteration of the sharp angle of the fornices but maintenance of papillary impressions in the majority of calices; and V has gross dilatation and tortuosity of the ureter.[32] Comparing the VCUG with the IC, Grade I would represent mild reflux, Grades II and III moderate, and Grades IV and V severe VUR.

For direct IC, ^{99m}Tc-pertechnetate and saline are infused into the bladder through a catheter. The bladder is filled with saline to a volume of:

$$\text{total volume (in mL)} = (\text{age in years} + 2) \times 30$$

Images are obtained in the posterior projection with the patient in the supine position. When the bladder is full, imaging continues while the patient voids, either lying on the table or sitting on a bedpan (Fig. 7).

The indirect IC is an alternative technique, but is not widely used because of frequent false-negative results. After intravenous injection of the radiopharmaceutical, usually ^{99m}Tc-DTPA, the patient is imaged until the bladder has filled and the collecting system has emptied. At this point, the patient is instructed to void and further images are obtained. This method has limited clinical utility for several reasons. The patient must have good bladder control, both to keep from voiding while the bladder fills and then to void on command. Furthermore, reflux is only identified during the voiding phase, and the radiation dose is higher than with the IC. In general, the rate of false-negative studies is high.[33] However, one group has found that compared to direct IC the indirect study has a sensitivity of 74% and a specificity of 91% compared to VCUG.[34]

IC is recommended as the first study in girls, who have normal physical examinations, because of their extremely low incidence of urethral anomalies.[35] IC is preferred to VCUG whenever possible, because the radiation exposure is much lower for IC, by a factor of 50 to 100.[36,37,38] VCUG is the first study for boys and for girls with other genitourinary anomalies, to evaluate abnormalities of the urethra. All follow-up studies should utilize the IC, again because of the much lower radiation absorbed dose. In addition, screening examinations for VUR in children with functional bladder disorders (eg, neurogenic bladder secondary to myelomeningocele) should be done with IC rather than VCUG because the nuclear study can yield quantitative information about residual volume, volume of reflux, and bladder volume at the time of reflux.

If fever is associated with the UTI, further diagnostic evaluation is required because neither clinical evaluation nor standard laboratory tests, such as a complete blood count or sedimentation rate, is reliable in identifying renal parenchymal infection in children.[39,40] Renal cortical scintigraphy (RCS) is the current "gold standard" for the diagnosis of pyelonephritis, based on recent animal experiments that have demonstrated a high sensitivity and specificity of DMSA for identifying the renal parenchymal changes of pyelonephritis when correlated with histopathology.[40–43] Studies have shown RCS to be more sensitive and specific than either sonography or intravenous urography in the identification of renal parenchymal infection, because both of these modalities underestimate the degree of involvement, and have high false-negative rates.[39,44–51]

When patients have a febrile UTI, RCS, utilizing either ^{99m}Tc-DMSA or ^{99m}Tc-GHA, should be performed to look for the renal parenchymal changes of pyelonephritis, so that appropriate therapy can be given. Delayed images should be obtained with a pinhole collimator to better evaluate the cortical architecture. Single photon emission tomography (SPECT) images may give additional information.

Although the majority of children with UTI have no anatomic or functional anomalies, there is an association with UTI and obstructive uropathy. Causes of obstruction include posterior urethral valves, UPJ, ureterovesical junction obstruction, and an obstructed upper moiety in a duplicated collecting system. Renal sonography should be used to evaluate the kidneys and ureters for evidence of dilatation of the collecting systems. If hydronephrosis is found, diuretic renography can determine if obstruction is present.

Testicular scintigraphy is discussed in Chapter 30 and in references 52-56.

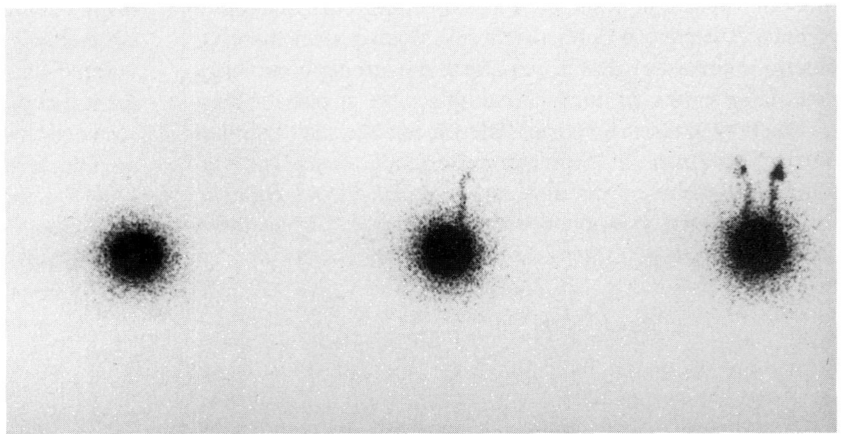

Figure 7. Isotope cystogram demonstrating bilateral vesicoureteral reflux.

HEPATIC SCINTIGRAPHY

Liver-spleen imaging in children is performed with ^{99m}Tc-sulfur colloid, which is taken up by the reticuloendothelial system. Images of the liver and spleen are evaluated for shape, homogeneity of uptake, colloid shift to the spleen, and the size of the liver and spleen. The liver size (vertical length on the anterior projection) is about 5 cm at birth, and increases by approximately 1 cm per year until age 12. The spleen is usually measured in the posterior projection in the longest dimension. A commonly used formula for average spleen size is:

$$\text{Size} = 5.7 + (0.31\ x)$$

where x is the age in years.[59]

With the increasing use of CT and MRI studies, liver-spleen imaging is seldom requested for patients with diffuse or focal disease of the liver and/or spleen. However, it is still helpful in the evaluation of patients with visceroatrial situs abnormalities. The diagnosis of asplenia (right isomerism) or polysplenia (left isomerism) may be aided by the liver-spleen scintigraphy. If, after imaging, the diagnosis of asplenia is still in question, further evaluation with ^{99m}Tc-labeled heat-damaged red blood cells to evaluate functioning splenic tissue may also be done (see Chapter 32). Careful work-up of these infants is indicated because antibiotic prophylaxis is recommended for asplenia syndrome. Severe cyanotic congenital heart lesions may also be associated with asplenia syndrome. Infants with polysplenia syndrome may have abdominal heterotaxia, with partial or complete failure of rotation of the intestinal tract.[58]

Hepatobiliary Scintigraphy—Biliary Atresia

Neonates with cholestasis, defined as a direct bilirubin level over 2.0 mg/dL, may have an underlying hepatic disease. Causes of cholestasis include infections (bacterial, viral, syphilis), metabolic disorders—either inherited (alpha-1-antitrypsin deficiency, cystic fibrosis, galactosemia, tyrosinemia, fructosemia) or acquired (secondary to hemolysis or total parental nutrition), idiopathic disorders (neonatal hepatitis, Byler's disease, Zellweger's syndrome), and biliary tract anomalies. In this last group are disorders involving hypoplasia or paucity of intrahepatic bile ducts (Watson-Alagille syndrome; asyndromic) and extrahepatic biliary atresia.[59] Imaging with ^{99m}Tc-iminodiacetic acid (IDA) analogs can differentiate between these etiologies. It is essential to confirm the diagnosis of biliary atresia early, to insure timely surgical intervention. If a Kasai procedure (hepatic portoenterostomy) is performed within the first 60 days of life, the chance of a successful outcome is nearly 90%. However, if surgery is delayed beyond 90 days, the percentage of those with sustained bile drainage falls to 17%.[60]

Prior to hepatobiliary scintigraphy, the patient should be given phenobarbital to increase hepatic excretion and decrease false-positive studies.[61] IDA compounds are extracted from the blood, excreted into the biliary tract, and then pass from the common bile duct into the bowel. Mebrofenin (trimethyl-bromo-IDA) is frequently chosen because it has the fastest blood clearance. It also demonstrates high hepatic uptake, rapid hepatic excretion, and great resistance to displacement by bilirubin from serum proteins.[62]

In infants less than 3 months of age with biliary atresia, hepatic extraction is usually adequate to visualize the liver well, while patients with neonatal hepatitis often have decreased extraction. With biliary atresia, no excretion into the bowel is seen, even on delayed imaging up to 24 hours. Renal excretion may be increased in cases of hepatocellular disease, intrahepatic cholestasis, or biliary obstruction. Images should be carefully evaluated for activity in the kidneys to differentiate this from bowel activity. Lateral views of the abdomen may be helpful for this purpose. If the hepatobiliary study is equivocal, it should be repeated after 1 to 2 weeks.

CARDIAC SHUNT SCINTIGRAPHY

Left-to-right shunts

One of the most important applications of radionuclide angiocardiography is the detection, localization, and quantification of intracardiac shunts and shunts between the great vessels. During the performance of the study, left-to-right shunts may be recognized by prolonged activity in the lungs and the right side of the heart, along with poor visualization of the left ventricle and aorta. This is caused by the shortened recirculation time of the tracer through the pulmonary system, resulting in a pulmonary blood flow, *Qp*, which is greater than the systemic blood flow, *Qs*.

When the ratio of *Qp/Qs* is greater than 1.4, the level of left-to-right shunting, atrial or ventricular, can usually be detected by analysis of time activity curves. The radiopharmaceutical most commonly used is ^{99m}Tc-DTPA. After the tracer is injected into the right external jugular vein in a rapid bolus, a normal lung time-activity curve demonstrates a single peak. However, if left-to-right shunting is present, recirculation causes a second peak.[63,64] In the most commonly used method to calculate the *Qp/Qs* ratio, a computer program fits the pulmonary time-activity curve with a gamma variate function (Fig. 8). The area, A1, under the computer-generated curve represents a normal first pulmonary transit. The area under the recirculation curve, A2, is also fitted to a gamma variate function.

Comparison with experimental results has shown that the ratio A1/(A1—A2) is a good approximation of the *Qp/Qs* ratio.[65] If the first gamma variate function is assumed to represent the initial passage of tracer, any deviation of the original data from this fitted curve, before sufficient time has passed for the second pulmonary passage of the radioactivity, can be attributed to left-to-right shunting. This deviation is directly related to A2. Therefore, when no shunt exists, *Qp/Qs* is close to 1.0. The results indicate that this method can detect shunts with *Qp/Qs* greater than 1.2, and the correlation with catheterization data is excellent when the ratio is between 1.2 and 3.0.[66,67] Calculations assume that there is no valvular incompetence or large bronchial or intercostal collaterals.

In left-to-right shunts at the atrial level, the images show reappearance of activity in the right atrium, as well as prolonged lung activity. Analysis of time-activity curves shows recirculation in the right atrium preceding the recirculation peak in the right ventricle. In left-to-right shunts at the ventricular level, ventricular recirculation is apparent, whereas atrial recirculation occurs in normal sequence following systemic return. For patients with patent ductus arteriosus, prolonged lung activity is evident without abnormal right atrial or ventricular recirculation.

Right-to-Left Shunts

While the same gamma variate analysis described for left-to-right shunts can theoretically be applied to left ventricular time-activity curves to quantify the degree of right-to-left shunting, there have been few reports on this application. Once the diagnosis of a right-to-left shunt is made, the progress of the cardiac disease is best followed directly by oxygen saturation studies. Another approach to measuring right-to-left shunting involves the use of intravenously injected ^{99m}Tc-macroaggregated albumin (MAA). These particles, measuring more than 10 μm in diameter, are almost completely trapped in the first capillary system they encounter, which is the pulmonary bed in the case of an intravenous injection. Under normal circumstances, between 3 to 10% of intravenously injected particles find their way to the systemic circulation. Any excess over 10% can usually be attributed to right-to-left shunting. If whole body and total lung counts are obtained, the percentage of shunting can be calculated.

$$\%\ \text{shunting} = \frac{(\text{total body counts} - \text{pulmonary counts})}{\text{total body counts}} \times 100$$

When a right-to-left shunt is present, activity in the brain and kidneys should be apparent.

THYROID SCINTIGRAPHY

For the majority of pediatric patients, initial thyroid imaging may be performed with ^{99m}Tc-pertecnetate, which is trapped by the thyroid but not organified. Alternatively, ^{123}I may be used. Diagnostic imaging with ^{131}I is not routinely recommended in children, although the relatively high radiation dose may be useful in the treatment of thyroid carcinoma (see Chapter 40).

Congenital Hypothyroidism

Congenital hypothyroidism is seen in approximately 1 out of 4000 live births.[69,70] The causes, in order of prevalence, include: (1) dysgenesis of the thyroid gland (aplasia, hypoplasia, ectopia); (2) dyshormonogenesis (defects in TSH receptors, iodide trapping, organification, or thyroglobulin, and iodotyrosine deiodinase deficiency), (3) hypothalamic-pituitary hypothyroidism (hypothalamic-pituitary anomaly, panhypopituitarism, and isolated TSH deficiency); (4) transient neonatal hypothyroidism (drug-induced, maternal antibody-induced, and idiopathic).[71] Signs and symptoms of neonatal hypothyroidism include prolonged jaundice, hoarse cry, macroglossia, enlarged posterior fontanelle ($>$1 cm), umbilical hernia, constipation, and failure to thrive.

Prior to the advent of newborn screening programs, most infants had suffered irreversible brain damage by the time the diagnosis of congenital hypothyroidism was made.[72] Currently, the majority of cases are discovered on neonatal screening tests prior to the onset of symptoms. Once the diagnosis is confirmed, treatment with hormone replacement should be initiated immediately to prevent intellectual impairment. Therapy does not need to be delayed for nuclear medicine imaging, because TSH levels will remain elevated for several days after treatment is begun.[73] A pinhole collimator should be utilized to evaluate the area from the mouth down to the sternal notch. If ectopic uptake is identified, a

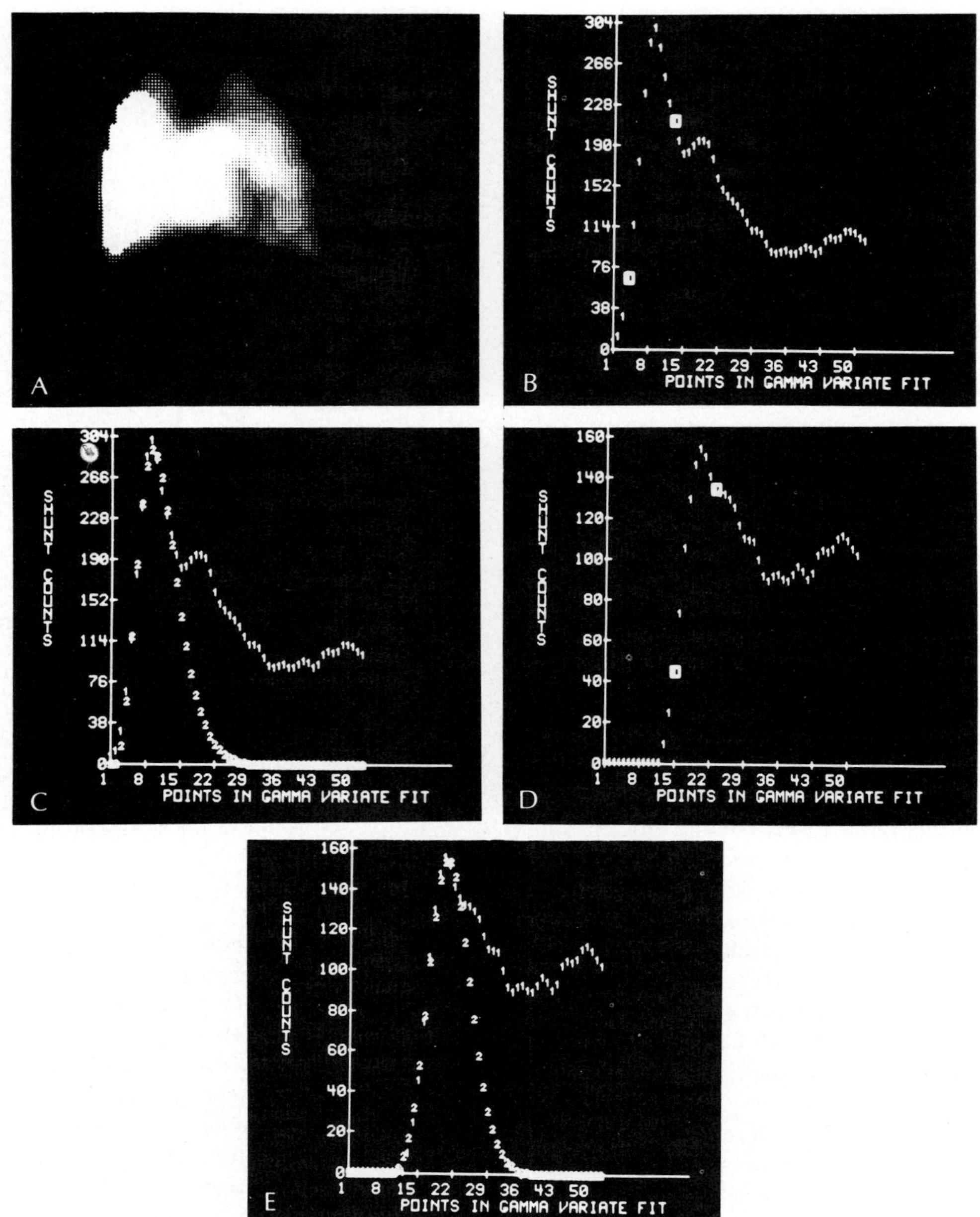

Figure 8. Computer analysis of left-to-right shunting. **(A).** Region of interest over right lung is highlighted over image that represents a composite of all frames. **(B).** Time-activity curve of raw data with computer-selected points at 10% of upslope and 70% of downslope just before recirculation. **(C).** Curve 2 is gamma variate fit of curve 1. **(D).** Computer-generated recirculation curve from raw data. **(E).** Curve 2 is gamma variate fit of recirculation data.

lateral view should also be obtained to aid in localization and help to distinguish normal salivary gland activity.

Of those infants with thyroid dysgenesis, approximately one third will have no thyroid tissue visualized on nuclear scintigraphy.[74] Rudimentary thyroid tissue may be located from the base of the tongue down to the normal position in the neck. Although most children with lingual thyroid glands have no functioning tissue present, approximately 25% will have some thyroid tissue that can respond to elevated serum TSH levels by increasing in size. This may lead to difficulty swallowing or airway obstruction.

Thyroglossal Duct Cyst

During development, the embryonic thyroid gland descends from the base of the tongue, where it is connected to the thyroglossal duct, to its position in the lower cervical region anterior to the trachea. Thyroglossal duct cysts arise from the partial persistence of the embryonic tract between the foramen cecum of the tongue and the pyramidal lobe of the thyroid gland. They are usually located at the level of the hyoid bone. When the tract remains patent, a cystic structure may result. This cyst fills with mucinous secretions, producing swelling in the midline of the anterior neck. Occasionally, draining sinuses may communicate with either the base of the tongue or the skin. Thyroid imaging should be performed prior to surgical removal of the cyst to insure that functioning thyroid tissue is not present in the mass.

Acknowledgments. Figures 1–8 courtesy of Massoud Majd, M.D., Department of Diagnostic Imaging, Children's National Medical Center, Washington, D.C.

REFERENCES

1. Kelleher JF. Pulse Oximetry. *J Clin Monit* 1989;5:37–62.
2. Trackler RT, Miller KE, Sutherland DH, Chadwick DL. Childhood pelvic osteomyelitis presenting as a "cold" lesion on bone scan: Case report. *J Nucl Med* 1976;17:620–622.
3. Russin LD, Staab EV. Unusual bone-scan findings in acute osteomyelitis: Case report. *J Nucl Med* 1976;17:617–619.
4. Murray IPC. Photopenia in skeletal scintigraphy of suspected bone and joint infection. *Clin Nucl Med* 1982;7:13–20.
5. Ash JM, Gilday DL. The futility of bone imaging in neonatal osteomyelitis: Concise communication. *J Nucl Med* 1980; 21:417–420.
6. Bressler EL, Conway JJ, Weiss SC. Neonatal osteomyelitis examined by bone scintigraphy. *Radiology* 1984;152:685–688.
7. Myers PA. Malignant bone tumors in children: osteosarcoma. *Hem/Onc Clin North Am* 1987;1:655–664.
8. Myers PA. Malignant bone tumors in children: Ewing's sarcoma. *Hem/Onc Clin North Am* 1987;1:667–673.
9. Caldicott WJH. Diagnosis of spinal osteoid osteoma. *Radiology* 1967;92:1192–5.
10. Edeburn GF, Mortensson W. Value of bone scan in the McCune-Albright syndrome. *Acta Radiol Diagn* 1986;27: 719–721.
11. Pfeffer S, Molina E, Feuillan P, Simon TR. McCune-Albright syndrome: the patterns of scintigraphic abnormalities. *J Nucl Med* 1990;31:1474–1478.
12. ter Meulen DC, Majd M. Bone scintigraphy in the evaluation of children with obscure skeletal pain. *Pediatrics* 1987; 79:587–592.
13. Museles M, Gaudry CL, Bason WM. Renal anomalies in the newborn found by deep palpation. *Pediatrics* 1971;47:97–100.
14. Perlman M, Williams J. Detection of renal anomalies by abdominal palpation in newborn infants. *Br Med J* 1976;2: 347–349.
15. Sherwood DW, Smith RC, Lemmon RH, Vrabel I. Abnormalities of the genitourinary tract discovered by palpation of the abdomen of the newborn. *Pediatrics* 1956;18:782–789.
16. Anand SK. Clinical evaluation of renal disease, in Taeusch HW, Ballard RA, Avery ME (eds.): *Schaffer and Avery's Diseases of the Newborn*, 6th edition, Philadelphia, WB Saunders Co., 1991, p 848.
17. Wedge JJ, Grosfeld JL, Smith JP. Abdominal masses in the newborn: 63 cases. *J Urol* 1971;106:770–775.
18. Clarke NW, Gough DCS, Cohen SJ. Neonatal urological ultrasound: Diagnostic inaccuracies and pitfalls. *Arch Dis Child* 1989;64:578–580.
19. Kirks DR, Merten DF, Grossman H, Bowie JD. Diagnostic imaging of pediatric abdominal masses: An overview. *Radiol Clin North Am* 1981;19:527–545.
20. Wilson DA. Ultrasound screening for abdominal masses in the neonatal period. *Am J Dis Child* 1982;136:147–151.
21. Dejter SW, Gibbons MD. The fate of infant kidneys with fetal hydronephrosis but initially normal postnatal sonography. *J Urol* 1989;142:661–662.
22. Homsy YL, Saad F, Laberge I, Williot P, Pison C. Transitional hydronephrosis of the newborn and infant. *J Urol* 1990; 144:579–583.
23. Sfakianakis GN. Nuclear medicine in congenital urinary tract anomalies. Nuclear Medicine Annual, 1991;129–192.
24. Kunin CM. The natural history of recurrent bacteriuria in schoolgirls. *N Engl J Med* 1970;282:1443–1448.
25. Randolph MF, Morris KE, Gould EB. The first urinary tract infection in the female infant. Prevalence. recurrence, and prognosis: a 10-year study in private practice. *J Pediatri* 1975; 86:342–348.
26. Winberg J, Andersen HJ, Bergstrom T, Jacobsson B, Larson H, Lincoln K. Epidemiology of symptomatic urinary tract infection in childhood. *Acta Paediatr Scand* (suppl) 1974; 252:2–20.
27. The Newcastle Asymptomatic Bacteriuria Investigation (Cain ARR, Furness JA, Selkon JB, Simpson W, et al.): Asymptomatic bacteriuria in school children in Newcastle-upon-Tyne. *Arch Dis Child* 1975;50:90–102.
28. Strife JL, Bisset GS, Kirks DR, Schlueter FJ, Gelfand MJ, Babcock DS, Han BK. Nuclear cystography and renal sonography: Findings in girls with urinary tract infection. *AJR* 1989;153:115–119.
29. Bisset GS, Strife JL, Dunbar JS. Urography and voiding cystourethrography: findings in girls with urinary tract infection. *AJR* 1987;148:479–482.
30. Ransley PG. Vesicoureteral reflux: continuing surgical dilemma. *Urology* 1978;12:246–255.
31. Skoog SJ, Belman AB, Majd M. A nonsurgical approach to the management of primary vesicoureteral reflux. *J Urol* 1987;138:941–946.
32. Lebowitz RL, Olbing H, Parkkulainen KV, Smellie JM, Tamminen-Mobius TE. International reflux study in children: international system of radiographic grading of vesico-ureteric reflux. *Pediatr Radiol* 1985;105–109.
33. Majd M, Kass EJ, Belman AB. The accuracy of the indirect (intravenous) radionuclide cystogram in children. *J Nucl Med* 1983;24:P23.
34. Gordon I, Peters AM, Morony S. Indirect radionuclide cystography: a sensitive technique for the detection of vesico-ureteral relux. *Pediatr Nephrol* 1990;4:604–606.
35. Bisset GS, Strife JL, Dunbar JS. Urography and voiding cystourethrography: Findings in girls with urinary tract infection. *AJR* 1987;148:479–482.
36. Lerner GR, Fleischmann LE, Perlmutter AD. Reflux nephropathy. *Pediatr Clin North Am* 1987;34:747–770.
37. Willi U, Treves S. Radionuclide voiding cystography. *Urol Radiol* 1983;5:161–173.
38. Conway JJ, King LR, Belman AB, Thorson T. Detection of vesicoureteral reflux with radionuclide cystography. A comparison study with roentenographic cystography. *AJR* 1972;115: 720–727.
39. Majd M, Rushton HG, Jantausch B, Wiedermann BL. Relationship among vesicoureteral reflux, P-fimbriated *Escherichia coli*, and acute pyelonephritis in children with febrile urinary tract infection. *J Pediatr* 1991;119:578–585.
40. Majd M, Rushton HG. Renal cortical scintigraphy in the diagnosis of acute pyelonephritis. *Semin Nucl Med* 1992;22:98–11.
41. Arnold AJ, Brownless SM, Carty HM, Rickwood AMK. Detection of renal scarring by DMSA scanning—an experimental study. *J Pediatr Surg* 1990;25:391–393.
42. Parkhouse HF, Godley ML, Cooper J, Risdon RA, Ransley PG. Renal imaging with 99Tcm-labelled DMSA in the detection of acute pyelonephritis: an experimental study in the pig. *Nucl Med Commun* 1989;10:63–70.
43. Rushton HG, Majd M, Chandra R, Yim D. Evaluation of 99m-technetium-dimercapto-succinic acid renal scans in experimental acute pyelonephritis in piglets. *J Urol* 1988;140:1169–1174.
44. Bjorgvinsson E, Majd M, Eggli KD. Diagnosis of acute pyelo-

nephritis in children: comparison of sonography and 99mTc-DMSA scintigraphy. *AJR* 1991;157:539–543.

45. Farnsworth RH, Rossleigh MA, Leighton DM, Bass SJ, Rosenberg AR. The detection of reflux nephropathy in infants by 99mTechnetium dimercaptosuccinic acid studies. *J Urol* 1991;145:542–546.
46. Conway JJ. The role of scintigraphy in urinary tract infection. *Semin Nuc Med* 1988;18:308–319.
47. Verber IG, Strudley MR, Meller ST. 99mTc dimercaptosuccinic acid (DMSA) scan as first investigation of urinary tract infection. *Arch Dis Child* 1988;63:1320–1325.
48. Monsour M, Azmy AF, MacKenzie JR. Renal scarring secondary to vesicoureteric reflux. Critical assessment and new grading. *Br J Urol* 1987;60:320–324.
49. Sty JR, Wells RG, Starshak RJ, Schroeder BA. Imaging in acute renal infection in children. *AJR* 1987;148:471–477.
50. Stoller ML, Kogan BA. Sensitivity of 99mTechnetium-dimercaptosuccinic acid for the diagnosis of chronic pyelonephritis: Clinical and theoretical considerations. *J Urol* 1986; 135:977–980.
51. Traisman ES, Conway JJ, Traisman HS, Yogev R, Firlit C, Shkolnik A, Weiss S. The localization of urinary tract infection with 99mTc glucoheptonate scintigraphy. *Pediatr Radiol* 1986;16:403.
52. Gelfand MJ, Williams PJ, Rosenkrantz. Pinhole Imaging: Utility in Testicular Imaging in Children. *Clin Nucl Med* 1980;5: 237–240.
53. Chen DCP, Holder LE, Melloul M. Radionuclide scrotal imaging: further experience with 210 patients. Part I: Anatomy, pathophysiology, and methods. *J Nucl Med* 1983;24:735–742.
54. Chen DCP, Holder LE, Melloul M. Radionuclide scrotal imaging: further experience with 210 new patients. Part 2: Results and discussion. *J Nucl Med* 1983;24:841–853.
55. Dunn EK, Macchia RF, Solomon NA. Scintigraphic pattern in missed testicular torsion. *Radiology* 1981;139:175–180.
56. Holland JM, Graham JB, Ignatoff JM. Conservative management of twisted testicular appendages. *J Urol* 1981;125: 213–214.
57. Treves ST. *Pediatric Nuclear Medicine*. New York, Springer-Verlag, 1985, p 131.
58. Tonkin ILD, Allen AK. Visceroatrial situs abnormalities: sonographic computed tomographic appearance. *AJR* 1982; 138:509–515.
59. Rudolph AM, Hoffman JIE, Rudolph CD, Sagan P, (eds): Rudolph's Pediatrics. Appleton & Lange, Norwalk, CT 1991, 1064–5.
60. Kasai M, Suzuki H, Ohashi E, Ohi R, Chiba T, Okamoto A: Technique and results of operative management of biliary atresia. *World J Surg* 1978;2:571–580.
61. Massoud M, Reba RC, Altman RP. Effect of phenobarbital on 99mTc-IDA scintigraphy in the evaluation of neonatal jaundice. *Semin Nucl Med* 1981;XI:194–204.
62. Krishnamurthy S, Krishnamurthy GT. Technetium-99m-iminodiacetic acid organic anions: review of biokinetics and clinical application in hepatology. *Hepatology* 1989;9:139–153.
63. Parker JA, Treves S. Radionuclide detection, localization and quantitation of intracardiac shunts and shunts between the great arteries. *Prog Cardiovasc Dis* 1977;20:121–150.
64. Treves S. Detection and quantitation of cardiovascular shunts with commonly available radionuclides. *Semin Nucl Med* 1980;10:16–26.
65. Maltz DL, Treves S. Quantitative radionuclide angiography: determination of Qp:Qs in children. *Circulation* 1973;47: 1049–1056.
66. Alderson PO, Jost RG, Strauss AW, Boonvisut S, Markham J. Radionuclide angiography: Improved diagnosis and quantitation of left-to-right shunts in children using area ratio techniques. *Circulation* 1975;51:1136–1143.
67. Askenazi J, Ahnberg DS, Korngold E, LaFarge CG, Maltz DL, Treves S. Quantitative radionuclide angiocardiography: Detection and quantitation of left-to-right shunts. *Am J Cardiol* 1976;37:382–387.
68. Beekhuis H, Piers DA. Radiation risk of thyroid scintigraphy in newborns. *Eur J Nucl Med* 1983;8:348–350.
69. Fisher DA. Second International Conference on Neonatal Thyroid Screening: progress report. *J Pediatr* 1983;103:653–654.
70. New England Congenital Hypothyroidism Collaborative (RZ Klein, coordinator): Characteristics of infantile hypothyroidism discovered on neonatal screening. *J Pediatr* 1984; 104:539–544.
71. Polk DH, Fisher DA. Disorders of the thyroid gland, in Taeusch HW, Ballard RA, Avery ME (eds.): *Schaffer and Avery's Diseases of the Newborn*, 6th edition. Philadelphia, WB Saunders Co., 1991, p 958.
72. Jacobsen BB, Brandt NJ. Congenital hypothyroidism in Denmark. *Arch Dis Child* 1981;56:134–136.
73. New England Congenital Hypothyroidism Collaborative: Effects of neonatal screening for hypothyroidism: prevention of mental retardation by treatment before clinical manifestations. *Lancet* 1981;2:1095–1098.
74. Fisher DA, Klein AH. Thyroid development and disorders of thyroid function in the newborn. *N Engl J Med* 1981; 304:702–712.

38 Methods for Evaluating New Tests

Barbara J. McNeil, Carolyn M. Rutter

The rising costs of health care have put increasing pressures on clinicians to be parsimonious in their use of health-care resources. And, although diagnostic medicine is not a large component of total health care costs, *new* technologies are a significant part of new operating expenses in hospitals; capital costs are also high. Both of these factors cause policy makers and administrators to view diagnostic medicine, particularly imaging, as expensive. In addition, increased emphasis on the development of practice guidelines by the American Medical Association, the Agency for Health Care Policy and Research, and private organizations has caused many to look more critically at the contribution of each step in the diagnostic or therapeutic process.

As a result of these pressures, it is increasingly important to know the relative benefits and absolute benefits of new diagnostic tests. These benefits must also be related to their financial costs. In this chapter, we review basic approaches to measure the value of diagnostic tests. There are several textbooks now available that expand on these areas, in particular work by Sox et al.[1] Because of the continued importance of cost considerations, we briefly review approaches to measuring the costs of medical interventions.

GENERAL PRINCIPLES

There are several methods for evaluating diagnostic procedures.[1–4] The following discussion summarizes the 2 methods used most frequently when analyzing radiological and scintigraphic data: the decision matrix and the receiver operating characteristic (ROC) curve.

The Decision Matrix

The decision matrix, shown in Table 1, relates results of a dichotomous diagnostic test (normal or abnormal outcome) to dichotomous clinical or pathological findings, which also have a binary outcome (disease or no disease). Five ratios can be derived from this table and are used to characterize such binary tests:

1. The true-positive (*TP*) ratio is the proportion of positive tests in all patients with disease, $a/(a + b)$, and is the *sensitivity* of the test.
2. The false-positive (*FP*) ratio is the proportion of positive tests in all patients without disease, $c/(c + d)$.
3. The true-negative (*TN*) ratio is the proportion of negative tests in all patients without disease, $d/(c + d)$, and is the *specificity* of the test.
4. The false-negative (*FN*) ratio is the proportion of negative tests in all patients with disease, $b/(a + b)$.
5. The likelihood ratio (*L*) of a test is the ratio of the *TP* ratio to the *FP* ratio:

$$\frac{a}{(a + b)} \times \frac{(c + d)}{c}$$

Because a perfect test correctly identifies all diseased patients without incorrectly including patients without disease, it has a *TP* ratio of 1 and a *FP* ratio of 0. Tests with high likelihood ratios are better discriminators of disease than those with low ones.

All five ratios are independent of the *prevalence* of disease, or the *prior probability* of disease in the study group, $P(D+)$; as such, they characterize the test per se. Another proportion, $(a + d)/(a + b + c + d)$, is frequently used, and is called the *accuracy* of the test; it is the ratio of correct outcomes to all outcomes. Inspection of its formula reveals that, unlike the above 5 ratios, it *is* dependent on the prevalence of disease in the study group.

Although these ratios characterize the test, they alone do not determine the significance of a positive or negative diagnostic test in a particular patient, nor do they indicate the consequences of introducing a screening test with given characteristics into a large asymptomatic patient population. Extended analyses are necessary in both cases. Bayes' theorem is the basis of one of the most common analyses.

Bayes' Theorem

In examining a patient's test result, two questions arise: (1) What is the probability that the patient has disease if the test result is positive? and, (2) What is the probability that the patient is disease-free if the test result is negative? These questions are answered using *Bayes' theorem*, a technique whereby the test ratio characteristics 1 through 5 and the prior probability of disease in the patient population being studied are combined to give posterior probabilities (ie, the answers to the above two questions).[1–4] A major difficulty with this approach is accurate estimation of the prior probability. In general, disease prevalence rates can be applied to a large population but, for a particular patient, other historic, clinical, or laboratory findings may modify such population

Table 1. A General Decision Matrix

TEST RESULTS	DISEASE PRESENT ($D+$)	DISEASE ABSENT ($D-$)	TOTAL
Abnormal (T+)	a	c	$a + c$
Normal (T−)	b	d	$b + d$
Total	$a + b$	$c + d$	$a + b + c + d$
True-positive ratio = (sensitivity)	$\frac{a}{a+b}$		
True-negative ratio = (specificity)	$\frac{d}{c+d}$		

$$\text{Accuracy} = \frac{a + d}{a + b + c + d}$$

Table 2A. A Decision Matrix for a Hypothetic Scintigraphic Staging Test Performed in 500 Patients, 300 of Whom Have Known Metastatic Disease

SCAN RESULTS	METASTATIC DISEASE *Present* ($D+$)	METASTATIC DISEASE *Absent* ($D-$)	TOTAL
Abnormal (T+)	270 ($TP = 0.90$)	30 ($FP = 0.15$)	300
Normal (T−)	30 ($FN = 0.10$)	170 ($TN = 0.85$)	200
Total	300	200	500

Table 2B. A Decision Matrix for a Hypothetic Scintigraphic Staging Test Performed in 500 Patients, 30 of Whom Have Known Metastatic Disease

SCAN RESULTS	METASTATIC DISEASE *Present* ($D+$)	METASTATIC DISEASE *Absent* ($D-$)	TOTAL
Abnormal (T+)	27 ($TP = 0.90$)	70 ($FP = 0.15$)	97
Normal (T−)	3 ($FN = 0.10$)	400 ($TN = 0.85$)	403
Total	30	470	500

rates. Therefore, the possible combinations of such modifiers make estimation of the prior probability extremely difficult.

One approach to this problem is to use factors that have been shown to be related to disease status to estimate patients' prior probability of disease.[5] Based on results from several sources, including the Framingham study on cardiovascular disease, Diamond and Forrester were able to estimate prior probabilities of coronary artery disease with reasonable accuracy using a patient's laboratory results (eg, cholesterol levels), ECG changes, age, sex, etc. Such data made it possible to estimate which patients would most benefit from additional noninvasive tests (eg, thallium studies).

When the patient population used to form the decision matrix has the same prevalence of disease as the larger general population, the posterior probability of disease, given a positive test result of $P(D+|T+)$, can be obtained directly from Table 1. In this case, $P(D+|T+)$ is $a/(a + c)$. Similarly, the probability of no disease given a negative test result , $P(D-|T-)$, is $d/(b + d)$.

The decision matrix, Bayes' theorem, and the influence of the prior probability on posterior probabilities can best be illustrated through a specific example. Consider a hypothetical staging test used to search for metastatic disease in a group of 500 patients, 300 of whom actually have metastatic disease (Table 2A). Assume that the test has a sensitivity of 0.90 and a specificity of 0.85. In this situation, the probability that a patient with an abnormal test actually has disease is 270/300 = 0.90, and that a patient with a normal test actually has no disease is 170/200 = 0.85. In this case, a positive test has changed the probability of disease from 0.60 to 0.90 (a factor of 1.5), and a negative test changes the probability of no disease from 0.40 to 0.85 (a factor of 2.1). This situation might occur in searching for metastatic disease in patients with oat cell carcinoma because, on average, a large percentage of them (here estimated at 60%) actually have distant disease at the time their primary malignancy is discovered.

If this same test is applied to another group of 500 patients, only 30 (6%) of whom have metastatic disease, the decision matrix would change to that depicted in Table 2B. Now, the probability of disease in a patient with an abnormal test is 27/97 = 0.28, and the probability of no disease in a patient with a normal test is 400/403 = 0.99. In this case, a positive test changes the probability of disease from 0.06 to 0.28 (a factor of 4.7), and a negative test changes the probability of no disease from 0.94 to 0.99 (a factor of 1.05). This situation might occur in searching for metastatic disease in patients with early testicular carcinoma, because only a small percentage of them actually have distant (extranodal) metastatic disease.

In the preceding examples, the influence of prior probability on posterior probability was determined by drawing a new decision matrix. The same results could have been obtained using Bayes' theorem in two of its formulations:

$$P(D+|T+) = \frac{TP \cdot P(D+)}{TP \cdot P(D+) + FP \cdot P(D-)} \quad (1)$$

$$P(D-|T-) = \frac{TN \cdot P(D-)}{TN \cdot P(D-) + FN \cdot P(D+)} \quad (2)$$

where $TP = P(T+|D+)$, $FP = P(T+|D-)$, $TN = P(T-|D-)$, and $FN = P(T-|D+)$. For example, for the data in Table 2A [$P(D+) = 0.60$], using equation (1):

$$P(D+|T+) = \frac{(0.90)\,(0.60)}{(0.90)\,(0.60) + (0.15)\,(0.40)} = 0.90$$

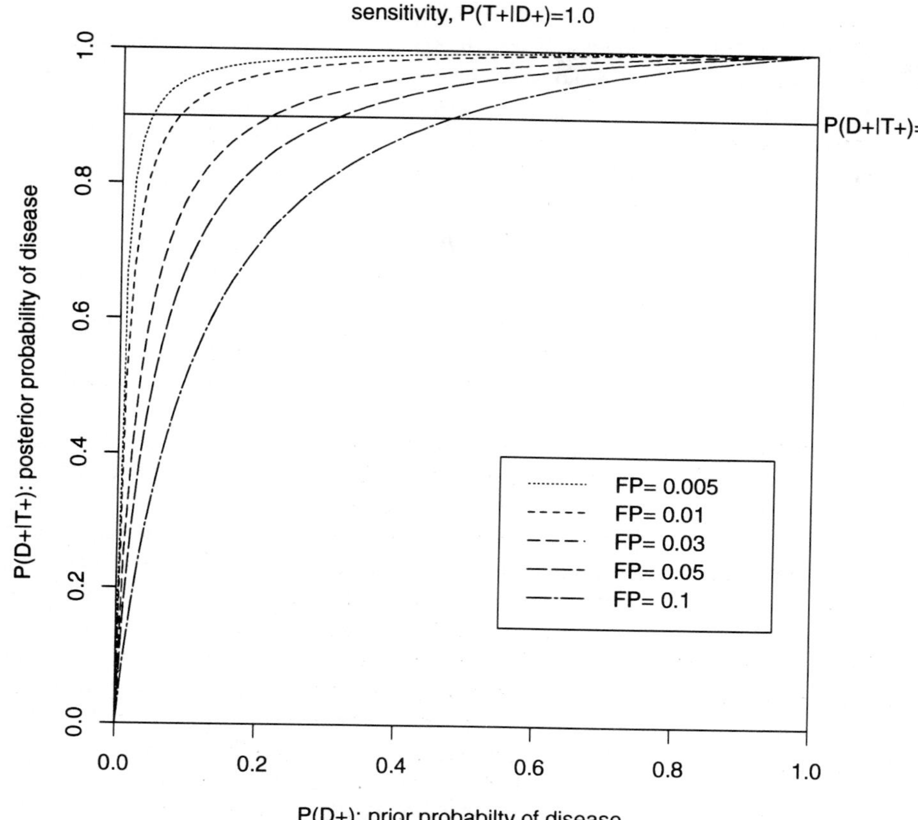

Figure 1. Diagnostic value of a test: prior probability versus posterior probability of disease given a positive test result for a perfectly sensitive test, adapted from Katz, reference 6.

and for the data in Table 2B [$P(D+) = 0.06$], using equation (1):

$$P(D+|T+) = \frac{(0.90)\ (0.06)}{(0.90)\ (0.06) + (0.15)\ (0.94)} = 0.28$$

Similar calculations can be made using equation (2).

A drop in the prevalence of disease for the same pair of *TP* and *FP* ratios decreases the reliability with which a positive test result can be used to indicate the presence of disease. This relationship is expressed graphically in Figure 1 for a perfectly sensitive test (*TP* ratio = 1.00) with varying false-positive ratios. The series of hyperbolic curves shows that increasingly higher prevalence rates are required as the false-positive ratio increases to achieve the same probability of disease given a positive test result, $P(D+|T+)$.[6] When false-positive ratios are greater than 0.10, positive test results are associated with a high probability of disease [$P(D+|T+) > 0.90$] only when the prevalence of disease is greater than 45%. Similarly, when the *FP* rate is held constant, higher prevalence rates are required as the true-positive ratio decreases to achieve the same probability of disease given a positive test result. In other words, to achieve the same level of diagnostic information, diagnostic tests performed on patients from a population with a lower prevalence of disease must be much more accurate than tests performed on patients from a group with a higher prevalence. A current illustration of this point is the fact that exercise stress testing of young women at low risk for cardiac disease is not considered a useful procedure.

Bayes' theorem is frequently expressed in terms of likelihood ratios. For an abnormal test result:

$$\frac{P(D+|T+)}{P(D-|T+)} = L \times \frac{P(D+)}{P(D-)} \qquad (3)$$

where $P(D+)/P(D-)$ is the prior odds of disease and $P(D+|T+)/P(D-|T-)$ is the posterior odds of disease, given a positive test result.

According to equation (3), the odds of disease after a test is performed varies linearly with the odds before the test is performed and has a slope of L. L is also known as the odds ratio, because it is the ratio of the posterior odds of disease to the prior odds of disease. When the posterior odds of disease given a positive test are equal to the prior odds of disease ($L = 1$) the test has provided no new information.

Biases and Their Impact on Results

Ransohoff and Feinstein summarized several biases that, when present, can markedly distort the ability to measure correctly a test's performance.[7] For a more general review of these biases, see also Sox et al.,[1] and Begg and McNeil.[8] *Spectrum* bias is a common bias that usually leads to inflation in estimates of sensitivity and specificity. Spectrum bias occurs when tests are evaluated on the "sickest of the sick and the wellest of the well,"[1] though it may also occur in a less pronounced way when investigators "grab" patients for study. For example, this would happen when estimating sensitivities of SPECT studies using patients who have a thallium test instead of a more clearly defined population, say, all patients who have chest pain one week after a myocardial infarction.

Test-referral or *verification* bias can be introduced when test results influence the chance that a patient will go on and have other tests, particularly ones that will give definitive information about his/her disease status. For example, patients with a positive test result may be more likely to undergo biopsy than those with a negative result. Verification bias can also occur when study samples are restricted to patients with confirmed disease because these patients are likely to differ from patients whose disease has not been confirmed. Either sensitivity or specificity can be altered when verification bias occurs. When the only factor influencing referral is the test result itself (not, for example, concomitant clinical factors), methods developed by Begg and Greenes can be used to adjust estimates of sensitivity and specificity to account for simple verification bias.[9] However, as imaging tests are perceived to become more and more accurate, clinicians may be less inclined to refer patients to a "gold standard" measure of truth, and initial estimates of sensitivity and specificity as well as those corrected for verification bias will become more difficult to obtain.

Test interpretation or *test review* bias arises when the reader of the test has information beyond the test itself that may influence their interpretation of the test. Knowing, for example, the results of another test believed to be more definitive may cause a reader to alter his opinion about a less definitive test. In nuclear medicine, knowledge of angiography results could influence interpretation of a thallium study.

Diagnostic review bias occurs when the test result affects the interpretation of the data used to establish the diagnosis. *Inclusion* or *incorporation* bias occurs when the results of the test being evaluated are used to define the "gold standard." In the past, both of these biases were much more common than now.

In addition to these, another type of bias influencing test results occurs when a test has a large number of uninterpretable results. In this case, a true measure of a test's performance should account for these uninterpretable data. Excluding uninterpretable test results artificially elevates measures of a test's true sensitivity or specificity. This is particularly true if the probability of an uninterpretable result is related to disease status.

Thoughtful study design reduces the potential for bias.[8,10] For example, prospective studies with 'reasonable' follow-up can reduce verification bias and problems encountered when there is not a "gold standard." Test interpretation bias can be avoided by controlling the amount of information made available to readers participating in a study.

Receiver Operating Characteristic Curve

When tests have no binary outcomes but, rather, a continuum of values (any one of which can be selected as the boundary between normal and abnormal), the true- and false-positive ratios vary with the value selected as the cutoff point. Routine chemistry tests and radioimmunoassays are examples of such tests. The effect of changes in the cutoff point on test sensitivity can be graphically visualized by using a *receiver operating characteristic* (ROC) *curve*, a plot of the true-positive ratio against the false-positive ratio for various cutoff points (Fig. 2). For example, when test results larger than those corresponding to the value at point A are considered abnormal, fewer than 40% of the diseased patients are detected, but the false-positive rate is 0.01. At this point, the test has great specificity but poor sensitivity. At the other extreme, when a low cutoff value (point E) is used to separate those with disease from those without, nearly all (99%) patients with disease are identified, but at the expense of including a larger proportion (60%) of patients without disease. The location of a cutoff point along an ROC curve is called an *operating position*. In general, cutoff points corresponding to point A are used in screening tests in which a large number of false-positive tests would lead to many unnecessary secondary confirmatory tests. On the other hand, cutoff points corresponding to point E are used when a high morbidity is associated with failure to diagnose and treat disease and a low morbidity is associated with treating unnecessarily; patients suspected of having hypothyroidism would fall into the latter category.

Similar ROC curves can be constructed for situations that do not involve a single test with a continuous scale of outcomes. For example, this plot can be used to evaluate criteria of image interpretations (e.g., radiographic or scintigraphic) in which the observer rates his or her confidence that some characteristic (eg, tumor) is present, usually on a five-point scale. ROC curves are obtained by varying the degree of confidence corresponding to a positive reading; each threshold corresponds to a different pair of true-positive and false-positive ratios. This technique has been applied in several investigations of comparative imaging systems.[11–14] When data for 2 radiographic systems are plotted on ROC curves (Fig. 3), curves that lie closer to the upper left-hand corner of the graph (curve A) are better discriminators of disease than those located closer to the positive diagonal (curve B). For every *TP* ratio, the *FP* ratio found on curve B is lower than the *FP* ratio found on curve A. The statistical significance of observed differences depends on both the size and variability of the estimated differences. Small differences can be statistically significant when variability is small, and large differences may not be significant if variability is also large. Testing issues are discussed further in the following section.

In the past, evaluation of imaging methods has focused on detection. Current research has shifted emphasis to diagnosis, which combines detection of abnormalities and discrimination of particular characteristics. For example, a re-

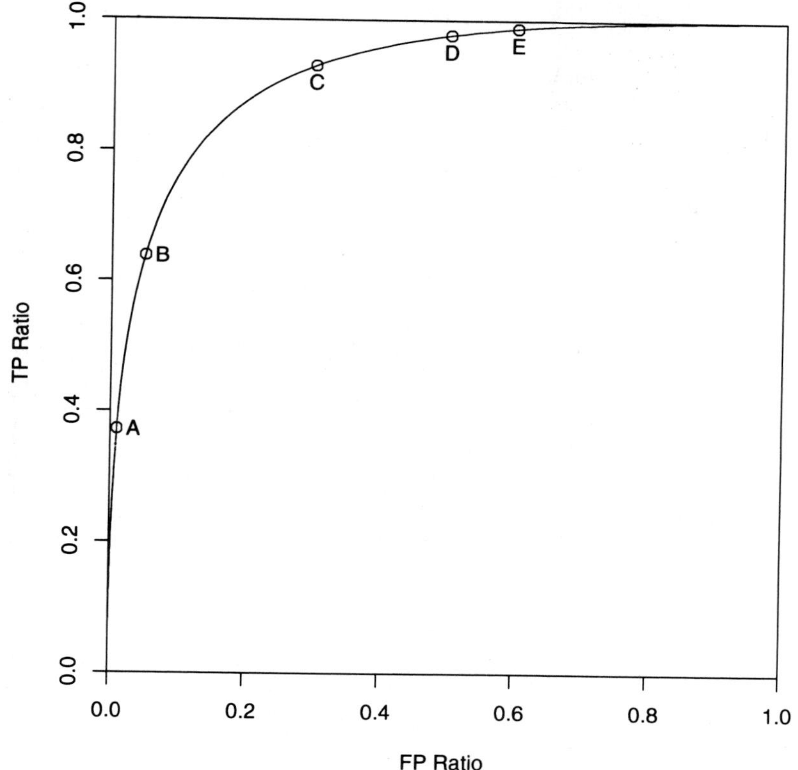

Figure 2. Receiver operating characteristic (ROC) curve: *TP* versus *FP* rates, with operating points.

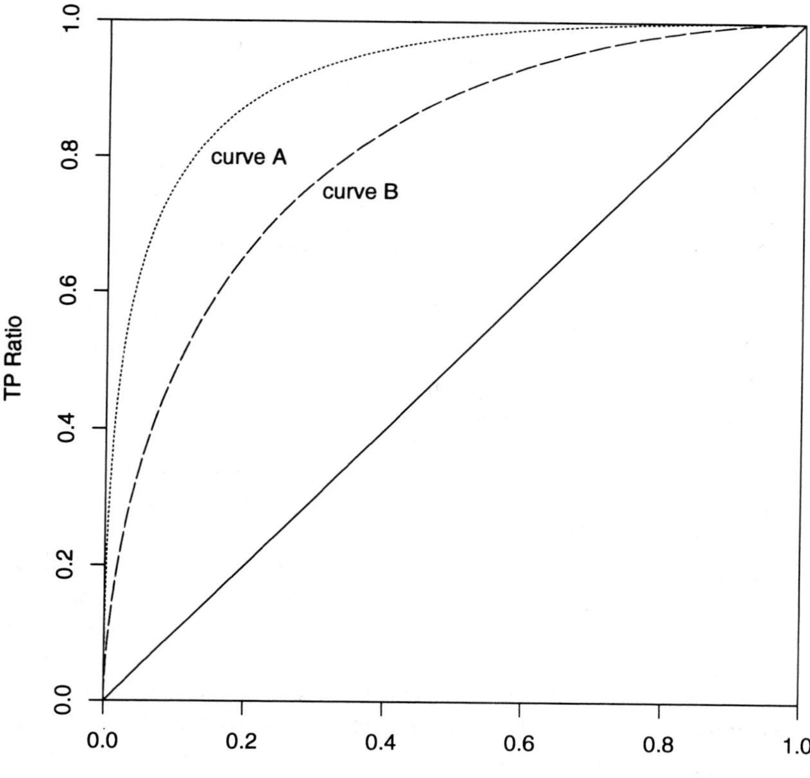

Figure 3. Comparison between two ROC curves: curves closer to the upper left-hand corner are more accurate than those closer to the diagonal.

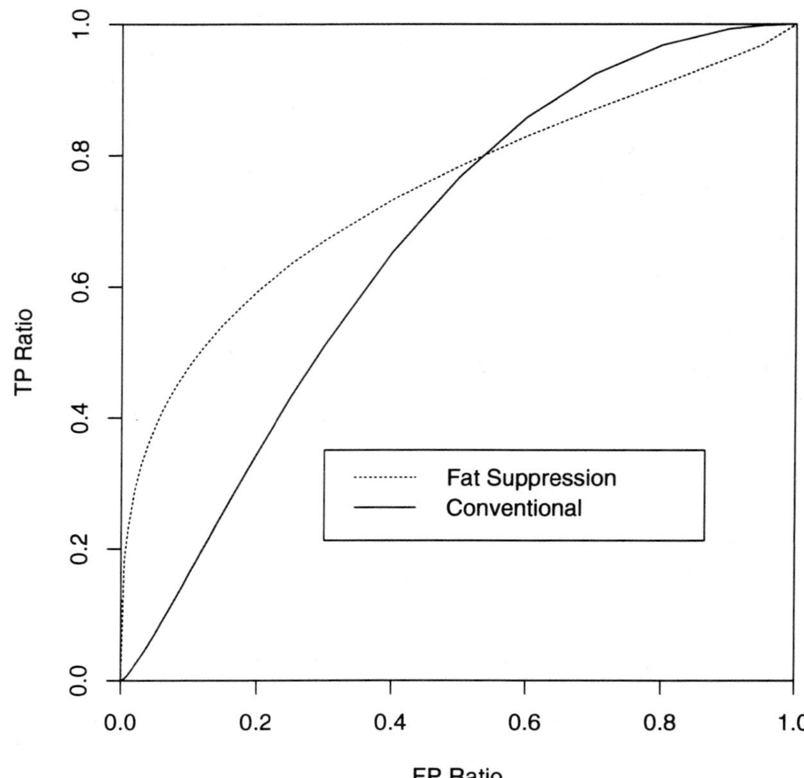

Figure 4. ROC curves for conventional MRI and MRI with fat suppression for detection of periprostatic invasion in patients with prostate cancer. All patients (n = 79) were evaluated with both methods and these images were read independently by different radiologists.

cent study of colorectal cancer examines the ability of CT and magnetic resonance (MR) readers to detect a tumor and determine whether it has extended into extracolonic tissue. This approach is likely to become increasingly important as clinicians demand that new imaging modalities do more than detect disease (ie, that they provide accurate diagnosis as well).

Another use of ROC curves in differential diagnosis that is gaining popularity is for the comparison of a basic modality (mammography is the example commonly used) interpreted in its traditional fashion and then interpreted with the addition of enhancements or aids to improve the accuracy of diagnosis. Figure 4 illustrates such an example with ROC curves fit to reader ratings of periprostatic invasion using conventional MRI, versus MRI with fat suppression. Readings of MRI with fat suppression are observed to be more accurate than conventional MRI for low false-positive rates. Statistical tests for differences between these curves are discussed in the following section.

ROC CURVE ANALYSIS

Use of the ROC curve has increased in popularity, particularly over the past ten years as CT, ultrasound, and magnetic resonance imaging (MRI) "compete" for similar patients with similar diagnostic problems. New statistical approaches for comparing the information obtained from competing imaging modes have been required for evaluations in the ROC format.[10,15–17] Several theoretic measures have been proposed to reduce an entire ROC curve into a single quantitative index of diagnostic accuracy; these include estimated *TP* and *FP* pairs, the area under the entire ROC curve, and the area under the ROC for a clinically significant range of *FP* values.[18] All of these measures assume that the underlying distributions representing normal and abnormal groups of patients are Gaussian.

The most popular current index is the area under a ROC curve; this area is used for most statistical approaches. The area under the ROC curve can be interpreted as the "probability of correctly ranking a (normal, abnormal) pair."[19] Hanley and McNeil (1982) discuss the interpretation of the area under ROC curves in detail. Areas range from 0.5 for worthless tests to 1.00 for perfect tests. Using the trapezoidal rule to calculate the area under the fitted ROC curve results in underestimation because the curve is concave. The area under the smooth ROC curve based on maximum likelihood estimates[20] can be obtained with an estimate of its standard error using available software. Metz's programs are also commonly used.[21]

For ROC data collected on unpaired data (eg, CT images on one set of subjects, MRI or nuclear medicine images on another set), the area and its standard error can be used directly in the traditional test between two proportions. These tests should not be applied blindly; fitted ROC curves should be examined first. Because the area under the ROC curve is an overall measure, 2 curves with different shapes that behave differently for different *FP* values can have the same area although they may not have the same clinical value. An example of this is shown in Figure 4. There is no statistical difference between the area under the 2 ROC curves (0.75 for fat suppression versus 0.67 for conventional MR, based on 79 patients). However, the difference between the 2 methods at a *FP* rate of 0.2, estimated to be 0.34 for conventional MRI and 0.59 for MRI with fat suppression, *is* statistically significant (one sided p-value 0.04). Typically, the performance of diagnostic tests at low false-positive rates is of greater interest than performance at high false-positive rates.

When the same patients are used to evaluate 2 or more imaging modalities, comparisons become more complex. Information is needed, not only on the areas and their standard errors, but also on the *correlations* between areas.[17] The correlations between areas, in turn, depend upon correlations between the rankings obtained for normal and abnormal patients by each of the imaging modes under investigation. Hanley and McNeil have described means for obtaining these correlations and have illustrated their use.[17]

An important problem regarding ROC curves is that of determining the proper sample size necessary to demonstrate the superiority of one imaging method over another. This problem can be stated somewhat differently. If an investigator does *not* detect a significant difference between 2 imaging techniques, what is the chance that a difference *could* have been detected, given the sample size used? Should the sample size have been larger? The relationship between areas under the ROC curve and the well-known *Wilcoxon* statistic, makes it possible to answer these questions. Table 3 summarizes sample sizes needed to detect a difference between areas ranging from 0.70 to 0.975 for *unpaired* data using a one sided t-test at the 0.05 level with 80%, 90%, and 95% power.[17] (The power of the test is the probability of detecting the difference.) Required sample sizes increase with increasing power and decrease as the difference between areas increases.

Consider the specific example that follows. If an investigator has a technique with an area of 0.925 and has a new test believed to be better (almost perfect, 0.975), how many patients should be studied, assuming that no patient can be studied by both techniques (ie, unpaired data). Table 3 indicates that 165 normal patients and 165 abnormal patients are needed for each test to detect a difference between these two areas (at power of 80%). Suppose that the investigator realizes that each patient studied could have been studied by both techniques (ie, paired data). What happens to the estimates of sample size? Overall sample size is reduced and decreases with increasing positive correlation between test results. For example, when comparing 2 different imaging modes, sample sizes can decrease by approximately 30%. An example supporting the need for large numbers of patients, even with a paired experimental design, comes from a recent study comparing MRI and ultrasound (US) in staging patients with prostate cancer.[22] An interim analysis of about 200 patients showed that the sensitivities of MRI and CT were 77 and 66%, respectively, and the specificities were 57 and 46%. These differences were not statistically significant, apparently due to variability in reading accuracy across those interpreting the films. A more detailed discussion of the relationship between sample size requirements and correlation may be found in Hanley and McNeil.[17]

REGRESSION METHODS FOR ROC CURVES

Although most work using ROC curves for the assessment of diagnostic tests has involved using parametric approaches suggested by Dorfman and Alf,[20] Metz[21] and others, investigators have long realized the limitations of these approaches, specifically in their inability to include covariates that may influence a test's accuracy. Adjustment for covariates with these approaches requires that patients be placed into subgroups according to the covariate(s) of interest; this obviously leads to subgroups with sample sizes that may be too small for most analyses. An example of an important covariate in nuclear medicine is type of cancer (eg, breast versus colon) and its effect on the ability of liver scintigraphy to detect metastases.[23] About the time the imaging community realized the potential importance of covariates, advances in statistics allowed inclusion of covariates in ROC analyses. Specifically, regression models were developed for ordinal data[24] and extended to ROC data.[25] Tosteson and Begg[26] describe the use of ordinal regression models to fit ROC curves in general and illustrate these methods using ultrasound data in patients with either breast or colon cancer.[26] The use of ordinal regression approaches for ROC analysis allows the inclusion of several covariates, including *continuous* ones (eg, CEA levels, year in which test was performed), in a way that is analytically parsimonious and methodologically flexible. The significance of particular covariates can be tested using t-tests based on the ratio of the estimate to its standard error. Further work is needed to explore methods for assessing how well ordinal regression models explain observed data.

Further extension of ordinal regression models include using a random effects approach to analyze the effects of having different readers.[27] This approach allows generalization of results from a particular group of readers to a broader group of readers.

Financial Considerations

In discussing the financial costs associated with the delivery of health care, it is necessary to consider several kinds of costs: commonly discussed are total financial costs, average costs, and marginal costs, as well as several components of costs, both direct and indirect factors.

Direct (health care) costs can be measured in several ways: (1) amounts billed by providers, (2) amounts paid by insurers and patients for health care, (3) the costs of the resources (professional labor, supplies, equipment, etc.) used in providing the care and, (4) resource costs at constant factor prices.[28] The first of these is relatively readily obtained, but of limited value because amounts charged are fairly arbitrary, particu-

Table 3. Number of Normal and Abnormal Subjects Required for Estimation of Each ROC Curve to Provide 80% (top number), 90% (middle number), and 95% (bottom number) Power to Detect the Difference Between Areas θ_1 and θ_2 under two ROC curves Based on Independent Samples Using a One Sided t-Test at the 0.05 Significance Level. Reproduced from Hanley and McNeil[17]

	θ_2									
θ_1	0.750	0.775	0.800	0.825	0.850	0.875	0.900	0.925	0.950	0.975
0.700	652 897 1131	286 392 493	158 216 271	100 135 169	68 92 115	49 66 82	37 49 61	28 38 46	22 29 36	18 23 29
0.725		610 839 1057	267 366 459	148 201 252	93 126 157	63 85 106	45 61 75	34 45 55	26 34 42	20 27 33
0.750			565 776 976	246 337 423	136 185 231	85 115 143	58 77 96	41 55 68	31 41 50	23 31 38
0.775				516 707 889	224 306 383	123 167 209	77 104 129	52 69 86	37 49 60	27 36 44
0.800					463 634 797	201 273 342	110 149 185	68 92 113	46 61 75	33 43 53
0.825						408 557 699	176 239 298	96 129 160	59 79 97	40 52 64
0.850							350 477 597	150 203 252	81 108 134	50 66 81
0.875								290 393 491	123 165 205	66 87 107
0.900								960 1314 1648	228 308 383	96 127 156
0.925									710 966 1209	165 220 272
0.950										457 615 765

larly for new procedures like stereotactic diagnosis. Also, amounts charged often do not reflect amounts actually paid, particularly for hospital services. The second measure, amounts paid, is the total that the rest of society transfers to the health care system in exchange for care and is, therefore, an important measure for public attention. However, amounts paid somewhat reflect the vagaries of differential mark-ups and different payment policies by different payors. For example, Medicare typically pays less than other payors for the same services yet, for estimating costs, it seems unreasonable to count the cost of the same diagnostic services as less because Medicare, rather than another payor, is paying for them. The third measure, "costs of resources used" adjusts for these problems by measuring the cost of each service as the cost of the resources used in producing the service (ie, the hourly compensation of each type of worker involved multiplied by the time that type of worker expends in the service). Alternatively known as "opportunity costs," this measure captures how much else society might have produced if the health care service in question was not used. Measuring resource costs, however, is difficult: it requires measuring direct input (such as labor hours and machine time), making throughput and depreciation assumptions for equipment and physical plant, and allocating overhead through imputations. A somewhat simpler procedure for measuring resource costs, which relies on average charge-to-cost ratios for entire hospital departments, such as radiology or pharmacy, is used by Medicare but is not always suitable because it assumes patients use a wide mix of services, while technology assessment studies in nuclear medicine or radiology are typically restricted to a small number of specific procedures. The fourth measure, resource costs at constant factor prices, adjusts the resource costs for facility-to-facility variation (for example, differences in wages for the same type of workers).

Indirect health care costs are important because death or

disability may prevent patients from supporting themselves or others, which results in additional costs to society and insurers for support of these patients or their dependents. The use of direct medical costs alone to determine the cost of diagnosis and treatment underestimates total financial costs. Even if these support costs cannot be determined exactly, they must be taken into consideration. Other indirect costs include the work-loss costs associated with the time involved in the performance of and recovery from diagnostic procedures. Ideally, these would be measured as the patient's actual compensation rate (including both wages and fringe benefits) multiplied by the hours he/she lost from work. However, given the reluctance of individuals to report their wages, researchers generally need to impute compensation as the average for persons of the age, education, and gender of the patient.

REFERENCES

1. Sox HC Jr, Blatt MA, Higgins MC, Marton KI. *Medical Decision Making*, Boston, Butterworths, 1988, chapts 4 & 5.
2. McNeil BJ, Keeler E, Adelstein SJ. Primer on certain elements of medical decision making. *N Engl J Med* 1975;293:211–215.
3. Fletcher RW, Fletcher SW, Wagner EH. *Clinical Epidemiology-The Essentials*. Baltimore, Williams and Wilkins, 1982.
4. Griner PF, Mayewski RJ, Mushlin AI, Greenland P. Selection and interpretation of diagnostic tests and procedures. *Ann Intern Med* 1981;94:557–592.
5. Diamond GA, Forrester JS. Analysis of probability as an aid in the clinical diagnosis of coronary artery disease. *N Engl J Med* 1979;300:1350.
6. Katz MA. A probability graph describing the predictive value of a highly sensitive diagnostic test. *N Engl J Med* 1974; 291:115.
7. Ransohoff DF, Feinstein AR. Problems of spectrum and bias in evaluating efficacy of diagnostic tests. *N Engl J Med* 1978;299:926–930.
8. Begg CB, McNeil BJ. Assessment of radiologic tests: control of bias and other design considerations. *Radiology* 1988; 167:565–569.
9. Begg CB, Greenes R. Assessment of diagnostic tests when disease verification is subject to selection bias. *Biometrics* 1983;39:207–216.
10. Gatsonis CG, McNeil BJ. Collaborative evaluations of diagnostic tests: experience of the radiology diagnostic oncology group. *Radiology* 1990;175:571–575.
11. McNeil BJ, Weber E, Harrison D, Hellman S. Use of a signal detection theory in examining the results of a contrast examination: A case study using the lymphangiogram. *Radiology* 1977;123:613–618.
12. Hessel SJ, Siegelman SS, McNeil BJ, et al. A prospective evaluation of computed tomography and ultrasound of the pancreas. *Radiology* 1982;143:129–133.
13. Webb WR, Gatsonis C, Zerhouni EA, Helan RT, Glazer GM, Francis IR, McNeil BJ. CT and MR imaging in staging non-small cell bronchogenic carcinoma: report of the Radiology Diagnostic Oncology Group. *Radiology* 1991;178:705–713.
14. D'Orsi CJ, Getty DJ, Swets JA, Pickett RM, Seltzer SE, McNeil BJ. Reading and decision aids for improved accuracy and standardization of mammographic diagnosis. *Radiology* 1992; 184:619–622.
15. Hanley JA. Receiver operating characteristic (ROC) methodology: the state of the art. *Crit Rev Diagn Imaging* 1989; 29:307–569.
16. Hanley JA, McNeil BJ. The measuring and use of the area under a receiver operating characteristic (ROC) curve. *Radiology* 1982;143:29–36.
17. Hanley JA, McNeil BJ. A method of comparing the areas under receiver operating characteristic curves derived from the same cases. *Radiology* 1983;148:839–843.
18. Thompson ML, Zucchini W. On the statistical analysis of ROC curves. *Stat Med* 1989;8:1277–1290.
19. Bamber D. The area above the ordinal dominance graph and the area below the receiver operating graph. *J Math Psych* 1975;12:387–415.
20. Dorfman DD, Alf E. Maximum likelihood estimation of parameters of signal detection theory and determination of confidence intervals-rating-method data. *J Math Psychol* 1969;6:487–496.
21. Metz CE, Kronman HB, Shen JH, Wang PL: *ROCFIT, INDROC, CORROC2, ROCPWRPC. Programs for ROC Analysis*. Chicago, Department of Radiology, The University of Chicago, 1989.
22. Rifkin MD, Zerhouni EA, Gatsonis CA, Quint LE, et al. Comparison of MRI and US in staging early prostate cancer: results of a multi-institutional cooperative trial. *N Engl J Med* 1990;323:621–626.
23. Alderson PO, Adams DF, McNeil BJ, et al. Computed tomography, ultrasound and scintigraphy of the liver in patients with colon or breast carcinoma: prospective comparison. *Radiology* 1983;149:225–230.
24. McCullagh P. Regression models for ordinal data, with discussion. *J Roy Stat Soc* 1980; series B, 422:109–142.
25. Altham PME. Discussion of Dr. McCullagh's paper. *J Roy Stat Soc* 1980; series B, 422:129–130, 1980.
26. Tosteson ANA, Begg CB. A general regression methodology for ROC curve estimation. *Med Decis Making* 1988;8: 204–215.
27. Gatsonis CG. Random effects in ordinal regression, with applications to ROC analysis, unpublished manuscript, 1990.
28. Sunshine J, McNeil BJ. *Estimation of Costs in Diagnostic Medicine*. American College of Radiology, working paper, 1993.

Section Three

Therapy

39 Radioiodine Therapy of Hyperthyroidism

John C. Harbert

Hyperthyroidism, or *thyrotoxicosis,* is the clinical state that results from hypersecretion of thyroid hormones, principally triiodothyronine (T_3) and thyroxine (T_4). The wide spectrum of symptoms and signs associated with hyperthyroidism represents the effects of these hormones upon the many tissues that are responsive to them. The most common cause of hyperthyroidism in developed countries is *toxic diffuse goiter* or *Graves' disease* (Table 1).[1] This is a disease of genetic origin involving the immune surveillance system, often associated with specific skin and eye changes. A less common cause, *toxic nodular goiter* or *autonomous functioning thyroid nodules* (AFTN), involves islands of acinar tissue that function independently of thyroid stimulating hormone (TSH), surrounded by *suppressed* normal thyroid tissue and is unassociated with skin and eye changes. To understand the role of ^{131}I therapy in the management of these diseases, the pathophysiology of hyperthyroidism will be reviewed briefly.

PATHOPHYSIOLOGY

Graves' Disease

The cause of Graves' disease is not established; it appears to be a disease limited to humans. There is a striking familial incidence; however, its expression in mono- and dizygotic twins suggest both genetic and environmental factors in its causation.[2] The disease is 4 to 8 times more prevalent in women than men. It is associated with disturbances in the immune surveillance system and onset may be associated with infections (*Yersinia enterocolitica* is a candidate), rapid weight reduction, or severe emotional stress.[3–5] This disease can occur from birth to old age, but peak incidence occurs in the third and fourth decades.[6]

In Graves' disease the gland is usually hypertrophied diffusely and functions at an accelerated rate. Serum levels of thyroid hormones are increased while serum TSH is depressed. The clearance of plasma iodide by the gland increases from the normal rate of 10 to 20 ml/min to over 100 ml/min. For this reason the ^{131}I uptake at 24 hours is usually elevated and is not suppressed by the administration of T_3 or T_4. Thyroid hormone and thyroglobulin (Tg) production are increased and the accelerated production results in the appearance of protein-bound ^{131}I (PB^{131}I) more rapidly and at higher levels than in normal persons following administration of ^{131}I. Accelerated T_4 turnover is also observed, probably as a result of hypermetabolism.[7] With the general hyperactivity of the thyroid, excess Tg is released and serum levels are elevated.

The clinical manifestations of Graves' disease appear to result from the effects of autoantibodies on the thyroid tissue TSH receptors. When these antibodies bind to TSH receptors, they activate them which, in turn, stimulates thyroid hormone biosynthesis. Antibodies against thyroglobulin and thyroid peroxidase can also be identified.[2]

The metabolism of iodine is distinctly abnormal in Graves' disease. Administration of as little as 2 mg of potassium iodide per day decreases ^{131}I uptake. This is known as the *Wolff-Chaikoff block.*[8] In fact, Graves' disease can be temporarily, and in some cases permanently, controlled by iodine administration.[9] The effect appears to be one of inhibition of organification because the administration of perchlorate results in discharge of accumulated ionic ^{131}I.[10] Coincident with the block in iodine uptake, iodine administration causes a marked reduction in the release of previously formed thyroid hormone.[11] This is thought to be responsible for the beneficial clinical effects of iodine administration in Graves' disease. It has also been proposed that this phenomenon be used as a means of increasing the radiation dose to the thyroid from therapeutic doses of ^{131}I. Iodine administration inhibits iodine uptake and hormone release, but it does not inhibit hormone synthesis and, in many patients, prolonged iodine administration is accompanied by a gradual buildup of glandular thyroid hormone and thyroid enlargement.

Toxic Nodular Goiter (Plummer's Disease)

Multinodular goiter is thought to evolve from long-continued, low-grade, intermittent stimulus to thyroid hyperplasia.[12] Marine postulated that periods of iodine deficiency alternating with iodine repletion cause cyclic hyperplasia and colloid involution, and that eventually nodular hyperplasia results.[13] Other possible mechanisms include dietary goitrogens, defects of T_4 synthesis, or such thyroid-stimulating factors as *thyroid growth immunoglobulin.*[14]

Another concept advanced by Studer[15] is that, unlike Graves' disease in which all of the follicles are more or less uniform, the follicular pattern in multinodular goiter is distinctly nonhomogeneous (Fig. 1). Each follicle contributes its own highly variable share of the total hormone

Table 1. Causes of Thyrotoxicosis

TYPE	CAUSE
Autoimmune	Graves' disease Hashimoto's thyroiditis
Autonomous	Toxic multinodular goiter Autonomous functioning thyroid nodule(s) (AFTN)
Transient	Postpartum thyroiditis Subacute thyroiditis Thyroid destruction (postsurgical storm)
Drug-induced	Iodine-induced (Jod-Basedow) Thyroxine-induced (factitious) Lithium carbonate (long-term therapy)
Secondary	TSH-secreting tumor Inappropriate TSH secretion Trophoblastic tumors
Ectopic	Struma ovarii Metastatic follicular carcinoma

production. The individual activity of each follicle depends upon its own degree of autonomous function; that is, the follicles have different sensitivities to TSH. The variable scintigraphic pattern (Fig. 2) is caused by cohorts of follicles that produce little hormone (and thus appear "cold"), interspersed with more active cohorts that have abundant colloid formation (and thus appear "hot"). Thyrotoxicosis develops slowly and is often preceded by subclinical hyperthyroidism.[16] The total thyroid hormonal output in multinodular goiter depends on the total number of follicles and their relative activity. When the number of follicles with at least some degree of autonomous function grows large enough to produce hormone in excess of daily requirements, thyrotoxicosis becomes manifest. Some of the clinical and morphological differences between Graves' disease and toxic nodular goiter are listed in Table 2. If careful histological sections of these glands are made, from 4 to 17% are found to harbor microscopic papillary carcinoma, similar to nonhyperthyroid glands.[17,18] On the other hand, development of clinical thyroid cancer in patients with toxic nodular goiter is rare.[19]

Thyrotoxicosis develops in a substantial number of patients with multinodular goiter and the incidence increases with the duration of the disease. In one study, 60% of patients with nodular goiter who were over 60 years of age had developed thyrotoxicosis.[20] With time, these glands become autonomous and independent of TSH control. From this point on, they behave clinically much like Graves' disease, with a few notable exceptions.[1,21]

1. Exophthalmos is rare in toxic nodular goiter. When it does occur, the condition is more likely to be underlying Graves' disease in which nodularity has developed secondarily;
2. Patients with toxic nodular goiter are generally older; the thyrotoxicosis is usually less severe and generally requires larger doses of ^{131}I to control;
3. Recurrent thyrotoxicosis is less common following surgery of toxic nodular goiter and few patients become hypothyroid.

Graves' Disease with Incidental Nodularity

A distinction should be made between toxic nodular goiter and Graves' disease with incidental nodularity (Fig. 3). In the latter, nodules contain less radioiodine and usually resemble multinodular goiter in appearance. Although the underlying condition is Graves' disease, patients with nodular goiters may require higher doses of ^{131}I to achieve remission of symptoms.[22]

Manifestations of Hyperthyroidism

The classic symptoms of hyperthyroidism are weight loss despite increased appetite, weakness, dyspnea, palpitations, sweating, heat intolerance, tremor, and irritability. In older patients, cardiovascular symptoms predominate, often with signs of cardiac failure, and often associated with atrial fibrillation and tachyarrythmias. Special features of Graves' disease not often associated with other causes of hyperthyroidism include pretibial myxedema and exophthalmos. Both are caused by excessive deposition of mucopolysaccharide—subcutaneously in the legs in the former, and retroorbitally in the latter. Exophthalmos is mild in about 60% of cases, moderate in about 10%, and severe in about 3%.[13]

Acropachy, clubbing of the terminal phalanges, also results from subcutaneous deposition of mucopolysaccharide.

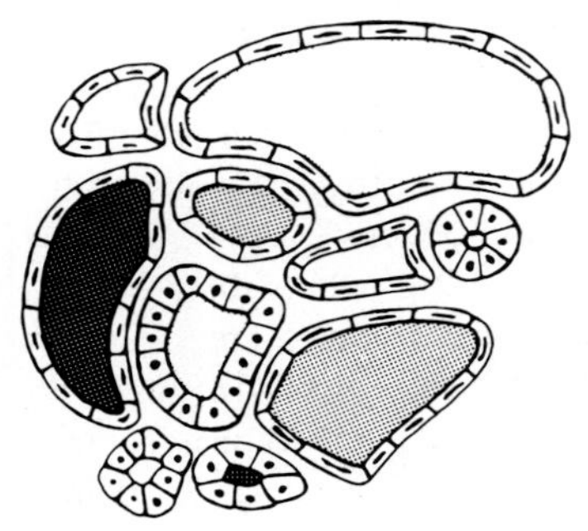

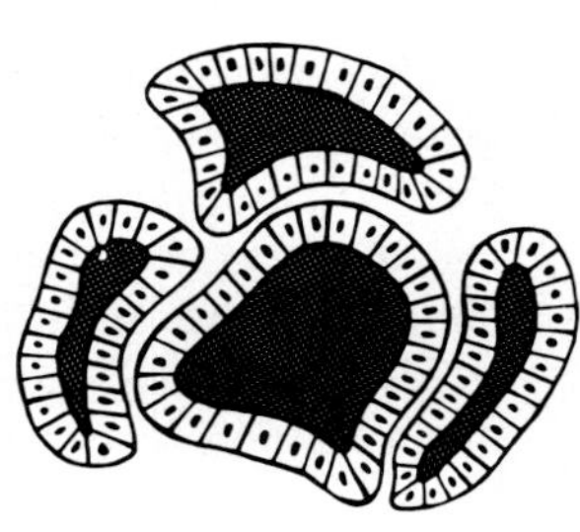

Fig. 1. Morphological and functional characteristics of Graves' goiter (right) and multinodular hyperthyroid goiter (left). *In Graves' goiter,* all follicles are lined by the same type of highly columnar epithelial cells and contain weakly PAS-positive colloid in the small- or medium-sized follicular lumina. Autoradiographically, all follicles have the same iodine turnover. *In multinodular goiters,* tiny follicles may coexist with giant ones. The follicular epithelium varies from flat to highly columnar, but there is no correlation between morphology of cells or follicles and their widely varying iodine turnover. Iodine turnover is also unrelated to follicle size. (From: Studer H: Pathogenesis of goiter: a unifying hypothesis, *Thyroid Today,* Travenol Laboratories, Deerfield IL. Vol 8, No 4, 1984. With permission.)

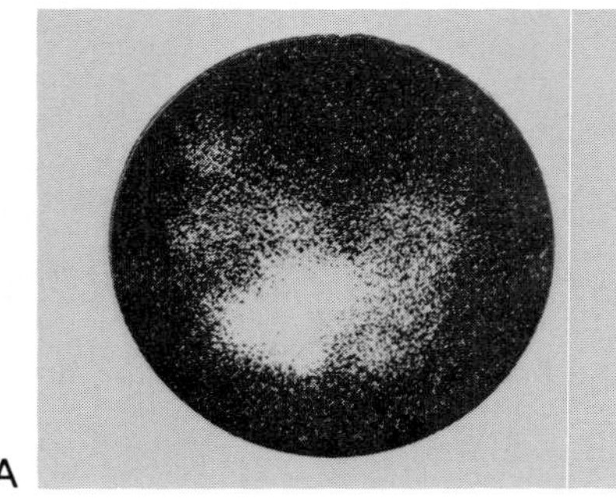
A

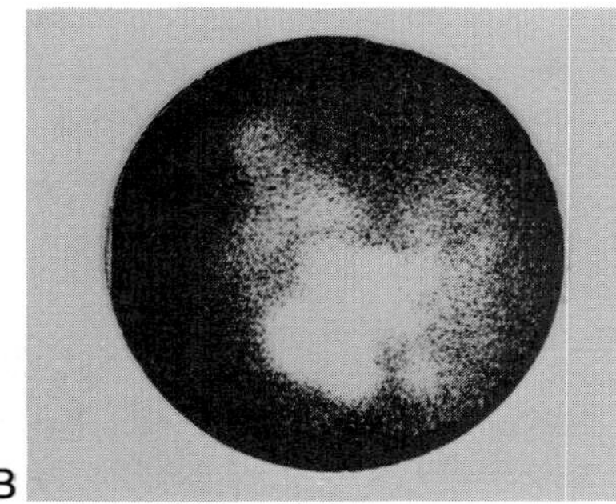
B

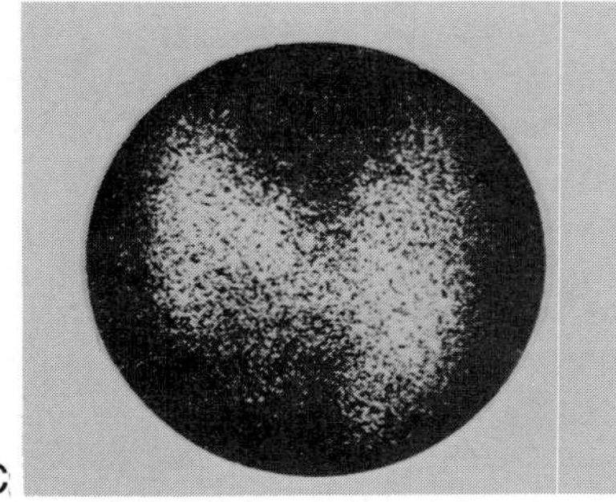
C

Figure 2. Toxic nodular goiter. **(A).** Irregular hot nodule imaged with ^{123}I. **(B).** TSH stimulation of suppressed thyroid tissue. **(C).** Image 5 months following ^{131}I therapy showing substantial ablation of the hyperfunctioning nodules and stimulation of previously suppressed tissue.

The pretibial edema usually clears with treatment, but exophthalmos often persists.

The symptoms associated with hyperthyroidism may be so mild that they are barely distinguishable from anxiety, or so severe that they require emergency medical management. Most manifestations of hyperthyroidism relate to the effects of thyroid hormone on organ systems.

CENTRAL NERVOUS SYSTEM

Central-nervous-system stimulation causes anxiety, tremor, and emotional lability; insomnia is also a frequent complaint.

METABOLISM

Increased heat production leads to heat intolerance, sweating, and vasodilation, which produce warm, moist skin. The basal metabolic rate is significantly elevated. Often, loss of weight occurs despite a good appetite. Thinning of the hair, skin, and nails may also occur.

Table 2. Clinical and Morphological Differences Between Graves' Disease and Toxic Nodular Goiter

GRAVES' DISEASE	TOXIC NODULAR GOITER
Diffuse	Diffuse initially, becoming multinodular with progression
Usually small, <40 g	Frequently large
Grows rapidly (weeks or months)	Grows slowly over years
Always associated with rapidly developing hyperthyroidism	Hyperthyroidism develops slowly and at a later age
Histologically and metabolically follicles are uniform	Very heterogeneous follicle size and iodine turnover
Microscopic carcinoma rare	Microscopic carcinoma common

OTHER EFFECTS

Gastrointestinal effects include hyperperistalsis and diarrhea. Cardiovascular effects include tachycardia, increased cardiac output and, occasionally, congestive heart failure, especially in older patients. Menses may be excessive or scant, and are often irregular.

Laboratory Diagnosis

While the clinical manifestations and history are often sufficient to create a strong impression of hyperthyroidism, laboratory data are required to verify the diagnosis, to estimate the disease severity, and to distinguish among the causes listed in Table 1. For practical purposes, the most appropriate tests are the serum T_4, TSH, the free thyroxine index (FTI), and the radioactive iodine uptake test. Values of serum T_4 above about 14 μg/dL are consistent with hyperthyroidism and the degree of elevation above this level correlates well with disease severity (Table 3).

When the total T_4 is elevated it is necessary to exclude thyroid binding globulin (TBG) excess by measuring the T_3 uptake and FTI. In TBG–excess states, such as pregnancy, estrogen therapy, acute hepatitis, and congenital TBG excess, the T_3 uptake is depressed. The FTI (T_3 uptake $\times$ T_4) is usually in the upper normal range, or slightly above the upper limit of normal in cases of TBG excess. Measurements of total T_3 (by radioimmunoassay) are variable in hyperthyroidism. Triiodothyronine is elevated in the majority of patients with hyperthyroidism; it may be normal or depressed, however, if the patient is severely ill or is receiving drugs that inhibit T_4 to T_3 conversion (glucocorticoids, propranolol, propylthiouracil, and other drugs listed in Table 3). In 2 to 4% of patients with hyperthyroidism, the predominant form

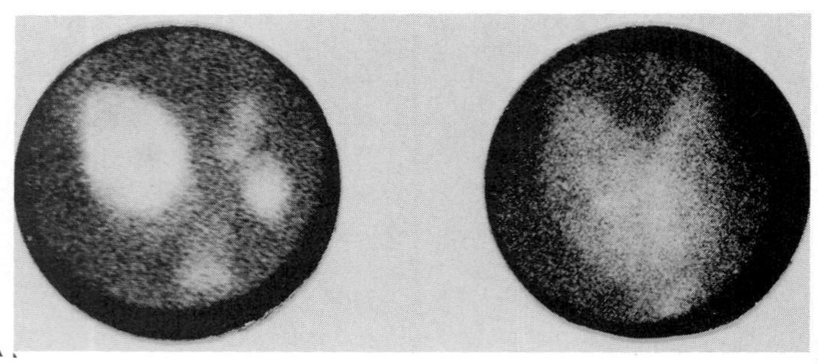

Figure 3. **(A).** Thyroid scintigram with ^{99m}Tc-pertechnetate in a patient with toxic nodular goiter. **(B).** ^{99m}Tc-pertechnetate scintigram in Graves' disease with nodularity.

of thyroid hormone produced by the thyroid is T_3. In these patients, serum T_4 is normal or low, and the T_3 resin uptake is normal because serum T_3 concentration is not sufficiently high to compete for T_3 in the in vitro uptake assay.[23,24]

The serum TSH is suppressed in patients with thyrotoxicosis, but a highly sensitive TSH assay is necessary to achieve clear-cut differentiation between euthyroid and hyperthyroid levels. With the introduction of high-sensitivity TSH assays, assays of thyrotropin releasing hormone (TRH) have generally been superseded.

The thyroid uptake may be normal in patients with *apathetic* hyperthyroidism and hyperthyroid patients with expanded iodide pool. In these patients, a negative response to TRH stimulation may be the best means of diagnosing underlying hyperthyroidism.

Rarely, in patients with greatly increased hormone synthesis and rapid thyroid hormone turnover, the 24-hour uptake is normal, but the 4- to 6-hour uptake is elevated. Since assays of thyroid hormones have become so reliable, there has been a tendency to dispense with the thyroid uptake unless ^{131}I therapy is planned. The problem with such oversight is that cases of transient thyrotoxicosis, such as subacute thyroiditis, may be missed. In these diseases, the 24-hour uptake is depressed and serum T_3 and T_4 may be elevated.

Thyroid scintigraphy is usually performed with ^{99m}Tc-pertechnetate, ^{123}I, or ^{131}I. In Graves' disease, thyroid scintigraphy characteristically demonstrates a pattern of uniform distribution within an enlarged gland, with all of these radiopharmaceuticals (Fig. 4). In some patients, the gland is not palpably enlarged and the thyroid image is normal. In toxic nodular goiter and AFTN, the nodule(s) are hyperfunctioning and are not suppressed following T_3 administration.

Autoantibodies to thyroid peroxidase can be detected in about 90% of patients with Graves' disease, and are useful to confirm the autoimmune nature of the disease (Table 4). Thyroglobulin antibodies are less frequently elevated. Autoantibodies to TSH receptors are elevated in Graves' disease, although their routine measurement is not generally indicated.

Table 3. Drugs that Interfere with Thyroid Hormone Synthesis and Metabolism

MECHANISM AFFECTED	DRUG OR CONDITION
Iodine trapping	Thiocyanate Perchlorate Nitroprusside
Organification	Propylthiouracil Tapazol Sulfonylureas Sulfonamides p-Aminosalicylic acid Phenylbutazone Aminoglutethimide
Hormone synthesis	Iodine
Hormone release	Iodine Lithium
Conversion of T_4 to T_3	Propylthiouracil Glucocorticoids Propranolol Iopanoic acid Amiodarone
	Fasting Significant illness Hepatic disease

TREATMENT OF GRAVES' DISEASE

The use of ^{131}I for treating hyperthyroidism dates from 1942.[25] Now, after more than 50 years and millions of hyperthyroid patients treated, it is recognized as the simplest, safest, least expensive, and most effective form of therapy

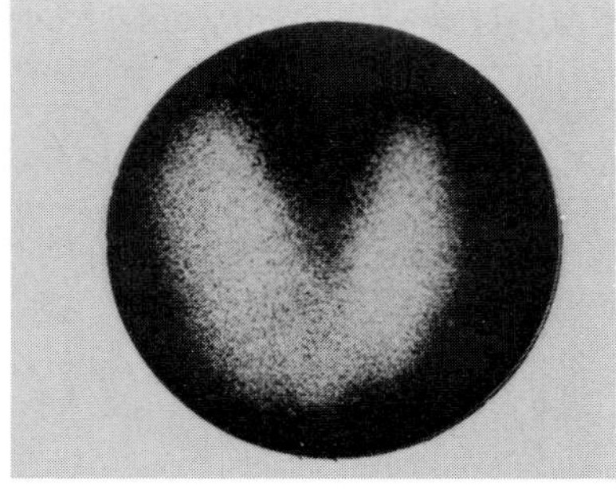

Figure 4. Thyroid scintigram in Graves' disease (^{99m}Tc-pertechnetate) showing characteristic glandular fullness.

Table 4. Laboratory Diagnosis of Thyrotoxicosis

CAUSE	TPO Ab	TSH Ab	UPTAKE	SCINTIGRAPHY
Graves' disease	+	+	↑	Diffuse symmetrical
"Hashitoxicosis"	+++	±	↑	Irregular
Postpartum thyroiditis	+	0	↓	Diffuse
Subacute thyroiditis	0	0	↓	Diffuse
Toxic multinod. goiter	0	0	↑	Hot and cold nodules
Toxic adenoma	0	0	↑	Single hot nodule
Iodine or T_4 ingestion	±	0	↓	Diffuse

TPO Ab = Thyroid peroxidase antibody; TSH Ab = TSH antibody.

for most patients. It has largely replaced surgery as the definitive therapy of this disorder.

Selection of Patients

Because the treatment of hyperthyroidism with ^{131}I is relatively inexpensive, convenient, and effective, it is the first line of therapy for most patients, except for those who are pregnant or lactating, who have severe ophthalmopathy, or who are very young. It is suggested by some that mild Graves' disease may be better treated with antithyroid drugs, because the chance of permanent remission is high.[2] Patients with very large goiters are probably better treated by thyroidectomy, because radioiodine is unlikely to shrink the goiter to a normal size, and successful treatment with a single dose is unlikely.

Patients with severe hyperthyroidism, ophthalmopathy, or cardiac failure are generally treated with antithyroid drugs for 2 months before ^{131}I therapy. Antithyroid drugs should be discontinued 3 to 4 days before administration of ^{131}I, to ensure adequate thyroid uptake of ^{131}I. Since ophthalmopathy may increase in severity following ^{131}I therapy, treatment with corticosteroids has been advised. Bartalena and colleagues found that patients with mild to moderate ophthalmopathy improved with corticosteroid therapy, while in those who received only ^{131}I ophthalmopathy frequently increased in severity.[26] They recommended prednisone 0.4 to 0.5 mg/kg of body weight for 1 month following ^{131}I administration, with gradual tapering of the dose over the next 3 months.

Hyperthyroidism that relapses following treatment with thyroidectomy is usually retreated with ^{131}I. These patients tend to have a higher sensitivity to ^{131}I and a higher incidence of early hypothyroidism.[27] However, the long-term incidence of hypothyroidism remains the same as for populations that have not undergone thyroidectomy.

Dose Determination

The biological basis for radioiodine therapy of hyperthyroidism lies in the high thyroidal concentration of iodine and in the radiation-induced damage that inhibits thyroid follicle cell function. The effectiveness of a particular dose of radioiodine in the gland depends on several factors: the fractional iodine uptake, gland weight, effective half-life of iodine in the gland, the tissue distribution of radioactivity, and the radiosensitivity of the follicle cells. Since some of these factors can be easily evaluated and others cannot, perhaps no single formula can be applied in determining an optimum therapeutic dose for a given individual. At least three general dose strategies have been advanced: the fixed-dose method, the microcurie (Bequerel) per gram method, and the delivered thyroidal radiation dose method.

1. FIXED-DOSE METHOD

Some physicians administer a fixed dose of 3 to 5 mCi (110 to 185 MBq) of ^{131}I orally. According to Werner,[28] about 60% of patients thus treated become euthyroid within 3 to 4 months. Those who fail to respond are given a second dose, after which about 85% are euthyroid or hypothyroid. Since the dose administered has no relation to gland size, uptake, or severity of disease, this strategy ignores all of the variables that affect the radiation changes desired. Others modify the fixed dose by giving larger total doses to larger glands.[29] Although a definite uncertainty exists regarding the outcome of any therapeutic dose of radioiodine, a better understanding of dose-response relationships is unlikely to emerge from such empirical treatment strategies.

2. MICROCURIE (BEQUEREL) PER GRAM METHOD

By this strategy, the administered dose is based on gland size and radioiodine uptake and is calculated as a fixed-dose per gram of functioning thyroid:

$$(1)\ \text{Dose } (\mu\text{Ci}) = \frac{\mu\text{Ci/g selected} \times \text{estimated gland weight (g)} \times 100}{\%\ \text{uptake at 24 hours}}$$

Most practitioners have given 55 to 110 μCi/g (~1.5 to 3.0 MBq/g), which will deliver 5000 to 10,000 cGy to the gland.

This strategy can be modified by several clinical factors. For example, larger doses usually are given to patients who have nodular goiter, rapid ^{131}I turnover,[30,31] or elevated levels of PB^{131}I,[32] or to patients who have severe hyperthyroidism or fibrillation, in whom it is desirable to achieve rapid control.[33] Several authors have used a scaled dosage depending on the

Table 5. Dosage Schedule for ^{131}I Therapy Based on Gland Size

THYROID WEIGHT (g)	DESIRED μCi RETAINED PER GRAM OF THYROID AT 24 h	ESTIMATED AVERAGE DOSE IN RADS (ASSUMING A 5.9-DAY THYROID ^{131}I HALF-TIME)
10–20	40	3,310
21–30	45	3,720
31–40	50	4,135
41–50	60	4,960
51–60	70	5,790
61–70	75	6,200
71–80	80	6,620
81–90	85	7,030
91–100	90	7,440
100–	100	8,270

DeGroot LJ, Larsen PR, Reietoif S, et al: *The Thyroid and Its Diseases,* Ed. 5. New York, Wiley, 1984. With permission.

size of the gland.[34–36] This strategy is adapted out of the conviction that large glands are more resistant to radioiodine. Such a dose schedule is given in Table 5.

3. DELIVERED RADIATION DOSE METHOD

This strategy is based on absorbed radiation dose calculations. An administered dose of ^{131}I is calculated to deliver a predetermined radiation dose to the thyroid using, for example, the Quimby-Marinelli formula[37]:

$$(2)\ \text{Dose}\ (\mu\text{Ci}) = \frac{\text{cGy selected} \times \text{estimated gland weight (g)} \times 100}{\%\ \text{uptake at 24 h} \times 90}$$

where 90 is a constant based on tissue-absorbed fractions and biologic half-life of 24 days (effective half-life of 6 days). This formula yields results within approximately 3% of the absorbed-dose estimates using medical internal radiation dose (MIRD) formulations.[36]

It has been argued that this formula is no more effective in curing hyperthyroidism nor avoiding hypothyroidism than a fixed-dose strategy. A method based on dosimetric considerations, however, has the advantage of providing a consistent framework that uses universally accepted units and measurements and provides a sounder base for comparing results from different institutions.[38]

If the biologic half-life of intrathyroidal iodine is shortened, as in patients who have previously undergone thyroidectomy or treatment with antithyroid drugs, the effective half-life can be determined from the following:

$$(3)\qquad T_{1/2(\text{eff})} = \frac{T_{1/2\,\text{biol}} \times T_{1/2\,\text{phys}}}{T_{1/2\text{biol}} + T_{1/2\text{phys}}}$$

Equation (2) can then be modified to:

$$(4)\ \text{Dose}(\mu\text{Ci}) = \frac{\text{cGy selected} \times \text{estimated gland weight (g)} \times 6.67}{T_{1/2\text{eff}}(\text{days}) \times \%\ \text{uptake at 24 h}}$$

The biologic half-life is determined by serially measuring gland activity over several days following an appropriate tracer dose of ^{131}I. Such measurements require repeated visits to the laboratory. Becker and Hurley contend that satisfactory estimates can be derived from two measurements made 5 to 7 days apart, the first at 24 hours.[39] Extrapolation to time zero gives the uptake value from which the half-life is determined. Using this method, the rapidly changing activity under the initial rising portion of the uptake curve is neglected for the sake of simplicity. This slightly overestimates accumulated activity but, since the biologic half-life is long relative to the time to reach peak thyroid activity, only a small error is imposed. In most of their pretherapy measurements, Becker and Hurley[39] found the biologic half-life averaged about 33 days in hyperthyroid patients. However, a small group of patients (about 15%) had very rapid turnover of radioiodine; the average biologic half-life was only 2.8 days. These patients are believed to have an unusually small thyroidal iodine pool, the so-called "small pool syndrome."[40,41] This phenomenon is commonly encountered after prolonged administration of antithyroid drugs, which tends to deplete the thyroid of iodine. It may also be found in recurrent hyperthyroidism following surgery.[40] The effect of such rapid turnover is to greatly reduce the radiation absorbed dose to the thyroid per unit of ^{131}I administered, and to increase the radiation dose to the blood, since most of the administered radioiodine circulates as $PB^{131}I$.

Table 6 lists characteristic parameters for a group of seven patients with "small pool syndrome" compared to those of a large group of unselected hyperthyroid patients. The dose of ^{131}I calculated to deliver 7000 cGy to these patients' thyroids averaged 28.4 mCi (1.05 GBq), which would have delivered 154 cGy to the blood because of the very high levels of circulating $PB^{131}I$. This is a high radiation dose for a benign condition and surgery may be more appropriate in these patients. On the other hand, a "fixed dose" of 5 mCi (185 MBq) would only have delivered about 1700 cGy to the average thyroid gland in this group, and these patients would most likely have been recorded as treatment failures. Such patients may benefit from lithium therapy prior to ^{131}I administration, which is most effective in prolonging thyroid retention of ^{131}I in patients with rapid turnover.

Use of equation (2) or (4) is probably the best method for calculating the administered dose of ^{131}I. As a guideline to selecting the most appropriate radiation absorbed dose for specific clinical circumstances, the following radiation doses appear reasonable:

1. For young patients and patients with small glands and mild or moderate hyperthyroidism: 5000 to 7000 cGy.

Table 6. Comparison of Biological Half-Life and Radiation Dose Estimates in Hyperthyroid Patients with Normal and Small Thyroid Iodine Pools

	MEASURED		CALCULATED	
HYPERTHYROID PATIENTS	*Thyroid* $T_{\frac{1}{2}biol}$ *(days)*	*PB* ^{131}I *48-h (% dose/L)*	*Thyroid mCi* ^{131}I *to deliver 7,000 cGy*	*Blood Radiation dose (cGy)*
Group A: unselected (50)	32.2 ± 4	0.57 ± 0.5	4.8 ± 0.6	5.3 ± 0.7
Group B: small pool (7)	2.8 ± 0.7	4.4 ± 0.3	28.4 ± 2	154 ± 34

Becker DV, Hurley JR: Current status of radioiodine (I-131) treatment of hyperthyroidism, in Freedman LM, Weissman HS (eds): *Nuclear Medicine Annual, 1982.* New York, Raven, 1982, p 275.

This dose is equivalent to 55 to 74 μCi (1.5 to 2.0 MBq) of ^{131}I deposited per gram.

2. For patients with larger glands or more severe disease: 7500 to 10,000 cGy. This is equivalent to 75 to 110 μCi (2 to 3 MBq) of ^{131}I deposited per gram.
3. For patients who have toxic nodular goiter: 10,000 to 12,000 cGy (110 to 133 μCi/g). Hamburger recommends that patients with very large toxic multinodular goiters (greater than 100 g) receive 200 μCi/g or 18,000 cGy.[19]
4. For AFTNs: 10,000 to 12,000 cGy to the nodule.
5. For patients with cardiac disease: 10,000 to 18,000 cGy (110 to 200 μCi/g). The object of therapy in patients with heart disease and thyrotoxicosis is to control the hypermetabolism as quickly as possible. This is best accomplished by the use of β-adrenergic blocking agents, such as propranolol, and digitalization in patients with congestive heart failure, followed by relatively large doses of ^{131}I in an attempt to induce hypothyroidism quickly. Scott et al found that reversion of atrial fibrillation accompanying thyrotoxicosis was much more likely when patients became hypothyroid soon after ^{131}I therapy, than when ^{131}I therapy rendered the patient euthyroid.[33] There is no indication that ^{131}I therapy exacerbates cardiac disease if the patient is adequately treated medically, that is, after normalization of thyroid hormone levels by antithyroid drugs or adequate β-adrenergic blockade. Since use of the latter may be contraindicated in patients with congestive heart failure, an adequate period of pretreatment with antithyroid drugs is often recommended.

Thyroid Gland Weight

The thyroid gland weight (mass) can be estimated by several methods, none having very high accuracy. Most clinicians estimate gland weight by palpation, which they "learn" from their mentors. Becker and Hurley suggest that greater accuracy can be achieved by comparing estimates from presurgical palpation with measured weights of pathologic specimens when total thyroidectomy is performed.[39] Several formulas have been offered for estimating thyroid weight from anterior thyroid scans.[42,43] An example is that suggested by Mandart and Erbsman,[43] which relates scintigraphic area, A, with gland mass in grams, M, as: $M = 0.86A$.[1,26] The use of computer and digital scintigraphy is recommended because the results can be determined automatically, with no operator decisions, and the problem of edge determination inherent in film is avoided. Estimates based on scintigraphic area are relatively simple with rectilinear scanners; but, few institutions have them. With pinhole collimators, calibration markers must be carefully placed to avoid inaccuracies due to parallax.[44] In the best circumstances, such estimates correlate within 25% of the weights of surgical specimens in about 70% of patients and within 50% in more than 90% of patients.[39] However, palpation is about as accurate. Computed tomography and ultrasound may lend greater accuracy to these estimates,[45] but currently such expensive tests are not widely used.

Response to Therapy

With doses of 80 μCi/g (2.2 MBq/g) early investigators reported that the incidence of hypothyroidism at the end of the first year was between 4 and 7%[46–48] and rose to 20% or greater with higher doses.[49–52] Without doubt, the lesser incidence of hypothyroidism was achieved at a cost of prolonged hyperthyroidism and the need for multiple doses in many patients. After the first year, the increase in hypothyroidism progresses at about the same rate regardless of the dose used, averaging about 3%/year (Fig. 5). Glennon, Gordon, and Sawin reported 48% hypothyroidism in patients 17 years after low-dose therapy.[53] Dunn and Chapman reported about 40% of patients were hypothyroid after 10 years using intermediate doses,[49] and Nofal[54] found 70% of patients were hypothyroid 10 years after high doses.

Following the early recognition of postradioiodine hypothyroidism,[55–58] there was a trend toward using lower doses of ^{131}I.[34,41,46,59,60] This strategy, while decreasing the early appearance of hypothyroidism, did not reduce significantly the progressive appearance of later hypothyroidism; it also greatly prolonged the period of hyperthyroidism and increased the cost of treatment.[59] Thus, for some time there has been a trend toward administering larger doses of ^{131}I to quickly bring patients under control and begin long-term thyroid hormone replacement.[61–63] By the philosophy of this therapeutic approach, hypothyroidism would not be viewed as a complication, but rather the therapeutic objective. Hypothyroidism is easily compensated for, and its treatment is much more economic than multiple visits to the physician, prolonged testing, and repeated therapeutic doses of ^{131}I. Still, many clinicians today prefer to aim for a euthyroid

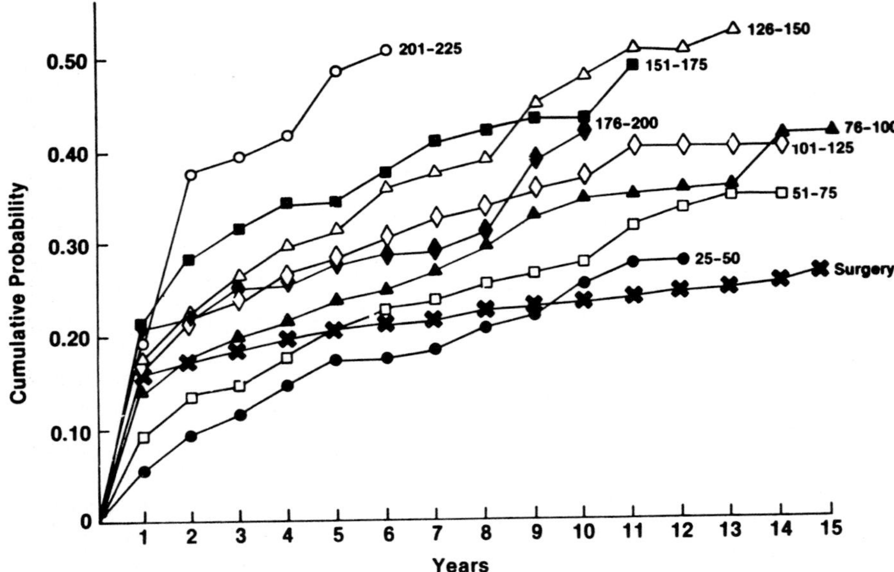

Figure 5. Probability of developing hypothyroidism in patients receiving varying doses of ^{131}I. This chart shows the cumulative probability of becoming hypothyroid (ordinate) as determined by standard life table techniques. The data were obtained from 6,000 patients without prior therapy for Graves' disease who received a single treatment with radioiodine. The abscissa shows the interval in years from the time of administration of radioiodine. Each curve indicates the radioiodine delivered to the thyroid (in microcuries per gram) based on measured thyroid uptake and estimated thyroid weight. The heavy line indicates the annual probability of becoming hypothyroid after surgical thyroidectomy. (From ref 221, with permission of the Thyrotoxicosis Follow-up Study of the Bureau of Radiological Health. U.S. Department of Health, Education and Welfare.)

state. They remain basically opposed to the concept of inducing one disease while curing another. When given the alternatives, most patients will probably elect to invest some additional expense and inconvenience at the time of therapy to avoid a lifelong dependence on pills—even one a day. The treatment regimens outlined above seem to be a reasonable compromise in assuring a relatively low incidence of repeat therapeutic doses and an acceptable incidence of early hypothyroidism.

Primary thyroid ablation for hyperthyroidism may, however, be the best treatment strategy for many patients, especially those who are felt to be unreliable in maintaining a long-term follow-up plan, or who depend on others for their care. Primary thyroid ablation is also recommended for patients in whom, for any reason, it is appropriate to reduce the number of tests. For these patients, 240 μCi/g is usually effective for prompt thyroid ablation.

Often the most appropriate treatment strategy will be determined by patients themselves after being informed of the consequences of each alternative. For many patients, the prospect of a long symptom-free medication-free period in their lives will serve as a strong incentive to disregard cost and inconvenience to achieve it. For others, the prospect of the insidious development of hypothyroidism may seem like an intolerable Sword of Damocles. Whatever strategy is adopted, long-term compliance by the patient and a commitment to life-long follow-up by the physician are essential. The danger of undiagnosed and untreated hypothyroidism cannot be overestimated.

During the first few months after therapy, antithyroid drugs or propranolol should be administered to reduce symptoms of hyperthyroidism until the therapeutic effect of ^{131}I becomes evident, in 2 to 4 months. Often the gland size decreases before hyperthyroidism is brought under control. This is a favorable indication that a clinical response will follow within 6 to 9 months.

If no change in gland size is observed and no abatement of symptoms occurs, retreatment should be considered 3 to 4 months after the initial dose. When a subsequent dose is required, it should be calculated to deliver the same radiation dose as the initial therapy. Often, with this calculation, a larger total dose of ^{131}I is required because of reduced $T_{1/2\text{eff}}$ of ^{131}I.[39] Beierwaltes recommends that subsequent doses of ^{131}I should deposit 20 to 30% more ^{131}I in the gland.[64]

Evaluation of the functional thyroid state soon after ^{131}I therapy is often difficult. Correlations between clinical status and various laboratory parameters are variable. Diminished serum T_4 does not necessarily signify hypothyroidism, because a preferential secretion of T_3 may exist. On the other hand, some patients who appear clinically hypothyroid may have normal or elevated serum T_4 levels.[65] A substantial number of these patients later become hypothyroid and they must be followed carefully. Connell et al found that 5 of 55 hyperthyroid patients (9%) developed hypothyroidism within 8 months of ^{131}I therapy.[66] In all of these patients, iodide trapping was preserved as evidenced by a normal 20-min ^{123}I uptake. By contrast, in all patients who went on to become permanently hypothyroid, iodide trapping was markedly impaired and did not recover. Thus, early iodine uptake studies appear to be useful in identifying transient hypothyroidism for which permanent thyroid hormone replacement may be avoided.

Although TSH is usually a reliable indicator of thyroid hormone production, Toft et al occasionally found elevated levels in euthyroid patients, probably because of reduced thyroid hormone reserve following therapy.[67] In some patients, a better functional test is achieved with TRH stimulation, which identifies patients at high risk of becoming hypothyroid.[68] Patients with diminished thyroid reserve may have a normal TSH response to TRH, but a blunted response in T_3 and T_4 secretion.

^{131}I *Therapy for Toxic Multinodular Goiter*

Toxic multinodular goiter (TMG) is not an autoimmune disease, but rather a goitrous condition in which many autonomously functioning nodules are found. The goiter and autonomous function often precede the onset of hyperthyroidism by several years.[69] In patients with TMG, the thyroid is generally more resistant to ^{131}I therapy than in patients with Graves' disease. For this reason, the standard dose of ^{131}I often is increased by 20 to 50%. Because the gland is frequently large, doses of 15 to 25 mCi (555 to 925 MBq) are not uncommon.[57] On the other hand, hypothyroidism results much less commonly than following ^{131}I therapy of Graves' disease; this is probably because follicles with low ^{131}I uptake are relatively protected. When endogenous TSH increases following therapy, these follicles begin to function; this process is reflected in the scintigraphic sequence of Figure 2.

In patients with severe cardiac problems, pretreatment with antithyroid drugs and β-adrenergic drugs, as discussed above for Graves' disease, is appropriate. Alternatively, smaller, divided doses may be warranted; for example, a dose that will deliver 4000 to 5000 cGy every 7 to 8 days may be tried. Because thyroid storm usually has its onset at about 6 days following ^{131}I administration, in the rare cases that it occurs, the effects of the initial dose can be carefully observed before the next dose is given.

Adjuncts to ^{131}I *Therapy*

Potassium iodide has long been used as an adjunct to radioiodine because it inhibits the release of thyroid hormone.[54,70] It must be administered after ^{131}I therapy because it competitively interferes with ^{131}I uptake. The hyperthyroid gland is especially sensitive to iodine, possibly because of its increased concentrating capacity. Thompson[71] found that 6 mg produces a maximum metabolic effect; this amount is contained in a single drop of Lugol's solution (one drop of SSKI contains 38 mg iodine). The usual practice is to wait 24 hours after ^{131}I therapy and then administer two drops of Lugol's solution or one drop of SSKI orally per day. Symptoms of hyperthyroidism are usually brought under control within a few days. With the advent of β-adrenergic blocking agents, however, iodide therapy is seldom used. It is probably most useful in patients who cannot tolerate antithyroid and β-blocking drugs.

The thionamide group of drugs, carbimazole, methimazole, and propylthiouracil (PTU), have long been used in conjunction with ^{131}I therapy. These drugs block thyroid hormone biosynthesis by inhibiting iodide oxidation and organification and by blocking the coupling of iodotyrosines to form T_4 and T_3. Often, these drugs are administered before radioiodine to bring symptoms under control more rapidly. Since they do not affect release of thyroid hormone, there is some delay in clinical response; they usually result in symptomatic improvement in 7 to 10 days. The choice of antithyroid drug often depends more on the incidence of sensitivity reactions than relative potency. With PTU, the usual starting dose is 300 to 600 mg/day; doses of 1 to 2 g/day may occasionally be necessary for control. The dose can often be reduced as hyperthyroidism abates. After the patient is euthyroid, or at least markedly improved, the drug is withdrawn for 3 days before administering ^{131}I. Prolonged use of antithyroid drugs may inhibit thyroid uptake and alter ^{131}I kinetics; therefore $T_{1/2\mathrm{eff}}$ should be measured and equation (4) used to determine the administered dose.

Steinbach found that simultaneous treatment of Graves' disease with ^{131}I and antithyroid drugs—PTU or methimazole—significantly reduced the posttherapeutic incidence of hypothyroidism: 8% at 12 months versus 36% at 12 months for control subjects treated without antithyroid drugs.[72] The authors postulate that the sulfhydryl moieties of these antithyroid drugs somehow impart radioresistance to thyroid cells. This effect had long been noted by others,[73,74] who advised against this combination therapy. They perceived the apparent radioresistance as interfering with the effects of ^{131}I, rather than being protective against subsequent hypothyroidism. Studies with larger numbers of patients are necessary before recommendations for this kind of treatment can be made.

PROPRANOLOL

The most effective group of drugs used to control the symptoms of hyperthyroidism are the β-adrenergic blocking agents, particularly propranolol, metoprolol, and atenolol.[75] These drugs act peripherally on the beta receptor sites of adrenergic action. The patient may be rendered eumetabolic while remaining functionally hyperthyroid.[76,77] The drugs have a rapid action (hours), and do not interfere with measurements of thyroid function or with the uptake of radioiodine. They may therefore be used before radioiodine therapy and need not be discontinued at the time of therapy. The principal clinical effects are cardiac: reduced cardiac output, heart rate, and myocardial oxygen consumption and increased myocardial efficiency.[78,79] Propranolol is usually given in doses of 20 to 80 mg every 6 hours, which may be increased to more than 600 mg/day in exceptional cases. Doses every 3 to 4 hours may be necessary in patients with accelerated clearance of the drug. Side effects include emotional depression, hypoglycemia, bronchospasm, gastrointestinal symptoms and, occasionally, increased heart block and congestive failure in cardiac patients. These symptoms usually disappear when dosage is reduced. Therapy is usually continued for 1 to 2 months or until euthyroidism is confirmed by functional thyroid tests. All β-blocking agents must be used with caution in patients with congestive heart failure, asthma, advanced grades of heart block, unstable insulin-dependent diabetes, or in patients taking quinidine, quinine, or psychotropic drugs, which augment adrenergic activity and the potential for arrhythmias.

LITHIUM

The use of lithium carbonate, although still experimental, may prove a useful adjunct to ^{131}I therapy. The lithium ion inhibits the proteolysis of thyroglobulin.[80] It therefore has two potentially beneficial effects: it prevents release of thyroid hormones, thus reducing the effect of transiently increased thyrotoxicosis which occasionally follows ^{131}I administration; and it increases thyroid retention of ^{131}I, thus increasing the effective radiation to the thyroid and reducing the circulating level of $PB^{131}I$.[81–87] Turner found that low-dosage lithium therapy (400 mg daily) significantly prolonged ^{131}I retention in the thyroid of patients with thyrotoxicosis, as compared with control patients treated with ^{131}I alone.[87] In addition, the mean 48-hour $PB^{131}I$ level fell from 1.21 to 0.55% dose/L in treated patients.

COMPLICATIONS OF RADIOIODINE THERAPY

Early Complications

EXACERBATION OF HYPERTHYROIDISM AND THYROID STORM

Following ^{131}I therapy, serum Tg may be elevated[88] and serum levels of thyroid hormones may transiently increase.[89,90] These elevations are thought to result directly from the effects of radiation on the thyroid follicle; they occur within the initial 2 weeks after ^{131}I administration and last a similar length of time. Usually no exacerbation of clinical symptoms occurs.

Thyroid storm is a rare complication of ^{131}I therapy[91–93] and occasional deaths have been reported.[94,95] The pathogenesis of storm in these patients is presumed to be rapid outpouring of thyroid hormones secondary to radiation thyroiditis. Of a total of 2975 patients reviewed by McDermott et al,[92] thyroid storm occurred in 10 patients, an incidence of 0.34%. In the same review, 16 case reports of thyroid storm following ^{131}I therapy were analyzed. This complication generally occurred in older patients (mean age = 53 years) with all but two over 40 years old, and the mortality was 25%. The mean interval between ^{131}I administration and onset of storm (fever and tachycardia) was 6 days. There appeared to be little correlation with the amount of ^{131}I given: 3.3 to 35 mCi; mean = 11.2 mCi (414 MBq). Most of the glands were large and 5 of 16 (31%) were nodular. Becker and Hurley[91] have noted that in some patients thyroid storm has occurred when patients have been taken off antithyroid drugs prior to administration of ^{131}I. Nevertheless, from their review, McDermott and colleagues[92] were not able to define a group of patients clearly at risk for developing thyroid storm.

Thyroid storm is usually of abrupt onset. Fever is the most important feature and, if storm is untreated, fever mounts progressively and may be lethal in 48 hours. Tachycardia and often auricular fibrillation are also present. The diagnosis is not always apparent, especially since laboratory tests are of little assistance. The levels of serum T_3 and T_4 may not be appreciably different from those found in thyrotoxicosis without crisis, nor from pretherapeutic baseline levels. Furthermore, common precipitating factors, especially infection, may present with the same features as storm: fever, abdominal pain, nausea, vomiting, diarrhea, and leukocytosis. The physician must then select among these possibilities: intercurrent illness incidental to thyrotoxicosis, but without storm; storm with manifestations suggesting intercurrent illness; and storm precipitated by intercurrent illness. The importance of differentiating among these entities stems both from the urgency of treating the intercurrent illness and determining whether full treatment for storm should be instituted. In acutely ill patients, it is usually not possible to exclude thyroid storm, and the patient should be treated for both storm and any coincident illness.

Once thyroid storm is recognized, treatment must be undertaken with the greatest urgency. These are four key elements to therapy that have been reviewed by Ingbar[96] and Wartofsky[97]:

1. The most important of these is beta-adrenergic blockade using propranolol.[98–100] The major effect of propranolol is to alleviate cardiac abnormalities, by reducing tachycardia, heart block, cardiac output, and cardiac work. Propranolol also helps lower body temperature, possibly by interfering with the peripheral conversion of T_4 to T_3.
2. Iodine in large doses (30 drops of SSKI per day) is given to reduce thyroid hormone release.
3. Propylthiouracil (900 to 1200 mg/day) is given to block hormone synthesis as well as to inhibit peripheral conversion of T_4 to T_3. Antithyroid drugs are administered prior to iodide, so that organification of iodide is blocked.
4. Thermoregulation, physiological support, and treatment of coexistent illness complete the therapy.

Exacerbation of preexisting illnesses has been reported in about 1% of hyperthyroid patients treated with ^{131}I.[92] Patients at risk for exacerbation in general include the elderly, those with severe thyrotoxicosis, very large goiters, multinodular goiters, and those with thyrotoxic-related cardiovascular or cerebrovascular diseases.[101–103] Precautions against thyroid storm and exacerbations include several general measures:

1. Adequate treatment of underlying illness prior to ^{131}I therapy;
2. Bed rest to decrease circulating thyroid hormone levels[36];
3. Hospitalization of high-risk patients;
4. The use of multiple small doses of ^{131}I may avoid acute discharge of thyroid hormones[55,91,101];
5. Prior administration of antithyroid drugs for 2 to 8 weeks may be effective in reducing symptoms of hyperthyroidism and depleting the thyroid gland of stored hormone.[64,91,94,95,104–106] These drugs should be discontinued 2 to 3 days prior to ^{131}I therapy, since maximum ^{131}I uptake occurs about 2 days after termination of PTU.[18] The antithyroid medication can be reinstituted 2 to 3 days after

^{131}I therapy to decrease renewed synthesis of thyroid hormone, and because PTU acts to decrease peripheral conversion of T_4 to T_3.

In patients who have been treated recently for thyroid storm, ^{131}I therapy will probably have to be delayed for 4 to 5 weeks because large doses of oral iodine block thyroid uptake.

OTHER COMPLICATIONS

Radiation thyroiditis, occurring 1 to 3 days following ^{131}I therapy, may be manifested by sore throat, usually minor. This symptom is more common in patients with toxic nodular goiter than with Graves' disease. Three cases of vocal cord paralysis following ^{131}I therapy for hyperthyroidism have been reported.[107–109] Presumably it is caused by perineural edema of the recurrent laryngeal nerve. Complete vocal cord paralysis requires that both recurrent laryngeal nerves be involved; in such cases, an airway problem may develop, necessitating intubation and tracheostomy. When only one side is involved, the airway is adequate and only stridor develops until one cord compensates by adducting over to the opposite cord.

Late Complications

HYPOTHYROIDISM

From necropsy and surgical specimens following ^{131}I therapy of the thyroid, the sequential changes of radiation thyroiditis can be described.[110] Following moderate to high doses given for thyroid ablation, 30 to 150 mCi (1.1 to 5.5 GBq), stromal edema, nuclear pyknosis, and granularity of the epithelial cytoplasm develop by 4 days.[111] Between 14 and 24 days after therapy follicular necrosis, exudation of neutrophils and fibrin, and acute vasculitis with thrombosis and hemorrhage develop.[112] By 40 days, reduction in follicular size and early replacement of follicles by connective tissue are observed. Lymphocytic infiltration occurs between 40 and 80 days after treatment. These changes are followed by laying down of dense fibrous stroma with some remaining follicles, often containing atypical cells and fragmented colloid. Autoradiographs reveal highly nonuniform distribution of radioiodine.[111] Regeneration of the thyroid parenchyma may follow if ^{131}I doses are not too large[110,113] and the pattern of regeneration is just as focal and irregular as the initial damage. Postradiation fibrosis in the thyroid is progressive over several years. The balance between regeneration and fibrosis appears to determine, in part, whether hypothyroidism will ensue. In animal studies, a shortened follicle cell life span can be demonstrated.[114] If damage to DNA synthesis occurs, follicle cells may not be replaced after normal attrition, which may also explain the progressively rising incidence of hypothyroidism following radiation.[115]

The substantial incidence of hypothyroidism within the first year following ^{131}I therapy has been mentioned earlier.

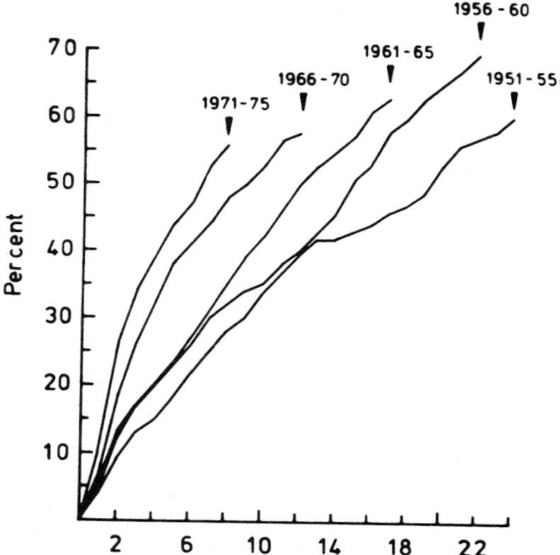

Figure 6. Cumulative incidence of hypothyroidism (in years) after ^{131}I therapy for hyperthyroidism in relation to treatment period. (From Holm L-E: Changing annual incidence of hypothyroidism after iodine-131 therapy for hyperthyroidism, 1951–1975. *J Nucl Med* 23:108, 1982. With permission.)

The incidence increases progressively with time and appears to be dose dependent (Fig. 5).

Recent evidence suggests that hypothyroidism following ^{131}I therapy is increasing.[63,116] In a large study reported from Sweden, Holm found the incidence rose progressively from 1951 to 1955 and from 1971 to 1975 (Fig. 6).[117] The reason for such large increases is not apparent. Cunnien et al observed the same trend at the Mayo Clinic.[118] In the earliest group, 3% of patients were hypothyroid 3 months after ^{131}I administration and 40% were hypothyroid at 1 year. In the last group, 1977 to 1978, 35% were hypothyroid at 3 months and 91% were hypothyroid at 1 year. In that interval, the same general pretherapeutic regimens were used and doses were calculated in an identical manner. The only trends observable in this population were that the average dose of ^{131}I increased and the percentage of patients requiring retreatment declined. Since the average dose calculated in microcuries per gram by the treating physician remained unchanged, the authors surmised that physicians may have been inflating, either consciously or unconsciously, their estimates of gland size.

At least one study has reported a lower incidence of early hypothyroidism among patients who were treated with corticosteroids before and after receiving ^{131}I.[119] These patients had lower levels of serum thyroid peroxidase antibody and thyroglobulin antibody as well as lower levels of circulating thyroid hormone following ^{131}I therapy, compared with control patients who received no steroids. These preliminary findings suggest a possible protective effect of steroids in reducing radiation-induced inflammation.

At this time, no clinical or laboratory factor or set of factors reliably predicts the development of hypothyroidism following ^{131}I therapy. Many studies have shown that such factors as larger goiters, longer effective half-lives of ^{131}I, negative antimicrosomal antibodies, lower ^{131}I doses, and possibly concurrent treatment with corticosteroids and antithyroid drugs *tend* to reduce the incidence of posttherapeutic hypothyroidism. However, statistical significance remains elusive.

HYPOPARATHYROIDISM

Hypoparathyroidism has been reported as a rare complication of ^{131}I therapy of hyperthyroidism.[120–123] When reported, its usual manifestation is decreased serum calcium. Tetany is very rare.[124] Of 60 patients treated with ^{131}I studied by Adams and Chalmers, serum calcium was normal in all patients.[125] However, in 12 patients challenged by EDTA infusion, the calcium level fell further and returned more slowly than in control subjects, suggesting reduced parathyroid reserve. In the few studies in which parathyroids have been examined at autopsy, no morphological changes as a result of radiation have been observed.[124,126]

The radiation dose absorbed by the parathyroid glands from therapeutic doses of ^{131}I is difficult to estimate and must be highly variable. A dose of ^{131}I estimated to deliver 9000 cGy to the thyroid has been calculated to deliver 400 to 500 cGy to the parathyroids.[125] Doniach calculated a dose of 1650 cGy from an administered dose of 5 mCi (185 MBq).[115] If such dose rates are correct, observable radiation effects can be readily understood.

HYPERPARATHYROIDISM

Sporadic cases of hyperparathyroidism associated with external radiation to the head and neck have been reported.[127,128] In 1982, Esselstyn et al described four patients who developed hyperparathyroidism following ^{131}I therapy for Graves' disease.[129] Rosen et al reported a series of 8 patients who presented with hyperparathyroidism and gave a history of radioiodine therapy.[130] These patients had received from 4.5 to 100 mCi (166 MBq to 3.7 GBq) for thyroid ablation; hyperparathyroidism developed from 4 to 20 years later. Surgical specimens revealed parathyroid adenomas in 5 patients and hyperplasia in 2. One of the 8 patients was found also to have a mixed papillary and follicular carcinoma of the thyroid in addition to a parathyroid adenoma.

More recently, Bondeson et al[131] analyzed 600 consecutive cases of primary hyperparathyroidism and found 10 patients who had received ^{131}I for the treatment of hyperthyroidism or thyroid ablation. The majority were women aged 21 to 72 years and the interval to detection of hypercalcemia was 3 to 27 years. In this small group, there was a trend toward an age-dependent effect, with patients treated with ^{131}I at younger ages at greater risk for developing hyperparathyroidism.

From these studies, it is likely that the development of hyperparathyroidism following ^{131}I therapy is more than coincidental and that it must be accepted as a risk factor in ^{131}I therapy.

CALCITONIN DEFICIENCY

Calcitonin is produced by intrathyroidal C cells. While the C cells do not trap radioiodine, they may be indirectly damaged due to their contiguity to follicular cells. At least one study has shown significant calcitonin deficiency among patients treated with ^{131}I for hyperthyroidism.[132] Patients rendered hypothyroid following ^{131}I had lower calcitonin levels than those who were rendered euthyroid. None of these patients had significantly lowered serum calcium levels. The long-term implications of these findings for effects on bone mass have not been determined. However, this may be one more reason not to treat hyperthyroidism with ablative doses of ^{131}I.

LEUKEMIA

The possibility of inducing leukemia has been examined because of the fact that significant radiation (8 to 16 cGy) is delivered to the blood in the course of ^{131}I therapy for hyperthyroidism.[133] This question was carefully reviewed by the United States Public Health Service Cooperative Thyrotoxicosis Follow-up Study Group.[134] This consortium of 26 hospitals compared the incidence of leukemia in 18,000 patients treated by ^{131}I to that in 1000 patients treated by surgery and antithyroid drugs. No differences were found during a follow-up that totaled more than 100,000 patient years.

In another large Swedish study that examined the records of 10,552 patients treated for hyperthyroidism (mean dose = 506 MBq), no increase in the incidence of leukemia over the expected rate was observed.[134] These and other studies[135] should lay to rest any suspicion of leukemia resulting from ^{131}I therapy of hyperthyroidism.

Carcinogenesis

The concern that ^{131}I therapy may induce thyroid adenomas and cancer stems from four sources:

1. The increased incidence of thyroid cancer following external beam therapy to the neck for thymic, facial, and nasopharyngeal lesions in both children and adults[136,137];
2. The increased incidence of thyroid cancer in atomic bomb survivors and those exposed to test explosion radiation[138,139];
3. Thyroid tumors in rats given radioiodine[140,141]; and
4. Sporadic reports of thyroid malignancy following ^{131}I therapy.[142,143]

This question was addressed by the Thyrotoxicosis Follow-Up Study Group.[144] Among 16,000 patients treated by ^{131}I for hyperthyroidism, the incidence of thyroid cancer was one sixth that which might be predicted based upon the incidence found in patients who had undergone thyroid sur-

Table 7. Gonadal Radiation Dose (in cGy) from Diagnostic Procedures and ^{131}I Therapy

PROCEDURE	MALES *Median*	MALES *Range*	FEMALES *Median*	FEMALES *Range*
Barium meal	0.03	0.005–0.23	0.34	0.06–0.83
Intravenous pyelogram	0.43	0.015–2.09	0.59	0.27–1.16
Retrograde pyelogram	0.58	0.15–2.09	0.52	0.085–1.4
Barium enema	0.3	0.095–1.59	0.87	0.46–1.75
Femur x-ray film	0.92	0.23–1.71	0.24	0.058–0.68
^{131}I therapy (5 mCi)	0.4	—	<2.0	

Robertson JM, Gorman CA: Gonadal radiation dose and its genetic significance in radioiodine therapy of hyperthyroidism. *J Nucl Med* 17:826, 1976.

gery. The lower incidence of thyroid neoplasm following ^{131}I therapy is thought to be due to follicle cell destruction that reduces or eliminates the capacity of the cells to respond to TSH.

Another large Swedish study examined the incidence of cancer in 10,552 patients treated with ^{131}I for hyperthyroidism and found a *possible* radiogenic excess for stomach cancer.[134] The risk for malignant lymphoma was significantly below expectation. These and other studies have concluded that ^{131}I imposes no risk for the development of thyroid cancer.[135,145,146] There appears at this time to be no or only minimal risk of increased incidence of any cancer type as a consequence of ^{131}I therapy for hyperthyroidism.

GENETIC DAMAGE

With all therapeutic applications of radionuclides, the genetic risk must be assessed for individuals of childbearing age in order to provide intelligent family counseling. The assessment of risk is somewhat easier for females than for males, because the ova are nonrenewing. Robertson and Gorman[147] have estimated that the radiation dose received by the ovaries is approximately the same as that for the whole body. Given a peak PB^{131}I level of 1.0% of the administered dose per liter, the gonadal dose is about 0.4 cGy/mCi or about 0.01 cGy/MBq. For an administered dose of 5 mCi (185 MBq), this would result in about 2 cGy to the ovaries. This gonadal dose is about the same as that delivered during such diagnostic radiological procedures as barium enemas and intravenous pyelograms (Table 7). To examine the genetic consequences of this dose, it is interesting to relate the reasoning and analysis of DeGroot et al (Ref.1, p.423):

"If the radiation data derived from Drosophila and lower vertebrates are applied to human radiation exposure (a tenuous but not illogical assumption in the light of present limited knowledge), the increased risk of visible mutational defects in the progeny can be calculated. On the basis of administration to the entire population of sufficient ^{131}I to deliver 2 cGy or 2% of the doubling dose (assumed to be the same as in the mouse), the increase in the rate of mutational defects would ultimately be about 0.04%, although only one-tenth would be seen in the first generation. Obviously only a minute fraction of the population will ever receive therapeutic ^{131}I. The incidence of thyrotoxicosis is perhaps 0.03% per year, or 1.4% for the normal life span. At least one-half of these persons will have their disease after the childbearing age has passed. Although most of them will be women, this fact does not affect the calculations after a lapse of a few generations. Assuming that the entire exposed population receives ^{131}I therapy in an average amount of 5 mCi, the increase in congenital genetic damage would be on the order of 0.02 (present congenital defect rate) × 0.02 (^{131}I radiation to the gonads as a fraction of the doubling dose) × 0.014 (the fraction of the population ever at risk) × 0.5 (the fraction of patients of childbearing age) = 0.0000028."

This relatively crude estimate, which has been derived from several sources, implies that if all patients with thyrotoxicosis were treated with ^{131}I, the number of birth defects might ultimately increase from 4% (the rate of birth defects in the general population) to 4.0003%. From the same source:

"Unfortunately, it is more difficult to provide a reliable estimate of the increased risk of genetic damage in the offspring of any given treated patient. Calculations such as the above simply state the problem for the whole population. Since most of the mutations are recessive, they appear in the children only when paired with another recessive gene derived from the normal complement carried by all persons. The increased chance of a treated mother having an abnormal child would certainly be higher than the 0.00028% noted above for the entire population, but how much higher is uncertain. Assuming that only one parent receives radiation from ^{131}I therapy amounting to 2% of the doubling dose, the risk of apparent birth defects in the patient's children might increase from the present 4.0% to 4.004%: 0.02 (present genetic defect rate) × 0.02 (fraction of the doubling dose) × 0.1 (fraction of defects appearing in the first generation) = 0.00004, or an increase from 4.0 to 4.004%."

Obviously, with such low rates of genetic expression, it is unlikely that any clinical study will demonstrate a genetic effect. Hayek et al studied 150 children delivered by 110 mothers who had previously received ^{131}I therapy.[148] There was no increase in congenital abnormalities, prematurity, or birth mishaps in this group compared with an age-matched

Table 8. Radiation Dose Estimates for ^{131}I in Hyperthyroid Patients* as a Function of Maximum Thyroid Uptake

ORGAN	ESTIMATED RADIATION DOSE (mGy/MBq)				
	20†	*40†*	*60†*	*80†*	*100†*
Bladder	0.94	0.79	0.66	0.59	0.61
Ovaries	0.047	0.045	0.044	0.043	0.043
Red marrow	0.076	0.12	0.14	0.16	0.15
Testes	0.039	0.037	0.036	0.035	0.035
Thyroid	400	760	1040	1200	1100
Uterus	0.063	0.058	0.055	0.052	0.053
Total Body	0.17	0.30	0.39	0.45	0.42

*Adult female (58 kg).
†Indicates thyroid uptake (%) and thyroid uptake half-time = 6.1 h.

control group. Other studies have also failed to demonstrate any genetic effect from ^{131}I for either hyperthyroidism or thyroid cancer.[149–152] Sarkar and colleagues[153] also found no abnormalities of fertility or birth defects among children and adolescents treated with ^{131}I. Given these considerations, it is fair to counsel patients that the risk of genetic abnormalities in subsequent offspring, while calculable, is not demonstrable.

There is very little information available concerning the induction of genetic damage in males. However, it is obvious that sperm cells are renewable. Thus, if conception is delayed (eg, 6 months) after treatment to allow for replacement of sperm mature and maturing at the time of exposure, the risk of transmitting mutations must approach zero.

It is especially important to counsel patients in such a manner that they are left in a state free of anxiety. Each physician must examine these arguments and the data that support them if she or he has any doubt about the efficacy and safety of ^{131}I, before addressing these issues with patients or referring physicians. Physicians must never explore their own attitudes nor resolve their own uncertainties while engaged with patients. To do so would be analogous to a priest wrestling with his own moral conflicts while hearing confession.

Radiation Dosimetry

The radiation absorbed dose to various organs has been calculated for euthyroid individuals for several iodine isotopes by the MIRD Committee.[154] However, more reliable dose estimates for hyperthyroid patients have been calculated by Stabin et al[155] and are presented in Table 8. These authors have also calculated absorbed doses to the fetus in pregnant women who have inadvertently received ^{131}I.

Pregnancy

Pregnancy is an absolute contraindication to administration of ^{131}I because of the danger of substantial radiation to the fetus. In women of childbearing age, ^{131}I may usually be administered within 10 days of the onset of the last menses without a pregnancy test. However, since some patients are not reliable in this regard, it is prudent policy to require a negative pregnancy test before administering therapeutic doses of ^{131}I. Using immunoenzymetric assays for urine human chorionic gonadotropin (HCG), most hospital laboratories today can provide an accurate determination of pregnancy within 15 to 30 minutes. There are also commercial kits available that can be used by technologists in small laboratories. Therefore, pregnancy testing is inexpensive and widely available and should be used routinely prior to ^{131}I therapy. Women of childbearing age should be advised to avoid pregnancy for at least 1 year following ^{131}I therapy in case retreatment is required.

Since ^{131}I is excreted in human breast milk, it should not be given to lactating women.

OTHER TREATMENT

Surgery

Subtotal thyroidectomy, once the principal treatment for hyperthyroidism, has declined greatly, partly because of the safety and success of ^{131}I therapy, partly because of unavoidable surgical complications, and a tendency for hyperthyroidism to recur.[59,156,157] Complication rates, particularly hypoparathyroidism and recurrent laryngeal nerve injuries, are low in the hands of experienced surgeons.[158,159] However, with the declining number of operations, the experience needed to acquire a high level of surgical skill becomes more elusive. Surgical therapy at the Mayo Clinic in recent years has been associated with only a 1% recurrence rate of hyperthyroidism.[160] However, to achieve this, thyroidectomies have become so extensive as to entail a 75% rate of hypothyroidism. In fact, some surgeons now routinely perform near-total thyroidectomy to control hyperthyroidism.[159,161] With such high postsurgical hypothyroidism, there would appear to be no advantage over ^{131}I therapy, and a definite risk of serious long-term hypoparathyroidism. Once hyperthyroidism has recurred following initial surgery, ^{131}I therapy is usually the only practicable therapy because of the high complication rate associated with reoperation in the neck.[162,163]

DeGroot et al[1] list the following clear-cut indications for surgery:

1. Patients who have not responded to antithyroid drugs and who, for whatever reason, are not suitable candidates for ^{131}I therapy;
2. Patients with large toxic nodular goiters that are unlikely to shrink sufficiently with ^{131}I therapy to avoid unsightly appearance or tracheal obstruction (they are more resistant to ^{131}I therapy and cancer is more difficult to recognize in the large, irregular residual goiter);
3. When a suspicion of thyroid cancer exists.

Some would include in this list the presence of severe Graves' ophthalmopathy likely to worsen with ^{131}I therapy. However, progressive ophthalmopathy may be just as frequent following surgery as following ^{131}I therapy.[164]

Antithyroid Drugs

The thionamide drugs carbimazole, methimazole, and propylthiouracil act by inhibiting iodide oxidation and organification and by blocking the coupling iodotyrosines to form T_3 and T_4. They are much more commonly employed as first-line therapy in Europe than in the United States.[165] Antithyroid drugs are most successful in achieving long-term remissions among young patients with small glands and less severe disease. Patients with these characteristics should probably be given a trial of drug therapy for 6 to 12 months before administering ^{131}I. Permanent remission is achieved in 25 to 30% of these patients, but there is evidence that the rate of permanent remissions has been decreasing over the last 40 years, and most thyroidologists avoid long-term antithyroid drug regimens.[1,166] Therapy with antithyroid drugs is generally less effective in toxic nodular goiter than in Graves' disease.

Toxicity due to antithyroid drugs develops in 3 to 12% of patients and consists of fever, pruritus, arthralgia, urticaria, and granulocytopenia.[167–170] The development of hypothyroidism in patients maintained on long-term antithyroid drugs was found by Lamberg to be 0.6% per year.[58]

Therapeutic Applications of ^{125}I

The use of ^{125}I in the treatment of hyperthyroidism stems largely from attempts to reduce the incidence of posttherapeutic hypothyroidism.[171,172] The rationale for using ^{125}I was that its weaker energy gamma and Auger electron emissions originating from within the follicular lumen would deposit more energy in the apex of the cells, which is responsible for hormonogenesis, and spare the more distant follicle cell nucleus.[173] By this means, it was hoped that follicle cell reproductive capacity might be preserved. In practice, however, approximately the same rate of hypothyroidism is found in patients treated with ^{125}I as in those treated with ^{131}I. ^{125}I appears to have no advantage over ^{131}I and it is much more expensive.

Autonomously Functioning Thyroid Nodules (AFTN)

A second type of hyperthyroidism, distinct from Graves' disease, was recognized in 1913 by Henry Plummer[20] and has since been widely referred to as Plummer's disease. This is a type of hyperthyroidism associated with AFTN rather than tissue stimulation by thyroid-stimulating immunoglobulins as in Gravess' disease.

Hamburger[69], in a persuasive revisionist review, makes a good case for the eponymous *Goetsch's disease,* arguing that the surgeon, Emil Goetsch, was the first, in 1918[174] to recognize that:

1. The nodules themselves were responsible for the hyperthyroidism and that their removal cures the hyperthyroidism;
2. The hyperfunctioning nodules began as mitochondria-rich fetal rest cells that gradually develop into toxic nodules as they increase in size; and
3. Removal of hyperfunctioning nodules with cure of hyperthyroidism may be followed by subsequent hypertrophy of other nodules and recurrence of hyperthyroidism.

Goetsch was thus the first to recognize most of the pathologic and physiological characteristics of AFTN that have since become well accepted.

AFTN are uncommon and they are far more often nontoxic than toxic.[175] Hamburger reported an incidence of only 0.9% among all thyroid referrals to his practice in Michigan accounted for only 2% of patients with thyrotoxicosis.[176] In goitrous Switzerland, on the other hand, they are much more common and account for about one-third of all patients with thyrotoxicosis.

PATHOPHYSIOLOGY

The natural history of toxic AFTN is that they are no different from nontoxic AFTN until they reach a critical mass of about 2.5 cm, when they produce sufficient hormone to suppress extranodular tissue.[177] By this time, the TRH stimulation test produces a negligible response. As these nodules increase in size, they produce hormone in excess of daily metabolic needs and hyperthyroidism results. With increasing size, there is a greater likelihood of central degeneration resulting from acute hemorrhagic infarction and this, in itself, may give rise to transient hyperthyroidism.[178] The long-term residual effect may be the presence of a thyroid cyst. Thyroid scintigraphy then reveals a so-called "owl eye" appearance of a central cyst surrounded by a rind of better-perfused peripheral nodular tissue.[69] If sufficient tissue is destroyed by hemorrhage into a toxic AFTN, the thyrotoxicosis may be spontaneously cured. This phenomenon has

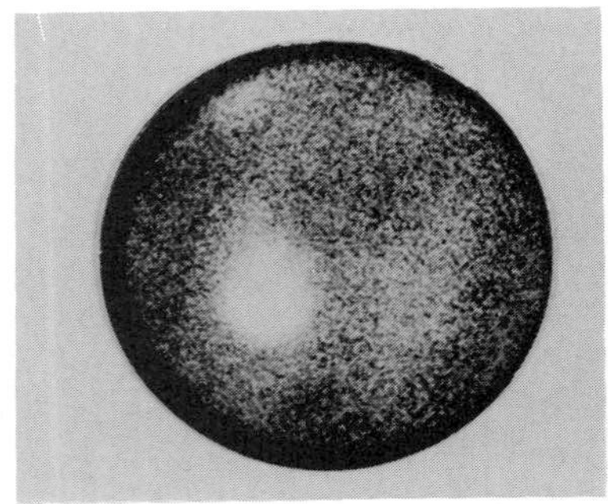

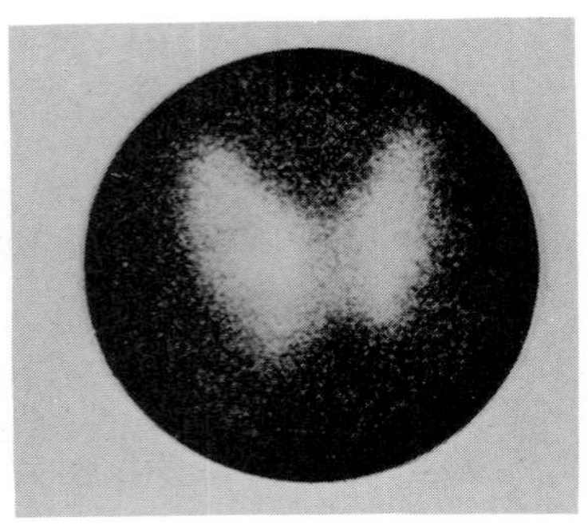

Figure 7. **(A).** Autonomous functioning thyroid nodule with suppression of normal thyroid tissue. (B). Following 8-mCi dose (300 MBq) of ^{131}I, the remainder of the thyroid functions normally. Note that the nodule has not been destroyed, but appears to function at about the same level as normal tissue. The nodule remained palpable.

provided the stimulus for the injection (still experimental) of sclerosing agents as a treatment for AFTN.

While random reports have associated thyroid carcinoma with AFTN, it is now generally believed that this is coincidental and that the association is rare and too infrequent to influence clinical judgement.[69]

DIAGNOSIS

Thyroid scintigraphy reveals one, or occasionally more, discrete "hot" nodules within the thyroid gland (Fig. 7). The degree of suppression of surrounding tissue is thought to be a function of the thyroid hormone secretion of the nodules. In the case of toxic AFTN, circulating thyroid hormone levels are usually sufficient to suppress TSH and, thus, the surrounding normal thyroid tissue will demonstrate very little function. It is important to confirm AFTN with radioiodine scintigraphy, since ^{99m}Tc-pertechnetate is occasionally taken up by thyroid carcinomas that are cold to radioiodine.

It is also useful to distinguish AFTN from compensatory nodular hypertrophy in patients who are not toxic. The latter occur when thyroid hyperplasia develops regionally in response to TSH stimulation of a diseased thyroid gland. Compensatory nodular hypertrophy is suppressed by exogenous T_3. Administration of T_3 is not indicated in thyrotoxicosis, because the nonsuppressible AFTN secretion is additive to the exogenous hormone, thus increasing toxicity.

It is useful to demonstrate the presence of extranodular functioning thyroid tissue, since this tissue will take over hormone production as endogenous TSH rises following ablation of the AFTN. This used to be accomplished by imaging with radioiodine following exogenous TSH injection. Huysmans et al[174] argue against this strategy because the injected TSH can have a stimulating effect for several weeks on the suppressed tissue; this increases the likelihood of ^{131}I uptake by normal tissue during ^{131}I therapy and thus increases the chance of developing posttherapeutic hypothyroidism. Rather, they suggest using ultrasound or ^{201}Tl scintigraphy to visualize extranodular tissue. Ultrasound is also the most accurate means of determining nodule volume, if the therapy strategy depends upon dose per unit mass of tissue.

TREATMENT

^{131}I is the preferred therapy of AFTN.[69,174,179,180] The nature of the disease assures concentration of a large percentage of the dose in the tissue to be ablated, and endogenous suppression protects the normal gland tissue. Following ablation of the nodule(s), the thyroid-pituitary feedback mechanisms assure a return of function to the normal tissue and euthyroidism is usually restored (Fig. 7). Consequently, large doses (30 to 60 mCi) of ^{131}I were formerly recommended for toxic AFTN.[181–183] However, a high incidence of subsequent (and needless) hypothyroidism has forced a revision of this approach.[174,183–186]

Ross et al reported 45 patients with toxic AFTN treated with only 160 μCi/g (mean dose, 10.3 mCi or 380 MBq) of ^{131}I deposited in the thyroid.[186] After follow-up of 0.5 to 13.5 years (mean 4.9 years), no patient had become hypothyroid and 3 patients had borderline hypothyroidism manifested by elevated serum TSH, but normal serum T_4. Euthyroidism was established by 2 months for 77% of patients, by 6 months for 91%, and by 1 year for 93% of patients. Only 3 of 45 (7%) patients required more than one dose of ^{131}I. Late recurrent hyperthyroidism occurred at 4.5, 6, and 10 years in three patients who received single doses of ^{131}I.

Huysmans treated 52 patients with solitary AFTN using a fixed dose of 20 mCi (740 MBq).[174] They followed these patients for 10 ± 4 years. The failure rate (recurrent hyperthyroidism) was 2%. The incidence of hypothyroidism was 6% and was not related to the dose per gram of nodular tissue; thus, this fixed dose appeared to be simple and reliable. They stress that ^{131}I is inappropriate treatment for those patients with unsuppressed normal thyroid tissue, because of the much higher incidence of posttherapeutic hypothyroidism in this group. Rather, thyroid lobectomy is the more appropriate therapy.

In patients who require additional doses of ^{131}I, it is appropriate to retreat with the same dose as the initial one. Because AFTNs are frequently multiple and toxic nodules develop from nontoxic precursors, lifelong surveillance is important.

Surgery. Many respected thyroidologists of long experience believe that surgery for a *solitary* AFTN is the preferred treatment. Surgery reliably removes the lesion and risks of complications from simple lobectomy or nodulectomy are low. Irradiation is avoided and the incidence of postsurgical hypothyroidism is low. Others advise surgery only for patients under 50 years of age, and ^{131}I for older patients and those in whom surgery is contraindicated. We believe that the most appropriate indication for surgery is in patients with AFTN who have unsuppressed surrounding thyroid tissue that will concentrate ^{131}I, thus increasing the risk of hypothyroidism. Both surgery and ^{131}I appear to be safe and effective with few risks of complications when appropriately executed. The patient's preference will probably weigh most heavily in the ultimate decision. One issue that should be made clear to patients is that, with either therapy, the risk of thyroid cancer is low. Occult thyroid cancers are occasionally found in surgical specimens containing AFTN. However, it is well understood now that such occult cancers affect neither health nor longevity. Surgery for AFTN does not decrease the risk of subsequent clinical cancer, nor does ^{131}I therapy increase the risk.

Nontoxic Autonomous Functioning Thyroid Nodules

The question of ablating AFTNs that do not cause symptoms of hyperthyroidism nor elevated circulating thyroid hormones is a more subtle problem. The question arises because it is well recognized that some of these nodules progress and become clinically toxic, while others remain unchanged or undergo degeneration.[22,69,175,187–192] If one can identify those nodules likely to become toxic, it seems prudent to ablate them before a symptomatic disease develops and risks of therapy may be increased. Two questions thus arise: (1) which, if any, nontoxic AFTN should be ablated? and, (2) what is the most appropriate means of ablation? These questions have been reviewed extensively by Hamburger.[69,188] In his group of 147 patients with nontoxic AFTN followed for 6 years or longer, 31 (21%) became toxic or borderline toxic. These patients were predominantly males over 60 years of age, and also patients under 20 years old with nodules 2.5 cm or larger. Furthermore, no nodule that had not become toxic by 6 years after diagnosis later became toxic during 7 to 15 years of follow-up. These findings suggest a subset of patients with nontoxic AFTN that might benefit from prophylactic nodule ablation.

With regard to therapy, the same considerations that apply to toxic AFTN apply to nontoxic AFTN. However, if ^{131}I is elected, certain treatment precautions should be kept in mind:

1. If the remainder of the gland is not fully suppressed by the nodule, it is advisable to protect this tissue from radioiodine by the administration of T_3 (75 μg/day) for 1 week prior to and 3 weeks following the therapeutic dose, thereby reducing the risk of subsequent hypothyroidism. In the few patients made factitiously thyrotoxic by this regimen, the symptoms can usually be controlled with propranolol.
2. The presence of suppressed normal thyroid tissue should be demonstrated by means of ultrasound or by ^{201}Tl scintigraphy.[174]

Thyrotoxicosis in Thyroid Ectopia

Substernal and *intrathoracic* goiters occur when there is a predominant downward extension of a nodular goiter. De-Groot and colleagues distinguish these two conditions by their position relative to the sternal notch.[1] By their definition, "substernal" refers to goiters with the greatest diameter above the level of the sternal notch and "intrathoracic" refers to those in whom it is below the notch. About 70% of intrathoracic goiters are associated ultimately with respiratory symptoms, dysphagia, pain, or compression of intrathoracic veins.[193,194]

Intrathoracic goiters rarely manifest themselves by clinical or laboratory thyrotoxicosis. Rather, they are most often identified by routine radiography and confirmed by radioiodine (not pertechnetate) scintigraphy.[195,196] In a large series reported by Reeve et al only 2 of 161 (1.2%) intrathoracic goiters were thyrotoxic.[195] In most patients, intrathoracic goiters are direct extensions of enlarged thyroid glands in the neck. In rare instances, they may be connected to thyroid in the neck only by a fibrous band. In these cases, they occasionally appear as separate functioning masses and can be missed by a pinhole collimator image of the neck.[197] The treatment for intrathoracic goiter is surgical removal, especially when compression symptoms exist. If surgery is contraindicated, they may be treated with ^{131}I in a manner identical to AFTN.

Struma ovarii are ovarian teratomas derived from pluripotential embryonal cells. In one series of 297 ovarian teratomas, identifiable thyroid tissue was present in 2.7% of patients.[198] In rare cases, thyrotoxicosis may develop.[199] Such patients may be expected to have low serum TSH, low thyroid uptake, and small thyroid glands. The treatment is surgical removal because up to 20% of these tumors contain malignant elements[200] and some may develop metastases.[201]

Graves' Disease in Children and Adolescents

While thyrotoxicosis in childhood may be caused by AFTN, the vast majority of cases are due to Graves' disease and the pathogenesis is the same as that in adults (see above). Still, the disease is rare in childhood and is very rare before the age of 5 years; the peak incidence in children is at 11 to 15 years of age.[202]

CLINICAL MANIFESTATIONS

The clinical signs and symptoms of childhood Graves' disease are similar to those in adults: goiter, nervousness or restlessness, tachycardia, tremor, and weight loss. Exophthalmos is also common, although it is generally not as severe as in adults, and usually abates with treatment.[203] Behavioral changes, often quite subtle and easily attributable

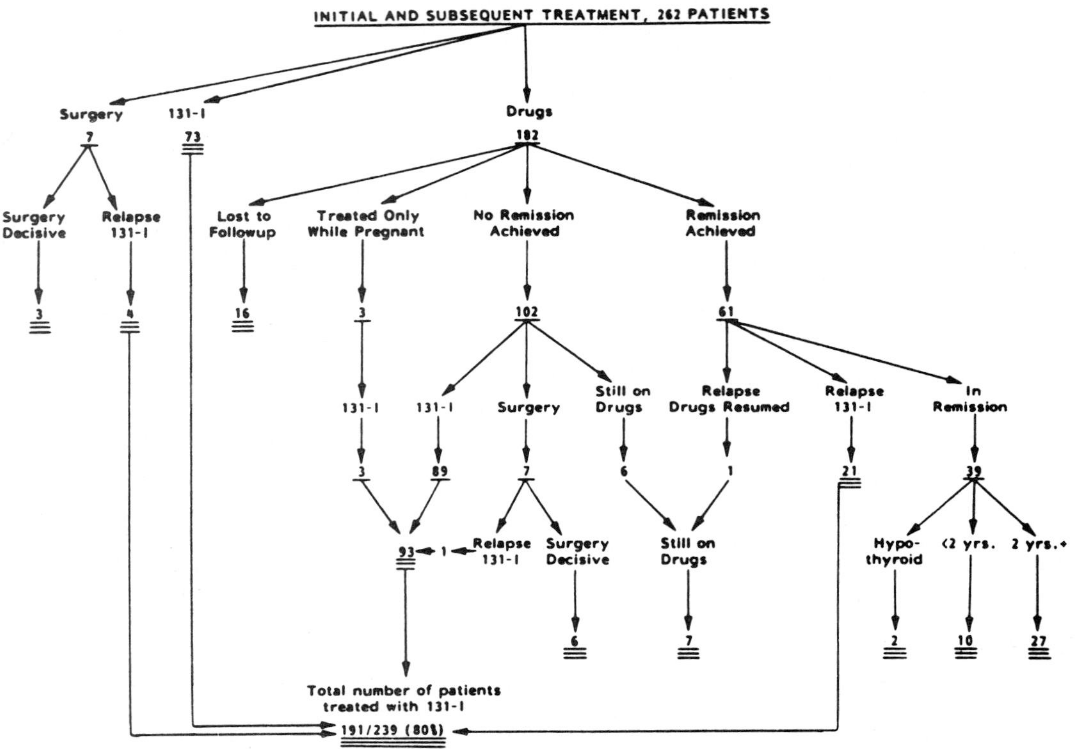

Figure 8. Course of treatment for 262 children and adolescents with Graves' disease. *Triple underlining* indicates the final treatment status of the patients. The three pregnant patients could not receive their first-choice therapy (^{131}I) until after pregnancy. (From Hamburger JI: Management of hyperthyroidism in children and adolescents. *J Endocrinol Metab* 60:109, 1985. With permission.)

to environmental factors, include declining school performance, temper tantrums, irritability, and excessive crying. The height and bone age of hyperthyroid children is usually advanced at the time of diagnosis, while weight is often decreased.[203] In addition, coexisting conditions are more frequently found in childhood Graves' disease, including diabetes, Down's syndrome, vitiligo, rheumatoid arthritis, acute nephritis, hyperlipidemia, and asthma.[204]

DIAGNOSIS

The laboratory diagnosis is essentially the same as in adults; both total and free T_3 and T_4 are elevated and TSH is low. Antithyroid immunoglobulins are elevated, but their measurement is usually not essential, unless another cause of thyrotoxicosis is contemplated. Thyroid scintigraphy is usually not necessary unless a nodule is palpable. The thyroid uptake is useful in determining the administered dose of ^{131}I.

TREATMENT

Pediatric thyroidologists traditionally have been reluctant to use ^{131}I in children for fear of inducing neoplasia and genetic abnormalities. Rather, they have preferred to rely on antithyroid drugs[1,204–210] or surgery,[211–213] despite generally discouraging results with both. However, with the ever-mounting experience of children treated with ^{131}I, prejudice against its use is declining.[148,149,152,203,214–216]

A good case for the use of ^{131}I in childhood Graves' disease can be made:

1. Several studies with long-term follow-up have shown no effect on the incidence of neoplasm, birth mishap, or congenital anomaly as a result of radioiodine therapy of hyperthyroidism. Actually, the radiation dose to the gonads is no higher than some diagnostic radiographic procedures (see Table 7).
2. Surgery for childhood Graves' disease is associated with a high rate of recurrence, a higher complication rate than in adults, and a small, but unavoidable mortality.[160,217–219] To achieve an acceptably low rate of recurrence, near-total thyroidectomy must generally be performed. Damage to the parathyroids necessitates a complicated, lifelong program of medical therapy. This is one of the chief reasons for avoiding surgery for this disease.
3. Antithyroid drugs have several drawbacks, the most conspicuous of which is failure to achieve remission in more than 50% of patients despite several years of therapy. In fact, some evidence suggests that patients under 20 years of age have a lower rate of remission; Hamburger found less than 5% sustained remission in this group.[177] Other problems include noncompliance (particularly among ad-

olescents); drug toxicity in up to 45% of patients, including granulocytopenia and a lupus-like syndrome[167]; enlarging goiter; and exacerbation of hyperthyroidism.

4. ^{131}I therapy is the most cost-effective of the three treatment modalities for hyperthyroidism.

If one accepts these arguments, ^{131}I becomes an attractive form of therapy for hyperthyroidism in children. A report of a large number of children treated with ^{131}I by Hamburger best amplifies this approach.[220] Figure 8 diagrams the primary and secondary therapeutic modalities and responses to them in 262 children with Graves' disease. The most important point illustrated here is that, of the patients treated with antithyroid drugs and not lost to follow-up, only 39 of 166 or 23% did not require a second treatment modality. Of 191 patients treated with ^{131}I, 163 (85%) were effectively treated with one dose, 17 (9%) required two doses, and one patient required three doses. Ten patients were lost to follow-up. Of these same patients, 161 of 191 (84%) became hypothyroid following ^{131}I therapy. These findings are nearly identical to the University of Michigan experience.[149] Of 51 children who received 100 to 150 μCi/g, 47 (92%) were hypothyroid an average of 14.6 years later. This high incidence of hypothyroidism underscores the necessity of lifelong follow-up in these patients and suggests that children should be started on thyroid hormone replacement as soon as the thyrotoxicosis is controlled.

A dose of 150 to 200 μCi/g of thyroid, equation (1), has most commonly been used for treating children.[149,203,220] Low-dose ^{131}I therapy has been abandoned because persistent hyperthyroidism is common in the early years following therapy and hypothyroidism is unavoidable in later years. The considerations regarding adjunctive therapy are essentially the same as described for adults, adjusted for smaller body size.

REFERENCES

1. DeGroot LJ, Larsen PR, Refetoff S, et al: *The Thyroid and Its Diseases,* Ed. 5. Wiley, New York, 1984.
2. Kendall-Taylor P: Thyrotoxicosis, in Grossman A, (ed) *Clinical Endocrinology.* Oxford, Blackwell Scientific, 1992, p 309.
3. Goodall JS, Rogers L: The effects of the emotions in the production of thyrotoxicosis. *Med J Rec* 1933;411.
4. Stewart T, Rochon J, Lenfestey R, et al: Correlation of stress with outcome of radioiodine therapy for Graves' disease. *J Nucl Med* 1985;26:592.
5. Volpé R: The pathogenesis of Graves' disease: An overview, in Volpé R (ed): *Clinics in Endocrinology and Metabolism.* W.B. Saunders, Philadelphia, PA, 1978, pp 3–29.
6. Werner SC, Ingbar S (eds): *The Thyroid,* Ed. 4. Harper & Row, Hagerstown, MD, 1978, pp 814–843.
7. Sterling K, Chodos RB: Radiothyroxine turnover studies in myxedema, thyrotoxicosis, and hypermetabolism without endocrine disease. *J Clin Invest* 1956;35:806.
8. Raben MS: The paradoxical effects of thiocyanate and of thyrotropin on the organic binding of iodine by the thyroid in the presence of large amounts of iodide. *Endocrinology* 1949;45:296.
9. Plummer HS: Results of administering iodine to patients having exophthalmic goiter. *JAMA* 1923;80:1955.
10. Suzuki H, Mashimo K: Significance of the iodide-perchlorate discharge test in patients with ^{131}I-treated and untreated hyperthyroidism. *J Clin Endocrinol Metab* 1972;34:332.
11. Greer MA, DeGroot LJ: The effect of stable iodide thyroid secretion in man. *Metabolism* 1956;5:682.
12. Taylor S: The evolution of nodular goiter. *J Clin Endocrinol Metab* 1953;13:1232.
13. Marine D: Etiology and prevention of simple goiter. *Medicine* 1924;3:453.
14. Drexhage HA, Bottazzo GF, Doniach D: Evidence for thyroid-growth-stimulating immunoglobulins in some goitrous disease. *Lancet* 1980;2:287.
15. Studer H: Pathogenesis of goiter: a unifying hypothesis. *Thyroid Today,* Travenol Laboratories, Deerfield, IL. Vol 8, No 4, 1984.
16. Gemsenjager E, Staub JJ, Girard J, et al: Preclinical hyperthyroidism in multinodular goiter. *J Clin Endocrinol Metab* 1976;43:810.
17. Cole WH, Majarahis JD, Slaughter DP: Incidence of carcinoma of the thyroid in nodular goiter. *J Clin Endocrinol* 1949;9:1007.
18. Ward R: Cancer of the thyroid. *Calif Med* 1948;68:170.
19. Hamburger JI, Hamburger SW: Diagnosis and management of large toxic multinodular goiters. *J Nucl Med* 1985;26:888.
20. Plummer HS: The clinical and pathologic relationship of hyperplastic and nonhyperplastic goiters. *JAMA* 1913;61:650.
21. Wiener JD: A systematic approach to the diagnosis of Plummer's disease (autonomous goitre) with a review of 224 cases. *Neth J Med* 1975;18:218.
22. Charkes ND: High dose I-131 treatment of Plummer's disease. *J Nucl Med* 1981;22:6.
23. Hollander CS, Nihei N, Burday SZ, et al: Clinical and laboratory observations in cases of triiodothyronine toxicosis confirmed by radioimmunoassay. *Lancet* 1972;1:609.
24. Sterling K, Refetoff S, Selenkow HA: T_3 thyrotoxicosis due to elevated serum triiodothyronine levels. *JAMA* 1970;213:571.
25. Hertz S, Roberts A: Radioactive iodine as indicator in thyroid physiology: Use of radioactive iodine in differential diagnosis of 2 types of Graves' disease. *J Clin Invest* 1942; 21:31.
26. Bartalena L, Marcocci C, Bogazzi F, et al: Use of corticosteroids to prevent progression of Graves' ophthalmopathy after radioiodine therapy for hyperthyroidism. *N Engl J Med* 1989;321:1349.
27. Vestergaard H, Laurberg P: Radioiodine treatment of recurrent hyperthyroidism in patients previously treated for Graves' disease by subtotal thyroidectomy. *J Intern Med* 1992; 231:13.
28. Werner SC: Radioiodine, in Werner SC, Ingbar SH (eds): *The Thyroid.* Harper & Row, Hagerstown, MD, 1978, pp 827–835.
29. Irvine WJ, Toft AD: The diagnosis and treatment of thyrotoxicosis. *Clin Endocrinol* 1976;5:687.
30. Becker DV: The role of radioiodine treatment in childhood hyperthyroidism. *J Nucl Med* 1979;20:890.
31. Spencer RP: Observations on radioiodine therapy of hyperthyroidism. *Int J Nucl Med Biol* 1978;5:195.
32. Rall JE, Sonenberg MS, Robbins J, et al: The blood levels as a guide to therapy with radioiodine. *J Clin Endocrinol Metab* 1953;13:1369.
33. Scott GR, Forfar JC, Toft AD: Graves' disease and atrial fibrillation: The case for even higher doses of therapeutic iodine-131. *Br Med J* 1984;289:399.
34. Roudebush CP, Hoye KE, DeGroot LJ: Compensated low-

dose ^{131}I therapy of Graves' disease. *Ann Intern Med* 1977;87:441.
35. Glanzmann C, Horst W, Madgeburg W: Results of radioiodine ($^{131/125}$I) therapy of hyperthyroidism. *Radiol Clin* 1975; 44:484.
36. Goolden AWG, Frazer R: Treatment of thyrotoxicosis with low doses of radioactive iodine. *Br Med J* 1969;3:442.
37. Silver S: *Radioactive Nuclides in Medicine and Biology,* Lea & Febiger, Philadelphia, 1968.
38. Becker DV, Hurley JR: The impact of technology on clinical practice in Graves' disease, *Mayo Clin Proc* 1972;47, 835.
39. Becker DV, Hurley JR: Current status of radioiodine (I-131) treatment of hyperthyroidism. In Freedman LM, Weissman HS (eds): *Nuclear Medicine Annual 1982.* Raven, New York, 1982, p 265–290.
40. Barandes M, Hurley JR, Becker DV: Implication of rapid intrathyroidal iodine turnover for ^{131}I therapy: The small pool syndrome. *J Nucl Med* 1973;14:379.
41. Jackson GL: Calculated low dose radioiodine therapy of thyrotoxicosis. *Int J Nucl Med Biol* 1975;2:80.
42. Malone JF: Recent developments in dosimetry of radionuclides in the thyroid, in Dumone JE, Malone JF, Van Herle AJ (eds): *Irradiation and Thyroid Disease (EU R–6713).* Commission of the European Communities, Luxembourg, 1980, pp 40–108.
43. Mandart G, Erbsman F: Estimation of thyroid weight by scintigraphy. *Int J Nucl Med Biol* 1975;2:185.
44. McKitrick WL, Park HM, Kosegi JE: Parallax error in pinhole thyroid scintigraphy: A critical consideration in the evaluation of substernal goiters. *J Nucl Med* 1985;26:418.
45. Rasmussen SN, Hjorth L: Determination of thyroid volume by ultrasonic scanning. *I. Clin Ultrasound* 1974;2:143–147.
46. Smith RN, Wilson GM: Clinical trial of different doses of ^{131}I in treatment of thyrotoxicosis. *Br Med J* 1967;1:129.
47. Rapoport B, Caplan R, De Groot L: Low dose sodium iodine ^{131}I therapy in Graves' disease. *JAMA* 1973;224:1610.
48. Hagen GA, Ouelette RP, Chapman EM. Comparison of high and low dosage levels of ^{131}I in treatment of thyrotoxicosis. *N Engl J Med* 1967;277:559.
49. Dunn JT, Chapman EM: Rising incidence of hypothyroidism after radioactive iodine therapy in thyrotoxicosis. *N Engl J Med* 1964;271:1037.
50. Green M, Wilson GM: Thyrotoxicosis treated by surgery or iodine ^{131}I, with special reference to development of hypothyroidism. *Br Med J* 1964;1:1005.
51. Goolden AWG, Stewart JSW: Long-term results from graded low dose radioactive iodine therapy for thyrotoxicosis. *Clinical Endocrinology* 1986;24:217.
52. Alevizaki CC, Alevizaki-Harzalzki MD, Ikkos DG: Radioiodine-131 treatment of thyrotoxicosis: dose required for and some factors affecting the early induction of hypothyroidism. *Eur J Nucl Med* 1985;10:450.
53. Glennon JA, Gordon ES, Sawin CT: Hypothyroidism after low dose ^{131}I treatment of hyperthyroidism. *Ann Intern Med* 1972;76:721.
54. Nofal MM, Beierwaltes WH, Patno ME: Treatment of hyperthyroidism with sodium iodine ^{131}I—a 16-year experience. *JAMA* 1966;197:605.
55. Beierwaltes WH, Johnson PC: Hyperthyroidism treated with radioiodine. *Arch Intern Med* 1967;97:393.
56. Beling U, Einhorn J: Incidence of hypothyroidism and recurrences following I^{131} treatment of hyperthyroidism. *Acta Radio* (Stockh), 1981;56:275.
57. Chapman EM, Maloof F: The use of radioactive iodine in the diagnosis and treatment of hyperthyroidism: Ten years' experience. *Medicine* 1955;34:261.
58. Lamberg BA, Salmi J, Wagar G, et al: Spontaneous hypothyroidism after antithyroid treatment of hyperthyroid Graves' disease. *J Endocrinol Invest* 1981;4:399.
59. Sridama V, McCormick M, Kaplan EL: Long-term follow-up of compensated low-dose ^{131}I therapy for Graves' disease. *New Engl J Med* 1984;311:426.
60. Rappaport B, Caplan R, DeGroot JJ: Low-dose sodium iodide I-131 therapy in Graves' disease. *JAMA* 1973;224:1610.
61. Hamburger JI: Intentional radioiodine ablation in Graves' disease (Letter to the Editor). *Lancet* 1976;1:492.
62. Safa AM, Skillern PG: Treatment of hyperthyroidism with a large initial dose of sodium iodide ^{131}I. *Arch Intern Med* 1975;135:673.
63. Wise PH, Ahmad A, Burnet RB, et al: Intentional radioiodine ablation in Graves' disease. *Lancet* 1975;2:1231.
64. Beierwaltes WH: The treatment of hyperthyroidism with Iodine-131. *Semin Nucl Med* 1978;8:95.
65. Goldsmith RE: Radioisotope therapy for Graves' disease. *Mayo Clin Proc* 1972;47:953.
66. Connell JMC, Hilditch TE, McCruden DC, et al: Transient hypothyroidism following radioiodine therapy for thyrotoxicosis. *Br J Radiol* 1983;56:309.
67. Toft AD, Seth J, Hunter WM, et al: Plasma-thyrotrophin and serum-thyroxine in patients becoming hypothyroid in the early months after iodine-131. *Lancet* 1974;1:704.
68. Bremner WF, et al: The assessment of ^{125}I treatment of thyrotoxicosis. *Clin Endocrinol* 1976;5:225.
69. Hamburger JI: The autonomously functioning thyroid nodule: Goetsch's disease. *Endocr Rev* 1987;8:439.
70. Lerman J: Iodine response and other factors in their relation to mortality in thyrotoxicosis. *N Engl J Med* 1937;217:1041.
71. Thompson WO, Thorp EG, Thompson PK, et al: The range of effective iodine dosage in exophthalmic goiter. II. The effect on basal metabolism of the daily administration of one-half drop of compound solution of iodine. *Arch Intern Med* 1930;45:420.
72. Steinbach JJ, Donoghue GD, Goldman JK: Simultaneous treatment of toxic goiter with I-131 and antithyroid drugs: A prospective study. *J Nucl Med* 1979;20:1263.
73. Crooks J, Buchanan WW, Wayne EJ, et al: Effect of pretreatment with methylthiouracil on results of ^{131}I therapy. *Br Med J* 1960;1:151.
74. Einhorn J, Saterborn NE: Antithyroid drugs in iodine-131 therapy of hyperthyroidism. *Acta Radiol* 1962;58:161.
75. Sterling K, Hoffenberg R: Beta blocking agents and antithyroid drugs as adjuncts to radioiodine therapy. *Semin Nucl Med* 1971;1:422.
76. Shanks RG, Hadden DR, Lowe DC, et al: Controlled trial of propranolol in thyrotoxicosis. *Lancet* 1969.
77. Mazzaferri EL, Reynolds JC, Young RL, et al: Propranolol as primary therapy for thyrotoxicosis. *Arch Intern Med* 1976;136:50.
78. Saunders J, Hall SEH, Crowther A, et al: The effect of propranolol on thyroid hormones and oxygen consumption in thyrotoxicosis. *Clin Endocrinol* 1978;9:67.
79. Wiener L, Stout BD, Cox JW: Influence of beta sympathetic blockade with propranolol on the hemodynamics of hyperthyroidism. *Am J Med* 1969;46:227.
80. Radvila A, et al: Inhibition of thyroglobulin biosynthesis and degradation by excess iodide synergism with lithium. *Acta Endocrinol* 1976;81:495.
81. Berens SC, Bernstein RS, Robbins J, et al: Antithyroid effects of lithium. *J Clin Invest* 1970;49:1357.
82. Burrow GN, et al: Effect of lithium on thyroid function. *J Clin Endocrinol Metab* 1971;32:647.
83. Kristensen O, Andersen HH, Pallisgaard G: Lithium carbonate in the treatment of thyrotoxicosis. *Lancet* 1976;1:603.
84. Spaulding SW, et al: The inhbiting effect of lithium on thyroid

hormone release in both euthyroid and thyrotoxic patients. *J Clin Endocrinol Metab* 1972;35:905.

85. Hagen GA: Treatment of thyrotoxicosis with ^{131}I and post-therapy hypothyroidism. *Med Clin N Am* 1968;52:417.
86. Temple R, Berman M, Robbins J, et al: The use of lithium in the treatment of thyrotoxicosis. *J Clin Invest* 1972;51:2746.
87. Turner JG, Brownlie BEW, Rogers TGH: Lithium as an adjunct to radioiodine therapy for thyrotoxicosis. *Lancet* 1976;1:614.
88. Uller RP, VanHerle AJ: Effect of therapy on serum thyroglobulin levels in patients with Graves' disease. *J Clin Endocrinol Metab* 1978;46:747.
89. Riggs DS: Elevation of serum protein bound iodine after large doses of radioactive iodine. *Fed Proc*1948;7:251.
90. Shafer RB, Nuttall FQ: Acute changes in thyroid function in patients treated with radioactive iodine. *Lancet* 1975;2:635.
91. Becker DV, Hurley JR: Complications of radioiodine treatment of hyperthyroidism. *Semin Nucl Med* 1971;1:442.
92. McDermott MT, Kidd GS, Dodson LE, et al: Radioiodine-induced thyroid storm. *Am J Med* 1983;75:353.
93. Meier D, Hamburger JI: When and how often is it necessary to prepare hyperthyroid patients for ^{131}I therapy with antithyroid drugs, in Hamburger JI, Miller JM (eds): *Controversies in Clinical Thyroidology.* Springer-Verlag, New York, 1981, pp 185–208.
94. Lamberg BA: The medical thyroid crisis. *Acta Med Scand* 1959;164:479.
95. Nelson RB, Cavenagh JB, Bernstein A: A case of fatal thyroid crisis occurring after radioactive iodine therapy. *Illinois Med J* 1952;101:265.
96. Ingbar SH: Thyroid storm or crisis, in Werner SC, Ingbar SH (eds): *The Thyroid.* Ed. 4. Harper & Row, New York, 1978, p. 800.
97. Wartofsky L: Thyrotoxic Storm, in Braverman LE and Utiger RD (eds): *Werner and Ingbars' The Thyroid.* Philadelphia, J.B. Lippincott, 1991, p 871.
98. Das G, Krieger M: Treatment of thyrotoxic storm with intravenous administration of propranolol. *Ann Intern Med* 1969;70:985.
99. Galaburda M, Rosman NP, Haddow JE: Thyroid storm in an 11-year-old boy managed by propranolol. *Pediatrics* 1974;53:920.
100. Riddle M, Schwartz TB: New tactics for hyperthyroidism: Sympathetic blockade. *Ann Intern Med* 1970;72:749.
101. Werner SC, Coelho B, Quimby EH: Ten year results of I^{131} therapy of hyperthyroidism. *Bull NY Acad Med* 1957; 33:783.
102. Edsmyr F, Einhorn J: Complications of radioiodine treatment of hyperthyroidism. *Acta Radiol [Ther]* (Stockh), 1966; 4:49–54.
103. Creutzig H, Kallfelz I, Haindl J, et al: Thyroid storm and iodine-^{131} treatment. *Lancet* 1976;1:145.
104. Davis PJ, David FB: Hyperthyroidism in patients over the age of 60 years. *Medicine* 1974;53:161.
105. Rubenfeld S, Lowenthal M, Kohn A, et al: Radioiodine in the treatment of hyperthyroidism: a seven-year evaluation. *Arch Intern Med* 1959;104:532.
106. Shafer RB, Nuttall FQ: Thyroid crisis induced by radioactive iodine. *J Nucl Med* 1971;12:262.
107. Craswell PW: Vocal cord paresis following radioactive iodine therapy. *Br J Clin Pract* 1972;26:571.
108. Robson AM: Vocal cord paralysis after treatment of thyrotoxicosis with radioiodine. *Br J Radiol* 1981;54:632.
109. Synder S: Vocal cord paralysis after radioiodine therapy. *J Nucl Med* 1978;19:975.
110. Rubin PR, Casarett GW: *Clinical Radiation Pathology,* Vol. 2. Saunders, Philadelphia, 1968, pp. 721–766.
111. Currant RC, Eckert H, Wilson GM: The thyroid gland after treatment of hyperthyroidism by partial thyroidectomy or iodine^{131}. *J Pathol Bacteriol* 1958;76:541.
112. Freedberg AS, Kurland GS, Blumgart HL: The pathologic effects of ^{131}I on the normal thyroid gland of man. *J Clin Endocrinol Metab* 1952;12:1315.
113. Vickery AL: Thyroid alterations due to irradiation, in Hazard JB, Smith DE (eds): *The Thyroid.* Williams & Wilkins, Baltimore, 1964, pp 184–206.
114. Sommers SC: Effects of ionizing radiation upon endocrine glands, in Berdjis CC (ed): *Pathology of Irradiation.* Williams & Wilkins, Baltimore, 1971, pp 408–446.
115. Doniach I: Biologic effects of radiation on the thyroid, in Werner SC, Ignbar SH (eds): *The Thyroid*, 4th ed. Harper & Row, New York, 1978, p 274.
116. Von Hofe SE, Dorfman SG, Carretta RF, et al: The increasing incidence of hypothyroidism within one year after radioiodine therapy for toxic diffuse goiter. *J Nucl Med* 1978;19:180.
117. Holm L-E: Changing annual incidence of hypothyroidism after iodine-131 therapy for hyperthyroidism, 1951–1975. *J Nucl Med* 1982;23:108.
118. Cunnien AJ, Hay ID, Gorman CA, et al: Radioiodine-induced hypothyroidism in Graves' disease: Factors influencing the increasing incidence. *J Nucl Med* 1982;23:978.
119. Gamstedt A, Karlsson A: Pretreatment with betamethasone of patients with Graves' disease given radioiodine therapy: thyroid autoantibody responses and outcome of therapy. *J Clin Endocrinol Metab* 1991;73:125.
120. Einhorn J, Einhorn N: Effects of irradiation of the endocrine glands. *Front Rad Ther Oncol* 1972; 6:386.
121. Fulop M: Hypoparathyroidism after 131-I therapy. *Ann Intern Med* 1971;75:868.
122. Klotz HO, Tomkiewicz S, Witchitz S, et al: L'insuffisance parathyroidienne et la tetanie chronique constitutionelle, in Klotz HO (ed): *L'Insuffisance Parathyroidienne.* L'Expansion Scientifique, Paris, 1962, pp 173–200.
123. Orme MCL'E, Conally ME: Hypoparathyroidism after iodine-131 treatment of thyrotoxicosis. *Ann Intern Med* 1971;75:1361.
124. Dunn JT: Choice of therapy in young adults with hyperthyroidism of Graves' disease. *Ann Intern Med* 1984;100:891.
125. Adams PH, Chalmers PM: Parathyroid function after ^{131}I therapy for hyperthyroidism. *Clin Sci* 1965;29:391.
126. Freedberg AS, et al: A critical analysis of the quantitative ^{131}I therapy of thyrotoxicosis. *J Clin Endocrinol* 1952;12:88.
127. Rosen IB, Strawbridge H, Bain J: Case of hyperparathyroidism associated with radiation of the head and neck area. *Cancer* 1975;36:111–114.
128. Tissell L-E: Irradiation to the neck and hyperparathyroidism, in Kaplan, E (ed): *Surgery of the Thyroid and Parathyroid Gland.* New York, Churchill Livingstone, 1983, pp 188–200.
129. Esselstyn CB, Schumacher O, Eversman J, et al: Hyperparathyroidism after radioactive iodine therapy for Graves' disease. *Surgery* 1982;92:811–814.
130. Rosen IB, Palmer JA, Rowen J, Luk, SC: Induction of hyperparathyroidism by radioactive iodine. *Am J Surg* 1984; 148:441.
131. Bondeson A-G, Bondeson L, Thompson NW: Hyperparathyroidism after treatment with radioactive iodine: Not only a coincidence? *Surgery* 1989;106:1025.
132. Body JJ, Demeester-Mirkine N, Corvilain J: Calcitonin deficiency after radioactive iodine treatment. *Ann Int Med* 1988;109:590.
133. Green M, Fisher M, Miller H, et al: Blood radiation dose after 131-I therapy of thyrotoxicosis. Calculations with reference to leukemia. *Br Med J* 1962;2:210.
134. Saenger EL, Thoma GE, Tompkins EA: Incidence of leuke-

mia following treatment of hyperthyroidism. Preliminary report of the Cooperative Thyrotoxicosis Therapy Follow-up Study. *JAMA* 1968;205:855.

135. Anno Y, Takeshita A, Iwamoto M: Medical use of radioisotopes in Japan, especially for treating hyperthyroidism and evaluation of the consequent radiation risk. *Gann Mono* 1970;9:241.
136. Clark DW: Association of irradiation with cancer of the thyroid in children and adolescents. *JAMA* 1955;159:1007.
137. Simpson CL, Hempelmann LH, Fuller LM: Neoplasia in children treated with x-rays in infancy for thymic enlargement. *Radiology* 1955;64:840.
138. Conard RA, Dobyns BM, Sutow W: Thyroid neoplasia as late effect of exposure to radioactive iodine in fallout. *JAMA* 1970;214:316.
139. Sampson RJ, Key CR, Buncher CR, Iijuma S: Thyroid carcinoma in Hiroshima and Nagasaki. *JAMA* 1969;209:65.
140. Doniach I: The effect of radioactive iodine alone and in combination with methylthiouracil upon tumour production in the rat's thyroid gland. *Br J Cancer* 1953;7:181.
141. Doniach I. Effects including carcinogenesis of ^{131}I and x-rays on the thyroid of experimental animals: A review. *Health Phys* 1963;9:1357.
142. McDougall IR, Nelsen TS, Kempson RL: Papillary carcinoma of the thyroid seven years after I-131 therapy for Graves' Disease. *Clin Nucl Med* 1981;6:368.
143. Holm LE, Dahlqvist I, Israelsson A, et al: Malignant thyroid tumors after iodine-131 therapy: A retrospective cohort study. *N Engl J Med* 1980;303:188.
144. Dobyns BM, Sheline GE, Workman JB, et al: Malignant and benign neoplasms of the thyroid in patients treated for hyperthyroidism. A report of the Cooperative Thyrotoxicosis. Follow-up Study. *J Clin Endocrinol Metab* 1974; 38:976.
145. Malone JF: The radiation biology of the thyroid. *Curr Top Radiat Res Q* 1975;10:263.
146. Maxon RR, Thomas SR, Saenger EL, et al: Ionizing irradiation and the induction of clinically significant disease in the human thyroid gland. *Am J Med* 1977;63:967.
147. Robertson JS, Gorman CA: Gonadal radiation dose and its genetic significance in radioiodine therapy of hyperthyroidism. *J Nucl Med* 1976;17:826.
148. Hayek A, Chapman E, Crawford JD: Long-term results of treatment of thyrotoxicosis in children and adolescents with radioactive iodine. *N Engl J Med* 1970;283:949.
149. Freitas JE, Swanson DP, Gross MD, et al: Iodine-131: Optimal therapy for hyperthyroidism in children and adolescents. *J Nucl Med* 1979;20:847.
150. Hollingsworth JW: Delayed radiation effects in survivors of the atomic bombings: A summary of the findings of the Atomic Bomb Casualty Commission, 1947–1959. *N Engl J Med* 1960;263:481.
151. Kitchin FD, Weinstein JB: Genetic factors in thyroid disease, in Werner SC, Ingbar SH (eds): *The Thyroid*, Ed. 4. Harper & Row, New York, 1978.
152. Safa AM, Schumacher OP, Rodriguez-Antunez A: Long term follow-up results in children and adolescents treated with radioactive iodine (131-I) for hyperthyroidism. *N Engl J Med* 1975;292:167.
153. Sarkar SD, Beierwaltes WH, Gill SP, et al: Subsequent fertility and birth histories of children and adolescents treated with ^{131}I for thyroid cancer. *J Nucl Med* 1976;17:460.
154. Berman M, Braverman LE, Burke J, et al: Summary of current radiation dose estimates to humans from I-123, I-124, I-125, I-126, I-130, I-131, and I-132 as sodium iodide. *J Nucl Med* 1975;16:857.
155. Stabin MG, Watson EE, Marcus CS, Salk RD: Radiation dosimetry for the adult female and fetus from iodine-131 administration in hyperthyroidism. *J Nucl Med* 1991;32:808.
156. Colcock BP, King ML: The morality and morbidity of thyroid surgery. *Surg Gynecol Obstet* 1962;114:131.
157. Maier WP, Derrick BM, Marks AD: Long-term follow-up of patients with Graves' disease treated by subtotal thyroidectomy. *Am J Surg* 1984;147:266.
158. Beahrs OH, Sakulsky SB: Surgical thyroidectomy in the management of exophthalmic goiter. *Arch Surg* 1968;96: 511.
159. Lee TC, Coffey RJ, Currier BM, et al: Propranolol and thyroidectomy in the treatment of thyrotoxicosis. *Ann Surg* 1982;195:766.
160. Farnell MB, van Heerden JA, McConahey WM, et al: Hypothyroidism after thyroidectomy for Graves' disease. *Am J Surg* 1981;142:535.
161. Perzik SL: The place of total thyroidectomy in the measurement of 909 patients with thyroid disease. *Am J Surg* 1976;132:480.
162. Crile G Jr: The treatment of hyperthyroidism. *World J Surg* 1978;2:279.
163. Hoffman DA, McConahey WM, Diamond EI, et al: Mortality in women treated for hyperthyroidism. *Am J Epidemiol* 1982;115:243.
164. Hamilton RD, Mayberry WE, McConahey WM, et al: Ophthalmopathy of Graves' disease: A comparison between patients treated surgically and patients treated with radioiodide. *Mayo Clinic Proc* 1967;42:812.
165. Wartofsky L, Glinoer D, Solomon B, Lagasse R: Differences and similarities in the treatment of diffuse goiter in Europe and the United States. *Exp Clin Endocrinol* 1991;97:243.
166. Wartofsky L: Low remission for therapy of Graves' disease: Possible relation of dietary iodine with antithyroid therapy results. *JAMA* 1973;226:1083.
167. Amrhein JA, Kenny FM, Ross D: Granulocytopenia lupus-like syndrome, and other complications of propylthiouracil therapy. *J Pediatr* 1980;76:54.
168. Chevalley J, McGavack TH, Kenigsberg S, et al: A four-year study of the treatment of hyperthyroidism with methimazole. *J Clin Endocrinol Metab* 1954;14:948.
169. Vanderlaan WP, Storrie VM: A survey of the factors controlling thyroid function, with special reference to newer views on antithyroid substances. *Pharmacol Rev* 1955;7:301.
170. Wiberg JJ, Nuttall FQ: Methimazole toxicity from high doses. *Ann Intern Med* 1972;77:414.
171. Gershengorn MC Izumi M, Robbins J: Use of lithium as an adjunct to radioiodine therapy in thyroid carcinoma. *J Clin Endocrinol Metab* 1976;42:105.
172. McDougall DR, Greig WR: ^{125}I therapy in Graves' disease—long term results in 355 patients. *Ann Intern Med* 1976;85:720–723.
173. Lewitus Z, et al: Treatment of thyrotoxicoses with ^{125}I and ^{131}I. *Semin Nucl Med* 1971;1:411.
174. Huysmans DA, Corstens FH, Kloppenborg PW: Long-term follow-up in toxic solitary autonomous thyroid nodules treated with radioactive iodine. *J Nucl Med* 1991;32:27.
175. Silverstein GE, Burke G, Cogan R: The natural history of the autonomous hyperfunctioning thyroid nodule. *Ann Intern Med* 1967;67:539.
176. Hamburger JI: Evolution of toxicity in solitary nontoxic autonomously functioning thyroid nodules. *J Clin Endocrinol Metab* 1980;50:1089.
177. Hamburger JI: Is long-term antithyroid drug therapy for Graves' disease cost-effective? In Hamburger JI, Miller JM (eds): *Controversies in Clinical Thyroidology.* Springer-Verlag, New York, 1981, p 119.

178. Hamburger JI: Transient thyrotoxicosis associated with acute hemorrhagic infarction of autonomously functioning thyroid nodules. *Ann Intern Med* 1979;91:406.
179. Doumith R, De Monteverde JP, Vallé G: Traitement par ^{131}I de 200 cas d'adenomes toxiques thyroidiens. *Nouv Presse Med* 1974;3:939.
180. Scandellari C: ^{131}I treatment of toxic autonomous adenoma of the thyroid, in Fiorentino M, Vangelisto R, Grigiolette E (eds): *Thyroid Tumors, Lymphomas, and Granulocytic Leukemia.* Piccin, Padua, 1972, p 89.
181. Miller JM: Radioiodine therapy of the autonomous functioning thyroid. *Semin Nucl Med* 1971;1:432.
182. Molnar GD, Wilber RD, Lee RD, et al: On the hyperfunctioning solitary thyroid nodule. *Mayo Clin Proc* 1976;40:665.
183. Skillern PG, McCullagh EP, Clamen M: Radioiodine in diagnosis and therapy of hyperthyroidism: Hyperthyroidism caused by hyperfunctioning thyroid adenoma. *Arch Intern Med* 1962;110:888.
184. Fontana B, Curti G, Biggi A, et al: The incidence of hypothyroidism after radioactive iodine (^{131}I) therapy for autonomous hyperfunctioning thyroid nodule evaluated by means of life-table method. *J Nucl Med Allied Sci* 1980;24:85.
185. Goldstein R, Hart IR: Follow-up of solitary autonomous thyroid nodules treated with ^{131}I. *N Engl J Med* 1983;309:1472.
186. Ross DS, Ridgway EC, Daniels GH: Successful treatment of solitary toxic thyroid nodules with relative low-dose iodine-131 with low prevalence of hypothyroidism. *Ann Intern Med* 1984;101:488.
187. Ferraz A, Medeiros-Neto GA, Toledo AC, et al: Autonomous thyroid nodules. I. A clinical classification and the use of a diagnostic index. *J Nucl Med* 1972;13:733.
188. Hamburger JI: Should all autonomously functioning thyroid nodules be ablated to prevent the subsequent development of thyrotoxicosis? In Hamburger JI, Miller JM (eds): *Controversies in Clinical Thyroidology.* Springer-Verlag, New York, 1981, p 69.
189. Lobo LCG, Rosenthal D, Fridman J: Evolution of autonomous thyroid nodules, in Cassano C, Andreoli M (eds): *Current Topics in Thyroid Research.* Academic Press, New York, 1965, p 892.
190. Holm L-E, Hall P, Wiklund K, et al: Cancer risk after iodine-131 therapy for hyperthyroidism. *J Nat Cancer Inst* 1991; 83:1072.
191. McCormack KR, Sheline G: Long-term studies of solitary autonomous thyroid nodules. *J Nucl Med* 1967;8:701.
192. Vague J, Simonin R, Miller G, et al: Diagnosis and evolution of autonomous secreting thyroid nodules, in Cassano C, Andreoli M (eds): *Current Topics in Thyroid Research.* Academic Press, New York, 1965, pp 883–891.
193. Rietz KA, Werner B: Intrathoracic goiter. *Acta Chir Scand* 1960;119:379.
194. Samaan HA, Murali R: Intrathoracic goiter. *J R Coll Surg Edinb* 1972;17:45.
195. Reeve TS, Rundle FF, Hales IB, et al: The investigation and management of intrathoracic goiter. *Surg Gynecol Obstet* 1962;115:223.
196. Lamke LO, Bergahl L, Lamke B: Intrathoracic goiter: A review of 29 cases. *Acta Chir Scand* 1979;145:83.
197. Fogelfeld L, Rubinstein U, Bar-on J, et al: Severe thyrotoxicosis caused by an ectopic intrathoracic goiter. *Clin Nucl Med* 1986;11:20.
198. Gusberg SB, Danforth DN: Clinical significance of struma ovarii. *Am J Obstet Gynecol* 1944;48:537.
199. Emge LA: Functional and growth characteristics of struma ovarii. *Am J Obstet Gynecol* 1940;40:738.
200. Kempers RD, Dockerty MB, Hoffman DL, et al: Struma ovarii—ascitic, hyperthyroid, and asymptomatic syndromes. *Ann Inter Med* 1970;72:885.
201. Wynne HMN, McCartney JS, McClendon JF: Struma ovarii. *Am J Obstet Gynecol* 1940;39:263.
202. LaFranchi S, Mandel SH: Graves' disease in the neonatal period and childhood, in Braverman LE and Utiger RD (eds): *Werner and Ingbar's The Thyroid.* Philadelphia, J.B. Lippincott, 1991, p 1237.
203. Levy WJ, Schumacher OP, Gupta M: Treatment of childhood Graves' disease, *Cleve Clin J Med* 1988;55:373.
204. Howard CP, Hayles AB: Hyperthyroidism in children. *Clin Endocrinol Metab* 1978;7:127.
205. Becker DV: Current status of radioactive iodine treatment of hyperthyroidism. *Thyroid Today* 1979;2:1.
206. Green W, Wessler S, Avioli LV: Management of juvenile hyperthyroidism. *JAMA* 1970;213:1652.
207. Lee WNP: Thyroiditis, hyperthyroidism, and tumors. *Pediatr Clin N Am* 1979;26:53.
208. Maenpaas J, Hiekkala H, Lamberg BA: Childhood hyperthyroidism. *Acta Endocrinol* (Copenh), 1966;51:321.
209. Kogut MD, Kaplan SA, Callipp PJ, et al: Treatment of hyperthyroidism in children. *N Engl J Med* 1965;272:217.
210. Vaidya VA, Bongiovanni AM, Parks JS, et al: Twenty-two years' experience in the medical management of juvenile thyrotoxicosis. *Pediatrics* 1974;54:565.
211. Bacon GE, Lowrey GH: Experience with surgical treatment of thyrotoxicosis in children. *J Pediatr* 1965;67:1.
212. Hedley AJ, Flemming C, Chesters MI, et al: The surgical treatment of thyrotoxicosis. *Br Med J* 1970;1:519.
213. Reeve TS, Hales IB, White B, et al: Thyroidectomy in the management of thyrotoxicosis in the adolescent. *Surgery* 1969;65:694.
214. Crile Jr G, Schumacher OP: Radioactive iodine treatment of Graves' disease. *Am J Dis Child* 1965;110:501.
215. Stanbury JB, Chapman EM: Nonoperative management of hyperthyroidism, in Varco RL, Delaney JP (eds): *Controversy in Surgery.* Saunders, Philadelphia, 1976, p 555.
216. Starr P, Jaffe HL, Oettinger L Jr: Late results of I-131 treatment of hyperthyroidism in seventy-three children and adolescents. *J Nucl Med* 1969;5:81.
217. Ching T, Warden MJ, Fefferman RA: Thyroid surgery in children and teenagers. *Arch Otolaryngol* 1977;103:544.
218. Foster RS Jr: Morbidity and mortality after thyroidectomy. *Surg Gynecol Obstet* 1978;146:423.
219. Hayles AB, Kennedy RLJ, Beahrs OH, et al: Exophthalmic goiter in children. *J Clin Endocrinol Metab* 1959;19:138.
220. Hamburger JI: Management of hyperthyroidism in children and adolescents. *J Clin Endocrinol Metab* 1985;60:1019.
221. Becker DV, McConahey WM, Dobyns BM, et al: The results of radioiodine treatment of hyperthyroidism. A preliminary report of the Thyrotoxicosis Therapy Follow-up Study. In Fellinger K, Hofer R (eds): *Further Advances in Thyroid Research, Vol. 1.* Verlage der Wiener Medizinischen Akademie, Wien, 1971, p 607.

40 Radioiodine Therapy of Differentiated Thyroid Carcinoma

John C. Harbert

The treatment of differentiated thyroid carcinoma has always sparked controversy. Physicians have long differed over the extent of initial surgical resection, over the proper use of adjuvant radioiodine to ablate residual thyroid remnants, and over the best method of treating recurrent disease. Much of this controversy stems from the long life expectancy associated with differentiated thyroid carcinoma, its low incidence in most populations, and its frustrating tendency to recur, often many years after initial therapy. Thus, the efficacy of any management protocol can be analyzed only after large numbers of patients have been treated and after long follow-up periods provide sound statistical bases for comparisons. Several long-term studies, many extending over 20 years, have now been published. Some conclusions are widely accepted and can enter the realm of textbook certitude. Other elements of management still reside within the arena of philosophical judgment and the scope of limited experience. This chapter will attempt to assess the underlying principles of evaluation and therapy and to present a best-reasoned approach to the postsurgical management of differentiated thyroid carcinoma.

INCIDENCE

The thyroid gland is a relatively uncommon site of cancer in the United States, accounting for 0.6% and 1.6% of all cancers among men and women, respectively.[1] During the past several decades the incidence of differentiated thyroid cancer in the United States has been increasing, although mortality has remained constant. The incidence rate in women is twice that in men and peaks earlier for papillary than for follicular carcinoma (Table 1). According to the Surveillance Epidemiology and End Results (SEER) Program of the National Cancer Institute, thyroid cancer is more common among whites than blacks and increased from 2.4 to 3.9 per 100,000 population between 1947 and 1971.[2] The incidence rose again between 1973 and 1977, probably as a result of the emergence of thyroid cancer induced by external irradiation of children for benign head and neck diseases 30 to 40 years earlier.[2,3] In the United States, papillary carcinomas outnumber follicular carcinomas by about 3:1.

PATHOLOGY

Malignant thyroid tumors of all types are grouped according to the classification in Table 2. Differentiated thyroid carcinomas comprise about 80% of these malignancies. Undifferentiated carcinomas makes up approximately 15%; they are not discussed here because radionuclide therapy has no place in their treatment unless they also contain follicular elements that concentrate radioiodine. About 5% of thyroid cancers are medullary carcinomas, which are discussed in Chapter 41.

Differentiated thyroid carcinomas may extend by direct invasion, lymphatic spread, or by angioinvasion and blood-borne metastases. Staging is determined by combined surgical and histopathologic examinations (Table 3).

PROGNOSTIC FEATURES OF DIFFERENTIATED THYROID CARCINOMA

One problem with many large epidemiological studies in determining mortality due to a specific cancer is a failure to compare the survival in the group studied with survival statistics from a population carefully matched in age and sex. For example, Woolner et al examined the survival of patients treated for papillary carcinoma by subtotal thyroidectomy, and followed over 40 years.[4] Patients were divided into 3 groups according to lesion progression: "occult" (now called microfollicular) tumors (<1.5 cm in diameter), intrathyroidal tumors (no capsular invasion), and extrathyroidal (capsular invasion or nodal metastases). Survival in these 3 groups was compared with a normal life table survival curve, the dotted line in Figure 1. From these comparisons, patients with occult and noninvasive papillary carcinomas had normal survival, and only patients with extrathyroidal extension had significantly reduced survival. However, Beierwaltes compared the same data with a survival curve appropriate for a population matched to the ages (20 to 60 years) and sex distribution (3:1 female/male ratio) of the study group.[5] This is the heavy solid line in Figure 1. When this curve is compared with Woolner's data from the Mayo Clinic, all of these cancer populations have subnormal survival. The point that Beierwaltes stresses is that, despite the benign characterization by some thyroidologists, well-differentiated thyroid

Table 1. Thyroid Cancer: Age-Adjusted Incidence Rates in the United States (1973–1977) per 100,000 Population

	MALES	FEMALES	TOTAL
White	2.3	5.2	3.8
Black	1.4	4.0	2.8
All races	2.4	5.5	4.0

SEER program, National Cancer Institute.

Table 2. Causes of Thyroid Nodules

Benign
- Cysts: simple, colloid, hemorrhagic
- Multinodular goiter
- Hashimoto's thyroiditis
- Follicular adenomas
  - Macrofollicular (simple colloid)
  - Microfollicular (fetal)
  - Embryonal (trabecular)
  - Hürthle-cell (oxyphil)
  - Atypical (signet-ring and adenomas with papillae)
- Rare types
  - Cystic hygroma
  - Dermoid
  - Teratoma
  - Subacute thyroiditis
  - Granulomatous disease

Malignant
- Papillary carcinoma (70%)
  - Follicular variant
  - Cystic
- Follicular carcinoma (15%)
  - Hürthle cell type (oxyphilic)
- Medullary carcinoma (5–10%)
- Anaplastic (5%)
- Primary lymphoma (5%)
- Metastatic carcinoma (eg, breast, renal cell carcinomas)

carcinoma is a potentially lethal disease and subtotal thyroidectomy by itself is not reliably curative.

Tumor Histology

Papillary carcinoma is the most common thyroid malignancy worldwide, and by convention includes both pure papillary and "mixed" papillary-follicular carcinomas because their clinical behavior and therapy are essentially the same. The incidence of papillary carcinoma varies with geographic location; in the United States, the incidence reported in two large series was 71% of all thyroid malignancies.[6,7] About 80% of papillary carcinomas are found to be multifocal when serial sections of surgical specimens are made.[8] In about half of all patients, they have spread to regional lymph nodes have occurred by the time of diagnosis.[9] Distant metastases develop in 4 to 25% of patients, depending on the type of therapy received, age at onset, geographic location, and other, less understood factors. Recent evidence suggests that the so-called "tall cell variant" of papillary carcinomas is a more aggressive carcinoma.[10]

Pure follicular carcinoma occurs in about 15% of thyroid cancers in the United States.[11] Both papillary and follicular carcinomas arise from thyroid follicle cells, but they have quite different manifestations. As a group, follicular carcinomas have a somewhat worse prognosis than papillary tumors and occur in an older age group. Distant metastases occur more frequently and mortality is higher.[12] Follicular carcinomas can be further subdivided according to their degree of histologic differentiation. Low-grade follicular carcinomas are well-differentiated and tend to occur at younger ages. Their prognosis is not greatly different from that of papillary carcinomas.[13,14] They are often difficult to distinguish histologically from benign follicular adenomas and are categorized as malignant only because of capsular or microvascular invasion. A second group of follicular carcinomas is less differentiated and displays obvious histologic malignancy; they occur at an older mean age and have a strong tendency for vascular invasion, even from small, nonpalpable primary tumors. Consequently, the relatively benign significance associated with small, "occult" (microfollicular) papillary carcinomas does not pertain to these follicular carcinomas.

Woolner reported 10-year survival rates of only 34% in patients with invasive follicular carcinoma as opposed to 97% in patients with noninvasive tumor[13] (Fig. 2). However, the comparison with an age- and sex-matched population (heavy solid line) again shows that so-called "noninvasive" disease has the potential to kill.[5]

Papillary thyroid carcinomas grow slowly as a rule. Usually, they are discovered incidentally by physical examination for unrelated complaints and appear as asymptomatic thyroid nodules or as a lateral neck mass. The prognosis of these tumors, when confined to the neck and given appropriate therapy and follow-up, is excellent. Woolner reported 3% mortality among 656 patients followed over 40 years.[13] Mazzaferri et al reported only 1% mortality in 576 patients followed over 10 years.[15] In the latter series, prognosis worsened with tumors greater than 1.5 cm in diameter and with invasion through the thyroid capsule. Curiously, the presence of lymph node metastases did not appear to influence the outcome. Even with distant metastases, survival is long, but the ultimate mortality is high with lung, bone, and brain metastases.[16,17] Larger papillary tumors pose a much graver prognosis. Hay found that patients with papillary

Table 3. Staging of Malignant Thyroid Tumors

Stage		
Stage I		
	A	Unilateral
	B	Bilateral or multifocal
Stage II		
	A	Unilateral lymph nodes
	B	Bilateral or mediastinal lymph nodes
Stage III		
		Local cervical invasion with or without positive lymph nodes
Stage IV		
		Distant metastases

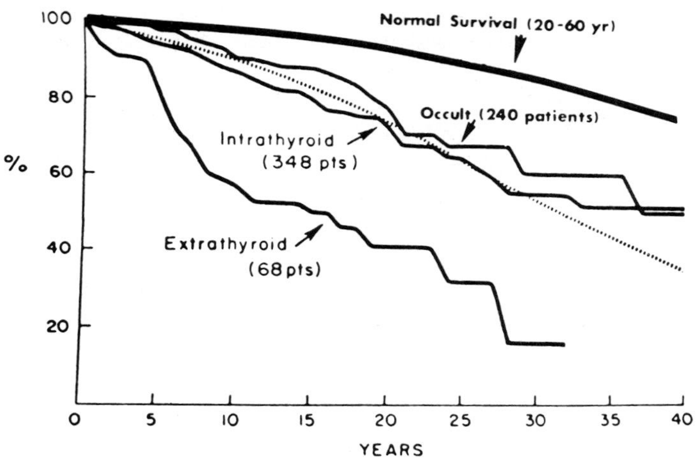

Figure 1. Survival curves in papillary thyroid carcinoma. The original study of Woolner et al[4] compared survivals in patients with occult and intrathyroidal carcinomas with "normal" survival curve (dotted line), which suggests that these two cancers did not significantly reduce survival. However, the survival of an age- and sex-matched normal population (heavy solid line) shows that occult and intrathyroidal papillary carcinomas do reduce survival. From Beierwaltes.[5]

tumors of advancing size, going from 2 to 3.9 cm to 4 to 6.9 cm, and to 7 cm or greater experienced cancer mortality rates of 6, 16, and 50%, respectively.[18]

Capsular Invasion

About 10% of papillary carcinomas have a well-defined capsule surrounding the tumor, which is a particularly favorable prognostic characteristic.[19,20] In such tumors, size may not be a factor in prognosis as long as the capsule remains unbreached.

Small papillary carcinomas occasionally arise in a thyroglossal duct remnant. Such tumors are usually well encapsulated by the cyst. However, even those that metastasize to local lymph nodes usually have a favorable prognosis.[21]

Most follicular carcinomas are encapsulated and, when there is no or only minimal invasion, a favorable outcome is the rule.[22]

Age

Almost all survival studies of both papillary and follicular carcinomas have shown increasing cancer mortality as the age at the time of diagnosis increased. Mazzaferri and colleagues found that tumor *recurrence* increased at both extremes of ages, giving a U-shaped curve.[23] Interestingly, mortality is not increased in well-differentiated thyroid carcinoma of childhood. Buckwalter et al reported only a single death among patients under age 20 at the time of diagnosis, even those followed for as long as 30 years.[24] Despite increased recurrence and increased distant metastases, children usually respond well to therapy.[25,26] In general, patients with well-differentiated thyroid cancer diagnosed after the age of 40 should be treated aggressively.[23]

Sex

Papillary carcinoma is 2 to 3 times more common in females but appears to be more aggressive in males. Some studies report higher mortality among males,[27] while others show no difference in mortality between males and females.[9,15] If sex has prognostic significance, it must be minor.

Multicentricity

As stated above, a large number of papillary carcinomas are found to show microscopic multicentricity on careful sectioning. During routine surgical sectioning, about 20%

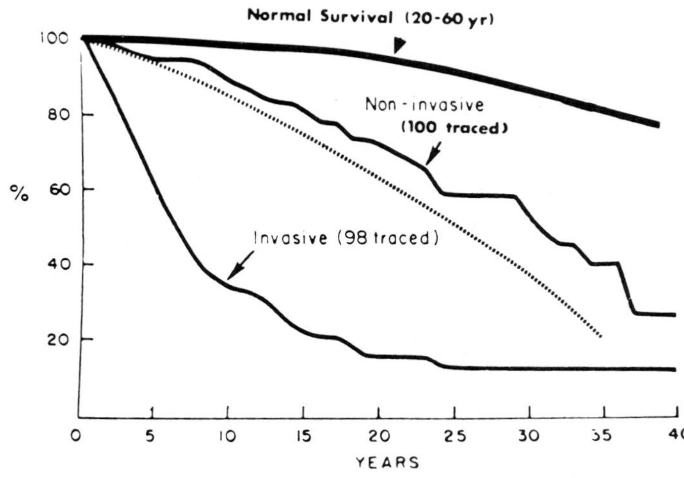

Figure 2. Survival curves for differentiated follicular thyroid carcinoma. The dotted line is the "normal" curve of Woolner.[13] Both noninvasive and invasive disease have reduced survival relative to a normal population matched for age and sex (heavy solid line). From Beierwaltes.[5]

are found to be multicentric.[28,29] Such tumors are thought to represent intraglandular metastases and are associated with greater recurrence rates in the unresected thyroid, more nodal and distant metastases, and more persistent disease.[28] This greater apparent aggressiveness should affect the extent of surgical resection.

DNA Aneuploidy

In recent years, the nuclear DNA content of tumor cells (*ploidy*) has come to be regarded as a good prognostic index of malignant potential.[30] Normal postmitotic diploid human cells contain 46 chromosomes (2n), measuring about 6×10^{-12} g DNA.[30] During cell growth, the amount of nuclear DNA doubles to 4n in preparation for the next cell division. *Euploidy* refers to the condition in which nuclear DNA content is either 2n or 4n. *Aneuploidy* represents a chromosome complement that is not an exact multiple of the haploid (n) number. Several studies have shown that tumor DNA aneuploidy is associated with higher morbidity and mortality.[31,32] Thus far, no recommendations for altered therapy on the basis of DNA content have come forth.

Graves' Disease

Belfiore et al reported a high incidence of thyroid carcinoma among patients who had both Graves' disease and a palpable nodule.[33] Furthermore, these tumors were larger and more aggressive than the same tumor type in patients without Graves' disease. There is some evidence from animal studies that thyroid-stimulating antibodies may accelerate tumor growth.[34] Such evidence suggests the need for vigorous treatment of these thyroid carcinomas.

PATHOPHYSIOLOGY

Normal thyroid physiology has been described earlier. The alterations that occur in differentiated thyroid carcinoma are important because the success of therapy with radioiodine depends upon the tumor capacity to concentrate iodine. Field and colleagues[35] found that both iodine transport and organification were reduced in papillary carcinomas and, to a lesser extent, in benign thyroid adenomas when tested in vitro. The difference between benign and malignant tissues was more pronounced when tested for thyroid stimulating hormone (TSH) response. Organification of iodine was stimulated by TSH equally in benign adenomas and normal thyroid tissues, but had little or no effect in 75% of malignant papillary carcinomas. Some possible reasons for these differences are discussed below.[36]

Impaired TSH Binding

In experimental animal thyroid tumors, Mandato et al[37] found reduced binding of ^{125}I-labeled TSH compared with normal thyroid. The same has been found in some human tumors.[38] Because TSH stimulates virtually all phases of thyroid cellular metabolism, impaired TSH binding might explain the failure of some thyroid tumors to trap or organify iodine.[39–41] Fragu et al[36] studied TSH stimulation of adenylcyclase activity in cell membranes from several primary and metastatic thyroid carcinomas. Such stimulation of adenylcyclase did not differ significantly between normal tissue and well-differentiated follicular carcinomas. However, the response was significantly lower in many moderately differentiated follicular carcinomas and in all papillary carcinomas analyzed. In the same study, there was significant correlation between TSH stimulation of adenylcyclase and TSH stimulation of in vitro ^{125}I uptake.[36] There was some relationship between adenylcyclase responsiveness and tissue content of stable ^{127}I. Most importantly, TSH stimulation of adenylcyclase was lower in human tumors that failed to concentrate ^{131}I in vivo than in tumors that did concentrate ^{131}I. These important studies suggest the possibility of tissue typing to determine the diagnostic and therapeutic efficacy of ^{131}I in individual patients.[42] Analysis of individual data showed some discrepancies; that is, about 25% of tumors responded with increased adenylcyclase activity, but did not concentrate radioiodine. Thus, the response of neoplastic cell membranes to TSH appears to be necessary for iodine transport, but is apparently not sufficient. Additional cellular defects may exist in some tumors to prevent iodine trapping and organification.

Altered Peroxidase Content

Thyroid peroxidase is responsible for oxidizing iodide to neutral iodine (I) or to hypoiodide (IO^{-2}), the only forms of iodine that can be utilized in organification.[43] At least one study has demonstrated a peroxidase deficiency in thyroid carcinoma.[44]

Altered Thyroglobulin Synthesis or Release

Tumor culture and protein extraction studies have demonstrated reduced thyroglobulin (Tg) content or reduced iodination in some thyroid tumors.[36,45–47] In such cases, radioiodine uptake is low and the iodine remaining in the tumor is in the form of iodide or monoiodotyrosine.[36]

Dralle et al[45] found several cases of thyroid carcinoma in which elevated serum Tg occurred with almost no Tg within tumor follicles. They assumed that, in such cases (which also showed no radioiodine concentration in the tumor tissue), Tg is released directly into the serum, bypassing follicular storage. Follicular carcinomas generally are associated with higher serum Tg levels than papillary carcinomas, while poorly differentiated and anaplastic tumors contain almost no Tg. Dralle et al[45] concluded:

1. There is a positive correlation between serum Tg levels and tumor synthesis of Tg;
2. Thyroglobulin synthesis and radioiodine uptake in differentiated thyroid carcinoma often function independently of one another; and

3. Pathomorphological studies suggest that serum Tg levels depend on the number of cells synthesizing Tg and the degree of cytological differentiation.

These studies also suggest the possible value of tissue typing through histochemical techniques to predict the efficacy of radioiodine therapy. Thus far, mechanisms to induce iodine uptake by unresponsive tumors have not been widely explored.

DIAGNOSIS OF DIFFERENTIATED THYROID CANCER IN THYROID NODULES

Prevalence

The most common presenting feature of papillary and follicular thyroid carcinomas is an asymptomatic thyroid nodule or neck mass. Thyroid nodules are common. In as many as 50% of autopsies, the glands contain nodules that had not been suspected clinically and in three fourths of these cases, multiple nodules are found.[48,49] By contrast, solitary nodules are 3 times more common than multinodular goiter in clinically palpable disease. In 2 large studies of children, the prevalence of palpable thyroid nodules was 0.22%[50] and 1.5%[51] Prevalence increases linearly with age, with spontaneous nodules occurring early in life and extending into late life.[52] In the United States, clinically palpable nodules are present in 4 to 7% of adults and are more common in women than men.[52–54]

The incidence of all thyroid cancers within thyroid nodules also varies with locale, age, and sex.[55] While nodular thyroid disease is 4 times more prevalent in females, the approximate female/male ratio for thyroid cancer is only 2:1. Thus, solitary cold nodules are more likely to be malignant in males than in females. Of all thyroid glands that on surgical resection prove to contain solitary nodules, 70 to 80% are benign adenomas and 10 to 30% are malignant.[56–58] This picture is complicated by the problem of truly *occult* thyroid carcinomas, cancer found at surgery or autopsy, but clinically unsuspected (nonpalpable). Sampson et al[59] found the incidence of occult thyroid cancer (<5 mm) in the United States to be 5.7% of all adults coming to autopsy when the thyroid was sectioned every 1 to 2 mm. However, the high incidence of occult thyroid cancers in patients who die from unrelated causes suggests that, in these individuals, it is a benign occurrence.

Presentation

The term "nodule," defined as a palpably discrete swelling within the thyroid gland, is nonspecific and embraces a variety of pathologic processes as outlined in Table 2. Most thyroid nodules are benign. In several recent studies of surgically removed nodules, an estimated 42 to 77% are benign colloid nodules, 15 to 40% are adenomas, and 8 to 17% are carcinomas.[60–65] Factors that increase the likelihood of cancer include a history of radiation exposure to the neck, voice changes suggesting vocal cord paresis, Horner's syndrome suggesting cervical nerve involvement, dysphagia suggesting esophageal compression, and superior vena cava syndrome. Fixation of the thyroid to surrounding neck structures and the presence of enlarged cervical or laryngeal lymph nodes is an ominous sign of invasive disease. Thyroid nodules in males under 20 or over 60 years of age have a high likelihood of malignancy.[66] Rapid tumor growth and nodules over 4 cm in diameter increase the suspicion of cancer. Finally, a family history of medullary carcinoma should always suggest the need for a prompt definitive tissue diagnosis. The sudden appearance of a nodule, especially when accompanied by local tenderness, is usually caused by hemorrhage into a benign lesion. Hemorrhage can occur in malignant lesions, however, especially in nodules greater than 2.5 cm in diameter.

The probability of malignancy increases in nodules that fail to decrease (or that actually increase in size) after several months of thyroid suppression, and in multinodular glands in males under 40 who did not live in a goitrous area and who do not have a history of thyroiditis.

Nodules that have a low incidence of malignancy include the following:

1. Nodules that involve an entire lobe are likely to be caused by subacute thyroiditis;
2. Large, soft nodules with smooth borders are most often benign cysts (Fig. 3);
3. Nodules associated with hyperthyroidism are most often benign cysts.[67,68]

The risk of malignancy is also lower in multinodular goiter than in solitary nodules among individuals unexposed to radiation—approximately 10%.[69] However, among patients who have received childhood neck irradiation, the risk is much higher, 18 to 30%.[70,71] Despite these many associations, all of the above findings are nonspecific. Therefore, additional diagnostic tests are essential. Figure 4 outlines a common diagnostic approach to evaluating thyroid nodules for thyroid cancer.

Laboratory Examination

The only biochemical test that is routinely required is serum TSH to identify patients with unsuspected hyperthyroidism, which increases the likelihood of a toxic adenoma and decreases the likelihood of cancer. Thyroid scintigraphy is then the next most logical test to determine nodule function. Elevated TSH suggests hypothyroidism and the possibility of nodular thyroid tissue enlarging under the stimulus of TSH. Aspiration biopsy will confirm this diagnosis, or one can use ultrasound as follow-up because such nodules usually shrink with thyroxine therapy.

Fine-Needle Aspiration Biopsy

Fine-needle aspiration biopsy (usually with a 25-gauge needle) has become the initial test of choice in the diagnosis

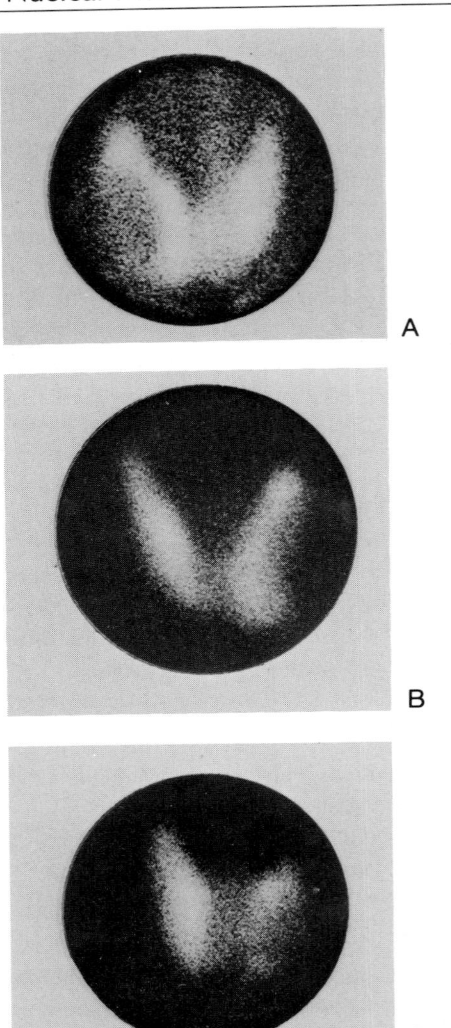

Figure 3. Cold thyroid nodules using ^{99m}Tc-pertechnetate: (A) colloid cyst in right lobe; (B) extrinsic lipoma compressing lateral margin of left lobe. Compare with large irregular thyroid carcinoma in the left lobe (C).

of thyroid nodules because it is safe and more accurately selects patients for surgery than other tests.[72–79] Fine-needle biopsies have had a substantial impact upon the management of thyroid nodules, virtually halving the number of patients who undergo surgery and doubling the incidence of malignant disease in surgically excised nodules.[63,80–82] As a result, the cost of managing thyroid nodules has been significantly reduced. This technique is simple and almost free of complications. Seeding of the biopsy tract is no longer considered likely,[83] and the rare complication of hemorrhage with tracheal obstruction is generally well controlled by external application of cold compresses. However, the participation of an interested pathologist with extensive experience in thyroid cytology is essential to proper interpretation of needle aspirates.

Most aspiration biopsies are negative. In a large series of over 9000 patients,[84] 74% of samples were benign, 4% were malignant, and 22% were indeterminant or the biopsy was inadequate. Of positive biopsies, about half are falsely positive.[84,85] These misdiagnoses are often caused by Hashimoto's thyroiditis.[86]

The reported accuracy of cytological diagnosis ranges from 70 to 97%.[86] These results are somewhat better than earlier reports,[29,72,74–77,80,87,88] most likely due to increasing experience. Most false-negative needle biopsies result from nodules under 1 cm or greater than 4 cm in diameter. Failure in the former case often results from missing the nodule, a rate that can be reduced using ultrasound guidance; in large nodules, fluid may be removed but malignant epithelium may be missed. False-negative aspiration biopsies are often due to sampling error. Depending on nodule size, it may be prudent to make up to five passes through the nodule to assure representative sampling.[89] Cystic lesions should be aspirated and then scanned by means of high-resolution ultrasound to identify a solid component that can then be biopsied.[90] Failure to obtain satisfactory specimens decreases with experience.[75,91]

Hürthle-cell neoplasms (oxyphilic type) are generally considered suspicious, because of the difficulty in differentiating invasive carcinoma from benign adenoma.[79,89]

In summary, if unsatisfactory smears and cores of normal thyroid tissue (occurring when the needle misses the lesion) are eliminated, and categorization is made merely on the basis of malignant versus nonmalignant nodules, the false-negative rate appears to be about 5% or less. Since approximately 20% of solitary cold nodules are malignant, only about 1% of malinant lesions would thus be missed. If these nodules are carefully followed, the risk of delayed surgery appears to be small. Under no circumstance should a negative biopsy dissuade either the physician or the patient from subsequent follow-up examinations at 6-month intervals.

Radionuclide Scintigraphy

Most thyroid scintigraphy is performed with ^{123}I-sodium iodide using a scintillation camera and pinhole collimator. Today scintigraphy is generally limited to patients with indeterminate cytological results after fine-needle biopsy (Fig. 4). The principal limitation of radionuclide scintigraphy is that it cannot distinguish benign from malignant nodules. Rather, it is used to assign a probability of malignancy on the basis of the number and apparent functional status of thyroid nodules. In a review of 22 series in which radioiodine scintigraphy was obtained and all patients underwent surgery regardless of nodular function, 84% of solitary nodules were cold, 10.5% were warm, and 5.5% were hot.[85,92] Of these, thyroid cancer was found in 16% of the cold nodules, 9% of the warm nodules, and 4% of hot nodules. Therefore, the radionuclide scan is useful for defining the functional status of nodules from which rough probabilities of malignancy can be assigned. On the other hand, the study neither excludes malignancy in hot nodules nor distinguishes benign from malignant cold nodules. Since the incidence of carcinoma

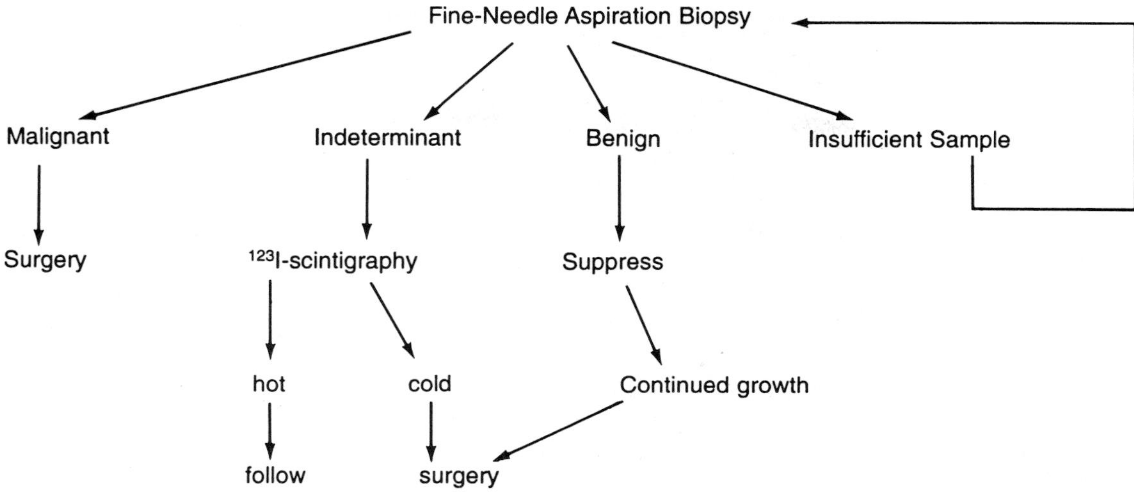

Figure 4. Diagnostic scheme for the diagnosis and management of palpable thyroid nodules.

in functioning thyroid nodules is quite low, they can generally be followed with ultrasound to monitor subsequent growth or involution.

Some endocrinologists prefer to document autonomous thyroid function in "warm" nodules. This is done by ^{123}I scintigraphy following TSH suppression. This technique is discussed in Chapter 39.

Ultrasound

Conventional gray-scale ultrasonography is accurate in determining the number, morphology, and size of thyroid nodules.[93,94] In a review of 16 series by Ashcraft and Van Herle, 69% of nodules were solid, 19% cystic, and 12% mixed solid and cystic.[85,92] Of the nodules operated in these series, malignancy was found in 21% of solid lesions, 12% of mixed lesions, and 7% of cystic lesions. By this classification, solid nodules are most often benign and, at the same time, have the highest likelihood of malignancy. Morphological characterization therefore appears unlikely to distinguish benign from malignant nodules.

With high-resolution real-time ultrasonography, nodules as small as 1 mm can be detected.[95,96] Using this technique, as many as 40% of patients with clinically apparent solitary nodules are found to have multiple "micronodules" (Fig. 5).[95] Thus, ultrasound is a valuable test to help surgeons select the most appropriate extent of resection.

The significance of these micronodules, when associated with solitary palpable nodules, has not been determined. Moreover, high-resolution ultrasonography demonstrates that lesions that appear cystic by gray-scale techniques are not true cysts, but contain some solid tissue that indicates their mixed character.[96] Thus, as noninvasive imaging becomes more refined, traditional classifications and their significance undergo continuing revision.

The attempt to distinguish sonographic patterns unique to cancers has also been frustrated. Most solid carcinomas are hypoechoic, but benign follicular adenomas may elicit the same pattern. It was once thought that the "halo sign", a sonolucent rim surrounding a solid lesion, might be diagnostic of benign adenomas.[97] However, this sign has since been found in association with both papillary and follicular carcinomas.[98] At this time, the principal value of ultrasound lies in the follow-up of suspicious lesions to determine whether growth is occurring, since this is the most accurate means of determining nodular volume.[78] Ultrasound is helpful in pregnant patients who should receive neither radionuclides nor contrast material intravenously. Ultrasound may also indicate whether or not cervical lymph nodes are enlarged.

Thyroid Hormone Suppression

The rationale for suppressing functioning thyroid nodules and aspirated cysts is to assess TSH dependence of the nodule tissue. Many benign neoplasms contain TSH receptors that, in part, regulate their growth. Most carcinomas do not have TSH receptors; that is, they are TSH independent.[99] It was once common to suppress most thyroid nodules in the belief that the majority, being benign, could regress or disappear completely and surgery would thereby be avoided.[100,101] However, the experience of most thyroidologists has shown that suppression of nodules as a routine is largely ineffective. Most nodules, with the exception of aspirated cysts, do not decrease substantially in size.[102,103] Furthermore, reduction in nodule size does not guarantee benignity, since carcinomas have occasionally been reported to regress partially following suppression, possibly due to shrinkage of surrounding normal tissue.[104,105] Today, most clinicians recommend a trial suppression of aspirated cysts containing no malignant cells and nontoxic hot nodules. Suppression must be sufficient (0.2 to 0.3 mg thyroxine per day) to completely suppress serum TSH. In 2 series in which all patients with solitary nodules that failed to respond to hormone suppression underwent surgery, the incidence of malignancy was 20 and 40%.[87,106] Thus, hormone suppression of carefully selected and observed thyroid nodules is war-

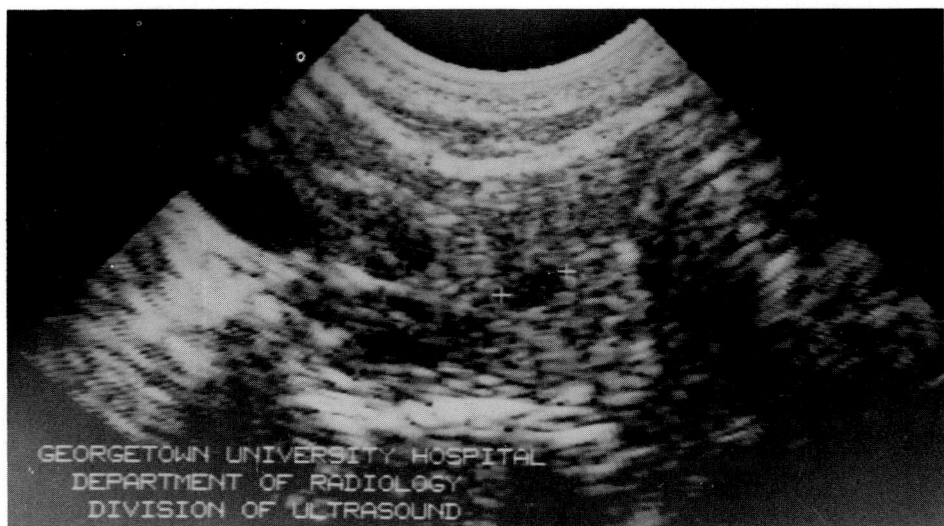

Figure 5. High-resolution real-time ultrasound image of thyroid showing multiple small solid nodules in a patient with a clinical diagnosis of solitary thyroid nodule.

ranted. The best technique for judging a response is to measure lesion diameter with ultrasound. Lesions that do not disappear completely should be removed surgically.[85]

Other Tests

Scintigraphy with ^{201}Tl-chloride has been explored as a means to distinguish primary thyroid carcinoma from benign adenomas.[107] The uptake and washout of this tracer depend largely on regional blood flow. Tenvall et al[107] found that benign adenomas and well-differentiated thyroid carcinomas, both appearing as cold nodules using pertechnetate, could be distinguished from carcinoma by the more rapid washout from carcinoma, but not by the intensity of ^{201}Tl uptake.

^{201}Tl may also be useful in identifying thyroid metastases that fail to concentrate ^{131}I.[108,109] The most likely use for this radiopharmaceutical is in postsurgical patients who have elevated serum Tg that suggests residual tumor, but have negative ^{131}I localization (see below).

Hürthle cell carcinomas, which often do not concentrate radioiodine, have been successfully visualized with ^{201}Tl,[110] ^{99m}Tc-sestamibi,[111] and ^{131}I-labeled anti-CEA antibody.[112] Because uptake of these tracers is not affected by thyroid function, hormone therapy need not be interrupted prior to scintigraphy.

^{131}Cs-chloride, ^{67}Ga-citrate, and ^{75}Se-selenomethionine have all been used to evaluate thyroid nodules. None has been reliable in differentiating benign from malignant disease.[91]

Patton and colleagues[113,114] measured the iodine content of solitary thyroid nodules by fluorescent scanning to distinguish benign from malignant lesions. They showed that a nodule iodine content 60% of normal adjacent thyroid tissue or greater was highly (99%) specific for benign lesions. However, the sensitivity was only 63%, that is, most malignant tumors and many benign lesions have a low iodine content.

Radiolabeled Antithyroglobulin

Scintigraphy with radiolabeled antithyroglobulin is a logical extension of the rapidly developing field of radioimmunometric detection. Fairweather et al[115] studied 12 patients with follicular and papillary carcinomas using IgG antibody to human thyroglobulin labeled with ^{131}I. They identified 34 of 40 tumor deposits (85%) by antibody scintigraphy, while only 16 (40%) were positive with ^{131}I. Thus, radiolabeled antibody scanning may replace or supplement ^{131}I scintigraphy for detecting thyroid metastases.[116]

Thyroid Nodules in Children

The significance of thyroid nodules in children is somewhat different from that in adults because infections and developmental abnormalities are more common.[117,118] Nevertheless, cancers occur; the incidence in excised solitary thyroid nodules ranges from 14 to 60%.[89,117] Fine-needle aspiration may be more difficult because young children are often uncooperative, short of anesthesia. Therefore, ultrasound to evaluate size and number of nodules and ^{123}I scintigraphy to exclude hyperfunctioning nodules are more common initial diagnostic studies. Solitary hypofunctioning nodules are usually surgically removed.

CLINICAL STAGING OF DIFFERENTIATED THYROID CARCINOMA

Multivariate Analysis

Given the large number of prognostic features, both tumor-related and patient-related, that appear to affect outcome, several studies have been reported using multivariate analysis to predict survival and to select the most appropriate therapy. Most of these studies find that age at diagnosis, sex, tumor size, principal cell type, and presence of metastases have been the most sensitive features in predicting survival.[119–130] These various studies are well reviewed by Mazzaferri.[23] Of note is that few of these analyses agree on either the most sensitive prognostic factors, or their order of importance. The probable reason for this is that none of these studies used treatment factors in analyzing outcome.

Several clinical staging systems have been devised to select the most important therapy and to facilitate comparative studies. These vary because there is no consensus about the relative importance of the above-described prognostic variables. Four of these systems will be described here.

AGES SYSTEM

Hay and colleagues[131] evaluated prognostic variables in 860 patients with papillary carcinoma and developed a prognostic scoring system, called AGES, based on patient *a*ge, tumor *g*rade, *e*xtent, and *s*ize. The AGES score, based on regression analysis, was equal to 0.05 × age in years if age 40 or more or 0 if less than 40 years of age; +1 if grade 2 histologic tumor or +3 if grade 3 or 4; +1 if extrathyroid or +3 if distant metastases; +0.02 × tumor size (maximum diameter in centimeters). Patients were then divided into four groups with AGES scores of 0 to 3.99 (739 patients), 4 to 4.99 (61 patients), 5 to 5.99 (30 patients), and 6+ (30 patients). The 25-year cancer mortality rates in the four groups were 2%, 7%, 49%, and 93%, respectively. As is apparent, this scoring system is highly age-dependent.

AMES SYSTEM

Cady and Rossi[132] analyzed 821 patients with differentiated thyroid carcinoma according to *a*ge at diagnosis, *m*etastases to distant sites other than lymph nodes, *e*xtent of primary tumor, and *s*ize larger than 5 cm. Patients were divided into *low-risk* and *high-risk* categories. The low-risk category included younger patients (men <41 and women <51 years) without distant metastases whose primary tumors were smaller than 5 cm, and were either intrathyroidal, or with minor capsular invasion. The high-risk category included all older patients, tumors larger than 5 cm, or with distant metastases. These groups were followed for a minimum of 5 years. In the low-risk category, there was a recurrence rate of only 5%, and 1.8% had died. These authors advocated conservative treatment for low-risk patients (ie, lobectomy with isthmectomy, provided the primary tumor is resected with wide margins. Few of these patients were treated with ^{131}I.

MAZZAFERRI SYSTEM

Mazzaferri[23] analyzed 1133 patients with differentiated thyroid carcinoma, dividing patients into 4 stages (Table 4) according to the size and extent of their local and distant disease, without regard to cervical lymph node involvement. These patients were followed from 3 to 10 years. As can be seen, the Stage IV patients were significantly older than other stages, and there is a generally increasing rate of local and distant recurrence and cancer death through the increasing stages. Mazzaferri believes that treatment is better based on tumor stage than primarily on age, because younger patients with relatively high risk tumors are more appropriately selected for aggressive treatment.

THERAPY

Surgery

The primary treatment of thyroid cancer is surgical and the outcome depends to a great extent upon the skill of the surgeon.[6] In the past, opinion varied widely as to the extent of excision, although today there is much greater agreement. Solitary thyroid nodules found to be malignant should be removed by total lobectomy and isthmectomy. If ultrasound has shown nodularity in the contralateral lobe, that affected tissue is resected as well. The specimens are submitted immediately for frozen section. If the tumor is multiple, if there is capsular or vascular invasion, extension beyond the thyroid, or if a solitary carcinoma is larger than 1.5 cm, most surgeons today advocate a "near-total" thyroidectomy: an effort to resect as much thyroid as possible while preserving the parathyroids and protecting the recurrent laryngeal nerves.[133] The morbidity associated with "total" thyroidectomy is high and is largely unnecessary, given the effectiveness of postoperative high-dose ablation with radioiodine in removing residual functioning thyroid from the neck.

The case for near-total thyroidectomy as opposed to lobectomy is enormously strengthened by the 38 to 87% prevalence of multifocal (often microscopic) thyroid cancer in the contralateral lobe of patients undergoing thyroidectomy for a lesion apparently confined to one lobe.[8,134] The incidence of recurrence following lobectomy alone varies from 2 to 40%, with most series reporting 5 to 10%.[134–139]

In the series of 800 patients with papillary thyroid carcinoma analyzed by McConahey et al,[140] the recurrence rates during the first 2 years were fourfold greater after unilateral lobectomy than after total or near-total thyroidectomy (26% versus 6%, $P = 0.01$). In the above cited series of 1133 patients analyzed by Mazzaferri,[23] recurrence rates were fivefold greater, distant metastases occurred with about twice the frequency, and cancer death rates were much more frequent after subtotal lobectomy compared with subtotal or near-total thyroidectomy. In fact, multivariate analysis indicated that subtotal lobectomy is an *independent variable* associated with both a higher cumulative recurrence rate ($P = 0.0001$) and a higher overall death rate ($P = 0.01$).

A second argument for near-total thyroidectomy is that postsurgical thyroid ablation with ^{131}I is more effective and requires smaller doses as the mass of residual thyroid remnant decreases.[141,142] Near-total thyroidectomy results in hypothyroidism and elevated TSH, which enhances early detection of functioning metastases. Finally, there is a well-documented tendency for recurrent thyroid cancer to progress to highly aggressive anaplastic carcinoma.[143–145]

Table 4. Mazzaferri Staging System

	STAGES			
	I	*II*	*III*	*IV*
Tumor Characteristics				
Diameter (cm)	<1.5	1.5–4.4	≥4.5	Any
Involvement	or one lobe	or two lobes	or entire gland	Any
Local invasion	none	none	yes	Any
Distant metastases	none	none	none	Yes
Group Characteristics				
Age (y ± SE)	35.1 ± 0.7	32.9 ± 0.5	37.1 ± 1.3	50.9 ± 19.5
Recurrences	6.8%	17.4%	36.2%	50.0%
Distant recurrences	0	2.9%	8.0%	16.7%
Cancer deaths	0.4%	1.3%	9.1%	60.0%
Follow-up (median y)	10	9.8	9	3

Data from Mazzaferri.[23]

The neck is, of course, carefully palpated at the time of surgery and any suspicious nodes are excised. Ultrasound is also useful in identifying enlarged cervical nodes. The pre- and paratracheal lymph nodes are the most common sites of nodal metastases and should be removed routinely.[146,147] If these nodes contain tumor, the superior mediastinal nodes approachable through the thyroidectomy incision should be removed and a modified neck dissection undertaken.[148] In the absence of demonstrable nodal metastases, the value of node dissection is unproven. In neither papillary nor follicular carcinoma is there a statistically greater rate of recurrence or death among patients who have no lymph node surgery when nodal metastases are not detected at surgery.[12,139,149] On the other hand, Mazzaferri and Young[149] found that the risk of recurrence in patients with positive nodes who are less than 40 years of age is twofold higher than in patients without nodal metastases, and fivefold higher in patients over 40 who have positive nodes.

POSTOPERATIVE MANAGEMENT

Figure 6 outlines a guide to the postoperative diagnosis and management of well-differentiated thyroid carcinoma; the protocol has been derived from several sources, and represents a reasonable approach to reducing recurrence rates and increasing the disease-free interval. Most authorities recommend that small, unifocal cancers be treated conservatively.[5,9,149–151] Woolner was the first to describe the relatively benign clinical behavior and excellent prognosis of occult papillary thyroid carcinoma (<1.5 cm in diameter with or without nodal metastases).[9] These lesions accounted for 26% of well-differentiated cancers studied by Mazzaferri and Young.[149] In their series, the difference in recurrence rates between patients who underwent subtotal versus total thyroidectomy was not significant, and no deaths from thyroid cancer occurred during 6 to 10 years of follow-up. Thyroid ablation is therefore not recommended in these patients unless disease recurs (4.8% in the review by Mazzaferri and Young[149]). Patients are followed with annual chest x-rays and careful physical examinations throughout their lifetime. Serum TSH levels should be completely suppressed by adequate thyroid hormone replacement.[27,99,149]

In patients with carcinomas larger than 1.5 cm, capsular or vascular invasion, multifocal disease, or with extrathyroidal extension, thyroid ablation and total body metastatic surveys are indicated. The same is recommended for small, follicular carcinomas that are less well differentiated and for Hürthle cell carcinomas.

Thyroid Ablation With ^{131}I

The value of postsurgical ablation of thyroid remnants with ^{131}I is now generally recognized in the management of well-differentiated thyroid carcinoma. This rationale stems from the following observations:

1. Excision of the thyroid gland is seldom complete, even when total thyroidectomy is attempted. Postoperative ^{131}I scans usually demonstrate some functioning thyroid tissue.[152,153]
2. Thyroid carcinoma, especially papillary, is multifocal in 20 to 30% of cases.
3. Ablation induces hypothyroidism, which, by stimulating secretion of TSH, increases the likelihood of demonstrating functioning thyroid metastases if they exist or should develop.[154,155] While near-total thyroidectomy usually induces hypothyroidism, sufficient residual tissue may remain and hypertrophy to maintain TSH within normal levels.[156]
4. Ablation eliminates intense uptake in normal or hypertrophied thyroid remnants that may conceal the development of functioning metastases.

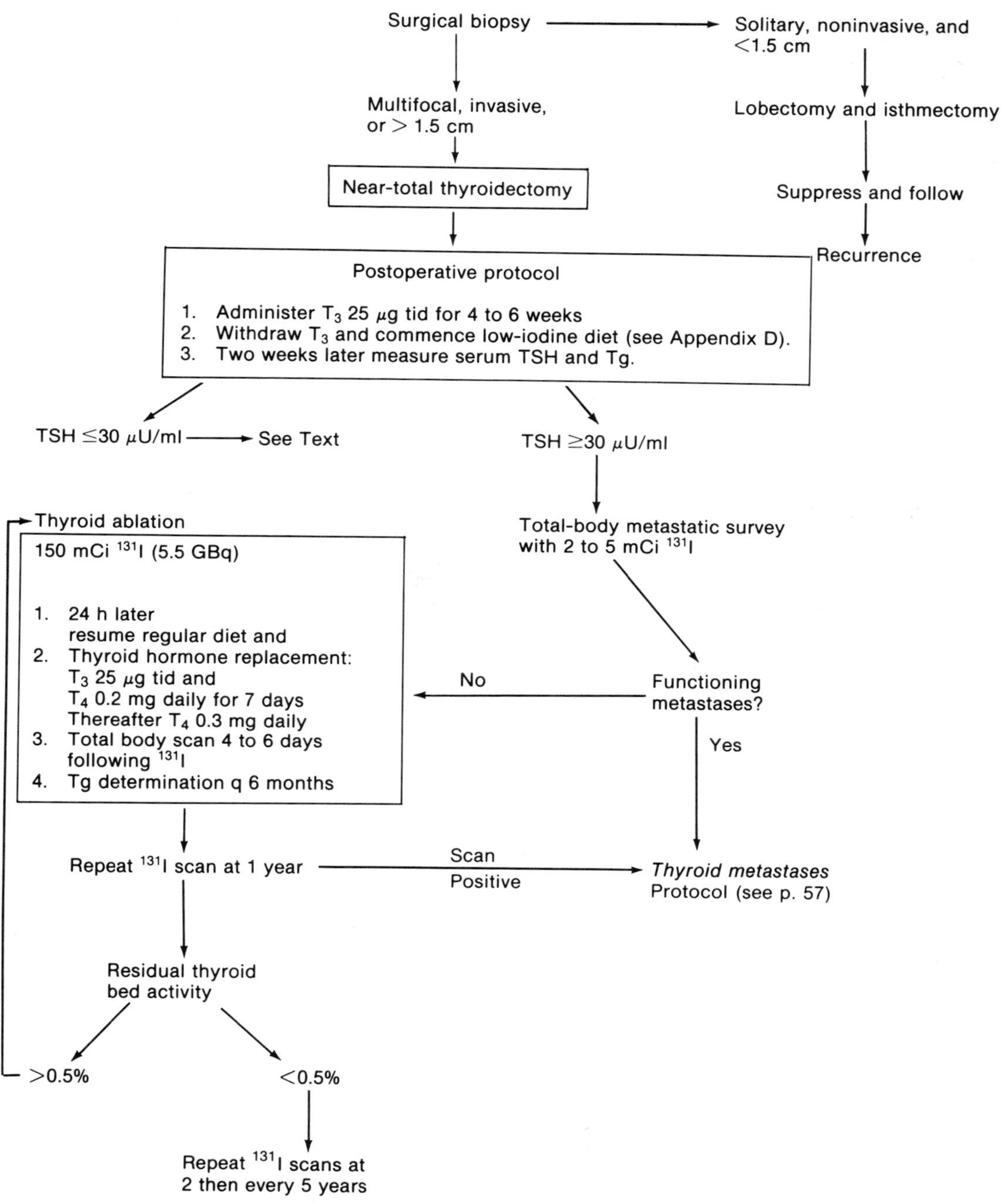

Figure 6. Postoperative management of differentiated thyroid carcinoma.

5. Occasionally, total-body imaging following large ablating doses of ^{131}I reveals the presence of functioning metastases that smaller, imaging doses of 2 to 5 mCi (74 to 185 MBq) fail to demonstrate.[157,158] (On the other hand, very few such sites, detected only with large-dose ^{131}I, are the sole metastatic deposits.[159])
6. Ablation eliminates residual normal thyroid tissue as a source of serum Tg, thus increasing the specificity of this marker in detecting recurrent thyroid cancer.
7. Tumor recurrence is reduced by ablation.[12,15,23,154,160,161]
8. Ablation may increase survival.[5,12,15,23,153,154,161,162]

INDICATIONS FOR ^{131}I ABLATION

Opinions vary about the indications for thyroid ablation. Among the options are:

1. Ablate detectable residual normal thyroid in all patients with well-differentiated cancer[154,163];
2. Ablate residual remnants with "significant" uptake of radioiodine (eg, >0.5%) in all except those patients who had solitary, noninvasive carcinomas (<1.5 cm in greatest dimension)[5,149];
3. Ablate residual thyroid tissue only in patients with unre-

sectable cancer in the neck or with distant metastases in preparation for possible treatment with $^{131}I^{6}$;
4. Ablate according to individual characteristics, such as the risk of recurrence.[164]

The recommendations outlined in Figure 6 lean toward the last approach. Ablation with any detectable uptake is recommended when:

1. The primary tumor is unresectable;
2. The primary tumor is >1.5 cm in its greatest dimension;
3. There is invasion of lymphatics, blood vessels, or thyroid capsule or if multiple intrathyroidal cancer foci can be demonstrated;
4. In most patients over 40 years of age with papillary carcinoma of any size because of increased risk of undetected metastases and recurrence in this group;
5. In all patients with follicular carcinoma of a less well-differentiated type, regardless of size of the primary tumor.

Moreover, a good case can be made for treating *patients who have no detectable neck uptake* automatically with 150 mCi (5.5 GBq) of ^{131}I in cases 2 through 5 on the basis that functioning, nondetectable micrometastases are thereby destroyed. If this practice is adhered to, the preablation whole-body survey can probably be eliminated if the TSH is greater then 30 μU/mL, because it is unlikely that a large residual thyroid remnant or significant functioning metastases are present. In this case, whole-body imaging should be performed 4 to 6 days following the ablation dose.

PATIENT PREPARATION FOR THYROID ABLATION AND THERAPY

It is generally recommended that following near-total thyroidectomy, thyroid replacement be withheld for 4 to 6 weeks until serum TSH rises sufficiently to stimulate ^{131}I uptake by functioning metastases.[5,164]

However, a better postoperative strategy may be to place the patient on full thyroid hormone replacement immediately after surgery. Euthyroidism during the postoperative period is thought by some to promote wound healing and avoid postsurgical complications.[70] After 4 to 6 weeks, the patient is switched to triiodothyronine (T_3) (25 μg tid) for 2 weeks. At the end of this period, all thyroid hormone is stopped for 11 to 14 days and the whole-body ^{131}I imaging and thyroid ablation are performed (Fig. 6). The rationale for this management stems from the following considerations:

1. Serum TSH rises more rapidly following withdrawal of T_3 than T_4.[144,165–167] The difference is shown in Figure 7. By extension, the duration of elevated TSH is shortened, thus decreasing the period of clinical hypothyroidism and the time tumor growth might be stimulated.

   The different responses are due to the markedly differing half-lives of circulating T_3 and T_4 (0.8 day versus 7 days, respectively).[168] Hilts et al[167] found that, in athyreotic patients, serum TSH reached 50 μU/mL an average of 11 days after withdrawal of T_3. Thus, 2 weeks off T_3 should be sufficient to raise TSH to a high level in most individuals. Although TSH continues to rise slowly after 2 weeks, Goldman et al[144] found no significant difference in ^{131}I uptake by whole-body imaging at 4 weeks following T_3 withdrawal compared to the uptake at 2 weeks.
2. In some patients, TSH does not rise substantially above normal following thyroidectomy, largely because of residual thyroid tissue or functioning metastases that produce sufficient thyroid hormone to suppress TSH. Edmonds et al[156] found that only about 50% of patients developed TSH levels exceeding 30 μU/mL. Even following thyroid ablation with 80 mCi (2.9 GBq) ^{131}I, 10% of patients failed to develop increased TSH levels. Faced with this dilemma, the physician must disregard TSH levels and be guided by whole body imaging and serum Tg in deciding management.

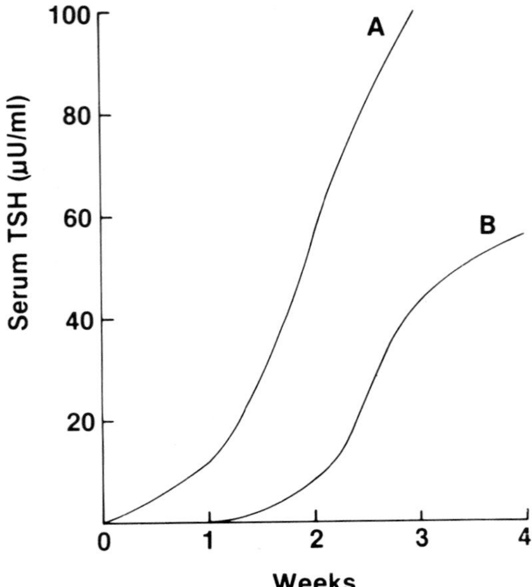

Figure 7. Curve A represents the serum TSH following withdrawal of replacement T_3 (75 μg daily) in athyreotic patients. (Data from Hershman and Edwards.[166]) Curve B represents serum TSH following withdrawal of replacement L-thyroxine in athyreotic patients. (Data from Edmonds et al[156] and Hilts et al.[167])

We recognize that there is insufficient evidence at this time to judge the relative merits of withholding T_4 for 6 weeks and withholding T_3 for 2 weeks. However, the latter strategy probably entails less discomfort for most patients and probably holds no real disadvantage by failing to detect functioning metastases.

At the time T_3 is withheld, the patient is placed on a low-iodine diet (see Appendix I). Two weeks later, serum TSH and Tg are measured. If serum TSH is >30 μU/mL, an ablation dose of 150 mCi (5.5 GBq) of ^{131}I can be administered directly because there is virtually no danger that a large volume of residual thyroid tissue or functioning metastases are present. If serum TSH is <30 μU/mL, whole-body images are obtained at 48 hours following 2 to 5 mCi (74 to 185 MBq) of ^{131}I. If only thyroid bed remnants are present, the same ablation dose of 150 mCi (5.5 GBq) is given. If significant functioning thyroid metastases are found, the physician proceeds as for the treatment of thyroid metastases.

Thyroid hormone replacement may be given 24 hours following administration of the ablation dose.[143] Postablation imaging is performed 2 to 6 days after the ablation dose, or when less than 10 mCi (370 MBq) of ^{131}I remains in the body. These images are important for prognostic reasons. If no metastases are found, the probability of recurrence is low.

If a subtotal thyroidectomy has been performed, it is probably preferable to ablate the remaining gland with ^{131}I rather than to reoperate, unless there is evidence of residual cancer in the neck. In the latter case, the thyroid should be reoperated. The calculation of the ^{131}I dose to be used for large thyroid remnants is discussed in the next section. In the case of unresectable cancer, ablation is necessary to prepare the patient for possible treatment with radioiodine.[5,6,14,149,151,154,163] When the patient becomes hypothyroid (usually 4 to 6 weeks following ablation) and serum TSH reaches 30 μU/mL or greater, whole-body imaging is performed 48 hours after giving 2 to 5 mCi (74 to 185 MBq) of ^{131}I. If functioning thyroid elements are found, 150 mCi (5.5 GBq) of ^{131}I is administered. If no functioning tissue is found, the patient is started on thyroid replacement, and the above procedure is repeated in 1 year, then at 3 years and thereafter at intervals of 5 years. Recurrent disease is treated with 150 to 200 mCi (5.5 to 7.5 GBq) of ^{131}I, but not more frequently than at 8- to 12-month intervals.

THE ABLATION DOSE

The appropriate dose of ^{131}I to use for thyroid ablation is a source of continuing controversy. High, fixed doses of ^{131}I (75 to 150 mCi or 2.8 to 5.5 GBq) have been advocated by most authors.[5,14,153,154,163,169–172] By this strategy, complete ablation (the elimination of all functioning activity in the thyroid bed) is achieved in more than 85% of patients with a single dose, thereby obviating the need for additional doses.[21] By extension of this reasoning, fewer tests, laboratory visits, and hospitalizations are required; fewer periods of debilitating hypothyroidism are imposed on the patient, who can sooner be placed on a symptom-free regimen of thyroid hormone replacement. There is also evidence that residual functioning tissue after initial low-dose ablation is more resistant to subsequent therapy because of decreased biologic half-life of ^{131}I.[172,173] There is no evidence that long-term effects of high-dose ablation, such as leukemia or second cancers, are increased as a result of the higher radiation exposure associated with 150 mCi (5.5 GBq) of ^{131}I.[174]

Low-dose ablation, that is, a fixed dose of 30 mCi (1.1 GBq) of ^{131}I, has been advocated by some authors[141,175,176] because:

1. Hospitalization in isolated rooms is avoided; the United States Nuclear Regulatory Commission requires monitored isolation of all patients as long as more than 30 mCi (1.1 GBq) of ^{131}I remain in the body.
2. The radiation dose to whole body and gonads is reduced, considerations most important to younger individuals who may wish to have children and who have a longer life expectancy during which potential tumorogenic effects may be expressed. The principal factors that determine whole-body dose from radioiodine are thyroid iodine turnover and renal clearance of iodine. After thyroidectomy, renal clearance is the dominant factor. Estimates of whole body radiation dose would be reduced from about 60 cGy (maximum) from a dose of 150 mCi (5.5 GBq) ^{131}I to about 12 cGy from a dose of 30 mCi (1.1 GBq).

The chief disadvantage with the low-dose regimen as perceived by its critics is that this dose ablates the thyroid in only about 53% of patients, which increases testing, inconvenience, and expense.[175–181] A still theoretical, yet increasingly persuasive, disadvantage is that micrometastases may receive inadequate radiation. The evidence for this supposition lies in the greatly increased recurrence of thyroid cancer among patients who do not receive adequate thyroid ablation.[15,149]

Still a third method of selecting the ablation dose is that proposed by Becker and colleagues, whereby the administered dose is determined by a dosimetric formula to achieve a predetermined radiation dose to the thyroid remnants.[164,182] The administered dose is calculated according to the equation:

$$\text{(1)} \quad \text{Administered } \mu\text{Ci} = \frac{\text{cGy desired} \times \text{gland weight (g)} \times 6.67}{T_{1/2\text{eff}}\text{ (days)} \times \%\text{ uptake (24 h)}}$$

They have arbitrarily selected a dose of 100,000 cGy, a conservative doubling of the 50,000 cGy that Goolden and Davey[183] found to reliably ablate the entire normal gland in patients with angina pectoris, and residual lobes in patients with thyroid cancer. The effective half-life is determined from the relationship:

$$\text{(2)} \quad T_{1/2\text{eff}} = \frac{T_{1/2\text{biol}} \times T_{1/2\text{phys}}}{T_{1/2\text{biol}} + T_{1/2\text{phys}}}$$

The biologic half-life is measured by sequential determinations of activity in the remnants over a 5- to 7-day period. A good approximation of this value can be made from 2 uptake measurements 5 to 7 days apart.[182] The gland weight is the estimate made by the surgeon in the operative report. The figure 6.67 is a constant that relates the various units used.

Example: To calculate the dose of ^{131}I required to deliver

100,000 cGy to a 2-g thyroid remnant, in which the uptake is 4% at 24 hours and $T_{1/2\text{eff}} = 5$ days:

$$(3)\quad \text{Administered dose } (\mu\text{Ci}) = \frac{100{,}000 \times 2 \times 6.67}{5 \times 4} = 66{,}700\ \mu\text{Ci} = 67\ \text{mCi} = 2.5\ \text{GBq}$$

Maxon advocates administering a dose calculated to deliver 30,000 cGy to the remnant, arguing that this delivered dose effectively ablates residual thyroid in 86% of patients (85 studied), and that delivering more radiation does not increase the efficacy of ablation.[184,185] Their criteria for successful ablation is visually negative images and less than 0.1% uptake in the neck. In their patient population, 37% could be satisfactorily treated with doses under 30 mCi of ^{131}I, thus avoiding hospitalization.

The objections to dose calculation methods, which are undeniably more elegant than using some arbitrary fixed dose, are these:

1. The determination of biologic half-time requires at least 4 days (during which the patient may be uncomfortably hypothyroid);
2. The preablation measurements using tracer doses of ^{131}I appear to overestimate the measurement of biologic half-times of therapeutic doses, which are shorter due to an outpouring of activity at days 3 to 5, presumably caused by radiation thyroiditis[182];
3. The determination of administered dose depends heavily on the surgeon's estimate of residual thyroid mass; such estimates may err by wide margins.

In Becker's study, the thyroid ablation dose ranged from 20 to 130 mCi with a median of 30 mCi (1.1 GBq).[182] The 24-hour uptake ranged from 2 to 38% (mean, 20%) which is a considerably higher average than the 6 to 7% usually expected after near-total thyroidectomy.[142,186] Because of the wide variation in remnant size and uptake and the variation in biologic half-time, pretherapeutic estimates did not correlate at all with the therapeutic dose estimates. Nevertheless, when tested 3 to 5 months later, all patients had TSH levels greater than 45 μU/ml and most had neck uptakes of less than 1%, although some had residual functioning foci in the neck when imaged 48 hours after administration of 2 mCi (74 MBq) ^{131}I. These results are about the same as those achieved using a fixed dose of 75 to 150 mCi (2 to 4 GBq). The advantages gained were less irradiation to most patients and the avoidance of hospitalization for 40% of patients. The comparison of cancer recurrence using this method will probably take several years to determine.

Among Maxon's patients, doses required to administer 30,000 cGy ranged from 25.8 to 246.3 mCi (mean ± 1 SD = 86.8 ± 62.1 mCi). Considering that they were calculating an absorbed radiation dose 3 times lower than Becker's, the great variability encountered in such estimates is clear.

We have recommended a standard dose of 150 mCi (5.5 GBq). Using a fixed-dose strategy (100 to 200 mCi), Beierwaltes and co-workers[142] eliminated all functioning thyroid activity from the neck, or reduced uptake to less than 1% in 92% of patients with one dose. Only 4.9% of patients required 2 doses; 1.6% of patients required 3 doses; and 1 patient required 6 doses.

We believe that a lower uptake limit of 0.5% in an apparently normal thyroid remnant is a good criterion for a second ablation dose. However, this criterion *should not* apply in the decision to ablate initially. The standard dose of 150 mCi (5.5. GBq) may be modified if the patient is under 20 years of age, or is a female of childbearing age and expresses a strong desire to bear children. In such cases, we quantify uptake and clearance and calculate a dose sufficient to deliver 100,000 cGy according to equation (1).

At the time of ablation, many hospital and radiological safety precautions must be taken. These are delineated in standard texts.[187] Informed consent is always obtained. The patient should be instructed to drink large quantities of water and empty the bladder frequently, to reduce bladder and whole-body irradiation. It is important to provide or to instruct patients to bring hard candy to the hospital to suck on for 2 to 3 days following administration of ^{131}I to reduce radiation sialadenitis.

Dosimetry Considerations in Patients with Renal Failure. As far as we know, the only report of a patient treated with ^{131}I while on renal dialysis, in which dosimetry is documented, is that of Morrish et al.[188] They found that the effective excretion half-life on four measurements ranged from 19.6 to 47.1 hours in their patient, a 36-year-old male. The effective excretion half-life of iodine in normal individuals is 72 to 96 hours.[189,190] Presumably, iodine is effectively cleared by dialysis, reducing the effective uptake by thyroid remnants and functioning tumor. These authors recommend administering ^{131}I immediately after dialysis and delaying the subsequent dialysis to increase tumor and thyroid uptake. In establishing the thyroid T_{eff}, the serial thyroid measurements after the tracer dose should be made more frequently, and with the same schedule in relation to dialyses as the treatment dose.

Interestingly, radiation safety considerations were not essentially different from other therapy cases, as they found little contamination of dialysis equipment.

EFFICACY OF SURGERY FOLLOWED BY ^{131}I ABLATION THERAPY

Beierwaltes illustrates the efficacy of ^{131}I ablation and more complete thyroid surgery by comparing recent with earlier experience at the University of Michigan, before the value of these measures was appreciated.[5] Between 1935 and 1955, with less aggressive surgery and little use of postoperative radioiodine in 255 patients, there was a 12.5% mortality rate from papillary carcinoma and 11.7% mortality from follicular carcinoma. In the period from 1957 to 1972, with more complete surgery and routine use of ^{131}I postoperatively, mortality was 2.4% from papillary carcinoma and 3.1% from follicular carcinoma. As with most other comparative studies in well-differentiated thyroid carcinoma, it is not easy to separate the effects of radioiodine ablation from improved or more extensive surgical removal. Nevertheless, no center that has adopted postoperative thyroid ablation has abandoned it.

In 1963, Haynie et al[191] treated 71 patients with postoperative thyroid ablation. None of these patients had evidence of residual or metastatic disease at the time of ablation. After a mean follow-up of 4 years, there was no evidence of recurrent disease in any patient.

In 1977, Krishnamurthy and Blahd[154] reported treating 52 patients with well-differentiated thyroid carcinoma by postoperative thyroid ablation. Two patients developed recurrences, which were successfully eradicated with radioiodine. No patient had died of thyroid cancer during a mean follow-up period of 8 years (range 2 to 20 years).

In a long-term follow-up study of 576 patients with papillary or mixed papillary-follicular cancer, Mazzaferri and colleagues found that, among patients who had surgery only (no postoperative medical therapy), the recurrence rate was 32%.[15] The recurrence rate was 11% in those given thyroid hormone postoperatively and only 2.7% in those who received ^{131}I therapy followed by hormone therapy after operation ($p < 0.001$ for all comparisons). In those patients treated with surgery and thyroid hormone alone, the recurrence rate was 15% if only a lobe or the isthmus was removed, and 9% if more extensive subtotal or total thyroidectomy was performed. These data support the concept, now generally accepted, that differentiated thyroid carcinoma should be treated by near-total thyroidectomy, which preserves the parathyroid glands and recurrent laryngeal nerves, followed by a well-defined program of ^{131}I treatment with long-term follow-up.

Hurley and Becker[164] speculate that the most probable benefit from ^{131}I ablation is not the destruction of the normal thyroid remnant, but rather the destruction of microscopic metastases in cervical lymph nodes and at distant sites. Papillary carcinoma spreads primarily by the lymphatics. At the time of surgery, microscopic foci of papillary carcinoma are present in the intraparenchymal or pericapsular lymphatics of the isthmus or opposite lobe in up to 87% of patients, and in the ipsilateral cervical lymph nodes in 90% of patients.[147,192] There is also some evidence that papillary carcinoma may reach the lungs via mediastinal lymphatic channels.[14] Although the fate of these microscopic metastases is not known, 10 to 30% of patients not treated with ^{131}I develop recurrences.[6,149] In patients with follicular carcinoma not treated with postoperative ^{131}I ablation, 10 to 40% develop a recurrence.[6,12] About half of these recurrences develop within 5 years. *The significant reduction of recurrences following postoperative* ^{131}I ablation may thus be due to a direct effect on the metastases rather than residual cancer in the small postoperative remnant.

More direct evidence for this concept lies in the fact that therapeutic doses of ^{131}I frequently reveal functioning metastases that small tracer doses miss.[17,158,193] Nemec and colleagues[17] found that nearly one fourth of the 206 patients imaged following therapeutic doses revealed tumor tissue, usually lymph-node metastases, not revealed by tracer doses.

There are at least 2 important implications to these findings. First, all patients might benefit from postoperative ^{131}I therapy, regardless of demonstrable residual uptake in the neck. We are not aware of any studies that have addressed this question, although the practice appears justifiable. Beierwaltes stated flatly in 1983 that he never gives ^{131}I to ablate remnants in the thyroid bed unless there is "significant" uptake of ^{131}I.[15] By significant, he meant >2% of the dose at 24 hours. By 1984, however, Beierwaltes[142] had amended the definition of "significant uptake" to >0.5% of the dose at 24 hours. Second, large doses (150 mCi) of ^{131}I may be more effective in lowering recurrence rates than more conservative doses (ie, 30 mCi).

Follow-Up

Thyroid hormone replacement is begun 24 hours following the ablation dose of ^{131}I. If smaller ablation doses than 150 mCi (5.5 GBq) are administered, thyroid replacement should be withheld until whole-body imaging confirms the absence of functioning metastases that would indicate the need for additional ^{131}I.

If postablation imaging reveals no evidence of thyroid metastases, fully suppressive doses of thyroid hormone are begun, usually 200 to 300 μg of L-thyroxine daily or sufficient amounts to maintain serum TSH below detectable levels by sensitive assays. One year later, thyroid hormone replacement is withdrawn and whole-body imaging using 2 to 5 mCi (74 to 185 MBq) of ^{131}I is repeated. If this is negative, the same routine is repeated at 3 years and subsequently every 5 years thereafter for life.[5]

Clinical examination should be performed every 6 months initially and should include serum TSH, to monitor effectiveness of suppression, and serum Tg, the most sensitive indicator of recurrent well-differentiated thyroid cancer. If subsequent examinations remain negative, the schedule can be increased to yearly intervals. It was previously recommended that chest radiographs be obtained yearly to rule out pulmonary metastases. It is unlikely, however, that lung metastases will become evident roentgenographically if serum Tg is normal.

If functioning thyroid cancer is found at the time of ^{131}I ablation, and less than 150 mCi (5.5 GBq) has been administered for ablation, additional ^{131}I should be given to a total of 200 mCi (7.4 GBq) before replacement thyroid hormone is initiated.[15] Such patients must be treated as if they had metastatic disease; they are placed on thyroid suppression and restudied 9 to 12 months later.

It should be noted that there are many respected clinicians who do not agree with repeated withdrawals of thyroid hormone after the initial one or two attempts to demonstrate tumor uptake. They believe that regular clinical examination, thyroglobulin assays, and chest x-rays constitute good follow-up in the absence of symptoms or palpable masses.

Table 5. Serum Thyroglobulin Levels in Normal Subjects and in Various Thyroid Abnormalities*

CONDITION	MEAN ± SEM (ng/mL)
Control subjects (blood donors)	5.1 ± 0.49
Cord blood	29.3 ± 4.7
Pregnancy (delivery)	10.1 ± 1.3
Active Graves' disease	176.0 ± 30.0
Euthyroid Graves' disease	6.8 ± 1.25
Non-Graves' disease thyrotoxicosis	145.0 ± 27.0
Subacute thyroiditis (acute phase)	136.8 ± 74.5
Differentiated thyroid carcinoma (all histological types)	103.4 ± 125.6
Differentiated thyroid carcinoma (post-thyroidectomy, without metastases)	4.9
Metastatic thyroid carcinoma (differentiated type)	464.9 ± 155.6
Medullary thyroid carcinoma	4.9 ± 1.6
Thyroid adenoma	424.6 ± 189.4
Endemic goiter	208.1 ± 19.8

*Data from several sources. See Van Herle.[203]

Indeed, repeated imaging with ^{131}I has largely gained acceptance because of the expertise of Dr. Beierwaltes and his colleagues at the University of Michigan, who have demonstrated recurrent functioning metastases after long latent periods of apparent inactivity.[174] This experience, combined with occasional reports of normal levels of serum thyroglobulin in patients with functioning metastases, have convinced most clinicians that a life-long imaging program is the more conservative approach to well-differentiated thyroid cancer.

THE ROLE OF SERUM THYROGLOBULIN (TG) IN FOLLOWING THYROID CANCER

The development of highly sensitive immunoradiometric and tissue-receptor assays has lead to the recognition of tumor marker substances in many cancers. Both Tg and carcinoembryonic antigen (CEA) have been identified as tumor antigens associated with differentiated thyroid carcinoma. Of these, Tg is the more important. While elevated CEA has been reported in some patients with well-differentiated thyroid carcinoma, it is an unreliable marker because it is neither a constant finding nor is it specific.[194]

Thyroglobulin was previously thought to be a secluded antigen, confined to the thyroid and only released under such pathologic conditions as thyroiditis and thyroid surgery. However, it is now known that this large glycoprotein is not only released in normal individuals, it is most likely under the control of TSH.[195,196] Entry into the serum is thought to be through the thyroidal lymphatics.[197] Normal serum levels vary considerably from one laboratory to another. Van Herle et al have reported normal values to vary from 0 to 30 ng/mL with a mean of 5 ng/mL.[198,199] Values are elevated in several thyroid diseases, including thyrotoxicosis, thyroiditis, and thyroid tumors (Table 5).

Several studies have shown elevated serum Tg levels in patients with differentiated thyroid cancer prior to surgery.[199–203] The highest levels are found in follicular cancer, followed by mixed papillary follicular cancer, and papillary cancer. Evidence suggests that the degree of elevation prior to surgery is proportional to the number of follicular elements in the tumor, as well as its mass, and that there is no significant difference in levels between patients with and without metastases.[200] There appear to be some physiochemical differences in salting out and ultracentrifugal patterns between Tg from cancers and Tg from normal follicles.[47] However, these differences have not yet proved diagnostic.[204]

The release of Tg from thyroid metastases appears also to be under the control of TSH. Schlumberger and colleagues[205] studied this effect in 19 patients with functioning metastases following surgery and total thyroid ablation (no ^{131}I uptake in the thyroid bed). After T_3 withdrawal, serial TSH and Tg levels were measured. As serum TSH rose, Tg rose in parallel, reaching a plateau ranging from 2 to 20 times the baseline suppression level. A second group of three patients without radioiodine uptake in their metastases were studied using the same protocol. Serum Tg levels rose only 1.7 to 2.8 times baseline levels. While there is a correlation with ^{131}I uptake, Tg may serve as a tumor marker even in the absence of radioiodine uptake.

Elevated Tg levels do not necessarily indicate the presence of cancer because Tg is elevated in most thyroid diseases. Rather, the value of measuring serum Tg lies in monitoring patients after surgery and thyroid ablation. The greater sensitivity of serum Tg compared with ^{131}I imaging for detecting recurrent disease has been documented by many studies.[202,206–216] However, early enthusiasm for limiting ^{131}I imaging to patients who demonstrate elevated serum Tg was dampened somewhat by several reports of positive ^{131}I imaging in patients with normal Tg levels.[203,217–221] Nevertheless, when Van Herle surveyed the world literature in 1981, such reports accounted for only 3.2% of all patients with metastatic disease.[200] In a large series of 1323 patients with differentiated thyroid carcinoma studied by Galligan et al,[211] 284 had documented metastases. Of these, 37 (13%) were not detected by ^{131}I imaging, but their presence was suggested by elevated serum Tg levels, clinical findings, or both. Only 12 of the 284 (4%) had positive images for metastases and undetectable or low-normal serum Tg. In another study by Brendel et al[221] comparing Tg levels with imaging following therapeutic doses of ^{131}I, they found that 8.5% of their patients had metastases despite having low serum Tg levels.

There is disagreement as to whether low or undetectable serum Tg levels reliably exclude the presence of functioning metastases in patients on suppressive T_4. Many studies have reported no false-negative Tg values during suppression.[209,212–214,222,223] However, other studies have shown a small percentage of patients with low or nondetectable Tg levels on T_4 suppression, who had raised levels of Tg when TSH became elevated and who had positive ^{131}I uptake in functioning metastases, particularly on posttherapeutic imaging.[220,221]

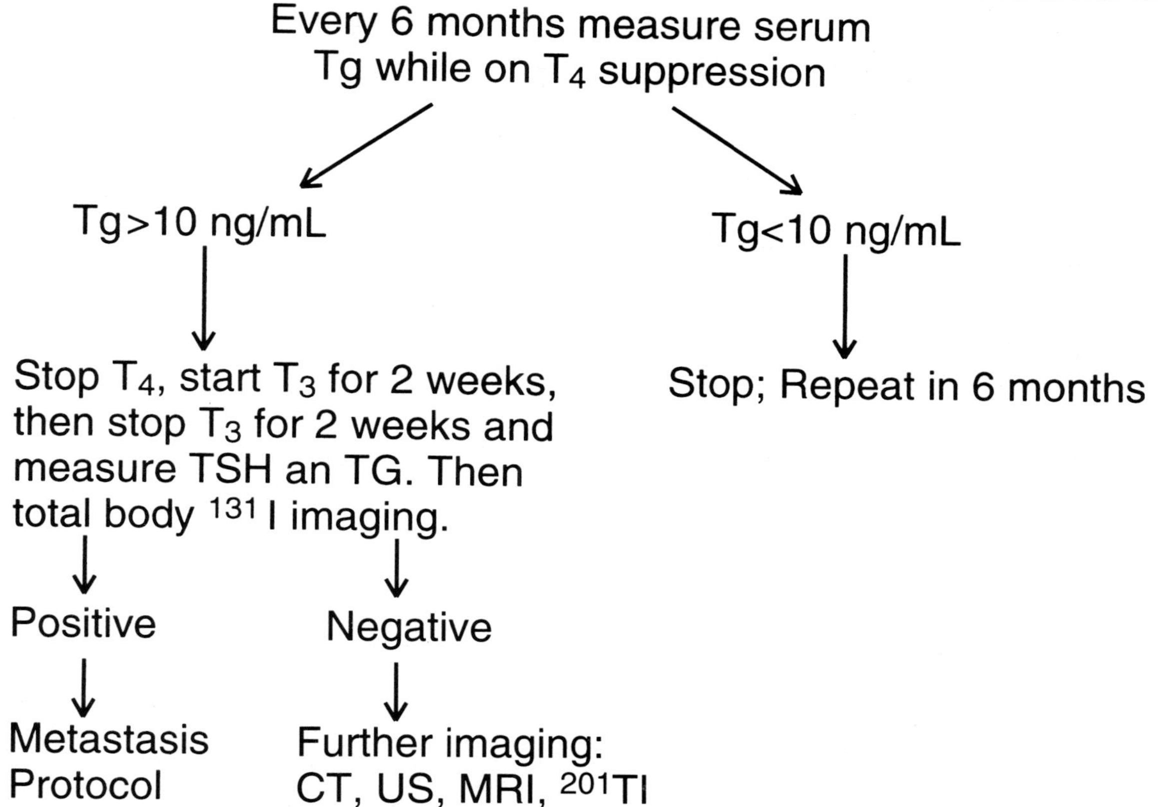

Figure 8. Clinical scheme for following patients with well differentiated thyroid cancer proposed by Van Herle.[224] Following near-total thyroidectomy and ablation of thyroid remnants and/or functioning metastases, serum Tg and TSH are measured while on T_4 suppression. Patients with Tg below 10 ng/mL are followed by serial measurements every 6 months and T_4 suppression continued. If serum Tg exceeds 10 ng/mL, T_4 is discontinued, serum Tg and TSH are both measured and ^{131}I total body imaging is performed. If images are positive, metastases are treated. If images are negative, further search for metastases is warranted. When antithyroglobulin antibodies are present in the serum, immunoradiometric assays (IRMA) that are less sensitive to interferences should be used to follow Tg levels.[228]

Most authorities today recognize that a follow-up program that combines serum Tg measurements with ^{131}I imaging is to be recommended. Furthermore, monitoring Tg while on T_4 suppression therapy is much more efficient, less costly, and more acceptable to patients. It seems to us that a follow-up scheme proposed by Van Herle[224] and illustrated in Fig. 8 provides an acceptable approach to thyroid cancer follow-up after surgery and thyroid ablation.

SIGNIFICANCE OF ANTITHYROGLOBULIN ANTIBODIES

Circulating antithyroglobulin antibodies (TgAbs) are present in 2 to 15% of patients with differentiated thyroid carcinoma.[225–227] TgAbs are usually measured to determine the sensitivity of serum Tg measurements in following tumor progression. However, newer immunoradiometric assays (IRMAs) for Tg are less influenced by the presence of TgAbs, despite some decreased sensitivity.[228,229] There is some evidence to suggest that TgAbs disappear after treating thyroid cancer and reappearance indicates recurrence.[225] In a study by Rubello and colleagues[230] of 43 patients treated for differentiated thyroid cancer, TgAbs became undetectable in 24 patients, all of whom were considered tumor-free by other diagnostic criteria. In the 19 patients in whom TgAbs remained elevated, there was disease progression or persistence in 5. The reason for elevation in the remaining 14 patients, considered tumor-free, could not be explained. It may be that longer follow-up will confirm residual metastases in these patients. Further studies will clarify the role of TgAbs as a tumor marker.

THALLIUM-201 SCINTIGRAPHY IN THE FOLLOW-UP OF THYROID CARCINOMA

Several studies have shown that ^{201}Tl-chloride scintigraphy is useful in detecting thyroid metastases, the detectability ranging from 35 to 91%.[231–235] The values of ^{201}Tl include:

1. Patients do not need to be made hypothyroid, because uptake of this blood flow tracer in tumor and metastases is unaffected by circulating TSH;
2. Imaging can be performed 10 minutes after injection;
3. The radiation absorbed dose is a fraction of that of ^{131}I; and
4. ^{201}Tl may be taken up in metastases when diagnostic

doses of ^{131}I show no, or more limited, disease, thus improving sensitivity of detection.[236]

The addition of (SPECT) imaging further improves sensitivity. Charkes et al[235] reported detecting foci as small as 1 cm in the neck and 1.5 cm in the lungs. They found SPECT most useful in detecting micronodular pulmonary metastases, especially in patients who had negative ^{131}I images. At this time, the principal value of ^{201}Tl imaging appears to be in conjunction with patients who are being followed with serial serum Tg measurements while on T_4 suppression treatment, since these two tests can be done at the same time. They are complementary,[236,237] in that the two are always more sensitive than either alone, and the patient avoids the discomfort of periodic hypothyroidism.

TSH SUPPRESSION

Thyroid hormone replacement following thyroidectomy and ^{131}I ablation serves both to maintain the patient euthyroid and to suppress pituitary TSH, which promotes the growth of papillary and follicular carcinomas.[99] The increased growth rate of well-differentiated thyroid carcinomas in hypothyroid patients is presumed to result from stimulation by endogenous TSH.[238,239] L-thyroxine is the replacement hormone preparation of choice because of the long serum half-life and uniform serum levels of T_3 (due to peripheral metabolism of T_4) and T_4 that result from a single daily dose.[240]

The dose of T_4 required to completely suppress serum TSH varies from 150 to 300 μg/day, with a mean of about 225 μg/day.[241,242] This dose is usually somewhat higher than that required to achieve clinical euthyroidism. The best means of assessing the adequacy of TSH suppression is by the thyrotropin-releasing hormone (TRH) stimulation test. The dose of L-thyroxine that eliminates all response to TRH stimulation and yet avoids clinical hyperthyroidism is deemed *ideal suppression.* If TSH can be detected following TRH stimulation, augmentation of the suppression dose by 50 μg/day usually corrects the dosage.[242]

Hurley and Becker[143] make an interesting observation about selecting the replacement dosage of T_4. They note that in all reported studies, the upper limit of T_4 required to produce a negative response to TRH is 300 μg/day. This is equivalent to 3 grains of desiccated thyroid, which was the standard dose for TSH suppression before the advent of TSH assays.[149,154] Therefore, if 300 μg/day T_4 is tolerated, TRH stimulation testing may not be necessary.

When T_4 replacement is withdrawn and serum TSH has risen to maximum levels, considerable time is required for the TSH to return to suppression levels after reinstitution of T_4 replacement alone. Some investigators have suggested an initial regimen of combined T_3 and T_4 following ^{131}I diagnostic studies and therapy, to suppress serum TSH in the shortest time possible.[164,243–245] Figure 9 shows the relative levels of TSH following initiation of suppressive thyroid hormone replacement using 4 different regimens. The data are from Busnardo and colleagues.[243] Curve A describes the TSH response to a daily dose of 3.8 μg/kg T_4. Note that TSH does not fall below 2.0 μU/mL until 25 days of therapy have elapsed. Curve B describes the response to a daily dose of 1.1 μg/kg of T_3, given in 3 divided doses. Curves C and D describe the TSH responses to "saturation" regimens developed by Mak and DeStefano[245] that are considered optimum for rapid saturation of T_3 and T_4 distribution spaces. Curve C describes the response of decreasing daily doses of T_4 according to the schedule: 24, 12, 6, 4, 3.7, 3.7, . . . μg/kg/day. The baseline level of 2.0 μU/mL of TSH is reached in 10 days. Curve D describes the response to a saturation regimen of T_3 based on the sequential daily schedule: 2.4, 1.8, 1.4, 1.2, 1.1, 1.1, . . . μg/kg/day. The TSH level of 2.0 μU/mL is reached in only 8 days.

Hurley and Becker[164] have chosen empirically an initial replacement regimen of 25 μg T_3 twice daily and 0.2 mg T_4 daily. This combination is begun 24 hours following therapy, under the presumption that the radiation delivered to the tumor in the first 24 hours causes sufficient cellular damage to preclude further uptake of ^{131}I. This regimen is continued for 7 days, after which the T_3 is eliminated and the optimum suppressive dose of T_4 is determined by TRH stimulation testing. From Figure 9 it is apparent that TRH stimulation testing should be deferred until at least 4 weeks have elapsed.

Treatment of Functioning Thyroid Metastases

Thyroid metastases, both in cervical lymph nodes and outside the neck, may be evident at the time of surgery or may only manifest themselves many years later. In a large study of distant metastases (ie, outside the neck), Beierwaltes found that 60% were present at the time of surgery and the remaining 40% were found on average 7.4 years after surgery.[174] The treatment of functioning metastases is somewhat different from thyroid ablation. However, patient preparation is similar; thyroid replacement must be stopped until serum TSH exceeds 30 μU/mL (see Fig. 6). A low-iodine diet (Appendix I) is begun at the same time the ^{131}I tracer dose is administered for whole-body imaging.

QUANTITY OF ^{131}I ADMINISTERED

As with the thyroid ablation dose, opinion and practice vary concerning the optimum dose of ^{131}I to be administered for functioning metastases found after thyroidectomy. However, most investigators agree that, following ablation, therapeutic ^{131}I should not be administered if ^{131}I imaging fails to reveal uptake in regions likely to be metastases.* One must not be misled by normal activity in nonthyroidal tissues.

*There are some who argue that even in the absence of discernable uptake with diagnostic doses of ^{131}I (10 mCi or less), the presence of elevated serum thyroglobulin may be an indication for additional ^{131}I treatment in high-risk patients. In most of these patients, imaging following therapeutic doses will reveal uptake in small metastases. (Personal communication of Dr. Jacob Robbins.)

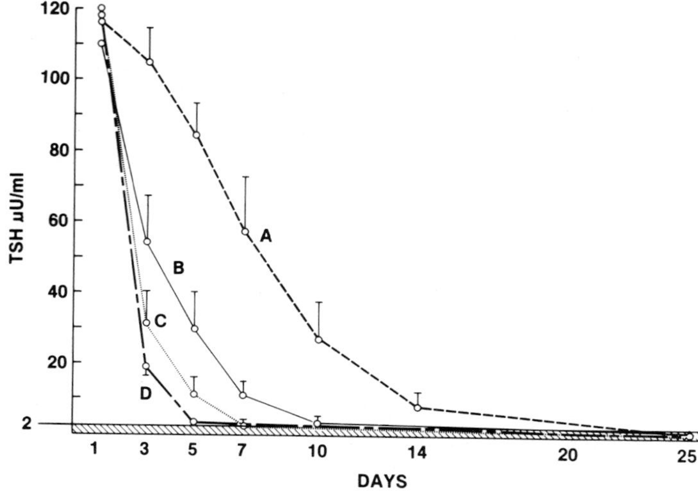

Figure 9. The decrease in serum TSH following reinstitution of four regimens of thyroid hormone replacement in athyreotic patients with thyroid cancer who had discontinued suppressive treatment with T_3 at least 18 days previously. See text for description of regimens. (From Busnardo et al.[243])

Two general approaches for determining administered dose are used:

1. Maximum "safe" administered dose. The approach to treating functioning thyroid metastases developed at Memorial Sloan-Kettering Center Institute is to administer a dose of ^{131}I that will deliver the maximum tumor radiation, yet avoid the most serious complication, namely, bone-marrow depression.[151,159,171,246] The limit of radiation dose to blood has been set at 200 cGy because doses up to this limit seldom produce clinically significant bone-marrow suppression. The radiation dose (measured in rads or cGy) to the blood per millicurie administered is estimated using the Marinelli formula, which assumes that all of the β^- energy is absorbed in whole blood and that both the ^{131}I and the critical organ (bone marrow) are uniformly distributed in the body. The Memorial protocol, formulas, and computer program are contained in Appendix J. They have not used the more rigorous Medical Internal Radiation Dose (MIRD) formula because of the complexities of determining marrow distribution. The Memorial group also recommends that body retention 48 hours after treatment not exceed 120 mCi (4.4 GBq).[246] Such high retention may lead to a dangerous outpouring of $PB^{131}I$ into the blood from damaged tumor that could not be predicted from the tracer studies. In the presence of lung metastases, lung retention should not exceed 80 mCi (3 GBq) to avoid radiation pneumonitis. In a review by Leeper, administered doses that would deliver 200 cGy to the blood ranged from 70 to 650 mCi (2.6 to 24 GBq), the average value being 300 mCi (11 GBq).[151]

Becker recommends the same dosimetric strategy, except that he limits the dose administered at any one time to 300 mCi (11 GBq).[164] Judged by this dose strategy, an arbitrary fixed dose of 200 mCi (7.4 GBq) would "undertreat" 54% of patients and overtreat about 3%.

2. Standard fixed dose. Most clinicians administer a fixed amount of ^{131}I that varies between 100 and 200 mCi (3.7 to 7.4 GBq).[5,163,172,247] As numerous studies with long-term follow-up have shown no or only minimal effects from large doses of ^{131}I, administered doses have generally increased. Beierwaltes varies the treatment dose according to the location of the cancer; 150 mCi (5.5 GBq) for functioning remnants in the thyroid bed, 175 mCi (6.5 GBq) for lymphnode metastases, and 200 mCi (7.4 GBq) for functioning metastases outside the neck.[6,174] The rationale for the lower and upper limits are:

1. The use of 150 mCi (5.5 GBq) for thyroid remnants or functioning metastases in the thyroid bed (this distinction cannot be made by ^{131}I imaging) has, in the experience of the University of Michigan group, been successful in eliminating functioning tissue in 95% of patients;
2. The Atomic Energy Commission Subcommittee on Human Use, in a study of dose-effect relationship, failed to find evidence that doses greater than 200 mCi (7.4 GBq) were more effective. They also found that radiation doses to the blood greater than 200 cGy were associated with an increased incidence of complications.[246]

We subscribe to this approach to therapy of well-differentiated thyroid carcinoma (Table 6), not only for the above reasons, but also because:

1. The large number of patients treated in this manner have proven it to be safe and efficacious;
2. It avoids time-consuming measurements of retention and biologic half-times of ^{131}I, which add a minimum of 4 days to the treatment program and increase the time period during which the patient is hypothyroid;
3. It reduces the cost of therapy;
4. No convincing evidence has been published that proves

Table 6. Recommended Doses of ^{131}I for Functioning Thyroid Metastases

SITE	Dose	
	mCi	*GBq*
Uptake in bed of thyroid or cervical neck nodes	150	5.5
Distant metastases	200	7.4
Lung metastases	200*	7.4

*(<80 mCi retained in lung)

more "rigorous" approaches to dose determinations are more effective.

Some exceptions to the above treatment protocol are:

- In patients with functioning pulmonary metastases, we advise an administered dose that limits to 80 mCi (3 GBq) the retained dose at 24 hours to avoid radiation pneumonitis.
- In patients with widespread extrapulmonary functioning metastases, the administered dose should not deliver >200 cGy radiation absorbed dose to the blood. Such high absorbed doses may be encountered in rare patients who retain more than 35% of a tracer dose. In such patients, we recommend the dosimetric studies outlined by Benua in Appendix J.
- In patients with nonresectable cancer in the neck, the protocol in Appendix J is also recommended because it provides the highest permissible doses of ^{131}I.

The experience of most investigators suggests that these exceptions will pertain to about 3% of patients treated. Therefore, a treatment plan that adequately serves 97% of patients seems appropriate for a standard protocol.

DOSIMETRY-BASED PROTOCOLS

While 70 to 80% of metastases of well-differentiated thyroid carcinomas concentrate ^{131}I when maximally stimulated, the degree of uptake is variable. It is considered important by some to determine from tracer studies whether an adequate radiation dose can be delivered to the metastases, before embarking on radioiodine therapy.[185,247]

The radiation absorbed dose to tumor can be estimated from measurements of ^{131}I uptake, tumor volume, and effective half-life.[164,172,248–250] From these values, absorbed dose (*D*) in small tumors can be approximated from the formula:

$$(4)\quad D\ (\text{cGy/mCi})\ \text{administered} = \frac{T_{1/2\text{eff}}\ (\text{days}) \times \%\ \text{uptake}\ (24\ \text{h}) \times 152}{\text{tumor mass (g)}}$$

where 152 is a constant that includes the deposited energy and relates the various units in the equation. It bears repeating that absorbed-dose estimates from tracer doses are thought generally to overestimate absorbed radiation from therapeutic doses because the $T_{1/2\text{eff}}$ is generally shorter following therapeutic doses.[246] The effective half-life is usually measured using a scintillation camera and area of interest analysis, taking daily measurements for 4 to 7 days following administration of the tracer dose. Appropriate background subtractions must be made. Alternatively, the biologic half-life can be assumed to be 4 days.[172] The effective half-life is then 2.67 days.* The mass is considered to be equivalent to volume and can thus be estimated from images taken in 2 planes. Normally the activity (except in the lungs) can be represented as an ellipse on both the anterior and lateral scans, with one axis common to both images. The volume of the lesion is then $4/3\ \pi\ abc$ (the volume of an ellipsoid with semiaxes a, b, and c). Tumor volume can also be estimated by SPECT or PET imaging using appropriate tissue attenuation parameters.[251] Useful information can occasionally be obtained by ultrasound or CT imaging. Very small regions of ^{131}I uptake may be arbitrarily assigned a mass of 1 g.[164]

The tumor uptake of ^{131}I is determined by computer analysis of scintillation camera images. Calibrations for depth attenuation must be made for each instrument used in these determinations. Figure 10 shows such a calibration curve for a scintillation camera fitted with a high-energy collimator. A 3-mL syringe was filled with 30 μCi ^{131}I and counted at successive depths in a water bath. For this camera, the 64 × 64 pixel dimensions are 0.38 cm × 0.38 cm. A simple program can be written to calculate specific tumor activity and absorbed dose automatically.[249] A method of determining lesion activity from conjugate scintillation camera views is described by Thomas et al.[250]

The purpose of estimating radiation absorbed dose to tumor is to determine those patients likely to benefit from ^{131}I therapy. For example, Becker suggests that, if the predicted dose to tumor is less than 5000 cGy, alternative means of treatment must be explored.[164] Assuming an effective half-life of 2.67 days, this requires an uptake of 0.06%/g or 120 μCi/g for an administered dose of 200 mCi (7.4 GBq). Since Becker and colleagues administer up to 300 mCi (11 GBq), presumably they treat uptakes as low as 0.04%/g.[164]

UPTAKE OF RADIOIODINE BY NONTHYROIDAL TISSUES

Uptake of radioiodine by tissues other than the thyroid or functioning thyroid carcinoma metastases is not uncommon. In some cases, benign focal localization can be mistaken for metastases. Such uptake can occur with or without a thyroid gland. Such uptake is more likely encountered in

*Equation 4 overestimates absorbed dose to the lesion somewhat because it assumes "instantaneous uptake" of the 24 h concentration. The more rigorous MIRD equation is:

$$D(\text{cGy}) = \frac{A}{m}\,\Sigma\Delta_i\Phi_i$$

Since $\Sigma\Delta_i\Phi_i$ for the penetrating and nonpenetrating radiations of ^{131}I for small (2 to 60g) unit density spherical masses is about 0.63, the equation thus simplifies to $D = 0.63A$. Equation 4 avoids having to integrate tumor uptake of ^{131}I during the early hours of rising concentration. Thomas found the overestimation to be only 10 to 15%, which is an acceptable error.[250]

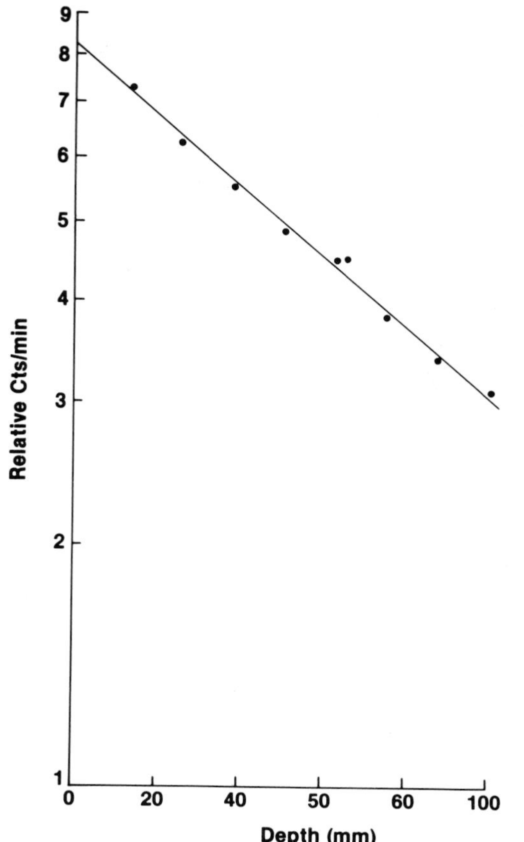

Figure 10. Relation between counting rate and ^{131}I source depth in water.

imaging for metastases after a therapeutic dose of ^{131}I, because of the very large doses administered.

Extrathyroidal localization is common in the mouth, salivary glands, stomach, intestines, urinary bladder, and liver, where the presence of radioiodine is a normal variation (Fig. 11). The correct identification of normal activity is usually made by follow-up imaging, in which either the localization or the intensity of activity changes. Activity in the oropharynx (eg, Zenker's diverticulum), esophagus, and stomach can often be washed out by swallowed water. Diffuse hepatic uptake may not change, but miliary thyroid metastases to the liver almost never occur, and the rare functioning hepatic metastases appear as focal hot lesions.[252]

Diffuse hepatic uptake is very common and is dose dependent.[253,254] Rosenbaum et al observed diffuse hepatic uptake in 13% of patients following diagnostic doses of 10 mCi (370 MBq), and in 52% of patients posttherapy.[253] Hepatic uptake does not correlate strongly with serum PB^{131}I or with serum thyroglobulin levels.[253,254] The most likely explanation is physiological uptake of ^{131}I-labeled thyroxine, because it is known that hepatic localization occurs soon after administration of ^{131}I-thyroxine, most likely because the liver is the principal site of deiodination of T_4 to T_3.[254,255] Such deiodination occurs more slowly in hypothyroidism, which many of these patients have, thus slowing release of the hormone from the liver. Hepatic visualization thus suggests the presence of functioning thyroid tissue, either from thyroid remnants or from functioning metastases. The fact that hepatic visualization sometimes occurs when no functioning remnants can be demonstrated may suggest that the functioning foci are too small to image.

Other causes of extrathyroidal uptake of radioiodine are listed in Table 7. Nearly all of these localizations involve:

1. body secretions;
2. pathologic transudates and inflammation;
3. neoplasms of nonthyroidal origin, or
4. nonspecific mediastinal uptake.

AUGMENTATION OF THE RADIATION DOSE

There are at least two ways of increasing the radiation absorbed dose to thyroid remnants and functioning metastases from ^{131}I in addition to merely increasing the dose administered. In fact, the doses of ^{131}I generally recommended are already at maxima consistent with acceptable incidences of such side effects as sialoadenitis, bone-marrow depression, and radiation sickness. Practical measures include first, increasing radioiodine uptake by increasing serum TSH *or* decreasing body iodide pool, and, second, prolonging thyroid retention of radioiodine.

A theoretical means of increasing the radiobiologic effect is to increase target tissue sensitivity to radiation. However, for thyroid cancer, such sensitization techniques have not been developed.

Increasing Serum TSH. Probably the most important means of increasing radioiodine uptake is to increase serum TSH, chiefly by increasing trapping and organification of ^{131}I. The easiest and safest means of increasing serum TSH is to withdraw or withhold thyroid replacement until serum TSH exceeds 30 μU/mL, as has already been described. After prolonged suppression with T_4, the rise in serum TSH may be retarded. Edmonds found that patients who had been on T_4 suppression continuously for more than 2 years had a pronounced delay in TSH response following withdrawal.[156] In many patients, there was no significant increase in serum TSH even after 4 weeks. Older patients (over 45 years of age) may never develop high levels of endogenous TSH in response to T_4 withdrawal.[205] They also appear to have reduced pituitary reserve when challenged by TRH stimulation. In such patients, therapeutic ^{131}I should be administered as soon as serum TSH ceases to rise. It is also prudent to measure serum T_3 and T_4. If these values are not very low, either the patient is surreptitiously continuing thyroid hormone medication, or else the tumor metastases are producing thyroid hormone in sufficient quantities to suppress TSH.

Exogenous TSH. Although recombinant human TSH has been developed, it is not at this writing approved for general use. Therefore, medical science must still rely upon bovine TSh (bTSH). Indeed, injections of bTSH do increase intake of ^{131}I in patients in whom endogenous TSH is suppressed by thyroid hormone replacement or by functioning thyroid

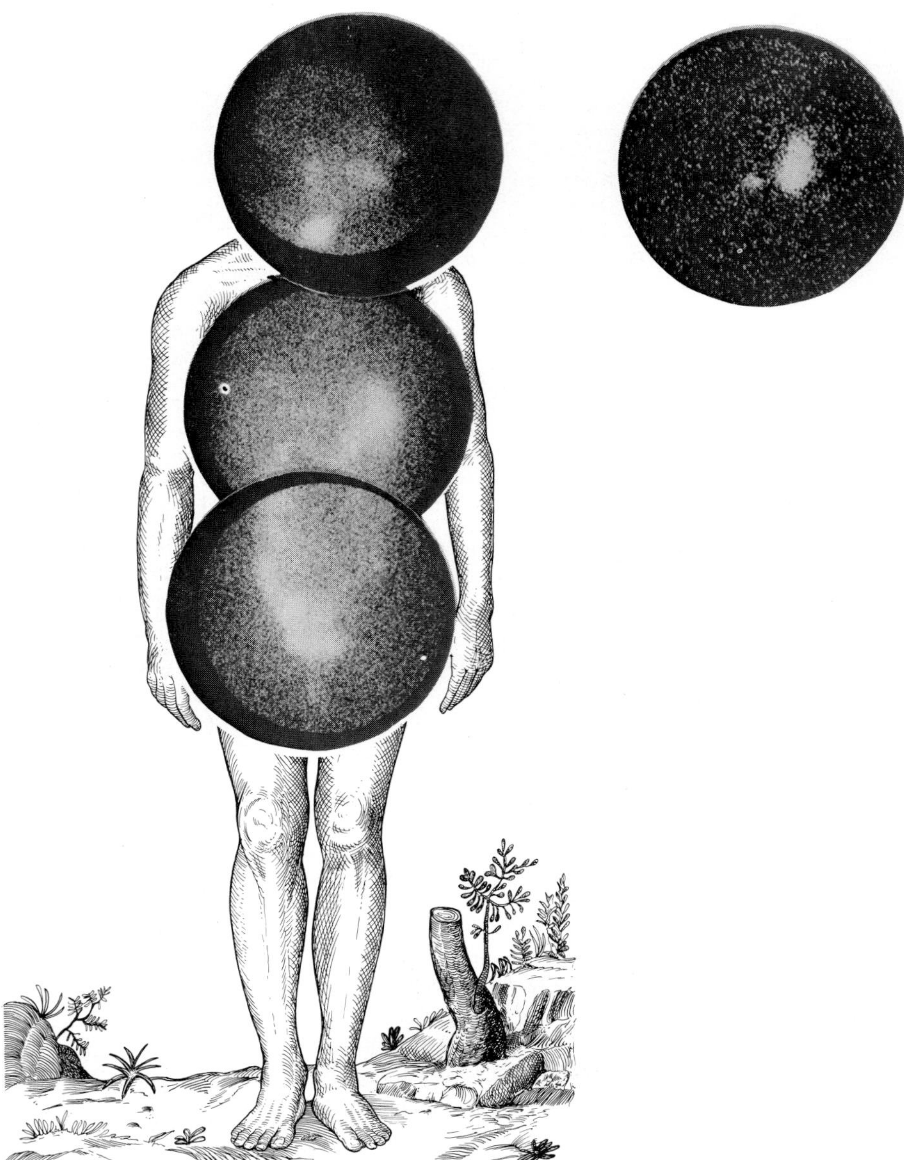

Figure 11. Normal distribution patterns of $Na^{131}I$. This whole body scan was performed 48 h following administration of 5 mCi (185 MBq) ^{131}I. Uptake in the thyroid bed representing postsurgical thyroid remnants imaged in the pinhole view at upper right. Uptake in the remnants measured 0.6% of the administered dose. Note normal uptake in salivary glands, oral cavity, orbits, stomach, liver, small bowel, colon, bladder, and vagina.

remnants.[14,276] However, there are more drawbacks than advantages in its use:

1. Blood levels of bTSH are only transiently elevated because of its short circulating half-life[131];
2. Allergic reactions have resulted from bTSH injection;
3. Injections of bTSH may induce antibody production against both bTSH and endogenous TSH, leading to TSH resistance[277];
4. Bovine TSH appears to be less effective in stimulating thyroid uptake than endogenous TSH.

Thus, it is preferable to rely upon endogenous TSH production to stimulate tumor uptake of ^{131}I. The usual reasons for using bTSH are not compelling. Functioning remnants of normal thyroid tissue that produce sufficient thyroid hormone to suppress endogenous TSH almost always take up enough ^{131}I to ablate them with 150 mCi (5.5 GBq). The same is true of functioning thyroid metastases. Perhaps the only circumstance that might warrant use of exogenous TSH is that in which pituitary reserve is reduced, as in older patients, and metastatic uptake is so low that a therapeutic effect is unlikely without such stimulation. In such cases, pre- and poststimulation uptake measurements should be made to determine the efficacy of further TSH stimulation.

The Use of TRH to Stimulate Endogenous TSH. The rise of serum TSH following intravenous injection of TRH is transient. However, a more sustained rise in TSH follows oral administration of TRH.[278–280] An oral dose of 80 μg TRH induces a maximum response in serum TSH and 80

Table 7. Extrathyroidal Uptake of Radioiodine

Common
1. Normal activity in salivary glands, oropharynx, urinary bladder, liver, and urinary tract
2. Normal activity in lactating breasts
3. Ectopic thyroid: substernal, sublingual, or intrathoracic
4. Metastatic differentiated thyroid carcinoma
5. Skin, hair, or clothing contamination by salivary, urinary, or sweat activity (especially common in high-dose ^{131}I metastatic surveys)

Rare
1. Postoperative colon interposition[256]
2. Barrett's esophagus[257]
3. Nonlactating breast[258]
4. Pulmonary infection[259,260]
5. Salivary gland tumor[261]
6. Intrathoracic gastric cyst[262]
7. Struma ovarii[263]; struma cordis[264]
8. Papillary meningioma[265]
9. Primary lung adenocarcinoma[266] and bronchogenic carcinoma[267]
10. Metastatic gastric adenocarcinoma[268]
11. Meckel's diverticulum[269]
12. Ovarian cyst[270]
13. Lymphoepithelial cyst of the parotid gland[271]
14. Scrotal hydrocele[271]
15. Renal cyst[272]
16. Nonspecific thymus uptake[273]
17. Gallbladder[274]
18. Skin burn[271]
19. Pelvic teratoma[275]

mg given every 12 hours for 5 doses can increase ^{131}I uptake in normal thyroid glands.[281] The important question is: Does TRH increase tumor uptake of ^{131}I? Samaan[282] showed that in patients already maximally stimulated by hypothyroidism, TRH does not increase serum TSH, nor does it increase ^{131}I uptake by tumor. However, it might be possible to give oral TRH shortly after withdrawing T_3 as a means of reducing the interval between T_3 withdrawal and ^{131}I therapy or whole-body imaging.[283] Thus far, studies designed to test this protocol have not been completed.

Decreasing Serum Iodide Pool. Reducing the concentration of serum inorganic iodine increases the uptake of radioiodine by thyroid carcinoma by increasing the ratio of radioactive to stable atoms. This can be accomplished in two ways: reducing intake and increasing excretion of iodine.

Several studies have shown that low-iodine diets reduce total-body iodine, increase ^{131}I uptake by functioning thyroid carcinoma, and increase estimated radiation dose to tumor.[284–287] Using a diet containing <25 μg/day, Goslings found that urinary excretion of iodine fell from 120 to 30 μg/day by the fourth day.[284] Following this regimen, tumor uptake of ^{131}I rose and the biologic half-time in the tumor rose. These effects combined to double the estimated radiation dose to the tumor. Similar findings are reported by Hurley and Becker[164] and Maruca.[287]

Diuretics also induce iodine depletion. Hamberger used ethacrynic acid (50 mg every 8 hours for 4 days).[285] Tumor uptake of ^{131}I increased in 19 of 25 patients, although the biologic half-time did not increase.

Hydrochlorothiazide is also a potent stimulator of renal iodine clearance.[148,287] Maruca[287] combined the administration of hydrochlorothiazide (100 mg bid) with a low-iodine diet in 4 patients. Total-body iodine decreased by 25 to 66% and estimated tumor absorbed dose increased 146% (range 48 to 243%). However, because iodine clearance decreased by an average of 56%, the total-body radiation per standard 150 mCi dose of ^{131}I increased by 68% (range 19 to 111%). These authors calculated that the increase in lesion irradiation relative to the incremental increase in total-body radiation was only 46% (range 24 to 82%). Nevertheless, this is a significant increase in lesion irradiation, and iodine depletion regimens should form a part of any carefully considered thyroid carcinoma treatment protocol. The value of adding diuretics to a low-iodine diet has not been determined. However, the complications likely to be encountered by such doses as 200 mg of hydrochlorothiazide daily for 4 days are minimal and may result in an augmented tumor uptake of ^{131}I.

Prolonging Tumor Retention of ^{131}I. The use of lithium to prolong tumor retention of ^{131}I has been investigated in only a few patients.[283,288–290] Ionic lithium, Li^+, has 3 effects on thyroid metabolism: it blocks thyroid release of iodide and of thyroid hormone and it inhibits peripheral conversion of T_4 to T_3. The first 2 effects have drawn attention to its use in thyroid cancer therapy. Increasing thyroid retention is especially important in ^{131}I therapy because of the 8-day physical half-life and the rapid release of iodine from thyroid cancer.[291] In the 4 patients reported by Robbins,[283] raising serum lithium levels to 0.6 to 1.0 mEq/L (usually by giving 300 mg lithium carbonate 3 to 4 times daily) slowed the rate of ^{131}I release from the tumor in every case. The effect was greatest in those patients in whom the biologic half-life of ^{131}I initially was shortest (Fig. 12). These findings have been corroborated by Rasmusson and colleagues[292] in 7 of 8 patients. However, Schraube et al found no prolongation of ^{131}I retention in 14 patients given Li^+ as an adjunct to ablation of postsurgical thyroid remnants.[293]

Because Li^+ is toxic and the range separating toxic and therapeutic levels is narrow, serum lithium levels must be monitored.[294] One important factor in toxicity is the adequacy of renal function. This is the principal route of Li^+ excretion and hypothyroid patients may have impaired renal excretory function. Further study of Li^+ is clearly warranted.

EFFICACY OF ^{131}I THERAPY FOR METASTASES

Locally Invasive, Nonresectable Disease. Local invasion to the extent that the primary tumor becomes unresectable carries a particularly grave prognosis. Smithers[295] reported 23 patients with unresectable cancer; of 10 patients with tumors that concentrated and could be treated with ^{131}I, 9

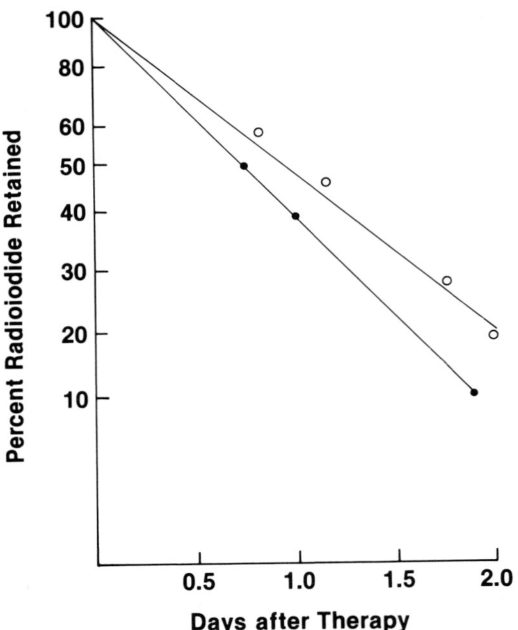

Figure 12. Retention of ^{131}I in thyroid remnants before (solid dots) and after (open circles) pretreatment with lithium carbonate. (From Robbins.[283])

had died of their disease within 11 years of resection. Of 13 patients with little or no ^{131}I uptake, 9 died within 5 years. Similar results have been reported by Tubiana.[247] Most of these tumors were treated with a combination of ^{131}I, if tumor concentration was satisfactory, and external beam radiotherapy. Follicular carcinomas appeared to respond to ^{131}I therapy somewhat more favorably than papillary carcinomas, but combined therapy was superior in both cases.[247,296]

Considering the poor prognosis of these tumors, it is appropriate to treat unresectable metastases in the neck vigorously. In such patients, the initial ablation should be carried out with a dose calculated to deliver 100,000 cGy to the remaining thyroid. Following ^{131}I therapy, T_4 suppression is started and external beam therapy is completed. Six months after the initial ^{131}I therapy, thyroid hormone is withheld and the Sloan-Kettering protocol described in Appendix J is followed to administer the highest permissible doses of ^{131}I.

METASTASES TO CERVICAL LYMPH NODES

The relatively benign significance of cervical lymph node metastases has already been mentioned. Nodal metastases are common in patients with papillary carcinoma; they are found in about 48% of patients under 40 years of age at the time of surgery and in about 17% of patients over the age of 40.[6] However, most studies have shown that nodal metastases do not increase mortality, and Cady reported a *lower* death rate among patients with nodal metastases.[6] Nodal metastases occur less frequently in follicular carcinoma and they appear to affect neither the rate of recurrence nor mortality.[12,276] Whether this is caused by some beneficial immunologic response, a higher association with papillary carcinoma, or merely the fact that their presence triggers an aggressive treatment regimen, has not been determined.

The most persuasive rationale for treating nodal metastases with ^{131}I is to decrease the incidence of recurrent metastases. Harwood et al found that recurrence of well-differentiated thyroid carcinoma is twice as common in patients with nodal metastases (32% vs. 14%).[297] Mazzaferri and Young showed that patients under the age of 40 have a twofold greater risk of recurrence and patients over 40 have a fivefold increased risk when cervical node metastases are found at surgery.[149]

Mazzaferri analyzed the impact of therapy on a group of 576 patients with papillary thyroid carcinoma.[15] Of these patients, 116 individuals were treated with ^{131}I for uptake in cervical nodes. During a mean follow-up period of 6 years, none of these patients had died and recurrent disease was found in only 3 (2.6%). These 3 patients had received less than 90 mCi (3.3 GBq) for their metastases, and nodal metastases were eradicated with additional ^{131}I in all. In a comparison group of 414 patients who received only thyroid suppression, the rate of recurrence was 11%; this difference was highly significant. Interestingly, there was no difference in mortality rates between the 2 groups.

DISTANT METASTASES

Patients with distant metastases (ie, outside the neck) have a significantly reduced survival rate compared with patients without metastases, or with a control population.[12,153,174,276] In the large series reported by Beierwaltes and co-workers,[174] 19% of patients with well-differentiated thyroid carcinoma who received ^{131}I therapy developed distant metastases (31% mediastinal, 44% lung, 23% bone, 2% liver). Of these, 60% were present at the time of surgery and the remaining 40% developed over an average of 7.4 years following ^{131}I therapy. The incidence of distant metastases was thought to be unusually high because the University of Michigan is a regional cancer center and because patients with well-differentiated thyroid cancer, who were not treated with ^{131}I, were not included in the analysis. Interestingly, there was no difference in survival rates between papillary and follicular cancers when compared with age-matched populations (Figs. 13 and 14).

In the same study, patients with mediastinal metastases were most likely to respond to ^{131}I therapy and most patients with bone and brain metastases died of their disease.[174] Patients who could be freed of metastases survived 3 times longer than patients with persistent disease. Therefore, the use of ^{131}I therapy in patients with functioning metastases is strongly indicated.

LUNG METASTASES

The incidence of lung metastases in all categories of differentiated thyroid carcinoma varies from 2% to 12%, depending upon the series reported and the treatment

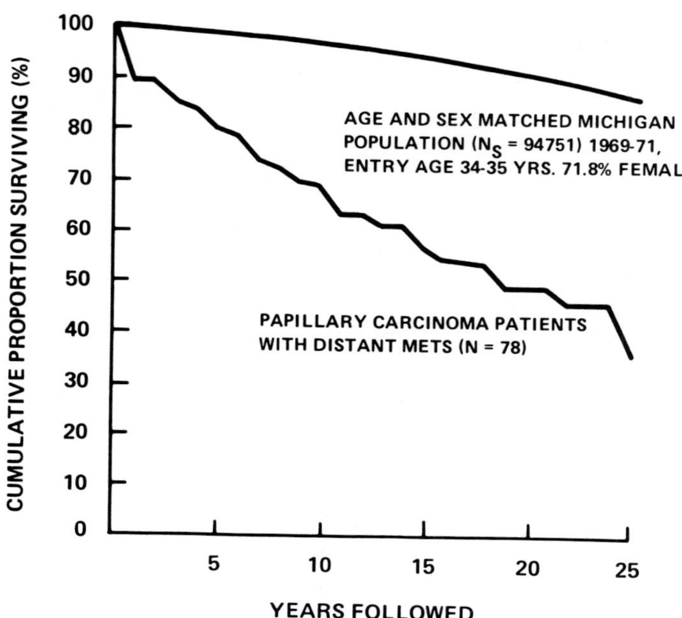

Figure 13. Survival of 78 patients having papillary thyroid carcinoma with distant metastases treated with ^{131}I compared with age- and sex-matched population. (From Beierwaltes et al.[174])

used.[9,12,17,142,174,298,299] Lower incidences are generally encountered among patients treated with total thyroidectomy and thyroid ablation with ^{131}I.[12,15,298,299] In a large series of patients reported by Massin et al,[298] among patients treated with total thyroidectomy plus ^{131}I, lung metastases developed in only 1.3%; with total thyroidectomy alone, in 3%; with incomplete thyroidectomy plus ^{131}I, in 5%; and with incomplete thyroidectomy alone, in 11%.

The presence of cervical lymph node metastases also appears to increase the probability of lung metastases. In the study of Massin and colleagues,[298] lung metastases occurred in 11% of patients with cervical lymph node involvement, but in only 5% of patients without ($p < 0.01$). Interestingly, in the same series of patients, there was a strong *inverse* correlation between cervical lymph node involvement and the development of bone metastases. These findings led Nemec to postulate that lung metastases reach the lungs by lymphatic channels and the thoracic duct, rather than through microvascular invasion and hematogenous spread, which is thought to characterize bone metastases.[17]

Treatment and Dosimetry. The treatment of functioning lung metastases with ^{131}I is the same as that for other distant metastases: 200 mCi (7.4 GBq) with a limit of 80 mCi (3 GBq) retained in the lungs at 48 hours.[246] Doses of ^{131}I may be repeated at 6- to 9-month intervals.

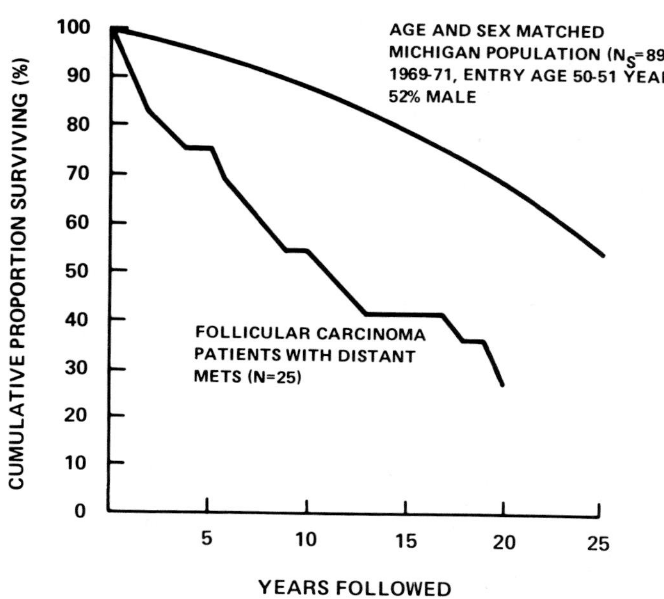

Figure 14. Survival of 25 patients having follicular carcinoma with distant metastases treated with ^{131}I, compared with age- and sex-matched population. (From Beierwaltes et al.[174])

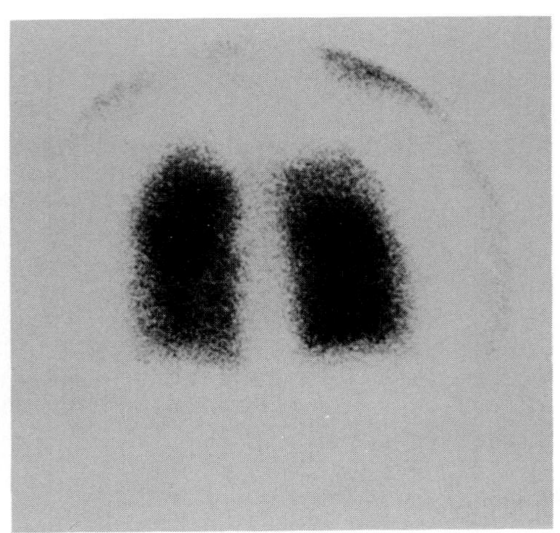

Figure 15. Pulmonary metastases from follicular thyroid cancer. **(A).** Whole-body ^{131}I scan using pinhole collimator 3 m from patient. **(B).** High-energy parallel-hole collimator images of ^{131}I uptake in miliary lung metastases in the same patient.

The lung uptake is measured by determining the ratio of activity retained at 48 hours with the activity administered. The denominator is obtained by counting the patient at a suitable distance (eg, 3 m) from a detector 1 to 2 hours following administration of the tracer dose, and without the patient voiding; this gives the 100% baseline count. The count is repeated using the same geometry at 48 hours, when nearly all of the retained activity will be in the lungs (Fig. 15). Correcting for decay, the lung uptake is:

$$\text{lung uptake } (\mu\text{Ci}) = \frac{\text{counting rate at 48 h}}{\text{counting rate at 2 h} \times 0.842 \times \text{administered dose } (\mu\text{Ci})}$$

The patient should void before the 48-hour count to eliminate bladder activity. If whole-body imaging demonstrates significant bowel activity, the abdomen can be shielded with lead when making the 48-hour count. Either a probe counter with flat-field collimator or a scintillation camera with pinhole collimator aimed at the patient's waist provides a suitable detector. The analyzer should be set to a narrow (20-keV) window to reduce the effects of scattered radiation.[292] Preliminary tests must be made to ensure that the tracer dose does not exceed the counting rate capacity of the detector and that, at the distance selected, the detector has a flat response over the length of the patient's body.[250]

It is useful to determine the radiation dose to the lungs as a guide to further therapy. This is easily accomplished by taking serial body counts to determine effective half-life. Application of linear regression and curve stripping resolves the clearance curve into fast and slow components (Fig. 16).

Example: The following example is borrowed from Nusynowitz and colleagues.[300] The patient was a 53-year-old man with pulmonary metastases from a medullary carcinoma that concentrated, but did not organify, radioiodine. Diagnostic whole-body imaging with 5 mCi (185 MBq) ^{131}I revealed lung uptake at 24 hours of 31.5%. Following this, 200 mCi (7.4 GBq) ^{131}I was administered orally; the whole-body retention curve is shown in Figure 16. The two clearance curves give biologic half-times of 0.63 and 7.95 days, respectively.

The radiation dose to the patient's lungs can be estimated from MIRD equations.[169] The cumulated activity $\tilde{A}$ is calcu-

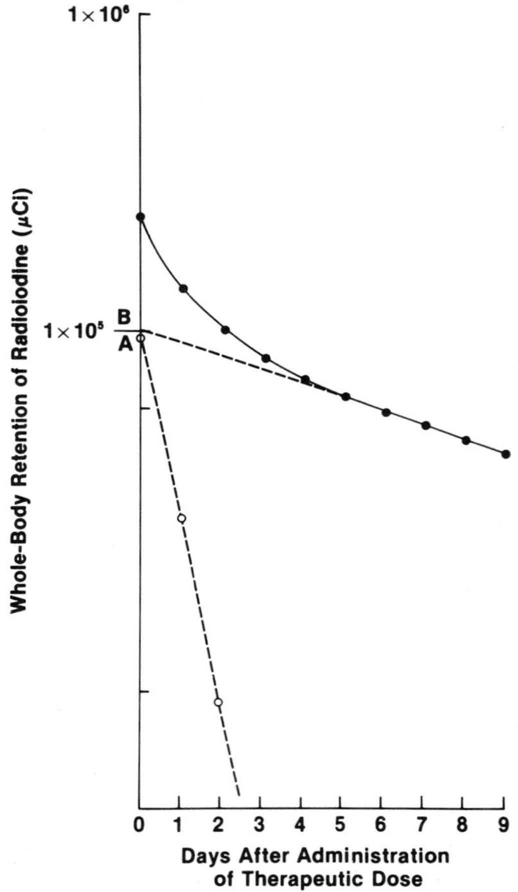

Figure 16. Whole-body retention of ^{131}I corrected for radioactive decay. The biexponential curve is resolved into its two functions with rate constants and initial concentrations. (Modified from Nusynowitz.[300])

lated by multiplying the zero-time activity of each of the 2 components from the clearance curves by their respective average effective half-time:

$$\tilde{A}_1 = (97{,}000\ \mu\text{Ci})\ (1.44)\left(\frac{0.63 \times 8.1}{0.63 + 8.1}\right)$$
$$= 1.96 \times 10^6\ \mu\text{Ci} \cdot \text{h}$$
$$\tilde{A}_2 = (103{,}000\ \mu\text{Ci})\ (1.44)\left(\frac{7.95 \times 8.1}{7.95 + 8.1}\right)$$
$$= 1.43 \times 10^7\ \mu\text{Ci} \cdot \text{h}$$

Based on the above data, it is assumed that 100% of component 1 is in the lung, and 31.5% of component 2 is in the lung. The remaining 68.5% of component 2 is in the "rest of body" (*RB*), defined as *RB* = [total body (*TB*) − lung]. The absorbed dose *S* factor[301] for ^{131}I located in and irradiating the lungs is:

$$S(\text{lung} \leftarrow \text{lung}) = 4.5 \times 10^{-4}\ \text{cGy}/\mu\text{Ci} \cdot \text{h}$$

and for *TB* activity irradiating lungs:

$$S(\text{lung} \leftarrow TB) = 1.0 \times 10^{-5}\ \text{cGy}/\mu\text{Ci} \cdot \text{h}$$

From this, the *S* factor for irradiating the lung from the *RB* is:

$$\begin{aligned} S(\text{lung} \leftarrow RB) & \\ &= S(\text{lung} \leftarrow TB)\ (70/69) - S(\text{lung} \leftarrow \text{lung})(1/69) \\ &= 1.0 \times 10^{-5}\ (70/69) - (4.5 \times 10^{-4})\ (1/69) \\ &= 3.6 \times 10^{-6}\ \text{cGy}/\mu\text{Ci} \cdot \text{h} \end{aligned}$$

The absorbed dose, $\overline{D}$ is then obtained:

$$\begin{aligned} \overline{D}(\text{lung} \leftarrow \text{lung}) & \\ &= [\tilde{A}_1 + (\tilde{A}_2 \times \text{fractional lung uptake})]\ [S(\text{lung} \leftarrow \text{lung})] \\ &= [1.96 \times 10^6 + (1.43 \times 10^7)\ (0.315)]\mu\text{Ci} \cdot \text{h} \times 4.5 \times 10^{-4}\ \text{cGy}/\mu\text{Ci} \cdot \text{h} \\ &= 2{,}909\ \text{cGy} \end{aligned}$$

$$\begin{aligned} \overline{D}(\text{lung} \leftarrow RB) &= [(RB\ \text{uptake})\ (\tilde{A}_2)]S\ (\text{lung} \leftarrow RB) \\ &= (0.685)\ (1.43 \times 10^7\ \mu\text{Ci} \cdot \text{h})\ (3.6 \times 10^{-6}\ \text{cGy}/\mu\text{Ci} \cdot \text{h}) \\ &= 35\ \text{cGy} \end{aligned}$$

$$\overline{D}(\text{lung}) = 2{,}909 + 35 = 2{,}944\ \text{cGy}$$

This absorbed dose, obviously, is an average for the lungs as a whole. Since the distribution of activity within the lung is nonuniform, so too is the distribution of the radiation absorbed dose. Furthermore, the tumor mass that concentrates the activity must have an attenuating influence on the dose absorbed by the lung parenchyma. Therefore, absorbed dose estimates, such as these, serve chiefly as a guide to the clinician concerning the most appropriate time to begin monitoring pulmonary function as it is affected by pulmonary fibrosis.

PROGNOSIS

Several factors appear to affect or, at least, to be related to outcome in patients with lung metastases from differentiated thyroid carcinoma. Some of these are listed in Table 6, taken from the study of Massin et al.[298]

Histological Characteristics. A more favorable prognosis is associated with lung metastases from papillary than from follicular carcinoma. This difference appears to be due to 3 factors; first, micronodular metastases occur more frequently in papillary than in follicular carcinomas. Radiographically, micronodular metastases appear as tiny miliary densities predominating in the lower lung fields or as diffuse reticular patterns (Fig. 17A). These, in turn, are usually associated with homogeneously diffuse uptake by radionuclide imaging (see Fig. 15). Macronodular metastases are characterized roentgenographically by irregular distribution of nodular masses varying between 0.5 and 3 cm in diameter (Fig. 17B). Radionuclide images of macronodular metastases are characterized by heterogeneous patterns of uptake, in which areas of activity are generally less numerous than the corresponding roentgenographic masses. Second, follicular carcinoma is more commonly encountered in older individuals in whom metastatic ^{131}I concentration is often reduced or absent. Third, follicular carcinoma is associated with a higher rate of lymph-node involvement. While these factors are interrelated to some extent, they each correlate with reduced survival.

^{131}I Uptake. Uptake of ^{131}I by lung metastases carries a favorable prognosis and is more characteristic of micronodular (86%) than macronodular (43%) metastases. There is generally no difference in ^{131}I uptake between papillary and follicular carcinomas. ^{131}I uptake is related to age; most patients with lung metastases who present under 30 years of age have positive ^{131}I uptake, while few patients over 80 years of age have positive uptake.

In the large series reported by Samaan et al, 42 (42%) of 101 patients had positive chest x-rays but negative ^{131}I scans, and 10 patients (10%) had positive ^{131}I scans and negative chest x-rays.[299] Uptake of radioactive iodine by lung metastases was a favorable prognostic factor, especially in patients with negative radiographic findings.

Tumor Invasion. The extent of tumor invasion greatly affects survival, as evidenced by the low survival in patients with mediastinal metastases (Table 8). We have already noted that cervical metastases do not appear to have an adverse effect on the outcome of patients. In the study of Massin and coworkers,[298] 30 patients had cervical and pulmonary metastases with an 8-year survival of 40%, and 28 patients without cervical metastases had a 25% survival; this difference was not significant. In the same study, 24 patients with pulmonary metastases were treated with ^{131}I; 10 of these patients (42%) were alive after 8 years, although 2 had died of unrelated causes, giving a cure rate of 50%. The 12 apparently cured patients received cumulative doses of between 100 and 500 mCi (3.7 to 18.5 GBq), with a mean of 280 mCi (10 GBq). These quantities include the ablation dose; the average number of therapeutic doses was 2.5. The results of ^{131}I therapy compared with other forms of therapy

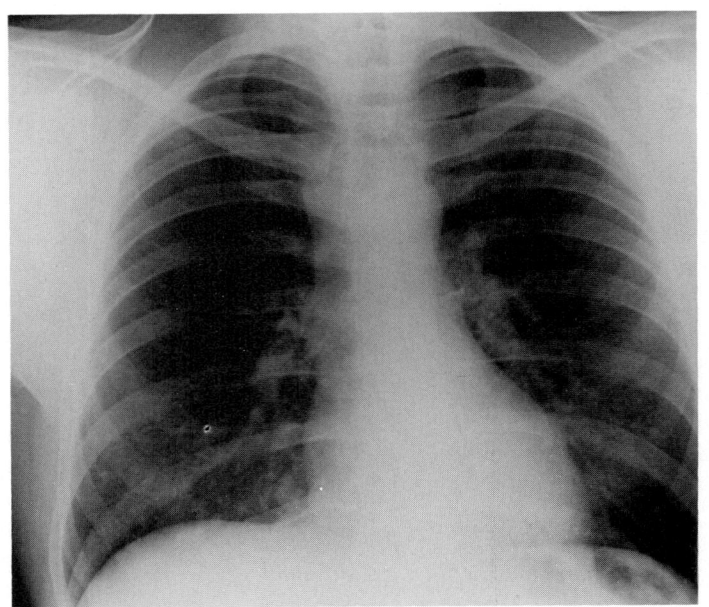

A

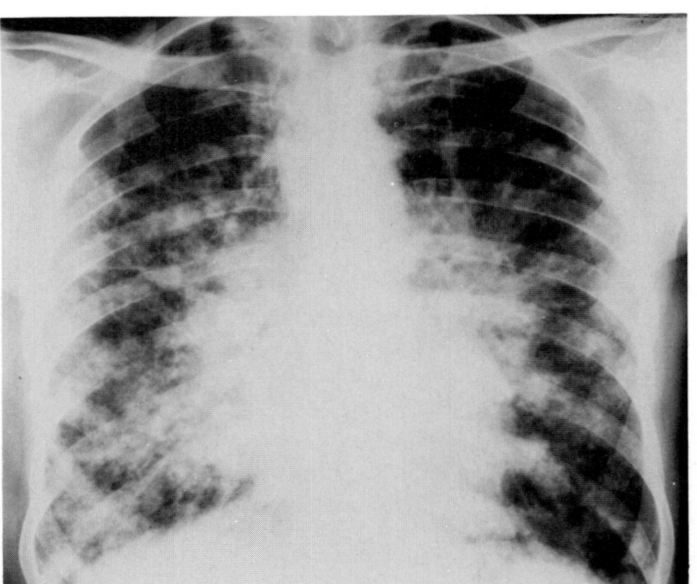

B

Figure 17. (A). Chest radiograph of patient with diffuse micronodular metastases from papillary thyroid carcinoma. **(B).** Chest radiograph of patient with macronodular metastases from follicular thyroid carcinoma.

shown in Figure 18 leave little doubt about the efficacy of ^{131}I therapy in patients with positive uptake.

Other investigators have also shown good results when sufficient ^{131}I concentrates in lung metastases. Benua and colleagues[246] found favorable responses in 11 of 14 (78%) patients, although survival rates for this group of patients were not given.

Němec and co-workers[301] found lung metastases in 12% of patients with well-differentiated thyroid carcinoma, and positive ^{131}I uptake in 50% of 66 patients. They found generally greater ^{131}I uptake in patients with micronodular metastases and in patients under 40 years of age. Ten- and 15-year survival rates were significantly higher in patients treated with ^{131}I. Similar findings have been reported by Beierwaltes.[174]

In summary, lung metastases from differentiated thyroid carcinoma are associated with significantly reduced survival. Better prognosis for prolonged survival or cure is associated with younger age, with papillary carcinoma, with micronodular metastases, and with intense, uniform uptake of ^{131}I. The probability of developing lung metastases is greatly reduced by near-total thyroidectomy and ^{131}I ablation.[298]

BONE METASTASES

Bone metastases carry a much more grave prognosis than lung metastases. Of 21 patients studied by Brown and associates[302] at the Royal Marsden Hospital in London, 95% died within 5 years of diagnosis and no patient lived longer than

Table 8. Factors Associated with Survival in Patients with Lung Metastases

FACTOR	NO. PATIENTS	SURVIVAL RATE AT 8 YEARS (%)
Micronodular metastases	14	77
Macronodular metastases	27	18
Mediastinal metastases	17	9
Bone and brain metastases	27	14
Cervical node metastases	30	40
Papillary carcinoma	27	51
Follicular carcinoma	30	11
Positive ^{131}I uptake	28	43
Negative ^{131}I uptake	23	26
All patients	58	28

Source: Massin JP, Savoie JC, Garnier H, et al: Pulmonary metastases in differentiated thyroid carcinoma. *Cancer* 53:982, 1984. With permission.

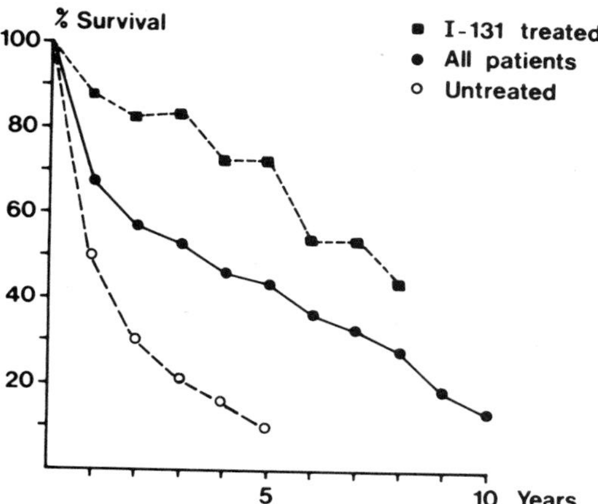

Figure 18. Survival among patients with pulmonary metastases from differentiated thyroid carcinoma is greatly increased by ^{131}I therapy. (From Massin et al.[298])

8 years (Fig. 19). Patients with bone metastases tend to be older, and follicular carcinoma is 5 times more likely to spread to bone than papillary carcinoma.[302] At least one half of all bone metastases from thyroid carcinoma are discovered at the time of initial diagnosis. The mode of spread is through the systemic circulation. Němec[17] postulated that bone metastases located in the skull, spine, or rib cage most likely spread by way of the vertebral venous system, and these patients usually do not have concurrent lung metastases. Patients with multiple bone metastases, without regard to location, more frequently have concurrent lung metastases and spread is thought to develop through the systemic circulation. These patients may also develop brain, liver, and kidney metastases, but the latter are far less frequent sites.

While nearly all patients with bone metastases die of their disease, ^{131}I therapy may prolong life.

CARCINOMA IN ABERRANT THYROID TISSUE

Developmental abnormalities may leave part or all of the thyroid in aberrant sites at the base of the tongue, along the thyroglossal duct, in the mediastinum, or in the lateral neck. While rare, carcinomas may develop in this tissue.[303–306] Ectopic tissue remnants undergo hyperplasia in response to inadequate T_4 production and increased serum TSH. It is thought that prolonged and intense TSH stimulation dispose toward the development of thyroid carcinoma. This association has been noted, for example, in patients with T_4 synthesis defects who have been inadequately treated with T_4.[307,308] Sublingual thyroid is the most common aberrancy; if left alone, such tissue frequently undergoes involution with eventual hypothyroidism.[309] The usual treatment of aberrant thyroid is with T_4 suppression, under which these tissues usually shrink.[310] If the mass fails to regress or if it enlarges, despite T_4 suppression, it should be removed surgically. In some patients, ^{131}I has been used to ablate aberrant thyroid that recurs after surgery; however, surgery should be the initial remedy because of the possibility of coexisting cancer.[311] Occasionally, aberrant thyroid tissue may give rise to thyrotoxicosis; in such rare cases ablation with ^{131}I is appropriate, although surgical removal should be the first consideration.

Papillary thyroid cancer may arise in the thyroglossal duct, and about 10% of these become invasive.[312] This always raises the question of how to approach the thyroid gland. DeGroot and colleagues suggest subtotal resection only for cervical node metastases, or if thyroid scanning demonstrates a thyroid lesion.[313] Since these cancers have all the potential for invasion and dissemination, an aggressive approach including ^{131}I ablation is warranted if cancer is found.

Another dilemma arises when lateral extranodal aberrant thyroid tissue is found. On rare occasions, histologically normal thyroid tissue is found along the internal carotid artery, in the supraclavicular fossa, or in the mediastinum.[314] Some authorities believe these represent remnants of normal thyroid tissue derived from the pharyngeal pouches, since this is a common location of thyroid in fish.[315] However, the prevailing view is that, in man, lateral aberrant thyroid represents cervical metastases from an occult primary thyroid cancer. DeGroot and colleagues suggest that if the aberrant mass is connected to the thyroid by a definite fibrous band and appears histologically normal, simple resection is adequate therapy.[313] If the tissue is entirely detached from the thyroid, and if the histologic appearance suggests carcinoma, then thyroidectomy and examination of regional lymph nodes is indicated. These aberrant thyroid masses should not be confused with small clusters of histologically normal thyroid follicles that may be found in perithyroid lymph nodes. The latter are believed to be benign and analogous to transport of endometrial tissue into abdominal structures in endometriosis.[316]

When thyroid tissue occurs in ovarian teratomas, it is known as *struma ovarii.* Such tissue arises *de novo* from

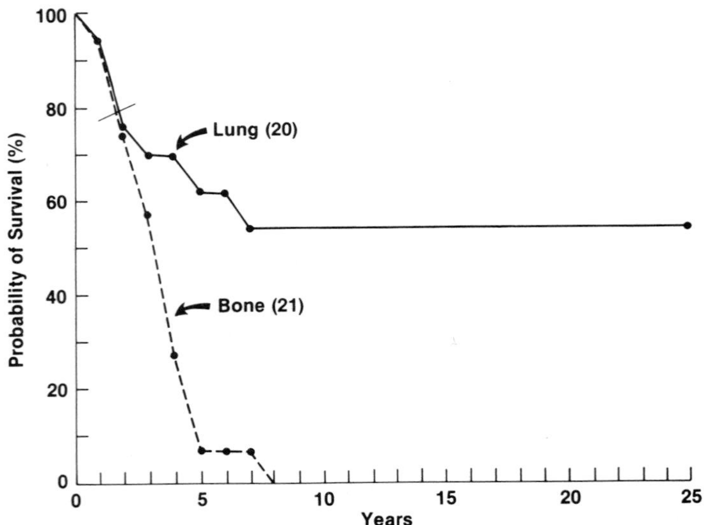

Figure 19. Comparison of survival among patients with lung and bone metastases. (From Brown et al.[302])

pluripotential embryonal cells. In one series, struma occurred in about 3% of ovarian teratomas.[317] Rarely, thyrotoxicosis develops and these teratomas concentrate ^{131}I. In 5 to 20% of struma, low-grade malignant tumors develop, some of which metastasize.[318,319] Benign tumors are usually treated by simple oophorectomy, although with malignant extension, total abdominal hysterectomy with bilateral salpingooophorectomy may be necessary.[320] Although little experience has been reported in these rare tumors, metastases would presumably be treated as though they arose from the thyroid gland. Thus, the best chance for effective therapy would include thyroid ablation and whole body imaging, in the hope that high TSH levels may increase ^{131}I uptake.

Radiation Safety Considerations

Federal regulations in the United States require hospitalization in private rooms for patients with body burdens of greater than 30 mCi (1110 MBq) of gamma-emitting radionuclides or until the radiation exposure is less than 5 mR/hr at a distance of 1 meter from the organ with the greatest radioactivity.[321] Because of these requirements, some have suggested using fractionated doses at weekly intervals in such amounts that body burdens exceeding 30 mCi are avoided.[322] However, this practice is seldom followed, chiefly because the radiation dose to thyroid and tumor is almost impossible to estimate.

Radiation exposure measurements are most appropriately taken with a calibrated survey meter held 1 meter from the anterior surface of the abdomen or neck.[323] Visitors and nursing staff can minimize their radiation exposure by reducing close contact with the patient. In most cases, patients can be discharged about 48 hours after administration. Other radiation safety practices are outlined in Chapter 54 and elsewhere.[324,325]

With regard to close personal contact with radioactive patients after hospital discharge, we have found no instances in which family members who were directly monitored with film badges ever exceeded 0.005 Sv, the maximum permitted dose for the general public.[326] In cases in which very close and prolonged contact might be an issue, guidelines for contact have been published.[327]

COMPLICATIONS OF ^{131}I

Short-Term Complications. Transient sialoadenitis is common following therapeutic doses of ^{131}I. In a study of 87 patients reviewed by Allweiss et al, acute and/or chronic sialoadenitis developed in 11.5% of patients.[328] The parotid and submandibular glands were affected about equally. The precipitating dose of I-131 varied between 10 mCi (370 MBq) and 164 mCi (6.1 GBq), and clinical symptoms occurred most frequently following repeat doses. The development of radiation sialoadenitis in patients receiving 100 to 200 mCi (3.7 to 7.4 GBq) is hardly surprising; Doniach estimated that the salivary glands receive as much as 50 cGy per millicurie administered (1.35 cGy/MBq).[329]

The salivary glands receive a significant radiation dose because of their ability to concentrate iodine. The effect is more pronounced during dehydration, which increases ^{131}I retention. The diagnosis is easily recognized by pain and swelling, usually bilateral, occurring in the first 3 days following therapy. Local pain and swelling is also encountered in the region of the thyroid bed. This local effect is more common in patients who have had only partial thyroidectomy than in patients who have undergone near-total thyroidectomy.[330] Posttherapeutic development of cystic degeneration has also been reported.[331]

Not infrequently, patients report dry mouth, hypogeusia, or dysgeusia (especially a metallic taste) following ^{131}I therapy. These symptoms may be transient, last several weeks, or may be permanent.[246,332,333] Salivary scans using ^{99m}Tc-pertechnetate following doses of 150 mCi (5.5 GBq) of ^{131}I demonstrate impaired clearance of pertechnetate.[334] Ample fluids and giving hard sour candy to promote salivary secretion during the first 24 hours after administration greatly reduces this complication.

Radiation gastritis is not uncommon when high doses are administered and is best prevented by ample fluid intake. With doses of ^{131}I larger than 200 mCi (7.4 GBq), vomiting occurs in about 5% of patients.[171]

Acute radiation sickness may occur within 12 hours of administration of high doses of ^{131}I. This syndrome is characterized by fatigue, headache, nausea and, rarely, vomiting. Older reports have cited the incidence as varying between 36%[246] and 73%[335] but the experience of most investigators using 150 to 200 mCi (5.5 to 7.4 GBq) has been that this syndrome is not common.

Thyroid storm is a rare occurrence in patients who have hyperthyroidism secondary to large masses of functioning metastases and high retained uptake.[336,337] Such patients should be controlled with antithyroid drugs and beta-blocking drugs prior to ^{131}I administration. For a more thorough discussion of thyroid storm, see Chapter 1.

Vocal cord paralysis is a rare complication that may require tracheostomy. Although this condition is more common following ^{131}I therapy for hyperthyroidism, at least one case has been reported following near-total thyroidectomy and ablation with 150 mCi (5.5 GBq).[338] Vocal cord paralysis only occurs in cases of bilateral injury to the recurrent laryngeal nerves. This patient had bilateral injury at surgery with recovery of one side during the postoperative period; the thyroid remnant lay on the recovered side. Three days following thyroid ablation, stridor recurred and intubation was again required; 2 months later, unilateral function returned and the tracheostomy was closed. The uptake of ^{131}I in the thyroid remnant was only 0.4%, yet with a dose of 150 mCi (5.5 GBq), the absorbed dose to a 1-g remnant would be 36,000 cGy. It was postulated that the resultant edema in close proximity to a compromised nerve could result in prolonged neuropraxia.

Bone-marrow depression may occur within 1 month of radioiodine therapy and is usually transient.[171] Haynie and Beierwaltes[170] reported transient anemia in 36% of patients, leukopenia in 10%, and thrombocytopenia in 3%. Severe bone-marrow suppression seldom occurs when the radiation dose to the blood is less than 200 cGy.[171] Bone-marrow depression occurs most often in patients who

1. receive a large cumulative amount of radioiodine;
2. receive external beam therapy in addition to ^{131}I;
3. have large functioning tumors that produce a high concentration of PB^{131}I; and
4. have extensive bony metastases.[169,170] The peripheral blood count should be monitored, but the anemia seldom requires transfusion.

Temporary Ovarian Failure. Raymond and colleagues studied ovarian function in 66 women who received ^{131}I for the treatment of thyroid carcinoma.[339] Of course, 18 (27%) developed temporary amenorrhea, accompanied by increased serum gonadotropin concentrations and, in some cases, hot flashes. The mean ages of the 18 was 38.9 ± 7.1 years. The ^{131}I administered was 270 ± 54 mCi and the estimated radiation dose to the ovaries was 1.76 ± 0.49 Gy. There was no correlation found between the radioactive iodine dose absorbed, thyroid uptake before treatment, oral contraceptive use, or thyroid autoimmunity. Only age was a determining factor, with older women being the most affected.

Local effects consisting of pain, hemorrhage, and edema may develop at the site of metastases. Such effects are caused by radiation inflammation.[169,246,340] Pain is especially likely following therapy of functioning bone metastases.[340] By far the most serious of these effects is cerebral hemorrhage or edema caused by functioning cerebral metastases.[341,342] Because of such a possibility, it is recommended that radioiodine in therapeutic doses not be administered to patients with functioning cerebral metastases, until such function is reduced or eliminated by external beam therapy.

A related case was recently reported by Sziklas, in which treatment of a functioning pituitary metastasis resulted in panhypopituitarism.[343]

Long-Term Complications. *Myelogenous leukemia* develops in about 2% of patients treated with ^{131}I for thyroid carcinoma metastases, whereas the number of cases expected would be less than 0.1%.[344,345] Of these patients, about 85% are acute and 15% are chronic; 85% of cases occur in women over 50 years of age. Of the cases reported by Brincker,[344] the average cumulative dose was 910 mCi (34 GBq). The mean interval between treatment and the onset of clinical leukemia was 3 years and the longest interval was 7 years.

Beierwaltes has reported a much lower incidence of leukemia; only 1 among 400 patients treated with radioiodine.[346] Most authorities believe that high doses frequently administered dispose toward development of leukemia. When radioiodine is administered no more often than once yearly (provided the patient's condition is stable) the incidence of leukemia is not increased.[15,56,153,154,347] Beierwaltes and colleagues suggest that the cumulative amount of ^{131}I administered should not exceed 800 mCi (~30 GBq) or 500 mCi (18.5 GBq) in patients under 30 years of age.[5,53,348]

Other malignancies appear to be associated with thyroid cancers.[349,350] Mazzaferri[15] reported a 3.5% incidence of at least one other cancer. However, in over half the patients, the second malignancy preceded the detection of the thyroid cancer. Beierwaltes[5] looked for other malignancies in their series of 400 patients that might develop cancer in other organs concentrating radioiodine. They found only 2 cases of parotid gland tumors; both were diagnosed prior to detection and treatment of their thyroid cancers. Wiseman[333] reported 2 cases of parotid gland lymphoma following ^{131}I therapy. One patient received 675 mCi (25 GBq) and the other 350 mCi (13 GBq). Parotid gland lymphomas developed 10 and 3 years, respectively, following ^{131}I therapy.

A slight excess of bladder cancers has been reported.[351] This cancer is most likely due to direct radiation exposure to the bladder wall.

Anaplastic transformation has been reported as a rare complication of ^{131}I therapy.[171,347] However, anaplastic carcinoma can develop in patients who have received no irradiation and a true causal relationship has not been established.[15,352]

Azoospermia was reported by Handelsman[353] in a 32-year-old man who received 350 mCi (13 GBq) in 3 doses over a 3-year period. The azoospermia was severe enough to cause sterility. The radiation dose to the testes was estimated at 175 to 525 cGy. While there is little that can be done to prevent this occurrence, male patients should be advised of its possibility. In a series of 33 patients including 20 women and 13 men treated before the age of 20, Sarkar[354] found no difference in infertility, miscarriage rate, or congenital abnormalities between patients who received 196 to 691 mCi (7.2 to 26 GBq) and the general population; the average follow-up period was 18.7 years.

Pulmonary fibrosis must always be considered as a potential complication when functioning lung metastases are treated with ^{131}I. Rall and colleagues[355] reported 15 patients with diffuse functioning pulmonary metastases who had been treated with ^{131}I. Two patients died of radiation pneumonitis 4 months after treatment; these patients had lung uptakes of 162 (6 GBq) and 193 mCi (7 GBq). Four other patients developed roentgenographic evidence of pulmonary fibrosis. Benua and co-workers[246] recommended that, in the presence of functioning lung metastases, the therapeutic dose be limited so that the 48-hour retention in the whole body not exceed 80 mCi (3 GBq). Following this guideline, Leeper and Shimaoka[171] reported no radiation fibrosis following ^{131}I therapy. Rall concluded that radiation fibrosis does not develop when less than 100 mCi (3.7 GBq) of ^{131}I concentrates within pulmonary metastases.[355] Since pulmonary uptake rarely exceeds 20% of the administered dose, cumulative administered doses up to 1 Ci (37 GBq) should not result in pulmonary fibrosis. After 1-Ci cumulative dose, periodic pulmonary function tests are prudent. Some investigators suggest the use of steroids following ^{131}I for lung metastases as an additional precaution against pulmonary pneumonitis.[169]

Hyperparathyroidism and hypoparathyroidism; both of these conditions can develop following ^{131}I ablation for thyroid cancer, although hypoparathyroidism is more common. These subjects are discussed in Chapter 1. Periodic monitoring of serum calcium is a prudent measure.[357]

Thyroid Cancer and Pregnancy. Pregnancy imposes a dilemma for patients with thyroid cancer and their attending physicians. The patient, of course, must be reassured both as to the effect of thyroid cancer, its diagnosis and its treatment, on the fetus and as to the effect of pregnancy upon the course of her disease.

The Fetus. Three factors relating to maternal thyroid cancer concern the well-being of the fetus: the effect of the thyroid cancer itself, the effect of exogenous thyroid hormone, and the effect of radioiodine inadvertently administered to the mother. As regards the first of these, there is little danger of thyroid cancer metastasizing to the fetus because of the placental barrier. Provided the nutritional health of the mother is maintained, no adverse effects upon the fetus are to be anticipated.

Table 9. Maturation of Human Fetal Thyroid Function

FETAL AGE (days)	FETAL WEIGHT (g)	THYROID WEIGHT (*mg*)	THYROID WEIGHT (*mg/g of body weight*)	THYROID ^{127}I CONTENT (μg)
95–100	75	80	1.07	1.1
105–120	146	131	0.97	3.9
122–138	203	139	0.69	1.8
145–165	465	261	0.59	7.1
166–230	1,080	728	0.68	22.0
Term	3,270	1,430	0.43	49.0

Costa A, Cottino F, Dellepiane M, et al: Thyroid function and thyrotropin activity in mother and fetus, in Cassano C, Andreoli M (eds.): *Current Topics in Hormone Research.* New York, Academic Press, 1965, pp 738–748.

During pregnancy, there is an increased demand for thyroid hormone. Maternal basal metabolic rate rises from 8 to 25% during the later stages of pregnancy.[358,359] The serum concentration of TBG rises, causing increased total, but not free, T_3 and T_4.[360,361] Therefore, replacement thyroid hormone may have to be increased to maintain maternal well-being. However, the placenta is relatively impermeable to maternal thyroid hormones, particularly in early pregnancy.[362,363] In the last trimester, placental permeability of thyronines increases but, by this time, the fetus is producing adequate quantities autonomously. Therefore, the fetus is relatively unaffected by maternal hypothyroidism or inadequate replacement.

A more subtle problem concerns the effect upon the fetus of inadvertent administration of ^{131}I to the mother. During the first trimester, there is no fetal thyroid hormone production and therefore no concentration of iodine. Consequently, the radiation dose absorbed by the whole fetus is the same as the maternal whole-body absorbed dose, ~0.47 cGy · mCi (~0.1 mGy/MBq) orally administered (MIRD 5, 1975).

By 11 to 12 weeks gestation, follicle organization is nearly complete and the ability of the fetal thyroid to concentrate iodine and synthesize hormone can be demonstrated.[364] Thereafter, colloid stores, iodine-concentrating capacity, and glandular stores of iodine and thyroid hormones increase progressively until term.[365–368] The course of fetal thyroid maturation is depicted in Table 9. The fetal thyroid has a greater avidity for radioiodine than does the adult gland; 12- to 48-hour uptakes by the fetal thyroid after maternal injection of radioiodine increase from very low levels at 12 to 14 weeks to 4 to 5%/g fetal thyroid during the last trimester.[365–367] Quantitative data regarding fetal thyroid hormone secretion is not available; however, the biologic half-time of ^{131}I must be longer in fetal than in adult thyroids because thyroid stores are increasing. Thus, in the second and especially in the third trimester, irradiation to the fetal thyroid by even small quantities of ^{131}I may be high. Halnan[369] estimated that a tracer dose of 50 μCi (1.85 MBq) ^{131}I given to the mother for thyroid imaging could deliver as high as 250 cGy to the fetal thyroid. This is of the same order of magnitude as the external radiation doses in infants and children implicated in causing thyroid cancer.[3,370,371] Therefore, there is a theoretical danger of inducing radiation-associated thyroid neoplasms as the child matures. In such event, Kudlow and Burrow[372] recommend that the child be followed by a surveillance program indefinitely. If a therapeutic dose of ^{131}I is given, the risk of serious thyroidal and genetic damage to the fetus exists and therapeutic abortion should be considered.[373]

Several cases of fetal thyroid ablation by ^{131}I have been reported.[373–377] If hypothyroidism is not suspected, cretinism and irreversible mental retardation may develop. Therefore, prolonged surveillance of patients exposed to ^{131}I in utero is prudent. Patients with reduced thyroid reserve found by TRH stimulation should probably be placed on T_4 replacement for life.

The Mother. There is no evidence at this time that pregnancy either alters the course or in any way hastens progression or recurrence of occult thyroid cancer metastases.[378,379] Rosvoll and Winship[379] studied 60 patients who had thyroid carcinoma diagnosed under the age of 15 years and who subsequently became pregnant. Of these, 38 were free of disease at the time of pregnancy, while 22 had active thyroid cancer when they became pregnant. These authors could detect no change in the manifestation of the existing tumor, regardless of the number of pregnancies, nor did they observe any complication of pregnancy related to the presence of tumor.

Hill and colleagues[378] studied 179 women between 10 and 45 years of age who had thyroid cancer; of these, 70 subsequently became pregnant. The remaining 109 patients were either never pregnant or had no pregnancy after the diagnosis of cancer. There was no significant difference in the recurrence rate between the 2 groups.

Sarkar[354] reported 33 young patients treated postsurgically with ^{131}I and followed for more than 14 years. The mean total dose of ^{131}I was 196 mCi (~7 GBq). The incidence of infertility (12%), miscarriage (1.4%), prematurity (8%), and major congenital anomalies (1.4%) found in this series did not differ from that in the general population. Thus, pregnancy is not contraindicated in patients with thyroid cancer, nor is the presence of thyroid cancer *per se* a compelling reason for abortion.

The effect of prior ^{131}I therapy on subsequent pregnancies is far less certain. Most patients with well-differentiated thyroid carcinoma receive a postsurgical ablation dose of 150 mCi (5.5 GBq) which, at 0.14 cGy/mCi (4 cGy/GBq), delivers approximately 21 cGy to the ovaries (MIRD no. 5, 1975). While the number of patients treated with ^{131}I for thyroid cancer who subsequently became pregnant is small, no increase in spontaneous abortion or increased frequency of congenital defects has been found.[354,380] However, cytogenetic analyses in the offspring studies by Einhorn and colleagues[380] revealed a higher incidence of chromosomal abnormalities than in age-matched control subjects who had received no ^{131}I. Second-generation data on these offspring are not available and, thus, no convincing evidence can be marshalled that pregnancy in such treated patients is contraindicated, nor can abortion be recommended in treated patients who become pregnant. Nevertheless, prudence dictates that these patients should be counseled that chromosomal aberrations can be expected in their offspring and that their family planning should take such risks, albeit undefined, into consideration. But, most importantly, the fear of mutation in future offspring should not in any way preclude radioiodine therapy in the management of this potentially fatal disease.[372]

Males Treated with ^{131}I. No studies have been published that bear upon the offspring of males treated with therapeutic amounts of ^{131}I. However, since the turnover of sperm is rapid with conception 6 months following ^{131}I therapy, no measurable effect should be seen.

Management of Thyroid Nodules During Pregnancy. From time to time thyroid nodules are discovered during pregnancy. Since radionuclide diagnostic procedures are contraindicated during pregnancy, the preliminary diagnosis rests primarily on physical and laboratory examinations, ultrasound, and fine-needle biopsy. Most nodules will fall into 1 of 3 categories (see Fig. 3):

1. Predominantly cystic. These nodules should be aspirated; if no malignant cells are found the patient is placed on T_4 suppression (0.2 to 0.3 mg L-thyroxine daily). If malignant cells are found by histological examination, the patient should be referred for surgery;
2. Patients with solid malignant nodules (approximately 20%) should be referred for surgery;
3. Patients with solid benign nodules should be placed on T_4 suppression and followed.

Surgery does impose some risk to the fetus and this increases with the extent and duration of surgery. Following surgery, the patient should be placed on T_4 suppression and whole-body ^{131}I scans delayed until after delivery. If the malignant lesion is small and nonfixed and there is no evidence of extension outside the thyroid, T_4 suppression may be elected with surgery following delivery. There is no evidence that pregnancy adversely affects tumor progression, nor that T_4 suppression adversely affects the fetus. In the case of frankly malignant nodules clinically, it is probably wise not to delay surgery.

THYROID CARCINOMA IN CHILDREN

Thyroid carcinoma is rare in childhood. Several decades ago, the incidence rose as a result of therapeutic neck irradiation for a variety of benign conditions.[3] Since this practice has stopped, the incidence has decreased to between 3 and 4% of childhood malignancies.[381,382] As with adults, the incidence in female children is twice that in males. However, thyroid carcinoma in children differs somewhat from that in adults. In children, thyroid carcinomas are usually papillary or mixed papillary-follicular; there is a high frequency (50 to 80%) of neck metastases, which are often multicentric (30 to 80%), and there is a generally favorable prognosis.[382] Lung metastases are common, while bone metastases are uncommon. Neck and lung metastases usually concentrate ^{131}I and they respond well to ^{131}I therapy.

Diagnosis and Treatment

The diagnosis of thyroid carcinoma in children does not differ appreciably from that in adults. Solid cold nodules should be biopsied and those found to be suspicious for malignancy are resected. Near-total thyroidectomy is performed when frozen section examination indicates invasive carcinoma. Solid functioning nonmalignant nodules should be suppressed and those nodules found to be autonomous should be removed.

Opinion regarding the use of ablation and whole-body ^{131}I imaging in children following thyroidectomy varies. Clayton and Kirkland[383] believe that serial ^{131}I imaging is not indicated because of the more serious consequences of periodic hypothyroidism on growth and development in children. Their policy at Baylor College of Medicine is to place the child on T_4 suppression following surgery without thyroid ablation and to observe closely until adult life, at which time assessment for metastases is undertaken.

We are of a different opinion. This is a malignant disease and the more favorable prognosis in children should encourage every effort to eradicate it, rather than to temporize on the basis of theoretical consequences. The high incidence of multifocal disease in children, especially, should encourage postsurgical ablation. We usually ablate thyroid remnants in children with invasive disease with smaller doses than used in adults. Following surgery, full thyroid hormone replacement is instituted for 6 weeks followed by T_3 for 3 weeks. Triiodothyronine is then withdrawn and 2 weeks later body imaging is performed with 30 μCi/kg of ^{131}I. Uptake within functioning remnants and metastases is determined, volume is estimated, and a dose administered calculated to deliver 50,000 cGy to all functioning tissue remnants. In patients with recurrent neck metastases, surgery is recommended. In the case of functioning, but inoperable, neck or mediastinal metastases, and in all cases of functioning lung metastases, ^{131}I therapy is obviously indicated. The doses to be administered depend on the age of the patient, the extent and location of metastases, and the percent uptake. It is prudent in these patients that the course of treatment be decided by the nuclear medicine physician, with the concurrence of a pediatric endocrinologist.

A GUIDELINE FOR SCREENING AND FOLLOW-UP OF PATIENTS WITH CHILDHOOD NECK IRRADIATION FOR NONMALIGNANT DISEASE

Radiation of the head and neck has long been recognized as predisposing to subsequent development of thyroid carcinoma.[3] The emergence of cancer is both slow and variable. DeGroot and Paloyan found clinical manifestations on an average of 20 years after initial radiation.[371] Several studies impressively document this association. Arnold and colleagues examined 1452 persons who had irradiation to the neck region, either documented or presumed, for benign conditions 18 to 35 years previously.[384] Thyroid abnormalities were found in 21% of these patients. Of those patients who underwent surgical exploration, 29% were found to have thyroid cancer. The overall incidence of thyroid cancer in these neck-irradiated patients was 7%. The same incidence of thyroid cancer was found in other series.[154,385]

Some evidence suggests that radiation-induced nodularity and thyroid cancer depend upon the patient's age at the time of irradiation. Among 553 patients studied by Straub who were irradiated at an average age of 17 years, the incidence of cancer found at follow-up was only 0.7%.[386] The lower emergence of cancer in this group of patients was thought to be due to the later age at the time of irradiation.

Favus and colleagues examined 1056 patients who had received irradiation to the tonsil-nasopharyngeal area, mostly for recurrent infections, 18 to 25 years previously.[387] Palpable thyroid nodules were found in 16.5%, and nonpalpable lesions were detected by ^{99m}Tc-pertechnetate scans in an additional 10.7%, for a total prevalence of 27.2%. Thyroid cancer was found in 33% of 182 patients with nodules who underwent a surgical procedure; the overall incidence of thyroid cancer in this group was 5.6%. Although many of these cancers are only microscopic foci, most are invasive malignancies with a clear potential to metastasize.[388]

The prognosis in irradiated patients appears to be similar to other patients with the same cancer type who have not been irradiated.[389]

The risk of thyroid cancer to individuals irradiated during childhood is therefore great. The need for a rational screening and follow-up program for these patients is obvious. In the study of Arnold and co-workers, ^{99m}Tc-pertechnetate imaging with a scintillation camera and pinhole collimator detected 96% of all nodules found at operation, 40% of which could not have been established unequivocally by physical examination alone.[384] The following guidelines have been prepared by Maxon and colleagues.[180]

1. Confirm the history of exposure to ionizing radiation. Patients with documented exposure records are at higher risk than those whose exposure cannot be documented. If the patient insists that he was irradiated but no documentation can be found, the patient must be considered at risk and must be evaluated.

2. Examination should include history and careful physical examination. Often, the field of radiation exposure extends from the umbilicus upward; thus, careful examination of the skin, breast, and particularly thyroid, are essential. This examination is followed by a thyroid scan utilizing ^{99m}Tc or ^{123}I, and a gamma camera with pinhole collimator.
3. If no nodules are palpable on physical examination of the thyroid, and if the thyroid scan is entirely normal, the patient should be reassured and advised to have yearly examinations that include pertechnetate thyroid scans.
4. Patients with a palpable nodule and an abnormality on the thyroid scan should have fine-needle biopsy. The presence of multiple lesions does not decrease the probability of thyroid carcinoma among patients who have been previously irradiated.
5. If the patient has a normal gland by palpation and a suspicious scan, he should be placed on full replacement doses of thyroid hormone to shrink normal tissue, and have physical examination and scan repeated at 6-month intervals. If the scan remains abnormal, even in the absence of any physical findings, the patient has approximately the same likelihood of having carcinoma as a patient with a palpable nodule and, thus, should have thyroid surgery.

A National Institutes of Health (NIH) task group [Department of Health, Education and Welfare (DHEW) Publication No. [NIH]77–1120] has identified a third category of patients, those with diffuse enlargement by palpation without palpable nodules. Usually, in patients with normal thyroid function, the enlargement is due either to benign hypertrophy or to Hashimoto's thyroiditis. In addition to receiving the appropriate workup for these conditions, these patients should also have a thyroid scan. The task group recommends the following (National Cancer Institute, 1977):

1. If the scan shows no areas of abnormal isotope concentration, the patient may be placed on suppressive therapy to shrink the hypertrophied tissue, since hypertrophy may conceal a nodule buried deep in the gland. The patient should be reexamined in 6 months. If a nodule(s) is then palpable, surgical exploration is indicated. If no nodule is found, the patient may be continued on thyroid therapy indefinitely and reexamined annually.
2. If the scan shows a definite cold area but no nodule is palpable, the patient should be placed on thyroid hormone and reexamined in 6 months. Surgical exploration is not indicated until or unless a nodule becomes palpable.

ROLE OF EXTERNAL BEAM RADIATION THERAPY IN WELL-DIFFERENTIATED THYROID CARCINOMA

Mazzaferri and Young have demonstrated quite clearly that external radiation therapy has no role as routine adjunctive therapy following surgery for well-differentiated thyroid carcinoma.[184] Among 18 patients treated with external radiation postoperatively, 11 (61%) developed recurrent tumors. This number was significantly higher than the recurrence rate in patients treated with no postoperative therapy whatever (40%). Furthermore, recurrent disease that could not be eradicated was significantly more frequent among patients treated with external irradiation (17%) than among patients treated with other forms of adjunctive therapy (2.3%).

Table 10. Indications for Radiation Therapy in Differentiated Thyroid Carcinoma

1. Any lesion that does not concentrate ^{131}I
2. Primary treatment if locally unresectable
3. Skeletal metastases
   a. Following ^{131}I therapy for lesions that concentrate ^{131}I
   b. To prevent pathologic fracture
4. Brain metastases
5. In cases of bulky tumor; for example, mediastinal nodes of such volume that they are unlikely to be controlled by ^{131}I alone
6. Recurrent metastases after maximum ^{131}I therapy
7. Superior vena cava obstruction
8. In combination with chemotherapy

The indications for external beam therapy in differentiated thyroid carcinoma are listed in Table 10. The primary indication is, of course, progressive or recurrent disease that is not controlled by ^{131}I. Both supervoltage x-rays and electrons are used because these modalities can deliver tumoricidal doses at depth before the skin tolerance is reached. The usual therapy consists of 5000 to 6000 cGy over 5 to 6 weeks.[301] The radiation dose may be limited by the tolerance of surrounding structures, such as trachea, esophagus, and spinal cord. Papillary and mixed papillary carcinomas are more radiosensitive than follicular carcinomas.[263]

The decision to use radiation therapy before or after ^{131}I therapy depends on the presenting clinical circumstances. If tumor concentrates ^{131}I, but concentration is inadequate or nonuniform, it is prudent to administer the ^{131}I first, because prior radiation may inhibit the cancer's iodine-trapping mechanism.[48] Radiation therapy can then commence a few days later, without waiting for the full effect of the ^{131}I to become manifest, because ^{131}I uptake in thyroid carcinoma is virtually complete by 48 hours.[22] In the case of brain metastases, radiation therapy should probably precede ^{131}I therapy because of occasional inflammatory edema and vascular rupture associated with ^{131}I therapy.

ROLE OF CHEMOTHERAPY IN THE MANAGEMENT OF WELL-DIFFERENTIATED THYROID CARCINOMA

The majority of patients with differentiated thyroid carcinoma are well managed by surgery, ^{131}I and, in exceptional cases, external beam radiation. However, in the small number of patients who manifest progressive disease following adequate surgery and in whom ^{131}I fails to halt disease progress, chemotherapy is warranted. Benkar and co-workers[24] have listed several criteria for patient selection:

1. The presence of thyroid carcinoma must be proven and classified according to well-accepted staging criteria;
2. All attempts at curative treatment must have been made, and nonresectable tumors should have been debulked to the greatest extent feasible;
3. The disease must be progressive; that is, there should be an increase in size of measurable lesions within an observation period of 3 to 6 months. If the lesions are life-threatening or may by progression lead to serious danger, chemotherapy should be instituted;
4. The patient should be in reasonably good general health and have a life expectancy, if untreated, of at least 10 weeks.

Because the effects of chemotherapy are usually not apparent before at least 2 courses have been completed, gravely ill patients are not likely to benefit from such treatment. Patients over 70 are generally poor candidates for chemotherapy.

Results of Chemotherapy

Of the several drugs and drug combinations evaluated in thyroid carcinoma, doxorubicin (adriamycin), bleomycin, cisplatin, dactinomycin, and methotrexate have been studied most extensively. The results of many of these studies are reviewed by Burgess and Stratton Hill[41] and Benkar and colleagues.[24] By far the largest experience has been reported with doxorubicin, and this drug appears to be most promising. In several studies,[23,41,164,215] response to doxorubicin has averaged about 35%. Response is usually partial; that is, reduction in size of metastases or reduction in symptoms without disappearance of clinical cancer. Nevertheless, mean survival time is significantly increased compared to that in patients with similarly staged cancer who do not undergo chemotherapy. Doxorubicin has significant cardiotoxicity and the total cumulative dose is usually restricted to 550 mg/m^2. At present, there is no satisfactory maintenance therapy when doxorubicin treatment has been completed.

REFERENCES

1. Silverberg E, Lubera JA: Cancer statistic, 1989. *CA* 1989;39:3.
2. Third National Cancer Survey. *Natl Cancer Inst* 1975;41.
3. Duffy BJ, Fitzgerald PJ: Cancer of the thyroid in children: a report of 28 cases. *J Clin Endocrinol Metab* 1950;10:1296.
4. Woolner LB, Beahrs OH, Black BM, et al: Thyroid carcinoma: General considerations and follow-up data on 1,181 cases. In: Young S, Inman DR (eds): *Thyroid Neoplasia.* New York, Academic Press, 1968, p 51.
5. Beierwaltes WH: The treatment of thyroid carcinoma with radioactive iodine. *Semin Nucl Med.* 1978;8:79.
6. Cady B: Thyroid neoplasms. In Sedgwick CG, Cady B (eds): *Surgery of the Thyroid and Parathyroid Glands.* Ed. 2. Philadelphia, Saunders, 1980, pp 131–158.
7. McConahey WM, Taylor WF, Gorman CA, et al: Retrospective study of 820 patients treated for papillary carcinoma of the thyroid at the Mayo Clinic between 1946 and 1971. In: Andreoli M, Moraco F, Robbins J (eds): *Advances in Thyroid Neoplasia.* Rome, Field Educational Italia, 1981, pp 245–262.
8. Clark RL, White EC, Russell WO: Total thyroidectomy for cancer of the thyroid: Significance of intraglandular dissemination. *Ann Surg* 1959;149:858.
9. Woolner LB, Beahrs OH, Black BM, et al: Classification and prognosis of thyroid carcinoma. *Am J Surg* 1961;102:354.
10. Johnson TL, Lloyd RV, Thompson NW, et al: Prognostic implications of the tall cell variant of papillary thyroid carcinoma. *Am J Surg Pathol* 1988;12:22.
11. Samaan NA, Maheshwari YK, Nader S, et al: Impact of therapy for differentiated carcinoma of the thyroid: an analysis of 706 cases. *J Clin Endocrinol Metab* 1983;56:1131.
12. Young RL, Mazzaferri EL, Rahe AJ, et al: Pure follicular thyroid carcinoma: Impact of therapy in 214 patients. *J Nucl Med* 1980;21:733.
13. Woolner LB: Thyroid carcinoma: pathologic classification with data on prognosis. *Semin Nucl Med* 1971;1:481.
14. Tubiana M: Thyroid cancer. In: Beckers C, et al (eds): *Thyroid Diseases.* Paris, Pergamon, 1982, pp 187–227.
15. Mazzaferri EL, Young RL, Oertel JE, et al: Papillary thyroid carcinoma: The impact of therapy in 576 patients. *Medicine* 1977;56:171.
16. Němec J, Pohunková D, Zamrasil V, et al: Pulmonary metastases of thyroid carcinoma. *Czech Med* 1979;2:78.
17. Němec J, Zamrazil V, Pohunková D, et al: Mode spread of thyroid cancer. *Oncology* 1979;36:232.
18. Hay ID: Papillary thyroid carcinoma. *Endocrinol Metab Clin North Am* 1990;19:545.
19. Evans HL: Encapsulated papillary neoplasms of the thyroid. A study of 14 cases followed for a minimum of 10 years. *Am J Surg Pathol* 1987;11:592.
20. Bocker W, Schroder S, Dralle H: Minimal thyroid neoplasia. *Recent Results Cancer Res* 1988;106:131.
21. McNicoll MP, Hawkins DB, England K, et al: Papillary carcinoma arising in a thyroglossal duct cyst. *Otolaryngol Head Neck Surg* 1985;99:50.
22. Crile G Jr: Factors influencing the survival of patients with follicular carcinoma of the thyroid gland. *Surg Gynecol Obstet* 1985;160:409.
23. Mazzaferri EL: Radioiodine and other treatment and outcomes. In: Braverman LE, Utiger RD (eds): *Werner and Ingbar's the Thyroid,* 6th ed. Philadelphia, JB Lippincott Co, 1991, p 1138.
24. Buckwalter JA, Gurll NJ, Thomas CG Jr: Cancer of the thyroid in youth. *World J Surg* 1981;5:15.
25. Goepfert H, Dichtel WJ, Samaan NA: Thyroid cancer in children and teenagers. *Arch Otolaryngol Surg* 1984;110:72.
26. Schlumberger M, De Vathaire F, Travagli JP, et al: Differentiated thyroid carcinoma in childhood: long-term follow-up of 72 patients. *J Clin Endocrinol Metab* 1987;65:1099.
27. Cady B, Sedgwick CE, Meissner WA, et al: Changing clinical, pathologic, therapeutic, and survival patterns in differentiated thyroid carcinoma. *Ann Surg* 1976;184:541.
28. Carcangiu ML, Zampi G, Pupi A, et al: Papillary carcinoma of the thyroid: a clinicopathologic study of 241 cases treated at the University of Florence, Italy. *Cancer* 1985;55:805.
29. Mazzaferri EL: Papillary thyroid carcinoma: factors influencing prognosis and current therapy. *Semin Oncol* 1987;14:315.
30. Hay ID: Prognostic factors in thyroid carcinoma. *Thyroid Today* 1989;12(1):1.

31. Cohn K, Backdahl M, Forsslund G, et al: Prognostic value of nuclear DNA content in papillary thyroid carcinoma. *World J Surg* 1984;8:474.
32. Zimmerman D, Hay ID, Gough IR, et al: Papillary thyroid carcinoma in children and adults: long-term follow-up of 1039 patients conservatively treated at one institution during three decades. *Surgery* 1988;104:1157.
33. Belfiore A, Garofalo MR, Giuffrida D, et al: Increased aggressiveness of thyroid cancer in patients with Graves' disease. *J Clin Endocrinol Metab* 1990;70:830.
34. Filetti S, Belfiore A, Amir SM, et al: The role of thyroid-stimulating antibodies of Graves' disease in differentiated thyroid cancer. *N Engl J Med* 1988;318:753.
35. Field JB, Larsen PR, Yamashita K, et al: Demonstration of iodide transport defect but normal iodide organification in nonfunctioning nodules of human thyroid glands. *J Clin Invest* 1973;52:2404.
36. Fragu P, Thomas-Morvan C, Vignal A, et al: Biochemistry of differentiated thyroid carcinoma. *Acta Endocrinol* 1983;(suppl 252):46.
37. Mandato E, Meldolesi MF, Macchia V: Diminished binding of thyroid-stimulating hormone in a transplantable rat thyroid tumor as a possible cause of hormone unresponsiveness. *Cancer Res* 1975;35:3089.
38. Ichikawa Y, Saito E, Abe Y, et al: Presence of TSH receptor in thyroid neoplasms. *J Clin Endocrinol Metab* 1976;42:395.
39. Hoffman GL, Thompson NW, Heffron C: The solitary thyroid nodule: A reassessment. *Arch Surg* 1972;105:379.
40. Kendall LA, Condon RD: Prediction of malignancy in solitary thyroid nodules. *Lancet* 1969;1:1071.
41. Shimaoka K and Sokal JE: Differentiation of benign and malignant thyroid nodules by scintiscan. *Arch Intern Med* 1964;114:36.
42. Abe Y, Ichikawa Y, Muraki T, et al: Thyrotropin (TSH) receptor and adenylate cyclase activity in human thyroid tumors: Absence of high affinity receptor and loss of TSH responsiveness in undifferentiated thyroid carcinoma. *J Clin Endocrinol Metab* 1981;52:23.
43. Taurog A: Thyroid peroxidase and thyroxine biosynthesis. *Recent Prog Horm Res* 1970;26:187.
44. Valenta LJ, Valenta V, Wang CA, et al: Subcellular distribution of peroxidase activity in human thyroid tissue. *J Clin Endocrinol Metab* 1973;37:560.
45. Dralle H, Schwarzrock R, Böcker W, et al: Thyroglobulin synthesis and radioiodine uptake in differentiated thyroid carcinoma. *Acta Endocrinol* 1983;(suppl 252):45.
46. Monaco F, Grimaldi S, Dominici R, et al: Defective thyroglobulin synthesis in an experimental rat thyroid tumor: Iodination and thyroid hormone synthesis in isolated tumor thyroglobulin. *Endocrinology* 1975;97, 347.
47. Valenta L, Lissitzky S, Aquaron R: Thyroglobulin iodine in thyroid tumors. *J Clin Endocrinol Metab* 1968;28:437.
48. Mortensen JD, Woolner LB, Bennet WA: Gross and microscopic findings in clinically normal thyroid glands. *J Clin Endocrinol Metab* 1955;15:1270.
49. Rice CO: Incidence of nodules in the thyroid: A comparative study of symptomless thyroid glands removed at autopsy and hyperfunctioning goiters operatively removed. *Arch Surg* 1932;24:505.
50. Trowbridge FL, Matovinovic J, McLaren GD, et al: Iodine and goiter in children. *Pediatrics* 1975;56:82.
51. Rallison ML, Dobyns BM, Keating FR Jr, et al: Thyroid nodularity in children. *JAMA* 1975;233:1069.
52. Vander JB, Gaston EA, Dawber TR: The significance of nontoxic thyroid nodules: Final report of a 15-year study of the incidence of thyroid malignancy. *Ann Intern Med* 1968;69:537.
53. Stoffer RP, Welch JW, Hellwig CA, et al: Nodular goiter, incidence, morphology before and after iodine prophylaxis, and clinical diagnosis. *Arch Intern Med* 1960;106:10.
54. Vander JB, Gaston EA, Dawber TR: Significance of solitary nontoxic thyroid nodules: Preliminary report. *N Engl J Med* 1954;251:970.
55. Tunbridge WMG, Evered DC, Hall R, et al: The spectrum of thyroid disease in an English community: The Wickham survey. *Clin Endocrinol* 1977;7:481.
56. Willems JS, Löwhagen T: Fine needle aspiration cytology in thyroid disease. *Clin Endocrinol Metab* 2:247, 1981.
57. Liechty RD, Stoffel PT, Zimmerman DE, et al: Solitary thyroid nodules. *Arch Surg* 1977;112:59.
58. Brown CL: Pathology of the cold nodule. *Clin Endocrinol Metab* 1981;10:235.
59. Sampson RJ, Woolner LB, Bahn RC, et al: Occult thyroid carcinoma in Olmstead County, Minnesota: Prevalence at autopsy compared with that in Hiroshima and Nagasaki, Japan. *Cancer* 1974;34:2072.
60. Murray D: The thyroid gland. In: Kovacs K, Asa SL (eds): *Functional Endocrine Pathology.* Cambridge, MA, Blackwell Scientific, 1991, pp 293–374.
61. Christensen SB, Bondeson L, Ericsson UB, Lindholm K: Prediction of malignancy in the solitary thyroid nodule by physical examination, thyroid scan, fine-needle biopsy and serum thyroglobulin: a prospective study of 100 surgically treated patients. *Acta Chir Scand* 1984;150:433.
62. Cusick EL, MacIntosh CA, Krukowski, et al: Management of isolated thyroid swellings: a prospective six-year study of fine needle aspiration cytology in diagnosis. *BMJ* 1991;301:318.
63. Giansanti M, Monico S, Fugiani P: Fine-needle aspiration cytodiagnosis of the "cold" thyroid nodule. *Tumori* 1989; 75:475.
64. Harsoulis P, Leontsini M, Economou A, et al: Fine needle aspiration biopsy cytology in the diagnosis of thyroid cancer: comparative study of 213 operated patients. *Br J Surg* 1986;73:461.
65. Pepper GM, Zwickler D, Rosen Y: Fine-needle aspiration biopsy of the thyroid nodule: results of a start-up project in a general teaching hospital setting. *Arch Intern Med* 1985;149:594.
66. Belfiore A, LaRosa GL, LaPorta GA, et al: Cancer risk in patients with cold thyroid nodules: Relevance of iodine intake, sex, age, and multinodularity. *Am J Med* 1992;93:363.
67. Dische S: The radioisotope scan applied to the detection of carcinoma in thyroid swellings. *Cancer* 1964;17:473.
68. Molnar GD, Wilber RD, Lee RE, et al: On the hyperfunctioning solitary thyroid nodule. *Mayo Clin Proc* 1965;40:665.
69. Cole WH, Majarakis JD, Slaughter DP. Incidence of carcinoma of the thyroid in nodular goiter. *J Clin Endocrinol Metab* 1949;9:1007.
70. DeGroot LJ, Reilly M, Pinnameneni K, et al: Retrospective and prospective study of radiation-induced thyroid disease. *Am J Med* 1983;74:852.
71. Rosen IB, Palmer JA, Bain J, et al: Efficacy of needle biopsy in postradiation thyroid disease. *Surgery* 1983;94:1002.
72. Block MA, Dailey GE, Robb JA: Thyroid nodules indeterminate by needle biopsy. *Am J Surg* 1983;146:72.
73. Gobien RP. Aspiration biopsy of the solitary thyroid nodule. *Radiol Clin North Am* 1979;17:543.
74. Hamaker RC, Singer MI, DeRossi RV, et al: Role of needle biopsy in thyroid nodules. *Arch Otolaryngol* 1983;109: 225.
75. Lowhagen T, Granberg PO, Lundell G, et al: Aspiration biopsy cytology (ABC) in nodules of the thyroid gland suspected to be malignant. *Surg Clin North Am* 1979;59:3.

76. Norton LW, Wangensteen SL, Davis JR, et al: Utility of thyroid aspiration biopsy. *Surgery* 1982;92:700.
77. Rosen IB, Wallace C, Strawbridge HG, et al: Reevaluation of needle aspiration cytology in detection of thyroid cancer. *Surgery* 1981;90:747.
78. Rojeski MT, Gharib H: Nodular thyroid disease: evaluation and management. *N Engl J Med* 1985;313:428.
79. Mazzaferri EL: Management of a solitary thyroid nodule. *N Engl J Med* 1993;328:553.
80. Gharib H, Goellner JR, Zinsmeister DR, et al: Fine-needle aspiration biopsy of the thyroid. *Ann Intern Med* 1984;101:25.
81. Hamburger B, Gharib H, Melton LJ III, et al: Fine-needle aspiration biopsy of thyroid nodules: Impact on thyroid practice and cost of care. *Am J Med* 1982;73:381.
82. Miller JM, Hamburger JI, Kini SR: The impact of needle biopsy on the preoperative diagnosis of thyroid nodules. *Henry Ford Hosp Med J* 1980;28:145.
83. Frable WJ: *Thin-needle Aspiration Biopsy.* Philadelphia, Saunders, 1983.
84. Caruso D, Mazzaferri EL: Fine needle aspiration biopsy in the management of thyroid nodules. *Endocrinologist* 1991;1: 194.
85. Ashcraft MW, Van Herle AJ: Management of thyroid nodules. II. Scanning techniques, thyroid suppressive therapy, and fine needle aspiration. *Head Neck Surg* 1981;3:297.
86. Hall TL, Layfield LJ, Philippe A, Rosenthal DL: Sources of diagnostic error in fine needle aspiration of the thyroid. *Cancer* 1989;63:718.
87. Blum M, Rothschild M: Improved nonoperative diagnosis of the solitary 'cold' thyroid nodule: Surgical selection based on risk factors and three months of suppression. *JAMA* 1980;243:242.
88. Miller TR, Abele JS, Greenspan FS. Fine-needle aspiration biopsy in the management of thyroid nodules. *West J Med* 1981;134:198.
89. McHenry C, Smith M, Lawrence AM, et al: Nodular thyroid disease in children and adolescents: a high incidence of carcinoma. *Am Surg* 1988;54:444.
90. Simeone JF, Daniels GH, Mueller P, et al: High resolution realtime sonography of the thyroid. *Radiology* 1982;145:431.
91. Van Herle AJ, Rich P, Ljung BME, et al: The thyroid nodule. *Ann Intern Med* 1982;96:221.
92. Ashcraft MW, Van Herle AJ: Management of thyroid nodules. I. History and physical examination, blood tests, x-ray tests, and ultrasonography. *Head, Neck Surg* 1981;3:216–30.
93. Thijs LG: Diagnostic ultrasound in clinical thyroid investigation. *J Clin Endocrinol Metab* 1971;32:709.
94. Lees WR, Vahl SP, Watson LR, et al: The role of ultrasound scanning in the diagnosis of thyroid swellings. *Br J Surg* 1978;65:681–684.
95. Scheible W, Leopold GR, Woo VL, et al: High-resolution real-time ultrasonography of thyroid nodules. *Radiology* 1979;133:413.
96. Simeone JF, Daniels GH, Mueller PR, et al: High-resolution real-time sonography of the thyroid. *Radiology* 1982;145:431.
97. Nassani SN, Bard R: Evaluation of solid thyroid neoplasms by gray scale and real-time ultrasonography: The halo sign. *Ultrasound Med Biol* 1978;4:323.
98. Propper RA, Skolnick ML, Weinstein BJ, et al: The nonspecificity of the thyroid halo sign. *J Clin Ultrasound* 1980;8:129.
99. Clark OH: TSH suppression in the management of thyroid nodules and thyroid cancer. *World J Surg* 1981;5:39.
100. Astwood EB, Cassidy CE, Auerbach GD: Treatment of goiter and thyroid nodules with thyroid. *JAMA* 1960;174:459.
101. Greer MA, Astwood EB: Treatment of simple goiter with thyroid. *J Clin Endocrinol Metab* 1953;13:1312.
102. Glassford GH, Fowler EF, Cole WH: The treatment of nontoxic nodular goiter with desiccated thyroid: Results and evaluation. *Surgery* 1965;58:621.
103. Taylor S: Limitations of thyrotropin suppression in the treatment of nodular goiter and thyroid carcinoma. In: Werner SC (ed): *Thyrotropin. Proceedings of Conference on Thyrotropin.* Springfield, IL, Charles C Thomas, 1963, p 353.
104. Getaz EP, Shimaoka K, Razack M, et al: Suppressive therapy for postirradiation thyroid nodules. *Can J Surg* 23:558, 1980.
105. Hill LD, Beebe HG, Hipp R, et al: Thyroid suppression. *Arch Surg* 1974;108:403.
106. Gershengorn MC, McClung MR, Chu EW, et al: Fine-needle aspiration cytology in preoperative diagnosis of thyroid nodules. *Ann Intern Med* 1977;87:265.
107. Tennvall J, Palmer J, Bjorklund A, et al: Well-differentiated carcinomas of the thyroid. A double isotope investigation with ^{99m}Tc and ^{201}Tl. *Acta Radiol Oncol* 1984;23:55.
108. Němec J, Zamrazil V, Pohunková D, et al: The rational use of ^{201}Tl scintigraphy in the evaluation of differentiated thyroid cancer. *Eur J Nucl Med* 1984;9:261.
109. Tonami N, Hisada K: ^{201}Tl scintigraphy in post-operative detection of thyroid cancer. A comparative study with ^{131}I. *Radiology* 1980;136:461.
110. Tsuda T, Kubota M, Iwakuba A, et al: A case of Hurthle cell carcinoma in the superior mediastinum. *Jpn J Nucl Med* 1990;27:741.
111. Balon HR, Fink-Bennett D, Stoffer SS: Technetium-99m-Sestamibi uptake by recurrent Hurthle cell carcinoma of the thyroid. *J Nucl Med* 1992;33:1393.
112. Abdel-Nabi H, Hinkle GH, Falko JM, et al: Iodine-131-labeled anti-CEA antibodies uptake by Hurthle cell carcinoma. *Clin Nucl Med* 1985;10:713.
113. Patton JA, Sandler MP, Partain CA: Prediction of benignancy of the solitary cold thyroid nodule by fluorescent scanning. *J Nucl Med* 1985;26:461.
114. Patton JA, Hollifield JW, Brill AB, et al: Differentiation between malignant and benign solitary thyroid nodules by fluorescent scanning. *J Nucl Med* 1976;17:17.
115. Fairweather DS, Bradwell AR, Watson-James SF, et al: Detection of thyroid tumors using radiolabelled anti-thyroglobulin. *Clin Endocrinol* 1983;18:563.
116. Shepherd PS, Lazarus CR, Mistry RD, et al: Detection of thyroid tumor using a monoclonal ^{123}I anti-human thyroglobulin antibody. *Eur J Nucl Med* 1985;10:291.
117. De Keyser LFM, Van Herle AJ: Differentiated thyroid cancer in children. *Head Neck Surg* 1985;8:100.
118. KGorlin JB, Sallan SE: Thyroid cancer in childhood. *Endocrinol Metab Clin North Am* 1990;19:649.
119. Byar DP, Green SB, Dor P, et al: A prognostic index for thyroid carcinoma a study of the E.O.R.T.C. Thyroid Cancer Cooperative Group. *Eur J Cancer* 1979;15:1033.
120. Fourquet A, Asselain B, Joly J: Cancer de la thyroide: Analyse multidimensionnelle des facteurs pronostiques. *Ann Endocrinol (Paris)* 1983;44:121.
121. Bacourt F, Asselain B, Savoie JC, et al: Multifactorial study of prognostic factors in differentiated thyroid carcinoma and a re-evaluation of the importance of age. *Br J Surg* 1986;73:274.
122. Joensuu H, Klemi PJ, Paul R, Tuominen J: Survival and prognostic factors in thyroid carcinoma. *Acta Radiol Oncol Radiat Phys Biol* 1986;25:243.
123. Kerr DJ, Burt AD, Boyle P, et al: Prognostic factors in thyroid tumors. *Br J Cancer* 1986;54:475.
124. Palestini N, Cappello N, Cottino F, et al: Multifactorial study of prognostic factors in differentiated thyroid carcinoma. *Ital J Surg Sci* 1989;19:137.
125. Schelfhout LJ, Creutzberg CL, Hamming JF, et al: Multivariate analysis of survival in differentiated thyroid cancer: the

prognostic significance of the age factor. *Eur J Cancer Clin Oncol* 1988;24:331.
126. Tennvall J, Biorklund A, Moller T, et al: Is the EORTC prognostic index of thyroid cancer valid in differentiated thyroid carcinoma? Retrospective multivariate analysis of differentiated thyroid carcinoma with long follow-up. *Cancer* 1986;57:1405.
127. DeGroot L, Paloyan E: Thyroid carcinoma and radiation. *JAMA* 1973;225:487.
128. Roudebush CP, DeGroot LJ: The natural history of radiation-associated thyroid cancer. In: DeGroot LJ, Frohman LA, Kaplan EL, et al (eds): *Radiation-Associated Thyroid Carcinoma.* New York, Grune & Stratton, 1977.
129. Tubiana M, Schlumberger M, Rougier P, et al: Long-term results and prognostic factors in patients with differentiated thyroid carcinoma. *Cancer* 1985;55:794.
130. Wanebo HJ, Andrews W, Kaiser KL: Thyroid cancer: some basic considerations. *Am J Surg* 1981;142:474.
131. Hay ID, Grant CS, Taylor WF, McConahey WM: Ipsilateral lobectomy versus bilateral lobar resection in papillary thyroid carcinoma: a retrospective analysis of surgical outcome using a novel prognostic scoring system. *Surgery* 1987;102:1088.
132. Cady B, Rossi R: An expanded view of risk-group definition in differentiated thyroid carcinoma. *Surgery* 1988; 104:947.
133. Buckwalter JA, Thomas CG Jr: Selection of surgical treatment for well differentiated thyroid carcinomas. *Ann Surg* 1972;176:565.
134. Tollefson HR, DeCosse JJ: Papillary carcinoma of the thyroid. Recurrence in the thyroid gland after initial surgical treatment. *Am J Surg* 1963;106:728.
135. Black BM, Kirk TA, Woolner LB: Multicentricity of papillary adenocarcinoma of the thyroid: Influence of treatment. *J Clin Endocrinol Metab* 1960;20:130.
136. Crile G: Late results of treatment for papillary cancer of the thyroid. *Ann Surg* 1964;160:178.
137. Hirabayashi RN, Lindsay S: Carcinoma of the thyroid gland: A statistical study of 390 patients. *J Clin Endocrinol Metab* 1961;21:1596.
138. Marchetta FC, Sako K: Modified neck dissection for carcinoma of the thyroid gland. *Surg Gynecol Obstet* 1974; 119:557.
139. Tollefson HR, Shah JP, Huvos AG: Follicular carcinoma of the thyroid. *Am J Surg* 1973;126:523.
140. McConahey WM, Hay ID, Woolner LB, et al: Papillary thyroid cancer treated at the Mayo Clinic, 1946 through 1970: initial manifestations, pathologic findings, therapy and outcome. *Mayo Clin Proc* 1986;61:978.
141. Synder J, Gorman C, Scanlon P: Thyroid remnant ablation: Questionable pursuit of an ill-defined goal. *J Nucl Med* 1983;24:659.
142. Beierwaltes WH, Rabbani R, Dmuchowski C, et al: An analysis of "Ablation of thyroid remnants" with I-131 in 511 patients from 1947–1984: Experience at University of Michigan. *J Nucl Med* 1984;25:1287.
143. Frazell EL, Foote FW: Papillary cancer of the thyroid: A review of 25 years of experience. *Cancer* 1958;11:895.
144. Goldman JM, Line BR, Aamodt RL, et al: Influence of triiodothyronine withdrawal time on ^{131}I uptake postthyroidectomy for thyroid cancer. *J Clin Endocrinol Metab* 1980;50:734.
145. Perez CA, Knapp RC, Young RC: Gynecologic tumors. In: DeVita VT, et al (eds): *Cancer Principles and Practice of Oncology.* Philadelphia, Lippincott, 1982, p 852.
146. Thompson NW, Nishiyama RH, Harkness JK: Thyroid carcinoma: Current controversies. *Curr Probl Surg* 1978;15(11):1.
147. Noguchi S, Noguchi A, Murakami N: Papillary carcinoma of the thyroid: I. Developing pattern of metastasis. *Cancer* 1970;26:1053.
148. Scanlon EF, Kellogg JE, Winchester DP, et al: The morbidity of total thyroidectomy. *Arch Surg* 1981;116:568.
149. Mazzaferri EL, Young RL: Papillary thyroid carcinoma: A 10 year follow-up report of the impact of therapy in 576 patients. *Am J Med* 1981;70:511.
150. Beierwaltes WH: Controversies in the treatment of thyroid cancer: The University of Michigan approach. *Thyroid Today* 1983;6(5).
151. Leeper R: Controversies in the treatment of thyroid cancer. The New York Memorial Hospital approach. In: Oppenheimer JH (ed): *Thyroid Today.* 1982;5(4):1–4.
152. Katz AD, Bronson D: Total thyroidectomy. The indications and results of 630 cases. *Am J Surg* 136:450, 1978.
153. Varma VM, Beierwaltes WH, Nofal MM, et al: Treatment of thyroid cancer. Death rates after surgery and after surgery followed by sodium iodine I 131. *JAMA* 1970;214:1437.
154. Krishnamurthy GT, Blahd WH: Radioiodine I-131 therapy in the management of thyroid cancer. *Cancer* 1977;40:195.
155. Hilton G, et al: The role of radioiodine in the treatment of carcinoma of thyroid. *Br J Radiol* 1956;29:297.
156. Edmonds CJ, Hayes S, Kermode JC, et al: Measurement of serum TSH and thyroid hormones in the management of treatment of thyroid carcinoma with radioiodine. *Br J Radiol* 1977;50:799.
157. Němec J, Röhling S, Zamrazil V, et al: Comparison of the distribution of diagnostic and thyroablative I-131 in the evaluation of differentiated thyroid cancers. *J Nucl Med* 1979;20:92.
158. Waxman A, Ramanna L, Chapman D, et al: The significance of I-131 scan dose in patients with thyroid cancer. Determination of ablation: Concise communication. *J Nucl Med* 1981;22:861.
159. Maxon HR, Thomas SR, Hertzberg VS, et al: Relation between effective radiation dose and outcome of radioiodine therapy for thyroid carcinoma. *N Engl J Med* 1983;309:937.
160. Simpson WJ, Panzarella T, Carruthers JS, et al: Papillary and follicular thyroid cancer: impact of treatment in 1578 patients. *Int J Radiat Oncol Biol Phys* 1988;14:1063.
161. DeGroot LJ, Kaplan EL, McCormic M, Straus FH: Natural history, treatment, and course of papillary thyroid carcinoma. *J Clin Endo Metab* 1990;71:414.
162. Greene R: Treatment of thyroid cancer. *Br Med J* 1969;4:787.
163. Maheshwari YK, Hill CS Jr, Haynie TP III, et al: ^{131}I therapy in differentiated thyroid carcinoma. *Cancer* 1981;47:664.
164. Hurley JR, Becker DV: The use of radioiodine in the management of thyroid cancer. In: Freeman LM, Weissman HS (eds): *Nuclear Medicine Annual.* New York, Raven Press, 1983, p 329.
165. Busnardo B, Girelli ME, Cimitan M, et al: Relationships between metastases of differentiated thyroid carcinoma and serum thyrotropin (TSH) levels. *J Clin Endocrinol Metab* 1977;44:1193.
166. Hershman JM, Edwards L: Serum thyrotropin (TSH) levels after thyroid ablation compared with TSH levels after exogenous bovine TSH: Implications for ^{131}I treatment of thyroid carcinoma. *J Clin Endocrinol Metab* 1972;34:814.
167. Hilts SV, Hellman D, Anderson J, et al: Serial TSH determination after T-3 withdrawal or thyroidectomy in the therapy of thyroid carcinoma. *J Nucl Med* 1979;20:928.
168. Nicoloff JT, Low JC, Dussault JH, et al: Simultaneous measurement of thyroxine and triiodo-thyronine. Peripheral turnover kinetics in man. *J Clin Invest* 1972;51:473.
169. Edmonds CJ: Treatment of thyroid cancer. *Clin Endocrinol Metab* 1979;8:223.

170. Haynie TP, Beierwaltes WH: Hematologic changes observed following I^{131} therapy for thyroid carcinoma. *J Nucl Med* 1963;4:85.
171. Leeper RD, Shimaoka K: Treatment of metastatic thyroid cancer. *Clin Endocrinol Metab* 1980;9:383.
172. Pochin EE: Radioiodine therapy of thyroid cancer. *Semin Nucl Med* 1971;1:503.
173. Rawson RW, Rall JE, Peacock W: Limitations and indications in the treatment of cancer of the thyroid with radioactive iodine. *J Clin Endocrinol* 1951;11:1128.
174. Beierwaltes WH, Nishiyama RH, Thompson NW, et al: Survival time and "cure" in papillary and follicular thyroid carcinoma with distant metastases: Statistics following University of Michigan therapy. *J Nucl Med* 1982;23:561.
175. McCowen KD, Adler RA, Ghaed N, et al: Low dose radioiodide thyroid ablation in postsurgical patients with thyroid cancer. *Am J Med* 1976;61:52.
176. Ramacciotti C, Pretorius HT, Line BR, et al: Ablation of nonmalignant thyroid remnants with low doses of radioactive iodine. Concise communication. *J Nucl Med* 1982;23:483.
177. DeGroot LJ, Reilly M: Comparison of 30- and 50-mCi doses of iodine-131 for thyroid ablation. *Ann Intern Med* 1982; 96:51.
178. Kline CC, Klingensmith WC III: Failure of low doses of ^{131}I to ablate residual thyroid tissue following surgery for thyroid cancer. *Radiology* 1980;137:773.
179. Kuni CC, Klingensmith WC: Failure of low doses of ^{131}I to ablate residual thyroid tissue following surgery for thyroid cancer. *Radiology* 1980;137:773.
180. Siddiqui AR, Edmondson J, Wellman HH, et al: Feasibility of low doses of ^{131}I for thyroid ablation in postsurgical patients with thyroid carcinoma. *Clin Nucl Med* 1981;6:158.
181. Sisson JC: Applying the radioactive eraser: I-131 to ablate normal thyroid tissue in patients from whom thyroid cancer has been resected. *J Nucl Med* 1983;24:743.
182. Becker DV, Hurley JR, Motazedi A, et al: Ablation of postsurgical thyroid remnants in patients with differentiated thyroid cancer can be achieved with less whole body radiation. *J Nucl Med* 1982;23:P43.
183. Goolden AW, Davey JB: The ablation of normal thyroid tissue with iodine 131. *Br J Radiol* 1963;36:340.
184. Maxon HR III: The role of ^{131}I in the treatment of thyroid cancer. *Thyroid Today* 1993;16(2):1.
185. Maxon HR, Englaro EE, Thomas SR, et al: Radioiodine-131 therapy for well-differentiated thyroid cancer—a quantitative radiation dosimetric approach: outcome and validation in 85 patients. *J Nucl Med* 1992;33:1132.
186. Black BM, YaDeau RE, Woolner LB: Surgical treatment of thyroidal carcinomas. *Arch Surg* 1964;88:610.
187. Shapiro J: *Radiation Protection,* Ed. 2. Cambridge, MA, Harvard University Press, 1981.
188. Morrish DW, Filipow LJ, McEwan AJ, et al: ^{131}I treatment of thyroid papillary carcinoma in a patient with renal failure. *Cancer* 1990;66:2509.
189. Koral KF, Adler RS, Carey JE, Beierwaltes WH: Iodine-131 treatment of thyroid cancer: absorbed dose calculated from post-therapy scans. *J Nucl Med* 1986;27:1207.
190. Maxon HR, Thomas SR, Hertzberg VS, et al: Relation between effective radiation dose and outcome of radioiodine therapy for thyroid cancer. *N Engl J Med* 1983;309:937.
191. Haynie TP, Nofal MM, Beierwaltes WH: Treatment of thyroid carcinoma with I^{131}. *JAMA* 1963;183:303.
192. Russell WO, Ibanez MI, Clark RI, et al: Thyroid carcinoma. *Cancer* 1963;16:1425.
193. Balachandran S, Sayle BA: Value of thyroid carcinoma imaging after therapeutic doses of radioiodine. *Clin Nucl Med* 1981;6:162.
194. Rochman H, deGroot LJ, Rieger CHL, et al: Carcinoembryonic antigen and humoral antibody response in patients with thyroid carcinoma. *Cancer Res* 1975;35:2689.
195. Unger J, Van Heuwyn B, Decoster C, et al: *J Clin Endocrinol Metab* 1980;51:590.
196. Van Herle AJ, Vassart G, Dumont JE: Control of thyroglobulin synthesis and secretion. *N Engl J Med* 1979;301:239, 307.
197. Van Herle AJ, Klandorf H, Uller RP: A radioimmunoassay for serum rat thyroglobulin. Physiologic and pharmacological studies. *J Clin Invest* 1975;56:1073.
198. Van Herle AJ, Uller RP: Elevated serum thyroglobulin, a marker of metastases in differentiated thyroid carcinomas. *J Clin Invest* 1975;56:272.
199. Van Herle AJ, Uller RP, Matthews N, et al: Radioimmunoassay for measurement of thyroglobulin in human serum. *J Clin Invest* 1973;52:1320.
200. Van Herle AJ: Serum thyroglobulin measurement in the diagnosis and management of thyroid disease. *Thyroid Today* 1981;4(2).
201. DeGroot LJ, Hoye K, Refetoff S, et al: Serum antigens and antibodies in the diagnosis of thyroid cancer. *J Clin Endocrinol Metab* 1977;45:1220.
202. Schlumberger M, Fragu P, Parmentier C, et al: Thyroglobulin assay in the follow-up of patients with differentiated thyroid carcinomas: Comparison of its value in patients with or without normal residual tissue. *Acta Endocrinol* 1981;98:215.
203. Shlossberg AH, Jacobson JC, Ibbertson HK: Serum thyroglobulin in the diagnosis and management of thyroid carcinoma. *Clin Endocrinol* 1979;10:17.
204. Dunn JT: Thyroglobulin: Structure, function and clinical relevance. *Thyroid Today* 1985;8(3):1.
205. Schlumberger M, Charbord P, Fragu P, et al: Circulating thyroglobulin and thyroid hormones in patients with metastases of differentiated thyroid carcinoma: Relationship to serum thyrotropin levels. *J Clin Endocrinol Metab* 1980;51:513.
206. Ashcraft MW, Van Herle AJ: The comparative value of serum thyroglobulin measurements and iodine 131 total body scans in the follow-up study of patients with treated differentiated thyroid cancer. *Am J Med* 1981;71:806–814.
207. Barsano CP, Skosey C, DeGroot LJ, et al: Serum thyroglobulin in the management of patients with thyroid cancer. *Arch Intern Med* 1982;142:763.
208. Black EG, Gimlette TMD, Maisey MN, et al: Serum thyroglobulin in thyroid cancer. *Lancet* 1981;2:443.
209. Blahd WH, Drickman MV, Porter CW, et al: Serum thyroglobulin, a monitor of differentiated thyroid carcinoma in patients receiving thyroid hormone suppression therapy. *J Nucl Med* 1984;25:673.
210. Charles MA, Dodson LE Jr, Waldeck N, et al: Serum thyroglobulin levels predict total body iodine scan findings in patients with treated well-differentiated thyroid carcinoma. *Am J Med* 1980;69:401.
211. Galligan JP, Winship J, Van Doorn T, et al: A comparison of serum thyroglobulin measurements and whole body I-131 scanning in the management of treated differentiated thyroid carcinoma. *Aust NZ J Med* 1982;12:248.
212. Jansch A, Heinze HG, Hast B: Serum thyroglobulin (S-HTG): A tumor marker in patients with differentiated thyroid carcinoma. *Strahlentherapie* 1981;157:381.
213. McDougall IR, Bayer MF: Follow-up of patients with differentiated cancer using serum thyroglobulin measured by immunoradiometric assay. Comparison with I-131 total body scan. *J Nucl Med* 1980;21:741.
214. Schatz H, Grebe SF, Norn W, et al: Follow-up of patients

with differentiated thyroid cancer: Determination of serum thyroglobulin in place of routine ^{131}I scintigraphy? *Wien Klin Wochenschr* 1984;96:389.

215. Schneider AB, Line BR, Goldman JM, et al: Sequential serum thyroglobulin determinations, ^{131}I scans, and ^{131}I uptakes after triiodothyronine withdrawal in patients with thyroid cancer. *J Clin Endocrin Metab* 1981;53:1199.
216. Tang Fui SCN, Hoffenberg R, Maisey MN, et al: Serum thyroglobulin concentration and whole-body radioiodine scan in follow-up of differentiated thyroid cancer after thyroid ablation. Br Med J 1979;2:298.
217. Bednar J, Němec J, Zamrazil V, et al: Serum thyroglobulin determinations in patients with differentiated thyroid carcinoma. *Nuklearmedizin* 1983;22:204.
218. Colacchio TA, Lo Gerfo P, Colacchio DA, et al: Radioiodine total body scan versus serum thyroglobulin levels in follow-up of patients with thyroid cancer. *Surgery* 1982;91:42.
219. Pincheria A, Pacini F, Mariotti S, et al: Recent studies on the application of serum thyroglobulin measurement in thyroid disease. In: Eggo MC, Burrow GN (eds): *Thyroglobulin—The Prothyroid Hormone.* New York, Raven Press, 1985, pp 307–316.
220. Moser E, Fritsch G, Braun S: Thyroglobulin and ^{131}I uptake of remaining tissue in patients with differentiated carcinoma after thyroidectomy. *Nucl Med Comm* 1988;9:262.
221. Brendel AJ, Lambert B, Guyot M, et al: Low levels of serum thyroglobulin after withdrawal of thyroid suppression therapy in the follow up of differentiated thyroid carcinoma. *Eur J Nucl Med* 1990;16:35.
222. Hufner M, Stumpf HP, Grussendorf M, et al: A comparison of the effectiveness of ^{131}I whole body scans and plasma TG determinations in the diagnosis of metastatic differentiated carcinoma of the thyroid: A retrospective study. *Acta Endocrinol (Copenh)* 1983;104:327.
223. Sulman C, Gosselin P, Carpenbier P, et al: Value of the estimation of thyroglobulin levels in the surveillance of treated differentiated thyroid carcinoma. *J Clin Chem Clin Biochem* 1984;22:215.
224. Van Herle AJ: Thyroglobulin. In: Braverman LE, Utiger RD (eds): *Werner and Ingbar's the Thyroid.* 6th ed. Philadelphia, JB Lippincott, 1991, p 493.
225. Pacini F, Mariotti S, Formica N, et al: Thyroid antibodies in thyroid cancer: incidence and relationship with tumor outcome. *Acta Endocrinol* 1988;119:373.
226. Amino N, Pysher Y, Cohen E, De Groot LJ: Immunological aspects of human thyroid cancer. *Cancer* 1975;36:963.
227. De Groot LJ, Hoye K, Refetoff S, et al: Serum antigen and antibodies in the diagnosis of thyroid cancer. *J Clin Endocrinol Metab* 1976;45:1220.
228. Schlumberger M, Fragu P, Gardet P, et al: A new immunoradiometric assay (IRMA) system for thyroglobulin measurement in the follow-up of thyroid cancer patients. *Eur J Nucl Med* 1991;18:153.
229. Rubello D, Girelli ME, Casara D, et al: Usefulness of the combined antithyroglobulin antibodies and thyroglobulin assay in the follow-up of patients with differentiated thyroid cancer. *J Endocrinol Invest* 1990;13:737.
230. Rubello D, Casara D, Girelli ME, et al: Clinical meaning of circulating antithyroiglobulin antibodies in differentiated thyroid cancer: a prospective study. *J Nucl Med* 1992; 33:1478.
231. Harada T, Ito Y, Shimaoka K, et al: ^{201}Thallium chloride scan for thyroid nodule. *Eur J Nucl Med* 1980;5:125.
232. Makimoto K, Ohmura M, Tamada A, et al: Combined scintiscans in the diagnosis of thyroid carcinomas. *Acta Otolaryngol* 1985;410(suppl):189.
233. Varma V, Reba R: Comparative study of T1-201 and I-131 scintigraphy in postoperative metastatic thyroid carcinoma. In: Raynard C (ed): *Nuclear Medicine and Biology. Proceedings 3rd World Congress of Nuclear Medicine and Biology,* Vol. I. Paris: Pergamon Press, 1982, p 103.
234. Brendel JJ, Gugot M, Jeandot R, et al: Follow-up of differentiated thyroid carcinoma. *J Nucl Med* 1988;29:1515.
235. Charkes ND, Vitti RA, Brooks K: Thallium-201 SPECT increases detectability of thyroid cancer metastases. *J Nucl Med* 1990;31:147.
236. Ramanna L, Waxman A, Braunstein G: Thallium-201 scintigraphy in differentiated thyroid cancer: comparison with radioiodine scintigraphy and serum thyroglobulin determinations. *J Nucl Med* 1991;32:441.
237. Iida Y, Hidaka A, Hatabu H, et al: Follow-up study of postoperative patients with thyroid cancer by thallium-201 scintigraphy and serum thyroglobulin measurement. *J Nucl Med* 1991;32:2098.
238. Crile G Jr.: The endocrine dependency of certain thyroid cancers and the danger that hypothyroidism may stimulate their growth. *Cancer* 1957;10:1119.
239. Goldberg LD, Ditchek NT: Thyroid carcinoma with spinal cord compression. *JAMA* 1981;245:953.
240. Van Middlesworth L: Metabolism and excretion of thyroid hormones. In: Greep RO, Astwood EB, Greer MA, et al (eds): *Handbook of Physiology: Endocrinology, Vol. 3, Thyroid.* Washington, DC, American Physiological Society, 1974, pp 215–231.
241. Hoffman DP, Surks MI, Oppenheimer JH, et al: Response to thyrotropin releasing hormone: An objective criterion for the adequacy of thyrotropin suppression therapy. *J Clin Endocrinol Metab* 1977;44:892.
242. Lamberg BA, Rantanen M, Saarinen P, et al: Suppression of the TSH response to TRH by thyroxine therapy in differentiated thyroid carcinoma patients. *Acta Endocrinol (Copenh)* 1979,91:248.
243. Busnardo B, Bui D, Girelli ME, et al: Rapid suppression of TSH secretion using an optimal saturation regimen of thyroid hormones in patients with thyroid cancer. In Andreoli M, et al (eds): *Advances in Thyroid Neoplasia.* Rome, Field Education of Italia, 1981, p 341.
244. Lamberg BA, Rantanen M, Saarinen P: Choosing thyroxine dose after treatment of thyroid cancer. *Lancet* 1977;2: 1290.
245. Mak PH, De Stefano JJ III: Optimal control policies for the prescription of thyroid hormone. *Math Biosci* 1978;42:159.
246. Benua RS, Cicale NR, Sonenberg M, et al: The relation of radioiodine dosimetry to results and complications in the treatment of metastatic thyroid cancer. *Am J Roentgenol* 1962;87:171.
247. Schlessinger T, Flower MA, McCready VR: Radiation dose assessments in radioiodine (131I) therapy. 1. The necessity for in vivo quantitation and dosimetry in the treatment of carcinoma of the thyroid. *Radiother Oncol* 1989;14:35.248.
248. Dagan J, Meyer JM: A simple method for determining isotope uptake in disseminated metastatic thyroid disease. *Eur J Nucl Med* 1981;6:23.
249. Scott JS, Halnan KE, Shimmins J, et al: Measurement of dose to thyroid carcinoma metastases from radio-iodine therapy. *Br J Radiol* 1970;43:256.
250. Thomas SR, Maxon HR, Kereiakes JG, et al: Quantitative external counting enabling improved diagnostic and therapeutic decisions in patients with well-differentiated thyroid cancer. *Radiology* 1977;122:731.
251. Flower MA, Schlesinger T, Hinton PJ, et al: Radiation dose assessment in radioiodine therapy. 2. Practical implementa-

tion using quantitative scanning and PET, with initial results on thyroid carcinoma. *Radiother Oncol* 1989;15:345.
252. Woolfenden JM, Waxman AD, Wolfstein RS, Siemsen JK: Scintigraphic evaluation of liver metastases from thyroid carcinoma. *J Nucl Med* 1975;16:669.
253. Rosenbaum RC, Johnston GS, Valente WA: Frequency of hepatic visualization during I-131 imaging for metastatic thyroid carcinoma. *Clin Nucl Med* 1988;13:657.
254. Ziessman HA, Bahar H, Fahey FH, Dubiansky V: Hepatic visualization on iodine-131 whole-body thyroid cancer scans. *J Nucl Med* 1987;28:1408.
255. Oppenheimer JH. Thyroid hormones in liver. *Mayo Clin Proc* 1972;47:854.
256. Lin DS: Thyroid imaging—mediastinal uptake in thyroid imaging. *Semin Nucl Med* 1983;13:395.
257. Berquist Th, Nolan NG, Stephens DM, Carlson HC: Radioisotope scintigraphy in diagnosis of Barrett's esophagus. *AJR* 1975;123:401.
258. Ganatra RD, Atmaram SH, Shanna SM: An unusual site of radioiodine concentration in a patient with thyroid cancer. *J Nucl Med* 1972;13:777.
259. Echenique RL, Kasi L, Haynie TP, et al: Critical evaluation of serum thyroglobulin levels and I-131 scans in post therapy patients with differentiated thyroid carcinoma. *J Nucl Med* 1982;23:235.
260. Hoschl R, Choy, DH-L, Gandevia B: Iodine-131 uptake in inflammatory lung disease: a potential pitfall in treatment of thyroid carcinoma. *J Nucl Med* 1988;29:701.
261. Burt RW: Accumulation of I-123 in a Warthin's tumor. *Clin Nucl Med* 1978;3:155.
262. Kamoi I, Nishitani H, Oshiumi Y, et al: Intrathoracic gastric cyst demonstrated by Tc-99m pertechnetate scintigraphy. *AJR* 1980;134:1080.
263. Yeh EL, Meade RC, Ruetz PP: Radionucleid study of struma ovarii. *J Nucl Med* 1973;14:118.
264. Rieser GD, Over P, Cowan RJ, Cordell AR: Radioiodide imaging of struma cordis. *Clin Nucl Med* 13:1988.
265. Preisman RA, Halpern SE, Shishido R, et al: Uptake of I-131 by a papillary meningioma. *AJR* 1977;129:349.
266. Fernandez-Ulloa M, Manon HR, Mehta S, Sholiton LJ: Iodine-131 uptake by primary lung adenocarcinoma, misinterpretation of I-131 scan. *JAMA* 1976;236:857.
267. Acosta J, Chitkara R, Khan F, et al: Radioactive iodine uptake by a large cell undifferentiated bronchogenic carcinoma. *Clin Nucl Med* 1982;8:368.
268. Wu SY, Kollin J, Coodley E, et al: I-131 total body scan: Localization of disseminated gastric adenocarcinoma. *J Nucl Med* 1984;25:1024.
269. Caplan RH, Gunnar A, Gundersen MD, et al: Meckel's diverticulum mimicking metastatic thyroid cancer. *Clin Nucl Med* 1986;11:760.
270. Nodine JH, Maldia G: Pseudostruma ovarii. *Obstet Gynecol* 1961;17:460.
271. Greenler DP, Klein HA: The scope of false-positive iodine-131 images for thyroid carcinoma. *Clin Nucl Med* 1989; 14:111.
272. Brachman MB, Rothman BJ, Ramanna L, et al: False-positive iodine-131 body scan caused by a large renal cyst. *Clin Nucl Med* 1988;13:416.
273. Jackson GL, Graham WP, Flickinger FW, et al: Thymus accumulation of radioactive iodine. *Penn Med* 1979;11:37.
274. Achong DM, Oates E, Lee SL, Doherty FJ: Gallbladder visualization during post-therapy iodine-131 imaging of thyroid carcinoma. *J Nucl Med* 1991;32:2275.
275. Lakshman M, Reynolds J: Unexpected pelvic radioiodine uptake in a young woman after thyroidectomy for papillary carcinoma. *Endocrinology* 1987;120:T-89.
276. Cady B, Sedgwick CE, Meissner WA, et al: Risk factor analysis in differentiated thyroid cancer. *Cancer* 1979; 43:810.
277. Hays MT, Solomon DH, Beall GN: Suppression of human thyroid function by antibodies to bovine thyrotropin. *J Clin Endocrinol Metab* 1967;27:1540.
278. Eastman CJ, Lazarus L: The effect of orally administered synthetic thyrotropin releasing factor on adenohypophyseal function. *Horm Metab Res* 1972;4:58.
279. Haigler ED, Hershman JM, Pittman JA: Response to orally administered synthetic thyrotropin-releasing hormone in man. *J Clin Endocrinol Metab* 1972;35:631.
280. Rabello MM, Snyder PJ, Utiger RD: Effects on the pituitary-thyroid axis and prolactin secretion of single and repetitive oral doses of thyrotropin-releasing hormone (TRH). *J Clin Endocrinol Metab* 1974;39:571.
281. Bangerter S, Weiss S, Staub JJ, et al: Effekt von peroral verabreichtem TRH auft die Radiojodaufnehme der Schilddrüse. *Schweiz Med Wochenschr* 1971;101:1269.
282. Samaan NA, Beceiro JR, Hill CS, et al: Thyrotropin-releasing hormone (TRH) studies in patients with thyroid cancer. *J Clin Endocrinol Metab* 1972;35:438.
283. Robbins J: The role of TRH and lithium in the management of thyroid cancer. In: Andreoli M, Monaco F, Robbins J (eds): *Advances in Thyroid Neoplasia.* Rome, Field Educational Italia, 1981, pp 233–234.
284. Goslings BM: Effect of a low iodine diet on ^{131}I therapy in follicular thyroid carcinomata. *J Endocrinol* 1975;64:30 P.
285. Hamburger JI, Desai P: Mannitol augmentation of ^{131}I uptake in the treatment of thyroid carcinoma. *Metabolism* 1966;15:1055–1058.
286. Hamburger JI: Diuretic augmentation of ^{131}I uptake in inoperable thyroid cancer. *N Engl J Med* 1969;280:1091–1094.
287. Maruca J, Santner S, Miller KI, et al: Prolonged iodine clearance with a depletion regimen for thyroid carcinoma. *J Nucl Med* 1984;25:1089.
288. Pons F, Carrio I, Estorch M, et al: Lithium as an adjuvant of iodine-131 uptake when treating patients with well-differentiated thyroid carcinoma. *Clin Nucl Med* 1987;8:644.
289. Turner JG, Brownlie BEW, Rogers TGH: Lithium as an adjunct to radioiodine therapy for thyrotoxicosis. *Lancet* 1976;1:614.
290. Brière J, Pousset G, Darsy P, et al: Intéret de l'association lithium-iode 131 dans le traitement des métastase captantes du cancer thyroidien. *Ann Endocrinol (Paris)* 1974;35:281.
291. Tata JR, Pochin EE: Thyroid cancer. In: Pitt-Rivers R, Pochin WR (eds): *The Thyroid Gland,* vol. 2. Washington, DC, Butterworths, 1964, p 208.
292. Rasmusson B, Olsen K, Rygård J: Lithium as an adjunct to ^{131}I-therapy of thyroid carcinoma. *Acta Endocrinol* 1983;(suppl 252):74.
293. Schraube P, Kimmig B, zum Winkel K: Lithium as an adjuvant in the radioiodine therapy of thyroid cancer. *Nuclearmedizin* 1984;23:151.
294. Vacaflor L: Lithium side effects and toxicity. The clinical picture. In: Johnson FN (ed): *Lithium Research and Therapy.* London, Academic Press, 1975, pp 211–226.
295. Smithers DW: Thyroid carcinoma treated with radioiodine. In: Hedinger CE (ed): *Thyroid Cancer.* Berlin, Springer-Verlag, 1969, pp 288–293.
296. Simpson WJ, Carruthers JS: The role of external radiation in the management of papillary and follicular thyroid cancer. *Am J Surg* 1978;136:457.
297. Harwood J, Diarck OH, Dunphy JE: Significance of lymph node metastasis in differentiated thyroid cancer. *Cancer* 1979;43:810.

298. Massin JP, Savoie JC, Garnier H, et al: Pulmonary metastases in differentiated thyroid carcinoma. *Cancer* 1984;53:982.
299. Samaan NA, Schultz PN, Haynie TP, Ordonoz NG: Pulmonary metastases of differentiated thyroid carcinoma: Treatment results in 101 patients. *J Clin Endocrinol Metab* 1985;65:376.
300. Nusynowitz ML, Pollard E, Benedetto AR, et al: Treatment of medullary carcinoma of the thyroid with I-131. *J Nucl Med* 1981;23:143.
301. Synder WS, Ford MR, Warner GG, et al: "S," Absorbed dose per unit cumulated activity for selected radionuclides and organs. Medical Internal Radiation Dose (MIRD) Committee Pamphlet No. 11. New York, Society of Nuclear Medicine, 1975.
302. Brown AP, Greening WP, McCready VR, et al: Radioiodine treatment of metastatic thyroid carcinoma: The Royal Marsden Hospital experience. *Br J Radiol* 1984;57:323.
303. Fish J, Moore RM: Ectopic thyroid tissue and ectopic thyroid carcinoma: A review of the literature and report of a case. *Ann Surg* 1963;157:212.
304. Jaques DA, Chambers RG, Oertal JE: Thyroglossal duct carcinoma. *Am J Surg* 1970;120:439.
305. LiVolsi VA, Perzin KH, Savetsky L: Carcinoma arising in median ectopic thyroid (including thyroglossal duct tissue). *Cancer* 1974;34:1303.
306. Potdar GG, Desai PB: Carcinoma of the lingual thyroid. *Laryngoscope* 1971;81:427.
307. McGirr EM, Clement WE, Currie AR, et al: Impaired dehalogenase activity as a cause of goitre with malignant changes. *Scot Med J* 1959;4:232.
308. Elman DS: Familial association of nerve deafness with nodular goiter and thyroid carcinoma. *N Engl J Med* 1958;259:219.
309. Little G, Meador CK, Cunningham R, et al: "Cryptothyroidism", the major cause of sporadic "athyreotic" cretinism. *J Clin Endocrinol Metab* 1965;25:1529.
310. Odell WD, Stevenson JK, Williams RH: Treatment of a lingual goiter with triiodothyronine. *J Clin Endocrinol Metab* 1959;19:363.
311. Richardson JR, Lineback M: Radioactive iodine in the diagnosis and treatment of lingual thyroid adenoma. *Laryngoscope* 1952;62:934.
312. Turner PL, Hill HF, Aberdeen JB: Papillary adenocarcinoma arising in a thyroglossal cyst. *Aust NZ J Surg* 1978;48:426.
313. DeGroot LJ, Larsen PR, Refetoff S, et al: *The Thyroid and Its Diseases*. 5th ed. New York, John Wiley & Sons, 1984, p 633.
314. Kingsbury BF: The question of a lateral thyroid in animals, with special reference to man. *Am J Anat* 1939;65:333.
315. Baker-Cohen KF: Renal and other heterotropic thyroid tissue in fishes. In: Gorbman A (ed): *Comparative Endocrinology.* New York, Wiley, 1959, p 283.
316. Nicastri AD, Foote FW, Frazell EL: Benign thyroid inclusions in cervical lymph nodes. *JAMA* 1965;194:1.
317. Gusberg SB, Danforth DN: Clinical significance of struma ovarii. *Am J Obstet Gynecol* 1944;48:537.
318. Teilum G: Strauma ovarii. In: *Special Tumors of Ovary and Testis—Comparative Pathology and Histological Identification.* Philadelphia, Lippincott, 1971, p 166.
319. Wynne HMN, McCartney JS, McClendon JF: Struma ovarii. *Am J Obstet Gynecol* 1940;39:263.
320. Fox H, Langley FA: *Tumors of the Ovary.* Heinemann Medical Books, England, 1976, p 236.
321. Title 10, Chapter 1, Code of Federal Regulations—Energy, Part 35, Section 35.75, October 31, 1986.
322. Arad E, Flannery K, Wilson GA, O'Mara RE: Fractionated doses of radioiodine for ablation of postsurgical thyroid tissue remnants. *Clin Nucl Med* 1990;10:676.
323. Kovalic JJ, Grigsby PW, Slessinger E: The relationship of clinical factors and radiation exposure rates from iodine-131 treated thyroid carcinoma patients. *Med Dosimetry* 1990;15:209.
324. NCRP: Precautions in the management of patients who have received therapeutic amounts of radionuclides. Report No. 37. Washington, DC, National Council on Radiation Protection and Measurements. 1 October 1970.
325. Becker DV, Siegel BA: Guidelines for patients receiving radioiodine treatment. New York, The Society of Nuclear Medicine, Inc, 1983.
326. Harbert JC, Wells SN: Radiation exposure to the family of radioactive patients. *J Nucl Med* 1974;15:887.
327. Culver CM, Dworkin HJ: Radiation safety considerations for post-iodine-131 thyroid cancer therapy. *J Nucl Med* 1992;33:1402.
328. Allweiss P, Braunstein GD, Katz A, Waxman A: Sialadenitis following I-131 therapy for thyroid carcinoma. *J Nucl Med* 1984;25:755.
329. Doniach I: Biologic effects of radiation on the thyroid. In: Werner SC, Ingbar SH (eds): *The Thyroid.* New York, Harper & Row, 1978, pp 274–283.
330. Burmeister LA, duCret RP, Mariash CN: Local reactions to radioiodine in the treatment of thyroid cancer. *Am J Med* 1991;90:217.
331. Morrish DW, Jackson FI, Lalani ZH, et al: Cystic thyroid mass following I-131 treatment of papillary thyroid carcinoma: an unusual complication. *Clin Nucl Med* 1989;14:894.
332. Blahd WH: Treatment of malignant thyroid disease. *Semin Nucl Med* 1979;9:95.
333. Wiseman JC, Hales IB, Joasoo A: Two cases of lymphoma of the parotid gland following ablative radioiodine therapy for thyroid carcinoma. *Clin Endocrinol* 1982;17:85.
334. Delprat CC, Hoefnagel CA, Marcuse HR: The influence of ^{131}I therapy in thyroid cancer on the function of salivary glands. *Acta Endocrinol* 1983;(suppl 252):73.
335. Abbatt JD, Court Brown WM, Farran HEA: Radiation sickness in man following the administration of therapeutic radioiodine: Relationship between latent period, dose-rate and body size. *Br J Radiol* 1955;28:358.
336. Cerletty JM, Listwan WJ: Hyperthyroidism due to functioning metastatic thyroid carcinoma: Precipitation of thyroid storm with therapeutic radioactive iodine. *JAMA* 1979; 242:269.
337. Cooper DS, Ridgway EC, Maloof F: Unusual types of hyperthyroidism. *Clin Endocrinol Metab* 1978;7:199.
338. Lee TC, Harbert JC, Dejter SW, et al: Vocal cord paralysis following I-131 ablation of a post-thyroidectomy remnant. *J Nucl Med* 21:1965.
339. Raymond JP, Izembart M, Marliac V, et al: Temporary ovarian failure in thyroid cancer patients after thyroid remnant ablation with radioactive iodine. *J Clin Endocrinol Metab* 1989;69:186.
340. Němec J, Zamrazil V, Pohunková D, et al: Bone metastases of thyroid cancer, biological behaviour and therapeutic possibilities. *Acta Univ Carol Med* 1978;83:1.
341. Holmquest DL, Lake P: Sudden hemorrhage in metastatic thyroid carcinoma of the brain during treatment with iodine-131. *J Nucl Med* 1976;17:307.
342. Datz FL: Ecrebal edema following iodine-131 therapy for thyroid carcinoma metastatic to the brain. *J Nucl Med* 1986;27:637.
343. Sziklas JJ, Mathews J, Spencer RP, et al: Thyroid carcinoma metastatic to pituitary. Letter. *J Nucl Med* 1985;26:1097.
344. Brincker H, Hansen HS, Andersen AP: Induction of leukaemia by ^{131}I treatment of thyroid carcinoma. *Br J Cancer* 1973;28:232.
345. Refetoff S, Harrison J, Kavanfilski BT, et al: Continuing oc-

currence of thyroid carcinoma after irradiation to the neck in infancy and childhood. *N Engl J Med* 1975;292:171.

346. Beierwaltes WH: The treatment of hyperthyroidism with iodine-131. *Semin Nucl Med* 1978;8:95.
347. Leeper RD: The effect of ^{131}I therapy on survival of patients with metastatic papillary or follicular thyroid carcinoma. *J Clin Endocrinol Metab* 1973;36:1143.
348. Harness JK, Thompson NW, Sisson JC, et al: Differentiated thyroid carcinomas. Treatment of distant metastases. *Arch Surg* 1974;108:410.
349. Shirndoka K, Tokeuchi S, Pickren JW: Carcinoma of thyroid associated with other primary malignant tumors. *Cancer* 1967;20:1000.
350. Wyse ED, Hill CS, Ibanez ML, et al: Other malignant neoplasms associated with carcinoma of the thyroid: Thyroid carcinoma multiplex. *Cancer* 1969;24:701.
351. Edmonds CJ, Smith T: The long-term hazards of the treatment of thyroid cancer with radioiodine. *Br J Radiol* 1986; 59:45.
352. Nishiyama RH, Dunn EL, Thompson NW: Anaplastic spindle-cell and giant-cell tumors of the thyroid gland. *Cancer* 1972;30:113.
353. Handelsman DJ, Conway AJ, Donnelly PE, et al: Azoospermia after iodine-131 treatment for thyroid carcinoma. *Br Med J* 1980;281:1527.
354. Sarkar SD, Beierwaltes WH, Gill SP, et al: Subsequent fertility and birth histories of children and adolescents treated with ^{131}I for thyroid cancer. *J Nucl Med* 1976;17:460.
355. Rall JE, Alpers JB, Lewallen CG, et al: Radiation pneumonitis and fibrosis: A complication of radioiodine treatment of pulmonary metastases from cancer of the thyroid. *J Clin Endocrinol Metab* 1957;17:1263.
356. Němec J, Zamrazil V, Pohunková E, et al: Radioiodide treatment of pulmonary metastases of differentiated thyroid cancer. *Nuklearmedizin* 1979;18:86.
357. Glazebrook MB: Effect of decicurie doses of radioactive iodine 131 on parathyroid function. *Am J Surg* 1987;154:368.
358. Root HF, Root HK: Basal metabolism during pregnancy and the puerperium. *Arch Intern Med* 1923;32:411.
359. Sandiford I, Wheeler T: The basal metabolism before, during and after pregnancy. *J Biol Chem* 1924;62:329.
360. Dowling JT, Freinkel N, Ingbar SH: Thyroxine binding by sera of pregnant women. *J Clin Endocrinol Metab* 1956;16:280.
361. Man EB, Reid WA, Hellegers AE, et al: Thyroid function in human pregnancy. III. Serum thyroxine binding prealbumin (TBPA) and thyroxine binding globulin (TBG) of pregnant women aged 14–43 years. *Am J Obstet Gynecol* 1969; 103:338.
362. Grumbach MM, Werner SC: Transfer of thyroid hormone across the human placenta at term. *J Clin Endocrinol* 1956;16:1392.
363. Osorio C, Myant NB: The passage of thyroid hormone from mother to foetus and its relation to foetal development. Br Med Bull 1960;16:159.
364. Shepard TH: Onset of function in the human fetal thyroid: Biochemical and radioautographic studies from organ culture. *J Clin Endocrinol* 1967;27:945.
365. Chapman EM, Corner GW Jr., Robinson D, et al: The collection of radioactive iodine by the human fetal thyroid. *J Clin Endocrinol* 1948;8:717.
366. Evans TC, Kretzschmar RM, Hodges RE, et al: Radioiodine uptake studies of the human fetal thyroid. *J Nucl Med* 1967;8:157.
367. Hodges RE, Evans TC, Bradbury JT, et al: The accumulation of radioactive iodine by human fetal thyroids. *J Clin Endocrinol* 1955;15:661.
368. Shepard TH, Andersen HU, Andersen H: The human fetal thyroid. I. Its weight in relation to body weight, crown-rump length, foot length and estimated gestation age. *Anat Rec* 1964;148:123.
369. Halnan KE: Radioiodine uptake of the human thyroid in pregnancy. *Clin Sci* 1958;17:281.
370. Braverman LE: Consequences of thyroid radiation in children. *N Engl J Med* 1975;292:204.371.
371. Duffy BJ Jr, Fitzgerald P: Thyroid cancer in childhood and adolescence: A report on 28 cases. *Cancer* 1950;3:1018.
372. Kudlow JE, Burrow GN: Thyroid cancer and pregnancy. In: Greenfield LD (ed): *Thyroid Cancer.* West Palm Beach, FL, CRC Press, 1978, p 199.
373. Stoffer SS, Hamburger JI: Inadvertent ^{131}I therapy for hyperthyroidism in the first trimester of pregnancy. *J Nucl Med* 1976;17:146.
374. Fisher WD, Voorhess ML, Gardner LI: Congenital hypothyroidism in infant following maternal ^{131}I therapy. *J Pediatr* 1963;62:132.
375. Green NG, Garsis FJ, Shepard TH, et al: Cretinism associated with maternal sodium iodide ^{131}I therapy during pregnancy. *Am J Dis Child* 1971;122:247.
376. Hamill GC, Jarman JA, Wynne MD: Fetal effects of radioactive iodine therapy in a pregnant woman with thyroid cancer. *Am J Obstet Gynecol* 1961;81:1018.
377. Russell KP, Rose H, Starr P: The effects of radioactive iodine on maternal and fetal thyroid function during pregnancy. *Surg Gynecol Obstet* 1957;104:560.
378. Hill CS Jr, Clark RL, Wolf M: The effect of subsequent pregnancy on patients with thyroid carcinoma. *Surg Gynecol Obstet* 1966;122:1219.
379. Rosvoll RV, Winship T: Thyroid carcinoma and pregnancy. *Surg Gynecol Obstet* 1965;121:1039.
380. Einhorn J, Hulten M, Lindsten J, et al: Clinical and cytogenetic investigation in children of parents treated with radioiodine. *Acta Radiol Ther Phys Biol* 11:193, 1972.
381. Silverberg E: Cancer statistics, 1977, from National Cancer Institute's Third National Cancer Survey. *CA* 1977;27:26.
382. Winship T, Rosvoll RV: Thyroid carcinoma in childhood: Final report on a 20 year study. *Clin Proc Child Hosp Natl Med Cent* 1970;26:327.
383. Clayton GW, Kirkland RT: Cancer of the thyroid in children. In: Greenfield LD (ed): *Thyroid Cancer.* West Palm Beach, FL. CRC Press, 1978, p 207.
384. Arnold J, Pinsky S, Ryo UY, et al: ^{99m}Tc-pertechnetate thyroid scintigraphy in patients predisposed to thyroid neoplasms by prior radiotherapy to the head and neck. *Radiology* 1975;115:653.
385. Shimaoka K, Bakri K, Sciascia M, et al: Thyroid screening program. *NY State J Med* 1982;82:1184.
386. Straub W, Miller M, Sanislow C, et al: Radiation and risk for thyroid cancer. Atypical findings of a community thyroid recall program. *Clin Nucl Med* 1982;6:272.
387. Favus MJ, Schneider AB, Stachura ME, et al: Thyroid cancer occurring as a late consequence of head-and-neck irradiation. Evaluation of 1056 patients. *N Engl J Med* 1976;294: 1019.
388. Wagner DH, Recant WM, Evans RH: A review of 150 thyroidectomies following prior irradiation to the head, neck and upper part of the chest. *Surg Gynecol Obstet* 1978;147:903.
389. Pacini F, Lippi F, Formica N, et al: Therapeutic doses of Iodine-131 reveal undiagnosed metastases in thyroid cancer patients with detectable serum thyroglobulin levels. *J Nucl Med* 1987;28:1888.390.
390. Maxon HR, Saenger EL, Goldsmith RE: Suggested guidelines for use by physicians in advising patients who received radiation therapy for nonmalignant diseases in childhood and ado-

lescence. With approval of the Council of the Cincinnati Academy of Medicine, 1975. *Bull Allegheny County Med Soc* 1976;269.

391. Tubiana M, Lacour J, Monnier JP, et al: External radiotherapy and radioiodine in the treatment of 359 cancers. *Br J Radiol* 1975;48:894.
392. Sheline GE, Galante M, Lindsay S: Radiation therapy in the control of persistent thyroid cancer. *Am J Roentgenol* 1966;97:923.
393. Carr EA, Jr, Dingledine WS, Beierwaltes WH: Premature resort to x-ray therapy. A common error in treatment of carcinoma of the thyroid gland. *Lancet* 1958;78:478.
394. Bell GO: Cancer of the thyroid. *Med Clin North Am* 1975;59:459.
395. Benkar G, Dabag S, Reinwein D: Chemotherapy of thyroid carcinoma: Benefits and side-effects. In Andreoli M, et al (eds): *Advances in Thyroid Neoplasia.* Rome, Field Educational Italia, 1981.
396. Burgess MH, Stratton Hill C: Chemotherapy in the management of thyroid cancer. In: Greenfield LD (ed): *Thyroid Cancer.* West Palm Beach, FL, CRC Press, 1978, pp 233–245.
397. Benkar G, Dabag S, Hackenberg K, et al: Adriamycin in der Behandlung metastasierender Schilddrüsenkarzinome. In: Fetzer J, Füllenbach D, Musill J (eds): *Adriamycin, Vol. 3: Solide Tumoren, Hamoblastosen.* Kehrer, Offset Freiburg, 1980, pp 17–23.
398. O'Bryan RM, Baker LH, Gottlieb JE, et al: Dose-response evaluation of adriamycin in human neoplasia. *Cancer* 1977;39:1940.

41 Medullary Carcinoma of the Thyroid

John C. Harbert

Medullary carcinoma of the thyroid is one of the neuroendocrine tumors or APUDomas, and derives from the calcitonin-secreting perifollicular, or C cells, of the thyroid (see Table 1, Chapter 42). The C cells derive embryologically from the neural crest via the ultimobranchial body, hence they are part of the diffuse neuroendocrine system. Medullary carcinoma comprises 3 to 10% of all thyroid cancers[1–4] and has its peak incidence in the fifth to seventh decade.[5–7] The familial type may occur in childhood.[7]

These tumors secrete calcitonin, a calcium-mobilizing hormone; elevated levels of circulating calcitonin can be detected by radioimmunoassay even before the tumors become palpable.[8] They also secrete a variety of other potent substances, including histamine, serotonin, vasoactive intestinal peptide (VIP), adrenocorticotropic hormone (ACTH), somatostatin, and prostaglandins. The familial variety, which accounts for 25% of medullary thyroid carcinomas, is associated with bilateral pheochromocytomas and hyperparathyroidism. This is the multiple endocrine neoplasia (MEN) type IIA syndrome, also known as Sipple's syndrome.[9]* Medullary thyroid carcinoma progresses by local neck invasion, lymph node metastases, and distant metastases, especially to the lungs, liver, and bone.

The natural history of medullary thyroid carcinoma is that of a moderately aggressive tumor compared with the more indolent papillary and follicular thyroid carcinomas. Tumor spread depends both on the patient's age and the type of tumor. Older patients have a greater likelihood of metastases beyond the confines of the thyroid gland. Metastases are present in about 64% of patients, with sporadic disease at the time of operation in about 60% of MEN IIB patients, and only 26% of MEN IIA patients.[11] In spite of relatively slow growth, the 5-year survival is only slightly better than 50%.[2]

The interest in these tumors in nuclear medicine is that a small number of them either concentrate radioiodine or are associated with a sufficient mass of follicular elements to make ^{131}I therapy feasible.[2,12–14] Furthermore, they are frequently multifocal, which demands that thyroid ablation be considered as adjunctive therapy.

DIAGNOSIS

The initial presentation is most often thyroid enlargement or a palpable thyroid nodule, with or without cervical adenopathy. In this respect, the differential diagnosis includes all of the entities associated with neck masses.[2,5] Thyroid images using ^{131}I, ^{123}I or ^{99m}Tc-pertechnetate have a variable appearance. Rasmusson[15] found that 6 (21%) of 29 primary lesions (1.5 to 8.0 cm diameter) showcd some tracer uptake. Most lesions, however, are "cold" to both radioiodine and pertechnetate. In lesions of long standing, both primary and metastatic tumors may demonstrate diffuse calcification on neck radiographs and CT scans. Mediastinal metastases are suggested by mediastinal widening on chest radiographs.[2]

Approximately 30% of patients present with persistent diarrhea and, in some patients, a full-blown carcinoid syndrome develops.[2,16] In rare cases, secretion of ACTH by these tumors may give rise to Cushing's syndrome.[17]

Ultimately, the diagnosis of medullary thyroid carcinoma rests on the demonstration of characteristic histological and histochemical findings. Most tumors can be divided into one of two cell types: round cell and spindle cell.[4] Stromal amyloid is nearly always present, although some tumor variants have been observed without amyloid.[3,18] Microscopic vascular invasion is commonly found and electron microscopy demonstrates neurosecretory granules.[19] Histochemical studies demonstrate the presence of immunoreactive calcitonin and high histaminase activity.[20] Spencer reported a case of "pseudomedullary" thyroid carcinoma that appeared by light and electron microscopic studies to be indistinguishable from medullary carcinoma, yet immunohistochemistry indicated the presence of thyroglobulin, and no calcitonin.[21] This was thought to be a variant tumor of follicular cell origin; it concentrated, but did not appear to organify radioiodine.

*There are two main varieties of MEN syndromes. MEN 1 (Werner's syndrome) is characterized by hyperparathyroidism, islet cell tumors of the pancreas (clinically apparent in 85% of patients), and pituitary tumors (clinically apparent in 65% of patients).[10] Patients with MEN II (Sipple's syndrome) have bilateral medullary thyroid carcinoma and about 50% have pheochromocytomas, also usually bilateral. There are two subgroups: MEN IIA is familial and often includes hyperparathyroidism. Patients with MEN IIB carry a specific phenotype with characteristic facies, multiple submucosal ganglioneuromas, and a Marfan-like syndrome; hyperparathyroidism is rare (about 4%). Multiple endocrine neoplasia is also known as multiple endocrine adenopathy (MEA).

Provocative tests for calcitonin secretion are recommended postoperatively to detect the presence of residual tumor and for asymptomatic close relatives to rule out the presence of occult familial medullary thyroid carcinoma. These challenge tests involve the intravenous infusion of calcium,[8,22] pentagastrin,[23–25] or the two combined, followed by serial measures of plasma calcitonin by radioimmunoassay.

Serum carcinoembryonic antigen (CEA) may also be elevated in the presence of metastases and measurements of this tumor marker have been used as a postoperative surveillance measure to detect recurrent disease.[26] At least one report has documented positive images of metastases using ^{111}In-labeled anti-CEA antibodies.[27]

In patients with elevated calcitonin levels postoperatively, every effort to locate metastases must be made. Sequential palpation of the neck may locate nodes missed at surgery. Chest radiographs may show diffuse interstitial infiltrates, particularly in the middle and lower lobes. Computed tomography of the lungs, mediastinum, and liver are useful, as is radionuclide bone imaging to search for bone metastases. About 25% of patients have bone and/or liver metastases at presentation.[28] Bone metastases appear to have a predilection for the vertebral bodies and ribs,[29] which suggests hematogenous spread by way of the vertebral veins. Soft tissue metastases may also concentrate radiophosphates, probably because of the tendency of metastases to calcify.[28,30] Norton used selective venous catheterization and serial calcitonin sampling following pentagastrin stimulation to localize metastases.[31]

Ohta and colleagues[32] used ^{99m}Tc-dimercaptosuccinic acid (DMSA) to localize primary and metastatic tumors in 4 patients. Other experimental diagnostic imaging techniques include the use of radiolabeled antibodies,[26,33] ^{131}I metaiodobenzylguanidine (MIBG),[34] ^{201}T1,[35] ^{99m}Tc-MIBI,[27] and ^{111}In-octreotide. Gautvik used an ^{131}I-labeled rabbit immunoglobulin against rat medullary carcinoma antibody and ^{113}In-transferrin as a blood pool marker[33]; they obtained tumor/nontumor ratios of 3:6.

Several reports have documented the use of ^{131}I-MIBG to image medullary thyroid carcinoma metastases.[34,36–41] Uptake of this tracer, however, has been quite variable.[34,39] In one series (9 patients), Clarke et al found positive uptake in 4 patients, equivocal uptake in 1 patient, and no uptake in 4 patients.

The uptake of ^{201}Tl in both primary[13,42] and metastatic medullary thyroid cancer has been reported. Hoefnagel reported positive uptake in 8 of 18 patients studied following total thyroidectomy.[43] All of these patients had abnormal calcitonin levels and negative ^{131}I uptake. Thus, ^{201}Tl imaging may be a useful diagnostic procedure when other tests fail to localize the tumor or to resolve ambiguous results.

When medullary thyroid cancer is discovered, the presence of other endocrine lesions must be ruled out. Serial calcium and phosphate determinations should be made to exclude hyperparathyroidism. Urinary catecholamines are measured to exclude the concurrent presence of pheochromocytoma. Because there is a familial history in some types of medullary carcinoma, a careful screening program for close family members is essential.

Screening for Occult Disease

The detection of occult medullary thyroid carcinoma has been greatly aided by measurements of basal and pentagastrin-stimulated serum calcitonin. Telander et al reviewed the Mayo Clinic experience in children under 16 years of age with first-degree relatives with MEN II[44], pentagastrin stimulation of calcitonin proved more sensitive than either basal calcitonin or calcium stimulation. Thirty-three children underwent total thyroidectomy; at surgery, 7 patients had C-cell hyperplasia, 19 patients had medullary thyroid carcinoma without metastases, and 7 patients had metastases. Thus, screening for familial medullary thyroid carcinoma appears to be highly effective and is recommended by 1 year of age for children with a first-degree relative having MEN-IIA and MEN-IIB.

TREATMENT

Both familial and sporadic forms of medullary thyroid carcinoma are treated by total thyroidectomy because of its aggressive and multifocal nature. If the initial operation has involved less than near-total thyroidectomy, reoperation with total thyroidectomy is imperative. Dissection and removal of all observable cervical nodes is mandated by the fact that nearly 50% of patients have cervical node involvement even with primary tumors as small as 1 mm in size.[2,8,45,46,47] Duh et al followed 40 patients with medullary thyroid carcinoma and 3 patients with C-cell hyperplasia using these guidelines.[48] The overall actuarial survival was 88 and 78% at 5 and 10 years, respectively. No deaths occurred in patients with C-cell hyperplasia or medullary thyroid carcinoma of the sporadic or familial non-MEN variants, if the disease was limited to the thyroid. Significantly more follow-up surgery was required in patients with more limited surgery.

Some authors recommend ipsilateral modified radical neck dissection, although more radical surgery has not been proved more effective.[49] Postoperative radiation therapy is an important adjunctive therapy. In one study, patients with residual cervical disease treated with neck and mediastinal radiation had a survival rate similar to patients without cervical disease treated by surgery alone.[50]

Thyroid Ablation with ^{131}I

Opinion regarding the use of ^{131}I to ablate residual thyroid and to treat medullary thyroid carcinoma metastases is divided. Most studies have found little or no iodine uptake by medullary carcinoma.[51,52] Saad compared the 5- and 10-year

42 Therapy of Neuroendocrine Tumors

John C. Harbert

Radionuclide therapy of neural crest tumors rests on the pioneering work of Beierwaltes and colleagues at the University of Michigan and the development of [^{131}I]Metaiodobenzylguanidine (^{131}I-MIBG), an analogue of norepinephrine. This analogue concentrates in the adrenergic vesicles of most pheochromocytomas and neuroblastomas, as well as in many of the other neural crest tumors, in amounts sufficient to deliver therapeutic doses of radiation.[1–5] Studies using ^{131}I-MIGB in other centers have confirmed the University of Michigan experience so that, at this time, the role of ^{131}I-MIBG in the diagnosis and treatment of pheochromocytoma and neuroblastoma is generally well-understood, and its role in the management of other neural crest tumors is promising.[6]

PATHOLOGY

In the 1960s, Pearse[7] came to realize that a miscellaneous group of cells, arranged diffusely and distributed widely throughout the body, had certain histological and histochemical features in common. All of these cells he regarded as neuroendocrine, with some derived from neuroectoderm, others from neural crest, and still others from more primitive cells of the ectoblast. Ultimately, more than 40 such cells have been recognized and given the acronym APUD, derived from their amine handling properties: they have high *Amine* content (A), a capacity for amine *Precursor Uptake* (PU), and the function of carrying out *Decarboxylation* (D) of these precursors to form potent amine substances (Table 1). These cells are divided into two principal groups: a central division of glandular structures that includes the pituitary, pineal, and hypothalamus, and a peripheral division that consists of cells in the gastrointestinal tract, pancreas, the C cells of the thyroid, the sympathetic nervous system, adrenal medulla, dermal melanocytes, Meckel cells, and certain cells in the lungs, carotid body, and urogenital tract.[8]

The APUD cells have similar immunofluorescent properties, they are labeled with peroxidase and other histochemical methods, and they contain the enzyme, neuron-specific enolase (NSE), previously thought to be unique to neurons.[9] All of these observations have led to the concept of a single neuroendocrine system that pervades nearly every tissue of the body.[10] Its cells synthesize amines and regulatory peptides which act through 3 different modes of action: *endocrine* (eg, ACTH and calcitonin), *paracrine*, secreted locally and acting on adjacent cells (eg, somatostatin and 5-hydroxytryptamine), and *neurocrine*, secreted at synapses and acting as neurotransmitters (eg, norepinephrine and vasoactive intestinal peptide). For this reason, the term "APUD system" is giving way to the term "neuroendocrine system," which connotes the common physiological rather than histochemical characteristics of the system.[11] Tumors derived from these cells are APUDomas, or more often *neuroendocrine*, and sometimes "neural crest" tumors, indicating their embryological precursor. Often these tumors occur in well-defined pluriglandular endocrinopathies, giving rise to several syndromes known as multiple endocrine neoplasia, MEN I and MEN II.

MIBG

Early work by Morales et al[12] showed that radiolabeled epinephrine and epinephrine precursors, such as ^{14}C-dopamine, concentrate in the adrenal medulla. However, *in vivo* imaging studies with such agents were not successful. Later, Wieland and colleagues[5,13] developed radioiodinated analogs of bretylium which concentrated in the myocardium and adrenal medulla. They combined the benzyl portion of bretylium with the guanidine groups of guanethidine to form ortho-, para-, and metaiodobenzylguanidine. The meta-isomer (MIBG) was the most stable and most subsequent work has concentrated on this tracer (Fig. 1).

The mechanism of MIBG uptake by sympathoadrenal tissues is not completely understood. However, the prevailing model suggests that the majority of MIBG enters the cytoplasm of these tissues by an active sodium and energy-dependent (uptake-one) mechanism.[14–16] A smaller fraction enters by passive diffusion. Once in the cytoplasm, the MIBG then enters the intracellular hormone storage vesicles by means of an active uptake mechanism.[14,15] Thus, MIBG acts as a tracer of catecholamine uptake and storage capacity by the sympathoadrenal system. The primary sites of normal uptake are the adrenal medulla, and in the sympathetic neuronal innervation of the heart, spleen, and salivary glands. Uptake in neuroendocrine tumors is based upon the same mechanisms.[2]

Pharmacological intervention studies in animals and clinical observations in humans show that MIBG uptake is blocked by such uptake-one inhibitors as tricyclic antidepressants, cocaine, reserpine, and phenylpropanolamine[13,17]; most

Table 1. Major APUDomas

NEUROENDOCRINE GLANDS	CELLS OF ORIGIN	SECRETIONS (PEPTIDES AND AMINES)	APUDOMAS	ENDOCRINE SYNDROMES
Central Division of Neuroendocrine System				
Anterior pituitary	c	Corticotropin	Corticotropinoma	Cushing's syndrome
	s	Somatotropin	Somatotropinoma	Giantism Acromegaly
	l	Prolactin	Prolactinoma	Forbes-Albright syndrome Hypopituitarism
Pineal	P	Melatonin	Pinealoma	Hypogonadism
Peripheral Division of Neuroendocrine System				
Pancreas	β	Insulin	Insulinoma Nesidioblastosis	Hyperinsulinism
	α	Glucagon	Glucagonoma	Glucagonoma
	δ	Somatostatin	Somatostatinoma	Somatostatinoma
	Neurons	VIP	Vipoma	WDHA (Verner-Morrison syndrome)
	PP(F)	PP	PP-oma	Nil
GI tract	EC	5-HT	Carcinoid (benign) Carcinoid (malignant)	Nil Malignant carcinoid
	G	Gastrin	Gastrinoma	Ulcerogenic (Zollinger-Ellison syndrome)
Thyroid	C	Calcitonin	Medullary carcinoma	Nil
Adrenal medulla	α	Epinephrine (adrenaline)		
			Pheochromocytoma	Hypertension, etc.
	NA	Norepinephrine (noradrenaline)		
			Ganglioneuroma	
	Ganglia	VIP	Neuroblastoma (vipoma)	WDHA

Welbourn RB, Manolas KJ, Khan O, et al: Tumors of the neuroendocrine system (APUD cell tumors—APUDOMAS). *Curr Prob Surg* 21:7, 1984. With permission.

Abbreviations: 5-HT, 5-hydroxytryptamine; GI, gastrointestinal; PP, pancreatic polypeptide; VIP, vasoactive intestinal polypeptide; WDHA, watery diarrhea, hypokalemia, and achlorhydria syndrome.

alpha- and beta-blocking drugs are without effect. MIBG is discharged from the adrenal medulla in response to insulin hypoglycemia.[18] Uptake is also decreased in the heart and salivary glands by denervation.[18] Obviously, the degree to which MIBG is useful in the therapy of neuroendocrine tumors depends on its uptake and retention and the dosimetry of the radiopharmaceutical.

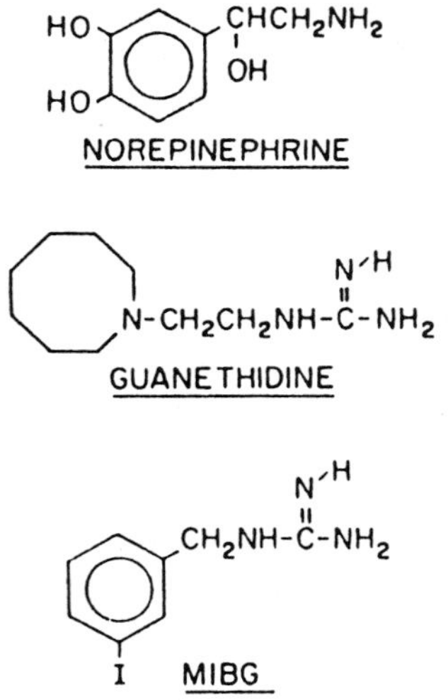

NOREPINEPHRINE

GUANETHIDINE

MIBG

Figure 1. Comparison of norepinephrine, guanethidine, and meta-iodobenzylguanidine. (From McEwan AJ, Shapiro B, Sisson JC, et al: Radio-iodobenzylguanidine for the scintigraphic location and therapy of adrenergic tumors. *Semin Nucl Med* 1985;15:154.)

Metabolism and Dosimetry of MIBG

Only about 2% of the injected dose of MIBG is taken up in tumor in patients with malignant pheochromocytoma.[4] In 8 patients studied by Lindberg et al, tumor uptake ranged from 0.0033 to 0.038%/g of tumor tissue.[19] The remainder is excreted largely undegraded into the urine with 40 to 55% in the first 24 hours and 70 to 90% within 4 days.[20] Radioactivity extracted from excised tumors also shows most in the form of MIBG.[20] Using a thyroid gland-blocking dose of 100 mg KI orally twice a day for 10 days, the absorbed radiation dose in (9) patients with suspected pheochromocytoma imaged with ^{131}I-MIBG is given in Table 2.[19]

Conditions Affecting MIBG Uptake and Distribution

There are numerous drugs that interfere with MIBG uptake in neuroendocrine tissues and tumors. These are reviewed by Khafagi et al[21] and listed in Table 3. The interference mechanisms in most cases are uptake-one inhibition and/

Table 2. Radiation Absorbed Dose in Major Organs from ^{131}I-MIBG

ORGAN	DOSE	
	cGy/MBq	*cGy/mCi*
Liver	0.083	3.07
Spleen	0.061	2.26
Salivary glands	0.022	0.81
Adrenals	0.02	0.74
Thyroid*	0.01	0.34

*Blocked with 100 mg KI twice daily for 10 days (Lindberg et al[19]).

or storage vesicle depletion. Related drugs that have *no* significant effect on MIBG uptake are listed in Table 4. A careful review of potentially interfering medications should be made prior to diagnostic, and especially therapeutic, administration of MIBG.

Because MIBG is primarily excreted in the urine, it is not surprising that both image quality and dosimetry are greatly affected by renal insufficiency.[22] It is prudent to check the plasma creatinine levels prior to administration of ^{131}I-MIBG. If elevated, delayed imaging may be useful to allow background levels to decline. Furthermore, reduced therapeutic doses may be indicated by virtue of increased bone-marrow radiation.[22] The radiation dosimetry of MIBG in specific tumors is discussed below.

TREATMENT OF MALIGNANT PHEOCHROMOCYTOMA

Pathophysiology

During early fetal life, primitive ectodermal stem cells migrate down from the neural crest to form the sympathetic nervous chain and ganglia and invade the developing mesodermal adrenal cortex to form the adrenal medulla. The mesodermal cells give rise to pheochromoblasts and catecholamine-producing chromaffin cells. The latter are so named because the intracellular catecholamine stores stain brown with chromic acid. Chromaffin cells are distributed not only within the adrenal medulla, but all along the sympathetic nerve chain and in the organ of Zukerkandl at the lower end of the aorta (Fig. 2). The distribution accounts for the wide dispersal of extra-adrenal sites; chromaffin tissue may even be drawn into the scrotum during descent of the testes. At birth, the adrenal medulla is small and medullary tissue function is due largely to the paraganglionic masses. During early childhood, the extramedullary sites normally undergo involution, but there is always the potential for stimulation and tumor development.

Incidence

Pheochromocytomas are rare; they occur in from 0.01% to 0.001% of the population and it has long been believed that, of these, from 10 to 13% exhibit malignancy.[23–25] However, with extended follow-up and with the introduction of MIBG scintigraphy, which localizes chromaffin tissue with high accuracy, this proportion has increased in recent years, and may reach as high as 50% with extended follow-up.[1,25–28] Bilateral tumors occur in about 10% of adults and 20% of children. Extramedullary pheochromocytomas occur in about 13% of patients.[29] In adults, about 90% of malignant pheochromocytomas occur within the adrenal gland.[30] In children, extra-adrenal tumors account for about 30% of pheochromocytomas and as many as 40% of these are malignant.[30]

Malignancy cannot be distinguished among pheochromocytomas by histlogical criteria; the sole criteria for malignancy is the presence of metastases in sites where chromaffin tissue is normally absent. The most frequent sites are bone (44%), lymph nodes and liver (37%) and lung (27%).[31]

Clinical Features

The symptoms and signs of malignant pheochromocytoma are generally the same as those encountered in benign pheochromocytoma: headache, palpitations, hyperhidrosis, and hypertension. The notable exception is pain often associated with bone metastases. The dominant feature is hypertension, which may be either paroxysmal or sustained. In the latter case, differentiation from other forms of hypertension is more difficult. Paroxysms may be triggered by emotional stress, physical exertion, as well as palpation of the tumor itself. The sudden release of catecholamines may precipitate very high blood pressure, ventricular fibrillation, cerebral hemorrhage, and pulmonary edema.

The onset of symptoms may occur at any time from childhood on to advanced years, although most tumors are diagnosed in the fourth or fifth decades of life. Tumor size varies from as small as 1 cm up to several kilograms, but average 5 to 6 cm in diameter. The spectrum of malignancy also varies, from relatively static with only local invasion, to highly aggressive tumors that behave as neuroblastomas with rapid dissemination.

Pheochromocytomas are part of the MEN type II (Sipple's syndrome) in which they may be associated with medullary thyroid carcinoma and parathyroid adenomas. They may also be associated with neurofibromatosis (von Recklinghausen's disease) or with cerebral hemangiomas, as in von Hippel-Lindau disease.

Diagnosis

The diagnosis of pheochromocytoma is based on the demonstration of elevated and/or nonsuppressible concentrations of the plasma catecholamines norepinephrine and epinephrine, and of elevated rates of catecholamine and catecholamine metabolite excretion in the urine.[32] In the majority of patients urine levels of the metabolites, vanillylmandellic acid (VMA), metanephrine, and normetanephrine, are elevated and additional testing is not necessary. Clonidine, a centrally acting agent that inhibits catecholamine secretion from the

Table 3. Drugs Known or Expected to Reduce MIBG Uptake

	DRUG	MECHANISM
A. **Known:**		
	Antihypertensive/cardiovascular	
	• Labetalol	• Uptake-1 inhibition • Depletion of storage vesicle contents
	• Reserpine	• Depletion of storage vesicle contents • Inhibition of vesicle active transport
	• Calcium-channel blockers • Diltiazem • Nifedipine • Verapamil	• Uncertain (Also enhance retention of previously stored NE and MIBG by blocking Ca^{++}-mediated release from vesicles)
	Tricyclic antidepressants • Amitriptyline and derivatives • Imipramine and derivatives • Doxepin • Amoxapine • Loxapine (antipsychotic agent)	• Uptake-1 inhibition
	Sympathomimetics • Phenylephrine • Phenylpropanolamine • Pseudoephedrine, ephedrine	• Depletion of storage vesicle contents These drugs occur in numerous nonprescription decongestants and "diet aids"—their use should be ruled out
	Cocaine	• Uptake-1 inhibition
B. **Expected:**		
	Antihypertensive/cardiovascular	
	• Adrenergic neurone blockers • Bethanidine, debrisoquine • Bretylium • Guanethidine	• Depletion of storage vesicle contents • Competition for transport into vesicles
	"Atypical" antidepressants • Maprotiline • Trazolone	• Uptake-1 inhibition
	Antipsychotics *("Major tranquilizers")* • Phenothiazines • Chlorpromazine,* triflupromazine,* promethazine* • Fluphenazine, acetophenazine, perphenazine* • Prochlorperazine,* thiethylperazine,* trifluoperazine • Thioridazine, mesoridazine • Thioxanthines • Chlorprothixene • Thiothixene • Butyrophenones • Droperidol • Haloperidol • Pimozide	• Uptake-1 inhibition
	Sympathomimetics • Amphetamine and related compounds • Amphetamine and derivatives • Diethylpropion • Fenfluramine • Mazindol • Methylphenidate • Phenmetrazine and derivatives • Phentermine and derivatives • Beta-sympathomimetics† • Albuterol (salbutamol) • Isoetharine • Isoproterenol • Metaproterenol • Terbutaline • Dobutamine • Dopamine • Metaraminol	• Depletion of storage vesicle contents

*Frequently used as antiemetic/antipruritic agents.

†Systemic use, effect unlikely with aerosol administration in conventional doses.

Table 4. Drugs That Do Not Affect MIBG Uptake in Neuroendocrine Tissues*

Cardiovascular
Alpha-blockers: clonidine, phenoxybenzamine, phentolamine, prazosin
Alphamethyldopa†
Angiotensin converting enzyme (ACE) inhibitors: captopril, enalapril
Beta-blockers
Digitalis glycosides
Diuretics
Analgesics and tranquilizers
Opiates
Aspirin
Acetaminophen
Alphamethylparatyrosine

*Modified from Khafagi et al.[21]

†Falsely elevates catecholamine and metabolite levels.

nervous system, can be given to differentiate between pheochromocytoma and other nonpheochromocytoma causes of elevated concentrations of catecholamine, such as essential hypertension and stress.[32] Failure of plasma catecholamine concentrations to decrease by 50% of the initial value after clonidine administration is strong evidence for the presence of pheochromocytoma.

The three imaging techniques, MRI, CT, and MIGB scintigraphy are all about equal in sensitivity (85 to 95%).[33] CT is less specific, as pheochromocytomas cannot be differentiated from adenomas and metastases. Both CT and MRI are less sensitive for extra-adrenal tumors. The sensitivity of scintigraphy with either ^{123}I or ^{131}I-MIBG is 85 to 90% and the specificity is over 95% in the correct clinical setting.[6] Thus, the fact that MIBG does not distinguish between pheochromocytoma and such other neuroendocrine tumors as carcinoid or neuroblastoma is of little clinical relevance.

The advantages of ^{123}I-MIBG over ^{131}I-MIBG, of course, lie in the characteristics of ^{123}I, which permit sharper images, while reducing radiation absorbed dose. A real clinical advantage, however, has yet to be proven.[6] With both tracers, it is essential to stop all interfering medication (Table 3) at least 2 to 3 weeks before injection. Figure 3 shows a large pheochromocytoma in the right adrenal gland.

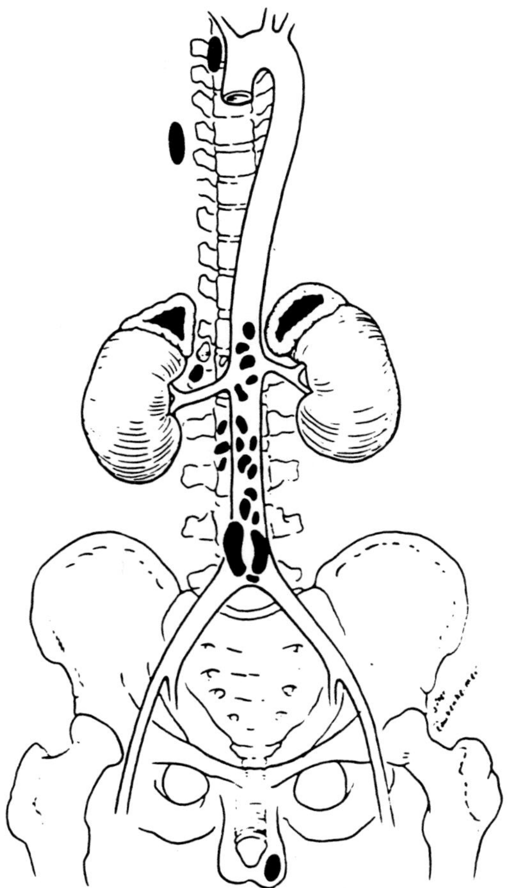

Figure 2. Extraadrenal sites of medullary tissue.

Treatment

SURGERY

Surgical removal of all tumor tissue is the first line of treatment, along with metastases and recurrences whenever feasible. In some cases, catheter embolization of the primary tumor or metastases is also indicated.[31] The use of α- and β-blocking drugs during surgery can help prevent cardiovascular and hypertensive crises during surgery. Even so, the overall mortality is significant with a five-year survival of about 44%.[26]

CHEMOTHERAPY

The combination of cyclophosphamide, vincristine, and dacarbazine has been shown to induce a tumor response in about 60% and an endocrine response in about 80% of patients.[34] However, such effects are transient and this treatment is reserved usually for those patients who respond to no other treatment.

EXTERNAL RADIOTHERAPY

Malignant pheochromocytoma is quite resistant to external beam therapy and it is reserved largely for palliation of bone pain.[31]

Treatment with ^{131}I-MIBG

Sufficiently large numbers of patients with malignant or nonresectable pheochromocytoma have now been treated with ^{131}I-MIBG, and adequate follow-up achieved to assert that this radiopharmaceutical has a definite (although by no means *fully* defined) therapeutic role.

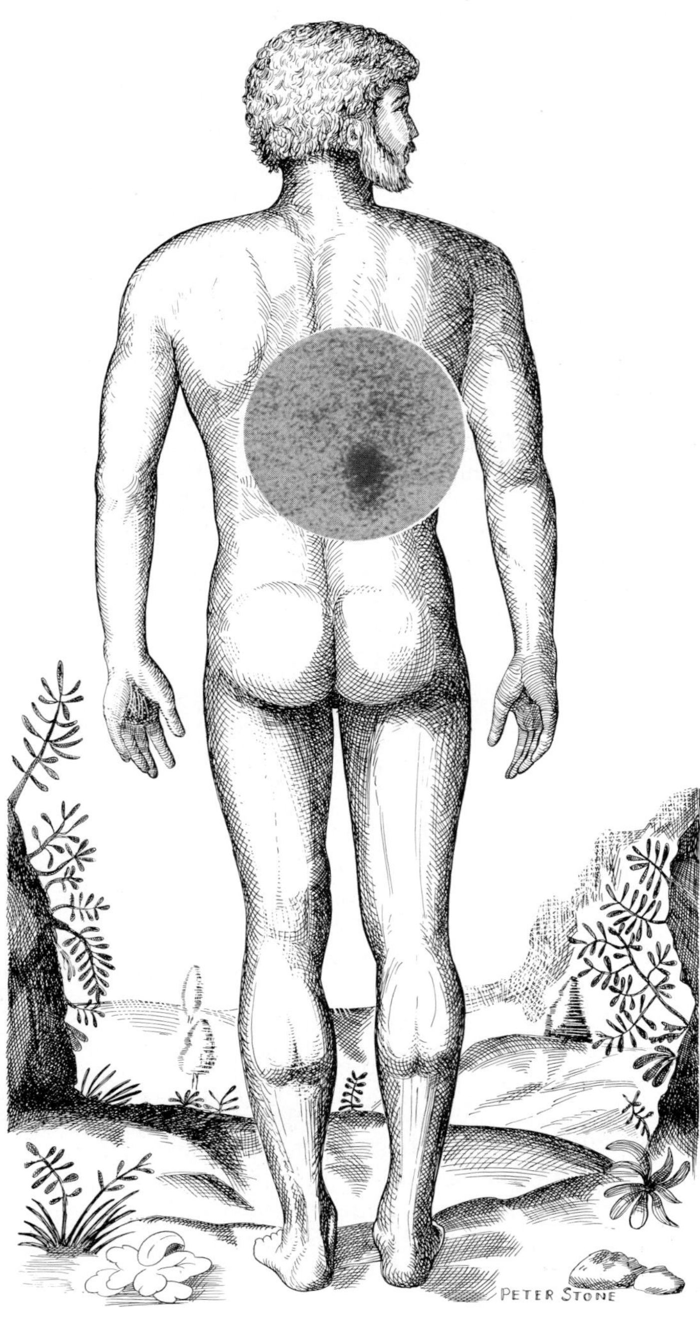

Figure 3. Posterior abdominal ^{131}I-MIBG scintiphoto showing a large focus of uptake in the right adrenal gland. Activity in left adrenal is completely suppressed. Surgery revealed a large right pheochromocytoma. (Courtesy of Dr. Harvey Ziessman.)

PATIENT SELECTION

The criteria for selection of patients for treatment of malignant pheochromocytoma with ^{131}I-MIBG used at the University of Michigan[35] appear to be typical of most centers. *Absolute criteria* include:

1. Malignant or otherwise unresectable pheochromocytoma proven by histology
2. Avid uptake and prolonged retention of ^{131}I-MIBG by all known sites of disease (see Dosimetry below)
3. Ability to return repeatedly for follow-up and retreatment
4. Ability to give informed consent (by legal guardian in the case of minors),
5. Anticipated survival of at least 1 year (Karnofsky performance status >50%);
6. Acceptable bone-marrow function (WBC $>3.5 \times 10^9$/L, platelets $>100 \times 10^9$/L), renal function (serum creatinine <2 mg/dL), and hepatic function (serum bilirubin <1.5 mg/dL).

Desirable criteria for therapy include:

1. Multiple abnormalities of biochemical tumor markers,
2. Objectively measurable tumor dimensions on at least one representative lesion,
3. Tumor dosimetry on at least one representative lesion to deliver >20 cGy/mCi (740 cGy/GBq) with a whole body radiation dose <1 cGy/mCi (37 cGy/GBq),
4. High or rising dopamine levels.

The patient work-up includes complete history, physical, and analysis of current medications. Laboratory measurements include plasma catecholamines and urinary catecholamines and metabolites, which are used as a guide to evaluating hormonal response to therapy. Hepatic and renal function are also assessed, as is hematologic status, used to gauge toxicity.

Diagnostic and dosimetric studies. The protocol described by Sisson and colleagues[3,35] is representative of most therapeutic approaches using MIBG. Tracer doses of 18.5 to 37 MBq (0.5 to 1.0 mCi) of high-specific activity ^{131}I-MIBG (5 to 10 Ci/mmol) are administered by slow intravenous injection. Whole-body imaging is obtained with a wide field-of-view scintillation camera, equipped with a high-energy collimator, at 24 and 48 hours from pelvis to skull to assess the distribution of tumor and metastases.

To estimate tumor dosimetry, additional conjugate views are obtained of representative tumor deposits, with and without an external ("mock tumor") source, placed in a region of similar background activity and attenuation.[36] Imaging is performed over 5 to 7 days to determine tumor uptake and retention. Generally, images are collected for 20 minutes or 100,000 counts.

Estimating precise radiation absorbed doses to tumor deposits remains difficult because of significant errors in measuring *in vivo* activity by means of planar imaging. As with ^{131}I therapy for thyroid cancer, the usual limiting dose of radiopharmaceutical is determined by self-radiation to blood (bone marrow).[37,38] Details of these measurement calculations are given in Appendix J; detailed tumor dosimetry is given in Reference 43. Nevertheless, the results of ^{131}I-MIBG have little relationship to the estimated dosimetry.

Treatment with ^{131}I-MIBG

The treatment protocol described by Sisson et al[3] has been widely used. The thyroid is blocked to prevent uptake of free ^{131}I. One drop of SSKI is given orally 3 times daily (150 mg iodine) beginning 1 day prior to tracer administration and continued for 1 month following treatment. Diagnostic and dosimetry studies are conducted as described above. Following these, ^{131}I-MIBG is administered using specific activities of 8 to 11 Ci/mmol. Infusions are delivered in a volume of 30 ml over 90 minutes by means of a syringe infusion pump. Doses range from 100 to 300 mCi (3.7 to 11 GBq).[3,35] Calculated tumor doses vary from about 3500 cGy to over 20,000 cGy.[3] With the high-specific activities of modern formulations of MIBG, no pharmacological effect should be noted.

During the infusion and for 24 hours thereafter, pulse, blood pressure, and EKG are monitored. Observations are made every 5 minutes during infusion and hourly for the next 24 hours. Patients are encouraged to drink plenty of fluids and empty their bladders frequently to avoid radiation cystitis. Posttherapy images are taken at about day 5 and often reveal tumor foci that were not present on diagnostic studies. In the University of Michigan experience, retreatment intervals varied from 13 to 115 weeks with a mean of 32 weeks.[35]

RESPONSE TO THERAPY

The classifications of patient responses have generally been based on modifications of those used for evaluating chemotherapeutic responses in malignant pheochromocytoma developed by Averbuch et al.[34] Responses to both tumor size and biochemical changes are recorded. Tumor response is recorded as follows:

1. *Complete response*: complete regression of all evidence of tumor by palpation and diagnostic studies.
2. *Partial response*: at least 50% reduction in measurable tumor bulk (determined from 2 measurements at least 4 weeks apart and based on the product of the greatest cross-sectional diameters of the lesions).
3. *Stable disease*: no significant change in measurable tumor diameter (less than 50% decrease or <25% increase) and no new lesions or tumor-related symptoms.
4. *Progression*: significant enlargement (>25% increase in tumor bulk and or appearance of new lesions).

Some investigators also record a *Minor response* in which there is from 25 to 50% decrease in tumor bulk.[35]

Biochemical response is similarly classified:

1. *Complete response*: complete normalization of all biochemical evidence of catecholamine hypersecretion.
2. *Partial response*: at least 50% reduction in the mean 24-hour urine excretion rate of the 2 most abnormal catecholamines and metabolites (based on the mean of at least 2 collections at each time point with at least 4 weeks between the series of collections).
3. *Stable disease*. No significant change in the mean 24-hour urine excretion rate of catecholamines and metabolites (less than 25% increase and less than 50% decrease).
4. *Progression*: greater than 25% increase in the mean 24-hour urine excretion rate of catecholamines and metabolites.

Table 5 lists the results of 8 studies totalling 87 patients with malignant pheochromocytoma treated with ^{131}I-MIBG. Only 1 patient experienced a complete tumor response and this patient was tumor-free 58 months after therapy.[41] Six patients (7%) experienced complete normalization of biochemical parameters, although most of these later relapsed.

Table 5. Responses to ^{131}I-MIBG Therapy of Malignant Pheochromocytoma Reported in Eight Studies

REF.	NO. PTS.	AGE MEAN (RANGE)	DOSE (mCi) MEAN (RANGE)	TOTAL DOSE (mCi)	TUMOR RESPONSE (HORMONAL RESPONSE) *Comp.*	*Part.*	*Stab.*	*Prog.*
35	28	40 (13–79)	181 (97–301)	111–916	0 (0)	2 (5)	16 (13)	9 (0)
36	15	48 (28–75)	100	300–1362	0 (4)	5 (3)	7 (6)	3 (2)
37	6	45 (27–66)	150 (100–200)	147–1022	0 (0)	2 (4)	3 (1)	1 (1)
38	6	37 (16–73)	— (65–210)	405–1055	0	1	2	3
39	9	51 (14–76)	— (100–200)	96–624	0 (0)	1 (1)	3 (3)	4 (4)
40	14	42 (13–73)	— (64–200)		0	2	11	1
41	5	36 (26–43)	— (65–200)	150–670	1 (2)	1	2	1
42	4	39 (40–61)	100	200–600	0		3	1
	87				1 (6)	14 (15)	47 (23)	23 (7)

Comp. = Complete response; Part. = Partial response; Stab. = Stable disease (no change); Prog. = Progressive disease.

A somewhat greater number of patients experienced partial response in both tumor bulk and biochemical parameters; however, the overall results as measured by bulk tumor and biochemical responses are not very impressive.

This is not to conclude that ^{131}I-MIBG therapy is not worthwhile. Symptomatic relief is often clinically gratifying.[35,40] The most significant include relief of pain, improved function (decreased sweating, relief of constipation), and reduction of medication, often for sustained periods of time. As Shapiro and colleagues note, a strong case can be made for dose escalation trials to determine the side effect-limiting dose of radiopharmaceutical.[35] The small number of toxic side effects reported in these 8 studies suggest that larger individual and cumulative doses can be tolerated, possibly with a better clinical response. Cumulative doses of ^{131}I-MIBG as high as 2322 mCi (85.9 GBq) have been well tolerated.[36] There is some preliminary evidence to suggest that pretreatment with the calcium channel antagonist, nifedipine, may be of value in increasing tumor blood flow to increase MIBG uptake.[47]

At least one study suggests that tumor uptake of ^{131}I-MIBG decreases after the initial treatment.[48] It may, therefore, be useful to increase the initial dose to achieve maximum effect.

TOXICITY

In the doses reported here, relatively few cases of toxicity have been observed. The rare alteration in pulse, blood pressure, or EKG usually responds to adrenergic blockade.[35] In the University of Michigan experience, about two thirds of patients experienced a mild syndrome of anorexia and nausea; this was occasionally accompanied by mild vomiting during the first posttherapy day, seldom lasting more than 3 days, and was managed by light diet and common antiemetics. This response is thought to represent a mild form of radiation sickness.

The bone marrow is the critical tissue following ^{131}I-MIBG treatment; myelosuppression with leukopenia and thrombocytopenia is commonly observed. This is rarely of clinical significance but, since toxicity is cumulative, the interval between treatments may be limited by the rate of platelet recovery. The risk of myelosuppression increases in patients who have extensive osseous metastases. Lewington et al[46] reported 1 patient with mediastinal compression and extensive marrow involvement who died 3 weeks after an infusion of 11 GBq (300 mCi) with marrow aplasia. This patient had received a cumulative dose of 26 GBq (702 mCi). These authors recommend that young patients who are likely to undergo repeated ^{131}I-MIGB treatments have bone marrow harvested for subsequent autologous rescue, if necessary.

TREATMENT OF NEUROBLASTOMAS

Neuroblastoma is the third most frequent malignant disease of childhood and the most common solid tumor found in infants under 1 year of age.[49] The overall incidence is 8.7 per million per year in children up to 15 years of age. Most primary tumors arise in the adrenal gland, although they can arise anywhere along the extra-adrenal sympathetic chain (Fig. 2); 15 to 20% arise in the thorax. Neuroectodermal tissue can even be pulled into the scrotum during testicular descent, from which neuroblastomas can arise.[55] About one third of tumors found in children over 1 year of age are disseminated at the time of diagnosis, most commonly to liver, lung, and bone. Therefore, the earlier the tumor is diagnosed, the better the prognosis. Even so, only 10 to 20% of children are alive 2 years after diagnosis.[50] The most common presenting signs and symptoms include a palpable mass or the secondary conditions associated with bone marrow involvement: anemia, thrombocytopenia, and leukopenia.

Diagnosis and Staging

An international committee has recently revised the diagnostic and staging criteria for neuroblastoma to provide more

Table 6. Diagnosis of Neuroblastoma

Established if:

(1) Unequivocal pathologic diagnosis* is made from tumor tissue by light microscopy (with or without immunohistology, electron microscopy, increased urine or serum catecholamines, or metabolites†);

OR

(2) Bone marrow aspirate or trephine biopsy contains unequivocal tumor cells* (eg, syncytia or immunocytologically positive clumps of cells) and increased urine or serum catecholamines or metabolites.†

NOTE. See text also for clarifications.

*If histology is equivocal, karyotypic abnormalities in tumor cells characteristic of other tumors [eg, 1(11;22)], then exclude a diagnosis of neuroblastoma, whereas genetic features characteristic of neuroblastoma (1p deletion, N-*myc* amplification) would support this diagnosis.

†Catecholamines and metabolites include dopamine, HVA, and/or VMA; levels must be >3.0 SD above the mean per milligram creatinine for age to be considered increased, and at least 2 of these must be measured.

Adapted from Brodeur et al.[51]

useful comparisons of treatment results.[51] Table 6 lists the current diagnostic criteria. Immunohistology is recommended to exclude such tumors as Ewing's sarcoma, primitive neuroectodermal tumor (PNET), rhabdomyosarcoma, and non-Hodgkin's lymphoma. The most common immunologic reagents available commercially are neuron-specific enolase (NSE), synaptophysin, and chromogranin A (CGA).[51]

The recommended staging procedures are listed in Table 7. CT or MRI are preferred over ultrasound in evaluating the abdomen, because of superior resolution and ease of assessing tumor mass. Imaging with MIBG is recommended whenever it is available, because it is particularly useful in assessing the extent of metastatic disease, in distinguishing residual active tumor from masses composed of scar tissue, and is more sensitive in detecting response of tumor involving cortical bone.[52] Approximately 90% of neuroblastomas concentrate MIBG,[52] although because most neural crest tumors do also, it is much more sensitive than specific. In general, MIBG uptake correlates well with elevated tumor markers, especially increased urinary VMA and dopamine and high serum NSE.[60] As with all neural crest tumors, the number of lesions identified by scintigraphy is dose-dependent; nearly twice as many lesions are identified when imaged after therapeutic doses (150+ mCi) as imaged following diagnostic doses (0.5 to 1.0 mCi).[61] In those cases in which MIBG scintigraphy is negative, bone scintigraphy with ^{99m}Tc- diphosphonate is recommended, even though small bone lesions may be missed in infants. This is especially true of those adjacent to epiphyses, which exhibit very high uptake of this radiopharmaceutical.[54]

The revised International Neuroblastoma Staging System (INSS) is shown in Table 8.

Table 7. Assessment of Extent of Neuroblastoma

TUMOR SITE	RECOMMENDED TESTS
Primary tumor	CT and/or MRI imaging* with 3D measurements; MIBG imaging, if available.†
Metastastic sites†	
Bone marrow	Bilateral posterior iliac crest marrow aspirates and trephine (core) bone marrow biopsies required to exclude marrow involvement. A single positive site documents marrow involvement. Core biopsies must contain at least 1 cm of marrow (excluding cartilage) to be considered adequate.
Bone	MIBG; ^{99m}Tc-MDP imaging required if MIBG imaging negative or unavailable, and plain radiographs of positive lesions are recommended.
Lymph nodes	Clinical examination (palpable nodes), confirmed histologically. CT scan for nonpalpable nodes (3D measurements).
Abdomen/liver	CT and/or MRI scan* with 3D measurements.
Chest	AP and lateral chest radiographs. CT/MRI necessary if chest radiograph positive, or if abdominal mass/nodes extend into chest.

See text for clarifications. AP = anteroposterior.

*Ultrasound considered suboptimal for accurate 3D measurements.

†MIBG imaging is applicable to all sites of disease.

From Brodeur et al.[51]

PROGNOSIS AS A FUNCTION OF TUMOR STAGE

Surgery alone is generally sufficient treatment for children with stage 1 neuroblastoma; they have a 95 to 100% 3-year survival regardless of age at diagnosis.[72] Surgery alone is also usually sufficient treatment for Stage 2 neuroblastoma. In selected cases, radiation or chemotherapy may be necessary if specific organ function is threatened or if neurological symptoms develop as a result of spinal cord compression. The overall 5-year survival for children with stage 2 neuroblastoma is 96%, with a progression-free survival of 90%.[73]

Patients with stage 4S neuroblastoma often undergo tumor regression spontaneously and have a disease-free survival of 85 to 90%. Since chemotherapy and extensive radiation therapy is not well tolerated in these very young patients, treatment is usually supportive.[74]

In contrast to stages 1, 2, and 4S, stages 3 and 4 carry a grave prognosis.[51,79] In addition, certain histochemical and genetic characteristics worsen prognosis. These include (1) undifferentiated histology[75]; (2) elevated serum ferritin levels;[76] and (3) increased copies of the *Nmyc* oncogene in the tumor.[77] In such patients, fewer than 10% would be expected to survive 1 year after recurrence despite reinstitution of conventional therapy.[78] It is in this group of patients that MIBG plays an effective role in management.

Table 8. International Neuroblastoma Staging System

STAGE	DEFINITION
1	Localized tumor with complete gross excision, with or without microscopic residual disease; representative ipsilateral lymph nodes negative for tumor microscopically (nodes attached to and removed with the primary tumor may be positive).
2A	Localized tumor with incomplete gross excision; representative ipsilateral nonadherent lymph nodes negative for tumor microscopically.
2B	Localized tumor with or without complete gross excision, with ipsilateral nonadherent lymph nodes positive for tumor. Enlarged contralateral lymph nodes must be negative microscopically.
3	Unresectable unilateral tumor infiltrating across the midline,* with or without regional lymph node involvement; or localized unilateral tumor with contralateral regional lymph node involvement; or midline tumor with bilateral extension by infiltration (unresectable) or by lymph node involvement.
4	Any primary tumor with dissemination to distant lymph nodes, bone, bone marrow, liver, skin and/or other organs (except as defined for stage 4S).
4S	Localized primary tumor (as defined for stage 1, 2A or 2B), with dissemination limited to skin, liver, and/or bone marrow† (limited to infants <1 year of age).

See text also for clarifications. Multifocal primary tumors (eg, bilateral adrenal primary tumors) should be staged according to the greatest extent of disease, as defined above, and followed by a subscript letter M (eg, 3_M).

*The midline is defined as the vertebral column. Tumors originating on one side and crossing the midline must infiltrate to or beyond the opposite side of the vertebral column.

†Marrow involvement in stage 4S should be minimal, ie, <10% of total nucleated cells identified as malignant on bone marrow biopsy or on marrow aspirate. More extensive marrow involvement would be considered to be stage 4. The MIBG scan (if performed) should be negative in the marrow.

From Brodeur et al.[51]

Treatment with ¹³¹I-MIBG

UPTAKE IN NEUROBLASTOMA CELLS

As discussed above, MIBG is taken up by adrenergic tissue and in pheochromocytoma by a high-affinity, saturable, sodium-temperature-, and energy-dependent system (specific or type-1 uptake). A much smaller amount enters these cells by a nonspecific passive diffusion mechanism. However, neuroblastoma cells are quite heterogeneous; several cell lines have been identified.[56] Recent studies suggest that some of these cell lines either do not take up MIBG at all, or else do so only on a passive diffusion basis.[57–59] Furthermore, few cell lines studied *in vitro* store MIBG in neurosecretory storage granules, a fact that may decrease cell retention.

In one *in vivo* study in which ^{125}I-MIBG was injected preoperatively and tumor tissues assayed postsurgically, tumor uptake within neuroblastoma measured 0.0013 to 0.071% of injected dose per gram of tissue. Uptake also varied between different parts of individual tumors. Interestingly, undifferentiated tumors took up more ^{125}I-MIBG than differentiated tumors.[62] Means of potentially increasing uptake and retention of MIBG *in vivo* are discussed below.

PATIENT SELECTION

The criteria for treating neuroblastoma with ^{131}I-MIBG at the University of Michigan are essentially the same as for pheochromocytoma, except that expected survival may be as short as 3 months.[63]

PROCEDURE AND DOSIMETRY

These considerations are essentially the same as described for the treatment of pheochromocytoma with ^{131}I-MIBG above.

RESULTS OF THERAPY

As of 1991, more than 250 patients with neuroblastoma had been treated with ^{131}I-MIBG.[63] Tumor responses are judged by follow-up CT scans, skeletal surveys, and ^{131}I-MIBG diagnostic imaging. Responses are categorized as follows:

- Complete response—disappearance of all symptoms and signs of disease;
- Partial response—greater than 50% decrease in all measurable tumor lesions. Some investigators also require a 50% decrease in VMA-HVA urinary excretion;
- Stable disease—less than 50% decrease in lesion size. (Some investigators record a *Minor Response*, indicating a decrease in lesion size between 20 and 50%);[64]
- Progressive disease—increase in any tumor size, or the appearance of new lesions.

Table 9 lists the results of 6 series of patients that have been well documented. As with pheochromocytoma, relatively few patients experienced a complete tumor response. A greater number had partial responses, although most of these were temporary, lasting from weeks to months. A great many more patients had improvement of their symptoms, including decreased analgesia requirement and improved quality of life. The conclusion of most investigators is that ^{131}I-MIBG is a worthwhile palliative measure in patients who do not respond to other forms of therapy.

Other findings that were general to most studies include:

1. There was no apparent correlation between tumor response and either total accumulative dose administered or the estimated radiation absorbed dose to tumor. Once again, this lack of correlation attests to the absence of reliable dosimetry.
2. The best responses occurred in patients without bone-marrow involvement.

Table 9. Long-term Results of ^{131}I-MIBG Therapy of Neuroblastoma

REF.	NO. PTS.	DOSE (mCi)	TOTAL DOSE (mCi)	TUMOR RESPONSE			
				CR	*PR*	*MR/SD*	*PD*
64	42	62–162		2	5	23	12
65	12	20 mCi/kg	130–560	2	6	4	
66	11	100–325	100–842	0	2	5	4
67	7	90–150	90–530	0	2		3
68	14	50–220	50–654	0	NR		
69	9	62–256	80–676	1		5	2
	—			—	—	—	—
	95			5	16	39	21

Note: CR, complete response; PR, partial response; MR, mild response; SD, stable disease; PD, progressive disease; NR, not reported

TOXICITY

No significant pharmacologic toxicity was found. Acute radiation sickness, characterized by anorexia, nausea, and vomiting occurred in some patients. The toxicity from ^{131}I-MIBG is similar to that experienced by patients treated for pheochromocytoma (above). Bone-marrow depression may be severe in children when extensive bone-marrow metastases are present. Prior bone-marrow transplantation appears to sensitize patients to this complication.[70] Some cases of hypothyroidism have been reported despite thyroid blockade with oral iodine.[63]

FUTURE DIRECTIONS

Attempts to improve the results of MIBG therapy have included:

Pharmacological Intervention. Rapid renal clearance is thought to be responsible for a significant waste of injected MIBG. Thus, antidiuretics administered before MIBG therapy may improve tumor uptake.[59] Pre-dosing with unlabeled MIBG to block uptake in normal target tissues, such as platelets and precursor megakaryocytes, may reduce toxicity and permit larger therapeutic doses.[59] The administration of nifedipine to provoke peripheral vasodilatation and consequently increase tumor blood supply may also be considered.[71]

Use of ^{125}I-MIBG. One hypothesis for the frequent failure of ^{131}I-MIBG to prevent recurrence is that its beta energy may be too widely dispersed in small (<2.5 mm) metastases.[80] The rationale for using ^{125}I to label MIBG is that the beta energy is more tightly dispersed and may, thus, be more cytodestructive to tumor cells that concentrate the radiopharmaceutical.[78,81]

Sisson et al[78] have reported treating 7 patients with 261 to 809 mCi (9.6 to 30 GBq) of ^{125}I-MIBG. Three of these patients experienced unexpectedly long remission-free survival of 1 to 3 years, which suggests that further study is warranted. They encountered serious bone-marrow toxicity (thrombocytopenia) with estimated whole-body absorbed doses of 85 to 135 cGy, which is lower than for estimated doses with ^{131}I. Again, this suggests a failure of accurate dosimetry, a recurring problem in radionuclide therapy.

MIBG Therapy at Diagnosis. The rationale for using MIBG as a first-line therapeutic modality includes: (1) less pre-existing morbidity with consequent reduced radiation toxicity, (2) reduction of small metastases may provide greater effectiveness of the subsequent primary surgery. Thus far, 3 reports have described the early use of ^{131}I-MIBG.[82–84] The preliminary results appear to be favorable; 1 patient with stage 3 disease was alive and disease-free 4 years after therapy.[84] Among 13 other patients treated and evaluable, partial responses were frequent and toxicity much less than among patients treated after radiation and chemotherapy protocols were exhausted.

TREATMENT OF OTHER NEUROENDOCRINE TUMORS

Paragangliomas

Paragangliomas are tumors that arise from extra-adrenal paraganglion tissue, a multicentric system of histologically similar organs known as paraganglia. Paragangliomas contain small amounts of catecholamines and may be "functional" or "nonfunctional," according to whether or not they secrete catecholamines in sufficient quantities to produce the clinical syndrome of a pheochromocytoma: hypertension, headache, and sweating.[85] Other names for these tumors include "chemodectoma" and "glomus tumor." As with pheochromocytomas (the same tumor arising in the adrenal medulla), malignancy is defined by either local invasion, spread to regional lymph nodes, or metastases to distant sites not associated with neuroendocrine tissue. Multicentric tumors occur in about 10% of cases.[86]

The mechanism of uptake of MIBG in paragangliomas is presumed to be the same as that in pheochromocytomas. Interestingly, the uptake of MIBG is unrelated to the secretory activity of the tumor, since "nonfunctional" paragangliomas have been shown to take up ^{131}I-MIBG in sufficient quantities to effectively treat these tumors.[87–91]

Table 10. ^{131}I-MIBG Therapy of Carcinoid Tumors

REF.	NO. PTS.	DOSE (mCi)	TOTAL DOSE (mCi)	SYMPTOM RESPONSE	TUMOR RESPONSE *PR*	*SD*	*PD*
98	20	200	400+	13	0	18	2
99	6	100–300	−798	4	0	5	1
100	2	150	743	2	1		
101	5	–	100–600	5	1	3	1

PR, partial response; SD, stable disease; PD, progressive disease

Relatively few patients with paraganglioma have been treated with ^{131}I-MIBG.[87–91] In general, the protocol is the same as that for the treatment of pheochromocytoma (see above) and the results appear to be the same, as far as can be judged from the very small number of patients treated to date.

Carcinoid Tumors

Carcinoid tumors occur widely throughout the gastrointestinal tract from the larynx to anus, including the pancreas, biliary tract, and many that obstruct the appendix.[92] The carcinoid syndrome, with clinical features of diarrhea, flushing, dyspnea, and bronchospasm, occurs in only about 10% of carcinoid tumors.[93] Many of these tumors secrete 5-hydroxytryptamine (serotonin), which causes elevated urinary levels of its metabolite, 5-hydroxyindolacetic acid (5-HIAA). Other tumors secrete the serotonin precursor 5-hydroxytryptophan, which gives rise to normal urinary 5-HIAA excretion, despite the occurrence of carcinoid syndrome.

The traditional treatment for carcinoids is surgical removal whenever feasible. The five-year survival rate for appendiceal tumors is 99%; however, from all sites it is about 70% and decreases to about 30% in patients with distant metastases, primarily in regional lymph nodes and liver.[94] Metastases are uncommon in tumors smaller than 1 cm, and are present in virtually 100% of tumors larger than 2 cm.[95]

The treatment of metastatic hormone-secreting tumors currently consists of hepatic artery embolization, interferon-α, somatostatin analogue (Sandostatin), with chemotherapy reserved for patients who are not controlled by other means.[96]

TREATMENT WITH ^{131}I-MIBG

Uptake of MIBG is documented in about 60% of carcinoid tumors.[97] Therefore, MIBG scintigraphy is not a useful diagnostic screening procedure but, once carcinoid has been documented, total body MIBG scintigraphy is useful to document the extent of disease and to evaluate the potential for therapeutic application. In general, the uptake within tumors is less than is found with neuroblastoma and pheochromocytoma.[98]

At least 4 small series of patients treated with ^{131}I-MIBG have been reported.[98–101] These patients were selected for treatment because of progressive disease, usually with carcinoid syndrome, and high uptake of diagnostic MIBG. Treatment doses ranged from 100 to 300 mCi (3.7 to 11 GBq), with doses repeated at intervals of about 2 months and with cumulative doses as high as 798 mCi (29.5 GBq). Side effects of therapeutic doses included occasional nausea. The pharmacological effects of MIBG are largely avoided with high-specific activity radiopharmaceutical.

The results of these series are detailed in Table 10. Note the very high percentage of patients (about 70%) who experienced relief of subjective symptoms, many lasting more than a year. No tumor disappearance was reported, and only a few documented partial reduction in tumor size. In many cases, decreased uptake of subsequent MIBG was recorded. Relatively few patients had an objective reduction in metabolite excretion. Thus, ^{131}I-MIBG appears to have a promising role in the palliation of carcinoid tumors.

REFERENCES

1. Ackery DM, Tippet P, Condon B, et al. New approach to the localization of phaeochromocytoma: Imaging with ^{131}I-MIBG. *Br Med J* 1984;288:1587.
2. Nakajo M, Shapiro B, Copp J, et al. The normal and abnormal distribution of the adrenomedullary imaging agent m[I-131]iodobenzylguanidine (131-I-MIBG) in man: Evaluation by scintigraphy. *J Nucl Med* 1983;24:672.
3. Sisson JC, Shapiro B, Beierwaltes WH: Radiopharmaceutical treatment of malignant pheochromocytoma. *J Nucl Med* 1984;25:198.
4. Sisson JC, Frager MS, Val TW, et al. Scintigraphic localization of pheochromocytoma. *N Engl J Med* 1981;305:12.
5. Wieland DM, Brown LE, Tobes MC. Imaging the primate adrenal medulla with ^{123}I and ^{131}I-meta-iodobenzylguanidine. Concise communication. *J Nucl Med* 1981;22:358.
6. Shapiro B: Summary, conclusions, and future directions of [^{131}I]metaiodobenzylguanidine therapy in the treatment of neural crest tumors. *J Nucl Biol Med* 1991;35:357.
7. Pearse AGE: Common cytochemical and ultrastructural characteristics of cells producing polypeptide hormones (the APUD series) and their relevance to thyroid and ultimobranchial C cells and calcitonin. *Proc R Soc Lond [Biol]* 1968;170:71.
8. Pearse AGE: The APUD concept: Embryology, cytochemistry and ultrastructure of the diffuse neuroendocrine system, in Friesen SR (ed): *Surgical Endocrinology; Clinical Syndromes*. Philadelphia, Lippincott, 1978, pp 18–34.
9. Schmechel D, Marangos PJ, Brightman M: Neurone-specific enolase is a molecular marker for peripheral and central neuroendocrine cells. *Nature* 1978;276:834.
10. Welbourn RB, Manolas KJ, Khan O, et al. Tumors of the

neuroendocrine system (APUD-cell tumors—APUDOMAS). *Curr Prob Surg* 1984;21:7.
11. Andrew A. The APUD concept: Where has it let us? *Br Med Bull* 1982;38:221.
12. Morales JO, Beierwaltes WH, Counsell RE, et al. The concentration of radioactivity from labeled epinephrine and its precursors in the dog adrenal medulla. *J Nucl Med* 1967;8:800.
13. Wieland DM, Swanson DP, Brown LE, et al. Imaging the adrenal medulla with an I-131-labeled antiadrenergic agent. *J Nucl Med* 1979;20:155.
14. Sisson JC, Wieland DM, Sherman P, et al. Metaiodobenzylguandidine as an index of the adrenergic nervous system integrity and function. *J Nucl Med* 1987;28:1625.
15. Sisson JC, Shapiro B, Meyers L, et al. Metaiodobenzylguanidine to map scintigraphically the adrenergic nervous system in man. *J Nucl Med* 1987;28:1625.
16. Tobes MC, Jaques S, Wieland DM, et al. Effect of uptake-one inhibitors on the uptake of norepinephrine and metaiodobenzylguanidine. *J Nucl Med* 1985;16:897.
17. Wieland DM, Wu JL, Brown LE, et al. Radiolabeled adrenergic neuron blocking agents: adrenomedullary imaging with [^{131}I]iodobenzylguanidine. *J Nucl Med* 1981;22:358.
18. Shapiro B, Wieland DM, Brown LE, et al. ^{131}I-metaiodobenzylguanidine (MIBG) adrenal medullary scintigraphy: Interventional studies, in: Spencer RP, (ed): *Interventional Nuclear Medicine*. New York, Grune and Stratton, Inc, 1984 pp 451.
19. Lindberg S, Fjalling M, Jacobsson L, et al. Methodology and dosimetry in adrenal medullary imaging with Iodine-131 MIBG. *J Nucl Med* 1988;29:1638.
20. Mangner TJ, Tobes MC, Wieland DW, et al. Metabolism of Iodine-131 metaiodobenzylguanidine in patients with metastatic pheochromocytoma. *J Nucl Med* 1986;27:37.
21. Khafagi FA, Shapiro B, Fig LM, et al. Labetalol reduces iodine-131 MIBG uptake by pheochromocytoma and normal tissues. *J Nucl Med* 1989;30:481.
22. Tobes MC, Fig LM, Carey J, et al. Alterations of Iodine-131 MIBG biodistribution in an anephric patient: Comparison to normal and impaired renal function. *J Nucl Med* 1989; 30:1476.
23. Scott WH, Reynolds V, Green N, et al. Clinical experience with malignant pheochromocytomas. *Surg Gynecol Obstet* 1982;154:801.
24. Scott WH, Halter SA. Oncologic aspects of pheochromocytoma: The importance of follow-up. *Surgery* 1984;96:1061.
25. Van Herdeen JA, Sheps SG, Hamberger B, et al. Pheochromocytoma: current status and changing trends. *Surgery* 1982; 91:367.
26. Shapiro B, Sisson JC, Lloyd R, et al. Malignant phaeochromocytoma: clinical, biochemical and scintigraphic characterization. *Clin Endicrinol (Oxf)* 1984;20:189.
27. Shapiro B, Copp JE, Sisson JC, et al. Iodine-131 metaiodobenzylguanidine for the locating of suspected pheochromocytoma: Experience in 400 cases. *J Nucl Med* 1985;26:576.
28. Beierwaltes WH: Update on basic research and clinical experience with metaiodobenzylguanidine. *Med Ped Oncol* 1987;15:163.
29. Schonebe CK. Malignant pheochromocytoma. *Scand J Urol Nephrol* 1969;3:64.
30. Manger WM, Gifford RW. *Pheochromocytoma*. New York, Springer-Verlag, 1972.
31. Shapiro B, Fig LM. Management of pheochromocytoma. *Endocrinol Metab Clin North Am* 1989;18:443.
32. Bravo EL, Tarazi RC, Fouad FM, et al. Clonidine-suppression test: A useful aid in the diagnosis of pheochromocytoma. *N Engl J Med* 1981;305:623.
33. Velchik MG, Alavi A, Kressel HY, Engelman K. Localization of pheochromocytoma: MIGB, CT, and MRI Correlation. *J Nucl Med* 1989;30:328.
34. Averbuch SD, Steakley CS, Young RC, et al. Malignant pheochromocytoma: effective treatment with a combination of cyclophosphamide, vincristine and decarbazine. *Ann Intern Med* 1988;109:267.
35. Shapiro B, Sisson JC, Wieland DM, et al. Radiopharmaceutical therapy of malignant pheochromocytoma with [^{131}I]Metaiodobenzylguanidine: Results from ten years of experience. *J Nucl Biol Med* 1991;35:269.
36. Krempf M, Lumbroso J, Mornex R, et al. Treatment of malignant pheochromocytoma with [^{131}I]Metaiodobenzylguanidine: A French multicenter study. *J Nucl Biol Med* 1991; 35:284.
37. Bestagno M, Pizzocaro C, Maira G, et al. Results of [^{131}]Metaiodobenzylguanidine treatment in metastatic malignant phaeochromocytoma. *J Nucl Biol Med* 1991;35:277.
38. Fisher M, Vetter H. Treatment of pheochromocytomas with ^{131}I-Metaiodobenzylguanidine, in C. Winkler, (ed): *Nuclear Medicine in Clinical Oncology*. Berlin, Springer-Verlag, 1986, 327.
39. Lumbroso J, Schlumberger M, Tenenbaum F, et al. [^{131}]Metaiodobenzylguanidine therapy in 20 patients with malignant pheochromocytoma. *J Nucl Biol Med* 1991;35:288.
40. Fischer M. Therapy of pheochromocytoma with [^{131}I]Metaiodobenzylguanidine. *J Nucl Biol Med* 1991;35:292.
41. Troncone L, Rufini V, Daidone MS, et al. [^{131}I]Metaiodobenzylguanidine treatment of malignant pheochromocytoma: Experience of the Rome group. *J Nucl Biol Med* 1991; 35:295.
42. Colombo L, Lomuscio G, Bignati A, Dottorini ME. Preliminary results of [^{131}I]Metaiodobenzylguanidine treatment in metastatic malignant pheochromocytoma. *J Nucl Biol Med* 1991;35:300.
43. Koral KF, Wang X, Sisson JC, et al. Calculating radiation absorbed dose for pheochromocytoma tumors in 131-I MIBG therapy. *Int J Radiat Oncol Biol Phys* 1989;17:211.
44. Leeper RD, Shimaoka K. Treatment of metastatic thyroid cancer. *Clin Endocrinol Metab* 1980;9:383.
45. Averbuch SD, Steakley CS, et al. Malignant pheochromocytoma: effective treatment with a combination of cyclophosphamide, vincristine and dacarbazine. *Ann Intern Med* 1988;109:267.
46. Lewington VJ, Zivanovic MA, Tristam M, et al. Radiolabelled metaiodobenzylguanidine targeted radiotherapy for malignant phaeochromocytoma. *J Nucl Biol Med* 1991;35: 280.
47. Blake GM, Lewington VJ, Fleming JS, et al. Modification by nifedipine of 131-I metaiodobenzylguanidine kinetics in malignant phaeochromocytoma. *Eur J Nucl Med* 1988;14: 345.
48. Aritake S: Radioisotope therapy of malignant pheochromocytoma with iodine-131 metaiodobenzylguanidine—absorbed dose assessments using SPECT. *Kaku Igaku* 1992;29:667.
49. Matthay KK. Congenital malignant disorders, in: Taeusch HF, Ballard RA, Avery ME, (eds): *Schaeffer and Avery's Diseases of the Newborn*. 6th ed. Philadelphia, Saunders, 1991, p 1025.
50. Breslow N, McCann B. Statistical estimation of prognosis for children with neuroblastoma. *Cancer Res* 1971;31:2098.
51. Brodeur GM, Pritchard J, Berthold F, et al. Revisions of the international criteria for neuroblastoma diagnosis, staging, and response to treatment. *J Clin Oncol* 1993;11:1466.
52. Voute PA, Hoefnagel CA, Marcuse HR, et al. Detection of neuroblastoma with ^{131}I-meta-iodobenzylguanidine, in Evans AE, D'Angio GJ, Seeger RC (eds): *Advances in Neuroblastoma Research*. New York, Liss, 1985, pp 389–398.

53. Hoefnagel CA. Radionuclide therapy revisited. *Eur J Nucl Med* 1991;18:408.
54. Gordon AM, Peters M, Morony S, et al. Skeletal assessment in neuroblastoma— the pitfalls of Iodine-123-MIBG scans. *J Nucl Med* 1990;31:129.
55. Shulkin BL, Geatti O, Hattner RS, et al. Bilateral testicular neuroblastoma. Scintigraphic depiction and therapy with I-131 MIBG. *Clin Nucl Med* 1992;17:638.
56. Ciccarone V, Spengler BA, Meyers MB, et al. Phenotypic diversification in human neuroblastoma cells: expression of distinct neural crest lineages. *Cancer Res* 1989;49:219.
57. Iavarone A, Lasorella A, Servidei T, et al. Biology of Metaiodobenzylguanidine interactions with human neuroblastoma cells. *J Nucl Biol Med* 1991;35:186.
58. Montaldo PG, Carbone R, Lanciotti M, et al. In vitro pharmacology of metaiodobenzylguanidine uptake, storage and release in human neuroblastoma cells. *J Nucl Biol Med* 1991;35:195.
59. Smets LA, Rutgers M. Model studies on metaiodobenzylguanidine (MIBG) uptake and storage: Relevance for ^{131}I-MIBG therapy of neuroblastoma. *J Nucl Biol Med* 1991;35:191.
60. Yeh SDJ, Helson L, Benua RS. Correlation between iodine-131 MIBG imaging and biological markers in advanced neuroblastoma. *Clin Nucl Med* 1988;13:46.
61. Parisi MT, Matthay KK, Huberty JP, Hattner RS. Neuroblastoma: dose-related sensitivity of MIBG scanning in detection. *Radiology* 1992;184:463.
62. Moyes JSE, Babich JW, Carter R, et al. Quantitative study of radioiodinated metaiodobenzylguanidine uptake in children with neuroblastoma: Correlation with tumor histopathology. *J Nucl Med* 1989;30:474.
63. Shapiro B. Imaging of catecholamine-secreting tumours: uses of MIBG in diagnosis and treatment. *Bailliere's Clin Endocrinol Metab* 1993;7:491.
64. Claudiani F, Garaventa A, Bertolazzi L, et al. [^{131}I]metaiodobenzylguanidine therapy in advanced neuroblastoma. *J Nucl Biol Med* 1991;35:224.
65. Klingebiel T, Feine U, Treuner J, et al. Treatment of neuroblastoma with [^{131}I]Metaiodobenzylguanidine: Long-term results in 25 patients. *J Nucl Biol Med* 1991;35:216.
66. Matthay KK, Huberty JP, Hattner RS, et al. Efficacy and safety of [^{131}I]Metaiodobenzylguanidine therapy for patients with refractory neuroblastoma. *J Nucl Biol Med* 1991;35:244.
67. Castellani MR, Rottoli L, Maffioli L, et al. Experience with palliative [^{131}I]Metaiodobenzylguanidine therapy in advanced neuroblastoma. *J Nucl Biol Med* 1991;35:241.
68. Hutchinson RJ, Sisson JC, Miser JS, et al. Long-term results of [^{131}I]Metaiodobenzylguanidine treatment of refractory advanced neuroblastoma. *J Nucl Biol Med* 1991;35:237.
69. Troncone L, Rufini V, Riccardi R, et al. The use of [^{131}I]Metaiodobenzylguanidine in the treatment of neuroblastoma after conventional therapy. *N Nucl Biol Med* 1991;35:232.
70. Sisson JC, Hutchinson RJ, Carey JE, et al. Toxicity from treatment of neuroblastoma with ^{131}I meta-iodobenzylguanidine. *Eur J Nucl Med* 1988;14:337.
71. Sisson JC, De Bernardi B. Session on the biology and treatment of neuroblastoma as related to metaiodobenzylguanidine. Chairmen's report. *J Nucl Biol Med* 1991;35:199.
72. Evans AE, D'Angio GJ, Sather HN, et al. A comparison of four staging systems for localized and regional neuroblastoma: a report from the Childrens Cancer Study Group. *J Clin Oncol* 1990;8:678.
73. Matthay KK, Sather HN, Seeger RC, Hasse GM, Hammond GD: Excellent outcome of stage II neuroblastoma is independent of residual disease and radiation therapy. *J Clin Oncol* 1989;7:236.
74. Haas D, Ablin AR, Miller C, et al. Complete pathologic maturation and regression of stage IVS neuroblastoma without treatment. *Cancer* 1988;62:818.
75. Shimada M, Chatten J, Newton WA, et al. Histopathologic prognostic factors in neuroblastoma tumors: definition of subtypes of ganglioneuroblastoma and age-linked classification of neuroblastoma. *JNCI* 1984;73:405.
76. Hahn H-WL, Evans AE, Siegel SE, et al. Prognostic importance of serum ferritin in patients with stages II and IV neuroblastoma: the Childrens Cancer Study Group experience. *Cancer Res* 1985;45:2843.
77. Seeger RC, Brodeur GM, Sather H, et al. Association of multiple copies of the N-myc oncogene with rapid progression of neuroblastomas. *N Engl J Med* 1985;313:1111.
78. Sisson JC, Shapiro B, Hutchinson RJ, et al. Treatment of Neuroblastoma with [^{125}I]Metaiodobenzylguanidine. *J Nucl Biol Med* 1991;35:255.
79. Matthay KK. An overview on the treatment of neuroblastoma. *J Nucl Biol Med* 1991;35:179.
80. Loevinger R, Japha EM, Brownell GL. Discrete radioisotope sources, in: Hine GJ, Brownell GL (eds): *Radiation Dosimetry.* New York, Academic Press, 1956, pp 713–44.
81. Sisson JC, Hutchinson RJ, Shapiro B, et al. Iodine-125-MIBG to treat Neuroblastoma: Preliminary report. *J Nucl Med* 1990;31:1479.
82. Mastrangelo R, Lasorella A, Troncone L, et al. [^{131}I]Metaiodobenzylguanidine in neuroblastoma patients at diagnosis. *J Nucl Biol Med* 1991;35:252.
83. Hoefnagel CA, De Kraker J, Voute PA, Valdés Olmos RA. Preoperative [^{131}I]Metaiodobenzylguanidine therapy of neuroblastoma at diagnosis ("MIBG de novo"). *J Nucl Biol Med* 1991;35:248.
84. Mastrangelo R, Troncone L, Lasorella A, et al. ^{131}I-Metaiodobenzylguanidine in the treatment of neuroblastoma at diagnosis. *Am J Pediatr Hematol Oncol* 1989;11:28.
85. Glenner GG, Grimley PM. Tumors of the extra-adrenal paraganglion system (including chemoreceptor), in *Atlas of Tumor Pathology*, second series, Fascicle 9. Washington, DC, Armed Forces Institute of Pathology, 1974.
86. Irons GB, Wieland LH, Brown WL. Paragangliomas of the neck: Clinical and pathological analysis of 116 cases. *Surg Clin North Am* 1977;15:897.
87. Khafagi F, Egerton-Vernon J, van Doorn T, et al. Localization and treatment of familial malignant nonfunctional paraganglioma with Iodine-131 MIBG: Report of two cases. *J Nucl Med* 1987;28:528.
88. Baulieu JL, Guilloteau D, Baulieu F, et al. Therapeutic effectiveness of Iodine-131 MIBG metastases of a nonsecreting paraganglioma. *J Nucl Med* 1988;29:2008.
89. Castellani MR, Rottoli L, Maffioli L, et al. [^{131}I]Metaiodobenzylguanidine therapy in paraganglioma. *J Nucl Biol Med* 1991;35:315.
90. Khafagi FA, Shapiro B, Fischer M, et al. Phaeochromocytoma and functioning paraganglioma in childhood and adolescence: role of iodine ^{131}metaiodobenzylguanidine. *Eur J Nucl Med* 1991;18:191.
91. Ball AB, Tait DM, Fisher C, et al. Treatment of metastatic para-aortic paraganglioma by surgery, radiotherapy and I-131 MIBG. *Eur J Surg Oncol* 1991;17:543.
92. Berge T, Linell F. Carcinoid tumors. *Acta Pathol Microbiol Immunol Scand (A)* 1976;84:322.
93. Davis Z, Moertel CG, McJirath DC. The malignant carcinoid syndrome. *Surg Gynecol Obstet* 1973;137:637.
94. Maton PN. The carcinoid tumor and the carcinoid syndrome, in: Becker KL (ed): *Principle and Practice of Endocrinology and Metabolism.* Philadelphia, Lippincott, 1990, pp 1640–3.
95. Vinik AI, Thompson NW, Eckhauser F, Moattari AR. Clinical